Principles and Practice of Geriatric Surgery

Ronnie Ann Rosenthal
Michael E. Zenilman
Mark R. Katlic

Editors

Principles and Practice of Geriatric Surgery

Second Edition

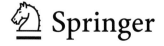 Springer

Editors

Ronnie Ann Rosenthal, MD
Professor
Department of Surgery
Yale University School of Medicine
New Haven, CT
and
Chief, Surgical Service
Department of Veterans Affairs
VA Connecticut Healthcare System
West Haven, CT, USA
ronnie.rosenthal@yale.edu

Michael E. Zenilman, MD
Department of Surgery
Johns Hopkins Medicine, Baltimore, MD
and
SUNY Downstate School of Public Health,
Brooklyn, NY
mzenilm1@downstate.edu

Mark R. Katlic, MD
Division of Thoracic Surgery
Director, Regional Ambulatory Campus
Geisinger Wyoming Valley Medical Center
Wilkes-Barre, PA, USA
mrkatlic@geisinger.edu

ISBN 978-1-4419-6998-9   e-ISBN 978-1-4419-6999-6
DOI 10.1007/978-1-4419-6999-6
Springer New York Dordrecht Heidelberg London

Library of Congress Control Number: 2011929046

Printed on acid-free paper

Springer is part of Springer Science+Business Media (www.springer.com)

Contents

Section III   Perioperative Issues

Section VI   Respiratory System

Section VII   Cardiovascular System

Section VIII   Gastrointestinal System

Section IX   Hepatobiliary System

Section X   Urogenital System

Contributors

Steven A. Ahrendt, MD
Associate Professor of Surgery, Department of Surgery, University of Pittsburgh, UPMC Cancer Center, Pittsburgh, PA, USA

Peter C. Albertsen, MD
Professor, Department of Surgery, Division of Urology, University of Connecticut Health Center, Farmington, CT, USA

Daniel Albo, MD, PhD
Department of Surgery, Baylor College of Medicine, Michael E. DeBakey Veterans Affairs Medical Center, Houston, TX, USA

Daniel A. Anaya, MD
Assistant Professor of Surgery, Michael E. DeBakey Department of Surgery, Baylor College of Medicine, Houston, TX, USA

Charlotte E. Ariyan, MD, PhD
Assistant Attending, Department of Surgery, Memorial Sloan-Kettering Cancer Center, New York, NY, USA

Wilbert S. Aronow, MD, FACC, FAHA
Cardiology Division, New York Medical College, Macy Pavilion, Valhalla, NY, USA

Stanley W. Ashley, MD
Frank Sawyer Professor and Vice Chair of Surgery, Department of Surgery, Brigham and Women's Hospital, Harvard Medical School, Boston, MA, USA

Lodovico Balducci, MD
Chief, Senior Adult Oncology Program, H. Lee Moffitt Cancer Center and Research Institute, Tampa, FL, USA

Asha G. Bale, MD
Assistant Professor of Surgery, Department of Surgery, New Jersey Medical School/ University Hospital, Newark, NJ, USA

Sheila R. Barnett, MD
Department of Anesthesiology, Beth Israel Deaconess Medical Center, Harvard Medical School, Boston, MA, USA

Hilary A. Beaver, MD
Associate Professor, Department of Ophthalmology, University of Iowa, Iowa City, IA, USA

Richard M. Bell, MD, FACS
Professor and Chairman, Department of Surgery, University of South Carolina School of Medicine, Columbia, SC, USA

David H. Berger, MD, MHCM
Professor and Vice Chair, Chief Division of General Surgery and Surgical Oncology;
Operative Care Line Executive, Michael E. DeBakey Department of Surgery,
Baylor College of Medicine, Houston, TX, USA; Michael E. DeBakey Veterans Affairs
Medical Center, Houston, TX, USA

Jack M. Berger, MS, MD, PhD
Professor of Clinical Anesthesiology, Department of Anesthesiology,
Keck School of Medicine, University of Southern California, LAC + USC Medical Center,
Los Angeles, CA, USA

Sarah E. Billmeier, MD
Resident, General Surgery, Brigham and Women's Hospital, Boston, MA, USA

Elisa H. Birnbaum, MD
Professor of Surgery, Department of Surgery, Barnes Jewish Hospital,
Washington University School of Medicine, St. Louis, MO, USA

Marie Boltz, PhD, RN
Assistant Professor, Hartford Institute for Geriatric Nursing,
New York University College of Nursing, New York, NY, USA

Daniel Borja-Cacho, MD
Hepatobiliary Fellow, Department of Surgery, University of Minnesota, Minneapolis,
MN, USA

C. Bryce Bowling, MD
Instructor/Fellow, Division of Women's Pelvic Medicine and Reconstructive Surgery,
Department of Obstetrics and Gynecology, University of Alabama at Birmingham
Medical Center, Birmingham, AL, USA

Wilbur B. Bowne, MD
Department of Surgery, SUNY Downstate Medical Center, Brooklyn, NY, USA

Elizabeth Breen, MD
Department of Surgery, Brigham and Women's Hospital, Harvard Medical School,
Boston, MA, USA

Murray F. Brennan, MD
Benno C. Schmidt Chair in Clinical Oncology, Department of Surgery,
Memorial Sloan-Kettering Cancer Center, New York, NY, USA

Nefertiti A. Brown, MD
Department of Surgery, SUNY Downstate Medical Center,
Brooklyn, NY, USA

F. Charles Brunicardi, MD
Professor and Chairman, Michael E. DeBakey Department of Surgery,
Baylor College of Medicine, Houston, TX, USA

Khalid M.H. Butt, MD, FRCS(Eng), FACS
Department of Surgery – Transplant Section, Westchester Medical Center,
Valhalla, NY, USA

Juan S. Calderon, MD
Department of Urology, VA Connecticut Healthcare System, West Haven, CT, USA

Margarita T. Camacho, MD
Surgical Director, Cardiac Transplantation and Mechanical Heart Program, Department
of Cardiothoracic Surgery, Newark Beth Israel Medical Center, Newark, NJ, USA

Edward J. Campbell, MD
Department of Internal Medicine, University of Utah Health Sciences Center, Salt Lake City, UT, USA

Elizabeth A. Capezuti, PhD, RN, FAAN
Hartford Institute for Geriataric Nursing, NYU College of Nursing,
New York, NY, USA

Tobias Carling, MD, PhD
Associate Professor of Surgery, Department of Surgery, Yale University School of Medicine, New Haven, CT, USA

Ara A. Chalian, MD
Department of Otorhinolaryngology: Head and Neck Surgery, Hospital of the University of Pennsylvania, Philadelphia, PA, USA

Gurkamal S. Chatta, MD
Associate Professor of Medicine, Division of Hematology-Oncology; Chief, Division of Hematology-Oncology, Department of Medicine, University of Pittsburgh Medical Center, Pittsburgh, PA, USA; Veterans Administration Public Health System, Pittsburgh, PA, USA

Neil N. Chheda, MD
Assistant Professor, Department of Otolaryngology, University of Florida, Gainesville, FL, USA

Anita Kit Wan Chiu, MD
Resident, Department of General Surgery, SUNY Downstate Medical Center, Brooklyn, NY, USA

Colleen Christmas, MD
Program Director, Johns Hopkins Bayview Medical Center,
Baltimore, MD, USA

Elizabeth B. Claus, MD, PhD
Attending Neurosurgeon, Department of Neurosurgery, Brigham and Women's Hospital, Boston, MA, USA

Leo M. Cooney, Jr. MD
Yale–New Haven Hospital, New Haven, CT, USA

Howard A. Crystal, MD
Professor of Neurology, Department of Neurology, SUNY Downstate Medical Center, Brooklyn, NY, USA

Kathryn M. Dalbec, MD
Department of Surgery, Indiana University Hospital, Indianapolis, IN, USA

Alan Dardik, MD, PhD
Associate Professor of Surgery, Department of Surgery, Yale University School of Medicine, New Haven, CT, USA

Susan M. Day, MD
Orthopaedic Surgeon; Clinical Instructor, Department of Surgery, Michigan State University College of Human Medicine, Grand Rapids, MI, USA

Edwin A. Deitch, MD
Professor and Chairman, Department of Surgery, New Jersey Medical School/University Hospital, Newark, NJ, USA

Dale A. Distant, MD
Professor of Clinical Surgery, Department of Transplant Surgery, SUNY Downstate Medical
Center, Brooklyn, NY, USA

George W. Drach, MD, FACS
Professor Emeritus of Urology in Surgery, Department of Surgery/Urology,
Hospital of the University of Pennsylvania, Philadelphia, PA, USA

Margaret Drickamer, MD
Professor of Medicine, Department of Medicine (Geriatrics), Yale University School
of Medicine, New Haven, CT, USA

Stanley J. Dudrick, MD
Professor of Surgery, Department of Surgery, Yale University School of Medicine,
Saint Mary's Hospital/Yale Affiliate, Waterbury, CT, USA

Kenneth A. Egol, MD
Associate Professor, Vice Chairman and Chief of Trauma, Department of Orthopaedic
Surgery, New York University Hospital for Joint Diseases, New York, NY, USA

Ben Eiseman, MD, MSc, FACS
Department of Surgery, Denver Vetarans Affairs Hospital, University Hospital,
Denver, CO, USA

David A. Etzioni, MD, MSHS
Department of Surgery, Mayo Clinic Arizona, Mayo Clinic College of Medicine,
Phoenix, AZ, USA

Amanda Feigel, MD
Department of Surgery, Yale University School of Medicine, New Haven, CT, USA

Yuman Fong, MD
Murray F. Brennan Chair in Surgery, Department of Surgery,
Memorial Sloan Kettering Cancer Center, New York, NY, USA

William H. Frishman, MD, MACP
Rosenthal Professor & Chairman Cardiology Division, New York Medical College,
Macy Pavilion, Valhalla, NY, USA

Shefali Gandhi, DO, MPH
Clinical Neurophysiology Fellow, Department of Neurology, SUNY Downstate Medical
Center, Brooklyn, NY, USA

Timothy J. Gardner, MD
Center for Heart & Vascular Health, Christiana Health Care System, Newark, DE, USA

Kimberly A. Gerten, MD
Instructor/Fellow, Division of Women's Pelvic Medicine and Reconstructive Surgery,
Department of Obstetrics and Gynecology, University of Alabama at Birmingham
Medical Center, Birmingham, AL, USA

Babak Givi, MD
Head & Neck Surgery Fellow, Head & Neck Surgery Section, Department of Surgery,
Memorial Sloan Kettering Cancer Center, New York, NY, USA

Philip J. Glassner, MD
Resident, Department of Orthopaedic Surgery, NYU Hospital for Joint Diseases,
New York, NY, USA

James S. Goodwin, MD
Mitchell Distinguished Chair in Geriatric Medicine, University of Texas Medical Branch,
Sealy Center on Aging, Galveston, TX, USA

Lazar J. Greenfield, MD
Professor of Surgery and Chair Emeritus, Department of Surgery, University of Michigan,
Ann Arbor, MI, USA

William B. Greenough, MD
Professor, Division of Geriatric Medicine, Johns Hopkins Bayview Medical Center,
Baltimore, MD, USA

W. Jerod Greer, MD
Instructor/Fellow, Division of Women's Pelvic Medicine and Reconstructive Surgery,
Department of Obstetrics and Gynecology, University of Alabama at Birmingham
Medical Center, Birmingham, AL, USA

Scott R. Gunn, MD
Associate Professor of Critical Care Medicine and Emergency Medicine,
Department of Critical Care Medicine, University of Pittsburgh Medical Center,
Pittsburgh, PA, USA

John W. Harmon, MD, FACS
Professor of Surgery, Department of Surgery, Johns Hopkins Bayview Medical Center,
Baltimore, MD, USA

Stefan D. Holubar, MD
Colon and Rectal Surgery Fellow, Division of Colon and Rectal Surgery,
Dartmouth Medical School, Dartmouth-Hitchcock Medical Center,
Lebanon, NH, USA

Bruce O. Hough, MD
Fellow, Division of Hematology/Oncology, University of Pittsburgh Medical Center,
Pittsburgh, PA, USA

John W. Hsu, MD
Transplant Surgery Fellow, Division of Surgery, University of Pennsylvania Transplant
Institute, Hospital of the University
of Pennsylvania, Philadelphia, PA, USA

Jonathan J. Hwang, MD
Associate Professor, Department of Urology, Georgetown University School of Medicine,
Washington Hospital Cancer/Georgetown University Hospital, Washington, DC, USA

Danny O. Jacobs, MD, MPH
David C. Sabiston, Jr. Professor and Chairman, Surgeon-in-Chief, Department of Surgery,
Duke University Hospital, Durham, NC, USA

Michael T. Jaklitsch, MD
Associate Professor of Surgery, Department of Thoracic Surgery,
Brigham and Women's Hospital, Boston, MA, USA

Sean M. Jeffery, PharmD
Associate Clinical Professor; Adjunct Assistant Professor, University of Connecticut
School of Pharmacy, Storrs, CT, USA; Yale University School of Medicine,
VA Connecticut Healthcare System, West Haven, CT, USA

Michael M. Johns, III MD
Director – Emory Voice Center; Assistant Professor, Department of Otolaryngology,
Emory University School of Medicine, Emory University Hospital, Atlanta, GA, USA

Sarah H. Kagan, PhD, RN
School of Nursing, University of Pennsylvania, Philadelphia, PA, USA

Kim U. Kahng, MD
Associate Director, Women's Health Education Program, Department of Medicine,
Drexel University College of Medicine, Philadelphia, PA, USA

Larry R. Kaiser, MD
President, Alkek-Williams Distinguished Physician Endowed Chair; Professor of
Cardiothoracic Surgery, University of Texas Health Science Center at Houston,
Houston, TX, USA

Prathima Kanumuri, MD
Department of Surgery, Baystate Medical Center, Springfield, MA, USA

Ilhan Karabicak, MD
Fellow, Department of Transplant Surgery, SUNY Downstate Medical Center, Brooklyn,
NY, USA

Ajay R. Kashi, DDS, MS
PhD Candidate, Department of Orthopaedic Surgery and Rehabilitation Medicine,
State University of New York Downstate Medical Center, Brooklyn, NY, USA

Mark R. Katlic, MD, MMM, FACS
Division of Thoracic Surgery, Director, Regional Ambulatory Campus Geisinger Wyoming
Valley Medical Center, Wilkes-Barre, PA, USA

Hongsoo Kim, PhD, MPH
Assistant Professor, Department of Health Policy and Management, Graduate School
of Public Health, Seoul National University, Seoul, South Korea

Sylvia S. Kim, MD
Assistant Professor of Surgery, Department of Colorectal and General Surgery,
SUNY Downstate Medical Center, Brooklyn, NY, USA

Denise C. King, RN, BSN, WCC
Wound Program Manager, Department of Wound Management, Johns Hopkins Bayview
Care Center, Baltimore, MD, USA

Joseph T. King Jr., MD, MSCE
Chief of Neurosurgery, VA Connecticut Healthcare System Chair, VA Neurosurgery
Surgical Advisory Board; Associate Professor of Neurosurgery, Director of Outcomes
Research, Department of Neurosurgery, Yale University School of Medicine,
West Haven, CT, USA

Clifford Y. Ko, MD, MS, MSHS, FACS
Professor of Surgery and Health Services, Robert and Kelly Chair in Surgical Outcomes,
Department of Surgery, David Geffen School of Medicine at UCLA, Los Angeles, CA, USA

Angela R. Kohli, BSN, WOCN, CWCN
Ambulatory Services Manager, Johns Hopkins Wound Healing Center/Dermatology,
Johns Hopkins Bayview Medical Center, Baltimore, MD, USA

John C. Kucharczuk, MD
Assistant Professor of Surgery, Department of Thoracic Surgery, University of Pennsylvania,
Philadelphia, PA, USA

Hiroko Kunitake, MD
Surgical Resident, Department of Surgery, Massachusetts General Hospital, Boston, MA, USA

Aaron N. LacKamp, MD
Clinical Associate, Department of Anesthesiology and Critical Care Medicine, Johns Hopkins Bayview Medical Center, Baltimore, MD, USA

Sandhya A. Lagoo-Deenadayalan, MD, PhD
Assistant Professor of Surgery, Department of Surgery, Duke University Hospital, Durham, NC, USA

Andrew G. Lee, MD
Professor of Ophthalmology, Neurology and Neurosurgery, Department of Ophthalmology, University of Iowa Hospitals and Clinics, Iowa City, IA, USA

David J. Leffell, MD
David Paige Smith Professor of Dermatology & Surgery, Yale New Haven Hospital, Department of Dermatology, Yale University School of Medicine, New Haven, CT, USA

Joshua L. Levine, MD
Director of Surgical Services, Department of Plastic and Reconstructive Surgery, New York Eye and Ear Infirmary, New York, NY, USA

Keith D. Lillimoe, MD
Jay L. Grosfeld Professor and Chairman, Department of Surgery, Indiana University School of Medicine, Indianapolis, IN, USA

Alexander Y. Lin, MD
Former Chief Resident, UCSF Plastic Surgery, University of California San Francisco, San Francisco, CA, USA; Assistant Professor of Surgery, Division of Plastic Surgery, Saint Louis University Director, St. Louis Cleft-Craniofacial Center, Cardinal Glennon Children's Medical Center at SLU, St. Louis, MO, USA

Lixin Liu, PhD
Postdoctoral Fellow, Department of Surgery, Johns Hopkins Bayside Medical Center, Baltimore, MD, USA

Kay O. Lovig, MD
Department of Internal Medicine, Greenwich Hospital, Greenwich, CT, USA

Frank E. Lucente, MD
Vice-Dean for Graduate Medical Education; Professor, Department of Otolaryngology, Downstate Medical Center, State University of New York, Brooklyn, NY, USA

Paul J. Maccabee, MD
Professor of Neurology, Department of Neurology, State University Hospital of Brooklyn, Brooklyn, NY, USA

Juan F. Macías-Núñez, MD, PhD
Titular Professor of Medicine, Department of Nephrology, Chief Section of Nephrology, University Hospital, Salamanca, Spain

Thomas H. Magnuson, MD
John's Hopkins Bayview Medical Center, Baltimore, MD, USA

Martin A. Makary, MD
The Mark Ravitch Chair, General Surgery, Associate Professor of Health Policy, Department of Surgery, Johns Hopkins Hospital, Baltimore, MD, USA

Richard A. Marottoli, MD, MPH
Associate Professor of Medicine, Department of Internal Medicine (Geriatrics)
Yale University School of Medicine, VA Connecticut Healthcare System,
New Haven, CT, USA

Gary T. Marshall, MD
Assistant Professor of Surgery, Department of Trauma Surgery, University of Pittsburgh
Medical Center, Pittsburgh, PA, USA

Guy P. Marti, MD
Department of Surgery, Johns Hopkins Bayview Medical Center, Baltimore, MD, USA

Manuel Martínez-Maldonado, MD
Executive Vice President for Research, University of Louisville; Professor of Medicine,
Professor of Pharmacology and Toxicology, University of Louisville Medical School,
Louisville, KY, USA

Marcus A. McFerren, MD, PhD
Resident Physician, Yale New Haven Hospital, Department of Dermatology,
Yale University School of Medicine, New Haven, CT, USA

Marcia L. McGory, MD
Resident Surgeon, Department of Surgery, David Geffen School of Medicine at the
University of California, Los Angeles, CA, USA

Mary H. McGrath, MD, MPH, FACS
Assistant Professor of Surgery, Division of Plastic Surgery,
University of California San Francisco, San Francisco, CA, USA

George H. Meier, MD
Professor and Chief, Department of Vascular Surgery, University Hospital of Cincinnati,
Cincinnati, OH, USA

Jay Menaker, MD
Assistant Professor, Department of Surgery, University of Maryland Medical Center,
R. Adams Cowley Shock Trauma Center, Baltimore, MD, USA

Manuel Mendizabal, MD
Staff Hepatologist, Division of Hepatology and Liver Transplantation, Austral University
Hospital Pilar, Buenos Aires, Argentina

William Min, MD, MS, MBA
Resident, Department of Orthopaedic Surgery, NYU Hospital for Joint Diseases,
New York, NY, USA

Monica Morrow, MD
Breast Service, Department of Surgery, Memorial Sloan-Kettering Cancer Center,
New York, NY, USA

Leigh Neumayer, MD, MS
Professor of Surgery, Department of Surgery, University of Utah and Huntsman
Cancer Hospital, Salt Lake City, UT, USA

Mark A. Newell, MD
Assistant Professor, Department of Surgery, Brody School of Medicine, East Carolina
University, Pitt County Memorial Hospital, Greenville, NC, USA

Andrew D. Norden, MD
Department of Neurology, Center for Neuro-Oncology, Dana-Farber Cancer Institute,
Brigham and Women's Hospital, Harvard Medical School,
Boston, MA, USA

Jack R. Oak, MD
Vascular Surgery Fellow, Department of Vascular Surgery, Barnes-Jewish Hospital,
University of Washington School of Medicine, St. Louis, MO, USA

Pat O'Donnell, MD
Department of Surgery, University of Arkansas for Medical Sciences,
Little Rock, AR, USA

Aundrea L. Oliver, MD
Resident, Department of Surgery, Brigham and Women's Hospital,
Harvard Medical School, Boston, MA, USA

John M. Olsewski, MD, FACS
Associate Professor of Orthopaedic Surgery, Department of Orthopaedic Surgery,
Albert Einstein College of Medicine, Bronx, NY, USA

Babak J. Orandi, MC, MSc
Halsted Surgery Resident, Department of Surgery, Johns Hopkins Hospital, Baltimore,
MD, USA

Darin L. Passer, MD
General Surgery Resident, Department of Surgery, University of South Carolina,
Palmetto Health Richland, Columbia, SC, USA

Toral R. Patel, MD
Neurosurgery Resident, Yale-New Haven Hospital, Yale University School of Medicine,
New Haven, CT, USA

Melissa F. Perkal, MD
Assistant Professor, Department of Surgery, Yale University School of Medicine,
West Haven, CT, USA; Surgical Service, Department of Veterans Affairs, VA Connecticut
Healthcare System, West Haven, CT, USA

Kitt F. Petersen, MD
Associate Professor, Department of Internal Medicine (Endocrinology), Yale University
School of Medicine, New Haven, CT, USA

Roshini C. Pinto-Powell, MD
Assistant Professor of Medicine, Department of General Internal Medicine, Dartmouth
Medical School, Dartmouth Hitchcock Medical Center, Lebanon, NH, USA

Walter E. Pofahl, MD
Vice Chairman, Department of Surgery, Brody School of Medicine, East Carolina University,
Pitt County Memorial Hospital, Greenville, NC, USA

Gregory N. Postma, MD
Director, Center for Voice and Swallowing Disorders; Professor, Department of
Otolaryngology, Medical College of Georgia, Augusta, GA, USA

Susan Pugliese, DDS, RN
Department of Dentistry, University Hospital of Brooklyn, State University of New York,
Downstate Medical Center, Brooklyn, NY, USA

Priyamvada Rai, PhD
Assistant Professor, Department of Medicine, Division of Gerontology and Geriatric
Medicine, Leonard M. Miller School of Medicine, University of Miami, Miami, FL, USA

Philip A. Rascoe, MD
Department of Thoracic Surgery, University of Pennsylvania,
Philadelphia, PA, USA

Pooja R. Raval, BA
Newark Beth Israel Hospital, Warren, NJ, USA

Maura Reinblatt, MD
Assistant Professor, Department of Plastic Surgery, John's Hopkins Bayview Medical Center, Baltimore, MD, USA

Jerry G. Reves, MD
Vice President for Medical Affairs; Dean, College of Medicine; Professor, Department of Anesthesia and Perioperative Medicine, Cell and Molecular Pharmacology & Experimental Therapeutic, Medical University of South Carolina, Charleston, SC, USA

Holly E. Richter, PhD, MD
Professor, Department of Obstetrics and Gynecology, Division Director, Women's Pelvic Medicine and Reconstructive Surgery, University of Alabama at Birmingham Medical Center, Birmingham, AL, USA

David Rispler, MD
Assistant Professor, Michigan State Orthopedic Residency Program, Grand Rapids Orthopedic Residency Program, Grand Rapids, MI, USA

Sanziana A. Roman, MD
Chief, Endocrine Surgery, Associate Professor, Yale University School of Medicine, New Haven, CT, USA

Carlos Rosales, MD
Vascular Surgery Fellow, Department of Vascular Surgery, University of Cincinnati, Cincinnati, OH, USA

Klara Rosenquist, MD
Department of Internal Medicine (Endocrinology), Yale University School of Medicine, New Haven, CT, USA

Ronnie A. Rosenthal, MD
Professor, Department of Surgery Yale University School of Medicine, New Haven; Chief Surgical Service, Department of Veterans Affairs, VA Connecticut Healthcare System, West Haven, CT, USA

Jesse Roth, MD
Professor of Medicine; Investigator; Former Professor and Chief, Geriatric Medicine and Gerontology; Former Scientific Director and Chief, Diabetes Branch, Feinstein Institute for Medical Research, Albert Einstein College of Medicine, North Shore-Long Island Jewish Health System, Whitestone, NY, USA`

Thomas J. Rutherford, MD, PhD
Associate Professor, Department of Obstetrics and Gynecology/Gynecologic Oncology, Yale University School of Medicine/Yale New Haven Hospital, New Haven, CT, USA

Thomas M. Scalea, MD
Physician in Chief, R. Adams Cowley Shock Trauma Center, Baltimore, MD, USA

Peter E. Schwartz, MD
Professor, Department of Obstetrics and Gynecology/Gynecologic Oncology, Yale University School of Medicine/Yale New Haven Hospital, New Haven, CT, USA

Seymour I. Schwartz, MD, FACS
Distinguished Alumni Professor of Surgery, Department of Surgery, University of Rochester, Strong Memorial Hospital, Rochester, NY, USA

Dorry L. Segev, MD, PhD
Associate Professor of Surgery, Department of Transplant Surgery, Johns Hopkins Hospital,
Baltimore, MD, USA

Neal E. Seymour, MD
Division Chief General Surgery; Professor, Department of Surgery, Baystate Medical Center,
Springfield, MA, USA; Tufts University School of Medicine, Springfield, MA, USA

Ashok R. Shaha, MD
Attending Surgeon, Professor of Surgery, Department of Surgery,
Memorial Sloan Kettering Cancer Center, New York, NY, USA

Abraham Shaked, MD, PhD
Professor of Surgery, Division of Surgery; Director, University of Pennsylvania
Transplant Institute, Hospital of the University of Pennsylvania, Philadelphia, PA, USA

Vadim Sherman, MD, MSc, FRCSC
Assistant Professor of Surgery, Michael E. DeBakey Department of Surgery,
Baylor College of Medicine, Houston, TX, USA

Gregorio A. Sicard, MD
Professor of Surgery, Vice Chair of the Department of Surgery, Barnes-Jewish Memorial
Hospital/Washington University School of Medicine, St. Louis, MO, USA

Frederick E. Sieber, MD
Associate Professor; Chairman, Department of Anesthesiology and Critical Care Medicine,
Johns Hopkins Bayview Medical Center, Baltimore, MD, USA

Dan-Arin Silasi, MD
Assistant Professor, Department of Obstetrics and Gynecology/Gynecologic Oncology,
Yale University School of Medicine/Yale New Haven Hospital, New Haven, CT, USA

Samir K. Sinha, MD, DPhil, FRCPC
Director of Geriatrics, Mount Sinai and the University Health Network Hospitals,
Division of Geriatric Medicine, University of Toronto, Suite 475 - 600 University Avenue,
Toronto, Ontario CANADA, M5G 1X5

James Slover, MD, MS
Assistant Professor, Department of Orthopaedic Surgery, NYU Hospital for Joint Diseases,
New York, NY, USA

Kelley A. Sookraj, MD
Department of Surgery, SUNY Downstate Medical Center, Brooklyn, NY, USA

Julie Ann Sosa, MA, MD
Associate Professor of Surgery, Department of Surgery, Maine Medical Center, Portland,
ME, USA

Dennis Spencer, MD
Harvey and Kate Cushing Professor and Chair, Department of Neurosurgery,
Yale University School of Medicine, Yale New Haven Hospital, New Haven, CT, USA

Raymond P. Stowe, PhD
Senior Scientist, Microgen Laboratories, La Marque, TX, USA

Catherine M. Straub, BS, MD
Department of General Surgery, University of Utah, Salt Lake City, UT, USA

John A. Taylor III, MD
Assistant Professor, Division of Urology, Department of Surgery, University of Connecticut
Health Center, Farmington, CT, USA

Roby C. Thompson Jr., MD
Department of Orthopaedic Surgery, University of Minnesota, Minneapolis, MN, USA

Scott C. Thornton, MD, FACS, FASCRS
Assistant Clinical Professor of Surgery, Department of General Surgery,
Bridgeport Hospital, Yale University, Bridgeport, CT, USA

Pedro J. Torrico, MD
Resident, Department of Neurology, SUNY Downstate Medical Center, Whitestone,
NY, USA

Courtney M. Townsend Jr., MD
Professor and John Woods Harris Distinguished Chairman, Department of Surgery,
University of Texas Medical Branch, Galveston, TX, USA

Bruce R. Troen, MD
Department of Medicine, Division of Gerontology and Geriatric Medicine,
Leonard M. Miller School of Medicine, University of Miami, Miami VA GRECC,
Miami, FL, USA

Donald D. Trunkey, MD
Professor Emeritus, Department of Surgery, Oregon Health & Science University,
Portland, OR, USA

Edward M. Uchio, MD
Chief of Urology; Assistant Professor of Surgery, Section of Urology, VA Connecticut
Healthcare System, West Haven, CT, USA; Department of Surgery, Yale University
School of Medicine, New Haven, CT, USA

Robert Udelsman, MD, MBA
William H. Carmalt Professor of Surgery and Oncology Chairman, Department of Surgery,
Yale University School of Medicine, New Haven, CT, USA

Frank J. Veith, MD, FACS
Professor of Surgery, Department of Surgery, New York University, Bronx, NY, USA

Selwyn M. Vickers, MD
Jay Phillips Professor and Chairman, Department of Surgery, University of Minnesota,
Minneapolis, MN, USA

Jennifer F. Waljee, MD, MPH, MS
House Officer, Plastic and Reconstructive Surgery, Department of Surgery,
University of Michigan Medical Center, Ann Arbor, MI, USA

Lisa M. Walke, MD
Associate Professor; Chief, Geriatrics Consult Service, Geriatrics & Extended Care Service,
Department of Medicine, Yale University School of Medicine, New Haven, CT, USA;
VA Connecticut Healthcare System, West Haven, CT, USA

Barbara A. Ward, MD
Medical Director, Department of Surgery, The Breast Center at Greenwich Hospital,
Greenwich, CT, USA

Jennifer A. Wargo, MD
Instructor of Surgery; Assistant in Surgery, Division of Surgical Oncology, Harvard Medical
School, Boston, MA, USA; Massachusetts General Hospital, Boston, MA, USA

Samuel A. Wells, Jr. MD
Professor of Surgery, Department of Surgery, Washington University Medical Center,
St. Louis, MO, USA

Thomas Wheeler II, MD, MSPH
Assistant Professor, Division of Women's Pelvic Medicine and Reconstructive Surgery, Department of Obstetrics and Gynecology, University of Alabama at Birmingham Medical Center, Birmingham, AL, USA

Lisa S. Wiechmann, MD
Department of Surgery, Memorial Sloan-Kettering Cancer Center, New York, NY, USA

Michael Wilderman, MD
Vascular Fellow, Division of Vascular Surgery, Barnes Jewish Hospital, Washington University, St. Louis, MO, USA

Earle W. Wilkins, Jr. MD
Clinical Professor of Surgery, Department of Surgery, Massachusetts General Hospital, Boston, MA, USA

Hugh L. Willcox, III MD
Resident, Department of General Surgery, Palmetto Health Richland Hospital, Columbia, SC, USA

Aaron M. Winnick, MD
Fellow, Department of Transplant Surgery, SUNY Downstate Medical Center, Brooklyn, NY, USA

Jordan M. Winter, MD
Department of Surgery, Johns Hopkins Hospital, Baltimore, MD, USA

Bruce G. Wolff, MD
Professor of Surgery, Department of Surgery; Chair, Division of Colon and Rectal Surgery, College of Medicine Mayo Clinic, Rochester, MN, USA

Leslie S. Wu, MD
Clinical Fellow, Department of Surgery, Maine Medical Center, Portland, ME, USA

Dongmei Xing, MD, PhD
Johns Hopkins University School of Medicine, Baltimore, MD, USA

Arash Yaghoobian, MD
Orthopaedic Resident, Department of Orthopaedic Surgery, Montefiore Medical Center, Albert Einstein College of Medicine, Bronx, NY, USA

Michael E. Zenilman, MD, FACS
School of Public Health, SUNY Downstate, Brooklyn, NY; Department of Surgery, Johns Hopkins School of Medicine, Baltimore, MD

Xianjie Zhang, MD, PhD
Post-doctoral Fellow, Department of Surgery, Johns Hopkins School of Medicine, Baltimore, MD, USA

Joseph D. Zuckerman, MD
Walter A. L. Thompson Professor of Orthopaedic Surgery and Chairman, Department of Orthopaedics, NYU Hospital for Joint Diseases, New York, NY, USA

Section I
Physiology of Aging

Chapter 1
Invited Commentary

Jesse Roth

Get in league with the future.

Horace Greeley

The Future

By reading this piece, you are identifying yourself as a part of the vanguard in geriatric surgery. Textbooks of surgery and textbooks of geriatrics cover geriatric surgery very sparingly. You have chosen to tackle a textbook on geriatric surgery.

Demographics and Dollars

The elderly are the fastest growing segment of the population, with the so-called old–old in the lead. The elderly are highly overrepresented in the hospital population and in the medical expenses column. The application more widely of basic well-established principles of care for the elderly will almost certainly reduce the number of elderly in the hospital and increase the return on money spent. Most important, we can expect better outcomes for the elderly patients, especially for those who were hospitalized. Hospitalization and surgery are each serious threats for the elderly patient.

Geriatrics Is a Frontier

"Go West, young man," [1] was an exhortation to move from the built up to the new, the frontier, the so-called cutting edge. Geriatrics as a branch of medicine is young and is having a growth spurt. The subspecialties in medicine are increasing their attention to issues related to care for the elderly. In geriatric surgery, the frontiers are open.

History provides us with some models. Harvey Cushing was one of the twentieth century's giants, a pioneer. In the early years of the twentieth century, with great daring and deep thought, he took principles of general surgery and very meticulously applied them to the brain. In addition to his skills in the operating theater, he gave his patients extraordinarily attentive care, before surgery as well as after. Indeed, infection rates on his patients in the pre-antibiotic area, would win a commendation medal today. Today we revere him as the father of neurosurgery [2].

Pediatrics emerged from adult medicine at about the same time [3]. Now pediatrics has a complete array of sub-specialists covering all aspects of care for the young. When I was a medical student 50 years ago, pediatric surgery was just coming into its own. Now it is a well-established subspecialty.

Quest for Excellence

As the age of the patient increases, the gap grows that separates the *good physician* from the *excellent physician*. A similar gap shows itself as the age of the child decreases. The premature baby and the frail elderly share many features. One very big difference – pediatrics, pediatric surgery, pediatric nursing, neonatology, pediatric gastroenterology, pediatric endocrinology, and their cousins are well-developed areas of expertise with highly trained practitioners. Their counterparts in the care of the elderly are fewer and are less deeply trained. It is much more difficult for physicians involved in the care of an elderly patient to get expert help than it is for the doctor caring for a child. Worse yet, the adult physicians (and other medical providers) who are inadequately trained in geriatric care are often unaware of their deficiencies.

J. Roth (✉)
Feinstein Institute for Medical Research, Albert Einstein College of Medicine, North Shore-Long Island Jewish Health System, 149-37 Powells Cove Blvd, Whitestone 11357, NY, USA
e-mail: jesserothmd@hotmail.com

R.A. Rosenthal et al. (eds.), *Principles and Practice of Geriatric Surgery*, DOI 10.1007/978-1-4419-6999-6_1, © Springer Science+Business Media, LLC 2011

Fifty years ago, all of us were deficient as well as unaware of our deficiencies in care of the elderly. I have clear memories of a man in his eighties cared for by me and by a surgeon. The surgery was successful but the patient had a series of complications and died. Today, I can think of many useful interventions that were unknown and unused by us in those days.

The Challenge

The elderly patient is intrinsically more complex and challenging than the equally ill youngster. The young patient typically has one disease – complications and medications are few. The older patient classically has multiple conditions and a long list of medications, co-conspirators that blur the diagnosis and complicate the therapy. Laboratory values in young patients have established norms developed in young people. Normal ranges for the elderly are much less reliable, often guesses, appropriated with little testing from a much younger age group. Family responsibility for the young patient has a well-defined societal pattern whereas family links to the elderly patient are very variable and may require high level diplomacy. Yet, optimal outcomes for the young patient and for the old often require skillful and energetic family involvement.

Medical decisions with an elderly patient require professional skills at their best. The physician may start with an evidence-based algorithm conceived on experience with younger patients but the plan needs to be custom made for the particular patient at hand. In addition to deciding which tests and which surgery should be done, an important part of the care is deciding which tests and which surgery should not be performed. Even when a patient fulfills all the criteria for surgery, good judgment may modify or veto that decision for an elderly patient.

Medical Care from Here to the Future

Someday, care for the elderly will be totally in the hands of skilled caregivers who are highly trained in geriatrics, as exists now in pediatrics. Today, individual caregivers must gain multiple skills in many aspects of caring for the elderly. There are unique opportunities at your medical center to be among the pioneers who are importing best geriatric practices into surgery. In addition, you need to search for and recruit as advisors the minority of health care deliverers in your community who are skilled in caring for the geriatric patient.

Learning, teaching, and research opportunities will abound.

Scientific Advances in Geriatrics

The opening chapters of this book tackle several important scientific areas related to aging and the elderly patient. I recall meetings in geriatrics 20 years ago when the papers dealing with lab studies on aging fit a single track for 1 day. Now multiple tracks on multiple days are needed. The scientific basis of bone health, muscle wasting, and longevity are each a rich lode of discovery. The coming age of science in geriatrics is best epitomized by studies of cell aging that led to the 2009 Nobel Prize for pioneer work on telomeres.

The Road Ahead for the Physician

Intense focus in a well-circumscribed area can add great value to the physician's effort. These efforts often translate into shorter less expensive stays in the hospital, a language understood by administrators. At a time when burnout is increasingly widespread among physicians, these efforts can also be very rewarding to the professional soul.

Treatment for burnout has a poor prognosis. Prevention is more likely to succeed. Given the large loan balances and uncertain retirement programs that burden young physicians, the journey ahead may be unexpectedly long. Passionate commitment to a segment of one's professional life may be the key to a long happy satisfying medical career at this difficult time. Care for the elderly is energized by a pioneer spirit that makes it especially attractive for a long career.

References

1. Ascribed to Horace Greeley
2. Bliss M (2005) Harvey cushing: a life in surgery. University of Toronto Press, Toronto
3. Markel H (2000) For the welfare of children: the origins of the relationship between us public health workers and pediatricians. Am J Public Health 90:893–899

Chapter 2
Cell and Molecular Aging*

Priyamvada Rai and Bruce R. Troen

Every day you get older – that's a law.
Butch Cassidy to the Sundance Kid

Aging seems to be the only available way to live a long life
Daniel Francois Esprit Auber

There is no such thing as a free lunch
Anonymous

Introduction

Discussions of aging invariably begin by establishing a satisfactory definition for the term *aging* and the related word *senescence*. Although the term *aging* is commonly used to refer to postmaturational processes that lead to diminished homeostasis and increased organismic vulnerability, the more correct term for this is *senescence* (derived from the Latin word "senescere," meaning to grow old or to diminish), which explicitly refers to the process of growing old and sustaining related deterioration. *Aging* on the other hand can refer to any time-related process. We will use *senescence* to refer to cellular phenomena and *aging* to refer to changes, as organisms grow old.

Gerontologists often categorize the process of aging into normal, usual, or successful aging. *Normal* aging involves inexorable and universal physiological changes, whereas *usual* aging includes age-related diseases. For example, menopause and the decline in renal function represent aspects of normal aging. In contrast, coronary artery disease is an example of usual aging and is not found in all older persons. *Successful* aging encompasses the concept of growing older without significant impairment of physiological, cognitive, and social function. This approach to aging enables the utilization of a conceptual framework that identifies intrinsic (developmental-genetic) versus extrinsic (stochastic) causes. However, accumulating evidence increasingly stresses the importance of both. Indeed, the altered homeostasis in older organisms is likely the result of a genetic program that determines the response to exogenous influences and thereby increases the predisposition to illness and death.

Life Span and Life Expectancy

The average/median life span (also known as life expectancy) is represented by the age at which 50% of a given population survives, and maximum life span potential (MLSP) represents the longest-lived member(s) of the population or species. The average life span of humans has increased dramatically over time, yet the MLSP has remained approximately constant (Fig. 2.1) [1]. For 99% of our existence as a species, the average life expectancy for human was very short compared to the present. During the Bronze Age (circa 3,000 B.C.), the average life expectancy was 18 years due to disease and accidents. Average life expectancy in 275 B.C. was still only 26 years. By 1900, improved sanitation helped to improve the average life expectancy at birth for humans to 47 years, but infectious disease was still a major killer. As of 2005, better diet, health care, and reduced infant mortality had resulted in an average life expectancy of 77.8 years [2]. The increase in the average life expectancy has resulted in a compression of morbidity (a squaring

*Portions of this chapter are reprinted with permission from Troen BR (2003) The biology of aging. Mt Sinai J Med 70(1):3–22.

P. Rai (✉) and B.R. Troen (✉)
Department of Medicine, Division of Gerontology and Geriatric Medicine, Leonard M. Miller School of Medicine, University of Miami, Miami VA GRECC, Miami, FL, USA
e-mail: prai@med.miami.edu; troen@miami.edu

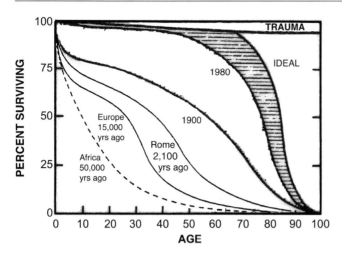

Figure 2.1 Percent survival curve for humans at different times in history with varying environments, nutrition, and medical care. The 50% survival values have improved, but maximum life-span potential has remained the same (From Troen BR (2003) The biology of Aging. Mt Sinai J Med 70(1):3–22. Reprinted with permission of John Wiley & Sons, Inc.).

of the mortality curve) towards the end of the life span (Fig. 2.1). Of note, the longest-lived human for whom documentation exists was Jeanne Calment, who died at the age of 122 in August 1997. The longest-lived male was Christian Mortensen, who died in 1998 at the age of 115. As causes of early mortality have been eliminated through public-health measures and improved medical care, more individuals have approached the maximum life span. Between 1960 and 2000, the population of those aged 85 years and over grew 356%, whereas the elderly population in general rose 111%, and the entire U.S. population grew only 57% [3].

A number of physiological functions begin a progressive decline from the fourth decade onward, including the cardiovascular, pulmonary, renal, and immune systems. In women, this correlates with a decline in reproductive capacity. Interestingly, one study has shown that women who are fertile in their forties are nearly four times as likely to survive to the age of 100 than women who are not [4], suggesting that reproductive fitness later in life may be an indicator of longevity. The age of menopause has also been linked to life span. Controlling for socioeconomic factors, women who undergo menopause before the age of 40 are twice as likely to die before those who experience menopause after the age of 50 [5, 6]. These findings hold true even when a history of estrogen replacement therapy is taken into account, suggesting that reduced estrogen alone is not responsible for the ostensible reduction in life span. Another study found that while late reproduction correlated with increased longevity in postreproductive Sami women, maternal age at first birth and total fecundity did not appear to impact female longevity [7]. In males, although spermatogenesis per se does not show a significant age-related decline, testosterone levels fall with advancing age, and a few studies have linked reduced bioavailability of testosterone to age-related functional

degeneration [8, 9]. Therefore, it would appear that there is a link between reproductive health, aging, and life span (see the disposable soma theory discussed below).

MLSP appears to be species-specific, implying a significant genetic component to the rate of aging. For example, humans have an MLSP 25- to 30-fold higher than mice. Some biodemographic estimates predict that elimination of most of the major killers such as cancer, cardiovascular disease, and diabetes would add no more than 10 years to the average life expectancy, but would not affect MLSP [10, 11]. This implies an upper limit to the MLSP. Some models suggest that genes operate by raising or lowering the relative risk of death by making cancer, coronary disease, or Alzheimer's disease more likely, rather than by fixing the life span. One mathematical model predicts that if participants in the Framingham Heart Study had been able to maintain the levels of 11 different risk factors similar to those of a typical 30 year old, the men and women would have survived to an average age of 99.9 and 97.0 years, respectively [10].

There are three known regimens that can extend life span. The first two involve lowering ambient temperature and reducing exercise and are effective in poikilotherms (cold-blooded species). A 10°C drop or the elimination of a housefly's capacity to fly extends the maximum life span approximately 250% [12]. Both of these manipulations decrease the metabolic rate and are accompanied by decreases in free radical generation and oxidative damage to protein and DNA.

The third intervention is caloric restriction, which can extend life span in yeast, worms, flies, grasshoppers, spiders, water fleas, hamsters, mice, rats, and dogs [13]. Dietary restriction without malnutrition can increase both the average and maximum life spans of mice and rats by more than 50% [14, 15]. Although calories are severely restricted (up to 40%), essential nutrients such as vitamins and minerals are maintained at levels equivalent to those found in ad libitum diets. The diet-restricted animals also exhibit a delay in the onset of physiological and pathological changes with aging [16]. These include hormone and lipid levels, female reproduction, immune function, nephropathy, cardiomyopathy, osteodystrophy, and malignancies. Size, weight, fat percentage, and some organ weights are markedly less in calorically restricted animals [17]. The specific metabolic rate, the amount of oxygen consumed per gram of tissue, decreased in rats subjected to caloric restriction [18, 19]. However, in one study, long-term food restriction did not alter the metabolic rate [20]. This finding suggests that the specific metabolic rate may not be a critical determinant of longevity. To date, life span extension in mammals by dietary restriction has been most convincingly demonstrated in rodents. However, dietary restriction in primates [21–24] and in humans [25, 26] does appear to improve a number of metabolic and cardiovascular disease risk parameters.

Characteristics of Aging

There is evidence supporting at least five common characteristics of aging in mammals (Table 2.1):

1. *Increased mortality with age after maturation*: In the early nineteenth century, Gompertz first described the exponential increase in mortality with aging due to various causes, a phenomenon that still pertains today [27]. In 2005, the death rate for all causes at the age of 25–34 was 104.4/100,000 and at the age of 35–44 was 193.3/100,000. Death rates at the age of 65–74, 75–84, and 85 and over were 2,137.1/100,000, 5,260.0/100,000, and 13,798.6/100,000 respectively: a greater than 130-fold increase from young adults to the oldest group [28]. Indeed, the pattern of age-related survival is similar across species, including invertebrates and single-cell organisms (Fig. 2.2).

2. *Changes in biochemical composition in tissues with age*: There are notable age-related decreases in lean body mass and total bone mass in humans [29, 30]. Although subcutaneous fat is either unchanged or declining, total fat remains the same [29]. Consequently, the percentage of adipose tissue increases with age. At the cellular level,

TABLE 2.1 Characteristics of aging

1. Increased mortality with age after maturation
2. Changes in biochemical composition in tissues with age
3. Progressive decrease in physiological capacity with age
4. Reduced ability to respond adaptively to environmental stimuli with age
5. Increased susceptibility and vulnerability to disease

many markers of aging have been described in various tissues from different organisms [31]. Two of the first to be described were increases in lipofuscin (age pigment) [32] and increased cross-linking in extracellular matrix molecules such as collagen [33, 34]. Recent studies have shown that DNA damage markers such as gamma-H2AX and 53BP1 are upregulated in tissues of aged primates [35, 36] and mice [37], presumably arising from DNA double-strand breaks (DSB) and/or dysfunctional chromosome ends called telomeres. Additional examples include age-related changes in both the rates of transcription of specific genes and the rate of protein synthesis and numerous age-related alterations in posttranslational protein modifications, such as glycation and oxidation [38, 39]. For instance, the p16INK4a gene product has been found to be upregulated in a number of tissues from aging individuals and animals (see below).

3. *Progressive decrease in physiological capacity with age*: Many physiologic changes have been documented in both cross-sectional and longitudinal studies. Examples include declines in glomerular filtration rate, maximal heart rate, and vital capacity [40]. These decreases occur linearly from about the age of 30; however, the rate of physiological decline is quite heterogeneous from organ to organ and individual to individual [41, 42].

4. *Reduced ability to respond adaptively to environmental stimuli with age*: A fundamental feature of senescence is the diminished ability to maintain homeostasis [43]. This is manifested, not primarily by changes in resting or basal parameters, but in the altered response to an external stimulus such as exercise or fasting. The loss of "reserve"

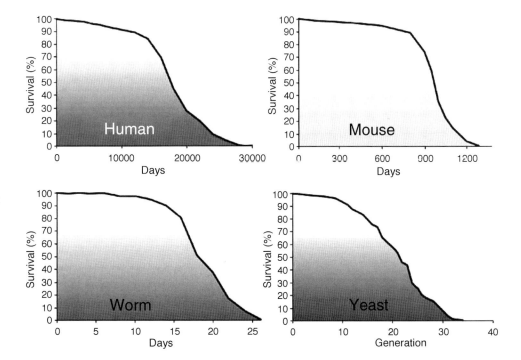

FIGURE 2.2 Viability curves from different model organisms have a similar characteristic shape. Representative mortality data are shown for *Homo sapiens*, *Mus musculus*, *Caenorhabditis elegans*, and *Saccharomyces cerevisiae* (From Troen BR (2003) The biology of Aging. Mt Sinai J Med 70(1):3–22. Reprinted with permission of John Wiley & Sons, Inc.).

can result in blunted maximum responses as well as in delays in reaching a peak level and in returning to basal levels. For example, the induction of hepatic tyrosine aminotransferase activity by fasting is both attenuated and delayed in old rodents [43]. The immune response also appears to be impaired in older individuals, leading to reduced ability to fight infections, less protection from vaccinations, higher incidences of autoimmunity, and impaired antigen affinity and class-switching by lymphocytes (reviewed by Dorshkind et al. [44]).

5. *Increased susceptibility and vulnerability to disease*: The incidence and mortality rates for many diseases increase with age and parallel the exponential increase in mortality with age [45]. For the five leading causes of death for people over 65 years of age, the relative increase in death rates compared to people aged between 25 and 44 is: heart disease – 92-fold, cancer – 43-fold, stroke – >100-fold, chronic lung disease – >100-fold, and pneumonia and influenza – 89-fold [46]. The basis for these dramatic rises in mortality is incompletely understood but presumably involves changes in the function of many types of cells that lead to tissue/organ dysfunction and systemic illness. Interestingly, a retrospective study of centenarians demonstrated that they live 90–95% of their lives in very good health and with a high level of functional independence [47]. The centenarians do suffer a 30–50% annual mortality at the end of their lives, but this represents a marked compression of morbidity towards the end of life and is close to the idealized survival curve in Figs. 2.1 and 2.2.

Mechanisms/Theories of Aging

In an effort to adequately explain the phenotype of aged organisms, many speculations about the cause(s) of aging have been proposed. However, what is known about the fundamental molecular mechanisms involved in aging remains controversial and largely unproven. A major reason for this is the obvious complexity of the problem. Aging changes are manifested from the molecular to the organismal level; environmental factors affect experimental observations; secondary effects complicate elucidation of primary mechanisms; there exist a dearth of easily measurable "biomarkers" that are consistent over different tissues and species. No one unifying theory may exist since the mechanisms of aging could be quite distinct in different organisms, tissues, and cells, although there appear to be certain mechanisms, such as DNA damage, that are broadly conserved despite differences in specific response.

Theories of aging have historically been divided into two general categories: developmental-genetic and stochastic (Table 2.2). The term "developmental-genetic" implies a more active genetic control of aging than likely exists. In

Table 2.2 Theories of aging

Developmental/genetic
Antagonistic pleiotropy theory
Longevity-associated genes
Disposable soma theory

Stochastic
Free radical/oxidative stress
Mitochondrial dysfunction theory
DNA damage theory of aging

addition, as described below, these categories are not mutually exclusive, particularly when considering the free radical/mitochondrial DNA theory of aging. Indeed, there is likely a spectrum from birth to senescence that reflects a decreasing influence of active genetic influences and an increasing effect of stochastic events. This would parallel the shift in importance in general versus species-specific genes.

Developmental/Genetic Theories

A general framework for a plausible theory of aging begins with attempting to understand the evolutionary basis of senescence. Developmental-genetic theories consider the process of aging to be part of the genetically programmed and controlled continuum of development and maturation. Although this is an attractive notion, the diverse expression of aging effects is in sharp contrast to the tightly controlled and very precise processes of development. Also, evolution selects for the optimization of reproduction; the effects of genes expressed in later life probably do not play a large role in the evolution of a species. This class of theories is supported by the observation that the maximum life span is highly species-specific. As noted above, the maximum life span for humans is 30 times that of mice. In addition, studies comparing the longevity of monozygotic and dizygotic twins and nontwin siblings have shown a remarkable similarity between monozygotic twins that is not seen in the other two groups.

However, it is also likely that the interplay of genetic responses to extrinsic stresses may modulate the extent of aging. An interesting example of this theory comes from a study by Niedernhofer et al. who demonstrated that aging mice as well as normal adult mice treated with mitomycin C to elevate DNA damage levels showed a shift in gene expression that was very similar to that observed in a mouse model of XPF-ERCC deficiency, a novel genetic disorder associated with accelerated aging [48]. The alterations in the transcriptome reflected enhanced antioxidant and anabolic pathways and reduced insulin growth factor (IGF-1) signaling (a known longevity assurance mechanism), suggesting a systemic shift of the somatotrophic axis from growth to maintenance under genotoxic stress. Thus, in the model of

XFE/ERCC$^{-/-}$ progeroid syndrome, the phenotypic outcomes depend not just on DNA damaging stimuli, which likely cause a functional decline, but also on the genetic adaptive response to the damage mediated by the IGF metabolic pathway [48].

Antagonistic Pleiotropy

Evolutionary pressures select for a minimum successful life: this includes the ability to reach reproductive age, procreate, and then care for offspring until weaned (so that they, in turn, will achieve reproductive age and continue the cycle) [49, 50]. Within this context, it is likely that the postreproductive/ parental physiology of an organism is an epigenetic and pleiotropic manifestation of the optimization for early fitness. Kirkwood proposes that three categories of genes may be involved in senescence [51]: (1) those that regulate somatic maintenance and repair, (2) negatively pleiotropic genes that enhance early survival but are disadvantageous later in life (antagonistic pleiotropy), and (3) harmful late-acting mutations upon which little evolutionary selection is exerted. The presence of these genes may represent a spectrum from general to species-specific. Genes involved in cell maintenance and repair are likely to be present in all (or most) organisms, since such essential processes are similar across species. Late-acting mutations are probably species-specific because they are likely to be individualistic and random. Nonmaintenance pleiotropic genes could be universally found within a population or species, but may not be shared between species. An example of antagonistic pleiotropy would be the high expression of testosterone in a male gorilla that could lead to increased aggression and strength that would allow the male to become dominant and mate more frequently, but may eventually lead to a shortened life span due to increased atherosclerosis. Recent studies at the molecular genetic level have suggested that cellular senescence may be antagonistically pleiotropic because it prevents tumorigenesis but also contributes to organismal aging (see below).

Longevity Genes

There is ample evidence in multiple species that MLSP is under genetic control, though the degree of heritability is likely to be less than 35% [52]. Despite this apparently low figure, genetic mutations can significantly modify senescence. In yeast, a number of genes affect both the average and maximum life span [53]. The products of these genes act in diverse ways, including modulating stress response, sensing nutritional status, increasing metabolic capacity, and silencing genes that promote aging. In the nematode (*C. elegans*), mutants with increased life span have revealed various genes

that appear to play a role [54]: *age*-1 – altered aging rate, *daf*-2 and *daf*-23 – activation of a delay in development, *spe*-26 – reduced fertility, and *clk*-1 – altered biological clock. These genes alter stress resistance (particularly in response to ultraviolet light), development, signal transduction, and metabolic activity. The *daf*-2 gene appears to encode an insulin receptor family member [55]. Mutations in *daf*-2 can double the life span but require the *daf*-16 gene [56]. A mutation in the daf-16 gene suppresses the UV resistance and increased longevity of the other gene mutants, suggesting that it acts at a critical point downstream of the other genes [54]. The *daf*-16 gene is a member of the hepatocyte nuclear factor-3/forkhead family of transcriptional regulators involved in a variety of signal transduction pathways, including insulin signaling [57]. A notable connection between single gene effects upon aging in yeast and higher eukaryotes was revealed by the finding that overexpression of the SIR2 gene and its homolog Sirt1 (sirtuin 1) extend life span in yeast and nematodes, respectively [58]. Sir2 (silent information regulator) is an NAD+-dependent histone deacetylase that silences transcription and stablizes repetitive DNA in yeast. Aging and DNA damage induce Sir protein complexes to relocalize to sites of genomic instability, resulting in desilencing of genes. Sirtuin genes can function as antiaging genes in yeast, worms, and flies [59]. There are seven mammalian sirtuin genes whose protein products function as histone deacetylases (SIRT1,2,3,5,6,7) and/or ADP-ribosyltransferases (SIRT4,6). SIR2 and its homologs appear to exert their effects by linking metabolism to aging and also enhancing mitochondrial biogenesis and efficiency [59, 60] (see below). SIRT1 modulates the activity of multiple critical transcriptional regulators of metabolism, including FOXO1, FOXO3a, PPARα, PPARγ, and PGC-1α, which in turn impacts fatty acid oxidation, gluconeogenesis and glycolysis, oxidative capacity, fat mobilization and adipogenesis, and insulin secretion.

A line of *Drosophila melanogaster* has been identified that exhibits an approximately 35% increase in average life span and enhanced resistance to various forms of stress, including starvation, high temperature, and dietary paraquat, a free-radical generator [61]. The mutation responsible, dubbed methuselah, appears to reside within a single gene that is homologous to GTP-binding transmembrane domain receptors. Another single-gene mutation leads to almost a doubling of the average adult *Drosophila* life span without a decline in fertility or physical activity [62]. This gene, named Indy (for I'm not dead yet), is homologous to a mammalian sodium dicarboxylate cotransporter, which is a membrane protein that transports Kreb's cycle intermediates. The investigators speculate that the mutation in the Indy gene may create a metabolic state that mimics caloric restriction. Previous studies have demonstrated that one group of long-lived flies is more resistant to oxidative stress [63], whereas another group exhibits resistance to starvation and desiccation [64].

Genetic analysis of longevity in mammals has not been as revealing. However, immune loci in mice and humans have been implicated in long-lived subjects [53]. In addition, a mutation in the gene encoding the signaling molecule p66(shc), which significantly enhances the resistance to oxidative stress, increases the mean life span of mice by 30% [65]. The Snell dwarf mouse contains a single-gene mutation that alters pituitary development and prevents the production of growth hormone, thyrotropin, and prolactin [66]. The dwarf mouse also exhibits an extended life span of 25–50% but is much smaller than normal mice. In contrast, the mice with the mutant p66 develop normally and are not significantly smaller than wild-type mice (see Table 2.3).

There does appear to be a genetic component to longevity in humans. A number of mitochondrial DNA polymorphisms and variants are associated with life span (reviewed by De Benedictis et al. [67] and by Salvioli et al. [68]). The J haplogroup was found in a significantly greater percentage of male centenarians in northern Italy than in younger subjects. Interestingly, this same mitochondrial haplotype is overrepresented in a number of complex diseases [69], raising the possibility of an antagonistically pleiotropic gene or genes that exert deleterious effects in younger patients, but lead to better health at later ages (successful aging). To complicate matters further, mitochondrial DNA polymorphisms are present in different frequencies in various aged populations from Italy, Ireland, and Japan [70].

Single-nucleotide polymorphisms in nuclear chromosomal DNA that appear to be linked to either increases or decreases in life span have been identified in a variety of populations (reviewed by Capri et al. [71] and by Glatt et al. [72]). An interesting pattern is emerging that strongly suggests that polymorphisms in genes implicated in metabolic signaling, inflammation, and stress response pathways play a role in aging and longevity. Metabolic genes implicated include the cholesterol ester transport protein [73], Foxo3A [74, 75], Foxo1A [76], SIRT3 [77, 78], the IGF1 receptor [79], and the insulin-degrading enzyme [80]. Inflammatory genes implicated include IL-6 [81, 82], IL-2 [83], CRP [84, 85], and TNF [86]. A number of genes from both of the previous categories fall into the stress response domain. It is important to stress that many gene association studies uncover modest relationships that may pertain to specific population groups. Individual genes may contribute in only small ways to aging or longevity, and it is highly likely that multigenic impacts and interactions play more significant roles in modulating longevity within the context of environmental stresses and lifestyle behaviors. Furthermore, there is intriguing evidence that a number of gene variants may play a more important role in increasing the human "health span," rather than extending actual life span [72].

Interestingly, the human epsilon 4 allele of apolipoprotein E (ApoE), which is associated with increased coronary disease and Alzheimer's disease, is inversely correlated with longevity [87]. In contrast, the epsilon 2 allele of ApoE and an angiotensin-converting enzyme (ACE) allele are found more frequently in French centenarians [87], although the ApoE2 allele is associated with type III and IV hyperlipidemia, and the ACE allele predisposes to coronary disease. These findings further suggest that genes can exert pleiotropic age-dependent effects upon longevity. Further support for a genetic contribution to human longevity is provided by data demonstrating that siblings and parents of centenarians live longer [88]. In addition, centenarian offspring are significantly less likely to experience myocardial infarction, stroke, and diabetes and to die than offspring of noncentenarians [89]. Linkage analysis implicates the presence of a gene or genes on chromosome 4 that are associated with exceptional longevity [88]. Perls et al. note that a high percentage of centenarians had children while in their 40s (well before assisted reproduction). They, therefore, postulate that an evolutionary force to prolong the period of childbearing would lead to the selection of longevity-enabling genes. Collectively, these studies also raise the question whether some genes affect susceptibility to disease rather than alter intrinsic aging.

In contrast to studies that uncover alterations in the expression of single genes during aging, Weindruch and Prolla and their colleagues have investigated the broad program of changes in gene expression that occur during aging and caloric restriction in mice and in monkeys [90–93]. A common theme is that aging induces a differential gene expression pattern in muscle and brain, consistent with inflammatory and oxidative stress and reduced expression of metabolic and biosynthetic genes. In muscle and brain from mice, caloric restriction either completely or partially prevented the age-related changes in gene expression. Interestingly, caloric restriction did not ameliorate the aging-induced alteration in the program of gene expression seen in muscle from aging monkeys. So, even though the age-related changes in gene expression may be similar across species, the response to caloric restriction may not.

Disposable Soma Theory

The disposable soma theory [94] postulates that indefinite maintenance of somatic cells and tissues is not favored by natural selection, which instead allots available energy and resources towards the reproductive health of the organism in the early years of life. The basic prediction of this theory is that while immortal germline cells are faithfully maintained, the reduced investment in somatic cells causes deterioration and accumulation of unrepaired damage. Thus, the primary genetic control of longevity operates through ability to modulate the investment in basic cellular maintenance systems in

TABLE 2.3 Genetic mouse models of life-span extension

Model	Improvement in aging phenotype	Life-span extension	Model of aging examined	Genetics	References
Catalase overexpression	Increase in median and maximum life span, delayed onset of cardiac pathology and cataracts, reduced oxidative damage, slightly reduced splenomegaly and splenic lymphoid neoplasia, reduced mitochondrial deletions in skeletal muscle	Life span extended by ~5 months	Free radical theory of aging	Targeted overexpression of human catalase (an antioxidant enzyme which detoxifies hydrogen peroxide)	[135]
Thioredoxin (TRX) overexpression	Increased life span, resistance to oxidative stress, higher splenic telomerase activity, higher resistance to UV damage	35% life-span extension	Free radical theory of aging	Transgenic mice generated via pronuclei microinjection of recombinant TRX, an enzyme involved in redox homeostasis and antioxidant defense	[136]
SuperARF/p53 overexpression	Delayed aging, increased cancer resistance, decreased oxidative damage, increased antioxidant expression	16% increase in median life span	DNA damage/free radical theory	Introduction of a single extra gene-dose each of ARF/INK4a/INK4b and p53 via bacterial artificial chromosome-mediated genomic DNA transgenesis	[380]
clk1−/−	Extended life span, reduced levels of ROS and oxidative damage in hepatocytes and ES cells from clk-deficient mice	15–30% life span extension with respect to wild-type littermates	Stochastic/free radical theory of aging	Homozygous inactivation of the mouse ortholog of the C. elegans gene, clk1 (an enzyme required for ubiquinone biosynthesis)	[402]
IGFR1+/−	Increased life span, without accompanying dwarfism, reduced metabolic signaling or fertility, derived fibroblasts show reduced sensitivity to oxidants	26% mean life span extension	Genetic/developmental/ free radical theory of aging	Inactivation of the insulin growth factor receptor 1 (IGFR1) gene by Cre-mediated recombination	[403]
Fat-specific insulin receptor knockout (FIRKO) mice (CR model)	Increased life span, protected against age-related obesity and glucose intolerance, lowered insulin levels	~18% increase in mean life span	Genetic/developmental	Cre-recombinase-mediated deletion of exon 4 of the insulin receptor, leading to loss of insulin signaling in adipose tissue	[404]
Heterozygotic reduction of IGF1 signaling in the brain	Increased mean life span, smaller adult size, low growth hormone (GH) levels	~2 month increase in mean life span, no change in maximal life span	Genetic/developmental/ neuroendocrine theory of aging	Conditional mutagenesis to generate brain-specific IGF-1 receptor heterozygous knockout mice	[104]
uPA overexpression	Increased life span, reduced body weight, reduced food consumption and blood sugar levels	~20% increase in life span	Genetic/developmental	Chimeric uPA overexpression	[405]
p66shc−/−	Increased life span, resistance to superoxide radical-mediated damage, increased cellular resistance to apoptosis and to p53/p21 pathway induction	30% increase in life span	Stochastic/free radical theory of aging	Targeted mutation of p66shc gene (a cytoplasmic signal transducer in the mitogenic Ras pathway)	[65]
CCAAT/enhancer binding protein (C/EBP) β	Increased life span, reduced lipid accumulation in white adipose tissue, higher mitochondrial biogenesis and energy expenditure	20% increase in life span	Mitochondrial/free radical theory of aging	Knock-in replacement of the C/EBP α gene with the C/EBP β gene to generate β/β mice	[406]

(continued)

TABLE 2.3 (continued)

Model	Improvement in aging phenotype	Life-span extension	Model of aging examined	Genetics	References
Adenylyl cyclase (type 5) knockout	Increased mean and median life span, increased antioxidant enzyme defense, reduced susceptibility to osteoporosis and fracture, protection against cardiomyopathy	~30% increase in median life span	Genetic/developmental/ free radical theory aging	Deletion knockout of the AC5 gene, which catalyses formation of the signaling molecule, cAMP, from ATP	[407]
Ames dwarf mouse (Prop-1)	Increased life span, reduced size, delayed puberty and sterility in females, lower body temperature, reduced insulin levels and circulating glucose, reduced age-related adiposity, increased antioxidant activity and reduced oxidative damage	35–70% increase in life span, depending on sex and diet	Genetic/developmental	Recessive mutation in the Prop-1 (Prophet of Pit1) gene which encodes a homeobox transcription factor involved in hormonal regulation	[408]
Snell dwarf mouse (Pit1^{dw})	Increased life span, reduced size, reduction in age-related immune dysfunction, delayed fertility, improved joint and cartilage health	~40% increase in life span	Genetic/developmental	Two noncomplement-ing point mutations in Pit-1, pituitary-specific transcription factor-1	[409]
Laron mouse (GHR/BP)	Increased life span, reduced size, reduced insulin signaling	~45% increase in life span	Genetic/developmental	Homozygous knockout of the growth hormone receptor	[410]
Little mouse (GHRHR)	Increased life span, small size, stunted growth, normal fertility, reduced insulin signaling	25% increase in mean life span, 15% increase in maximum life span relative to wild-type or heterozygous littermates	Genetic/developmental	Single nucleotide substitution (Asp60Gly) in the growth hormone releasing factor receptor	[408]

relation to the level of environment hazard. Accordingly, one claim of this theory would be that there is a tradeoff between fertility and longevity, with long-lived populations exhibiting reduced fertility. One study that assessed correlations between the number of children and age of members of British aristocratic families noted that the longest-lived members had the fewest children [95]; however, the oldest women studied had a mean age of 68 years. As noted above, middle-aged women who give birth tend to live longer. These two disparate observations do not necessarily need to be contradictory in the context of the disposable soma theory, as longer-lived individuals may possess a genetic advantage that allows the tradeoffs between longevity and reproductive ability to take place later in life.

Two other theories of longevity which may be broadly classed under the disposable soma theory of aging are the neuroendocrine theory and the immunologic theory of aging, both of which suggest aging is a result of declining somatic function. The neuroendocrine theory proposes that functional decrements in neurons and their associated hormones are central to the aging process [96]. An important version of this theory holds that the hypothalamic–pituitary–adrenal (HPA) axis is the master regulator of aging in the organism. Because the neuroendocrine system regulates early development, growth, puberty, control of the reproductive system, metabolism, and many other aspects of normal physiology, functional changes in this system could exert effects throughout the organism. The decline in female reproductive capacity is an obvious neuroendocrine age-related change. Mounting evidence suggests both the ovary and the brain play key roles in the menopause (rather than the previously held view of ovarian exhaustion) [97]. The neuroendocrine theory of aging is supported by experiments that show that hypophesectomy, followed by the replacement of known hormones, maintains (and may extend) life span in rodents [98]. In addition, reductions in brain dopaminergic neurotransmission are more prominent in a shorter-lived rat strain [99]. Levodopa, a dopaminergic drug can prolong the mean life span in mice [100]. Treatment of rats with deprenyl facilitates the activity of the nigrostriatal dopaminergic neurons and protects these neurons from their age-related decay [101], and deprenyl increases both the average and maximum life span [102, 103]. Many human studies demonstrate gradually decreasing levels of peripheral hormones accompanied by normal levels of trophic hormones [96]. This suggests either increased response to the peripheral hormones by the HPA axis or inappropriately low expression of the stimulating hormone. However, many organisms with aging phenotypes similar to those of higher vertebrates lack complex neuroendocrine systems. The changes that occur in the neuroendocrine system may be due to fundamental age-related changes in all cells and are therefore secondary manifestations of the aging phenotype.

However, the neuroendocrine theory received some validation via a study of aging phenotypes in a mouse model of reduced neuronal growth signaling. Partial inactivation of the IGF-1R receptor in the murine embryonic brain inhibits growth hormone and IGF signaling, leading to smaller size and an increased mean life span, apparently due to inhibition of the somatotrophic axis (see Table 2.3 [104]).

The immunologic theory of aging is based upon two main observations: (1) the functional capacity of the immune system declines with age, as evidenced by a decreased response of T cells to mitogens and reduced resistance to infectious disease and (2) autoimmune phenomena increase with age, such as an increase in serum autoantibodies [105]. There is a shift to increasing proportions of memory T cells, accompanied by enhanced expression of the multidrug resistance p-glycoprotein [106]. Humoral (B cell mediated) immunity also declines with age, as evidenced by decreased antibody production and a disproportionate loss in the ability to make high-affinity IgG, IgA antibodies. In addition, differences in the MLSP of different strains of mice have been related to specific alleles in the major histocompatibility gene complex [107]. The genes in this region also contribute to the regulation of mixed-function oxidases (P-450 system), DNA repair, and free radical scavenging enzymes. Caruso et al. suggest that mouse and human histocompatibility genes may be associated with longevity via different mechanisms: in mice via susceptibility to lymphomas and in humans via infectious disease susceptibility [108]. There is also evidence that cytokine gene polymorphisms may interact with histocompatibility genes to influence longevity [108]. Although the immune system obviously plays a central role in health maintenance and survival through the life span, similar criticism can be directed at the immunologic theory as at the neuroendocrine theory. Complex immune systems are not present in organisms that share aspects of aging with higher organisms. In addition, the inability to distinguish between fundamental changes occurring in many types of cells and tissues, not just those of the immune system, and the secondary effects mediated by the aging-altered immune system make interpretation of the theory difficult. Proposed mechanistic studies of the immune theory include producing transgenic mice carrying the histocompatibility complex from a longer-lived rodent species to determine effects on disease incidence and life span.

The discovery of caloric restriction as a means to extend organismal life span (at least in lower organisms and rodents) calls the disposable soma theory into question because it would predict reduced rather than increased life span in the face of limiting nutrient resources and consequently energy. Indeed, early studies of rodents fed on restricted diets reported a delay in the onset of puberty and lower reproductive capacity [109, 110]. A survey of the reproductive profiles of long-lived mice, including naturally long-lived variants such as the Snell dwarf mouse as well as transgenic models such as FIRKO mice (see Table 2.3) also suggests that, as a general rule, mice with longer life span show reduced fecundity (reviewed by Partridge et al. [111]). However, another study utilizing moderate caloric restriction (60% of normal dietary intake) of adult rodents discovered that CR conferred both increased fecundity in mice as well as increased survival of their pups [112], suggesting that an optimal balance in maintaining the reproductive axis without compromising the somatic axis may be achieved via nutritional interventions (see below).

Stochastic Theories

Free Radical/Oxidative Stress

Denham Harman proposed one of the oldest and most enduring theories of aging over 50 years ago when he postulated that most aging changes are due to molecular damage caused by free radicals [113, 114], which are incompletely reduced, highly reactive intermediates of oxygen. The term "free radical" is misleading because one of these intermediates is hydrogen peroxide, which contains no unpaired electrons and is therefore not a radical. The more accurate nomenclature for these intermediates is reactive oxygen species or ROS, and for the purposes of discussion herein and in the context of aging theories, we use the term free radical interchangeably with ROS, which likely is what Harman intended when he named his theory of aging.

Aerobic metabolism generates the superoxide radical ($O_2 \bullet^-$), which is metabolized by superoxide dismutases to form hydrogen peroxide (H_2O_2) and oxygen [115]. Hydrogen peroxide can go on to form the extremely reactive hydroxyl radical ($OH\bullet$). These oxygen-derived species can react with macromolecules in a self-perpetuating manner; they create free radicals out of subsequently attacked molecules, which in turn create free radicals out of other molecules thereby amplifying the effect of the initial free radical attack [12]. ROS appear to play a role in regulating differential gene expression, cell replication, differentiation, and apoptotic cell death (in part by acting as second messengers in signal transduction pathways) [116–118]. In addition, nonradical prooxidants, for instance metals such as iron and copper that catalyze formation of the hydroxyl radical, as well as high concentrations of certain antioxidants can together generate a retrograde redox regenerative cycle, leading to homeostatic imbalance and oxidative stress (reviewed by Valko et al. [119]).

In lower organisms, the role of antioxidants on life-span extension is also complex. Increasing expression of the mitochondrial Mn-superoxide dismutase (aka SOD2) in flies has yielded conflicting results, with one study reporting

approximately 15% extension in mean and maximum life span without changes in oxygen consumption [120] and another reporting no significant effect on life span [121]. However, SOD2 reduction in flies reduces life span and mimics aging-related defects; progressive reduction in SOD2 activity correlates with further shortening of life span [122]. This dose-dependent effect of SOD2 on life span is consistent with overexpression of SOD2 in flies [120].

Overexpression of Cu, Zn-superoxide dismutase (aka SOD1), the cytosolic superoxide dismutase, has been reported to extend life span in flies by around 40–50% [123, 124]; however, the significance of these results to the oxidative stress theory of aging are undercut by the facts that the majority of life extension was seen in the shortest-lived flies or by overexpressing SOD1 in tissues where there was a clear deficiency of the enzyme. In ant colonies, where large differences exist in life span between queens and workers, SOD1 activity correlates mostly negatively with life span with the shorter-lived males having higher SOD1 expression and activity compared to the long-lived queens [125]. Overexpression of catalase alone in transgenic flies also does not extend life span [126]. Some transgenic flies with increased expression of both Cu, Zn-superoxide dismutase and catalase, which act in tandem to remove superoxide and hydrogen peroxide, respectively, exhibit up to a one-third extension of average and maximum life span [126]. In addition, they exhibit increased resistance to oxidative damage and an increase in the metabolic potential (total amount of oxygen consumed during adult life per unit body weight). However, combinatorial overexpression of the major antioxidants, SOD1, SOD2, catalase, and thioredoxin reductase in relatively long-lived flies did not appear to enhance longevity [127]. It has also been shown that overexpressing glutathione reductase extends the life span of transgenic flies kept under hyperoxic or oxidant-treated conditions, but not under ambient conditions [128].

In *C. elegans*, a model system in which a number of long-lived mutants have been identified, the role of oxidants and antioxidants is similarly complicated. Although nutrient-sensing pathways appear to be a dominant mechanism of life-span determination in *C. elegans*, a causal role for oxidative stress in their aging still has neither been validated nor disproved. In long-lived worms that overexpress daf-2, ROS production was higher than in wild-type worms throughout the life span, but protein carbonylation was reduced [129]. The observed reduction in damage in the face of elevated ROS levels has been ascribed to compensatory protective effects due to enhanced enzymatic antioxidant activity from SOD proteins and glutathione-s-transferases [129–131]. However, treatment of wild-type *C. elegans* strains with SOD and catalase mimetics failed to extend life span despite increasing antioxidant activity [132]. Yet, the role of oxygen tension nevertheless appears to have an effect on life span and oxidative damage because worms kept at 1% oxygen have lower carbonyl levels and show approximately 24% increase in life span relative to counterparts kept at ambient oxygen [133].

Production of ROS in the heart, kidney, and liver of a group of mammals was found to be inversely proportional to the maximum life span, although the activities of individual antioxidant enzymes were not consistently related to maximum life span [134]. However, catalase overexpression targeted to the mitochondria does increase life span and improve functional health of the mice as they age [135]. Transgenic mice that overexpress thioredoxin, another antioxidant protein, also exhibit about a 30% improvement in mean life span [136]. A series of studies has demonstrated that oxidative stress resistance of dermal fibroblasts correlates with the longevity of the species [137–139].

The studies discussed above illustrate the complexity behind the free radical theory of aging. Antioxidants, in general, only appear to have a significant effect on life-span extension if their levels/function are limiting or under conditions of stress. Thus, overexpression of enzymes that are already present at robust levels are not likely to have an effect on life span simply because increasing expression does not enhance catalytic efficiency of these enzymes, which are already operating at near optimal rates. Furthermore, given the importance of antioxidant enzymes to survival of aerobically respiring organisms, there is a certain amount of redundancy between different antioxidants, and different tissues require their individual actions to different extents. This heterogeneity and overlap of function may also be obscuring the effects of altering antioxidant levels in animal models of life-span extension. Thus, rather than overexpressing antioxidants alone, a more viable strategy of life-span extension perhaps needs to center on reducing production of ROS by modulating mitochondrial function or the prooxidant factors, which contribute to the deleterious effects of oxygen radicals.

Mitochondrial Dysfunction Theory of Aging

The mitochondrial DNA/oxidative stress hypothesis represents a synthesis of several theories and therefore comprises elements of both stochastic and developmental-genetic mechanisms of aging (see below). It is proposed that ROS contribute significantly to the somatic accumulation of mitochondrial DNA mutations, leading to the gradual loss of bioenergetic capacity and eventually resulting in aging and cell death [140–142]. Ozawa has dubbed this the "redox mechanism of mitochondrial aging" [143]. Mitochondrial DNA (mtDNA) undergoes a progressive age-related increase in oxygen free radical damage in skeletal muscle [144–146], the diaphragm [147, 148], cardiac muscle [149–152], and the brain [153, 154]. This exponential increase in damage correlates with the increase in both point and deletional somatic mtDNA mutations seen with age. Interestingly, extrapolation of the curve to the point where 100% of cardiac mtDNA exhibits deletion mutations gives an age of 129 [143].

Mitochondrial DNA is maternally transmitted, continues to replicate throughout the life span of an organism in both proliferating and postmitotic (nonproliferating) cells and is subject to a much higher mutation rate than nuclear DNA. This is due, in large part, to inefficient repair mechanisms and its proximity to the mitochondrial membrane where reactive oxygen species are generated. Defects in mitochondrial respiration with age are found not only in normal tissues [155] but also in diseases that are increasingly manifested with age such as Parkinson's disease [156, 157], Alzheimer's disease [158, 159], Huntington's Chorea [160], and other movement disorders [161]. Diseases for which mtDNA mutations have been found include Alzheimer's [162, 163], Parkinson's [153, 163–166], and a large number of skeletal and cardiac myopathies [147, 167–171]. Apoptosis has also been associated with mtDNA fragmentation [172]. As noted above, mitochondrial haplotype J is associated with human longevity. However, the role of inherited and somatic mutations in mitochondrial DNA during human aging is clearly complex, and additional studies are required to gain further insight (reviewed by Salvioli et al. [68].)

The idea of mitochondrial involvement in aging postulates that accumulation of mtDNA damage leads to defective mitochondrial respiration, which in turn enhances oxygen free radical formation, leading to additional mtDNA damage. However, the reality appears not to be quite so simple. A mouse model has been developed to address the issue whether phenotypic aging of tissues depends on mitochondrial DNA mutations. These mice express an error-prone version of the major mitochondrial DNA polymerase, pol-gamma, generated by mutating the proofreading domain of the enzyme. The mutant mice show fairly uniform accumulation of both deletions and point mutations in the mitochondrial genomes of different tissues and an accelerated aging phenotype [173]. The observations from the mutant pol-gamma mouse model mirror previous findings regarding the role of mitochondrial mutations in aging. On the surface, these observations fit well with the free radical/oxidative stress theory of aging, since mutations in mitochondrial genes coding for respiratory chain enzymes could in principle result in leakier electron transfer, thus leading to increased accumulation of ROS. However, this does not appear to be the case in mouse embryonic fibroblasts derived from the mutant mice that, despite impaired respiration, show neither augmentation of ROS production nor sensitivity to oxidative stress-mediated cell death [174]. Lack of change in protein carbonylation levels is presented to support the idea that these mice suffer no elevation in oxidative stress, although these lesions may not be appropriate as the sole marker of cellular oxidative damage as they are detected only if they are present in a degradation-resistant state [175]. Furthermore, since mitochondrial deletions in the pol-gamma mutant mice lead to linearized mitochondrial genomes, another possibility is that the premature aging phenotype observed in these mice is the result of a DNA damage response (DDR) (see below) rather than accruing directly due to mitochondrial dysfunction. Nevertheless, the pol-gamma mice provide an elegant and useful system in which to further explore the role of mitochondrial mutations and ROS in engendering the aging phenotype.

In humans, specific mutations, while increasing with age, seldom account for more than several percent of the total mtDNA. However, some studies suggest that the total percentage of mtDNA affected by mutations is much greater, as much as 85%, and increases with age [143]. In addition, caloric restriction in mice retards the age-associated accumulation of mtDNA mutations [176]. Agents that bypass blocks in the respiratory chain such as coenzyme Q10, tocopherol, nicotinamide, and ascorbic acid would be predicted to ameliorate some of the effects of mitochondrial disease and aging. Withdrawal of coenzyme Q from the diet of nematodes extends the life span by approximately 60% [177]. Caloric restriction, which can extend life span, reduces oxidative damage in primates [178]. There are epidemiologic studies that appear to implicate dietary antioxidants in the reduction of vascular dementia, cardiovascular disease, and cancer in humans [179]. However, results to date, in treatment of patients with myopathies, have been variably or only anecdotally successful [143]. This suggests that a complex interaction exists between prooxidant and antioxidant forces in the cell and that regulation of the balance between the two may be the critical determinant in mitochondrial, and subsequently, cellular and tissue integrity during aging.

An increasing number of studies have implicated mitochondrial biogenesis and efficiency as playing significant roles to enhance cellular fitness and organismal longevity [180]. Maintenance of energy production and prevention and/or amelioration of oxidative stress by mitochondria are key to healthy aging. As previously discussed, caloric restriction is the most reliable intervention to extend life span in a number of species, including mammals such as rodents, dogs, and rhesus monkeys [13]. Multiple signals modulate PGC1α activity and subsequent mitochondrial production and efficiency, such as AMP kinase, sirtuins, and nitric oxide, all of which can be increased by caloric restriction [180]. Furthermore, caloric restriction increases mitochondrial biogenesis in healthy humans [181]. However, perhaps the best intervention to enhance mitochondrial production and function is exercise, which can at least partly normalize age-related mitochondrial dysfunction [182] and can significantly reverse age-related transcriptional alterations [183].

DNA Damage Theory of Aging: Somatic Mutation, DNA Repair, Error Catastrophe

Stochastic theories propose that aging is caused by random damage to vital molecules. The damage eventually accumulates to a level that results in the physiological decline associated with aging. The most prominent example is the somatic mutation theory of aging, which states that genetic damage from background radiation produces mutations that lead to functional failure and, ultimately, death [184, 185]. Exposure to ionizing radiation does shorten life span [186, 187]. However, analysis of survival curves of radiation-treated rodent populations reveals an increase in the initial mortality rate without an effect on the subsequent rate of aging [188]. The life-span shortening is probably due to increased cancer and glomerulosclerosis rather than accelerated aging per se [189].

The DNA repair theory is a more specific example of the somatic mutation theory. Impairment of genomic maintenance has been strongly implicated as a major causal factor in the aging process [190]. Defects in DNA repair mechanisms form the basis of a majority of human progeroid syndromes (see below). The ability to repair ultraviolet radiation-induced DNA damage in cell cultures derived from species with a variety of different life spans is directly correlated with the MLSP [191]. Unfortunately, there is not enough experimental support to conclude that these differences between species are a causative factor in aging. Although the prevailing belief has been that overall DNA repair capacity does not appear to change with age, several studies now indicate that repair of oxidative DNA damage lesions via base excision repair (BER) becomes more inefficient in aged mice [192, 193]. Caloric restriction can restore the age-related decline in BER [194]. Repair of DNA double-strand breaks (DSBs) is also compromised in replicatively senescent human fibroblasts [195] and in fibroblasts and lymphocytes taken from older humans [196].

Additionally, the site-specific repair of select regions of DNA appears to be important in several types of terminally differentiated cells [197]. Biochemically, oxidative DNA damage has been shown to affect specific DNA sequences more than others, with the most affected sequences corresponding to conserved motifs in transcriptional elements involved in the regulation of stress-response genes [198]. Studies in cultured human neurons show that promoters of genes involved in memory, stress protection, and neuronal survival sustain selective oxidative stress-mediated DNA damage and exhibit reduced BER [199]. Transcriptional profiling of the human frontal brain cortex reveals that the genes under the control of these promoter elements also show the most reduced function after the age of 40. Thus, DNA damage to specific areas of the neuronal genome appears to contribute to age-related cognitive decline. Future studies will need to focus upon repair rates of specific genes rather than indirect general measurements.

The error-catastrophe theory also centers on the role of DNA integrity in the aging process and proposes that random errors in synthesis eventually occur in proteins that synthesize DNA or other "template" molecules [200]. Generally, errors occurring in proteins are lost by natural turnover and simply replaced with error-free molecules. Error-containing molecules involved in the protein-synthesizing machinery, however, would introduce errors into the molecules that they produce. This could result in an amplification such that the subsequent rapid accumulation of error-containing molecules results in an "error catastrophe" that would be incompatible with normal function and life. Although there are numerous reports of altered proteins in aging, no direct evidence of age-dependent protein mis-synthesis has yet been reported. The altered proteins that do occur in aging cells and tissues are, instead, due to posttranslational modifications such as oxidation and glycation [201, 202]. The increases in altered proteins appear to be due to decreased clearance in older cells [203].

Models of Aging

Accelerated Aging Syndromes in Humans

Although no disease exists that is an exact phenocopy of normal aging, several human genetic diseases, including Hutchinson–Guilford syndrome (the "classic" early-onset progeria seen in children), Werner's syndrome ("adult" progeria), Cockayne's Syndrome or NFE Syndrome (another childhood-onset progeroid disease), and Down's syndrome exhibit features of accelerated aging.

Hutchinson–Guilford progeroid syndrome (HGPS) is an extremely rare autosomal recessive disease in which aging characteristics begin to develop within several years of birth [204]. These include wrinkled skin, stooped posture, early hair loss, and growth retardation. HGPS patients suffer from advanced atherosclerosis, and myocardial infarction is the usual cause of death by the age of 30. However, unlike Werner's Syndrome patients (see below), these patients do not typically suffer from cataracts, glucose intolerance, and skin ulcers. HGPS is a laminopathy resulting from a single-nucleotide substitution (1824 C>T) in the lamin A gene, which encodes two components of the nuclear envelope, lamins A and C (reviewed by Meshorer and Gruenbaum [205]). The mutation leads to activation of a cryptic splice site and production of a truncated version of the precursor protein, prelamin A, denoted progerin or $LA\Delta50$ [206, 207], which then leads to formation of abnormal nuclear lamina and delayed nuclear reassembly, as well as DNA damage and chromosomal abnormalities [208–212].

Werner's syndrome (WS) is an autosomally recessive inherited disease [204]. Patients prematurely develop arteriosclerosis, glucose intolerance, osteoporosis, early graying, loss of hair, skin atrophy, and hypogonadism (reviewed by Muftuoglu [213]). However, patients do not typically suffer from Alzheimer's disease or hypertension. WS patients have an increased predisposition to cancer with a higher than usual incidence of sarcomatous (mesenchymal) tumors and develop cataracts in the posterior surface of the lens, not in the nucleus as is usually seen in older people. In addition, they develop laryngeal atrophy and ulcerations on the arm and legs. Most patients die before the age of 50, usually of myocardial infarction or cancer [214, 215]. The gene responsible for WS has been localized to chromosome 8 [216] and appears to be a helicase [217], an enzyme involved in unwinding DNA. DNA helicases play a critical role in DNA replication and repair. Cells from WS patients display chromosomal instability, shortened telomeres, elevated rates of gene mutation, and nonhomologous recombination (reviewed by Brosh and Bohr [218]). Furthermore, WS is characterized by hypersensitivity to the chemical carcinogen, 4-NQO [219, 220], cross-linking agents [221], and the topoisomerase inhibitor, camptothecin [222, 223], suggesting impairment of DNA repair mechanisms.

Cockayne's syndrome (CS) is a congenital autosomal recessive disorder characterized by stunted growth, extreme sensitivity to sunlight, retinopathy, deafness, nervous system abnormalities, and premature aging (reviewed by Stevnsner et al. [224]). This is a progressive disease that becomes apparent after 1 year of age and leads to mortality by 12 years of age. There are rare variants, one of which manifests at birth and another which presents milder symptoms and appears in late childhood. CS results from mutations in the transcription-coupled repair (TCR) and global genomic (GG) repair proteins, ERCC6 and ERCC8, also known as Cockayne's Syndrome B (CSB) and Cockayne's Syndrome A (CSA), respectively. The CSA protein is a 396-amino acid protein with no known enzymatic activity [225] and is part of a multicomponent ubiquitin ligase complex that also includes the DNA damage binding protein DDB1 [226]. Not much is known about its specific role in producing the CS phenotype. CSB consists of 1,493 amino acids and is a member of the SWI2/SNF2 family of DNA-dependent ATPases [227]. Although there is no phenotypic difference in disease whether it arises from mutations in CSA or mutations in CSB, approximately 80% of CS cases have mutated CSB. Neither the site nor the specific nature of CSB mutations appears to correlate with severity of the disease, and in one patient, complete loss of the CSB gene product led to photosensitivity, but not CS [228], suggesting that there may be an environmental or epigenetic component to the disease. Surprisingly, unlike Werner's syndrome and other DNA repair defect diseases, Cockayne's syndrome patients do not have a significantly higher incidence of cancer unless they also suffer xeroderma pigmentosum (XP), which is linked to a strong predisposition to skin cancer.

People with Down's syndrome have trisomy or a translocation involving chromosome 21 [204, 229]. They suffer from the early onset of vascular disease, glucose intolerance, hair loss, degenerative bone and joint disease, and increased cancer. The life span is apparently 50–70 years (not as short as previously believed, since earlier mortality may have represented neglect of these individuals). Dementia occurs earlier and more often in patients with Down's syndrome than in the general population. Patients develop neuropathological changes similar to the changes seen in dementia of Alzheimer's type, including amyloid deposition and neurofibrillary tangles. This may be related to the presence of the β-amyloid gene on chromosome 21.

Although not strictly classified as progeroid syndromes, two diseases that bear mention are Fanconi anemia (FA) and dyskeratosis congenita (DC). Fanconi anemia is a rare autosomal recessive blood disorder, associated with multiple clinical symptoms [230]. Classified as a developmental rather than progeroid disorder, FA is nevertheless characterized by several aspects of premature aging syndromes, including childhood-onset bone marrow failure, susceptibility to squamous cell carcinomas, and congenital deformities. Furthermore, FA patients exhibit growth hormone and thyroid hormone deficiencies, glucose intolerance, and premature infertility. There are 13 FANC genes in which biallelic mutations lead to FA (reviewed by Neveling et al. [231]). Their protein products can aggregate into different core protein complexes in the nucleus; one of the complexes acts as a ubiquitin ligase to modify another FANC complex, thereby facilitating its recruitment to chromatin foci in conjunction with the BRCA1, BRCA 2, and Rad51 DNA repair proteins. Not surprisingly, FA cells exhibit chromosomal instability and are highly susceptible to several forms of DNA damage, particularly interstrand cross-links (ICL), therefore displaying acute sensitivity to cisplatin, mitomycin, and nitrogen mustard.

More significantly, cells derived from FA patients are uniquely sensitive to ambient air and show a definitive effect of oxygen concentration on formation of chromosomal aberrations [232]. Repeated hypoxia–reoxygenation cycles have been shown to induce premature senescence of bone marrow cells in a murine model of FA [233]. Together, these observations suggest that the dramatic bone marrow dysfunction and chromosomal aberrations observed in FA likely stem from ROS-mediated DNA damage to hematopoietic cells. Additionally, there is evidence that multimerization of FANC proteins and formation of nuclear complex 1 may be redox-dependent [234], suggesting that the observed sensitivity to DNA damage may be compounded by an inability of mutated FANC proteins to facilitate recognition and repair of DNA damage. Thus, with its progeroid features and the mechanistic convergence of oxidative stress and DNA damage in its etiology, FA appears to be the only human model for the stochastic theories of aging.

Dyskeratosis congenita is a rare syndrome associated with severe bone marrow failure around the age of 30 years [235]. In addition, DC patients suffer from aging-associated pathologies such as increased risk of cardiopulmonary failure and malignancy, early graying of hair, changes in skin pigmentation, brittle nails, and immune system failure which manifests itself as mucosal leukoplakia. DC is also characterized by chromosomal instability and telomere shortening at the cellular level [236]. The X-linked version of DC results from mutations in the dyskerin gene DKC1 that appear to impair its association with TERC, the RNA component of telomerase, whereas the autosomal form arises from mutations in the TERC gene itself [237]. Additionally, DC patients exhibit a uniform reduction in TERC itself. Thus, DC is unique in being the only human syndrome with progeroid features associated with telomere dysfunction, long considered a major causative biomarker of aging (see below).

Consistent with the classic theories of aging, the human progeroid syndromes discussed above suggest that the critical determinants of aging are likely to be oxidative stress levels, accumulation of DNA damage/chromosomal instability, and nonfunctional or reduced DNA repair mechanisms. These three features have formed the basis of a number of animal and cellular models of aging, which are discussed below and which recapitulate the phenomenon of aging to varying degrees.

Mouse Models of Aging

The major murine models of aging are summarized in Table 2.4. These encompass defects in a fairly comprehensive cross-section of biological processes implicated in aging including DNA damage/repair, metabolic, and developmental processes. Some of these models display the gamut of aging-related morphology and pathologies besides the obligatory reduction in mean and/or maximal life span. For instance, the *klotho* mouse suffers from a defect in a single gene that codes for a membrane protein and exhibits a plethora of marked age-related phenotypes that are also seen in humans. These include reduced life span, decreased activity, premature thymic involution, skin atrophy, arteriosclerosis, osteoporosis, emphysema, and lipodystrophy. There are a number of strains of senescence-accelerated mice (SAM) that exhibit a variable aging phenotype consistent with multigenic effects. Despite the fact that none of the mouse models displays all of the phenotypes associated with human aging, they are likely to be valuable tools in permitting delineation of some of the molecular mechanisms of aging. Significantly, some of the mouse models display a more

TABLE 2.4 Mouse models of aging

Model	Similarities to human aging	Life span and onset of aging	Differences from human aging	Genetics	References
Mutant p53 (p53 m/+)	Reduced life span, osteoporosis, lordokyphosis, organ degeneration, reduced wound healing, reduced subcutaneous adipose tissue, reduced ability to regrow hair	Median life span: 96 weeks. Onset of aging: >48 weeks	Resistance to late-onset spontaneous tumorigenesis, normal blood chemistry, no alopecia or graying hair	Deletion mutation in the first six exons that express a truncated RNA for the carboxy terminal of p53	[299]
p63-deficient (-/-, -/+)	Reduced life span, lordokyphosis, alopecia, weight loss, cellular senescence markers in vivo and in primary keratinocytes	Median life span: 95 weeks	Other aging phenotypes (i.e., bone density, muscle, subcutaneous fat) not examined/reported	Conditional disruption of p63 in an inducible and tissue-specific manner (using a flox/Cre system)	[392]
XPF/ERCC1-/-	Reduced life span, neurodegenerative symptoms, liver, skin and renal dysfunction, sarcopenia, kyphosis, premature senescence and sensitivity to oxidative insults in derived fibroblasts	Life span: ~4 weeks. Normal embryonic and initial postnatal development followed by dramatic reduction in growth in the second week	No reported enhancement in susceptibility to cancer	Insertional inactivation of ERCC-1 by gene targeting	[48]
Mutant pol-gamma	Reduced life span, weight loss, reduced subcutaneous fat, alopecia, anemia, kyphosis, osteoporosis, reduced fertility	Life span: <61 weeks. Onset of aging: ~25 weeks	Susceptibility to cancer not discussed, no observed increase in oxidative stress	Homozygous knock-in mice with a proof reading–deficient version of DNA polymerase gamma (the catalytic subunit of the mitochondrial polymerase)	[173]
SIRT6-/-	Significantly reduced life span, lymphopenia, reduced subcutaneous fat, lordokyphosis, osteopenia, reduced liver function and serum glucose	Life span: ~4 weeks. Onset of aging: ~3 weeks	Other aging phenotypes not discussed	Targeted deletion of SIRT6, a nuclear, chromatin-associated histone-deacetylase	[393]
Kl-/-	Shortened life span, infertility, growth retardation, decreased spontaneous activity, premature thymic involution, ectopic calcification, skin atrophy, arteriosclerosis, osteoporosis, pulmonary emphysema, lipodystrophy	Average life span: ~9 weeks. Onset of aging: ~4 weeks	Phenotypes not observed: neoplasms, cataracts, diabetes mellitus, brain atrophy	Loss of function mutations in the klotho gene (a single-pass membrane protein with homology to beta-glucosidase)	[394]
Senescence-accelerated mouse (SAM)	Amyloidosis, neoplasms, hyperinflation of the lung, hearing impairment, osteoporosis, defects in learning and memory, cataracts, brain atrophy	Average life span: ~10 months. Onset of aging: <8 months	Aging phenotypes are distributed among various SAMP strains	Not determined	[395]
WRN-/-	Premature loss of proliferative capacity in fibroblasts, sensitivity to topoisomerase inhibitors	Not reported	Mutant mice are apparently normal	Targeted disruption of the Werner syndrome gene (RecQ-like DNA helicase)	[396]
CSA-/- CSB-/-	Growth retardation, neurological defects	Almost normal life span	Other age-related phenotypes are not observed/examined	Targeted disruption of the Cockayne syndrome group A (CSA) or group B (CSB) gene (DNA helicase)	[397]
Atm-/-	Growth retardation, neurological dysfunction, infertility, malignant thymic lymphoma, sensitivity to X-ray irradiation	Develop thymic lymphoma before 4.5 months of age	Other age-related phenotypes are not observed or not examined	Targeted disruption of the ATM gene (a nuclear protein with PI-3-kinase-like domain)	[398]

(continued)

TABLE 2.4 (continued)

Model	Similarities to human aging	Life span and onset of aging	Differences from human aging	Genetics	References
Atr$^{-/-}$	Premature aging phenotype in adult mice relative to controls, including severe greying hair and alopecia, kyphosis, osteoporosis, organ fibrosis and thymic involution	No reported reduction in life span. Onset of aging phenotypes within 3 months after ATR inactivation in 8–12 week old mice. Severe stem cell attrition and loss of tissue homeostasis in a number of organs	Other age-related phenotypes are not reported	Cre-mediated deletion of ATR gene using a Cre-ERT2 transgenic mouse line	[399]
TERC$^{-/-}$	Infertility, graying of the hair, alopecia, skin lesions, impaired stress response, impaired proliferation of hematopoietic cells, neoplasms, delayed wound healing	Average life span: 18 months in the sixth generation	Aging phenotypes appear only in late-generation telomerase-deficient mice with extremely shortened telomeres. Phenotypes not observed: arteriosclerosis, osteoporosis, cataracts, diabetes mellitus, etc Enhanced aging seen with WRN–, POT1–/– and i ATM–/– double mutants	Targeted disruption of the gene for the telomerase RNA component	[339]
Over-expression of growth hormone	Scoliosis, weight loss, decline or reproductive capacity, insulin resistance, astrogliosis in the brain, glomerulonephritis, glomerulosclerosis, reduced replicative potential of fibroblasts	Life span: <50% of controls Onset of symptoms: 6–8 months of age	Growth hormone levels decline with age in humans and in experimental animals	Over-expression of rat, bovine, ovine or human growth hormone under the control of the metallothionein or phosphoenolpyruvate carboxykinase promoters	[400]
LMNA$^{L530P/L530P}$ (HGPS model)	Shortened life span, osteoporosis and bone malformation, reduced hair follicle density, poor muscle development, loss of subcutaneous fat, reduced life span and nuclear abnormality in derived fibroblasts	Life span: 4–5 weeks	Normal cholesterol/lipid levels, no obvious vascular defects, no reported predisposition to cancer	Knock-in of mutant Lamin A gene containing a leucine to proline substitution at residue 50	[401]

striking aging phenotype in conjunction with defects in other systems, for instance the mice jointly deficient in TERC and ATM or TERC and WRN [238, 239] experience accelerated premature aging relative to mice deficient in TERC alone.

Given the importance of the free radical/oxidative stress theory of aging (see above), a definitive mouse model for oxidative stress in aging is lacking, although several of the systems listed in Table 2.4 include elements of oxidative stress such as elevated oxidative DNA lesions, defects associated with ROS signaling (such as insulin resistance), and inflammation-related disorders. SOD1−/− mice show slightly reduced life span (~21 months relative to 28 months in the wild-type mice), elevated levels of 8-oxoguanine, a major oxidized DNA lesion, increased incidence of liver carcinogenesis [240], and increased retinal dysfunction [241]. SOD2−/− mice do not show a life span defect but do have increased age-related incidences of lymphomas and cardiac defects [242]. Mice deficient in catalase [243] and glutathione peroxidase [244] also appear to have a normal life span, with the former exhibiting tissue-specific sensitivity to hyperoxic insults and the latter showing some mild redox imbalance in platelets. The same is true for the mice in which SOD2 and glutathione peroxidase is jointly abrogated [245]. However, these results do not disprove the oxidative stress theory of aging but rather provide a caveat that laboratory mouse models, being protected from disease and fluctuations in living conditions and nutrition, perhaps do not accurately reflect the requirement for protection against oxidative stress that may alter life span. It is telling that despite a lack of longevity enhancement, many of the above model systems show a clear effect of altered redox status on stress resistance of the organism, which ultimately is a key benchmark in defining functional characteristics of the aging process. Given the importance of DNA damage and the pleiotropic effects of ROS in signaling pathways, perhaps a clearer picture of the role of oxidative stress will emerge by generating and studying mouse models deficient in antioxidant defenses as well as DNA repair/signaling mechanisms.

Cellular Senescence as a Model for Aging

The complexity of studying aging in organisms has led to the use of well-defined cell culture systems as models for cellular aging or senescence. Hayflick and Moorhead [246] pioneered the model of replicative senescence and identified normal human diploid fibroblasts in culture as an experimental system for aging by observing an initial period of rapid and vigorous proliferation, invariably followed by a decline in growth rate and proliferative activity, finally leading to cessation of proliferation. This model proposed that aging is a cellular as well as an organismal phenomenon and that the loss of functional capacity of the individual reflected the summation of the loss of critical functional capacities of individual cells. It is important to note that populations of senescent cells do not necessarily die and that, in fact, a number of senescent cell types (although not all) are thought to be resistant to apoptosis mediated by caspase 3 and inhibited by bcl-2 [247–249]. In culture, they can be maintained for years in a postmitotic (nonproliferating) state with regular changes of culture medium [250–252].

Although a majority of studies on cellular senescence have been conducted on skin and fetal lung fibroblasts, limited in vitro life span has been reported for glial cells [253], keratinocytes [254], vascular smooth muscle cells [255], lens cells [256], endothelial cells [257], lymphocytes [258], and human breast epithelial cells (HMECs) [259, 260]. In vivo, serial transplants of normal somatic tissues, such as skin and breast, from old donor mice to young genetically identical recipients show a decline in proliferative activity and eventual failure of the graft [261]. Similarly, skin from old donors retained an increased susceptibility to carcinogens whether transplanted to young or old recipients [262].

Do changes in cells in culture parallel changes in cells from aging organisms? The replicative life span of fibroblasts in culture is inversely related to the maximum life span of several diverse vertebrate species [263]. Studies suggest that the replicative life span of cells in culture is inversely related to the age of the donor in both humans and rodents [264–266]. This in vivo–in vitro relationship also holds for several different cell types, including skin fibroblasts [267], hepatocytes [268], keratinocytes [269], arterial smooth muscle cells [255], and T lymphocytes [270]. However, in these cross-sectional studies, there is a great deal of variability, and the correlation coefficient, though statistically significant, is low. Cells cultured from healthy individuals do not appear to exhibit a consistent age-related proliferative capacity [271]. Cells from people with Werner's syndrome do senesce more rapidly in culture than age-matched controls; however, a consistently similar relationship does not hold for cells from people with Hutchinson–Guilford syndrome [204]. Thus, under some circumstances, the proliferative characteristics of cells during aging in vivo are maintained in culture. There are several studies that point to an accumulation of senescent cells in vivo with advancing age of both humans and primates [35, 270, 272, 273].

The number of population doublings achieved before reaching a replicative limit is intrinsic to different cell types [246]. Even more significantly, cells rederived from animals that are the result of reproductive cloning via nuclear transfer show the same replicative proliferative capacity and rate of telomere shortening as the donor cells [274], suggesting an inherent mechanism of cellular life-span determination that is conserved even during the genetic reprogramming that occurs after nuclear transfer. The number of times the cells divide is more important in determining proliferative life span than the actual time the cells spend in culture [275]. Cells continuously passaged in culture until the end of their proliferative life span achieve approximately the same number of population doublings (PDLs) as cells that are held in a stationary phase for an extended period (months) and then recultured until senescence. Therefore, under a given set of culture conditions, cells seem to possess an intrinsic mechanism that "counts" the number of divisions and not the time that passes.

However, suboptimal culture conditions or environmental stresses can adversely affect cellular replicative life span, leading to accelerated loss of proliferative capacity that is referred to as premature senescence or stress-induced premature senescence (SIPS) [276–278]. A number of acute exogenous stresses can lead to premature senescence, including, but not limited to oxygen radical producers, radiation, chemotherapeutic drugs, and high oxygen tension culture. Additionally, creation of endogenous DNA damage due to failure of repair mechanisms and elevated ROS stemming from mitochondrial dysfunction or oncogene activation can also lead to rapid induction of a permanent proliferative arrest.

In morphological and biochemical respects, SIPS is almost identical to replicative senescence, leading to the idea that all exhaustion of replicative capacity may be a form of stress-induced proliferative arrest. In accordance with this idea, one pervasive common denominator between replicative and SIPS appears to be induction of a DDR ([279] and reviewed in [280]). In fact, a persistent DDR and elevated intracellular ROS production appear to play a critical role not only in the induction of the senescent phenotype but also in its maintenance [279, 281].

Products of the retinoblastoma (Rb) and p53 tumor suppressor genes have been identified as the major molecular pathways implicated in cellular senescence [282, 283]. The Rb gene product is not phosphorylated in senescent cells [284]. Simian virus 40 large T antigen, which is bound by the p53 and Rb gene products, can facilitate escape from senescence [285]. T-antigen deletion mutants that lack either Rb- or p53-binding domains are unable to mediate escape from senescence [286]. Furthermore, treatment with antisense oligonucleotides to the Rb and p53 tumor suppressor genes can extend the in vitro life span of human fibroblasts [287]. The p21 CIP1/WAF1 [288–290] and p16 INK4a [291–293] inhibitors of cyclin kinases (and therefore cell cycle progression) are overexpressed in senescent cells. The p21 protein appears to act by forming complexes with members of the family of E2F transcription factors in senescent cells (Rb/CDK2/cyclin E or with the Rb-related p107/CDK2/cyclin D), downregulating transcriptional activity, and thereby inhibiting progression through the cell cycle [288]. Targeted disruption of the p21 gene delays the onset of senescence in fibroblasts derived from human lung [294]. However, adrenocortical cells express high levels of p21 throughout their in vitro life span,

up to and including senescence [295]. Skin fibroblasts from patients with Li–Fraumeni syndrome are heterozygous for p53. These cells in culture lose the remaining p53 allele and are subsequently unable to express p21 but still undergo in vitro aging [296], suggesting that p53 and p21 are not required for senescence. In senescent cells, p16 complexes to and inhibits both the CDK4 and CDK6 cell cycle kinases [291]. Induction of expression of p16 by demethylation-dependent pathways or of p21 by demethylation-independent pathways can induce senescence in immortal fibroblasts that do not express p53 [297]. Of genes whose expression is required for G1/S cell cycle progression, senescent fibroblasts express no cdk2 and cyclin A and reduced amounts of the G1 cyclins, C, D1, and E, compared to young cells [298]. The expression of early G1 markers, but not late G1 markers, indicates that senescent cells may be blocked at a point in late G1 [299].

The p53/p21 and the p16/Rb pathways are not induced to equivalent extents during cell senescence and do not contribute equally to the senescent phenotype; the dominating pathway depends both on cell type and the nature of senescence-inducing stress. In general, the p53 pathway is activated in response to genotoxic stress, DNA damage, and telomere dysfunction, whereas the p16 arm of tumor suppression is engaged under conditions of oncogenic and other stresses. Skin fibroblasts typically enter senescence via the p53 pathway and have low levels of p16 even as they approach cellular senescence; in these cells, inhibition of the p53 pathway is sufficient to reverse the senescent phenotype [300]. Lung fibroblasts, on the other hand, tend to show elevated levels of both tumor suppressor proteins in a senescing population as a whole, although individual cells may show one pathway is more dominant than the other (reviewed by Itahana et al. [301]). Even so, a mosaicism has been reported in senescent cultures whereby both p53- and p16-mediated senescence programs are activated either in parallel or even jointly in individual cells [302].

The *ras* oncogene product can induce senescence that is accompanied by accumulation of p53 and p16 [303]. This occurs only in nonimmortalized cells and may reflect a tumor-suppressive response of the cell to a transforming stimulus, as discussed below. However, it has been reported that the RAS oncoprotein can only induce senescence in cells that have already upregulated levels of p16 [304]. Induction of a DDR and senescence by increasing oxidized nucleotides and accompanying genomic DNA damage in human skin fibroblasts also leads to upregulated levels of both p53 and p16, but the senescence response can be rescued by abrogation of the p53 (but not the p16) pathway [305]. In human mammary epithelial cells, there appear to be two different barriers to proliferation. After the initial four to five population doublings, these cells enter an early senescent-like arrest termed M0 that is mediated by p16, but a number of cells in a population are able to escape this proliferative barrier and continue to divide before reaching a p53-mediated senescence termed M1 [306]. In keratinocytes, abrogation of both p16 and p53 is needed to extend life span, but these cells still undergo senescence unless immortalized by introduction of hTERT. However, expression of hTERT alone does not immortalize these cells if one of the senescent pathways is still functional [307]. Together, these observations emphasize the presence of complex and incompletely understood overlapping networks regulating cell cycle progression and proliferation. Depending upon the balance of positive and negative influences, cell proliferation can continue or senescence may ensue.

Although many biochemical, metabolic, and phenotypic differences have been reported between senescent cells and their early passage counterparts, several characteristics appear to be shared across a majority of cells that have entered senescence and can therefore be accurately referred to as markers of senescence. These include a lack of proliferation and response to proliferative stimuli, absence of DNA replication, a marked morphological change involving a flattened appearance, accumulation of stress fibers and vacuoles as well as nuclear abnormalities, upregulation of p53 and/or p16 proteins, and beta-galactosidase activity detected at an acidic pH [308]. Senescent cells also exhibit autofluorescent globules of oxidized cellular proteins denoted as lipofuscin [309]. Additionally, heterochromatic nuclear DNA foci called SAHFs (senescence associated heterochromatic foci) have been observed in cell types in which Rb/p16 signaling is the dominant molecular mechanism of senescence [310]. These foci consist of a transcription-silencing variant macroH2A and various heterochromatic proteins and are believed to be formed by the action of chromatin regulator proteins, HIRA and ASF1a. They can be readily detected by their punctate appearance during DAPI staining of cell nuclei. Formation of DNA double-strand break (DSB) foci via activation of the ATM/ATR pathway has also been reported as a senescence marker, both in senescent cells as well as aging mice and primates [36, 37, 279, 302].

The senescence-associated (SA) beta-galactosidase activity, which is detected at pH 6.0, is commonly used in studies that assess induction of senescence both in cells and tissues [272]. Despite its common usage, conflicting data exists regarding the status of SA beta-gal activity as a specific marker for senescence. For instance, in situ expression of beta-galactosidase exists in confluent quiescent presenescent cells [311] and in cells undergoing crisis [312] or terminal differentiation [313]. The origin of SA beta-galactosidase activity appears to result from increases in lysosomal mass during the cellular aging process [314] or under cellular stresses that can induce senescence [311, 315]. Fibroblasts from patients with the lysosomal disorder GM1-gangliosidosis (in which lysosomal beta-galactosidase is defective) do not show SA beta-galactosidase activity [316]. Furthermore, beta-galactosidase activity at low pH is also observed in nonsenescent cells with high lysosomal content such as vascular smooth muscle cells and endothelial cells [314, 317]. Thus, it would appear that SA beta-galactosidase activity is not a direct measure of senescence but a reflection of the lysosomal alterations that commonly occur as a consequence of senescence. Nevertheless, in general, for most cell types, beta-galactosidase activity is still a reliable if nonspecific marker, although it is advisable to look for beta-galactosidase positivity in conjunction with the other markers of senescence.

The three markers most commonly used to assess senescence in vivo are lack of proliferation (measured by Ki67 staining), SA beta-galactosidase activity, and levels of p16 protein. In particular, p16 protein is likely to be a good marker for in vivo aging as well because it has been reported to be strongly upregulated (sevenfold to eightfold) in aging human skin and in islet cells from aged humans [273, 318] and in a number of tissues from aged rats and mice [319]. Additionally, a DNA microarray screen of oncogene-induced senescence in vitro identified three de novo markers of senescence which were validated in vivo, namely, p15INK4b, Dec1, and DcR2 [320].

Telomere length is another commonly used marker of senescence. The phenomenon of telomere shortening with aging represents a potential "clock" or counting mechanism for cellular lifespan [321]. Telomeres are structures at the end of chromosomes that prevent degradation and fusion with other chromosome ends [322]. The average length of the terminal restriction fragment of chromosomes decreases with both in vitro and in vivo aging of fibroblasts and peripheral blood lymphocytes [321, 323–327]. Indeed, telomere length in lymphocytes progressively declines as a function of donor age from newborn to great-grandparents in their eighties [328]. Immortalized and transformed cells and germline cells express telomerase, which prevents shortening of the telomeres [329, 330]. However, some immortal cells exist without detectable telomerase [331], whereas stem cells and some normal somatic cells express telomerase, yet continue to experience telomeric shortening [332–334]. Telomere length has been correlated with better health in centenarians [335]. Interestingly, telomere length also appears to be related to physical activity [336]; however, no correlation was found between telomere length and frailty in an elderly cohort [337].

Shortened telomeres are associated with the progeroid pathology of dyskeratosis congenita and Werner's syndrome (see earlier discussion; reviewed by Hofer et al. [338]) and also appear to lead to a form of premature aging in in vivo mouse models [339]. Mice lacking the RNA component of hTERT, TERC, do not show significant aging defects until the sixth generation [339]. Transgenic mice that overexpress

TERT exhibit increased tissue regeneration and a modest increase in maximal life span; however, these benefits are offset by the increased incidences of tumorigenesis suffered by these mice. Experimental nonenzymatic elongation of telomeres extends the life span of cells [340]. Furthermore, reactivation of telomerase, via the introduction of the telomerase reverse transcriptase unit into normal human cells, increased telomere length and extends the life span of a number of different cell types without inducing morphological or pretransformative abnormalities [341].

Furthermore, despite a clear ability to inhibit replicative senescence in a number of different cell types, telomerase cannot prevent or rescue many forms of SIPS, which are sometimes referred to as telomere-independent forms of senescence [342, 343]. However, it is not clear if telomeres are indeed not affected or whether telomerase is unable to heal certain types of damage to telomeres. Interestingly, while telomerase can readily immortalize adult lung fibroblasts under ambient culture conditions, fetal lung fibroblasts can only be immortalized under 3% oxygen and by addition of a number of chemical antioxidants to the culture medium [344], suggesting either that the integrity of the telomerase complex or its function may be affected by oxidative stress or that oxidative damage to telomeres may alter telomeric structure in a way that inhibits recognition/healing by telomerase.

Telomeric shortening has been attributed to inefficient repair of DNA single-strand breaks, which are hallmark lesions of oxidative damage [345]. Improvement of mitochondrial function, the major determinant of cellular ROS production, also slows down telomere shortening [346]. Although irrefutable in vivo proof for a causal role for oxidative stress in generating senescence-inducing telomere dysfunction is still lacking, telomeres appear to be excellent candidates for the missing link between DNA damage and oxidative stress that will allow us to achieve a complete understanding of the mechanism behind the internal "clock" that governs cellular life span.

Using the markers of senescence discussed above, senescent cells have been detected in tissues from aged rodents, primates, and humans [35, 36, 272, 273, 319]. Nevertheless, the question remains whether the in vivo presence of senescent cells in renewable tissue is coupled to any loss of organismal function. Presumably, such cells do not need to divide in vivo to the point of replicative exhaustion because they can be replenished by tissue progenitor cell populations. Thus, the role of cellular senescence in organismal aging, over and beyond its role as a tumor suppressor mechanism, may have greater functional relevance in stem cell populations than in more differentiated cells. The self-renewal and differentiation of stem cells is critical for the maintenance of tissue function, repair, and homeostasis. Hematopoietic stem cells (HSC) from older mice, which have deficiencies in self-renewal, repopulating, and homing mechanisms, accumulate high levels of p16 that impair their ability to undergo serial transplantation; HSCs displayed improved function and stress resistance in the absence of p16 [347]. There is also evidence to suggest that self-renewal ability of the lympho-hematopoietic stem cell system correlates with life span as a whole in mice ([348] and reviewed by Geiger and Van Zant [349]). Increasing p16 levels are also linked to decreased regenerative potential in pancreatic islet cells [318] and reduced proliferation of progenitor populations in the mouse forebrain [350].

Aging and Cancer

The idea that aging acts as a deterrent to tumorigenic transformation is one of the bases of the antagonistic pleiotropy theory of aging (discussed above). Within this context, traits that enhance the fitness of a younger organism (cellular senescence prevents cancer) may exert adverse effects later in life (increased predisposition to senescence leads to tissue aging and overall dysfunction). At a cellular level, senescence and tumorigenesis appear to be two sides of the same coin. Spontaneous transformation of normal primary human cells is an extremely rare event. Indeed, in the absence of telomerase activity or abrogation of the tumor suppressor pathways via viral oncoproteins, onset of senescence is an inevitable outcome of culturing primary cells, which must necessarily overcome this antiproliferative barrier before undergoing tumorigenic transformation. Cells that are immortalized via introduction of the catalytic subunit of telomerase, hTERT, and/or viral oncoproteins such as SV40 large T antigen or human papilloma virus proteins E6/E7, which block the p53 and p16 pathways, can continue to proliferate indefinitely [351], (reviewed by Vaziri and Benchimol [352]). These cells exhibit changes in morphology and growth rate and can be readily transformed by introduction of oncogenes [351, 353–355]. In contrast, introduction of activated oncogenes leads to premature senescence in primary cells [303, 356], again emphasizing the role of senescence in preventing tumorigenic transformation.

Significantly, senescent cells have been detected in tissue surrounding primary tumors, as well as in regions of nontumorigenic growths such as melanocytic nevi [357] and benign prostate hyperplasias [358, 359]. Similar results were observed with mice containing a conditionally expressed KRAS-V12 allele. Senescence markers were observed with far greater frequency in premalignant adenomas than in adenocarcinomas, which rarely exhibited senescence [320]. Together, these observations strongly suggest that senescence induction is a cellular response to hyperproliferative stimuli and that tumorigenic lesions are outgrowths of cells that have sustained further mutations/adaptations, thereby allowing this tumor-suppressive block to be circumvented. This theory is further substantiated by the finding that DNA damage and senescent markers are sharply increased in pre-neoplastic and early neoplastic tissue, but are not observed in late-stage tumors [356, 360]. Additionally, mouse models of oncogene activation exhibit in vivo induction of DNA damage-mediated senescence in response to the hypermitogenic signaling associated with oncogene stress [361, 362]. Similarly, short dysfunctional telomeres are able to induce a senescent response in pretumorigenic cells in Emu-myc transgenic mice (a model for Burkitt's lymphoma) crossed with TERC-null mice [363]. Interestingly, the tumor suppressor function of shortened telomeres can be rescued by abrogating p53, but not by expression of the antiapoptotic protein, bcl-2. In mouse models of inducible p53, restoring p53 expression in murine liver carcinomas leads to induction of senescence (rather than apoptosis) in the entire tumor and to its clearance by activation of an innate immune response [364]. Similarly, intact p53 and p16 senescence pathways are required for c-Myc inactivation-induced regression of lymphomas [365]. These results not only point to the importance of cell senescence as a major antitumorigenic barrier but also suggest that, at least in certain types of tumors, it may be a more dominant barrier than cell death.

Besides the obvious conclusion that in order to progress, tumors need to overcome senescence, these observations underscore another fact. Stimuli or stresses that lead to the induction of senescence in a majority of cells may also select for cells that are either inherently resistant to or are no longer responsive to such stresses. When p53 function is restored in established lymphoma cells, they experience rapid clearance; however, most of the treated animals eventually relapse due to the emergence of tumors with inactivated ARF or p53 [366]. In animal models of lung hyperplasia that experience sustained DNA damage signaling and genomic instability, progression to full-blown carcinoma is strongly associated with an increasing trend of p53 inactivation, suggesting that cells which have lost p53 function are strongly selected for in an environment where a functional DNA damage-induced tumor suppressor response is ongoing [367]. The notion of such stress-resistant cell populations is congruent with the emerging idea of tumor-initiating or cancer "stem cells" (reviewed by Eyler and Rich [368]). Investigations as to the behavior of such cells towards genotoxic stress or oncogene activation and changes in their population with advancing age should prove both interesting and instructive.

In addition to cell-autonomous means of senescence induction, stressed or senescent cells release growth-inhibitory soluble factors that may serve to engender or enforce the senescent phenotype in neighboring cells. These include upregulation of the secreted insulin-like growth factor IGFBP7 in response to oncogenic BRAF signaling [369], elevated expression of CXCR2 and cognate ligands leading to p53 induction and senescence [370], and oncogene-induced senescence mediated by the concerted action of C EBP transcription factors and the cytokines IL-6 and IL-8 [371]. Recently, a broader senescence-associated secretory phenotype (SASP) in response to genotoxic stress has been identified and includes IL-6, IL-8 and insulin-like growth factor proteins (although not IGFBP7) [372]. The SASP is found to be amplified by loss of p53, by introduction of oncogenic RAS, and, in vivo, by chemotherapeutic treatment of prostate tumors. Further study of the role of these factors in inhibiting outgrowths of resistant cells is required to understand the full extent of their tumor-suppressive function.

Consequently, these studies provide increasingly convincing evidence for a tumor suppressor function of in vivo cell senescence. However, the argument for whether organismal senescence is a tumor suppressor response is less clear. On the surface, a paradoxical observation in this context is that older organisms are more susceptible to cancer, not less so. Interestingly, studies of in vivo senescence in mouse models of tumorigenesis suggest that the link between cellular senescence and transformation mimic the observed link between organismal aging and cancer in that senescence precedes the onset of tumorigenesis. This can be interpreted in two ways – either that the process of aging/senescence creates conditions for tumorigenic transformation or the conditions that lead to aging or senescence can engender tumorigenesis in the absence of senescence induction. At an organismal level, the former hypothesis has been popular given that from 2001 to 2005, 55.2% of all cancers were diagnosed in people over the age of 65, suggesting cancer is a disease of the elderly [373]. Furthermore, the incidence rate of invasive cancers is almost tenfold greater in those over 65 years of age. However, at a cellular level, the latter theory is more strongly supported because the markers of senescence are most strongly upregulated in preneoplastic and early neoplastic tissue rather than in late-stage tumors (see above). However, even in a cellular context, there is evidence that once senescent cells are established, they can nevertheless encourage an environment that promotes carcinogenesis. To this end, it has been reported that senescent cells can foster the growth of premalignant and malignant epithelial cells in culture and the tumorigenesis of these cells in mice [374, 375] and that a genotoxic damage-invoked SASP in premalignant epithelial cells induced a potentially highly invasive and malignant mesenchymal phenotype in these cells [372].

These observations suggest that the role of senescence and indeed aging as an antitumor measure may be more complicated than initially believed. Just as activation of tumor suppressor pathways represents an example of antagonistic pleiotropy, the process of senescence itself may also become deleterious in later life, turning from a predominantly tumor suppressor mechanism, activated in response to isolated stresses that threaten immediate survival of the

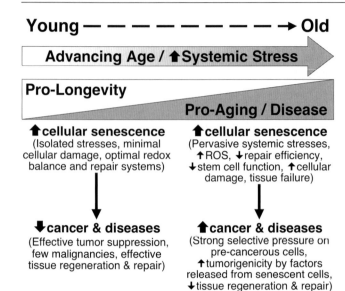

FIGURE 2.3 The cellular senescence paradox. In a background of low general damage and optimal stress responses, the process of cellular senescence can act as a prolongevity mechanism, activated in response to isolated stresses that threaten immediate survival of the young organism. However, in the context of mounting systemic stresses, cellular senescence may become deleterious in later life, turning from a predominantly tumor suppressor mechanism to a pervasive and ultimately degenerative response, paradoxically contributing to increased malignancies by allowing for selection and propagation of malignant cells that are able to evade of the senescence response.

young organism, to a pervasive and ultimately degenerative response to mounting systemic stresses (Fig. 2.3). Perhaps cancer is an aging-associated disease, not just because the stresses that induce aging also select from transformation-prone cells, but because the senescent tissue itself may be promoting tumorigenic growth in such cells.

From the mutant p53-expressing mouse model (see Table 2.4), the discouraging conclusion appeared to be that life span must be sacrificed to evade tumorigenesis [299, 376]. However, the above-mentioned models were the result of a genetic method that essentially led to elevated levels of p53 by eliminating its negative regulation by Mdm2. A more recent model of enhanced p53 function suggests that there need not be an inevitable tradeoff between increased cancer resistance and reduced life span. Transgenic mice that carry a genetic element containing the intact p53 gene [377] or the ARF gene [378], leaving these genes under normal physiologic regulation, or mice with moderately reduced Mdm2 activity [379] appear to benefit from the increased cancer protection accorded by elevated p53/ARF expression but without experiencing a concomitant reduction in life span. Even more significantly, using the same genetic technique, transgenic mice with combined enhanced p53 and ARF function have been generated that exhibit both an increased cancer resistance relative to the single gene-dose transgenic mice and also a 16% increase in median life span and improved stress

resistance (see Table 2.3, [380]). These results provide the first indication of an exciting new paradigm, namely, that longevity-assurance mechanisms (such as optimal levels of p53 function) exist that may cooperate with cancer protection mechanisms. Furthermore, similar to the two-hit hypothesis of tumorigenesis, the remarkable antiaging benefits that appear to accrue from enhancing both p53 and ARF functions suggest that perhaps the onset of aging is also triggered by coordinated dysfunction/dysregulation in more than one pathway. Thus, the genetic and stochastic components of aging may be explained by inherited deficiency in one or both of these pathways resulting in variable response to environmental stresses depending on the existing p53/ARF function.

Aging, Nutrition and Metabolism: A Modern-Day Elixir of Life?

Nearly every culture and civilization has its own mythic search for the elixir of life, from the desperate pursuit of immortality by Gilgamesh in ancient Babylon and by the Chinese emperor Qin Shi Huang before 200 B.C. to the European alchemists' attempts at creating the longevity-conferring philosopher's stone and the Spanish conquistador Ponce de Leon's quest for the fountain of youth. With an improved understanding of the molecular and biochemical pathways behind the aging process and the advent of nutraceuticals, there has been resurgence in the interest to generate scientifically validated interventions that can extend life span while minimizing the systemic disadvantages of aging.

Mouse models of life-span extension can be broadly categorized as either embodying alterations in metabolic/nutrient responsive-pathways or in mitochondrial/oxygen responsive pathways (Table 2.3). Most of these transgenic animal models exhibit a 15–30% life-span extension, with varied improvements in functional aging, such as low damage levels, increased tissue function and stress resistance at later stages of life, and reduced incidences of cancer. However, few of these models have more than a modest impact on MLSP, and almost none show the broad gamut of improved physiologic function that would translate to significant improvement in human quality-of-life aging issues. A valid criticism leveled at murine models of aging is that most of these organisms are studied under laboratory-controlled conditions that are unlikely to mimic the environmental vagaries that affect true aging [381]. Therefore, while these model systems offer mechanistic insights into the processes that may impact aging, the actual effects of these processes need to be assessed in human beings in a systematic and noninvasive manner.

The confluence of oxygen metabolism and nutritional signaling on life span observed in animal models ranging from

C. elegans to rodents suggests that dietary modifications are the most likely candidate for yielding maximal dividends when it comes to extending longevity and maintaining good health later in life. The ability to modulate diet is relatively simple, and accordingly, caloric restriction (CR) studies are at the forefront of life-span extension strategies. Caloric restriction in rhesus monkeys leads to reductions in body temperature and energy expenditure, consistent with changes seen in rodent studies in which aging is retarded by dietary restriction [21, 22]. Calorie restriction also increases high-density lipoprotein [23] and retards the postmaturational decline in serum dehydroepiandrosterone sulfate in the rhesus monkeys [382]. Levels of the aging biomarker, p16INK4a, are reduced in tissue from aging rodents fed a calorically restricted diet [319].

The Comprehensive Assessment of the Long-Term Effects of Reducing Intake of Energy (CALERIE) study is a randomized clinical trial to assess whether CR improves aging biomarkers in humans. After an initial 6-months of CR in 48 healthy men and women in the their 40s and 50s, the study found an improvement in two biomarkers of longevity, namely, reduction in fasting insulin levels and body temperatures in groups that underwent dietary restriction [25]. Other CALERIE studies have found that CR improves liver [383] and cardiovascular health [26] and increases muscle mitochondrial biogenesis and decreases oxygen consumption [181].

Population-based characterizations of aging have also identified diet and nutrition as likely major contributors to longevity. Long-lived human populations tend to share a few features in common, among them diets enriched in low-fat proteins such as fish and in fruits or beverages high in polyphenols and low in sugar and processed carbohydrates, often referred to as the Mediterranean Diet [384]. Consumption of red wine is also believed to be conducive to a healthy life span. In Sardinia and the south-western regions of France, longevity of the local population has been correlated with the high vasoactive polyphenol contents of the locally produced red wine [385].

Polyphenols such as quercetin, epigallocatechin gallate (EGCG), and resveratrol (3,5,4′-trihydroxystilbene) are naturally occurring protective compounds found in dark-green vegetables, fruits, green tea, dark chocolate, and red wine currently being included in a number of studies of aging and aging-related pathologies such as cancer and diabetes. Indeed, resveratrol is notable for its ability to activate sirtuins and to increase maximum life span in lower organisms, such as yeast, worms, and flies [386]. Resveratrol treatment improves the exercise capacity, insulin sensitivity, mitochondrial biogenesis, and survival of mice on a high fat, high calorie diet [387]. Resveratrol can prevent diet-induced obesity concurrently with improved mitochondrial production, insulin sensitivity, and exercise endurance by activating SIRT1 and PGC1α [388]. Resveratrol treatment of mice can also delay age-related changes in physical performance, bone mineral density, inflammation, and the vasculature [389] and concomitantly induces transcriptional profiles in a variety of tissues similar to those seen with dietary restriction [389, 390]. Consequently, there has been much interest in resveratrol as a supplement to enhance health and increase life span in humans. However, resveratrol does not appear to extend the maximum life span of mice, but can increase the mean life span of mice with cardiovascular- and obesity-related pathology who would otherwise die earlier.

Although nutritional interventions may be able to significantly impact aging, it is likely that the genetic background of the individual will determine just how effective any particular modification is likely to be. Both calorically restricted and long-lived mice share common longevity assurance mechanisms when compared to progeroid mice, although the efficacy of such mechanisms varies widely in the two sets of mice [391].

Conclusions

Despite the near-universal phenomenon of aging in living organisms, there is an extraordinarily varied phenotype that accompanies aging in specific individuals. Furthermore, it appears that evolutionary pressures have led to the development of a remarkable homeostatic complexity to the underlying mechanisms that cause us to grow old. The three quotations at the beginning of this chapter aptly represent these processes. Butch Cassidy recognized the inexorable forces that cause us to age. The concept of antagonistic pleiotropy is reflected in the other two insights. It seems that we clearly pay a price to maintain a high level of reproductive fitness – there is no free lunch. However, the ironic, yet ultimately satisfying, paradox may be that the only way that we can actually live as long as we do is, in fact, to grow old.

References

1. Cutler RG (1985) Evolutionary perspective of human longevity. In: Hazzard WR, Andres R, Bierman EL et al (eds) Principles of geriatric medicine and gerontology, 2nd edn. McGraw-Hill, New York, p 16
2. Kung HC, Hoyert DL, Xu JQ, Murphy SL (2008) Deaths: final data for 2005, vol 56. National Center for Health Statistics, Hyattsville, MD
3. He W, Sengupta M, Velkoff VA, DeBarros KA (2005) 65+ in the United States: 2005. Current Population Reports, P23-P209. U.S. Government Printing Office, Washington, DC
4. Perls TT, Alpert L, Fretts RC (1997) Middle-aged mothers live longer. Nature 389(6647):133

5. Snowden DA, Kane RL, Beeson WL (1989) Is early natural menopause a biological marker of health and ageing? Am J Public Health 79:709–714

6. van der Schouw YT, van der Graaf Y, Steyerberg EW, Eijkemans JC, Banga JD (1996) Menopause as a risk factor for cardiovascular mortality. Lancet 347(9003):714–718

7. Helle S, Lummaa V, Jokela J (2005) Are reproductive and somatic senescence coupled in humans? Late, but not early, reproduction correlated with longevity in historical Sami women. Proc R Soc B Biol Sci 272(1558):29–37

8. Morley JE, Haren MT, Kim MJ, Kevorkian R, Perry HM III (2005) Testosterone, aging and quality of life. J Endocrinol Invest 28(3 Suppl):76–80

9. Yeap BB (2008) Are declining testosterone levels a major risk factor for ill-health in aging men? Int J Impot Res 21(1):24–36

10. Roush W (1996) Live long and prosper? [news]. Science 273(5271): 42–46

11. Greville TN, Bayo F, Foster R (1975) United States life tables by causes of death: 1960-71, vol 1, Number 5, *Technical Report*

12. Sohal RS, Weindruch R (1996) Oxidative stress, caloric restriction, and aging. Science 273(5271):59–63

13. Mair W, Dillin A (2008) Aging and survival: the genetics of life span extension by dietary restriction. Annu Rev Biochem 77:727–754

14. Weindruch R, Walford RL (1982) Dietary restriction in mice beginning at 1 year of age: effect on life-span and spontaneous cancer incidence. Science 215(4538):1415–1418

15. Yu BP, Masoro EJ, McMahan CA (1985) Nutritional influences on aging of Fischer 344 rats: I. Physical, metabolic, and longevity characteristics. J Gerontol 40(6):657–670

16. Masoro EJ (1993) Dietary restriction and aging. J Am Geriatr Soc 41(9):994–999

17. Weindruch R, Sohal RS (337) Seminars in medicine of the Beth Israel Deaconess Medical Center. Caloric intake and aging. N Engl J Med 14:986–994

18. Dulloo AG, Girardier L (1993) 24 hour energy expenditure several months after weight loss in the underfed rat: evidence for a chronic increase in whole-body metabolic efficiency. Int J Obes Relat Metab Disord 17(2):115–123

19. Gonzales-Pacheco DM, Buss WC, Koehler KM, Woodside WF, Alpert SS (1993) Energy restriction reduces metabolic rate in adult male Fisher-344 rats. J Nutr 123(1):90–97

20. McCarter R, Masoro EJ, Yu BP (1985) Does food restriction retard aging by reducing the metabolic rate? Am J Physiol 248(4 Pt 1):E488–E490

21. Lane MA, Baer DJ, Rumpler WV et al (1996) Calorie restriction lowers body temperature in rhesus monkeys, consistent with a postulated anti-aging mechanism in rodents. Proc Natl Acad Sci USA 93(9):4159–4164

22. Ramsey JJ, Roecker EB, Weindruch R, Kemnitz JW (1997) Energy expenditure of adult male rhesus monkeys during the first 30 mo of dietary restriction. Am J Physiol 272(5 Pt 1):E901–E907

23. Verdery RB, Ingram DK, Roth GS, Lane MA (1997) Caloric restriction increases HDL2 levels in rhesus monkeys (Macaca mulatta). Am J Physiol 273(4 Pt 1):E714–E719

24. Mattison JA, Lane MA, Roth GS, Ingram DK (2003) Calorie restriction in rhesus monkeys. Exp Gerontol 38(1–2):35–46

25. Heilbronn LK, de Jonge L, Frisard MI et al (2006) Effect of 6-month calorie restriction on biomarkers of longevity, metabolic adaptation, and oxidative stress in overweight individuals: a randomized controlled trial. JAMA 295(13):1539–1548

26. Lefevre M, Redman LM, Heilbronn LK et al (2009) Caloric restriction alone and with exercise improves CVD risk in healthy non-obese individuals. Atherosclerosis 203(1):206–213

27. Gompertz B (1825) On the nature of the function expressive of the law of human mortality and on a new mode of determining life contingencies. Philos Trans R Soc Lond 115:513

28. Kung HC, Hoyert DL, Xu JQ, Murphy SL (2008) Deaths: final data for 2005. *National Vital Statistics Reports.* Vol 56. National Center for Health Statistics, Hyattsville, MD

29. Shock NW, Greulich RC, Andres R et al (eds) (1984) Normal human aging: the baltimore longitudinal study of aging. U.S. Department of Health and Human Services, Washington, DC

30. Riggs BL, Melton LJ III (1986) Involutional osteoporosis. N Engl J Med 314(26):1676–1686

31. Florini JR (ed.) (1981) Composition and function of cells and tissues. In: Handbook of biolochemistry in aging. CRC Press, Boca Raton

32. Strehler BL (1977) Time, cells, and aging, 2nd edn. Academic Press, New York

33. Bjorksten J (1974) Cross linkage and the aging process. In: Rothstein M (ed) Theoretical aspects of aging. Academic Press, New York, p 43

34. Kohn RR (1978) Aging of animals: possible mechanisms. In: Principles of mammalian aging, 2nd edn. Prentice-Hall, Englewood Cliffs, NJ

35. Herbig U, Ferreira M, Condel L, Carey D, Sedivy JM (2006) Cellular senescence in aging primates. Science 311(5765):1257

36. Jeyapalan JC, Ferreira M, Sedivy JM, Herbig U (2007) Accumulation of senescent cells in mitotic tissue of aging primates. Mech Ageing Dev 128(1):36–44

37. Sedelnikova OA, Horikawa I, Zimonjic DB, Popescu NC, Bonner WM, Barrett JC (2004) Senescing human cells and ageing mice accumulate DNA lesions with unrepairable double-strand breaks. Nat Cell Biol 6(2):168–170

38. Finch CE (1990) Introduction: gefinitions and concepts. In: Longevity, senescence, and the genome. University of Chicago Press, Chicago

39. Schneider EL, Rowe JW (eds) (1996) Handbook of the biology of aging, 4th edn. Academic Press, San Diego

40. Shock NW (1985) Longitudinal studies of aging in humans. In: Finch CE, Schneider EL (eds) Handbook of the biology of aging, 2nd edn. Van Nostrand Reinhold, New York, p 721

41. Lakatta EG (1990) Changes in cardiovascular function with aging. Eur Heart J 11(Suppl C):22–29

42. Lindeman RD, Tobin J, Shock NW (1985) Longitudinal studies on the rate of decline in renal function with age. J Am Geriatr Soc 33(4):278–285

43. Adelman RC, Britton GW, Rotenberg S (1978) Endocrine regulation of gene activity in aging animals of different genotypes. In: Bergsma D, Harrison DE (eds) Genetic effects on aging. Alan R. Liss, New York, p 355

44. Dorshkind K, Montecino-Rodriguez E, Signer RAJ et al (2009) The ageing immune system: is it ever too old to become young again? Nat Rev Immunol 9(1):57–62

45. Brody JA, Brock DB (1985) Epidemiological and statistical characteristics of the United States elderly population. In: Finch CE, Schneider EL (eds) Handbook of the biology of aging, 2nd edn. Van Nostrand Reinhold, New York, p 3

46. Rosenberg HM, Ventura SJ, Maurer JD et al (1996) Births and deaths: United States, 1995. Mon Vital Stat Rep 45(3 Suppl 2):31–33

47. Hitt R, Young-Xu Y, Silver M, Perls T (1999) Centenarians: the older you get, the healthier you have been. Lancet 354(9179):652

48. Niedernhofer LJ, Garinis GA, Raams A et al (2006) A new progeroid syndrome reveals that genotoxic stress suppresses the somatotroph axis. Nature 444(7122):1038–1043

49. Rose MR, Graves JL Jr (1989) What evolutionary biology can do for gerontology. J Gerontol 44(2):B27–B29

50. Kirkwood TB, Rose MR (1991) Evolution of senescence: late survival sacrificed for reproduction. Philos Trans R Soc Lond B Biol Sci 332(1262):15–24

51. Kirkwood TB (1996) Human senescence. Bioessays 18(12): 1009–1016

52. Finch CE, Tanzi RE (1997) Genetics of aging. Science 278:407–411
53. Jazwinski SM (1996) Longevity, genes, and aging. Science 273(5271):54–59
54. Murakami S, Johnson TE (1996) A genetic pathway conferring life extension and resistance to UV stress in Caenorhabditis elegans. Genetics 143(3):1207–1218
55. Kimura KD, Tissenbaum HA, Liu Y, Ruvkun G (1997) daf-2, an insulin receptor-like gene that regulates longevity and diapause in Caenorhabditis elegans [see comments]. Science 277(5328):942–946
56. Kenyon C, Chang J, Gensch E, Rudner A, Tabtiang R (1993) A C. elegans mutant that lives twice as long as wild type [see comments]. Nature 366(6454):461–464
57. Lin K, Dorman JB, Rodan A, Kenyon C (1997) daf-16: An HNF-3/forkhead family member that can function fo double the life-span of Caenorhabditis elegans. Science 278:1319–1322
58. Kaeberlein M, McVey M, Guarente L (2001) Using yeast to discover the fountain of youth. Science of aging and knowledge environment.http://sageke.sciencemag.org/cgi/content/full/sageke;2001/1/pe1:http://sageke.sciencemag.org/cgi/content/full/sageke;2001/1/pe1
59. Guarente L (2007) Sirtuins in aging and disease. Cold Spring Harb Symp Quant Biol 72:483–488
60. Schwer B, Verdin E (2008) Conserved metabolic regulatory functions of sirtuins. Cell Metab 7(2):104–112
61. Lin YJ, Seroude L, Benzer S (1998) Extended life-span and stress resistance in the Drosophila mutant methuselah. Science 282(5390):943–946
62. Rogina B, Reenan RA, Nilsen SP, Helfand SL (2000) Extended life-span conferred by cotransporter gene mutations in Drosophila. Science 290(5499):2137–2140
63. Dudas SP, Arking R (1995) A coordinate upregulation of antioxidant gene activities is associated with the delayed onset of senescence in a long-lived strain of Drosophila. J Gerontol A Biol Sci Med Sci 50(3):B117–B127
64. Rose MR, Vu LN, Park SU, Graves JL Jr (1992) Selection on stress resistance increases longevity in Drosophila melanogaster. Exp Gerontol 27(2):241–250
65. Migliaccio E, Giorgio M, Mele S et al (1999) The p66shc adaptor protein controls oxidative stress response and life span in mammals. Nature 402(6759):309–313
66. Flurkey K, Papaconstantinou J, Harrison DE (2002) The Snell dwarf mutation Pit1(dw) can increase life span in mice. Mech Ageing Dev 123(2–3):121–130
67. De Benedictis G, Rose G, Carrieri G et al (1999) Mitochondrial DNA inherited variants are associated with successful aging and longevity in humans. FASEB J 13(12):1532–1536
68. Salvioli S, Capri M, Santoro A et al (2008) The impact of mitochondrial DNA on human lifespan: a view from studies on centenarians. Biotechnol J 3(6):740–749
69. Rose G, Passarino G, Carrieri G et al (2001) Paradoxes in longevity: sequence analysis of mtDNA haplogroup J in centenarians. Eur J Hum Genet 9(9):701–707
70. Ross OA, McCormack R, Curran MD et al (2001) Mitochondrial DNA polymorphism: its role in longevity of the Irish population. Exp Gerontol 36(7):1161–1178
71. Capri M, Salvioli S, Sevini F et al (2006) The genetics of human longevity. Ann NY Acad Sci 1067:252–263
72. Glatt SJ, Chayavichitsilp P, Depp C, Schork NJ, Jeste DV (2007) Successful aging: from phenotype to genotype. Biol Psychiatry 62(4):282–293
73. Barzilai N, Atzmon G, Schechter C et al (2003) Unique lipoprotein phenotype and genotype associated with exceptional longevity. JAMA 290(15):2030–2040
74. Willcox BJ, Donlon TA, He Q et al (2008) FOXO3A genotype is strongly associated with human longevity. Proc Natl Acad Sci USA 105(37):13987–13992
75. Flachsbart F, Caliebe A, Kleindorp R et al (2009) Association of FOXO3A variation with human longevity confirmed in German centenarians. Proc Natl Acad Sci USA 106(8):2700–2705
76. Lunetta KL, D'Agostino RB Sr, Karasik D et al (2007) Genetic correlates of longevity and selected age-related phenotypes: a genome-wide association study in the Framingham Study. BMC Med Genet 8(Suppl 1):S13
77. Bellizzi D, Rose G, Cavalcante P et al (2005) A novel VNTR enhancer within the SIRT3 gene, a human homologue of SIR2, is associated with survival at oldest ages. Genomics 85(2):258–263
78. Rose G, Dato S, Altomare K et al (2003) Variability of the SIRT3 gene, human silent information regulator Sir2 homologue, and survivorship in the elderly. Exp Gerontol 38(10):1065–1070
79. Suh Y, Atzmon G, Cho MO et al (2008) Functionally significant insulin-like growth factor I receptor mutations in centenarians. Proc Natl Acad Sci USA 105(9):3438–3442
80. Hong MG, Reynolds C, Gatz M et al (2008) Evidence that the gene encoding insulin degrading enzyme influences human lifespan. Hum Mol Genet 17(15):2370–2378
81. Hurme M, Lehtimaki T, Jylha M, Karhunen PJ, Hervonen A (2005) Interleukin-6–174G/C polymorphism and longevity: a follow-up study. Mech Ageing Dev 126(3):417–418
82. Di Bona D, Vasto S, Capurso C et al (2009) Effect of interleukin-6 polymorphisms on human longevity: a systematic review and meta-analysis. Ageing Res Rev 8(1):36–42
83. Scola L, Candore G, Colonna-Romano G et al (2005) Study of the association with -330T/G IL-2 in a population of centenarians from centre and south Italy. Biogerontology 6(6):425–429
84. Hurme M, Kivimaki M, Pertovaara M et al (2007) CRP gene is involved in the regulation of human longevity: a follow-up study in Finnish nonagenarians. Mech Ageing Dev 128(10):574–576
85. Hindorff LA, Rice KM, Lange LA et al (2008) Common variants in the CRP gene in relation to longevity and cause-specific mortality in older adults: the Cardiovascular Health Study. Atherosclerosis 197(2):922–930
86. Cardelli M, Cavallone L, Marchegiani F et al (2008) A genetic-demographic approach reveals male-specific association between survival and tumor necrosis factor (A/G)-308 polymorphism. J Gerontol A Biol Sci Med Sci 63(5):454–460
87. Schachter F, Faure-Delanef L, Guenot F et al (1994) Genetic associations with human longevity at the APOE and ACE loci. Nat Genet 6(1):29–32
88. Perls T, Levenson R, Regan M, Puca A (2002) What does it take to live to 100? Mech Ageing Dev 123(2–3):231–242
89. Adams ER, Nolan VG, Andersen SL, Perls TT, Terry DF (2008) Centenarian offspring: start healthier and stay healthier. J Am Geriatr Soc 56(11):2089–2092
90. Lee CK, Klopp RG, Weindruch R, Prolla TA (1999) Gene expression profile of aging and its retardation by caloric restriction. Science 285(5432):1390–1393
91. Lee CK, Weindruch R, Prolla TA (2000) Gene-expression profile of the ageing brain in mice. Nat Genet 25(3):294–297
92. Kayo T, Allison DB, Weindruch R, Prolla TA (2001) Influences of aging and caloric restriction on the transcriptional profile of skeletal muscle from rhesus monkeys. Proc Natl Acad Sci USA 98(9):5093–5098
93. Weindruch R, Kayo T, Lee CK, Prolla TA (2001) Microarray profiling of gene expression in aging and its alteration by caloric restriction in mice. J Nutr 131(3):918S–923S
94. Kirkwood TB, Holliday R (1979) The evolution of ageing and longevity. Proc R Soc Lond B Biol Sci 205(1161):531–546
95. Westendorp RGJ, Kirkwood TBL (1998) Human longevity at the cost of reproductive success. Nature 396(6713):743–746
96. Mobbs CV (1996) Nueroendocrinology of aging. In: Schneider EL, Rowe JW (eds) Handbook of the biology of aging, 4th edn. Academic Press, San Diego, pp 234–282

97. Wise PM, Krajnak KM, Kashon ML (1996) Menopause: the aging of multiple pacemakers. Science 273(5271):67–70

98. Denckla WD (1975) A time to die. Life Sci 16(1):31–44

99. Gilad GM, Gilad VH (1987) Age-related reductions in brain cholinergic and dopaminergic indices in two rat strains differing in longevity. Brain Res 408(1–2):247–250

100. Cotzias GC, Miller ST, Tang LC, Papavasiliou PS (1977) Levodopa, fertility, and longevity. Science 196(4289):549–551

101. Knoll J (1992) (-)Deprenyl-medication: a strategy to modulate the age-related decline of the striatal dopaminergic system. J Am Geriatr Soc 40(8):839–847

102. Kitani K, Kanai S, Sato Y, Ohta M, Ivy GO, Carrillo MC (1993) Chronic treatment of (−)deprenyl prolongs the life span of male Fischer 344 rats. Further evidence. Life Sci 52(3):281–288

103. Milgram NW, Racine RJ, Nellis P, Mendonca A, Ivy GO (1990) Maintenance on L-deprenyl prolongs life in aged male rats. Life Sci 47(5).415–420

104. Kappeler L, De Magalhaes Filho CM, Dupont J et al (2008) Brain IGF-1 receptors control mammalian growth and lifespan through a neuroendocrine mechanism. PLoS Biol 6(10):e254

105. Walford RL (1974) Immunologic theory of aging: current status. Fed Proc 33(9):2020–2027

106. Miller RA (1996) The aging immune system: primer and prospectus. Science 273(5271):70–74

107. Yunis EJ, Salazar M (1993) Genetics of life span in mice. Genetica 91(1–3):211–223

108. Caruso C, Candore G, Romano GC et al (2001) Immunogenetics of longevity. Is major histocompatibility complex polymorphism relevant to the control of human longevity? A review of literature data. Mech Ageing Dev 122(5):445–462

109. Holehan AM, Merry BJ (1985) Lifetime breeding studies in fully fed and dietary restricted female CFY Sprague–Dawley rats. 1. Effect of age, housing conditions and diet on fecundity. Mech Ageing Dev 33(1):19–28

110. Merry BJ, Holehan AM (1979) Onset of puberty and duration of fertility in rats fed a restricted diet. J Reprod Fertil 57(2):253–259

111. Partridge L, Gems D, Withers DJ (2005) Sex and death: what is the connection? Cell 120(4):461–472

112. Selesniemi K, Lee H-J, Tilly JL (2008) Moderate caloric restriction initiated in rodents during adulthood sustains function of the female reproductive axis into advanced chronological age. Aging Cell 7(5):622–629

113. Harman D (1956) Aging: a theory based on free radical and radiation chemistry. J Gerontol 11:298

114. Harman D (1981) The aging process. Proc Natl Acad Sci USA 78(11):7124–7128

115. Fridovich I (1989) Superoxide dismutases. An adaptation to a paramagnetic gas. J Biol Chem 264(14):7761–7764

116. Sen CK, Packer L (1996) Antioxidant and redox regulation of gene transcription [see comments]. FASEB J 10(7):709–720

117. Suzuki YJ, Forman HJ, Sevanian A (1997) Oxidants as stimulators of signal transduction. Free Radic Biol Med 22(1–2):269–285

118. Finkel T (2003) Oxidant signals and oxidative stress. Curr Opin Cell Biol 15(2):247–254

119. Valko M, Morris H, Cronin TD (2005) Metals, toxicity and oxidative stress. Curr Med Chem 12(10):1161–1208

120. Sun J, Folk D, Bradley TJ, Tower J (2002) Induced overexpression of mitochondrial Mn-superoxide dismutase extends the life span of adult Drosophila melanogaster. Genetics 161(2):661–672

121. Mockett RJ, Orr WC, Rahmandar JJ et al (1999) Overexpression of Mn-containing superoxide dismutase in transgenic Drosophila melanogaster. Arch Biochem Biophys 371(2):260–269

122. Paul A, Belton A, Nag S, Martin I, Grotewiel MS, Duttaroy A (2007) Reduced mitochondrial SOD displays mortality characteristics reminiscent of natural aging. Mech Ageing Dev 128(11–12):706–716

123. Parkes TL, Elia AJ, Dickinson D, Hilliker AJ, Phillips JP, Boulianne GL (1998) Extension of Drosophila lifespan by overexpression of human SOD1 in motorneurons. Nat Genet 19(2):171–174

124. Sun J, Tower J (1999) FLP Recombinase-mediated induction of Cu/Zn-superoxide dismutase transgene expression can extend the life span of adult Drosophila melanogaster flies. Mol Cell Biol 19(1):216–228

125. Parker JD, Parker KM, Sohal BH, Sohal RS, Keller L (2004) Decreased expression of Cu-Zn superoxide dismutase 1 in ants with extreme lifespan. Proc Natl Acad Sci USA 101(10):3486–3489

126. Orr WC, Sohal RS (1994) Extension of life-span by overexpression of superoxide dismutase and catalase in Drosophila melanogaster. Science 263(5150):1128–1130

127. Orr WC, Mockett RJ, Benes JJ, Sohal RS (2003) Effects of overexpression of copper-zinc and manganese superoxide dismutases, catalase, and thioredoxin reductase genes on longevity in Drosophila melanogaster. J Biol Chem 278(29):26418–26422

128. Mockett RJ, Sohal RS, Orr WC (1999) Overexpression of glutathione reductase extends survival in transgenic Drosophila melanogaster under hyperoxia but not normoxia. FASEB J 13(13): 1733–1742

129. Brys K, Vanfleteren JR, Braeckman BP (2007) Testing the rate-of-living/oxidative damage theory of aging in the nematode model Caenorhabditis elegans. Exp Gerontol 42(9):845–851

130. Halaschek-Wiener J, Khattra JS, McKay S et al (2005) Analysis of long-lived C. elegans daf-2 mutants using serial analysis of gene expression. Genome Res 15(5):603–615

131. Murphy CT, McCarroll SA, Bargmann CI et al (2003) Genes that act downstream of DAF-16 to influence the lifespan of Caenorhabditis elegans. Nature 424(6946):277–283

132. Keaney M, Matthijssens F, Sharpe M, Vanfleteren J, Gems D (2004) Superoxide dismutase mimetics elevate superoxide dismutase activity in vivo but do not retard aging in the nematode Caenorhabditis elegans. Free Radic Biol Med 37(2):239–250

133. Adachi H, Fujiwara Y, Ishii N (1998) Effects of oxygen on protein carbonyl and aging in Caenorhabditis elegans mutants with long (age-1) and short (mev-1) life spans. J Gerontol A Biol Sci Med Sci 53(4):B240–B244

134. Sohal RS, Svensson I, Sohal BH, Brunk UT (1989) Superoxide anion radical production in different animal species. Mech Ageing Dev 49(2):129–135

135. Schriner SE, Linford NJ, Martin GM et al (2005) Extension of murine life span by overexpression of catalase targeted to mitochondria. Science 308(5730):1909–1911

136. Mitsui A, Hamuro J, Nakamura H et al (2002) Overexpression of human thioredoxin in transgenic mice controls oxidative stress and life span. Antioxid Redox Signal 4(4):693–696

137. Salmon AB, Murakami S, Bartke A, Kopchick J, Yasumura K, Miller RA (2005) Fibroblast cell lines from young adult mice of long-lived mutant strains are resistant to multiple forms of stress. Am J Physiol Endocrinol Metab 289(1):E23–E29

138. Harper JM, Salmon AB, Leiser SF, Galecki AT, Miller RA (2007) Skin-derived fibroblasts from long-lived species are resistant to some, but not all, lethal stresses and to the mitochondrial inhibitor rotenone. Aging Cell 6(1):1–13

139. Maynard SP, Miller RA (2006) Fibroblasts from long-lived Snell dwarf mice are resistant to oxygen-induced in vitro growth arrest. Aging Cell 5(1):89–96

140. Linnane AW, Zhang C, Baumer A, Nagley P (1992) Mitochondrial DNA mutation and the ageing process: bioenergy and pharmacological intervention. Mutat Res 275(3–6):195–208

141. Fleming JE, Miquel J, Cottrell SF, Yengoyan LS, Economos AC (1982) Is cell aging caused by respiration-dependent injury to the mitochondrial genome? Gerontology 28(1):44–53

142. Wallace DC (1992) Mitochondrial genetics: a paradigm for aging and degenerative diseases? Science 256(5057):628–632

143. Ozawa T (1997) Genetic and functional changes in mitochondria associated with aging. Physiol Rev 77(2):425–464

144. Katayama M, Tanaka M, Yamamoto H, Ohbayashi T, Nimura Y, Ozawa T (1991) Deleted mitochondrial DNA in the skeletal muscle of aged individuals. Biochem Int 25(1):47–56

145. Lee CM, Chung SS, Kaczkowski JM, Weindruch R, Aiken JM (1993) Multiple mitochondrial DNA deletions associated with age in skeletal muscle of rhesus monkeys. J Gerontol 48(6):B201–B205

146. Melov S, Shoffner JM, Kaufman A, Wallace DC (1995) Marked increase in the number and variety of mitochondrial DNA rearrangements in aging human skeletal muscle [published erratum appears in Nucleic Acids Res 1995 Dec 11;23(23):4938]. Nucleic Acids Res 23(20):4122–4126

147. Torii K, Sugiyama S, Tanaka M et al (1992) Aging-associated deletions of human diaphragmatic mitochondrial DNA. Am J Respir Cell Mol Biol 6(5):543–549

148. Hayakawa M, Torii K, Sugiyama S, Tanaka M, Ozawa T (1991) Age-associated accumulation of 8-hydroxydeoxyguanosine in mitochondrial DNA of human diaphragm. Biochem Biophys Res Commun 179(2):1023–1029

149. Sugiyama S, Hattori K, Hayakawa M, Ozawa T (1991) Quantitative analysis of age-associated accumulation of mitochondrial DNA with deletion in human hearts. Biochem Biophys Res Commun 180(2):894–899

150. Hayakawa M, Katsumata K, Yoneda M, Tanaka M, Sugiyama S, Ozawa T (1996) Age-related extensive fragmentation of mitochondrial DNA into minicircles [published erratum appears in Biochem Biophys Res Commun 1997 Mar 27;232(3):832]. Biochem Biophys Res Commun 226(2):369–377

151. Hayakawa M, Hattori K, Sugiyama S, Ozawa T (1992) Age-associated oxygen damage and mutations in mitochondrial DNA in human hearts. Biochem Biophys Res Commun 189(2):979–985

152. Hayakawa M, Sugiyama S, Hattori K, Takasawa M, Ozawa T (1993) Age-associated damage in mitochondrial DNA in human hearts. Mol Cell Biochem 119(1–2):95–103

153. Ikebe S, Tanaka M, Ohno K et al (1990) Increase of deleted mitochondrial DNA in the striatum in Parkinson's disease and senescence. Biochem Biophys Res Commun 170(3):1044–1048

154. Corral-Debrinski M, Horton T, Lott MT, Shoffner JM, Beal MF, Wallace DC (1992) Mitochondrial DNA deletions in human brain: regional variability and increase with advanced age. Nat Genet 2(4):324–329

155. Trounce I, Byrne E, Marzuki S (1989) Decline in skeletal muscle mitochondrial respiratory chain function: possible factor in ageing [see comments]. Lancet 1(8639):637–639

156. Schapira AH, Mann VM, Cooper JM et al (1990) Anatomic and disease specificity of NADH CoQ1 reductase (complex I) deficiency in Parkinson's disease. J Neurochem 55(6):2142–2145

157. Schapira AH, Cooper JM, Dexter D, Clark JB, Jenner P, Marsden CD (1990) Mitochondrial complex I deficiency in Parkinson's disease. J Neurochem 54(3):823–827

158. Hoyer S (1986) Senile dementia and Alzheimer's disease. Brain blood flow and metabolism. Prog Neuropsychopharmacol Biol Psychiatry 10(3–5):447–478

159. Sims NR, Finegan JM, Blass JP, Bowen DM, Neary D (1987) Mitochondrial function in brain tissue in primary degenerative dementia. Brain Res 436(1):30–38

160. Beal MF (1994) Neurochemistry and toxin models in Huntington's disease. Curr Opin Neurol 7(6):542–547

161. Schulz JB, Beal MF (1996) Mitochondrial dysfunction in movement disorders. Mech Dev 57(1):3–20

162. Lin FH, Lin R, Wisniewski HM et al (1992) Detection of point mutations in codon 331 of mitochondrial NADH dehydrogenase subunit 2 in Alzheimer's brains. Biochem Biophys Res Commun 182(1):238–246

163. Shoffner JM, Brown MD, Torroni A et al (1993) Mitochondrial DNA variants observed in Alzheimer disease and Parkinson disease patients. Genomics 17(1):171–184

164. Ozawa T, Tanaka M, Ino H et al (1991) Distinct clustering of point mutations in mitochondrial DNA among patients with mitochondrial encephalomyopathies and with Parkinson's disease. Biochem Biophys Res Commun 176(2):938–946

165. Ozawa T, Tanaka M, Ikebe S, Ohno K, Kondo T, Mizuno Y (1990) Quantitative determination of deleted mitochondrial DNA relative to normal DNA in parkinsonian striatum by a kinetic PCR analysis. Biochem Biophys Res Commun 172(2):483–489

166. Ikebe S, Tanaka M, Ozawa T (1995) Point mutations of mitochondrial genome in Parkinson's disease. Brain Res Mol Brain Res 28(2):281–295

167. Poulton J, Deadman ME, Ramacharan S, Gardiner RM (1991) Germ-line deletions of mtDNA in mitochondrial myopathy. Am J Hum Genet 48(4):649–653

168. Ionasescu VV, Hart M, DiMauro S, Moraes CT (1994) Clinical and morphologic features of a myopathy associated with a point mutation in the mitochondrial tRNA(Pro) gene. Neurology 44(5):975–977

169. Ozawa T, Tanaka M, Sugiyama S et al (1991) Patients with idiopathic cardiomyopathy belong to the same mitochondrial DNA gene family of Parkinson's disease and mitochondrial encephalomyopathy. Biochem Biophys Res Commun 177(1):518–525

170. Katsumata K, Hayakawa M, Tanaka M, Sugiyama S, Ozawa T (1994) Fragmentation of human heart mitochondrial DNA associated with premature aging. Biochem Biophys Res Commun 202(1):102–110

171. Ozawa T (1994) Mitochondrial cardiomyopathy. Herz 19(2):105–118, 125

172. Yoneda M, Katsumata K, Hayakawa M, Tanaka M, Ozawa T (1995) Oxygen stress induces an apoptotic cell death associated with fragmentation of mitochondrial genome. Biochem Biophys Res Commun 209(2):723–729

173. Trifunovic A, Wredenberg A, Falkenberg M et al (2004) Premature ageing in mice expressing defective mitochondrial DNA polymerase. Nature 429(6990):417–423

174. Trifunovic A, Hansson A, Wredenberg A et al (2005) Somatic mtDNA mutations cause aging phenotypes without affecting reactive oxygen species production. Proc Natl Acad Sci USA 102(50):17993–17998

175. Maisonneuve E, Ezraty B, Dukan S (2008) Protein aggregates: an aging factor involved in cell death. J Bacteriol 190(18):6070–6075

176. Melov S, Hinerfeld D, Esposito L, Wallace DC (1997) Multi-organ characterization of mitochondrial genomic rearrangements in ad libitum and caloric restricted mice show striking somatic mitochondrial DNA rearrangements with age. Nucleic Acids Res 25(5):974–982

177. Larsen PL, Clarke CF (2002) Extension of life-span in Caenorhabditis elegans by a diet lacking coenzyme Q. Science 295(5552):120–123

178. Zainal TA, Oberley TD, Allison DB, Szweda LI, Weindruch R (2000) Caloric restriction of rhesus monkeys lowers oxidative damage in skeletal muscle. FASEB J 14(12):1825–1836

179. Meydani M (2001) Nutrition interventions in aging and age-associated disease. Ann NY Acad Sci 928:226–235

180. Lopez-Lluch G, Irusta PM, Navas P, de Cabo R (2008) Mitochondrial biogenesis and healthy aging. Exp Gerontol 43(9):813–819

181. Civitarese AE, Carling S, Heilbronn LK et al (2007) Calorie restriction increases muscle mitochondrial biogenesis in healthy humans. PLoS Med 4(3):e76

182. Lanza IR, Short DK, Short KR et al (2008) Endurance exercise as a countermeasure for aging. Diabetes 57(11):2933–2942

183. Melov S, Tarnopolsky MA, Beckman K, Felkey K, Hubbard A (2007) Resistance exercise reverses aging in human skeletal muscle. PLoS ONE 2(5):e465

184. Failla G (1958) The aging process and carcinogenesis. Ann NY Acad Sci 71:1124

185. Szilard L (1959) On the nature of the aging process. Proc Natl Acad Sci USA 45:30

186. Casarett GW (1963) Concept and criteria of radiologic ageing. In: Harris RJ (ed) Cellular basis and aetiology of late somatic effects of ionizing radiation. Academic Press, New York, p 189

187. Walburg HE (1975) Radiation-induced life-shortening and premature aging. Adv Radiat Biol 5:145

188. Sacher CA (1977) Life table modification and life prolongation. In: Finch CE, Hayflick L (eds) Handbook of the biology of aging. Van Nostrand Reinhold, New York, p 582

189. Lindop PJ, Rotblat J (1961) Long-term effect of a single whoe-body exposure of mice to ionizing radiations. Proc R Soc Lond 154:350

190. Garinis GA, van der Horst GT, Vijg J, Hoeijmakers JH (2008) DNA damage and ageing: new-age ideas for an age-old problem. Nat Cell Biol 10(11):1241–1247

191. Hart RW, Setlow RB (1974) Correlation between deoxyribonu-cleic acid excision-repair and life-span in a number of mammalian species. Proc Natl Acad Sci USA 71(6):2169–2173

192. Cabelof DC, Raffoul JJ, Yanamadala S, Ganir C, Guo Z, Heydari AR (2002) Attenuation of DNA polymerase [beta]-dependent base excision repair and increased DMS-induced mutagenicity in aged mice. Mutat Res 500(1–2):135–145

193. Intano GW, Cho EJ, McMahan CA, Walter CA (2003) Age-related base excision repair activity in mouse brain and liver nuclear extracts. J Gerontol A Biol Sci Med Sci 58(3):B205–B211

194. Cabelof DC, Yanamadala S, Raffoul JJ, Guo Z, Soofi A, Heydari AR (2003) Caloric restriction promotes genomic stability by induction of base excision repair and reversal of its age-related decline. DNA Repair 2(3):295–307

195. Seluanov A, Mittelman D, Pereira-Smith OM, Wilson JH, Gorbunova V (2004) DNA end joining becomes less efficient and more error-prone during cellular senescence. Proc Natl Acad Sci USA 101(20):7624–7629

196. Sedelnikova OA, Horikawa I, Redon C et al (2008) Delayed kinetics of DNA double-strand break processing in normal and pathological aging. Aging Cell 7(1):89–100

197. Hanawalt PC, Gee P, Ho L (1990) DNA repair in differentiating cells in relation to aging. In: Finch CE, Johnson TE (eds) Molecular biology of aging. UCLA symposia on molecular and cellular biology, vol 123. Alan R. Liss, New York, p 45

198. Henle ES, Han Z, Tang N, Rai P, Luo Y, Linn S (1999) Sequence-specific DNA Cleavage by Fe2+-mediated Fenton reactions has possible biological implications. J Biol Chem 274(2):962–971

199. Lu T, Pan Y, Kao S-Y et al (2004) Gene regulation and DNA damage in the ageing human brain. Nature 429(6994):883–891

200. Orgel LE (1963) The maintenance of the accuracy of protein synthesis and its relevance to aging. Proc Natl Acad Sci USA 49:517

201. Kristal BS, Yu BP (1992) An emerging hypothesis: synergistic induction of aging by free radicals and Maillard reactions. J Gerontol 47(4):B107–B114

202. Levine RL, Stadtman ER (1996) Protein Modifications with Aging. In: Schneider EL, Rowe JW (eds) Handbook of the biology of aging, 4th edn. Academic Press, San Diego, pp 184–197

203. Gracy RW, Yuksel KU, Chapman MD et al (1985) Impaired protein degradation may account for the accumulation of "abnormal" proteins in aging cells. In: Adelman RC, Dekker EE (ed) Modern aging research, modification of proteins during aging. Alan R. Liss, New York, p 1

204. Brown WT (1990) Genetic diseases of premature aging as models of senescence. Annu Rev Gerontol Geriatr 10:23–42

205. Meshorer E, Gruenbaum Y (2008) Gone with the Wnt/Notch: stem cells in laminopathies, progeria, and aging. J Cell Biol 181(1):9–13

206. De Sandre-Giovannoli A, Bernard R, Cau P et al (2003) Lamin A truncation in Hutchinson–Gilford progeria. Science 300(5628):2055

207. Eriksson M, Brown WT, Gordon LB et al (2003) Recurrent de novo point mutations in lamin A cause Hutchinson–Gilford progeria syndrome. Nature 423(6937):293–298

208. Scaffidi P, Misteli T (2005) Reversal of the cellular phenotype in the premature aging disease Hutchinson–Gilford progeria syndrome. Nat Med 11(4):440–445

209. Cao K, Capell BC, Erdos MR, Djabali K, Collins FS (2007) A lamin A protein isoform overexpressed in Hutchinson–Gilford progeria syndrome interferes with mitosis in progeria and normal cells. Proc Natl Acad Sci USA 104(12):4949–4954

210. Dahl KN, Scaffidi P, Islam MF, Yodh AG, Wilson KL, Misteli T (2006) Distinct structural and mechanical properties of the nuclear lamina in Hutchinson–Gilford progeria syndrome. Proc Natl Acad Sci USA 103(27):10271–10276

211. Dechat T, Shimi T, Adam SA et al (2007) Alterations in mitosis and cell cycle progression caused by a mutant lamin A known to accelerate human aging. Proc Natl Acad Sci USA 104(12): 4955–4960

212. Liu B, Wang J, Chan KM et al (2005) Genomic instability in laminopathy-based premature aging. Nat Med 11(7):780–785

213. Muftuoglu M, Oshima J, von Kobbe C, Cheng W-H, Leistritz D, Bohr V (2008) The clinical characteristics of Werner syndrome: molecular and biochemical diagnosis. Hum Genet 124(4): 369–377

214. Epstein CJ, Martin GM, Schultz AL, Motulsky AG (1966) Werner's syndrome a review of its symptomatology, natural history, pathologic features, genetics and relationship to the natural aging process. Medicine (Baltimore) 45(3):177–221

215. Goto M (1997) Hierarchical deterioration of body systems in Werner's syndrome: implications for normal ageing. Mech Ageing Dev 98(3):239–254

216. Goto M, Rubenstein M, Weber J, Woods K, Drayna D (1992) Genetic linkage of Werner's syndrome to five markers on chromosome 8. Nature 355(6362):735–738

217. Yu CE, Oshima J, Fu YH et al (1996) Positional cloning of the Werner's syndrome gene [see comments]. Science 272(5259): 258–262

218. Brosh RM Jr, Bohr VA (2002) Roles of the Werner syndrome protein in pathways required for maintenance of genome stability. Exp Gerontol 37(4):491–506

219. Ogburn CE, Oshima J, Poot M et al (1997) An apoptosis-inducing genotoxin differentiates heterozygotic carriers for Werner helicase mutations from wild-type and homozygous mutants. Hum Genet 101(2):121–125

220. Poot M, Gollahon KA, Emond MJ, Silber JR, Rabinovitch PS (2002) Werner syndrome diploid fibroblasts are sensitive to 4-nit-roquinoline-N-oxide and 8-methoxypsoralen: implications for the disease phenotype. FASEB J 16(7):757–758

221. Poot M, Yom JS, Whang SH, Kato JT, Gollahon KA, Rabinovitch PS (2001) Werner syndrome cells are sensitive to DNA cross-linking drugs. FASEB J 15(7):1224–1226

222. Pichierri P, Franchitto A, Mosesso P, Palitti F (2000) Werner's syndrome cell lines are hypersensitive to camptothecin-induced chromosomal damage. Mutat Res 456(1–2):45–57

223. Poot M, Gollahon KA, Rabinovitch PS (1999) Werner syndrome lymphoblastoid cells are sensitive to camptothecin-induced apoptosis in S-phase. Hum Genet 104(1):10–14

224. Stevnsner T, Muftuoglu M, Aamann MD, Bohr VA (2008) The role of Cockayne Syndrome group B (CSB) protein in base excision repair and aging. Mech Ageing Dev 129(7–8):441–448

225. Henning KA, Li L, Iyer N et al (1995) The Cockayne syndrome group A gene encodes a WD repeat protein that interacts with CSB protein and a subunit of RNA polymerase II TFIIH. Cell 82(4):555–564

226. Groisman R, Polanowska J, Kuraoka I et al (2003) The ubiquitin ligase activity in the DDB2 and CSA complexes is differentially regulated by the COP9 signalosome in response to DNA damage. Cell 113(3):357–367

227. Troelstra C, van Gool A, de Wit J, Vermeulen W, Bootsma D, Hoeijmakers JH (1992) ERCC6, a member of a subfamily of putative helicases, is involved in Cockayne's syndrome and preferential repair of active genes. Cell 71(6):939–953

228. Horibata K, Iwamoto Y, Kuraoka I et al (2004) Complete absence of Cockayne syndrome group B gene product gives rise to UV-sensitive syndrome but not Cockayne syndrome. Proc Natl Acad Sci USA 101(43):15410–15415

229. Martin GM, Turker MS (1990) Genetic of human disease, longevity, and aging. In: Hazzard WR, Andres R, Bierman EL et al (eds) Principles of geriatric medicine and gerontology, 2nd edn. McGraw-Hill, New York, p 22

230. Fanconi G (1967) Familial constitutional panmyelocytopathy, Fanconi's anemia (F.A.). I. Clinical aspects. Semin Hematol 4(3):233–240

231. Neveling K, Bechtold A, Hoehn H (2007) Genetic instability syndromes with progeroid features. Z Gerontol Geriatr 40(5):339–348

232. Joenje H, Arwert F, Eriksson AW, de Koning H, Oostra AB (1981) Oxygen-dependence of chromosomal aberrations in Fanconi's anaemia. Nature 290(5802):142–143

233. Zhang X, Li J, Sejas DP, Pang Q (2005) Hypoxia-reoxygenation induces premature senescence in FA bone marrow hematopoietic cells. Blood 106(1):75–85

234. Park SJ, Ciccone SL, Beck BD et al (2004) Oxidative stress/damage induces multimerization and interaction of Fanconi anemia proteins. J Biol Chem 279(29):30053–30059

235. Drachtman RA, Alter BP (1992) Dyskeratosis congenita: clinical and genetic heterogeneity. Report of a new case and review of the literature. Am J Pediatr Hematol Oncol 14(4):297–304

236. Vulliamy T, Dokal I (2006) Dyskeratosis congenita. Semin Hematol 43(3):157–166

237. Marrone A, Dokal I (2004) Dyskeratosis congenita: molecular insights into telomerase function, ageing and cancer. Expert Rev Mol Med 6(26):1–23

238. Chang S, Multani AS, Cabrera NG et al (2004) Essential role of limiting telomeres in the pathogenesis of Werner syndrome. Nat Genet 36(8):877–882

239. Wong KK, Maser RS, Bachoo RM et al (2003) Telomere dysfunction and Atm deficiency compromises organ homeostasis and accelerates ageing. Nature 421(6923):643–648

240. Elchuri S, Oberley TD, Qi W et al (2005) CuZnSOD deficiency leads to persistent and widespread oxidative damage and hepatocarcinogenesis later in life. Oncogene 24(3):367–380

241. Hashizume K, Hirasawa M, Imamura Y et al (2008) Retinal dysfunction and progressive retinal cell death in SOD1-deficient mice. Am J Pathol 172(5):1325–1331

242. Van Remmen H, Ikeno Y, Hamilton M et al (2003) Life-long reduction in MnSOD activity results in increased DNA damage and higher incidence of cancer but does not accelerate aging. Physiol Genomics 16(1):29–37

243. Ho YS, Xiong Y, Ma W, Spector A, Ho DS (2004) Mice lacking catalase develop normally but show differential sensitivity to oxidant tissue injury. J Biol Chem 279(31):32804–32812

244. Ho YS, Magnenat JL, Bronson RT et al (1997) Mice deficient in cellular glutathione peroxidase develop normally and show no increased sensitivity to hyperoxia. J Biol Chem 272(26):16644–16651

245. Van Remmen H, Qi W, Sabia M et al (2004) Multiple deficiencies in antioxidant enzymes in mice result in a compound increase in sensitivity to oxidative stress. Free Radic Biol Med 36(12):1625–1634

246. Hayflick L, Moorhead PS (1965) The limited in vitro lifetime of human diploid cell strains. Exp Cell Res 37:614–636

247. Wang E (1995) Senescent human fibroblasts resist programmed cell death, and failure to suppress bcl2 is involved. Cancer Res 55(11):2284–2292

248. Marcotte R, Lacelle C, Wang E (2004) Senescent fibroblasts resist apoptosis by downregulating caspase-3. Mech Ageing Dev 125(10–11):777–783

249. Hampel B, Malisan F, Niederegger H, Testi R, Jansen-Dürr P (2004) Differential regulation of apoptotic cell death in senescent human cells. Exp Gerontol 39(11-12):1713–1721

250. Bayreuther K, Rodemann HP, Hommel R, Dittmann K, Albiez M, Francz PI (1988) Human skin fibroblasts in vitro differentiate along a terminal cell lineage. Proc Natl Acad Sci USA 85(14):5112–5116

251. Pignolo RJ, Rotenberg MO, Cristofalo VJ (1994) Alterations in contact and density-dependent arrest state in senescent WI-38 cells. In Vitro Cell Dev Biol Anim 30A(7):471–476

252. Matsumura T, Zerrudo Z, Hayflick L (1979) Senescent human diploid cells in culture: survival, DNA synthesis and morphology. J Gerontol 34(3):328–334

253. Ponten J (1973) Aging properties of glia. In: Bourliere F, Courtois Y, Macieira-Coelho A et al (eds) Molecular and cellular mechanisms of aging. INSERM, Paris, p 53

254. Rheinwald JG, Green H (1975) Serial cultivation of strains of human epidermal keratinocytes: the formation of keratinizing colonies from single cells. Cell 6(3):331–343

255. Bierman EL (1978) The effect of donor age on the in vitro life span of cultured human arterial smooth-muscle cells. In Vitro 14(11):951–955

256. Tassin J, Malaise E, Courtois Y (1979) Human lens cells have an in vitro proliferative capacity inversely proportional to the donor age. Exp Cell Res 123(2):388–392

257. Mueller SN, Rosen EM, Levine EM (1980) Cellular senescence in a cloned strain of bovine fetal aortic endothelial cells. Science 207(4433):889–891

258. Tice RR, Schneider EL, Kram D, Thorne P (1979) Cytokinetic analysis of the impaired proliferative response of peripheral lymphocytes from aged humans to phytohemagglutinin. J Exp Med 149(5):1029–1041

259. Stampfer MR (1985) Isolation and growth of human mammary epithelial cells. J Tissue Culture Methods 9:107–115

260. Yaswen P, Stampfer MR (2002) Molecular changes accompanying senescence and immortalization of cultured human mammary epithelial cells. Int J Biochem Cell Biol 34(11):1382–1394

261. Harrison DE (1985) Cell and tissue transplantation: a means of studying the aging process. In: Finch CE, Schneider EL (eds) Handbook of the biology of Aging, 2nd edn. Van Nostrand Reinhold, New York, p 332

262. Olsson L, Ebbesen P (1977) Ageing decreases the activity of epidermal G1 and G2 inhibitors in mouse skin independent of grafting on old or young recipients. Exp Gerontol 12(1–2):59–62

263. Rohme D (1981) Evidence for a relationship between longevity of mammalian species and life spans of normal fibroblasts in vitro and erythrocytes in vivo. Proc Natl Acad Sci USA 78(8):5009–5013

264. Martin GM, Sprague CA, Epstein CJ (1970) Replicative life-span of cultivated human cells. Effects of donor's age, tissue, and genotype. Lab Invest 23(1):86–92

265. Pignolo RJ, Masoro EJ, Nichols WW, Bradt CI, Cristofalo VJ (1992) Skin fibroblasts from aged Fischer 344 rats undergo similar changes in replicative life span but not immortalization with caloric restriction of donors. Exp Cell Res 201(1):16–22

266. Schneider EL, Mitsui Y (1976) The relationship between in vitro cellular aging and in vivo human age. Proc Natl Acad Sci USA 73(10):3584–3588

267. Goldstein S, Littlefield JW, Soeldner JS (1969) Diabetes mellitus and aging: diminished planting efficiency of cultured human fibroblasts. Proc Natl Acad Sci USA 64(1):155–160

268. Le Guilly Y, Simon M, Lenoir P, Bourel M (1973) Long-term culture of human adult liver cells: morphological changes related to in vitro senescence and effect of donor's age on growth potential. Gerontologia 19(5):303–313

269. Wille JJ Jr, Pittelkow MR, Shipley GD, Scott RE (1984) Integrated control of growth and differentiation of normal human prokeratinocytes cultured in serum-free medium: clonal analyses, growth kinetics, and cell cycle studies. J Cell Physiol 121(1):31–44

270. Effros RB, Boucher N, Porter V et al (1994) Decline in CD28+ T cells in centenarians and in long-term T cell cultures: a possible cause for both in vivo and in vitro immunosenescence. Exp Gerontol 29(6):601–609

271. Cristofalo VJ, Allen RG, Pignolo RJ, Martin BG, Beck JC (1998) Relationship between donor age and the replicative lifespan of human cells in culture: a reevaluation. Proc Natl Acad Sci USA 95(18):10614–10619

272. Dimri G, Lee X, Basile G et al (1995) A biomarker that identifies senescent human cells in culture and in aging skin in vivo. Proc Natl Acad Sci USA 92(20):9363–9367

273. Ressler S, Bartkova J, Niederegger H et al (2006) p16INK4A is a robust in vivo biomarker of cellular aging in human skin. Aging Cell 5(5):379–389

274. Clark AJ, Ferrier P, Aslam S et al (2003) Proliferative lifespan is conserved after nuclear transfer. Nat Cell Biol 5(6):535–538

275. Cristofalo VJ, Palaxxo R, Charpentier RL (1980) Limited lifespan of human fibroblasts in vitro: metabolic time or replications? In: Adelman RC, Roberts J, Baker GT et al (eds) Neural regulatory mechanisms during aging. Alan R. Liss, New York, p 203

276. Campisi J, D'Adda di Fagagna F (2007) Cellular senescence: when bad things happen to good cells. Nat Rev Mol Cell Biol 8(9):729–740

277. Toussaint O, Medrano EE, von Zglinicki T (2000) Cellular and molecular mechanisms of stress-induced premature senescence (SIPS) of human diploid fibroblasts and melanocytes. Exp Gerontol 35(8):927–945

278. Toussaint O, Remacle J, Dierick JF et al (2002) Stress-induced premature senescence: from biomarkers to likeliness of in vivo occurrence. Biogerontology 3(1–2):13–17

279. d'Adda di Fagagna F, Reaper PM, Clay-Farrace L et al (2003) A DNA damage checkpoint response in telomere-initiated senescence. Nature 426(6963):194–198

280. Hemann MT, Narita M (2007) Oncogenes and senescence: breaking down in the fast lane. Genes Dev 21(1):1–5

281. Takahashi A, Ohtani N, Yamakoshi K et al (2006) Mitogenic signalling and the p16INK4a-Rb pathway cooperate to enforce irreversible cellular senescence. Nat Cell Biol 8(11):1291–1297

282. Campisi J (1997) Aging and cancer: the double-edged sword of replicative senescence. J Am Geriatr Soc 45(4):482–488

283. Shay JW, Wright WE, Werbin H (1993) Toward a molecular understanding of human breast cancer: a hypothesis. Breast Cancer Res Treat 25(1):83–94

284. Stein GH, Beeson M, Gordon L (1990) Failure to phosphorylate the retinoblastoma gene product in senescent human fibroblasts. Science 249(4969):666–669

285. Ozer HL, Banga SS, Dasgupta T et al (1996) SV40-mediated immortalization of human fibroblasts. Exp Gerontol 31(1–2):303–310

286. Shay JW, Pereira-Smith OM, Wright WE (1991) A role for both RB and p53 in the regulation of human cellular senescence. Exp Cell Res 196(1):33–39

287. Hara E, Tsurui H, Shinozaki A, Nakada S, Oda K (1991) Cooperative effect of antisense-Rb and antisense-p53 oligomers on the extension of life span in human diploid fibroblasts, TIG-1. Biochem Biophys Res Commun 179(1):528–534

288. Afshari CA, Nichols MA, Xiong Y, Mudryj M (1996) A role for a p21-E2F interaction during senescence arrest of normal human fibroblasts. Cell Growth Differ 7(8):979–988

289. Noda A, Ning Y, Venable SF, Pereira-Smith OM, Smith JR (1994) Cloning of senescent cell-derived inhibitors of DNA synthesis using an expression screen. Exp Cell Res 211(1):90–98

290. Tahara H, Sato E, Noda A, Ide T (1995) Increase in expression level of p21sdi1/cip1/waf1 with increasing division age in both normal and SV40-transformed human fibroblasts. Oncogene 10(5):835–840

291. Alcorta DA, Xiong Y, Phelps D, Hannon G, Beach D, Barrett JC (1996) Involvement of the cyclin-dependent kinase inhibitor p16 (INK4a) in replicative senescence of normal human fibroblasts. Proc Natl Acad Sci USA 93(24):13742–13747

292. Palmero I, McConnell B, Parry D et al (1997) Accumulation of p16INK4a in mouse fibroblasts as a function of replicative senescence and not of retinoblastoma gene status. Oncogene 15(5):495–503

293. Reznikoff CA, Yeager TR, Belair CD, Savelieva E, Puthenveettil JA, Stadler WM (1996) Elevated p16 at senescence and loss of p16 at immortalization in human papillomavirus 16 E6, but not E7, transformed human uroepithelial cells. Cancer Res 56(13):2886–2890

294. Brown JP, Wei W, Sedivy JM (1997) Bypass of senescence after disruption of p21CIP1/WAF1 gene in normal diploid human fibroblasts. Science 277(5327):831–834

295. Yang L, Didenko VV, Noda A et al (1995) Increased expression of p21Sdi1 in adrenocortical cells when they are placed in culture. Exp Cell Res 221(1):126–131

296. Medcalf AS, Klein-Szanto AJ, Cristofalo VJ (1996) Expression of p21 is not required for senescence of human fibroblasts. Cancer Res 56(20):4582–4585

297. Vogt M, Haggblom C, Yeargin J, Christiansen-Weber T, Haas M (1998) Independent induction of senescence by p16INK4a and p21CIP1 in spontaneously immortalized human fibroblasts. Cell Growth Differ 9(2):139–146

298. Afshari CA, Vojta PJ, Annab LA, Futreal PA, Willard TB, Barrett JC (1993) Investigation of the role of G1/S cell cycle mediators in cellular senescence. Exp Cell Res 209(2):231–237

299. Tyner SD, Venkatachalam S, Choi J et al (2002) p53 mutant mice that display early ageing-associated phenotypes. Nature 415(6867):45–53

300. Beausejour CM, Krtolica A, Galimi F et al (2003) Reversal of human cellular senescence: roles of the p53 and p16 pathways. EMBO J 22(16):4212–4222

301. Itahana K, Zou Y, Itahana Y et al (2003) Control of the replicative life span of human fibroblasts by p16 and the polycomb protein Bmi-1. Mol Cell Biol 23(1):389–401

302. Herbig U, Jobling WA, Chen BP, Chen DJ, Sedivy JM (2004) Telomere shortening triggers senescence of human cells through a pathway involving ATM, p53, and p21(CIP1), but not p16(INK4a). Mol Cell 14(4):501–513

303. Serrano M, Lin AW, McCurrach ME, Beach D, Lowe SW (1997) Oncogenic ras provokes premature cell senescence associated with accumulation of p53 and p16INK4a. Cell 88(5):593–602

304. Benanti JA, Galloway DA (2004) Normal human fibroblasts are resistant to RAS-induced senescence. Mol Cell Biol 24(7):2842–2852

305. Rai P, Onder TT, Young JJ et al (2009) Continuous elimination of oxidized nucleotides is necessary to prevent rapid onset of cellular senescence. Proc Natl Acad Sci USA 106(1):169–174

306. Romanov SR, Kozakiewicz BK, Holst CR, Stampfer MR, Haupt LM, Tlsty TD (2001) Normal human mammary epithelial cells spontaneously escape senescence and acquire genomic changes. Nature 409(6820):633–637

307. Rheinwald JG, Hahn WC, Ramsey MR et al (2002) A two-stage, p16(INK4A)- and p53-dependent keratinocyte senescence mechanism that limits replicative potential independent of telomere status. Mol Cell Biol 22(14):5157–5172

308. Muller M (2009) Cellular senescence: molecular mechanisms, in vivo significance, and redox considerations. Antioxid Redox Signal 11(1):59–98

309. Sohal RS, Brunk UT (1989) Lipofuscin as an indicator of oxidative stress and aging. Adv Exp Med Biol 266:17–26; discussion 27–19

310. Narita M, Nunez S, Heard E et al (2003) Rb-mediated heterochromatin formation and silencing of E2F target genes during cellular senescence. Cell 113(6):703–716

311. Severino J, Allen RG, Balin S, Balin A, Cristofalo VJ (2000) Is beta-galactosidase staining a marker of senescence in vitro and in vivo? Exp Cell Res 257(1):162–171

312. Litaker JR, Pan J, Cheung Y et al (1998) Expression profile of senescence-associated beta-galactosidase and activation of telomerase in human ovarian surface epithelial cells undergoing immortalization. Int J Oncol 13(5):951–956

313. Untergasser G, Gander R, Rumpold H, Heinrich E, Plas E, Berger P (2003) TGF-beta cytokines increase senescence-associated beta-galactosidase activity in human prostate basal cells by supporting differentiation processes, but not cellular senescence. Exp Gerontol 38(10):1179–1188

314. Kurz DJ, Decary S, Hong Y, Erusalimsky JD (2000) Senescence-associated (beta)-galactosidase reflects an increase in lysosomal mass during replicative ageing of human endothelial cells. J Cell Sci 113(Pt 20):3613–3622

315. Yang NC, Hu ML (2005) The limitations and validities of senescence associated-beta-galactosidase activity as an aging marker for human foreskin fibroblast Hs68 cells. Exp Gerontol 40(10):813–819

316. Lee BY, Han JA, Im JS et al (2006) Senescence-associated beta-galactosidase is lysosomal beta-galactosidase. Aging Cell 5(2):187–195

317. Matthews C, Gorenne I, Scott S et al (2006) Vascular smooth muscle cells undergo telomere-based senescence in human atherosclerosis: effects of telomerase and oxidative stress. Circ Res 99(2):156–164

318. Krishnamurthy J, Ramsey MR, Ligon KL et al (2006) p16INK4a induces an age-dependent decline in islet regenerative potential. Nature 443(7110):453–457

319. Krishnamurthy J, Torrice C, Ramsey MR et al (2004) Ink4a/ARF expression is a biomarker of aging. J Clin Invest 114(9):1299–1307

320. Collado M, Gil J, Efeyan A et al (2005) Tumour biology: senescence in premalignant tumours. Nature 436(7051):642

321. Harley CB (1991) Telomere loss: mitotic clock or genetic time bomb? Mutat Res 256(2–6):271–282

322. Greider CW (1990) Telomeres, telomerase and senescence. Bioessays 12(8):363–369

323. Harley CB, Futcher AB, Greider CW (1990) Telomeres shorten during ageing of human fibroblasts. Nature 345(6274):458–460

324. Allsopp RC, Vaziri H, Patterson C et al (1992) Telomere length predicts replicative capacity of human fibroblasts. Proc Natl Acad Sci USA 89(21):10114–10118

325. Chang E, Harley CB (1995) Telomere length and replicative aging in human vascular tissues. Proc Natl Acad Sci USA 92(24):11190–11194

326. Lindsey J, McGill NI, Lindsey LA, Green DK, Cooke HJ (1991) In vivo loss of telomeric repeats with age in humans. Mutat Res 256(1):45–48

327. Vaziri H, Schachter F, Uchida I et al (1993) Loss of telomeric DNA during aging of normal and trisomy 21 human lymphocytes. Am J Hum Genet 52(4):661–667

328. Frenck RW Jr, Blackburn EH, Shannon KM (1998) The rate of telomere sequence loss in human leukocytes varies with age. Proc Natl Acad Sci USA 95(10):5607–5610

329. Counter CM, Hirte HW, Bacchetti S, Harley CB (1994) Telomerase activity in human ovarian carcinoma [see comments]. Proc Natl Acad Sci USA 91(8):2900–2904

330. Sugihara S, Mihara K, Marunouchi T, Inoue H, Namba M (1996) Telomere elongation observed in immortalized human fibroblasts by treatment with 60Co gamma rays or 4-nitroquinoline 1-oxide. Hum Genet 97(1):1–6

331. Bryan TM, Englezou A, Gupta J, Bacchetti S, Reddel RR (1995) Telomere elongation in immortal human cells without detectable telomerase activity. EMBO J 14(17):4240–4248

332. Chiu CP, Dragowska W, Kim NW et al (1996) Differential expression of telomerase activity in hematopoietic progenitors from adult human bone marrow. Stem Cells 14(2):239–248

333. Broccoli D, Young JW, de Lange T (1995) Telomerase activity in normal and malignant hematopoietic cells. Proc Natl Acad Sci USA 92(20):9082–9086

334. Counter CM, Gupta J, Harley CB, Leber B, Bacchetti S (1995) Telomerase activity in normal leukocytes and in hematologic malignancies. Blood 85(9):2315–2320

335. Terry DF, Nolan VG, Andersen SL, Perls TT, Cawthon R (2008) Association of longer telomeres with better health in centenarians. J Gerontol A Biol Sci Med Sci 63(8):809–812

336. Ludlow AT, Zimmerman JB, Witkowski S, Hearn JW, Hatfield BD, Roth SM (2008) Relationship between physical activity level, telomere length, and telomerase activity. Med Sci Sports Exerc 40(10):1764–1771

337. Woo J, Tang NL, Suen E, Leung JC, Leung PC (2008) Telomeres and frailty. Mech Ageing Dev 129(11):642–648

338. Hofer AC, Tran RT, Aziz OZ et al (2005) Shared phenotypes among segmental progeroid syndromes suggest underlying pathways of aging. J Gerontol A Biol Sci Med Sci 60(1):10–20

339. Rudolph KL, Chang S, Lee HW et al (1999) Longevity, stress response, and cancer in aging telomerase-deficient mice. Cell 96(5):701–712

340. Wright WE, Brasiskyte D, Piatyszek MA, Shay JW (1996) Experimental elongation of telomeres extends the lifespan of immortal × normal cell hybrids. EMBO J 15(7):1734–1741

341. Bodnar AG, Ouellette M, Frolkis M et al (1998) Extension of lifespan by introduction of telomerase into normal human cells [see comments]. Science 279(5349):349–352

342. Gorbunova V, Seluanov A, Pereira-Smith OM (2002) Expression of human telomerase (hTERT) Does not prevent stress-induced senescence in normal human fibroblasts but protects the cells from stress-induced apoptosis and necrosis. J Biol Chem 277(41):38540–38549

343. Naka K, Tachibana A, Ikeda K, Motoyama N (2004) Stress-induced premature senescence in htert-expressing ataxia telangiectasia fibroblasts. J Biol Chem 279(3):2030–2037

344. Forsyth NR, Evans AP, Shay JW, Wright WE (2003) Developmental differences in the immortalization of lung fibroblasts by telomerase. Aging Cell 2(5):235–243

345. Petersen S, Saretzki G, Zglinicki Tv (1998) Preferential accumulation of single-stranded regions in telomeres of human fibroblasts. Exp Cell Res 239(1):152–160

346. Passos JF, Saretzki G, von Zglinicki T (2007) DNA damage in telomeres and mitochondria during cellular senescence: is there a connection? Nucleic Acids Res 35(22):7505–7513

347. Janzen V, Forkert R, Fleming HE et al (2006) Stem-cell ageing modified by the cyclin-dependent kinase inhibitor p16INK4a. Nature 443(7110):421–426

348. de Haan G, Van Zant G (1999) Dynamic changes in mouse hematopoietic stem cell numbers during aging. Blood 93(10):3294–3301

349. Geiger H, Van Zant G (2002) The aging of lympho-hematopoietic stem cells. Nat Immunol 3(4):329–333

350. Molofsky AV, Slutsky SG, Joseph NM et al (2006) Increasing p16INK4a expression decreases forebrain progenitors and neurogenesis during ageing. Nature 443(7110):448–452

351. Hahn WC, Counter CM, Lundberg AS, Beijersbergen RL, Brooks MW, Weinberg RA (1999) Creation of human tumour cells with defined genetic elements. Nature 400(6743):464–468

352. Vaziri H, Benchimol S (1999) Alternative pathways for the extension of cellular life span: inactivation of p53/pRb and expression of telomerase. Oncogene 18(53):7676–7680

353. Elenbaas B, Spirio L, Koerner F et al (2001) Human breast cancer cells generated by oncogenic transformation of primary mammary epithelial cells. Genes Dev 15(1):50–65

354. Kendall SD, Linardic CM, Adam SJ, Counter CM (2005) A network of genetic events sufficient to convert normal human cells to a tumorigenic state. Cancer Res 65(21):9824–9828

355. Lundberg AS, Randell SH, Stewart SA et al (2002) Immortalization and transformation of primary airway epithelial cells by gene transfer. Oncogene 21(29):4577–4586

356. Bartkova J, Horejsi Z, Koed K et al (2005) DNA damage response as a candidate anti-cancer barrier in early human tumorigenesis. Nature 434(7035):864–870

357. Michaloglou C, Vredeveld LCW, Soengas MS et al (2005) BRAFE600-associated senescence-like cell cycle arrest of human naevi. Nature 436(7051):720–724

358. Castro P, Giri D, Lamb D, Ittmann M (2003) Cellular senescence in the pathogenesis of benign prostatic hyperplasia. Prostate 55(1):30–38

359. Chen Z, Trotman LC, Shaffer D et al (2005) Crucial role of p53-dependent cellular senescence in suppression of Pten-deficient tumorigenesis. Nature 436(7051):725–730

360. Bartkova J, Rezaei N, Liontos M et al (2006) Oncogene-induced senescence is part of the tumorigenesis barrier imposed by DNA damage checkpoints. Nature 444(7119):633–637

361. Di Micco R, Fumagalli M, Cicalese A et al (2006) Oncogene-induced senescence is a DNA damage response triggered by DNA hyper-replication. Nature 444(7119):638–642

362. Mallette FA, Gaumont-Leclerc M-F, Ferbeyre G (2007) The DNA damage signaling pathway is a critical mediator of oncogene-induced senescence. Genes Dev 21(1):43–48

363. Feldser DM, Greider CW (2007) Short telomeres limit tumor progression in vivo by inducing senescence. Cell 11(5):461–469

364. Xue W, Zender L, Miething C et al (2007) Senescence and tumour clearance is triggered by p53 restoration in murine liver carcinomas. Nature 445(7128):656–660

365. Wu C-H, van Riggelen J, Yetil A, Fan AC, Bachireddy P, Felsher DW (2007) Cellular senescence is an important mechanism of tumor regression upon c-Myc inactivation. Proc Natl Acad Sci USA 104(32):13028–13033

366. Martins CP, Brown-Swigart L, Evan GI (2006) Modeling the therapeutic efficacy of p53 restoration in tumors. Cell 127(7): 1323–1334

367. Gorgoulis VG, Vassiliou L-VF, Karakaidos P et al (2005) Activation of the DNA damage checkpoint and genomic instability in human precancerous lesions. Nature 434(7035):907–913

368. Eyler CE, Rich JN (2008) Survival of the fittest: cancer stem cells in therapeutic resistance and angiogenesis. J Clin Oncol 26(17):2839–2845

369. Wajapeyee N, Serra RW, Zhu X, Mahalingam M, Green MR (2008) Oncogenic BRAF induces senescence and apoptosis through pathways mediated by the secreted protein IGFBP7. Cell 132(3):363–374

370. Acosta JC, O'Loghlen A, Banito A et al (2008) Chemokine signaling via the CXCR2 receptor reinforces senescence. Cell 133(6): 1006–1018

371. Kuilman T, Michaloglou C, Vredeveld LCW et al (2008) Oncogene-induced senescence relayed by an interleukin-dependent inflammatory network. Cell 133(6):1019–1031

372. Coppe J-P, Patil CK, Rodier F et al (2008) Senescence-associated secretory phenotypes reveal cell-nonautonomous functions of oncogenic RAS and the p53 tumor suppressor. PLoS Biol 6(12):e301

373. Ries LAG, Melbert D, Krapcho M, Stinchcomb DG, Howlader N, Horner MJ, Mariotto A, Miller BA, Feuer EJ, Altekruse SF, Lewis DR, Clegg L, Eisner MP, Reichman M, Edwards BK (eds) (2008) SEER cancer statistics review, 1975-2005, National Cancer Institute. Bethesda, MD, http://seer.cancer.gov/csr/1975_2005/, based on November 2007 SEER data submission, posted to the SEER web site

374. Krtolica A, Parrinello S, Lockett S, Desprez PY, Campisi J (2001) Senescent fibroblasts promote epithelial cell growth and tumorigenesis: a link between cancer and aging. Proc Natl Acad Sci USA 98(21):12072–12077

375. Liu D, Hornsby PJ (2007) Senescent human fibroblasts increase the early growth of xenograft tumors via matrix metalloproteinase secretion. Cancer Res 67(7):3117–3126

376. Maier B, Gluba W, Bernier B et al (2004) Modulation of mammalian life span by the short isoform of p53. Genes Dev 18(3):306–319

377. Garcia-Cao I, Garcia-Cao M, Martin-Caballero J et al (2002) 'Super p53' mice exhibit enhanced DNA damage response, are tumor resistant and age normally. EMBO J 21(22):6225–6235

378. Matheu A, Pantoja C, Efeyan A et al (2004) Increased gene dosage of Ink4a/Arf results in cancer resistance and normal aging. Genes Dev 18(22):2736–2746

379. Mendrysa SM, O'Leary KA, McElwee MK et al (2006) Tumor suppression and normal aging in mice with constitutively high p53 activity. Genes Dev 20(1):16–21

380. Matheu A, Maraver A, Klatt P et al (2007) Delayed ageing through damage protection by the Arf/p53 pathway. Nature 448(7151): 375–379

381. Partridge L, Gems D (2007) Benchmarks for ageing studies. Nature 450(7167):165–167

382. Lane MA, Ingram DK, Ball SS, Roth GS (1997) Dehydroepiandrosterone sulfate: a biomarker of primate aging slowed by calorie restriction. J Clin Endocrinol Metab 82(7): 2093–2096

383. Larson-Meyer DE, Newcomer BR, Heilbronn LK et al (2008) Effect of 6-month calorie restriction and exercise on serum and liver lipids and markers of liver function. Obesity 16(6):1355–1362

384. Trichopoulou A, Vasilopoulou E (2000) Mediterranean diet and longevity. Br J Nutr 84(Suppl 2):S205–S209

385. Corder R, Mullen W, Khan NQ et al (2006) Oenology: red wine procyanidins and vascular health. Nature 444(7119):566

386. Allard JS, Perez E, Zou S, de Cabo R (2009) Dietary activators of Sirt1. Mol Cell Endocrinol 299(1):58–63

387. Baur JA, Pearson KJ, Price NL et al (2006) Resveratrol improves health and survival of mice on a high-calorie diet. Nature 444(7117):337–342

388. Lagouge M, Argmann C, Gerhart-Hines Z et al (2006) Resveratrol improves mitochondrial function and protects against metabolic disease by activating SIRT1 and PGC-1alpha. Cell 127(6):1109–1122

389. Pearson KJ, Baur JA, Lewis KN et al (2008) Resveratrol delays age-related deterioration and mimics transcriptional aspects of dietary restriction without extending life span. Cell Metab 8(2):157–168

390. Barger JL, Kayo T, Vann JM et al (2008) A low dose of dietary resveratrol partially mimics caloric restriction and retards aging parameters in mice. PLoS ONE 3(6):e2264

391. Schumacher B, van der Pluijm I, Moorhouse MJ et al (2008) Delayed and accelerated aging share common longevity assurance mechanisms. PLoS Genet 4(8):e1000161

392. Keyes WM, Wu Y, Vogel H, Guo X, Lowe SW, Mills AA (2005) p63 deficiency activates a program of cellular senescence and leads to accelerated aging. Genes Dev 19(17): 1986–1999

393. Mostoslavsky R, Chua KF, Lombard DB et al (2006) Genomic instability and aging-like phenotype in the absence of mammalian SIRT6. Cell 124(2):315–329

394. Kuro-o M, Matsumura Y, Aizawa H et al (1997) Mutation of the mouse klotho gene leads to a syndrome resembling ageing. Nature 390(6655):45–51

395. Takeda T, Hosokawa M, Higuchi K (1997) Senescence-accelerated mouse (SAM): a novel murine model of senescence. Exp Gerontol 32(1–2):105–109

396. Lebel M, Leder P (1998) A deletion within the murine Werner syndrome helicase induces sensitivity to inhibitors of topoisomerase and loss of cellular proliferative capacity. Proc Natl Acad Sci USA 95(22):13097–13102

397. van der Horst GT, Meira L, Gorgels TG et al (2002) UVB radiation-induced cancer predisposition in Cockayne syndrome group A (Csa) mutant mice. DNA Repair (Amst) 1(2): 143–157

398. Barlow C, Hirotsune S, Paylor R et al (1996) Atm-deficient mice: a paradigm of ataxia telangiectasia. Cell 86(1):159–171

399. Ruzankina Y, Pinzon-Guzman C, Asare A et al (2007) Deletion of the developmentally essential gene ATR in adult mice leads to age-related phenotypes and stem cell loss. Cell Stem Cell 1(1): 113–126

400. Bartke A, Brown-Borg HM, Bode AM, Carlson J, Hunter WS, Bronson RT (1998) Does growth hormone prevent or accelerate aging? Exp Gerontol 33(7–8):675–687

401. Mounkes LC, Kozlov S, Hernandez L, Sullivan T, Stewart CL (2003) A progeroid syndrome in mice is caused by defects in A-type lamins. Nature 423(6937):298–301

402. Liu X, Jiang N, Hughes B, Bigras E, Shoubridge E, Hekimi S (2005) Evolutionary conservation of the clk-1-dependent mechanism of longevity: loss of mclk1 increases cellular fitness and lifespan in mice. Genes Dev 19(20):2424–2434

403. Holzenberger M, Dupont J, Ducos B et al (2003) IGF-1 receptor regulates lifespan and resistance to oxidative stress in mice. Nature 421(6919):182–187

404. Bluher M, Kahn BB, Kahn CR (2003) Extended longevity in mice lacking the insulin receptor in adipose tissue. Science 299(5606): 572–574

405. Miskin R, Masos T (1997) Transgenic mice overexpressing urokinase-type plasminogen activator in the brain exhibit reduced food consumption, body weight and size, and increased longevity. J Gerontol A Biol Sci Med Sci 52(2):B118–B124

406. Chiu CH, Lin WD, Huang SY, Lee YH (2004) Effect of a C/EBP gene replacement on mitochondrial biogenesis in fat cells. Genes Dev 18(16):1970–1975

407. Yan L, Vatner DE, O'Connor JP et al (2007) Type 5 adenylyl cyclase disruption increases longevity and protects against stress. Cell 130(2):247–258

408. Flurkey K, Papaconstantinou J, Miller RA, Harrison DE (2001) Lifespan extension and delayed immune and collagen aging in mutant mice with defects in growth hormone production. Proc Natl Acad Sci USA 98(12):6736–6741

409. Brown-Borg HM, Borg KE, Meliska CJ, Bartke A (1996) Dwarf mice and the ageing process. Nature 384(6604):33

410. Coschigano KT, Clemmons D, Bellush LL, Kopchick JJ (2000) Assessment of growth parameters and life span of GHR/BP gene-disrupted mice. Endocrinology 141(7):2608–2613

Chapter 3
Cancer, Carcinogenesis, and Aging

Lodovico Balducci

Cancer is mainly a disease of aging. At present 50% of all cancers occur in the 12% of the population aged 65 and older [1]. By the year 2030, individuals over 65 years will represent 20% of the population of the United States and account for 70% of all cancers [1, 2]. The management of cancer in the older age group is going to become the most common practice of oncology.

The interactions of cancer and age are multiple and complex. They include carcinogenesis, tumor biology, as well as cancer prevention and treatment. We will explore these interactions after reviewing the extent of the problem.

Epidemiology of Cancer in the Aged

The incidence and prevalence of most cancers increase with age (Fig. 3.1). The association of cancer and age elicits a number of important questions: Is there a linear association between age and the incidence of cancer? Is the patient going to die or suffer from cancer? Does the presentation of cancer differ in older and in younger individuals? What are the consequences of cancer and its treatment for the older person? Epidemiology may provide important insights into these questions.

The Age Window

The incidence of most cancers increases steeply between ages 55 and 80, plateaus between 80 and 85, and declines thereafter. The prevalence of cancer, even occult cancer discovered only at autopsy, is negligible after age 95 [3]. This observation suggests a number of explanations including the possibility that the so-called longevity genes confer a protection against cancer or alternatively that an increasingly catabolic status prevents cancer growth after age 95.

Variations in the Incidence of Different Cancers in Older Individuals

Whereas the incidence of most cancers increases with age, the pattern of increase varies from one neoplasm to another. For example, the incidence of melanoma peaks at the age of 55 in men and plateaus thereafter; the incidence of breast cancer plateaus around the age of 80, whereas the incidences of cancer of the prostate and of the large bowel seem to increase without plateau even beyond the age of 80 [2]. These different incidence patterns suggest that a lesser number of carcinogenic stages are involved in the cancers whose incidence peaks earlier and also that some tissues, including the prostate and the colonic mucosa, become more susceptible to environmental carcinogens as the patient ages.

The case of lung cancer is of particular interest. In the last 20 years, the median age of lung cancer has changed from age 55 to age 71 [4]; the incidence of the disease has decreased for those younger than 50 years but has increased for individuals aged 65 and older, and the incidence of lung cancer in ex-smokers or non-smokers has increased. The likely explanation involves a decreased rate of cardiovascular deaths after smoking cessations, the development of a less aggressive type of lung cancer in ex-smokers, and a persistent susceptibility of the bronchial mucosa to environmental carcinogens in ex-smokers or non-smokers exposed to passive smoke. This hypothesis is supported in part by the change in lung cancer histology that includes higher incidence of adenocarcinoma and lower incidence of the most aggressive histologies, such as small cell and squamous cell.

Cancer Epidemics

Between 1950 and 1970, the incidence of non-Hodgkin lymphoma has increased by 80% among individuals aged 60 and over, and the incidence of malignant brain tumors (anaplastic carcinoma and glioblastoma multiforme) has increased sevenfold in those aged 70 and over [4]. These findings

L. Balducci (✉)
Senior Adult Oncology Program, H. Lee Moffitt Cancer Center
and Research Institute, Tampa, FL, USA
e-mail: Lodovico.balducci@moffitt.org

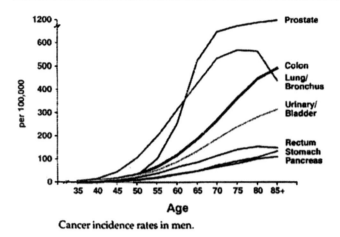

Cancer incidence rates in men.

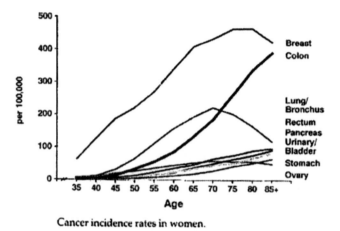

Cancer incidence rates in women.

FIGURE 3.1   The incidence of cancer increases with age (from Yancik [2]. Reprinted with permission of John Wiley & Sons, Inc.).

similar age without cancer to be independent and to have fewer comorbid conditions. The low prevalence of cancer among long term nursing home residents also supports this suggestion [7]. Obviously, cancer is a cause of mortality for older individuals and the prevention and treatment of cancer in the elderly can prolong life and preserve function.

Presentation of Cancer in the Older Person

A number of studies in the 1980s, on the basis of statewide tumor registries, indicated that some cancers present at a more advanced stage in older individuals [8]. These included cancer of the breast, of the colon, and of the bladder, whereas lung cancer was diagnosed at an early stage in older individuals. More recent studies of the issue are wanted. The increased use of early detection might have increased the diagnosis of breast and colon cancer. At least three explanations may account for the presentation of some cancer at a more advanced stage: increased aggressiveness of cancer with age (unlikely), lesser use of cancer screening and early detection by older individuals, and delayed recognition of cancer symptoms. It is well known that older individuals may harbor many comorbid conditions at the same time. Comorbidity may delay the diagnosis of cancer because early cancer symptoms may be mistakenly ascribed to preexisting conditions.

Multiple Malignancies

Approximately 20% of individuals aged 70 and over with cancer may carry a diagnosis of two or more malignancies [9]. It is not clear whether multiple malignancies may be attributed to increased susceptibility to cancer. In some cases, the use of diagnostic tests for monitoring the first malignancies may precipitate the diagnosis of a second one. For example, the association of non-Hodgkin's lymphoma and renal cell carcinoma may be explained through this mechanism. The frequent scanning of the abdomen to monitor the lymphoma may lead to early diagnosis of kidney cancer. In other cases, the treatment of a previous cancer may be responsible for the second one: for example adjuvant chemotherapy of breast cancer may increase the incidence of myelodysplasia and acute myelogenous leukemia in women aged 65 and older [10–13]. In the majority of cases, the association appears simply casual and because of the fact that age is a risk factor for multiple cancers.

suggest one of two possibilities. The first is that the improved life expectancy of the population has allowed the survival of individuals predisposed to develop these neoplasias. The second is that older individuals are natural monitoring systems for new environmental carcinogens. In other words, when exposed to new environmental carcinogens, older people are likely to develop cancer earlier than younger people. An epidemic of cancer in older individuals may herald an epidemic of cancer in the general population at a later time.

Who Are the Elderly with Cancer?

In studying the National Cancer Institute's Surveillance Epidemiology and End Results (SEER) data, Diab et al. determined that breast cancer did not shorten the survival of women aged 75–80 and was associated with an increased survival when it was diagnosed at the age of 80 and over [5]. These findings suggest that cancer is a prevalent disease among healthy elderly people. This suggestion is supported by the findings of Repetto et al. [6], indicating that older individuals with cancer were more likely than individuals of

Cancer Behavior and Age

Some cancers become more aggressive and others more indolent with age. For example, breast cancer in older women is more likely to metastasize to bone and skin rather than to the viscera and the brain [14]. Likewise, older studies showed that the metastases from non-small cell lung cancer had a longer doubling time in older individuals [14]. Conversely, age is a poor prognostic factor for acute leukemia, lymphomas, and ovarian cancer. The potential mechanisms of these differences will be discussed in the biology of aging and cancer.

Consequences of Cancer and Its Treatment in the Older Person

Cancer has become the most common cause of death up to age 85 since 2000 [15]. Surprisingly, in the same period of time, the overall cancer-related mortality has decreased, but not as rapidly as mortality from cardiovascular disease.

A number of recent studies have also shown that age is a risk factor for the development of acute myelogenous leukemia [10–13] and of late congestive heart failure after chemotherapy [16–18]. A recent study based on the SEER data also suggested an association between chemotherapy and dementia [19]. Prolonged castration with LH-RH analogs for prostate cancer has been associated with increased incidence of osteoporosis and bone fractures and possibly also with increased incidence of diabetes and coronary artery disease [20, 21].

Are cancer and its treatment causes of disability? The answer to this important question is still wanted. Older studies suggested an inverse relationship between incidence and prevalence of disability and cancer, probably related to the fact that cancer was associated with an early death which prevented the emergence of chronic disabling conditions [22]. This situation might have changed, however, with the emergence of more effective cancer treatment that results in prolonged survival from many malignancies.

In conclusion, the epidemiology of cancer and age provides important information that allows the formulation of appropriate clinical and research questions (Table 3.1).

TABLE 3.1 The lessons from epidemiology

1. Cancer has become the main cause of mortality in the older aged person: it is likely, but yet unproven that cancer is a major cause of disability
2. Cancer affects predominantly older individuals in good health, for whom cancer is a cause of morbidity and mortality. Effective prevention and treatment of cancer may prolong the life and preserve the function of older individuals
3. Cancer may be diagnosed at a later time in older than in younger individuals, as a result of decreased use of cancer screening and neglect of the initial symptoms of cancer
4. Multiple malignancies are found in as many as 20% of cancer patients aged 70 and older. In the majority of cases, the association appears casual; in some cases it may be related to treatment of a previous cancer
5. The prognoses of some cancers change with age. The underlying biology of these changes is described in the section of cancer biology and aging

Biologic Interactions of Cancer and Age

Aging and Carcinogenesis

The association of cancer and age may be explained by three non-mutually exclusive mechanisms: duration of carcinogenesis, increased susceptibility of aging tissues to environmental carcinogens, and environmental changes that favor the development of cancer.

As carcinogenesis is a time-taking process, it is reasonable to expect that cancer will become more common with advanced age. Again, the example of lung cancer is compelling. Smoking cessation has been associated with a spate of lung cancer in older ex-smokers [4]. Apparently, smoking cessation resulted in reduced mortality from cardiovascular complications of smoking, and this allowed ex-smokers to live long enough to develop cancer.

The application of the same dose of a carcinogen to the skin of younger and older mice causes more cancers in the older than in the younger animal, suggesting that the older skin is in a condition of advanced carcinogenesis and consequently more susceptible to "late stage carcinogens." The lymphatic system, the liver, and the central nervous system of older animals also display increased susceptibility to environmental carcinogens [23].

For obvious reasons, these experiments cannot be performed in humans. Epidemiological observations suggest however that this may be the case in older humans as well. As already discussed in the epidemiology section, the incidence of prostate cancer, colonic cancer, and non-melanomatous skin cancer increases geometrically with age, and this finding suggests accelerated carcinogenesis. Likewise, one possible mechanism for the increased incidence of lymphoma and malignant brain tumors in older individuals includes enhanced susceptibility of the aged to environmental carcinogens [4]. In addition, age is a risk factor for acute myelogenous leukemia and myelodysplasia following adjuvant chemotherapy of breast cancer [11–13].

The contribution of the body environment to carcinogenesis is less clear. Chronic inflammation may cause the formation of carcinogens from the adipose tissue [24–26]. Adiponectin, a hormone produced by the adipose tissues, appears to stimulate the growth of colonic cancer in predisposed individuals [27]. Proliferative senescence of the stromal cells may facilitate tumor growth and metastases and possibly may influence carcinogenesis [28, 29]. Of special interest is the fact that the small molecules thalidomide and lenalidomide are able to reconstitute a normal hemopoiesis in some patients with myelodysplasia and to abrogate, for some time at least, the neoplastic clone involving the 5q-mutations [30]. As these agents act mainly at the level of the marrow microenvironment, their effectiveness suggests that the stroma has a role in carcinogenesis.

Aging and Tumor Growth

If one thinks of cancer as a plant, the growth of the plant depends on the seed (the tumor cell) and the soil (the tumor host). The importance of the tumor host was illustrated by a now classical experiment by Ershler et al. [31] These investigators injected the same doses of Lewis Lung Carcinoma and B16 melanoma into both older and younger mice [31]. The younger animals died earlier and with many more lung metastases than the older ones. As the seed in this case was exactly the same, only the diversity of the tumor bearers could explain the different outcome.

Age related differences in the neoplastic cells are well known. In older individuals, acute myelogenous leukemia (AML) presents a number of negative prognostic and predictive factors, including mutations in flt-3, wild type nucleophosmin, and multidrug-resistant 1 (MDR-1) [32]. In addition, AML in older individuals appears to be a disease of the pluripotent stem cells, which renders its eradication all but impossible. Breast cancer presents a more favorable proteomic and genomic profile in older than in younger patients. It has been known for a long time that the prevalence of hormone receptor positive breast cancer was higher among older women, whereas the prevalence of HER-2 positive or triple negative breast cancers was more common among the younger ones. More recently, a study from Duke University showed that a cluster of 24 genes purporting a particularly bad prognosis was more common in breast cancers occurring in women aged 35 and younger [33]. In breast cancer, the characteristics of the tumor bearer may also lead to a more indolent disease in older women. These include endocrine senescence and possibly immune senescence. Through mechanisms that have not been completely clarified, immune senescence may also be a favorable prognostic factor in the case of breast cancer [34].

Age is a poor prognostic factor in both follicular and large cell lymphoma. In the case of large-cell lymphoma, the prevalence of unfavorable genomic abnormalities does not seem to change with age, so that the seed does not seem different with age [35]. Increased concentration of IL6 in the circulation may explain in part the poorer prognosis in older individuals, because IL-6 is a lymphocytic growth factor. A recent study showed that the stromal pattern (stromal II), rich in new vessels, heralds a poor prognosis [36]. It is not clear whether this pattern becomes more common with age.

In conclusion, aging is associated with a different behavior and prognosis in a number of common neoplasms. These changes may be explained by fairly well defined genomic and proteomic changes in the tumor cell (seed effect) and less well defined but equally well established changes in the tumor host (soil effect). The exploration of soil effects in tumor growth appears as a promising research area in geriatric oncology.

Aging and Cancer Prevention

Aging has contrasting effects on cancer prevention [22]. On one side, the increasing prevalence of cancer in the older person makes the aged an ideal target of cancer prevention; on the other side, reduced life-expectancy, increased risk of treatment complications, and the less aggressive course of some tumors, such as breast cancer, may lessen the benefits of prevention in older individuals. We'll briefly describe two common forms of cancer prevention: chemoprevention and early detection.

Chemoprevention

Chemoprevention involves offsetting carcinogenesis with chemical substances. Older individuals appear as ideal targets for chemoprevention because of their condition of advanced tissue carcinogenesis and increased susceptibility to late stage carcinogens. A number of chemopreventative agents are available (Table 3.2), but none of them has widespread clinical use. The selective estrogen receptor modulators (SERM) tamoxifen and raloxifen prevent the occurrence of hormone-receptor positive breast cancer, but neither has been associated with a decreased risk of breast cancer mortality [37]. Both may exacerbate menopausal symptoms such as hot flashes and vaginal dryness and may cause deep vein thrombosis (more common in women 70 years and older who are overweight). Unlike tamoxifen, raloxifen does not cause endometrial cancer. Both substances prevent osteoporosis. Given the lack of demonstrable survival advantage and the substantial compromise of quality of life, the majority of practitioners do not recommend this form of cancer prevention.

Finasteride reduces the incidence of prostate cancer but it may increase the risk of aggressive prostate cancer [38]. Until this issue is properly addressed, the value of finasteride as a chemopreventative agent remains dubious. Furthermore, the treatment may cause gynecomastia and decreased libido. An ongoing trial explores the chemoprevention of prostate cancer with a dual 5alpha reductase inhibitor, dutasteride [39].

Retinoids may reduce the risk of smoking-related cancer of the upper digestive tract and airways, but the high incidence of serious complications prevents the general use of these agents [40].

TABLE 3.2 Chemopreventative substances

Selective estrogen receptors modulators (SERMs)	Breast cancer
Retinoids	Upper airways
Finasteride	Prostate
Non-steroidals (NAS)	Large bowel
Statins	Multiple cancers

A number of retrospective studies support a reduction in the incidence of colorectal cancer with aspirin and other non-steroidal agents [41]. A small prospective study showed that Vioxx, no longer clinically available, reduced the number and the size of colonic polyps in patients with familial colonic polyposis. The clinical applications of these findings are problematic; in the absence of prospective studies, the dose and the treatment duration are unknown. The cancer-preventing ability of statins is controversial [42].

In conclusion, some human cancers may be prevented with chemoprevention, but the benefits of this cancer-preventing strategy are marginal at best.

Screening and Early Detection of Cancer

Early detection of cancer by screening asymptomatic individuals at risk has reduced cancer-related mortality from breast cancer among women aged 50–65, the mortality from cervical cancer for sexually active women, and the colon cancer-related mortality for people aged 50–80 [22]. The benefits of early detection may decline with age, given the patient's limited life expectancy and increased susceptibility to treatment complications. Is screening beneficial in older individuals? Data from randomized controlled studies are nonexistent and probably will never be obtained. Given the rapid development of new diagnostic techniques, randomized studies would become obsolete by the time they have been terminated. Retrospective analysis based on SEER data suggests that mammographic screening for breast cancer may be beneficial up to the age of 85, even in women with moderate degrees of comorbidity [43, 44]. Some form of screening for colorectal cancer appears reasonable in individuals with a life expectancy of 5 years and longer. Indiscriminate screening in older individuals is not advisable as it may have more complications than benefits [45]. In this respect, it is useful to remember that the United State Preventive Service Task Force (USPSTF) recently issued a recommendation against screening men aged 75 and older for prostate cancer because the risk of complications from unnecessary treatment appears to overwhelm the potential benefits of early detection [46].

Aging and Cancer Treatment

It has already been highlighted that aging involves a reduced life expectancy and reduced tolerance of stress, including cancer and cancer treatment. The risk/benefit ratio of preventive and therapeutic interventions may become smaller with age. The risk of therapeutic complications may mandate the enactment of measures that may ameliorate these complications, such as the administration of myelopoietic growth factors following cytotoxic chemotherapy or adjustment of the doses of chemotherapy to the glomerular filtration rate (GFR) [47].

In addition to prolongation of survival and preservation of quality of life, preservation of function is another major goal of cancer treatment in older individuals (which is often referred to as "active life expectancy") [48]. Functional dependence purports a decline in a person's life expectancy and quality of life, and substantially increases costs of management of the older aged person. Cancer treatment in older persons should therefore be undertaken with these considerations in mind.

Assessing the Geriatric Patient for Cancer Treatment

Clearly, elderly cancer patients may benefit from an array of treatment modalities. The practitioner is often faced with the vexing decision of whether to recommend a toxic treatment to patients with compromised functional status. While aging is universal, the rate of aging is highly individualized. For the purpose of clinical decisions, it is thus important to estimate each person's physiologic age rather than relying on chronological age alone. As the prevalence of age-related changes increases rapidly after the age of 70, it appears reasonable to estimate the physiologic age of individuals aged 70 and older [49–51]. In this estimate, it is important to remember that social support is instrumental to overcome some age-related limitations in a person's activities. For example, a reliable home caregiver may provide adequate access to care to a person unable to use transportation and to mitigate the complications of treatment.

The time honored methods to assess the physiologic age of an individual is a comprehensive geriatric assessment (CGA) that includes ability to perform activities of daily living and instrumental activities of daily living, comorbidity, presence of geriatric syndromes, nutrition, and social support [47, 52, 53]. Activities of daily living (ADL) include transferring, continence, feeding, grooming, dressing, and ability to use the bathroom alone. Instrumental activities of daily living (IADL) include use of transportation, ability to take medications, to provide to one's nutrition, to go shopping, using the telephone, and to manage one's finances. The geriatric syndromes are conditions that become more common with aging, although they are not specific of age, and include dementia, severe depression, delirium triggered by diseases and drugs that do not affect the central nervous system, spontaneous bone fractures, falls, dizziness, failure to thrive, and neglect and abuse.

The CGA provides an estimate of life expectancy on the basis of age, function, and co-morbidity. Using the CGA, 4 year mortality of patients of different ages (Fig. 3.2) can also

a

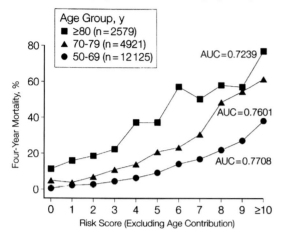

Four-year Mortality by Risk Score in Differing Age Groups

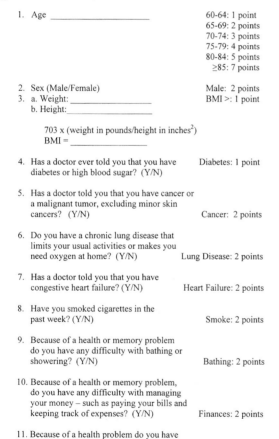

b **Four-Year Mortality Index for Older Adults**

1. Age _____   60-64: 1 point
                                        65-69: 2 points
                                        70-74: 3 points
                                        75-79: 4 points
                                        80-84: 5 points
                                        ≥85: 7 points

2. Sex (Male/Female)   Male: 2 points
3. a. Weight: _____   BMI >: 1 point
   b. Height: _____

   703 x (weight in pounds/height in inches²)
   BMI = _____

4. Has a doctor ever told you that you have   Diabetes: 1 point
   diabetes or high blood sugar? (Y/N)

5. Has a doctor told you that you have cancer or
   a malignant tumor, excluding minor skin
   cancers? (Y/N)   Cancer: 2 points

6. Do you have a chronic lung disease that
   limits your usual activities or makes you
   need oxygen at home? (Y/N)   Lung Disease: 2 points

7. Has a doctor told you that you have
   congestive heart failure? (Y/N)   Heart Failure: 2 points

8. Have you smoked cigarettes in the
   past week? (Y/N)   Smoke: 2 points

9. Because of a health or memory problem
   do you have any difficulty with bathing or
   showering? (Y/N)   Bathing: 2 points

10. Because of a health or memory problem,
    do you have any difficulty with managing
    your money – such as paying your bills and
    keeping track of expenses? (Y/N)   Finances: 2 points

11. Because of a health problem do you have
    any difficulty with walking several blocks?
    (Y/N)   Walking: 2 points

12. Because of a health problem do you have any
    Difficulty with pulling or pushing large
    Objects like a living room chair? (Y/N)   Push or Pull: 1 point

                Total Points   _____

FIGURE 3.2 (a) The relationship between age, geriatric assessment, and 4-year mortality in a home dwelling population. (b) Mortality index: each element of the geriatric assessment receives a score. The total score provides an estimate of the 4-year mortality for individuals of different ages (from Lee et al. [49] Copyright © 2006 American Medical Association. All rights reserved).

be estimated [49]. The CGA also provides information on treatment tolerance on the basis of function and co-morbidity, as well as of family support and cognition (information of how treatment and cancer affect quality of life). According to recent studies, the CGA may also provide an estimate of the risk of chemotherapy-related complications [54]. An ongoing study, the Chemotherapy Risk Assessment Score in High Age Patients (CRASH) is aimed to assess the contribution of the various components of the CGA to an individual's risk of myelotoxicity and other complications.

The CGA also provides a profile of potentially reversible conditions, such as malnutrition, limited mobility, inadequate social support, and unrecognized geriatric syndromes, which may compromise treatment outcome.

Perhaps most importantly, the CGA translates the diversity of the elderly population into objective categories that may be used when planning clinical trials of cancer treatment in old persons.

Systemic Therapy

Hormonal Therapy

The major forms of hormonal cancer treatment are listed in Table 3.3. In the management of breast cancer, both adjuvant and metastatic, the aromatase inhibitors have proven more active than the SERMs and are now the management of choice. The main complications of these agents include severe arthralgias and osteoporosis [55]. The SERMs tamoxifen and toremifene may delay osteoporosis, but do cause endometrial cancer and deep vein thrombosis and the risk of these complications increases with age and in the presence of obesity. They may still represent valid options for the occasional patient for whom arthralgia causes severe impairment of movements. The role of the pure estrogen antagonist, Faslodex®, is not clear at present. This agent does not cause endometrial cancer and deep vein thrombosis. Progestin, estrogen in high doses,

TABLE 3.3 Common hormonal treatment of cancer

Tumor	Cancer
Breast	Aromatase inhibitors
	Selective Estrogen Receptor Modulators (SERMs)
	Pure estrogen antagonists (Faslodex)
	Progestins
	Estrogen in high doses
	Androgen
Prostate	Orchiectomy
	Estrogen
	LH-RH analogs
	Ketoconazol
	Abiraterone

and androgen are rarely used, although they may still have a role, especially in patients without visceral disease who have experienced a prolonged response to hormonal treatment.

Castration, surgical or chemical (LH-RH analogs, estrogen, ketoconazol, abiraterone), is the treatment of choice for metastatic prostate cancer and for locally advanced prostate cancer in combination with radiation therapy. The benefits of treating patients experiencing a chemical recurrence (elevated PSA) after prostatectomy or radiation have not been established, although this approach has become a common practice. Prolonged castration with LH-RH may cause increased risk of bone fractures, diabetes, and coronary artery disease [20, 21]. Intermittent medical castration may be as effective as continuous castration, and is associated with fewer complications [56]. Estrogens are now seldom used, because of the risk of deep vein thrombosis, but they had significant benefits over LH-RH analogs, including preservation of libido, as well as prevention of osteoporosis and hot flushes.

Ketoconazol blocks steroidogenesis throughout the body. Without a supplement of corticosteroids, it would cause renal insufficiency. It may also cause hepatitis. It is generally used after disease progression with LH-RH analogs. Abiraterone, currently in clinical trials, has two advantages over current treatment [57]. Unlike ketoconazol, it selectively blocks the production of sexual steroids in the testicles and the adrenal. Also, it seems to prevent steroidogenesis within the neoplastic tissue which is a major cause of resistance to current hormonal treatment. Androgen antagonists are mainly used in combination with castration; as single agents, they are less effective than castration. As single agents, they may represent the treatment of choice for patients who do not want to lose their libido.

Cytotoxic Chemotherapy

Cytotoxic chemotherapy is still the mainstay systemic cancer treatment. Individuals over the age of 70 appear to benefit from cytotoxic chemotherapy in terms of cure, survival prolongation, and palliation. It is important to recognize, however, that the information related to patients aged 80 and older is very limited [58].

A number of complications of chemotherapy become more common with aging (Table 3.4). This is due in part to age-related alterations in pharmacokinetics and in part to decreased functional reserve of normal tissues. The most common pharmacokinetic change is reduction in GFR. Other changes of interest that are more difficult to assess include decreased intestinal absorption and hepatic metabolism, and decreased volume of distribution of hydrosoluble agents.

Myelotoxicity and febrile neutropenia may be prevented in more than 50% of older individuals with prophylactic myelopoietic growth factors (filgrastim, pegfilgrastim, and lenograstim). Prevention of malnutrition and anemia may also ameliorate the complications of chemotherapy to some extent.

Table 3.4 Age and complications of chemotherapy

A. Acute complications
Neutropenia and neutropenic infections
Mucositis
Cardiomyopathy
Neuropathy

B. Chronic complications
Myelodysplasia (MDS) and Acute Myelogenous Leukemia (AML)
Chronic cardiomyopathy and congestive heart failure
Neuropathy
Dementia

Cardiotoxicity may be prevented by avoidance of cardiotoxic anthracyclines, by combining anthracyclines with dexrazoxane, a drug that chelates the iron in the heart sarcomeres and prevents the release of free radicals responsible for the cardiac damage, or by substituting doxorubicin with pegylated liposomal doxorubicin that causes minimal cardiac damage. The use of anthracyclines has decreased dramatically in recent years and is largely restricted to the management of lymphomas and leukemias.

Mucositis is mainly a complication of methotrexate and intravenous fluorinated pyrimidines. There is no proven antidote to mucositis, but the utilization of the oral prodrug of fluorouracil, capecitabine, in lieu of intravenous fluorouracil may minimize this complication.

Peripheral neuropathy is a complication of alkaloids, platinum derivatives, and tubulin modulators (taxanes and epothilones), and may restrict considerably the independence of older individuals. The only prevention is early detection and dose-reduction. The substitution of cisplatin with carboplatin and of paclitaxel with docetaxel may minimize the risk of peripheral neuropathy.

The long term complications of chemotherapy in older individuals have been described only in the last 5 years [10–13, 16–19]. Age is a risk factor for anthracyclines induced myelodysplasia and acute leukemia. The reduced role of these drugs in the adjuvant treatment of breast cancer will minimize the risk of this complication; likewise, age is a risk factor for a chronic cardiomyopathy, incidence of which increased over the years since the chemotherapy was terminated, and has been described in patients treated for breast cancer, lymphoma, and small cell cancer of the lung. According to a SEER study, the incidence of dementia increases progressively in breast cancer patients treated with chemotherapy beginning 3 years from the termination of the treatment [19].

Unfortunately, there is no information concerning the most undesirable chronic complications of chemotherapy in older individuals, loss of independent living, and decreased active life-expectancy. Prospective studies of survivors are necessary to establish the risk and the prevention of this complication.

The NCCN has issued a number of guidelines for the safe management of older individuals with chemotherapy (Table 3.5) [47].

TABLE 3.5 NCCN guidelines for the management of older patients with chemotherapy

1. A geriatric assessment is necessary in all individuals aged 70 and older with cancer. This may provide an estimation of life expectancy and tolerance of treatment, and it may unearth conditions such as comorbidity or inadequate social support that may interfere with treatment
2. All patients aged 65 and older receiving moderately toxic chemotherapy should receive prophylactic filgrastim or peg-filgrastim
3. Hemoglobin should be maintained around 12 g/dl
4. In patients aged 65 and over, the dose of chemotherapy should be adjusted to the GFR
5. When possible the less toxic forms of chemotherapy should be utilized including capecitabine, pegylated liposomal doxorubicin, gemcitabine, vinorelbine, weekly taxanes, and pemetrexed

Targeted Therapy

An exhaustive review of the subject is beyond the scope of this chapter. We'll describe here commonly used products relevant to the management of older patients [59].

Imatinib is the quintessential form of targeted therapy. This small molecule is an inhibitor of the cytoplasmic tyrosine kinase, and has prolonged the survival of patients with chronic myelogenous leukemia, who now rarely need bone marrow transplantation. It is also effective against the tyrosine kinase encoded by c-Kit and for this reason, it is effective in gastro-intestinal stromal tumors (GIST). Complications are rare and reversible, and include myelosuppression and fluid retention.

Rituximab is a monoclonal antibody with CD20 specificity that has improved the survival in virtually all B-cell malignancies. Besides rare allergic reactions, the incidence of complications is minimal, although it has been reported that long term use may lead to demyelinating disorders.

Alentuzumab is also a monoclonal antibody with CD52 specificity that is very effective in some of the most therapy-refractory B-cell malignancies such as chronic lymphocytic leukemia with 17p (-) mutation. This agent has considerable myelotoxicity and should be used with prophylactic antimicrobial coverage.

Trastuzumab has revolutionized the history of the 25% of breast cancers that over-express HER2neu. It is a monoclonal antibody with specificity for Epidermal growth factor 2 (EGFR2). In combination with chemotherapy in the adjuvant setting, it almost doubles the number of patients who are free of disease 5 years from mastectomy. Trastuzumab causes myocardial freezing by interfering with myocardial trophism. Age is a risk factor for this complication that is generally reversible upon discontinuance of the treatment.

Bevacizumab is a monoclonal antibody directed against the endothelial growth factor, which inhibits tumor angiogenesis and decreases intratumoral pressure, thus allowing better chemotherapy diffusion. As a single agent, bevacizumab is active only in renal cell carcinoma, but it enhances the effects of chemotherapy in cancer of the colon, of the lung, and of the breast. Bevacizumab is associated with hypertension, bleeding, and deep vein thrombosis. It should not be used within 4 weeks of surgery, because it interferes with healing. Rarely, after abdominal surgery, bevacizumab has caused visceral perforation. All complications of bevacizumab are more common in the aged.

Receptor bound tyrosine kinase is critical to the signal transduction. This enzyme is the target of a number of agents, both monoclonal antibodies and small molecules. A common complication of all these agents is a maculopapular rash, that is more common and severe in the elderly, in whom necrolytic epidermolysis occasionally may be fatal.

Conclusions

Age is a risk factor for cancer because carcinogenesis is a lengthy process, older tissues are more susceptible to environmental carcinogens, and changes in the body environment favor cancer growth. Changes in cancer behavior are seen in some common malignancies. These are partly because of a change in the neoplastic cell and of changes in the tumor host. Although the elderly appear as ideal targets for chemoprevention, the benefits of this form of prevention have not been conclusively demonstrated. Screening and early detection of breast and colon cancer may be beneficial in older individuals with a life expectancy of at least 5 years. Systemic cancer treatment is effective in older patients. Although the complications become more common with age, most of the time they may be minimized with appropriate interventions.

References

1. Balducci L, Ershler WB (2005) Cancer and ageing: a nexus at several levels. Nat Rev Cancer 5:655–662
2. Yancik R (2005) Population aging and cancer: a cross national problem. Cancer J 11(6):437–441
3. Stanta G (2004) Morbid anatomy of aging. In: Balducci L, Lyman GH, Ershler WB, Extermann M (eds) Comprehensive geriatric oncology, 2nd edn. Taylor & Francis, London, pp 187–193
4. Jemal A, Thun MJ, Ries LA et al (2008) Annual report to the nation on the status of cancer: 1975–2005. Featuring trend in lung cancer, tobacco use and tobacco control. J Natl Cancer Inst 100(23): 1672–1694
5. Diab SG, Elledge RM, Clark GM (2000) Clinical characteristics and outcome of elderly women with breast cancer. J Natl Cancer Inst 92(7):550–556
6. Repetto L, Venturino A, Gianni W (2004) Prognostic evaluation for the older cancer patient. In: Balducci L, Lyman GH, Ershler WB, Extermann M (eds) Comprehensive geriatric oncology, 2nd edn. Taylor & Francis, London, pp 309–322

7. Kanapuru B, Posani K, Muller D, Ershler WB (2008) Decreased cancer prevalence in the nursing home. J Am Geriatr Soc 56(11):2165–2166

8. Goodwin JS, Osborne C (2004) Factors affecting the diagnosis and treatment of older patients with cancer. In: Balducci L, Lyman GH, Ershler WB, Extermann M (eds) Comprehensive geriatric oncology, 2nd edn. Taylor & Francis, London, pp 56–66

9. Luciani A, Balducci L (2004) Mutiple primary malignancies. Semin Oncol 31:264–273

10. Schaapveld M, Visser O, Lowman MJ et al (2008) Risk of new primary non-breast cancers after breast cancer treatment: a Dutch population-based study. J Clin Oncol 26(8):1239–1246

11. Muss HB, Berry DA, Cirrincione C et al (2007) Toxicity of older and younger patients treated with adjuvant chemotherapy for node-positive breast cancer: the Cancer and Leukemia Group B Experience. J Clin Oncol 25(24):3699–3704

12. Patt DA, Duan Z, Fang S et al (2007) Acute myeloid leukemia after adjuvant breast cancer therapy in older women: understanding risk. J Clin Oncol 25(25):3871–3876

13. Hershman D, Neugut AI, Jacobson JS et al (2007) Acute myeloid leukemia or myelodysplastic syndrome following use of granulocyte colony-stimulating factors during breast cancer adjuvant chemotherapy. J Natl Cancer Inst 99(3):196–205

14. Holmes FF (2004) Clinical evidence for change in tumor aggressiveness with age: a historical perspective. In: Balducci L, Lyman GH, Ershler WB, Extermann M (eds) Comprehensive geriatric oncology, 2nd edn. Taylor & Francis, London, pp 180–186

15. Jemal A, Siegel R, Ward E et al (2008) Cancer statistics. CA Cancer J Clin 58(2):71–96

16. Hershman DL, McBride RB, Eisenberger A (2008) Doxorubicin, cardiac risk factors, and cardiac toxicity in elderly patients with diffuse B cell non-Hodgkin's lymphoma. J Clin Oncol 26(19):3159–3165

17. Doyle JJ, Neugut AI, Jacobson JS (2005) Chemotherapy and cardiotoxicity in older breast cancer patients: a population based study. J Clin Oncol 23(34):8597–8605

18. Swain SM, Whaley FS, Ewer MS (2003) Congestive heart failure in patients treated with doxorubicin: a retrospective analysis of three trials. Cancer 97(11):2869–2879

19. Heck JE, Albert SM, Franco R, Gorin SS (2008) Pattern of dementia diagnosis in surveillance, epidemiology and end results breast cancer survivors who use chemotherapy. J Am Geriatr Soc 56(9):1687–1692

20. Shainian VB, Kuo YE, Freeman JL et al (2005) Risk of bone fracture after androgen deprivation in prostate cancer. N Engl J Med 352:154–164

21. Leahy Y (2008) Risk of metabolic syndrome, cardiovascular diseases and diabetes in androgen deprivation therapy. Clin J Oncol Nurs 12(5):771–776

22. Balducci L, Beghé C (2002) Prevention of cancer in the older aged person. Clin Geriatr Med 18(3):505–528

23. Anisimov VN (2009) Carcinogenesis and aging 20 year after: escaping horizon. Mech Ageing Dev 130(1–2):105–121

24. Schwartsburd PM (2004) Aging-promoted creation of a pro-cancer microenvironment by inflammation: pathogenesis of dyscoordinated feed-back control. Mech Ageing Dev 125(9):581–590, Review

25. Khatami M (2008) Yin and Yang in inflammation: duality in immune cell function and tumorigenesis. Expert Opin Biol Ther 8(10):1461–1472

26. Vasto S, Carruba G, Lio D (2008) Inflammation, ageing and cancer. Mech Ageing Dev 130(1–2):40–45

27. Kaklamani VG, Wisinski KB, Sadim M et al (2008) Variants of adiponectin and adiponectin receptor 1 genes and colorectal cancer. JAMA 300(13):1523–1531

28. Campisi J (2008) Aging and cancer cell biology. Aging Cell 7(3):281–284

29. Campisi J, d'Adda di Fagagna F (2007) Cellular senescence: when bad things happen to good cells. Nat Rev Mol Cell Biol 8(9):729–740

30. List AF (2008) Treatment strategies to optimize clinical benefits in patients with myelodysplastic syndromes. Cancer Control 15(Suppl):29–39

31. Ershler WB (2004) Tumor-host interactions, aging, and tumor growth. In: Balducci L, Lyman GH, Ershler WB, Extermann M (eds) Comprehensive geriatric oncology, 2nd edn. Taylor & Francis, London, pp 147–157

32. Gingerich J, Bow EJ (2006) Approach to the complications of treatment of acute leukemia in the elderly. Semin Hematol 43(2):134–143, Review

33. Anders CK, Hsu DS, Broadwater G et al (2008) Young age at diagnosis correlated with worse prognosis and defines a subset of breast cancers with shared patterns of gene expression. J Clin Oncol 26(20):3324–3330

34. Nixon AJ, Neuberg D, Hayes DF et al (1994) Relationship of patient age to pathologic features and prognosis for patients with stage I or II breast cancer. J Clin Oncol 12:888–894

35. Jacobi N, Peterson BA (2008) Non-Hodgkin lymphoma. In: Balducci L, Ershler WB, DeGaetano G (eds) Blood disorders in the elderly. Cambridge University Press, Cambridge, pp 290–310

36. Lenz G, Wright G, Dave SS et al (2008) Stromal gene signatures in large cell lynphomas. N Engl J Med 359(22):2313–2323

37. Vogel VG, Costantino JP, Wickerham DL et al (2006) Effects of Tamoxifen vs Raloxifen on the risk of development of invasive breast cancer and other disease outcome: the NSABP study of Tamoxifen vs Raloxifen (STAR) P2 trial. JAMA 295(23):2727–2741

38. Thompson IM, Goodman PJ, Tangen CM et al (2003) The influence of finasteride on the development of prostate cancer. N Engl J Med 349(3):215–224

39. Masquera M, Fleshner NE, Finelli A et al (2008) The REDUCE trial: chemoprevention in prostate cancer using a dual 5alpha-reductase inhibitor, dutasteride. Expert Rev Anticancer Ther 8:1073–1079

40. Klass CM, Shin DM (2007) Current status and future perspectives of chemoprevention of head and neck cancer. Curr Cancer Drug Targets 7(7):623–632

41. Antonakopoulos N, Karamanolis DG (2007) The role of NSAID in colon cancer prevention. Hepatogastroenterology 54(78):1694–1700

42. Browning DR, Martin RM (2007) Statins and risk of cancer: a systematic review and meta-analysis. Int J Cancer 120:833–843

43. McCarthy EP, Burns RB, Freund KM (2000) Mammography use, breast cancer stage at diagnosis and survival among older women. J Am Geriatr Soc 48(10):1226–1233

44. McPherson CP, Swenson KK, Lee MW (2002) The effects of mammographic detection and comorbidity on survival of older women with breast cancer. J Am Geriatr Soc 50(6):1061–1068

45. Walter LC, Lewis CL, Barton MB (2005) Screening for colorectal, breast, and cervical cancer in the elderly: a review of the evidence. Am J Med 118(10):1078–1086

46. U.S. Preventive Services Task Force (2008) U.S. Preventive Services Task Force: screening for prostate cancer. USPSTF recommendations. Ann Intern Med 149(3):185–191

47. Balducci L, Cohen HJ, Engtrom P et al (2005) Senior adult oncology clinical practice guidelines in oncology. J Natl Compr Canc Netw 3:572–590

48. Manton KG, Gu X, Lowrimore GR (2008) Cohort changes in active life expectancy in the US elderly population: experience from the

1982–2004 National Long Term Care Survey. J Gerontol B Psychol Sci Soc Sci 63(5):S269–S281

49. Lee SJ, Lindquist K, Segal MR et al (2006) Development and validation of a prognostic index for 4-year mortality in older adults. JAMA 295(7):801–808

50. Carey EC, Covinsky KE, Lui LY et al (2008) Prediction of mortality in community-living frail elderly people with long-term care needs. J Am Geriatr Soc 56(1):68–75

51. Rockwood K, Mitnitski A, Song X et al (2006) Long-term risks of death and institutionalization of elderly people in relation to deficit accumulation at age 70. J Am Geriatr Soc 54(6):975–979

52. Maas HA, Janssen-Heijnen ML, Olde Rikkert MG et al (2007) Comprehensive geriatric assessment and its impact in oncology. Eur J Cancer 43(15):2161–2169

53. Rodin MB, Mohile SG (2007) A practical approach to geriatric assessment in oncology. J Clin Oncol 25(14):1936–1944

54. Extermann M, Chen A, Cantor AB et al (2002) Predictors of tolerance of chemotherapy in older patients. Eur J Cancer 38: 1466–1473

55. Ozair S, Iqbal S (2008) Efficacy and safety of aromatase inhibitors in early breast cancer. Expert Opin Drug Saf 7(5):547–558, Review

56. Boccon-Gibod L, Hammerer P, Madersbacher S et al (2007) The role of intermittent androgen deprivation in prostate cancer. BJU Int 100(4):738–743

57. Harzstark AL, Ryan CJ (2008) Novel therapeutic strategies in development for prostate cancer. Expert Opin Investig Drugs 17(1):13–22

58. Carreca I, Balducci L (2009) Cancer chemotherapy in the older cancer patient. Oncology 27(6):633–642

59. Balducci L (2007) Molecular insights in cancer treatment and prevention. Int J Biochem Cell Biol 39(7–8):1329–1336

Chapter 4
Effects of Aging on Immune Function

Raymond P. Stowe and James S. Goodwin

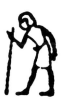

Physiologic changes with age – immune system

Parameter	Change with age	Functional impact of change
T-cells		Increased susceptibility to acute viral infections; increased latent herpesvirus reactivation along with clonally expanded CD8+ T-cells
Memory T cells	Increase	
Thymus gland	Decrease (involutes)	
Naïve T cells	Decrease	
DTH	Decrease	
IL-2 production	Decrease	
Proliferation	Decrease	
Cytotoxicity	Decrease	
B-cells		Increased autoantibodies; decreased antibody production following vaccination
Number	Decreased	
High-affinity antibodies	Decreased	
Non-specific antibodies	Increased	
Inflammation		Increased morbidity and mortality; may play a role in age-related diseases (Alzheimer's, Parkinson's, osteoporosis, atherosclerosis, and type-2 diabetes)
Low-grade inflammation		
Circulating IL-6	Increased	
Circulating TNF-α	Increased	
CRP	Increased	

In this chapter we describe changes in the immune system that are thought to be related to age per se. We subsequently review the clinical implications of these changes, including the effects of surgical trauma on immune function (see the physiology table at beginning of chapter). We then discuss how stress modifies many of these changes. We also describe recent information on persistent infections, in particular latent viral infections and how they may be partly responsible for shaping the aging immune system. We conclude with a discussion of some of the latest research on ways to restore or stimulate immune function in the elderly.

R.P. Stowe (✉)
Microgen Laboratories, La Marque, TX, USA
e-mail: rpstowe@microgenlabs.com

Changes in Immune Cell Function with Age

T Lymphocytes

Quantitative changes in T cell populations in aging humans and experimental animals include declines in "virgin" (reactive) T cells and increases in "memory" (primed) T cells [1–5]. It is not clear which subpopulations account for the accumulation of memory cells. Some studies have described increases in the population of CD4+ T-helper memory cells [6] and others reported increases in CD8+ T suppressor memory cells as well [1]. Although the number of naive T cells declines in old animals, they appear to produce larger amounts of interleukin-2 (IL-2) than naive cells from young animals [7]. Memory T cells normally produce IL-2; and although aged animals have larger proportions of memory

R.A. Rosenthal et al. (eds.), *Principles and Practice of Geriatric Surgery*,
DOI 10.1007/978-1-4419-6999-6_4, © Springer Science+Business Media, LLC 2011

cells, many studies have described decreased IL-2 production by aged memory lymphocytes. This paradox of low production of IL-2 despite increased proportions of IL-2-producing cells may be related to a lack of other regulatory cytokine signals, such as IL-4 [8].

A decrease in the proliferative response of lymphocytes to specific antigens or nonspecific mitogens was one of the earliest age-related changes in immune function to be reported [9–12]. Decreased responsiveness to mitogens is due to a number of variables, including reduced numbers of mitogen-responsive cells and decreased vigor of the proliferative response [10]. A smaller percentage of T splenocytes from old mice respond to mitogenic stimulation by entering active phases of cell replication, a defect noted with CD4+ T-helper cells and to a lesser extent with CD8+ T suppressor/cytotoxic cells [13]. Some studies suggest that the type of stimulus may affect the degree of decreased proliferation of lymphocytes from old animals [14]. T-helper cells from old mice generate fewer cytotoxic effector cells involved in delayed hypersensitivity skin reactions [15].

The ability of T cells to support antibody production changes with increasing age. Lymphocytes from old subjects display increased helper activity in vitro for nonspecific antibody production [16, 17], and they proliferate more to nonspecific stimulation [14]. Studies comparing suppressor cells from young and old mice have shown that cells from aged animals have more difficulty in recognizing and exerting suppressive effects against specific antigens from self and other old animals [17–20]. The increased incidence of autoantibodies seen during aging (antibodies directed against parts of the self) may be related to a failure of tonic inhibition by suppressor T cells [21] and has been correlated with the decreased proliferation of T cells to mitogen [22] (i.e., the lower the proliferation of T cells to mitogens, the higher was the level of autoantibodies).

One mechanism that is believed to contribute to the decline in T cell immunity is involution of the thymus, which precedes the age-related decline in T cell function and decreased thymic hormone levels (Fig. 4.1). Thymic function gradually starts declining from the first year of life [23, 24]. The thymic epithelial space, in which thymopoiesis occurs, shrinks to less than 10% of the total thymus tissue by age 70. Despite the reduction in functional thymic area, the aging thymus still demonstrates T-cell output although at a lesser rate [25]. The continual presence of T-cell receptor excision circle-positive T-cells, which represent recent thymic emigrants, were found in the peripheral blood of elderly adults [26]. Thymic atrophy has been speculated to be the result of aging of the T-cell progenitor population [27], loss of self-peptide expressing thymic epithelium [28], defects in TCRβ gene rearrangement [29], and aging of the thymic microenvironment with loss of trophic cytokines such as IL-7 [30].

Another mechanism contributing to T cell immunosenescence is "replicative senescence" [31]. Senescent T cells

in vitro exhibit a loss of CD28, a costimulatory molecule critical to the outcome of antigen recognition and signal transduction induced by the T-cell receptor [32]. Similarly, during aging, there is a progressive accumulation of memory CD8 T cells that are CD28-negative, with some elderly adults having more than 50% of their total CD8 T cells being CD28-negative [33, 34]. Notably, CD28 is involved in a number of critical T-cell functions such as lipid raft formation, IL-2 gene transcription, apoptosis, stabilization of cytokine mRNA, and cell adhesion [35–37].

Another observation of CD28-negative T cells is their inability to proliferate, even when using phorbol esters to bypass cell-surface receptors and directly signal proliferation [38]. Extensive research on a variety of cell types have attributed this to the irreversible nature of the proliferative block, which is linked to the upregulation of cell-cycle inhibitors and p53 checkpoints [39]. Once generated, these T cells do not disappear, but show increased expression of bcl2 and are resistant to apoptosis *ex vivo* [40]. Moreover, increased CD8+CD28- T cells are often present as a result of oligoclonal expansions that may reduce the overall spectrum of antigenic specificities within the T cell pool [31, 41].

A clinically important implication of large expansions of antigen-specific CD8 T cells in the elderly is that they appear to function as suppressor T cells and affect a number of immune parameters. Poor antibody responses to influenza vaccination in the elderly were significantly correlated with high proportions of CD8+CD28- T cells [42, 43]. High levels of CD8+CD28- T cells also correlate with greater disease severity in patients with ankylosing spondylitis [44]. CD8+CD28- T cells have been implicated as the critical subset in allogeneic organ transplant tolerance, whereby donor-specific CD8+CD28- T cells can be found in peripheral blood of stable transplant recipients but not in patients with acute rejection [45]. Notably, CD8+CD28- T cells have been shown to induce antigen-presenting cells to become tolerogenic to helper T cells with cognate antigen specificity [45]. Importantly, increased numbers of CD8+CD28- T cells (along with low CD4 and poor proliferative responses) were found to predict higher 2-year mortality in a Swedish longitudinal study [46].

B Lymphocytes

Age-related quantitative changes in B cells have become apparent more recently than those described in T cells. The absolute number of B cells does not appear to change appreciably with age [47]. Studies in aged mice have shown a decrease in bone marrow B-cell precursors [48–50] and structural changes in B-cell membranes [51]. B cells from old individuals proliferate less efficiently in response to mitogen stimulation, similar to what has been described for T cells [21]. Also similar to T cells [52], activation of PKC

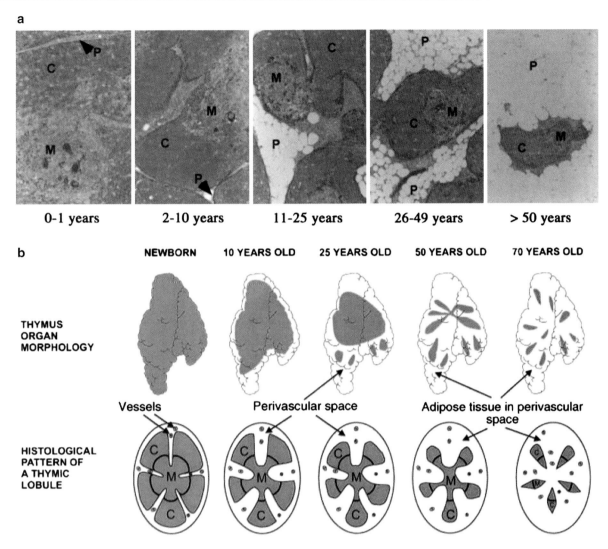

FIGURE 4.1 The human thymus across the lifespan. (**a**) Representative views of human thymus morphology throughout aging. All tissue was formalin-fixed, paraffin-embedded, and sections stained with haematoxylin and eosin and anti-keratin antibody [*brown*] to determine the percentage thymic epithelial space [each panel, ×25]. C, cortex; M, medulla; P, perivascular space. (**b**) Graphical depiction of the impact of age on human thymus morphology. Thymic epithelial space, *pink*; perivascular space, *white* (reprinted with permission from [267], copyright 2000, The American Association of Immunologists, Inc).

and protein tyrosine kinases is reduced in B cells from old humans [53]. The expression of PKC was not reduced in B cells in this study [54].

The generation of antibody responses by B cells does change with age [55], although much of it is related to changes in T cell function. The distinction between antibody responses to T cell-dependent and T cell-independent antigens is made on the basis of whether there is an absolute requirement for T cell help in the antibody response. The decrease in T cell-dependent antibody responses is obvious in experimental animals, with 80% fewer antibody-forming cells in older animals [2]. The accumulation of anti-idiotypes (antibodies directed against other antibodies) with increasing age may interfere with the production of specific antibody [56].

The ability to respond to specific antigenic challenge with specific antibody production decreases with age [55].

This phenomenon has been described in studies of both primary and secondary antibody responses. When subjects of different ages were immunized with the primary antigen flagellin, similar levels of anti-flagellin antibody were found in both old and young subjects, but the older subjects were unable to maintain the response [57]. In contrast, De Greef et al. immunized old and young subjects with the primary antigen *Helix pomatia* hemocyanin. Compared to young subjects, old subjects had similar numbers of antibody-producing cells after in vitro stimulation with the antigen [58].

Although most investigators agree that changes in antibody production with age are primarily the result of declines in T lymphocyte function, there is also evidence for a decline in intrinsic B cell function. Some studies suggest a diminished ability of purified human B cells to respond to purified T-helper cells, or to T cell-derived helper factors [59, 60].

Studies with murine cells have shown that certain subsets of B cells from old animals function at a much lower level than the same cells from young mice, whereas other subsets produce comparable levels of antibody [61]. Cerny et al. found that the antiphosphorylcholine antibody produced by aged mice did not protect animals against lethal doses of *Streptococcus pneumoniae,* although old animals produced levels of antibody comparable to those in young animals [62]. The genes encoding the variable heavy portions of the antibody molecule were different in the old mice. The resulting antibody had lower affinity for the bacterial antigen and conferred less protection [62, 63].

Macrophage Function

Macrophage function during aging is particularly relevant to the theme of this book, suggesting that "old" macrophages are comparable to "young" macrophages in terms of producing similar levels of cytokines. Differences in function appeared to be modulated through changes in T and B cell responses to the cytokines [64, 65]. Studies of human monocytes have shown decreased secretion of IL-1 with mitogen stimulation [66]. Bone marrow stem cells from senescence-accelerated mice are defective in their ability to generate granulocyte/macrophage precursor cells [67]. In vivo function of macrophages illustrated by cutaneous wound healing in mice, showed that wounds in aged control animals took twice as long to heal as in young ones [68]. When peritoneal macrophages from animals of different ages were added to wounds on old mice, healing was accelerated regardless of the age of the source animal, although, macrophages from young mice accelerated the healing process to the greatest degree [68].

Studies of macrophage function in aged mice and humans suggest defects in macrophage–T cell interactions. Antigen-sensitized macrophages from old mice stimulated significantly lower levels of T cell proliferation than sensitized macrophages from young mice [14]. Dendritic cells are tissue-fixed macrophages that stimulate formation of germinal centers in lymph follicles where B cell memory develops; they thus play an important role in the secondary immune response. Szakal et al. described serious age-related compromise in this pathway [69]. When macrophages were replaced with other sources for activation (e.g., IL-2, or an activator such as phorbol-12-myristate-13-acetate), T cells from old adults displayed enhanced responses [70]. Macrophages from young adults were able to restore old T cell responses to the level seen in young adults in 70% of the subjects studied. Because the "old" macrophages effectively supported "young" T cells, the authors postulated that the defect resulted from impaired macrophage–T cell communication [70].

In other studies, monocytes from old adults displayed less cytotoxicity against certain tumor cell lines, decreased production of reactive oxygen intermediates (H_2O_2 and NO_2), and lower IL-1 secretion than monocytes from young adults [66, 71].

Natural Killer Cells

Natural killer (NK) cells are cytotoxic cells with the ability to lyse targets without the need for antigenic sensitization, a characteristic that distinguishes them functionally from cytotoxic T cells. Lymphokine-activated killer (LAK) cells, thought to be highly activated NK cells, are able to lyse certain cell lines that are resistant to NK cells. NK cells from mice display a declining ability to lyse spleen cells with increasing age [72, 73]. Most studies using old human subjects have shown little or no change in NK cell cytotoxic ability [74]. There do appear to be differential requirements for maximal activation of NK cells by interferon-α (IFNα). Young NK cells show maximal responses when stimulated with low concentrations of IFNα [75]. The activity of LAK cells from old humans appears to be reduced compared to that of LAK cells from young humans [74, 75].

Changes in Production and Response to Regulatory Factors

Prostaglandins

Prostaglandin E$_2$ (PGE$_2$), a metabolite of cell membrane arachidonic acid, is a feedback inhibitor of T cell proliferation in humans [76]. T cells from adults over 70 years of age are a magnitude more sensitive to inhibition by PGE$_2$ than those from adults less than 40 years of age [9, 77]. Thus PGE$_2$ may interfere with expansion of antigen-specific T-helper cell clones. T cells from aged mice are not only more sensitive to inhibition by PGE$_2$, their splenocytes appear to produce more PGE$_2$ than splenocytes from young mice [78]. Meydani et al. have continued to provide evidence that macrophage production of excess PGE$_2$ is a significant mechanism in the suppression of T cell proliferation and IL-2 production in old mice [79].

Delfraissey et al. found that PGE$_2$ suppressed the primary antibody response to trinitrophenylated polyacrylamide beads by lymphocytes from old adults [65]. Removing the monocytes that were the source of PGE$_2$ production or adding drugs that blocked production of PGE$_2$, partially reversed the depressed response [9, 65]. Using a different system of lipopolysaccharide-stimulated versus unstimulated lymphocytes, other investigators have not found increased PGE$_2$ production in old versus young donors [80]. Polyclonal antibody production was not suppressed by PGE$_1$ when added to lymphocytes from donors of any age [80].

The increased sensitivity to PGE$_2$ with age does not appear to be part of a general increase in sensitivity to all immunomodulators. Lymphocytes from subjects over 70 years of age are less sensitive to inhibition by substances such as histamine and hydrocortisone [77].

Interleukins

Interleukins-1 and -2 play a primary role in activation, recruitment, and proliferation of T lymphocytes. Activated T cells then go on to produce a variety of growth and differentiation factors. T-helper (Th) cells can be classified based on the profile of the cytokines they produce and by distinct surface receptors. Th1 cells elaborate IFN-γ, IL-2, IL-12, and tumor necrosis factor-β (TNF-β), leading to the induction of cytotoxic T cells and cellular immunity; Th2 cells elaborate IL-4, IL-5, IL-6, IL-10, and IL-13, which ultimately results in antibody production [81, 82].

A decreased response to IL-2 has been studied extensively as a potential mechanism underlying the age-related defect in cellular immunity. Work from various investigators has demonstrated decreased production of IL-2 after mitogen stimulation, decreased density of IL-2 receptor expression, and decreased proliferation of T cells in response to IL-2 [83–88]. The picture is complicated by variable sensitivity to IL-2 depending on the activation signal [3, 89]. Human memory T cells generally produce low levels of IL-2 when stimulated by mitogen, in contrast to high IL-2 production by young memory T cells [8]. However, production of IL-2 by old cells was greater when a different stimulus was employed [8]. Studies from Nagelkerken's group found no differences in T cell proliferation or IL-2 production when memory T cells from old and young humans were stimulated with a variety of activation signals [3]. CD4$^+$ T cells from old mice accumulate similar levels of IL-2 transcripts, though secretion of IL-2 is lower than that seen in cells from young mice [90].

Increasing evidence has been accumulating that there are age-related declines in lymphocyte production and response to cytokines other than IL-2 [2, 91]. Monocytes from aged humans produce levels of IL-1 precursor comparable to monocytes from young humans, although they secrete less IL-1 [67]. Lymphocytes from old individuals produce higher levels of IL-1, IL-2, and TNF-α than those from healthy young individuals in mixed lymphocyte culture [92].

Li and Miller found a threefold decline in IL-4 production with age when activated murine T cells were immobilized with antibody to the T cell receptor, CD3, and cultured with anti-CD3 and IL-2 [93]. Memory T cells from old donors displayed a sixfold deficit in IL-4 production compared to cells from young donors [93]. In a similar system, CD4$^+$ T cells from young mice were more sensitive to stimulation with exogenous IL-4, producing much higher levels of IL-2 than old CD4$^+$ T cells [8]. Blocking endogenous IL-4 boosted "old" lymphocyte production of specific anti-influenza IgM and IgG1 to levels seen in young animals during a primary antibody response [94]. A similar effect was achieved by blocking endogenous IFN-γ and IL-10 [94]. We have shown that lymphocytes from old adults produce less IL-4 when stimulated with specific antigen than lymphocytes from young adults [95]. When IL-4 is added early during the course of stimulation, old lymphocytes are less inhibited to produce specific antibodies [95], similar to findings described earlier in mice [8].

Other investigators have found no differences between lymphocytes from old and young adults in terms of their ability to produce IL-4 or IL-6 when stimulated with the mitogen phytohemagglutinin [96]. In this system, lymphocytes from old adults produced significantly less IFN-γ [96]. With variation in the activating signals, old human T cells produce larger amounts of IL-4 and IFN-γ [3, 97].

Proinflammatory Cytokines

Aging is associated with elevated levels of circulating inflammatory cytokines such as TNF-α, IL-6, IL-1ra, and the acute phase protein CRP [98–100]. The plasma levels of TNF-α were positively correlated with IL-6, sTNF-RII, and CRP in 126 centenarians indicating an interrelated activation of the entire inflammatory cascade [101]. However, the increased proinflammatory cytokines in healthy elderly adults is not very marked and far from levels observed during acute infection. Thus, aging is associated with chronic low-grade inflammation.

In agreement with low-grade inflammation in aging, aged T cells produce much higher levels of the proinflammatory cytokines TNF-α and IL-6 [102]. Increased production of TNF-α by unstimulated mononuclear cells has been shown [103]. Increased production of IL-6 and IL-1ra by unstimulated mononuclear cells was demonstrated, but no difference was found in levels of TNF-α and IL-1β [104]. However, cells in tissues other than peripheral blood may also contribute to the increased levels of circulating proinflammatory cytokines such as endothelial cells, adipose cells, and macrophage-derived cells in CNS and peripheral tissues.

Clinical Implications of Age-Related Immune Changes

All-Cause Mortality

We have described a variety of immunologic changes with aging. What are the implications of these changes for the occurrence of disease and maintenance of health in older adults? There is little direct causal evidence linking specific changes in immunity to specific clinical diseases or mortality. Most authorities simply assume that a decline in immune function is deleterious, or use theoretic arguments to support this belief. The question of whether decreased immune responses contribute to morbidity and mortality in elderly persons has been addressed mostly by cross-sectional studies looking for associations between a particular abnormal immune response and general health status [105]. For example, the Baltimore Longitudinal Aging Study found that declines in absolute lymphocyte counts predicted mortality after 3 years in aging men [106]. Ferguson et al. found that the presence of two or more suppressed immune parameters predicted poor 2-year survival in a group of adults over the age of 80 [46].

The response to delayed-type hypersensitivity skin tests has been associated with mortality in a number of studies. Delayed-type hypersensitivity skin testing is thought to be the in vivo correlate of in vitro mitogen-stimulated proliferation. Elderly subjects who respond poorly or not at all to a battery of antigens placed intradermally (anergy), have an increased risk of mortality compared to elderly subjects who respond well to one or more antigens [12, 107]. We found a twofold higher mortality rate and incidence of pneumonia during 10 years of follow-up in the one-third of healthy elderly individuals who were anergic at initial testing [107, 108].

We and others have examined mitogen-stimulated lymphocyte proliferation in community-dwelling adults over age 65 years [46, 105, 108, 109]. One study found that 18% of adults seen in an outpatient geriatric clinic had lymphocytes that did not respond to any of the three mitogens [109]. These nonresponders had a 26% mortality rate at 3-year follow-up versus 13% mortality in those whose lymphocytes proliferated to at least one mitogen. The increase in all-cause mortality remained significant after controlling medication use, an indirect indicator of health status. Our own studies showed slightly higher all-cause mortality in old adults with low proliferative responses to the mitogen phytohemagglutinin [105].

Response to Immunization and Infections

Adults over the age of 65 experience greater morbidity and mortality in association with common infections, providing a basis for targeting this population with preventive immunization. Unfortunately, elderly people respond less well to preventive immunizations against common infections compared with young individuals because of the waning of immunity. Epidemiologic evidence suggests that despite decreased efficacy in the elderly, immunizations do reduce morbidity and mortality. The next section focuses on influenza, pneumococcal pneumonia, tetanus, tuberculosis, and herpes zoster, because information is available on disease epidemiology and aging immune responses specific to these entities.

Influenza

Influenza is a common viral respiratory illness that becomes clinically important when complicated by bacterial pneumonia, or when it occurs in debilitated or elderly patients (reviewed by Burns et al.) [110] Individuals who suffer from one or more chronic, systemic illnesses (e.g., chronic obstructive pulmonary disease, diabetes, chronic renal insufficiency) experience a 40- to 150-fold increase in the basal incidence rate for influenzal pneumonia of four cases per 100,000 persons per year. More than 80% of deaths related to influenza epidemics occur in the elderly [111], and the risk of developing influenzal pneumonia or superimposed bacterial pneumonia increases with increasing age. Individuals living in long-term care facilities are at particularly high risk of morbidity and mortality.

After vaccination with influenza, old mice display impaired cytotoxic T cell function and ineffective antibody generation against the virus [112]. When an intranasal viral load is administered after vaccination, old animals are more likely to develop influenzal pneumonia than young animals [112]. Studies in humans have described impaired production of anti-influenza antibodies and impaired influenza-specific cytotoxic activity in old adults compared to that in young adults [113]. Some of the mechanisms mediating this response include reduced IL-2 production and T cell activation in vivo and in vitro [85]. NK cell cytotoxicity is unchanged in old adults after vaccination against influenza, in contrast to increased NK cell activity in young adults [114]. Elderly individuals who do display a significant response to influenza vaccine have increased numbers of T cells capable of responding to the specific viral stimulus, whereas nonresponders have low numbers of such cells [115]. After immunization, IgG and IgG1 antibody production and agglutinating ability were decreased in the elderly compared to that in young subjects [116]. The investigators were able to restore the responses of the elderly subjects to the levels seen in young subjects by doubling the dose of vaccine [116].

Although influenza vaccination is less effective in the higher risk population of old adults, the incidence and severity of influenza infections is clearly reduced by annual usage of the standard preparation [117]. The vaccine confers the highest degree of protection when the epidemic strains are similar to those in the vaccine [118]. Even when the antigenic determinants of the wild virus have drifted over the course of a year, vaccine utilization can still have a substantial impact on morbidity and mortality [117].

Pneumococcal Pneumonia

An increased incidence of morbidity and mortality due to pneumonia has been recognized in the elderly for years [110]. Hospitalization necessitated by a diagnosis of pneumonia is most often caused by bacteria, primarily (about two-thirds of cases) *S. pneumoniae*. High mortality rates result from the increased incidence of bacteremia and meningitis seen in old adults. Similar to influenza, patients with one or more chronic systemic diseases are at increased risk of complications and mortality from pneumococcal infection.

Most of the information on the immunologic response to pneumococcal vaccination derives from murine studies. After vaccination with phosphocholine, old mice produced levels of antibody similar to those in young mice, but with a molecular shift in the antibody repertoire [62]. The antibody produced by old animals has a lower affinity for its target and is less effective in preventing infection [62]. In old mice, many of the antibodies produced after pneumococcal vaccination cross-react with self-antigens [62]. In humans, serum antibody levels fade more rapidly in old individuals, prompting recommendations to re-vaccinate after 6 years in elderly patients [119]. The vaccine has been estimated to be about 70% effective for reducing morbidity and mortality in the elderly [120].

Tuberculosis and Intracellular Infections

For more than 20 years the risk of active tuberculosis in the Western world is increasingly confined to two populations: those with immunocompromising diseases (e.g., AIDS) and the very elderly [121, 122]. Animal studies show that old mice display increased susceptibility to infection with *Mycobacterium tuberculosis* [123]. The infection containment rate in old mice is similar to that in young animals; but once pulmonary infection is established, there is increased hematogenous spread to other organs [123]. Old animals display decreased CD4+ T cell function, significantly lower levels of IL-12 in the lung [123], and delayed emergence of protective, IFN-γ-secreting CD4+ T cells [124]. The protective cells from old animals were slower to express surface adhesion markers necessary for migration across endothelial linings to sites of active infection [124]. The increased spread of disease in old animals may also be related to alterations in other cytokine levels [123]. Orme has shown that CD4+ cells from young mice protect old mice from infection, suggesting that old macrophages function adequately and the major defect lies in the T cell population [123, 124].

Herpes Zoster

There is a clear positive correlation between age and the incidence of herpes zoster, with an annual incidence rate of 400 cases per 100,000 adults over age 75 [125]. Other surveys suggest an even higher overall incidence [126]. The varicella-zoster virus (VZV) is harbored in dorsal root ganglia for many decades following childhood illness; and when it is reactivated it causes a cutaneous, varicella-type vesicular eruption involving the dermatome of the involved dorsal root ganglion.

Cellular immunity, measured by cutaneous delayed hypersensitivity to varicella zoster, wanes with increasing age, although other factors may be involved in controlling viral latency [127]. Cutaneous zoster is often an indication of immune-compromised status in young persons and those with early recurrence [126], but is not associated with occult malignancy in old adults [128].

Stress, Immunity, and Aging (Table 4.1)

Physical Stress

A number of studies have described the effects of physical stress on the immune system, although most have not analyzed outcomes by age. Time-limited physical stress, such as hypoxia, head-up tilt challenge (approximating conditions of acute hemorrhage), hyperthermia, and exercise, tend to enhance measures of immunity on a transient basis (e.g., increased lymphocyte numbers and increased NK cell activity) [129]. Physical stress associated with tissue injury (e.g., trauma, burns, surgery) is generally characterized by suppressed immune function. CD4+

TABLE 4.1 Immunologic changes during stress

Type of stress	Parameter	Functional impact of change
Physical (e.g., surgical, trauma, burns)	↓ T-cell number and function	↑ Post-op infections
	↓ NK cell number and function	Delayed wound healing
	↓ PMN function	
	↑ Inflammatory cytokines	
Psychological (e.g., academic exams, major life events, caregiving, spaceflight)	↓ T-cell function	↑ Herpesvirus reactivation
	↓ NK cell function	Delayed wound healing
	↓ Th1 cytokines (e.g., IL-2)	↓ Vaccine responses
	↑ Th2 cytokines (e.g., IL-10)	

and CD8[+] cells have been reported to decrease in number [130–132], and T cell activation is decreased [133]. Mitogen-induced lymphocyte proliferation is decreased after surgery and trauma [134–136], and anergy is increased [137]. The presence of anergy has been associated with an increased incidence of postoperative infections [137]. Neutrophil function is adversely affected by surgery, with decreased chemotaxis [137, 138], decreased intracellular killing [139], and disruption of superoxide release [138, 139].

One of the most consistently demonstrated findings is decreased cytotoxicity of NK cells [129, 130, 140–142]. In murine studies, decreased NK activity following surgery is associated with increased tumor metastases [143]. Levels of IL-2, mRNA for IL-2, IFN IL-10, and IL-12 are decreased [131, 135, 137, 144], whereas IL-4 and IL-6 levels are generally increased [131, 133, 136, 137, 144], although some investigators have reported decreased IL-6 [133, 145]. Of clinical relevance are observations that the degree of immune suppression correlates positively with the duration of surgery and volume of blood loss [137, 139].

The mechanisms underlying immune suppression with physical stress are slowly becoming elucidated. Tissue damage results in release of inflammatory substances, including TNF, IL-1, and IL-2 [146–148]. Hypothalamic production of corticotropin-releasing hormone (CRF) and arginine vasopressin (AVP) is stimulated by the locally produced cytokines and by afferent nerve signals from the site of injury. CRF and AVP stimulate pituitary adrenocorticotropic hormone (ACTH) release and subsequent adrenal glucocorticoids, the latter two of which are also directly stimulated by the cytokines from the site of injury [149, 150]. Activation of the hypothalamic–pituitary–adrenal (HPA) axis stimulates transformation of uncommitted Th cells to Th2 cells and inhibits transformation to Th1 cells [151]. The cellular immune responses are thus suppressed partly due to a lack of Th1 cells. The cytokines secreted by the Th2 cells (e.g., IL-1, IL-6, TNF-α) further stimulate the HPA axis and glucocorticoid production [152] and subsequently cause immune suppression [153, 154]. Given the extensive age-related changes in immunity, it is not surprising that old age in surgical patients has been associated with increased postoperative immune suppression and septic complications [139]. It is interesting to speculate that postsurgical immune suppression might be less pronounced in the elderly than expected because of decreased sensitivity to glucocorticoids [76], as mentioned previously.

Psychological Stress

In addition to physical stress from trauma or surgery, psychological stress can have a significant impact on immune system function. Complex and direct links have been described between the immune system and the perceptual capabilities of the central nervous system. Ader and Cohen demonstrated that it was even possible to condition specific immune responses with sensory cues [47]. In a series of taste-aversion learning experiments in rats, saccharin water was initially administered to the animals along with a dose of cyclophosphamide. The rats were subsequently injected with sheep red blood cells with or without readministration of the saccharin solution. Animals who received the saccharin along with the injection had profound suppression of the hemagglutinin response to sheep red blood cells [47].

Carefully controlled experiments with rodents and primates have demonstrated the neurohumorally mediated effects of stress on the immune system [155, 156]. Similar findings are seen in cross-sectional studies with humans, though it is impossible to achieve the same degree of control as in the animal studies. Clusters of illness, from the common cold to cancer, have been reported to occur around the time of major life changes [157]. Strong negative correlations have been seen between loneliness and the proliferative response of lymphocytes to mitogens, NK cell activity, and DNA splicing and repair [157, 158]. We found that healthy old adults with a strong social support system had greater total lymphocyte counts and a stronger mitogen-induced proliferation of lymphocytes than those without a close confidant [159].

Studies of individuals in "naturally occurring" stressful situations have also demonstrated links to suppressed immune function and illness. Mitogen-induced lymphocyte proliferation is suppressed after bereavement [160] and with depression [161]. The stress of taking final examinations has been correlated with recurrence of cold sores, rises in serum antibody titers against herpes simplex type I virus [162], and decreased proliferation of memory T cells [163]. Caregiving for a demented spouse is associated with a poor response to influenza vaccination [164]. Lymphocytes from the caregivers produced less IL-1β and IL-2 when stimulated with influenza virus in vitro compared to age-matched, non-care-giving controls [164]. Caregivers displayed slower wound healing after skin biopsy than did matched controls [165].

Spaceflight

Many studies have reported similarities between spaceflight and aging. The average age of NASA astronauts is early to mid 40s [166–169]. In 1998, however, former Senator John Glenn flew on STS-95 at the age of 77 as a payload specialist (PS2). This afforded a unique opportunity to compare the effects of stress and microgravity in an aged individual to those of six younger astronauts under identical spaceflight conditions. After the 9-day mission, blood and urine samples were collected and neuroendocrine and immune responses were compared to those before flight. As shown in Fig. 4.2, variable levels of plasma and urinary cortisol were observed

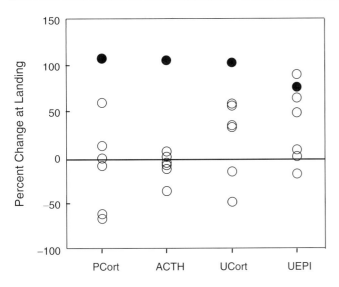

Figure 4.2 Postflight change in plasma cortisol (PCort), ACTH, urinary cortisol (UCort) and urinary epinephrine (UEPI). *Filled circles* indicate values for PS2. *Open circles* indicate individual values for the remaining six STS-95 crewmembers. Data are expressed as the percent change at landing as compared to L-10 values.

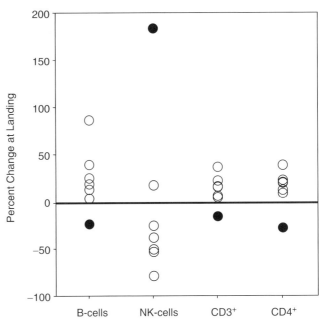

Figure 4.3 Postflight change in circulating lymphocytes. *Filled circles* indicate values for PS2. *Open circles* indicate individual values for the remaining six STS-95 crewmembers. Data are expressed as the percent change at landing as compared to L-10 values.

after spaceflight for all seven crew members. However, PS2 had the greatest increase in both plasma and urinary cortisol. Little change was found in ACTH for the younger astronauts, but once again a significant increase was found in PS2. Postflight levels of urinary epinephrine were mostly increased for the seven astronauts. Again, the aged astronaut had one of the highest epinephrine levels.

Given prior studies of psychological and physical stress on circulating leukocytes and lymphocytes, it would be expected that spaceflight would also result in significant changes in these white blood cell populations. As expected, significant increases in neutrophils were found postflight for all seven astronauts [170]. Excluding PS2 from data analysis, there was a significant increase in circulating B-cells (Fig. 4.3). A non-significant decrease was found in NK cells at landing, while significant increases were found in CD3+ T-cells and CD4+ T-cells. Notably, the magnitude (≥20% difference) and the direction of the shift in lymphocyte subsets for PS2 was opposite from that of the other six crew members. Given the recent explosion in commercial spaceflight and associated opportunities for adults (both young and old) to fly in space, this will be an important area of future research.

Reactivation of Latent Herpesviruses: A Potential Role in Shaping the Aged Immune System

Herpesviruses commonly establish latent infections in the majority of adults. The best known members of this family

include herpes simplex virus (HSV), VZV, cytomegalovirus (CMV), and Epstein-Barr virus (EBV). Herpesviruses are medically important viruses; HSV-1 infects 70–80% of all adults and is classically associated with oropharyngeal lesions such as cold sores, pharyngitis, and tonsillitis [171]. EBV infects over 85% of the adult population and is the causative agent of infectious mononucleosis, Burkitt's lymphoma, undifferentiated nasopharyngeal carcinoma, and diffuse polyclonal B-cell lymphoma [172]. Most CMV infections in adults are asymptomatic, but may result in an infectious mononucleosis-like syndrome, central nervous system infections, and febrile illnesses [173]. Notably, CMV infections can be severe in immunocompromised individuals such as AIDS and post transplant patients [174]. VZV causes chicken pox on primary infection and remains latent thereafter; VZV may reactivate resulting in episodes of zoster or "shingles" [175].

Recent work on has focused on herpesviruses, in particular CMV. Numbers of CD8+CD28- T cells have been found to positively correlate with CMV seropositivity independent of age [176]. This correlation was also found in the OCTO study [177] as well as the subsequent NONA study [178].

The recent development of MHC tetramers, which allows direct detection of T cells carrying receptors for single peptide epitopes [179], has yielded new information on the way that CMV shapes the immune system. Using tetramers, numerous studies have demonstrated detectable levels of CMV-specific CD8+ T cells present in both healthy and diseased individuals [180–184]. Notably, studies of CMV tetramer-positive cells have demonstrated the following: (a) CMV tetramer-positive cells are mainly pp65-specific, owing to the fact that pp65 is the most abundant structural protein throughout CMV infection and it is regarded as the dominant antigen recognized by CD8 T cells [185, 186]; (b) the frequency of pp65 tetramer-positive cells can reach 25–50% in healthy individuals and are often present as oligoclonal expansions as determined by TCR-Vβ analysis [181, 187–189]; (c) CMV-specific T cells increase in direct proportion with age [189, 190]; and (d) pp65-positive cells are CD28⁻CD57⁺ indicating a fully differentiated effector T cell [178, 181, 187, 188, 191].

Importantly, high levels of CMV pp65-specific T cells may downregulate immune responses to other herpesviruses. Recently, Khan and coworkers [192] who found that CMV infection in the elderly impaired the CD8 T cell immunity against EBV, another important member of the herpesvirus family that is known to cause numerous diseases including carcinomas and lymphomas. The authors found aged related increases in the number of EBV-specific T-cells. However, the frequency of EBV-specific CD8⁺ T cells never exceeded 3% in CMV seropositive individuals, whereas in CMV sero-negative individuals it was a high as 14%. Additionally, they also found that the proportion of functional EBV-specific CD8⁺ T cells was significantly lower than for CMV-specific CD8⁺ T cells. This study confirmed an earlier report that also demonstrated reduced IFN-γ production by EBV-specific CD8⁺ T cells in the elderly [193]. Subsequently, Vescovini and coworkers [194] showed that several elderly subjects had a predominance of CD8⁺ T cells specific for EBV latent epitopes rather than lytic epitopes typically found in younger subjects. Collectively, these observations suggest a lack of immune control over EBV in the elderly.

It was not known until recently whether the clonally expanded herpesvirus-specific T-cells represented increased viral reactivation or simply reflected an accumulation over time. We showed for the first time direct evidence of increased viral reactivation in the elderly which included increased antiviral antibodies and increased viral load (EBV) in peripheral blood B-cells [195]. In addition, we found plasma viremia (EBV DNA), which was supported by a program of viral gene transcription (e.g., LMP-1, gp350) similar to that found in patients with infectious mononucleosis. CMV DNA was not found in peripheral blood mononuclear cells; however, we did frequently detect CMV DNA in urine. These results were accompanied by clonal expansions of CD8⁺ and CD4⁺ T-cells directed against EBV (Fig. 4.4) and CMV (Fig. 4.5).

Notably, recent reports have suggested a link between herpesviruses and inflammation. Elevated levels of CMV antibodies have been associated with increased IL-6 and TNF-α levels in older adults [196–198]. The EBV-encoded dUTPase has also been shown to upregulate TNF-α, IL-1β, and IL-6 [199, 200]. EBV and CMV infection also result in a clonal expansion of virus-specific CD8⁺ T-cells [181, 187, 192, 195, 201]. Thus, activation or an increase in the numbers of virus-specific CD8⁺ T-cells, as well as direct interaction with viral antigens, may result in increased levels of circulating inflammatory cytokines. Consistent with this notion, we found increased urinary IL-6 levels in elderly subjects with plasma viremia as compared to those without viremia (Fig. 4.6, unpublished data).

The increased levels of proinflammatory cytokines associated with herpesvirus infection may have important health consequences. CMV, and more recently, EBV have been implicated in the development of coronary artery disease [202, 203]. Strandberg and coworkers [204] found that HSV and CMV were associated with cognitive impairment in elderly adults with cardiovascular disease. A subsequent study identified CMV as a predictor of cognitive impairment even after controlling for numerous covariates including age, education, and health conditions [205]. In perhaps the most striking study, Wikby et al. [197] found that the immune risk phenotype, characterized in part by co-infection with EBV and CMV, was significantly associated with cognitive impairment; the individuals with cognitive impairment were all deceased at follow-up, which was attributed to allostatic overload due in part to multiple herpesvirus infections. Future studies are needed to investigate the role of herpesvirus reactivation in healthy aging.

Reversal of Age-Related Declines in Immune Function

When considering physiologic changes of aging it is important to keep in mind that the changes described do not appear to be synchronized with each other [2, 206]. Defects occur to varying degrees in different systems within a given individual, and immune modulatory substances may affect some systems and not others. It is increasingly clear that there are complex interactions between the nervous, endocrine, and immune systems, although no "global" mechanism has been found that might be the common underlying cause of immune senescence [207]. We conclude with a brief discussion of potential ways to stimulate a failing immune system in elderly persons and review a number of investigations reporting attenuation or reversal of surgically induced immune suppression in animals and humans.

One of the most obvious organ changes that occur with aging is involution of the thymus, loss of thymic hormones, and a subsequent decline in T cell function [208]. In humans and experimental animals, involution begins during adolescence; and the lymphatic mass, particularly in the cortical area, decreases with age [209]. These observations stimulated a number of experiments attempting to enhance lymphocyte function by reestablishing "young" levels of thymic hormone. Exposing lymphocytes of old individuals to thymic hormones in vivo or in vitro, or transplanting young thymic tissue into

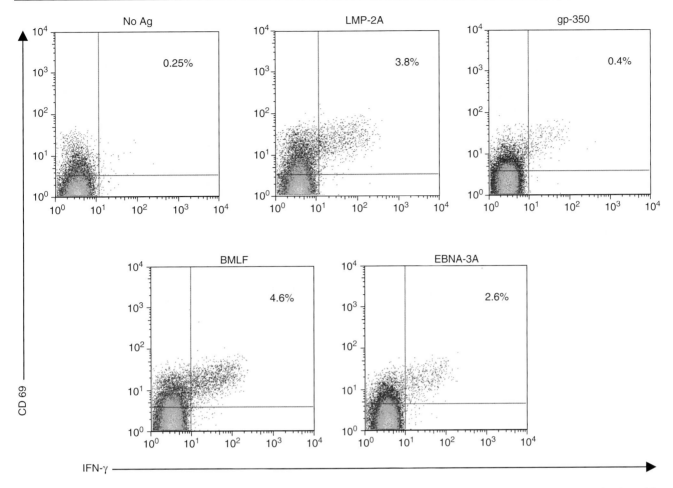

Figure 4.4 Frequency of EBV-specific CD8 T cells in healthy elderly subjects. Fifty thousand cells were included in each analysis. The frequency of CD8$^+$ T cells shown indicate the percentage of CD69 and IFN-γ-positive cells after pulsing with A*0201-restricted peptides to EBV lytic (gp-350; BMLF) and latent proteins (LMP-2A; EBNA-3A).

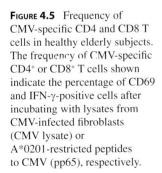

Figure 4.5 Frequency of CMV-specific CD4 and CD8 T cells in healthy elderly subjects. The frequency of CMV-specific CD4$^+$ or CD8$^+$ T cells shown indicate the percentage of CD69 and IFN-γ-positive cells after incubating with lysates from CMV-infected fibroblasts (CMV lysate) or A*0201-restricted peptides to CMV (pp65), respectively.

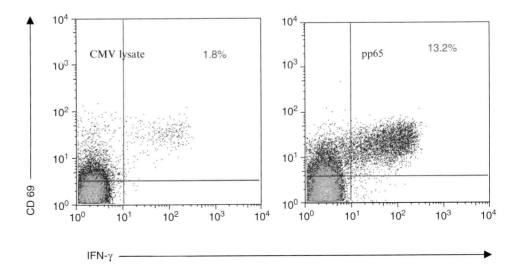

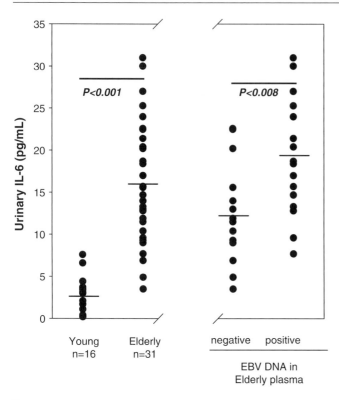

Figure 4.6 Levels of urinary IL-6 in: young versus elderly subjects, and elderly subjects with viremia versus non-viremic subjects.

including stimulation of phagocyte activity and cytokine production, both of which may help protect against bacterial infection [226]. Elderly patients with GH deficiency have low NK cell activity, but it can be at least partially restored in vitro by exposing NK cells to IGFI [227]. However, healthy old women who were not GH-deficient did not display changes in immune parameters after receiving 6 months of daily supplements [228]. VaraThorbeck et al. gave hypocaloric parenteral nutrition with or without growth hormone supplements to patients undergoing the stress of open cholecystectomy [229]. Those receiving GH had improved responses to delayed hypersensitivity skin testing, a lower incidence of wound infection, and shorter duration of hospital stay than the nonsupplemented group [229, 230]. In a series of experiments by Hinton et al., rats were given total parenteral nutrition with or without IGF-I and were subjected to the stress of a surgical incision or treatment with the synthetic glucocorticoid dexamethasone [231]. IGF-I treatment was associated with restoration of splenic B cell numbers in surgically stressed animals and increased mitogen-stimulated thymocyte proliferation and lymphyocyte-produced IL-6 in the dexamethasone-stressed animals [231].

The adrenal androgen dehydroepiandrosterone (DHEA) has been evaluated as a potential immune stimulant because it antagonizes the actions of cortisol, stimulating increased production of IL-2 and IFN-γ [153]. In vivo administration also augments antibody production by upregulating T cell subsets that are associated with increased antibody production [232]. When aged mice are primed with DHEA, the response to hepatitis B surface antigen vaccination and influenza vaccination is enhanced [233, 234], and the animals are more resistant to infection with influenza [234]. Old humans who received oral DHEA supplements before receiving influenza vaccine displayed a fourfold increase in hemagglutinin inhibition titers compared to elderly individuals who did not take supplements [235].

A few studies in mice have explored the effect of administering cytokines to animals after surgical or burn trauma. In one study, administration of the recombinant cytokine IL-1α 20 h after surgery showed restoration of suppressed NK and LAK cell activity [236]. In another study, mice with 20% burn injuries were treated in vivo with IL-12, which increased splenocyte production of IFN and significantly decreased mortality [144].

The 1990s saw a rapid accumulation of studies investigating links between nutrition and immune function (reviewed by Chandra [237] and Burns and Goodwin) [238]. Work on the effects of nutritional deprivation showed that starvation of experimental animals at young ages results in preservation of normal immune function into old age [238]. It is now known that caloric restriction rather than starvation can achieve the same results [239, 240]. The possibility that lesser amounts of caloric restriction supplemented with

old animals has resulted in at least partial restoration of immunity on a temporary basis [210–216]. IL-7 therapy alone in old mice can rejuvenate the thymus, but never to the point of the thymic size and output observed in young mice [217, 218]. Although production of IL-7 by thymic epithelial cells and dendritic cells clearly plays a role in murine thymocyte proliferation, attempts to show an age-related change in IL-7 in human studies have failed [219]. Other growth factors have been studied including IL-12, which appears to slow down thymic involution [220], while keratinocyte growth factor may provide critical survival signals for the thymic epithelium [221].

Other hormonal substances being studied for their potential to reverse age-related declines in immunity include melatonin, growth hormone, and adrenal androgens. The pineal hormone melatonin has free-radical-scavenging properties, and its production declines with age [222]. When melatonin has been administered to individuals with a variety of cancers, improved measures of immunity after surgery have been observed (increased number of lymphocytes, T cells, and Th cells) [223] as have partial tumor regression and enhanced 1-year survival of patients with metastatic solid tumors [224]. When melatonin is injected into old mice, it enhances antibody production and increases Th cell activity and IL-2 production [225].

Growth hormone (GH) and its precursor insulin-like growth factor-I (IGF-I) have immune-enhancing effects,

essential nutrients might have similar beneficial effects in humans is being formally tested in primate models [241].

In contrast to findings in the experimental setting, nutritional deficiencies in the clinical setting are generally associated with poor immune responses [237]. In both nutritionally deficient and healthy elderly adults caloric, vitamin, and trace element supplementation has been associated with enhanced immune responses, better responses to vaccines, and fewer days of infectious illness [242, 243]. NK cell activity correlates negatively to the level of polyunsaturated fatty acids in the diet, but there was no effect on NK activity in men who ingested high levels of polyunsaturated fatty acids for 5 weeks [244]. Nutritional supplements given by the enteral or parenteral route have been associated with improved surgical outcomes, but the effects on immune function are not well characterized. Rats receiving total parenteral nutrition display deficits in gut immunity and lymphocyte proliferation [245–249]. In humans, most studies have focused on the role of lipid additives in depressing immune function [247, 249–253]. In contrast to the immune suppression associated with surgery, patients with closed head trauma who receive early parenteral nutrition have preserved or increased CD4+ cell counts and improved lymphocyte proliferation to mitogen stimulation [254].

Antioxidants such as vitamins C (ascorbic acid) and E (tocopherol) have been studied intensively as potential "anti-aging" treatments [255, 256]. When healthy elderly subjects were supplemented with 400–800 IU of vitamin E, delayed-type hypersensitivity skin testing and in vitro lymphocyte production of IL-2 increased [257, 258]. Vitamin E may cause these effects via inhibition of PGE_2 or other suppressive factors [255] (see below). In vitro exposure of T cells from mice to another antioxidant, glutathione, enhanced T cell proliferation at all ages owing at least in part to blockade of eicosanoid production [259]. A placebo-controlled, double-blind trial of vitamin E and β-carotene supplementation in healthy old adults was associated with marked increases in various parameters of immunity, 50% fewer days with infection, and 40% fewer days taking antibiotics during the 1-year trial [242]. Although there is concern over the findings of a higher incidence of lung cancer in heavy smokers, taking β-carotene [260, 261], supplementation with vitamin E was not associated with an increased incidence of lung cancer [260].

Administering drugs or vaccines that in one way or another stimulate immune function are other potential ways of preventing age-related declines in immunity. Nonsteroidal antiinflammatory drugs (NSAIDs) inhibit cyclooxygenase and reduce production of PGE_2, thus stimulating immune responses in vitro and in vivo [76]. For example, an early case report of two anergic patients with an acquired immunodeficiency state showed restoration of the response to delayed-type hypersensitivity skin testing after treatment with indomethacin [262]. The proportion of adults over age 75, displaying a fourfold rise in anti-A/Beijing antibody after influenza immunization was significantly increased by aspirin supplementation [263]. The use of NSAIDs might be especially relevant to elderly persons because their T cells are more sensitive to inhibition by PGE_2 [9].

Cyclooxygenase inhibitors might also reduce the excess autoantibody production that occurs with age [264] and stimulate primary antibody responses to new antigens [22]. Unfortunately, the use of NSAIDs is not without risk, and older adults are at greater risk for experiencing the potential adverse effects of medications.

Suppression of immunity due to psychological stress has been reversed with psychological interventions. Simple relaxation exercises and writing about traumatic events enhanced the measured immune response compared to that in control subjects [265, 266]. The duration of these effects and the mechanisms that underlie them are not fully understood.

References

1. Jackola DR, Ruger JK, Miller RA (1994) Age-associated changes in human T cell phenotype and function. Aging (Milano) 6(1):25–34
2. Miller RA (1991) Aging and immune function. Int Rev Cytol 124:187–215
3. Nijhuis EW, Remarque EJ, Hinloopen B et al (1994) Age-related increase in the fraction of CD27-CD4+ T cells and IL-4 production as a feature of CD4+ T cell differentiation in vivo. Clin Exp Immunol 96(3):528–534
4. Philosophe B, Miller RA (1990) Diminished calcium signal generation in subsets of T lymphocytes that predominate in old mice. J Gerontol 45(3):B87–B93
5. Xu X, Beckman I, Ahern M, Bradley J (1993) A comprehensive analysis of peripheral blood lymphocytes in healthy aged humans by flow cytometry. Immunol Cell Biol 71(Pt 6):549–557
6. Kudlacek S, Jahandideh-Kazempour S, Graninger W, Willvonseder R, Pietschmann P (1995) Differential expression of various T cell surface markers in young and elderly subjects. Immunobiology 192(3–4):198–204
7. Dobber R, Tielemans M, Nagelkerken L (1995) Enrichment for Th1 cells in the Mel-14+ CD4+ T cell fraction in aged mice. Cell Immunol 162(2):321–325
8. Dobber R, Tielemans M, de Weerd H, Nagelkerken L (1994) Mel14+ CD4+ T cells from aged mice display functional and phenotypic characteristics of memory cells. Int Immunol 6(8):1227–1234
9. Goodwin JS, Messner RP (1979) Sensitivity of lymphocytes to prostaglandin E2 increases in subjects over age 70. J Clin Invest 64(2):434–439
10. Inkeles B, Innes JB, Kuntz MM, Kadish AS, Weksler ME (1977) Immunological studies of aging. III. Cytokinetic basis for the impaired response of lymphocytes from aged humans to plant lectins. J Exp Med 145(5):1176–1187
11. Murasko DM, Weiner P, Kaye D (1987) Decline in mitogen induced proliferation of lymphocytes with increasing age. Clin Exp Immunol 70(2):440–448
12. Roberts-Thomson IC, Whittingham S, Youngchaiyud U, Mackay IR (1974) Ageing, immune response, and mortality. Lancet 2(7877):368–370

13. Ernst DN, Weigle WO, McQuitty DN, Rothermel AL, Hobbs MV (1989) Stimulation of murine T cell subsets with anti-CD3 antibody. Age-related defects in the expression of early activation molecules. J Immunol 142(5):1413–1421
14. Kirschmann DA, Murasko DM (1992) Splenic and inguinal lymph node T cells of aged mice respond differently to polyclonal and antigen-specific stimuli. Cell Immunol 139(2):426–437
15. Vissinga C, Nagelkerken L, Zijlstra J, Hertogh-Huijbregts A, Boersma W, Rozing J (1990) A decreased functional capacity of CD4+ T cells underlies the impaired DTH reactivity in old mice. Mech Ageing Dev 53(2):127–139
16. Crawford J, Oates S, Wolfe LA 3rd, Cohen HJ (1989) An in vitro analogue of immune dysfunction with altered immunoglobulin production in the aged. J Am Geriatr Soc 37(12):1140–1146
17. Kishimoto S, Tomino S, Mitsuya H, Fujiwara H (1979) Age-related changes in suppressor functions of human T cells. J Immunol 123(4):1586–1593
18. Doria G, Mancini C, Frasca D, Adorini L (1987) Age restriction in antigen-specific immunosuppression. J Immunol 139(5):1419–1425
19. Grossmann A, Ledbetter JA, Rabinovitch PS (1989) Reduced proliferation in T lymphocytes in aged humans is predominantly in the CD8+ subset, and is unrelated to defects in transmembrane signaling which are predominantly in the CD4+ subset. Exp Cell Res 180(2):367–382
20. Russo C, Cherniack EP, Wali A, Weksler ME (1993) Age-dependent appearance of non-major histocompatibility complex-restricted helper T cells. Proc Natl Acad Sci USA 90(24):11718–11722
21. Hara H, Negoro S, Miyata S et al (1987) Age-associated changes in proliferative and differentiative response of human B cells and production of T cell-derived factors regulating B cell functions. Mech Ageing Dev 38(3):245–258
22. Hallgren HM, Buckley CE 3rd, Gilbertsen VA, Yunis EJ (1973) Lymphocyte phytohemagglutinin responsiveness, immunoglobulins and autoantibodies in aging humans. J Immunol 111(4):1101–1107
23. Steinmann GG (1986) Changes in the human thymus during aging. Curr Top Pathol 75:43–88
24. Steinmann GG, Klaus B, Muller-Hermelink HK (1985) The involution of the ageing human thymic epithelium is independent of puberty. A morphometric study. Scand J Immunol 22(5):563–575
25. Douek DC, McFarland RD, Keiser PH et al (1998) Changes in thymic function with age and during the treatment of HIV infection. Nature 396(6712):690–695
26. Jamieson BD, Douek DC, Killian S et al (1999) Generation of functional thymocytes in the human adult. Immunity 10(5):569–575
27. Tyan ML (1977) Age-related decrease in mouse T cell progenitors. J Immunol 118(3):846–851
28. Hartwig M, Steinmann G (1994) On a causal mechanism of chronic thymic involution in man. Mech Ageing Dev 75(2):151–156
29. Aspinall R (1997) Age-associated thymic atrophy in the mouse is due to a deficiency affecting rearrangement of the TCR during intrathymic T cell development. J Immunol 158(7):3037–3045
30. Plum J, De Smedt M, Leclercq G, Verhasselt B, Vandekerckhove B (1996) Interleukin-7 is a critical growth factor in early human T-cell development. Blood 88(11):4239–4245
31. Effros RB (2004) Replicative senescence of CD8 T cells: potential effects on cancer immune surveillance and immunotherapy. Cancer Immunol Immunother 53(10):925–933
32. Lenschow DJ, Walunas TL, Bluestone JA (1996) CD28/B7 system of T cell costimulation. Annu Rev Immunol 14:233–258
33. Boucher N, Dufeu-Duchesne T, Vicaut E, Farge D, Effros RB, Schachter F (1998) CD28 expression in T cell aging and human longevity. Exp Gerontol 33(3):267–282
34. Effros RB (2000) Costimulatory mechanisms in the elderly. Vaccine 18(16):1661–1665
35. Holdorf AD, Kanagawa O, Shaw AS (2000) CD28 and T cell costimulation. Rev Immunogenet 2(2):175–184
36. Sansom DM (2000) CD28, CTLA-4 and their ligands: who does what and to whom? Immunology 101(2):169–177
37. Shimizu Y, van Seventer GA, Ennis E, Newman W, Horgan KJ, Shaw S (1992) Crosslinking of the T cell-specific accessory molecules CD7 and CD28 modulates T cell adhesion. J Exp Med 175(2):577–582
38. Effros RB, Allsopp R, Chiu CP et al (1996) Shortened telomeres in the expanded CD28-CD8+ cell subset in HIV disease implicate replicative senescence in HIV pathogenesis. AIDS 10(8):F17–F22
39. Campisi J (2001) From cells to organisms: can we learn about aging from cells in culture? Exp Gerontol 36(4–6):607–618
40. Posnett DN, Edinger JW, Manavalan JS, Irwin C, Marodon G (1999) Differentiation of human CD8 T cells: implications for in vivo persistence of CD8+ CD28– cytotoxic effector clones. Int Immunol 11(2):229–241
41. Posnett DN, Sinha R, Kabak S, Russo C (1994) Clonal populations of T cells in normal elderly humans: the T cell equivalent to "benign monoclonal gammapathy". J Exp Med 179(2):609–618
42. Goronzy JJ, Fulbright JW, Crowson CS, Poland GA, O'Fallon WM, Weyand CM (2001) Value of immunological markers in predicting responsiveness to influenza vaccination in elderly individuals. J Virol 75(24):12182–12187
43. Saurwein-Teissl M, Lung TL, Marx F et al (2002) Lack of antibody production following immunization in old age: association with CD8(+)CD28(−) T cell clonal expansions and an imbalance in the production of Th1 and Th2 cytokines. J Immunol 168(11):5893–5899
44. Schirmer M, Goldberger C, Wurzner R et al (2002) Circulating cytotoxic CD8(+) CD28(-) T cells in ankylosing spondylitis. Arthritis Res 4(1):71–76
45. Cortesini R, LeMaoult J, Ciubotariu R, Cortesini NS (2001) CD8+CD28- T suppressor cells and the induction of antigen-specific, antigen-presenting cell-mediated suppression of Th reactivity. Immunol Rev 182:201–206
46. Ferguson FG, Wikby A, Maxson P, Olsson J, Johansson B (1995) Immune parameters in a longitudinal study of a very old population of Swedish people: a comparison between survivors and nonsurvivors. J Gerontol A Biol Sci Med Sci 50(6):B378–B382
47. Makinodan T (1977) Biology of aging: retrospect and prospect. In: Makinodan T, Yunis E (eds) Immunology and aging. Plenum, New York, pp 1–8
48. Ben-Yehuda A, Szabo P, Dyall R, Weksler ME (1994) Bone marrow declines as a site of B-cell precursor differentiation with age: relationship to thymus involution. Proc Natl Acad Sci USA 91(25):11988–11992
49. Viale AC, Chies JA, Huetz F et al (1994) VH-gene family dominance in ageing mice. Scand J Immunol 39(2):184–188
50. Zharhary D (1988) Age-related changes in the capability of the bone marrow to generate B cells. J Immunol 141(6):1863–1869
51. Callard RE, Basten A, Blanden RV (1979) Loss of immune competence with age may be due to a qualitative abnormality in lymphocyte membranes. Nature 281(5728):218–220
52. Whisler RL, Newhouse YG, Bagenstose SE (1996) Age-related reductions in the activation of mitogen-activated protein kinases p44mapk/ERK1 and p42mapk/ERK2 in human T cells stimulated via ligation of the T cell receptor complex. Cell Immunol 168(2):201–210
53. Whisler RL, Grants IS (1993) Age-related alterations in the activation and expression of phosphotyrosine kinases and protein kinase C (PKC) among human B cells. Mech Ageing Dev 71(1–2):31–46
54. Whisler RL, Newhouse YG, Grants IS, Hackshaw KV (1995) Differential expression of the alpha- and beta-isoforms of protein kinase C in peripheral blood T and B cells from young and elderly adults. Mech Ageing Dev 77(3):197–211
55. Delafuente JC (1985) Immunosenescence. Clinical and pharmacologic considerations. Med Clin North Am 69(3):475–486

56. Arreaza EE, Gibbons JJ Jr, Siskind GW, Weksler ME (1993) Lower antibody response to tetanus toxoid associated with higher auto-anti-idiotypic antibody in old compared with young humans. Clin Exp Immunol 92(1):169–173

57. Whittingham S, Buckley JD, Mackay IR (1978) Factors influencing the secondary antibody response to flagellin in man. Clin Exp Immunol 34(2):170–178

58. De Greef GE, Van Staalduinen GJ, Van Doorninck H, Van Tol MJ, Hijmans W (1992) Age-related changes of the antigen-specific antibody formation in vitro and PHA-induced T-cell proliferation in individuals who met the health criteria of the Senieur protocol. Mech Ageing Dev 66(1):1–14

59. Ennist DL, Jones KH, St Pierre RL, Whisler RL (1986) Functional analysis of the immunosenescence of the human B cell system: dissociation of normal activation and proliferation from impaired terminal differentiation into IgM immunoglobulin-secreting cells. J Immunol 136(1):99–105

60. Whisler RL, Williams JW Jr, Newhouse YG (1991) Human B cell proliferative responses during aging. Reduced RNA synthesis and DNA replication after signal transduction by surface immunoglobulins compared to B cell antigenic determinants CD20 and CD40. Mech Ageing Dev 61(2):209–222

61. Hu A, Ehleiter D, Ben-Yehuda A et al (1993) Effect of age on the expressed B cell repertoire: role of B cell subsets. Int Immunol 5(9):1035–1039

62. Borghesi C, Nicoletti C (1994) Increase of cross(auto)-reactive antibodies after immunization in aged mice: a cellular and molecular study. Int J Exp Pathol 75(2):123–130

63. Miller C, Kelsoe G (1995) Ig VH hypermutation is absent in the germinal centers of aged mice. J Immunol 155(7):3377–3384

64. Delfraissy JF, Galanaud P, Dormont J, Wallon C (1980) Age-related impairment of the in vitro antibody response in the human. Clin Exp Immunol 39(1):208–214

65. Delfraissy JF, Galanaud P, Wallon C, Balavoine JF, Dormont J (1982) Abolished in vitro antibody response in elderly: exclusive involvement of prostaglandin-induced T suppressor cells. Clin Immunol Immunopathol 24(3):377–385

66. McLachlan JA, Serkin CD, Morrey-Clark KM, Bakouche O (1995) Immunological functions of aged human monocytes. Pathobiology 63(3):148–159

67. Izumi-Hisha H, Ito Y, Sugimoto K, Oshima H, Mori KJ (1990) Age-related decrease in the number of hemopoietic stem cells and progenitors in senescence accelerated mice. Mech Ageing Dev 56(1):89–97

68. Danon D, Kowatch MA, Roth GS (1989) Promotion of wound repair in old mice by local injection of macrophages. Proc Natl Acad Sci USA 86(6):2018–2020

69. Szakal AK, Kapasi ZF, Masuda A, Tew JG (1992) Follicular dendritic cells in the alternative antigen transport pathway: microenvironment, cellular events, age and retrovirus related alterations. Semin Immunol 4(4):257–265

70. Beckman I, Dimopoulos K, Xu XN, Bradley J, Henschke P, Ahern M (1990) T cell activation in the elderly: evidence for specific deficiencies in T cell/accessory cell interactions. Mech Ageing Dev 51(3):265–276

71. McLachlan JA, Serkin CD, Morrey KM, Bakouche O (1995) Antitumoral properties of aged human monocytes. J Immunol 154(2):832–843

72. Ho SP, Kramer KE, Ershler WB (1990) Effect of host age upon interleukin-2-mediated anti-tumor responses in a murine fibrosarcoma model. Cancer Immunol Immunother 31(3):146–150

73. Itoh H, Abo T, Sugawara S, Kanno A, Kumagai K (1988) Age-related variation in the proportion and activity of murine liver natural killer cells and their cytotoxicity against regenerating hepatocytes. J Immunol 141(1):315–323

74. Kutza J, Kaye D, Murasko DM (1995) Basal natural killer cell activity of young versus elderly humans. J Gerontol A Biol Sci Med Sci 50(3):B110–B116

75. Kutza J, Murasko DM (1994) Effects of aging on natural killer cell activity and activation by interleukin-2 and IFN-alpha. Cell Immunol 155(1):195–204

76. Goodwin JS, Webb DR (1980) Regulation of the immune response by prostaglandins. Clin Immunol Immunopathol 15(1):106–122

77. Goodwin JS (1982) Changes in lymphocyte sensitivity to prostaglandin E, histamine, hydrocortisone, and X irradiation with age: studies in a healthy elderly population. Clin Immunol Immunopathol 25(2):243–251

78. Hayek MG, Meydani SN, Meydani M, Blumberg JB (1994) Age differences in eicosanoid production of mouse splenocytes: effects on mitogen-induced T-cell proliferation. J Gerontol 49(5):B197–B207

79. Beharka AA, Wu D, Han SN, Meydani SN (1997) Macrophage prostaglandin production contributes to the age-associated decrease in T cell function which is reversed by the dietary antioxidant vitamin E. Mech Ageing Dev 93(1–3):59–77

80. Riancho JA, Zarrabeitia MT, Amado JA, Olmos JM, Gonzalez-Macias J (1994) Age-related differences in cytokine secretion. Gerontology 40(1):8–12

81. Del Prete G, Maggi E, Romagnani S (1994) Human Th1 and Th2 cells: functional properties, mechanisms of regulation, and role in disease. Lab Invest 70(3):299–306

82. Romagnani S (1992) Induction of TH1 and TH2 responses: a key role for the 'natural' immune response? Immunol Today 13(10):379–381

83. Goonewardene IM, Murasko DM (1993) Age associated changes in mitogen induced proliferation and cytokine production by lymphocytes of the long-lived brown Norway rat. Mech Ageing Dev 71(3):199–212

84. Hara H, Tanaka T, Negoro S et al (1988) Age-related changes of expression of IL-2 receptor subunits and kinetics of IL-2 internalization in T cells after mitogenic stimulation. Mech Ageing Dev 45(2):167–175

85. McElhaney JE, Beattie BL, Devine R, Grynoch R, Toth EL, Bleackley RC (1990) Age-related decline in interleukin 2 production in response to influenza vaccine. J Am Geriatr Soc 38(6):652–658

86. Chopra RK, Holbrook NJ, Powers DC, McCoy MT, Adler WH, Nagel JE (1989) Interleukin 2, interleukin 2 receptor, and interferon-gamma synthesis and mRNA expression in phorbol myristate acetate and calcium ionophore A23187-stimulated T cells from elderly humans. Clin Immunol Immunopathol 53(2 Pt 1): 297–308

87. Negoro S, Hara H, Miyata S et al (1986) Mechanisms of age-related decline in antigen-specific T cell proliferative response: IL-2 receptor expression and recombinant IL-2 induced proliferative response of purified Tac-positive T cells. Mech Ageing Dev 36(3):223–241

88. Vissinga C, Hertogh-Huijbregts A, Rozing J, Nagelkerken L (1990) Analysis of the age-related decline in alloreactivity of CD4+ and CD8+ T cells in CBA/RIJ mice. Mech Ageing Dev 51(2):179–194

89. Ajitsu S, Mirabella S, Kawanishi H (1990) In vivo immunologic intervention in age-related T cell defects in murine gut-associated lymphoid tissues by IL2. Mech Ageing Dev 54(2):163–183

90. Hobbs MV, Ernst DN, Torbett BE et al (1991) Cell proliferation and cytokine production by CD4+ cells from old mice. J Cell Biochem 46(4):312–320

91. Bradley SF, Vibhagool A, Kunkel SL, Kauffman CA (1989) Monokine secretion in aging and protein malnutrition. J Leukoc Biol 45(6):510–514

92. Molteni M, Della Bella S, Mascagni B et al (1994) Secretion of cytokines upon allogeneic stimulation: effect of aging. J Biol Regul Homeost Agents 8(2):41–47

93. Li SP, Miller RA (1993) Age-associated decline in IL-4 production by murine T lymphocytes in extended culture. Cell Immunol 151(1):187–195

94. Dobber R, Tielemans M, Nagelkerken L (1995) The in vivo effects of neutralizing antibodies against IFN-gamma, IL-4, or IL-10 on the humoral immune response in young and aged mice. Cell Immunol 160(2):185–192

95. Burns EA, L'Hommedieu GD, Cunning JL, Goodwin JS (1994) Effects of interleukin-4 on antigen-specific antibody synthesis by lymphocytes from old and young adults. Lymphokine Cytokine Res 13(4):227–231

96. Candore G, Di Lorenzo G, Melluso M et al (1993) Gamma-Interferon, interleukin-4 and interleukin-6 in vitro production in old subjects. Autoimmunity 16(4):275–280

97. Nagelkerken L, Hertogh-Huijbregts A, Dobber R, Drager A (1991) Age-related changes in lymphokine production related to a decreased number of CD45RBhi CD4+ T cells. Eur J Immunol 21(2):273–281

98. Ballou SP, Lozanski FB, Hodder S et al (1996) Quantitative and qualitative alterations of acute-phase proteins in healthy elderly persons. Age Ageing 25(3):224–230

99. Bruunsgaard H, Andersen-Ranberg K, Jeune B, Pedersen AN, Skinhoj P, Pedersen BK (1999) A high plasma concentration of TNF-alpha is associated with dementia in centenarians. J Gerontol A Biol Sci Med Sci 54(7):M357–M364

100. Catania A, Airaghi L, Motta P et al (1997) Cytokine antagonists in aged subjects and their relation with cellular immunity. J Gerontol A Biol Sci Med Sci 52(2):B93–B97

101. Bruunsgaard H, Pedersen M, Pedersen BK (2001) Aging and proinflammatory cytokines. Curr Opin Hematol 8(3):131–136

102. O'Mahony L, Holland J, Jackson J, Feighery C, Hennessy TP, Mealy K (1998) Quantitative intracellular cytokine measurement: age-related changes in proinflammatory cytokine production. Clin Exp Immunol 113(2):213–219

103. Saurwein-Teissl M, Blasko I, Zisterer K, Neuman B, Lang B, Grubeck-Loebenstein B (2000) An imbalance between pro- and anti-inflammatory cytokines, a characteristic feature of old age. Cytokine 12(7):1160–1161

104. Roubenoff R, Harris TB, Abad LW, Wilson PW, Dallal GE, Dinarello CA (1998) Monocyte cytokine production in an elderly population: effect of age and inflammation. J Gerontol A Biol Sci Med Sci 53(1):M20–M26

105. Goodwin JS (1995) Decreased immunity and increased morbidity in the elderly. Nutr Rev 53(4 Pt 2):S41–S44, discussion S44–S46

106. Bender BS, Nagel JE, Adler WH, Andres R (1986) Absolute peripheral blood lymphocyte count and subsequent mortality of elderly men. The Baltimore Longitudinal Study of Aging. J Am Geriatr Soc 34(9):649–654

107. Wayne SJ, Rhyne RL, Garry PJ, Goodwin JS (1990) Cell-mediated immunity as a predictor of morbidity and mortality in subjects over 60. J Gerontol 45(2):M45–M48

108. Goodwin JS, Searles RP, Tung KS (1982) Immunological responses of healthy elderly population. Clin Exp Immunol 48(2): 403–410

109. Murasko DM, Weiner P, Kaye D (1988) Association of lack of mitogen-induced lymphocyte proliferation with increased mortality in the elderly. Aging Immunol Infect Dis 1:1–6

110. Burns EA, Goodwin JS (1990) Immunology and infectious disease. In: Cassel CK, Riesenberg DE, Sorensen LB, Walsh JR (eds) Geriatric medicine, 2nd edn. Springer, New York, pp 312–329

111. Sullivan KM, Monto AS, Longini IM Jr (1993) Estimates of the US health impact of influenza. Am J Public Health 83(12): 1712–1716

112. Ben-Yehuda A, Ehleiter D, Hu AR, Weksler ME (1993) Recombinant vaccinia virus expressing the PR/8 influenza hemagglutinin gene overcomes the impaired immune response and increased susceptibility of old mice to influenza infection. J Infect Dis 168(2):352–357

113. Fagiolo U, Amadori A, Cozzi E et al (1993) Humoral and cellular immune response to influenza virus vaccination in aged humans. Aging (Milano) 5(6):451–458

114. Kutza J, Gross P, Kaye D, Murasko DM (1996) Natural killer cell cytotoxicity in elderly humans after influenza immunization. Clin Diagn Lab Immunol 3(1):105–108

115. Swenson CD, Cherniack EP, Russo C, Thorbecke GJ (1996) IgD-receptor up-regulation on human peripheral blood T cells in response to IgD in vitro or antigen in vivo correlates with the antibody response to influenza vaccination. Eur J Immunol 26(2):340–344

116. Remarque EJ, van Beek WC, Ligthart GJ et al (1993) Improvement of the immunoglobulin subclass response to influenza vaccine in elderly nursing-home residents by the use of high-dose vaccines. Vaccine 11(6):649–654

117. Gross PA, Quinnan GV, Rodstein M et al (1988) Association of influenza immunization with reduction in mortality in an elderly population. A prospective study. Arch Intern Med 148(3):562–565

118. Smith NM, Bresee JS, Shay DK, Uyeki TM, Cox NJ, Strikas RA (1997) Prevention and control of influenza: recommendations of the Advisory Committee on Immunization Practices (ACIP). MMWR Recomm Rep 46(RR-9):1–25

119. Stein BE (1993) Adult vaccinations: protecting your patients from avoidable illness. Geriatrics 48(9):46, 49–52, 55

120. Sims RV, Steinmann WC, McConville JH, King LR, Zwick WC, Schwartz JS (1988) The clinical effectiveness of pneumococcal vaccine in the elderly. Ann Intern Med 108(5):653–657

121. Stead WW, Lofgren JP, Warren E, Thomas C (1985) Tuberculosis as an endemic and nosocomial infection among the elderly in nursing homes. N Engl J Med 312(23):1483–1487

122. Stead WW, To T (1987) The significance of the tuberculin skin test in elderly persons. Ann Intern Med 107(6):837–842

123. Cooper AM, Callahan JE, Griffin JP, Roberts AD, Orme IM (1995) Old mice are able to control low-dose aerogenic infections with Mycobacterium tuberculosis. Infect Immun 63(9):3259–3265

124. Orme IM (1993) The response of macrophages from old mice to Mycobacterium tuberculosis and its products. Aging Immunol Infect Dis 4:187–195

125. Ragozzino MW, Melton LJ 3rd, Kurland LT, Chu CP, Perry HO (1982) Population-based study of herpes zoster and its sequelae. Medicine (Baltimore) 61(5):310–316

126. Donahue JG, Choo PW, Manson JE, Platt R (1995) The incidence of herpes zoster. Arch Intern Med 155(15):1605–1609

127. Burke BL, Steele RW, Beard OW, Wood JS, Cain TD, Marmer DJ (1982) Immune responses to varicella-zoster in the aged. Arch Intern Med 142(2):291–293

128. Ragozzino MW, Melton LJ 3rd, Kurland LT, Chu CP, Perry HO (1982) Risk of cancer after herpes zoster: a population-based study. N Engl J Med 307(7):393–397

129. Pedersen BK, Kappel M, Klokker M, Nielsen HB, Secher NH (1994) The immune system during exposure to extreme physiologic conditions. Int J Sports Med 15(Suppl 3):S116–S121

130. Tonnesen E, Brinklov MM, Christensen NJ, Olesen AS, Madsen T (1987) Natural killer cell activity and lymphocyte function during and after coronary artery bypass grafting in relation to the endocrine stress response. Anesthesiology 67(4):526–533

131. Vallina VL, Velasco JM (1996) The influence of laparoscopy on lymphocyte subpopulations in the surgical patient. Surg Endosc 10(5):481–484

132. Zedler S, Faist E, Ostermeier B, von Donnersmarck GH, Schildberg FW (1997) Postburn constitutional changes in T-cell reactivity occur in CD8+ rather than in CD4+ cells. J Trauma 42(5):872–880, discussion 880–871

133. Horgan AF, Mendez MV, O'Riordain DS, Holzheimer RG, Mannick JA, Rodrick ML (1994) Altered gene transcription after burn injury results in depressed T-lymphocyte activation. Ann Surg 220(3):342–351, discussion 351–342

134. Keel M, Schregenberger N, Steckholzer U et al (1996) Endotoxin tolerance after severe injury and its regulatory mechanisms. J Trauma 41(3):430–437, discussion 437–438

135. Miller-Graziano CL, De AK, Kodys K (1995) Altered IL-10 levels in trauma patients' M phi and T lymphocytes. J Clin Immunol 15(2):93–104

136. Wlaszczyk A, Adamik B, Durek G, Kubler A, Zimecki M (1996) Immunological status of patients subjected to cardiac surgery: serum levels of interleukin 6 and tumor necrosis factor alpha and the ability of peripheral blood mononuclear cells to proliferate and produce these cytokines in vitro. Arch Immunol Ther Exp (Warsz) 44(4):225–234

137. Meakins JL (1989) Host defense mechanisms in surgical patients: effect of surgery and trauma. Acta Chir Scand Suppl 550:43–51, discussion 51–43

138. Redmond HP, Watson RW, Houghton T, Condron C, Watson RG, Bouchier-Hayes D (1994) Immune function in patients undergoing open vs laparoscopic cholecystectomy. Arch Surg 129(12):1240–1246

139. Shigemitsu Y, Saito T, Kinoshita T, Kobayashi M (1992) Influence of surgical stress on bactericidal activity of neutrophils and complications of infection in patients with esophageal cancer. J Surg Oncol 50(2):90–97

140. Blazar BA, Rodrick ML, O'Mahony JB et al (1986) Suppression of natural killer-cell function in humans following thermal and traumatic injury. J Clin Immunol 6(1):26–36

141. Pollock RE, Lotzova E, Stanford SD (1991) Mechanism of surgical stress impairment of human perioperative natural killer cell cytotoxicity. Arch Surg 126(3):338–342

142. Pollock RE, Lotzova E, Stanford SD (1992) Surgical stress impairs natural killer cell programming of tumor for lysis in patients with sarcomas and other solid tumors. Cancer 70(8):2192–2202

143. Oka M, Hazama S, Suzuki M et al (1994) Depression of cytotoxicity of nonparenchymal cells in the liver after surgery. Surgery 116(5):877–882

144. O'Sullivan ST, Lederer JA, Horgan AF, Chin DH, Mannick JA, Rodrick ML (1995) Major injury leads to predominance of the T helper-2 lymphocyte phenotype and diminished interleukin-12 production associated with decreased resistance to infection. Ann Surg 222(4):482–490, discussion 490–482

145. Trokel MJ, Bessler M, Treat MR, Whelan RL, Nowygrod R (1994) Preservation of immune response after laparoscopy. Surg Endosc 8(12):1385–1387, discussion 1387–1388

146. Hauser CJ, Zhou X, Joshi P et al (1997) The immune microenvironment of human fracture/soft-tissue hematomas and its relationship to systemic immunity. J Trauma 42(5):895–903, discussion 903–894

147. Traynor C, Hall GM (1981) Endocrine and metabolic changes during surgery: anaesthetic implications. Br J Anaesth 53(2):153–160

148. Wilmore DW (1991) Homeostasis: bodily changes in trauma and surgery. In: Sabiston DC (ed) Textbook of surgery: the biological basis of modern surgical practice, 14th edn. Saunders, Philadelphia, pp 19–33

149. Besedovsky HO, del Rey A, Klusman I, Furukawa H, Monge Arditi G, Kabiersch A (1991) Cytokines as modulators of the hypothalamus-pituitary-adrenal axis. J Steroid Biochem Mol Biol 40(4-6):613–618

150. Gaillard RC (1994) Neuroendocrine-immune system interactions the immune-hypothalamo-pituitary-adrenal axis. Trends Endocrinol Metab 5(7):303–309

151. Rook GA, Hernandez-Pando R, Lightman SL (1994) Hormones, peripherally activated prohormones and regulation of the Th1/Th2 balance. Immunol Today 15(7):301–303

152. Blalock JE (1994) The syntax of immune-neuroendocrine communication. Immunol Today 15(11):504–511

153. Hassig A, Wen-Xi L, Stampfli K (1996) Stress-induced suppression of the cellular immune reactions: on the neuroendocrine control of the immune system. Med Hypotheses 46(6):551–555

154. Ottaviani E, Franceschi C (1996) The neuroimmunology of stress from invertebrates to man. Prog Neurobiol 48(4–5):421–440

155. Borysenko M, Borysenko J (1982) Stress, behavior, and immunity: animal models and mediating mechanisms. Gen Hosp Psychiatry 4(1):59–67

156. Rosenberg LT, Coe CL, Levine S (1982) Complement levels in the squirrel monkey (Saimiri sciureus). Lab Anim Sci 32(4):371–372

157. Minter RE, Kimball CP (1978) Life events and illness onset: a review. Psychosomatics 19(6):334–339

158. Glaser R, Thorn BE, Tarr KL, Kiecolt-Glaser JK, D'Ambrosio SM (1985) Effects of stress on methyltransferase synthesis: an important DNA repair enzyme. Health Psychol 4(5):403–412

159. Thomas PD, Goodwin JM, Goodwin JS (1985) Effect of social support on stress-related changes in cholesterol level, uric acid level, and immune function in an elderly sample. Am J Psychiatry 142(6):735–737

160. Schleifer SJ, Keller SE, Camerino M, Thornton JC, Stein M (1983) Suppression of lymphocyte stimulation following bereavement. JAMA 250(3):374–377

161. Bartoloni C, Guidi L, Antico L et al (1991) Psychological status and immunological parameters of institutionalized aged. Panminerva Med 33(3):164–169

162. Glaser R, Kiecolt-Glaser JK, Speicher CE, Holliday JE (1985) Stress, loneliness, and changes in herpesvirus latency. J Behav Med 8(3):249–260

163. Glaser R, Pearson GR, Bonneau RH, Esterling BA, Atkinson C, Kiecolt-Glaser JK (1993) Stress and the memory T-cell response to the Epstein-Barr virus in healthy medical students. Health Psychol 12(6):435–442

164. Kiecolt-Glaser JK, Glaser R, Gravenstein S, Malarkey WB, Sheridan J (1996) Chronic stress alters the immune response to influenza virus vaccine in older adults. Proc Natl Acad Sci USA 93(7):3043–3047

165. Kiecolt-Glaser JK, Marucha PT, Malarkey WB, Mercado AM, Glaser R (1995) Slowing of wound healing by psychological stress. Lancet 346(8984):1194–1196

166. Stowe RP, Pierson DL, Barrett AD (2001) Elevated stress hormone levels relate to Epstein-Barr virus reactivation in astronauts. Psychosom Med 63(6):891–895

167. Stowe RP, Pierson DL, Feeback DL, Barrett AD (2000) Stress-induced reactivation of Epstein-Barr virus in astronauts. Neuroimmunomodulation 8(2):51–58

168. Stowe RP, Sams CF, Mehta SK et al (1999) Leukocyte subsets and neutrophil function after short-term spaceflight. J Leukoc Biol 65(2):179–186

169. Stowe RP, Sams CF, Pierson DL (2003) Effects of mission duration on neuroimmune responses in astronauts. Aviat Space Environ Med 74(12):1281–1284

170. Stowe RP, Mehta SK, Ferrando AA, Feeback DL, Pierson DL (2001) Immune responses and latent herpesvirus reactivation in spaceflight. Aviat Space Environ Med 72(10):884–891

171. Miller CS, Danaher RJ, Jacob RJ (1998) Molecular aspects of herpes simplex virus I latency, reactivation, and recurrence. Crit Rev Oral Biol Med 9(4):541–562

172. Okano M, Thiele GM, Davis JR, Grierson HL, Purtilo DT (1988) Epstein-Barr virus and human diseases: recent advances in diagnosis. Clin Microbiol Rev 1(3):300–312

173. Alford CA, Britt WJ (1993) Cytomegalovirus. Raven, New York

174. Komanduri KV, Feinberg J, Hutchins RK et al (2001) Loss of cytomegalovirus-specific CD4+ T cell responses in human immunodeficiency virus type 1-infected patients with high CD4+ T cell counts and recurrent retinitis. J Infect Dis 183(8):1285–1289

175. Arvin AM (1996) Varicella-zoster virus. Clin Microbiol Rev 9(3):361–381

176. Looney RJ, Falsey A, Campbell D et al (1999) Role of cytomegalovirus in the T cell changes seen in elderly individuals. Clin Immunol 90(2):213–219

177. Olsson J, Wikby A, Johansson B, Lofgren S, Nilsson BO, Ferguson FG (2000) Age-related change in peripheral blood T-lymphocyte subpopulations and cytomegalovirus infection in the very old: the

Swedish longitudinal OCTO immune study. Mech Ageing Dev 121(1–3):187–201

178. Wikby A, Johansson B, Olsson J, Lofgren S, Nilsson BO, Ferguson F (2002) Expansions of peripheral blood CD8 T-lymphocyte subpopulations and an association with cytomegalovirus seroposi- tivity in the elderly: the Swedish NONA immune study. Exp Gerontol 37(2–3):445–453

179. Altman JD, Moss PA, Goulder PJ et al (1996) Phenotypic analysis of antigen-specific T lymphocytes. Science 274(5284):94–96

180. Komanduri KV, Viswanathan MN, Wieder ED et al (1998) Restoration of cytomegalovirus-specific CD4+ T-lymphocyte responses after ganciclovir and highly active antiretroviral therapy in individuals infected with HIV-1. Nat Med 4(8):953–956

181. Gillespie GM, Wills MR, Appay V et al (2000) Functional hetero- geneity and high frequencies of cytomegalovirus-specific CD8(+) T lymphocytes in healthy seropositive donors. J Virol 74(17): 8140–8150

182. Jin X, Demoitie MA, Donahoe SM et al (2000) High frequency of cytomegalovirus-specific cytotoxic T-effector cells in HLA- A*0201-positive subjects during multiple viral coinfections. J Infect Dis 181(1):165–175

183. Komanduri KV, Donahoe SM, Moretto WJ et al (2001) Direct measurement of CD4+ and CD8+ T-cell responses to CMV in HIV-1-infected subjects. Virology 279(2):459–470

184. Sester M, Sester U, Gartner B et al (2002) Sustained high frequen- cies of specific CD4 T cells restricted to a single persistent virus. J Virol 76(8):3748–3755

185. Wills MR, Carmichael AJ, Mynard K et al (1996) The human cytotoxic T-lymphocyte (CTL) response to cytomegalovirus is dominated by structural protein pp 65: frequency, specificity, and T-cell receptor usage of pp65-specific CTL. J Virol 70(11): 7569–7579

186. Kern F, Bunde T, Faulhaber N et al (2002) Cytomegalovirus (CMV) phosphoprotein 65 makes a large contribution to shaping the T cell repertoire in CMV-exposed individuals. J Infect Dis 185(12):1709–1716

187. Khan N, Shariff N, Cobbold M et al (2002) Cytomegalovirus sero- positivity drives the CD8 T cell repertoire toward greater clonality in healthy elderly individuals. J Immunol 169(4):1984–1992

188. Lang KS, Moris A, Gouttefangeas C et al (2002) High frequency of human cytomegalovirus (HCMV)-specific CD8+ T cells detected in a healthy CMV-seropositive donor. Cell Mol Life Sci 59(6):1076–1080

189. Ouyang Q, Wagner WM, Wikby A et al (2003) Large numbers of dysfunctional CD8+ T lymphocytes bearing receptors for a single dominant CMV epitope in the very old. J Clin Immunol 23(4): 247–257

190. Komatsu H, Sierro S, Cuero AV, Klenerman P (2003) Population analysis of antiviral T cell responses using MHC class I-peptide tetramers. Clin Exp Immunol 134(1):9–12

191. Papagno L, Appay V, Sutton J et al (2002) Comparison between HIV- and CMV-specific T cell responses in long-term HIV infected donors. Clin Exp Immunol 130(3):509–517

192. Khan N, Hislop A, Gudgeon N et al (2004) Herpesvirus-specific CD8 T cell immunity in old age: cytomegalovirus impairs the response to a coresident EBV infection. J Immunol 173(12): 7481–7489

193. Ouyang Q, Wagner WM, Walter S et al (2003) An age-related increase in the number of CD8+ T cells carrying receptors for an immunodominant Epstein-Barr virus (EBV) epitope is counter- acted by a decreased frequency of their antigen-specific respon- siveness. Mech Ageing Dev 124(4):477–485

194. Vescovini R, Telera A, Fagnoni FF et al (2004) Different contribu- tion of EBV and CMV infections in very long-term carriers to age-related alterations of CD8+ T cells. Exp Gerontol 39(8): 1233–1243

195. Stowe RP, Kozlova EV, Yetman DL, Walling DM, Goodwin JS, Glaser R (2007) Chronic herpesvirus reactivation occurs in aging. Exp Gerontol 42(6):563–570

196. Trzonkowski P, Mysliwska J, Szmit E et al (2003) Association between cytomegalovirus infection, enhanced proinflammatory response and low level of anti-hemagglutinins during the anti-influenza vaccination – an impact of immunosenescence. Vaccine 21(25–26):3826–3836

197. Wikby A, Ferguson F, Forsey R et al (2005) An immune risk phe- notype, cognitive impairment, and survival in very late life: impact of allostatic load in Swedish octogenarian and nonagenarian humans. J Gerontol A Biol Sci Med Sci 60(5):556–565

198. Wikby A, Nilsson BO, Forsey R et al (2006) The immune risk phenotype is associated with IL-6 in the terminal decline stage: findings from the Swedish NONA immune longitudinal study of very late life functioning. Mech Ageing Dev 127(8):695–704

199. Glaser R, Litsky ML, Padgett DA et al (2006) EBV-encoded dUT- Pase induces immune dysregulation: implications for the pathophys- iology of EBV-associated disease. Virology 346(1): 205–218

200. Glaser R, Padgett DA, Litsky ML et al (2005) Stress-associated changes in the steady-state expression of latent Epstein-Barr virus: implications for chronic fatigue syndrome and cancer. Brain Behav Immun 19(2):91–103

201. Tan LC, Gudgeon N, Annels NE et al (1999) A re-evaluation of the frequency of CD8+ T cells specific for EBV in healthy virus carri- ers. J Immunol 162(3):1827–1835

202. Kendall TJ, Wilson JE, Radio SJ et al (1992) Cytomegalovirus and other herpesviruses: do they have a role in the development of accelerated coronary arterial disease in human heart allografts? J Heart Lung Transplant 11(3 Pt 2):S14–S20

203. Waldman WJ, Williams MV Jr, Lemeshow S et al (2007) Epstein- Barr virus-encoded dUTPase enhances proinflammatory cytokine production by macrophages in contact with endothelial cells: evi- dence for depression-induced atherosclerotic risk. Brain Behav Immun 22(2):215–223

204. Strandberg TE, Pitkala KH, Linnavuori KH, Tilvis RS (2003) Impact of viral and bacterial burden on cognitive impairment in elderly per- sons with cardiovascular diseases. Stroke 34(9):2126–2131

205. Aiello AE, Haan M, Blythe L, Moore K, Gonzalez JM, Jagust W (2006) The influence of latent viral infection on rate of cognitive decline over 4 years. J Am Geriatr Soc 54(7):1046–1054

206. Cinader B, Thorbecke GJ (1990) "Aging and the Immune System". Report on Workshop #94 held during the 7th international con- gress of immunology in Berlin on August 3, 1989. Aging Immunol Infect Dis 2:45–53

207. Fabris N (1990) A neuroendocrine-immune theory of aging. Int J Neurosci 51(3–4):373–375

208. Song L, Kim YH, Chopra RK et al (1993) Age-related effects in T cell activation and proliferation. Exp Gerontol 28(4-5):313–321

209. Lewis VM, Twomey JJ, Bealmear P, Goldstein G, Good RA (1978) Age, thymic involution, and circulating thymic hormone activity. J Clin Endocrinol Metab 47(1):145–150

210. Cillari E, Milano S, Perego R et al (1992) Modulation of IL-2, IFN-gamma, TNF-alpha and IL-4 production in mice of different ages by thymopentin. Int J Immunopharmacol 14(6):1029–1035

211. Duchateau J, Servais G, Vreyens R, Delespesse G, Bolla K (1985) Modulation of immune response in aged humans through different administration modes of thymopentin. Surv Immunol Res 4(Suppl 1):94–101

212. Ershler WB, Moore AL, Hacker MP, Ninomiya J, Naylor P, Goldstein AL (1984) Specific antibody synthesis in vitro II. Age- associated thymosin enhancement of antitetanus antibody synthe- sis. Immunopharmacology 8(2):69–77

213. Frasca D, Adorini L, Doria G (1987) Enhanced frequency of mitogen- responsive T cell precursors in old mice injected with thymosin alpha 1. Eur J Immunol 17(5):727–730

214. Goso C, Frasca D, Doria G (1992) Effect of synthetic thymic humoral factor (THF-gamma 2) on T cell activities in immunodeficient ageing mice. Clin Exp Immunol 87(3):346–351

215. Hirokawa K, Utsuyama M, Kasai M, Kurashima C (1992) Aging and immunity. Acta Pathol Jpn 42(8):537–548

216. Meroni PL, Barcellini W, Frasca D et al (1987) In vivo immunopotentiating activity of thymopentin in aging humans: increase of IL-2 production. Clin Immunol Immunopathol 42(2):151–159

217. Aspinall R (2006) T cell development, ageing and Interleukin-7. Mech Ageing Dev 127(6):572–578

218. Plum J, De Smedt M, Leclercq G (1993) Exogenous IL-7 promotes the growth of CD3-CD4-CD8-CD44+CD25+/- precursor cells and blocks the differentiation pathway of TCR-alpha beta cells in fetal thymus organ culture. J Immunol 150(7): 2706–2716

219. Henson SM, Pido-Lopez J, Aspinall R (2004) Reversal of thymic atrophy. Exp Gerontol 39(4):673–678

220. Li L, Hsu HC, Stockard CR et al (2004) IL-12 inhibits thymic involution by enhancing IL-7- and IL-2-induced thymocyte proliferation. J Immunol 172(5):2909–2916

221. Min D, Taylor PA, Panoskaltsis-Mortari A et al (2002) Protection from thymic epithelial cell injury by keratinocyte growth factor: a new approach to improve thymic and peripheral T-cell reconstitution after bone marrow transplantation. Blood 99(12): 4592–4600

222. Reiter RJ (1994) Pineal function during aging: attenuation of the melatonin rhythm and its neurobiological consequences. Acta Neurobiol Exp (Wars) 54(Suppl):31–39

223. Lissoni P, Brivio F, Brivio O et al (1995) Immune effects of preoperative immunotherapy with high-dose subcutaneous interleukin-2 versus neuroimmunotherapy with low-dose interleukin-2 plus the neurohormone melatonin in gastrointestinal tract tumor patients. J Biol Regul Homeost Agents 9(1):31–33

224. Lissoni P, Barni S, Fossati V et al (1995) A randomized study of neuroimmunotherapy with low-dose subcutaneous interleukin-2 plus melatonin compared to supportive care alone in patients with untreatable metastatic solid tumour. Support Care Cancer 3(3):194–197

225. Caroleo MC, Frasca D, Nistico G, Doria G (1992) Melatonin as immunomodulator in immunodeficient mice. Immunopharmacology 23(2):81–89

226. Saito H, Inoue T, Fukatsu K et al (1996) Growth hormone and the immune response to bacterial infection. Horm Res 45(1–2):50–54

227. Auernhammer CJ, Feldmeier H, Nass R, Pachmann K, Strasburger CJ (1996) Insulin-like growth factor I is an independent coregulatory modulator of natural killer (NK) cell activity. Endocrinology 137(12):5332–5336

228. Bonello RS, Marcus R, Bloch D, Strober S (1996) Effects of growth hormone and estrogen on T lymphocytes in older women. J Am Geriatr Soc 44(9):1038–1042

229. Vara-Thorbeck R, Guerrero JA, Rosell J, Ruiz-Requena E, Capitan JM (1993) Exogenous growth hormone: effects on the catabolic response to surgically produced acute stress and on postoperative immune function. World J Surg 17(4):530–537, discussion 537–538

230. Vara-Thorbeck R, Ruiz-Requena E, Guerrero-Fernandez JA (1996) Effects of human growth hormone on the catabolic state after surgical trauma. Horm Res 45(1–2):55–60

231. Hinton PS, Peterson CA, Lo HC, Yang H, McCarthy D, Ney DM (1995) Insulin-like growth factor-I enhances immune response in dexamethasone-treated or surgically stressed rats maintained with total parenteral nutrition. JPEN J Parenter Enteral Nutr 19(6): 444–452

232. Swenson CD, Gottesman SR, Belsito DV, Samanich KM, Edington J, Thorbecke GJ (1995) Relationship between humoral immunoaugmenting properties of DHEAS and IgD-receptor expression in young and aged mice. Ann N Y Acad Sci 774:249–258

233. Araneo BA, Woods ML 2nd, Daynes RA (1993) Reversal of the immunosenescent phenotype by dehydroepiandrosterone: hormone treatment provides an adjuvant effect on the immunization of aged mice with recombinant hepatitis B surface antigen. J Infect Dis 167(4):830–840

234. Danenberg HD, Ben-Yehuda A, Zakay-Rones Z, Friedman G (1995) Dehydroepiandrosterone (DHEA) treatment reverses the impaired immune response of old mice to influenza vaccination and protects from influenza infection. Vaccine 13(15):1445–1448

235. Araneo B, Dowell T, Woods ML, Daynes R, Judd M, Evans T (1995) DHEAS as an effective vaccine adjuvant in elderly humans. Proof-of-principle studies. Ann N Y Acad Sci 774: 232–248

236. Shen RN, Wu B, Lu L, Kaiser HE, Broxmeyer HE (1994) Recombinant human interleukin-1 alpha: a potent bio-immunomodifier in vivo in immunosuppressed mice induced by cyclophosphamide, retroviral infection and surgical stress. In Vivo 8(1):59–63

237. Chandra RK (1990) Nutrition is an important determinant of immunity in old age. Prog Clin Biol Res 326:321–334

238. Burns EA, Goodwin JS (1994) Aging: nutrition and immunity. In: Forse RA, Bell SJ, Blackburn GL (eds) Diet, nutrition and immunity. CRC, Boca Raton, FL, pp 57–72

239. Effros RB, Walford RL, Weindruch R, Mitcheltree C (1991) Influences of dietary restriction on immunity to influenza in aged mice. J Gerontol 46(4):B142–B147

240. Ershler WB, Sun WH, Binkley N et al (1993) Interleukin-6 and aging: blood levels and mononuclear cell production increase with advancing age and in vitro production is modifiable by dietary restriction. Lymphokine Cytokine Res 12(4):225–230

241. Kemnitz JW, Weindruch R, Roecker EB, Crawford K, Kaufman PL, Ershler WB (1993) Dietary restriction of adult male rhesus monkeys: design, methodology, and preliminary findings from the first year of study. J Gerontol 48(1):B17–B26

242. Chandra RK (1992) Effect of vitamin and trace-element supplementation on immune responses and infection in elderly subjects. Lancet 340(8828):1124–1127

243. Chandra RK, Puri S (1985) Nutritional support improves antibody response to influenza virus vaccine in the elderly. Br Med J (Clin Res Ed) 291(6497):705–706

244. Rasmussen LB, Kiens B, Pedersen BK, Richter EA (1994) Effect of diet and plasma fatty acid composition on immune status in elderly men. Am J Clin Nutr 59(3):572–577

245. Alverdy JA, Aoys E, Weiss-Carrington P, Burke DA (1992) The effect of glutamine-enriched TPN on gut immune cellularity. J Surg Res 52(1):34–38

246. Alverdy JC, Aoys E, Moss GS (1988) Total parenteral nutrition promotes bacterial translocation from the gut. Surgery 104(2):185–190

247. Hamawy KJ, Moldawer LL, Georgieff M et al (1985) The Henry M Vars Award. The effect of lipid emulsions on reticuloendothelial system function in the injured animal. JPEN J Parenter Enteral Nutr 9(5):559–565

248. Mainous M, Xu DZ, Lu Q, Berg RD, Deitch EA (1991) Oral-TPN-induced bacterial translocation and impaired immune defenses are reversed by refeeding. Surgery 110(2):277–283, discussion 283–274

249. Shou J, Lappin J, Daly JM (1994) Impairment of pulmonary macrophage function with total parenteral nutrition. Ann Surg 219(3):291–297

250. Gogos CA, Kalfarentzos FE, Zoumbos NC (1990) Effect of different types of total parenteral nutrition on T-lymphocyte subpopulations and NK cells. Am J Clin Nutr 51(1):119–122

251. Jensen GL, Mascioli EA, Seidner DL et al (1990) Parenteral infusion of long- and medium-chain triglycerides and reticuloendothelial system function in man. JPEN J Parenter Enteral Nutr 14(5):467–471

252. Salo M (1990) Inhibition of immunoglobulin synthesis in vitro by intravenous lipid emulsion (Intralipid). JPEN J Parenter Enteral Nutr 14(5):459–462

253. Sedman PC, Somers SS, Ramsden CW, Brennan TG, Guillou PJ (1991) Effects of different lipid emulsions on lymphocyte function during total parenteral nutrition. Br J Surg 78(11):1396–1399

254. Sacks GS, Brown RO, Teague D, Dickerson RN, Tolley EA, Kudsk KA (1995) Early nutrition support modifies immune function in patients sustaining severe head injury. JPEN J Parenter Enteral Nutr 19(5):387–392

255. Meydani M (1995) Vitamin E. Lancet 345(8943):170–175

256. Meydani M, Hayek M (1992) Vitamin E and immune response. In: Chandra RK (ed) Proceedings of international conference on nutrition and immunity. ARTS Biomedical, St. John's Newfoundland, pp 105–128

257. Meydani SN, Barklund MP, Liu S et al (1990) Vitamin E supplementation enhances cell-mediated immunity in healthy elderly subjects. Am J Clin Nutr 52(3):557–563

258. Meydani SN, Meydani M, Blumberg JB et al (1997) Vitamin E supplementation and in vivo immune response in healthy elderly subjects. A randomized controlled trial. JAMA 277(17): 1380–1386

259. Wu D, Meydani SN, Sastre J, Hayek M, Meydani M (1994) In vitro glutathione supplementation enhances interleukin-2 production and mitogenic response of peripheral blood mononuclear cells from young and old subjects. J Nutr 124(5): 655–663

260. Albanes D, Heinonen OP, Taylor PR et al (1996) Alpha-Tocopherol and beta-carotene supplements and lung cancer incidence in the alpha-tocopherol, beta-carotene cancer prevention study: effects of base-line characteristics and study compliance. J Natl Cancer Inst 88(21):1560–1570

261. Omenn GS, Goodman GE, Thornquist MD et al (1996) Risk factors for lung cancer and for intervention effects in CARET, the Beta-Carotene and Retinol Efficacy Trial. J Natl Cancer Inst 88(21):1550–1559

262. Goodwin JS, Bankhurst AD, Murphy SA, Selinger DS, Messner RP, Williams RC Jr (1978) Partial reversal of the cellular immune defect in common variable immunodeficiency with indomethacin. J Clin Lab Immunol 1(3):197–199

263. Hsia J, Tang T, Parrott M, Rogalla K (1994) Augmentation of the immune response to influenza vaccine by acetylsalicylic acid: a clinical trial in a geriatric population. Methods Find Exp Clin Pharmacol 16(9):677–683

264. Ceuppens JL, Rodriguez MA, Goodwin JS (1982) Non-steroidal anti-inflammatory agent inhibit the synthesis of IgM rheumatoid factor in vitro. Lancet 1(8271):528–530

265. Kiecolt-Glaser JK, Glaser R, Williger D et al (1985) Psychosocial enhancement of immunocompetence in a geriatric population. Health Psychol 4(1):25–41

266. Pennebaker JW, Kiecolt-Glaser JK, Glaser R (1988) Disclosure of traumas and immune function: health implications for psychotherapy. J Consult Clin Psychol 56(2):239–245

267. Sempowski GD, Hale LP, Sundy JS et al (2000) Leukemia inhibitory factor, oncostatin M, IL-6, and stem cell factor mRNA expression in human thymus increases with age and is associated with thymic atrophy. J Immunol 164(4):2180–2187

Chapter 5
Hematological Changes, Anemia, and Bleeding in Older Persons

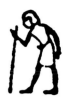

Bruce O. Hough and Gurkamal S. Chatta

Hematological changes, anemia, and bleeding in older persons

Change observed	Key points	Clinical implications
Anemia	Anemia is the most common hematologic abnormality observed in the elderly	Look for underlying cause, in particular occult gastrointestinal bleed and/or neoplasm
	Age per se is not associated with a change in baseline blood counts	
Propensity for bleeding	Bleeding disorders are more common in the elderly	Clotting factor and blood product support prior to and after surgery
Thrombophilia	Hypercoagulable states are more common in the elderly	Appropriate prophylaxis prior to and after surgery
Reduced hematopoietic reserve	Hematopoietic reserve diminishes with advancing age	Blood product support and growth factor support as indicated
	– Rate of restoration of hemoglobin levels after blood loss may be decreased	
	– Granulocyte responses to stress may be decreased	
Primary marrow disorders	Marrow disorders like myelodysplasia (MDS) and clonal hematological diseases like acute myeloid leukemia (AML), polycythemia vera (PV), essential thrombocythemia (ET), and idiopathic myelofibrosis (IMF) have a predilection for the elderly	Appropriate diagnosis and treatment

Introduction

Age-related changes in the human hematopoietic system are subtle, are often difficult to separate from coexistent comorbidities, and are of clinical import under conditions that stress hematopoiesis. Anemia is the most common age-related hematologic abnormality, and in the elderly surgical patient, proper management of disorders of hemostasis and thrombosis is particularly important. These are covered in detail in the chapter that follows. Marrow disorders such as myelodysplasia (MDS), acute myeloid leukemia (AML), monoclonal gammopathies (MG), polycythemia vera (PV), essential thrombocythemia (ET), and idiopathic myelofibrosis (IMF), all of which have a predilection for the elderly, are also discussed.

B.O. Hough (✉)
Division of Hematology/Oncology, University of Pittsburgh Medical Center, Pittsburgh, PA, USA
e-mail: houghbo@upmc.edu

Hematopoiesis [1]

The hematopoietic system derives from a small pool of hematopoietic stem cells (HSCs), which can either self-renew or differentiate along specific lineages to form mature leukocytes, erythrocytes, or platelets. HSCs differentiate into mature cells through an intermediate set of committed progenitors and precursors, each with decreasing self-renewal potential and increasing lineage commitment. Hematopoiesis is tightly regulated by a complex series of interactions between HSCs, their stromal microenvironment, and diffusible regulatory molecules, the hematopoietic growth factors (HGFs) that effect cellular proliferation. The orderly development of the hematopoietic system in vivo and the maintenance of homeostasis require that a strict balance be maintained between self-renewal, differentiation, maturation, and cell loss. A major question with regard to the aging hematopoietic system is whether or not the pluripotent hematopoietic stem cell has a finite replicative capacity. Currently, it is thought that although

R.A. Rosenthal et al. (eds.), *Principles and Practice of Geriatric Surgery*,
DOI 10.1007/978-1-4419-6999-6_5, © Springer Science+Business Media, LLC 2011

finite, the life span of HSCs is thought to be well in excess of the potential life span of a species. Accumulated DNA damage has been proposed as the principle and unifying mechanism underlying age-dependent HSC decline [2].

Evaluation of the effect of age on human hematopoiesis at the organ or cellular level demonstrates evidence of a diminished reserve capacity. Abnormalities in function, not evidenced in the basal state, become apparent in the stimulus-driven state. In addition to being lower, the aging response tends to be more variable. Given a comparable stress, hematologic abnormalities are likely to occur earlier and to be of greater severity in elderly than in younger persons. Thus, the rate of return of the hemoglobin level to normal following phlebotomy may be blunted, and the ability to mount a granulocyte response to infection may be reduced. Data from earlier studies suggest that in the setting of severe infection, older patients may have normal or suppressed granulocyte counts. However, the precise definition of "elderly" and the impact of coexistent comorbidities and concomitant medications were not accounted for in these studies [3, 4]. Based on contemporary literature, it is true that a blunted hematopoietic response to different insults may be seen in the elderly [5, 6]. However, this can be overcome by the administration of exogenous growth factors [7, 8]. Furthermore, the relative contributions of age per se and age-related comorbidities to this suboptimal response are unclear. Several elegant animal studies have shown a reduced ability of the aged hematopoietic system to respond to a sustained insult [1]. Similar studies in humans are either not feasible or have been inconclusive. It is currently believed that HSC function in humans, though finite, is well in excess of human life span. Thus, diminutions in hematopoietic reserve capacity in aging humans may only be of clinical relevance in the presence of other comorbidities (occult or latent)[1] or under conditions of extreme hematopoietic stress [1].

Thus, as we age, changes occur in multiple components of the hematologic system. In this chapter, we discuss the more commonly observed age-associated phenomena and the likely clinical consequences in the elderly surgical patient. The emphasis is on anemia and disorders of hemostasis and thrombosis.

Anemia [9, 10]

Clearly, the most common age-related hematologic abnormality, anemia, occurs in both older men and women. According to World Health Organization (WHO) criteria, anemia is diagnosed if the hemoglobin concentration (Hb) is <13 g/dL in men and <12 g/dL in women. Studies have shown a high prevalence of anemia in hospitalized older persons, patients attending geriatric clinics, and institutionalized older persons. However, if stringent criteria are employed for the selection of apparently normal subjects, the prevalence drops. Results from the third National Health and Nutrition Examination Survey (NHANES III) in the United States indicated that the prevalence of anemia was 11% in community-dwelling men and 10.2% among women over 65 years of age. Survey findings indicated further that most anemia among the elderly were mild; only 2.8% of women and 1.6% of men had a Hb<11 g/dL. NHANES III data also indicated that about 35% of all anemia among elderly individuals in the U.S. results from nutrient deficiencies (iron, vitamin B12, and/or folate); 45% of all anemia in the elderly was attributable to chronic disease/s; and in 15–20%, despite an exhaustive workup, the anemia was unexplained. In the elderly patient, extra caution must be exercised to exclude subtle iron deficiency due to either occult gastrointestinal (GI) blood loss or a GI malignancy or both.

There are few reports on the incidence of new cases of anemia in the elderly population. In the general population, the annual incidence of anemia is estimated to be 1–2%. Compared with this, the incidence of anemia in a well-defined population of elderly (>65 years of age) Whites attending the Mayo Clinic was reported to be four- to sixfold higher [11]. In this study, in every age group over 65 years, the incidence of anemia in men was higher than that in women. This has been attributed to a reduced sensitivity of erythroid progenitors to erythropoietin (EPO), secondary to declining testosterone concentrations. In several studies, the prevalence of anemia in the population over 80 years of age is reported as being 12–16% in women and 18–22% in men. At the time of diagnosis, over 50% of the patients had mild anemia (Hb>11.0 g/dL), and only 2% had a hemoglobin concentration lower than 10 g/dL [12]. In the latter cohort, over 80% of patients had a normocytic anemia, with the etiology being multifactorial.

Significantly, despite an exhaustive workup, in 15–20% of elderly persons, the cause of the anemia remained uncertain [9]. Several theories have been put forward to explain this: reduced pluripotent HSC reserve, decreased production of HGFs, reduced sensitivity of HSCs to HGFs, marrow microenvironment abnormalities, unrecognized anemia of chronic disease, occult renal failure, and undiagnosed myelodysplasia. It is also possible that age-associated increases in levels of proinflammatory cytokines, such as interleukin-6 (IL-6), may reduce the responses of stem cells to growth factors, including EPO. Results from the InChianti study have examined levels of Hb, EPO, and inflammatory molecules (C-reactive protein [CRP], IL-6, IL-1, IL-1b, and TNF-a) in 1453 elderly individuals. In this population, the inflammatory score based on the upper tertile results of the following increased with age: CRP, >3.8 mg/L; IL-6, >1.75 pg/mL; IL-1b, >0.12 pg/mL; TNF-a, >2.52 pg/mL. There was a commensurate increase in the EPO level in individuals with a normal Hb and an inappropriately low EPO level in those with anemia [13, 14].

Presentation of Anemia

The presence of multiple pathologic conditions in older persons often makes the evaluation of anemia challenging. The possibility of a multifactorial etiology – including blood loss, malnutrition, folate deficiency, or hemolysis – should always be considered when the anemia of chronic disease or inflammation is associated with a hemoglobin level below 10 g/dL. In this circumstance, laboratory investigations commonly give equivocal results; hence, a bone marrow examination may be required. Clinical judgment is critically important in deciding how aggressive the workup for anemia ought to be.

Workup of Anemia

For practical purposes, we recommend 12 g/dL as a lower limit of normal for hemoglobin for both elderly men and women. Attempting to define the cause of anemia when the hemoglobin concentration is between 12 and 14 g/dL rarely yields a cause. Even at a level of 12 g/dL, a decision as to how aggressively should a patient with borderline low hematocrit be evaluated must rest on clinical judgment. In the surgical patient, subtle changes in hemoglobin should always prompt a thorough search for subtle GI blood loss and/or an early GI malignancy, both of which increase exponentially with increasing age. Once a decision has been made to investigate low hemoglobin in an older person, the principles involved in assessment and evaluation are very similar to those that would be used in patients of any age.

The causes of the various anemias seen in elderly persons are summarized in Table 5.1 [15]. The initial approach to the patient with anemia must include a complete history and physical examination, including a rectal exam, as well as a complete blood cell count to allow evaluation of the production rate of red blood cells. Microcytosis (mean corpuscular volume [MCV] < 84) indicates an impairment of hemoglobin synthesis, and macrocytosis (MCV > 100) may be caused by

reticulocytosis or more commonly by an abnormality in nuclear maturation. Red cell production is estimated from the reticulocyte production index. Hemolytic anemia usually has a reticulocyte index greater than 3, whereas a failure of production is indicated by a reticulocyte index of less than 2. Decreased production is caused by the hypoproliferative anemias or by ineffective erythropoiesis. An elevated lactate dehydrogenase (LDH) level and indirect hyperbilirubinemia result from the increased destruction of red cell precursors in the marrow and may be used to distinguish ineffective erythropoiesis from hypoproliferative anemia. A systematic approach to the laboratory workup of anemia is illustrated in Fig. 5.1. A significantly elevated reticulocyte count, indirect hyperbilirubinemia, and an elevated LDH level are diagnostic of hemolytic anemia. A low reticulocyte count, elevated indirect bilirubin, and an elevated LDH level suggest ineffective erythropoiesis. In older persons with ineffective erythropoiesis, macrocytosis strongly suggests vitamin B_{12} or folate deficiency [16], and microcytosis should suggest sideroblastic anemia [17]. However, as alluded to earlier, anemia in the elderly may have complex pathophysiology. Hence, one must maintain a high index of suspicion for the existence of GI pathology, and every effort should be made to exclude GI blood loss and/or a GI neoplasm as the cause of the anemia.

The Hypoproliferative Anemias [9]

These are categorized as being due to (a) iron-deficient erythropoiesis, (b) lack of erythropoietin, or (c) stem cell dysfunction and/or aplastic anemia (Table 5.1)

Iron-Deficient Erythropoiesis

Inadequate iron supply for erythropoiesis is the commonest cause of anemia in the elderly. Absolute iron deficiency (blood loss) is the usual cause of iron-deficient erythropoiesis in younger persons. Blood-loss anemia, the anemia of inflammation or chronic disease, and the anemia associated with protein-energy malnutrition are the most prevalent anemias in older populations. Nutritional iron deficiency is very rare in the older age group, despite the prominence of other nutritional problems. When unexplained iron deficiency does occur, it is almost exclusively due to blood loss from the GI tract. Typical findings in blood-loss anemia are low serum iron, low serum ferritin, and high total iron-binding capacity (TIBC), reflecting absence of iron stores. Angiodysplasia of the large bowel and diverticular disease are common causes in the elderly but should be considered only after a neoplasm has been excluded. Rarely, iron deficiency can result from malabsorption or urinary losses of iron, which occurs in the face of intravascular hemolysis.

TABLE 5.1 Physiologic classification of anemia

Hypoproliferative	Ineffective	Hemolytic
1. *Iron-deficient erythropoiesis* Iron deficiency Chronic disease	1. *Macrocytic* Vitamin B12 Folic acid MDS (RA)	1. *Immunologic* Idiopathic Secondary
2. *Erythropoietin lack* Renal Endocrine	2. *Microcytic* Thalassemia Sideroblastic	2. *Intrinsic* Metabolic Abnormal Hb
3. *Stem cell dysfunction*	3. *Normocytic* MDS	3. *Extrinsic* Mechanical /toxic/viral
4. *Aplastic anemia*		

Source: Data from Chatta [15]

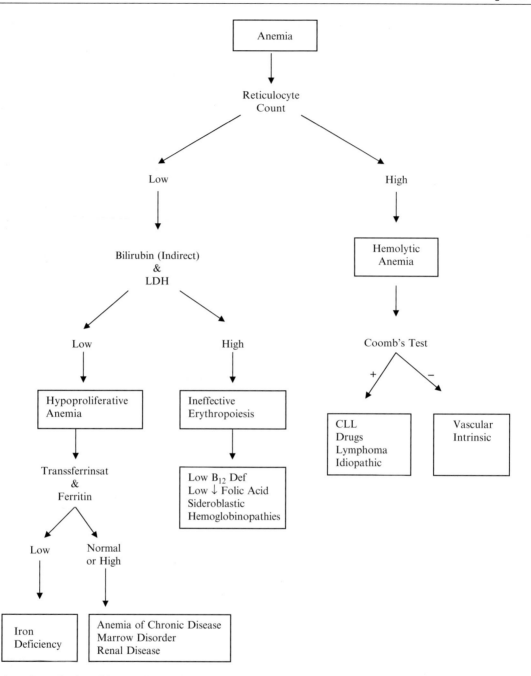

Figure 5.1 Workup of anemia (from Chatta et al. [1] Adapted with permission from The McGraw Hill Companies).

Iron-deficient erythropoiesis as opposed to absolute iron deficiency is much more common in the elderly. The former reflects a defective ability of the reticuloendothelial system to reutilize iron derived from senescent red cells. This is diagnosed by the presence of a decreased serum iron and a reduced transferrin saturation (serum iron divided by the TIBC, expressed as a percentage). Thus, tissue iron stores are normal or increased, resulting in a serum ferritin concentration above 50 ng/mL. In contrast, in the setting of blood-loss anemia, iron stores are absent or low, with a low serum ferritin and high TIBC.

The terms *anemia of inflammation* or *anemia of chronic disease* are often used to explain the anemia associated with iron-deficient erythropoiesis [18]. This occurs in major disease processes including cancer, collagen vascular disorders, rheumatoid arthritis, inflammatory bowel disease, and protein-energy malnutrition. However, laboratory parameters often can be equivocal, and it may be difficult to distinguish between iron deficiency and defective iron utilization. Hepcidin [18], a 25-amino-acid peptide produced in the liver, has been implicated in the pathogenesis of anemia of chronic disease. Hepcidin functions as a direct mediator of iron homeostasis, regulating both intestinal iron absorption as well as release of macrophage iron to erythroid progenitors. Although hepcidin levels have been reported to be increased nearly 100-fold in association with anemia of chronic disease, studies on the clinical utility of hepcidin are limited by the availability of a suitable clinical assay. The possibility of a multifactorial causation, including blood loss, malnutrition, folate deficiency, or hemolysis, should always be considered when the anemia of inflammation or chronic disease is associated with a Hb < 10 g/dL.

Lack of Erythropoietin

Decreased erythropoietin (EPO) production accounts for the anemia of end-stage renal disease and is implicated in some anemias of cancer and chronic diseases [19]. Depending on symptoms, erythroid support is recommended for patients with hemoglobin concentrations <10 g/dL. EPO has been in clinical use since 1985 for patients with end-stage renal disease. EPO treatment should be instituted after excluding hemolysis and iron deficiency. Typically, the starting dose of EPO ranges from 20,000 to 40,000 units subcutaneously every week. If required, the dosage can be escalated to 60,000 units per week. Conversely, some patients require treatment only every 2–3 weeks. Hemoglobin levels should be monitored weekly, to avoid the vascular sequelae of an iatrogenic polycythemia. This is even more true in the elderly given the higher incidence of hypertension and cerebrovascular disease. A target hemoglobin level of 11 g/dL is usually safe. The 2007 revision of the National Kidney Foundations Outcomes Quality Initiative [20] has specifically recommended targeting the hemoglobin between 11 and 12 g/dL with the recommendation to stay below 13 g/dL. No distinction is made between aged and nonaged populations in their recommendations. Most patients respond within 4–6 weeks. Iron should be added to the regimen if ferritin levels fall below 50 ng/mL.

Many cancer patients have anemia independent of any myelosuppressive therapy. The anemia is characterized by an inability to use iron stores and an inadequate EPO response, indicated by inappropriately low EPO levels. In addition, a component of the erythroid suppression is mediated by cytokines such as interleukin-1, TNF-αF, and transforming growth factor beta (TGF-β). Although the precise incidence of cancer-related anemia is not known, a number of studies have documented a decrease in transfusion frequency after treatment with EPO. If there is no reticulocyte response after 4–6 weeks of EPO treatment, therapy should be discontinued. Although it is difficult to prospectively identify responders, it has been reported that patients with endogenous EPO levels of <200 mU/mL are most likely to respond to treatment with EPO [21].

Stem Cell Dysfunction and/or Aplastic Anemia

Marrow failure due to interference with the proliferation of hematopoietic cells is seen in older adults. The disorder is generally associated with suppression of all marrow elements and is suggested by the presence of peripheral pancytopenia. Common causes include medications, immune damage to the stem-cell population, intrinsic marrow lesions, and marrow replacement by malignant cells or fibrous tissue. The latter is usually associated with a myelophthisic blood picture (nucleated RBCs, giant platelets, and metamyelocytes) as a reflection of the disruption of marrow stromal architecture. The presence of pancytopenia and the absence of iron-deficient erythropoiesis is an indication for bone marrow aspiration and biopsy. Occasionally, isolated suppression of erythropoiesis occurs, which is referred to as *pure red cell aplasia*. This disorder can be related to medication or caused by benign or malignant abnormalities of lymphocytes, including thymoma. These patients have isolated anemia, an increased serum iron, and an absence of erythroid precursors on bone marrow examination [22].

Ineffective Erythropoiesis [16]

Ineffective erythropoiesis and *macrocytic anemias* in the elderly person result from vitamin B_{12} and folate deficiency. The prevalence of pernicious anemia increases with advancing age. The disorder results from malabsorption of vitamin B_{12} as a consequence of the action of antibodies against gastric parietal cells and intrinsic factor. Atrophic gastritis and decreased secretion of intrinsic factor occur, resulting in failure of vitamin B_{12} absorption. The presence of pancytopenia, macrocytosis, hypersegmented neutrophils in the peripheral smear, a decreased reticulocyte index, an increased LDH level, and indirect hypobilirubinemia suggests a diagnosis of megaloblastic anemia. Chronic pancreatitis and diseases of the distal ileum (blind loop syndrome) may also cause vitamin B_{12} deficiency. Folate deficiency of sufficient severity to cause anemia in the elderly person is rare. Alcohol and various other drugs are also known to interfere with folate absorption and metabolism. Vulnerability to deficiency is significantly greater when folate requirements are increased as a result of inflammation, neoplastic disease, or hemolytic anemia.

Vitamin B_{12}, Folate, and Homocysteine [16]

In epidemiologic studies, approximately 10% of apparently healthy persons aged 70 years and over were found to have vitamin B_{12} levels that are deficient, and 5–10% were found to have low folate values. These low values may be clinically important, and there is evidence that even low normal vitamin B_{12} levels may contribute to cognitive decline in older adults. Hence, vitamin B_{12} and folate should be aggressively replaced in the elderly. Even in patients with atrophic gastritis, oral vitamin B_{12} is generally adequate; 10% will be absorbed by mass action alone and not require the presence of intrinsic factor. Thus, a daily dose of 1 mg (1,000 mcg) of vitamin B_{12} will replete a person with concentrations in the low-to-normal range. Parenteral replacement should be used in severe deficiencies with vitamin B_{12}, i.e., concentrations <100 pg/mL.

In older adults with low normal (≤350 pg/mL) B_{12} concentrations, methylmalonic acid (MMA) concentrations may be more sensitive for excluding metabolically active B_{12} deficiency. Renal failure can artificially increase the serum MMA concentration. In patients with low-normal B_{12} concentrations and macrocytosis (with or without anemia), vitamin replacement should be considered, particularly if the MMA concentration is increased. Low concentrations of vitamin B_{12} or folate are also accompanied by increased concentrations of homocysteine. In recent years, studies have focused on the role of raised homocysteine levels in coronary artery disease risk. A relationship may exist between coronary artery disease and low vitamin B_{12} and elevated homocysteine in older persons. Levels of homocysteine can be reduced by prescribing 400 µg of folic acid once or twice daily. Empiric prescription of vitamin B_{12} or folate for older persons with ischemic heart disease may be reasonable.

The major causes of ineffective erythropoiesis and *microcytosis* are thalassemia and the sideroblastic anemias. Although thalassemia is generally diagnosed at an earlier age, there are reports of its initial detection in older people. Mild anemia, a disproportionately low MCV, and the absence of iron deficiency usually points to a diagnosis of thalassemia trait, a condition of little or no clinical consequence. Iron supplements have no role in the treatment of thalassemia trait; on the contrary, they can be detrimental. Acquired sideroblastic anemia, although uncommon, is primarily a disease of elderly persons [18]. It is a heterogeneous group of disorders characterized by the presence of iron deposits in the mitochondria of normoblasts. The disorder is a consequence of impaired heme synthesis. It usually reflects an intrinsic marrow lesion (idiopathic) but may be secondary to inflammation, neoplasia, or drug ingestion. The common finding is the presence of a dimorphic red cell population, in part markedly hypochromic and in part well filled with hemoglobin. The diagnosis is made by the demonstration of ringed sideroblasts in the bone marrow as well as the presence of maturation abnormalities of myeloid and erythroid precursors. A fraction of elderly patients (<5%) with sideroblastic anemia show some response to pharmacologic doses of pyridoxine (200 mg three times daily).

The *myelodysplastic syndromes (MDS)* [17, 23] are a group of stem-cell disorders characterized by disordered hematopoiesis that occur primarily in the elderly age group. Refractory anemia and refractory anemia with ringed sideroblasts account for 25–30% of the MDS syndromes. Refractory anemia commonly presents as a macrocytic anemia with marrow erythroid hyperplasia and relatively normal myeloid and megakaryocytic lineages. Cytogenetic abnormalities are relatively common in MDS, and one of particular interest in elderly patients is deletion of the long arm of chromosome 5 (5q−). The median age at presentation of the 5q− syndrome is 68 years with a female:male ratio of 7:3 [24]. The syndrome is characterized by macrocytic anemia, modest leukopenia, normal or increased platelet counts, and marrow erythroid hypoplasia or hyperplasia. Di Guglielmo's syndrome is another stem-cell disorder that is more common in older people; patients present with anemia that is characterized by megaloblastic erythroid precursors, dysplastic myeloid cells, and hyperplasia in the marrow. The disease usually evolves into an erythroleukemia, with an associated pancytopenia and the presence of nucleated red cells, and immature myeloid and megakaryocytic precursors in the circulation.

Treatment of MDS in the elderly person till now has been primarily supportive. However, recent advances in elucidating the molecular basis of MDS have identified hypermethylation of the promoter region as an important mechanism of gene silencing. Treatment with hypomethylating agents can restore gene expression and induce differentiation of hematopoietic progenitors in MDS. Thus far, 5-azacytidine and decitabine (both hypomethylating agents) have been FDA-approved for the treatment of MDS [25, 26]. Immunomodulatory agents such as lenalidomide are also currently being evaluated for high-risk MDS patients (especially those with a 5q− abnormality) [27].

Hemolytic Anemias [9]

The causes of hemolytic anemia in elderly persons are somewhat different than in younger persons. Autoimmune hemolytic anemia (AHA) is the commonest cause in the elderly age group; the diagnosis is made by the presence of a positive Coombs' test. In an elderly population, the anemia is likely to be associated with a lymphoproliferative disorder (non-Hodgkin's lymphoma or chronic lymphocytic leukemia), collagen vascular disease, or drug ingestion. Corticosteroids and splenectomy are usually effective in patients with red cell antibodies of the immunoglobulin G (IgG) type.

A disorder of some importance in older adults is microangiopathic hemolytic anemia [28], secondary to either disseminated intravascular coagulation (DIC) or occurring as a manifestation of the syndrome of thrombotic thrombocytopenic purpura (TTP). DIC is usually associated with severe infections or disseminated neoplasm and presents not only with hemolysis but also with a consumptive coagulopathy [29]. The presence of red cell fragmentation, thrombocytopenia, a prolonged prothrombin time and prolonged partial thromboplastin time, and hemosiderinuria suggests this diagnosis. Treatment of DIC entails treating the underlying disorder, as well as blood product support (including fresh frozen plasma and cryoprecipitate as needed). TTP is characterized by the pentad of fever, intravascular hemolysis, thrombocytopenia, neurologic symptoms, and renal dysfunction [30, 31]. In contrast to DIC, in TTP, both the prothrombin time and partial thromboplastin time are normal. Early diagnosis is imperative, as TTP responds very well to treatment with plasmapheresis [29, 32].

Hemolysis is also associated with prosthetic heart valves. In different series, the incidence of hemolysis varies from 5 to 35% and is conditioned by a variety of factors, most of which relate to the type of valve implanted and to the hemodynamic conditions following implantation [33]. However, the anemia is seldom severe, and both the presence and degree of hemolysis is assessed on the basis of the level of serum lactic dehydrogenase and serum haptoglobin and the presence and amount of reticulocytes and schistocytes in the peripheral blood. Treatment of hemolysis includes the supplementation of iron and folate when their deficiency is evident. The use of β-blockers appears to decrease the severity of hemolysis, likely because of the induction of bradycardia and of their negative inotropic effects. In a recent report of 278 patients, for both mitral and aortic valves, at 12 months, mild subclinical hemolysis was identified in 26% of patients with a mechanical prosthesis and 5% with a bioprosthesis ($P<0.001$) [33].

Hemostasis and Thrombosis

Platelet counts do not change with aging, but the concentrations of a large number of coagulation enzymes have been shown to increase with age [34]. These include factors VII, VIII, and fibrinogen. In centenarians, highly significant increases in the concentrations of these factors are noted, as are levels of factors IX, X, and thrombin–antithrombin complexes. Fibrin formation is also increased, as evidenced by higher concentrations of fibrinopeptide A. In addition, elevated levels of d-dimers suggest increased hyperfibrinolysis. Hyperhomocysteinemia, secondary to low B_{12} levels, is also more common in the elderly. Thus, aging may be accompanied by increased hypercoagulability, as supported by Silverstein's retrospective review, demonstrating an increase in the incidence of deep vein thrombosis (DVT) and pulmonary embolism (PE) in the elderly [35].

The coagulation cascade can be viewed as two intimately related processes. The *first* is the formation of the *platelet*

Table 5.2 Disorders of bleeding and clotting

Disorders of bleeding	
Acquired	**Congenital**
Common	von Willebrand's disease
Drugs-iatrogenic	
Sepsis	
DIC	
Malnutrition, vitamin K deficiency	
End-stage liver disease	
Loss of elastin/structural	
Chronic renal insufficiency	
Unusual	
ITP	
Factor VIII inhibitor	
Fibrinolysis after bladder or liver surgery	

Disorders of clotting in the elderly	
Acquired	**Congenital**
Common	Prothrombin Gene mutation
Lupus anticoagulant	Factor V Leiden
Central venous catheters	
Drugs-estrogens	
Heparin-induced thrombocytopenia	
Malignancy, especially pancreatic, ovarian, glioblastoma Multiforme (GBM)	
Immobility, venous stasis	
Unusual	
Essential thrombocytosis	
Paroxysmal Nocturnal Hemoglobinuria	
Polycythemia Vera	

plug that occurs with vascular injury when the basement membrane is exposed to blood and platelets. Adherent platelets attract fibrinogen to bind together multiple platelets along with von Willebrand Factor (vWF) that attaches to platelet glycoprotein IIB/IIIA. This process causes *primary hemostasis*. The second simultaneous process is activation of the clotting cascade, which results in conversion of fibrinogen to fibrin by thrombin, allowing the fibrin to crosslink, thereby making the primary plug stronger. A comprehensive review of the clotting cascade is beyond the scope of this chapter, but it is well summarized in Alving and Kitchens [36]. There are multiple sites along this cascade that both drugs and disease act to either disrupt or facilitate hemostasis. We first discuss the most common causes of excessive bleeding in the elderly surgical patient and then follow with the most common causes of excessive clotting or thrombophilia. Table 5.2 lists the most common causes of bleeding and clotting in the elderly.

Bleeding Diathesis

Unexplained bruises, repeated nosebleeds, gastrointestinal losses, or excessive blood loss during surgery or following dental extraction are common presentations. In these patients, screening platelet counts and coagulation studies should be obtained.

Platelets

Thrombocytopenia is a common cause of bleeding problems in older persons [32]. A level less than 100,000 per μL is considered significant, but bleeding usually occurs at much lower levels. Common causes include decreased production of platelets in the bone marrow, sequestration in enlarged spleens, and increased peripheral destruction. Decreased production of platelets in older persons is most commonly associated with drugs that suppress platelet production. The major cause of increased peripheral destruction is immune thrombocytopenia, secondary to either drugs or an underlying lymphoproliferative disorder [37, 38]. Tests of platelet aggregation are useful in detecting disorders of platelet function.

Treatment of thrombocytopenia depends upon the cause. For decreased production, platelet transfusion should be considered if there is significant blood loss, irrespective of the platelet count. Generally, spontaneous bleeding occurs when the count drops to 20,000 per μL or less. Immune thrombocytopenia is typically treated with a trial of corticosteroids and/or IVIG. Isolated thrombocytopenia in the elderly person should prompt a workup to exclude MDS. DIC and TTP are also important causes of thrombocytopenia in the elderly group, which ought to be recognized and treated appropriately. For most surgical procedures, the platelet count should be maintained over 75,000–100,000 per μL (see under "Blood Products and Transfusions") [39]. Platelet function disorders, although uncommon, can cause significant bleeding and are often medication-related. Patients on treatment with either vitamin K antagonists or oral direct thrombin inhibitors are also prone to bleeding in the context of supratherapeutic dosing. The common offending agents include:

(i) *Aspirin (ASA)*, which causes irreversible, noncompetitive inhibition of cyclooxygenase (COX), an enzyme necessary for the formation of thromboxane, a prostaglandin that activates platelets. ASA is a more potent inhibitor of COX-1 than it is of COX-2. COX-1 is the enzyme that catalyzes thromboxane, while COX-2 is the enzyme that catalyzes prostacyclin, a prostaglandin that causes platelet inhibition and vascular dilation. Given that this action is irreversible and given that platelets have a half-life of 5–7 days, aspirin should be held for 7 days prior to an intervention expected to cause bleeding. NSAIDS inhibit both COX-1 and COX-2, and given that they are competitive inhibitors, their action is shorter than that of aspirin. Additionally, the NSAIDs do not cause the same degree of platelet inhibition as aspirin does.

(ii) *Clopidogrel (Plavix)* is a medication used for platelet inhibition in atherosclerotic disease of the heart, brain, or peripheral arteries. It acts by inhibiting the binding of ADP to the platelet which normally results in platelet activation. This inhibition remains for the life of the platelet and thus the action of clopidogrel is irreversible [40]. Hence, in the event of bleeding, the only available treatment is platelet transfusion.

(iii) *Vitamin K antagonists* (VKA) such as Coumadin are medications used to inhibit the production of clotting factors II, VII, IX, and X, as well as protein C and protein S. Bleeding secondary to overanticoagulation is not uncommon. Fortunately, VKAs can be reversed either immediately by giving the patient fresh frozen plasma or nonemergently by giving excess vitamin K orally or intravenously.

(iv) *Thrombin inhibitors*: these are new medications [41] including lepirudin, argatroban, and bivalirudin which directly inhibit thrombin rather than acting through antithrombin as heparin does. They are used in patients who have been diagnosed with heparin-induced thrombocytopenia (HIT). As discussed below, HIT is paradoxical in that despite a declining platelet count, the risk for thrombosis is increased. This is due to an immune reaction resulting in platelet clumping. In these patients, it is necessary to give anticoagulants until the platelet count rises above 150,000 or longer if the patient has a resultant clot.

Hereditary Factor Deficiencies

Unprovoked bleeding may also be caused by hereditary von Willebrand's disease, which may present initially in older persons. The disease is caused by a reduction in concentration of von Willebrand's factor (vWF) that is accompanied by reductions in factor-VIII concentrations. vWF is essential for normal platelet function, and so bleeding occurs because of a platelet function defect. Acquired von Willebrand's disease, although rare, is a disease of older persons. It is commonly associated with monoclonal gammopathies, lymphomas, or myeloma [42, 43]. When treatment is necessary, desmopressin acetate (DDAVP) may be used for type I vWF. Type II disease, which is characterized by normal concentration of an abnormal protein, requires individualized treatment. DDAVP is a synthetic analog of arginine vasopressin that stimulates endothelial cells to release stored vWF. Treatment is often successful, but adverse effects are common. In this instance, factor VIII concentrates that have high doses of vWF should be used [44].

Acquired Factor Deficiencies

Bleeding can also occur because of clotting factor deficiencies, which in the elderly person are usually acquired and caused by the presence of circulating clotting factor inhibitors. The most common is an acquired inhibitor to factor VIII. The onset is often sudden, titers to anti-factor VIII antibodies can be very high, and presentation is with bleeding into joints and muscle, similar to that in hemophilia A [45]. The characteristic laboratory abnormality is a prolonged PTT that does not correct with a mixing test. Treatment involves factor replacement. Depending on the severity, prednisone or cyclophosphamide may also be needed.

Deficiency of the vitamin K-dependent clotting factors tends to occur in older persons with major illnesses. Disorders of the hepatobiliary tree, antibiotics that neutralize bowel bacteria (a major source of the vitamin), malabsorption, and severe malnutrition are the causes. Even if the patient was not prescribed warfarin, inappropriate use must be considered. The deficits are readily treated with vitamin K. Liver disease must always be considered in patients who present with excessive bleeding. The prothrombin time is prolonged even in mild to moderate liver disease. The partial thromboplastin time remains normal until liver disease becomes severe. With the exception of factor VIII (which is produced by endothelial cells), liver disease causes reductions in all clotting factors. Liver disease is also associated with DIC. Fibrin degradation products are not cleared as well, and platelet function may be affected. The treatment of a bleeding diathesis in liver disease is fresh frozen plasma [44]. A bleeding disorder will be thought of only if it is appropriately included in a differential diagnosis. This particularly applies to chronic blood loss from the gastrointestinal system. In patients for whom endoscopic evaluation does not identify a cause, careful evaluation of platelets, including platelet functions and coagulation, should always be considered.

Workup of a Patient with a Bleeding Disorder

The cornerstone of the workup remains a thorough personal and family history. This helps narrow the differential into an acquired or congenital coagulopathy. In the elderly patient without a history of bleeding, a coagulopathy is likely to be acquired if hemostatic stress has been tolerated in the past. To that end, care must be taken to ask about childbirth, types of prior surgery including dental extraction, and any blood products required after any surgical procedure.

All patients with a new bleeding disorder should have a CBC and PT/PTT performed. If those tests are unrevealing, hematology consultation should be requested to evaluate for more unusual problems. If the PT or PTT is prolonged, a mixing study should be obtained to determine if there is a factor deficiency or the presence of a circulating inhibitor. If the CBC reveals a thrombocytopenia that is a potential contributor, care must be taken with both current and recent medications to exclude an iatrogenic cause.

Thrombophilia

The risk for unprovoked venous thromboembolism increases with age [34, 46]. There is a constant balance in our body between clotting and fibrinolysis to maintain homeostasis. Aging and the diseases associated with it alter this balance through several different mechanisms. The LITE study (Longitudinal Investigation of Thromboembolism etiology) evaluated cohorts from two separate studies to determine the risk factors for thromboembolism: Atherosclerosis Risk In Communities (ARIC) study and the Cardiovascular Health Study (CHS). Analysis of those combined cohorts identified a clear increase in incidence of venous thromboembolism with age [47, 48]. A detailed discussion regarding the inherited causes of thrombophilia (including Protein C, S, and Antithrombin C deficiency) are beyond the scope of this review and may not be especially pertinent to the elderly population. However, the acquired causes of thrombophilia are pertinent and are especially helpful to determine the risk of postoperative venous thrombosis in an elderly surgical patient. Some of the common causes of acquired thrombophilia in the elderly are listed in Table 5.3.

Acquired thrombophilia may be either drug-related (estrogens, heparin, thalidomide, lenalidomide, etc.) or secondary to disease. Cancer increases the risk of thrombosis through increased production and expression of tissue factor and other procoagulable factors, which trigger the coagulation cascade. Some malignancies, such as pancreatic adenocarcinoma, ovarian cancer and glioblastoma multiforme have especially high rates of thrombosis, approaching a 5–6% incidence

Table 5.3 Common causes of acquired thrombophilia in the elderly

Malignancy – all, but especially ovarian, pancreatic, glioblastoma multiforme (GBM)
Immobility, venous stasis
Smoking
Thalidomide treatment for myeloma
Lupus anticoagulant
Paroxysmal nocturnal hemoglobinuria (PNH)
Lupus anticoagulant
Nephrotic syndrome with ATIII deficiency/loss
Central venous catheters
Intimal injury
Myeloproliferative disorders (CML, ET, PV, IMF)
Hormone replacement therapy (maybe)
Heparin-induced thrombophilia

among patients with metastatic disease [47]. These tumors occasionally present with thrombosis as the sentinel event in their cancer diagnosis. Moreover, once diagnosed, the several treatments for malignancy increase the risk of thrombosis. One such example is the use of thalidomide and lenalidomide (Revlimid) for the treatment of multiple myeloma [49]. Cytotoxic chemotherapy through the destruction of tumor and the resultant spillage of tissue factor into the circulation may increase the risk of thrombosis. Immobility and venous stasis further increase the risk of clot, as does venous stasis from a bulky pelvic lymphadenopathy and/or tumor.

Heparin-Induced Thrombocytopenia [50]

HIT is an immune disorder that causes platelet clumping and activation. This clumping and activation causes a reduction in the circulating platelet count while increasing the risk for both arterial and venous clotting. Patients who are on chronic heparin are the least likely to develop HIT, while those undergoing large joint repair or replacement with postoperative heparin are the most likely to develop HIT. Definitive diagnosis is challenging in that the most available test, the platelet factor 4 antibody test, has a high false positive rate. Therefore, the patient's pretest probability has to be taken into account when interpreting the test. The pretest probability is derived by evaluating four factors – *timing* of heparin (usually 5–10 days after initiation), rate and magnitude of *thrombocytopenia* (a 50% drop in platelets and a count of >20,000), *thrombosis* or skin necrosis, and lack of alternative causes of *thrombocytopenia* [51]. This 4 T's scoring system for the evaluation of HIT has recently been validated both retrospectively and prospectively (Table 5.4). If the diagnosis of HIT is likely, patients should be started on a direct thrombin inhibitor while waiting for the result of the test. If the PF4 antibody test is discordant with the clinical picture, a confirmatory test, the serotonin release assay, can be done. It has a high specificity, but a low sensitivity. Unfortunately, this test is done in only a few reference laboratories in the country and seldom impacts clinical management in real time.

The Lupus Anticoagulant [52, 53]

The Lupus anticoagulant (LAC) is a contradictory term in that it gives rise to a procoagulant state and can occur in patients without lupus. It is due to acquired antibodies to phospholipids that can cause an increase in laboratory parameters (PT and PTT) used for assaying time to clotting. These circulating antibodies interfere with the phospholipids reagents used in the in vitro assays, causing a prolongation of the PT and/or PTT. In contrast, "in vivo," these antibodies have the potential of binding procoagulation factors and triggering the clotting cascade. The classic presentation is that of a patient with prolonged aPTT, either asymptomatic or in the setting of a recently diagnosed unprovoked clot. While the diagnosis of LAC in a patient with thrombosis should prompt initiation of anticoagulation, the asymptomatic presence of a LAC does not require prophylactic anticoagulation. In terms of surgical prophylaxis, patients with a clear history of a clot in the past and a positive LAC need aggressive postoperative DVT prophylaxis if they are not already on anticoagulation. Management of perioperative anticoagulation is beyond the scope of this text, but the reader is directed towards an excellent review of the recently published guidelines from the ACCP [54], summarized in Table 5.5.

Myeloproliferative Disorders [55]

The Philadelphia chromosome-negative chronic myeloproliferative disorders, namely, polycythemia vera (PV), essential thrombocythemia (ET), and idiopathic myelofibrosis (IMF), occur primarily in the elderly age group and are characterized by the involvement of a multipotent hematopoietic progenitor cell. Marrow hypercellularity, overproduction of one or more marrow lineages, thrombotic and hemorrhagic diatheses, exuberant extramedullary hematopoiesis, and a slow rate of spontaneous transformation to acute leukemia are hallmarks of these disorders. Thus, PV [56] (excess production of red cells), ET [55] (excess production of platelets), and IMF [57] (extramedullary hematopoiesis) have a long natural history, distinguishing them from chronic myeloid leukemia, the

TABLE 5.4 Pretest probability of HIT: the 4 T's score

Points	2	1	0
Thrombocytopenia	>50% drop; nadir>20K	30–50% drop; nadir 10–19K	<30% drop; nadir<10K
Timing of drop in platelets	5–10 Days	>10 days	<4 Days (1st exposure)
Thrombosis	Yes	Suspected	None
OTher causes of low platelets	None	Possible	Definite

Source: Adapted from Pouplard et al. [51], with permission from Wiley-Blackwell
Score 0–3: <5% likelihood of HIT
Score 4–5: 10–30% likelihood of HIT
Score 6–8: 40–80% likelihood of HIT

TABLE 5.5   AACP guidelines for prevention of venous thrombosis

Type of surgery	Recommendation
Hip or knee replacement	LMWH or Arixtra starting 12–24 h after surgery, or VKA started the evening before surgery
Hip-fracture surgery	LMWH, LDUH, or VKA
Length of anticoagulant for hip or knee surgery	>10 Days up to 35 days
General surgery low risk	Early ambulation
General surgery mod-high risk	LMWH, LDUH tid, Arixtra
At risk for both bleeding/thrombosis	Mechanical thromboprophylaxis with GCS and IPC

LMWH low-molecular-weight heparin, i.e., enoxaparin (Lovenox) or dalteparin (Fragmin); *LDUH* low-dose unfractionated heparin; *VKA* vitamin K antagonist, i.e., Coumadin; *GCS* graduated compression stockings; *IPC* intermittent pneumatic compression; *ACCP* American College of Chest Physicians
Source: Data from Geerts et al. [54]

Philadelphia chromosome-positive myeloproliferative disorder, which progresses and transforms much more rapidly. The main cause of morbidity and mortality in PV and ET is thrombosis, which occurs more commonly in older patients or in those with previous vascular complications. Severe bleeding is rare and limited to patients with a very high platelet count or to those taking antiplatelet drugs. Since there is no curative therapy for PV and ET, the goals of therapy are to minimize thrombotic and bleeding risk and prevent progression to marrow fibrosis or acute leukemia, or both.

The risk of thrombotic events in PV is highest in patients aged 60 years or older and those with a prior history of thrombosis. The Italian PV study group demonstrated a 3.4% yearly risk of thrombosis following diagnosis. The recommendations for the treatment of PV are as follows: (a) phlebotomy in all patients to keep the hematocrit below 45% and (b) myelosuppressive agents in patients at high risk of thrombosis (>60 years of age) and in those with excessive phlebotomy requirements. Finally, all patients with PV should be treated with low-dose aspirin, as there is a 59% reduction in cardiovascular mortality, with a nonsignificant risk of increased bleeding. The incidence of thrombotic and hemorrhagic complications in ET ranges from 7 to 17% and 8 to 14%.respectively. Age over 60 years, a prior thrombotic event, and a long duration of thrombocytosis are the major risk factors for thrombotic events. A very high platelet count (1.5 million/cmm) is a risk factor for both thrombosis and bleeding. Consensus-based practice guidelines for ET include: (a) observation in asymptomatic low-risk patients with platelet counts below 1.5 million/cmm, (b) hydroxyurea plus aspirin in high-risk patients with a platelet count over 1.5 million/cmm. Anagrelide, a new antiplatelet agent, is also very effective at reducing high platelet counts. However, its efficacy as compared with hydroxyurea in reducing thrombotic events remains to be proven in a randomized controlled trial. An elderly patient with PV or ET should have a hematology consultation prior to surgery. Management for the elderly surgical patient with PV or ET has to be individualized based on prior thrombosis history, current platelet count, type of surgery, risk of anticoagulation, etc.

Mechanical Causes

Central venous catheters (CVC) also increase the risk of thrombosis through several mechanisms including foreign body reaction, local stasis, and intimal injury. For patients with symptomatic clot, most clinicians treat by first removing the catheter. The current ACCP (American College of Chest Physicians) guidelines [54] recommend treating an upper extremity clot in the same manner as a lower extremity clot. Therefore, catheter removal is most often supplemented with anticoagulation. For symptomatic patients in whom the CVC is critical, catheters may be left in place and the clot treated with anticoagulants, usually delivered through the line. Since many of these cases are complex, decision making about catheter removal and anticoagulation needs to be individualized.

Two other important questions often arise when discussing central venous catheters. The first is whether patients with CVCs benefit from prophylaxis with low-dose Coumadin prior to the formation of a clot. Unfortunately, data regarding primary prevention with Coumadin is conflicting [58]. The second centers on whether patients with asymptomatic clots should be treated. Treatment of asymptomatic clots is also controversial, given the high frequency with which the ends of catheters become clogged with fibrinous debris. The ACCP [54] makes a distinction between those clots that *do not cause swelling* and those clots *that do* and recommends treating clots that cause swelling. What is less clear is what do to about large, asymptomatic clots found on routine imaging that do not cause swelling. Most clinicians would treat patients with symptomatic clot in a CVC and remove the catheter if the indication for placement has expired. However, the most common scenario is a patient who continues to require a CVC and develops a symptomatic clot.

Workup of a Patient with a Clotting Disorder

In a patient with a new unprovoked clot, attention should be given to finding an underlying cause for clotting. In the elderly patient, this is most likely to be due to an acquired cause (Table 5.2). The first course of action is to check a CBC and PT/PTT. A prolonged PTT in a patient with a recent clot is highly suggestive of the antiphospholipid syndrome (aka lupus anticoagulant). However, 40% of patients with a LAC do not have a prolonged PTT, so additional testing is required for evaluation. A high hemoglobin or platelet count in a patient with a recent clot is suggestive of one of the myeloproliferative disorders mentioned above (PV or ET). Lastly, pancytopenia with a recent unexplained clot should prompt concern for paroxysmal nocturnal hemoglobinuria (PNH), a stem cell disorder. Ideally, testing for thrombophilias should be ordered prior to anticoagulation. If there is a concern about what tests to send, draw three blue top tubes from the patient and set aside on ice prior to initiating anticoagulation. Anticoagulation is typically initiated with a heparin, either unfractionated (intravenous) or low-molecular-weight heparin (LMWH) [59]. LMWH is easy to administer (subcutaneous), can be given in an outpatient setting, and does not require regular monitoring like heparin. However, its half-life is much longer and it cannot be reversed as easily with protamine. Therefore, the specific clinical situation will dictate which initial heparin is used to eventually bridge to Coumadin [60]. In the presence of a history of HIT, initial anticoagulation needs to be initiated with a direct thrombin inhibitor (DTI). The choice of a DTI is often dictated by the presence or absence of normal renal and liver function [41].

Blood Products and Transfusions [32, 39, 44, 61, 62]

Blood products commonly available for transfusion include packed red blood cells (pRBC), platelets, plasma, cryoprecipitate, and recombinant clotting factors. These products are made by separating single units of blood from donors. Platelets acquired from one donation are pooled into a larger unit along with 3–4 other donors. One unit of pRBCs is expected to increase the hemoglobin of a 70-kg patient by 1 g/dL. One 4–5 pack of platelets is expected to increase the platelet count of a 70-kg patient by 10×10^9 cells/L).

The indications for transfusion have changed over the last decade, bear repetition, and are summarized in Table 5.6 [61]. It has been previously felt to be advantageous for sicker patients to have a hemoglobin level closer to 10 g/dL, to allow for maximum oxygen exchange. Hebert et al. have recently compared an aggressive versus a restrictive

transfusion regimen in critically ill patients and found the restrictive strategy to be at least as effective and possibly superior with a lower hospital mortality rate among those in the restrictive group (22.2% vs. 28.1%, $P = 0.05$) Therefore, most clinicians feel that in patients who are not actively bleeding, who have not received myelotoxic treatment, and who are not having active cardiac or cerebral ischemia, the transfusion threshold should be closer to or below 8 g/dl [32, 61] However, in the elderly patient with compromised cardiac function, a higher hemoglobin threshold for transfusion may be appropriate, i.e., Hb at or around 10 g/dl.

Platelet transfusions occur in two broad categories – prophylactic, to prevent spontaneous bleeding or bleeding during a procedure, and therapeutic, when a patient is actively bleeding with a low platelet count. The current consensus is that the platelet count should be over 50×10^9/L for surgical procedures and over 100×10^9/L for neurologic and ophthalmologic procedures. Most consensus papers adhere to these guidelines [39].

Transfusion of plasma products for prophylaxis for a procedure is another common hematologic question in the surgical setting. Thus, fresh frozen plasma (FFP) contains normal levels of all coagulation factors and is typically administered at a dose of 10–20 mL/kg (3–6 units), to correct a significant coagulopathy. Indications for the use of FFP include: (a) active bleeding/invasive procedure with PT > 3 s above normal (INR > 1.5), (b) massive transfusion and bleeding with proven coagulopathy, (c) congenital deficiency of factors II, V, X, XI, XII, or XIII, (d) emergency reversal of warfarin overdose, since immediate oral or intravenous vitamin K reversal takes 6–8 h, and (e) in the setting of plasmapheresis for TTP. The volume of one unit of plasma is approximately 220 mL. Since plasma stays in the vascular space, caution should be used in those patients prone to volume overload [44].

Other types of blood products include cryoprecipitate as well as factor replacements and most recently activated factor VII, which can be used to overcome factor VIII inhibitors found in patients with hemophilia or in the elderly. Each unit of cryoprecipitate (15–20 mL) contains (a) fibrinogen (150–250 mg), (b) vWF, factor VIII (80–100 units), (c) factor XIII, and (d) fibronectin. Typically, it is administered as a pool of 6 units. Indications for the use of cryoprecipitate include: severe DIC, congenital or acquired hypofibrinogenemia, and uremic bleeding diathesis unresponsive to DDAVP [44, 63]. It is no longer used for von Willebrand's Disease or hemophilia due to availability of factor concentrates. Evidence-based guidelines for blood product administration are reviewed in more detail in the references listed above.

In summary, aging is associated with an increasing incidence of anemia and an increasing frequency of problems associated with hemostasis and thrombosis. The latter, particularly in the perioperative setting, can be challenging and require timely hematologic consultation.

TABLE 5.6 Indications for transfusion

Transfusion type	Trigger	Grade of evidence
Anemia in the steady state	7 g/dL	RCT[a]
Plasma for coagulopathy	INR ≥ 1.5	Lab/correlative
Platelets for major surgery	50×10^9/L	Consensus
Platelet for neuro- or ophthalmologic surgery	100×10^9/L	Consensus
Platelets for prophylaxis in AML	10×10^9/L	RCT[b,c]

RCT randomized clinical trial
[a]Hebert et al. [61]
[b]Rebulla et al (1997) NEJM 337(26):1872–1875
[c]Wandt et al (1998) Blood 91(10):3601–3606

References

1. Chatta GS, Lipschitz DA (2008) Anemia. In: Hazzard W et al (eds) Principles of geriatric medicine and gerontology. McGraw-Hill, New York
2. Rossi DJ et al (2007) Deficiencies in DNA damage repair limit the function of haematopoietic stem cells with age. Nature 447(7145): 725–729
3. Corberand J et al (1981) Polymorphonuclear functions and aging in humans. J Am Geriatr Soc 29(9):391–397
4. Sasso RD, Hanna EA, Moore DL (1970) Leukocytic and neutrophilic counts in acute appendicitis. Am J Surg 120(5):563–566
5. Hodkinson CF et al (2006) Whole blood analysis of phagocytosis, apoptosis, cytokine production, and leukocyte subsets in healthy older men and women: the ZENITH study. J Gerontol A Biol Sci Med Sci 61(9):907–917
6. Plackett TP et al (2004) Aging and innate immune cells. J Leukoc Biol 76(2):291–299
7. Chatta GS et al (1994) Effects of in vivo recombinant methionyl human granulocyte colony-stimulating factor on the neutrophil response and peripheral blood colony-forming cells in healthy young and elderly adult volunteers. Blood 84(9):2923–2929
8. Smith TJ et al (2006) 2006 update of recommendations for the use of white blood cell growth factors: an evidence-based clinical practice guideline. J Clin Oncol 24(19):3187–3205
9. Eisenstaedt R, Penninx BW, Woodman RC (2006) Anemia in the elderly: current understanding and emerging concepts. Blood Rev 20(4):213–226
10. Spivak JL (2005) Anemia in the elderly: time for new blood in old vessels? Arch Intern Med 165(19):2187–2189
11. Ania BJ et al (1997) Incidence of anemia in older people: an epidemiologic study in a well defined population. J Am Geriatr Soc 45(7):825–831
12. Guralnik JM et al (2004) Prevalence of anemia in persons 65 years and older in the United States: evidence for a high rate of unexplained anemia. Blood 104(8):2263–2268
13. Ferrucci L et al (2007) Unexplained anaemia in older persons is characterised by low erythropoietin and low levels of pro-inflammatory markers. Br J Haematol 136(6):849–855
14. Ferrucci L et al (2004) Circulating erythropoietin (EPO) and pro-inflammatory markers in elderly (>/=65) persons with and without anemia. Blood ASH Annu Meet Abstr 104:453a, Abstract 1629
15. Chatta G (2009) In: Geriatrics Review Syllabus (GRS), MKSAP
16. Clarke R et al (2004) Vitamin B12 and folate deficiency in later life. Age Ageing 33(1):34–41
17. Tefferi A, Vardiman JW (2009) Myelodysplastic syndromes. N Engl J Med 361(19):1872–1885
18. Weiss G, Goodnough LT (2005) Anemia of chronic disease. N Engl J Med 352(10):1011–1023
19. Drueke TB et al (2006) Normalization of hemoglobin level in patients with chronic kidney disease and anemia. N Engl J Med 355(20):2071–2084
20. KDOQI; National Kidney Foundation (2006) KDOQI Clinical Practice Guidelines and Clinical Practice Recommendations for Anemia in Chronic Kidney Disease. Am J Kidney Dis 47(5 Suppl 3):S11–S145
21. Lichtin A (2005) The ASH/ASCO clinical guidelines on the use of erythropoietin. Best Pract Res Clin Haematol 18(3):433–438
22. Renoult E et al (2006) Recurrent anemia in kidney transplant recipients with parvovirus B19 infection. Transplant Proc 38(7): 2321–2323
23. Estey E (2007) Acute myeloid leukemia and myelodysplastic syndromes in older patients. J Clin Oncol 25(14):1908–1915
24. Mathew P et al (1993) The 5q- syndrome: a single-institution study of 43 consecutive patients. Blood 81(4):1040–1045
25. Kantarjian H et al (2006) Decitabine improves patient outcomes in myelodysplastic syndromes: results of a phase III randomized study. Cancer 106(8):1794–1803
26. Silverman LR et al (2002) Randomized controlled trial of azacitidine in patients with the myelodysplastic syndrome: a study of the cancer and leukemia group B. J Clin Oncol 20(10):2429–2440
27. List A et al (2006) Lenalidomide in the myelodysplastic syndrome with chromosome 5q deletion. N Engl J Med 355(14):1456–1465
28. Moake JL (2002) Thrombotic microangiopathies. N Engl J Med 347(8):589–600
29. Levi M (2004) Current understanding of disseminated intravascular coagulation. Br J Haematol 124(5):567–576
30. Moake J (2009) Thrombotic thrombocytopenia purpura (TTP) and other thrombotic microangiopathies. Best Pract Res Clin Haematol 22(4):567–576
31. Zhan H et al (2010) Thrombotic thrombocytopenic purpura at the Johns Hopkins Hospital from 1992 to 2008: clinical outcomes and risk factors for relapse. Transfusion 50(4):868–874
32. Drews RE (2003) Critical issues in hematology: anemia, thrombocytopenia, coagulopathy, and blood product transfusions in critically ill patients. Clin Chest Med 24(4):607–622
33. Mecozzi G et al (2002) Intravascular hemolysis in patients with new-generation prosthetic heart valves: a prospective study. J Thorac Cardiovasc Surg 123(3):550–556
34. Mari D et al (1995) Hypercoagulability in centenarians: the paradox of successful aging. Blood 85(11):3144–3149
35. Silverstein MD et al (1998) Trends in the incidence of deep vein thrombosis and pulmonary embolism: a 25-year population-based study. Arch Intern Med 158(6):585–593
36. Kitchens C, Alving B (eds) (2007) Consultative hemostasis and thrombosis. Saunders/Elsevier, Philadelphia
37. Aster RH et al (2009) Drug-induced immune thrombocytopenia: pathogenesis, diagnosis, and management. J Thromb Haemost 7(6): 911–918
38. Warkentin TE (2007) Drug-induced immune-mediated thrombocytopenia – from purpura to thrombosis. N Engl J Med 356(9): 891–893
39. Slichter SJ (2007) Evidence-based platelet transfusion guidelines. Hematology Am Soc Hematol Educ Program 172–178
40. Kapetanakis EI et al (2006) Effect of clopidogrel premedication in off-pump cardiac surgery: are we forfeiting the benefits of reduced hemorrhagic sequelae? Circulation 113(13):1667–1674
41. Laux V et al (2009) Direct inhibitors of coagulation proteins – the end of the heparin and low-molecular-weight heparin era for anticoagulant therapy? Thromb Haemost 102(5):892–899
42. Dispenzieri A, Kyle RA (2005) Multiple myeloma: clinical features and indications for therapy. Best Pract Res Clin Haematol 18(4):553–568
43. Kyle RA et al (2002) A long-term study of prognosis in monoclonal gammopathy of undetermined significance. N Engl J Med 346(8):564–569
44. Stanworth SJ (2007) The evidence-based use of FFP and cryoprecipitate for abnormalities of coagulation tests and clinical coagulopathy. Hematology Am Soc Hematol Educ Program 179–186
45. Franchini M (2006) Acquired hemophilia A. Hematology 11(2): 119–125
46. Rosendaal FR, VAN Hylckama Vlieg A, Doggen CJ (2007) Venous thrombosis in the elderly. J Thromb Haemost 5(Suppl 1):310–317
47. Blom JW et al (2006) Incidence of venous thrombosis in a large cohort of 66,329 cancer patients: results of a record linkage study. J Thromb Haemost 4(3):529–535
48. Cushman M et al (2004) Deep vein thrombosis and pulmonary embolism in two cohorts: the longitudinal investigation of thromboembolism etiology. Am J Med 117(1):19–25
49. Zangari M et al (2001) Increased risk of deep-vein thrombosis in patients with multiple myeloma receiving thalidomide and chemotherapy. Blood 98(5):1614–1615

50. Warkentin TE (2003) Heparin-induced thrombocytopenia: pathogenesis and management. Br J Haematol 121(4):535–555

51. Pouplard C et al (2007) Prospective evaluation of the '4Ts' score and particle gel immunoassay specific to heparin/PF4 for the diagnosis of heparin-induced thrombocytopenia. J Thromb Haemost 5(7):1373–1379

52. Devreese K, Peerlinck K, Hoylaerts MF (2010) Thrombotic risk assessment in the antiphospholipid syndrome requires more than the quantification of lupus anticoagulants. Blood 115(4): 870–878

53. Metjian A, Lim W (2009) ASH evidence-based guidelines: should asymptomatic patients with antiphospholipid antibodies receive primary prophylaxis to prevent thrombosis? Hematology Am Soc Hematol Educ Program 247–249

54. Geerts WH et al (2008) Prevention of venous thromboembolism: American College of Chest Physicians evidence-based clinical practice guidelines (8th edition). Chest 133(6 Suppl):381S–453S

55. Tefferi A (2008) Essential thrombocythemia, polycythemia vera, and myelofibrosis: current management and the prospect of targeted therapy. Am J Hematol 83(6):491–497

56. Tefferi A (2007) JAK2 mutations in polycythemia vera – molecular mechanisms and clinical applications. N Engl J Med 356(5):444–445

57. Tefferi A (2007) Primary myelofibrosis and its paraneoplastic stromal effects. Haematologica 92(5):577–579

58. Shivakumar SP, Anderson DR, Couban S (2009) Catheter-associated thrombosis in patients with malignancy. J Clin Oncol 27(29):4858–4864

59. Lee AY et al (2003) Low-molecular-weight heparin versus a coumarin for the prevention of recurrent venous thromboembolism in patients with cancer. N Engl J Med 349(2):146–153

60. Bates SM, Ginsberg JS (2004) Clinical practice. Treatment of deep-vein thrombosis. N Engl J Med 351(3):268–277

61. Hebert PC et al (1999) A multicenter, randomized, controlled clinical trial of transfusion requirements in critical care. Transfusion Requirements in Critical Care Investigators, Canadian Critical Care Trials Group. N Engl J Med 340(6):409–417

62. Kuter DJ (2009) Thrombopoietin and thrombopoietin mimetics in the treatment of thrombocytopenia. Annu Rev Med 60:193–206

63. Boccardo P, Remuzzi G, Galbusera M (2004) Platelet dysfunction in renal failure. Semin Thromb Hemost 30(5):579–589

Chapter 6
Invited Commentary

Stanley J. Dudrick

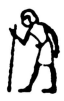

Optimal nutritional support in the geriatric population, of which I am a grateful living member, is obviously important not only for the maintenance of optimal structure, body composition, cellular and system function, health, well-being, and life style, but also for productive longevity and vitality. Life itself, the quality of life, and living life to its full capacity are all clearly dependent upon, and related to, the quality of all aspects of nutritional support and fitness.

Nutrition support is an amalgamation of art and science, as is the rest of the broad field of medicine including geriatrics. Both had their origins in curiosity, empirical observations, ideals, concepts, philosophy, innovation, experimentation, and the application of newly accumulated and evaluated knowledge to practical use. This has been the basis for the practice of medicine for millennia, and advances have been made arithmetically and tediously for hundreds of years until the late nineteenth century and early twentieth century, when discovery, creativity, science, and technology virtually exploded, and have continued to advance logarithmically to the current day. Moreover, this rapid increase in knowledge and technology is likely to continue in the foreseeable future and has a significant influence on the application of nutritional support to the practice of geriatrics, especially geriatric surgery.

When I was a first year surgical resident in 1962 at the Hospital of the University of Pennsylvania, I experienced an epiphany from which I have not recovered nor deviated to this day. While caring for the complex, critically ill patients of my chair and mentor, Dr. Jonathan E. Rhoads, on a particularly devastating weekend, I was unable to support them adequately after technically successful major operations performed earlier that week, and despite my best efforts to provide them with the highest possible state-of-the-art care available in that venerable tertiary care academic institution at that time, three of the patients, all elderly in their seventh

and eighth decades of life, died. I was disheartened, disappointed, and discouraged by my helplessness and ineffectiveness in achieving success in our therapeutic goals, and I unabashedly expressed my frustrations to Dr. Rhoads on rounds afterward. Indeed, I informed him that this series of ultimate failures indicated to me that I was not likely to become an effective surgeon and that I was seriously considering leaving the surgical residency to train in another specialty or even a different profession. Dr. Rhoads listened patiently to my lamentations, and then gave me the most significant tutorial of my life. He explained to me that surgical operations were only one important part of patient care: that the procedures undertaken might have been maximally technically proficient, but that the patients could not withstand the sum of the series of insults imposed by the pathophysiologic condition, the major operative injury (sometimes multiple within a short time period), the general anesthetic side effects, the associated comorbidities, complications including pneumonia and sepsis, and the resultant poor nutritional and metabolic state. Indeed, he pointed out to me that the common denominator contributing to the death of these patients was clearly malnutrition, which severely compromised their ability to recover, to restore normal cellular function, and to survive, and even though the operation was a technical success, the overall functional reserve capacity of the patient was exhausted beyond the requirements essential to provide endogenous substrates to support immunocompetence, healing, and vital bodily functions. Essentially, although the patients starved to death, they manifested their malnutrition clinically and functionally by serial failure of their cellular and system functions. This concept, of which I had not previously been aware, was not only surprising, but also foreign and difficult for me to accept initially. After all, the surgical mantra at that time was, "cut well, sew well, do well." The master had patiently and skillfully converted what started out to be quite a negative encounter to the most positive turn-around in my embryonic career. My life was forever transformed from that moment, and I have pursued the "holy grail" of providing optimal nutrition to all patients from that point forward and will likely be obsessed with attempting to perfect the technology and results until my own end.

S.J. Dudrick (✉)
Department of Surgery, Yale University School of Medicine, Saint Mary's Hospital/Yale Affiliate, 40 Beechter Street, Naugatuck, 06770 Waterbury, CT, USA
e-mail: stanteri@comcast.net; sdudrick@stmh.org

R.A. Rosenthal et al. (eds.), *Principles and Practice of Geriatric Surgery*,
DOI 10.1007/978-1-4419-6999-6_6, © Springer Science+Business Media, LLC 2011

I owe much to the many geriatric individuals I have had the privilege of having as patients throughout my career for all that they have taught me in so many ways. My experiences with them have served to forge a body of knowledge, skills, expectations, and more importantly, an attitude that if you give them the opportunity and a little help and direction, that there is virtually no limit to what they can accomplish within the realm of human possibility. Contrarily, in a manner analogous to premature infants, if you ignore their needs, are inattentive to them for too long a time, or do not provide them with the critical support they require in adequate amounts and for critical periods of time, then they are likely to slip through your fingers and be irretrievably lost. Nowhere is the old adage more relevant, "be where you are supposed to be, when you are supposed to be there, fully prepared and willing to do what you are expected to do, as well as you can do it." Without an appropriate attitude and timing, all of the skills acquired from mastery of the "six competencies" of education and training will fall short of expectations, and of the potentials both of the patient and the caregiver.

Early in my training, I met a 97-year-old woman in the emergency department with acute upper abdominal distress. She proved to have multiple gallstones in an inflamed gallbladder together with secondary pancreatitis. The medical service consulted our surgical service pro forma, indicating that this "ancient" lady had an obviously lethal situation from which she would not likely recover, and that a surgical procedure would only accelerate her demise. But they, nonetheless, consulted us out of courtesy and for reinforcement of their decision rather than for surgical intervention. However, she was an intelligent, strong, and delightful lady with a positive outlook and supportive family who all wanted our best help and services. I admitted her, resuscitated her, started her on antibiotics, initiated pulmonary toilette procedures, and confirmed the adequacy of her hematologic and biochemical indices, together with an appraisal of her renal, kidney and cardiopulmonary functions. She responded to the supportive measures much to our satisfaction, and the next day I removed her gallbladder under local anesthesia supplemented by mild analgesics and sedatives. She rebounded amazingly well and left the hospital for home in 5 days. All she needed was adequate supportive preoperative and postoperative care and the chance to show that she had the strength, will, and reserve to overcome this major threat to her life. She was "the talk of the hospital" for quite some time and a great source of satisfaction to me and the surgical service. She celebrated her 100th birthday anniversary with us a few years later to our mutual great joy.

In a cadre of 39 patients with end-stage malignancies and malnutrition secondary to their pathophysiologic processes, and compounded further by surgical procedures, chemotherapy, radiotherapy, and combinations thereof, we undertook a study of the feasibility of attempting to meet nutritional requirements by infusing moderately hypertonic (5–15%) nutrient solutions by peripheral vein in volumes of 5 L per day while giving intravenous diuretics to help excrete the excess water administered as a vehicle for infusing the nutrients. The vast majority of these patients were in their seventh, eighth, and ninth decades of life, many of them were cathectic, and all of them were aware that they would not likely benefit from the study and perhaps might even be harmed by fluid and electrolyte aberrations, pulmonary edema, congestive heart failure, infection, thrombophlebitis, sepsis, etc. Nonetheless, this seemingly fragile, debilitated, incurable group of mostly geriatric patients demonstrated the courage, strength, determination, hope, and desire to be useful in the generation of new medical knowledge and experience, such that they participated willingly, conscientiously, and enthusiastically in this clinical experiment.

They all improved their strength, sense of well-being, ambulation, self-help, hygiene, and overall quality of hospital life to the point that several of the patients and/or their families began to express the thought that the parenteral feeding solution might be "curing" their cancers. This was most likely related to the anabolic effect of the nutrient energy substrates on their body cell mass and systems, but also in part, secondary to the fact that the health care team was much more involved with them, was keenly interested in them, spent much more time with them, and obviously cared about them. In some instances, we felt morally and ethically obligated to inform the patient and/or family sadly that the improved mental, physical, and emotional response they were witnessing was a caloric and balanced nutrient effect rather than an anticancer effect so as not to promote false hope or unfairly raise their expectations for a cancer cure. I remain grateful to this courageous, caring, unselfish group of patients and their families to this day. Furthermore, my experiences with them have convinced me of the importance of providing optimal nutrition and support to geriatric patients, even when they are likely to succumb imminently or ultimately to their underlying nonneoplastic or neoplastic pathologic disorder.

Thus, I have developed the philosophy over the years that there is more to the nutritional support of the cancer patient, especially the geriatric cancer patient, than the current science and clinical practice of medicine and surgery mandate or justify unequivocally. The emotional and psychological support of the patient and their significant others and the socially important aspects of food or nutrient intake and "breaking bread" with family and friends cannot be denied. These needs do exist, and we must address and do something about them rather than ignore them, as is all too often done. After we have exhausted all possibilities of providing reasonable, rational, or justifiable specific antineoplastic, and/or nutritional, therapy for the patient with an inexorably lethal cancer, it is of utmost importance that we never abandon the patient or the family, and at the very least, continue to support them, bond with them, relieve their guilt, and above all, reinforce their faith in our humane and core values simply by "being there" for them and providing a feeling of comfort and hope that cannot otherwise be accomplished. The frontiers for specialized nutritional support of geriatric patients, especially geriatric cancer patients await our exploration, discovery, and judicious clinical applications.

Another illustrative vignette that I would like to share is related to the importance of will and determination on the part of seriously ill elderly patients in making difficult clinical judgment decisions. Even if we cannot cure them, and might actually accelerate their demise by our interventions, we must discuss all of the options with the patient and family and be tolerant of their right to make choices that may expose the patient to significant risks with major surgical treatment. This is especially true when taking no action will inevitably result in death. For example, at the Philadelphia VA Hospital, I had an 80-year-old patient with COPD who developed a squamous cell carcinoma in his left mainstem bronchus. His split pulmonary functions indicated that he would have marginally adequate ability to survive with only his right lung if he underwent left pneumonectomy. He was an avid Pennsylvania deer hunter who enjoyed hunting with his sons and his grandsons virtually as a family tradition. He knew from our discussions that he had a highly lethal condition, might not survive a pneumonectomy procedure, and certainly could not entertain rationally the thought that he would be capable afterward of withstanding the rigors of hunting deer in the cold winter season. However, he pleaded with me to give him a chance to have just one more deer season hunting with his boys, and I could not look into his pleading eyes and deny him his fervent wish. He tolerated the left pneumonectomy surprisingly well after having stopped smoking for a week or so, and his recovery was uncomplicated, reinforcing to me that patient goals and motivations are invaluable assets to surgeons and to surgical outcomes. Later that winter he not only hunted with his sons, but shot a deer while having to place the heavily padded butt of his rifle against his shoulder only 4 months post pneumonectomy. I shall never forget how happy he was to see me afterward and relate the details of his successful hunt in the snow to me and share pictures of the event. Subsequently, he rejoined his bowling team, and much to my delight, hunted again and bowled again the following year. He died more than 2 years later at age 82, but he did it his way, with our consideration, understanding, support, and love, all of which he and his wonderful family appreciated. Even though we have much more to learn regarding geriatric surgery, geriatric nutrition, and the complexities introduced by malignancies, we can take useful actions and accomplish satisfactory results while producing and/or awaiting new data, simply by exercising compassion, common sense, good judgment, and "giving a damn." Those of us who have helped caring for geriatric surgical patients have learned first-hand that age of the patient is not uniformly an independent risk factor and

that physiologic changes associated with the normal aging process occur at different rates among individuals.

I have very little patience or tolerance for those of my colleagues who "write off" geriatric patients and deny them optimal care simply because they are elderly. This is the most unprofessional, disrespectful, and demeaning attitude that is anathema to me, but I am fearful that it is already creeping insidiously and increasingly into our culture and society and beginning to corrupt not only our healthcare system, but our morals, ethics, and core values. We are obligated to treat all patients, especially geriatric patients, as individuals and with respect, dignity, and compassion rather than as inanimate entry items in a computerized management algorithm.

With improved medical care delivery and effectiveness, people are living longer, and the population of patients with whom general surgeons interact is becoming progressively older at an unprecedented rate. Currently, in 2009, there are more than 38 million people in the USA who are 65 years of age or older. By the year 2030, more than 20% of the population will be over the age of 65 years, and one-half of these individuals will be admitted to a hospital during their remaining lifetime for an operative procedure. Caring for these individuals requires an awareness and understanding by the surgeons of the global changes that take place as an individual ages, as well as a clinical acumen and ability to assess accurately their relative needs, both as inpatients and as outpatients.

Issues in overall geriatric management and in geriatric surgery and nutritional support will continue to challenge us in the future and must be addressed expeditiously. The most compelling reality is that the geriatric population will continue to grow both in numbers and in longevity. This will require a major sea-change in the manner in which their health, fitness, and function will be supported, literally on an individual basis, and the means by which the fundamental social, professional, medical, ethical, financial, and other costs thereof will be embraced and met by our society.

We must develop and carry out relevant meticulously controlled study protocols specifically designed for the various cohorts of the geriatric populations to provide the data essential to understanding and solving their unique nutritional, functional, and surgical problems. We must recognize and allow for the difficulties associated with carrying out studies in aged patients with seemingly inevitable comorbidities. Moreover, we must understand that the physiologic changes that accompany the normal aging process, especially those related to nutritional needs, occur at different rates among human beings. The difference between chronologic age and physiologic age in the elderly patients must be determined clinically in a scientific manner in order to help guide prudent decision-making in their management. Although the old adage is that the chronologic age of the patient is not an independent risk factor for surgical procedures or actions, the age of the elderly patient can, indeed, become an independent risk factor in some patients in whom a great disparity exists between their chronologic age and their physiologic age. Furthermore, establishing nutrient requirements for a heterogeneous population is not an easy task even when the group is healthy, much less when accompanied by a wide variety of health conditions, comorbidities, fitness, disabilities, nutritional status, etc.

Prior to the latter part of the twentieth century, people in the 50–65 years age range were defined as the geriatric or elderly population, and a reasonable amount of useful clinical data had been accrued to justify various aspects of their health and nutritional recommendations for management. However, it has become obvious to nutritionists, surgeons and others that it is not valid to extrapolate from the data that exist for the 50–65-year-old age group upward to the eighth, ninth, and tenth decades of life. This problem must be solved by the systematic collection of data specifically for the older groups from 65 to 100 years of age if they are to receive optimal care based on their scientifically determined requirements, potentials, and tolerances. The challenges involved will be difficult enough in determining nutrient requirements and assessing nutritional and physiological status, but will become increasingly more difficult and complex when evaluating nutritional interventions and appraising the success of other outcomes of implementing ambitious nutritional and/or surgical therapies among the patients in these deciles. The most difficult group, and those who are most vulnerable from a nutritional standpoint, are the elderly who are institutionalized, have little or no family support, have multiple health problems, have neurological challenges, cannot perform the activities of daily living competently, and require assistance not only with feeding, but also with total custodial care. The rather steady loss of lean body mass [about 1% per year, which has been documented to occur in the elderly (>50 years age)] is greatest in those who are not able or willing to ambulate or exercise, while ingesting diets adequate in protein, thus resulting in a compounding of the usual sarcopenia that occurs in such patients. Nowhere is the "chicken or egg" phenomenon more evident than in this group of elderly persons. In addition to protein deficiencies, energy, macronutrient, micronutrient, and fluid deficiencies are also relatively more common in geriatric patients than in younger adults, although their daily requirements per kilogram body weight are not dissimilar. A major problem in the elderly is the difficulty in convincing them to drink more water and fluids, thus resulting in dehydration and its untoward consequences. Examples of other nutrient aberrations that occur commonly in the elderly are calcium and vitamin D deficiencies, which can lead to significant increases in morbidity and mortality, and these essential nutrients must be provided in larger doses in the diet or as supplements. Preventive health measures regarding the intake of these important nutrients are likely to result in significant reductions in morbidity, mortality, and health care costs, which remain to be confirmed in future studies.

As the current saga regarding health care funding and regulation unfolds, and as the vested interests of the various private and governmental power groups become more "transparent," debated, and compromised or modified, it will be particularly critical to the welfare of the geriatric population that the highest moral and ethical values be followed, that all age groups receive the respect and quality health care appropriate to their needs, and that the financial burdens be shared equitably among the citizens of this nation not only as a compassionate and caring duty, but also as a fulfillment of humane responsibility to humanity and to society.

Of paramount importance is the right of self-determination of elderly individuals and their families in the provision, modification, and cessation of all aspects of nutritional support not only from the ethical and religious points of view but from the legal mandate. A government that guarantees the rights of women to decision-making regarding their bodies and fetuses must guarantee the equivalent rights of the elderly to decision-making regarding their nutrition, surgical management, and life support. How we nourish and treat our elderly population during the next decade or two will influence greatly how we define our character as a society, culture, and nation.

I would like to close this commentary with one of my favorite anecdotal recollections from my long-time friend and fellow surgeon, Dr. David Heimbach. "It was a busy morning, about 8:30 a.m., when an elderly gentleman in his 80s, arrived to have stitches removed from his thumb. He said he was in a hurry as he had an appointment at 9 a.m. I took his vital signs and had him take a seat, knowing it would be over an hour before someone would be able to see him. I saw him looking at his watch, and decided, since I was not busy with another patient, that I would evaluate his wound. On examination, it was well healed, so I talked to one of the doctors and got the needed supplies to remove his sutures and redress his wound. While taking care of his wound, I asked him if he had another doctor's appointment this morning as he was in such a hurry. The gentleman told me no, that he needed to get to the nursing home to eat breakfast with his wife. I inquired as to her health; he told me that she had been there for a while and that she was a victim of Alzheimer's disease. As we talked, I asked if she would be upset if he was a bit late. He replied that she no longer knew who he was, that she had not recognized him in 5 years now. I was surprised, and asked him, "And you still go every morning, even though she doesn't know who you are?" He smiled as he patted my hand and said, "She doesn't know me, but I still know who she is." I had to hold back the tears as he left; I had goose bumps on my arms, and thought, "That is the kind of love I want in my life." True love is neither physical, nor romantic. True love is an acceptance of all that is, has been, will be, and will not be." Such is the human condition from my perspective.

Chapter 7
Nutrition

Sandhya A. Lagoo-Deenadayalan and Danny O. Jacobs

Nutrition in the Elderly

Throughout most of adult life, our bodies maintain near-perfect metabolic balance interrupted only by disease. This equilibrium lasts a finite period – until the inevitable aging process begins. Aging is a complex phenomenon that includes molecular, cellular, physiologic, and psychological changes. Individual aging is influenced primarily by a person's genetic makeup, lifestyle, and environment. Of these factors, the first is predetermined and constant; the other two are optional, variable, and therefore modifiable. Some very old individuals can stay healthy and have a good nutritional status [1, 2], but physiologic decline and health problems are expected for most of us before death. Aging of cellular function results in a natural decline in physiologic performance and reserve capacity. Thus elderly individuals have increased susceptibility and are less resistant to illness [3].

These factors contribute to an increased prevalence of illness and increased risk for primary and secondary malnutrition. There is an estimated 5–10% prevalence of protein-calorie malnutrition among community-dwelling elderly. In the USA, approximately 85% of the noninstitutionalized elderly suffer from at least one condition that could be improved by proper nutrition [1]. Physicians often fail to recognize its presence. Malnutrition in this population may predispose the elderly to prolonged hospitalization.

Many studies have documented a high prevalence of malnutrition among the elderly residents of nursing homes. Surveys have shown incidences of malnutrition that range from 30 to 85% and increased mortality rates [4, 5]. Hypoalbuminemia is also common: a 37% incidence of this disorder was documented in a Veterans Administration nursing home. In elderly medical patients, nutritional status during acute illness is a determinant of morbidity, length of hospital stay, and mortality [1, 6]. In older surgical patients

malnutrition is associated with high morbidity and mortality, particularly when emergency surgery is necessary. In addition, malnutrition negatively affects postoperative functional recovery and rehabilitation [3]. Nutritional screening and intervention in the elderly has been proposed as a cost-effective measure [1], as approximately 30% of the health-care budget is spent on this age group.

Physical and Psychosocial Issues in Nutrition

A combination of physical, social, and psychological factors contributes to primary malnutrition in the elderly. Physical deterioration with age can influence nutritional status. As years pass, the elderly become frail, have diminished visual function, increased cognitive impairment, and gait and balance disorders that affect mobility and decrease their ability to obtain and prepare food. The US National Health and Nutrition Examination Survey (NHANES) III cohort study evaluated the hypothesis that socio-economic status is consistently and negatively associated with levels of biological risk. The nine parameters known to predict health risk are diastolic and systolic blood pressure, pulse, HDL and total cholesterol, glycosylated hemoglobin, C-reactive protein, albumin, and waist–hip ratio. Education and income effects were each independently and negatively associated with cumulative biological risks, independent of age. However, older age was associated with significantly weaker education and income gradients [7].

Adherence to lifestyle guidelines has been shown to markedly reduce mortality in middle-aged women in a study that observed them for 24 years. Guidelines addressed five lifestyle factors, namely cigarette smoking, being overweight, little to moderate exercise, light to moderate alcohol intake and low diet quality score [8].

Malnourishment is common in home-bound adults due to a variety of causes. These include various co-morbidities, medications, economic, social, religious, and psychological problems. Men are more likely to be undernourished than women and the higher the patients' body mass index, the

S.A. Lagoo-Deenadayalan (✉)
Department of Surgery, Duke University Hospital,
Durham, NC, USA
e-mail: lagoo002@mc.duke.edu

R.A. Rosenthal et al. (eds.), *Principles and Practice of Geriatric Surgery*,
DOI 10.1007/978-1-4419-6999-6_7, © Springer Science+Business Media, LLC 2011

greater the odds of under eating, defined as not consuming enough calories to maintain their current body weight [9].

Dental diseases are common in the elderly. There is a direct relationship between poor dentition and difficulty ingesting certain food items, such as meat and hard foods such as nuts, raw vegetables in salads, and multigrain bread or rolls. This may result in changes in choice and the quality of food intake. Taste and smell are also affected. A progressive loss of taste buds occurs, predominantly affecting the anterior tongue. This region has taste buds that detect sweet and salt. Because the remaining buds detecting bitter and sour are relatively increased with aging, elderly people have a greater sensitivity to these tastes. This could explain their preference for high sugar foods. The elderly need a greater concentration change to perceive a difference in intensity. They also have a reduction in taste intensity (hypogeusia) and an increase in taste distortion (dysgeusia). These conditions can be exacerbated by medications and concurrent disease states [10, 11]. Use of food flavors (roast beef, ham, natural bacon, maple, and cheese) has been found to increase intake and nutritional status in elderly institutionalized patients.

The presence of multiple diseases can also affect nutritional status. Disorders that interfere with eating include neurological diseases, such as Parkinson's disease, cerebrovascular disease, chronic obstructive pulmonary disease, congestive heart failure, and chronic renal insufficiency. Some of these diseases require dietary restrictions that affect the palatability or variety of the food offered. Swallowing disorders are not uncommon in the elderly, and nutritional disorders are frequently associated with dysphagia in institutionalized persons (refer to Chap. 43 on swallowing disorders).

Disturbances of mood and affect are common in the elderly. Anorexia is a common symptom during depression, and these depressed patients often become malnourished. The prevalence of malnutrition among older patients hospitalized for depression can be as high as 20–35% [5]. One of the most difficult situations in geriatric medicine is to determine if the refusal of food is due to a curable depression or is the will of a mentally healthy individual. In particular, the death of a spouse can dramatically influence appetite and food intake. Depressed patients may put less effort into caring for themselves and may lose the symbolism of warmth and sharing associated with eating. The anorexia of aging is neither depression nor willfulness yet it is also a major cause of poor nutrition (see below).

Cognitive impairment such as dementia may also significantly decrease nutrient intake. To study this, a prospective study of 349 patients with a mean age of 85.2 years admitted to a Geriatric Rehabilitation center was carried out. Patients included those with no dementia, mild cognitive dysfunction or dementia. Although there was no significant difference in co-morbidities between older demented vs. nondemented patients, there was a considerable deterioration in nutritional and functional status in the patients with dementia [12]. Routine nutritional assessments, functional assessment and review of medications should therefore be performed more often in patients with dementia so that appropriate interventions can be instituted.

Approximately 30% of elderly Americans live alone, and 25% of free-living elderly need assistance with activities of daily living. Social isolation can lead to problems of obtaining and preparing food. Timing of meals in hospitals and nursing homes may be disadvantageous, as meals may be separated by short periods of time. Appetite may be poor for each meal when they are offered too close together. Food presentation is key for patients to accept the meals offered. Food intake can increase by 25% if the environment is changed to a familiar one (home cooked meals, family and friends visiting during meal times, favorite music). Pureed food is not readily accepted, so imaginative ways of presenting such meals should be tried [13].

Age-Related Changes in Body Composition

Lean Body Mass

Presently, the most widely used body composition model is a two-compartment model in which the body is divided into lean body mass and fat. Aging is accompanied by a net loss of lean body mass. As a consequence, the elderly becomes debilitated and lose an important portion of their tissue amino acid and energy reserves. The lean body mass declines by approximately 6.3% every 10 years. Thus it decreases by an average of 0.45 kg/year after age 60. By age 70 muscle mass may be 20% less than that in young adults. This loss occurs disproportionately more from skeletal muscle than from viscera. Studies have suggested that changes in growth hormone metabolism may mediate age-related changes in body composition. People deficient in growth hormone have a decrease in lean body mass similar to that experienced by the healthy elderly [14, 15]. In addition, treatment with growth hormone or insulin-like growth factor-I (IGF-I) increases lean body mass, nitrogen retention, and muscle strength in the elderly [16]. Androgens have also been proposed to play a role in the body composition changes of aging. Plasma levels of testosterone may decrease with aging, and testosterone supplementation in aging individuals may increase their lean body mass.

Serum total testosterone and the calculated free testosterone correlate well with each other and are superior in defining a group of elderly men with suspected androgen deficiency. In contrast, free testosterone measured by direct

RIA reflects gonadal function poorly. Repetitive use of total testosterone is therefore recommended when screening for androgen deficiency in elderly men [17]. A study investigating the association between various testosterone measures and clinical and biochemical parameters of the aging male was undertaken. The parameters included serum levels of sex hormone-binding globulin, estradiol, and lipid profile after an overnight fast; questionnaires assessing clinical symptoms, erectile function and mood; bone mineral density and body composition. Testosterone values did not correlate with clinical signs and symptoms of hypogonadism. It is therefore critical that symptoms of the aging male be considered multifactorial and not be indiscriminately assigned to the age-associated decrease in testosterone levels [18].

Age-associated decline in growth hormone and androgen secretion contributes to the alterations in body composition and organ function seen during the normal aging process. Despite all these changes, the elderly may continue to function adequately but may have decreased capacity to adapt and to mobilize endogenous protein stores during the catabolic stress imposed by infection or trauma.

Body Fat

The proportion of body fat increases with age and is redistributed from subcutaneous to intramuscular sites. Body fat increases at a rate of 0.4–1.5% per year, beginning at around age 30. As with lean body mass, growth hormone and androgen administration appear to minimize alterations in body fat. The impact of testosterone supplementation on body fat is less dramatic. Testosterone appears to decrease the uptake of triglycerides and increase triglyceride turnover while reducing lipoprotein lipase activity. Furthermore, growth hormone and androgens may act together in the regulation of fat metabolism during adult life.

Energy Requirements

The total energy expenditure (TEE) can be divided into three parts: resting energy expenditure (REE, the energy expended at rest after overnight fasting), thermic effect of feeding (TEF, the increase in energy expenditure above baseline due to the consumption and processing of food), and energy expenditure for physical activity and arousal (EEPAA). Daily energy expenditure declines progressively throughout adult life. REE is approximately 15% lower (7.35 vs. 6.20 mega Joules (MJ)/day) in elderly subjects than that in the young. Changes in REE and EEPAA, which account for most of the energy consumed during daily activity, account for most

(73%) of the decline in TEE observed in elderly individuals [19]. Interestingly, body weight, rather than fat-free mass, appears to best predict the REE (Fig. 7.1). Aging is also associated with a significant decrease in energy expenditure per unit of fat-free mass and body weight. Changes in muscle mass affect energy consumption and utilization. Creatinine excretion, which is an index of muscle mass and is closely related to the basal metabolic rate, decreases with aging; thus the reduction in energy expenditure is in large part due to a decrease in lean body mass (fat-free mass) and to a more sedentary life style. These changes are reflected in a decreased total energy requirement in men from 2,700 kcal/day at age 30 to 2,100 kcal/day by age 80 [20]. These observations suggest that preservation of muscle mass and prevention of muscle atrophy could help prevent the decrease in metabolic rate associated with advancing age [21].

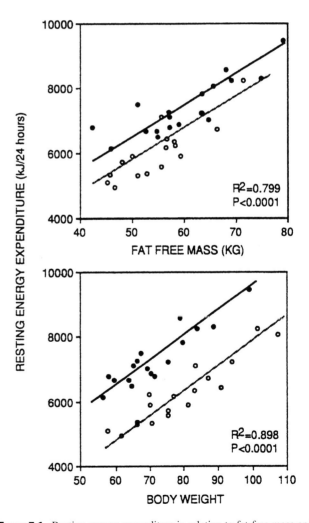

Figure 7.1 Resting energy expenditure in relation to fat-free mass and body weight in young men (*filled circles*) and elderly men (*open circles*) (from Roberts et al. [18], with permission).

Nutritional Assessment

Nutritional assessment is a key aspect of elderly patient care. With so many physiologic changes due to aging that heighten the susceptibility to disease, the importance of proper nutrition grows. It is a challenge, however, to identify elderly persons who would benefit from dietary intervention. Not every elderly patient needs to undergo a cascade of anthropometric, dietary, and laboratory tests to assess their nutritional status in the perioperative period. Simplified nutritional assessment can be done quickly (see Chap. 22) and will provide the caregivers with the appropriate perspective to plan for perioperative nutritional needs. This knowledge can drastically influence therapy and outcome. Key elements of a full nutritional assessment are defined below.

History and Physical Examination

A detailed social, nutritional, and medical history is an essential first step in assessing the nutritional status of the elderly. Particular attention should be paid to the presence of chronic diseases. Cancer by itself impairs nutritional status. Other diseases such as chronic obstructive pulmonary disease and congestive heart failure may make feeding difficult. Neurological illnesses that interfere with the eating process place patients at particular risk. Swallowing function and absorptive capacity should be specifically assessed. Disturbances of mood and affect (e.g., depression) are not uncommon and should be considered during the evaluation.

A social history is equally important. The degree of independence can influence the capacity to purchase and prepare food. Information about who lives with the patient, cooking facilities, and income is also needed. Particular attention should be paid to patients who live in nursing homes and institutions. The physical and cognitive conditions of these patients and the eating environment and food presentation may be unsuitable, placing them at risk of undernourishment. Elderly patients commonly take multiple medications. These drugs should be listed, as should alcohol use; and possible drug–nutrient interactions must be considered. Drugs that may interfere with nutrition are listed in Table 7.1.

The physical examination should always include body weight and height. Oral health, dentition, and swallowing capability should be assessed. Because dehydration may present subtly and atypically in the elderly, hydration status must be carefully evaluated. Orthostatic hypotension or tachycardia may indicate dehydration. Physical signs of malnutrition include muscle wasting and dermatitis associated with deficiency syndromes as well as perioral stomatitis and hair loss due to zinc deficiency. Cognitive impairments could

TABLE 7.1 Drug therapy that interferes with nutritional support

Drug therapy	Subject of interference or effect
Drugs that interfere with nutrient assimilation	
AlOH and MgOH	Phosphorus
H_2 antagonists	Vitamin B_{12}
Cholesterol-binding agents	Fat-soluble vitamins, folate
Phenytoin	Vitamins D and K, folate
Drugs interfering with nutrient delivery	
Sucralfate	Forms clogs in the feeding tube
Digoxin, phenytoin, theophylline, potassium chloride	Diarrhea due to hyperosmolarity
Nutrients affecting drug therapy	
Calcium	Phenytoin absorption
Vitamin K	Anticoagulants

Source: Data are from Rolandelli and Ullrich [3]

TABLE 7.2 Screening tools at the time of hospital admission for assessing nutritional risk

Screening tool
Nutritional risk index (NRI)
Malnutrition universal screening tool (MUST)
Nutritional risk screening tool 2002 (NRS-2002)
Subjective global assessment (SGA)
Mini nutritional assessment (MNA)

Source: Reprinted from Kyle et al. [25], with permission from Elsevier

indicate a deficiency of vitamin B_{12}, which should always be considered in the elderly if mentation is affected. The presence of decubitus ulcers is a common sign of malnutrition in institutionalized elderly and can indicate protein or vitamin C deficiency.

Nutrition Screening Initiative

Evaluation of nutritional status is an especially important aspect of the surgical evaluation. Many attempts have been made to standardize nutritional risk assessment in the elderly. Screening tools are shown in Table 7.2. The Malnutrition Universal Screening Tool (MUST) classifies malnutrition risk as low, medium, or high based on body mass index, unintentional weight loss, and acute illness. This test is for community-based ambulatory populations but also has high validity in a hospital setting [22]. Another test, the Mini Nutritional Assessment (MNA) has been developed to evaluate the risk of malnutrition in the elderly in home-care programs, nursing homes, or hospitals [23]. The factors included in the evaluation are shown in Table 7.3. The MNA-SF (Mini Nutritional Assessment – Short Form) was developed and validated to allow a two-step screening process. The MNA-SF and MNA are both sensitive, specific, and accurately identify nutrition at risk. The MNA detects risk of malnutrition before severe change in weight or serum protein. In hospital settings,

TABLE 7.3 Mini-nutritional assessment (MNA): (Short Form – 6 questions)

Question	Ratings	Score
Has food intake declined over the past 3 months due to loss of appetite, digestive problems, chewing or swallowing difficulties?	0 = Severe loss of appetite 1 = Moderate loss of appetite 2 = No loss of appetite	
Weight loss during the last 3 months?	0 = Weight loss greater than 3 kg 1 = Does not know 2 = Weight loss between 1 and 3 kg 3 = No weight loss	
Mobility?	0 = Bed or chair bound 1 = Able to get out of bed/chair but does not go out 2 = Goes out	
Has the patient suffered psychological stress or acute disease during the past 3 months?	0 = Yes 1 = No	
Neuropsychological problems?	0 = Severe dementia or depression 1 = Mild dementia 2 = No psychological problems	
Body mass index (BMI) = weight(kg)/height(m²)	0 = BMI less than 19 1 = BMI 19 to less than 21 2 = BMI 21 to less than 23 3 = BMI 23 or greater	

Maximum screening score: Total score of 12 or more: not at risk for malnutrition; no need to complete the remainder of MNA

Total score less than 12: may be at risk for malnutrition; complete the full MNA assessment

Additional questions for full MNA (12 questions)

Question	Ratings	Score
Lives independently (not in a nursing home or hospital?	0 = No; 1 = Yes	
Takes more than 3 prescription drugs per day?	0 = Yes; 1 = No	
Pressure sores or skin ulcers?	0 = Yes; 1 = No	
How many full meals does the patient eat daily?	0 = 1 meal; 1 = 2 meals; 2 = 3 meals	
At least 1 serving of daily products per day? Yes or No	0 = If 0 or 1 Yes answers	
2 or more servings of legumes or eggs per week? Yes or No	0.5 = If 2 Yes	
Meat, fish, or poultry every day? Yes or No	1.0 = If 3 Yes	
Consumes 2 or more servings of fruits or vegetables per day?	0 = No; 1 = Yes	
How much fluid is consumed per day?	0 = Less than 3 cups 0.5 = 3–5 cups 1.0 = More than 5 cups	
Mode of feeding?	0 = unable to eat without assistance 1 = Self-fed with some difficulty 2 = Self-fed without any problem	
Self view of nutritional status?	0 = View self as malnourished 1 = Uncertain of nutritional state 2 = Views self without nutritional problems	
In comparison with other people of the same age, how do they consider their health status?	0 = Not as good 0.5 = Does not know 1.0 = As good 2.0 = Better	
Mid-arm circumference (MAC) in cm?	0 = MAC less than 21 0.5 = MAC 21 or 22 1.0 = MAC 22 or greater	
Calf circumference in cm?	0 = CC < 31; 1 = CC > 31	
Maximum full assessment score = 16	*Total score ≥ 23.5* – normal nutrition, no further action required	
Combine screening + full assessment scores = maximum of 30	*Total score ≤ 23.5* – risk of malnutrition *Total score ≤ 17* – protein and calorie	

a low MNA score is associated with increased mortality, prolonged length of stay, and a greater likelihood of discharge to a nursing home [24]. Other screening tools include nutritional risk index (NRI), nutritional risk screening tool 2002 (NRS-2002) and subjective global assessment (SGA) (Table 7.2). NRS-2002 has been shown to have higher sensitivity and specificity than the MUST and NRI. In general, nutritional status and risk can be assessed by SGA, NRS-2002, and MUST in patients at hospital admission [25].

Anthropometrics

Anthropometric measurements are a convenient tool for evaluating nutritional status. They are inexpensive, safe, and easily performed in any outpatient clinic or surgery ward. They do have some drawbacks. First, anthropometric data are affected by age and severity of illness more than any other index of nutritional status [26]. Second, they are subject to individual variation depending on who monitors the measurements. Third, they must be compared to normal standards; and in the case of the elderly, there are few normative anthropometric data. Change of a specific parameter over time is generally more important than comparing it to standards. Various tables of weight per height that include elderly populations have been suggested by various investigators [27, 28], and a more valid ideal weight can be assigned using these age-specific tables. Weight loss of 5% over 4 weeks or 10% over 3 months is a sensitive indicator of malnutrition.

If the patient is not able to stand upright, height can be calculated from knee-height measurements using a normogram or the following height formulas [29].

$$\text{Stature for men} = (2.02 \times \text{knee height})$$
$$- (0.04 \times \text{age}) + 64.19$$

$$\text{Stature for women} = (1.83 \times \text{knee height})$$
$$- (0.24 \times \text{age}) + 84.88$$

Calculation of ideal body weight provides a valid weight reference for the individual. Percent of ideal weight is calculated as follows:

$$\text{Actual weight} / \text{ideal weight} \times 100$$

An ideal body weight of less than 90% is an indicator of malnutrition. Weight/height ratios can be expressed as the body mass index (BMI) – weight in kilograms/height in square meters. A normogram for body mass index is shown in Fig. 7.2. The Euronut–Seneca survey, which studied apparently healthy elderly individuals aged 70–75 years, found a mean BMI that ranged from 24.4 to 30.3 in men and from 23.9 to 30.5 for women. Results of the Third National Health and Nutrition Examination Surveys (NHANES III) include BMI data from men and women over 60 years of age in 10-year increments [30]. BMI, however, correlates more strongly with body fat than with lean body mass and may not be a sensitive index of muscle or body protein stores, except in the presence of emaciation.

Other anthropometric measures can determine body fat and lean body mass. Body fat can be assessed by measuring the triceps and subscapular skinfold thickness, and at other sites [31]. Lean body mass can be estimated in women and men by measuring the mid-arm muscle circumference and by the creatinine height index. Equations that use these indexes have been developed to relate anthropometric measurements to body composition [32]. In 1989 Frisancho reported standards for the elderly 64–74 years of age [33], the anthropometric data for European elderly over 90 years old were completed later [34].

Biochemical Markers

Use of serum laboratory values is an integral part of nutritional assessment in the adult population, although aging itself can affect test results. The most commonly used parameter, albumin, has been reported to be modified in the elderly. Albumin concentration decreases 3–9% each decade after age 70 in the community-dwelling elderly [35, 36].

In these individuals, the albumin loss is close to 0.8 g/l per decade [35], and in institutionalized individuals, the albumin has been observed to decrease by 1.3 g/l per decade. Of course, relative hypoalbuminemia may indicate poor nutritional status. Serum albumin is positively correlated with muscle mass in the elderly, and the relation may reflect shared changes with age in protein synthesis [37]. This decrease may be attributed to the decrease in skeletal muscle mass. Because of the minimal decline in albumin levels with age, hypoalbuminemia should not be ascribed solely to aging, and other causes should be considered [1]. Albumin is an important predictor of length of hospitalization, morbidity, and mortality among elderly people [37]. Severe hypoalbuminemia (<20 g/l) strongly predicts 90-day mortality and extended hospitalization in the elderly. It requires focused clinical attention regardless of the elderly patient's admitting diagnosis [38]. In the VA National Surgical Quality Improvement Program (a prospective analysis of surgical risk factors), low serum albumin was the single factor most predictive of poor postoperative outcome [39].

Because of their shorter half-lives compared to that of albumin, prealbumin, transferring, and retinal-binding protein are better markers for acute changes in nutritional status. The serumconcentration of these proteins, especially prealbumin, are better maintained in the geriatric population [39].

Level II Screen

Complete the following screen by interviewing the patient directly and/or by referring to the patient chart. If you do not routinely perform all of the described tests or ask all of the listed questions, please consider including them but do not be concerned if the entire screen is not completed. Please try to conduct a minimal screen on as many older patients as possible, and please try to collect serial measurements, which are extremely valuable in monitoring nutritional status. Please refer to the manual for additional information.

Anthropometrics

Measure height to the nearest inch and weight to the nearest pound. Record the values below and mark them on the Body Mass Index (BMI) scale to the right. Then use a straight edge (paper, ruler) to connect the two points and circle the spot where this straight line crosses the center line (body mass index). Record the number below; healthy older adults should have a BMI between 22 and 27; check the appropriate box to flag an abnormally high or low value.

Height (in): _____
Weight (lbs): _____
Body Mass Index
(weight/height²): _____

Please place a check by any statement regarding BMI and recent weight loss that is true for the patient.

❑ Body mass index <22

❑ Body mass index >27

❑ Has lost or gained 10 pounds (or more) of body weight in the past 6 months

Record the measurement of mid-arm circumference to the nearest 0.1 centimeter and of triceps skinfold to the nearest 2 millimeters.

Mid-Arm Circumference (cm): _____
Triceps Skinfold (mm): _____
Mid-Arm Muscle Circumference (cm): _____

Refer to the table and check any abnormal values:

❑ Mid-arm muscle circumference <10th percentile

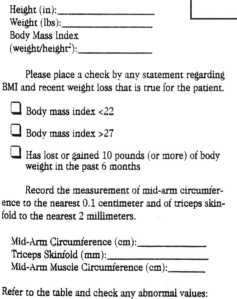

❑ Triceps skinfold <10th percentile

❑ Triceps skinfold >95th percentile

Note: mid-arm circumference (cm) - {0.314 x triceps skinfold (mm)}= mid-arm *muscle* circumference (cm)

For the remaining sections, please place a check by any statements that are true for the patient.

Laboratory Data

❑ Serum albumin below 3.5 g/dl

❑ Serum cholesterol below 160 mg/dl

❑ Serum cholesterol above 240 mg/dl

Drug Use

❑ Three or more prescription drugs, OTC medications, and/or vitamin/mineral supplements daily

FIGURE 7.2 Normogram for body mass index (from the Nutrition Screening Initiative, a project of the American Academy of Family Physicians, the American Dietetic Association, and the National Council on the Aging, with permission. Funded in part by a grant from Ross Products Division, Abbott Laboratories).

Serum prealbumin protein appears to be a more sensitive marker of protein malnutrition than transferrin, although its use as a predictor of clinical outcome has yet to be determined [39, 40].

Iron stores (ferritin) usually increase with aging, which can cause circulating transferrin levels to diminish. Other conditions that may decrease transferrin levels include the anemia associated with chronic disease, acute inflammation,

Clinical Features

Presence of (check each that apply):

❏ Problems with mouth, teeth, or gums

❏ Difficulty chewing

❏ Difficulty swallowing

❏ Angular stomatitis

❏ Glossitis

❏ History of bone pain

❏ History of bone fractures

❏ Skin changes (dry, loose, nonspecific lesions, edema)

Percentile	Men 55-65 y	65-75 y	Women 55-65 y	65-75 y
Arm circumference (cm)				
10th	27.3	26.3	25.7	25.2
50th	31.7	30.7	30.3	29.9
95th	36.9	35.5	38.5	37.3
Arm muscle circumference (cm)				
10th	24.5	23.5	19.6	19.5
50th	27.8	26.8	22.5	22.5
95th	32.0	30.6	28.0	27.9
Triceps skinfold (mm)				
10th	6	6	16	14
50th	11	11	25	24
95th	22	22	38	36

From: Frisancho AR. New norms of upper limb fat and muscle areas for assessment of nutritional status. Am J Clin Nutr 1981; 34:2540-2545. © 1981 American Society for Clinical Nutrition.

Eating Habits

❏ Does not have enough food to eat each day

❏ Usually eats alone

❏ Does not eat anything on one or more days each month

❏ Has poor appetite

❏ Is on a special diet

❏ Eats vegetables two or fewer times daily

❏ Eats milk or milk products once or not at all daily

❏ Eats fruit or drinks fruit juice once or not at all daily

❏ Eats breads, cereals, pasta, rice, or other grains five or fewer times daily

❏ Has more than one alcoholic drink per day (if woman); more than two drinks per day (if man)

Living Environment

❏ Lives on an income of less than $6000 per year (per individual in the household)

❏ Lives alone

❏ Is housebound

❏ Is concerned about home security

❏ Lives in a home with inadequate heating or cooling

❏ Does not have a stove and/or refrigerator

❏ Is unable or prefers not to spend money on food (<$25-30 per person spent on food each week)

Functional Status

Usually or always needs assistance with (check each that apply):

❏ Bathing

❏ Dressing

❏ Grooming

❏ Toileting

❏ Eating

❏ Walking or moving about

❏ Traveling (outside the home)

❏ Preparing food

❏ Shopping for food or other necessities

Mental/Cognitive Status

❏ Clinical evidence of impairment, e.g. Folstein<26

❏ Clinical evidence of depressive illness, e.g. Beck Depression Inventory>15, Geriatric Depression Scale>5

Patients in whom you have identified one or more major indicator (see pg 2) of poor nutritional status require immediate medical attention; if minor indicators are found, ensure that they are known to a health professional or to the patient's own physician. Patients who display risk factors (see pg 2) of poor nutritional status should be referred to the appropriate health care or social service professional (dietitian, nurse, dentist, case manager, etc.).

FIGURE 7.2 (continued)

and chronic infection. High transferrin levels may be found with iron deficiency.

Plasma IGF-I concentration is considered a valuable index of PEM in young and middle-aged adults. As mentioned previously, because IGF-I levels decrease with age, it may not be valid to extrapolate these results to the elderly. However, changes in IGF-I strongly predict the likelihood of life-threatening complications in the elderly [41]. Furthermore, in one study IGF-I was well correlated with markers of nutritional status, including (1) serum albumin, transferrin, and cholesterol; (2) triceps skinfold thickness; and (3) percentage of ideal body weight. These changes may reflect the detrimental effects of low IGF-I concentrations. Despite these findings, the validity of

IGF-I as a nutritional marker in the elderly still must be determined.

Various signaling pathways are influenced by reactive oxygen species. The glutathione precursor cysteine has been shown to decrease insulin responsiveness in the fasted state. Supplementation with cysteine in clinical trials leads to improvement of various conditions that deteriorate with aging. These include skeletal muscle function, immune functions and plasma albumin levels. It also causes a decrease in body fat/lean body mass ratio. These data suggest that aging may also be associated with a deficiency in cysteine [42].

Immune Markers

Total lymphocyte count is a nonspecific indicator of protein-energy malnutrition (PEM). An absolute lymphocyte count of less than $1,500/mm^3$ indicates malnutrition if other causes of lymphopenia can be excluded. The lymphocyte count appears to decrease in the elderly, although it remains above $1,500/mm^3$ [43].

Delayed hypersensitivity skin testing is a parameter used to assess relative immune competence. An anergic response has been linked to both increasing age and malnutrition. As yet it is unclear whether PEM-Associated changes in immune competence can be distinguished from those due to aging alone. In general, anergy is a poor predictor of malnutrition in the elderly and may be less reliable than in younger patients.

Functional Assessment

Functional assessment of the elderly helps detect physical and cognitive alterations that may increase the risk of malnutrition. Nutritional well-being is related to the ability of elders to perform the activities of daily life. The BMI, used as a standard measure of overall nutrition, is related to the functional capabilities of community-dwelling elderly. Elderly individuals with a low BMI are at greater risk for functional impairment [44]. Among other methods for evaluating capacity, direct measurements of neuromuscular performance, including motor strength, vibratory sense, gait and balance, and gait speed, are strongly related to disability [45]. In addition, many evaluation scales for cognitive and physical assessment that vary in simplicity have been developed [46]. These include the Activities of Daily Living (ADL) and Instrumental Activities of Daily Living (IADLs). ADL include bathing, dressing, toileting, transfer in and out of bed/chair, bowel and bladder continence, and the ability to feed oneself. Instrumental activities of daily living include the ability to use the telephone, shopping, food preparation, laundry, transportation, responsibility for medications, and ability to handle finances. Poor performance scores on these tests should be carefully evaluated because deficits may result from malnutrition or may render the patient susceptible to malnutrition. Depressive symptoms and cognitive impairment are independent predictors of decline in functional status and increased dependence in activities of daily living [47]. These, in turn, can lead to inadequate food intake and malnutrition.

Nutritional Requirements of the Elderly

Energy requirements in the elderly decrease because of a reduction in muscle mass and a reduction in physical activity. Subjects over the age of 70 consume about a third less calories than their younger counterparts. Without adequate supplementation, this results in a reduction of all nutrients. Unfortunately, the requirements for these nutrients does not decrease. Nutrient dense foods can decrease mortality and decrease LOS in hospitals [48]. The modified MyPyramid (Fig. 7.3) was developed by researchers at Tufts University

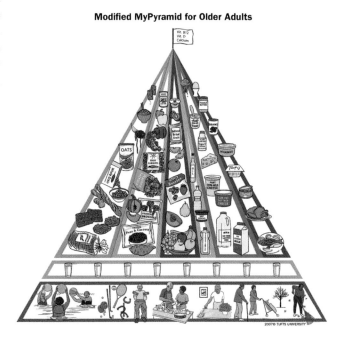

Figure 7.3 The major features of the modified MyPyramid for Older Adults graphic that are different from MyPyramid are the expanded presentation of food icons throughout the pyramid highlighting good choices within each category, a foundation depicting a row of water glasses and physical activities emphasizing the increased importance of both fluid intake and regular physical activity in older adults, and a flag on the top to suggest that some older adults, due to biological changes, may need supplemental vitamins B-12 and D, and calcium (reprinted from Lichtenstein A (2008) Modified pyramid of older adults. J Nutr 138(1):5–11, with permission from the American Society for Nutrition).

in Boston and emphasizes the importance of nutrient and fiber-rich foods and provides guidance about alternate food forms and the importance of regular exercise and adequate fluid intake [49]. The pyramid is most useful when used in combination with the US Department of Agriculture's general MyPyramid food guide.

Fluid Requirements

Dehydration is one of the main discharge diagnoses in patients over age 65 [50]. Inadequate intake is one of the most common reasons for water and electrolyte disorders in this age group. Possible explanations include a decrease in the thirst sensation with increasing age. Age-related decreases in vasopressin secretion and an alteration in the opioid system may also impair fluid regulation [51]. Renal function decreases with age, as does the kidney's capacity to adapt to changes in hydration status and electrolyte intake, thereby interfering with regulatory mechanisms. Stress and infection are often associated with decreased fluid intake and hydration. Fluid losses may be further increased by fever, vomiting, diarrhea, fistulas, and open surgical wounds, and they should be accounted for. In addition, fluid intake may be restricted owing to chronic renal insufficiency or congestive heart failure. The above factors predispose the elderly patient to hydration and fluid overload. Thus a more gradual approach to fluid delivery is appropriate. Dehydration may lead to confusion, resulting in decreased fluid intake. Patients and their families should be informed about the importance of adequate fluid intake and the need for monitoring intake and output during stressful periods.

Various formulas can be used to predict baseline fluid requirements, although some formulas do not account for obesity and low body weight and may give unrealistic estimates [52]. The following formula is appropriate for establishing fluid recommendations, as it adjusts for height and weight: 100 ml fluid/kg for the first 10 kg of body weight, 50 ml/kg for the next 10 kg of body weight, and 15 ml/kg for the remaining kilograms of body weight. A goal of at least 1,500–2,000 ml fluid is recommended. Given the reduced volume of formula required to meet the decreasing energy needs of the elderly, patients receiving the tube feeding may need additional fluid to maintain adequate hydration [1].

Energy Requirements

Several formulas are available to estimate energy requirements of the elderly. The Harris and Benedict equations (HBEs), which take into consideration sex, age, height, and weight, can be used to estimate the resting energy expenditure (REE).

$$\text{Men} = 66.47 + [13.75 \times W\,(\text{kg})]$$
$$+ [5.0 \times H\,(\text{cm})] - [6.76 \times A\,(\text{years})]$$
$$\text{Women} = 66.51 + [9.6 \times W\,(\text{kg})]$$
$$+ [1.85 \times H\,(\text{cm})] - [4.68 \times A\,(\text{years})]$$

W is the weight, H is the height, and A is the age. The REE obtained is expressed in kilocalories per day. Unfortunately, the HBEs are performed poorly in some instances, and they can underestimate the actual REE in malnourished and critically ill patients [53]. The same is true in undernourished nursing home residents [54]. In these instances, direct measurement of REE is more appropriate. REE can also be predicted without height with only a minor loss of accuracy [1].

$$\text{Men} = 13.5(W) + 487$$

$$\text{Women} = 19.5(W) + 596$$

A correlation factor should be added to the REE depending on the degree of metabolic stress of the patient (Table 7.4).

Currently, recommendations for energy requirements in the elderly are based on assumed levels of physical activity relative to the basal metabolic rate (BMR). However, substantial error is found when total energy expenditure is derived from measurements or predictions of BMR [55]. Furthermore, current recommended daily allowances (RDAs) may significantly underestimate the energy requirements for physical activity in healthy elderly persons. Accurate estimation of energy needs is important for delivering adequate nutritional care and preventing disability. Human aging has been associated with reduced ability to regulate energy balance. This might explain the vulnerability of older persons to unexplained weight gain and weight loss [56]. Thus in some older individuals, successful weight maintenance may require increased control over food intake and energy requirements.

Table 7.4 Adjustment factors for resting energy expenditure

Correction factor	Stress
1.0–1.1	Postoperative
1.1–1.3	Multiple fractures
1.2–1.5	Weight gain/replenishment
1.3–1.6	Severe infection/bullet wounds
1.6	Sepsis
1.5–2.1	Third-degree burns
1.2	Confined to bed
1.3	Out of bed
1.5	Active

Source: Data from Nelson and Franzi [13]

Protein Requirements

Although the recommended daily allowance for protein is 0.8 mg/kg/day, recent studies have shown that the protein requirement in the elderly should be as much as 1.5 g/kg/day, i.e., 15–20% of total caloric intake [57]. This may increase muscle mass and function leading to greater activity. This is particularly important in patients with co-morbidities such as diabetes, low-grade inflammation, etc. that cause anorexia. A 24-h urine urea nitrogen (UUN) can determine the amount of total nitrogen excreted and can be used to estimate protein requirements, though it is rarely used in clinical practice. Rather, nitrogen losses are more commonly estimated or extrapolated. The following formula accounts for insensible and fecal losses and can be used to estimate total nitrogen loss.

$$\text{Total nitrogen loss} = 24\text{ h UNN (g / day)}$$
$$+ (0.20 \times 24\text{ UNN}) + 2\text{ g / day}$$

$$\text{Nitrogen (N) balance} = N\text{ intake}$$
$$- [\text{urine N} + \text{stool N} + \text{insensible}$$
$$N\text{ losses}]$$

Generally a positive nitrogen balance of 4–6 g is necessary for anabolism. During the metabolic response to trauma, proteins are broken down to amino acids and are used for hepatic gluconeogenesis. The decrease in lean body mass that occurs with aging reduces tissue protein reserve and may diminish the body's capacity to resynthesize proteins. However, excluding burn patients, it seems prudent that during periods of stress such as infection, surgical trauma, or cancer, the daily protein intake should be increased to 1.5 g/kg/day [7].

Vitamin Requirements

As we have discussed, it is a combination of physical, social, and psychological factors that make the elderly population particularly susceptible to malnutrition. Aging alone might be accompanied by a decrease in some vitamin levels. These modifications may lead to an increased risk of vitamin deficiencies and disease. In the following sections, we review the most important vitamins and the role their supplementation may play in the nutritional status of aged individuals.

Vitamin A

Special consideration should be given to vitamin A supplementation in elderly subjects. In contrast to other vitamin levels, serum concentrations of vitamin A are usually within the normal range in the elderly. The liver has a great capacity to store vitamin A, and hepatocellular levels of vitamin A are maintained through life. In addition, older individuals have an increased capacity to absorb vitamin A, and they have decreased renal excretion. Thus, over supplementation could predispose the elderly to vitamin A toxicity [58]. Increased vitamin A intake by the elderly can raise serum retinyl ester concentrations, which are an index of vitamin A overload. Elderly subjects with elevated fasting plasma retinyl esters were shown to have elevated liver function tests, indicative of liver damage. In view of the above findings, the current RDA for vitamin A of 5,000 IU for men and 4,000 IU for women may be too high for the elderly and should probably be reduced.

Vitamin B$_6$

Vitamin B$_6$ appears to play an important role in the regulation of homocysteine metabolism. Vitamin B$_6$ plasma concentrations inversely correlate with homocysteine concentrations, and elevated levels of homocysteine are associated with the development of occlusive vascular disease [59]. In addition, plasma pyridoxal-5′-phosphate (the coenzyme of vitamin B$_6$) concentrations have been linked to stenosis [60]. At this time, it cannot be concluded that lowering plasma homocysteine by increasing vitamin intake reduces the risk of vascular disease. It is not uncommon to encounter low vitamin B$_6$ plasma levels among the elderly, so it is probable that vitamin B$_6$ requirements are insufficient [60, 61]. Considering the above findings, a vitamin B$_6$ intake of 1.9–2.0 mg/day is adequate.

Vitamin B$_{12}$

Serum vitamin B$_{12}$ levels decline with advancing age. Prevalence of vitamin B$_{12}$ deficiency varies among countries, from none in the United Kingdom up to 7.3% in the rest of Europe [62]. In the USA, the prevalence of vitamin B$_{12}$ deficiency was shown to be more than 12% in a large sample of free-living elderly. By measuring serum homocysteine, a vitamin B$_{12}$ metabolite, many elderly people with normal serum vitamin concentrations were found to be metabolically deficient in cobalamin [63]. The reasons for the high prevalence of vitamin B$_{12}$ deficiency is probably a major etiologic factor. The vitamin B$_{12}$ level may also be affected by the high prevalence of atrophic gastritis (a partial decrease in fundic glands and of parietal cell mass) in the elderly population. There is a significant association between age and the prevalence of atrophic gastritis, which is as high as 24% after age 50 and 37% after age 80 [64]. In addition, gastric and intestinal bacterial overgrowth may contribute to vitamin B$_{12}$ malabsorption.

In view of these findings, the current RDA may underestimate the need for vitamin B_{12} in the elderly. Low B12 concentrations were less prevalent among persons consuming B12-containing supplements. Biochemical B12 deficiency has been found to be higher in adults over 50 years of age. Current recommended daily allowance for B12 of 2.4 mug may be insufficient for those aged >50 years [65]. Clinically, the hematological changes typical of megaloblastic anemia can be absent in most subjects with evidence of deficiency.

Neuropsychiatric symptoms of vitamin B_{12} deficiency may be present even with normal serum levels of vitamin B_{12}. Any elderly patient who is, or is suspected to be, vitamin B_{12}-deficient, based on the neurologic symptoms of vitamin B_{12} deficiency, should receive a course of parenteral vitamin B_{12} to replete stores [1]. Once the etiology of the deficiency is determined, appropriate maintenance therapy can be initiated.

Calcium and Vitamin D

With aging, serum vitamin D levels decline as a result of less-efficient synthesis of vitamin D by the skin, less-efficient intestinal absorption, and possibly reduced sun exposure and intake of vitamin D [66]. Sun exposure is essential for maintaining vitamin D levels and institutionalized elderly who do not receive enough sun are at particular risk of vitamin D deficiency. [67] Note that exposure of skin to sunlight that has passed through windowpane glass or Plexiglas does not produce cholecalciferol [68]. Sunscreen use and dark skin pigmentation can also substantially influence cutaneous production of vitamin D. Latitude influences the amount of vitamin D as well. In northern latitudes and during winter, ultraviolet B rays do not reach the earth's surface. People in these regions are entirely dependent on dietary sources of vitamin D during this season. In the USA, the major dietary source of vitamin D is milk. Elderly individuals with lactose intolerance may avoid milk products that contain vitamin D and may be dependent on endogenous synthesis of this vitamin.

Intestinal calcium absorption is independently reduced with age and after menopause as estrogen levels decrease [69]. This might be due to age-related changes in the metabolism of vitamin D. Although antifracture efficacy is of primary interest, change in bone mineral density (BMD) is widely used in clinical trials because it is a strong predictor of fracture risk; with its use, a far smaller number of patients are required for a study [68]. Data have shown that calcium supplements significantly reduce bone mineral loss and increased bone density. In addition, calcium combined with vitamin D supplements have reduced hip and other nonvertebral fracture rates in nursing home residents [70]. However, vitamin D supplements alone do not decrease the incidence of hip fractures, which suggest that only the combination of calcium and vitamin D is beneficial [71]. *The current vitamin D RDA*

of 200 IU may not be sufficient to minimize bone loss. An intake of 400–800 IU/day appears to be needed for healthy postmenopausal women [1, 62, 72]. A randomized placebo-controlled double blind study in patients greater than or equal to 64 years of age revealed that in greater than 97.5% of these individuals, the requirement for vitamin D is met by intake between 7.9 and 42.8 mug/day of Vitamin D. Factors influencing this requirement include summer sun exposure at an adequacy of 25(OH)D [73]. Calcium intakes of 1,000 mg/day for postmenopausal women taking estrogen and 1,500 mg/day for women not taking estrogen are now considered optimal by many [54, 61, 68]. Calcium intake should not exceed 2,400 mg/day, because of the risk of nephrolithiasis [1].

Nutritional Problems in the Elderly

Obesity

Obesity is a major problem worldwide. In the USA, 74% of men and 66% of women aged 60 and older in are overweight or obese based on body mass index. A recent study showed that increased body mass index did not correlate with increased mortality in the elderly. Instead, it was the waist circumference that served as a more significant marker of increased mortality in the elderly [74]. It is therefore felt that both body mass index and waist circumference should be taken into account when evaluating obesity in the elderly. Obesity has also been shown to relate to functional disability in the elderly. In women, waist circumference has been found to be a better predictor of functional disability than BMI [75]. Obesity may exacerbate cardiovascular disease through several mechanisms including systemic inflammation, hypercoagulopathy and activation of the renin–angiotensin mechanisms [76].

Anorexia of Aging

Anorexia commonly occurs with aging. The decrease in appetite can be due to a decrease in basal metabolic rate, most likely secondary to a decrease in lean body mass and to a more sedentary lifestyle. Drugs can also cause anorexia as well as interfere with the intake, absorption, and metabolism of nutrients. Because of their use of multiple medications, the elderly are at increased risk of drug interactions, which may interfere with nutrient assimilation. Decreased food intake is more common in men than in women [4]. It is also seen in healthy elderly individuals. Psychosocial factors, such as depression and isolation also influence food intake.

The physiological decrease in food intake in the elderly is termed anorexia of aging and can be attributed to several factors. Among these are an increase in peripheral satiating systems, decreased compliance of the fundus of the stomach, an increase in basal levels of cholecystokinin and in secretion of cholecystokinin in response to intraduodenal fat. Decrease in testosterone in males results in increased levels of leptin and this in turn may accentuate anorexia.

Cachexia

Cachexia may result from an adaptation to an underlying illness such as cancer. A diagnosis of cachexia is made when there is a weight loss of at least 5% in a period of 12 months accompanied by three of the five following factors: decreased muscle strength, fatigue, anorexia, low fat-free mass index and abnormal biochemistry such as increased CRP or IL-6, anemia or low serum albumin. These factors help to distinguish cachexia from anorexia alone. Cachexia can result from problems with oral intake due to mucositis, or due to gastrointestinal concerns such as nausea and vomiting, bowel obstruction due to tumor burden, or delayed gastric emptying. Increased levels of TNF-α and IL-1 can cause cachexia, nausea, and vomiting. Central nervous system mediated effects result from pain and altered sense of smell and taste. Treatment options are limited. The use of androgens, selective androgen receptor modulators, antimyostatin drugs, growth hormone, insulin-like growth factor, and ghrelin have yet to show significant efficacy [77]. Megestrol acetate has been shown to improve appetite and decrease nausea in some cases, by causing a reduction of IL-1, IL-6, and TNF-α [78]. Data is still sparse for geriatric recommendations with nutriceutical repletion using Omega-3 fatty acids, co-essential/essential aminoacids.

Sarcopenia

Decreased food intake coupled with decreased activity leads to decreased muscle mass, which is termed sarcopenia. Cytokines play a role in both anorexia and sarcopenia. Chronic inflammatory conditions lead to an increase in cytokines such as IL-1β, IL-6, and TNF-α. Several cytokines belong to the same family as leptin and exert their effects by stimulating the leptin receptor. IL-I causes a decrease in luteinizing hormone, resulting in decreased testosterone levels and worsening anorexia and sarcopenia. Recently, a specific dietary approach has been found to prevent or slow down muscle loss with ageing. Rather than suggesting a large global increase in protein intake, it has been

found that ingestion of a sufficient amount of protein with each meal is more beneficial. Dietary plans that include 25–30 g of protein with each meal can maximize muscle protein synthesis [79].

Unintentional Weight Loss

Unintentional weight loss is a common problem in elderly patients and should be recognized and evaluated without undue delay. Several studies have shown that weight loss of 4–5% of body weight or more within 1 year or 10% over 5–10 years is associated with increased morbidity and mortality [80]. Low BMI (body mass index of less than 18.5) is an indication of protein-calorie malnutrition [81]. In nursing home residents 65 years of age or older, low BMI has a negative impact on the quality of life [82].

Although a quarter of these patients may not have any identifiable cause to explain the weight loss, the etiology can be detected in others by specific symptom-related investigation. Common causes of unintentional weight loss include malignant diseases (16–36%), psychiatric disorder (9–42%), gastrointestinal disease (6–19%), hyperthyroidism (4–11%), nutritional disorders or alcoholism (4–8%), and respiratory disease (6%) or renal disease (4%) [83] (Table 7.5). A thorough history and physical examination and the mini-nutritional assessment are used to assess unintentional weight loss. Attention should also be paid to medications that cause anorexia, dry mouth, nausea or vomiting, and dysphagia. Psychological and psychosocial causes should be identified and addressed. Nonpharmacological interventions include minimizing dietary restrictions [84] adding favorite foods to the diet, adding nutritional supplements, and involving nutritional programs such as meals on wheels. Pharmacological therapies are used to either stimulate appetite or cause weight gain. These include megestrol, acetate, ornithine, oxoglutarate, recombinant human growth hormone and dronabinol.

Table 7.5 Meals on wheels pneumonic for weight loss in older adults

Medications
Emotions – depression
Alcoholism
Late life paranoia
Swallowing problems

Oral factors
Nosocomial infections

Wandering
Hyperthyroidism, hypercalcemia, hypoadrenalism
Enteral
Eating problems
Low salt, low cholesterol diets
Stones

They are associated with multiple side effects and there are no prospective randomized trials that justify their use in elderly patients.

Frailty

Both undernutrition and obesity should be viewed as indicators of frailty in the older adult. The definition proposed by Fried [85] includes the presence of three or more of the following factors: unintentional weight loss, self-reported exhaustion, weakness, slow gait speed, and low physical activity. Severity and duration of weight loss and enquiry into activities of daily living (ADL) such as cooking and meal preparation are important. Frail older people may show low leptin levels and increased levels of IL-6 and C-reactive protein [86]. Other markers include 25-hydroxyvitamin D, IGF-1, and D-Dimer, suggesting a state that is pro-inflammatory [87].

Anemia

It has been shown that there is a significant association between anemia and malnutrition in the elderly. A third of anemia cases can be attributed to deficiency of nutritional factors such as iron, vitamin B12, and folic acid [88]. A cross-sectional study of 60 elderly hospitalized patients showed a 36.7% incidence of anemia. In this study, mid-arm muscle circumference (MAMC), albumin, and prealbumin correlated with hemoglobin in the bivariate analysis. MAMC and albumin were found to be significant predictors of hemoglobin in patients without inflammation (estimated by erythrocyte sedimentation rate) and prealbumin was found to be a predictor of hemoglobin in patients with inflammation [89].

Calorie Restriction

Changes with age include a gradual build up of degradative agents such as reactive oxygen and nitrogen species. Gene stability and function at fat-soluble and water-soluble sites within the mitochondria are affected by these reactive species [90]. The only intervention that has been shown to alter this phenomenon is calorie reduction. Restriction of total caloric intake has been shown to delay the rate of primary aging in many species such as worms, flies, and mice [91] although the mechanism responsible for this is not clear. Candidate mechanisms of calorie restriction in these species include decreased oxidative damage due to a reduction of reactive oxygen species generation and increased removal, altered neuroendocrine function and decreased incidence of

chronic diseases such as obesity, diabetes and cardiovascular diseases [92].

In overweight nonobese humans, caloric restriction improves whole body metabolic efficiency and lowers markers of oxidative stress [93]. Studies in mice and rats have shown that caloric restriction leads to a delay in immunosenescence – the expected decline in humoral and cell-mediated immune function associated with aging. The phenomenon may account for the delay in the development of certain neoplasms in these animals. Caloric restriction has also been shown to decrease the oxidative damage to proteins, lipids, and DNA resulting in decreased production of free oxygen radicals. Surrogate measures show that calorie restriction in humans reduces the risk factor for atherosclerosis and diabetes [94]. These include a very low level of inflammation as evidenced by low circulatory levels of c-reactive protein and TNFα, serum triiodothyronine levels at the low end of the normal range, and a more elastic "younger" left ventricle (LV), as evaluated by echo-Doppler measures of LV stiffness.

Nutritional Supplementation

Acute Care

Nutritional support in elderly patients is particularly important during admission for acute illness. Attention should be focused on the initial medical or surgical management of the acute problem. Strategies to counteract decreased consumption, poor appetite, and chewing problems are particularly critical in the elderly [95].

Enteral Nutrition

Physicians should be careful with orders that prohibit or limit oral intake. Such orders should be temporary in nature, with specific plans for nutritional supplementation in the event that the oral intake has to be withheld longer than anticipated. Fast-track rehabilitation may be possible in elderly patients following laparoscopic or open colonic surgery. In a small nonrandomized study, early enteral feeding and mobilization coupled with pain relief and management of postoperative nausea and vomiting (PONV) was feasible in patients over the age of 70 and resulted in improved organ function and improved outcomes [96].

There is a need to determine values or markers that can help assess prognostic factors of 6-month mortality in patients admitted in the post-acute care setting. Functional and nutritional changes following an acute health crises can help determine such outcomes [97]. The INTERACTIVE trial combines nutrition (recommendations of nutrient dense foods, provision of recipes and referral to community meal programs and supplementation with commercial liquid diets, protein supplements or multi-vitamins where deemed necessary by a dietitian) and exercise therapy (exercise and fall prevention information) as an early intervention to address deconditioning, weight loss, and the ability to return to pre-admission status in elderly patients following proximal femur fractures. The study will be completed in September 2009, following which the results will become available [98].

Meal replacement products are often used to supplement oral intake in older adults. Liquid products, more than solid replacements, blunt the postprandial decline in hunger and therefore increase subsequent food intake in older adults [99].

Enteral nutrition is a preferred form of nutritional supplementation in the postoperative period. It helps to maintain epithelial cell structure and function and also helps in maintenance of mucosal immunity. Enteral tube feeding may be necessary in elderly patients hospitalized for an acute illness when they are unable to eat or swallow but have a functioning gut. Short-term feeding is possible through a small bore nasogastric feeding tube that does not interfere with the patient's ability to swallow. Radiographic evidence of proper placement of tubes is important before starting feeds. Full strength formulas should be used, starting at 25 ml/h and gradually increasing to reach the goal in 24–48 h.

Gastrostomy tube and jejunostomy tubes are used for long-term feeding, especially in patients who may require nutritional support for greater than 6–8 weeks. Temporary feeding tubes help maintain nutrition with the perioperative period. However, there is concern about placing feeding tubes in elderly patients who will not benefit from its intervention and whose quality of life in terminal stages of illness is adversely affected. Problems encountered include need for placement in nursing homes, lack of social interaction, need for restraints to protect the feeding tube and cellulites at the tube sites. Multidisciplinary approaches and frank discussions between the patient, the patient's family, and physicians can help with informed decision-making [100].

In patients with the prerenal disease, the BUN:plasma creatinine ratio may be greater than 20:1 due to an increased absorption of urea. BUN also increases with increased nitrogen intake. Adequate attention needs to be paid to high protein administration in elderly patients with impaired renal function [101]. These patients can retain excessive fluid resulting in peripheral edema and cardiac failure.

Fiber supplementation is important in enteral feeding. Although it does not have any effect on nutrition, it results in improved bowel function. In a study of 183 patients (mean age = 82 years), randomized to enteral feeds with and without fiber, the patients who received fiber had reduced stool frequency and more solid stool [102].

Total Parenteral Nutrition

Elderly patients tolerate total parenteral nutrition (TPN) well and are not at greater risk of complications than their younger counterparts [103]. If oral feeds have to be withheld for greater than 7 days due to a nonfunctioning gut as in paralytic ileus, then TPN should be considered, through a centrally or peripherally inserted central venous catheter. There is no data showing any significant advantage of peripherally inserted central catheters over centrally inserted central venous catheters. A recent study showed that while peripherally inserted lines were not superior to centrally inserted lines, the incidence of thrombotic complications was higher in peripherally placed lines. Other studies show that peripherally placed lines have a lower cost of insertion, lower rate of infection, and lower complication rate [104].

Irrespective of the site of the intravenous catheter, parenteral nutrition can be associated with metabolic, infectious, and technical complications [105]. It should therefore be used for the shortest period possible and every attempt made to start enteral or oral feeding as soon as possible. Protein and caloric requirements can be provided and are calculated using the Harris–Benedict Equation. The goal is to achieve a positive nitrogen balance using amino acids, 10% dextrose and intralipids. Calorie requirements should be calculated carefully and patients should not be given excessive calories. Metabolic complications include hyper- or hypoglycemia, hyperlipidemia, hypercapnia, acid-base disturbances, and refeeding syndrome. Older patients are particularly susceptible to overfeeding with resultant azotemia, hypertonic dehydration, and metabolic acidosis [106].

Liver dysfunction can occur when patients are on TPN. Liver function tests are monitored on a weekly basis. In a prospective cohort study of patients in 40 Intensive Care Units, administration of TPN within the first 24 h after admission was found to have a protective effect on liver function [107]. Once the patient is able to tolerate 50% oral intake or enteral feeds, TPN can be weaned off. Percutaneous lines should be left in place until there is assurance that the patient can continue to tolerate oral intake.

Frequent accuchecks are critical to avoid hypoglycemia. Patients are usually given 10% Dextrose at 50 cc/h during the weaning period. Inability to tolerate oral intake should be an indication of failure to wean and the patient should be restarted on TPN. The importance of glycemic control in older sick surgical patients, particularly in the ICU cannot be overemphasized. Hyperglycemia (glucose > 10 mmol/l) contributes to mortality seen in critically ill ICU patients. The incidence of infectious complications also increases with hyperglycemia. Currently glucose levels between 4.5 and 6.1 mmol/l are recommended, as there is a significant risk of hypoglycemia in patients treated to tighter limits [108].

Nutritional Issues in Specific Disease States

Few changes in the gastrointestinal system occur with aging and therefore signs and symptoms should be attributed to specific disease processes. Table 7.6 summarizes age-related alterations in the GI tract. The information is helpful in the evaluation and management of understanding nutritional needs in the elderly in the perioperative period [109].

Pancreatitis

Nutrition in the setting of acute pancreatitis is a challenging problem. Most of these patient present with abdominal pain, nausea, and vomiting. A metaanalysis of 11 randomized controlled trials showed that enteral nutrition in comparison with parenteral nutrition resulted in a statistically significant (59%) decrease in infectious complications and a statistically non-significant (40%) decrease in mortality [110]. A subsequent metaanalyses evaluated the effect of timing of the commencement of feeds in patients with acute pancreatitis. When started within 48 h of admission, enteral nutrition as compared to parenteral nutrition showed a statistically significant reduction in the risk of multiple organ failure, infectious complications, and mortality. There was no decrease in multiple organ failure risk, infectious complications or mortality if initiation of enteral nutrition was delayed to greater than 48 h following admission. This shows that timing of artificial nutrition is critical in patients with pancreatitis [111].

When enteral feeding is started, it is usually through a Dophoff tube with the tip positioned as distally to the ampulla of Vater as possible. Once the pancreatitis has resolved, low fat oral intake is encouraged.

Enterocutaneous Fistula

Maintenance of fluid and electrolyte balance is critical in the initial management of small bowel fistulas. Nutritional disturbances are present in 55–90% of patients with enterocutaneous fistulae [112]. Parenteral nutrition maybe initiated and should include trace elements and vitamins. Enteral nutrition should be administered in small bowel fistulas that are not expected to close spontaneously, in colocutaneous fistulas and when fistula output does not interfere with wound care [113]. Clear fluid up to 500 cc/day can be ingested. Enteral nutrition should consist of low residue diets [114].

Pressure Ulcers

Pressure ulcers can be a significant drain on energy reserves. Advanced stage pressure ulcers cause a catabolic and this state is influenced by the volume of the ulcers [115]. Specific instructions should be followed by the nursing staff to prevent development of pressure ulcers during hospitalizations for an acute problem. MNA is a useful screening and assessment tool in multimorbid geriatric patients with pressure ulcers [116]. Identification and management of nutritional deficiencies can decrease the risk of developing pressure ulcers.

TABLE 7.6 Gastrointestinal changes of senescence by segment

Segment of GI tract	Age-related alterations in GI tract	Diseases with nutritional consequences
Esophagus	Minor alterations in UES	Dysphagia
		GERD
Stomach	↓ Pepsin activity	Gastritis type A
	↓ Prostaglandin synthesis	Gastritis type B
	↓ Mucosal blood flow	Delayed gastric emptying
	↓ Gastric fluid secretion	Achlorhydria
Small intestine	↓ Lactase activity	Bacterial overgrowth
	↓ Intestinal blood flow	Lactose intolerance
	↓ Sodium/glucose co-transport	Inflammatory bowel disease
Colon	↓ In neuronal density	Constipation
	↓ Wall elasticity from collagen deposition	Diverticulosis
	↓ Resting pressure of internal sphincter	Angiodysplasia
Liver	↓ Liver size and blood flow	Hepatic encephalopathy cirrhosis (hepatitis C, ethanol,
	↓ Dynamic liver function	primary biliary cirrhosis)
Pancreas	↓ Pancreatic mass	Pancreatic cancer
	Ductular changes/fibrosis	Chronic pancreatitis
		Diabetes

Source: Adapted with permission from Dryden and McClave [110]

CASE STUDY

A 74-year-old man presented with an incarcerated ventral hernia. At exploratory laparotomy he was found to have a small bowel perforation within the hernia sac. Following small bowel resection and anastomoses, his fascial defect was too large to be repaired primarily. It was therefore repaired with a double layer of vicryl mesh and wound vacuum device. His past medical history was significant for diabetes, hypertension, and remote history of left hemicolectomy for diverticular disease.

Nutrition Assessment included weight 125 kg, height 175 cm, ideal body weight (IBW): 75 kg, percent IBW:167%, BMI=41. Duration of inadequate nutrition: 7 days. He was eating adequately until a week prior to admission. His albumin (1.9) was severely depleted but likely represented a stress response rather than long-term nutritional status. Preoperatively, it was recommended that he receive: 1,875–2,250 cal/day to maintain weight. As part of the weekly nutritional assessment, he was weighed three times a week, and visceral protein labs were checked once a week.

The patient was kept NPO following surgery. The nasogastric tube placed prior to surgery was removed on postoperative day 2; he was given clear liquids on postoperative day 3; and advanced to a regular diet on postoperative day 5 after return of bowel function. He was subsequently discharged home on postoperative day 6.

He was readmitted 2 weeks later following increased drainage from abdominal wound and found to have an enterocutaneous fistula with an output of 1,200 cc/day. He was kept NPO and started on total parenteral nutrition (TPN) through a PICC line. Three weeks later, examination of his abdominal wound revealed small bowel mucosa at the site of the enterocutaneous fistula. At this time it was felt that the fistula would not close spontaneously and that he would need to undergo an exploratory laparotomy with small bowel resection and anastomoses. He was started on a low residue diet and weaned off his TPN. He was allowed 1,000 ml of free water per day to avoid dehydration. Calorie counts performed over a 2-day period showed an average calorie intake of 1,600 cal/day, with 80 g of protein per day. A higher protein intake of 113–135 g/day (1.3–1.5 g/kg) was advised.

At the time of his preoperative evaluation 5 months later, he weighed 125 kg.

His nutritional lab findings revealed an albumin of 3.3. He underwent a successful takedown of his enterocutaneous fistula and repair of his ventral hernia with bilateral separation of components. Five days following his surgery he was tolerating a regular diet.

Correcting zinc and calcium deficiencies and increasing the protein intake to 25% of total caloric intake increases the rate of healing of pressure ulcers.

Palliative Care

Artificial nutrition is considered medical treatment and not basic care [117]. The distinction is important because patients have a right to avail themselves of, or deny, medical treatment. Whenever possible, patient's wishes regarding enteral nutrition, parenteral nutrition, and the acceptable length of time for such intervention should be elicited. The "TLC" model of palliative care encourages a timely and team-oriented, longitudinal, collaborative, and comprehensive approach [118]. Artificial nutritional support is indicated in patients with head and neck cancers or esophageal cancer who are unable to swallow but continue to have an appetite. However, it has not been shown to improve survival in patients with advanced cancer. Megestrol acetate can be used in these patients to stimulate appetite, as can a short course of corticosteroids. The patient's condition, prognosis, and treatment goals should be discussed with patient and family. Treatment options should include curative treatment and palliative care. Treatment withdrawal should be discussed. Specific details of comfort care afforded to terminally ill patients should be shared with patients. In a study of patients who had cancer or stroke as their terminal diagnosis, patients were offered food and assistance with feeding but without force. Fifty three percent of patients did not experience hunger; 34% initially felt hunger but this resolved. Sixty two percent of patients did not experience thirst or did so only initially [119]. When a terminally ill patient cannot make decisions, the advance directive should be consulted to obtain information regarding the patient's wishes. If this does not exist, the legal guardian or first order relative of the patient will need to make decisions based on the patient's known wishes. In unbefriended patients, the physician's judgment should be used to determine a care plan [120].

References

1. Saltzman E, Mason JB (1997) Enteral nutrition in the elderly. In: Rombeau JL, Rolandelli RH (eds) Enteral and tube feeding. Saunders, Philadelphia, PA, pp 385–402
2. Garry PJ, Vellas BJ (1996) Aging and nutrition. In: Ziegler EE, Filer LJ (eds) Present knowledge in nutrition. ILSI Press, Washington, DC, pp 414–419
3. Rolandelli RH, Ullrich JR (1994) Nutritional support in the frail elderly surgical patient. Surg Clin North Am 74:79–92
4. Morley JE, Silver AJ (1995) Nutritional issues in nursing home care. Ann Intern Med 123:850–859
5. Keller HII (1993) Malutrition in institutionalized elderly: how and why? J Am Geriatr Soc 41:1212–1218
6. Giner M, Laviano A, Meguid MM (1996) In 1995 a correlation between malnutrition and poor outcome in critically ill patients still exists. Nutrition 12:23–29
7. Seeman T, Merkin SS, Crimmins E et al (2008) Education, income and ethnic differences in cumulative biological risk profiles in a national sample of US adults: NHANES III (1988–1994). Soc Sci Med 66(1):72–87
8. Van Dam RM, Li T, Spiegelman D et al (2008) Combined impact of lifestyle factors on mortality: Prospective cohort study in US women. BMJ 337:a1440
9. Locher JL, Ritchie CS, Robinson CO et al (2008) A multidimensional approach to understanding under-eating in homebound older adults. The importance of social factors. Gerontologists 48(2):223–234
10. Schiffman SS, Sattely-Miller EA, Taylor EL, Graham BG, Landerman LR, Zervakis J, Campagna LK, Cohen HJ, Blackwell S, Garst JL (2007) Combination of flavor enhancement and chemosensory education improves nutritional status in older cancer patients. J Nutr Health Aging 11(5):439–454
11. Rapin CH (1995) Nutrition support and the elderly. In: Payne-James J, Grimble G, Silk D (eds) Artificial nutrition support in clinical practice. Little, Brown, Boston, MA, pp 535–544
12. Zekry D, Herrmann FR, Grandjean R et al (2008) Demented versus non-demented very old inpatients: the same comorbidities but poorer functional and nutritional status. Age and Ageing 37:83–89
13. Nelson RC, Franzi LR (1989) Nutrition and aging. Med Clin North Am 73:1531
14. Toogood AA, Adams JE, O'Neill PA et al (1996) Body composition in growth hormone deficient adults over the age of 60 years. Clin Endocrinol (Oxf) 45:339–405
15. Boonen S, Lesaffre E, Aerssens J et al (1996) Deficiency of the growth hormone-insulin-like growth factor-I axis potentially involved in age-related alterations in body composition. Gerontology 42:330–338
16. Rudman D, Feller AG, Nagraj HS et al (1990) Effects of human growth hormone in men over 60 years old. N Engl J Med 323:1–6
17. Christ-Crain M, Meier C, Huber P, Zimmerli L, Trummler M, Müller B (2004) Comparison of different methods for the measurement of serum testosterone in the aging male. Swiss Med Wkly 134(13–14):193–197
18. Christ-Crain M, Mueller B, Gasser TC et al (2004) Is there a clinical relevance of partial androgen deficiency of the aging male? J Urol 172(2):624–627
19. Roberts SB, Fuss P, Heyman M et al (1995) Influence of age on energy requirements. Am J Clin Nutr 62(Suppl):1053S–1058S
20. McGrandy RB, Barrows CH, Spanias A et al (1966) Baltimore Longitudinal Study. Nutrient intakes and energy expenditure in men of different ages. J Gerontol 21:581–587
21. Taaffe DR, Pruitt L, Pyka G et al (1996) Comparative effects of high- and low-intensity resistance training on thigh muscle strength, fiber area, and tissue composition in elderly women. Clin Physiol 16:381–392
22. Stratton RJ, Hackston A, Longmore D, Dixon R, Price S, Stroud M, King C, Elia M (2004) Malnutrition in hospital outpatients and inpatients: prevalence, concurrent validity and ease of use of the 'malnutrition universal screening tool' ('MUST') for adults. Br J Nutr 92(5):799–808
23. Berner YN (2003) Assessment tools for nutritional status in the elderly. Isr Med Assoc J 5(5):365–367, Review
24. Guigoz Y (2006) The Mini Nutritional Assessment (MNA) review of the literature – what does it tell us? J Nutr Health Aging 10(6):466–485
25. Kyle UG, Kossovsky MP, Karsegard VL, Pichard C (2006) Comparison of tools for nutritional assessment and screening at hospital admission: a population study. Clin Nutr 25(3):409–417
26. Jacobs DO, Scheltinga M (1993) Metabolic assessment. In: Rombeau JL, Caldwell MD (eds) Clinical nutrition: parenteral nutrition. Saunders, Philadelphia, PA, pp 245–274
27. De Onis M, Hablicht JP (1996) Anthropometric reference data for international use: recommendations from a World Health Organization expert committee. Am J Clin Nutr 64:650–658
28. Weight by height by age for adults 18–74 years: U.S., 1971–74. DHEW Publ No (PHS)79-1656, September 1979
29. Chumlea WC, Roche AF, Steinbaugh ML (1989) Anthropometric approaches to the nutritional assessment of the elderly. In: Munro HN, Danford DE (eds) Nutrition, aging, and the elderly. Plenum, New York, NY, p 335
30. Kuczmarski RJ, Flegal KM, Campbell SM et al (1994) Increasing prevalence of overweight among US adults: the national health and nutrition examination surveys, 1960 to 1991. JAMA 272:205–211
31. Durning JVGA, Womersley J (1974) Body fat assessment from total body density and its estimation from skinfold thickness. Br J Nutr 32:77–79
32. Herrmann VM (1995) Nutritional assessment. In: Torosian MH (ed) Nutrition for the hospitalized patient. Marcel Dekker, New York, NY, pp 233–253
33. Frisancho AR (1989) New norms of upper limb fat and muscle areas for assessment of nutritional status. Am J Clin Nutr 34:2540–2545
34. Ravaglia G, Morini P, Forti P et al (1997) Anthropometric characteristics of healthy Italian nonagenarians and centenarians. Br J Nutr 77:9–17
35. Salive ME, Cornoni-Huntley J, Phillips CL et al (1992) Serum albumin in older persons: relationship with age and health status. J Clin Epidemiol 45:213
36. Baumgartner RN, Koelher KM, Romero L (1996) Serum albumin is associated with skeletal muscle in elderly men and women. Am J Clin Nutr 64:552–558
37. Sahyoun NR, Jacques PF, Dallal G et al (1996) Use of albumin as a predictor of mortality in community dwelling and institutionalized elderly populations. J Clin Epidemiol 49:981–988
38. Ferguson RP, O'Connor P, Crabtree B et al (1993) Serum albumin and prealbumin as predictors of clinical outcomes of hospitalized elderly nursing home residents. J Am Geriatr Soc 41:545–549
39. Butters M, Straub M, Kraft K et al (1996) Studies on nutritional status in general surgery patients by clinical, anthropometric and laboratory parameters. Nutrition 12:405–410
40. Cals MJ, Devanlay M, Desveaux N et al (1994) Extensive laboratory assessment of nutritional status in fit, health-conscious, elderly people living in the Paris area. J Am Coll Nutr 13:646–657
41. Sullivan DH, Carter WJ (1994) Insulin-like growth factor I as an indicator of protein-energy undernutrition among metabolically stable hospitalized elderly. J Am Coll Nutr 13:184–191
42. Dröge W (2005) Oxidative stress and ageing: Is ageing a cysteine deficiency syndrome? Phil Trans R Soc B 360:2355–2372

43. McArthur WP, Taylor BK, Smith WT (1996) Peripheral blood leukocyte population in the elderly with and without periodontal disease. J Clin Periodontol 23:846–852

44. Galanos AN, Pieper CF, Cornoni-Huntley JC (1994) Nutritional and function: is there a relationship between functional capabilities of community-dwelling elderly? J Am Geriatr Soc 42:368–373

45. Ensrud KE, Nevitt MC, Yunis C et al (1994) Correlates of impaired function in older women. J Am Geriatr Soc 42:481–489

46. Applegate WB, Blass JP, Williams TF (1990) Instruments for the functional assessment of older patients. N Engl J Med 322:1207–1213

47. Mehta KM, Yaffe K, Covinsky KE (2002) Cognitive impairment, depressive symptoms, and functional decline in older people. J Am Geriatr Soc 50:1045–1050

48. Milne AC, Potter J, Avenell A (2002) Protein and energy supplementation in elderly people at risk from malnutrition [Cochrane review]. In: The Cochrane Library, Issue 3. Update Software, Oxford

49. Lichtenstein AH, Rasmussen H, Yu WW et al (2008) Modified MyPyramid for older adults. J Nur 138:78–82

50. Weinberg AD, Minaker KL et al (1995) Dehydration: evaluation and management in older adults. JAMA 274:1552–1556

51. Campbell WW, Evans WJ (1996) Protein requirements of elderly people. Eur J Clin Nutr 50(suppl 1):S180–S185

52. National Research Council (1989) Recommended dietary allowances, 10th edn. National Academy Press, Washington, DC

53. Roza AM, Shizgal HM (1984) The Harris Benedict equation reevaluated: resting energy requirements and the body cell mass. Am J Clin Nutr 40:168–182

54. Hoffman P, Richardson S, Giacoppe J (1995) Failure of the Harris-Benedict equation to predict energy expenditure in undernourished nursing home residents. FASEB J 9:A438

55. Fuller NJ, Sawyer MB, Coward WA (1996) Components of total energy expenditure in free-living elderly men (over 75 years of age): measurement, predictability and relationship to quality-of-life indices. Br J Nutr 75:161–173

56. Roberts SB, Fuss P, Heyman MB (1994) Control of food intake in older men. JAMA 272:1601–1606

57. Wolfe RR, Miller SL, Miller KB (2008) Optimal protein intake in the elderly. Clin Nutr 27:675–684

58. Krasinski SD, Russell RM, Otradovec CL (1989) Relationship of vitamin A and vitamin E intake to fasting plasma retinol, retinol-binding protein, retinyl esters, carotene, alpha-tocopherol, and cholesterol among elderly people and young adults: increased plasma retinyl esters among vitamin A-supplement users. Am J Clin Nutr 49:112–120

59. Selhub J, Jacques PF, Wilson PF et al (1993) Vitamin status and intake as primary determinants of homocysteinemia in an elderly population. JAMA 270:2693–2698

60. Ribaya-Mercado JD, Rusell RM, Sahyoun N (1991) Vitamin B-6 requirements of elderly men and women. J Nutr 121:1062–1074

61. Bailey AL, Maisey S, Southon S et al (1997) Relationships between micronutrient intake and biochemical indicators of nutrient adequacy in "free-living" elderly UK population. Br J Nutr 77:225–242

62. Haller J, Weggemans RM, Lammi-Keefe CJ, Ferry M (1996) Changes in the vitamin status of elderly Europeans: plasma vitamins A, E, B-6, B-12, folic acid and carotenoids. SENECA Investigators. Eur J Clin Nutr 59(Suppl 2):S32–S46

63. Lindenbaum J, Rosenberg IH, Wilson P et al (1994) Prevalence of cobalamin deficiency in the Framingham elderly population. Am J Clin Nutr 60:2–11

64. Krasinski SD, Russell RM, Samloff M (1986) Fundic atrophic gastritis in an elderly population: effect on hemoglobin and several serum nutritional indicators. J Am Geriatr Soc 34:800–806

65. Evatt ML, Terry PD, Ziegler TR, Oakley GP (2009) Association between vitamin B12-containing supplement consumption and prevalence of biochemically defined B12 deficiency in adults in NHANES III (Third National Health and Nutrition Examination Survey). Public Health Nutrition. Public Health Nutr 11:1–7

66. Dawson-Hughes B (1996) Calcium and vitamin D nutritional needs of elderly women. J Nutr 126:1165S–1167S

67. Webb AR, Pilbeam C, Hanafin N (1990) An evaluation of the relative contributions of exposure to sunlight and of diet to the circulating concentrations of 25-hydroxyvitamin D in an elderly nursing home population in Boston. Am J Clin Nutr 51:1075–1081

68. Holick MF (1994) McCollum award lecture, 1994: vitamin D – new horizons for the 21st century. Am J Clin Nutr 60:619–630

69. Lovat LB (1996) Age related changes in gut physiology and nutritional status. Gut 38:306–309

70. Chapuy MC, Arlot E, Delmas PD et al (1994) Effect of calcium and cholecalciferol treatment for three years on hip fractures in elderly women. Br Med J 308:1081–1082

71. Lips P, Graafmans WC, Ooms ME et al (1996) Vitamin D supplementation and fracture incidence in elderly persons: a randomized, placebo controlled clinical trial. Ann Intern Med 124:400–406

72. Dawson-Hughes B, Harris SS, Krall EA (1995) Rates of bone loss in postmenopausal women randomly assigned to one of two dosages of vitamin D. Am J Clin Nutr 61:1140–1145

73. Cashman KD, Wallace JM, Horigan G et al (2009) Estimation of the dietary requirement for vitamin D in free-living adults >=64 y of age. Am J Clin Nutr 89:1366–1374

74. Visscher TLS, Seidell JC, Molarius A, van der Kuip D, Hofman A, Witteman JCM (2001) A comparison of body mass index, waist–hip ratio and waist circumference as predictors of all cause mortality among the elderly: The Rotterdam study. Int J Obes 25:1730–1735

75. Chen H, Guo X (2008) Obesity and functional disability among elder Americans. J Am Geriatr Soc 56(4):689–694

76. Zalesin KC, Franklin BA, Miller WM, Peterson ED, McCullough PA (2008) Impact of obesity on cardiovascular disease. Endocrinol Metab Clin North Am 37(3):663–684, ix. Review

77. Evans WJ, Morley JE, Argilés J et al (2008) Cachexia: A new definition. Clin Nutr 27(6):793–799

78. Mantovani G, Maccio A, Esu S, Lai P et al (1997) Medroxyprogesterone acetate reduces the in vitro production of cytokines involved in anorexia/cachexia and emesis by peripheral blood mononuclear cells of cancer patients. Eur J Cancer 33:602–607

79. Paddon-Jones D, Rasmussen BB (2009) Dietary protein recommendations and the prevention of sarcopenia. Curr Opin Clin Nutr Metab Care 12(1):86–90

80. Losonczy KG, Harris TB, Cornoni-Huntley J et al (1995) Does weight loss from middle age to old age explain the inverse weight mortality relation in old age? Am J Epidemiol 141(4):312–321

81. Olschewski U, Haupt CM, Löschmann C, Dietsche S (2009) Study of malnutrition with residents of nursing homes. Interviews of relatives, nursing staff and survey of nursing documentation. Pflege Z 62(1):28–32

82. Crogan NL, Pasvogel A (2003) The influence of protein-calorie malnutrition on quality of life in nursing homes. J Gerontol A Biol Sci Med Sci 58(2):159–164

83. Alibhai SM, Greenwood C, Payette H (2005) An approach to the management of unintentional weight loss in elderly people. CMAJ 172(6):773–780

84. Bouras EP, Lange SM, Scolapio JS (2001) Rational approach to patients with unintentional weight loss. Mayo Clin Proc 76(9):923–929

85. Fried LP, Tangen CM, Walston J, Newman AB, Hirsch C, Gottdiener J, Seeman T, Tracy R, Kop WJ, Burke G, McBurnie MA, Cardiovascular Health Study Collaborative Research Group (2001) Frailty in older adults: evidence for a phenotype. J Gerontol A Biol Sci Med Sci 56(3):M146–M156

86. Hubbard RE, O'Mahony S, Calver BL, Woodhouse KW (2008) Nutrition, inflammation, and leptin levels in aging and frailty. J Am Geriatr Soc 56:279–284

87. Topinková E (2008) Aging, disability and frailty. Ann Nutr Metab 52(suppl 1):6–11

88. Guralnik JM, Ershler WB, Schrier SL, Picozzi VJ (2005) Anemia in the elderly: a public health crisis in hematology. Hematology Am Soc Hematol Educ Program 528–532

89. Ramel A, Jonsson PV, Bjornsson S, Thorsdottir I (2008) Anemia, nutritional status, and inflammation in hospitalized elderly. Nutrition 24:1116–1122

90. Pierson RN (2003) Body composition in aging: a biological perspective. Curr Opin Clin Nutr Metab Care 6:15–20

91. Weindruch R, Naylor PH, Goldstein AL, Walford RL (1988) Influences of aging and dietary restriction on serum thymosin alpha 1 levels in mice. J Gerontol 43(2):B40–B42

92. Smith JV, Heilbronn LK, Ravussin E (2004) Energy restriction and aging. Curr Opin Clin Nutr Metab Care 7(6):615–622

93. Civitarese AE, Carling S, Heilbronn LK, Hulver MH, Ukropcova B, Deutsch WA, Smith SR, Ravussin E, CALERIE Pennington Team (2007) Calorie restriction increases muscle mitochondrial biogenesis in healthy humans. PLoS Med 4(3):e76

94. Holloszy JO, Fontana L (2007) Caloric restriction in humans. Exp Gerontol 42(8):709–712, Review

95. Feldblum I, German L, Castel H et al (2007) Characteristics of undernourished older medical patients and the identification of predictors for undernutrition status. Nutr J 6:37

96. Scharfenberg M, Raue W, Junghans T, Schwenk W (2007) "Fast track" rehabilitation after colonic surgery in elderly patients – is it feasible? Int J Colorectal Dis 22:1469–1474

97. Espaulella J, Arnau A, Cubi D et al (2007) Time-dependent prognostic factors of 6-month mortality in frail elderly patients admitted to post-acute care. Age Ageing 36:407–413

98. Thomas SK, Humphreys KJ, Miller MD et al (2008) Individual nutrition therapy and exercise regime: A controlled trial of injured, vulnerable elderly (INTERACTIVE trial). BMC Geriatr 8:4

99. Stull AJ, Apolzan JW, Thalacker-Mercer AE et al (2008) Liquid and solid meal replacement products differentially affect postprandial appetite and food intake in older adults. J Am Diet Assoc 108(7):1226–1230

100. Monteleoni C, Clark E (2004) Using rapid-cycle quality improvement methodology to reduce feeding tubes in patients with advanced dementia: before and after study. BMJ 329:491–494

101. Shavit L, Lifschitz M, Plaksin J et al (2007) Acute increase in blood urea nitrogen caused by enteric nutrition. J Am Geriatr Soc 55(4):631–632

102. Vandewoude MF, Paridaens KM, Suy RA et al (2005) Fibre-supplemented tube feeding in the hospitalised elderly. Age Ageing 34(2):120–124

103. DeLegge MH, Sabol DA (2004) Provision for enteral and parenteral support. In: Handbook of clinical nutrition and aging, pp 583–595

104. Pittiruti M et al (2009) ESPEN Guidelines on Parenteral Nutrition: central venous catheters (access, care, diagnosis and therapy of complications). Clin Nutr 28:365–377. doi:10.1016/J.clnu.2009.03.015

105. Btaiche IF, Khalidi N (2004) Metabolic complications of parenteral nutrition in adults, part 1. Am J Health Syst Pharm 61(18):1938–1949

106. Klein CJ, Stanek GS, Wiles CE 3rd (1998) Overfeeding macronutrients to critically ill adults: metabolic complications. J Am Diet Assoc 98(7):795–806

107. Grau T, Bonet A, Rubio M et al (2007) Liver dysfunction associated with artificial nutrition in critically ill patients. Critical Care 11:R10

108. Singer P, Berger MM, Berghe GV et al (2009) ESPEN Guidelines on Parenteral Nutrition: intensive care. Clin Nutr 28(4):387–400. doi:10.1016/J.clnu.2009.04.024

109. Dryden GW, McClave SA (2004) Gastrointestinal senescence and digestive diseases of the elderly. In: Bales CW, Ritchie CS (eds) Handbook of clinical nutrition and aging. Humana, Totowa, NJ, pp 569–581

110. Petrov MS, Pylypchuk RD, Uchugina AF (2008) A systematic review on the timing of artificial nutrition in acute pancreatitis. Br J Nutr 19:1–7

111. Petrov MS, Pylypchuk RD, Uchugina AF (2009) A systematic review on the timing of artificial nutrition in acute pancreatitis. Br J Nutr 101:787–793. doi:10.1017/S0007114508123443

112. Berry SM, Fischer JE (1996) Classification and pathophysiology of enterocutaneous fistulas. Surg Clin North Am 76(5):1009–1018, Review

113. Gonzalez-Pinto I, Gonzalez E (2001) Optimising the treatment of upper gastrointestinal fistulae. Gut 49(Suppl 4):iv21–iv28

114. Visschers RG, Damink SW, Winkens B et al (2008) Treatment strategies in 135 consecutive patients with enterocutaneous fistulas. World J Surg 32(3):445–453

115. Sergi G, Coin A, Mulone S et al (2007) Resting energy expenditure and body composition in bedridden institutionalized elderly women with advanced-stage pressure sores. J Gerontol A Biol Sci Med Sci 62(3):317–322

116. Hengstermann S, Fischer A, Steinhagen-Thiessen E, Schulz RJ (2007) Nutrition status and pressure ulcer: What we need for nutrition screening. JPEN J Parenter Enteral Nutr 31(4):288–294

117. Annas GJ, Arnold B, Aroskar M et al (1990) Bioethicist's statement on the US Supreme Court Cruzan decision. N Engl J Med 323:686–687

118. Jerant AF, Azari RS, Nesbitt TS, Meyers FJ (2004) The TLC model of palliative care in the elderly: Preliminary application in the assisted living setting. Ann Fam Med 2:54–60

119. McCann RM, Hall WJ, Groth-Juncker A (1994) Comfort care for terminally ill patients: the appropriate use of nutrition and hydration. JAMA 272:1263–1266

120. Furman C, Ritchie C (2004) Nutrition and end of life care. In: Bales C, Ritchie C (eds) Handbook of clinical nutrition in aging. Humana, Totowa, NJ, pp 367–375

Chapter 8
Wound Healing in the Elderly

Guy P. Marti, Lixin Liu, Xianjie Zhang, Dongmei Xing, Denise C. King, Angela R. Kohli, Maura Reinblatt, William B. Greenough, and John W. Harmon

Introduction

Wound healing impairment in the elderly has been accepted as a medical reality for many years now. The most devastating wounds in the elderly include pressure ulcers, diabetic foot ulcers, venous stasis ulcers, and poorly healing surgical wounds. Recently, improved wound care products (see Table 8.1) and best practice guidelines (see Table 8.2) have helped to improve care of elderly patients with these types of wounds.

However, to date there is no compelling clinical study that proves that increased age impairs wound healing. The best evidence available is from studies, performed four decades ago which reported an increase in the incidence of wound dehiscence after laparotomy in older men [1, 2]. Likewise, the incidence of anastomotic complications was reported to increase with age [3, 4]. None of these studies is definitive owing to the variability of patient co-morbidities such as nutrition, vascular insufficiency, and the presence and severity of diabetes. Furthermore, human wounds cannot be precisely matched. These factors make it extremely difficult to carry out a conclusive clinical study. In contrast, animal studies have successfully demonstrated age related defects in wound healing.

However, these classical studies, along with fundamental histological findings and, more recently, in-depth descriptions of cellular functions and interactions remain the basis for future studies at a molecular and genetic level.

From a biological point of view, wound healing, tumor development and suppression, and aging are processes involving common mechanisms. Hayflick showed in 1961 that cultured cells in vitro had a limited lifespan, thus giving rise to the term cellular senescence [5]. New and powerful methods, which are now routinely available, have introduced the concepts of telomeric attrition and DNA damage by oxidative stress [6]. Despite the growing body of knowledge and exciting fundamental research, cellular senescence and its mechanisms in vitro have only tenuous links with the aging of a whole organism [7]. Therefore, animal models remain our best option to study the physiology of wound healing in the elderly.

Physiology of Wound Healing

From the moment of injury, the body responds with a series of complex interactions that culminate in the restoration of integrity. Under normal conditions, healing can be divided into four specific stages: coagulation, inflammation, fibroplasia, and remodeling. Although described in a sequential fashion, healing is an active, dynamic process that proceeds through a series of mechanisms that are often redundant and simultaneous.

Coagulation

Coagulation initiates the process that leads to healing. Injury disrupts tissues and cells and induces local hemorrhage. Vasoconstriction occurs almost immediately as a response to catecholamine release to limit blood loss. Tissue destruction induces mast cells to release various vasoactive compounds including bradykinin, serotonin, and histamine, which initiate the process of diapedesis. Platelets from the hemorrhage help form the hemostatic plug by releasing clotting factors that produce fibrin and form the fibrin mesh onto which inflammatory cells migrate. Fibrin deposition is followed by fibrinolysis and the release of chemoattractive peptides, particularly fibrinopeptide E, which attracts monocytes, and fibrinopeptide B, which is angiogenic. In addition, platelet degranulation releases platelet-derived growth factor (PDGF), platelet factor IV, transforming growth factor 1 (TGF-1), and insulin-like growth factor 1 or somatomedin C (IGF-1), all of which stimulate fibroblast replication. Platelets

G.P. Marti (✉)
Department of Surgery, Johns Hopkins Bayview Medical Center, Baltimore, MD, USA
e-mail: gmarti1@jhmi.edu

R.A. Rosenthal et al. (eds.), *Principles and Practice of Geriatric Surgery*,
DOI 10.1007/978-1-4419-6999-6_8, © Springer Science+Business Media, LLC 2011

Table 8.1 Wound care products categories

Product classification	Most common brands
Antimicrobial dressings	

Topical wound products derived from _silver, iodine, and/or polyhexeth-ylene biguanide_
Available in
  Foams
  Alginates
  Hydrogels
  Hydrocolloids
  Barrier layers
May or may not need secondary dressing
Use in draining, and non-healing wounds where protection from bacterial contamination is desired
	Silver products
	  Acticoat absorbent dressing
	*Aquacel Silver
	  Contreet foam dressing
	  Contreet Hydrocolloid
	  Silva Sorb (silver hydrogel)
	*Silverlon
	*Silver Med (silver hydrogel)
	Iodines
	  *Cadexomer Iodines
	*Iodosorb Gel
	  Iodoflex Pad

Calcium alginate	

Absorbs moderate to heavy drainage
Origin – brown seaweed
Non-woven fibers
  Ropes
  or pads
Absorbent and conforms to the shape of the wound
Absorbs up to 20 times its weight
	*Aquacel is a hydrofiber, not a Ca alginate but performs in a similar fashion
	Curasorb
	Kaltostat
	SeaSorb alginate
	3M Tegagen
	Genteel calcium alginate
	Restore calcicare
	Sorbsan

Collagens	

Promotes the deposition of newly formed collagen fibers and granulation tissue in the wound bed. Stimulates new tissue development and wound debridement
Available in
  Sheets
  Pads
  Particles
  Gels
	Fibracol + collagen with alginate
	*Promogran Matrix
	*Promogran Prisma Matrix (collagen + silver)

Composite dressings	
Combination of two or more different products into one dressing, i.e., absorptive layer with an adhesive border for ease of application	*Alldress – low-adherent layer + absorbent pad + tape border Covaderm DermaDress Stratasorb 3M Tegaderm Plus
Compression	
Used to manage edema, promote venous return to the heart and manage wounds caused by venous insufficiency. Multilayered. Available in individual layers or packaged as a multi-layer system	Alto press (single-layer system) Coban2 compression system DYNA-FLEX (multi-layer system) Profore (multi-layer system) Seto press (single-layer system) *Zinc Unna Boot + cotton padding + Flex wrap or Coban
Debriding agents	

Debridement of necrotic tissue and liquefaction of slough
Dry eschar must be scored before applying debriding gel
Gels available by prescription only
Mesalt available in:
  Squares
  Ribbons
	*Accuzyme (gel Rx)
	  Gladase (gel Rx)
	*Mesalt
	  Panafil (gel Rx)
	  Santyl (gel Rx)

(continued)

TABLE 8.1 (continued)

Product classification	Most common brands
Foams	
Absorbs moderate to heavy drainage	Allevyn
Provide a moist environment and thermal insulation	*Biatain
Primary dressing for absorption and insulation, or secondary dressing for wounds with packing. Also effective to treat hypergranulation tissue. May be used under compression	Curafoam
	Hydrasorb
	Polyderm
Available:	PolyMem
With adhesive border	3M Tegaderm Foam
Without adhesive border	Tielle
Varied shapes and sizes	
Hydrocolloids	
Absorbs light to moderate exudates	Combiderm
Occlusive or semi occlusive dressings composed of gelatin, pectin, and carboxymethylcellulose	Comfeel Plus
	*DuoDerm CGF or -DuoDerm Extra Thin
Provide a moist healing environment	RepliCare Hydrocolloid
Promotes granulation in clean wounds	Restore
Helps debride necrotic wounds autolytically	*3M Tegasorb
Used as primary or secondary dressing	*3M Clear Acrylic Dressing – new product that performs similar to a hydrocolloid. Absorbs more than a hydrocolloid. Clear acrylic that allows visualization of the wound. May extend wear time due to visualization
Available in:	
Thin or thick	
Varied shaped wafers	
May or may not have transparent film border	
May be used under compression	
May be opaque or translucent	
Also available in pastes and powders	
Hydrogels	
Can absorb minimal drainage. Water or glycerin-based gels. Helps to maintain moist wound environment. Promotes granulation and epithelialization and facilitates removal of necrotic tissue or slough by autolytic debridement	Curafil Gel
	Curasol Gel
	*DuoDerm Gel
	IntraSite Gel
	Purilon Gel
Available in:	SAF-Gel
Amorphous gels	TenderWet Gel Pad
Impregnated gauze	Curagel
Sheets	DermaGel
	Hypergel
	Normlgel
	*Restore Hydrogel
	SoloSite Wound Gel
	3M Tegagel
Non-adherent layer	
Wound contact layers used to prevent dressing from sticking to the wound bed	*Adaptic
	Mepitel
May or may not be impregnated with gel, petroleum jelly, or other compounds	*Vaseline gauze
	*Xeroform Gauze
Also used over hydrogel to keep gel in place and prevent secondary dressing from absorbing gel	
Transparent films	
Non-absorbent	Clearsite
Adhesive, semi permeable, polyurethane membrane dressings that vary in thickness and size	Dermaview
	OpSite
Waterproof and impermeable to bacteria and contaminants, yet permit water vapor to cross the barrier	*3M Tegaderm
Maintain a moist healing environment, promoting granulation tissue and autolysis of necrotic tissue	
Not recommended for infected wounds	
Available in varied sizes	

When writing orders, refer to the product classification and not the brand name

TABLE 8.2 Pressure ulcer prevention best practices

Interventions	Reason
Get resident out of bed if condition allows. Residents with skin breakdown, should be up a maximum of 2 h at a time	Redistributes weight bearing sites and minimizes the risks of immobility
Teach and encourage resident to shift weight every 15 min, assisting as necessary, while up in chair	Prevents pressure points from developing and allows blood flow to return. Helps prevent pressure ulcers from developing on the lower portion of the buttocks
Assist or provide resident with devices to maintain mobility, i.e., passive ROM, splint, hand cones	Lessens resident's risk for development of a pressure ulcer or contracture
Turn and/or reposition non-ambulatory residents every 2 h minimum	Rotates the sites of pressure and allows blood flow to return to an area where blood flow had been restricted
• Lift resident off bed, do not drag when moving, especially heels and sacrum • Use a draw sheet to help when moving or turning resident • Place socks or heel protectors on resident • Place pajama top or elbow protectors on resident to protect elbows	Minimizes shear and friction which can tear the skin and damage the capillaries supplying blood to the skin
Elevate heels by placing a pillow lengthwise under the residents calves	Decreases pressure on the heels and may decrease shear and friction
Place resident on pressure reducing mattress	Reduces effects of pressure
Place resident on pressure reducing cushion in chair	Reduces effects of pressure
Use maximum of two incontinent pads under resident in bed	Too many layers of linen between resident and pressure reducing mattress, will decrease the effectiveness of the mattress
Avoid incontinent pads over wheelchair cushion, use drawsheet or pillowcase for cover	Incontinent pads reduce effectiveness of pressure reduction provided by cushion
Inspect resident's skin during bath, when changing clothes, etc.	Identify any redness or skin break so that appropriate treatment or prevention measures can begin immediately
Apply lotion to bony prominences, back, and dry, flaky skin at bath time and prn	Keeps skin soft and supple
Apply moisture barrier ointment to the skin of an incontinent resident	Helps prevent incontinence from making the skin soft and prevents burning of the skin
Report frequent incontinence to ensure that appropriate methods of containment or treatment will be promptly implemented	Decreases the chance of complications from incontinence
Encourage resident to drink prescribed supplements and adequate amounts of water between and/or with meals. Report if resident refuses supplements	Helps maintain and/or improve nutritional status and hydration
Keep linen neat and wrinkle free	Helps prevent shear and friction

Prevention is part of every aspect of wound care, regardless if a wound exists or not. Many recommended practices regarding pressure ulcer prevention are nothing more than "good old common sense." Prevention requires a holistic approach from all members of the health care team
Source: Reprinted with permission from the Wound Care Education Institute

are critical in wound healing because they are the first to produce several essential cytokines thought to modulate many subsequent wound healing events [8].

Inflammation

The inflammatory stage is characterized by an increased migration of mast cells, polymorphonuclear leukocytes (PMNs), and lymphocytes into the wound. Within 24 h of injury, PMNs predominantly populate the wound area. Their role is more important for antibacterial defense than for repair. These cells are progressively replaced by macrophages, which are predominant by 48 h after injury. Macrophages stimulate replication and movement of fibroblasts and vascular endothelial cells, which in turn regulate the repair of the connective tissue. When stimulated by injured tissue, fibrin, foreign bodies, low oxygen, and high lactate concentrations, macrophages have been shown to secrete IL-1 (Interleukine-1), IL-6, IL-8, tumor necrosis factor-α (TNF-α), transforming growth factor-β (TGF-β), IGF-1, and fibroblast growth factor-like molecules (LDGF). These factors regulate cell growth and chemotaxis of inflammatory cells, new fibroblasts, and endothelial cells. Inflammation is aggravated by the release of free radicals. The damaging effect of free radicals is enhanced by reactive hyperemia.

Fibroplasia

Fibroplasia is the stage where wound strength increases and integrity is restored. Fibroblasts originate locally, and replication rates are proportional to oxygen availability. By 72 h fibroblasts migrate into the wound and synthesize collagen and proteoglycans. The latter are important extracellular compounds that stabilize and support cells and fibrous components of tissue. Collagen synthesis starts as early as 10 h after injury and reaches a peak between the first and second week before stabilizing. Initially, the collagen within a wound is comprised of large amounts of type III collagen but relatively little type I collagen. Collagen III provides strength during the late phase of wound healing by crosslinking. Vitamin C plays an important role in this process.

During this stage, the production of ground substance in the matrix increases, and vessels proliferate. Neovascularization occurs along the steep oxygen gradient that characterizes wounds. Regrowth of sympathetic nerve fibers is also associated with angiogenesis. Along with invading fibroblasts, fibronectin appears and promotes cell adhesion and phagocytosis, and it may be involved in matrix remodeling. Fibrinogen, laminin, and fibronectin constitute a framework from which new vessels can form and reepithelialization can occur. Reepithelialization is a complex phenomenon in which resting G_0 cells (cells in the inactive phase of mitosis) are recruited from the margins of the wound, followed by migration of epidermal cells. This process is essential for reconstitution of cutaneous barrier function [9]. It has been suggested that as the wound epithelializes, inflammation is downregulated owing to the presence of apoptotic cells at the advancing epithelial wound edge [10–12].

Remodeling

Remodeling is an extensive phase during which collagen is produced and remodeled to reach an equilibrium between collagen formation and destruction by collagenases. The type III/type I collagen ratio decreases allowing the mature type I collagen fibers to cross-link, organize, and rearrange along the tension lines of the skin. Acute and chronic inflammatory cells gradually diminish, and fibroplasia ends. Fibronectin that guided the migration of multiple cells during earlier phases is removed within a few weeks [13].

The first migration of epithelial cells has been observed 6–48 h following an injury, and epidermal proliferation reaches maximum values at 12–48 h. Neovascularization regresses, and a mature scar is formed.

Aging and Wound Healing

While clinical studies have not been able to clearly demonstrate an isolated age related defect in healing in humans, animal studies have shown this age related defect. In human studies, confounding variables of nutrition and vascular insufficiencyand the difficuty in identifying sufficient numbers of identical wounds, make a definitive study impossible. On the other hand numerous animal studies demonstrate very clearly an impairment of wound healing in the elderly compared to the young.

Coagulation and Inflammation

Specific age-related alterations in both the coagulation and immune system have been shown to influence wound healing. Older patients show signs of vascular fragility or risk of hemorrhage. However, the cellular and molecular events that could support these clinical findings are unclear. Frequent comorbidities and impaired renal function are the primary reasons for hemostasis dysfunction [14–16].

Platelet and macrophage adhesion to substrates within the wound increases while macrophage function declines [17]. Old mice display a slower wound healing rate when compared to young mice [18]. Furthermore, wound healing is accelerated when macrophages from young mice are added locally to wounds of old mice. It is possible that the migratory capacity of macrophages in addition to other macrophage functions are affected by age, and the correction of such dysfunction might stimulate wound healing [19]. In accordance with the above reports, Ashcroft et al. observed a similar phenomenon. At 7 days after injury, wounds of young animals consisted of mature granulation tissue and scattered inflammatory cells, whereas the wounds of middle-aged and old mice showed persistent inflammation and immature granulation tissue [20].

Any study of macrophages is affected by their source (spleen, liver, brain, bone, mice, humans) and their state of activation and the experimental conditions (circulating macrophages, peritoneal exudates, in vivo, in vitro) leading to contradictory results in the cellular functions like chemotaxis and phagocytosis. However, there is a general consensus that macrophages are impaired by aging at a molecular level including a decrease in cytokine production and dysfunction of intracellular signaling pathways like NF-KappaB [21].

T cell-mediated immune function also deteriorates during aging. There is a loss of T cell proliferative capacity, a decline in the synthesis and release of IL-2, and a decrease in IL-2 receptor expression. A major factor responsible for the loss of T cell function is the inability of the T cell to respond to activation signals transmitted through the membrane binding of specific stimulatory signals [22]. An IL-2 deficit alone cannot explain these effects because exogenous administration of IL-2 does not completely restore the decreased T cell proliferative response of the elderly. A defect in the IL-2 receptor expression or function may exist. In addition to IL-2, T cells have an increased ability to produce interferon-γ (IFN-γ), IL-4, IL-6, and TGF [23, 24]. Aging is associated with a decrease in cytotoxic lymphocyte activity and a reduction in lytic capacity. A significant portion of the age-related decline in CD8$^+$ T cell-mediated cytotoxic activity is secondary to age-related alterations in the CD4$^+$ T cell subset. The well-documented diminution in IL-2 production with age may contribute to the defect seen in the CD4$^-$ cells [25].

Proliferation

Cell proliferation is affected by aging in a number of ways. Fibroblast migration in vitro is reduced, but the number of cells within an acute wound is not altered. Fibroblast proliferation declines as well. It seems that the mitogenic and stimulatory effects of growth factors, hormones, and other agents are significantly reduced during aging [26, 27]. The in vitro loss of responsiveness to specific stimulatory cytokines also occurs, with no changes in response to inhibitors [28]. In addition, fibroblast cultures from premature aging syndromes such as Werner syndrome, show a significantly reduced mitogenic response to PDGF, fibroblast growth factor (FGF), and serum [29, 30].

In addition to these intrinsic alterations, a detrimental microenvironment such as hypoxia has been demonstrated to have a dramatic effect on the migration of fibroblasts impeding even further the healing capacity of the elderly [31].

Studies show that epidermal behavior in elderly subjects differs from that of young subjects. Reepithelialization has shown to be delayed in wounds of old mice [32]. The rate of epithelialization of open wounds is slowed in elderly patients compared to that in young individuals [33, 34]. This is due, in part, to a longer migration time for the kera-

tinocytes to migrate from the basal layer to the epidermal surface [35].

Moreover, in vitro studies have revealed a decline in keratinocyte responsiveness to stimulatory cytokines, an increased response to inhibitory cytokines, and a decline in IL-1 production in elderly patients. This physiologic delay, when coupled with other factors that impair epithelial repair, may result in significant healing problems in the elderly.

Several studies have described changes in angiogenesis during aging. Elements of the microvasculature in young rats are periodic acid-Schiff (PAS)-negative and become increasingly PAS-positive beyond the halfway life-span. This observation reflects an increase in the carbohydrate content of blood vessels with aging. During acute wound repair in old animals the microvasculature is PAS-negative after injury and intensely PAS-positive after 8 weeks, reproducing the process of aging in an accelerated manner [36].

Aged endothelium may exhibit an increased adhesive response to leukocytes and TNF-α. Furthermore, IL-1 production increases and subsequently endothelial cell proliferation declines but vascular smooth muscle cell proliferation increases.

Recent work may guide the way to understanding the precise biological processes that are impaired in the elderly. Instability of hypoxia inducible factor I alpha (HIF) seems to be involved in the impairment of neovascularization and wound healing in elderly mice [37, 38]. HIF is a transcription factor that upregulates the expression of numerous angiogenic peptides including vascular endothelial growth factor (VEGF), platelet-derived growth factor (PDGF), Angiopoietin 1 and 2, as well as placental growth factor [38, 39]. Delivery of a constitutively stable form of HIF can improve wound healing in diabetic mice (see Fig. 8.1), and this improvement in wound healing is associated with increased angiogenesis [38]. Recently it has been shown that aged mice had significant upregulation of hydroxylases

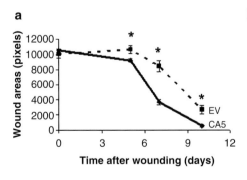
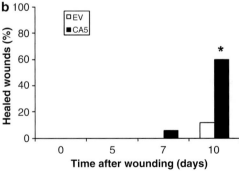
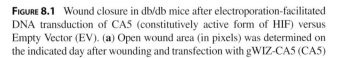

Figure 8.1 Wound closure in db/db mice after electroporation-facilitated DNA transduction of CA5 (constitutively active form of HIF) versus Empty Vector (EV). (**a**) Open wound area (in pixels) was determined on the indicated day after wounding and transfection with gWIZ-CA5 (CA5) or gWIZ-EV (EV). Mean ± SEM is shown ($n = 48$ for CA5; $n = 20$ for EV). *$P < 0.05$, ANOVA with Tukey Test. (**b**) Percentage of wounds achieving ≥95% closure after transfection with CA5 versus EV is shown. *$P < 0.001$, Mann–Whitney Rank Sum Test (from [38], with permission).

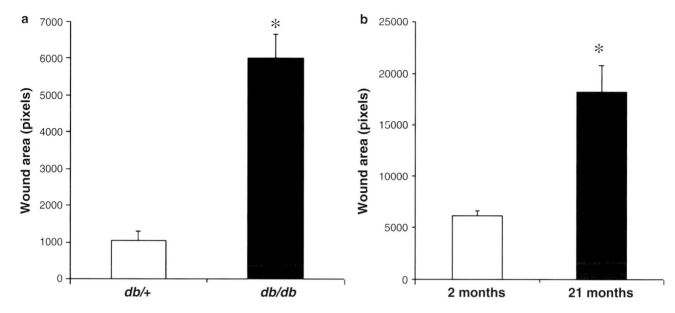

Figure 8.2 Wound healing characteristics of *db/db* mice. (**a**) Excisional wound closure in 2-month-old diabetic mice (*db/db*) and their heterozygous littermates (*db/+*). The bar graph shows the wound area (in pixels) measured by computer assisted plannimetry on day 9 (mean±SEM, *n*=20 for each group). *P<0.01, Student's *t* test. (**b**) The effect of age on wound healing in *db/db* mice. For mice of the indicated age, the bar graph shows wound area on day 9 (mean±SEM, *n*=20 for each group). *P<0.01, Student's *t* test (from [38], with permission).

which degrade HIF. The aged mice had significantly delayed wound healing (see Fig. 8.2) with reduced levels of HIF and downstream transcription products (see Fig. 8.3) as well as decreased neovascularization, compared with younger mice. Inhibitors of hydroxylation of HIF tended to improve wound healing in the older mice [37]. These studies provide an interesting insight into the biology of impaired wound healing in the elderly and suggest strategies for directly addressing the problem with targeted treatments. In addition to this recent work on the role of HIF in the impairment of wound healing in the elderly, defects in other aspects of wound healing have also been demonstrated.

Remodeling and Collagen Deposition

The structure of the extracellular matrix changes with age. Aging is associated with significantly reduced levels of wound matrix constituents, including collagen, basement membrane components, glycosaminoglycans, and fibronectin [40].

It is assumed that anastomotic strength and collagen metabolism are primarily determined by assessing collagen synthesis and content [36]. Collagen metabolism also seems to be altered by aging, with decreased production and increased degradation, although animal studies have reported conflicting findings and no general agreement has been reached [40–42]. In healthy human volunteers, intrinsic aging can be studied excluding extrinsic aging like UV light exposure. In covered skin, age will show a decrease in collagen content when, in contrast, this content will be increased in exposed tissue. In both situations, age will constantly show a disorganization of the collagen and elastin fibers and architecture [43].

Wounds have been reported to change with age. The tensile strength of skin is positively correlated with collagen fiber diameter. During normal wound healing, the tensile strength of wounds increases with time, despite a decrease in the rate of collagen synthesis. The breaking strength of wounds in old animals has been found to be lower than that of young animals [44, 45]. This difference is believed to be due to less organized collagen fiber arrangement [46]. Tensile strength and energy absorption of abdominal incisional wounds are lower in old rats than in young rats by the fourth postoperative day. If wound strength is in fact impaired in the elderly, collagen might not be the only element involved in this phenomenon. A defect in the synthesis of noncollagenous proteins such as glycosaminoglycans, laminin, enzymes, and cytokines may affect the mechanical properties of wounds in the elderly. Imbalance between matrix metalloproteinases and their inhibitors [tissue inhibitors of metalloproteinases (TIMPs)] has been shown in humans but, to complicate things further, this phenomenon seems tissue and cell type dependent [27, 47].

Skin Stem Cells

Different types of adult stem cells have been found in the skin and are protected within a specific niche by a group of

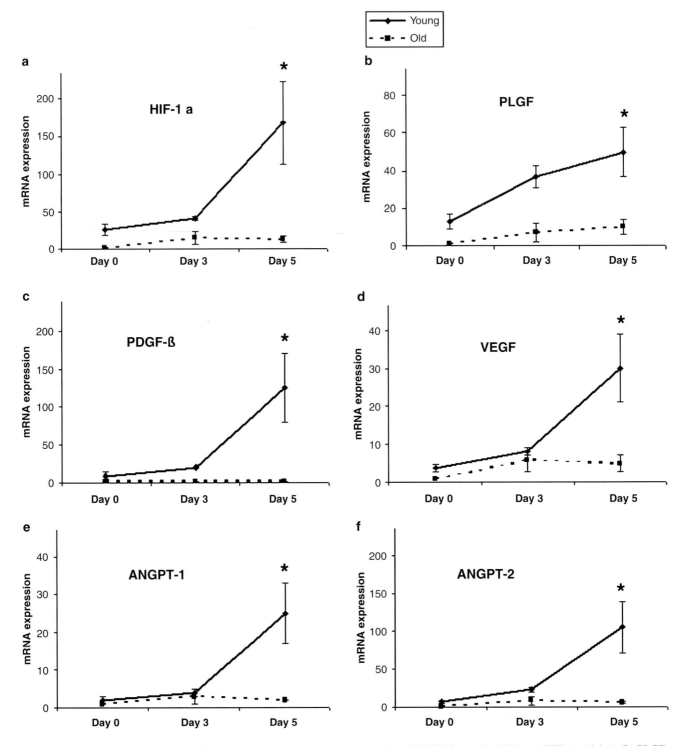

Figure 8.3 Expression of mRNAs for HIF-1α (alpha) and angiogenic cytokines in wounds of 2- and 6-month-old db/db mice. Total RNA was extracted from normal skin (day 0) and wounds on day 3 and day 5 and assayed by qRT-PCR for each mRNA. (**a**) HIF-1α (alpha); (**b**) PLGF; (**c**) PDGF-B; (**d**) VEGF; (**e**) ANGPT1; (**f**) ANGPT2. *$P < 0.01$, ANOVA with Tukey Test, $n = 3$ for each group (from [38], with permission).

specialized niche-cells from extrinsic trauma. It has been observed that the number and self-renewal capacity of these stem cells are not affected by age, but their specific role, which is the ability to produce differentiated effector cells, declines [48].

Muscle and hepatic production of progenitor cell also decline with age. Exposure to young animals' systemic factors (serum) has increased, in vitro, the capacity of niche-cells from liver tissue of aged animals to proliferate and increased the gene expression of specific remodeling pathways to levels seen in younger animal tissues [49]. These findings, together with the study of dermal gene expression, suggest that epidermal stem cells are resistant to intrinsic aging, but sensitive to changes in the local environment. Recently, strong data supports the new idea of stem cells within hair follicule bundles homing into epidermal scar tissue. This finding opposes a common paradigm that hair follicules do not regenerate [50]. This whole new field in medicine holds great promise for future treatment in tissue repair and cell-based therapies.

Co-morbidities

Co-morbidities can further impair the healing process in the elderly. Often co-morbidities appear to be the primary impediment to successful wound healing. Careful clinical evaluation of the patient can reveal the presence of disease processes that require intervention.

Nutrition

Frequent minor deglutition accidents, loss of appetite, and loss of social interaction are the major causes of malnutrition in the aging population. Poor nutrition is associated with impaired wound healing [51], with decreased wound tensile strength, decreased T-cell function, decreased phagocytic activity, and decreased complement and antibody levels.

However, the nutritional status will affect the healing course differently depending on the type of wound. A wound such as a surgical incision or colonic anastomosis that heals by primary intention could heal in a malnourished patient in a reasonable time if protected from infection. On the contrary, a wound like a bed sore or a large burn that heals by secondary intention will be severely affected by a poor nutritional status and could trigger a state of catabolism [52].

Animal studies have helped us understand this relation. A commonly encountered degree of malnutrition, insufficient to affect nutritional indices used for clinical assessment, may interfere with colonic healing. Early feeding to enhance nutrition during the postoperative period may be able to reverse this effect [53]. Daly et al. showed that rats deprived of protein for only 1 week exhibited a 17% reduction in mean bursting strength of colonic anastomoses compared to that of controls. They also observed a correlation between serum albumin and bursting strength with prolonged malnutrition [54]. These studies were later confirmed by Irving, who showed that severe protein deprivation reduced the breaking strength of abdominal wall wounds. A recent animal study from 2009 confirmed these original findings. Malnutrition impairs the healing of colonic anastomosis and a proper food intake given to malnourished rats 7 days prior to surgery will normalize the anastomosis tensile strength and its collagen contents [55].

In humans the wound healing response has been assessed by measuring the collagen content (hydroxyproline) of subcutaneously inserted Gore-Tex tubes. In this respect, a delay in the wound healing response is also seen in malnourished elderly surgical patients; but contrary to what happens in animals, it occurs even with mild degrees of protein–calorie malnutrition [56]. In addition, low serum levels of nutritional markers such as albumin and transferrin correlate with a high incidence of wound complications in elderly patients undergoing vascular operations [57].

The wound healing response, measured by hydroxyproline accumulation, is improved by intravenous nutrition in surgical patients. This improvement is seen after only 1 week of nutritional therapy and before the indices of nutritional status are significantly changed [58]. In the latest meta-analysis update from the Cochrane collaboration on nutritional supplementation for hip fracture aftercare, oral multinutrient feeds seem to reduce the risk of unfavourable outcomes, but data are insufficient to recommend nasogastric feeding, whereas protein-rich supplementation may reduce long-term complications and the number of days spent in hospital [59]. ESPEN guidelines on parenteral nutrition are in agreement with this review and conclude that a time limited parenteral support is beneficial only to severe malnourished patients and should be quickly replaced by intraoral intake [60].

Diabetes

Diabetes has been shown to impair wound healing and increase the potential for infection. Cruse and Foord demonstrated that diabetic patients have five times the risk of infection in a clean surgical wound compared to nondiabetic patients. Obesity, insulin resistance, and hyperglycemia all contribute significantly and independently to the wound impairment observed in diabetics [61, 62].

In experimental animals, insulin restores collagen synthesis and granulation tissue formation to normal levels if given during the early phases of healing [63]. However, this is not the case in phenotypically obese mice [38, 64]. In humans with juvenile-onset diabetes, insulin treatment ensures normal wound collagen accumulation. Specific phases of wound healing involving collagen metabolism and cellular proliferation as well as chemotactic, phagocytic, and adherence properties of neutrophils have been shown to improve with insulin administration or lowering of the blood glucose level below 200 mg/dl. Careful preoperative correction of blood glucose levels can improve the outcome of wounds in diabetic patients [65].

Future approaches in diabetic wound treatments will probably take into account the critical role played by advanced glycoxidation products that seem to act negatively both on the vascular and peripheral nerve injuries sustained by diabetic patients [66].

Hypoxia and Hypoperfusion

Local tissue perfusion and oxygenation are key elements in wound healing [67]. Unfortunately, the elderly experience a progressive decline in health and are more prone to develop diseases that compromise tissue perfusion. Diabetes, arteriosclerosis, venous insufficiency, and cardiac failure are among the major diseases that can affect local oxygen delivery. It is even possible that a substantial portion of surgical patients are hypoperfused [68]. Healing of ischemic wounds in old animals is impaired by 40–65% (wound shrinkage) compared to similar wounds in young animals [69]. Tissues from older animals are less tolerant to ischemia with increasing age. Consequently, limiting ischemia time during surgical procedures in older patients is beneficial [70].

Collagen synthesis requires oxygen as a cofactor, especially during hydroxylation of proline. Oxygen tensions in surgical wounds are often below what is desirable [71]. Perfusion during the first postoperative days seems to be crucial for collagen accumulation. In fact, collagen deposition is directly proportional to wound oxygen tension and other measurements of perfusion [72]. Interestingly, moderate anemia does not influence collagen deposition. Thus replacing fluid postoperatively based on the results of tissue oxygen tension measurements rather than clinical criteria may improve the overall wound healing response [67, 73]. The use of a transcutaneous oxymeter device has proven useful in predicting a successful wound closure but no consensus has been reached in clinical practice [74].

Infections

Infection of surgical sites and healing of secondarily infected wounds, are two wound problems commonly affecting aged patients with various co-morbidities.

Surgical site infection is the most frequent nosocomial infection in hospitalized patients and will affect at least 2% of all surgical patients and up to 20% of patients undergoing some specific surgical procedures. Local wound infection represents the most frequent cause of defective wound healing. These numbers are very likely underestimated because of a lack of documentation concerning patients prematurely discharged in the context of private insurance coverage [75]. The transfer of the cost of disabilities, depression, and death due to these infections to the community is therefore very high [76].

For classification purposes, these infections have been classified according to the initial incision (superficial, deep, organ/space) and the preexisting infectious risk (clean, contaminated, dirty, infected). This classification is now essential to determine a risk index, to study various risk factors, and suggest specific practice guidelines [77] including the use of general measures, skin preparation, and surgical environment and eventually antimicrobial prophylaxis. These measures can be found in extensive reviews [78, 79].

The clinical examination is the first most important element to recognize a wound that is being challenged by a bacterial infection. The loss of bacterial balance can affect the wound superficially or within deeper tissues. The most important evidence of this imbalance is the delay in wound closure and the presence of an exudate. Odor, pain, and surrounding tissue inflammation will indicate uncontrolled infection, but these signs may be less obvious in the elderly patient [80]. Therefore, it may be necessary to study the bacterial contents of the wound.

The mere presence of organisms in a wound is less important than the level of bacterial growth. Experimental data have shown that bacterial growth of more than 100,000 organisms per gram of tissue is necessary to delay or inhibit wound healing. The bacterial growth can be measured in the clinic by performing a biopsy for culture. It is more reliable than a bacterial swab that can isolate superficial noninvasive bacteria and miss the anaerobes responsible for the infection [81].

Recently, the pathophysiology of infections associated with chronic wounds has begun to be better defined. Many more microorganism species have been identified [such as methicillin resistant *Staphylococcus aureus* (MRSA)] but most of them develop in the form of biofilms. This complex structure supports colony growth, retention of nutrients, and formation of water channels and allows cell–cell communication and even gene transfer through transduction [82]. In addition, bacterial cells in these structures are protected from antimicrobial agents and host defenses, explaining the frequent inability to eradicate them in infections. In addition, developing molecular microbiology techniques (nucleic acid amplification-PCR and metagenomic methods) have shown that chronic wounds from different etiologies will display a different microorganism population and therefore require different treatment regimens. These molecular techniques are indeed reserved for the research community but should become a standard for resistant wounds [83].

Drugs

The major effect of steroids is to inhibit the inflammatory phase of wound healing. The stronger the anti-inflammatory effect of the steroid used, the greater is the inhibitory effect on wound healing [84, 85]. Large doses of steroids reduce collagen synthesis and wound strength. Dexamethasone increases the frequency of colonic anastomotic rupture 5 days postoperatively [86]. In addition, long-term perioperative steroids have a deleterious effect on colonic anastomoses and skin healing [87, 88]. Short-term high preoperative and postoperative steroid therapy does not decrease the strength of the anastomoses as measured by bursting pressure. Treatment with a single preoperative high dose of methylprednisolone may improve pulmonary function and reduce the inflammatory response without having a detrimental effect on collagen accumulation in the wound [89].

Cancer therapies have long been known to affect wound healing adversely. Chemotherapeutic antimetabolite drugs inhibit early cell proliferation, which is crucial to the onset of successful wound repair. Radiation therapy also has unwanted effects, as it can induce fibrosis, strictures, and ischemia in adjacent tissues. It can also generate an early decrease in seromuscular blood flow in colorectal anastomoses, although single preoperative doses may not compromise healing [90].

Other drugs may also have unexpected adverse effects on wound healing. Octreotide, a somatostatin analogue commonly used in surgical patients, has been shown to decrease wound breaking strength in experimental animals; these effects are comparable in magnitude to those caused by steroids [91].

Therapeutic Approaches

The healing impairment in aged individuals is a combination of intrinsic and extrinsic factors that act at multiple levels of the healing cascade. As a result, a multifaceted therapeutic approach is necessary. In addition, the incomplete success in translating animal research results to human clinical applications demonstrates the complexity of human biology in which, identification of relevant subtypes will be the next avenue to explore.

The correct assessment and correction of co-morbidities will be the first major step to take to achieve success. Each co-morbidity will have a specific age-related treatment to render with the relevant medical specialties.

Nutritional Support

Nutritional support will have to be adapted to the degree of malnutrition, the urgency in closing the wound, and the ability of the patient to tolerate nutritional intake. General nutritional support can be started by mouth if there is no deglutition problem, which generally manifests itself as a pulmonary infection in the elderly. Enteral nutrition is a very effective way to correct malnutrition and should not be delayed for patients with even a moderate 10% weight loss. Specific nutritional supplementation such as arginine, vitamin A, vitamin C, and zinc have been shown to be effective experimentally, but their mechanisms of action are still unclear. Again, subpopulations of patients have responded differently to specific supplements depending on their comorbidities and the type of wound.

Growth Hormone

In wound healing research studies, growth hormone (GH) has been shown to increase the strength of incisional wounds [92]. Rats treated with preoperative and postoperative GH experienced an increase in breaking strength and collagen content of colonic anastomoses. The increments in these parameters were accompanied by an increase in collagen deposition in the anastomotic segment. These effects were seen only when GH was given during the healing phase [93]. GH seems to stimulate structural organization of the anastomotic collagen fibrils into fibers [94]. In addition, GH administration significantly improves skin wound strength in malnourished rats [95].

GH appears to exert its favorable effect in part by stimulating IGF-1 synthesis; in turn, IGF-1 mediates the anabolic effects of GH. IGF-1 is released early during wound healing by the lysis of platelet alpha granules and later by fibroblasts. This molecule stimulates fibroblast and endothelial cell proliferation as well as collagen synthesis [96]. IGF-1 appears to be critical for effective wound healing.

Rats depleted of IGF-1 experience a 50% decrease in wound protein, DNA, hydroxyproline, and macrophage concentrations. Moreover, infusion of IGF-1 into the wounds restores these variables [97]. Similar to GH, IGF-1 increases wound breaking strength in rats. However, its effect is evident only when it is combined with one of its specific binding proteins, such as IGFBP-1 [98, 99].

In clinical studies including those on burn patients, growth hormone can significantly reduce wound closure times and the length of hospitalization. In addition, it may accelerate donor site wound healing rates by 25%. With this increase in healing, patients with massive (>60% total body surface area) burn wounds can undergo further skin grafting procedures earlier [100–102]. The good results obtained with GH therapy in terms of the healing rates for donor sites and burn wounds are encouraging. The adverse effects of GH are multiple and potentially severe: carpal tunnel syndrome, peripheral edema, joint pain and swelling, gynecomastia, glucose intolerance, and possibly increased cancer risk. Caution should be exercised when considering treatment with growth-hormone [103–105].

Oxygen

Chronic wounds are hypoxic and arterial and venous diseases are not sufficient to fully explain the phenomenon. Using new models, mathematical models [106], hypoxia chambers models [39, 107], or local ischemia animal models [108], new tools to improve oxygen availability in wounds are being developed.

In a systematic review of human trials hyperbaric oxygen has been found to be efficient in treating diabetic foot ulcers but has not proven effective on arterial ulcers [109]. Reports of successful topical application of oxygen are encouraging but not completely convincing [110–112].

Gene Therapy

Growth factors are proteins that act as regulators of the cellular mechanisms and are intensely involved in the wound healing process. As some of these growth factors have been found deficient in elderly animal wounds, it has been postulated that the addition of growth factors should be sufficient to stimulate an adequate healing response. Topical application of growth factors has been shown to have a healing effect in animal experiments. PDGF (Regranex, Ortho-McNeil) has been approved by the FDA for the treatment of diabetic neuropathic ulcers [113]. Because of the presence of the wound eschar and proteases, daily application is required and only a marginal effect has been demonstrated, compared to placebo (50 versus 37% of complete healing). Direct injection of naked DNA in the wound requires repeated

injections of high doses, which can actually impair wound healing [114].

In some instances topical application and direct injection can be inappropriate, and hence new methods of delivering the DNA into the cells had to be developed. These methods can be classified as chemical, mechanical, and virally mediated methods. Liposomes directly interact with the cell membranes to transfect the plasmid load [115]. The Gene Gun uses high air pressure to fire gold beads coated with DNA plasmids through the skin [116]. Liposomes and Gene Gun techniques have shown very variable transfection results. Electroporation might be the delivery method, which will be used in clinical settings in the near future. With the application of an electrical field through the skin, the cell membranes are made transiently permeable to charged macromolecules such as plasmid DNA. The cellular uptake is less than with a viral vector but better than the other chemical or mechanical methods and has not shown any associated risk. Electroporation has been used in human beings to treat specific cancers and to improve the efficacy of DNA vaccines [117–119]. Virally mediated transfer (called transduction) has a high transduction efficacy but there are serious concerns about its safety and pathogenicity [120]. The use of Lentiviruses instead of adenoviruses might reduce these risks.

Tissue Engineering

After more than a decade of progress in biomaterials and cell cultures, bioengineered skin substitutes are now available. Different types can be used: Cultured epidermal graphs (Epicel* Genzyme Tissue Repair), dermal substitutes (AlloDerm* LifeCell), dermal and synthetic epidermal substitutes (Integra*, Integra Life Sciences), and bilayered living skin constructs (Apligraph*, Novartis). The primary indications are life-saving immediate coverage of burn wounds, reducing the need for autographs, and closing chronic wounds. The products will improve as the understanding of their mechanism of action increases [121].

Conclusion

It is apparent that the wound healing response is altered in the elderly compared to that in young individuals. Inflammation, angiogenesis, epithelialization, and remodeling show changes that may consequently impair wound healing. However, in elderly patients not suffering from concomitant diseases, the rate of wound healing is normal or slightly reduced. It is still difficult to reach definite conclusions on certain wound healing processes such as collagen metabolism, and the influence the above changes may have on morbidity and mortality.

Nonetheless, a clear relation is observed between wound healing and certain disease states (i.e., malnutrition, infections, hypoxia and reoxygenation, diabetes, and drug interactions). Patients with these conditions should be carefully evaluated and supplementation with growth factors and nutrient supplements considered. The potential uses of these factors may be of importance for wound healing in critically ill patients.

Local Wound Management in the Elderly

This chapter has reviewed the patho-physiology of wound healing impairment in the elderly and outlined systemic approaches to improve wound healing by improving blood flow, nutrition, oxygenation, and metabolic status. Now attention is turned to the local management of the wound. There are now consensus-based practice guidelines which provide a basis for management of all the major wound types in the elderly. Pressure ulcers are of such importance that the staging system for categorizing these wounds and guidelines for their prevention are included (see Fig. 8.4 and Table 8.1). In addition, we have categorized frequently used wound dressings in Table 8.2. The best practices for the care of chronic wounds including pressure ulcers, diabetic foot ulcers, and venous ulcers are available on line at the website of the Wound Healing Society [122–124]. The best practices in caring for acute wounds and avoiding impediments to wound healing in the elderly are currently only available as a journal article [125]. These guidelines are based on the consensus of experts and the authors of this chapter consider them to be the best guidance available for the care of wounds in patients of any age.

As surgeons, the most important principle to follow is the complete debridement of necrotic tissue. Adequate debridement of a large pressure ulcer often requires a trip to the operating room with adequate anesthesia to debride not only skin, but muscle and frequently bone as well. The days of performing these types of debridements at the bedside, or in the clinic should be behind us. Inadequate debridement will doom an elderly patient to failed healing, chronic wounds, and associated morbidity and mortality.

Surgeons also have to be vigilant in identifying and treating deep necrotizing soft tissue infections. Here, the decision to go to the operating room and excise the area of infection can be lifesaving. Erythema, pain, and swelling may be all that are required to make the diagnosis. Performing a CT scan, which shows air bubbles in muscle, or a needle aspiration to identify bacteria by gram stain or culture can waste valuable time and lead to poor outcomes, including mortality.

The availability of new dressings has improved outcomes for elderly patients with wounds. The important features of these new dressings include the capacity to hydrate the wound with a gel or alginateand antimicrobial effectiveness based on the presence of silver ion in the dressing. User choice determines which of the many types of dressings is preferable for a given patient.

Negative pressure dressing is an important advance that has been introduced over the past decade. Negative pressure dressing has been engineered to be applicable to open wounds ranging from small to large, including even the open abdomen. The system has revolutionized the nursing care of wounds, making the three times a day dressing changes a thing of the past. Negative pressure dressing can be applied and left in place for up to 3 days with good results. Importantly infection must be controlled in the wound prior to deploying it. Negative pressure dressing does not replace the need for surgical debridement. The wound must be debrided and clean for the negative pressure dressing to be effective. Infection can advance under such a dressing, even with a silver antimicrobial in place, if adequate debridement has not been performed.

Pressure ulcers remain a significant problem in the elderly and preventive methods can decrease their incidence. For this reason the pressure points where bony prominences lie under the soft tissue are highlighted in Fig. 8.5 (see Fig. 8.5). These areas must be carefully protected using the best practice guidelines in Table 8.1. When a stage I ulcer appears with erythema, this is a dangerous signal that ulceration is about to begin. Efforts should be re-doubled to avoid weight bearing on the vulnerable tissue. Pressure reducing strategies include frequent turning and off-loading with pillows as well as the other modalities listed Table 8.1. Prevention of pressure ulcers requires diligent nursing care and may sometimes be impossible for the extremely vulnerable patient with poor nutrition, cachexia, and contractures. Pressure reducing and air-flow mattresses are expensive and their cost effectiveness is unclear. These beds play a role in the management of the very vulnerable patient. Occasionally a colostomy is required to prevent tissue maceration in patients with incontinence. This strategy will sometimes achieve healing of a recalcitrant ulcer, or it may be performed prior to a major surgical tissue transfer procedure to cover a particularly severe pressure ulcer.

Absent from the list of treatment options, is a means to specifically accelerate wound healing. The only FDA approved treatment option of this type is Regranex*

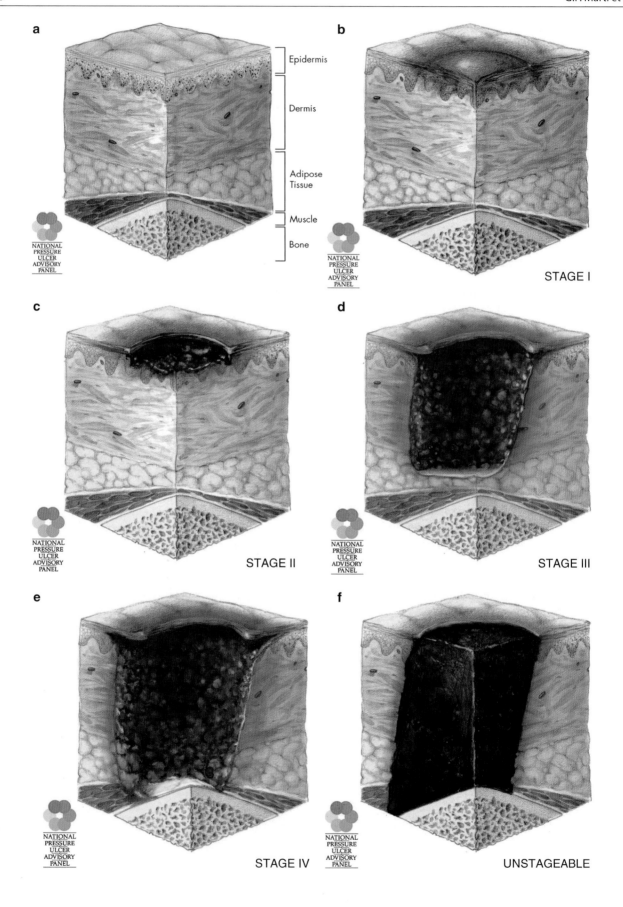

a

Epidermis

Dermis

Adipose
Tissue

Muscle

Bone

b

STAGE I

c

STAGE II

d

STAGE III

e

STAGE IV

f

UNSTAGEABLE

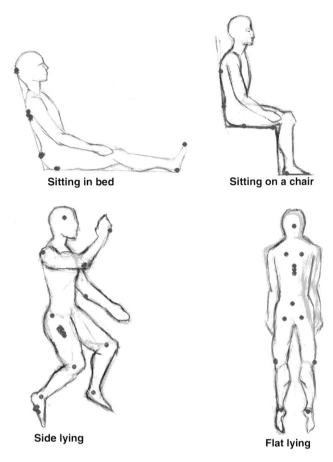

Sitting in bed   **Sitting on a chair**

Side lying   **Flat lying**

Figure 8.5 Pressure points.

(Becaplermin), Systagenix Wound Management, Gargrove England, which is platelet derived growth factor in a gel for topical application. Most clinicians have found it to be only minimally effective, but it may have a place restoring healing, particularly of a diabetic foot ulcer where healing has stalled, and all efforts necessary to off-load weight-bearing and restore blood flow have been exhausted. There are a number of promising agents including VEGF, KGF, and hypoxia inducible factor 1 alpha that are in preclinical and clinical trials. The delivery of these agents as well as PDGF, using DNA plasmids, or even viral vectors, has the potential to keep therapeutic levels elevated over relevant time periods without requiring frequent applications. In addition these types of delivery systems can place the agent deep in the wound tissue, obviating the need for transfer across a wound eschar. In the coming years as more studies are performed, some of these promising agents will be available in clinics.

◀

Figure 8.4 Staging system for decubitus ulcers. (**a**) Normal tissue. (**b**) Stage I: An observable pressure related alteration of intact skin whose indicators as compared to the adjacent or opposite area on the body may induce changes in one or more of the following: skin temperature (warmth or coolness), tissue consistency (firm of toggy feel), and/or sensation (pain, itching). The ulcer appears as a defined area of persistent redness in lightly pigmented skin, whereas in darker skin tones, the ulcer may appear with persistent red, blue, or purple hues. (**c**) Stage 2: Partial thickness skin loss involving epidermis, dermis, or both. The ulcer is superficial and presents clinically as an abrasion, blister, or shallow crater. (**d**) Stage III: Full thickness skin loss involving damage to, or necrosis of, subcutaneous tissue that may extent down to, but not through, underlying fascia. The ulcer presents clinically as a deep crater with or without undermining of adjacent tissue. (**e**) Stage IV: Full thickness skin loss with extensive destruction, tissue necrosis, or damage to muscle, bone, or supporting structures (e.g., tendon, joint capsule). Undermining and sinus tracts may also be associated with Stage IV pressure ulcer. (**f**) Unstageable: Eschar: Thick dry black necrotic tissue.

CASE STUDY: GERIATRIC WOUND HEALING

Background

Medical History

This 67-year old gentlemen was referred to our service with a complex wound. Two years prior to admission he had a sigmoid colectomy for removal of a polyp at an outside hospital. He developed MRSA wound infection requiring extensive debridement and reoperation. He was left with the bowel covered with skin graft with a 20 cm diameter ventral hernia (Fig. 8.6). His abdominal wound was complicated by the fact that he has alcoholic cirrhosis with ascites. His co-morbidities include coronary artery disease with a myocardial infarction managed with four coronary artery stents. He has COPD with periodic bronchitis requiring hospitalization. He does not use home oxygen, but he is severely short of breath after climbing one flight of stairs.

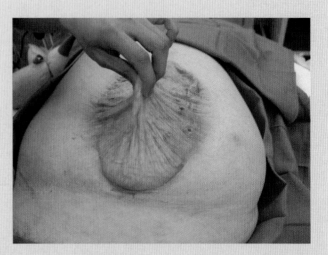

FIGURE 8.7 Case report: "Pinch Test" showing that the skin graft was not densely adherent to the underlying bowel.

(Fig. 8.7). This meticulous dissection was carried out without creating an enterotomy. A subcutaneous flap was raised to the mid axillary line bilaterally to perform component separation and myofascial transfer of the internal oblique to be able to close the defect primarily. With the prior MRSA we elected not to implant a mesh of any type.

The Wound

The wound with which this patient presented is ischemic necrosis at the midline of his abdominal flaps. This necrosis was evident 5 days after the repair of the hernia. This wound was 4 cm wide and extended for a distance of 20 cm along the midline incision.

The management of this wound is a classic problem in geriatric surgery.

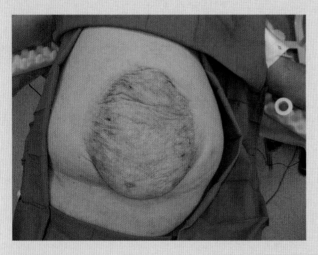

FIGURE 8.6 Case report: The ventral hernia with skin graft. There was an ascites leak through a punctuate ulceration in the skin graft.

He has insulin dependent Type 2 diabetes.

Considering his life threatening co-morbidities, and the benign status of his hernia, our initial approach was to simply monitor his situation and treat his hernia with a binder. But when he developed an ascites leak we proceeded to urgent repair of the hernia. The repair was carried out excising the skin graft from the bowel

Management Strategies

Surgical Debridement

When it became clear that the wound was necrosing, surgical debridement was carried out. Full thickness skin and subcutaneous tissue were excised. The necrotic tissue was excised back to bleeding tissue and a VAC drain was placed (Fig. 8.8).

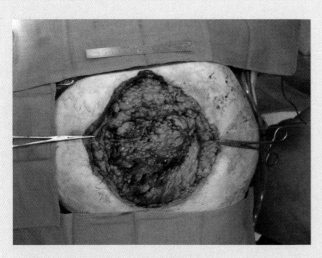

FIGURE 8.8 Case report: The wound after debridement of the necrotic skin flaps. Skin and full thickness subcutaneous tissue were debrided to the fascial level to remove the tissue that had suffered ischemic necrosis.

Diabetes

This patient has insulin dependent diabetes. Blood sugars was greater than 200 mg% in the face of the sepsis from the wound. Tight glucose control was instituted with continuous IV glucose drip to bring the blood sugar under 150 mg%.

Infectious Disease

The necrosis of the wound appeared to be ischemic, secondary to the raising of the lateral flaps, coupled with his overall debilitated condition. Nonetheless infection was a potential problem. He was covered with intravenous clindamycin to which his prior MRSA had been sensitive. This coverage was maintained for his initial hernia repair for 24 h and likewise at the time of his debridement.

Nutritional Support

During the post operative period after his hernia repair his nutrition was maintained with a Dobhoff feeding tube. The tube was carefully placed in the duodenum using fluoroscopic guidance. Initially a nasogastric tube was placed in the stomach to check gastric residuals. When residuals were greater than 200 cc with feeding at the rate of 60 cc per hour the feedings were discontinued. After 24 h they were reinstituted at 30 cc per hour. They were gradually returned to 60 cc per hour over 4 days.

Ascites

His ascites from alcoholic cirrhosis was managed initially with an intra-peritoneal JP drain following the primary hernia repair. This was to protect the closure from the pressure of intra-abdominal ascitic fluid. The ascities was also controlled medically with Lasix and Aldactone. When drainage from the JP drain was less than 100 cc per day, 72 h after surgery the JP drains were removed. Fortunately the re-accumulation of ascites was less of a problem than expected for this patient.

COPD

This patient developed ARDS with typical patchy infiltrate on chest X-ray and desaturation of O_2 accompanied by CO_2 retention. He required intubation and mechanical ventilation. After 10 days he was converted to a tracheostomy tube. He had gradual remission of his ARDS with this approach.

Coronary Artery Disease

After both surgeries the patient was ruled out for myocardial infarction. Serial troponins and EKG's confirmed that he did not sustain a myocardial infarction

Delirium

The patient developed florid delirium with agitation within 24 h of the initial surgery. The family asserts that he had discontinued alcohol intake; however, he appeared to be suffering from Delirium tremens. He was treated with Atavan and Haldol, and he also required four point restraints briefly. This delirium gradually cleared over 3 weeks of hospitalization.

Outcome

With this multi-pronged approach this patient survived a high risk scenario of ulcerated ventral hernia with ascites leak. After the debrided wound was treated with the VAC it granulated, and after 12 days was closed in the operating room (Fig. 8.9). It healed in a satisfactory manner, and the patient was discharged to a rehabilitation unit after 4 weeks of hospitalization.

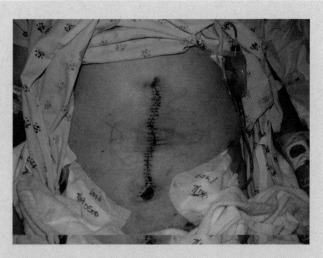

FIGURE 8.9 Case report: Closure of the wound after it had granulated. Open wound was treated with VAC* dressing. After it had granulated the wound was closed as shown.

References

1. Halasz NA (1968) Dehiscence of laparotomy wounds. Am J Surg 116:210–214
2. Mendoza CB Jr, Postlethwait RW, Johnson WD (1970) Veterans administration cooperative study of surgery for duodenal ulcer. II. incidence of wound disruption following operation. Arch Surg 101:396–398
3. Irvin TT, Goligher JC (1973) Aetiology of disruption of intestinal anastomoses. Br J Surg 60:461–464
4. Schrock TR, Deveney CW, Dunphy JE (1973) Factor contributing to leakage of colonic anastomoses. Ann Surg 177:513–518
5. Hayflick L, Moorhead PS (1961) The serial cultivation of human diploid cell strains. Exp Cell Res 25:585–621
6. Tollefsbol TO (2007) Techniques for analysis of biological aging. Methods Mol Biol 371:1–7
7. Jeyapalan JC, Sedivy JM (2008) Cellular senescence and organismal aging. Mech Ageing Dev 129:467–474
8. Hunt TK, Hopf HW (1996) Nutrition in wound healing. In: Fischer JE (ed) Nutrition and metabolism in the surgical patient, 2nd edn. Lippincott Williams & Wilkins, Philadelphia, pp 423–441
9. Van de Kerkhof PC, Van Bergen B, Spruijt K, Kuiper JP (1994) Age-related changes in wound healing. Clin Exp Dermatol 19:369–374
10. Brown DL, Kao WW, Greenhalgh DG (1997) Apoptosis downregulates inflammation under the advancing epithelial wound edge: delayed patterns in diabetes and improvement with topical growth factors. Surgery 121:372–380
11. Carter R, Sykes V, Lanning D (2009) Scarless fetal mouse wound healing may initiate apoptosis through caspase 7 and cleavage of PARP. J Surg Res 156:74–79
12. Chowdhury I, Tharakan B, Bhat GK (2006) Current concepts in apoptosis: the physiological suicide program revisited. Cell Mol Biol Lett 11:506–525
13. Ashcroft GS, Horan MA, Ferguson MW (1995) The effects of ageing on cutaneous wound healing in mammals. J Anat 187(Pt 1):1–26
14. Spyropoulos AC, Merli G (2006) Management of venous thromboembolism in the elderly. Drugs Aging 23:651–671
15. Brotman DJ, Jaffer AK (2008) Prevention of venous thromboembolism in the geriatric patient. Cardiol Clin 26:221–234, vi
16. Robert-Ebadi H, Le Gal G, Righini M (2009) Use of anticoagulants in elderly patients: practical recommendations. Clin Interv Aging 4:165–177
17. Toogood AA, Adams JE, O'Neill PA, Shalet SM (1996) Body composition in growth hormone deficient adults over the age of 60 years. Clin Endocrinol (Oxf) 45:399–405
18. Swift ME, Burns AL, Gray KL, DiPietro LA (2001) Age-related alterations in the inflammatory response to dermal injury. J Invest Dermatol 117:1027–1035
19. Danon D, Kowatch MA, Roth GS (1989) Promotion of wound repair in old mice by local injection of macrophages. Proc Natl Acad Sci USA 86:2018–2020
20. Ashcroft GS, Horan MA, Ferguson MW (1997) Aging is associated with reduced deposition of specific extracellular matrix components, an upregulation of angiogenesis, and an altered inflammatory response in a murine incisional wound healing model. J Invest Dermatol 108:430–437
21. Gomez CR, Nomellini V, Faunce DE, Kovacs EJ (2008) Innate immunity and aging. Exp Gerontol 43:718–728
22. Faunce DE, Palmer JL, Paskowicz KK, Witte PL, Kovacs EJ (2005) CD1d-restricted NKT cells contribute to the age-associated decline of T cell immunity. J Immunol 175:3102–3109
23. Thompson JL, Butterfield GE, Marcus R et al (1995) The effects of recombinant human insulin-like growth factor-I and growth hormone on body composition in elderly women. J Clin Endocrinol Metab 80:1845–1852
24. Jorgensen JO, Vahl N, Hansen TB, Fisker S, Hagen C, Christiansen JS (1996) Influence of growth hormone and androgens on body composition in adults. Horm Res 45:94–98
25. Bloom ET (1991) Functional importance of CD4+ and CD8+ cells in cytotoxic lymphocytes activity and associated gene expression. Impact on the age-related decline in lytic activity. Eur J Immunol 21:1013–1017
26. Rattan SI, Derventzi A (1991) Altered cellular responsiveness during ageing. Bioessays 13:601–606
27. Reed MJ, Ferara NS, Vernon RB (2001) Impaired migration, integrin function, and actin cytoskeletal organization in dermal

fibroblasts from a subset of aged human donors. Mech Ageing Dev 122:1203–1220

28. Phillips PD, Kaji K, Cristofalo VJ (1984) Progressive loss of the proliferative response of senescing WI-38 cells to platelet-derived growth factor, epidermal growth factor, insulin, transferrin, and dexamethasone. J Gerontol 39:11–17

29. Bauer EA, Silverman N, Busiek DF, Kronberger A, Deuel TF (1986) Diminished response of Werner's syndrome fibroblasts to growth factors PDGF and FGF. Science 234:1240–1243

30. Maier AB, Westendorp RG (2009) Relation between replicative senescence of human fibroblasts and life history characteristics. Ageing Res Rev 8:237–243

31. Mogford JE, Tawil N, Chen A, Gies D, Xia Y, Mustoe TA (2002) Effect of age and hypoxia on TGFbeta1 receptor expression and signal transduction in human dermal fibroblasts: impact on cell migration. J Cell Physiol 190:259–265

32. Mogford JE, Sisco M, Bonomo SR, Robinson AM, Mustoe TA (2004) Impact of aging on gene expression in a rat model of ischemic cutaneous wound healing. J Surg Res 118:190–196

33. Holt DR, Kirk SJ, Regan MC, Hurson M, Lindblad WJ, Barbul A (1992) Effect of age on wound healing in healthy human beings. Surgery 112:293–297, discussion 297–298

34. Grove GL, Kligman AM (1983) Age-associated changes in human epidermal cell renewal. J Gerontol 38:137–142

35. Gilchrest BA, Murphy GF, Soter NA (1982) Effect of chronologic aging and ultraviolet irradiation on langerhans cells in human epidermis. J Invest Dermatol 79:85–88

36. Sobin SS, Bernick S, Ballard KW (1992) Acute wound repair in an aged animal: a model for accelerated aging of the microvasculature? J Gerontol 47:B121–B125

37. Chang EI, Loh SA, Ceradini DJ et al (2007) Age decreases endothelial progenitor cell recruitment through decreases in hypoxia-inducible factor 1alpha stabilization during ischemia. Circulation 116:2818–2829

38. Liu L, Marti GP, Wei X et al (2008) Age-dependent impairment of HIF-1alpha expression in diabetic mice: correction with electroporation-facilitated gene therapy increases wound healing, angiogenesis, and circulating angiogenic cells. J Cell Physiol 217:319–327

39. Semenza GL (2007) Vasculogenesis, angiogenesis, and arteriogenesis: mechanisms of blood vessel formation and remodeling. J Cell Biochem 102:840–847

40. Rudman D, Feller AG, Nagraj HS et al (1990) Effects of human growth hormone in men over 60 years old. N Engl J Med 323:1–6

41. Petersen TI, Kissmeyer-Nielsen P, Laurberg S, Christensen H (1995) Impaired wound healing but unaltered colonic healing with increasing age: an experimental study in rats. Eur Surg Res 27:250–257

42. Johnson BD, Page RC, Narayanan AS, Pieters HP (1986) Effects of donor age on protein and collagen synthesis in vitro by human diploid fibroblasts. Lab Invest 55:490–496

43. El-Domyati M, Attia S, Saleh F et al (2002) Intrinsic aging vs. photoaging: a comparative histopathological, immunohistochemical, and ultrastructural study of skin. Exp Dermatol 11:398–405

44. Holm-Pedersen P, Zederfeldt B (1971) Strength development of skin incisions in young and old rats. Scand J Plast Reconstr Surg 5:7–12

45. Sussman MD (1973) Aging of connective tissue: physical properties of healing wounds in young and old rats. Am J Physiol 224:1167–1171

46. Holm-Pedersen P, Viidik A (1972) Tensile properties and morphology of healing wounds in young and old rats. Scand J Plast Reconstr Surg 6:24–35

47. Ashcroft GS, Herrick SE, Tarnuzzer RW, Horan MA, Schultz GS, Ferguson MW (1997) Human ageing impairs injury-induced in vivo expression of tissue inhibitor of matrix metalloproteinases (TIMP)-1 and -2 proteins and mRNA. J Pathol 183:169–176

48. Sharpless NE, DePinho RA (2007) How stem cells age and why this makes us grow old. Nat Rev Mol Cell Biol 8:703–713

49. Conboy IM, Conboy MJ, Wagers AJ, Girma ER, Weissman IL, Rando TA (2005) Rejuvenation of aged progenitor cells by exposure to a young systemic environment. Nature 433:760–764

50. Ito M, Yang Z, Andl T et al (2007) Wnt-dependent de novo hair follicle regeneration in adult mouse skin after wounding. Nature 447:316–320

51. Lau HC, Granick MS, Aisner AM, Solomon MP (1994) Wound care in the elderly patient. Surg Clin North Am 74:441–463

52. Howard L, Ashley C (2003) Nutrition in the perioperative patient. Annu Rev Nutr 23:263–282

53. Ward MW, Danzi M, Lewin MR, Rennie MJ, Clark CG (1982) The effects of subclinical malnutrition and refeeding on the healing of experimental colonic anastomoses. Br J Surg 69:308–310

54. Daly JM, Vars HM, Dudrick SJ (1972) Effects of protein depletion on strength of colonic anastomoses. Surg Gynecol Obstet 134:15–21

55. Goncalves CG, Groth AK, Ferreira M, Matias JE, Coelho JC, Campos AC (2009) Influence of preoperative feeding on the healing of colonic anastomoses in malnourished rats. JPEN J Parenter Enteral Nutr 33:83–89

56. Haydock DA, Hill GL (1986) Impaired wound healing in surgical patients with varying degrees of malnutrition. JPEN J Parenter Enteral Nutr 10:550–554

57. Casey J, Flinn WR, Yao JS, Fahey V, Pawlowski J, Bergan JJ (1983) Correlation of immune and nutritional status with wound complications in patients undergoing vascular operations. Surgery 93:822–827

58. Haydock DA, Hill GL (1987) Improved wound healing response in surgical patients receiving intravenous nutrition. Br J Surg 74:320–323

59. Avenell A, Handoll HH (2004) Nutritional supplementation for hip fracture aftercare in the elderly. Cochrane Database Syst Rev (1):CD001880

60. Braga M, Ljungqvist O, Soeters P, Fearon K, Weimann A, Bozzetti F (2009) ESPEN guidelines on parenteral nutrition: surgery. Clin Nutr 28:378–386

61. Cruse PJ, Foord R (1973) A five-year prospective study of 23, 649 surgical wounds. Arch Surg 107:206–210

62. Israelsson LA, Jonsson T (1997) Overweight and healing of midline incisions: the importance of suture technique. Eur J Surg 163:175–180

63. Goodson WH III, Hunt TK (1986) Wound collagen accumulation in obese hyperglycemic mice. Diabetes 35:491–495

64. Marti G, Ferguson M, Wang J et al (2004) Electroporative transfection with KGF-1 DNA improves wound healing in a diabetic mouse model. Gene Ther 11:1780–1785

65. McMurry JF Jr (1984) Wound healing with diabetes mellitus. Better glucose control for better wound healing in diabetes. Surg Clin North Am 64:769–778

66. Peppa M, Stavroulakis P, Raptis SA (2009) Advanced glycoxidation products and impaired diabetic wound healing. Wound Repair Regen 17:461–472

67. Heiner S, Whitney JD, Wood C, Mygrant BI (2002) Effects of an augmented postoperative fluid protocol on wound healing in cardiac surgery patients. Am J Crit Care 11:554–566

68. Stotts NA, Wipke-Tevis D (1996) Nutrition, perfusion, and wound healing: an inseparable triad. Nutrition 12:733–734

69. Quirinia A, Viidik A (1991) The influence of age on the healing of normal and ischemic incisional skin wounds. Mech Ageing Dev 58:221–232

70. Cooley BC, Gould JS (1993) Influence of age on free flap tolerance to ischemia: an experimental study in rats. Ann Plast Surg 30:57–59

71. Hartmann M, Jonsson K, Zederfeldt B (1992) Effect of tissue perfusion and oxygenation on accumulation of collagen in healing

wounds. Randomized study in patients after major abdominal operations. Eur J Surg 158:521–526

72. Jonsson K, Jensen JA, Goodson WH III et al (1991) Tissue oxygenation, anemia, and perfusion in relation to wound healing in surgical patients. Ann Surg 214:605–613

73. Wipke-Tevis DD, Williams DA (2007) Effect of oral hydration on skin microcirculation in healthy young and midlife and older adults. Wound Repair Regen 15:174–185

74. Fife CE, Smart DR, Sheffield PJ, Hopf HW, Hawkins G, Clarke D (2009) Transcutaneous oximetry in clinical practice: consensus statements from an expert panel based on evidence. Undersea Hyperb Med 36:43–53

75. Klevens RM, Edwards JR, Richards CL Jr et al (2007) Estimating health care-associated infections and deaths in U.S. hospitals, 2002. Public Health Rep 122:160–166

76. Fry DE (2002) The economic costs of surgical site infection. Surg Infect (Larchmt) 3(Suppl 1):S37–43

77. Edwards JR, Peterson KD, Andrus ML et al (2008) National healthcare safety network (NHSN) report, data summary for 2006 through 2007, issued november 2008. Am J Infect Control 36:609–626

78. Hedrick TL, Anastacio MM, Sawyer RG (2006) Prevention of surgical site infections. Expert Rev Anti Infect Ther 4:223–233

79. Kirby JP, Mazuski JE (2009) Prevention of surgical site infection. Surg Clin North Am 89:365–89, viii

80. Gardner SE, Frantz RA, Doebbeling BN (2001) The validity of the clinical signs and symptoms used to identify localized chronic wound infection. Wound Repair Regen 9:178–186

81. Lipsky BA, Berendt AR, Deery HG et al (2004) Diagnosis and treatment of diabetic foot infections. Clin Infect Dis 39:885–910

82. Davis SC, Ricotti C, Cazzaniga A, Welsh E, Eaglstein WH, Mertz PM (2008) Microscopic and physiologic evidence for biofilm-associated wound colonization in vivo. Wound Repair Regen 16:23–29

83. Martin JM, Zenilman JM, Lazarus GS (2009) Molecular microbiology: new dimensions for cutaneous biology and wound healing. J Invest Dermatol 130(1):38–48

84. Beer HD, Fassler R, Werner S (2000) Glucocorticoid-regulated gene expression during cutaneous wound repair. Vitam Horm 59:217–239

85. Schacke H, Docke WD, Asadullah K (2002) Mechanisms involved in the side effects of glucocorticoids. Pharmacol Ther 96:23–43

86. Eubanks TR, Greenberg JJ, Dobrin PB, Harford FJ, Gamelli RL (1997) The effects of different corticosteroids on the healing colon anastomosis and cecum in a rat model. Am Surg 63:266–269

87. Del Rio JV, Beck DE, Opelka FG (1996) Chronic perioperative steroids and colonic anastomotic healing in rats. J Surg Res 66:138–142

88. Hunt TK, Ehrlich HP, Garcia JA, Dunphy JE (1969) Effect of vitamin A on reversing the inhibitory effect of cortisone on healing of open wounds in animals and man. Ann Surg 170:633–641

89. Schulze S, Andersen J, Overgaard H et al (1997) Effect of prednisolone on the systemic response and wound healing after colonic surgery. Arch Surg 132:129–135

90. Ensrud KE, Nevitt MC, Yunis C et al (1994) Correlates of impaired function in older women. J Am Geriatr Soc 42:481–489

91. Waddell BE, Calton WC Jr, Steinberg SR, Martindale RG (1997) The adverse effects of octreotide on wound healing in rats. Am Surg 63:446–449

92. Belcher HJ, Ellis H (1990) Somatropin and wound healing after injury. J Clin Endocrinol Metab 70:939–943

93. Christensen H, Oxlund H (1994) Growth hormone increases the collagen deposition rate and breaking strength of left colonic anastomoses in rats. Surgery 116:550–556

94. Christensen H, Chemnitz J, Christensen BC, Oxlund H (1995) Collagen structural organization of healing colonic anastomoses and the effect of growth hormone treatment. Dis Colon Rectum 38:1200–1205

95. Zaizen Y, Ford EG, Costin G, Atkinson JB (1990) Stimulation of wound bursting strength during protein malnutrition. J Surg Res 49:333–336

96. Herndon DN, Nguyen TT, Gilpin DA (1993) Growth factors. Local and systemic. Arch Surg 128:1227–1233

97. Mueller RV, Hunt TK, Tokunaga A, Spencer EM (1994) The effect of insulinlike growth factor I on wound healing variables and macrophages in rats. Arch Surg 129:262–265

98. Jyung RW, Mustoe JA, Busby WH, Clemmons DR (1994) Increased wound-breaking strength induced by insulin-like growth factor I in combination with insulin-like growth factor binding protein-1. Surgery 115:233–239

99. Meyer NA, Barrow RE, Herndon DN (1996) Combined insulin-like growth factor-1 and growth hormone improves weight loss and wound healing in burned rats. J Trauma 41:1008–1012

100. Herndon DN, Barrow RE, Kunkel KR, Broemeling L, Rutan RL (1990) Effects of recombinant human growth hormone on donor-site healing in severely burned children. Ann Surg 212:424–429, discussion 430–431

101. Nguyen TT, Gilpin DA, Meyer NA, Herndon DN (1996) Current treatment of severely burned patients. Ann Surg 223:14–25

102. Herndon DN, Pierre EJ, Stokes KN, Barrow RE (1996) Growth hormone treatment for burned children. Horm Res 45(Suppl 1): 29–31

103. Harman SM, Blackman MR (2004) Use of growth hormone for prevention or treatment of effects of aging. J Gerontol A Biol Sci Med Sci 59:652–658

104. Liu H, Bravata DM, Olkin I et al (2007) Systematic review: the safety and efficacy of growth hormone in the healthy elderly. Ann Intern Med 146:104–115

105. Munzer T, Harman SM, Sorkin JD, Blackman MR (2009) Growth hormone and sex steroid effects on serum glucose, insulin, and lipid concentrations in healthy older women and men. J Clin Endocrinol Metab 94(10):3833–3841

106. Flegg JA, McElwain DL, Byrne HM, Turner IW (2009) A three species model to simulate application of hyperbaric oxygen therapy to chronic wounds. PLoS Comput Biol 5:e1000451

107. Semenza GL (2009) Regulation of oxygen homeostasis by hypoxia-inducible factor 1. Physiology (Bethesda) 24:97–106

108. Said HK, Hijjawi J, Roy N, Mogford J, Mustoe T (2005) Transdermal sustained-delivery oxygen improves epithelial healing in a rabbit ear wound model. Arch Surg 140:998–1004

109. Goldman RJ (2009) Hyperbaric oxygen therapy for wound healing and limb salvage: a systematic review. PM R 1:471–489

110. Banks PG, Ho CH (2008) A novel topical oxygen treatment for chronic and difficult-to-heal wounds: case studies. J Spinal Cord Med 31:297–301

111. Tawfick W, Sultan S (2009) Does topical wound oxygen (TWO2) offer an improved outcome over conventional compression dressings (CCD) in the management of refractory venous ulcers (RVU)? A parallel observational comparative study. Eur J Vasc Endovasc Surg 38:125–132

112. Kim HS, Noh SU, Han YW et al (2009) Therapeutic effects of topical application of ozone on acute cutaneous wound healing. J Korean Med Sci 24:368–374

113. Papanas N, Maltezos E (2008) Becaplermin gel in the treatment of diabetic neuropathic foot ulcers. Clin Interv Aging 3:233–240

114. Byrnes CK, Khan FH, Nass PH, Hatoum C, Duncan MD, Harmon JW (2001) Success and limitations of a naked plasmid transfection protocol for keratinocyte growth factor-1 to enhance cutaneous wound healing. Wound Repair Regen 9:341–346

115. Jeschke MG, Richter G, Hofstadter F, Herndon DN, Perez-Polo JR, Jauch KW (2002) Non-viral liposomal keratinocyte growth factor (KGF) cDNA gene transfer improves dermal and epidermal regeneration through stimulation of epithelial and mesenchymal factors. Gene Ther 9:1065–1074

116. Williams RS, Johnston SA, Riedy M, DeVit MJ, McElligott SG, Sanford JC (1991) Introduction of foreign genes into tissues of living mice by DNA-coated microprojectiles. Proc Natl Acad Sci USA 88:2726–2730

117. Pavselj N, Preat V (2005) DNA electrotransfer into the skin using a combination of one high- and one low-voltage pulse. J Control Release 106:407–415

118. Lin MP, Marti GP, Dieb R et al (2006) Delivery of plasmid DNA expression vector for keratinocyte growth factor-1 using electroporation to improve cutaneous wound healing in a septic rat model. Wound Repair Regen 14:618–624

119. Marti GP, Mohebi P, Liu L, Wang J, Miyashita T, Harmon JW (2008) KGF-1 for wound healing in animal models. Methods Mol Biol 423:383–391

120. Thomas CE, Ehrhardt A, Kay MA (2003) Progress and problems with the use of viral vectors for gene therapy. Nat Rev Genet 4:346–358

121. Garcia M, Escamez MJ, Carretero M et al (2007) Modeling normal and pathological processes through skin tissue engineering. Mol Carcinog 46:741–745

122. Robson MC, Barbul A (2006) Guidelines for the best care of chronic wounds. Wound Repair Regen 14:647–648

123. Steed DL, Attinger C, Colaizzi T et al (2006) Guidelines for the treatment of diabetic ulcers. Wound Repair Regen 14:680–692

124. Whitney J, Phillips L, Aslam R et al (2006) Guidelines for the treatment of pressure ulcers. Wound Repair Regen 14: 663–679

125. Franz MG, Robson MC, Steed DL et al (2008) Guidelines to aid healing of acute wounds by decreasing impediments of healing. Wound Repair Regen 16:723–748

Chapter 9
Frailty and Surgery in the Elderly

Babak J. Orandi, Jordan M. Winter, Dorry L. Segev, and Martin A. Makary

Introduction

Conventional surgical wisdom has long held that the elderly do not tolerate surgery as well as their younger counterparts. Numerous case series comparing outcomes such as morbidity and length of stay often corroborate that viewpoint. However, the older surgical population displays great heterogeneity, and that heterogeneity is not always obvious from preoperative morbidities and preoperative testing criteria. In fact, we have on numerous occasions been surprised by the elderly patient who beats the odds following surgery, and the patient who, ostensibly, should recover well, but does not.

Among older surgical patients, it can be quite challenging to predict who will thrive and who will develop a complication that can trigger a cascade of events that may lead to unexpected demise or permanent disability. In this chapter, we explore the emerging concept that frailty adds significant information to outcome prediction in elderly surgical candidates, beyond that of conventional preoperative criteria.

Limitations of Age as a Predictor

The effect of advanced age on surgical outcomes, independent of other patient-specific factors, is not well understood. The geriatric literature is replete with large series documenting comparable excellent surgical outcomes in the elderly [1–3]. Indeed, the risk factors for poor outcomes in the elderly are the same as for younger patients, namely comorbid illness and poor baseline functional status [4]. These factors have an increased prevalence in the elderly, though not uniformly across the entire elderly population. This varied distribution gives rise to the concept of the heterogeneity of aging.

Selection bias and the failure to account for a heterogeneous elderly population may explain why many other studies have shown that such good surgical outcomes are possible in older patients. This is particularly important because for many diseases, especially malignancies, age is often a major, if not the most important, risk factor for the development of the disease. With many groups publishing papers on their successful experience operating on octogenarians and nonagenarians, the indications for surgery in the elderly are expanding. For example, after adjusting for preoperative comorbidities, we found that age was not an independent risk factor for perioperative mortality and morbidity following pancreaticoduodenectomy [1]. Filsoufi and colleagues reached the same conclusion for patients over 80 years of age following aortic valve replacement [2]. Another group found that in elderly patients with minimal comorbid illness undergoing colon resection, there was no mortality difference in those over 70 years of age compared with younger patients [3]. In general, age is no longer an absolute contraindication to surgery.

Clinical Decision Making

A major challenge for surgeons in caring for the elderly is to determine which patients are good operative candidates. This estimation requires assessing potential operative candidates for a number of patient-specific factors, particularly comorbidities, disability, and frailty. These three factors, which are frequently used interchangeably in the common vernacular and might demonstrate overlap, are distinct clinical phenomena. In fact, there is near unanimous agreement in the gerontology community that disability and frailty are distinct clinical entities [5]. The conceptual model for frailty maintains that although disability and comorbidity may sometimes coexist with frailty, there is a significant group of frail individuals who present with neither disability nor comorbidity (Fig. 9.1). Disability is defined as difficulty in carrying out those activities that are essential for independent living, such as bathing, dressing, eating, shopping, and preparing meals. Comorbidity is the clinical manifestation of illness in an individual, such as congestive heart failure, osteoarthritis, or chronic obstructive pulmonary disease. The last factor, frailty, is a newer concept in the geriatrics literature.

M.A. Makary (✉)
Department of Surgery, Johns Hopkins Hospital, Baltimore, MD, USA

R.A. Rosenthal et al. (eds.), *Principles and Practice of Geriatric Surgery*,
DOI 10.1007/978-1-4419-6999-6_9, © Springer Science+Business Media, LLC 2011

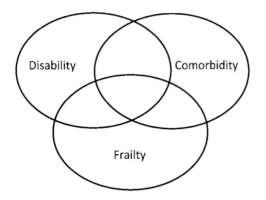

Figure 9.1 A conceptual framework for frailty, in the context of comorbidity and disability.

Frailty

Frailty in the elderly generally refers to patients with poor physiologic reserve who are at an increased risk of adverse events following exposure to stressors such as anesthesia and surgery. These clinically important adverse events include institutionalization in a long-term care facility, falls, and mortality. In 2001, Fried et al. published a standardized definition of frailty using five criteria (Table 9.1) [6]:

1. Slow gait speed
2. Low physical activity
3. Unintentional weight loss
4. Self-reported exhaustion
5. Muscle weakness

Frailty is defined as the presence of at least three of these five criteria. *Gait speed* is measured over a distance of 15 ft, with the criteria based on gender and height. The level of *physical activity* is based on the patient's kilocalorie expenditure over the prior 2 weeks using the Minnesota Leisure Time Activities Questionnaire [7]. *Unintentional weight loss* is present when the patient affirms that he or she has unintentionally lost more than 10 pounds over the preceding year. *Self-reported exhaustion* is based on the Center for Epidemiologic Studies Depression Scale (CES-D), and asks the patient to agree or disagree with these two statements: in the past week, "I felt that everything I did was an effort," and "I could not get going" [8]. Finally, *muscle weakness* is based on grip strength as measured by a hand-held dynamometer. This criterion varies by gender and body mass index. Of note, all of these criteria are quickly and inexpensively assessed in the clinic setting, lending them to easy adoption, even in a busy clinical practice.

Within the gerontology community, there remains considerable debate as to the appropriate definition of frailty. Some

Table 9.1 Frailty criteria

Criteria	Notes				
Slow gait speed	Timed 15 foot walk			*Height (cm)*	*Time (s)*
			Men		
				≤173	≥7
				≤173	≥6
			Women		
				≤159	≥7
				≤159	≥6
Low physical activity	Based on Minnesota Leisure Time Activity Questionnaire			*Weekly kcal expenditure*	
			Men	<343	
			Women	<270	
Unintentional weight loss	>10 lb weight loss in past year				
Self-reported exhaustion	Based on CES-D Depression Scale; quantifies the amount of time in the past week the patient felt the following		I felt that everything I did was an effort I could not get going		
Muscle weakness	Based on grip strength			*BMI*	*Force (kg)*
			Men		
				≤24	≤29
				24.1–26	≤30
				26.1–28	≤30
				>28	≤32
			Women		
				≤23	≤17
				23.1–26	≤17.3
				26.1–29	≤18
				>29	≤21

of the Fried criteria have been validated, while certain new ones have been proposed. Generally speaking, there is strong agreement amongst experts that the clinical syndrome represents a constellation of diseases, impairments, and/or symptoms, rather than simply the presence of one disease or condition [5]. Rothman and colleagues provided good preliminary evidence to support the use of slow gait speed, low physical activity, weight loss, and cognitive impairment as important indicators of frailty, but not self-reported exhaustion and muscle weakness [9]. In addition, they and others advocate including a number of different domains in the definition of frailty aside from just physical function, such as psychological characteristics and psychosocial factors. Rothman recommends integrating cognitive function into the frailty assessment as it is a strong predictor of adverse outcomes. While the exact definition of frailty may be in flux, there is no doubt that the presence of frailty portends a number of adverse clinical outcomes. We have found the above definition of frailty by Fried to be standardized and easy to implement.

Clinical Outcomes of Frailty

In the longitudinal Cardiovascular Health Study, which included over 5,000 community-dwelling Medicare-eligible people, subjects who met frailty criteria at baseline were more likely to be older, female, and African-American [6]. They also tended to have lower levels of education and income. Frail patients had a significantly higher mortality rate than their nonfrail counterparts at 3 and 7 years (18 vs. 3% and 43 vs. 12%, respectively). Frailty was also predictive of a number of other clinically relevant geriatric outcomes, including injurious falls, hospitalizations, and worsening disability, both in terms of performance of activities of daily living and in mobility.

In a separate longitudinal study of community-dwelling people over the age of 70 who were initially disability-free, frail individuals were also noted to experience increased mortality and incidence of chronic disability [9]. The study also found that 22% of frail patients had a long-term nursing home stay (>90 days) over 7.5 years of follow-up. Clearly, the presence of frailty has a number of ramifications in terms of clinical, economic, and quality-of-life outcomes.

Biologic Basis of Frailty

While the biologic basis of frailty remains uncertain, it likely results from multiple etiologies, rather than from one underlying cause, and affects multiple physiologic systems (Fig. 9.2) [10]. A multifactorial basis for frailty is more probable given the broad spectrum of clinical manifestations of the frailty syndrome.

While a detailed review of the current understanding of the biological underpinnings of frailty is beyond the scope of this chapter, it appears that inflammation is central to its pathogenesis. C-reactive protein (CRP), a nonspecific serum marker of inflammation, has been shown to be elevated in frail elderly patients compared to their nonfrail counterparts [11]. This finding holds true across gender and racial lines, as well as across the age spectrum over 65, and is independent of diabetes mellitus and cardiovascular disease status, two disease states associated with chronic inflammation. That same report, part of the Cardiovascular Health Study, found that frail patients were significantly more likely to have congenital heart disease, congestive heart failure, diabetes, and hypertension (Table 9.2). There was no statistically significant increase in cancer rates amongst frail patients, though that likely has more to do with study exclusion criteria, as

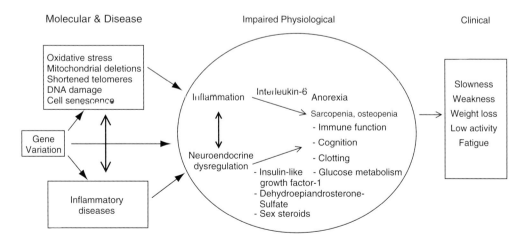

FIGURE 9.2 Overview of hypothesized molecular, physiological, and clinical pathway to frailty. *Arrows* pointing in both directions illustrate potential interactions between systems (from [5] reprinted with permission from The McGraw Hill Companies).

Frailty indicator	Prevalence					
	Frailty	CHD[a]	CHF	Cancer	Diabetes[a]	Hypertension[a]
Not frail (n=2289)	48.3	15	1	14.8	18.8	37.9
Intermediate (n=2147)	45.3	21	4	15.5	24.5	43.9
Frail (n=299)	6.3	30.8	14	16.4	32.4	48.5

patients actively being treated for a malignancy were not included in the study.

In addition to CRP, the major proinflammatory cytokine Interleukin-6 (IL-6) been shown to be predictive of mortality in the elderly [12]. IL-6 has also been extensively linked to, amongst other adverse clinical entities, osteopenia, sarcopenia (muscle loss), anemia, and insulin resistance, all of which contribute to the frailty syndrome [13] Leng et al. [29] demonstrated that elderly frail patients have significantly higher IL-6 levels than nonfrail elderly subjects, suggesting that IL-6 may also play a direct role in the pathogenesis of frailty.

Like serum IL-6 and CRP levels, plasma hypertonicity has been linked to adverse outcomes in the frail. Several theories have been proposed to explain this observation. Stookey et al. suggest that abnormalities in any of the myriad organs involved in regulating plasma homeostasis and thirst, from the pituitary to the kidneys, or states of glucose intolerance, as seen in such conditions as cancer, cachexia, diabetes, and chronic renal insufficiency, can lead to plasma hypertonicity [14]. These same underlying conditions may also play a simultaneous role in the development of frailty. As the understanding of frailty's pathogenesis improves, it is likely that biomarkers will become useful tools in screening patients and in predicting medical and surgical outcomes in the frail, similar to the MELD score for predicting 3-month mortality in surgical patients with end-stage liver disease [15].

Clinical Utility

A frailty index has many applications, including epidemiology, policy, and research. However, the most useful application may be at the bedside. In a prospective study of elderly surgical patients, we found that frail patients had a 2.5-fold increased odds of developing complications after surgery compared with their nonfrail counterparts [16]. Their hospital length of stay was twice as long as nonfrail patients for minor surgical procedures and over 80% longer for major operations. The odds of discharge to a skilled or assisted care facility were over 20 times higher in frail patients. Frailty also significantly augmented the predictive ability of other preoperative risk assessment systems, specifically the American Society of Anesthesiologists (ASA) score, and the Lee and Eagle [17–19] preoperative cardiac risk-stratification

tools, in terms of postoperative complications, length of hospital stay, and discharge disposition.

Frailty may be helpful in selecting appropriate patients for surgery, particularly in settings where selection tools are vague and not validated. Clinicians have traditionally used age as a rough surrogate for triaging patients. For instance, the elderly are less likely to receive organ-directed surgery for malignancies of the breast, esophagus, stomach, pancreas, and rectum, as well as for sarcoma and non-small-cell lung cancer [20]. Moreover, a referral bias from nonsurgeons to surgeons has been observed for elective surgical procedures [21]. In a survey of Dutch cardiologists, age was the most important determinant of whether or not referrers would recommend surgery to patients with aortic stenosis 40% of the time [22]. Frailty status, rather than age, would be more helpful in the determination of overall fitness. Nonfrail individuals with resilient physiologic reserve could be selected for surgery, while frail ones could be identified to prevent operations in those patients at highest risk of a catastrophic clinical outcome.

In addition to aiding the selection of appropriate surgical candidates, a frailty index may identify patients who could, with additional interventions, become candidates for elective operations. One's frailty status is not a fixed, permanent entity; rather, frailty can have a waxing and waning course. Studenski and colleagues have developed a measure of change in frailty that quantifies patient mobility, balance, strength, endurance, nutrition, and neuromotor performance over time [23]. While its application for optimizing the timing of an operation has yet to be validated, the concept that frailty is a dynamic condition is an important one. One can imagine a related application as a measuring stick after completing a preoperative intervention aimed at medical optimization.

Indeed, there are a number of possible targets for preoperative intervention that may particularly benefit the frail elderly. Aggressive physical therapy may be of benefit. For major abdominal operations performed on the elderly, better preoperative physical performance status almost invariably predicts better recovery and a faster return to the activities of daily living (ADLs) and the instrumental activities of daily living (IADLs) [24]. While the study that demonstrated this finding was not exclusively focused on the frail, it seems logical that the frail may stand to gain the most from increased physical activity as the syndrome is characterized by low physical activity, slow gait speed, and muscle weakness.

Preoperative nutritional supplementation is another attractive preoperative intervention for the frail. In a Cochrane review of preoperative enteral supplementation in the elderly, there was an overall weight gain for participants in the 31 included trials, as well as a decrease in mortality and a shorter length of hospital stay for those patients who received preoperative supplementation [25]. Just as with preoperative physical therapy, it remains to be seen in clinical trials whether the frail elderly will benefit from this preoperative intervention, though it does seem likely given the tight association between weight loss and the frailty syndrome.

Congestive heart failure (CHF) has been shown to be an independent predictor of postoperative complications in the elderly [26]. This suggests that, given a sufficiently lengthy window of opportunity preoperatively, frail patients, and elderly patients in general, who suffer from symptomatic CHF may benefit from pharmacologic optimization of their heart function prior to surgery in an effort to prevent postoperative complications.

Given that frail patients are more likely to suffer from postoperative, hospital-acquired complications, a frailty score may help identify which patients ought to be the subject of rigorous preventive measures to avoid the development of delirium, falls, infections, pressure sores, worsened malnutrition, and functional impairment. A number of strategies that are beyond the scope of this chapter have been described to prevent these complications, and identification of those most vulnerable to these complications using the frailty index will likely benefit from these measures.

Better risk assessment through the application of a frailty index has implications beyond just identifying opportunities to intervene: it also has implications for counseling of patients in the informed consent process. The decision to proceed with surgery should balance risk with the probability of survival and a meaningful quality of life as determined by the patient and the patient's family. Important to this discussion is the risk of discharge to a skilled nursing facility, as opposed to the patient's home. While not traditionally viewed as a surgical complication, discharge to a skilled nursing facility has a tremendous impact on patients and their families.

While a number of previously mentioned studies have demonstrated good surgical outcomes in elderly patients, a major criticism of these studies is their inherent selection bias. Patients who receive operations have been vetted by the referral process to a surgeon, as well as the surgeon's decision as to proceed with the surgery. Additionally, many of these results are from centers of excellence that have high patient volumes, as well as the resources, staff, and protocols necessary to care for these patients perioperatively.

It should be pointed out, however, that although frailty status can be an important aide in making decisions about management of patients, the heterogeneity of aging, the dearth of data regarding surgical outcomes in the frail, and the broad spectrum of patients' goals from surgery necessitate a highly individualized approach to care for the frail elderly.

Research Utility

Frailty may demonstrate particular utility in research, as its criteria become more standardized and its prognostic implications better defined. It has been well documented that the elderly are underrepresented in oncology clinical trials. In a study of 15 types of malignancies, Hutchins et al. found that while 63% of the US population comprises individuals over the age of 65, only 25% of cancer clinical trial participants are elderly [27]. While the reasons for this disparity are many, there is no doubt that clinician bias, at least in some part, is to blame. One half of surveyed oncologists stated that they deem elderly patients inappropriate for referral to clinical trials based on chronologic age alone [28]. A standardized frailty scoring system with predetermined cutoff points could be used as exclusion criteria in place of some of the more subjective and sometimes arbitrary considerations that are widely used, and thereby boost enrollment of elderly patients into clinical trials. Vulnerable elderly patients would still be excluded, while an important subgroup of suitable elderly candidates could be included.

Aside from using frailty to make clinical trial enrollment more equitable and representative of the population, knowledge about the aging process and frailty itself may be the endpoint of many future studies. An aging population and its incumbent economic considerations will likely drive research aimed at delaying or preventing the development of frailty, as well as trials to test interventions intended to minimize the effect of frailty on patient longevity, resource utilization, and quality of life.

Conclusion (Table 9.3)

Frailty is a multidomain syndrome that reflects poor physiologic and functional reserve and predicts a number of adverse clinical outcomes in surgery. We have found that the use of frailty as a clinical predictor adds significant value beyond other preoperative predictors, augmenting their ability to anticipate untoward postoperative events. Utilizing a standardized definition of frailty for future research in this highly vulnerable population may ultimately allow patients to be better risk-stratified for preoperative decision making. Increased awareness of the frailty syndrome and its clinical implications will undoubtedly improve care in older patients and improve their overall health outcomes.

TABLE 9.3 Frailty summary

Frailty is a multifactorial syndrome of poor physiologic reserve that puts patients at increased risk of adverse events following exposure to stressors

The standard definition of frailty uses the following five criteria slow gait speed, low physical activity, unintentional weight loss, self-reported exhaustion, and muscle weakness

Frailty is a better predictor of postoperative complications than a number of commonly used risk-stratification tools

Frailty can help with patient selection, risk stratification, and identification of patients who would benefit from preoperative risk-reduction interventions

References

1. Makary MA, Winter JM, Cameron JL, Campbell KA, Chang D, Cunningham SC et al (2006) Pancreaticoduodenectomy in the very elderly. J Gastrointest Surg 10(3):347–356

2. Filsoufi F, Rahmanian PB, Castillo JG, Chikwe J, Silvay G, Adams DH (2008) Excellent early and late outcomes of aortic valve replacement in people aged 80 and older. J Am Geriatr Soc 56(2):255–261

3. Boyd JB, Bradford B Jr, Watne AL (1980) Operative risk factors of colon resection in the elderly. Ann Surg 192:743–746

4. Hamel MB, Henderson WG, Khuri SF, Daley J (2005) Surgical outcomes for patients aged 80 and older: morbidity and mortality from major noncardiac surgery. J Am Geriatr Soc 53(93):424–429

5. Fried LP, Walston J (1993) Frailty and failure to thrive. In: Principles of geriatric medicine and gerontology, 3rd edn. McGraw-Hill, New York, pp 241–248

6. Fried LP, Tangen CM, Walston J, Newman AB, Hirsch C, Gottdiener J et al (2001) Frailty in older adults: evidence for a phenotype. J Gerontol A Biol Sci Med Sci 56:M146–M156

7. Taylor HL, Jacobs DR Jr, Schuker B, Knudsen J, Leon AS, Debacker G (1978) A questionnaire for the assessment of leisure-time physical activities. J Chronic Dis 31:745–755

8. Orme J, Reis J, Herz E (1986) Factorial and discriminate validity of the Center for Epidemiologic Studies depression (CES-D) scale. J Clin Psychol 42:28–33

9. Rothman RD, Leo-Summers L, Gill TM (2008) Prognostic significance of potential frailty criteria. J Am Geriatr Soc 56(12):2211–2216

10. Walston J, Hadley EC, Ferrucci L, Guralnik JM, Newman AB, Studenski SA et al (2006) Research agenda for frailty in older adults: toward a better understanding of physiology and etiology: summary from the AGS/NIA on Aging Research Conference on Frailty in Older Adults. J Am Geriatr Soc 54(6):991–1001

11. Walston J, McBurnie MA, Newman A, Tracy RP, Kop WJ, Hirsch CH et al (2002) Frailty and activation of the inflammation and coagulation systems with and without clinical comorbidities: results from the Cardiovascular Health Study. Arch Intern Med 162:2333–2341

12. Harris TB, Ferrucci L, Tracy RP, Corti MC, Wacholder S, Ettinger WH Jr et al (1999) Associations of elevated IL-6 and C-reactive protein levels with mortality in the elderly. Am J Med 106:506–512

13. Ershler WB, Keller ET (2000) Age-associated increased interleukin-6 gene expression, late-life diseases, and frailty. Annu Rev Med 51:245–270

14. Stookey JD, Purser JL, Pieper CF, Cohen HJ (2004) Plasma hypertonicity: another marker of frailty? J Am Geriatr Soc 52:1313–1320

15. Kamath PS, Wiesner RH, Malinchoc M et al (2001) A model to predict survival in patients with end-stage liver disease. Hepatology 33(2):464–470

16. Makary MA, Segev DL, Fried LP, Syin D, Bandeen-Roche K, Patel P et al (2006) Frailty as a predictor of surgical outcomes in older

17. Saklad M (1941) Grading of patients for surgical procedures. Anesthesiology 2:281–284

18. Lee TH, Marcantonio ER, Mangione CM, Thomas EJ, Polanczyk CA, Cook EF et al (1999) Derivation and prospective validation of a simple index for prediction of cardiac risk of major noncardiac surgery. Circulation 100(10):1043–1049

19. Fleisher LA, Beckman JA, Brown KA, Calkins H, Chaikof EL, Fleischmann KE et al (2007) ACC/AHA 2007 guidelines on perioperative cardiovascular evaluation and care for noncardiac surgery: executive summary a report of the American College of Cardiology/American Heart Association Task Force on Practice Guidelines (Writing Committee to Revise the 2002 Guidelines on Perioperative Cardiovascular Evaluation for Noncardiac Surgery). Circulation 116:1971–1996

20. O'Connell JB, Maggard MA, Ko CY (2004) Cancer-directed surgery for localized disease: decreased use in the elderly. Ann Surg Oncol 11(11):962–969

21. Ryynanen OP, Myllykangas M, Kinnunen J, Takala J (1997) Doctors' willingness to refer elderly patients for elective surgery. Fam Pract 14(3):216–219

22. Bouma BJ, van der Meulen JH, van den Brink RB, Arnold AE, Smidts A, Teunter LH et al (2001) Variability in treatment advice for elderly patients with aortic stenosis: a nationwide survey in The Netherlands. Heart 85(2):196–201

23. Studenski S, Hayes RP, Leibowitz RQ, Bode R, Lavery L, Walston J, Duncan P, Perera S (2004) Clinical global impression of change in physical frailty: development of a measure based on clinical judgment. J Am Geriatr Soc 52:1560–1566

24. Lawrence VA, Hazuda HP, Cornell JE, Pederson T, Bradshaw PT, Mulrow CD, Page CP (2004) Functional independence after major abdominal surgery in the elderly. J Am Coll Surg 199(5): 762–772

25. Milne AC, Potter J, Avenell A (2002) Oral protein and energy supplements reduce all-cause mortality in elderly persons. Cochrane Database Syst Rev (3):CD003288

26. Leung JM, Dzankic S (2001) Relative importance of preoperative health status versus intraoperative factors in predicting postoperative adverse outcomes in geriatric surgical patients. J Am Geriatr Soc 49:1080–1085

27. Hutchings LF, Unger JM, Crowley JJ, Coltman CA JR, Albain KS (1999) Underrepresentation of patients 65 years of age or older in cancer-treatment trials. New Engl J Med 34:2061–2067

28. Benson AB III, Pregler JP, Bean JA, Rademaker AW, Eshler B, Anderson K (1991) Oncologists' reluctance to accrue patients onto clinical trials: an Illinois Cancer Center study. J Clin Oncol 9:2067–2075

29. Leng S, Chaves P, Koenig K, Walston J. Serum interleukin-6 and hemoglobin as physiological correlates in the geriatric syndrome of frailty: a pilot study. J Am Geriatr Soc 50(7):1268–1271

patients. Paper presented at first annual academic surgical congress, San Diego, CA, 7–10 February 2006

Section II
Social/Societal Issues

Chapter 10
Invited Commentary

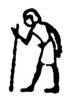

Michael E. Zenilman

Introduction

In this new section of our textbook, topics which have been in the background of surgery in elderly patients are now spotlighted. In the 10 years since publication of our first edition, it has been very gratifying for me to watch as more interest in the ramifications of surgery in the older patients – not just technical prowess – has developed; it brings us to the basics of medicine – "*Primum Non Nocere.*"

The increased interest has two mutually-non-exclusive sources. First, there has been more academic attention to the older surgical patient. For example, in 1976, the nine surgical journals I typically read published a total of 358 articles in which patients aged greater than 65 or 85 years were operated, in 1989 there were 368, in 1999 the number was 513, and in 2009 there were 893 articles. My impression is that the quality of the papers has drastically improved. Early articles proved – using simple and then more complex analyses – that we could do surgery safely, and discussed how to deal with the older patients, sometimes via editorial comments. The message was that chronologic age was not equal to physiologic age – especially if we controlled comorbid illnesses and emergency surgery. In fact, these concepts were the main message of our first edition.

Now papers are more scientific, and highly complex statistical analyses of large databases have allowed researchers to focus on outcomes and quality measures. We are only now on the cusp of defining that consequence of chronologic age and the aging process on surgical outcomes, and there is a real effect. The impact of frailty and disability, two non-reversible aging processes, on surgical outcomes is significant. Because of them and not comorbidity, the ultimate outcomes of major interventions may not be as good as we hope. While not reversible, these two processes are to some extent preventable; lifestyle changes can delay their onset.

Second, the sheer increase in number of patients in the older group has affected the population of patients we care for; the baby boomers have come of age. The predictions of the past – that the percentage of patients older than 65 and 85 in our population will grow – are coming true. While some papers wrongly predicted that Medicare would be financially insolvent by now, it is getting there. The shape of the age distribution in the USA has changed from a classic pyramid – where the small number of older population rest on top with increasing numbers of persons at the bottom – to a more rectangular (or trapezoidal) shape, where similar proportions of younger and older persons exist at multiple age levels. As our population pyramid changes, the demands on health care are changing too.

The societal burden for the expansion of the elderly patient population is intuitive, impressive, and expensive. An Institute of Medicine report in 2008 from the National Academy of Sciences entitled "Retooling for an Aging America: Building the Health Care Workforce" showed that the bulk of acute and chronic disease – diabetes, cardiac, hypertension, and cancer – rests in patients over 75 years of age. The older patient population uses more services. For example, 12% of our population uses up to one-third of total hospitalizations, and a similar percentage uses emergency medical responses and prescriptions for medication. The expanding use of nursing homes, short term rehabilitation facilities, and home care also has a cost.

The report suggested three goals to enhance the care of elderly patients: use education to improve the competence of health care providers, increase the number of geriatric specialists, and establish new models of care.

Achieving these goals will not be cheap. The IOM report noted that not only are chronic disease management, multidisciplinary care, and transitional care important for the elderly population, but also that to date, they have been underfunded. Bluntly, reimbursements for geriatricians, home care nurses, and even surgical care in this population is not very high, and the combination of low funding in all three areas is also problematic.

While surgical training programs have been asked to focus on education in geriatrics, to date it is mostly theoretical, and

M.E. Zenilman (✉)
School of Public Health, SUNY Downstate, Brooklyn, NY
and
Department of Surgery, Johns Hopkins School of Medicine,
Baltimore, MD
e-mail: mzenilman@downstate.edu

very few hospitals or institutions have active geriatric services which work closely with surgeons. The foundation of surgical training is to care for patients, not to just perform procedures. But there is very little in the surgical training for the topics described below.

The American Geriatrics Society has been an advocate in retooling the education practice of surgeons. Through their Jahnigan Scholars program, over 20 surgical specialists, in all disciplines, have been selected to do research, publish scholarly work, and teach geriatrics. Some basic curricula have been developed, and there is even one geriatric surgery fellowship available in the USA.

The real future of geriatric surgery is embedded in the chapters of this section; the foundation of education is evolving to a level of complexity higher than that described in the first edition of this textbook, and the need for multidisciplinary management is clear. To provide the elderly patient with quality care, we must be well versed in recognizing and addressing frailty and disability, not just controlling the established comorbidities of cardiac, pulmonary, kidney, and endocrine systems. Palliative care, do-not-resuscitate orders, and use of rehabilitation facilities and hospice need to be integrated early in a patient's care. As you will read, the American College of Surgeons, through the National Surgical Quality Improvement Project and the Task Force on Geriatric Surgery, is establishing quality indicators for the elderly patient, which will likely lead the change. In the future, these indicators will be just as important as the "core measures" we now follow.

Last, what about the elderly surgeon? While society has not yet mandated removal of driving licenses from older drivers, the elderly surgeon still has the same mandate as the younger "above all, do no harm."

Chapter 11
The Demography of Aging and Disability

Samir K. Sinha and Colleen Christmas

Over the previous century, there has been an extraordinary demographic shift which will no doubt persist well into this one. The lengthening of life span by over 50% and consequent increase in the proportion of the population that we refer to as the "elderly" has created a new and different social, economic, and medical imperative. We are now faced with the daunting task of providing health and social care for a huge number of persons living well into old age with more chronic illnesses, and increased needs and expectations. Anticipating the kinds of health care services, this population requires coordinated and creative efforts by many sectors of society and considerable educational and research activities to determine the best methods to deliver services. Indeed, this textbook has been written to respond to some of these challenges by addressing the specialized needs of older persons facing surgery.

The Demography of Aging

In the USA, as in other developed countries, the absolute numbers and relative proportions of older populations have continually increased to the point where there is now a higher percentage of older people than at any time in history. Indeed, while the overall US population had almost quadrupled in size over the course of the twentieth century, the portion of the population 65 years and older had increased 11-fold. The older population has grown from 3.1 million (4.1% of the overall population) in 1900 to 35 million (12.4%) in 2000 [1]. Among this latter figure, 18.4 million (53%) were aged 65–74, 12.4 million (35%) aged 75–84, and 4.2 million (12%) age 85 and older [2]. While it is predicted that these figures will increase slowly over the next few years, what follows is a period of marked accelerated growth in the second and third decades of this century. This pattern of shifting demographics largely reflects the impact of birth rates; the slower change in the near future reflecting low fertility rates during World War II and the preceding worldwide economic depression, while the subsequent growth surge stems from the "baby boom" that characterized the postwar years (1946–1964) in many nations. The first members of this "baby boom generation" will reach age 65 in 2011. As a result, by 2030 the older population is projected to be twice as large as in 2000, growing from 35 million to 72 million, which will then represent nearly 20% of the total US population. Predictions are that this trend persists at least until the mid-century. In 2050, the older population is projected to number 86.7 million [1].

The most rapid and profound change in numbers has been seen among the oldest old individuals, defined here as those aged 85 years and older. In 1900, there were only 122,000 of these individuals, but by 2000, their number had increased 34-fold to 4.2 million. This trend is expected to continue with this population doubling to 9.6 million by 2030 and then more than doubling again to 20.9 million by 2050 [1].

The USA, despite the growth projections for its older population, remains a relatively young population when compared with other developed countries. While its proportion of older adults stood at 12.4% in 2000, at least a dozen developed countries were reporting proportions ranging between 15 and 18% (Table 11.1). Part of what explains this difference is that the USA has experienced higher levels of fertility and immigration in recent decades than those of other developed countries [1]. In 2000, while average life expectancy at birth in the USA reached a high of 76.9 years, the highest rates were being reported for Swedish males and Japanese females at 77.6 and 84.1 years, respectively [1].

Causes and Consequences of Population Aging

The term *population aging* refers to the process through which the proportions of older individuals within an overall population age structure increase. Changes in the age structures of populations principally result from changes over

C. Christmas (✉)
Program Director, Johns Hopkins Bayview Medical Center,
4940 Eastern Avenue, B1-114E, Baltimore, MD 21224, USA
e-mail: cchristm@jhmi.edu

R.A. Rosenthal et al. (eds.), *Principles and Practice of Geriatric Surgery*,
DOI 10.1007/978-1-4419-6999-6_11, © Springer Science+Business Media, LLC 2011

TABLE 11.1 Countries with significant elderly (65 years and over) populations as a percentage at 2000, 2030, and 2050

	2000	2030	2050		2000	2030	2050
Africa				**Europe**			
Ghana	3.4	6.6	11.8	Albania	7.1	17.3	22.1
Mauritius	6.1	16	21.6	Austria	15.5	26	30.1
Reunion	5.6	11.4	17.1	Belgium	16.8	25	27.7
South Africa	4.7	11.6	13.6	Bosnia and Herzegovina	8.6	20.6	26
Algeria	4.3	10.3	21.3	Bulgaria	16.6	24.6	33.8
Egypt	4	8.8	14.8	Croatia	15.1	24.4	29.6
Libya	3.9	7.6	15.7	Czech Republic	13.8	24.3	33.1
Morocco	4.6	9.1	16.2	Denmark	14.8	22.7	24.6
Tunisia	6.1	12.9	23.8	Finland	14.9	26	27.3
Near East				France	16	23.7	26.8
Iraq	3.1	5	10.9	Germany	16.4	27.5	30
Israel	9.9	14.9	20.1	Greece	17.4	24.9	32.1
Jordan	3.2	7.7	16.4	Hungary	14.6	21.9	29.4
Lebanon	6.7	10.2	23.2	Ireland	11.3	18.4	25.1
Qatar	2.3	16.3	19.6	Italy	18	27.2	33.5
Syria	3.2	6.1	13	Macedonia	9.8	18.2	25.1
Turkey	6	12.9	22.4	Netherlands	13.6	23.5	26
United Arab Emirates	2.2	16.8	16.2	Norway	15.2	22.4	25
Asia				Poland	12.3	22.2	29.6
Bangladesh	3.3	6	11	Portugal	16	23.2	30.6
Burma	4.7	9.8	18.3	Romania	13.3	19.6	30
China	6.9	16.4	24.5	Slovakia	11.4	21.3	30
East Timor	2.6	6.9	10.7	Slovenia	14	26.3	34
Hong Kong SAR	11.5	29.3	39.3	Spain	17	25.3	34.5
India	4.6	9	14.6	Sweden	17.2	24.4	25.7
Indonesia	4.5	10.9	18	Switzerland	15.1	24.7	29
Iran	4.6	9.3	21.3	UK	15.6	22.5	25.7
Japan	17.1	28.8	34.3	Yugoslavia	14.1	20.8	27.2
Korea, North	6.3	14.6	21.4	**Latin America and the Caribbean**			
Korea, South	7	20.6	29.2	Argentina	10.2	14.8	21.2
Malaysia	4.1	9.4	13.4	Bolivia	4.5	8	13.8
Mongolia	3.7	8.1	16.2	Brazil	5.3	13.1	21.9
Pakistan	4	6	10.8	Chile	7.2	16.4	22.1
Phillipines	3.7	7.7	12.9	Colombia	4.7	11.5	16.6
Singapore	7	24.4	37.1	Costa Rica	5.2	12.8	19.7
Sri Lanka	6.5	15.2	23.1	Cuba	9.5	20.3	28.1
Thailand	6.4	16.2	23.7	Dominican Republic	4.8	10.2	14
Taiwan	8.7	21	29.3	Ecuador	4.6	9.7	16.3
Vietnam	5.5	11	19.2	El Salvador	5	7.7	12.7
Central Asia				Honduras	3.5	6.2	10.3
Estonia	15	24.5	32.2	Jamaica	6.8	12.5	22.3
Latvia	14.7	23.1	31.2	Mexico	5	11.5	19
Lithuania	13.7	23.7	32	Nicaragua	2.8	6.6	13.8
Armenia	8.9	16.1	25.2	Panama	5.8	12.1	18.5
Azerbaijan	6.9	11.4	16.2	Paraguay	4.7	7.9	10.8
Belarus	13.7	19.5	26.6	Peru	4.7	10.4	17.2
Georgia	13.5	23.4	28.8	Puerto Rico	11.2	22.8	30.3
Kazakhstan	6.5	14	20.4	Trinidad and Tobago	7.3	24.2	33.9
Kyrgyzstan	5.8	8.5	12.4	Uruguay	12.9	17	23.2
Moldova	9.8	14.9	20	Venezuela	4.6	11.6	18.5
Russia	12.5	21.5	28.3	**Oceania**			
Turkmenistan	4	6.6	10.4	Australia	12.4	21.1	24.6
Ukraine	13.9	19.7	26	Fiji	3.4	9.5	14.1
Uzbekistan	4.6	7.5	12.1	New Zealand	11.5	17.8	24.1
North America				Papua New Guinea	3.6	6.1	10.8
Canada	12.7	22.9	24.9	Solomon Islands	3	5.4	11.4
USA	12.4	19.6	20.6				

Source: Data from [1], Current Population Reports, P23–209 (Table A–1)

time in fertility, mortality, and migration patterns [3]. Measures of population aging that can also be used to compare populations and assess changes over time include the median age, aged-dependency ratios or, most commonly, the proportion of a given population that is aged 65 and older. It has been the combined effects of declines in *both* mortality and fertility rates during more recent times that have largely been responsible for the demographic transition that led to the aging of human populations.

The earliest and most important causes of the decline of human mortality during the past few centuries were the general improvements in living conditions resulting from social and economic developments. Innovations in industrial and agricultural production and distribution methods led to significant improvements in nutrition [4]. Industrialization also brought about enhanced standards of living by improving the quality and quantity of available housing, running water, and electricity, which enabled individuals to be protected from the hazards of nature. Thereafter, a complex interplay of advancements in public health efforts, particularly sanitation, and later in medical and preventative health care, coupled with new modes of familial, social, economic, and political organization helped to promote and sustain further gains in human longevity [5].

The decline in human mortality has been the main driver of increased life expectancy throughout the world. The rapid mortality decline particularly among infants, children, and women of childbearing age increased average life expectancy from 47.3 years in 1900 to 68.2 years in 1950 [6]. The need to replace children lost to early mortality waned as the risk of death at younger ages declined rapidly [7]; this eventually led to declines in total fertility rates. Death rates from chronic diseases were stable in the USA from 1954 to 1968; thereafter, research programs around chronic diseases intensified and reductions in mortality from chronic diseases followed. In recent years, continued advances in the management and treatment of chronic diseases are now largely driving reductions in mortality at older ages.

Sex and Racial Differences

Interestingly, reduced mortality rates have not benefited men and women equally, with women having gained several more years of life expectancy than men (Table 11.2). For example, in the USA over the past century, life expectancy had increased by 31.2 years for women (from 48.3 to 79.5 years)

TABLE 11.2 Life expectancy at birth, at age 65, 75, and 85 by race and sex: selected years, 1900–2000

Age and year	All races			White		Black [a]	
	Both sexes	Male	Female	Male	Female	Male	Female
At Age 0							
1900[b,c]	47.3	46.3	48.3	46.6	48.7	32.5	33.5
1950[c]	68.2	65.6	71.1	66.5	72.2	59.1	62.9
1960[c]	69.7	66.6	73.1	67.4	74.1	61.1	66.3
1970	70.8	67.1	74.7	68.0	75.6	60.0	68.3
1980	73.7	70.0	77.4	70.7	78.1	63.8	72.5
1990	75.4	71.8	78.8	72.7	79.4	64.5	73.6
2000	76.9	74.1	79.5	74.8	80.0	68.2	74.9
At Age 65							
1900–1902[b,c]	11.9	11.5	12.2	11.5	12.2	10.4	11.4
1950[c]	13.9	12.8	15.0	12.8	15.1	12.9	14.9
1960[c]	14.3	12.8	15.8	12.9	15.9	12.7	15.1
1970	15.2	13.1	17.0	13.1	17.1	12.5	15.7
1980	16.4	14.1	18.3	14.2	18.4	13.0	16.8
1990	17.2	15.1	18.9	15.2	19.1	13.2	17.2
2000	17.9	16.3	19.2	16.3	19.2	14.5	17.4
At Age 75							
1980	10.4	8.8	11.5	8.8	11.5	8.3	10.7
1990	10.9	9.4	12.0	9.4	12.0	8.6	11.2
2000	11.3	10.1	12.1	10.1	12.1	9.4	11.2
At Age 85							
2000	6.3	5.6	6.7	5.5	6.6	5.7	6.5

[a] Data shown for 1900–1960 are for the non-White population
[b] Death registration area only. The death registration area increased from ten states and the District of Columbia in 1900 to the contiguous USA in 1933
[c] Includes deaths of nonresidents of the USA
Source: Data from [1], Current Population Reports, P23–209 (Table 3-1); National Center for Health Statistics 2003 (Tables 11 and 28). For full citations, see references at the end of the chapter

but by only 27.8 years for men (from 46.3 to 74.1 years). It appears that women may have a natural advantage over men that should imply a difference of about 2 years in terms of life expectancy at birth. Several hypotheses have been proposed to explain sex differences in longevity, including more active female immune functioning, the protective effect of estrogen, compensatory effects of the second X chromosome, and the influence of oxidative stress on aging and disease. At present, none of these hypotheses are strongly supported, although weak support is available for the oxidative stress hypothesis [8]. Nevertheless, other factors are thought to contribute to the much larger gap now being commonly observed between the sexes. Differences in life expectancy are attributed to differences in behaviors, social roles, attitudes, and biological risks between men and women, with the near-elimination of maternal mortality in developed countries explaining only a small fraction of this trend [9–12]. While these differential gains have been typical of developed countries, the gap has started to decline in recent years. Between 1900 and 1970, overall life expectancy in the USA increased by 26.4 years for women and 20.8 years for men, thereby increasing the gender gap in life expectancy from 2.0 to 7.6 years. This increase has been largely attributed to higher male mortality due to ischemic heart disease and lung cancer, both of which are related to the widespread and early practice of cigarette smoking among men [13, 14]. However, between 1970 and 2000, overall life expectancy rose by 4.8 years for women and 7.0 years for men, thereby narrowing the gender gap from 7.6 to 5.4 years. This subsequent decrease has been related to the proportionately larger increases in lung cancer mortality among women than men and a proportionately greater decline in heart disease mortality among men than women [13, 14].

In addition to the expected growth of the older population, demographic studies predict that the racial and ethnic diversity of this population in the USA also increases over the coming decades. Comparisons between racial groups in 2003 to what is predicted for 2050 suggest that while non-Hispanic whites decrease from representing 83–61% of the older population, the proportion of Blacks grows from 8 to 12%, Hispanics from 6 to 18%, and Asians from 3 to 8% [15]. While this growing diversity largely reflects the aging of a more diverse younger population, there is evidence that it also represents, to a small degree, the enhanced immigration of older individuals [16]. These demographic changes continue to have important implications, especially since mortality rates among the elderly have also been shown to be unevenly distributed across racial and ethnic groups. These differences appear to reflect different disease profiles for underlying populations, unequal access to health care, and likely other socio-demographic factors, such as income and education that have yet to be completely understood.

What partly explains our lack of understanding is that "minority" older adults have largely been excluded from studies or categorized together as "non-White," ignoring the significant heterogeneity that also characterize these groups, their differences in physiological aging, access to health care, educational levels, health habits, disease prevalence and progression, response to treatments, and social contributors to health. Indeed, the increasing heterogeneity of the older population in the coming decades will certainly have important implications for the delivery of health and social care services and associated research studies.

Shifting Mortality Patterns

With individuals now being better able to survive acute illnesses, increasing longevity has contributed to the rising incidence of chronic illness and greater likelihood that individuals die as a result of complications associated with chronic conditions. While the proportion of elderly fatalities caused by heart disease, strokes, and cancer fell over the last 25 years, this decrease was partially offset by a concurrent increase in the number of deaths attributable to other chronic diseases, such as diabetes, chronic lung disease, renal disease, and dementia. Today, the pattern of death at older ages generally reflects that of the population as a whole. However, while the leading causes of death are essentially the same, differences in the rankings become apparent when mortality rates across age groups are considered (Table 11.3). While heart disease and cancer remain the leading two causes of death across all older age groups, over the past 25 years the

TABLE 11.3 Changes in most common causes of death in the USA at all ages and those 65 years and older cohorts

Causes of death	Rank in 1900	Rank in 2005			
	All ages	All ages	65+	65–75	75–85	85+
Heart disease	4	1	1	2	1	1
Cancer	8	2	2	1	2	2
Stroke	5	3	3	4	4	3
Chronic lung diseases	9	4	4	3	3	5
Alzheimer's dementia	10	7	5	10	5	4
Diabetes	–	6	7	5	6	7
Influenza/ pneumonia	1	8	6	8	7	6
Nephritis	6	9	8	7	8	8
Accidents	7	5	9	6	9	9
Septicemia	2	10	10	9	10	10
Diarrhea and enteritis	3	–	–	–	–	–

Source: Data for 2005 from National Vital Statistics Report, Vol. 56, No. 10, April 24, 2008

largest decrease in heart disease mortality (−55.5%) was experienced by individuals between the ages of 65 and 74 years, followed by those between the ages of 75 and 84 years (−49.7%), and those 85 years and over (−37.0%). While cancer mortality has increased slightly for individuals 75 years and over (+3.8%), it decreased somewhat for the 65–74 age group (−7.7%). The more significant drop in heart disease as opposed to cancer mortality within the 65–74 age group has meant that cancer mortality is now the most common cause of death among individuals in this subgroup. Further shifts in mortality rates has meant that chronic lung disease and diabetes-related mortality now have their greatest impact among the youngest older age groups, while stroke, dementia, influenza, and pneumonia-related mortality have their greatest impact among the oldest age groups.

Fertility

Historically, the decline in human mortality has been followed, in most regions of the world, with a decline in fertility. This has caused some concern as extremely low levels of fertility, sustained over a period of time, are causing some populations to decline. The implications of population decline in conjunction with population aging can be significant. Governments, for example, may encounter the challenge of financing social security programs and health care costs while facing possible labor shortages. Further, these labor shortages may disproportionately impact low-wage work, such as those providing personal care to the elderly. These concerns have led some countries to develop progressive immigration policies in recent decades to help counter declining fertility rates and fuel overall population growth.

Developing Countries

Fertility and mortality rates have fallen in most developing countries, but usually not to the same degree as with their developed counterparts. These falls are partly due to economic growth but are mostly due to the adoption of modern medical and public health practices. While the populations of virtually every nation are aging, the level and pace with which they are doing so varies within regions (Fig. 11.1). Surprisingly, the most rapid proportionate increases among older populations are and will continue to be in the developing world. In 2000, 249 million people 65 and older living in developing countries represented 59% of the world's older population; their proportion of the global elderly is projected to rise to nearly 80% or 1.2 billion elderly people living in developing nations by 2050. In contrast, 171 million people were aged 65 and older in developed countries in 2000, and they are projected to grow to 327 million by 2050. Although developing regions had lower overall proportions of older people than developed regions in 2000, these proportions are

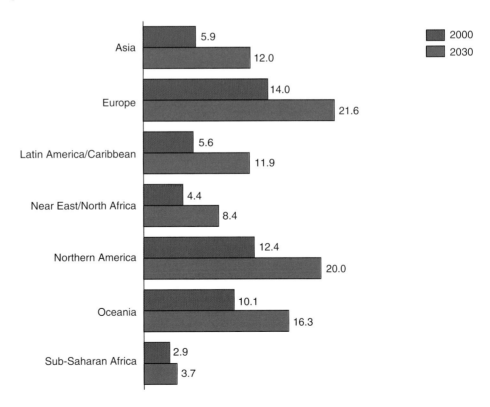

FIGURE 11.1 Percentage of the population aged 65 and over for regions of the world: 2000 and 2030 (from US Census Bureau 2004, International Programs Center, International Data Base, at http://www.census.gov/ipc/www/idbnew.html.).

expected to double in Asia and the Latin America/Caribbean regions by 2030. Sub-Saharan Africa has the youngest of the world's regions, with only 2.9% of its population being older than 65 years in 2000. It continues to remain the youngest region as the proportion of its older population grows slowly owing to the combined effects of high fertility rates coupled with an overall population decline due to the impact of AIDS. Nevertheless, population aging in many developing countries means they eventually encounter the same debates around intergenerational equity, social security, and increasing health care costs that have already emerged in Europe, the USA, and Canada [17].

Concepts in Individual Aging

Individual aging refers to the length of life for individuals, measured most often in years. A summary measure of individual aging for a population is most often represented by life expectancy [7]. Life expectancy is calculated from death probabilities observed throughout the age range over a selected time period, usually one calendar year, and may be estimated for a given birth cohort or for a population reaching any age or age range [7]. With individuals now living longer on average than ever before, there is growing interest around the degree to which life expectancies at birth and older ages can increase. While the risk of death remains relatively high at birth, it rapidly declines to its lowest point during sexual maturity, followed by an exponential rise until around 85 years of age. Thereafter, it has been demonstrated that the rate at which the risk of death increases actually begins to decelerate [18–21].

Complicating any discussion about individual aging is the idea that there may be some maximal lifespan that is biologically determined for every species, including humans. This belief, interestingly, had its nonscientific origins in biblical references to a human lifespan of 120 years (Genesis 6:6). Indeed, if there is some age *x* beyond which no one could survive, arguably there must be some eventual limit to the rise in life expectancy. The existence of such a maximal age is becoming increasingly questioned [22]. First, if it is possible to survive to age *x*, surely it must also be possible to survive to age *x* plus 1 day. Following this logic, there may be no finite limit, even though survival to very old age is already, from a statistical standpoint, highly unlikely. The oldest individuals whose ages have been reliably documented are a Frenchwoman, Jeanne Calment, who died in 1997 at the age of 122, and an American, Sarah Knauss, who died in 1999 at the age of 119 [23, 24]. Because the chance of death is high at such ages, the probability of observing significantly older individuals in the near future is exceedingly small. Nevertheless, these records are likely to be broken eventually.

Differential, Usual, and Successful Aging

Chronological age (age in number of years) and *physiological age* (age in terms of functional capacity) do not always coincide, and often the physical appearance and health status of an individual belie their chronological age. Increasingly, it is being observed that disparities in the timetable of aging may occur among individuals or among selected populations, or in other words, that some individuals "age" at much slower or faster rates than others. Furthermore, changes with aging are heterogeneous not only among individuals within a select group, but also among various organs within each individual person. The onset, rate, and magnitude of the changes vary depending on the cell, tissue, organ, system, or laboratory evaluation of several parameters [25–27] and the manifestations of aging are a complex interplay between genetic variables, disease states, and environmental exposures.

Attempts to define in humans a physiological "norm" inevitably disclose a range of functional decrements with advancing age. In earlier studies, the comparison of several functions from younger to older age focused on a gradation of decrements with increasing age [25]. However, as the prevalence of chronic diseases increase with age, the functional loss that was noted with age in these early studies, may have been due to the effects of disease rather than the natural concomitants of aging itself. More recent research has further continued to challenge the inevitability of functional impairment with chronological aging. While significant changes in laboratory evaluation of some physiological functions may be erroneously attributed to aging, normal aging changes may also be misinterpreted as evidence of disease. Laboratory values are generally interpreted with reference to a normal range. Many of the age-related levels do not change on average, but the variance (i.e., the deviation from average) tends to increase [26], making deviation from the norm increasingly common with aging.

Regulation of certain functions may remain efficient until advanced age, whereas in others it declines at an early age. Examples of such differential aging may be inferred from fasting blood glucose levels and acid–base balance, which remain stable as late as 70–90 years of age in a nonstressed state. In contrast, the basal metabolic rate declines continuously throughout the life-span, while certain sensory modalities, such as vision and hearing, show functional decrements beginning during early adulthood. Although fasting blood glucose values are minimally affected by aging, when these levels are determined after increased physiological demand, the ability of the organism to maintain normal levels and the rate at which the levels return to normal are markedly different in mature and aged subjects. Similarly, cardiac index parameters, renal function, respiratory function, and conduction velocity in nerves have been demonstrated to tolerate less stress in the elderly than in younger individuals but are seemingly unimpaired in nonstressed states. Such declining ability of the aging organism to withstand or respond adequately to stress reveals an age difference not otherwise obvious.

Aging is believed to be a slow, continuous process. Therefore, some of its effects can be observed only when they have progressed sufficiently to induce identifiable alterations that can be validated by available testing methods. An illustrative example is atherosclerosis, the consequences of which manifest during middle and old age even though the atherosclerotic lesion may start early in infancy. Whatever organ or tissue is considered, timetables of aging represent an approximation, as the onset of aging cannot be pinpointed precisely by a specific physiological sign.

While a number of functions undoubtedly decline as we age, the extreme heterogeneity of overall functional status even in the oldest cohorts supports the view that aging must be evaluated on an individual basis. In addition to genetic makeup, the elderly individual's health, social status, and economic and environmental conditions all contribute to how they age [28]. Aging processes have thus been categorized as *usual aging,* referring to the average physiological changes associated with some decrements in function, and *successful aging,* referring to advanced chronological age with minimal physical decrements [29].

Accordingly, individuals who age successfully are those who do not exhibit pathology and have minimal functional decrements. The concept of *successful aging* was formulated as "a reconceptualization of the aging process, one that provides a significant and necessary counterbalance to previous research that tended to emphasize age-related declines in functioning and health" [30]. It distinguishes three modalities of aging (1) disease/disabled, characterized by the presence of pathology, disability, or both; (2) "usual" (normal) aging, characterized by the absence of overt pathology but the presence of functional declines; and (3) "successful" aging, characterized by few or none of the physiological losses seen in the usual aging group. The concept is based on (1) the substantial heterogeneity among aged individuals; (2) the observation that aging is not a uniform or inevitable process of disease or disability; (3) the persistence of plasticity well into advanced age, that is, a continuing capacity for adaptive and compensatory rehabilitation; and (4) the identification of predictors of various patterns of aging, especially factors that contribute to more successful trajectories of aging.

Current studies of successful aging provide evidence for continuing good functional competence and recuperative plasticity into old age [31, 32]. The distinction among successful groups supports the hypothesis that extrinsic factors play an important role in age-associated functional decline. In one study, factors promoting maintenance or improvement of functioning included younger age, higher income, being Caucasian, low body weight, good lung function, the absence of diabetes or hypertension, higher education, and high cognitive performance. Other correlates of high functioning were the absence of hospitalization, participation in moderate/strenuous exercise, and receiving emotional support [30]. Taking all such factors into account, the prospects for avoidance, or eventual reversal, of functional loss with age are vastly improved, and the risks of adverse consequences are reduced [29].

Consequences of Successful Aging

By focusing on the various modalities of aging, the heterogeneity of the aging process is emphasized, and the validity of this concept is extended to all biomedical branches. Interventions may be beneficial at all ages provided they are customized to the individual [33, 34]. The potential for rehabilitation at advanced age is much greater than previously supposed [27, 35–37], and there is a significant probability of regaining function at all levels of disability. Physical exercise, dietary, surgical, and pharmacological interventions have proved successful in enhancing health even at older ages. Identification of "predictors" designed to maximize health and physiological competence enhances the quality of life of the elderly, reduces their burden of disease and disability, and decreases the socioeconomic need for health care resources. This previously underestimated the ability to significantly recover, though sometimes incompletely, portends even more benefit to surgical therapies into advanced age for certain individuals than once anticipated.

Future Trends

Rather than converging toward some biological limit, it seems that mortality trends are now pointing in the direction of further gains in human longevity. Mortality rates continue falling across the age ranges in most developed countries, where the pace of decline has accelerated among the elderly in particular. There is no sign in most demographic data that humans are approaching a mortality plateau imposed by some fixed biological limit [38]. The rapid increases in life expectancy witnessed during the first half of the twentieth century has slowed because the earlier increase resulted from the near-elimination of deaths during infancy and childhood which ultimately yields a much larger increment in average life expectancy than reducing deaths in later life. As measured by the chance of death at any given age, however, the reduction in mortality has been remarkably stable over the past century and shows no sign of decelerating [39].

Current projections based on trend extrapolation antici-pate that life expectancy at birth in developed countries will be around 85 years in 2050 [40, 41]. Given the long-term stability of mortality trends and the multiplicity of factors that have contributed to the historical change, it seems naive to believe that the pace of change in the future will be substantially different from that in the past. Thus, it seems unlikely either that the increase in human longevity will end abruptly in the near future or that medical innovations will lead to a significant acceleration in the pace of change. Rather, we should expect continued slow improvements in life expectancy, which will be accompanied by the continued aging of the population and therefore an associated increase in the demand for health and social services.

Aging and Disability

The extent to which a longer life will be a healthier one, rather than one that contains more years of chronic illness or disability will have a significant impact on the future demand for health and long-term care services. While controversy exists among studies in this area, recent studies have gener-ally concluded that most of the gains in life expectancy seem to be occurring without growth in disability and potentially less disability for a given age with time. Thus, the increase in total life expectancy does not specifically correspond to increased time living in severe disability [42–46]. This reflects what Fries [47] described as a progressive com-pression of morbidity that seems to be characterizing aging populations. Likewise, Manton et al. [48] have characterized the declining rates of disability and associated health care expenditures among the elderly population in the USA. According to Manton [49], what is largely responsible for this continuing trend is that rate of decline in disability prevalence continues to be a faster one than the increase in total expected years of life. For instance, while disability prevalence among older people declined 0.26% per year between 1982 and 1989, the rate of decline increased to 0.38% per year between 1989 and 1994, and further to 0.56% per year between 1994 and 1999 [45]. Multiple factors have been attributed to this progressive decline in the prevalence of disability, and including improvements in medical treatments, overall socioeconomic status, positive behavioral changes, and the more widespread use of assistive technologies. The overall result is illustrated in Fig. 11.2 which demon-strates how the prevalence of chronic disability among older people fell from 26% in 1982 through 23% in 1994 to 20% in 1999 [45]. This, it is argued, not only lessens the upward pressure of demographic change on health expenditures, but also has the potential to lower per capita demands on health and social services as well [50].

Thus, if in addition to living longer, the current generation of older people is healthier and less disabled than their predecessors, the important question then becomes – what level of disability is present in those extra years? With disability representing the inability to perform a specific task because of health or age, resulting in impaired functional performance, the concept of active life expectancy has been developed to measure the number of years that people can expect to live on average without disability. Manton and Land [51] estimate that a woman of 65 with a life expectancy of 22.2 years remains fit and active for 15.7 years and a man of the same age, with a life expectancy of 15.7 years for 13.7 years.

In the classification of functional dependency, the Activities of Daily Living (ADLs) and Instrumental Activities of Daily Living (IADLs) are two classes of measures, based on an individual's ability to perform specific tasks, that are widely utilized in home-dwelling populations to determine the capability for independent living or, vice versa, as indica-tors of disability. ADL tasks refer to those that are required to carry out basic self-care activities, such as transferring out of a bed or a chair, walking, toileting, bathing, and eating [52–54]. IADL tasks refer to those that are required to maintain an independent household, such as doing light housework, preparing meals, using the telephone, shopping for personal items, managing money, and getting around the community [55]. Within older populations, ADL dependency is less common than IADL dependency, and in the commu-nity dwelling population, 85 years of age and older, only 16% required help with one ADL, 10% with two or three ADLs, and 9% with four or more ADLs [56]. More than half of the community dwelling population, 80 years of age and over can still perform IADL tasks independently [56] which generally demand a combination of both cognitive and physical abilities.

Kane et al. [56] note that because health care profes-sionals tend to see the sick, they may form a distorted picture of the health and functional status of older individuals. Indeed, most older people are self-sufficient and able to function on their own or with minimal assistance. Even though they carry a greater burden of chronic conditions and impairments, 72% of older people report being in good to excellent health. Among all older adults, 95% are able to move about within their homes independently, 80% are able to leave their homes without assistance and had no difficulty with any personal care task, 68% had no difficulty with any domestic task, and 69% had no difficulty with any locomotor task [57]. As well, of those ages 75 and over, about one-fifth report taking no medication on a regular basis, two-fifths report needing medication regularly to control medical problems, while the remainder report having multiple medical problems and using three or four medicines on a regular basis [58].

Figure 11.2 Percentage of people aged 65 and over with chronic disability: 1982–1999 [45].

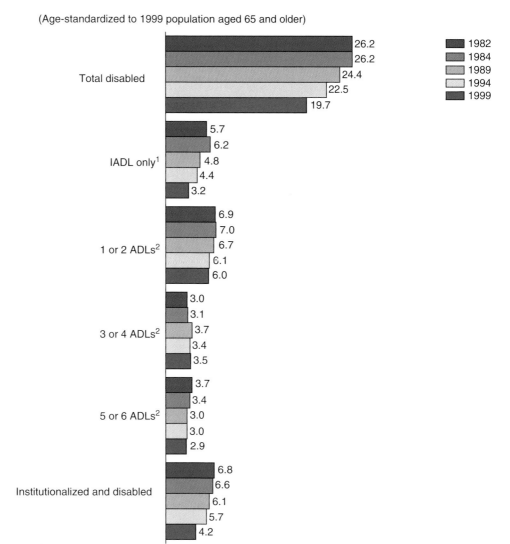

(Age-standardized to 1999 population aged 65 and older)

[1] Instrumental activities of daily living.
[2] Activities of daily living.
Note: The reference population for these data is the Medicare enrollees aged 65 and older.

Aging and Health Services Utilization

Notwithstanding the low degree of dependency among the majority of older people, this 12.4% of the population are the principal users of health care systems. In being the predominant user of more expensive institutional services, they account for over one-third of health expenditures in the USA [56]. The 1997 National Medical Expenditure Survey demonstrated that the annual per capita costs of health care for older persons in the USA was $5,947 as compared to $3,226 for those aged 45–64 years and $1,666 for those aged 18–44 years. Increasingly, questions are being raised around whether societies with aging populations are able to cope with the concomitant ever-increasing costs that seem to be associated in providing care for them. Clearly, new cost-conscious models of care delivery to meet the needs of the aging populations are needed.

While expenditure projections have traditionally examined the effect of age on health care costs, it is being increasingly argued that well-founded estimates should account for the influence of remaining life expectancy, declining disability rates and the concentration of costs that often occurs toward the end of life. Lubitz and Riley [59] demonstrated that just under a third of annual Medicare payments are made on behalf of persons in their last year of life, with over half of their costs being incurred in the last 60 days of life, reflecting the fact that over half the deaths among elderly persons occur in the hospital [60]. In considering remaining life expectancy on future health care spending, Seshamani and Gray [61] demonstrated that the despite the pressure of population increases and aging demographic structures on overall hospital expenditures, these will be partially countered by the postponement of death-related hospital costs later in life. The heterogeneous pattern of health care expenditures was further demonstrated when Lubitz et al. [62] determined that the average calculated Medicare expenditure for those who died at age 70 was $35,511 compared to $65,633 for those who survived to age 101 in the USA. Thus, the average Medicare expense per year from age 65 on for those who died at age 70 was $7,100 per year compared to only $1,823 for centenarians. While overall Medicare expenditures continue to increase, this should be properly attributed to the combined forces of cost inflation, therapeutic advances, and a growing number of beneficiaries with chronic illness requiring long-term maintenance therapy as opposed to aging itself.

When it was implemented, Medicare was designed to deal primarily with the effects of acute illness, which was then seen as the major threat to the health and financial security of older individuals. Now, the implications of having increasing numbers of older people living increasingly longer with chronic illness is becoming readily apparent, when 68% of current Medicare spending is accounted for by the 23% of Medicare beneficiaries having five or more chronic conditions [63]. Furthermore, federal outlays for Medicaid and Medicare are expected to grow substantially, from 21% of current government spending to an estimated 31% in 2017 [64]. The increasing cost pressures associated with financing public health insurance programs likely affect public spending around other priorities, and overall economic growth, especially as the ratio of nonelderly taxpayers to elderly beneficiaries contracts. It is likely that unless the financing mechanism for Medicare is changed, or its benefit structure altered, the Medicare Trust Fund will be depleted in 2019 [65]. Increasing consideration is being given to determine to what extent the government will be willing to shift the costs of providing care to current recipients and to what extent it will look at shifting resources to support the provision of preventive care or health promotion services – not currently covered by Medicare or Medicaid – that may help to lessen the burdens associated with managing chronic disease. Finally, the significant indirect costs associated with treating chronic diseases in the elderly should also be noted when relatives may shoulder an enormous personal and economic burden when caring for an older spouse, parents, or other relations unable to live independently.

The pattern of increasing Medicare expenditures, however, remains in distinct contrast to the accumulated liability that increased life expectancies have on Social Security expenditures, without any foreseeable countering mechanisms. While the Social Security trust fund will have resources until

2041, the more critical dates are when Social Security and Medicare begin paying out more in benefits than they are receiving in taxes because that represents the time the government must start redeeming the bonds in the trust funds that support these programs. To do that, the government will have to increase its borrowing on financial markets, raise taxes or divert money from other government programs. For Medicare, the threshold when benefits exceed program income already occurred a few years ago. For Social Security, it is estimated that this threshold will be crossed in 2017.

Effective Interventions in the Elderly

With the growing expectation that future older cohorts will live longer and be in better health at later ages, greater consideration is being given to how treatment interventions can be extended to mitigate morbidity and mortality within older populations. While more comprehensive evaluations of the efficacy of treatment interventions at later ages will better inform practitioners about how and for whom these interventions should be extended, overcoming agism around treating illness at later ages will be just as important.

Agism is a term that describes the negative stereotyping of older adults and discrimination because of older age. As Salzman [66] notes, health concerns and symptoms in the elderly are sometimes overlooked or dismissed as part of the normal aging process. Consequently, several conditions in older adults continue to go significantly underdiagnosed and undertreated which continues to provide further evidence of age discrimination still occurs in the delivery of health care [67–69].

While health care professionals do not necessarily intend to behave in a discriminatory fashion, it is clear that a lack of skills and confidence in working with older people can lead to behavior which may be perceived as discriminatory. Nevertheless, the quality of the care older individuals receive has also been demonstrated to be affected at times by negative staff attitudes in a number of settings [70, 71].

Denying access to services on the basis of age alone is not acceptable. Decisions about treatment and health care should be made on the basis of a patient's health needs, the overall health status of the individual, their own wishes and aspirations and, where appropriate, those of their carers, and the patient's ability to benefit as even complex treatments, used appropriately, can benefit older people.

The extension of surgical interventions to individuals at increasingly later ages is an area of active research. Largely, this body of literature demonstrates that the benefits of surgery in advanced age may have been underestimated. Hosking et al. [72] examined how intraoperative mortality rates in patients over 90 years of age had significant declined from 29 to 8%

over a 20-year period. Furthermore, the 5-year survival rate of this group at 21%, which had a mean age of 93.5 years, was determined to better than that of the comparable general population cohort at 16%. Elayda et al. [73] demonstrated similar results in demonstrating the efficacy and improved 5-year survival rates in patients 80 years of age and over undergoing aortic valve replacement. Ko et al. [74] demonstrated the increasing efficacy of elective coronary artery bypass surgery versus conventional medical treatment in patients 80 years of age and over with coronary artery disease.

Interventions with low mortality risks that have been demonstrated to significantly improve function and thus disability burden in older patients include cataract extractions and joint replacements. In regards to cataract extractions, Lundstrom et al. [75] demonstrated in one of few studies that looked specifically at individuals 85 and over that about 85% of patients achieved improved visual acuity from the surgery. Therefore, despite the higher risk of complications, cataract extraction remains a highly effective procedure for the very elderly [76]. In a recent review of 36,711 hip and knee replacement performed among nonagenarians and centenarians, the low in-hospital mortality data suggest that arthroplasties should not be denied to centenarians solely because of their relatively short remaining life expectancy estimates, when they can significantly improve functional status in these individuals [77].

The ability of pacemakers to improve survival and quality of life outcomes in elderly patients has become well established [78, 79]. In reviewing patients 80 years and over receiving pacemakers, Schmidt et al. [80], determined that pacemaker therapy is both a clinically and economically effective therapeutic option to control bradyarrhythmia-related symptoms, considering the median survival time of their patients stood at 8 years. Interestingly, while practice guidelines recommend dual rather than single-chamber pacing for patients with high-grade atrioventricular (AV) block, Toff et al. [81] noted that not only were elderly patients less likely than younger patients to receive more sophisticated dual-chamber pacemakers, but also 51% of elderly patients with this diagnosis were receiving them, despite their perceived association with improved quality of life and lower mortality risk. Nevertheless, their UKPACE trial, the first to evaluate and compare the long-term clinical impact and cost utility of dual versus single chamber pacing in patients aged 70 years and over with high-grade AV block, suggested no mortality benefit of dual over single-chamber pacing in this population [82].

In the field of organ transplantation, common practice has been to exclude older recipients because of the chronically limited supply of organs and lower expected survival of older patients after transplantation. While consensus guidelines for the selection of transplant recipients often recommend an upper age limit of 65 years, the number of people 65 years and older in the USA who have received organ transplants nearly tripled between 1996 and 2005, going from 1,145 to 3,154 [83]. Currently, elderly patients including those into their early 80s have come to represent 12% of the annual transplant recipients. Furthermore, Mahidhara et al. [84] have suggested that the idea that younger patients do better than older patients may not actually be valid after demonstrating that 73.6% of their elderly lung recipients were alive 3 years after surgery, compared with 74.2% of younger patients.

There is increasing evidence to support the greater use of nonsurgical interventions in the management of conditions common to the elderly patient as well. While the benefits of treating of hypertension in the very elderly were unclear as to whether they could be countered by an increased risk of death, the HYVET Trial demonstrated that treating hypertension in patients 80 years and older to a target of 150/80 was associated with a 64% reduction in the rate of heart failure, a 23% reduction in the rate of death from cardiovascular causes, a 30% reduction in the rate of fatal or nonfatal stroke, a 39% reduction in the rate of death from stroke, and a 21% reduction in the rate of death from any cause [85].

The increased recognition of osteoporosis as a preventable and treatable disease common in older individuals would aid in the dissemination of proven medical therapies that could significantly impact on the excess morbidity and mortality associated with this disease. Nevertheless, Kamel et al. [86] demonstrated that the failure of surgical and medical specialists to diagnose and initiate the treatment of osteoporosis in elderly patients hospitalized with hip fracture remains problematic when those treating the consequences of osteoporosis may often be ignoring the underlying condition [87].

Even though near complete vaccination coverage rates have been achieved in children, significantly fewer adults are being vaccinated against serious and even deadly diseases, such as influenza, pneumonia, and shingles. The CDC has established a goal to vaccinate at least 90% of individuals 65 years of age and over against influenza and pneumococcal disease, however, coverage estimates in this age group were just 69 and 66%, respectively in 2007. Despite being available for 1 year and having been integrated into the US Preventive Services Task Force guidelines as a recommendation for all elderly, only about 2% of eligible older adults appeared to have been vaccinated against shingles by 2007. While their effectiveness with aging is debated, estimates are that many of the 63,000 deaths in the USA in 2005 due to influenza and pneumonia could have been prevented by immunization against influenza and pneumococcal infections [88].

Because the aging population carries the greatest burden of illness and disability, it not only poses the most complex diagnostic and therapeutic problems, but also reaps the most benefit from medical and nursing care. The health problems

37. Kaplan GA, Wilson TW, Cohen RD (1994) Social functioning and overall mortality: prospective evidence from the Kuopio Ischemic Heart Disease Risk Factor Study. Epidemiology 5:495–500

38. Kannisto V, Lauritsen J (1994) Reduction in mortality at advanced ages. Popul Dev Rev 20:793–810

39. Wilmoth JR (1997) In search of limits. In: Wachter KW, Finch CE (eds) Between zeus and the salmon: the biodemography of longevity. National Academy Press, Washington, DC, pp 38–64

40. Lee RD, Carter LR (1992) Modeling and forecasting U.S. mortality. J Am Stat Assoc 87:659–675

41. Wilmoth JR, Skytthe S, Friou D (1996) The oldest man ever? A case study of exceptional longevity. Gerontology 36:783–788

42. Crimmins EM, Saito Y, Ingegnari D (1997) Trends in disability-free life expectancy in the United States, 1970–90. Popul Dev Rev 23(3):555–572

43. Manton KG, Corder L, Stallard E (1997) Chronic disability trends in elderly United States populations: 1982–1994. Proc Natl Acad Sci USA 94:2593–2598

44. Freedman VA (1998) Understanding trends in functional limitations among older Americans. Am J Public Health 10:1457–1462

45. Manton KG, Gu X (2001) Changes in the prevalence of chronic disability in the United States black and non-black population above age 65, from 1982 to 1999. Proc Natl Acad Sci USA 98: 6354–6359

46. Freedman VA, Martin LG, Schoeni RF (2002) Recent trends in disability and functioning among older adults in the United States. J Am Med Assoc 288(24):3137–3146

47. Fries JF (1980) Aging, natural death, and the compression of morbidity. N Engl J Med 303(3):130–135

48. Manton KG, Stallard E, Corder LS (1998) The dynamics of dimensions of age-related disability 1982 to 1994 in the U.S. elderly population. J Gerontol A Biol Sci Med Sci 53(1):B59–B70

49. Manton K, XiLiang G (2005) Disability declines and trends in Medicare expenditures. Ageing Horiz 2:25–34

50. Singer BH, Manton KG (1998) The effects of health changes on projections of health service needs for the elderly population of the United States. Proc Natl Acad Sci USA 95(26):15618–15622

51. Manton KG, Land KC (2000) Active life expectancy estimates for the U.S. elderly population: a multi-dimensional continuous-mixture model of functional change applied to completed cohorts, 1982–1996. Demography 37(3):253–265

52. Katz SJ, Ford AB, Moskowitz RW, Jackson BA, Jaffe MW (1963) Studies of illness in the aged. The index of ADL: a standardized measure of biological and psychosocial function. J Am Med Assoc 185:914–919

53. Katz SJ (1983) Assessing self-maintenance: activities of daily living, mobility and instrumental activities of daily living. J Am Geriatr Soc 31(12):721–726

54. Katz SJ, Stroud M (1989) Functional assessment in geriatrics: a review of progress and directions. J Am Geriatr Soc 37:267–271

55. Lawton MP, Brody EM (1969) Assessment of older people: self-maintaining and instrumental activities of daily living. Gerontologist 9:179–186

56. Kane RL, Ouslander JC, Abrass IB (2003) Essentials of clinical geriatrics, 5th edn. McGraw Hill, New York

57. Jarvis C (1996) Getting around after 60: a profile of Britain's older population. Age Concern Institute of Gerontology, Gerontology Data Service, HMSO, London

58. Martin J, Elliot D, Meltzer H (1988) The prevalence of disability among adults. Government Social Survey Department, HMSO, London

59. Lubitz JD, Riley GF (1993) Trends in Medicare payments in the last year of life. N Engl J Med 328(15):1092–1096

60. McMillan A, Mentnech RM, Lubitz JD, McBean AM, Russell D (1990) Trends and patterns in place of death for Medicare enrollees. Health Care Financ Rev 12:1–7

61. Seshamani M, Gray A (2004) Time to death and health expenditure: an improved model for the impact of demographic change on health care costs. Age Ageing 33(6):556–561

62. Lubitz JD, Beebe J, Baker C (1995) Longevity and Medicare expenditures. N Engl J Med 332(15):999–1003

63. Anderson GF (2005) Medicare and chronic conditions. N Engl J Med 353(3):305 309

64. US Congressional Budget Office (2007) The budget and economic outlook: fiscal years 2008 to 2017. US Congressional Budget Office, Washington, DC

65. Federal Hospital Insurance and Federal Supplementary Medical Insurance Trust Funds (2007) Annual report of the board of trustees of the Federal Hospital Insurance and Federal Supplementary Medical Insurance Trust Funds. Federal Hospital Insurance and Federal Supplementary Medical Insurance Trust Funds, Washington, DC

66. Salzman B (2006) Myths and realities of aging. Care Manag J 7(3):141–150

67. Alexander KP, Newby LK, Armstrong PW et al (2007) Acute coronary care in the elderly, Part II: ST-segment-elevation myocardial infarction: a scientific statement for healthcare professionals from the American Heart Association Council on Clinical Cardiology in collaboration with the Society of Geriatric Cardiology. Circulation 115(19):2570–2589

68. Bouchardy C, Rapiti E, Blagojevic S, Vlastos AT, Vlastos G (2007) Older female cancer patients: importance, causes, and consequences of undertreatment. J Clin Oncol 25(14):1858–1869

69. Grant PT, Henry JM, McNaughton GW (2000) The management of elderly blunt trauma victims in Scotland: evidence of ageism? Injury 31(7):519–528

70. Health Advisory Service 2000 (1998) "Not because they are old": an independent inquiry into the care of older people on acute wards in general hospitals. Health Advisory Service 2000, London

71. Lookinland S, Anson K (1995) Perpetuation of ageist attitudes among present and future health care personnel: implications for elder care. J Adv Nurs 21(1):47–56

72. Hosking MP, Warner MA, Lodbell CM (1989) Outcomes of surgery in patients 90 years of age and older. J Am Med Assoc 261: 1909–1915

73. Elayda MAA, Hall RJ, Reul RM (1993) Aortic valve replacement in patients 80 years and older: operative risks and long-term results. Circulation 88:11–16

74. Ko W, Gold JP, Lazzaro R (1992) Survival analysis of octogenarian patients with coronary artery disease managed by elective coronary artery bypass surgery versus conventional medical treatment. Circulation 86(Suppl II):191–197

75. Lundstrom M, Stenevi U, Thorburn W (2000) Cataract surgery in the very elderly. J Cataract Refract Surg 26:408–414

76. Wong TY (2001) Effect of increasing age on cataract surgery outcomes in very elderly patients. Br Med J 322:1104–1106

77. Krishnan E, Fries JF, Kwoh CK (2007) Primary knee and hip arthroplasty among nonagenarians and centenarians in the United States. Arthritis Rheum 57(6):1038–1042

78. Bush DE, Finucane TE (1994) Permanent cardiac pacemakers in the elderly. J Am Geriatr Soc 42:326–334

79. Shen WK, Hayes DL, Hammill SC (1996) Survival and functional independence after implantation of a permanent pacemaker in octogenarians and nonagenarians: a population-based study. Ann Intern Med 125:476–480

80. Schmidt B, Brunner M, Olschewski M, Hummel C, Faber T (2003) Pacemaker therapy in very elderly patients: long-term survival and prognostic parameters. Am Heart J 146:908–913

81. Toff WD, Skehan JD, De Bono DP, Camm AJ (1997) The United Kingdom pacing and cardiovascular events (UKPACE) trial. Heart 78:221–223

82. Toff WD, Camm AJ, Skehan JD (2005) Single-chamber versus dual-chamber pacing for high-grade atrioventricular block. N Engl J Med 353:145–155

83. Health Resources and Services Administration (2007) Annual report of the U.S. Organ Procurement and Transplantation Network and the Scientific Registry of Transplant Recipients: transplant data 1997–2006. Division of Transplantation, Health Resources and Services Administration, Healthcare Systems Bureau, Rockville, MD

84. Mahidhara R, Bastani S, Ross D, Saggar R, Lynch J (2008) Lung transplantation in older patients? J Thorac Cardiovasc Surg 135(2):412–420

85. Beckett NS, Peters R, Fletcher A, Staessen JA (2008) Treatment of hypertension in patients 80 years of age or older. N Engl J Med 358(18):1887–1898

86. Kamel HK, Hussain MS, Tariq S (2000) Failure to diagnose and treat osteoporosis in elderly patients hospitalized with hip fracture. Am J Med 109:326–328

87. Bauer DC (2000) Osteoporotic fractures: ignorance is bliss? Am J Med 109:338–339

88. Kung HC, Hoyert DL, Xu J, Murphy SL (2008) Deaths: final data for 2005. Natl Vital Stat Rep 56(10):1–120

Chapter 12
Providing Surgical Care to an Aging Population: Implications for the Surgical Workforce

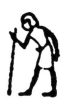

David A. Etzioni and Clifford Y. Ko

Introduction

The demographic trends underlying the "aging population" have already been discussed in Chap. 12. As a result of increasing life expectancy and the aging of the baby boomers, the United States (US) population will see a dramatic increase in the number of older individuals. Between 2010 and 2030, those aged 65 years and older are projected to rise by 78%, an absolute increase of over 30 million individuals. These unprecedented changes in the demographics of the US population will lead to significant growth in the demand for surgical treatment.

This chapter comes with an acknowledgement. In the interest of simplicity, we examine these trends within the context of the US population only. Furthermore, we focus more on general surgery and its subspecialties than on other areas of surgical specialization. This is in the interest of developing a succinct, circumscribed report. The analyses described here are easily applicable within other fields of medicine, as well as to other countries.

Another acknowledgement is also important. This chapter could easily be its own textbook. In selecting which points should be made, we focus on a survey of existing opinions and concepts that are driving policy. We will also offer some original analysis regarding how the aging population will affect the delivery of surgical treatment. Our hope is at the end of this chapter, the reader will be familiar with the methods used to forecast the impact of the aging population on the healthcare delivery system, and be able to differentiate the relative importance of the various factors that will drive health care expenditure in the immediate and more distant future.

D.A. Etzioni (✉)
Department of Surgery, Mayo Clinic Arizona, Mayo Clinic College of Medicine, 5777 E Mayo Blvd, Phoenix, AZ 85054, USA
e-mail: etzioni.david@mayo.edu

Older Individuals in the US Population: Disproportionately High Use of Resources

In general, older individuals use medical and surgical services at higher rates than do younger individuals. To illustrate and characterize this fact, we will rely on analyses of the National Hospital Discharge Survey (NHDS), a data source which deserves at least a brief explanation. Since 1965, the National Center for Health Statistics has conducted an annual survey (sampling) of domestic discharges. Each year, over 350,000 discharges from approximately 500 hospitals within the US are sampled, and the sampling strategy is designed to yield a dataset that is representative of the universe of domestic discharges [1]. The NHDS reports specific information about each discharge, including age, gender, race/ethnicity, diagnoses, procedures, diagnosis-related grouping (DRG) admission source (emergency room, home, etc.), and admission type (emergency, elective, etc.). At several points in this chapter, we will rely on analyses of the NHDS to give a quantitative analysis of historical and projected trends in the patterns of hospital-based health care delivery in the US.

Hospital-Based Care

According to data from the US census, in 2006, individuals over the age of 65 comprised 12.5% of the US population [2]. However, according to data from the NHDS, individuals over the age of 65 were responsible for:

- 32% of cholecystectomies
- 38% of hospitalizations
- 43% of hospital days of care
- 54% of colon resections
- 55% of total hip replacements
- 60% of total knee replacements

This disproportionate use of services can be considered in terms of an incidence rate curve, demonstrating the likelihood of an individual in the population requiring a specific

Figure 12.1 Incidence rate curves: admissions for medical vs. surgical DRGs.

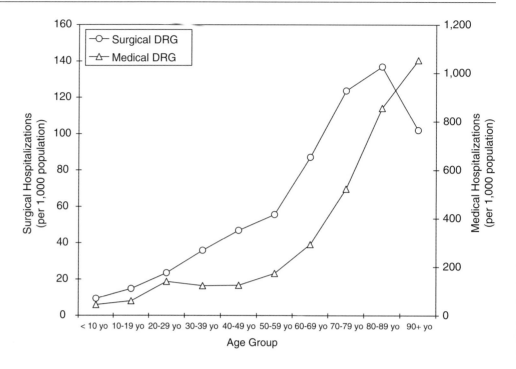

type of hospital-based medical or surgical service. Figure 12.1 represents such an analysis based on data from the 2006 NHDS. We categorized admissions as "surgical" or "medical" based on DRG, according to nomenclature used by the Centers for Medicare and Medicaid Services (CMS) [3]. Admissions for children in their first year of life or those related to childbirth were excluded.

These incidence rate curves clearly demonstrate the difference in the rates at which younger vs. older individuals are hospitalized. Compared with an individual aged 40–50, an individual aged 70–79 is 2.6 times more likely to be hospitalized for a surgical cause and 4.2 times more likely to be admitted for a medical reason. The duration of hospitalization also varies widely across different age groups, with average lengths of stays (LOS) being higher in older individuals admitted for both surgical and medical DRGs (Fig. 12.2).

Inpatient Procedures

The demand for specific types of inpatient surgical procedures can also be conceptualized as an incidence rate curve. Several examples are illustrated below, namely for knee replacement, coronary artery bypass graft (CABG), colectomy, cholecystectomy, carotid endarterectomy (CEA), and hysterectomy (vaginal or trans-abdominal) (Fig. 12.3). These curves illustrate very clearly the higher rates at which older individuals undergo surgical treatment. In fact, for each of these procedures (except for hysterectomy), individuals in their eighth or ninth decade of life have the highest frequency of surgery.

Outpatient Procedures

Outpatient surgical procedures are, in general, also performed much more commonly in older individuals. The following graph (Fig. 12.4) examines rates of seven of the most frequently performed outpatient procedures based on data from the State of Florida [4]. Two procedures – myringotomy tubes and tonsillectomy/adenoidectomy – are performed more commonly in younger patients and less so in older individuals. For the remaining five procedures, the age range with the highest rates of surgery is individuals aged 60 years and older. This is particularly true for cataract operations, which could not be included in the figure below for reasons of scale. The rate of cataract surgery among individuals aged 70–79 is 74 per 1,000 population, greater than the other seven procedures combined.

Older Patients are Different

In this section, we will explore how an older domestic population will affect not only the numbers of procedures, but also the types of procedures and the intensity of care provided for them.

A brief examination of the "top ten" surgical procedures performed on patients over vs. under the age of 65 tells some of this story. For this analysis, we once again turn to data from the NHDS and examine only the primary procedure performed during each hospitalization [5]. For patients under the age of 65, the most commonly performed procedures were hysterectomy (abdominal), followed by cholecystectomy then

Figure 12.2 Mean LOS: medical vs. surgical DRGs.

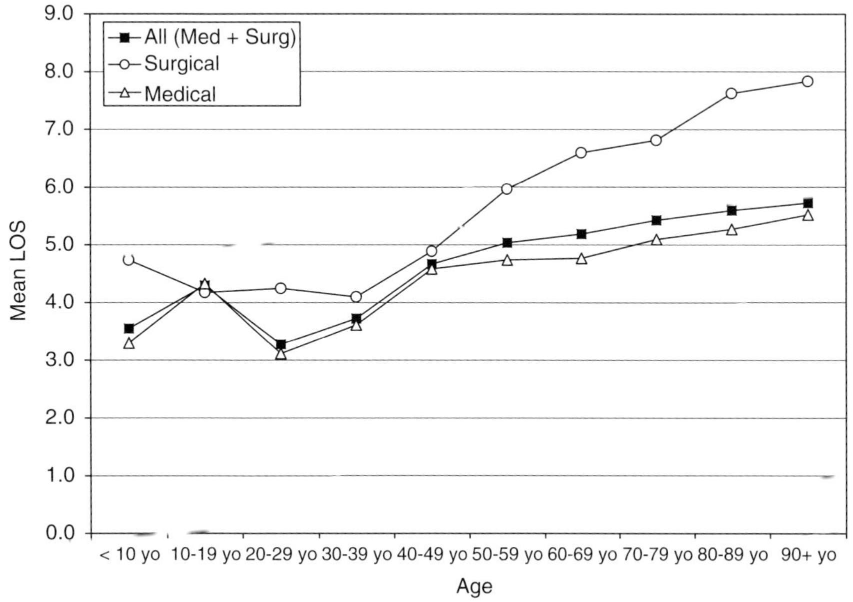

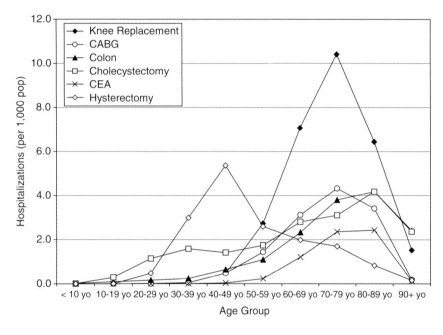

Figure 12.3 Incidence rate curves: commonly performed inpatient procedures.

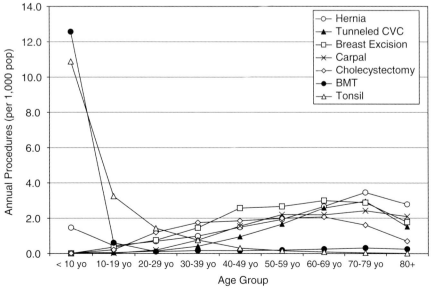

Figure 12.4 Incidence rate curves: commonly performed outpatient procedures.

knee replacement. For older patients, the top four inpatient procedures were all orthopedic. Seven out of these top ten procedures were orthopedic or neurosurgical in nature.

In addition to generating an increased demand for surgical procedures, the aging population presents a more fragile population of patients (Tables 12.1–12.3). As shown below

TABLE 12.1 Top ten procedures performed in individuals <65 years old

ICD code	Procedure description	Procedures in 2006
68.4	Total abdominal hysterectomy	418,588
51.23	Laparoscopic cholecystectomy	386,444
81.54	Total knee replacement	309,341
47.01	Laparoscopic appendectomy	288,023
47.09	Other appendectomy	212,380
79.36	Operative reduction/internal fixation tibia/fibula	157,726
81.51	Total hip replacement	154,469
68.59	Other vaginal hysterectomy	148,806
68.51	Laparoscopically assisted vaginal hysterectomy	91,169
45.76	Sigmoidectomy	65,892

TABLE 12.2 Top ten procedures performed in individuals ≥65 years old

ICD code	Procedure description	Procedures in 2006
81.54	Total knee replacement	574,021
79.35	Open reduction internal fixation	239,019
81.52	Partial hip replacement	221,981
81.51	Total hip replacement	218,685
51.23	Laparoscopic cholecystectomy	178,053
38.12	Endarterectomy	123,047
79.15	Operative reduction/internal fixation femur	114,949
45.73	Right hemicolectomy	96,556
03.09	Other exploration and decompression of spinal canal	76,415
81.08	Lumbar and lumbosacral fusion, posterior technique	60,645

in Table 12.3, older patients require a greater amount of care. The average length of stay was higher for older patients (4.8 vs. 3.3), and the likelihood of an in-hospital myocardial infarction (MI) was approximately ten times greater (0.7 vs. 0.07%). The greatest difference in outcomes is mortality, with patients over the age of 65 having an in-hospital mortality rate nearly 15 times higher (1.1 vs. 0.07%). Longer lengths of stay and higher rates of myocardial infarction and postoperative mortality only tell part of this story. In order to minimize the impact of medical comorbidity on peri-operative outcomes, surgeons will need to work closely with non-surgeon physicians to optimize medical management. There is already evidence that medical hospitalists are increasingly involved in the care of surgical patients. In a recent analysis of Medicare claims data, Kuo et al. found a more than fivefold increase in the percent of surgical admissions that involved care from a medical hospitalist [6]. A new paradigm of inpatient care may be emerging, with surgeons and non-surgical physicians working together to manage patients who are elderly and/or morbid.

As the number of elderly individuals in the US population continues to increase, another area that will require focused attention is the clinical effectiveness/appropriateness of different types of treatment in older patients. Many types of major surgery that historically were considered too risky to undertake in elderly patients are now widely considered safe [7–9]. The bias against aggressive surgical treatment for patients considered empirically "too old" appears to be diminishing, and the rates at which elderly individuals are undergoing several types of major surgical procedures are increasing [10]. There is still, however, evidence that elderly patients are under-treated for many types of conditions, especially oncologic diseases [11–13]. These findings are behind a movement advocating more focused research on clinical outcomes in elderly patients [14].

TABLE 12.3 Top ten procedures performed in individuals of all ages

ICD code	Procedure description	Procedures 2006	Patients <65 years			Patients ≥65 years		
			Mean LOS	% Mortality	% MI	Mean LOS	% Mortality	% MI
81.54	Total knee replacement	195,453	3.7	0	0	3.9	0.2	0.3
51.23	Laparoscopic cholecystectomy	138,699	3.2	0.05	0.03	5.4	0.03	0.2
81.51	Total hip replacement	93,636	3.8	0	0.02	3.9	0.2	0.2
47.01	Laparoscopic appendectomy	75,546	2.3	0	0	3.5	0	0.3
79.35	Operative reduction/internal fixation femur	63,882	5.5	0.3	0	6.3	0.5	0.1
47.09	Other appendectomy	60,345	3.5	0.03	0.2	6.0	0.3	2.6
81.08	Lumbar/lumbosacral fusion, posterior technique	54,270	4.1	0	0.07	5.2	0	0.1
79.36	Operative reduction/internal fixation tibia/fibula	53,028	4.3	0.4	0.4	4.6	0.8	1.4
81.52	Partial hip replacement	49,842	6.1	0.2	0	6.5	0.2	2.2
68.59	Other vaginal hysterectomy	41,796	1.6	0	0	2.2	0	0
Unadjusted totals		826,947	3.3	0.07	0.07	4.8	1.1	0.7

Current Capacity

As the number of older individuals in the US rises, it should be intuitive that the use of medical resources will increase at a rate faster than population growth. Before discussing the impact of *forthcoming* demographic changes on the surgical workforce, we will first consider the capacity of the *current* health care delivery system to provide surgical care. In doing so, we examine capacity in terms of two complementary components – physician workforce and hospital infrastructure.

Physician Workforce Capacity

Two main types of research have emerged to gauge the adequacy of the current physician work force relative to population-based demand, yielding conflicting results. The first type is a "macro" analysis, examining regional relationships between physician density and quality of care. A classic example of this type of research was performed by Baicker et al., who analyzed state-level measures of the quality of medical care provided to Medicare recipients and found *poorer* quality of care delivered to patients in states with *higher* per capita Medicare expenditures and physician density [15]. Furthermore, they found that quality of care was proportional to the density of general practitioners and *inversely* proportional to the concentration of specialist physicians. These findings were refuted by Cooper et al. who examined within-state variations, and concluded that states with more spending and more physicians – both generalist and specialists – had better quality of care [16, 17].

The second type of research examines the ability of the health care workforce to meet the demands of the regional population at a "micro" level. Several studies have examined hospital-based care, using the ability of emergency departments (EDs) to obtain consultations from surgical specialists as a measure of access to care. In a study of ED directors at over 4,000 US hospitals, the American College of Emergency Physicians found that 73% of EDs had problems with inadequate on-call coverage by specialist physicians [18]. Also, this figure had increased from 67% only the previous year. Difficulties with obtaining specialist consultations are also documented as worsening, both in terms of the ability to access on call specialists, and in the ability of EDs to initiate transfers to hospitals where a higher level of care can be provided [19]. Areas with lower mean zip code income had a lower likelihood of timely response to a request for surgical consultation [20].

If the network of available surgical specialists begins to fray, and access to care is compromised, how will we know? Is a state-level analysis sufficiently sensitive to capture life-threatening shortages in the availability of surgeons capable and willing to tackle acute surgical problems in the middle of the night? In considering these issues, it should be readily apparent that the areas of the country that are likely to experience the most acute shortages are rural areas of the US. Within the US, rural areas represent 75% of the country's land mass and 17–20% of the population, but only 10% of the domestic workforce of general surgeons [21]. Two recent front-page articles, one in the *Washington Post* and one in the *Wall Street Journal*, have highlighted the difficulties facing rural general surgeons and their surrounding communities [22, 23]. The departure of these physicians from the workforce – resulting either from harsh conditions/job dissatisfaction or simple age-related attrition – stands to have a significant impact on patient access to care and the financial viability of community hospitals [21, 24].

Several physician leaders within the field of general surgery have called attention to the growing problem of surgeon shortages in rural areas [24–28]. We refer the reader to this literature for a thorough discussion of this emerging issue, and plans to address it. In considering the plight of the rural communities, however, it is important to bear in mind that the rural surgical workforce does not exist separately from the non-rural surgical workforce, but rather in equilibrium with it. The acute shortage of surgeons in these areas is probably best considered as the first manifestation of a growing national problem.

Hospital Capacity

The ability of the existing hospital infrastructure to meet increased demand for inpatient care is an often-overlooked consideration. According to 2007 data from the American Hospital Association, there are currently 4,897 hospitals and 800,892 staffed hospital beds in the US [29]. Longitudinal trends in the number of beds and number of beds per 1,000 population between 1981 and 2006 are shown in Fig. 12.5.

Over the last decade, the use of hospital-based care has remained remarkably constant, in terms of age-specific rates of hospitalization (Fig. 12.6a). The annual number of hospitalizations and inpatient days of care used per year in the US between 1996 and 2006 are presented using data from the NHDS (Fig. 12.6b). Forecasts between 2006 and 2030 were calculated based on 2006 patterns of hospitalization in terms of age-specific rates of admission and lengths of stay.

Between 1996 and 2006, numbers of hospitalizations increased by 12.8% and inpatient days of care by 5.0%. The differential rates of growth are explained by an overall trend in decreased LOS. Based on the patterns of hospitalization from 2006, between 2006 and 2030 we forecast that the number of annual hospitalizations will increase by 39% and days of inpatient care by 43% (Fig. 12.6b).

Figure 12.5 Number of hospital beds in the US, 1987–2007 (data from the American Hospital Association Annual Survey, 2007, for community hospitals, Avalere Health, Washington, DC).

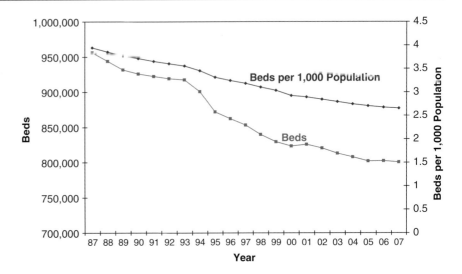

Given that the number of beds per population is decreasing and the population-based demand is increasing, the capacity of the current hospital network to cope with future growth in the numbers of domestic hospitalizations is worthy of investigation. At the time of writing this chapter, the authors know of no comprehensive studies of the occupancy rates within US hospitals. One study of New Jersey hospitals found occupancy rates on average well below 80%, implying ample capacity [30]. Are these levels of utilization representative of other communities in the US? The ability of hospitals to handle growing demand for inpatient care engendered by the aging population needs to be examined at every level.

Forecasting Utilization

The fact that older individuals use more health care resources than younger individuals is important, but other important forces also drive changes in utilization of medical services. These forces include population growth, changes in health care delivery, and economic expansion. In the past, several approaches have been applied to project the amount by which population-based use of medical resources will increase in the future. The methods behind these approaches are rooted in varying methodologies, and have yielded conflicting results over time. Broadly speaking, models used in forecasting medical expenditure can be categorized as needs-based, demands-based, or economic in terms of the approach taken.

of this discussion, we will first define the "need" for medical services based on an existing definition:

> That quantity of medical services which expert medical opinion believes ought to be consumed over a relevant time period in order for its members to remain or become as "healthy" as is permitted by existing medical knowledge [31].

Translating a needs-based model into prediction requires two main steps. First, an epidemiological estimate of disease frequency is developed. Second, the amount and type(s) of care necessary to adequately treat the disease is compiled. A needs-based model can also be "adjusted" to reflect predicted changes in either of the two elements of the model. The Graduate Medical Education National Advisory Committee (GMENAC) report, published in 1980, is an example of a needs-based approach [32]. In the GMENAC report, a panel of medical experts (6–10 for each specialty) estimated the profile of care required by the general population. The estimation was targeted at predicting patterns of care as they "should be," rather than as they actually were at some baseline point in time. Based on this needs-based model, the GMENAC report suggested that by the year 2000, there would be approximately a 25% physician surplus.

Inherent in any needs-based model is a prediction regarding what patterns of treatment will be in the future. This type of estimation can be a strength or a weakness, depending on its ability to move a prediction model in a way that makes it more or less accurate. While in retrospect it is easy to dismiss the GMENAC model as poorly conceived, in its time this effort was a significant driver of health policy.

Needs-Based Models

A needs-based model is predicated on estimating the population-based need for medical services and applying this estimate of need to the population as it will be in the future. For the purpose

Demands-Based Models

A demands-based model is based on interpreting the desires or "wants" of a population, and placing these motivations in the context of market forces, especially price. We defer, once

FIGURE 12.6 (**a**) Age-specific rates of hospitalization: 1996–2006; (**b**) annual hospitalizations and days inpatient care: 1996–2030.

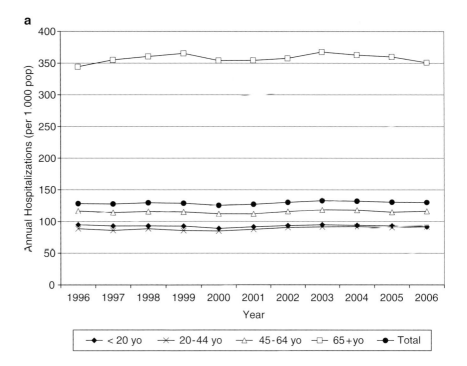

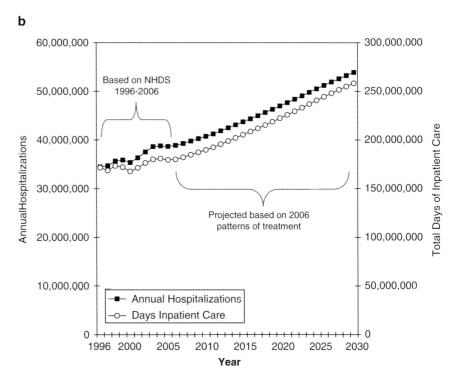

again, to a preexisting definition for "demand" in order to ground this discussion:

A multivariate functional relationship between the quantities of medical services that its members desire to consume over a relevant time period at given levels of prices of goods and services, financial resources, size and psychological wants of the population as reflected by consumer tastes and preferences for (all) goods and services [31].

Generating a demands-based model for predicting use of medical services is relatively straightforward, and relies on two core components. First, rates of surgical procedures can be calculated based on any one of a number of existing data sources. Second, these rates can then be applied to forecasted population changes in order to project trends in the use of different types of surgical procedures. A demands-based approach benefits from simplicity and objectivity. The major

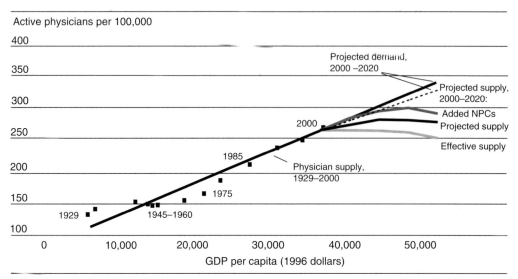

Sources: Physician supply: R.I. Lee and L.W. Jones, *The Fundamentals of Good Medical Care* (Chicago: University of Chicago Press, 1933); W.H. Stewart and M. Pennell, "Health Manpower, 1930–75," *Public Health Reports 75*, no. 3 (1960): 274–280; American Osteopathic Association; and Bureau of Health Professions. Population: Bureau of the Census. Gross domestic product: Bureau of Economic Analysis. Supply projections based on authors' model; see Note 4 in text.

Notes: "Physician supply 1929–2000" includes active physicians only (r^2 = 0.94). "Projected supply" includes all active physicians. "Effective supply" represents the number of active physicians reduced by the decrements in work effort associated with increasing numbers of female and older physicians in the workforce. "Added NPCs" represents the sum of "effective supply" plus the incremental contributions of nonphysician providers (NPCs). Per capita GDP is expressed in chained 1996 dollars. "Physician demand" is projected based on average annual GDP growth rates of 1.5 percent (dotted rule) and 2 percent (continued solid rule).

Figure 12.7 Physician supply and gross domestic product, 1929–2000 and projected to 2020 (from Cooper et al. [34]).

shortcoming of this approach stems from the underlying assumption that per capita demand will remain constant over the time period of interest.

In 1989, a private consulting firm (ABT Associates) was contracted by the Bureau of Health Professions to conduct a follow-up to the GMENAC study. The methods used in this report were demands-based, and findings included a projected increase in the use of general surgical care of 32.7% between 1990 and 2010. We published the results of a similar type of model in 2003, and found a projected increase in the demand for general surgical procedures of 31% between 2001 and 2020 [33].

Economic Models

Economic models add another important dimension to the science of forecasting growth in the use of medical resources. The arguments underlying a need to consider economic factors are elegant. In the US, the per capita use of medical resources has risen steadily over time, and this rate of rise is linear when compared with increases in gross domestic product (GDP). Economic models attempt to account for the

impact of economic factors, and incorporate projected growth in GDP into a predictive model. The use of economic models in physician workforce forecasts has been predominantly advocated by Cooper et al., and published initially in 2002 [34]. Their approach, termed a "trend model," incorporates four factors (1) economic expansion, (2) population growth, (3) physician work effort, and (4) services provided by nonphysician clinicians (NPCs) (Fig. 12.7).

This model is notably different from demands-based and needs-based models in that it (1) defines and quantifies a direct relationship between economic expansion [gross domestic product (GDP)] and physician supply, and (2) assumes that this relationship will remain constant into the future. An economic model also has special usefulness in characterizing the relationship between economic growth and specific subtypes of physician services. Based on a cross-sectional analysis of States (in the US) in 1995, this model documents a relationship between regional per-capita income and the supply of three types of physicians: general practitioners, surgical specialists, and medical specialists (Fig. 12.8). The implication of this finding is that continued economic growth will lead to a relatively greater growth in the demand for medical and surgical specialists than for general practitioners.

FIGURE 12.8 Physician supply in States, by major specialty group and State per capita income, 1995 (from Cooper et al. [34]).

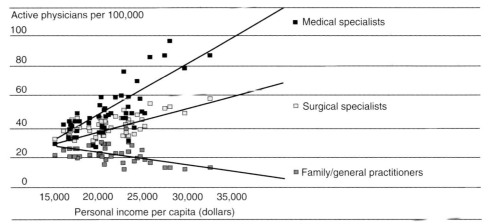

Sources: Bureau of Economic Analysis; American Medical Association; and Bureau of the Census.

FIGURE 12.9 US population age distribution: 2000–2050.

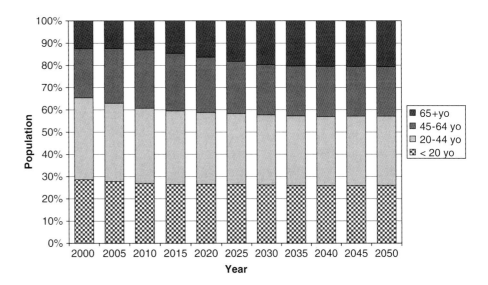

In forecasting the demand for physician services, economic models make an explicit assumption which might also be considered a weakness – that economic expansion will continue at rates that are roughly similar to those in recent history. At the time of the writing of this chapter, that assumption might be called into question. In a period of lesser economic growth or even recession, the actual demand for physicians (according to this type of model) would be lower than forecasted. It is also notable that this model explicitly fails to incorporate any acknowledgement of the aging of the US population. The extent to which the aging of the population is a significant driver of future expenditures is a topic of great debate. Several notable economists have argued that population aging is *not* a primary driver of growth in expenditures [35, 36]. Their argument is based on demonstrating that the demographic profile of the US population will not actually change dramatically in the coming decades (Fig. 12.9).

While at first glance, the demographic shift toward an aging population might appear minimal or modest, this type of display hides a subtle but important truth. Based on figures from the US census, in 2000 12.4% of the US population were aged 65 years or older; by 2030, this figure will increase to 19.7%, and between 2030 and 2050 the proportion of the population 65 years and older will remain stable at approximately 20%. Meanwhile, the overall US population is forecasted to increase by 29% between 2000 and 2030, and 49% by 2050. In the future, what proportion of growth in medical expenditures can be accounted for by population growth as opposed to population aging?

In Fig. 12.10a, b, we address this question looking at medical/surgical admissions and procedures using a forecasting method that is based on data from the 2006 NHDS. During a 25-year period that sees 22% growth in the US population, there will be a projected 44% increase in medical admissions and a 38% increase in surgical admissions for

FIGURE 12.10 (a) Projected growth in population and medical vs. surgical admissions: 2006–2030; (b) projected growth in selected surgical procedures: 2006–2030.

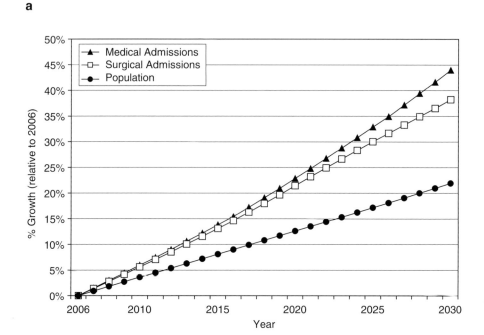

a

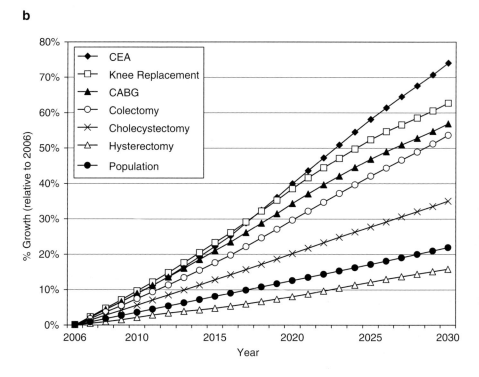

b

hospital-based care. Growth in specific surgical procedures varies widely, from 16% (hysterectomy) to 74% (CEA). In general, these rates of procedure-based growth are significantly greater than simple population growth.

So why do economists de-emphasize the aging of the US population in their forecasting models? The answer may lie in that their perspective encompasses a more global view of health care finance. In recent years and in the near future,

domestic health spending has grown by an estimated 6–7% per year [37–39]. From the perspective of national policy planning, it is clear that population expansion and aging are not the only (and perhaps not even one of the most important) drivers of growth in expenditures. This point of view – while valid – has the potential to overlook problems related to the adequacy of the supply of specific types of physicians relative to the projected demand for their care.

The Surgical Workforce

The forecasting models described above all predict a significant increase in the demand for health care services. These models tend to group all physicians together in considering workforce, or at best into "surgical specialists." In this section, we will describe the training pipeline that produces physicians in the US, and examine the general surgery workforce as a case in point.

Training: Medical Schools

Medical education is the first gateway through which physicians must pass en route to independent practice, and there are finite means through which this can occur. Between 1980 and 2005, the number of graduates from domestic medical schools (allopathic plus osteopathic) has remained at approximately 16,000–18,000 per year [40]. A significant number of physicians practicing in the US did not attend a domestic medical school. Physicians who graduated with a medical degree from a school listed in the World Health Organization directory of medical schools or the Foundation for the Advancement of International Medical Education and Research (FAIMER) are eligible to obtain licensure within the US. In 2007, 29% of entrants into graduate medical education (GME) training programs were international medical graduates (IMGs) [41]. The Association of American Medical Colleges recently recommended increasing the number of medical school positions in the US by 30% in the decade starting 2005 [42]. Recent projections place the estimated actual growth in positions at 21% [43].

Residency Training

Graduate (residency) medical education is funded both directly and indirectly through a variety of sources, most notably Medicare. The adequacy of these training programs is supervised by the American Council for Graduate Medical Education (ACGME) through Residency Review Committees (RRCs). The vast majority of physicians working in the US are trained through an ACGME-accredited residency program, and gauging the output of this pipeline over time is important to understand the current and future physician workforce.

Between 1980 and 1993, the number of residency training positions in the US increased from 61,819 to 97,370 (58%), a rate significantly more rapid than population growth [44]. By the early 1990s, however, general and academic consensus was that a period of physician oversupply was imminent

[45, 46]. The Balanced Budget Act (BBA) of 1997 placed limits on the number of such training positions that would be funded by Medicare, and this cemented a halt in the increase of graduate medical education. In the 10-year period after the passage of the BBA, there has been an 8% increase in training positions, primarily the result of increased trainees, but also due to increased sub-specialization and longer training programs [41].

The number of fully-trained physicians that can be trained each year in the US is a function primarily of the number of residency training positions. An increase in the number of qualified domestic medical school graduates without accompanying growth in residency slots will only result in a lower proportion of IMGs in domestic GME programs or a body of domestic graduates who are unable to find appropriate training positions. Despite the significant movement toward expanding the number of medical school slots, there has not yet been a co-existing mandate to increase GME expenditures or positions. In the context of a recessionary economy, it seems unlikely that Federal spending on GME will increase.

Work Effort

The work output per surgeon is another important element of the workforce equation. The economic model developed by Cooper et al. forecasts a decrease in work effort over the next 15–20 years as a result of an aging surgical workforce and the rising number of female physicians [34]. They assumed a reduction in work effort of 10% for physicians aged 55–65, and 20% for those aged >65, and that female physicians work output is 20% lower than male physicians. Within their model, these assumptions resulted in a net 5% reduction in overall physician effort in 2010, and 10% in 2020 (relative to 2000).

Another important factor affecting physician work effort/efficiency is the shifting paradigm of work hours during surgical training. In July 2003, the ACGME issued standards for all accredited residency programs, mandating an 80-h work week. Most recently, in December 2008, the Institute of Medicine (IOM) released a report entitled "Resident Duty Hours: Enhancing Sleep, Supervision, and Safety" [47]. While this report did not go beyond the ACGME standards in further limiting the number of hours worked by residents, it advocated significant changes to how those hours should be structured. As part of this report, the IOM commissioned an analysis of how many additional physicians would be required to meet staffing needs if its recommendations were implemented. This analysis found a need for an additional 5,001 attending physicians and 8,247 resident physicians.

It may also be a matter of time before the hours worked by surgeons in practice are reduced. This may be a result of the decreased hours in training carrying over into a desire by graduates to work less, or a more global shift on the part of medical students towards a desire for a controllable lifestyle [48, 49]. Another emerging trend that may affect the work output per surgeon in the US is the trend away from independent physician practice. According to data from the Center for Studying Health System Change, in 1996–1997 the proportion of surgical specialists who are full or partial owners of their practice was 75.5%, but by 2004–2005 this figure had decreased to 68.4% [50]. How does a shift away from independent practice affect overall clinical productivity? The relative productivity of surgeons in independent practice compared with surgeons in other types of practice environments is unknown. Regardless of the impact of this emerging trend on physician productivity, the loss of surgeon practice autonomy may have significant implications for the field which should be addressed at the highest level of leadership.

The aging of the surgical workforce is a significant challenge not only in terms of declining work effort, but also in terms of exit from the workforce. According to data from the American Medical Association, over 40% of active general surgeons, urologists, thoracic surgeons, and orthopedic surgeons are over the age of 55 [51]. Estimating the likelihood of retirement is difficult, given that physician self-report of retirement plans may not be entirely predictive of actual behavior [52]. Also, there is evidence that practice environment and work satisfaction can impact plans for retirement vs. continued practice [53].

General Surgery: A Case in Point

The American Board of Surgery (ABS) has certified diplomates in general surgery since 1938, and over the last 70 years, the field has changed dramatically. In the year 1938, 102 surgeons were board-certified, and in 2005 this number had increased to 1,026. Over the last 25 years, however, the number of general surgeons certified per year has been remarkably constant. Based on data obtained through the ABS regarding historical rates of certification, we have developed a basic model to estimate the number of general surgeons in practice. This model is based on the following assumptions (1) 1,000 annual certifications after 2005, (2) 30-year career in active clinical practice, and (3) 0.5% annual attrition rate. Based on this model, between 2005 and 2025 the number of active general surgery diplomates will increase by 2.1% (Fig. 12.11a). The numbers of active diplomates relative to the US population are shown in Fig. 12.11b.

The ratio of active general surgeons to the US population was highest in 1988, and declined by 7–8% by 2006. Based on our model, in 2025 the general surgical workforce relative to population-based demand will have decreased by 26%

relative to 1988. Importantly, this figure is refractory to immediate changes in rates of surgical training. If in 2010, the number of diplomates per year is increased to 1,100 per year, the ratio of workforce to population-based demand will be only 5% higher in 2025 than if the rates of graduation remain at 1,000 per year.

These estimates and projections are limited in that all board-certified general surgeons are considered "general surgeons," regardless of sub-specialization in training/practice. A recent study based on data from the American Medical Association's Physician Masterfile estimated that between 1981 and 2005 the number of active general surgeons decreased precipitously from 7.68 to 5.69 per 100,000 [25]. This estimate only included surgeons who listed their primary area of specialty as general surgery, abdominal surgery, trauma surgery, or critical care. Over the last two decades, the proportion of graduating general surgical residents who pursue additional subspecialty training has grown, and is currently over 70% [54]. The amount of general surgery performed by diplomates with subspecialty training is largely unknown and difficult to measure.

Health Care Reform: Will It Solve the Problem?

There is no argument that US residents pay a greater amount for health care than any other country in the world. According to recent statistics, the annual per capita expenditure was $6,401, and between 1970 and 2005 the rate of increase in the proportion of GDP directed toward health care spending was faster in the US than in any other country [55]. In return for its investment, it does not seem that the US population receives a concomitantly higher quality of care [56]. Waste is considered rampant:

> As much as $700 billion dollars a year in health care services are delivered in the US that do not improve health outcomes.
>
> Peter Orszag, Director of Congressional Budget Office [57].

The $700 billion figure listed above represents approximately 5% of the GDP. It has been further estimated that reducing the administrative overhead costs associated with healthcare expenditures would save an estimated $400 billion (2003 dollars) per year [58].

Given these dramatic figures, it seems reasonable to consider ways in which the US health care system might reduce waste and improve the value returned on spent health care dollars. In this section, we will focus on three key areas (access to care, regional variation, and technological change) that are targeted by policy makers in their quest to improve the value and effectiveness of health care, and consider the impact of changes in these areas on the supply and demand for surgical services.

FIGURE 12.11 (**a**) ABS
certifications: 1965–2025;
(**b**) active general surgeons in
US: 1965–2025.

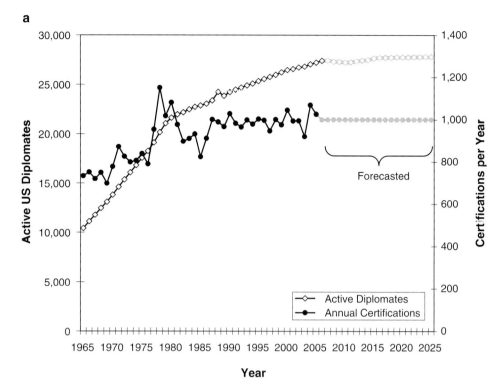

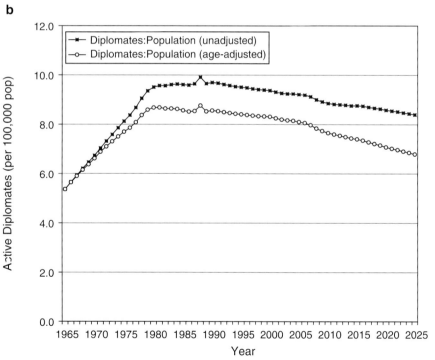

Access to Care

Changes in the type of health insurance held by the US population have the potential to dramatically alter the way in which individuals access surgeons and surgical treatment. Two main ways in which this might occur is (1) through increased use of managed care models for health care delivery or (2) through universal (or expanded) health coverage.

The managed care boom of the 1990s led to a growing belief that these new systems would regulate the inefficient and fee-driven use of specialist care. In one controversial prognostication, Weiner et al. in a 1994 *JAMA* article anticipated that the increased use of managed care (to 40–65% penetration) would lead to a 60% surplus of "specialists" in the year 2000 [59]. As with some of the prediction models discussed earlier, these forecasts were based on assumptions that proved erroneous.

In a similar vein, universal health coverage (or simply improved access to health care) has the capacity to nearly instantaneously improve the ability of millions of US residents to access surgical care. What would be the effect of these changes on population-based demand for surgical procedures? In an AAMC report published in 2008, the impact of universal health coverage on the number of full-time physicians was modeled [60]. Their model found a 3.6% estimated increase in the physician workforce. This relatively small effect stems from the fact that the uninsured population is relatively young and healthy. It should also be noted that a significant amount of surgical care for nonelective conditions is already provided to this population through safety-net institutions. Expanded health care coverage may, however, result in increased demand for elective procedures, especially those performed in younger, healthier patients.

The impact of a burgeoning elderly population on Medicare – the primary payor for healthcare delivery for individuals over the age of 65 years in the US – also needs to be considered. In the 2008 annual report, the Social Security and Medicare Boards of Trustees painted a grim picture of the financial health of both of these entitlement programs. Beginning in 2008, the Medicare Hospital Insurance Trust Fund will pay out more in hospital benefits than it receives in taxes and revenues. As more and more baby boomers enter retirement age, this trend will accelerate, and the Medicare reserves may be exhausted before 2020. In 2008 there were an estimated 3.3 workers per retiree; by 2020 this ratio is projected to decrease to 2.1 by 2031 [61]. Several approaches have been proposed to help cope with the emerging problem of funding healthcare for a growing population of retirees. One mechanism that generated initial enthusiasm was the Medicare advantage plans, whereby Medicare beneficiaries could enroll in private health insurance plans [62]. The privatization of portions of the care provided through the Medicare benefit has thus far failed to produce significant cost savings. Innovative practice plans and chronic disease management models have shown some promise, but not yet sizable enough to make an impact on forecasted deficits. New types of payment models, including the prospective payment system have some benefits, but have resulted in the shifting of in-hospital care to pre- and post-hospital environments. Other proposals, such as the Breaux–Thomas proposed legislation to increase the eligibility of age to 67 or increase co-payments/deductibles have proven politically difficult [63]. It is safe to say that the costs associated with providing healthcare to the aging US population will be an issue of growing importance for politicians, payors, and providers.

Regional Variation in Procedure Utilization

The rate at which physicians provide services to the population varies widely from region to region. This concept of regional variation was originally described by Wennberg and colleagues at Dartmouth, and continues to be a core concern of health policy makers at all levels [64, 65]. The annual Dartmouth Atlas of Health Care uses Medicare data to describe variation in care, and spur health care reform efforts.

Figure 12.12 shows an analysis of publicly available data from the 2005 Dartmouth Atlas, which reports regional utilization using hospital referral regions (HRR) as the geographic unit of interest. Within the Atlas, each patient is assigned to one of 306 HRRs. The boundaries that encompass each HRR are derived based on documenting the referral patterns of

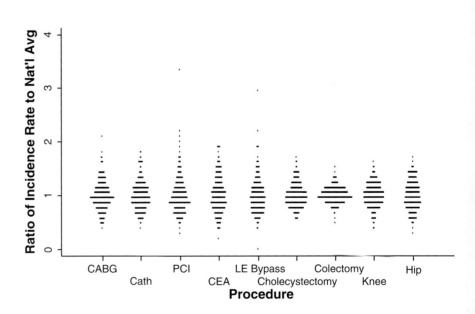

Figure 12.12 Regional (HRR) variation by procedure. Data from the Dartmouth Atlas of Health Care 2005.

patients who are referred for major cardiovascular procedures and for neurosurgery. In order to provide some data for a discussion regarding regional variation in procedure use, we will provide some preliminary data analysis.

Broadly speaking, these variations can only be the result of regional differences in either (1) the rates of disease or (2) the patterns of care received, and the extent to which each of these two explanations is responsible for the observed variations is difficult to assess. Why are there differences in the amount of variation between procedures? An elegant answer has been proffered by Birkmeyer et al., who note that procedures where the diagnosis does not linearly lead to a procedure (e.g., peripheral arterial disease ⇒ lower extremity bypass) may have greater variation than one where a procedure is the only logical next step (e.g., non-metastatic colon cancer ⇒ colectomy) [66].

For many, these variations are the manifestation of physician-induced demand, with subspecialists driving higher rates of potentially unnecessary procedures [67]. The extent to which this phenomenon exists has been hotly debated for decades. Another way of conceptualizing the debate over physician-induced demand is to consider part of the regional variations in rates of care as resulting from differences in the relative rates of underuse and/or overuse of surgical treatment. In moving forward with this concept, some definitions are important:

> Overuse: Occurs when a health care service is provided under circumstances in which its potential for harm exceeds the possible benefit
>
> Underuse: Failure to provide a health care service when it would have produced a favorable outcome for a patient
>
> Chassin and Galvin [68]

In determining the potential for a surgical procedure to provide an acceptable ratio of likelihood of benefit to possibility of harm – one estimate of value – the best available resources are evidence-based guidelines developed by professional organizations and consensus panels. The extent to which these guidelines reflect a significant body of evidence is not always perfect, but they are at least a starting point [69].

Generally speaking, it is much easier to accurately assess the presence of overuse than it is to quantify underuse. This is simply due to the availability of the denominator population. In a recent study by Keyhani et al., the appropriateness of tympanostomy tubes for otitis media in five New York hospitals was examined [70]. Of 682 pediatric patients who underwent the procedure, a majority (70%) were considered inappropriate overuse based on existing guidelines. In this study, the denominator population was easily identified – patients undergoing tympanostomy placement. A study examining underuse of tympanostomy tubes would be much more challenging, as it would involve examining primary care physicians' records for all patients with confirmed or suspected otitis media in a large population. If one was to examine the population-based need for tympanostomy tubes within New York, what would the actual use of the procedure be if there was no (or minimal) underuse or overuse?

Studies examining underuse yield dramatic findings as well. One classic study examined rates of coronary angiography after acute myocardial infarction (MI) within the Veterans Affairs (VA) system and Medicare [71]. The study cohort (denominator population) was defined a needed angiography based on American College of Cardiology guidelines. Cohort patients within the VA system received a needed angiography 43% of the time, whereas those in Medicare 51%.

Why are these types of studies important? As the demand for value in health care delivery increases, so will the expectation that procedure-based specialties justify the work they perform, in terms of outcomes for their patient population.

Technological Advance

The possibility that advancing medical technology will obviate the need for surgical care (and surgeons) is a source of great intuitive appeal and worthy of mention. Rates of surgical treatment for specific disease processes have been dramatically reduced, some nearly eliminated by innovation in medical (non-surgical) treatment. Some examples include peptic ulcer disease, tuberculosis, and coronary artery disease. The war on cancer also appears to be having some significant recent successes in reducing the incidence of certain malignancies, most notably lung, colorectal, breast, and prostate cancer [72].

On the other hand, minimally invasive surgical technology has resulted in a lower clinical threshold to perform specific surgical procedures (e.g., cholecystectomy) [73, 74]. With the increasing use of laparoscopic and other minimally invasive surgical approaches, more latent demand for procedures may be unlocked. Some surgical disease processes are actually becoming much more common (e.g., diverticulitis) [75]. And, surgical treatment is being applied to conditions that may have been historically managed only medically, for example obesity, with an estimated 113,000 inpatient surgical procedures for obesity per year in 2005 (800% increase from 1998) [76].

What is the overall impact of evolving technology on the profile and quantity of surgical procedures? In one study based on California data from 1990 to 2000, Liu et al. quantified trends in the volumes of 32 inpatient surgical procedures [77]. Total procedural volume increased by 20.4%, during a period in which the State population increased by 13.8%. Technological advance has the capacity to increase, decrease, and change the demand for surgical treatment.

Summary: Looking Toward the Future

The task of predicting what health care delivery will look like in the near (or distant) future is potentially foolhardy. In this chapter, we have demonstrated some of the most important variables that need to be considered in estimating the ability of the current and future systems of care to provide treatment to the US population. Despite the obvious difficulty in making accurate predictions and the historical problems with them, there is a growing consensus that the aging of the US population represents a looming crisis. Whatever magnitude of crisis evolves, efforts to minimize its impact on patient care will require action on multiple fronts and at multiple levels.

First and foremost, there is strong evidence that in the future demand for surgical procedures will outstrip the supply of surgeons. Solutions to this emerging problem will need to occur on multiple fronts. Training more surgeons is the most apparent solution, but this can only be part of the answer to the problem. In the immediate and near-term future (10–15 years) growth in surgical training programs can provide only a minimal boost to the active surgical workforce. Other informal pathways, such as allowing trained surgeons from other countries to become licensed in the US after an abbreviated domestic training may have some appeal, but the idea of draining these resources from less developed countries is ethically untoward [27, 78, 79]. In addition to increasing the number of new surgical trainees, attention may need to be focused on retaining those in practice. While the current state of the economy (and most retirement investment portfolios) may cause this even without any policy planning, steps may be taken to encourage physicians to remain in practice. This may call for developing means for surgeons in or near retirement to maintain reduced workloads with only proportionate reductions in professional income. Also, vanishingly little research has been conducted examining the relative efficiency of surgeons employed in private practice vs. academic practice vs. health maintenance organizations. The use of non-physician clinicians may have an important and widening role in enabling surgeons to focus more completely on operative and associated responsibilities and a reduced role in administrative and non-essential clinical activities.

The aging population will result not only in an increased demand for surgical procedures, but also in a different profile of surgical patients. Operations for disease processes specific to older patients will become more frequent, especially orthopedic and spinal operations. Patients will be older and more comorbid, and will require an increased focus on optimizing medical management. A greater partnership with medical hospitalists is already occurring, and will almost certainly continue to grow. In order to care for these patients in a way that provides the greatest benefit to the population at hand, surgeons need to be proactive in analyzing the outcomes, effectiveness and appropriateness of the surgical treatment provided to elderly patients. Rigorous quality monitoring and improvement efforts are a key part of how our field can rise to meet these demands.

In considering the impact of these forthcoming changes, surgeons of all specialties need to have a seat at the leadership table. The perspective of prominent health care economists envisions the physician workforce *en masse*, and in doing so may completely ignore crises within a particular field. Surgeons of all types will need to ensure that their needs and the needs of their patients are heard.

References

1. Dennison C, Pokras R (2000) Design and operation of the National Hospital Discharge Survey: 1988 redesign. Vital Health Stat 1 39:1–42
2. http://quickfacts.census.gov/qfd/states/00000.html. Accessed 20 Dec 2008
3. http://www.cms.hhs.gov-MedicareFeeforSvcPartsAB-Downloads-DRGDesc05.pdf. Accessed 20 Dec 2008
4. Reported figures based on original analysis of data from the 2005 Florida State Ambulatory Surgery Database
5. Reported figures based on original analysis of data from the 2006 National Hospital Discharge Survey
6. Kuo YF, Sharma G, Freeman JL, Goodwin JS (2009) Growth in the care of older patients by hospitalists in the United States. N Engl J Med 360(11):1102–1112
7. Ballarin R, Spaggiari M, Di Benedetto F et al (2009) Do not deny pancreatic resection to elderly patients. J Gastrointest Surg 13(2):341–348
8. Menon KV, Al-Mukhtar A, Aldouri A et al (2006) Outcomes after major hepatectomy in elderly patients. J Am Coll Surg 203(5):677–683
9. Shimada H, Shiratori T, Okazumi S et al (2007) Surgical outcome of elderly patients 75 years of age and older with thoracic esophageal carcinoma. World J Surg 31(4):773–779
10. Etzioni DA, Liu JH, O'Connell JB et al (2003) Elderly patients in surgical workloads: a population-based analysis. Am Surg 69(11):961–965
11. Chang GJ, Skibber JM, Feig BW, Rodriguez-Bigas M (2007) Are we undertreating rectal cancer in the elderly? An epidemiologic study. Ann Surg 246(2):215–221
12. Schrag D, Cramer LD, Bach PB, Begg CB (2001) Age and adjuvant chemotherapy use after surgery for stage III colon cancer. J Natl Cancer Inst 93(11):850–857
13. Schrag D, Gelfand SE, Bach PB et al (2001) Who gets adjuvant treatment for stage II and III rectal cancer? Insight from surveillance, epidemiology, and end results – Medicare. J Clin Oncol 19(17):3712–3718
14. Siu LL (2007) Clinical trials in the elderly – a concept comes of age. N Engl J Med 356(15):1575–1576
15. Baicker K, Chandra A (2004) Medicare spending, the physician workforce, and beneficiaries' quality of care. Health Aff (Millwood) Suppl Web Exclusives:W184–W197
16. Cooper RA (2009) States with more health care spending have better-quality health care: lessons about Medicare. Health Aff 28:w103–w115
17. Cooper RA (2009) States with more physicians have better-quality health care. Health Aff 28:w91–w102
18. American College of Emergency Physicians (2006) On-call specialist coverage in U.S. Emergency Departments: ACEP survey

of emergency department directors. American College of Emergency Physicians (Emergency Medicine Foundation). http://www3.acep.org/WorkArea/showcontent.aspx?id=33266. Accessed Apr 2006

19. Menchine MD, Baraff LJ (2008) On-call specialists and higher level of care transfers in California emergency departments. Acad Emerg Med 15(4):329–336

20. Mohanty SA, Washington DL, Lambe S et al (2006) Predictors of on-call specialist response times in California emergency departments. Acad Emerg Med 13(5):505–512

21. Shively EH, Shively SA (2005) Threats to rural surgery. Am J Surg 190(2):200–205

22. Fuhrmans V (2009) Surgeon shortage pushes hospitals to hire temps. Wall St J:A1

23. Brown D (2009) Shortage of general surgeons endangers rural Americans. Washington Post:A1

24. Fischer JE (2007) The impending disappearance of the general surgeon. JAMA 298(18):2191 2193

25. Lynge DC, Larson EH, Thompson MJ et al (2008) A longitudinal analysis of the general surgery workforce in the United States, 1981–2005. Arch Surg 143(4):345–350, discussion 351

26. Doty B, Zuckerman R, Finlayson S et al (2008) General surgery at rural hospitals: a national survey of rural hospital administrators. Surgery 143(5):599–606

27. Cofer JB, Burns RP (2008) The developing crisis in the national general surgery workforce. J Am Coll Surg 206(5):790–795, discussion 795–797

28. Finlayson SR (2005) Surgery in rural America. Surg Innov 12(4):299–305

29. http://www.aha.org/aha/resource-center/Statistics-and-Studies/fast-facts.html. Accessed 20 Jan 2009

30. DeLia D (2006) Annual bed statistics give a misleading picture of hospital surge capacity. Ann Emerg Med 48(4):384–388

31. Jeffers JR, Bognanno MF, Bartlett JC (1971) On the demand versus need for medical services and the concept of "shortage". Am J Public Health 61(1):46–63

32. McNutt DR (1981) GMENAC: its manpower forecasting framework. Am J Public Health 71(1081279592):1116–1124

33. Etzioni DA, Liu JH, Maggard MA, Ko CY (2003) The aging population and its impact on the surgery workforce. Ann Surg 238(2):170–177

34. Cooper RA, Getzen TE, McKee HJ, Laud P (2002) Economic and demographic trends signal an impending physician shortage. Health Aff (Millwood) 21(121896737):140–154

35. Reinhardt UE (2003) Does the aging of the population really drive the demand for health care? Health Aff (Millwood) 22(6):27–39

36. Strunk BC, Ginsburg PB, Banker MI (2006) The effect of population aging on future hospital demand. Health Aff (Millwood) 25(3):w141–w149

37. Poisal JA, Truffer C, Smith S et al (2007) Health spending projections through 2016: modest changes obscure part D's impact. Health Aff (Millwood) 26(2):w242–w253

38. Catlin A, Cowan C, Heffler S, Washington B (2007) National health spending in 2005: the slowdown continues. Health Aff (Millwood) 26(1):142–153

39. Smith C, Cowan C, Heffler S, Catlin A (2006) National health spending in 2004: recent slowdown led by prescription drug spending. Health Aff (Millwood) 25(1):186–196

40. Dill MJ, Salsberg E (2008) The complexities of physician supply and demand: projections through 2025. AAMC, Washington, DC

41. Salsberg E, Rockey PH, Rivers KL et al (2008) US residency training before and after the 1997 Balanced Budget Act. JAMA 300(10):1174–1180

42. American Association of Medical Colleges Statement on the Physician Workforce (2006). http://www.aamc.org/workforce/workforceposition.pdf. Accessed 26 Aug 2008

43. AAMC (2008) Medical school enrollment plans: analysis of the 2007 AAMC survey. AAMC, Washington, DC

44. Dunn MR, Miller RS, Richter TH (1998) Graduate medical education, 1997–1998. JAMA 280(9):809–812, 836–845

45. Council on Graduate Medical Education (1994) Fourth report: recommendation to improve access to health care through physician workforce reform. U.S. Health Resources and Services Administration, Rockville, MD

46. Pew Health Professions Commission (1995) Critical challenges: revitalizing the health professions for the twenty-first century. The Third Report of the Pew Health Professions Commission. U.C.S.F. Center for the Health Professions, San Francisco

47. Institute of Medicine (2008) Resident duty hours: enhancing sleep, supervision, and safety. Institute of Medicine, Washington, DC

48. Dorsey ER, Jarjoura D, Rutecki GW (2005) The influence of controllable lifestyle and sex on the specialty choices of graduating U.S. medical students, 1996–2003. Acad Med 80(9):791–796

49. Hyman NH (2009) Attending work hour restrictions: is it time? Arch Surg 144(1):7–8

50. Liebhaber A, Grossman JM (2007) Physicians moving to mid-sized, single-specialty practices. Tracking Report, Center for Studying Health System Change, Washington, DC

51. Colleges Center for Workforce Studies (2006) Physician specialty data: a chart book. Center for Workforce Studies, American Association of Medical Colleges, Washington, DC

52. Rittenhouse DR, Mertz E, Keane D, Grumbach K (2004) No exit: an evaluation of measures of physician attrition. Health Serv Res 39(5):1571–1588

53. Kletke PR, Polsky D, Wozniak GD, Escarce JJ (2000) The effect of HMO penetration on physician retirement. Health Serv Res 35(5 Pt 3):17–31

54. Stitzenberg KB, Sheldon GF (2005) Progressive specialization within general surgery: adding to the complexity of workforce planning. J Am Coll Surg 201(6):925–932

55. Anderson GF, Frogner BK (2008) Health spending in OECD countries: obtaining value per dollar. Health Aff (Millwood) 27(6):1718–1727

56. Hussey PS, Anderson GF, Osborn R et al (2004) How does the quality of care compare in five countries? Health Aff (Millwood) 23(3):89–99

57. Address delivered to the annual meeting of the Retirement Research Consortium, 7 August 2008.

58. Himmelstein DU, Woolhandler S, Wolfe SM (2004) Administrative waste in the U.S. health care system in 2003: the cost to the nation, the states, and the District of Columbia, with state-specific estimates of potential savings. Int J Health Serv 34(1):79–86

59. Weiner JP (1994) Forecasting the effects of health reform on US physician workforce requirement. Evidence from HMO staffing patterns. JAMA 272(3):222 230

60. AAMC (2008) The complexities of physician supply and demand: projections through 2025. AAMC, Washington, DC

61. http://www.socialsecurity.gov/policy/docs/chartbooks/fast_facts/2003/fast_facts03.html#chart36. Accessed 30 Mar 2009

62. Berenson R, Hash M, Ault T et al (2008) Cost containment in medicare: a review of what works and what doesn't. AARP Policy Institute, Washington, DC

63. http://thomas.loc.gov/medicare/. Accessed 30 Mar 2009

64. Wennberg J, Gittelsohn A (1973) Small area variations in health care delivery. Science 182(117):1102–1108

65. Wennberg J, Gittelsohn A (1982) Variations in medical care among small areas. Sci Am 246(482199381):120–134

66. Birkmeyer JD, Sharp SM, Finlayson SR et al (1998) Variation profiles of common surgical procedures. Surgery 124(599040741): 917–923

67. Grumbach K (2002) The ramifications of specialty-dominated medicine. Health Aff (Millwood) 21(1):155–157

68. Chassin MR, Galvin RW (1998) The urgent need to improve health care quality. Institute of Medicine National Roundtable on Health Care Quality. JAMA 280(11):1000–1005

69. Sanghavi D (2008) Plenty of guidelines, but where's the evidence? New York Times, 9 December 2008

70. Keyhani S, Kleinman LC, Rothschild M et al (2008) Overuse of tympanostomy tubes in New York metropolitan area: evidence from five hospital cohort. BMJ 337:a1607

71. Petersen LA, Normand SL, Leape LL, McNeil BJ (2003) Regionalization and the underuse of angiography in the Veterans Affairs Health Care System as compared with a fee-for-service system. N Engl J Med 348(2222658539):2209–2217

72. Jemal A, Thun MJ, Ries LA et al (2008) Annual report to the nation on the status of cancer, 1975–2005, featuring trends in lung cancer, tobacco use, and tobacco control. J Natl Cancer Inst 100(23):1672–1694

73. Chen AY, Daley J, Pappas TN et al (1998) Growing use of laparoscopic cholecystectomy in the national Veterans Affairs Surgical Risk Study: effects on volume, patient selection, and selected outcomes. Ann Surg 227(198105850):12–24

74. Escarce JJ, Chen W, Schwartz JS (1995) Falling cholecystectomy thresholds since the introduction of laparoscopic cholecystectomy. JAMA 273(2095264520):1581–1585

75. Etzioni DA, Mack TM, Beart RW Jr, Kaiser AM (2009) Diverticulitis in the United States: 1998–2005: changing patterns of disease and treatment. Ann Surg 249(2):210–217

76. Maggard MA, Yermilov I, Li Z et al (2008) Pregnancy and fertility following bariatric surgery: a systematic review. JAMA 300(19):2286–2296

77. Liu JH, Etzioni DA, O'Connell JB et al (2003) Inpatient surgery in California: 1990–2000. Arch Surg 138(10):1106–1111, discussion 1111–1112

78. Hooper CR (2008) Adding insult to injury: the healthcare brain drain. J Med Ethics 34(9):684–687

79. Wright D, Flis N, Gupta M (2008) The 'Brain Drain' of physicians: historical antecedents to an ethical debate, c. 1960–79. Philos Ethics Humanit Med 3:24

Chapter 13
Defining Quality of Care in Geriatric Surgery

Marcia L. McGory, Hiroko Kunitake, and Clifford Y. Ko

Introduction

Emphasis on Patient Safety and Quality of Care

Since the Institute of Medicine (IOM) reports *To Err is Human* and *Crossing the Quality Chasm* were released a great deal of attention has been focused on improving both patient safety and the quality of care. The IOM estimates that 98,000 people die per year in hospitals due to preventable medical errors, with higher error rates and more serious consequences occurring in intensive care units, operating rooms, and emergency departments [1, 2]. Surgeons not only care for patients in high-risk environments including intensive care units and operating rooms but also care for high-risk patients who may require a procedure under emergency circumstances or have multiple comorbid medical conditions. These patients are at the greatest risk for adverse outcomes and will likely have the largest benefit from improvements in the quality of health care. Elderly patients undergoing surgery are one example of such a population at risk and therefore attention has been focused on elderly surgical patients and the potential importance of geriatric surgery as a surgical specialty.

The IOM also recently addressed the health-care issues of our aging population through the Committee on the Future Healthcare Workforce for Older Americans in their 2008 report entitled *Retooling for an Aging America: Building the Healthcare Workforce* [3]. The committee proposed three mechanisms for improving the ability of our health-care system to care for older Americans: (1) Enhance the competence of all individuals in the delivery of geriatric care; (2) increase the recruitment and retention of geriatric specialists and caregivers; and (3) redesign models of care and broaden patient and provider roles to achieve greater flexibility. In addition, the committee noted that although general surgeons treat large numbers of older patients, there is no specific requirement for geriatric training or subspecialty certificate available in geriatric surgery. In contrast, there is a requirement for education in pediatrics within general surgery, as well as the subspecialty of pediatric surgery. The IOM recommendations are timely given the aging of the population and recent research efforts to improve the quality of care for elderly surgical patients.

Quality of Care Definitions

The conceptual framework driving quality improvement is based on the Donabedian model of quality evaluation, where care can be categorized into three types: structure, process, and outcomes [4]. As shown in Fig. 13.1, structural items are thought to influence both process and outcomes. Specifically, structural items include characteristics of the clinician (e.g., board certification), hospital (e.g., staffing patterns, procedure volume), and patients (e.g., insurance type, severity of comorbidities). Process items are the activities that occur between the patient and practitioner. Process refers to whether the medically appropriate decisions are made and whether care is provided in an effective and skillful manner. Outcomes data apply directly to patients and include mortality, morbidity, functional status, and quality of life. With respect to quality of care in geriatric surgery, examples of structural items include presence of a hospital ward designed for elderly patients or presence of a geriatric care coordinator. Examples of process items unique to geriatric surgery may include co-management of a geriatric surgery patient by a geriatrician or internist, and preoperative completion of a comprehensive geriatric assessment (CGA). Examples of outcomes unique to the geriatric surgery population may include postoperative delirium, change in functional status, and discharge to a skilled nursing facility.

M.L. McGory (✉)
Department of Surgery, David Geffen School of Medicine at the University of California, Los Angeles, CA, USA
e-mail: mmcgory@mednet.ucla.edu

R.A. Rosenthal et al. (eds.), *Principles and Practice of Geriatric Surgery*,
DOI 10.1007/978-1-4419-6999-6_13, © Springer Science+Business Media, LLC 2011

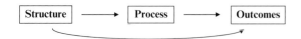

Figure 13.1 Donabedian model of quality of care.

The Impact of the Aging Population

The aging of the US population will place significant stress on the current health-care system. According to the US Census Bureau, in the last century the rate of growth of the elderly population (aged 65 and older) greatly exceeded the growth rate of the population as a whole. Between 1900 and 1994, while the total population tripled, the elderly population increased by a factor of 11. This rapid growth is expected to continue. In 2010, the elderly are predicted to account for 13% of the US population but by 2050 the elderly will comprise 20% of the US population. In addition, the elderly population is responsible for a disproportionate amount of health-care utilization and cost. According to the National Hospital Discharge Survey in 2006, patients aged 65 years and older contributed to 38% of hospital discharges and 43% of days of inpatient care [5].

The impact of the aging population has become especially apparent within the surgical disciplines. The field of surgery is undergoing a largely unrecognized paradigm shift due to the expanding and aging population in combination with an increasing emphasis on patient safety and quality of care. Patients aged 65 and older currently make up 60% of cases within general surgery and this is expected to increase 13% by 2010 and 31% by 2020 [6]. The impact of the aging population will be even more significant in some of the surgical subspecialties. The proportion of work performed on patients aged 65 and older is highest for ophthalmology (88%), cardiothoracic surgery (70.3%), and urology (64.8%) [6]. The anticipated increases in the number and proportion of elderly surgical patients are likely due to multiple factors – not only has the elderly population increased in absolute numbers, but the threshold for performing surgery in the elderly has likely decreased with time [7]. These two factors will significantly increase the demand for surgical services and surgeons must develop strategies to maintain high quality care despite an increased and increasingly complex workload.

While the performance of the surgeon may largely be identical in the operating room with respect to surgical technique, there are a significant number of unique aging-related issues that must be addressed when caring for an elderly surgical patient. The potential needs of an elderly surgical population include increased attention to preoperative risk assessment, explicit communication with the patient and family regarding functional outcomes, and an emphasis on postoperative rehabilitation. The new focus on patient safety and quality no longer revolves solely around conventional surgical morbidity and mortality but probably should include the equally important issues of quality of life and return to preoperative level of functioning for the elderly surgical patient. The combination of these forces has created significant demand for the development of a new model for elderly surgical care which would improve efficiency and provide optimum care for this vulnerable population.

Unique Processes of Care and Outcomes in Geriatric Surgery

One of the first steps to improve the quality of care in geriatric surgery revolves around the concepts of preoperative assessment as well as prevention of perioperative complications. The comorbid disease burden is higher in elderly patients and in combination with decreased physiologic reserves requires closer attention to preoperative assessment and optimization of cardiovascular, pulmonary, renal, and endocrine status. Prevention of untoward events (e.g., infection, myocardial ischemia, delirium) should become the emphasis for this vulnerable population. In addition, preoperative assessment should not be limited to traditional comorbid disease but should extend to include geriatric issues such as cognitive impairment, malnutrition, risk of falls, and pressure ulcer development. Assessment of baseline functional, nutritional, and cognitive status will not only guide the perioperative care of the elderly patient but may influence patient–provider discussions regarding the aggressiveness of surgical intervention. Appropriate goals of surgery may range from palliation of malignant bowel obstruction to curative colorectal cancer resection. Further work is needed to identify processes of care unique to the geriatric surgery population that address preoperative assessment, optimization of comorbidities, and prevention of complications.

The second step to improve the quality of care in geriatric surgery may involve expanding the traditional outcome measures in surgery (e.g., morbidity and mortality) to include items that emphasize quality of life, functional outcomes and symptoms rather than solely prolongation of life. This move to identify such outcomes would highlight and emphasize the importance of these priority issues in the geriatric patient. The typical definition of postoperative morbidity might be expanded to include such postoperative events as episodes of postoperative delirium, in-hospital falls, development of pressure ulcers, and maintenance vs. decline of functional or cognitive status. One of the primary outcomes of interest after surgical intervention in the elderly population could also be return of the patient to their previous environment as well as their functional level prior to surgery. Therefore, the location of discharge after surgery (e.g., home vs. skilled nursing facility) as well as the functional status as measured by activities of daily living (ADL), instrumental activities of daily living (IADL), or ambulation might be important to include as outcomes for the elderly patient undergoing surgery.

Potential Mechanisms for Improving the Quality of Elderly Surgical Care

The discipline of geriatrics is becoming an important part of the daily perioperative care of elderly patients on the surgical ward which has implications for how to restructure the surgical unit and train and teach both surgeons and other healthcare providers. A multitude of tools exist for restructuring surgical training and include involvement of the surgical boards and societies, pay-for-performance, the use of risk-adjusted outcomes, voluntary restructuring of the way we care for surgical patients, and feedback.

First, surgical boards and societies may need to become more directly involved with this paradigm shift. Similar changes have been performed in the field of Internal Medicine. The Residency Review Committee for Internal Medicine (RRC-IM) of the Accreditation Council for Graduate Medical Education (ACGME) recently proposed an outcomes-based accreditation strategy which shifts the emphasis from an external audit of education to a continuous assessment and improvement of the trainee's clinical competence [8]. The overarching goal of the change in the accreditation process of residency programs is to ensure that the emphasis on quality of care is also translated into quality of training [9]. Similar opportunities exist for surgical boards and societies to become leaders in this necessary paradigm shift. A partnership between the American College of Surgeons (ACS) and the American Geriatrics Society may help to address the necessary training and education issues of this intersection between the fields of geriatrics and surgery. Certainly, the Residency Review Committee (RRC) and ACGME are important in these endeavors as well. The ACS has already identified geriatric surgery as an important topic area through the development of a Geriatric Surgery Task Force, development of an online web portal with a geriatric surgery community, and identification of potential "geriatric-specific" variables for inclusion in the ACS National Surgery Quality Improvement Program (NSQIP) in order to help measure and improve the quality of care for geriatric surgery. More collaborative efforts of groups such as these are needed if we are to make headway with a paradigm shift toward the uniqueness, necessity, and importance specific to geriatric surgical care.

A second tool includes the potential use of incentivization for better care, or what is more commonly known as pay-for-performance. The Center for Medicare and Medicaid Services (CMS) is currently performing a Hospital Quality Incentive demonstration project utilizing widely accepted process and outcome measures for the conditions of acute myocardial infarction, heart failure, pneumonia, coronary artery bypass graft, and hip and knee replacement. Hospitals scoring in the top 10% for a given condition will receive a financial bonus while hospitals scoring in the second 10% receive a lesser bonus [10]. Potentially, Medicare could opt to reward hospitals for the presence of structural items such a geriatric care unit or process items such as adherence to geriatric surgery-related process measures (see below), or even outcomes. To date, many of the quality metrics in surgery are derived from the Surgical Care Improvement Project (SCIP), which has identified specific process measures related to surgical site infection, thromboembolism, cardiac complications, and ventilator associated pneumonia. What has been demonstrated is a substantial increase in process measure adherence – from around 40% adherence at the start of the project – to rates well above 80%, with many measures gaining adherence above 90%. Identifying important measures whether structural, process, or outcomes, goes a long way toward recognition and improvement.

A third tool includes the use of risk-adjusted outcomes. The current prototype for the assessment of risk-adjusted surgical outcomes is the Department of Veterans Affairs (VA) NSQIP, an ongoing quality improvement program that relies on the accurate and timely collection of prospective data by trained clinical nurse reviewers. The analysis of data within NSQIP provides the information necessary to create predictive models for morbidity and mortality for specific surgical procedures as well as compare the expected and observed numbers of deaths/complications across VA hospitals [11]. Since the inception of NSQIP in the mid-1990s, the 30-day mortality rate in the VA Medical Centers has decreased by 27% and the 30-day morbidity has decreased by 45%. These results demonstrate the usefulness of providing risk-adjusted outcomes as a benchmark, which assists with identification of areas for surgical quality improvement.[12]

Similarly, the ACS NSQIP has demonstrated that providing risk-adjusted outcomes also results in improvement in private sector hospitals. For example, an analysis of the most recent 3 years of data shows that 66% of hospitals were able to reduce their risk-adjusted mortality rates while 83% of hospitals reduced their risk-adjusted complication rates. Prior internal analyses by the ACS has also demonstrated interesting results regarding risk-adjusted outcomes in the elderly. While it is not surprising that the elderly had up to three times higher rates of complications and up to 20 times higher rates of mortality compared to nonelderly cohorts, it was interesting to note how the complications differed between the elderly and nonelderly. Specifically, the rates of surgical site infection, thromboembolism, postoperative bleeding, and return to the OR did not differ by age while the elderly had significantly higher rates of acute myocardial infarctions, pneumonias, unplanned reintubations, urinary tract infections, and renal failure. These specific complications may lend themselves to identifying important processes of care to reduce these untoward events. Further stratification by age as part of the risk-adjustment analysis may also help identify procedures and age groups (e.g., octogenarians) with the most variability in morbidity and mortality which could potentially lead to large improvements in the outcomes of surgical procedures performed in the elderly [13].

A fourth option is a voluntary restructuring of the way we take care of surgical patients. In the traditional surgical model, surgeons often round on their patients twice a day while the nursing staff traditionally has been trained to a large degree to care for the technical aspects of the patient's post-op recovery. A new model for elderly surgical care may be required which incorporates more of a collaborative team approach with the integration of providers including surgeons, anesthesiologists, geriatricians, general internists, medical specialists, rehabilitation medicine, and nursing. Additional services will also play a critical role including physical/occupational therapists, nutritionists, and others. The team approach is central to the success of this model because the elderly surgical patient often brings a complex mix of both medical and surgical comorbid disease in addition to a variable level of functionality with respect to cognition, ambulation, and degree of independent self-care. Few, if any, single providers can give the optimal care needed for an elderly patient undergoing a major surgical procedure and completely address the interwoven issues of nutrition, cognition, rehabilitation, management of comorbid disease burden and postoperative surgical care. The prevention of postoperative delirium, for example, may include specialized nursing care with minimal use of restraints and specialized equipment for hearing or visual impairment. Physical and occupational therapy may start in the immediate postoperative period with specific goals set based on the results of the preoperative functional assessment. Specialized geriatric care units could increase the role for the elderly patient's family in the preoperative, in-hospital, and postdischarge aspects of care. Physicians should probably limit certain medications such as narcotics. Family assistance with self-care and rehabilitation while the elder is in the hospital can ultimately facilitate the discharge planning process and transition to home.

However, none of these options for implementation of a new model for elderly surgical care will likely be as successful without some sort of level of feedback mechanism (transparent or not) to return information to the providers and hospitals. The concept of quality improvement relies on the return of information to the provider so that outcomes are acknowledged (e.g., rates of postoperative delirium, percentage of patients with a change in functional status requiring discharge to a skilled nursing facility), improvements are noted and changes can be implemented.

Current Research on Geriatric Surgery Quality of Care

A review of the literature demonstrates multiple ongoing research efforts on the topic of geriatric surgery quality of care. Potential mechanisms for quality improvement include the use of quality indicators specific to geriatric surgery, preoperative assessment of geriatric surgery patients, co-management of these patients by geriatricians, a geriatric surgery consult service for nursing home patients and nursing programs focused on the needs of hospitalized elderly patients.

The first avenue of research to improve geriatric surgery quality of care is the development of quality indicators. Health-care regulatory agencies are now beginning to use quality indicators, defined as process measures that signify or result in higher quality, to measure quality of care. CMS and JCAHO are using quality indicators to evaluate care in nonsurgical diseases but the main reason for their lack of use in the surgical domain is that appropriate surgery-related quality indicators are still being developed. The quality of medical care for the elderly population has been the target of a significant amount of research through the RAND Health Assessing Care of Vulnerable Elders (ACOVE) project [14, 15]. The most recent update to the ACOVE project specifically identified quality indicators for elderly surgical patients including quality indicators for hospitalization and surgery in vulnerable elders [16] and quality indicators for the treatment of colorectal cancer in vulnerable elders [17].

In another effort to identify both necessary and important process measures that must be performed when taking care of an elderly surgical patient, McGory et al. gathered a twelve member expert panel consisting of physicians in surgery, geriatrics, anesthesia, internal medicine, pulmonary and critical care, and rehabilitation medicine to identify important processes of care for elderly patients undergoing major abdominal surgery [18]. The validity of the process measures was assessed using a modification of the RAND/UCLA Appropriateness Methodology [19–25]. Eighty-nine candidate indicators were identified and categorized into seven domains: comorbidity assessment (e.g., cardiopulmonary disease), elderly issues (e.g., cognition), medication use (e.g. polypharmacy), patient-to-provider discussions (e.g., life-sustaining preferences), intraoperative care (e.g., preventing hypothermia), Postoperative management (e.g., preventing delirium), and discharge planning (e.g., home health care). Of the 89 candidate indicators, 76 were rated as valid by the expert panel. Importantly, the majority of indicators rated as valid address processes of care not routinely performed in younger surgical populations (Table 13.1). Currently, with support from the National Institute on Aging, this research group is attempting to identify process measures that are applicable to all of inpatient elderly surgery (rather than just major abdominal surgery) in addition to elderly specific structure and outcome measures.

A second avenue of research involves the comprehensive preoperative assessment of elderly surgical patients. The preoperative assessment in elderly cancer patients (PACE) was a prospective study of patients 70 years and older undergoing elective cancer surgery [26]. PACE components included a mini-mental state exam (MMSE), ADLs, IADLs, Geriatric Depression Scale (GDS), brief fatigue inventory (BFI), performance status, American Society of Anesthesiology Scale (ASA), and Satariano's index of comorbidities (SIC). Multivariate analysis demonstrated that IADL, BFI, and ASA were the most important components of PACE to explain postsurgical complications. Further work is needed to determine if PACE can predict postoperative outcomes including length of stay, morbidity, and mortality. Similarly, Harari et al. evaluated proactive care of older people undergoing

TABLE 13.1 Process measures unique to the elderly undergoing surgery vs. perioperative care items universal to all surgical patients

Domain of care	Process measures unique to elderly undergoing surgery	Process measures universal to all surgical patients
Comorbidity assessment	Complete standardized cardiovascular risk evaluation per ACC/AHA guidelines Estimation of creatinine clearance	Standardized preoperative lab panel Pulmonary physical exam/review of systems Obtain history of diabetes Assess use of tobacco/alcohol Smoking cessation
Evaluation of elderly issues	Screen for nutrition, cognition, delirium risk, pressure ulcer risk Assess functional status including ambulation, vision/hearing impairment, and ADLs/IADLs Referral for further evaluation for impaired cognition or functional status, high risk for delirium, or polypharmacy	Not applicable
Medication use	Indications for inpatient bowel preparation Evaluation of medication regimen and polypharmacy Avoid delirium-triggering medications and other potentially inappropriate medications (e.g., Beers criteria)	Instruction on preoperative medication management Perioperative beta blockade Intravenous antibiotic prophylaxis Endocarditis prophylaxis Deep venous thrombosis prophylaxis
Patient–provider discussions	Assess patient's decision-making capacity Specific discussion on expected functional outcome, life-sustaining preferences, and surrogate decision maker	Informed consent about treatment options, and risks/benefits of surgery Treatment preferences (e.g., do not resuscitate) should be followed
Intraoperative care	Not applicable	Prevent hypothermia Proper positioning
Postoperative management	Prevent malnutrition, delirium, deconditioning, pressure ulcers Daily screen for postoperative delirium and standardized workup for delirium episode Make staff aware if hearing/vision impairment Patient access to glasses, hearing aid, dentures Consider home health for assistance for ostomy care Infection prevention with daily assessment of central line and indication for use, early foley catheter removal, and standardized fever workup	Appropriate restraint use Measure daily input/output Aspiration precautions Use of incentive spirometer Use of translator or interpreted materials for deaf or non-English speaking Education about ostomy self-care Pain assessment with each set of vital signs
Discharge planning	A discussion with the patient or caretaker about purpose of drug, how to take it, and expected side effects/adverse effects for all medications prescribed for outpatient use Assess social support and need for home health prior to surgery Assess nutrition, cognition, ambulation, and ADLs prior to discharge	A complete list of medications and dosages to continue upon discharge from the hospital Assess need for medical equipment, home health, skilled nursing facility prior to discharge Written and oral discharge instructions Discharge summary to indicate follow-up labs, tests, appointments Follow-up visit within 6 weeks Communication to primary-care doctor

Source: Reprinted with permission from [17]. Copyright Elsevier 2005

elective surgery (POPS), a CGA service for older elective surgical patients [27]. The POPS team consisted of a geriatrician, geriatric nurse specialist, physical and occupational therapists, and social worker. The preoperative assessment included the abbreviated mental test score, GDS, Barthel index, timed up and go, 180° degree run, body mass index, continence screen, orthostatic blood pressure, numeric pain score, and peak expiratory flow rate. A comparison of outcomes before and after the POPS intervention revealed significantly decreased rates of delirium, pneumonia, wound infection, uncontrolled pain, presence of a urinary catheter for more than 4 days without indication, pressure sores, bedridden patients, and length of stay.

A third avenue of research is the use of a dedicated geriatric service for the co-management of geriatric surgery patients. Friedman et al. evaluated the outcomes of a geriatric fracture center co-managed by orthopedic surgeons and geriatricians [28]. The principles of the geriatric fracture center included the following: (1) most patients benefit from surgical stabilization of the fracture; (2) timely surgical intervention decreases the time in the hospital for development of iatrogenic illness; (3) co-management and frequent communication between the orthopedic surgery and geriatric teams decreases iatrogenesis; (4) standardized protocols decrease variability in care; and (5) discharge planning starts at the time of admission. During a 1-year time period, the geriatric fracture center managed 195 patients. The average time to the operating room was 24.1 h, length of stay was 4.6 days (expected length of stay was 5.2 days using a large healthcare database that determined expected outcomes while adjusting for patient characteristics), readmission within 30 days was 9.7% (expected 19.4%), and in-hospital mortality was 1.5% (expected 3.2%). Similarly, Fallon et al. evaluated the outcomes of geriatric trauma patients when evaluated by a geriatrician within 24 h of admission [29]. A standardized geriatric trauma consultation was utilized which included the following components: demographics, clinical information (e.g., trauma mechanism, primary and secondary diagnoses), physical function (e.g., ADLs, ability to ambulate), cognitive function (e.g., orientation-memory concentration exam, MMSE, confusion assessment method), mood (e.g., geriatric depression scale), medications (focus on potentially inappropriate medication), and pain control. In addition to providing input on geriatric trauma patient management, the geriatric trauma team participated in weekly multidisciplinary rounds as well as monthly performance improvement meetings. During a 1-year time period, 114 out of 285 geriatric trauma patients were seen in consultation by the geriatric trauma team. The most common issues addressed by the geriatricians were pain control, rehabilitation, delirium/dementia, hypertension, and decreased use of adverse drugs. The geriatric trauma patients seen by geriatricians had higher rates of discharge to rehabilitation and a

statistically significant lower mortality rate (4% vs. 18%). Both of these studies clearly demonstrate the benefits of geriatric assessment and co-management for two diverse patient populations (hip fracture and trauma) suggesting that routine geriatric co-management should be an essential component of improving the quality of care in geriatric surgery.

A fourth avenue of research is the use of a geriatric surgery consult service for frail nursing home patients requiring surgical intervention. This model was evaluated by Zenilman et al. [30]. Maintenance surgical care included monitoring of pressure ulcers, stomas, and enteral feeding tubes. However, abdominal, breast, and vascular disease were also commonly treated. The goals and indications of consultation for surgical intervention in an elderly patient vary widely and must be explicitly stated. The goals of surgery could potentially range from palliation to curative resection. Common procedures such as placement of a feeding tube may be secondary to severe malnutrition, cognitive decline (severe dementia), or loss of the ability to care and feed oneself. In addition, many procedures such as those relating to access (e.g., enteral, vascular) or wound care may be chronic in nature. The success of a geriatric surgery consult service depends on the ability to focus on the patient's goals for treatment rather than solely on a surgical cure.

Finally, a fifth avenue of research is the development of a nursing program that specifically addresses the needs of hospitalized geriatric patients. Nurses Improving Care for HealthSystem Elders (NICHE) was developed through the Hartford Institute for Geriatric Nursing at New York University College of Nursing. Components of NICHE include a geriatric institutional assessment profile, staff development tools, nursing care models (e.g., use of a geriatric resource nurse and acute care of the elderly unit model), and research-based clinical protocols (e.g., improving detection and management of delirium). Boltz et al. evaluated the changes in the geriatric care environment associated with NICHE in a sample of eight acute care hospitals in the USA [31]. After NICHE implementation, both perceptions of the geriatric nursing practice environment by nurses and the quality of geriatric care increased. This research is vitally important because of the important role of nurses as part of the team approach to delivering high quality geriatric care.

Conclusion

Just as pediatric surgery became a specialty unto itself, the expanding and aging population has created a potential niche for the specialty of geriatric surgery at the opposite end of the age spectrum. The field of geriatric surgery may indicate a focus on elderly patients for the surgeon, but more importantly the specialty of geriatric surgery represents a collaboration between surgeons, geriatricians, internists, and many other health-care providers who together will address the complex interdisciplinary issues unique to the growing elderly surgical patient population. A great deal of effort is currently being spent on the means of improving the quality of care for geriatric surgery patients through the process measures of developing appropriate quality indicators, improving preoperative assessments and collaboration between surgeons and geriatricians in novel ways such as co-management of elderly surgical patients and surgical consult services in nursing homes. However, to evaluate the quality of care for these elderly surgical patients we must have quality metrics. One possibility is to use adherence to process measures as representative of quality. However, adherence to these process measures may not correlate well with the outcomes of lower morbidity and mortality and improved quality of life which are the ultimate goals of the patient and providers.

Another option is to use outcomes to measure quality – the question becomes which outcomes should we employ to evaluate the quality of elderly surgical care? Should we use traditional outcomes such as mortality and complications or patient reported items such as quality of life and functional status? An important limitation to the use of any quality metric is the ability to measure the quality metric. Some outcomes such as mortality are easily quantified and measured while others such as quality of life are difficult to define and evaluate. And with all quality measures, are there potential unintended consequences to their use as a quality measure? If we decide to use urinary tract infection as a quality measure, is everyone then required to have a urinalysis or urine culture to ensure there is no urinary tract infection? Finally, when we decide on our quality measures, who will be held responsible for the quality of care – the surgeon, the geriatrician, or one of the many other members of the team caring for the elderly surgical patient? Certainly, there are a number of issues to address with the use of quality metrics, but progress in evaluating and improving geriatric surgical care should not be stalled.

Defining quality of care in geriatric surgery is an evolving process with many yet unresolved issues. However as increasing attention and effort is focused on the growing population of elderly surgical patients, we will better understand how to improve and define the quality of surgical care for this unique patient group.

References

1. Kohn LT, Corrigan JM, Donaldson MS. To err is human: building a safer health system. National Academy Press, Washington, DC
2. Institute of Medicine (2001) Crossing the quality chasm, a new health system for the 21st Century. National Academy Press, Washington, DC
3. Institute of Medicine (2008) Retooling for an Aging America: building the healthcare workforce. National Academy Press, Washington, DC
4. Donabedian A (1980) The definition of quality and approaches to its assessment, vol 1. Health Administration Press, Washington, DC, pp 163
5. DeFrances CJ, Lucas CA Buie VC Golosinskiy A. National Health Statistics Reports: 2006 National Hospital Discharge Survey. http://www.cdc.gov/nchs/data/nhsr/nhsr005.pdf. Accessed 7 June 2009
6. Etzioni DA, Liu JH, Maggard MA, Ko CY (2003) The aging population and its impact on the surgery workforce. Ann Surg 238:170–177
7. Etzioni DA, Liu JH, O'Connell JB, Maggard MA, Ko CY (2003) Elderly patients in surgical workloads: a population-based analysis. Am Surg 69:961–965
8. Goroll AH, Sirio C, Duffy FD, LeBlond RF, Alguire P, Blackwell TA et al (2004) A new model for accreditation of residency programs in internal medicine. Ann Intern Med 140:902–909
9. Cassel CK (2004) Quality of care and quality of training: a shared vision for internal medicine? Ann Intern Med 140:927–928
10. Medicare pay-for-performance demonstration shows significant quality of care improvement at participating hospitals. http://www.cms.hhs.gov/media/press/release.asp?Counter=1441. Accessed 13 May 2005
11. Khuri SF, Daley J, Henderson W, Hur K, Demakis J, Aust JB et al (1998) The Department of Veterans Affairs' NSQIP: the first national, validated, outcome-based, risk-adjusted, and peer-controlled program for the measurement and enhancement of the quality of surgical care. National VA Surgical Quality Improvement Program. Ann Surg 228:491–507
12. Khuri SF, Daley J, Henderson WG (2002) The comparative assessment and improvement of quality of surgical care in the Department of Veterans Affairs. Arch Surg 137:20–27
13. Hamel MB, Henderson WG, Khuri SF, Daley J (2005) Surgical outcomes for patients aged 80 and older: morbidity and mortality from major noncardiac surgery. J Am Geriatr Soc 53:424–429
14. Wenger NS, Shekelle PG (2001) Assessing care of vulnerable elders: ACOVE project overview. Ann Intern Med 135:642–646
15. Shekelle PG, MacLean CH, Morton SC, Wenger NS (2001) Assessing care of vulnerable elders: methods for developing quality indicators. Ann Intern Med 135:647–652
16. Arora VM, McGory ML, Fung CH (2007) Quality indicators for hospitalization and surgery in vulnerable elders. J Am Geriatr Soc 55(Suppl 2):S347–S358
17. McGory ML (2007) Quality indicators for the care of colorectal cancer in vulnerable elders. J Am Geriatr Soc 55(Suppl 2): S277 S284
18. McGory ML, Shekelle PG, Rubenstein LZ, Fink A, Ko CY (2005) Developing quality indicators for elderly patients undergoing abdominal surgery. J Am Coll Surg 201(6):870–883
19. Brook RH (1994) "The RAND/UCLA appropriateness method," clinical practice guideline development: methodology perspectives. Public Health Service: AHCR, Rockville, MD
20. Hemingway H, Crook AM, Feder G, Banerjee S, Dawson JR, Magee P et al (2001) Underuse of coronary revascularization procedures in patients considered appropriate candidates for revascularization. N Engl J Med 344:645–654
21. Kravitz RL, Laouri M, Kahan JP, Guzy P, Sherman T, Hilborne L et al (1995) Validity of criteria used for detecting underuse of coronary revascularization. J Am Med Soc 274:632–638
22. Merrick NJ, Fink A, Park RE, Brook RH, Kosecoff J, Chassin MR et al (1987) Derivation of clinical indications for carotid endarterectomy by an expert panel. Am J Public Health 77:187–190
23. Shekelle P (2004) The appropriateness method. Med Decis Making 24:228–231

24. Shekelle PG (2001) Are appropriateness criteria ready for use in clinical practice? N Engl J Med 344:677–678

25. Higashi T, Shekelle PG, Adams JL et al (2004) Vulnerable older patients receiving higher quality medical care have lower mortality. J Gen Intern Med 19:236

26. Audisio RA, Pope D, Ramesh HS, Gennari R, van Leeuwen BL, West C et al (2008) Shall we operate? Preoperative assessment in elderly cancer patients (PACE) can help. A SIOG surgical task force prospective study. Crit Rev Oncol Hematol 65:156–163

27. Harari D, Hopper A, Dhesi J, Babic-Illman G, Lockwood L, Martin F (2007) Proactive care of older people undergoing surgery ('POPS'): designing, embedding, evaluating and funding a comprehensive geriatric assessment service for older elective surgical patients. Age Ageing 36:190–196

28. Friedman SM, Mendelson DA, Kates SL, McCann RM (2008) Geriatric co-management of proximal femur fractures: total quality management and protocol-driven care result in better outcomes for a frail patient population. J Am Geriatr Soc 56:1349–1356

29. Fallon WF Jr, Rader E, Zyzanski S, Mancuso C, Martin B, Breedlove L et al (2006) Geriatric outcomes are improved by a geriatric trauma consultation service. J Trauma 61:1040–1046

30. Zenilman ME, Bender JS, Magnuson TH, Smith GW (1996) General surgical care in the nursing home patient: results of a dedicated geriatric surgery consult service. J Am Coll Surg 183:361–370

31. Boltz M, Capezuti E, Bowar-Ferres S, Norman R, Secic M, Kim H et al (2008) Changes in the geriatric care environment associated with NICHE (Nurses Improving Care for HealthSystem Elders). Geriatr Nurs 29:176–185

Chapter 14
Ethics in Clinical Practice

Margaret Drickamer

Introduction

Normative ethics addresses the criteria or standards by which we judge whether an action is considered to be right or wrong. Medical ethics is built on a utilitarian ethical structure; it bases what we *ought* to do on competing principles that are applied in the context of the clinical setting and not on overarching deontological moral imperatives. The guiding principles of American medical ethics are those of respect for autonomy, nonmaleficence, beneficence, and justice (Table 14.1). Autonomy is defined as the right to self-determination, the right to make one's own choices. The principle of nonmaleficence, often equated with the phrase primum non nocere, first do no harm, is better described as the obligation not to knowingly do harm by either an action or the omission of an action. Beneficence is the act of doing the most possible good; to take the action which will result in the most beneficial outcome for the patient. Justice, in the context of health care, refers to equality of medical treatment and the access to care. For any given clinical situation, the application of each of these principles may give different answers to what is right or wrong [1].

Weighing these competing principles in cultural, societal, and the individual contexts may lead to different actions. Not all cultures approach ethics in the same manner. For example, some religion-based cultures may feel that there are specific rules or god-given imperatives that may never be compromised and therefore all competing interests are secondary. The relative value of the four stated principles may be different for someone in a family-centered culture where individual autonomy may be less important than it is for American culture [2]. In this chapter, we discuss how these principles are applied in modern, mainstream American medicine with a special focus on the geriatric population.

Appropriate treatment of the geriatric patient involves a shift in perspective and priorities. The physician must recognize the multifactorial nature of illnesses, the need to fully understand the goals of care prior to initiating workup, and the need to continually review these goals as events unfold. Most illness states in older patients do not follow the paradigm of a unifying pathologic event. There may be many factors that need to be identified and addressed; factors that have predisposed the individual to the event, changes that have precipitated the event, and consequences of the situation. With age, the patient's perspective on the relative values of quantity and quality of life may change. A patient might wish to live a full, vital life to the age of 100, but may not want to merely survive that long in an incapacitated state. What is seen as a benefit, what weighs heavier as a burden, or what risks that individual is willing to take may change with time and experience.

Truth-Telling

The principle of nonmaleficence has, for millennium, been cited to justify the withholding of "bad news" from patients. The edict to withhold bad news was little challenged until the 1950s when the validity of this assumption came under scrutiny. In surveys conducted during the late 1950s and early 1960s, less than one-third of responding physicians stated that they always tell the truth to their patients about the diagnosis of cancer [3]; and in one survey 69% stated that they usually do not or never tell the patient the diagnosis of cancer [4]. By 1979, a similar survey revealed that 97% of responding physicians thought that a patient should be told the diagnosis of cancer [5].

This profound shift in practice in less than 20 years reflects both advances in medical knowledge and shifts in the emphasis in medical ethics. The development of treatment options for cancer initially drove this shift in communication. Patients could not undergo chemotherapy or irradiation unless they consented to the treatment and in order for them to be able to consent they needed to be informed of their diagnosis.

M. Drickamer (✉)
Department of Medicine (Geriatrics), Yale University School of Medicine, 874 Howard Avenue, New Haven, CT 06519, USA
e-mail: margaret.drickamer@yale.edu

R.A. Rosenthal et al. (eds.), *Principles and Practice of Geriatric Surgery*,
DOI 10.1007/978-1-4419-6999-6_14, © Springer Science+Business Media, LLC 2011

Table 14.1 Definitions in medical ethics

Respect for autonomy	Maximize the individual's ability for self-determination
Nonmaleficence	Do no harm by direct action or negligence
Beneficence	The weighing of benefits, risks, and burdens for the greatest good
Justice	The fair and equitable distribution of resources, greatest good for the greatest number of people

Table 14.2 Principles of informed consent

Assess the patient's ability to understand the consequences of the decision

If the patient is incapable, identify an appropriate surrogate

Document the goals/values of the patient (or surrogate) expressed as the most important for the decision

Explain how the goals would be affected by the benefits/burdens/risks of the intervention

Document the decision and those present for the discussion

In this case, recognizing the patients' autonomous right to choose treatments, or to forego treatments, was felt to be stronger than what was perceived to be the avoidance of the catastrophic harm that would be done by telling them their diagnosis (nonmaleficence). Interestingly, disclosure of information has not been found, in and of itself, to do harm. It does, in fact, allow the patient to discuss their goals and preferences more fully, as well as their emotional reactions, and to plan how they wish to approach this phase of their life.

Even when treatment options are still limited or nonexistent, as is the case with patients diagnosed with Alzheimer's disease, the weight of the argument is in favor of autonomy and therefore for truth-telling [6]. As we place an increasing emphasis on advance health care planning, the obligation to inform patients while they are capable of making decisions about their own future has become paramount. This is especially true when there is a risk of the patient becoming incapable of participating in decision-making, whether the patient is in the early stages of cognitive decline or facing the possibility of complications during surgery which might render them incapable of decision-making.

Older patients may have their right to know their diagnosis subverted by family members who feel that the patient would be unable to handle by knowing the information. On occasion, because of cultural values or for other personal reasons, a patient may not wish to be told a diagnosis. Patients may waive their right to be informed, but this must be an explicit decision between the patient and the physician [7]. Surveys have shown that 90–95% of elderly patients would want to know their diagnosis if they have cancer, which is not different than the percentages for younger patients.

Informed Consent

Every adult patient who has decisional capacity has the right to accept or decline any treatment that is offered. Informing the patient of the benefits, side effects, and alternatives of even common and simple therapies (such as medications) is the first step toward the patient's consent as represented by their compliance with that therapy [8]. The process of informed consent when obtaining consent for invasive procedures is

Table 14.3 Proposed communication skills for discussing evidence with patients

Ability to communicate complex information using nontechnical language

Tailoring the amount and pace of information to the patient's needs and preferences

Drawing diagrams to aid comprehension

Considering the values of the patient while weighing choices

Explanation for the probability and the risk for each option

Facilitative skills to encourage patient involvement

Evaluation of internet information that patients might bring to them

Creating an environment in which patients feel comfortable to ask questions

Giving patients time to take in the information

Declaration of equipoise when present

Checking patient understanding

Negotiation

Source: Adapted from [10] with permission from Elsevier

much more complex, but the same principles hold true (Table 14.2). The patient must understand the benefits of the procedure and the possible risks and burdens associated with it. The patient should also be informed of the benefits, risks, and burdens of all alternative therapies, including doing nothing. The quality of this discussion is as important as the content [9] (Table 14.3) [10]. Long lists of unlikely complications may not serve a useful purpose [11]. The discussion should be based on patients' values, fears, and goals and should inform them about the risks that either are common or, although rare, devastating. Documentation of the discussion should reflect the entire discussion, including the basis on which patients agreed or declined intervention and their ability to make the decision.

What information individual patients will want to know about their condition and possible treatments may differ with age. The 5-year prognosis may no longer be of as much significance as the quality of life to be had with different treatment options. The trade-offs between the burden of an intervention and its benefits will shift with different patient priorities [12]. An older person, or their surrogate, may wish to forego a diagnostic workup if they have already decided that they would not act on that information even if it was positive for disease. For example, a 90-year-old patient with multiple other medical conditions may decide to forego a biopsy of a lung lesion, having decided that she would not agree to surgery, radiation, or chemotherapy.

Many interventions other than those traditionally referred to as invasive are now requiring formal informed consent. The use of physical and chemical restraints in psychiatric and long-term care settings requires documentation of acceptance either by the patient or a surrogate. Appropriately informing patients of the meaning (i.e., positive and negative predictive value) of screening tests has been a recent focus, especially for cancer screening, in view of the patients' prognosis and preferences.

The corollary to a patient's right to informed consent is their right to decline treatment. In the 1991 case, *Cruzan v. the State of Missouri* the US Supreme Court ruled that patients have a right to refuse interventions and expanded this to include the right to refuse treatment for future care [13]. Chief Justice William H. Rehnquist wrote that a competent patient has a "constitutionally protected liberty interest in refusing unwanted treatment." The ethical conflict that the practitioners find themselves in is between the autonomous right of the patient to choose and practitioner's wish to do what they see as beneficent or nonmaleficent. This conflict often causes discomfort in the clinical setting. For example, a patient may choose to decline the repair of an abdominal aortic aneurysm despite what the physician knows is a very high risk of rupture and death.

The patient may decline a treatment before the intervention has been initiated or after it has been instituted. There is no legal or ethical distinction made between discontinuing and not initiating the same intervention [14], although frequently there is a stronger emotional component to the former. For example, if a patient has end-stage kidney disease and opts to forego dialysis, he or she will die from uremia. If patients who have been on dialysis for a period of time decide to stop dialysis, they too will die from their kidney disease.

Two areas often present a particular difficulty in the clinical setting: the discontinuation of ventilatory support and the discontinuing or noninitiation of artificial food or hydration. The discontinuation of ventilatory support parallels that of dialysis. The intervention has been instituted to maintain the patient through artificial means because of the failure of a vital organ to function. The patient will die from the effects of the underlying disease and resultant organ failure [15]. The conflicts cited in the case of discontinuation of ventilatory support are threefold: (1) that it is an active act (an act of commission) versus a passive act (act of omission) causing the demise of the patient; (2) that the proximity of the action to the death of the patient causes discomfort for the person stopping the ventilator; and (3) that the physician may not have a comfort level with palliation of the symptoms that may occur when ventilatory support is discontinued.

Much has been made of the arguments of "passive" versus "active" acts. Neither the legal nor the ethical literature supports it as a valid distinction [1], but it can make a major difference in the physician's level of comfort. Although the proximity of an action to the patient's death is uncomfortable for the physician, the need to discontinue invasive treatments for a patient who does not desire them is the more compelling duty. Being familiar with a routine of dignity and comfort care at the time of withdrawal of ventilatory support is crucial.

Discontinuing or foregoing artificial food or hydration in a dying patient also may cause discomfort on the part of physicians or patients' families, but not necessarily to the patients themselves [16]. Neither nutrition nor fluid support is necessary for comfort care, and there is evidence that fluids near the end of life cause discomfort by increasing secretions and suppressing the patient's endogenous endorphin responses. The duty to withhold artificial food and hydration if it is the patient's wish has been upheld in both state and federal courts and was confirmed in the *Cruzan* case. See the section below on "Decisions Near the End of Life" for more discussion of this topic.

Assessment of Decisional Capacity

Decisional capacity refers to the patients' ability to understand the consequences of the decision they are making, to make that decision, and to communicate the reasons for the decision. Understanding the consequences of the decision includes both the ability to understand the relevant information and to appreciate the situation and the impact of the decision [17, 18] (Table 14.4). Decisional capacity is decision specific, i.e., there are different standards of decisional ability needed to make different types of decisions (e.g., medical or financial) as well as different levels of complexity involved in the decision (e.g., simple procedure versus a complex procedure).

The ability to understand may be impaired because of temporary conditions such as delirium, transient coma, intoxication, or depression; or it may be permanently impaired by cognitive damage or psychiatric illness. Whatever the cause of the impairment, the key to the determination of capacity is the patient's ability to comprehend the advantages and disadvantages of treatment options and to make a decision. Whether we believe that the patient's decision is rational is not a determinant of capacity. Our society allows people to make what most would label as "irrational" decisions but, as part of our respect for autonomy, we cannot force what we would see as the right decision on others [19]. For example, we cannot prohibit alcoholics from drinking, even when it has been shown to impair their health or shorten their longevity. Patients' religious or ethnic beliefs may conflict strongly with our own beliefs, but they have the right to refuse any treatment option they believe is in conflict with their beliefs.

TABLE 14.4 Legally relevant criteria for decision-making capacity and approaches to assessment of the patient

Criterion	Patient's task	Physician's assessment approach	Questions for clinical assessment*	Comments
Communicate a choice	Clearly indicate preferred treatment option	Ask patient to indicate a treatment choice	Have you decided whether to follow your doctor's [or my] recommendation for treatment? Can you tell me what that decision is? [If no decision] What is making it hard for you to decide?	Frequent reversals of choice because of psychiatric or neurologic conditions may indicate lack of capacity
Understand the relevant information	Grasp the fundamental meaning of information communicated by physician	Encourage patient to paraphrase disclosed information regarding medical condition and treatment	Please tell me in your own words what your doctor [or I] told you about: The problem with your health now The recommended treatment The possible benefits and risks (or discomforts) of the treatment Any alternative treatments and their risks and benefits The risks and benefits of no treatment	Information to be understood includes nature of patient's condition, nature and purpose of proposed treatment, possible benefits and risks of that treatment, and alternative approaches (including no treatment) and their benefits and risks
Appreciate the situation and its consequences	Acknowledge medical condition and likely consequences of treatment options	Ask patient to describe the views of medical condition, proposed treatment, and likely outcomes	What do you believe is wrong with your health now? Do you believe that you need some kind of treatment? What is the treatment likely to do for you? What makes you believe it will have that effect? What do you believe will happen if you are not treated? Why do you think your doctor has [or I have] recommended this treatment?	Courts have recognized that patients who do not acknowledge their illnesses (often referred to as "lack of insight") cannot make valid decisions about treatment Delusions or pathologic levels of distortion or denial are the most common causes of impairment
Reason about treatment options	Engage in a rational process of manipulating the relevant information	Ask patient to compare treatment options and consequences and to offer reasons for selection of option	How did you decide to accept or reject the recommended treatment? What makes [chosen option] better than [alternative option]?	This criterion focuses on the process by which a decision is reached, not the outcome of the patient's choice, since patients have the right to make "unreasonable" choices

Source: Appelbaum [18] Copyright © 2007 Massachusetts Medical Society. All rights reserved

*Patients' responses to these questions need not be verbal

On the other hand, understanding the patient's goals and preferences, their priorities as they age, is of fundamental importance to helping the physician to be comfortable and understand the decisions a patient may make as well as giving them the appropriate options from which to choose. Respect for each individual's unique point of view, needs, and desires is fundamental not just for respecting their autonomy, but for truly doing no harm with and maximizing the benefit of interventions.

Every physician obtaining informed consent should be able to do a basic assessment of decisional capacity. The physician should be able to diagnose delirium and, if needed, assess basic cognitive function. Tools focused on parietal lobe function, as do many of the commonly used cognitive mental status tests, are relatively poor predictors of the ability to make decisions, per se, but instruments that have a larger emphasis on frontal lobe or executive function, such as the clock drawing and other executive function examinations, may be more useful. What is most important is the physician's thoughtful discussion with the patient and the real-time assessment of the patients' understanding of the consequences of the decision they are making. Since the standard for decisional capacity is situation specific, it is important that one is able to assess their ability to understand the level of information needed for the decision at hand.

There are many other decisions that a patient may need to make other than informed consent where their capacity will need to be assessed and differing standards met. For example, a very high standard for decisional capacity must be met for a patient to agree to participate in a research study [20, 21], whereas a very low standard is applied to their ability to make a last will and testament. Of particular concern to the clinician is deciding whether patients retain the ability to decide on care options and whether they can return home or need a more intense environment in order to remain safe [22, 23] (Table 14.5) [24].

If the physician is unsure of a patient's capacity, a psychiatric consultation may be requested if the question arises from a psychiatric illness; or a neuropsychologist or geriatrician may be consulted about cognitive or functional problems. The patient's decisional capacity at the time of any decision, whether they decide to accept treatment or to decline treatment, should be recorded in the medical record.

Competence is a term that has legal implications beyond what a physician judges on examination. Physicians should avoid using this term unless a court has ruled on the patient's competence. The court recognizes two major categories of competence; competence for financial decisions and competence to make decisions of person. Only if the court has ruled the individual to be incompetent *of person* should the individual be assumed to lack decisional capacity for medical decisions.

Decision-Making for Incapacitated Patients (Table 14.6)

If a patient is found to lack the capacity to make an informed decision, a surrogate decision maker must be identified. The principle of autonomy guides us to seek a surrogate who is the person most capable of representing the patient's wishes. If the patient has completed an Advance Directive that names a proxy decision maker, this is the person to whom questions should be deferred if the patient has lost decisional capacity. This designee may be variously referred to as the Durable Power of Attorney for Health Affairs or the Health Care Proxy, Surrogate, or Agent. It needs to be emphasized that this person can only make decisions for the patient if the patient no longer has decisional capacity. A patient may also choose a person in a less formal manner, and documentation of such a choice should help to guide the decision. A person who holds Power of Attorney for Finances does not, simply by having this limited power of attorney, have the ability to make other decisions for the person.

If the patient's choice of surrogate is not known, usually the next-of-kin is utilized. The hierarchy of authority is

TABLE 14.5 Levels of decisional capacity

Medical decisions

Ability to understand relevant information
Ability to understand the consequences of the decision
Ability to communicate a decision

Research subject

Ability to understand the probability of a lack of benefit
Appreciation of risks and the uncertainty of the risks
Appreciate their right to withdraw from the study

Decisions of self-care

Ability to care for oneself *or*
Ability to accept the needed help to keep oneself safe

Finances

Ability to manage bill payment
Ability to appropriately calculate and monitor funds

Last will and testament

Ability to remember estate plans
Ability to express logic behind choices

Source: Modified from [24]

TABLE 14.6 Hierarchy of decision-making

Patient's current wishes

If the patient has decisional capacity, this ALWAYS takes precedence

Substituted judgment

Done by the surrogate decision maker only when the patient is not fully capable of making the decision
Based on the patient's prior values and wishes
Advance directive is used as a guide
Patient input is used when possible even if the patient is not fully capable of making the decision

Beneficence

Done by the surrogate decision maker when the patient lacks decisional capacity and evidence does not exist for substituted judgment
Weighing of benefits and burdens as based on the patient's present indications of pleasures and burdens
Input from caregivers is very important

Source: Modified from [24]

spouse, adult children, parents, siblings, nieces, or nephews. Adult friends may sometimes be able to act as surrogate if the relationship with the patient is such that they can act on his or her behalf. If it is thought that the person identified by this procedure cannot, in fact, act as an appropriate surrogate, if there is conflict about identifying a decision maker, if there is a lack of consensus among individuals, or if there is no one to take on this role, the court may need to decide who will act for the patient. In emergent situations, where the decision-making process is unclear, physicians should apply the "best interest rule" and proceed with any interventions necessary to save the patient's life or preserve function until the situation is clarified. Each institution may have different procedures for obtaining such permission to act, such as an agreement to act by the Chief of Staff. If there is time, emergency conservatorship from a court can be sought. As the situation and the patient's wishes become clear, and an intervention that had been started as an emergency procedure is found to be against the patient's wishes, then the intervention must be discontinued.

The task of making the decision for the incapacitated patient should honor the patient's autonomy by maximizing the individual's continued influence on the ultimate decision. If a patient gave explicit directives that apply to the situation at hand at a time when he or she was capable of decision-making, they must be followed. For example, if a patient with a terminal illness requests that no further interventions be done, including artificial food and hydration, a family member cannot reverse this directive once the patient is in a coma.

If patients have not been explicit about their wishes, the surrogate decision maker and the physician are then obliged to apply substituted judgment. This term is defined as "the application of the patient's preferences and values … trying to choose as the patient would have wanted" [25]. In studies comparing hypothetical decisions made by would-be surrogates and patients with decisional capacity, there is a 66% correlation. Previous discussions between the patient and the surrogate help to make these decisions much more representative of the patient's wishes [26]. Helping a family to understand that their obligation is to do what their relative would have wanted often relieves them of some of the burden of decision-making and helps clarify their thinking. Living Wills may be useful in this context. Living Wills may be formal documents executed by a lawyer, but they may also be readily available forms completed by the patient with or without assistance or simply a written statement or narrative. If patients are still capable of making decisions, all treatments must still be discussed with them even if they have a Living Will.

The Living Will is a "what if" statement – a hypothetical situation. The patient is saying, "*If* one of these conditions occurs to me (e.g., permanent coma), *then* do not attempt resuscitation." It does not necessarily mean that the patient does not desire this intervention in their present state of health. For example, a patient who is fully capable of making decisions has a Living Will that states that he or she would decline resuscitation if in a vegetative state. If this patient was to have a cardiac arrest in their present state, resuscitation should be attempted. If after the resuscitation the patient is found to be vegetative, the Living Will would take effect and no further resuscitation attempts should be made were the patient to arrest again.

Frequently, the exact circumstances outlined in a Living Will are not met, but it can still give a good indication of the patient's preferences and values, which then can be applied to the current situation [27]. Living Wills cannot cover all circumstances that may arise, and most patients wish to have a proxy decision maker to interpret their intent. State laws vary as to whether the Living Will or the proxy decision maker takes precedence when there is a conflict with the decisions. Encouraging the family to remember other health care decisions or comments the patient made when other family members were ill is also helpful in trying to define what someone "would have said."

If there is no information that helps the surrogate decision maker to reconstruct what the patient would have said, the guiding principle becomes that of beneficence, defined as weighing the benefits, risks, and burdens of an intervention in the context of the individual. With beneficence, although a patient may no longer be fully capable of making a decision, their voice can still be an important one. Their stated preferences and fears can be used to guide the decision about relative benefits and burdens [28]. This can be true for even markedly demented patients.

For example, the relative burden of an intervention in two patients, equally cognitively impaired, can be quite different. One patient may not become agitated when an intravenous line is started, and intravenous treatment would not be a great burden. Another patient may fight such an intervention, repeatedly pulling out the intravenous catheter and needing restraints. Although the second patient is not making an informed decision to forego intravenous therapy, the relative burden of the intervention is greater in this patient and therefore the relative benefit would need to be greater than other less noxious alternatives for the burden/benefit ratio to be the same.

There can, at times, be conflicting interests in adhering to this hierarchy as circumstances change and the patient's condition alters what is a burden and what is a benefit. Surrogate decision-making often uses a combination of substituted judgment and beneficence to arrive at a treatment decision [29]. What is most important is that these discussions occur as they can have major impact both on patients' quality of life and on the bereavement adjustment of the relatives [30].

As previously stated, decisional capacity is decision specific and capacity is often not black or white. Utilizing an Assent/Consent modal is commonly being accepted.

This allows for different levels of patient involvement in the decision-making process. If the patient seems to be capable of making the decision but, due to memory problems or waxing and waning mental status, there is some question as to their ability to retain information, the family may be asked for their "assent," i.e., they agree that it is what the patient wants. If the patient cannot make the decision, the family may give the formal consent but the patient may need to "assent" in order to carry out the procedure. For example, a family may consent to chemotherapy but the patient must be willing to cooperate. The consent/assent modal balances the prior statements of the patient (future-looking autonomy) with beneficence for the person they are at this moment in time [31].

DNR Orders in the Operating Room

A patient's previously stated wish to forego intubation or attempts to resuscitate may be suspended at the time a patient undergoes surgery. Elective intubation in order to perform surgery or a cardiac arrest that occurs under general anesthesia where an immediate response is possible and where the cause may be readily reversible is different from a cardiopulmonary arrest under other circumstances. It may therefore be perfectly compatible with a patient's goals to have these procedures done in the operating room but not want them initiated in other circumstances. Indeed, intubation may be necessary if a procedure which the person does desire is to occur.

If a decision is made to reverse a do-not-resuscitate or do-not-intubate order during surgery, there must be a clear understanding prior to surgery of how postoperative events should be handled in case the patient is not then capable of making decisions. How long should an intubation continue if the patient is not quickly able to be extubated? If the patient does arrest and is resuscitated but has lost decisional capacity, what other treatment modalities would be an unwanted burden? Discussions with the patient, surgeon, anesthesiologist, and primary care physician can help safeguard against confusing and distressful situations [32].

Confidentiality

The Health Insurance Portability and Accountability Act (HIPAA) of 1996 has greatly enhanced the confidentiality of written records and communications [33]. It has also impacted verbal communication, but not to the same extent.

Sharing information with patients' relatives or friends is appropriate in only two circumstances: when patients have specifically stated that the physician may discuss their condition with the individual or when the patient has lost decisional capacity and a surrogate decision must be made. It is advisable to ask patients well in advance who they wish to have informed and how much they wish to have told.

The sharing of information among colleagues should be done in private and with respect for the patient's right to confidentiality. Casual conversations in public places, rounds in the hallways, and discussions in lobbies or waiting rooms with multiple families present can be a breach of a patient's right to privacy. Our sensitivity to this issue must be heightened, and the policing of each other should become everyone's responsibility.

Sharing medical information among health care providers without the patient's explicit authorization, if the clinical circumstances so require, is permitted. The use of clinical material for teaching purposes can be done only with sufficient safeguards to anonymity so the individuals involved are not identifiable. Other information can be released only with the patient's or surrogate's authorization unless it is required by law, as in the case of public health reporting of communicable and sexually transmitted diseases.

Limits to Autonomy and Choice (Futility)

The previous sections have dealt heavily with the respect for and safeguards of the patient's right to exercise autonomy. There are circumstances where this autonomy is tempered by other forces. Autonomy may be limited if the patient is a danger to others, a danger to self, or for the good of society. Laws may govern what procedures or interventions may be available to an individual. For instance, physician-assisted suicide is explicitly illegal in most states in the USA.

Although the US Supreme Court has affirmed an individual's right to refuse treatment, there is no corollary right to demand treatment [34]. In addition to the healthcare professionals' responsibility to understand the patient's goals of treatment and respect patient's own assessment of their quality of life, they also have the responsibility of knowing if an intervention is futile and not offering such treatments to the patient.

There are two perspectives on the definition of futility; referred to as quantitative and qualitative. An intervention is said to be quantitatively futile if it cannot achieve its physiologic objective. Because it is difficult to know what level of evidence is needed for what cut-off to call something physiologically futile, this concept has limited utility. A therapy is said to be qualitatively futile if it is unlikely to help patients achieve their primary goal even if it has a physiologic effect [35, 36]. An example is the foregoing of antibiotic therapy in a patient who is in the terminal phase of an illness. Although the antibiotics might have the physiologic effect of treating the infection, it would have no effect on comfort and a negative effect if it prolongs the patient's suffering. This concept, of futility in the light of the treatment goals, is paramount to the appropriate treatment of the geriatric patient.

If a procedure is judged futile, the physician does not have to offer the intervention to the patient or the surrogate. The very act of offering conveys the sense that there must be some benefit, some chance of success. Why else would it be offered? Therapies the patient and family might expect to have performed but that have become futile, such as an attempt to resuscitate a patient when circumstances clearly demonstrate that it would be futile, should be discussed in the context of their futility. For example, the patient or family should be told that where the patient's heart to stop, attempts to restart it would be futile and therefore would not be initiated. Simply ignoring the subject may engender mistrust, as most individuals are aware of the spectrum of treatments available. One in 20 patients who die in the ICU do not have a surrogate decision maker. The majority of the time physicians decide to cease life-sustaining interventions on the basis of their futility [37].

Defining a therapy as futile is simple under some circumstances and more difficult under others. The decision that someone is "not a surgical candidate" is frequently made when the relative risks and benefits clearly demonstrate that the treatment is not indicated. The decision to stop a therapy may also be made on the grounds of professional judgment. For example, if a tumor is not responding to chemotherapy, it can be unilaterally stopped by the clinician. The difficulty lies more in defining which therapies near the end of life still hold enough of an advantage for the patient that they should be offered.

Prognostication

In order for patients to be able to set goals, they need to be able to understand their prognosis and how interventions may or may not change that prognosis. Unfortunately, we are not very accurate in being able to prognosticate. Being able to predict short-term mortality in the acute care and intensive care unit setting has been explored through the SUPPORT Study [38] and through the use of the APACHE III instrument [39]. These instruments use a combination of diagnosis, cause of illness, and a scale for physiologic parameters to predict mortality risk, but the ability to apply them clinically remains a challenge [40]. The patients' physical and cognitive function prior to their hospitalization is the strongest predictors of outcome after an intervention [41].

Such legislative acts as the Medicare Hospice Benefits, and the Oregon Death with Dignity Act define the terminal phases of disease as the last 6 months of life. Our ability to accurately prognosticate this length of time is relatively poor, with only one-third of predictions being within 50% confidence intervals (i.e., if prognosis is 3 months, "accurate" would be from 1.5 to 6 months). Most physician prognoses are too optimistic [42].

Individuals in their eighth and ninth decades may define their goals similarly to patients with terminal diagnoses. Quality of life and relief from the burdens of illness and interventions may be more important than longevity per se. On the other hand, it should not be assumed that this is true for all individuals of advanced age. Although some elderly patients may look forward to more years of life, they may not wish to do so under any or all circumstances. In surveys of patients with and without terminal illnesses about why they might be motivated to avail themselves of physician-assisted suicide, fear of disability and dependence are the two most common motivators for wishing to end one's life. Predicting the risk or progression of disability is even more difficult than predicting death [43].

Decisions Near the End of Life

As has been emphasized in previous sections of this chapter, goal-oriented care is of the utmost importance to all geriatric care, but it is the sine quo non of end of life care. When a patient has a terminal illness or is faced with chronic, disabling, and progressive disease, decision-making must become very goal-focused. We have already discussed foregoing and discontinuing interventions when they no longer meet the goals of care. Treatment of suffering, physical, mental emotional or spiritual may lead to actions where the physician is seen as hastening death, either inadvertently or deliberately.

The potential for hastening the death of a patient is highest where there is a narrow therapeutic window between the dose of medication needed to control a symptom and the dose that could cause suppression of respiratory drive. The underlying ethical principle of "double effect" rests on the physician's intention and an acknowledgement that treatment may have two effects: one on symptoms and one on longevity. This is an acceptable risk to take if the physician and patient or surrogate have agreed that comfort is more important than longevity and the medica-tion or treatment is given with the *intention* of relieving symptoms.

At some point in the patient's clinical course, interventions that we normally think of as prolonging life may have shifted to prolonging death. An example of this may be antibiotics for pneumonia. The symptoms of pneumonia can be treated (e.g., with scopolamine to control secretions and morphine for dyspnea) without treating the underlying pathophysiology of the pneumonia. Since every patient will, eventually, die of something, there comes a time when it makes sense to allow the clinical course to determine the mode of death. Aggressively treating the symptoms is often preferable to a prolonged dying process with the occurrence of increasingly hard-to-control symptoms.

Physician-assisted suicide and euthanasia (physician-assisted death) are instances when a therapy is prescribed, provided, or administered with the *intention* of ending that patient's life. The acceptability of such actions from both a moral and a practical point of view is under wide debate within the profession and in society in general. Those who argue for the practice of physician-assisted death point out that there are some symptoms that cannot be alleviated short of death (e.g., the discomfort and indignity of destructive head and neck cancer), and individuals should have the right to determine the time and mode of their death. Arguments against physicians assisting in suicide point out that the medical profession's obligation is to "care and to cure" and not to end life [44]. The four principles of autonomy, nonmaleficence, beneficence, and justice are active parts of this debate. Some argue that out of respect for autonomy, individuals should be allowed to determine the time and mode of their death, especially if it is within the last 6 months of their "natural" lives. Others argue that if there is unbearable suffering that cannot be relieved by other means, then the principle of beneficence tells us that they should be allowed to end their lives. Many feel that physicians prescribing or acting with the intent of ending a patient's life would be professionally wrong because it would mean intentionally doing harm to the patient (nonmaleficence). Finally, many fear that the practice will be a "slippery slope" leading to the premature death of certain segments of society such as the elderly and the disabled. As of now, physician-assisted dying is legal in two states in the USA (Oregon and Washington) and many countries in Europe. Although the debate remains open, the fear of abuse has not proven to be a reality in any locale where it is legal, where it has remained a small minority of patients (less than 5% of deaths) who decide to actively end their lives.

Conclusion

As an individual ages and the accumulation of both life experience and illness burden increase, decisions need to be made on the basis of the individual's goals and preferences. Patients need to be informed of their situation, their prognosis and their options as best we can define them. They have a right to decide their course of action within choices that are not futile and they have a right to influence decisions made for them if they have become incapacitated. Weighing autonomy and

beneficence is often hard for the patient who has lost the ability to make decisions. Finding appropriate surrogate decision makers and helping them to understand their role is paramount to this process.

References

1. Beauchamp TL, Childress JF (2009) Principles of biomedical ethics, 6th edn. Oxford University Press, New York, NY, p 15
2. Blackhall LJ, Murphy ST, Frank G, Michel V, Azen S (1995) Ethnicity and attitudes toward patient autonomy. JAMA 274:820–825
3. Fitts WT, Ravdin IS (1953) What Philadelphia physicians tell patients with cancer. JAMA 153:901–904
4. Oken D (1961) What to tell cancer patients: a study of medical attitudes. JAMA 175:1120–1128
5. Novack DH, Olumer R, Smith RL, Ochitill H, Morrow GR, Bennett JM (1979) Changes in physicians' attitudes toward telling the cancer patient. JAMA 241:897–900
6. Drickamer MA, Lachs LS (1992) Should patients with Alzheimer's disease be told their diagnosis? N Engl J Med 336:947–951
7. Drickamer MA, Lachs LS (1993) Telling the diagnosis of Alzheimer's disease. N Engl J Med 328:442
8. Braddock CH, Edwards KA, Hasenber NM, Laidley TL, Levinson W (1999) Informed decision making in outpatient practice: time to get back to basics. JAMA 282:2313–2320
9. Epstein RM, Alper BS, Quill TE (2004) Communicating evidence for participatory decision making. JAMA 291:2359–2366
10. Ford S, Scofield T, Hope T (2003) What are the ingredients for a successful evidence-based patient choice consultation? A qualitative study. Soc Sci Med 56:589–602
11. Meisel A, Kuczewski M (1996) Legal and ethical myths about informed consent. Arch Intern Med 156:2521–2526
12. Fried TR, McGraw S, Agostini J, Tinetti ME (2008) Views of older persons with multiple morbidities on competing outcomes and clinical decision-making. J Am Geriatr Soc 56(10):1839–1944
13. Lo B, Steinbrook R (1991) Beyond the Cruzan case: the U.S. Supreme Court and medical practice. Ann Intern Med 114:895–901
14. Calvert GM, Hornung RW, Sweeney MH, Fingerhut MA, Halperin WE (1992) Hepatic and gastrointestinal effects in an occupational cohort exposed to 2, 3, 7, 8-tetrachlorodibenzo-para-dioxin. JAMA 267(16):2209–2214
15. Schneiderman LJ, Spragg RG (1988) Ethical decisions in discontinuing mechanical ventilation. N Engl J Med 318:984–988
16. Sullivan RJ (1993) Accepting death without artificial nutrition or hydration. J Gen Intern Med 8:220–224
17. Applebaum PS, Grisso T (1988) Assessing patients' capacities to consent to treatment. N Engl J Med 319:1635–1638
18. Appelbaum PS (2007) Assessment of patients' competence to consent to treatment. N Engl J Med 357:1834–1840
19. Brock DW, Wartman SA (1990) When competent patients make irrational choices. N Engl J Med 322:1595–1599
20. Jefferson AL, Lambe S, Moser DJ, Byerly LK, Ozonoff A, Karlawish JH (2008) Decisional capacity for research participation individuals with mild cognitive impairment. J Am Geriatr Soc 56:1236–1243
21. Stocking CB, Hougham GW, Danner DD, Patterson MB, Whitehouse PJ, Sachs GA (2008) Variable judgements of decisional capacity in cognitively impaired research subjects. J Am Geriatr Soc 56:1893–1897
22. Naik AD, Teal CR, Pavlik VN, Dyer CB, McCullougy LB (2008) Conceptual challenges and practical approaches to screen capacity

for self-care and protection in vulnerable older adults. Geriatr Soc 56:S266–S270

23. Lai J, Karlawish J (2007) Assessing the capacity to make everyday decisions: a guide for clinicians and an agenda for future research. Am J Geriatr Psychiatry 15(2):101–111

24. Drickamer MA (2009) Legal and ethical issues. In: Pacala JT, Sullivan GM (eds) Geriatric review syllabus: a core curriculum in geriatric medicine, 7th edn. American Geriatrics Society, New York, NY

25. Hastings Center (1987) Guidelines on the termination of life-sustaining treatment and the care of the dying. Indiana University Press, Bloomington, IN

26. Sulmasy DP, Terry PB, Weisman CS, Miller EJ, Stallings RY, Vettese MA, Haller KB (1998) The accuracy of substituted judgments in patients with terminal diagnoses. Ann Intern Med 128:621–629

27. Schneiderman LJ, Pearlman RA, Kaplan RM et al (1992) Relationship of general advance directive instructions to specific life-sustaining treatment preferences in patients with serious illness. Arch Intern Med 152:2114–2122

28. AGS Ethics Committee (1996) Making treatment decisions for incapacitated older adults without advance directives. J Am Geriatr Soc 44:986–987

29. Berger JT, DeRenzo EG, Schwartz J (2008) Surrogate decision making: reconciling ethical theory and clinical practice. Ann Intern Med 149:48–53

30. Wright AA, Zhang B, Ray A, Mack JW, Trice E, Balboni T et al (2008) Associations between end-of-life discussions, patient mental health, medical care near death, and caregiver bereavement adjustment. JAMA 300:1665–1673

31. Smyer M, Schaie KW, Kapp MB (eds) (1996) Older adults' decision making and the law. Springer, New York, NY

32. Walker RM (1991) DNR in the OR: resuscitation as an operative risk. JAMA 266:2407–2412

33. Gostin LO (2001) National health information privacy regulations under the Health Insurance Portability and Accountability Act. JAMA 285:3015–3021

34. Quill TE, Brody H (1996) Physician recommendations and patient autonomy: finding a balance between physician power and patient choice. Ann Intern Med 125:763–769

35. Schneiderman LJ (1994) The futility debate: effective versus beneficial intervention. J Am Geriatr Soc 42:883–886

36. Schneiderman LJ, Jecker NS, Jonsen AR (1996) Medical futility: response to critiques. Ann Intern Med 125:669–674

37. White DB, Curtis R, Wolf LE, Predergast TJ et al (2007) Life support for patients without a surrogate decision maker: who decides? Ann Intern Med 147:34–40

38. Knaus WA, Harrell FE, Lynn J et al (1995) The SUPPORT prognostic model. Objective estimates of survival for seriously ill hospitalized adults. Ann Intern Med 122:191–203

39. Knaus WA, Wagner DP, Draper EA et al (1991) The APACHE III prognostic system: risk predication of hospital mortality for critically ill hospitalized adults. Chest 100:1619–1636

40. Lynn J, Teno JM, Harrell FE Jr (1995) Accurate prognostication of death: opportunities and challenges for clinicians. West J Med 163:250–257

41. Teno JM, Harrell FE, Knaus W, Phillips RS, Wu AW et al (2000) Prediction of survival for older hospitalized patients: The HELP survival model. J Am Geriatr Soc 48:S16–S24

42. Christakis NA, Lamont EB (2000) Extent and determinants of error in doctors' prognoses in terminally ill patients: prospective cohort study. BMJ 320:469–473

43. Wu AW, Yasui Y, Alzola C, Galanos AN et al (2000) Predicting functional status outcomes in hospitalized patients aged 80 years and older. J Am Geriatr Soc 48:S6–S15

44. Quill TE, Meier DE, Blovk S, Billings A (1998) The debate over physician assisted suicide: empirical data and convergent views. Ann Intern Med 128:552

Chapter 15
Teaching Geriatrics to Surgeons

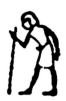

Hugh L. Willcox III, Darin L. Passer, and Richard M. Bell

Introduction

The 1970s is considered by many as the rise of geriatrics as a specialty – what Solomon refers to as the beginning of the "geriatrics renaissance." [1] At that time, a few individuals recognized the need for improved care of the elderly and the opportunity for a specialty to encompass its principles. Over time, geriatrics has grown into a recognized branch of medicine that has its own society, multiple journals, thousands of fellows, and hundreds of teaching attendings. Now, the ideals that led to this renaissance are spreading into the surgical and medical subspecialties. However, this growth is meeting with some resistance. Many surgeons have the attitude of "I already know how to take care of older patients – that's half of my practice." And, many do take care of the aged patient well. However, improvement in the care of the elderly can be realized through utilization of the available resources discussed in this chapter.

Like the pediatric patient, the geriatric patient is unique. The development of a curriculum addressing the perioperative care of the elderly surgical patient needs to embrace the fact that the normal end points of therapy should be adjusted to a population that is nearing the end of life. These patients respond differently and unpredictably to interventions that have been tested primarily on younger patients.

With the work hour restrictions firmly in place and potentially subject to further limitations, one of the challenges facing surgical residency program directors is how to incorporate all that has been the traditional purview of the general surgeon. The addition of new information, including the principles of geriatric care for the surgical patient, complicates the issue. Fortunately, many tools already exist. The John A. Hartford Foundation, the Donald W. Reynolds Foundation, and the American Geriatrics Society in particular have invested time and money for the development of programs to increase the exposure of surgical residents to geriatric issues.

The goal of this chapter is to serve as a reference for program directors and academicians as they begin modifying their own curriculum by integrating geriatric issues. What follows is a summary of the available resources and content that may be helpful for teaching geriatrics to surgeons.

Assessment of Need

"What makes me mad is how aging, in our language and culture, is equated with deterioration and impairment. I don't know how we're going to root that out, except by making people more aware of it." – Dr. Erdman Palmore from an interview with the Detroit News, September 5, 2004.

Though the assertion may be made that every surgical resident needs more exposure to geriatrics issues, determining what barriers exist, particularly in the form of subtle, and sometimes not so subtle, "ageism," is essential when targeting learners for a change in curriculum. Assessing the attitudes of the individual residents will help program directors delineate existing barriers to learning about geriatric issues and to maximize the benefit gained from changes to their curriculum.

Palmore's publication "The Facts on Aging Quiz" in 1977 is considered by many the landmark effort to address the issue of attitudes towards aging. His survey has been modified by many authors, and additional attitude assessment tools have been developed. Although these have been tested mostly on primary-care residents, they are applicable to residents in the surgical and medical subspecialties.

Palmore's survey has been updated, most recently by Breytspraak et al., of the University of Missouri-Kansas City, and can be found at the web site http://cas.umkc.edu/cas/AgingFactsQuiz.htm. Debate continues as to whether Palmore's tool and subsequent iterations are valid for research purposes, but the qualification of learner attitude should be helpful when developing a curriculum [2].

H.L. Willcox III (✉)
Department of General Surgery,
Palmetto Health Richland Hospital,
2 Medical Park, Columbia, SC 29203, USA
e-mail: hugh_willcox@yahoo.com

R.A. Rosenthal et al. (eds.), *Principles and Practice of Geriatric Surgery*,
DOI 10.1007/978-1-4419-6999-6_15, © Springer Science+Business Media, LLC 2011

Table 15.1 UCLA Geriatrics Attitude Scale (GAS): answers using the Likert scale 1 to 5

1. Most old people are pleasant to be with
2. The federal government should reallocate money from Medicare to research on AIDS or pediatric disease
3. If I have the choice, I would rather see younger patients than elderly ones
4. It is society's responsibility to provide care for its elderly persons
5. Medical care for older people uses up too much human and material resources
6. As people grow older, they become less organized and more confused
7. Elderly patients tend to be more appreciative of the medical care I provide than are younger patients
8. Taking a medical history from elderly patients is frequently an ordeal
9. I tend to pay more attention to and have more sympathy for my elderly patients than my younger patients
10. Old people in general do not contribute much to society
11. Treatment of chronically ill old patients is hopeless
12. Old persons do not contribute their fair share towards paying for their health care
13. In general, older people act too slow for modern society
14. It is interesting listening to old people's accounts of their past experiences

1 = Strongly disagree, 2 = somewhat disagree, 3 = neutral, 4 = somewhat agree, 5 = strongly agree

Table 15.2 University of Michigan's Geriatrics Clinical Decision Making Assessment quiz topics

1. Postoperative pain management
2. Constipation
3. Metastatic abdominal pain
4. Analgesia in presence of confusion
5. Assessment of in-hospital mortality
6. Competency and patient wishes
7. Delirium diagnosis
8. Reducing subsequent hospital utilization
9. Causes of incontinence
10. Medical management-only requests
11. Recognition of depression
12. Prevalence of mood disorders
13. Elder abuse suspicion
14. Postoperative respiratory distress
15. Return of ambulatory function predictors
16. Evaluation of syncope
17. Foot pain following immobility
18. Postoperative delirium and agitation
19. Medication-induced acute renal insufficiency
20. Evaluation of alcohol withdrawal

A lengthy and more detailed survey was constructed by Maxwell and Sullivan in 1980 [3]. Subsets of questions from this survey have been abstracted, decreasing the length of the survey but hopefully maintaining the accuracy of the responses to quantify an individual's attitude regarding the elderly.

Another commonly used and validated assessment tool for determining the attitude of a resident towards geriatric issues is the UCLA Geriatrics Attitude Scale (GAS) [4]. Like the Maxwell and Sullivan survey, the GAS uses the Likert scale but consists only of 14 questions. Initially published in 1998, Dr. Reuben and colleagues have evaluated this device for validity and reproducibility, publishing their results in 2005 [5] (see Table 15.1).

Once the attitude of the residents towards the elderly have been established, determining the geriatrics knowledge base of the residents can provide a starting point for program directors when making curriculum changes. In order to better gauge what that knowledge base is, the University of Michigan has developed a questionnaire consisting of 20 items that range from acute abdominal pain to palliative-care options and appropriate pain control. This test can be found at http://www.med.umich.edu/geriatrics/educationalprograms/gme.htm. Table 15.2 lists the topics covered by this test.

Krain et al. from the University of Michigan utilized the UCLA's Geriatrics Attitude Scale and the University of Michigan's Geriatrics Clinical Decision Making Assessment tools to determine the effectiveness of their faculty

development program [6]. The program was designed to increase the knowledge and to improve the attitude of the nonprimary-care residents towards the elderly. This was accomplished by identifying faculty within the nonprimary-care departments and giving them resources to incorporate geriatric issues into their curriculum. The program demonstrated an improvement in both knowledge and attitude toward the aged.

Establishing the attitude and knowledge of the residents prior to initiating any new curricular changes, and then measuring the effects of the interventions, can help guide whether the changes were successful or other changes are needed. Additionally, these tools can be used in completing research, as shown by Krain et al. [6].

Integrating Geriatrics into a General Surgery Curriculum

Many difficulties exist to insert geriatrics into an already overloaded general surgery curriculum. What is the best approach? What is sufficient time and coverage? How do you assess the effectiveness of the modality chosen? While there are many different approaches and tools such as didactic lectures in multiple formats, small group discussion tools, case-based simulation, and others, how best to integrate these tools into the tight educational schedule is a challenge.

To try to help surgical and medically related training programs (Emergency Medicine, Anesthesia, and Physical Medicine and Rehabilitation) meet this challenge, the

American Geriatrics Society in partnership with the John A. Hartford Foundation introduced a grant program, titled Geriatrics Education for Specialty Residents (GSR). Beginning in 2001, as a part of the larger Geriatrics for Specialists Initiative, the GSR began funding programs to develop educational models to improve the care that residents in surgical and medical subspecialties give to elderly patients. Every 2 years, a new round of grants was given to these specialty programs. To find out more about the Geriatrics Education for Specialty Residents, such as descriptions of projects that have received grants, please go to The American Geriatrics Society home page and follow the link to the Geriatrics for Specialists section. The web site address is http://www.americangeriatrics.org/specialists/gsr/default.asp.

Funding from the GSR has been used by several recipients to develop projects focusing specifically on how to integrate geriatrics into a surgical curriculum. One such example comes from Dr. Cox et al. at East Carolina University, which in 2002 used the grant to include geriatric issues into the 4th edition of the *Surgical Residency Curriculum*, published by the Association of Program Directors in Surgery. The authors provide a "structural basis for increasing resident expertise in caring for the special needs of elderly patients." Specific curriculum goals include understanding the principles of normal aging, pathophysiology in the elderly patient, preoperative assessment, operative management, and perioperative care of the aged patient, long-term recovery and rehab, financial and reimbursement issues, and lastly, analyzing outcomes of the geriatric surgical patient. To achieve these goals, each section of the curriculum has "geriatric objectives" associated with it and is clearly delineated in the table of contents where those objectives can be found within that specific section. This curriculum can be found at the web site of the Association of Program Directors in Surgery.

The curriculum mentioned above provides an outline of specific goals to obtain competence in caring for older patients. However, other grant recipients of the GSR have developed products to teach the specific geriatric issues. Bell et al. at the University of South Carolina designed "Top Blade," a simulation, case-based project used to cover the major geriatric topics at the learner's own pace. The learner is given a scenario and asked to develop an evidence-based response to complete the task. The solution to the scenario, which is to be written as if it is to be published as a case presentation, is reviewed by a faculty member with an interest in geriatrics who then provides feedback to the resident. There are a total of 22 different Top Blade cases to choose from. This type of integration takes a fair amount of time from one individual faculty member to review the cases but can be completed by the residents in between their clinical duties and does not use valuable conference or lecture time. Each time the project has been completed, feedback has been received from the residents that has been, overall, positive. To access Top Blade, please go to http://topblade.med.sc.edu and request a password to begin.

In another effort, also supported by the AGS and the Hartford Foundation, Sharon Levine, MD, at Boston University Medical Center, in association with the Association of Directors of Geriatric Academic Programs (ADGAP), has developed an intensive 2 and a half-day program for chief residents of nonprimary-care specialties, known as the CRIT (Chief Resident Immersion Training) program. This program, which is conducted off campus at an attractive location in one weekend, allows specialty chief residents to combine some time with family with concentrated interactive learning of geriatric principles with enhancing leadership skills and teaching skills. By the end of the weekend, the residents will have designed a simple project to bring geriatrics education back into their training programs. Information about the CRIT program can be found at http://www.americangeriatrics.org/adgap/crit/default.asp.

Individual universities have also developed their own programs to teach geriatric issues. The University of Chicago has made available its Curriculum for the Hospitalized Aging Medical Patient (CHAMP) program, which is described below. Also included is the E-Learning for Licensed Professionals from the University of Iowa, the Texas Tech Medcast series, and the Elder Care project from the University of Iowa.

Champ

The CHAMP Program (Curriculum for the Hospitalized Aging Medical Patient) is a 12-week faculty development program aimed primarily at primary-care faculty to help teach geriatric issues. However, each module has been separated out from the program and is available at http://champ.hsd.uchicago.edu. The topics covered include Foley catheter use, delirium/dementia/depression, drugs and aging, falls, wound care, identifying frail elders, nausea, deconditioning, palliative care, pain control, advance directives, nursing-home care, and discharge plans. Also included is a module on teaching techniques and a module regarding OSTEs (Observed Structured Teaching Exercise). Each module has a PowerPoint slide presentation, a bedside teaching triggers section, a pocket teaching card (where applicable), references, links, and a session evaluation form.

E-Learning for Licensed Professionals

The University of Iowa Geriatric Education Department has developed a variety of tools to advance geriatric education.

Under the heading of E-learning, five different types of products are available. The first is GeriaSims. GeriaSims is an interactive case-based tool that has a virtual mentor who guides you through the care of a geriatric patient, focusing on a specific topic of interest. Topics of interest to surgeons include delirium, functional assessment, polypharmacy, and palliative care.

The second product is a video streaming lecture series with slides that covers a variety of geriatric topics. Pain control, delirium, peripheral arterial disease, polypharmacy, pressure ulcers, and renal failure among many are presented here.

The third product consists of didactic modules from the Geriatric Consult Service Inpatient Curriculum at the University of Iowa. The residents that rotate on this service must complete these modules. Nutrition, delirium, adverse drug events, and an overview of aging are included in this product. Adobe Acrobat Reader is required for these modules.

The last two products deal with oral hygiene and train the preceptor in functional assessment. By going to the following web site, http://www.healthcare.uiowa.edu/igec/index.html, the user has access to the E-learning products as well as other resources. Many of the individual products can also be accessed through portals such as POGOe (see below).

Texas Tech Medcast Reynolds Geriatrics Series

This is a series of podcasts that covers subjects from polypharmacy, falls, incontinence, and functional assessment of the elderly. They come with a fact sheet as well as the podcasts themselves. These can be found at POGOe.

Elder Care

The University of Arizona has a series of articles in a journal format that review contents such as delirium/depression/dementia, urinary incontinence, falls, elder abuse, and health literacy. These are succinct and concise explanations of these topics. Access to these can be found at POGOe.

These are a few broad examples of how to begin integrating geriatrics into a surgical curriculum. However, once a program director has completed a needs assessment and has evaluated what the specific residency program may need, or if an academician or resident decides that a certain issue needs to be addressed, there exist topic-specific resources. The following section describes, in general, where these resources can be found, such as POGOe, and then lists specific products based on the disease process.

TABLE 15.3 Seventeen frequent and preventable hazards

1.	Acute renal failure
2.	Adverse drug events
3.	Inappropriate bladder catheterization
4.	Deconditioning and immobility
5.	Dehydration
6.	Delirium
7.	Depression
8.	Electrolyte disturbances
9.	Falls
10.	Functional decline
11.	Incontinence
12.	Infection
13.	Malnutrition
14.	Pressure ulcers
15.	Stress-induced gastrointestinal ulceration
16.	Thromboembolism
17.	Untreated or undertreated pain

Resources

The John A. Hartford Foundation and the American Geriatrics Society, along with representatives from ten surgical and medical subspecialties, compiled a list of the 17 frequent and preventable hazards of the inpatient care of the elderly (see Table 15.3) [7]. Educational resources have been developed to facilitate the recognition, treatment, and most importantly, the prevention of these occurrences. Included in this section is a discussion of the broad resources available for improving geriatric education followed by specific geriatric issues and the tools that are available for each one.

General Online Resources

The internet has become an easily accessible repository for educational materials. The geriatrics community is amassing a set of portals to access these educational tools. The Portal of Geriatric Online Education (POGOe), developed by the Mount Sinai School of Medicine in partnership with Vanderbilt University School of Medicine, is a free resource of educational materials that cover the gamut of geriatric topics. Many are evidence-based and are relevant to surgical and medical specialty patients. Many of the products listed below can be found on this site, located at http://www.pogoe.org/front2. Access to the site requires registration, which is easily completed at no cost.

The Consortium of E-Learning in Geriatrics Instruction (CELGI) is also a web site devoted to providing access and awareness of geriatric educational materials on the internet. By going to http://www.celgi.org, the user can read discussions regarding advances made in E-learning and also find

TABLE 15.4 GeriatricWeb topics

1. *Geriatric syndromes* – Dementia, delirium, urinary incontinence, osteoporosis, falls/gait disorders, decubitus ulcers, sleep disorders, failure to thrive
2. *Organ specific disease/syndrome* – Ear, eye, cardiovascular, musculoskeletal, neurological, communicable diseases, respiratory, oral, gastrointestinal, endocrinological, sexual dysfunction and gynecology, hematology and oncology, kidney/prostate, skin diseases
3. *Geriatric psychiatry* – Mood disorders, anxiety disorders, personality disorders, substance-related disorders, memory disorders (nondementia)
4. *Patient care* – Geriatric assessment, hospitalization, emergency medical services, surgical procedures, long-term care, preventive health services, rehabilitation, pain management/palliative care
5. *Aging* – Age distribution/demography, basic sciences, pharmacology/polypharmacy
6. *Economics* – Organizations/Medicare, health service research
7. *Medical ethics* – Advance directives/decision capacity, artificial nutrition/feeding tubes
8. *Miscellaneous topics* – Elder abuse, automobile driving, geriatric medical education

links to other learning resources. CELGI was established with the support of the Miami Jewish Home and Hospital for the Aged, Florida's teaching nursing home and is also affiliated with the VA Medical Center in Miami. Membership in CELGI is free.

GeriatricWeb is a resource for practitioners that have access to guidelines for treating many of the geriatric syndromes. Found at http://geriatricweb.sc.edu/, it is a collaborative effort between the Division of Geriatrics at Palmetto Health Richland Hospital and the University of South Carolina School of Medicine and its medical library. It is funded by a grant from the National Library of Medicine. Its web-based geriatric digital library is broken down into eight broad topics (see Table 15.4), and it is free to access.

MedEdPortal is a peer-reviewed resource for general medical information but includes geriatric topics. It is funded by the AAMC and is found at http://www.aamc.org/mededportal. Several universities have developed their own web sites with access to geriatric topics.

Resources by Topic

When making changes to a curriculum, the program director may have identified particular areas of need, or an academician or resident may have a particular interest in a certain geriatric topic. Provided below is a list of specific geriatric issues and the educational tools that are available to learn about them. Each item that follows will contain how to find the tool, a description of the type of learning

method used – lecture vs. standardized patient vs. interactive video presentation, etc., the author and institution where the product originated, and a brief summary of the product.

Delirium

1. *An Unfolding Case of Delirium, Dementia, and Depression* – University of California at San Francisco; Author – Bree Johnston, MD

This is a problem-based learning exercise in a Word document to be used in small groups. The case explores the concept of recognizing and managing the cognitive impairment in the hospitalized elderly patient and is suitable for learners from medical students to faculty. Find this at POGOe.

2. *Delirium in the Perioperative Elderly* – University of Nebraska Medical Center; Author – Ed Vandenberg, MD

The University of Nebraska Medical Center has two case-based tools that reviews perioperative delirium – diagnosis, pathophysiology, risk factors, prevention, and management. These are designed for M3 and M4 and PGY-1 learners. Find this tool at http://app1.unmc.edu/geriatricsed/delirium, or through POGOe – http://www.pogoe.org/productid/18401.

3. *Postoperative Delirium in the Elderly Patient* – Saint Louis University; Author – Miguel Paniagua, MD

This is an interactive video lecture series with exercises imbedded in the presentation that expounds on the breadth of the topic of delirium in the surgical patient – from preoperative risk factors to diagnosis and management options. This is found at POGOe – http://www.pogoe.org/productid/20118.

4. *Delirious: You or the Patient?* – University of North Carolina; Author – Debra Bynum, MD

This is a lecture presented in a PowerPoint format. The lecture has a few slides regarding delirium in the perioperative patient but with a primary focus on recognition of patients at risk, diagnosis, and management. The lecture can be found at POGOe – http://www.pogoe.org/productid/18928.

5. *Delirium: An Interactive Learning Experience* – Emory University; Author – Ugochi Ohuabunwa, MD

This is an interactive case presented in a Word format designed to facilitate discussion among small groups. Initially developed for medical students but can be applied to residents as well. This product has been peer-reviewed at MedEdPortal and can be accessed through that portal, as well as POGOe – http://www.pogoe.org/productid/20184.

Additional materials on delirium can be found at the CHAMP program and the E-Learning for Licensed Professionals web sites (see above).

Adverse Drug Events and Polypharmacy

1. *Health Promotion for Older Adults: Drug Use and Misuse* – University of Washington; Author – Shelly Gray, PharmD

This is described as a curricular module that is essentially a very extensive review of drug use in the elderly, looking at the epidemiology of adverse drug events, treatment strategies to prevent these, and a case study and self-study questions to put into practice the concepts presented. This can be found at GeriatricWeb http://geriatricweb.sc.edu/.

2. *Management of Polypharmacy in Community Dwelling Older Persons* – Spital Bern Ziegler, Switzerland; Author – Andreas Stuck, MD

Dr. Stuck presents this topic in a PowerPoint presentation that is accessible at GeriatricWeb. He discusses definitions, risk factors, risk reduction strategies, compliance issues, and overall polypharmacy management options. This can be found at http://www.healthandage.com.

3. *Geriatric Pharmacology* – Texas Tech University; Author – Kathryn McMahon, PhD

Dr. McMahon provides a case-based exercise for use in small groups to evaluate pharmacology issues in the elderly. There are three segments to this product – a didactic handout, the cases, and then a posttest. This can be found at POGOe – http://www.pogoe.org/productid/20116.

4. *Pharmacology Exercises For Small Groups of Medical Students* – University of California San Francisco; Author – Bree Johnston, MD

Initially designed for medical students, this device is made up of three cases. The second and third cases in particular may be of use to surgery residents as they discuss topics such as the impact of renal function on drug clearance and how to compensate for this as well as prescribing concerns. This can be found at POGOe – http://www.pogoe.org/productid/18817.

Polypharmacy and adverse drug events are topics also covered by both the CHAMP program and E-Learning for Professionals (see above).

Renal and Prostate Disorders

1. *Renal Failure in the Older Adult* – University of Iowa; Author – Rebecca Hegeman, MD

This is a video streaming lecture that is available from the University of Iowa Geriatrics Education web site – http://www.healthcare.uiowa.edu/igec/index.html, and is one of many video lectures available from them regarding geriatric issues. This is also available through POGOe – http://www.pogoe.org/productid/18472. The lecture addresses four objectives: To describe how to evaluate a patient's GFR from readily available clinical information, to identify the timing of referral to a nephrologist, to understand drug use in chronic kidney disease/end-stage renal disease, and to provide primary care in patients with end-stage renal disease.

2. *Renal and Prostate Disease* – University of Nebraska; Author – William Lyons, MD

Three PowerPoint modules are dedicated to discussing renal and prostate disease, with a focus on the association with elderly patients. Module #1 deals with chronic kidney disease, while modules #2 and #3 are concerned with BPH and prostate cancer respectively. This is not a peer-reviewed resource, but the recommendations are made from evidence-based sources. It is found on POGOe – http://www.pogoe.org/productid/18990.

Urinary Incontinence and Inappropriate Bladder Catheterization

1. *Incontinence and Urinary Catheters for the Inpatient Physician* – University of Colorado Denver; Author – Jeannette Guerrasio, MD

This is a product from Guerrasio et al. that is a "small group, preceptor-mediated, PowerPoint-guided workshop," designed to educate participants about the indications and pitfalls of catheterization. There are four different sections – one is a PowerPoint lecture, with the other three being devoted to facilitating the small group discussion on incontinence and urinary catheter use. This can be found at POGOe – http://www.pogoe.org/productid/20296.

2. *Urinary Incontinence in Older Adults for Practicing Physicians* – University of Cincinnati; Author – Gregg Warshaw, MD

There are six segments to this tool, including a PowerPoint didactic lecture, a patient handout, references, and a facilitators guide. This can be found on POGOe.org – http://www.pogoe.org/productid/19042.

Electrolyte Disturbances

1. *Evaluation and Management of Hyponatremia in the Elderly* – The University of North Carolina; Author – Debra Bynum, MD

Dr. Bynum has tackled the topic of hyponatremia in the elderly through the use of a case-based PowerPoint presentation. The recognition, management, and understanding of the etiologies of hyponatremia is the focus of this tool. Find this on the Web at http://www.med.unc.edu/aging/documents/gercurhyponatremia_000.ppt, or through POGOe – http://www.pogoe.org/productid/18931.

Falls

1. *Falls* – Mount Sinai School of Medicine; Author – Christine Chang, MD

From Mount Sinai School of Medicine comes a teaching tool that has five different components. First is the case of a 70-year-old female presenting in the outpatient setting with arm pain after a fall. To better use this case, a faculty guide explanation is included. Also included is a PowerPoint lecture discussing falls, as well as a resource for other information regarding falls and a comprehensive handout. This can be found at POGOe – http://www.pogoe.org/productid/20200.

2. *Falls and Gait Assessment: A Must for the Aging Population* – Ohio State University; Author – Bonnie Kantor, Sc.D

Instead of using a virtual patient or a fictional case patient, this product utilizes a "senior partner," a patient designated to the learner for which the learner has a list of assignments to accomplish. The learner is required to then go through their findings with the senior partner. The assignments cover the basics of falls and gait assessments, the significance of the findings, management, and prevention options. The concept is to learn about the concept of falls in the context of real-time patient care. This can be found at POGOe – http://www.pogoe.org/productid/18832.

3. *Falls and Mobility Problems in Older Adults* – University of Kansas Medical Center; Author – Shelley B. Bhattacharya, DO

Dr. Bhattacharya has developed a PowerPoint lecture that evaluates falls by looking at the 12 ACOVE (Assessing Care of Vulnerable Elderly) indicators. This is the one of the few presentations that uses the ACOVE indicators as the primary teaching tool. Also included is a brief discussion of the epidemiology of falls. Find this at POGOe – http://www.pogoe.org/productid/20273.

4. *Falls for the Inpatient Physician: Translating Knowledge Into Action* – University of Colorado; Author – Ethan Cumbler, MD

This is a PowerPoint module that is unique in that it discusses falls primarily in the elderly inpatient. Dr. Cumbler also briefly discusses the barriers to treating complex geriatric syndromes like falls, referencing the concepts of "multiple alternative bias" and "possibility paralysis." He includes a facilitator's manual in a Word document that gives suggestions as to how to lead group discussions with the use of the PowerPoint presentation. This can be found on POGOe – http://www.pogoe.org/productid/20212.

Both the CHAMP program and the E-Learning for Licensed Professionals have modules regarding falls in the elderly (see above).

Functional Decline

1. *Functional Assessment in the Older Adult* – University of Cincinnati College of Medicine; Author – E. Gordon Margolin, MD

Included is a case, a detailed discussion of the functional assessment of older patients, including definitions for ADLs and IADLs, and a document that explains the rehab services available at the University of Cincinnati. After the student has learned about the functional assessment, he or she is videotaped interviewing a standardized patient and her daughter, then critiqued by a geriatrician. This can be found at POGOe – http://www.pogoe.org/productid/18715.

2. *Functional Assessment WebCt Module for Medical Students* – University of New Mexico; Author – Carla Herman, MD

This is a module in PDF format for the third year medical students at the University of New Mexico that defines the functional assessment. Included is a thorough explanation of all aspects of the function assessment, from ADLs to recognizing cognitive dysfunction, and how to use the assessment tools, such as the clock drawing task. This can be found on POGOe – http://www.pogoe.org/productid/18486.

Malnutrition

1. *Involuntary Weight Loss in the Elderly* – Mount Sinai School of Medicine; Author – Beatriz Korc, MD

This is a PowerPoint lecture that discusses the significance of malnutrition for the aged patient. The etiology, management options, and overall importance are expounded upon. This can be found at POGOe – http://www.pogoe.org/productid/20367.

Pressure Ulcers

1. *Pressure Ulcers* – University of Kansas; Author – Shelley Bhattacharya, DO

Using the ACOVE-3 guidelines, Dr. Bhattacharya has developed a PowerPoint presentation focusing on risk factors, prevention, and treatment strategies. This can be found at POGOe – http://www.pogoe.org/productid/20274.

Preoperative Evaluation of the Elderly Patient

1. *Geriatric Anesthesia Modules for Perioperative Evaluation and Management* – University of Nebraska Medical Center; Author – Ed Vandenberg, MD

The University of Nebraska has provided five modules that look at a variety of different aspects of the perioperative evaluation of a geriatric patient, ranging from cardiac evaluation to assessing for delirium risk factors. These can be found at the web site through POGOe – http://www.pogoe.org/productid/18967.

2. *Five Practical Tips for the Older Surgical Patient: From a Geriatrician's Perspective* – University of South Carolina School of Medicine; Author – G. Paul Eleazer, MD

Dr. Eleazer has developed a PowerPoint lecture designed to give tips to physicians taking care of the older surgical patient. He describes the change in the physiology of older patients as well as topics such as postoperative delirium, polypharmacy, and fluid management. It can be found at POGOe – http://www.pogoe.org/productid/18530.

Pain Control

1. *Postoperative Pain Management in the Elderly* – University of Nebraska Medical Center; Author – Ed Vandenberg, MD

This is one of several modules from the University of Nebraska Medical Center that addresses perioperative issues in the geriatric patient. In the same format as the other modules, this particular module focuses on postoperative pain control using a case-based approach. The module is broken up into segments. To move onto each segment, the learner must answer a question, which is then given an explanation for the correct answer. At the end of the case are links to topics related to pain control. Also within the module itself are links to related topics. This can be found on POGOe – http://www.pogoe.org/productid/18774.

Summary

As the patient population ages, patients on surgical services will grey and present unique management challenges not commonly seen in a younger cohort. Issues for the elderly are complex, and the margin for error is small. Educators, surgical as well as nonsurgical, have begun to recognize the need to construct an infrastructure to insure that the surgeons graduating from training programs have the knowledge base and skills to recognize and manage these problems. Curricula must be designed to incorporate the problems associated with senescence, the response of the elderly patient to surgical stress, and the special needs of these patients after hospitalization. End-of-life questions and issues concerning palliative care have taken common place in dealing with the elderly surgical patient. Education in these areas cannot be left to chance.

Steps have been taken to begin the acquisition of resources to assist in this process. While the initial efforts are promising, they are far from complete. This chapter has been developed to serve as a general guide, not as a detailed road map. By the time this textbook has been published, additional resources will be available. The links found in this chapter will lead to some of the new materials, e.g., POGOe, but others will be available as well. The Association of Programs Directors in Surgery and the Association for Surgical Education will no doubt continue to develop resources for the education of tomorrow's surgeon that will include geriatric-specific topics. It is hoped that surgical educators will recognize the importance of specific educational curricula for surgical trainees that address the unique needs of an older population, introduce these objectives into their training programs, and develop new programs and ideas that can be shared with the entire surgical community.

References

1. Solomon DH, Burton JR, Lundebjerg NE, Eisner J (2000) The new frontier: increasing geriatrics expertise in surgical and medical specialties. J Am Geriatr Soc 48:702–704
2. Lusk SL, Williams RA, Hsuing S (1995) Evaluation of the facts on aging quizzes I & II. J Nurs Educ 34(7):317–324
3. Maxwell AJ, Sullivan N (1980) Attitudes toward the geriatric patient among family practice residents. J Am Geriatr Soc 28:341–345
4. Reuben DB, Lee M, Davis JW Jr, Eslami MS, Osterweil DG, Melchiore S, Weintraub NT (1998) Development and validation of a geriatrics attitudes scale for primary care residents. J Am Geriatr Soc 46(11):1425–1430
5. Lee M, Reuben DB, Ferrell BA (2005) Multidimensional attitudes of medical residents and geriatrics fellows toward older people. J Am Geriatr Soc 53(3):489–494
6. Krain LP, Fitzgerald JT, Halter JB, Williams BC (2007) Geriatrics attitudes and knowledge among surgical and medical subspecialty house officers. J Am Geriatr Soc 55(12):2056–2060
7. American Geriatrics Society, John A. Hartford Foundation (2000) A statement of principles: toward improved care of older patients in surgical and medical specialties. J Am Geriatr Soc 48(6):699–701

Chapter 16
Palliative Care and Decision Making at the End of Life

Melissa F. Perkal

CASE STUDY

Mr. O is an 82-year-old man living independently with his wife of 57 years. He presented to the surgery clinic with 2–3 months of left lower quadrant pain radiating to his groin, a mild increase in abdominal girth, and a small nontender umbilical hernia. Computerized tomography revealed a 24×17×7 cm retroperitoneal mass consistent with a liposarcoma, a moderate left-sided pleural effusion and atelectasis of left lower lobe. He described his bowel movements as normal and his pain was well-controlled with Tylenol. He had some early satiety, mild shortness of breath but was ambulating comfortably for 1–2 blocks with a walker. After a long discussion regarding the risks and benefits of surgery, he wished to proceed. His wife was identified as the surrogate decision maker.

His son had died many years prior and he felt that the son had suffered pain and indignity. At that time, Mr. O was the decision maker to decide to withdraw care (he states he had to "pull the plug") and he did not want to place his family in the same position. Therefore, he was given the opportunity to meet with the palliative care team preoperatively with his daughter-in-law and wife. He was adamant that if his surgery did not go well that he would opt for a transition to palliative care.

The patient underwent an 8 hr en-block resection of the tumor with positive margins and placement of a left chest tube. Postoperatively he remained intubated for 1 day in the surgical intensive care unit. He developed some

mild delirium which cleared by postoperative day 5. He then did well, ambulating, his diet was advanced, and the chest tube was removed. Postoperatively he was followed by both the geriatrics and palliative care teams. His pain was well-controlled with codeine products.

He was working with physical therapy, ambulating, tolerating a regular diet, and ready for discharge to short-term rehab by postoperative day 11. He had lengthy discussions with his care team, understood his diagnosis, and was looking forward to eventually returning home. He made sure that everyone knew his long-term wishes.

On postoperative day 12, he developed new shortness of breath, increased work of breathing, a pulmonary infiltrate, and leukocytosis consistent with pneumonia. After discussion with his family and the patient, he was intubated for short-term treatment of the acute problem. On postoperative day 15, he self-extubated and stated that he wanted no further intubation if needed; a DNR/DNI order was written. He received continued antibiotics, nutritional support, and was transferred to the stepdown unit. Again he developed some mild delirium treated with haldol. He again improved and was looking forward to discharge to a rehab facility. However, on a Sunday, postoperative day 26, he developed the acute onset of bradycardia, hypotension, and depressed mental status. Family visiting from the West Coast insisted on transfer to an increased level of care. The wife and primary surgeon felt pressured and Mr. O was transferred back to the intensive care unit for closer observation and

(continued)

M.F. Perkal (✉)
Department of Surgery, Yale University School of Medicine,
950 Campbell Avenue, West Haven, CT 06517, USA
and
Department of Veterans Affairs, VA Connecticut Healthcare System,
West Haven, CT, USA
e-mail: melissa.perkal@yale.edu

R.A. Rosenthal et al. (eds.), *Principles and Practice of Geriatric Surgery*,
DOI 10.1007/978-1-4419-6999-6_16, © Springer Science+Business Media, LLC 2011

Palliative Care

Palliative care is the interdisciplinary care focused on improving the quality of life for patients and families who face life-threatening illness. It provides pain and symptom relief, spiritual and psychological support from diagnosis to the end of life, and bereavement [1]. Palliative care is offered simultaneously with life-prolonging and curative therapies for persons living with serious, complex, and advanced illness [2]. Ideally, palliative care is provided at the same time as curative care. As a disease progresses and the goals of care change, the proportion of palliative care increases (see Fig. 16.1). Palliative medicine treats serious illness regardless of prognosis and patients can receive it at any point in their illness, with or without curative treatments [3]. It should provide care for the patient over time and not just crisis management at the end of life [4]. There is increasing support for the idea that having surgeons actively involved in the process provides the most effective means of helping surgical patients who need palliative care [5]. Surgeons bring unique expertise to palliative medicine because surgeons have a special relationship with their patients; this helps them in providing total care in complex medical circumstances [6]. Providing palliative care has become more universally accepted and palliative care programs are expanding dramatically. According to the Center for Advancement of Palliative Care, there has been an almost 50% increase in hospital-based palliative care programs from 2000 to 2008 (632 programs to 1,299 programs) [3]. Nearly 50% of hospitals located in cities with populations larger than one million have these services. However, research in and clinical guidelines for palliative care have predominantly focused on younger adults, especially those with cancer.

The proportion of the US population past the age of 80 has increased dramatically. At the age of 80, about four of every ten men and three of every ten women will die within 5 years [7]. National data reveal that marked variations were found in the number of days spent in the hospital in the last 6 months of life for the population over the age of 80. The local availability of hospital beds is the most powerful predictor of site of death in this age group according to a study by Goodlin et al. [7]. In general, regions with high rates of inpatient care were located in the states of New York, Pennsylvania, New Jersey, West Virginia, Kentucky, Maryland, South Carolina, Mississippi, Alabama, and Arkansas. Those with low rates were likely to be in the West (Oregon, Utah, and Washington). In this study, physicians reported the most significant difficulties for many patients included assistance with self-care, pain, need for emotional support, and cognitive impairment.

Older patients are still systematically disadvantaged in their access to palliative care. Although death occurs far more commonly in older people than in any other age group, the evidence base for palliative care in older adults is sparse [8]. A study of palliative care consultations comparing patients aged 80 and older to younger patients gives insight into how caring for these older adults is unique and challenging [9]. The researchers studied 1,184 patients referred to an academic palliative care service over a 38-month period. The three most common conditions for seeking consultation were: dementia, stroke or coma, and heart disease; only 38% of the elderly patients had cancer. Results showed that 37% of patients aged 80 and older already had a DNR order present at the time of consultation and that the remaining patients were more likely to have a DNR order issued at the time of consultation (73%) when compared with younger patients. There were significantly more recommendations (34–43%) to withhold or withdraw artificial nutrition, hydration, phlebotomy, and antibiotics in this age group when compared with those less than 80 years. In addition, there were fewer interventions for pain, nausea, anxiety, and other symptoms in the 80 and over age group. These significant results may be the result of the palliative care team communicating with the patient families and not with the patient directly in designing goals of care.

In 2001, the Assessing Care of Vulnerable Elders project (ACOVE) [10] published quality indicators for the end of life care. The 14 indicators aim to achieve a "good death" by focusing attention on patient preferences for care and on palliation. Nine of these measures tailor care so that it is matched

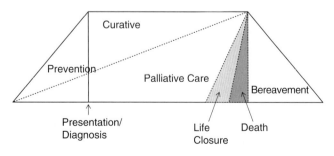

Figure 16.1 The continuum of palliative care: from presentation to death (from [2] with permission from Elsevier).

with the patients' preferences. The first guideline recommends that all vulnerable elders have an advance directive with a surrogate decision maker identified on their chart. "When a vulnerable elder is admitted to the hospital and survives 48 h then the patient's prior preferences regarding life-sustaining therapies should be documented in the medical record" [10]. Out-patient advance directives should be acknowledged when the patient changes care settings and honored in the new care setting. The remaining measures address ventilator withdrawal, treatment of dyspnea and pain, spiritual issues, and searching for next of kin.

Geriatric care and palliative care have many similar areas of concern and have much to offer in improving the care to this fragile population. Both emphasize the quality of life as the key determinant of choices in care and treatment options; both make "the person" and "the family" the unit-of care; and both have placed a strong emphasis on multidisciplinary models of care [11]. Both disciplines also have difficulty in establishing prognosis and time course in noncancer illnesses. Elderly people have distinct needs when providing palliative care. At a time when social support is most needed, many of our elderly patients have diminished financial resources and a lack of caregivers. The potential for isolation and loneliness is increased because of the deaths of loved ones, adult children (with their own medical problems) taking care of elderly parents, and families that are now spread over wide geographic areas [12].

Most elderly patients have at least two chronic medical disorders, which complicates palliative care. By the age of 74, the most common comorbid ailments are hypertension, angina and coronary artery disease, respiratory disease, diabetes mellitus, and previous solid tumors [13]. Symptoms associated with comorbid diseases need to be integrated into the overall palliative care plan. In addition, Bernard Isaac described the "giants of geriatric medicine" (dementia, delirium, urinary incontinence, and falls), which need to be taken into account when delivering high-quality palliative care. The more recently described syndrome of frailty adds an additional diagnosis to be considered in providing palliative care. Frailty manifests the following core clinical features: loss of strength, weight loss, low levels of activity, poor endurance or fatigue, and slowed performance. The presence of three or more of these features is associated with adverse outcomes including falls, new or worsened functional impairment, hospitalization, and death [14]. However, a recent study has shown that while patients with the diagnosis of frailty have a steady decline in functional ability in the last 2 years preceding death, there is only a slight acceleration in decline as death approaches. This study found there was no clear point before death where there was a marked increase in the prevalence of functional impairment [15]. Therefore, the hospice model which relies on a short-term period of decline and on the ability to care for oneself before death does not work for this population [15]. Older palliative care patients are more likely to suffer and die from chronic illnesses preceded by lengthy periods of decline and functional impairments [9].

Symptom Management

The transition from "cure" to "comfort" encompasses shifts in philosophy and practice for both physicians and patients. As the traditional medical model shifts to palliation and end-of-life care, aggressive care comes to a halt. Disease progression is no longer a focus of attention and the reduction of symptoms assumes primacy. Families and patients need to know that as the dying process continues, the frequency of contacts with the health care system will stay the same (or may even increase) as care shifts from curative to palliative. Assessing symptoms can be challenging in patients who have difficulty in verbalizing their needs. The most common physical symptoms in terminally ill elderly patients include pain, dyspnea, nausea and vomiting, anorexia, constipation, and fatigue. Certain symptoms are common no matter what the cause of death; nearly three quarters of all dying patients experience pain and half have difficulty in breathing and loss of appetite [16]. Physical symptom management is as important in elderly dying patients as in younger patients [9, 17]. Many symptoms near the time of death are more common with advancing age. Those aged 85 years and older are more than twice as likely as those younger than age 55 to experience confusion (52% vs. 21%) or loss of bladder control (51% vs. 24%) [17]. Elderly patients are also more likely to experience dizziness or loss of bowel control.

Pain

A full discussion of the physiology and treatment of pain can be found in Chap. 26. However, because pain is one of the most distressing and disabling problems which palliative medicine addresses, several points deserve repeating here [18].

The goals of a clinical assessment for pain in the elderly may be similar to those established for younger patients; however, unique characteristics of aging make this assessment more challenging for clinicians. These characteristics include the reluctance of older individuals to report pain, the assumption that pain is a normal part of aging, sensory and cognitive impairments, and fear of the consequences of acknowledging pains (such as further testing and hospitalization). In addition, older adults often have multiple comorbidities that may have an impact on the pain presentation. The pain experience can influence mood, physical functioning, and social interactions. The many factors that can contribute to pain in the older, dying adult are summarized by Gibson and presented in Table 16.1 [19].

TABLE 16.1 Factors that contribute to pain in the older, dying patient

Chronic conditions	Malignant disease	Breakthrough pain
• Musculoskeletal disorders	• Cardiac decompensation	• Incident pain
• Cardiovascular diseases	• Vascular compromise	• End of dose failure
• Diabetes	• Nerve involvement	
• Neurological disorders	• Bone infiltration	
• Herpes zoster		
• Temporal arteritis		
• Chronic constipation		

Care procedures	Emotional/ cognitive state	Response of others
• Medication side effects	• Depression	• Denial
• Intravenous starts	• Anxiety	• Distancing
• Venapunctures	• Helplessness	• Social isolation
• Chemotherapy	• Anger	• Miscommunication
• Surgery	• Denial	
• Thoracentesis	• Fear	
• Radiation sequelea	• Confusion	
• Personal care	• Vulnerability	
	• Dependency	

Source: Reprinted with permission from [19]

However, despite an increasing focus on pain research over the past decade, the precise incidence and prevalence of pain in older people is still not well described. It has been suggested that 45–80% of nursing residents have substantial pain and that many of these patients have multiple pain complaints and multiple potential sources of pain [20]. Studies have suggested that the prevalence of pain in community-dwelling older adults may be as high as 25–56%. In addition, a body of research indicates that pain is often present prior to death [21]. In one retrospective study, interviews with survivors representing 200 deceased older community residents, randomly selected from the death certificate list in a large American city, indicated that pain increased over the final year of life when compared with a matched comparison group of living persons [22].

Pain is also common in hospitalized elder patients. The Hospitalized Elderly Longitudinal Project (HELP) was a subset analysis of a controlled prospective study of hospitalized patients 80 years and older with one or more high-mortality diseases [23]. HELP evaluated the prognosis, symptoms, and decision making in these adults. Pain was reported by 45.8% of patients in the hospital with 12.9% being dissatisfied with their pain control while they were in the hospital. Pain was moderate to severe in 16.8–19% of the patients. Pain persisted after discharge, with 49.8% having pain for 2 months and 53.6% for 1 year follow-up [23].

In patients with terminal cancer, the high prevalence of pain is well documented. Treatment for pain in this population is commonly inadequate. A multicenter study of outpatients with metastatic cancer done by the Eastern Cooperative Oncology Group found that nearly half those with pain did not receive the type of analgesics recommended by the guidelines of standard cancer-pain management. Elderly patients, particularly those older than 70 years of age, and women from minority racial groups were at greatest risk of inadequate analgesia [24].

Pain assessment in older adults with delirium is extremely challenging. No single diagnostic test exists to determine the presence of either pain or delirium. Since there is considerable overlap between delirium behaviors and nonverbal pain behaviors, clinicians may need multiple assessment tools in addition to their own assessment and caregiver input to assess pain accurately. Close attention must be paid to nonverbal signs (vocalizations, grimacing, bracing, restlessness, rubbing, and agitation) in addition to the usual cues. Guidelines to pain assessment in nonverbal adults include: obtain self-report if possible, investigate for possible pathologies that could produce pain, observe for behaviors that may indicate pain, solicit surrogate report, and use analgesics to evaluate whether pain management causes a reduction in the behavioral indicators thought to be related to pain [25].

However, many patients with dementia can express that they are experiencing pain, and most are able to complete a pain assessment instrument [26]. In one study, 65 of 66 patients with moderate dementia [mean mini-mental status exam (MMSE) score of 16] were able to respond to at least one of the three scales including the Iowa pain Thermometer, the Verbal Descriptor Scale, and the Numeric Rating Scale [27]. Even in the most demented patients (MMSE < 11), 59% were able to complete a pain tool [28, 29].

Gibson et al. provide an excellent guideline for alleviating pain in the older dying patient. These management strategies do not rely only on medication (see Table 16.2). Non-pharmacologic interventions that may potentiate the analgesic effect or improve subjective well-being for older individuals with chronic pain include relaxation techniques, cutaneous stimulation (i.e., heat, cold, and vibration), modulated exercise, distraction and relaxation, and cognitive-behavioral therapy [19].

Once medication is needed, the American Geriatric Society (AGS) Guidelines for the management of chronic pain in older persons is an excellent resource to pain management [30]. The AGS guidelines caution to "start low, and go slow" allowing for the safe titration of effective pain treatment while avoiding adverse effects. These guidelines emphasize the optimization of the analgesic regimen and provision of medication "around the clock," rather than "as needed" for constant pain. A critical component of pain management is anticipation of breakthrough pain due to incident pain (pain related to specific events such as movement, coughing, and personal care or treatment procedures) and end of dose failure.

TABLE 16.2 Factors that alleviate pain in the older, dying patient

Chronic conditions	Malignant disease	Breakthrough pain
• Optimal analgesic management • Around-the-clock dosing for constant pain • Modulated exercise • Relaxation • Cutaneous stimulation (e.g., heat and cold vibration) • Cognitive-behavior therapy	• Optimal analgesic management • Comfort measures (e.g., positioning) • Nonpharmacologic interventions	• Treatment of underlying causes • Optimal analgesic regimen • Rescue dosing • Education • Participation

Care procedures	Emotional/ cognitive state	Response of others
• Preemptive analgesia/ anesthesia • Education • Distraction • Modified care routines	• Treatment of depression • Reassurance • Compassion • Hope	• Support • Permission • Therapeutic diversion • Practical assistance

Source: Reprinted with permission from [19]

The guidelines recommend acetaminophen as the initial and on-going pharmacotherapy in the treatment of persistent pain, unless the patient has liver failure. The maximum daily recommended dosages of 4 g per 24 h should not be exceeded and must include "hidden sources" such as from combination pills. Nonselective nonsteroidal anti-inflammatory drugs (NSAIDs) and COX-2 selective inhibitors may be considered rarely, and with extreme caution, in highly selected individuals [30]. Older patients taking these agents should use a proton pump inhibitor or misoprostol for gastrointestinal protection. The risk of gastrointestinal bleeding increases with age from 1% in the general population to 4% in those over the age of 60 [31, 32]. Older persons are also known to be at greater risk for NSAID-related renal toxicity [33]. Nonopioid agents are usually effective for mild pain (1–4 on a 0–10 scale) while opioids are often needed for moderate [5, 6] or severe (>7) pain.

Opioids are the mainstay of therapy with pain of moderate or greater intensity. Doses must be high enough to relieve pain and given frequently enough to prevent pain recurrence. Clinicians should anticipate the potential for opioid-associated adverse effects. For all patients on opioids, a stool softener and laxative is needed on a regular schedule. Fiber should be discouraged because it can exacerbate opioid-induced constipation in patients with poor oral intake [34]. The nausea and sedation often associated with the initiation of opioids usually abates within a few days; if these symptoms persist, a trial of a different opioid is warranted [35] (see Chap. 26). When switching between opioids, the dose of the new agent should be 50–67% of the calculated equianalgesic dose because patients are incompletely tolerant to the respiratory and sedative effects of the new opioid [36]. Methadone should be initiated and titrated cautiously only by clinicians well versed in its use and risks [30]. When long-acting opioid preparations are prescribed, breakthrough pain should be anticipated, assessed, prevented, and treated using short acting immediate-release opioid medications. For breakthrough pain, a "rescue" dose of an immediate-release opioid at 10% of the total daily opioid dose to be given every 2 h as necessary is indicated [37].

Dyspnea

One of the most common and distressing symptoms found in many end-stage disease processes is dyspnea. Dyspnea is the subjective sense of breathlessness or the uncomfortable awareness of breathing. It occurs at the end of life with a prevalence of 21–70% [38]. Dyspnea is not well correlated with the degree of hypoxemia or hypercarbia on arterial blood gas, airway obstruction on pulmonary function tests, or the presence of cyanosis or tachypnea on physical exam [38]. Initially, all reversible causes should be sought and aggressively managed (e.g., pleural effusion, pericardial effusion, congestive heart failure, bronchospasm, and bronchial obstruction). However, it remains a significant symptom even after maximal disease treatment. Nonpharmacologic interventions for dyspnea, such as positioning, dehumidification of ambient air, the use of fans, and soothing environmental changes, are often highly effective adjuncts to pharmacologic treatment.

Opioids, particularly morphine, provide highly effective relief for most patients and are the mainstay of therapy. For severe dyspnea, a dose of morphine of 5–15 mg orally is used. For breakthrough dyspnea, a dose can be repeated every 2 h. The mechanism of action is poorly understood but is likely the suppression of the central ventilatory drive in addition to the central effects of analgesia and euphoria that palliate dyspnea [38]. Fear and anxiety are often a component of dyspnea and the use of an anxiolytic can be beneficial. Benzodiazepines, and to a lesser extent phenothiazines, have also been used to treat dyspnea. These should be started at very low doses with frequent repeat administration to titrate for the reduction of symptoms. Benzodiazepines will occasionally contribute to delirium in the elderly and need to be used carefully. There is no clear evidence as to which category of medication will be most effective in any given patient, and clinical judgment combined with therapeutic trials is the best approach.

The use of oxygen is common in the treatment of dyspnea, but is not always effective. Hypoxemia does not necessarily correlate with the subjective symptom of dyspnea and its correction may not produce symptom relief. The drawbacks of oxygen therapy include cost, the intrusive and noisy apparatus, restrictions on activity, and difficulties in keeping tubing or masks in place in many elderly patients. Oxygen should only be used if the patient finds it to be of benefit. [39].

Constipation and Obstruction

Decreased gastrointestinal motility occurs frequently near the end of life and is also a common condition in the elderly. Ileus, mechanical obstruction, and metabolic abnormalities can lead to constipation. In addition, constipation is a frequent adverse drug effect of many drugs including opioids and those with anticholinergic side effects. Routine laxative therapy should not be initiated in patients with severe constipation until fecal impaction has been excluded.

Regular administration of stimulant laxatives (e.g., senna and bisacodyl) or osmotic agents (e.g., milk of magnesia, sorbitol, lactulose, and polyethylene glycol) is often necessary for the management of constipation in the terminally ill. It is important to titrate to an effective dose of a single agent before adding additional agents [39]. Recent studies have shown encouraging results relieving constipation with administration of the μ-opioid-receptor antagonists: methylnaltrexone and naloxone. Oral naloxone accelerates transit through the transverse and rectosigmoid colon and is poorly bioavailable; therefore, very little naloxone appears in the systemic circulation. Methylnaltrexone has a limited ability to cross the blood–brain barrier. Therefore, treatment does not affect central analgesia or precipitate opioid withdrawal. Methylnaltrexone given subcutaneously often results in relief of constipation within 4 h [40].

Differentiating bowel obstruction from constipation is an important consideration. For patients with a history of either completely resected abdominal malignancy or an earlier nonabdominal malignancy with known potential for intra-abdominal metastatic disease (breast cancer, lung cancer, and melanoma), malignant obstruction should be high on the differential diagnosis list if bowel obstruction is seen on radiographic evaluation. There are no comparative studies comparing cost, patient comfort, and diagnostic accuracy of different radiographic techniques but the data currently suggest that CT scanning should be used in the evaluation of malignant bowel obstruction [41]. One must remember that a large percentage of bowel obstructions even in patients with intra-abdominal malignancies are from benign causes, such as simple adhesions, and may have a straightforward surgical solution.

Although surgical approaches can be an option to treat malignant bowel obstruction, this does not mean that every patient should undergo surgery [41]. Appropriate patient selection is imperative because operative mortality is frequent (5–32%), morbidity is common (42%), and reobstruction after operation is high (10–50%) [41]. The primary goals of treatment are to relieve obstruction-related nausea and vomiting, to allow the patient to eat and to permit the patient to return home or to a nursing facility under hospice care. Literature suggests that patients less likely to obtain a benefit from surgery include those with ascites, carcinomatosiss, palpable intra-abdominal masses, multiple bowel obstructions, and very advanced disease with poor overall clinical status [41]. Surgical options should provide the quickest and safest procedure that can alleviate the obstruction (resection, intestinal bypass, or stoma).

Nasogastric suction is the mainstay for temporary treatment of bowel obstruction where surgical intervention may be indicated, however, it is poorly suited to the management for those patients where surgical intervention is not an option. Numerous endoscopic options provide more durable and comfortable benefit. Endoscopic stent placement has successfully relieved obstruction at many sites of malignant bowel obstruction in both the upper and lower GI tracts. Percutaneous endoscopic gastrostomy (PEG) tubes can alleviate the symptoms of intractable nausea and vomiting. This method has proved quite useful for patients with end-stage gynecologic malignancies even in the face of ascites [42].

There are many pharmacologic therapies available to relieve the signs and symptoms of bowel obstruction. Opioids can effectively alleviate pain related to intestinal obstruction. If cramping is not present, prokinetic agents such as metoclopramide can provide temporary relief of partial obstruction. Macrolide antibiotics have been shown to be beneficial for improving gastrokinesis by acting as a motilin receptor agonist [43]. Erythromycin which stimulates gastrointestinal motility has been useful in patients with both gastroparesis and colonic pseudo-obstruction [43]. Octreotide, a somatostatin analog, is one of the most effective medications for the relief of nausea, vomiting, abdominal distension, and pain in patients with permanent obstruction [44]. Somatostatin inhibits gastrointestinal hormones decreasing acid secretion, bile flow, mucous production, and splanchnic blood flow. Octreotide stimulates myoelectric activity within the gut leading to faster esophageal contractions and greater motility within the rectosigmoid [45]. The inhibitory effect of octreotide on secretion seems to reduce pain and vomiting by decreasing distension. Control of vomiting is rapid, often 2–4 h within achieving the correct daily dose of octreotide. Typical doses are from 0.3 to 0.6 mg per day, usually given subcutaneously. There are few side effects, mostly pain at the injection site.

Anorexia and Nutritional Concerns

Elderly patients are at risk for malnutrition. An estimated 35–65% of hospitalized older persons are malnourished and almost half have decreased appetite [46, 47]. This leads to negative nitrogen balance and then to significant muscle loss which reduces patient mobility, decreases respiratory function, and is associated with poor performance status and outcomes. Early in the course of palliative care, adequate nutrition to stabilize muscle loss or regain lean tissue mass is the goal in sustaining functional status, quality of life, and preventing events such as skin breakdown and pressure ulcers. Therefore, efforts should be made to assess the potential for nutritional intervention. Reversible causes of reduced food intake should be treated. These include inadequately treated pain, nausea, an inability to swallow, poor fitting dentures, malabsorption, gastroparesis from autonomic dysfunction, and clinical depression [46, 47]. However, data supporting the use of commercial nutritional supplements are varied. A systematic review of 31 randomized controlled trials of nutritional supplementation, involving 2,464 elderly hospitalized or community-dwelling participants, found that supplements containing protein and calories had a small effect on weight gain but no effect on strength, function, quality of life, or morbidity [48]. However, the rate of mortality was reduced in the supplemented group when compared with the control group.

There is little evidence of a benefit for artificial nutritional support in the context of cancer cachexia. Studies on cancer patients using oral or parenteral nutrition have found no difference in body weight, quality of life, or survival, despite a significant increase in nutritional intake [46, 47]. Therefore, the most cost effective and easy solution would be to encourage the patient to attempt small frequent meals and add easy to eat snacks that are energy-dense. This may provide help to patients experiencing early satiety and reduced appetite.

No drugs are approved by the US Food and Drug Administration to promote weight gain in older people. Corticosteroids have been used to improve appetite and general well-being in patients with advanced cancer, but they do not improve muscle mass [49]. A study on hypertensive women receiving ACE inhibitors reported superior muscle strength when compared with women treated with other antihypertensives [50]. Progestins, such as megastrol acetate and medroxyprogesterone, are the best established drugs for increasing appetite and reversing weight loss in patients with cancer, end-stage AIDs, and in frail nursing home residents [49–53]. Responses to megastrol acetate are observed up to a dose of 800 mg/day [49]. Testosterone levels drop in both elderly men and women. In the acute surgical setting, testosterone replacement was associated with a significant improvement in the ability to stand after knee replacement [54]. Many clinical studies report that testosterone and its analogs can facilitate muscle growth, yet the results of anabolic therapy in wasting disorders remain equivocal [49]. It seems a reasonable approach to determine the patient's hormonal status and to offer testosterone to patients with abnormal levels and clinical evidence of androgen deficiency [49].

At the end of life, persistent anorexia and inanition are markers for the terminal stage of several illnesses and may reflect a final common pathway to death. Unfortunately, anorexia is a common source of distress for caregivers. Many families worry that their loved one will "die of thirst" or "starve to death." In our food-centered culture, feeding is seen as a sign of love and many worry that withholding food and hydration will hasten death. A study of 32 mentally aware, terminally ill patients who were receiving minimum nourishment revealed that 63% never expressed feelings of hunger and 34% expressed feelings of hunger only initially [55]. Discomfort was noted when patients ate to please their families. By contrast thirst was expressed by 37% of study participants until death. Reassurance from the physician that it is natural to lose interest in eating in advanced illness is usually well-received and an important source of relief and comfort [55, 56]. Nonoral administration of fluids or calories in actively dying patient does not prolong life and it may make the time remaining less comfortable by increasing pulmonary congestion and peripheral edema or by enhancing tumor growth [57].

In patient with advanced dementia, tube feeding has been shown not to be beneficial [55]. It is unlikely to prevent aspiration, prolong survival, reduce the risk of pressure sores or infections, improve function, or provide palliation [58]. However, in most cases, the decision falls to family members, and their choice is then influenced more by cultural factors and family dynamics than by clinical benefit.

Delirium

Delirium is an acute change in a patient's level of consciousness and thought processes that develop over a short period of time; it is often waxing and waning and is a significant change from previous functioning. Attention, concentration, speech, memory, or perceptions may be impaired. Patients with delirium can be agitated or quietly confused [18]. Delirium is a common syndrome that affects sick or frail older adults at high rates. Approximately 30% of all hospitalized older adults [59] and as many as 50% of older patients undergoing surgery may develop delirium [60]. Greater than 70% of all patients admitted to the medical intensive unit experience delirium [61]. More than 80% of dying palliative care patients become delirious as part of the syndrome of imminent death [62].

The diagnosis of delirium is made clinically at the bedside. One useful and validated diagnostic tool is the confusion assessment method (CAM) [63]. To meet the criteria for delirium using the CAM, a patient must have an acute onset of a change in mental status, a fluctuating course, and an inability to hold attention. In addition, the patient must display one of the two criteria: disorganized thinking or altered level of consciousness [64].

Differentiation between delirium and dementia is not always clear, and the features of the two syndromes sometimes overlap. The onset of delirium is rapid; dementia usually develops slowly. In delirium, the ability to attend is primarily affected. In early stages of dementia, memory rather than attention is affected, although in late stages attention may be severely impaired.

Delirium is best treated by addressing the underlying cause (i.e., a urinary tract infection, dehydration, or untreated pain). Multicomponent nonpharmocologic interventions are effective and should be utilized first [65]. These include frequent reorientation with voice, calendars, and clocks, maintaining a quiet calm environment, eliminating the use of restraints, having familiar objects in the room, and ensuring that the patient has the use of assistive devices (glasses and hearing aids). Pharmacologic therapy should be saved for those patients who are suffering from agitation and hallucinations. Haloperidol starting at low doses (0.5–1.0 mg) is the first line of therapy. It is fast acting and can be administered orally, intramuscularly, or intravenously.

Adverse Drug Reactions

Management of many different symptoms creates an additional burden for clinicians who must also be vigilant for adverse drug reactions and interactions resulting from polypharmacy. Adverse drug reactions are more frequent and severe in the elderly population [66]. Elderly people may be more susceptible to adverse drug reactions because of age-related changes in body composition, metabolic rate, hepatic mass, blood flow, and glomerular filtration rate which affect how the body absorbs, distributes, and eliminates exogenous chemicals. For example, antibiotics commonly cause gastrointestinal side effects including nausea and antibiotic-associated diarrhea. Antibiotic-associated diarrhea has an incidence ranging between 2 and 25%. However, in older patients, the incidence of positive assays for *Clostridium difficile* toxin can be 20–100 times more frequent than in those 10–20 years of age [67]. Another example of the effect of age on adverse drug reactions is with the use of nonsteroidal anti-inflammatory drugs. Perforated peptic ulcer disease secondary to the use of nonsteroidal anti-inflammatory drugs in patients over 65 years is statistically higher than in younger people [68]. However, in order to avoid inadequate symptom management, it is more important for clinicians to monitor for the occurrence of adverse effects rather than withhold medications to avoid these potential side effects.

Prognosis

Understanding prognosis is particularly important in older patients because it can be the key piece of information affecting how the individual makes decisions. In addition, miscommunication about prognosis in older patients often occurs [69]. Even though predictive models can result in an accurate survival curve for a large group of people with various conditions such as organ failure and cancer, these models cannot accurately predict prognosis for individual patients [83, 84]. This becomes even more complicated in geriatric patients, who may have multiple illnesses, making it even more difficult to predict the ultimate cause and timing of death [8].

The National Hospice and Palliative Care Organization (NHPCO) guidelines for noncancer diagnoses were published in 1996 [70] as an attempt to help clinicians decide when it was appropriate to refer patients for hospice care based on a prediction of less than 6 months survival. The committee developing the guidelines used the best medical evidence at the time to establish clinical prognostic indicators. Hospice programs across the country have adopted these guidelines at the time of referral into the admission process to decide if the patient meets reimbursement criteria under the Medicare hospice benefit. Insurers have similarly adopted most aspects of the guidelines as criteria to use for determining payment eligibility. However, since 1996 many quality research projects looking at the validity of these prognostic criteria have shown that the disease-specific NHPCO guidelines are not accurate in determining whether a patient with end-stage heart or lung disease or dementia will survive more or less than 6 months. For example, both heart failure and chronic end-stage pulmonary disease have unpredictable disease trajectories. In addition, advances in medication and device therapies have changed the prognostic factors used in the NHPCO guidelines [70]. The palliative performance scale (Table 16.3) is a reliable and valid tool that correlates well with actual survival and median survival for a heterogeneous group of palliative care patients and may present more accurate information than individual disease prognoses [71–73].

Advance Directives

Advance directives, referred to as living wills, are applicable when individuals are terminally ill and unable to make their wishes known. Advance directives authorize another individual to execute a treatment directive that specifies which life-sustaining procedures would be "offensive and unwanted" and are based on the Congressional Uniform Rights of the Terminally Ill [74]. Another form of advance directive is the durable power of attorney for health care. A person can appoint another individual to make medical decisions. This delegation of authority over health care decisions becomes effective when individuals are incompetent to make decisions for themselves. Since a primary goal of palliative medicine is patient centered care, determining the patient's ability to make decisions is fundamental to respecting their true wishes.

TABLE 16.3 Palliative performance scale

Percentage	Ambulation	Activity level *Evidence of disease*	Self-care	Intake	Level of consciousness	Estimated median survival in days		
						(a)	(b)	(c)
100	Full	Normal *No disease*	Full	Normal	Full	N/A	N/A	108
90	Full	Normal *Some disease*	Full	Normal	Full			
80	Full	Normal with effort *Some disease*	Full	Normal or reduced	Full			
70	Reduced	Cannot do normal job or work *Some disease*	Full	As above	Full	145		
60	Reduced	Cannot do hobbies or housework *Significant disease*	Occasional assistance needed	As above	Full or confusion	29	4	
50	Mainly sit/lie	Cannot do any work *Extensive disease*	Considerable assistance needed	As above	Full or confusion	30	11	41
40	Mainly in bed	As above	Mainly assistance	As above	Full or drowsy or confusion	18	8	
30	Bed bound	As above	Total care	Reduced	As above	8	5	
20	Bed bound	As above	As above	Minimal	As above	4	2	6
10	Bed bound	As above	As above	Mouth care only	Drowsy or coma	1	1	
0	Death	–	–	–	–			

(a) Denotes survival postadmission to an inpatient palliative unit, all diagnoses
(b) Denotes days until inpatient death following admission to an acute hospice unit, diagnoses not specified
(c) Denotes survival postadmission to an inpatient palliative unit, cancer patients only
Source: Reprinted with permission from [71]

The distinction between competency and decision-making capacity is important. Competency is a legal term in which an individual retains their legal rights; decision-making capacity is a medical determination, made for a particular situation and at a particular point in time [2]. Capacity determinations are based on four key aspects: a person's ability to understand the relevant information and the decision at hand, appreciate the significance of the decision and relate it to his or her own life, reason through the options and potential outcomes of a decision, and make and articulate a choice [18]. In the elderly with cognitive impairment, impairment of capacity may be temporary as a result of delirium or depression. Even people with dementia may still participate in their decision making. One study showed that the majority of mildly to moderately demented patients had acceptable decision-making capacity [75]. In another study, 92% of patients with mild-to-moderate dementia indicated that they wanted to be involved in their treatment decisions, and the majority of caregivers supported this [76].

When the patient lacks decisional capacity, a surrogate is held to these same standards. A surrogate is asked to apply substituted judgment, that is, promote the patient's wishes and express the beliefs that the patient holds. The surrogate is encouraged to act as an advocate by being a voice for the patient. The distinction of substituted judgment is important not only to maintain the ethic of patient autonomy, but also to avoid the burden of the question of deciding to end the patient's life. Instead, the surrogate can be the advocate for the patient's interests in avoiding prolonged suffering [2]. For a more complete discussion of decision-making capacity, see Chap. 14.

Hospice

Current hospice care is modeled on patients who have diseases that are characterized by rapid declines in the ability to care for oneself shortly before death. Hospice provides a multidisciplinary team of professionals including physicians, nurses, home health aides, chaplains, social workers, and volunteers working in collaboration to provide for the needs of the patient and family during the last stage of an illness. The benefit includes care that can be provided in the home setting, skilled nursing facility, or inpatient hospice unit. Hospice provides symptom control, pain management, and emotional and spiritual support expressly tailored to the patient's needs and wishes. Family members also receive support, caregiver training, and help coping with the loss of their loved one.

Experts agree that hospice is most beneficial when provided for at least 3 months. NHPCO reports that the median length of service was 26 days in 2005 with 30% of people served by hospice in the USA dying in 7 days or less. Furthermore, while eight out of ten Americans have indicated they would prefer to spend their final days at home, those who received hospice for 7 days or less were more likely to be cared for outside of their homes. Families who felt their dying loved ones were referred "too late" to hospice care reported more unmet needs and lower satisfaction with the quality of care provided at the end of life. One of the ten families (11.4%) indicated that hospice care was not provided soon enough according to the research recently published in the Journal of Pain and Symptom Management. Inadequate symptom management, poor care coordination, and insufficient emotional support were some of the problems associated with late referrals [77].

The hospice Medicare benefit was introduced in the USA in 1982. To qualify for the Medicare hospice benefit, a patient must have Medicare and be terminally ill; the physician must choose to receive hospice care reimbursement instead of the standard Medicare benefits for the illness; and the care must be provided by a Medicare-participating hospice program [78]. Medicare reimbursement requires careful documentation and considers the patient to be terminally ill if one of the following conditions applies [79]:

1. "The medical documentation meets the criteria in the NHPCO prognosticating guidelines that the patient is terminally ill (i.e., there is no conflicting or inconsistent information in the record to suggest that the patient is not terminally ill even though the guidelines are met).
2. The medical documentation in the record supports that the patient is terminally ill even though the NHPCO guidelines are not met or the patient's condition is not covered by the NHPCO guidelines.
3. The patient dies from the illness for which he or she elected the hospice benefit."

The hospice medical director or attending physician provide clinical documentation to support the certification of terminal illness. Documentation may include results of tests or narrative descriptions of the clinical indicators or progression of disease. The patient must have a prognosis of 6 months or less for most hospice programs, including those under Medicare [80]. Unfortunately, older people dying with progressive frailty are poorly suited to taking advantage of this benefit because the course of their illness can be protracted beyond the 6-month limit and there is no clear point where a rapid decrease in functional abilities predicts imminent death [15].

Communication and Establishing Goals of Medical Care

One of the best ways to incorporate palliative care medicine and end-of-life issues into the care of the elderly patient is with a systematic approach at the time of diagnosis or when planning surgical care. Formal advanced care planning including a conversation regarding goals of treatment, living wills, power of attorney for health care decision making, surrogate decision making, and preferences for life-support measures, such as cardiac resuscitation and ventilator support, should be incorporated into the overall care plan of every patient undergoing major surgery, particularly the elderly. A discussion of goals of care is a core competency of geriatric medicine and palliative medicine, and it should be one in surgical specialties as well. As the burden of therapies increase, the patient's wishes for therapy and outcome become more relevant. Patient preferences can and should be formulated into therapeutic goals, for example, the desire to be discharged to home, surviving to a particular event, being able to communicate and say goodbye, or achieving a more rapid and certain death [2]. Once goals of care are established, they can be used to construct advance directives about specific care interventions, such as cardiopulmonary resuscitation, ventilator support, hospitalization, and appointment of a health care proxy. It is in the initial phase of working with a patient and family that the groundwork is laid for palliation and adherence to a person's goals and preferences [2]. Goodlin et al. [80] developed a process to improve the medical care for the very old. This involves clarifying and stating the goals of care with the family and patient, documenting that plan on the chart, and then carrying out that plan with careful attention to the patient's symptoms (see Fig. 16.2). This same process could apply to any surgeon and patient at any entry point into the medical system.

With the increasing age of the population and more complicated treatment regimens, increased communication is needed regarding disease trajectory, goals of care, and transitioning to an end of life setting. Patient's families are more likely to have overall satisfaction with their loved ones care if they are regularly informed about the patient's condition, if they are provided with emotional support, if they are given accurate information about the patient's medical treatment, and if they can identify one medical practioner as being in charge of their loved one's care [81]. The addition of a palliative care specialist, if available, could be an effective addition to the team in helping to negotiate patient-directed goals of care and facilitate dialogue regarding the complex issues surrounding care at the end of life. No matter who is in charge, our goals should focus on what the Institute of Medicine defines as a good death: "one who is free from avoidable distress and suffering for patients, families, and

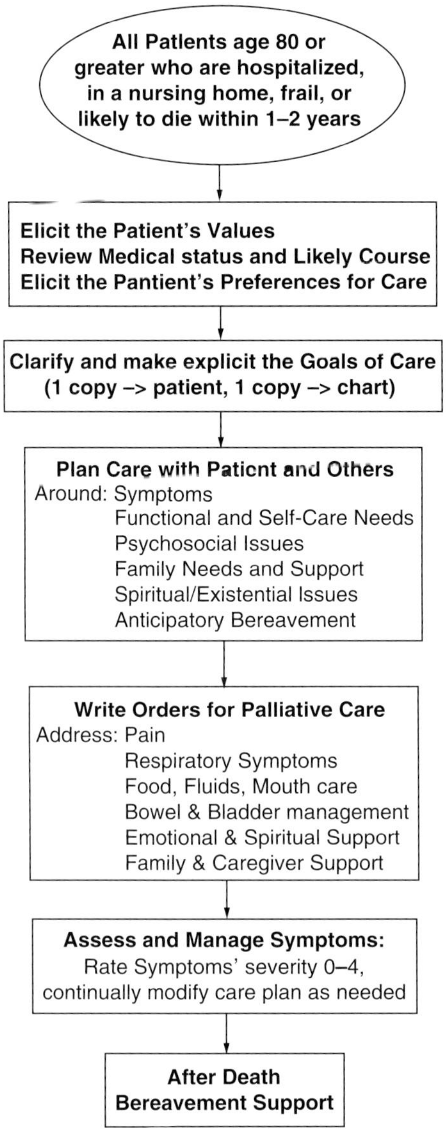

FIGURE 16.2 A process diagram for improving care of dying patients (from [7] Copyright © 1998 American Medical Association. All rights reserved).

caregivers; in general accord with the patients' and families' wishes; and reasonably consistent with clinical, cultural, and ethical standards" [82].

References

1. National Consensus Project for Quality Palliative Care (2009) Clinical practice guidelines for quality palliative care, 2nd edn. http://www.nationalconsensusproject.org2
2. Mularski RA, Osborne ML (2003) End of life in the critically ill geriatric population. Crit Care Clin 19:789–810
3. Center for the Advancement of Palliative Care New Analysis Shows Hospitals Continue to Implement Palliative Care Programs at Rapid pace: New Medical Subspecialty Fills Gap for Aging Population 2008. http://www.capc.org/news-and-events/relaeases/news-releases-4-14-08
4. Meyers FJ, Linder J (2003) Simultaneous care: disease treatment and palliative care throughout illness. J Clin Oncol 21(7):1412–1415
5. Dunn GP (2001) The surgeon and palliative care: an evolving perspective. Surg Oncol Clin N Am 10(1):7–24
6. Adolph MD, Dunn GP (2009) Postgraduate palliative medicine training for the surgeon: an update on ABMS subspecialty certification. Bull Am Coll Surg 94(2):6–13
7. Goodlin SJ, Winzelberg GS, Teno JM, Whedon M, Lynn J (1998) Death in the hospital. Arch Intern Med 158(14):1570–1572
8. Goldstein NE, Morrison RS (2005) The intersection between geriatrics and palliative care: a call for a new research agenda. J Am Geriatr Soc 53(9):1593–1598
9. Evers MM, Meier DE, Morrison RS (2002) Assessing differences in care needs and service utilization in geriatric palliative care patients. J Pain Symptom Manage 23:424–432
10. Wenger NS, Rosenfeld K (2001) Quality indicators for end of life care in vulnerable elders. Ann Intern Med 135:677–685
11. Seymour J (2001) Palliative care and geriatric medicine: shared concerns, shared challenges. Palliat Med 15:26–270
12. American Geriatrics Society Ethics Committee (1995) The care of dying patients: a position statement from the American Geriatrics Society. J Am Geriatr Soc 45:577–578
13. Piccirillo JF, Vlahiotis A, Barrett LB, Flood KL, Spitznage EL, Steyerberg EW (2008) The changing prevalence of comorbidity across the age spectrum. Crit Rev Oncol Hematol 67(2):124–132
14. Rockwood K, Fox RA, Stolee P, Roberston D (1994) Fraility in elderly people: an evolving concept. Can Med Assoc J 150(4):489–495
15. Covinsky KE, Eng C, Lui LY, Sands LP, Yaffe K (2003) The last 2 years of life: functional trajectories of frail older people. J Am Geriatr Soc 51(4):492–498
16. Ellershaw J, Ward C (2003) Care of the dying patient: the last hours of life. BMJ 326:30–34
17. Sheehan DK, Schirm V (2003) End of life care of older adults: debunking some common misconceptions about dying in old age. Am J Nurs 103(11):48–58
18. Kapo J, Morrison LJ, Liao S (2007) Palliative care of the older adult. J Palliat Med 10(1):185–209
19. Gibson MC, Schroder C (2001) The many faces of pain for older, dying adults. Am J Hosp Palliat Care 18(1):19–25
20. Ferrell B (1995) Pain evaluation and management in the nursing home. Ann Intern Med 123:681–687
21. Helme RD, Gibson SJ (2001) The epidemiology of pain in elderly people. Clin Geriatr Med 17:417–431
22. Moss MS, Lawton MP, Glicksman A (1991) The role of pain in the last year of life of older persons. J Gerontol 46(2):P51–P57
23. Desbiens NA, Mueller-Rizner N, Connors AF et al (1997) Pain in the oldest-old during hospitalization and up to one year later. J Am Geriatr Soc 45:1167–1172
24. Cleeland CS, Gonin R, Hatfield AK (1994) Pain and its treatment in outpatients with metastatic disease. N Engl J Med 330:592–596
25. Herr K, Bjoro K, Decker S (2006) Tools for assessment of pain in nonverbal older adults with dementia: a state of the science review. J Pain Symptom Manage 31(2):170–192
26. Chibnall JT, Tait RC (2001) Pain assessment in cognitively impaired and unimpaired older adults: a comparison of four scales. Pain 92:173–186
27. Taylor LJ, Harris J, Epps CD, Herr K (2005) Psychometric evaluation of selected pain intensity scales for use with cognitively impaired and cognitively intact older adults. Rehabil Nurs 30:55–61
28. Krulewitch H, London MR, Skakel VJ, Lundstedt GJ, Thomason H, Brummel-Smith K (2000) Assessment of pain in cognitively

impaired older adults: a comparison of pain assessment tools and their use by nonprofessional caregivers. J Am Geriatr Soc 48:1607–1611

29. Pautex S, Hermann F, LeLous P, Fabjan M, Michel JP, Gold G (2005) Feasibility and reliability of four pain self-assessment scales and correlation with an observational rating scale in hospitalized elderly demented patients. J Gerontol A Biol Sci Med Sci 60:524–529

30. American Geriatrics Society panel on the Pharmacological Management of Persistent Pain in Older Persons (2009) Pharmacological management of persistent pain in older persons. J Am Geriatr Soc 57(8):1331–1346

31. McCarthy D (1998) Nonsteroidal anti-inflammatory drug-related gastrointestinal toxicity: definitions and epidemiology. Am J Med 105:3S–9S

32. Greenberger NJ (1997) Update in gastroenterology. Ann Intern Med 127:827–834

33. Cheng HF, Harris RC (2005) Renal effects of non-steroidal anti-inflammatory drugs and selective cyclo-oxygenase-2 inhibitors. Curr Pharm Des 11:1795–1804

34. Abrahm JL (2003) Update in palliative medicine and end of life care. Annu Rev Med 54:53–72

35. Indelicato RA, Portenoy RK (2002) Opioid rotation in the management of refractory cancer pain. J Clin Oncol 20:348–352

36. Gammaitoni AR, Fine P, Alvarez N, McPherson ML (2003) Clinical applications of opioid equianalgesic data. Clin J Pain 198:286–297

37. Jacox A, Carr DB, Payne R et al (1994) Management of cancer pain: clinical practice guideline No. 9. AHCPR pub 94-0592. US Dept Health Hum Serv, Pub Health Serv, Rockville, MD

38. Mosenthal AC, Lee KF (2002) Management of dyspnea at the end of life: relief for patients and surgeons. J Am Coll Surg 194(3):377–386

39. Ogle KS, Hopper K (2005) End of life care for older adults. Prim Care 32(3):811–828

40. Thomas J, Karver S, Cooney GA, Chamberlain BH, Watt CK, Slatkin NE, Stambler N, Kremer AB, Israel RJ (2008) Methylnaltexone for opioid-induced constipation in advanced illness. N Engl J Med 358:2332–2343

41. Krouse RS, McCahill LE, Easson AM, Dunn GP (2002) When the sun can set on an unoperated bowel obstruction: management of malignant bowel obstruction. J Am Coll Surg 196(1):117–128

42. Marks WH, Perkal MF, Schwartz PE (1993) Percutaneous endoscopic gastrostomy for gastric decompression in metastatic gynecologic malignancies. Surg Gynecol Obstet 177:573–576

43. Janssens J, Peeters TL, Vantrappen G, Urbain JL, Roo MDe, Muls E, Bouillon R (1990) Improvement of gastric emptying in diabetic gastroparesis by erythromycin. N Engl J Med 322:1028–1031

44. Mercadente S, Caraceni A, Simonetti MJ (1993) Octreotide in relieving gastrointestinal symptoms due to bowel obstruction. Palliat Med 7:295–299

45. Dean A (2001) The palliative effects of octreotide in cancer patients. Chemotherapy 47(2):54–61

46. Omram MI, Morley JE (2000) Assessment of protein energy malnutrition in older persons. Part 1: history, examination, body composition, and screening tools. Nutrition 16:131–140

47. Easson AM, Hinshaw DB, Johnson DL (2002) The role of tube feeding and total parenteral nutrition in advanced illness. J Am Coll Surg 194(2):225–228

48. Milne AC, Potter J, Avenell A (2002) Protein and energy supplementation in elderly people at risk from malnutrition. Cochrane Database Syst Rev (3): CD003288

49. MacDonald N, Easson AM, Mazurak VC, Dunn GP, Baracos VE (2003) Understanding and managing cancer cachexia. J Am Coll Surg 197(1):143–161

50. Onder G, Penninx BW, Balkrishnan R, Fried L, Chaves P, Williamson J, Carter C, DiBari M, Guralnik J, Pahor M (2002) Relation between use of angiotensin converting enzyme inhibitors and muscle strength and physical function in older women: an observational study. Lancet 359:926–930

51. Reuben DB, Hirsch SH, Zhou Z, Greendale GA (2005) The effects of megestrol acetate suspension for elderly patients with reduced appetite after hospitalization: a Phase II randomized clinical trial. J Am Geriatr Soc 53(6):970–975

52. Oster MH, Enders SR, Samuels SJ et al (1994) Megestrol acetate in patients with AIDS and cachexia. Ann Intern Med 121:400–408

53. Raney MS, Anding R, Fay V (2000) A pilot study to assess the use of megestrol acetate to promote weight gain in frail elderly persons residing in long-term care. J Am Med Dir Assoc 1:154–158

54. Amory JK, Chansky HA, Chansky KL, Camuso MR, Hoey CT, Anawalt BD, Matsumoto AM, Brenner WJ (2002) Preoperative supraphysiological testosterone in older men undergoing knee replacement surgery. J Am Geriatr Soc 50:1698–1701

55. McCann RM, Hall WJ, Groth-Juncker A (1994) The appropriate use of nutrition and hydration. JAMA 272(16):1263–1266

56. Billings JA (1985) Comfort measures for the terminally ill: is dehydration painful? J Am Geriatr Soc 33:808–810

57. Finucane TE, Christmas C, Travis K (1999) Tube feeding in patients with advanced dementia. JAMA 282(14):1365–1370

58. Clay AS, Abernathy AP (2008) Total parenteral nutrition for patients with advanced life-limiting cancer; decision making in the face of conflicting evidence. Prog Palliat Care 16:69–77

59. Cole MG, Dendukuri N, McCusker J, Han L (2003) An empirical study of different diagnostic criteria for delirium among elderly inpatients. J Neuropsychiatry Clin Neurosci 15:200–207

60. Dyer CB, Ashton CM, Teasdale TA (1995) Postoperative delirium. A review of 80 primary data-collection studies. Arch Intern Med 155:461–465

61. McNicoll L, Pisani MA, Zhang Y, Ely EW, Siegel MD, Inouye SK (2003) Delirium in the intensive care unit: occurrence and clinical course in the intensive care unit. J Am Geriatr Soc 51:591–598

62. Casarett DJ, Inouye SK, American College of Physicians-American Society of Internal Medicine End-of-Life Care Consensus Panel (2001) Diagnosis and management of delirium near the end of life. Ann Intern Med 135:32–40

63. Inouye SK (2006) Delirium in older persons. N Engl J Med 354:1157–1165

64. Inouye SK, van Dyck CH, Alessi CA (1990) Clarifying confusion: the confusion assessment method: a new method for detection of delirium. Ann Intern Med 113:941–948

65. Inouye SK, Bogardus ST, Charpentier PA, Leo-Summers L, Acampora D, Holford TR, Cooney LM Jr (1999) A multicomponent intervention to prevent delirium in hospitalized older patients. N Engl J Med 340:669–676

66. Tangiisuran B, Wright J, Van der Cammen T, Rajkumar C (2009) Adverse drug reactions in the elderly: challenges in identification and improving preventive strategies. Age Ageing 38(4):358–359

67. Bartlett JG (2002) Antibiotic-associated diarrhea. N Engl J Med 346:334–339

68. Collier DS, Pain JA (1985) Non-steroidal anti-inflammatory drugs and peptic ulcer perforation. Gut 26:359–363

69. Fried TR, Bradley EH, O'Leary J (2003) Prognosis communication in serious illness. Perceptions of older patients, caregivers, and clinicians. J Am Geriatr Soc 51:1398–1403

70. Standards and Accreditation Committee, Medical Guidelines Task Force (1996) Medical guidelines for determining prognosis in selected non-cancer diseases, 2nd edn. National Hospice and Palliative Care Organization, Alexandria, VA

71. Wilner LS, Arnold R. The palliative performance scale (PPS). Fast facts #125. November 2004. http://www.eperc.mcw.edu/fastfacts

72. Rickerson HJ, Carroll JT, McGrath J, Morales K, Kapo J, Casarett D (2005) Is the palliative performance scale a useful predictor of

mortality in a heterogeneous hospice population? J Palliat Care 8(3):503–509

73. Lau F, Downing M, Lesperance M, Karlson N, Kuziemsky C, Yang J (2009) Using the palliative performance scale to provide meaningful survival estimates. J Pain Symptom Manage 38(1):134–144

74. Congressional Research Service (1997) The right to die: constitutional and statutory analysis (97-244A). Library of Congress, Washington, DC

75. Gabany JM (2000) Factors contributing to the quality of end of life care. J Am Acad Nurse Pract 12(11):472–474

76. Moye J, Karel MJ, Azar AR, Gurrera RJ (2004) Capacity to consent to treatment: empirical comparison of three instruments in older adults with and without dementia. Gerontologist 44:166–175

77. Hirschman KB, Joyce CM, James BD, Xie SX, Karlawish JH (2005) Do Alzheimer's disease patients want to participate in a treatment decision, and would their caregivers let them? Gerontologist 45:381–388

78. Teno JM, Shu JE, Casarett D, Spence C, Rhodes R, Connor S (2007) Timing of referral to hospice and quality of care: length of stay and bereaved family member's perceptions of the timing of hospice referral. J Pain Symptom Manage 34(2):780–787

79. Marelli TM, Williams MA (2004) Hospice and palliative care handbook, 2nd edn. Mosby, FL, p 71

80. Goodlin SJ, Fisher E, Patterson JW, Wasson J (1998) End of life care for persons age 80 years or older. J Ambul Care Manage 21(3):34–39

81. Rhodes RL, Mitchell SL, Miller SC, Connor SR, Teno JM (2008) Bereaved family members' evaluation of hospice care: overall satisfaction with services? J Pain Symptom Manage 35(4):365–371

82. Field MJ, Cassell CK (eds) (1997) Approaching death: improving care at the end of life. National Academy Press, Washington, DC

83. Reisfield GM, Wilson GR. Prognostication in heart failure. Fast fact #143. October 2005. http://www.eperc.mcw.edu/fastfacts

84. Childers JW, Arnold B, Curtis JR. Prognosis in end-stage COPD. Fast facts #141. August 2005. http://www.eperc.mcw.edu/fastfacts

Chapter 17
Surgery in Centenarians

Mark R. Katlic

Ninety years is old, but 100 is news.

Belle Boone Beard [1]

The 100th anniversary of an individual's birth still bestows an aura, a mystique, as the centenarian is as close to immortality as a human can be. This special prestige has been afforded the imprimatur of scientific study by Baker [2], who found that centenarians represented a striking exception to the inverted U curve of status across the life-span in Western culture. Baker's data, derived from factorial survey analysis, fit the postulate that there is an "American arc of life" that gives maximum prestige to middle age and least prestige to young and old persons. Centenarians, however, were given unique status nearly equal to that of middle-aged individuals (Fig. 17.1), because "like four leaf clovers or quintuplets, centenarians are rare."

Even those who care for centenarians are affected. Nishikawa [3] found that family members who care for centenarians had a lower accumulated fatigue level, despite being older themselves and despite their subjects' worse performance status, than those who cared for individuals aged 70–90 years. Webb and Williams described a case of acute tenosynovitis of the right wrist and hand (centenarian hand syndrome) resulting from the congratulatory handshakes of many friends and relatives on a man's 100th birthday [4].

We have an inherent curiosity about our oldest old. What does he eat? What is her secret? Can it be bottled and sold? Decades ago one entrepreneur, Dr. Marie Davenport, became a professional centenarian, offering to teach her secrets of longevity to others for a fee [1]. Jeanne Calment, the world's presumed oldest person when she died at 122 years, was interviewed weekly by the foreign press who sought her out in Arles, France [5]. In 1997, a popular magazine devoted its cover story to "How to Live to 100" [6].

The mystique may wane, however, as more of us reach this milestone. The present paucity of centenarians results from high mortality rates and a much smaller overall population a century ago. Over the past 40–50 years the number of centenarians has nearly doubled every decade, owing chiefly to improved survival from the age of 80–100 years [7]. When Beard began her monumental, sedulous study of centenarians in 1940, there were 3,700 possible subjects living in the United States; when she ended it during the late 1970s there were at least 14,000 [8]. This number had reached 50,000 by the year 2000 [9], and may be over 200,000 in 2020, and 500,000 to 4 million in 2050 [10]. Some authors argue that even these projections are too conservative because they discount the possibility of future baby booms and assume slow rates of mortality decline and low levels of immigration [11]. Vaupel and Gowan calculated that if mortality is reduced 2% per year, by the year 2080, the number of centenarians in the United States would approach 19 million [12].

Surgical problems do not end on a person's centennial. Surgeons will become increasingly familiar with these most senior citizens.

History

Surgeons have written with increasing frequency about operations in the elderly, but the definition of "elderly" has changed. A report in 1907 listed 167 operations performed on patients older than 50 years [13], and even 20 years later Ochsner taught that "an elective operation for inguinal hernia in a patient older than 50 years was not justified" [14]. Brooks used a limit of 70 years as "advanced age" in his series of 293 operations reported in 1937 [15], and over the next few decades most authors considered patients above age 60–70 years to be elderly. More recent studies show that good results can be expected in octogenarians and

M.R. Katlic (✉)
Division of Thoracic Surgery,
Director, Regional Ambulatory Campus Geisinger Wyoming Valley Medical Center, Wilkes-Barre, PA, USA
e-mail: mrkatlic@geisinger.edu

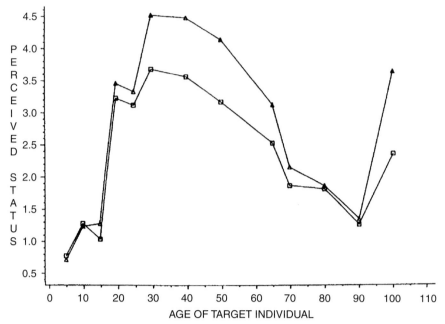

Figure 17.1 Perceived status by age and sex of target individual. *Triangles*, men; *squares*, women. (Reprinted with permission from Baker [2]).

nonagenarians [16, 17], even in those undergoing complex vascular [18, 19], cardiac [20], and cancer operations [21].

An occasional centenarian is included in these series, but most papers devoted to centenarians per se are case reports, some written 40 years ago. Welch and Whittemore [22] in 1954 presented a 100-year-old woman who recovered well from abdominoperineal resection of the rectum for carcinoma. The next year Maycock and Burns [23] discussed prostate surgery in two patents in this age group, and in 1957 Childress [24] successfully treated three femoral fractures under spinal anesthesia. In 1971, isolated cases of pacemaker placement [25] and below-knee amputation [26] were reported. A basket-size ovarian leiomyoma was excised from a 103-year-old woman because of bowel obstruction in 1979, allowing her to live at least two additional years [27]. Six patients aged 100–106 underwent pacemaker procedures with good results in the 1989 report of Cobler et al. [28].

During the 1990s greater numbers of patients were reported. There were three deaths (12.5% mortality) in McCann and Smith's series of 24 patients undergoing a variety of operations, such as colon resection, ruptured aortic aneurysm repair, and hip prosthesis placement [29]. Cogbill's 1992 series of 16 patients reported perioperative mortality of 6% and a 1-year survival of 69% after a variety of small operations [30].

In 1998, Warner [31] reported 42 procedures in 31 patients aged 100–107 years. There was one major complication

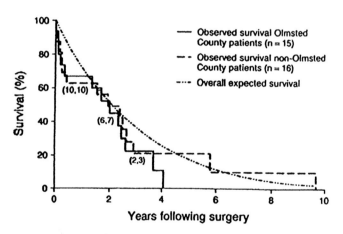

Figure 17.2 Survival following surgery for patients ≥100 years of age. *Numbers in parentheses* represent number of patients alive and followed at yearly intervals during the first 3 years after surgery. (Reprinted with permission from Warner [31]).

(3%) and no mortality within 48 h of operation; 30-day mortality was 16.1%, none directly related to the operative procedure or perioperative morbidity. Subsequent mortality of these patients equaled that of matched peers from the general population (Fig. 17.2). Grey [32] reported a case of revision total hip arthroplasty. This author reported a series of major and minor procedures in six patients aged 100–104 years, all of whom survived (Table 17.1) [33]. The illustrative cases below are from that series.

TABLE 17.1 Clinical summary of centenarians undergoing an operation

Patient no./sex	Age (years)	Medical problems	Operation	Status	Anesthesia	Complications	Death	Follow-up
1/M	100	Old MI, sick sinus syndrome with pacemaker, CHF, prostatectomy, cataract extraction, gout, arthritis, chronic renal failure	Pacemaker generator replacement	Urgent	Local	None	No	Died, age 102 years of CHF
2/F	100	Old MI, left radical mastectomy (13 years), arthritis	Excision of right femoral head, cemented Moore prosthesis	Urgent	General	None	No	Died, age 102 years of cerebrovascular disease
3/M	100	Hypertension, severe peripheral vascular disease, prostatectomy, chronic lung disease	Above-knee amputation	Urgent	General	None	No	Died, age 101 years of "old age"
4/F	100	Old MI, CHF, aortic stenosis, cataract extraction, cystocele repair, left hip open reduction internal fixation, arthritis, hiatus hernia	Open reduction, internal fixation of right hip fracture	Urgent	General	Acute gangrenous cholecystitis, protruding Enders rod pins	No	Died, age 102 years of "old age"
			Cholecystectomy	Emergency	General	Pneumonia, resolved; abdominal abscess, percutaneously drained		
			Removal of Enders rod pins	Elective	Local	None		
	101		Colonoscopic resection of villous adenoma	Elective	Local	Bleeding at excision site		
			Suture ligation of bleeding rectal polypectomy site	Emergency	General	None		
5/F	101	CHF, atrial fibrillation, blind, basal cell carcinoma of face excised, adult-onset diabetes	Right inguinal herniorrhaphy	Elective	Local	None	No	Died, age 102 years of CHF
6/M	104	Squamous cell carcinoma of neck excised, basal cell carcinoma of nose excised and irradiated	Gastroscopy with biopsy	Emergency	Local	None	No	Died, age 105 years of gastric carcinoma

Source: Reprinted with permission from Katlic [33]. Copyright © American Medical Association. All rights reserved

MI myocardial infarction, *CHF* congestive heart failure

CASE STUDIES

Case 1

A 100-year-old woman fractured her right hip in a nursing-home fall. She had a history of myocardial infarction, congestive heart failure, aortic stenosis, arthritis, and hiatus hernia. She had previously undergone cataract surgery, cystocele repair, and open reduction/internal fixation of a left hip fracture. Open reduction/internal fixation of her new fracture was performed under general anesthesia. During her second postoperative week she developed acute gangrenous cholecystitis, requiring emergency cholecystectomy. This episode was complicated by left lower lobe pneumonia, which resulted in antibiotic treatment, and by a localized intra-abdominal abscess, which was successfully treated with percutaneous drainage and antibiotics. Six weeks after admission she returned to her nursing home. Protruding Enders rod pins in her right leg led to pin removal under local anesthesia 8 months later. At 101 years of age, she underwent elective endoscopic resection of a rectal villous adenoma containing carcinoma in situ. Postoperative bleeding from the resection site mandated suture ligation under general anesthesia. She returned to her nursing home, where she lived two years. She died two weeks before her 103rd birthday.

Case 2

A 100-year-old retired laborer was ambulatory at his nursing home until his toes became painful. He had a history of hypertension, chronic lung disease, and severe peripheral vascular disease and had undergone prostatectomy. On examination, he had a gangrenous right foot with *Proteus* cellulitis extending to the calf and an absence of leg pulses below the femoral arteries. He underwent amputation of the right leg above the knee while under general anesthesia (spinal anesthesia was aborted because of the patient's agitation) and was discharged 11 days later. He had one later 4-day admission for bronchitis and died at age 101 years of "old age."

Case 3

A 101-year-old woman was ambulatory and independent at home, but suffered from a large right inguinal hernia. Her past history included congestive heart failure, atrial fibrillation, adult-onset diabetes mellitus, blindness, and a resected basal-cell carcinoma of the face. Elective right inguinal herniorrhaphy was completed under local anesthesia in the outpatient surgical unit. Postoperatively, stating that she would "rather wear out than rust out," she took a 3-month cruise around the world and later lectured at a local college geriatric course. On the penultimate day of her life she completed a political poll. She died of congestive heart failure at age 102.

Discussion

Centenarians recover surprisingly well from surgery, leading one to speculate that the 100-year-old patient who has not already succumbed to a myocardial infarction or pulmonary embolus is less likely to do so, even in the perioperative milieu. The Mayo Clinic study of surgery in nonagenarians supports this finding, as neither pneumonia nor atherosclerosis with myocardial infarction was a major cause of postoperative death [15].

Certainly all that has been learned about surgery in the elderly should be applied to the centenarian. Clinical presentation of surgical problems may be subtle, preoperative preparation is essential, and scrupulous attention to detail intraoperatively and perioperatively yields great benefit. Virtually all studies of surgery in the elderly have also shown an up to threefold greater risk for emergency surgery than elective surgery. The worst complications in the author's series, pneumonia and intraabdominal abscess, did occur after emergency surgery, but the patients generally tolerated even urgent operations well.

Centenarians may be considered a natural model of successful aging. What is it about the 100-year-old that allowed him or her to enter this select age group?

Physiologic Changes in Centenarians

The oldest-old manifest low frequencies of the E4 form of gene coding for apolipoprotein E, a protein linked to an increased risk of acquiring Alzheimer's disease. Among healthy subjects age 90–103 years, 14% had at least one E4 gene, in contrast to 25% of subjects younger than age 65 [10]. It may be that many of those with E4 suffer early Alzheimer's disease and do not survive to become centenarians. This *cohort effect* may explain some of the other physiologic and pathologic changes in centenarians described below. Silver found that dementia is not inevitable with aging and that dementia in centenarians is often not attributable to Alzheimer's disease [34–36].

Morphologic changes occur in the brain with age – decreased brain weight, atrophy of the cerebral hemispheres, fall in the number of Purkinje cells in the cerebellum – but healthy aged subjects show little difference from young adults with respect to cerebral blood flow and oxygen uptake [37]. Hubbard et al. studied electroencephalograms in centenarians and found slowing of the posterior dominant rhythm, but there was no evidence of a progressive decrease in frequency between the ages of 80–100 years [38]. Well-preserved mucociliary clearance in the lung of a centenarian was documented by Pavia and Thomson despite 80 years of smoking history [39].

An even more paradoxical finding was described by Mari's group [40]. They found that a high proportion of 25 healthy centenarians had laboratory evidence of activation of the coagulation system, shown by high levels of enzymes, activation peptides, and enzyme-inhibitor complexes. Levels of factor X activation peptide were equal to those found in patients with disseminated intravascular coagulation. Even procoagulant proteins such as fibrinogen and factor VIII – predictors of cardiovascular disease in young adults – were elevated in centenarians; yet these individuals had no current or past thrombotic events. The authors concluded that significant alterations of these markers are still compatible with health and long life. A more recent study by this group found that the 4G allele and 4G/4G genotype associated with elevated levels of plasminogen activator inhibitor 1 (PAI-1), which predicts recurrence of myocardial infarction in young men, were even more frequent in centenarians than young adults.

The homozygous genotype for the deletion of polymorphism of the angiotensin converting enzymes, which predisposes to coronary artery disease, is also paradoxically more frequent in centenarians than in adults of age 20–70 years [41]. Mannucci et al. speculated that occult factors compensate for these putatively unfavorable genotypes in centenarians (e.g., linkage dysequilibrium with a locus counteracting the bad effect of elevated PAI-1 levels offsets the risk of hypofibrinolysis). It may be that if an elderly person has already escaped thrombotic disease, it is advantageous to have decreased fibrinolysis [42]. A different genetic finding in centenarians – decreased frequency of the E4 allele of the gene, which encodes apolipoprotein E – would go along with decreased risk of ischemic heart disease [41].

Laboratory values in healthy centenarians may differ even from those of younger elderly adults: widening of the range for sodium levels to 132–146 mmol/L, slightly higher potassium and chloride, decreased total calcium, slight increase in ionized calcium, increased blood glucose, increased alkaline phosphatase and lactate dehydrogenase, slightly decreased

bilirubin and total protein, increased amylase likely due to decreased renal function, increased serum urea nitrogen and slightly increased creatinine, increased urinary albumin, elevated urate, decreased albumin, elevated carcinoembryonic antigen, decreased cholesterol and triglycerides, decreased vitamin B_{12}, decreased zinc, slightly decreased thyroxine, increased prolactin, no change in corticotropin, decreased testosterone and estradiol, marked decrease in dehydroepiandrosterone, decreased progesterone, unchanged cortisol, slightly higher gastrin, lower erythrocyte, leukocyte, and platelet counts, slight decreases in hemoglobin, hematocrit, and iron [43]. Higher functioning centenarians appear to have higher levels of serum albumin [44]. Discussion of possible mechanisms for these findings is beyond the scope of this chapter.

Franceschi asserted that a complex remodeling of the immune system occurs in healthy centenarians in contrast to the presumed progressive deterioration (especially with the T-cell branch) [45, 46]. Peripheral blood T cells and major T cell subsets are only slightly decreased despite age-related thymic involution. B lymphocytes are deceased despite data that several immunoglobulin classes are elevated in the serum. Interestingly, peripheral blood lymphocytes in centenarians appear resistant to the oxidative stress that causes irreversible cell damage in younger individuals; such stress may retard entrance into the cell cycle rather than cause permanent damage [47].

Centenarians are more likely to have low body weight [48, 49], possibly due to loss of muscle and fat [50]; a number of investigators have reported short stature even when the effects of aging are considered. Decreased bone mass, however, is not universally present [51]. Both male and female centenarians are more likely to have feminine or androgynous personality traits, rather than masculine ones and are more likely to have a type B behavior pattern (easygoing) [52].

Pathology in Centenarians

Although atherosclerosis has been found in coronary, cerebral, femoral, and abdominal aortas of centenarians [53], the ascending aorta may be spared [48, 54]. Myocardial fibrosis is located chiefly in the left ventricle and septum, and cardiac amyloid deposition is characteristic [53]. Coronary disease at autopsy is common [55, 56], though perhaps less so in Japanese centenarians [57]. Pneumonia was found in 15 of 23 patients in Ishii and Sternby's series and was also the most common cause of death [53]. Alveolar ectasia and decreased elastic fiber were also seen in the lungs. Interestingly, recent or old thromboembolism in the pulmonary arterial tree was common at autopsy despite the absence of clinical pulmonary emboli during life [53].

In the kidney, chronic pyelonephritis and atherosclerosis are usually pronounced; and the testes, ovaries, and uterus show atrophic changes [58]. In the gastrointestinal tract, the liver also shows atrophy and colonic diverticula are common. Gallstones are common (13/23 patients), and peptic ulcer is rare [58]. Osteoporosis is common [59], but not universal [51]. Similarly, in the brain, changes of Alzheimer's disease are common but not universal; when present these may not correlate with clinical neurologic findings [60, 61].

Cancer as a cause of death was unusual in Ishii and Sternby's autopsy series [59]; it represented 7.1% of Stanta's 99 autopsies in centenarians [62], and 31% of Klatt and Meyer's 32 patients [54]. The 7.1% rate in Stanta's series was significantly different ($p < 0.001$) from that in age groups 75–90 years (25%) and 95–99 years (9.5%). Metastases in this series were found in 23.5% of the centenarians with cancer and 63.2% of those 75–90 years old; local infiltration did not differ among groups. Many of the cancers in centenarians (70%) were undiagnosed during life, a fact that may explain the exceptionally low incidence of cancer (4%) as a cause of death in epidemiologic studies [63]. Of all the types of cancer, only the prevalence of gallbladder adenocarcinoma was increased in Stanta's series [62]. Germ-line polymorphisms may play a role in the decreased susceptibility of centenarians to cancer [64]. In exploring an animal model of extreme longevity, Cooley found that only 19% of extreme aged dogs died of cancer versus 82% of dogs with usual longevity ($p < 0.0001$) [65] (Fig. 17.3). In summary, cancer in the oldest-old is less frequent and less aggressive.

Centenarians, like younger individuals, die of specific organ failure, not "old age" [66]. Berzlanovich [67] reviewed autopsy records of forty Austrian centenarians, 60% of whom had been described as healthy before death; all had a specific cause of death, including cardiovascular in 68%, respiratory 25%, gastrointestinal 5%, and cerebrovascular 2%.

Determinants of Extreme Longevity

Despite our fascination with centenarians, little is known about the influences – genetic, environmental, and medical – on their longevity. Vaupel's group, in extensive studies of nearly 3,000 Danish twin pairs born during 1870–1900 estimated the heritability of longevity to be 0.26 for men and 0.23 for women; the sex difference resulted from the greater impact of unshared environmental factors in the women [68]. Other family studies have shown weak correlations for life-span between parents and offspring (0.01–0.05) and somewhat higher correlations between siblings (0.15–0.35) [69, 70] (Fig. 17.4) suggesting either that the genetic factors are nonadditive (genetic intralocus interaction) or there is a higher degree of shared environmental influences among sib-

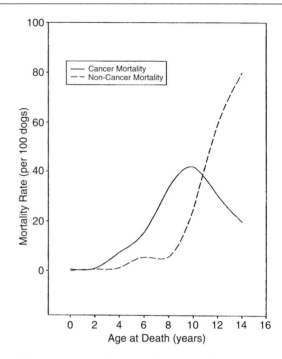

FIGURE 17.3 Comparison of age-specific cancer and noncancer mortality for 345 Rottweiler dogs. Age-specific cancer and noncancer mortality rates were calculated at 2-year intervals from 0 to 14 years of age and expressed as the number of cancer or noncancer deaths per 100 dogs that entered the interval. (Reprinted with permission from Cooley [65]).

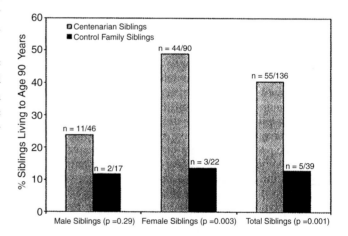

FIGURE 17.4 Percentage of siblings of centenarians and controls who reached age 90 years, when controlling for extrinsic or unknown causes of mortality. (Reprinted with permission from Willcox [70]).

lings than parents. The offspring of centenarians nevertheless manifest less cardiovascular disease than the general population at similar age [71–73], and, in one study, less cancer-specific mortality [73].

Several specific genetic factors have been associated with extremely long life [74]. In a study of Japanese centenarians, Takata et al. [75]. showed a significantly lower frequency of HLA-DRw9 and a higher frequency of HLA-DR1 among centenarians compared to younger adults; these antigens are negatively associated with autoimmune diseases in Japan, suggesting mediation of the genetic influence through a lower incidence of disease. The low prevalence of the E4 allele of apolipoprotein E (APOE) and increased prevalence of the DD genotype for angiotensin-converting enzyme (ACE) have been mentioned above [42]; neither of these, however, was associated with longevity in a Korean study [76]. Puca reported evidence for a specific locus (D451564) on chromosome 4 associated with longevity in a sibling pair linkage study [77]. The role of inherited and somatic mutations of mitochondrial DNA (mtDNA) in centenarians remains unclear [78]. Short chromosomal telomeres have been associated with increased mortality in persons over the age of 60 [79], but this has not held true for the oldest old [80, 81]; nevertheless, Terry [82] found that healthy centenarians have significantly longer telomeres than unhealthy centenarians (Fig. 17.5).

The mediation of genetic influences on longevity via genetic influences on smoking and body mass index – two factors associated with longevity in epidemiologic studies – was disproved by Herschind [83]. Even smoking status has shown no definite association with extreme longevity, nor has alcohol consumption, diet, or exercise [84]. Such "lifestyle" factors may, however, influence one's functional status at the age of 100 [44]. Environmental factors such as socioeconomic status and early life nutrition appear to have little influence [85]. Although no "fountain of youth" medicine has been discovered, the inverse correlation of blood levels of dehydroepiandrosterone (DHEA) with mortality has prompted ongoing clinical trials of its administration [86],

Table 17.2 Posulated Determinants of extreme life-span in the industrialized world

Genetics: genes coding for

Human leukocyte antigens HLA-DR

Apolipoprotein E

Angiotensin-converting enzyme (ACE)

Environment

Year of birth

Smoking

Alcohol

Diet

Locale cf. Sardinia, Okinawa

Medicine

Dehydroepiandrosterone (DHEA)

Other

Long-lived sibling

Long-lived parent

not all of them salutary [87]. Some environments, e.g., Sardinia and Okinawa, appear to be conducive to extreme longevity as do personal factors such as activity, discipline, altruism, spiritual faith [88], musical instruments, and humor. In a study of 483 Italian centenarians, 88.6% had never smoked cigarettes [89]. Centenarians themselves attribute their longevity to God, singing, pickled herring, shochu (sugar cane liquor), honey, port, abstinence, boiled onions, whiskey, red wine, fish, luck, chocolates, olive oil, weakness for women (or men), and more.

In summary, it is likely that a large number of factors interact to determine longevity, three-fourths of them being environmental (Table 17.2). The involvement of a number of genes, each contributing a little, might influence longevity directly or, more likely, through determining susceptibility to disease at different ages.

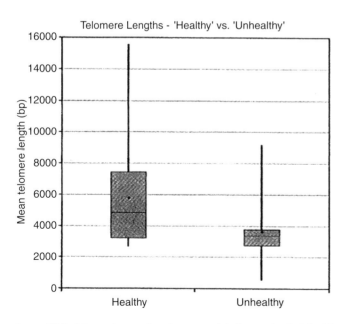

Figure 17.5 Mean telomere length measured in base pairs (bp) in 19 healthy versus 19 unhealthy centenarians. *Bars*: interquartile ranges (Q75% to Q25%) of telomere length. *Diamonds*: mean; *horizontal line within bars*: median telomere lengths; *Vertical lines*: overall range of telomere lengths. (Reprinted with permission from Terry [82]).

Selective Survival Hypothesis

A 100-year-old is as likely to survive surgery as are his sons and daughters, and one may speculate that he is even more likely to do so. The man or woman who has endured ten decades of life's labors enters a select group whose physiological resilience is greater than that of many who are chronologically younger. – M.R. Katlic, 1985 [33]

This selective survival concept was discussed by Thomas Perls, principal investigator with the New England Centenarian Study [10]. Perls postulated, supported by his research and that of others, that certain individuals are resistant to the diseases that cripple and kill most people before age 90. These individuals – although 95% have some form of chronic disease [90], including cardiovascular disease [91] – not only live longer lives, they also live relatively free of debilitating infirmities.

Mortality rates for centenarians, for example, are lower than would be anticipated by extrapolating the death rates of younger adults. Mortality can be reasonably predicted up to approximately age 80, but the linear decline in health not only slows at advanced age, but varies more among individuals, thus selecting the most fit [92]. Selection is more than sufficient to overcome the effects of aging and is greater in men, probably because of their higher mortality at younger ages [93, 94]. This "gender crossover" resulting from the selection of fit men can be seen as early as age 80, but is more evident in centenarians: men make up 20% of 100-year-olds and 40% of 105-year-olds. Female-to-male ratios, however, may range from 2:1 to 7:1 in different provinces within the same country [95]. Age 95–97 years appears to be the age at which a person's chance of dying increases in a linear rather than an exponential manner with time (Fig. 17.6) [10]. Carey [96] found the same phenomenon in medflies.

Whether due to compositional change in the cohort (selection of the fittest) or better intrinsic cellular defense mechanisms (see peripheral blood lymphocyte data above), the very old have a higher threshold for acquiring disease and a decreased mortality rate, allowing them not only to survive, but to do so in relatively good health (Fig. 17.7). In 1990, the Medicare costs for those who died at age 70 was $6475 during each of the last 5 years of life compared to $1,800 per year for those who died at age 100 [97]. In 1995 medical

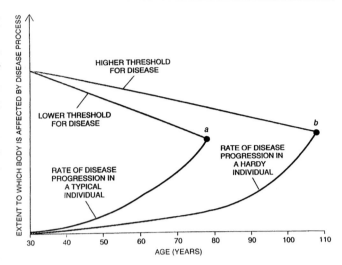

Figure 17.7 High threshold for acquiring disease and slow aging process may promote survival because of the good health of centenarians. (From Perls [10]. Copyright© 1995 by Scientific American, Inc. All rights reserved).

expenses for the last 2 years of life average $22,600 for people who died at age 70 and $8,300 for those who died after age 100 [6].

Perls' group has described three morbidity profiles for centenarians [98]. *Survivors* had an age-associated illness prior to age 80 years (24% of men and 43% of women); *Delayers* experienced an age-associated illness after 80 years (44% of men and 42% of women); *Escapers* reached age 100 without a diagnosis of common age-associated illness (32% of men and 15% of women). With respect to the most lethal diseases – heart disease, cancer, and stroke – 87% of male centenarians and 83% of female centenarians either delayed or escaped. Motta [99], who studied 602 Italian centenarians, writes that even those who are free of disease, autonomous, and bright should not be considered prototypes of "successful aging", as they have not maintained any social or productive activities. Most consider centenarians to be models of healthy aging from which we can learn, in order to improve the health of all elderly [100].

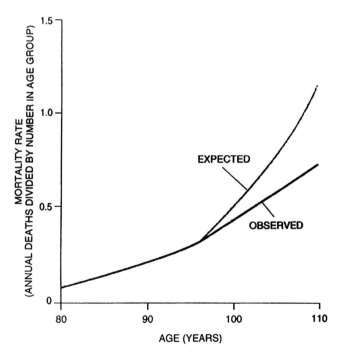

Figure 17.6 Observed mortality rate slows after age 97 years compared to the expected mortality rate. (From Perls [10]. Copyright© 1995 by Scientific American, Inc. All rights reserved).

Supercentenarians

Supercentenarians, those aged 110 years or more, likely number less than 500 worldwide; most are women [101]. Schoenhofen [102] studied 32 such individuals, 84% of them women. Cardiovascular disease and stroke were rare, Parkinson's disease absent, and cancer successfully treated in 25%; 41% were independent or required minimal assistance. The parents and siblings of supercentenarians also manifest a survival advantage [103].

Conclusions

All that has been learned about surgery in the elderly should be applied to the centenarian: clinical presentation of surgical problems may be subtle, preoperative preparation is essential, emergency surgery carries high risk compared to elective operation, and scrupulous attention to detail intraoperatively and perioperatively yields great benefit. It is not unreasonable to speculate that the 100-year-old who has not already succumbed to a myocardial infarction or pulmonary embolus is unlikely to do so, even during the perioperative period. Survival to the centenary indicates that one has been tested by life and has been found exceptionally fit. Elective surgery should not be deferred nor emergency surgery denied the centenarian on the basis of chronologic age.

References

1. Beard BB (1991) Centenarians: the new generation. Greenwood, Westport, CT, 3
2. Baker PM (1985) The status of age: preliminary results. J Gerontol 40(4):506–508
3. Nishikawa K, Harada Y, Fujimori J et al (2003) Possible model for successful care: burden of caregivers of centenarians. J Am Geriatr Soc 51(4):577–578
4. Webb R, Williams LM (1985) Centenarian hand syndrome. N Engl J Med 313(3):188
5. Matalon J (1997) World's oldest person dies. The Times Leader
6. Cowley G (1997) How to live to 100. Newsweek 30:56–67
7. Vaupel J, Jeune B (1995) The emergence and proliferation of centenarians. In: Jeune B, Vaupel J (eds) Exceptional longevity: from prehistory to the present. Odense University Press, Odense, Denmark
8. United States Bureau of the Census (1987) America's centenarians, vol Series P-23, Current population reports. US Government Printing Office, Washington, DC
9. Bureau USC. Census 2000: States and puerto rico ranked by population 100 years and over. www.census.gov/population/www/cen2000/briefs/phc-t13/index.html. Accessed 8 Oct 2008
10. Perls TT (1995) The oldest old. Sci Am 272(1):70–75
11. Ahlburg DA, Vaupel JW (1990) Alternative projections of the U.S. population. Demography 27(4):639–652
12. Vaupel JW, Gowan AE (1986) Passage to Methuselah: some demographic consequences of continued progress against mortality. Am J Public Health 76(4):430–433
13. Smith O (1907) Advanced age as a contraindication to operation. Med Rec (NY) 72:642–644
14. Ochsner A (1967) Is risk of indicated operation too great in the elderly? Geriatrics 22(11):121–130
15. Brooks B (1937) Surgery in patients of advanced age. Ann Surg 105(4):481–495
16. Warner MA, Hosking MP, Lobdell CM, Offord KP, Melton LJ 3rd (1988) Surgical procedures among those greater than or equal to 90 years of age. A population-based study in Olmsted County, Minnesota, 1975–1985. Ann Surg 207(4):380–386
17. Cohen JR, Johnson H, Eaton S, Sterman H, Wise L (1988) Surgical procedures in patients during the tenth decade of life. Surgery 104(4):646–651
18. Coyle KA, Smith RB 3rd, Salam AA, Dodson TF, Chaikof EL, Lumsden AB (1994) Carotid endarterectomy in the octogenarian. Ann Vasc Surg 8(5):417–420
19. Chalmers RT, Stonebridge PA, John TG, Murie JA (1993) Abdominal aortic aneurysm in the elderly. Br J Surg 80(9):1122–1123
20. Blanche C, Matloff JM, Denton TA et al (1997) Cardiac operations in patients 90 years of age and older. Ann Thorac Surg 63(6):1685–1690
21. Alexander HR, Turnbull AD, Salamone J, Keefe D, Melendez J (1991) Upper abdominal cancer surgery in the very elderly. J Surg Oncol 47(2):82–86
22. Welch CE, Whittemore WS (1954) Carcinoma of the rectum in a centenarian. N Engl J Med 250(24):1041–1042
23. Maycock P, Burns C (1955) Prostatic surgery in centenarians. J Urol 74:546–548
24. Childress HM (1957) Hip fractures in patients over one hundred years of age. NY State J Med 57(9):1604–1606
25. Grayzel J (1971) Pacemaker in a centenarian. JAMA 218(1):95
26. Milliken RA, Milliken GM (1971) Centenarian surgery. JAMA 218(9):1435–1436
27. Sapala JA, Sapala MA (1983) Clinical note: excision of a large ovarian leiomyoma in a centenarian. Henry Ford Hosp Med J 31(1):37–39
28. Cobler JL, Akiyama T, Murphy GW (1989) Permanent pacemakers in centenarians. J Am Geriatr Soc 37(8):753–756
29. McCann WJ, Smith JW (1990) The surgical care of centenarians. Curr Surg 47(1):2–3
30. Cogbill TH, Strutt PJ, Landercasper J (1992) Surgical procedures in centenarians. Wis Med J 91(9):527–529
31. Warner MA, Saletel RA, Schroeder DR, Warner DO, Offord KP, Gray DT (1998) Outcomes of anesthesia and surgery in people 100 years of age and older. J Am Geriatr Soc 46(8):988–993
32. Grey MA, Keggi KJ (2006) Revision total hip arthroplasty in a centenarian: a case report and review of the literature. J Arthroplasty 21(8):1215–1219
33. Katlic MR (1985) Surgery in centenarians. JAMA 253(21):3139–3141
34. Silver M, Newell K, Hyman B, Growdon J, Hedley-Whyte ET, Perls T (1998) Unraveling the mystery of cognitive changes in old age: correlation of neuropsychological evaluation with neuropathological findings in the extreme old. Int Psychogeriatr 10(1):25–41
35. Silver MH, Jilinskaia E, Perls TT (2001) Cognitive functional status of age-confirmed centenarians in a population-based study. J Gerontol B Psychol Sci Soc Sci 56(3):P134–P140
36. Perls T (2004) Dementia-free centenarians. Exp Gerontol 39(11–12):1587–1593
37. Brody H (1973) Aging of the vertebrate brain. In: Rockstein M, Sussman ML (eds) Development and aging in the nervous system. Academic, San Diego, pp 121–133
38. Hubbard O, Sunde D, Goldensohn ES (1976) The EEG in centenarians. Electroencephalogr Clin Neurophysiol 40(4):407–417
39. Pavia D, Thomson ML (1970) Unimpaired mucociliary clearance in the lung of a centenarian smoker. Lancet 1(7663):101–102
40. Mari D, Mannucci PM, Coppola R, Bottasso B, Bauer KA, Rosenberg RD (1995) Hypercoagulability in centenarians: the paradox of successful aging. Blood 85(11):3144–3149
41. Schacter F, Faure-Delanef L, Guenot F (1994) Genetic associations with human longevity at the APOE and ACE loci. Nat Genet 6:29–32
42. Mannucci PM, Mari D, Merati G et al (1997) Gene polymorphisms predicting high plasma levels of coagulation and fibrinolysis proteins. A study in centenarians. Arterioscler Thromb Vasc Biol 17(4):755–759

43. Tietz NW, Shuey DF, Wekstein DR (1992) Laboratory values in fit aging individuals – sexagenarians through centenarians. Clin Chem 38(6):1167–1185

44. Gondo Y, Hirose N, Arai Y et al (2006) Functional status of centenarians in Tokyo, Japan: developing better phenotypes of exceptional longevity. J Gerontol A Biol Sci Med Sci 61(3):305–310

45. Franceschi C, Monti D, Sansoni P, Cossarizza A (1995) The immunology of exceptional individuals: the lesson of centenarians. Immunol Today 16(1):12–16

46. Paolisso G, Barbieri M, Bonafe M, Franceschi C (2000) Metabolic age modelling: the lesson from centenarians. Eur J Clin Invest 30(10):888–894

47. Franceschi C, Monti D, Cossarizza A, Fagnoni F, Passeri G, Sansoni P (1991) Aging, longevity, and cancer: studies in Down's syndrome and centenarians. Ann NY Acad Sci 621:428–440

48. Lowbeer L (1987) Autopsy pathology in centenarians. Arch Pathol Lab Med 111(9):784

49. Chan YC, Suzuki M, Yamamoto S (1997) Dietary, anthropometric, hematological and biochemical assessment of the nutritional status of centenarians and elderly people in Okinawa, Japan. J Am Coll Nutr 16(3):229–235

50. Ravaglia G, Morini P, Forti P et al (1997) Anthropometric characteristics of healthy Italian nonagenarians and centenarians. Br J Nutr 77(1):9–17

51. Mellibovsky L, Bustamante M, Lluch P et al (2007) Bone mass of a 113-year-old man. J Gerontol A Biol Sci Med Sci 62(7):794–795

52. Shimonaka Y, Nakazato K, Homma A (1996) Personality, longevity, and successful aging among Tokyo metropolitan centenarians. Int J Aging Hum Dev 42(3):173–187

53. Ishii T, Sternby NH (1978) Pathology of centerarians. I. The cardiovascular system and lungs. J Am Geriatr Soc 26(3):108–115

54. Klatt EC, Meyer PR (1987) Geriatric autopsy pathology in centenarians. Arch Pathol Lab Med 111(4):367–369

55. Lie JT, Hammond PI (1988) Pathology of the senescent heart: anatomic observations on 237 autopsy studies of patients 90 to 105 years old. Mayo Clin Proc 63(6):552–564

56. Roberts WC (1998) The heart at necropsy in centenarians. Am J Cardiol 81(10):1224–1225

57. Bernstein AM, Willcox BJ, Tamaki H et al (2004) First autopsy study of an Okinawan centenarian: absence of many age-related diseases. J Gerontol A Biol Sci Med Sci 59(11):1195–1199

58. Ishii T, Sternby NH (1978) Pathology of centenarians. II. Urogenital and digestive systems. J Am Geriatr Soc 26(9):391–396

59. Ishii T, Sternby NH (1978) Pathology of centenarians. III. Osseous system, malignant lesions, and causes of death. J Am Geriatr Soc 26(12):529–533

60. Silver MH, Newell K, Brady C, Hedley-White ET, Perls TT (2002) Distinguishing between neurodegenerative disease and disease-free aging: correlating neuropsychological evaluations and neuropathological studies in centenarians. Psychosom Med 64(3):493–501

61. Imhof A, Kovari E, von Gunten A et al (2007) Morphological substrates of cognitive decline in nonagenarians and centenarians: a new paradigm? J Neurol Sci 257(1–2):72–79

62. Stanta G, Campagner L, Cavallieri F, Giarelli L (1997) Cancer of the oldest old. What we have learned from autopsy studies. Clin Geriatr Med 13(1):55–68

63. Smith DW (1996) Cancer mortality at very old ages. Cancer 77(7):1367–1372

64. Bonafe M, Barbi C, Storci G et al (2002) What studies on human longevity tell us about the risk for cancer in the oldest old: data and hypotheses on the genetics and immunology of centenarians. Exp Gerontol 37(10–11):1263–1271

65. Cooley DM, Schlittler DL, Glickman LT, Hayek M, Waters DJ (2003) Exceptional longevity in pet dogs is accompanied by cancer resistance and delayed onset of major diseases. J Gerontol A Biol Sci Med Sci 58(12):B1078–B1084

66. John SM, Koelmeyer TD (2001) The forensic pathology of nonagenarians and centenarians: do they die of old age? (The Auckland experience). Am J Forensic Med Pathol 22(2):150–154

67. Berzlanovich AM, Keil W, Waldhoer T, Sim E, Fasching P, Fazeny-Dorner B (2005) Do centenarians die healthy? An autopsy study. J Gerontol A Biol Sci Med Sci 60(7):862–865

68. Herskind AM, McGue M, Holm NV, Sorensen TI, Harvald B, Vaupel JW (1996) The heritability of human longevity: a population-based study of 2,872 Danish twin pairs born 1870–1900. Hum Genet 97(3):319–323

69. Wyshak G (1978) Fertility and longevity in twins, sibs, and parents of twins. Soc Biol 25(4):315–330

70. Willcox BJ, Willcox DC, He Q, Curb JD, Suzuki M (2006) Siblings of Okinawan centenarians share lifelong mortality advantages. J Gerontol A Biol Sci Med Sci 61(4):345–354

71. Terry DF, Wilcox M, McCormick MA, Lawler E, Perls TT (2003) Cardiovascular advantages among the offspring of centenarians. J Gerontol A Biol Sci Med Sci 58(5):M425–M431

72. Terry DF, Wilcox MA, McCormick MA, Perls TT (2004) Cardiovascular disease delay in centenarian offspring. J Gerontol A Biol Sci Med Sci 59(4):385–389

73. Terry DF, Wilcox MA, McCormick MA et al (2004) Lower all-cause, cardiovascular, and cancer mortality in centenarians' offspring. J Am Geriatr Soc 52(12):2074–2076

74. Gonos ES (2000) Genetics of aging: lessons from centenarians. Exp Gerontol 35(1):15–21

75. Takata H, Suzuki M, Ishii T, Sekiguchi S, Iri H (1987) Influence of major histocompatibility complex region genes on human longevity among Okinawan-Japanese centenarians and nonagenarians. Lancet 2(8563):824–826

76. Choi YH, Kim JH, Kim DK et al (2003) Distributions of ACE and APOE polymorphisms and their relations with dementia status in Korean centenarians. J Gerontol A Biol Sci Med Sci 58(3):227–231

77. Puca AA, Daly MJ, Brewster SJ et al (2001) A genome-wide scan for linkage to human exceptional longevity identifies a locus on chromosome 4. Proc Natl Acad Sci U S A 98(18):10505–10508

78. Salvioli S, Capri M, Santoro A et al (2008) The impact of mitochondrial DNA on human lifespan: a view from studies on centenarians. Biotechnol J 3(6):740–749

79. Cawthon RM, Smith KR, O'Brien E, Sivatchenko A, Kerber RA (2003) Association between telomere length in blood and mortality in people aged 60 years or older. Lancet 361(9355):393–395

80. Martin-Ruiz CM, Gussekloo J, van Heemst D, von Zglinicki T, Westendorp RG (2005) Telomere length in white blood cells is not associated with morbidity or mortality in the oldest old: a population-based study. Aging Cell 4(6):287–290

81. Bischoff C, Petersen HC, Graakjaer J et al (2006) No association between telomere length and survival among the elderly and oldest old. Epidemiology 17(2):190–194

82. Terry DF, Nolan VG, Andersen SL, Perls TT, Cawthon R (2008) Association of longer telomeres with better health in centenarians. J Gerontol A Biol Sci Med Sci 63(8):809–812

83. Herskind AM, McGue M, Iachine IA et al (1996) Untangling genetic influences on smoking, body mass index and longevity: a multivariate study of 2,464 Danish twins followed for 28 years. Hum Genet 98(4):467–475

84. Christensen K, Vaupel JW (1996) Determinants of longevity: genetic, environmental and medical factors. J Intern Med 240(6):333–341

85. McGue M, Vaupel JW, Holm N, Harvald B (1993) Longevity is moderately heritable in a sample of Danish twins born 1870–1880. J Gerontol 48(6):B237–B244

86. Herbert J (1995) The age of dehydroepiandrosterone. Lancet 345(8959):1193–1194
87. Nair KS, Rizza RA, O'Brien P et al (2006) DHEA in elderly women and DHEA or testosterone in elderly men. N Engl J Med 355(16):1647–1659
88. Zhang W (2008) Religious participation and mortality risk among the oldest old in china. J Gerontol B Psychol Sci Soc Sci 63(5):S293–S297
89. Nicita-Mauro V, Lo Balbo C, Mento A, Nicita-Mauro C, Maltese G, Basile G (2008) Smoking, aging and the centenarians. Exp Gerontol 43(2):95–101
90. Takayama M, Hirose N, Arai Y et al (2007) Morbidity of Tokyo-area centenarians and its relationship to functional status. J Gerontol A Biol Sci Med Sci 62(7):774–782
91. Galioto A, Dominguez LJ, Pineo A et al (2008) Cardiovascular risk factors in centenarians. Exp Gerontol 43(2):106–113
92. Economos AC (1982) Rate of aging, rate of dying and the mechanism of mortality. Arch Gerontol Geriatr 1(1):3–27
93. Barrett JC (1984) Longevity of selected centenarians. Lancet 2(8410):1032
94. Barrett JC (1985) The mortality of centenarians in England and Wales. Arch Gerontol Geriatr 4(3):211–218
95. Franceschi C, Motta L, Valensin S et al (2000) Do men and women follow different trajectories to reach extreme longevity? Italian Multicenter Study on Centenarians (IMUSCE). Aging (Milano) 12(2):77–84
96. Carey JR, Liedo P, Orozco D, Vaupel JW (1992) Slowing of mortality rates at older ages in large medfly cohorts. Science 258(5081):457–461
97. Lubitz J, Beebe J, Baker C (1995) Longevity and medicare expenditures. N Engl J Med 332(15):999–1003
98. Evert J, Lawler E, Bogan H, Perls T (2003) Morbidity profiles of centenarians: survivors, delayers, and escapers. J Gerontol A Biol Sci Med Sci 58(3):232–237
99. Motta M, Bennati E, Ferlito L, Malaguarnera M, Motta L (2005) Successful aging in centenarians: myths and reality. Arch Gerontol Geriatr 40(3):241–251
100. Franceschi C, Bonafe M (2003) Centenarians as a model for healthy aging. Biochem Soc Trans 31(2):457–461
101. Robine J, Vaupel JW (2001) Supercentenarians: slower ageing individuals or senile elderly? Exp Gerontol 36(4–6):915–930
102. Schoenhofen EA, Wyszynski DF, Andersen S et al (2006) Characteristics of 32 supercentenarians. J Am Geriatr Soc 54(8):1237–1240
103. Perls T, Kohler IV, Andersen S et al (2007) Survival of parents and siblings of supercentenarians. J Gerontol A Biol Sci Med Sci 62(9):1028–1034

Chapter 18
The Effect of Advancing Age on Physician Performance

Jennifer F. Waljee and Lazar J. Greenfield

Introduction

Regardless of profession, aging is ubiquitous and profoundly influences performance throughout one's career. Often, advanced age is considered to bring wisdom and knowledge through longitudinal experience. A common quote is frequently heard in the hallways of hospitals on rounds and at morbidity–mortality teaching conferences: "Good judgment comes from experience, and often experience comes from bad judgment."

However, there is considerable evidence to suggest that advanced age is associated with a decline in an individual's performance. One of the earliest examples of such research that has changed public policy is the ability to operate a motor vehicle. Prior research indicates that older adults have less visual field acuity and visuospatial attention compared with younger individuals, which has been correlated with a decreased ability to operate a motor vehicle [1]. Age-related factors associated with motor vehicle collisions include decreased attention, reaction time, memory, executive function, mental status, visual function, and physical function. Such individuals frequently lack insight into their cognitive, sensory, and physical limitations [2].

In recent years, there has been increasing interest in the effects of age on physician performance and healthcare quality. While not only a sensitive and controversial topic, understanding the effects of the aging process on medical practitioners is important for the assessment of competence and the mechanisms and timing for retirement. This review will examine recent data regarding the effects of age on physician performance and consider the implications for physicians in practice and for those who develop healthcare policy.

The Physiology of Aging in Relation to Performance

The physiologic effects of aging are complex and multifactorial. Previous studies have demonstrated that advancing age is correlated with a decline in motor skills (both gross and fine), decreased visual acuity, and impaired cognitive functioning. However, in practice, it is difficult to assess any individual factor in isolation, as they work in concert to enable an individual to complete a task. For example, over time, older individuals are not only less adept at learning a new motor skill by practice, but also less able to integrate these with cognition and to coordinate movement sequences. Older individuals also have slowed cognitive and motor responses to stimuli compared with younger individuals. Similarly, individuals who err in cognitive tasks are more likely to err in concurrent motor tasks as well [3].

Several aspects of cognition have been shown to decline with age. For example, older individuals are less able to learn new tasks through repeated training and subsequently to execute complex tasks. Additionally, age-related declines exist in several aspects of attentive skills, such as sustained attention, selective attention, and inhibition tasks [4, 5]. Previous studies have documented age differences with respect to memory retrieval, but not necessarily memory encoding or motor memory [3]. For example, new motor memories can be retained for at least 2 years without rehearsal in individuals up to 95 years in age [6].

Of interest to surgeons and those physicians in procedural subspecialties, hand dexterity and visual acuity are significantly influenced by the aging process [7, 8]. Older adults have more difficulty maintaining and varying manual force compared with younger individuals. Changes in ocular optics and neural pathways with age result in decreased visual perception, and an individual's ability to discriminate color, contrast, and motion. Older individuals may also have slower visual processing speeds compared with their younger counterparts [9, 10]. Recent encouraging studies indicate that some age-related declines in visual acuity and hand functioning can be prevented with more extended practice which may allow the development of training protocols to prevent age-related decline in skills for practicing physicians [11, 12].

J.F. Waljee (✉)
Plastic and Reconstructive Surgery, Department of Surgery,
University of Michigan Medical Center, Ann Arbor, MI, USA
e-mail: filip@med.umich.edu

R.A. Rosenthal et al. (eds.), *Principles and Practice of Geriatric Surgery*,
DOI 10.1007/978-1-4419-6999-6_18, © Springer Science+Business Media, LLC 2011

The Effect of Age on Physician Skill

Several studies have looked specifically at the effect of aging on physicians. In 1994, Powell et al. demonstrated a progressive decline in cognitive function among aging physicians, with a notable decline after age 65. These authors assessed physicians and age-matched controls using the Assessment of Cognitive Function (ACF) test, a series of neuropsychological tests assessing one's ability to process and retrieve new information, attention and language ability, visuospatial operations, and reasoning [13, 14]. The study demonstrated that age-related declines occur in both physicians and non-physician control subjects affecting verbal memory, reasoning, attention span, and visuospatial ability.

Bieliauskas et al. recently surveyed 359 surgeons over a 6-year period to identify an association between aging and cognitive functioning. Unlike previous studies addressing the effects of physician aging on performance, this study is longitudinal in design. These authors used the Cambridge Neuropsychological Test Automated Battery (CANTAB) instrument to assess several aspects of physician performance. First, surgeons were tested on measures of rapid visual information processing (RVIP), which also assesses stress tolerance. Surgeons were also tested on reaction time (RTI), and visual learning and memory (paired associates learning, PAL). The authors found age-related declines across all domains. Figure 18.1 demonstrates the effect of age on the RVIP task. There was a nearly linear decline in mean rapid visual processing response with advancing age. Additionally, older surgeons had notably slower movement and reaction time with response to stimuli (Fig. 18.2). Finally, with respect to visual learning and memory, older subjects experienced more incorrect responses per trial, and a lower proportion of correct responses on the first attempt of each

exercise (Fig. 18.3). Of note, these effects were more pronounced among those surgeons who had voluntarily decreased their operative caseloads compared with higher volume surgeons, implying that procedural volume may be an important factor in the correlation between aging and technical skill (Fig. 18.4).

Interestingly, recent data suggest that physicians may adapt to the aging process differently due to the technical and cognitive demands of their profession. Physicians may retain some skills that decline faster in age-matched counterparts. Boom-Saad et al. used CANTAB to determine the effect of age on psychomotor functioning among surgeons and trainees, specifically looking at efficiency of motion, reaction time, sustained visual attention, and visuospatial memory [15]. These authors also demonstrated a linear decline in functioning with respect to RTI, RVIP, and the visual paired associates learning test (PAL). However, compared with age-matched controls, surgeons outperformed age-matched controls despite the decline in age. Surgeons had greater efficiency of movement, shorter response time, and greater accuracy with PAL tasks compared with age-matched controls (Figs. 18.5–18.7), despite the overall decline with age.

To what extent these phenomena represent innate abilities compared acquired skill through the practice of surgery is not clear. However, it is encouraging that studies have shown that many cognitive and motor tasks can be learned and modified with practice. Wanzel et al. and Risucci et al. have studied the relationship between visuospatial ability and competency to perform surgical procedures. These authors have shown that visuospatial ability is easily tested and improves with practice and feedback. Such observations suggest that these and similar tasks could be an important tool for systematically assessing physician competence and skill [11, 12].

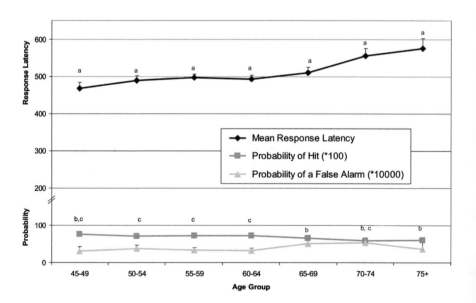

FIGURE 18.1 Correlation between subject age and rapid visual information processing (reprinted with permission from Bieliauskas et al. [31]).

FIGURE 18.2 Correlation between subject age and five choice movement and reaction time (reprinted with permission from Bieliauskas et al. [31].

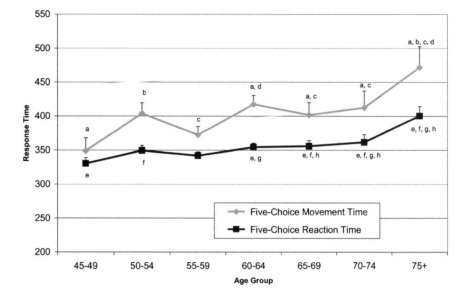

FIGURE 18.3 Correlation between subject age and paired associate learning to assess visual learning and memory (reprinted with permission from Bieliauskas et al. [31]).

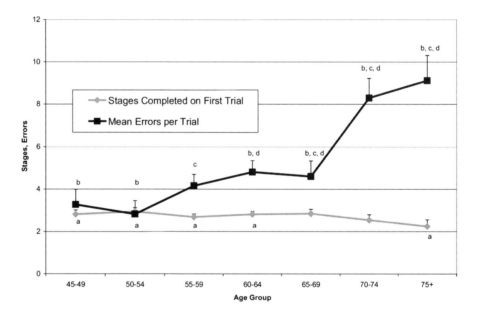

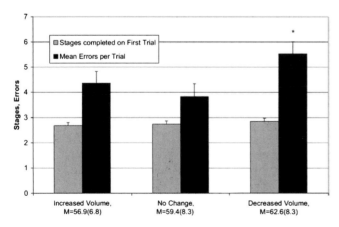

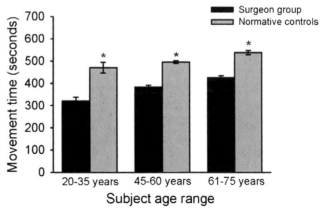

FIGURE 18.4 Correlation between surgeon case volume and paired associate learning (reprinted with permission from Bieliauskas et al. [31]).

FIGURE 18.5 Comparison of movement time between surgeons and normative controls stratified by age (reprinted with permission from Boom-Saad et al. [15]).

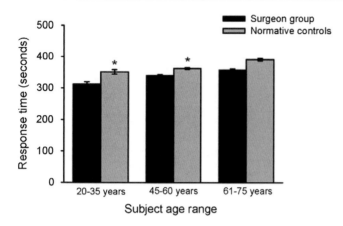

Figure 18.6 Comparison of response time between surgeons and normative controls stratified by age (reprinted with permission from Boom-Saad et al. [15]).

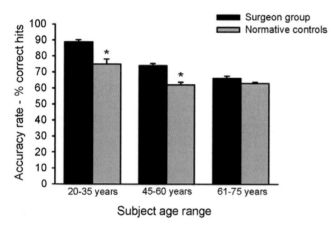

Figure 18.7 Comparison of visual information processing between surgeons and normative controls stratified by age (reprinted with permission from Boom-Saad et al. [15]).

The Effect of Physician Age on Patient Outcomes

Clearly, age-related declines in functioning exist, but to what extent these changes influence patient outcomes is less clear. A recent systematic review demonstrated that older physicians may have less up-to-date factual knowledge and may have poorer patient outcomes [16]. Older physicians are less likely to adhere to established screening guidelines or to standards of therapy use [17, 18]. Some authors have postulated that the effect of age may be related to difficulties in adapting to new techniques, such as laparoscopy or endovascular therapies. For example, Neumayer et al. studied 1,629 patients who underwent laparoscopic herniorrhaphy [19]. These authors found that surgeon age (≥45 years) was correlated with a higher incidence of hernia recurrence following laparoscopic hernia repair, particularly among surgeons inexperienced in laparoscopic repair. Conversely, surgeon age was not correlated with recurrence among patients undergoing open herniorrhaphy.

Previous studies have demonstrated a correlation between physician age and procedural mortality. O'Neill et al. evaluated the association between surgeon characteristics such as age, procedural volume and specialty training, and operative morbidity and mortality following carotid endarterectomy (CEA) [20]. Patients cared for by older surgeons, defined as surgeons in practice longer than 20 years since licensure, experienced a higher operative mortality rate following CEA compared with patients treated by younger surgeons, after adjustment for patient age and mortality risk. Hartz et al. also identified a significant correlation between advanced surgeon age and higher operative mortality following coronary artery bypass grafting (CABG) [21]. Waljee et al. examined the correlation between surgeon age and operative mortality following both cardiovascular and oncologic surgical procedures in a sample of Medicare patients in the USA. In this study, patients cared for by surgeons older than 60 years had a small but significantly higher risk of perioperative death following CEA, CABG, and pancreatectomy (Fig. 18.8) [22]. Conversely, surgeon age was not correlated with operative mortality for elective aortic aneurysm repair, aortic valve replacement, esophagectomy, cystectomy, and lung resection. Of note, for those procedures in which older surgeon age was correlated with higher patient operative mortality, this association was limited to those surgeons with low procedural volumes (Fig. 18.9). These findings suggest that procedural volume may have a protective effect against age-related decay in performance, and those surgeons who remain active with high operative caseloads may attenuate the effects of advancing age on their skill set. Conversely, surgeons who recognize diminishing skills may begin to voluntarily reduce their caseload.

In contrast to these findings, other authors have demonstrated that increasing physician age confers better outcomes for some procedures. Risucci et al. demonstrated that surgeon age and years since graduation were positively correlated with lower procedural times and better acquisition of laparoscopic skills [23]. Prystowsky et al. evaluated morbidity and mortality following complex alimentary tract procedures by physician age. In this study, patients of younger surgeons were more likely to have higher morbidity and mortality rates following highly complex alimentary tract procedures compared with older surgeons [24].

Implications for Practicing Physicians and Policy Makers

Although many studies have examined the relationship between physician aging, professional performance, and patient outcomes, it is unclear how best to utilize these data with respect to

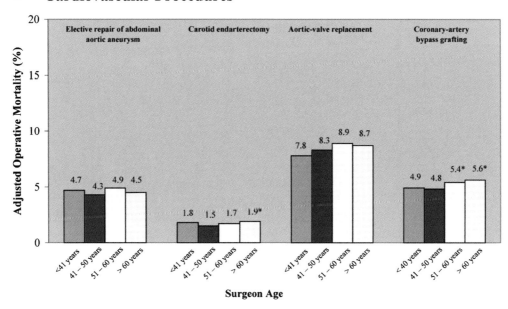

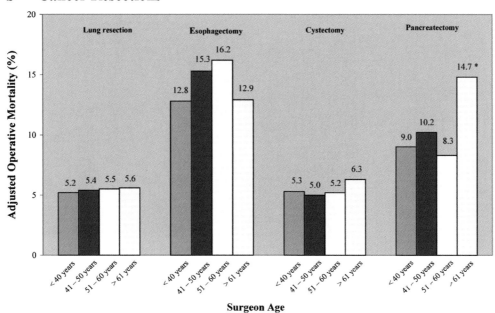

Figure 18.8 Adjusted operative mortality among Medicare patients in 1998 and 1999, according to surgeon age, for four cardiovascular procedures (**a**) and four cancer resections (**b**)[†]. (Reprinted with permission from Waljee et al. [22].) [†]Adjusted for patient severity, race, gender, age, surgeon volume, hospital volume, and hospital teaching status. *$p<0.05$.

health policy and guidelines for physicians approaching retirement age. We do not know the age limits of physician performance nor the role of other provider and practice setting characteristics on the effects of aging, such as acquiring subspecialty training or practicing in a teaching hospital. Previous studies are often limited by a lack of longitudinal data or reliance on administrative data which may not identify subtle factors that influence the relationship of age and performance.

Regardless, there have been efforts to improve healthcare quality through assessment of physician performance throughout one's career. Many fields in medicine today require recertification examinations at periodic intervals to ensure competence and test medical knowledge. However, written evaluation may not suffice for those in procedural-based fields. In recent years, the Society of American Gastrointestinal and Endoscopic Surgeons (SAGES) has

Figure 18.9 Adjusted operative mortality among Medicare patients in 1998 and 1999, according to surgeon age, and stratified by surgeon volume.[†] (**a**) Cardiovascular procedures; (**b**) cancer resections. (From Waljee et al. [22]). [†]Adjusted for patient gender, race, admission acuity, age, and Charlson score. *p<0.05.

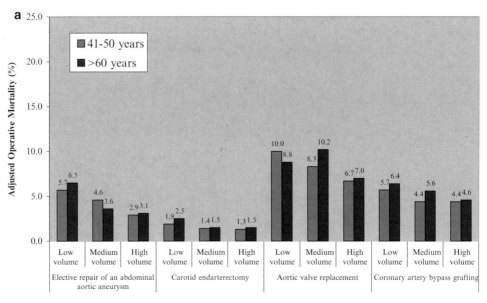

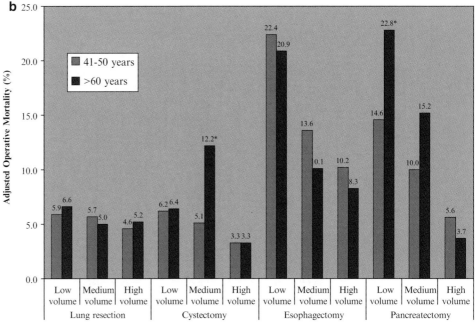

developed a standardized curriculum and assessment of surgical trainees acquiring laparoscopic skills, the Fundamentals of Laparoscopic Surgery (FLS) curriculum. The FLS program is designed to teach both the cognitive and psychomotor aspects of laparoscopy through didactic teaching modules as well as specific technical skill sets [25]. Early studies have shown these programs to be successful in improving performance, and they are increasingly becoming a requirement for surgeons seeking credentialing at certain hospitals [12, 26, 27]. Similar concepts could be applied to the recertification process for surgeons in practice to assess both medical knowledge and technical skill. However, there is no current

systematic assessment for the technical aspects of surgery for surgeons in practice, and few guidelines for surgeons considering or nearing retirement.

This research has also prompted debate regarding the optimal timing of and approach to retirement. A recent survey of surgeons revealed that many surgeons in practice begin to decrease their workload after the age of 60, but a substantial number continue to operate well beyond the age of 70 [28]. The reasons for retirement commonly cited relate to the medical business climate and fear of malpractice, rather than an innate sense of waning competence or inability to complete tasks. In fact, younger surgeons may be more likely to consider retirement due to increased rates of self-reported burnout, emotional exhaustion, depersonalization, and sense of reduced personal accomplishment [29, 30]. In addition to variation in timing of retirement, physicians also vary in their approach to retirement. Many surgeons gradually taper off their clinical practices and operative volumes [28, 31]. However, recent data indicate that those surgeons who maintain high procedural volumes can preserve their technical skills and have improved patient outcomes. It is well established that surgeons who perform certain procedures less frequently have poorer outcomes compared with those who perform these operations more frequently [32–34].

Physicians may lack self-awareness regarding the effects of aging on their professional skills. Recent data indicate that physicians do not report difficulties with memory recall or name recognition, despite age-related changes demonstrated on testing. Interestingly, self-awareness of cognitive changes may be the marker surgeons expect to use for the decision to retire. [31] Approximately 40% of surgeons report that they will retire when they feel their skills are waning, but only 27% report that they will retire at a predetermined age. In fact, there may be a significant delay between the onset of cognitive changes and retirement, and the extent to which this affects patient care is not known. It is also unclear what mechanisms should be in place for those surgeons who may not recognize deterioration in their skills. Greenfield and Proctor found that the majority of surgeons believe that withdrawing operating privileges should be based on peer-review measures or the onset of disability, and not on the basis of age alone [28]. However, this approach may be problematic for several reasons. In community hospital settings, senior surgeon influence and medicolegal concerns regarding disclosure of surgeon performance can inhibit objective peer review. Although an external reviewer could provide an objective viewpoint, the most appropriate method to assess performance has not been established. Instead, data on adherence to best processes of care, length of procedures, length of stay, and specific postoperative complication rates may be more helpful to assess the quality of patient care and could be used in conjunction with standardized tests of knowledge and technical skills to guide retirement.

In conclusion, current research has only begun to define the effects of aging on physician performance, but has raised important questions concerning physician competence and quality of healthcare delivered. While current data may not support the use of age alone as an indicator of performance, understanding the effects of aging and the mechanisms behind decline in performance can provide valuable insight for future policy decisions regarding recertification and retirement. Efforts to refine cognitive and procedural tests should continue with emphasis on confidentiality so that ultimately, surgeons will be able to track their own performance over time facilitating appropriate decisions regarding retirement.

References

1. Perryman KM, Fitten LJ (1996) Effects of normal aging on the performance of motor-vehicle operational skills. J Geriatr Psychiatry Neurol 9:136–141
2. Anstey KJ, Wood J, Lord S, Walker JG (2005) Cognitive, sensory and physical factors enabling driving safety in older adults. Clin Psychol Rev 25:45–65
3. Sawaki L, Yaseen Z, Kopylev L, Cohen LG (2003) Age-dependent changes in the ability to encode a novel elementary motor memory. Ann Neurol 53:521–524
4. Mani TM, Bedwell JS, Miller LS (2005) Age-related decrements in performance on a brief continuous performance test. Arch Clin Neuropsychol 20:575–586
5. Armstrong C (1997) Selective versus sustained attention: A continuous performance test revisited. Clinical Neuropsychologist 11:18–33
6. Smith CD, Walton A, Loveland AD, Umberger GH, Kryscio RJ, Gash DM (2005) Memories that last in old age: motor skill learning and memory preservation. Neurobiol Aging 26:883–890
7. Hackel ME, Wolfe GA, Bang SM, Canfield JS (1992) Changes in hand function in the aging adult as determined by the Jebsen Test of Hand Function. Phys Ther 72:373–377
8. Keogh J, Morrison S, Barrett R (2006) Age-related differences in inter-digit coupling during finger pinching. Eur J Appl Physiol 97:76–88
9. Jackson GR, Owsley C (2003) Visual dysfunction, neurodegenerative diseases, and aging. Neurol Clin 21:709–728
10. Jackson GR, Owsley C, Cordle EP, Finley CD (1998) Aging and scotopic sensitivity. Vision Res 38:3655–3662
11. Wanzel KR, Hamstra SJ, Anastakis DJ, Matsumoto ED, Cusimano MD (2002) Effect of visual-spatial ability on learning of spatially-complex surgical skills. Lancet 359:230–231
12. Risucci DA (2002) Visual spatial perception and surgical competence. Am J Surg 184:291–295
13. Powell D, Whitla DK (1994) Profiles in cognitive aging. In: Cognitive changes across the life-span. Harvard Press, Boston, Massachusettes
14. Greenfield LJ (1994) Farewell to surgery. J Vasc Surg 19:6–14
15. Boom-Saad Z, Langenecker S, Bieliauskas LA et al (2008) Surgeons outperform normative controls on neuropsychologic tests, but age-related decay of skills persists. Am J Surg 195:205–209
16. Choudhry NK, Fletcher RH, Soumerai SB (2005) Systematic review: the relationship between clinical experience and quality of health care. Ann Intern Med 142:260–273
17. Beaulieu MD, Blais R, Jacques A, Battista RN, Lebeau R, Brophy J (2001) Are patients suffering from stable angina receiving optimal medical treatment? QJM 94:301–308
18. Czaja R, McFall SL, Warnecke RB, Ford L, Kaluzny AD (1994) Preferences of community physicians for cancer screening guidelines. Ann Intern Med 120:602–608
19. Neumayer LA, Gawande AA, Wang J et al (2005) Proficiency of surgeons in inguinal hernia repair: effect of experience and age. Ann Surg 242:344–348, discussion 8–52
20. O'Neill L, Lanska DJ, Hartz A (2000) Surgeon characteristics associated with mortality and morbidity following carotid endarterectomy. Neurology 55:773–781
21. Hartz AJ, Kuhn EM, Pulido J (1999) Prestige of training programs and experience of bypass surgeons as factors in adjusted patient mortality rates. Med Care 37:93–103
22. Waljee JF, Greenfield LJ, Dimick JB, Birkmeyer JD (2006) Surgeon age and operative mortality in the United States. Ann Surg 244:353–362
23. Risucci D, Geiss A, Gellman L, Pinard B, Rosser J (2001) Surgeon-specific factors in the acquisition of laparoscopic surgical skills. Am J Surg 181:289–293

24. Prystowsky JB (2005) Are young surgeons competent to perform alimentary tract surgery? Arch Surg 140:495–500, discussion 2

25. Soper NJ, Fried GM (2008) The fundamentals of laparoscopic surgery: its time has come. Bull Am Coll Surg 93:30–32

26. Risucci D, Geiss A, Gellman L, Pinard B, Rosser JC (2000) Experience and visual perception in resident acquisition of laparoscopic skills. Curr Surg 57:368–372

27. Dath D, Regehr G, Birch D et al (2004) Toward reliable operative assessment: the reliability and feasibility of videotaped assessment of laparoscopic technical skills. Surg Endosc 18:1800–1804

28. Greenfield LJ, Proctor MC (1994) Attitudes toward retirement. A survey of the American Surgical Association. Ann Surg 220:382–389, discussion 7–90

29. Campbell DA Jr, Sonnad SS, Eckhauser FE, Campbell KK, Greenfield LJ (2001) Burnout among American surgeons. Surgery 130:696–702, discussion 5

30. Maslach C, Jackson S (1986) Maslach burnout inventory. Consulting Psychologists Press, Palo Alto, California

31. Bieliauskas LA, Langenecker S, Graver C, Lee HJ, O'Neill J, Greenfield LJ (2008) Cognitive Changes and Retirement among Senior Surgeons (CCRASS): Results from the CCRASS Study. J Am Coll Surg 207:69–79

32. Birkmeyer JD, Stukel TA, Siewers AE, Goodney PP, Wennberg DE, Lucas FL (2003) Surgeon volume and operative mortality in the United States. N Engl J Med 349:2117–2127

33. Hannan EL, Kilburn H Jr, Bernard H, O'Donnell JF, Lukacik G, Shields EP (1991) Coronary artery bypass surgery: the relationship between inhospital mortality rate and surgical volume after controlling for clinical risk factors. Med Care 29:1094–1107

34. Luft HS (1980) The relation between surgical volume and mortality: an exploration of causal factors and alternative models. Med Care 18:940–959

Section III
Perioperative Issues

Chapter 19
Invited Commentary

Ben Eiseman

Since the publication of the first edition of this book, geriatric surgery has achieved recognition of its professional independence. Like an adolescent youngster or an equivalent recently liberated nation, it now faces a number of policy decisions as it matures and seeks stability. This invited commentary is therefore for the founding mothers and fathers of Surgical Geriacistan. It comes from a veteran of similar wars of independence of Thoracic, Pediatric, and Vascular Surgcalistan, and many years ago as an invited outside founding father of Family Practistan.

Defining the Borders of Your Professional Turf

An essential early step in the maturing process for a person, a nation, or a clinical specialty is to define where it differs – and excels – from everyone else: to define its borders. This is of practical importance if, as for Surgical Geriacistan, it is surrounded by aggressive neighbors such as Intensivistan, Hospitalistan, and the bearded mullahs of Fundamentalistan. The political paradigm for Surgical Geriacistan resembles the diplomatic Great Game of Central Asia, the Balkans, and Central Africa.

Geriatric surgery has a unique focus: its primary concern is the elderly and those near the end of life when operation is under consideration. Such patients have a diminished life expectancy, suffer multiple comorbidities and most of their diseases are incurable and, therefore, palliation is the best that can be expected. Their quality of life is limited; their physiologic reserves and defensive mechanisms compromised, and they are uniquely dependent on support of family and society. Finally, their management is enormously expensive. Skills required to provide operative care to such a population requires special training, which must be codified by the founders of geriatric surgery.

Unique Skills

Essential skills for geriatric surgery are familiar to its practitioners but include familiarity with the following unique features of the elderly and the oldest old.

- Response to the stress of operation.
- Cumulative effects of comorbidities.
- Risks of polypharmacy.
- Communication skills with the elderly and their families.
- Economic implication of the cost of care in this high-risk, high-cost, low-outcome benefit population.

Once requirements for achieving these and other essential skills are identified, definition of the content and duration of the required training period will follow.

Defending Your Borders

Leaders of geriatric surgery must be skilled practitioners and good politicians because they are surrounded by acquisitive competitors with whom they must work in harmony. Sharing authority is seldom an inherent charm for most surgeons who prefer unity of command but such are the rules of engagement in geriatric surgery. The fact that their neighbors are often the source of patient referrals asserts a modulating force on authoritarian instincts.

Geriatric surgeons like any good diplomat should be prepared to protect their turf when all else fails. Clearly defined and accepted boundaries help avoid misunderstandings, but inoffensive traffic through gates in the fence should be encouraged. Poaching is unacceptable, but recent diplomatic experiments involving hubris have clearly demonstrated its destructive folly.

B. Eiseman (✉)
Department of Surgery, Denver Vetarans Affairs Hospital, University Hospital, 1055 Clermont St., Denver, CO 80220-112, USA
e-mail: Ben.eiseman@va.gov

R.A. Rosenthal et al. (eds.), *Principles and Practice of Geriatric Surgery*,
DOI 10.1007/978-1-4419-6999-6_19, © Springer Science+Business Media, LLC 2011

Allies

Warfare with neighbors, as mentioned, is to be avoided, but allies in peaceful negotiation should be cultivated by a newly independent specialty. The most obvious ally for the geriatric surgeon are the geriatricians who themselves only recently achieved their own independence. Even more powerful support, however, can come from those who pay the enormous cost of geriatric health care. The two big payers are the government and health insurers. Once they are convinced that geriatric surgical specialists are cost-effective, the war for specialty survival is assured. Subsequent bloody battles may be necessary, but independence will follow. Geriatric surgeons are well advised to improve and document their cost-effectiveness.

Internal Stability

Independence inevitably creates temporary turbulence and instability. Examples such as internal conflicts of the Sunnis and Shias or the Tutsis and Hutus abound in foreign affairs. The health care specialty equivalents are the internal disputes among vascular surgeons or invasivist vs. noninvasivist gastroenterologists or cardiologists.

Founders of surgical geriatrics should promptly settle self-destructive internal disputes among tribal leaders and present a united front to professional competitors.

The Slippery Slope of Health Care Specialization

Pioneer health care specialists routinely deny intent to become involved in the complexities that characterize administration of other new specialties. They inevitably fail and so will surgical geriatricians who might as well resign themselves to the frustrations and pangs of the required rites of transition. Steps on this slippery slope are familiar. An early manifestation is a web page, which now serves to advertise a new faith and as did the church door for Martin Luther. Subsequent steps include definition of training requirements for the new specialty. Fellowships precede specialty residencies which soon follow. This leads to Residency Review Committees, formal requirements for accreditation, an examination, one's very own Board, a Central Office, a Director and his or her staff, annual meetings and dues, and endless black-tie dinners and speeches. Soon thereafter, a large multiauthored textbook appears. A separate journal inevitably follows.

This formal professional minuet absorbs an unbelievable amount of time, energy, and stress on one's family but apparently is unavoidable.

Health Policy Decisions

Founders of geriatric surgery struggling for recognition can benefit from realizing their unique opportunity to influence US health-care policy at a moment when it is anticipating significant change. The high cost, low societal and personal yield of their patient population constitutes a particularly vulnerable segment of health- care patients whose most cost-effective care would be ideal for critical review and change when our society is ready to include cost–benefit analysis in the formulae dictating government reimbursement. Involvement in such medical political pioneering by the leadership in geriatric surgery would have enormous collateral benefit to this new specialty.

You are well launched and will thrive. You also predictably will resent future efforts of young whippersnappers who will suggest further separation from your then established authority.

Chapter 20
Principles of Geriatric Surgery

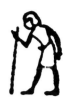

Mark R. Katlic

With a few obvious exceptions, those of us who are surgeons must become geriatric surgeons. The population as a whole is aging, with the most explosive growth in the over 85 year group, and the conditions that require surgery (atherosclerosis, cancer, arthritis, prostatism, cataract, and others) increase in incidence with increasing age. Improving our care of the elderly surgical patient – the *raison d'etre* of this book – will become progressively more important to us all.

Admittedly, surgeons have always cared for the elderly, but the definition of "elderly" has changed. A threshold of 50 years was chosen for the 167 patients described in a paper in 1907 [1], and 20 years later influential surgeons still wrote that elective herniorrhaphy in this age group was not warranted [2]. Now, though, we are performing complex operations in octogenarians, nonagenarians, and occasionally centenarians [3–7]. In addition, the salutary results of such surgery can even influence general sentiment about medical care of the elderly. Linn and Zeppa's study [8] of junior medical students reported that the surgery rotation, in contrast to other clerkships, positively influenced the students' attitudes about aging regardless of the students' career choices, as the elderly surgical patients were admitted and treated successfully.

Surgery therefore has much to offer the geriatric patient, but that patient must be treated with appropriate knowledge and attention to detail. Discussions of physiologic changes in the elderly and results of specific operations comprise the bulk of this book and are not presented here. The author's quarter-century study in this area, in addition to caring for an elderly thoracic oncology population, has led to a distillate of several general principles (Table 20.1) which are relevant to all who care for the aged. These principles are worthwhile chiefly for propaedeutic purposes, as they can-

TABLE 20.1 Principles of geriatric surgery

I. The *clinical presentation* of surgical problems in the elderly may be subtle or somewhat different from that in the general population. This may lead to delay in diagnosis

II. The elderly handle stress satisfactorily but handle severe stress poorly because of *lack of organ system reserve*

III. Optimal *preoperative preparation* is essential, because of Principle II. When preparation is suboptimal, the perioperative risk increases

IV. The results of elective surgery in the elderly are reproducibly good; the results of emergency surgery are poor though still better than nonoperative treatment for most conditions. The risk of *emergency surgery* may be many times that of similar elective surgery because of Principles II and III

V. Scrupulous *attention to detail* intraoperatively and perioperatively yields great benefit, as the elderly tolerate complications poorly (because of Principle II)

VI. A patient's age should be treated as a *scientific fact, not with prejudice*. No particular chronologic age, of itself, is a contraindication to operation (because of Principle IV)

M.R. Katlic (✉)
Division of Thoracic Surgery,
Director, Regional Ambulatory Campus Geisinger Wyoming Valley
Medical Center, Wilkes-Barre, PA, USA
e-mail: mrkatlic@geisinger.edu

R.A. Rosenthal et al. (eds.), *Principles and Practice of Geriatric Surgery*,
DOI 10.1007/978-1-4419-6999-6_20, © Springer Science+Business Media, LLC 2011

FIGURE 20.1 Operative mortality in the national Medicare population has declined for some, but not all, procedures. Adjusted odds ratios (average change in mortality) and 95% confidence intervals for the 6-year period 1994–1999. Adjusted for age, gender, race, comorbidities, admission acuity, income, and hospital volume (from Goodney et al. [10], reprinted with permission from Elsevier).

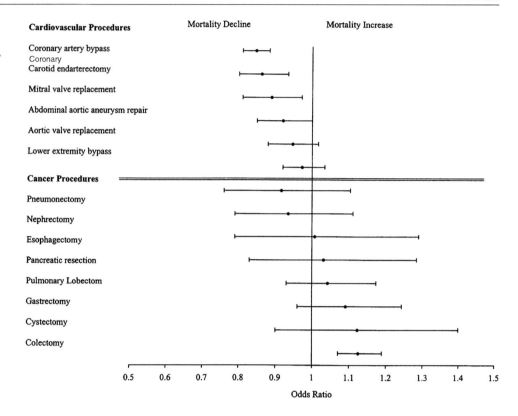

not apply to every patient or every clinical situation. Some principles also apply to surgery in the young patient, but the quantitative differences in the elderly are significant enough to approach qualitative status. Risks of many emergency operations in the young, for example, are indeed greater than the risks of similar elective operations, but the differences are small compared with the threefold increase in the elderly. With respect to these principles, the elderly need not be treated as a separate species but perhaps as a separate genus or order within the same larger group of surgical candidates.

Although our results have generally improved over the years [9], this improvement has not been universal [10] (Fig. 20.1), and emergency surgery is still risky (Fig. 20.2). So, how do we do better?

Principle I: Clinical Presentation

The clinical presentation of surgical problems in the elderly may be subtle or somewhat different from that in the general population. This may lead to delay in diagnosis.

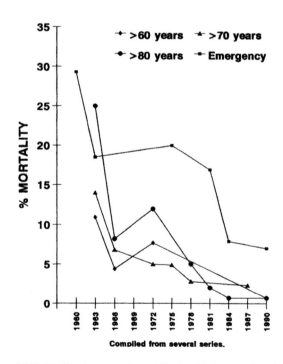

FIGURE 20.2 Decline in surgical mortality in elderly over time (emergency always much higher) (from Thomas and Ritchie [9], with permission from Blackwell Publishing).

CASE STUDY

This brief case report illustrates several of the six Principles of Geriatric Surgery outlined in this chapter.

An 88-year-old man was referred for evaluation and treatment of a right lung mass. He had been a cigarette smoker for 40 years but quit 25 years prior to evaluation. He had fully recovered from a cerebrovascular accident 8 years before – playing golf several times each week, had undergone inguinal herniorrhaphy, and took only nifedipine. A chest radiograph ordered because of a nagging cough showed a hazy perihilar density that, on computed tomogram (Fig. 20.3), proved to be a 4-cm right lower lobe mass. His family physician told him that he was too old for surgery, but he and his wife wanted another opinion.

Examination showed a tall man with a strong regular pulse and blood pressure 140/82 mmHg. Lungs were clear, heart without murmur, abdomen benign. Computed tomograms showed no adenopathy and no evidence of metastatic disease. Pulmonary function was greater than 100% of predicted. Bronchoscopy was grossly and cytologically unremarkable. After a discussion of risks and alternatives, he chose to undergo resection.

Right lower lobectomy was performed for what proved to be a 3-cm squamous cell carcinoma with negative hilar and mediastinal nodes. Stapled vessel and bronchial closures were reinforced with sutures. Venous compression stockings and monitoring of oxygen saturation and cardiac rhythm were maintained overnight. He had an uncomplicated postoperative course.

He resumed golfing and social life. I saw the patient and his wife of 70 years having dinner on Valentine's Day 1 month prior to his death from pneumonia, without evidence of cancer, at an age of 92.

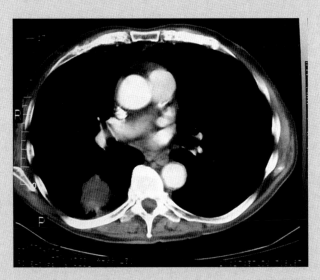

Figure 20.3 Computed tomogram of 88-year-old patient with right lower lobe cancer.

Classic symptoms of appendicitis are present in a minority of elderly patients, as few as 26% in Horattas' series over 20 years [11] (Table 20.2). Rebound tenderness was present in fewer than half the patients in another series [12] and leukocytosis in only 42.9% in a third series [13]. Clouding the picture further, objective tests may suggest alternative diagnoses: one in six patients has an elevated bilirubin and one in four has signs of ileus, bowel obstruction, gallstones, or renal calculus on abdominal radiographs [14]. Even astute diagnosis may not prevent perforation, present in 42–60% of elderly patients despite operation within 24 h of symptom onset [11, 13].

Biliary tract disease is the most common entity requiring abdominal surgery in the elderly, yet the diagnosis is often delayed. More than one-third of patients with acute cholecystitis are afebrile, one-fourth are nontender, and one-third are without leukocytosis [15–17]. Cholangitis may appear only as fever of unknown origin or as confusion [18]. Consequently, the elderly predominate in series of patients with complications of biliary disease (gallbladder perforation, empyema, gangrene, gallstone ileus, and cholangitis) [19],

Table 20.2 Classic symptoms of appendicitis are present in a minority of elderly patients, resulting in perforation despite expeditious operation

Twenty-year comparison and compilation

Characteristic	1978–1988 ($n=96$)	1988–1998 ($n=113$)	1978–1998 ($n=209$)
Classic presentation	(19) 20%	(36) 30%	(55) 26%
Delayed presentation (>48 h)	(32) 33%	(36) 30%	(68) 33%
Imaging			
AAS	(81) 84%	(86) 76%	(167) 80%
Sensitivity	(22) 27%	(22) 25%	(44) 26%
CT		(50) 44%	
Sensitivity		(45) 90%	
Correct admitting diagnosis	(49) 51%	(52) 46%	(101) 48%
Surgery within 24 h	(80) 83%	(97) 85%	(177) 85%
Perforation	(60) 72%	(58) 51%	(127) 61%
Complications	(30) 32%	(24) 21%	(54) 26%
Those with perforation	(25) 83%	(15) 72%	(40) 76%
Deaths	(4) 4%	(4) 4%	(8) 4%

From Storm-Dickerson [11]. Reprinted with permission from Elsevier

and the complication may result in the first apparent symptom [16, 20]. Saunders [21] reported that abdominal pain was a less prominent symptom and that the bilirubin level was nearly double in elderly patients presenting with bile duct carcinoma, compared with the findings in young patients seen during the same time period.

Peptic ulcer disease may present as confusion, malaise, anemia, or weight loss as opposed to pain [22]; even with perforation pain may be absent or minimal. Rabinovici and Manny [23] found a discrepancy between "severe intraoperative findings" and preoperative objective findings such as heart rate (mean 88/min), temperature (37.2°C), and white blood cell count (10,900/dl). Some have suggested that the elderly and possibly their physicians become tolerant over the years to abdominal pain, loss of energy, and other symptoms, resulting in a delay in diagnosis or an emergency presentation. In Mulcahy's [24] series of patients with colorectal carcinoma, for example, elderly patients were nearly twice as likely (18%) as younger patients (11%) to present emergently. Elderly patients with perforated diverticulitis are three times more likely to have generalized peritonitis at operation than young patients [25].

Gastroesophageal reflux disease in the elderly is less likely to cause heartburn and more likely to cause regurgitation or cough ($p=001$) [26]. In Pilotto's study of 840 consecutive patients [27], typical heartburn/acid reflux, pain, and indigestion were more likely in the young ($p<0.001$); older patients more often experienced dysphagia, anorexia, anemia, or vomiting ($p<0.001$ each) or weight loss ($p<0.007$) (Table 20.3).

Head and neck disease may also present differently in the elderly. Sinusitis may lead to subtle signs such as delirium or fever of unknown origin [28, 29]; and head and neck cancers are less likely to be associated with smoking ($p<0.01$) [30] and alcohol use ($p<0.001$) [30, 31]. Hyperparathyroidism is more likely to cause dementia or skeletal complaints and less likely to cause renal stones [32]. In Thomas and Grigg's series [33] of patients with carotid artery disease, stroke was

the most common indication for surgery in octogenarians and was the least common indication in younger patients. Unstable angina is as likely to present with dyspnea, nausea, or diaphoresis as it is with classic chest pain [34].

Even the eureka moments that keep us energized as diagnosticians [35] may be "subtler and less electric" [36] in the elderly.

The clinician who understands that classic presentations of surgical disease occur in a minority of elderly patients will maintain the high index of suspicion needed to minimize delay in diagnosis.

Principle II: Lack of Reserve

> The elderly handle stress satisfactorily but handle severe stress poorly because of lack of organ system reserve.

Functional reserve may be considered the difference between basal and maximal function (Fig. 20.4); it represents the capacity to meet increased demands imposed by disease or trauma. Although there is variability among individuals, this organ system reserve inexorably declines in one's 70s, 80s, and 90s (Fig. 20.5). With excellent anesthetic and perioperative care, the aged patient may tolerate the stress of even complex surgery – particularly if elective – but not the added stress of exceptional or emergency surgery.

The elderly patient with lung cancer, like our case report patient, can undergo routine pulmonary lobectomy with results nearly indistinguishable from those of the general population [37, 38], but the added stress of concomitant chest wall resection leads to a disparate increase in risk. In Keagy's series [39], the one death and two of the three respiratory

Table 20.3 Symptoms of gastroesophageal reflux disease may be different and more subtle in the elderly

| Symptoms | Number (%) of patients | | |
	Group A (<65 years) (n=241)	Group B (≥65 years) (n=63)	p-value
Heartburn	209 (86)	45 (47)	0.001
Dysphagia	92 (38)	28 (35)	0.77
Regurgitation	113 (47)	46 (71)	0.001
Chest pain	97 (39)	18 (28)	0.13
Cough	89 (37)	42 (67)	0.001
Response to proton pump inhibitors[a]	70	75	0.53

[a]Percentage of patients

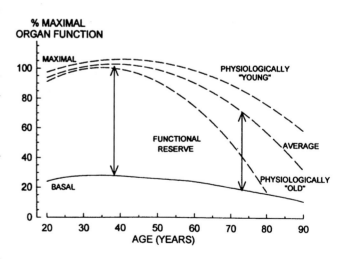

Figure 20.4 Organ system functional reserve is the difference between maximal function and basal function; reserve declines with age (reprinted with permission from Muravchick [192], copyright Elsevier 2000).

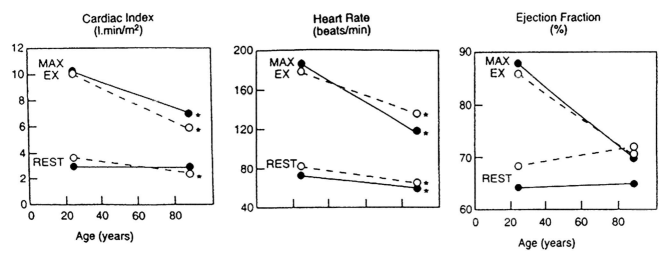

FIGURE 20.5 Lack of reserve: with increasing age cardiac function is maintained at rest but not under stress. Linear regression at rest and during maximal cycle ergometry in healthy sedentary men (*solid lines*) and women (*dotted lines*). All subjects are healthy, community-dwelling volunteers screened to exclude hypertension and occult coronary artery disease (reprinted with permission from Lakatta [193]).

failures were in patients who underwent the *en bloc* chest wall resection. An elderly patient, entering the operating room with decreased chest wall compliance and strength and decreased elastic recoil as a baseline, may tolerate lung resection but lacks the reserve to tolerate an extended operation. Other researchers have reported increased mortality in septuagenarians and octogenarians following pneumonectomy, especially right pneumonectomy or completion pneumonectomy [40–42].

On the other side of the spectrum, more limited procedures, such as video-assisted thoracic surgery, may decrease stress further by preserving respiratory muscle strength [43–46]. Yim [46] reported no deaths or pulmonary complications following thoracoscopic surgery in 22 patients over an age of 75, 5 with major resections; and Jaklitsch et al. [44] found decreased mortality, length of hospital stay, and postoperative delirium after 307 video-assisted procedures in patients aged 65–90 compared with that associated with open thoracotomy. Video assisted pulmonary lobectomy in half of a group of elderly lung cancer patients resulted in fewer complications ($p=0.04$) and decreased length of stay ($p<0.001$) compared with the half who underwent open (thoracotomy) lobectomy [47]. Patel et al. [48] reported shorter hospitalization and similar late outcomes following endovascular thoracic aortic procedures in patients greater than 75 years, compared with open procedures.

Left ventricular functional reserve assumes critical importance in elderly patients undergoing cardiac surgery. In general, results in the elderly diverge from those of young age groups only in the worst functional classes. Bergus et al. [49], for example, found that the length of stay following aortic valve replacement was significantly longer ($p<0.05$)

in septuagenarians in New York Heart Association class IV but not in class III, compared with patients under the age of 70. Patients over an age of 75 in Salomon's large series [50] had significantly higher mortality after coronary artery bypass grafting if they had suffered a myocardial infarction less than 3 weeks preoperatively compared with more than 3 weeks (14.1 vs. 5.2%); there was much less difference in patients younger than age 75 (3.5 vs. 2.3%). When patients over an age of 70 undergo a third coronary reoperation, only those in the worse Canadian Functional Class experience increased mortality, an increase not seen in young patients in a similar class [51]. Elayda et al. [52] reported that mortality for isolated aortic valve replacement in patients over an age of 80 was acceptable (5.2%), but addition of concomitant procedures increased this figure significantly (27.7%).

Similar findings pertain to major abdominal surgery. Fortner and Lincer [53] found that the increased number of deaths among elderly patients undergoing hepatic resection for liver cancer were nearly all in the extended-resection group (i.e., extended right hepatectomy or trisegmentectomy), among whom 60% of deaths were due to hepatic insufficiency. In another group of hepatic resections done for metastatic colon cancer, where cirrhosis and functional hepatic reserve are less important factors, there was no difference in mortality between young and old patients [54]. Even the addition of common duct exploration to open cholecystectomy significantly increased mortality in the elderly (3.5 vs. 1.8%, $p<0.05$) [55]. For some oncology cases (e.g., gastric cancer and lung cancer), a more limited operation in the elderly need not decrease survival [56–59].

The elderly can return to normal function after stressful operations (such as colectomy and hepatectomy), but after

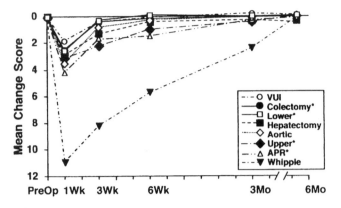

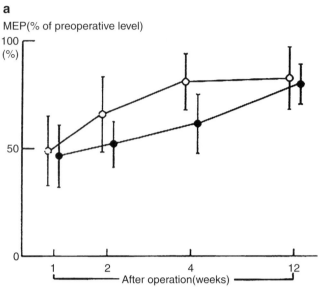

Figure 20.6 Return to activities of daily living after major surgery (function returns rapidly after stressful operations but not the most stressful, speaking to lack of reserve). From Lawrence et al. [60], reprinted with permission from Elsevier.

the most stressful operations (such as Whipple pancreaticoduodenectomy) it will take longer [60] (Fig. 20.6).

With modern anesthetic and critical care management, an elderly patient can tolerate the stress of even complex operations. However, if the most extended procedures are contemplated, a comprehensive preoperative evaluation of functional reserve is recommended.

Principle III: Preoperative Preparation

Optimal preoperative preparation is essential because of Principle II. When preparation is suboptimal the perioperative risk increases.

A patient's advanced age is immutable but some factors can be improved preoperatively, with benefits in excess of those to a younger patient. No universal threshold of blood hemoglobin applies to every patient, but correction of anemia and dehydration do assume greater importance in the elderly because of their general lack of reserve and particularly the physiology of the aged heart and kidney. Among the predictors of an overall good postoperative course in Seymour's series of 288 elderly general surgery patients were a hemoglobin level of more than 11.0 g/dl and absence of volume depletion [61]. Contrary to this, Dzankic found that routine blood testing in the elderly surgical patient rarely showed abnormal results and even when abnormal did not correlate with adverse postoperative outcome [62].

Few would argue that pulmonary problems are among the most common perioperative complications in the elderly, in part due to decreased respiratory muscle strength. Nomori et al. [45] showed that following thoracotomy patients older than 70 years experience significant reductions in both maximum inspiratory and expiratory pressures, unlike their younger counterparts; this effect persists for 12 weeks

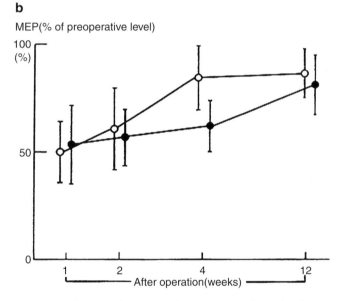

Figure 20.7 Postoperative changes in mean (**a**) maximum inspiratory pressure (MIP, percent of preoperative level) and (**b**) maximum expiratory pressure (MEP, percent of preoperative level) following pulmonary resection in 36 patients younger than 69 years (*open circles*) and 12 patients older than 70 years (*closed circles*). From Nomori et al. [45], reprinted with permission from Elsevier).

(Fig. 20.7). Although few data exist to support the routine use of preoperative pulmonary conditioning or rehabilitation, most authors strongly advocate smoking cessation [63] and treatment of bronchitis and reactive airways disease such as asthma [64, 65]. Prophylaxis against deep vein thrombosis (DVT), clearly a risk in the elderly [66], and against pulmonary embolism should be routine [67].

The value of preoperative optimization of cardiac function (e.g., via placement of a pulmonary artery catheter) is controversial. Some authors have shown clear benefit [68], whereas others [69, 70], citing methodologic flaws in the former studies, reported no reduction in perioperative morbidity or mortality. These studies do not include exceptionally high risk or very elderly patients, who could well be helped by such treatment. Another unsettled issue concerns the value of aggressive preoperative screening for coronary and carotid artery disease, particularly in patients scheduled for peripheral vascular surgery. Leppo [71] considered age over 70 years to be one of the several risk factors (the others being a history of angina, congestive heart failure, diabetes mellitus, prior myocardial infarction, and ventricular ectopy) that should trigger further cardiac assessment. Echocardiogram and dobutamine stress testing have been shown to bear incremental value over clinical evaluation [72] (Fig. 20.8).

There is some evidence that performance testing may hold value. Maximal oxygen consumption (VO_2 Max) tests

may not be readily available in all hospitals, but reasonable surrogates – stair climbing [73, 74], shuttle walk [75], long distance corridor walk [76], metabolic equivalent (MET) – have been shown to correlate. Weinstein [77] reported prolonged length of stay following thoracic cancer surgery in those patients with METs ≤4 (equating to calisthenics or walking briskly). The International Society of Geriatric Oncology has studied a standardized Preoperative Assessment in Elderly Cancer Patient (PACE); postoperative complications were associated with poor preoperative performance status and lower score on Instrumental Activities of Daily Living but major complications correlated only with American Society of Anesthesiologists (ASA) Physical Status ≤2 [78] (Table 20.4). However, as Internullo et al. recently concluded that "a practical and reliable individual risk assessment tool is still lacking" [79].

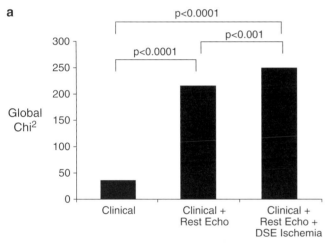
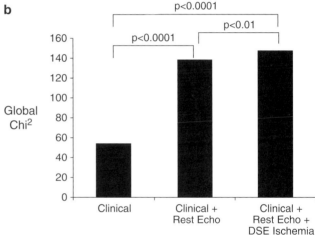

Figure 20.8 Incremental value of echocardiogram and dobutamine stress echocardiogram (DSE) over clinical evaluation for the prediction of cardiac events (**a**) and all-cause mortality (**b**) in the elderly (from Biagini et al. [72], reprinted with permission from the American Gerontological Society of America).

Table 20.4 Univariate association between components of preoperative assessment of cancer in the elderly (PACE) with 30-day morbidity (any and major complication) adjusted for age, sex, type, and stage of cancer and severity of surgery

Component of PACE	Any complication		Major complication	
	RR[a]	95% CI	RR[a]	95% CI
MMS abnormal (<24)	1.23	0.81–1.88	1.08	0.48–2.44
ADL dependent (>0)	1.41	0.95–2.10	1.87	0.95–3.69
IADL dependent (<8)	*1.43*	1.03–1.98	1.65	0.88–3.08
GDS depressed (>4)	1.30	0.93–1.81	1.69	0.93–3.08
BFI mod/severe fatigue (>3)	*1.52*	1.09–2.12	1.24	0.67–2.27
ASA abnormal (≥2)	1.00	0.73–1.38	*1.96*	1.09–3.53
PS abnormal (>1)	*1.64*	1.07–2.52	1.97	0.92–4.23
Satariano's index (1)	1.11	0.78–1.59	1.29	0.68–2.44
Satariano's index (2+)	1.58	0.88–2.85	1.95	0.74–5.18

From Audisio [78]. Reprinted with permission from Elsevier
MMS mini mental status, *ADL* activities of daily living, *IADL* instrumental activities of daily living, *GDS* geriatric depression scale, *BFI* brief fatigue inventory, *ASA* American society of anesthesiologists physical status, *PS* eastern cooperative oncology group performance status
[a]Bold italics represent significant relationship ($p < 0.05$)

Preoperative antibiotics are not necessary for every type of elective surgery, but researchers agree that advanced age is a risk factor for nosocomial infection. Iwamoto et al. [80] studied 4,380 patients who underwent general anesthesia for thoracic, abdominal, or neurologic surgery and concluded that advanced age is a risk factor for nosocomial pneumonia, especially after thoracic surgery. Age greater than 70 years has been shown to be a risk factor for both positive bile cultures ($p < 0.001$) [81] and septic complications of biliary surgery compared with younger patients [82]; antibiotic prophylaxis can reduce these complications [83].

Efforts to improve our elderly patients' preoperative nutritional state would seem desirable – even active, community-dwelling older adults manifest impaired recovery of strength after major surgery [84] – but it is unclear how to do this. Low levels of serum albumin, for example, correlate strikingly with postoperative problems [85] (Fig. 20.9), but cannot be improved to a great degree preoperatively. Souba [86] reviewed the literature on nutritional support and concluded that preoperative support should be reserved for severely malnourished patients scheduled to undergo major elective surgery and then should be provided for no more than 10 days.

In addition to those already cited, a number of surgeons have attributed their improved results in elderly patients to compulsive preoperative preparation. Bittner et al. [87] believed that the significant decrease in mortality after total

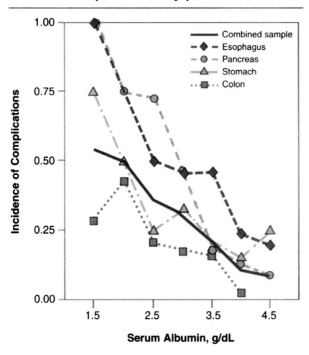

Albumin levels and incidence of surgical complications by procedure

FIGURE 20.9 Preoperative albumin level and major postoperative complications (from Kudsk et al. [85], reprinted with permission from the American Society for Parenteral and Enteral Nutrition).

gastrectomy in septuagenarians (32% in 1979 to 4.4% in 1996) was the result of standardized perioperative antibiotics, thromboembolic prophylaxis, "a systemic analysis of risk factors and their thorough preoperative therapy," and nutritional support for the malnourished. Our presented patient was neither anemic nor an active smoker; he received preoperative antibiotics and perioperative DVT prophylaxis.

Hypovolemia is tolerated poorly by the elderly patient and it must be corrected. Smoking should be stopped. Treating other correctable aberrations such as anemia, bronchitis, and hypertension preoperatively increases the elderly patient's chance for a smooth postoperative course.

Principle IV: Emergency Surgery

> The results of elective surgery in the elderly are reproducibly good; the results of emergency surgery are poor though still better than non-operative treatment for most conditions. The risk of emergency surgery may be many times that of similar elective surgery because of Principles II and III.

The results of elective surgery in the elderly are good, frequently indistinguishable from the results in younger counterparts [88–90]. Coyle [91] reported the results of carotid endarterectomy in 79 octogenarians and summarized the results of five other series (634 total patients); mortality and morbidity were similar to those in a younger cohort. Maehara et al. [92] had 0% operative mortality in 77 patients over an age of 70 who underwent resection of gastric carcinoma, and Jougon's [93] results for esophagectomy in 89 patients of age 70–84 years were identical to those in 451 younger patients. Our 88-year-old patient with lung cancer could anticipate mortality and survival after pulmonary lobectomy statistically identical to that of younger patients with similar stage disease [64, 88, 94–96]. Identical operations performed emergently in the elderly, however, carry at least a threefold (and as much as a tenfold) increased risk [97] (Fig. 20.10). Keller [98], for example, reported 31% morbidity and 20% mortality in 100 patients over an age of 70 who underwent emergency operations, which is significantly more ($p < 0.0005$) than the 6.8% morbidity and 1.9% mortality following elective operation in 513 similar patients. Elective cholecystectomy can be performed in young and old patients with the risk of death approaching 0% [20, 99, 100]; the risk of mortality for emergency cholecystectomy increases somewhat in the younger group (1–2%) but increases greatly in the elderly (5–15%) [20]. Surgical priority clearly affects cardiac surgery risk [101, 102]. Elective operative mortality for colorectal surgery is as low as 1.5–3.0%, rising to over 20% for emergency operation [103, 104].

A patient's advanced age therefore weighs in favor of commencing rather than deferring needed elective surgery.

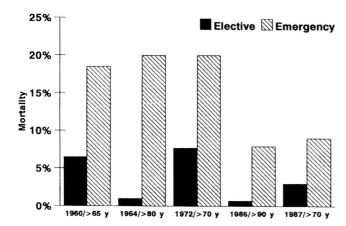

FIGURE 20.10 Elective vs. emergency surgery in the elderly (from Thomas and Ritchie [9], reprinted with permission of Blackwell Publishing).

Principle V: Attention to Detail

Scrupulous attention to detail intraoperatively and perioperatively yields great benefit, as the elderly tolerate complications poorly (because of Principle II).

Perioperative blood loss is the *bete noire* of geriatric surgery, as the elderly lack the responsive compensatory mechanisms necessary to restore equilibrium. Fong et al. [54] reported that the only independent predictor of postoperative complications in 138 patients over an age of 70 who underwent pancreatic resection was intraoperative blood loss exceeding 2 l. This finding has been mirrored in reports from cardiac surgery and neurosurgery. Sisto et al. [105] reported that 6 of 23 octogenarian coronary bypass patients who required reexploration for tamponade died; Logeais et al. [106] found that reoperation for tamponade following aortic valve replacement placed the elderly patient at high risk for mortality ($p < 0.001$). Hemostasis is exceptionally important in the elderly craniotomy patient, possibly because the elderly brain is less likely to expand to obliterate dead space. Maurice-Williams and Kitchen [107] reported that postoperative bleeding following resection of meningioma occurred in 20% of 46 elderly patients and 0% of 38 young patients ($p < 0.05$).

Meticulous surgical technique is important in any patient, but it becomes crucial in those of advanced age. Anastomotic leak after esophageal or gastric resection, a dreaded complication in any patient, embodies an exceptional risk of mortality in the elderly [108]; yet this complication can be minimized by careful technique [109, 110]. Only one of Bandoh's [111] elderly patients who underwent gastrectomy for cancer experienced a leak, as did only 2 of 163 patients over an age of 70 in Bittner's series [87]. Despite having significantly greater preoperative comorbidity, the elderly patients undergoing gastrectomy in Gretschel's series experienced no greater

postoperative morbidity [57]. The elderly cardiac surgery patient may benefit from extra care when they have a calcified aorta (e.g., intraoperative ultrasound or modified clamping and cannulation technique) or a fragile sternum (e.g., additional or pericostal wires) [112]. Operative speed is less important than technique: in Cohen's series of 46 nonagenarians undergoing major procedures [7], the duration of operation did not correlate with mortality.

Perioperative monitoring is more important in the elderly, since they may manifest few signs or symptoms of impending problems (see Principle I above). Bernstein [113] credits intensive hemodynamic monitoring in his lack of mortality among 78 patients over an age of 70 who underwent abdominal aortic aneurysmectomy. Such monitoring and intensive care were also emphasized by Alexander et al. [3], who reported excellent results for 59 octogenarians having major upper abdominal cancer operations, and by Lo [114] for 85 elderly patients undergoing adrenal surgery at the Mayo Clinic. Giannice [115] credits attention to perioperative care (DVT prophylaxis, antibiotics, monitoring, respiratory care, pain management, and early mobilization) for his group's improved recent results in gynecologic oncology patients. Our case report patient had reinforcement of vascular and bronchial closures in addition to compulsive hemostasis and minimization of parenchymal air leaks. He was monitored postoperatively. If he had developed an atrial arrhythmia, it would have been aggressively treated; if he had developed tracheobronchial secretions, he would have promptly undergone therapeutic bronchoscopy.

We should continue to teach the surgical aphorism, "Elderly patients tolerate operations but not complications" (Table 20.5).

TABLE 20.5 Importance of postoperative complications in failure of octogenarians to return to normal function following major abdominal surgery

All cases	Odds ratio	95% confidence interval
Emergency operation	2.7	0.99–7.24
ASA III or IV	1.0	0.29–3.56
Comorbidity index >5	1.8	0.48–6.66
Dependence on activities of daily living	1.8	0.42–7.73
Preexisting cardiac disease	1.9	0.69–5.44
Preexisting chronic pulmonary disease	2.0	0.54–7.47
Preexisting cerebrovascular disease	2.0	0.43–9.06
Development of postoperative complications	24.5	3.08–194.88
Elective cases only		
Comorbidity index >5	11.2	1.08–116.26
Development of postoperative complications	10.6	3.08–194.88

From Tan et al. [108]. Reprinted with permission from Springer Science + Business Media

Principle VI: Age is a Scientific Fact

> A patient's age should be treated as a scientific fact, not with prejudice. No particular chronologic age, of itself, is a contraindication to operation (because of Principle IV).

Great biologic variability exists among the elderly, with some octogenarians and nonagenarians proving to be healthier than their sons and daughters. Even our 88-year-old patient has a life expectancy exceeding 4 years [116, 117], so why not offer him resection of his lung cancer? No other treatment is likely to give him those 4 years. Yet even in 2005, this does not always happen: prejudice against the elderly, so-called "ageism" exists.

Despite the fact that elderly patients treated for lung cancer have survival equal to their younger matched counterparts, Nugent et al. [118] found that patients older than 80 years

colon cancer are less likely to undergo extensive lymph node dissection ($p<0.0001$) [132]. Selection bias in the elderly may also lead to delay in referral for abdominal aortic aneurysm surgery [133] and coronary artery bypass surgery [134].

Some studies do report increased operative mortality [97, 135, 136] (Fig. 20.11), increased complications [137, 138] (Fig. 20.12), and increased lengths-of-stay in the elderly [139–143], but overall results do not differ from the young for a wide variety of procedures: neurosurgery [107, 144], head and neck surgery [30, 145, 146], carotid endarterectomy [147, 148], cardiac surgery [52, 112, 134, 149–153], esophagectomy [79, 93, 109, 154–156] (Fig. 20.13), gastrectomy [3, 92, 157, 158] (Fig. 20.14), colectomy [159–161] (Fig. 20.15), hepatectomy [54, 162–165] (Fig. 20.16), pancreaticoduodenectomy [54, 166, 167], radical hysterectomy [168], total knee/hip replacement [169–171], microvascular free tissue transfer [172], cardiac transplant [173], lung

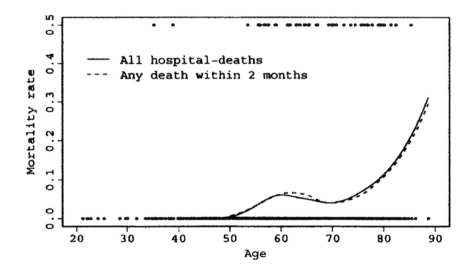

Figure 20.11 Linear logistic regression analysis of mortality rate by age as a continuous variable for all in-hospital deaths and any death within 2 months of esophagectomy (reprinted with permission from Moskovitz et al. [136], copyright Elsevier 2006).

were significantly less likely ($p<0.05$) to be treated surgically. Kuo et al. [119] similarly reported that octogenarian patients with lung cancer were more likely ($p<0.01$) to receive only palliative care; when offered chemotherapy they tolerate it [120]. Elderly patients with ovarian cancer are less likely to undergo aggressive chemotherapy and surgery [121, 122], despite results equal to the young [123]. Older women with breast cancer were less likely to have had screening mammograms [124, 125] and were more likely to present in advanced stages than younger women [125]; once diagnosed, they tolerated surgery well [126, 127]. Guadagnoli et al. [128] presented evidence against ageism in the treatment of early breast cancer, but Hebert-Croteau et al. [129] found that only the use of tamoxifen was similar in women over and under an age of 70 ($p<0.41$), while all other treatments (breast-conserving surgery, radiotherapy, axillary node dissection, and chemotherapy) differed significantly ($p<0.0001$). When elderly patients do receive chemotherapy for breast cancer they tolerate it [130] and they benefit from it [131]. Elderly patients with

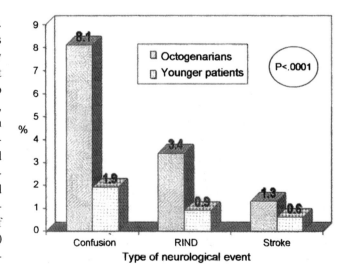

Figure 20.12 Early postoperative neurologic complications after coronary artery bypass surgery and valve surgery in octogenarians (*RIND* reversible ischemic neurological deficit) (from Ngaage et al. [137], reprinted with permission from Elsevier).

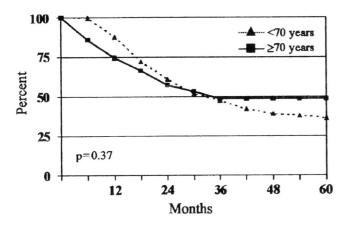

Figure 20.13 Esophagectomy following neoadjuvant chemoradiation. Kaplan–Meier survival curves (including postoperative deaths) plotted for patients age <70 vs. ≥70 years (from Ruol et al. [156], reprinted with permission from Springer Science+Business Media).

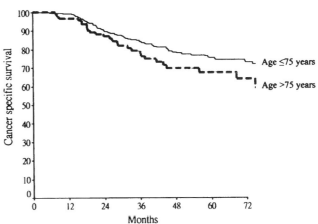

Figure 20.15 Cancer-specific survival of elderly and younger patients treated for mid-to-distal colorectal cancer ($p=0.061$), $n=612$ (from Law et al. [161], reprinted with permission from Springer Science+Business Media).

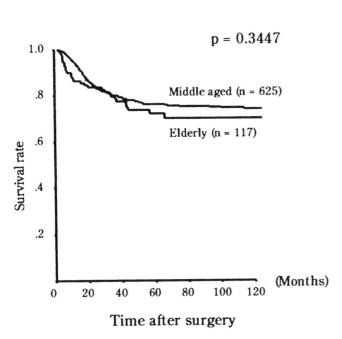

Figure 20.14 Surgical outcome in elderly (≥75 years) and middle-aged (45–65 years) patients with gastric cancer (from Kunisaki et al. [158], reprinted with permission from Elsevier).

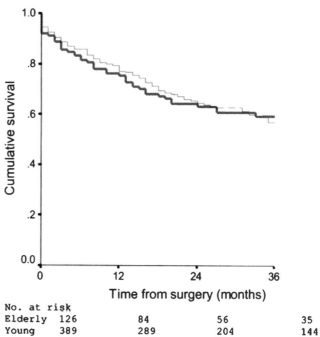

Figure 20.16 Major hepatectomy. Overall survival for patients ≥70 years (*solid line*) and <70 years (*dashed line*), $p=0.89$; $n=517$ (from Menon et al. [165], reprinted with permission from Elsevier).

transplant [174], endovascular surgery [175], gastric bypass [176], laparoscopic colectomy [177], and hernia [178]. Return to preoperative quality of life (QOL) is gratifying after elective surgery for gastric or colorectal surgery [179], joint replacement [171], thoracic aneurysm [180] (Fig. 20.17), and aortic valve replacement [181, 182] (Fig. 20.18).

For most patients, general medical condition and associated medical problems are more important than age. Dunlop et al. [183] studied 8,889 geriatric surgical patients in Canada and concluded that severity of illness on admission was a

much better predictor of outcome than was age; Akoh et al. [184] had similar findings in 171 octogenarians undergoing major gastrointestinal surgery. Comorbidities were a greater influence on survival than age in several series of elderly patients with lung cancer [37, 38, 185]. Mehta et al. [186] reported that separation of mitral valve replacement patients into low-, medium-, and high-risk medical groups was more important than stratification by age within these three groups. Within the American Society of Anesthesiologists Physical Status system [187], the ASA status influences results more

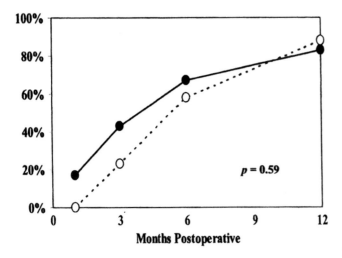

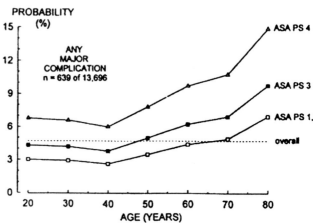

FIGURE 20.17 Return to normal functional activity after thoracic aneurysm repair depending on age: <70 years (*solid circles*) and ≥70 years (*open circles*); n=110 (from Zierer et al. [180], copyright Elsevier 2006).

FIGURE 20.19 Probability of a major postanesthesia complication based on age and the American Society of Anesthesiologists Physical Status (ASA) system (reprinted with permission from Muravchick [194]).

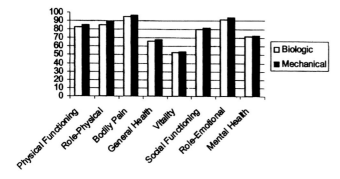

than age (Fig. 20.19). For elderly patients undergoing surgery for cancer, the stage of malignancy also influences outcome more than age [38, 188–191].

Many geriatric surgery patients, including nonagenarians, have survival rates equal to those expected in the general population; even the sobering results of emergency surgery in the elderly are better than the results of nonoperative treatment for the same conditions. A patient's age should therefore be considered but not feared.

FIGURE 20.18 Scores for the domains of the Medical Outcomes Survey Short-Form 36 Health Survey following aortic valve replacement in octogenarians; biologic (*open boxes*) and mechanical (*filled boxes*) valve prostheses; n=345 (reprinted with permission from de Vincentiis et al. [181], copyright Elsevier 2008).

CASE STUDY: FOLLOW-UP

Following his death, our patient's wife wrote me this note: "Dear Dr. Katlic – on 3/2/99 you removed part of Bob's lung – on 3/1/03 he died of pneumonia – four lovely years – he played golf was independent and happy (Fig. 20.20). I was with him when he died and he was peaceful and in no pain. I am grateful to you for every moment of those four 'extra' years."

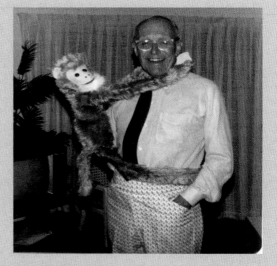

FIGURE 20.20 Eighty-eight-year-old man following right lower lobectomy for lung cancer. "I am grateful to you for every moment of those four 'extra' years".

Conclusion

Surgical problems abound in the elderly and the numbers of elderly are increasing worldwide. Surgeons must become students of the physiologic changes that occur with aging and, guided by a few general principles, apply this knowledge to daily clinical care. The results of surgery in the elderly do not support prejudice against advanced age. We owe it to our elders to become good geriatric surgeons and in so doing we will become better surgeons to patients of all ages.

References

1. Smith OC (1907) Advanced age as a contraindication to operation. Med Rec (NY) 72:642–644
2. Ochsner A (1967) Is risk of operation too great in the elderly? Geriatrics 22:121–130
3. Alexander HR, Turnbull AD, Salamone J, Keefe D, Melendez J (1991) Upper abdominal cancer surgery in the very elderly. J Surg Oncol 47(2):82–86
4. Bridges CR, Edwards FH, Peterson ED, Coombs LP, Ferguson TB (2003) Cardiac surgery in nonagenarians and centenarians. J Am Coll Surg 197(3):347–356, discussion 356–347
5. Katlic MR (1985) Surgery in centenarians. JAMA 253(21): 3139–3141
6. Ullery BW, Peterson JC, Milla F et al (2008) Cardiac surgery in select nonagenarians: should we or shouldn't we? Ann Thorac Surg 85(3):854–860
7. Cohen JR, Johnson H, Eaton S, Sterman H, Wise L (1988) Surgical procedures in patients during the tenth decade of life. Surgery 104(4):646–651
8. Linn BS, Zeppa R (1987) Student attitudes about surgery in older patients before and after the surgical clerkship. Ann Surg 205(3):324–328
9. Thomas DR, Ritchie CS (1995) Preoperative assessment of older adults. J Am Geriatr Soc 43(7):811–821
10. Goodney PP, Siewers AE, Stukel TA, Lucas FL, Wennberg DE, Birkmeyer JD (2002) Is surgery getting safer? National trends in operative mortality. J Am Coll Surg 195(2):219–227
11. Storm-Dickerson TL, Horattas MC (2003) What have we learned over the past 20 years about appendicitis in the elderly? Am J Surg 185(3):198–201
12. Elangovan S (1996) Clinical and laboratory findings in acute appendicitis in the elderly. J Am Board Fam Pract 9(2):75–78
13. Lau WY, Fan ST, Yiu TF, Chu KW, Lee JM (1985) Acute appendicitis in the elderly. Surg Gynecol Obstet 161(2):157–160
14. Horattas MC, Guyton DP, Wu D (1990) A reappraisal of appendicitis in the elderly. Am J Surg 160(3):291–293
15. Adedeji OA, McAdam WA (1996) Murphy's sign, acute cholecystitis and elderly people. J R Coll Surg Edinb 41(2):88–89
16. Hafif A, Gutman M, Kaplan O, Winkler E, Rozin RR, Skornick Y (1991) The management of acute cholecystitis in elderly patients. Am Surg 57(10):648–652
17. Parker LJ, Vukov LF, Wollan PC (1997) Emergency department evaluation of geriatric patients with acute cholecystitis. Acad Emerg Med 4(1):51–55
18. Chen Y, Zheng M, Hu X et al (2008) Fever of unknown origin in elderly people: a retrospective study of 87 patients in China. J Am Geriatr Soc 56(1):182–184
19. Stewart L, Grifiss JM, Jarvis GA, Way LW (2008) Elderly patients have more severe biliary infections: influence of complement-killing and induction of TNFalpha production. Surgery 143(1):103–112
20. Magnuson TH, Ratner LE, Zenilman ME, Bender JS (1997) Laparoscopic cholecystectomy: applicability in the geriatric population. Am Surg 63(1):91–96
21. Saunders K, Tompkins R, Longmire W Jr, Roslyn J (1991) Bile duct carcinoma in the elderly. A rationale for surgical management. Arch Surg 126(10):1186–1190, discussion 1190–1181
22. Hilton D, Iman N, Burke GJ et al (2001) Absence of abdominal pain in older persons with endoscopic ulcers: a prospective study. Am J Gastroenterol 96(2):380–384
23. Rabinovici R, Manny J (1991) Perforated duodenal ulcer in the elderly. Eur J Surg 157(2):121–125
24. Mulcahy HE, Patchett SE, Daly L, O'Donoghue DP (1994) Prognosis of elderly patients with large bowel cancer. Br J Surg 81(5):736–738
25. Watters JM, Blakslee JM, March RJ, Redmond ML (1996) The influence of age on the severity of peritonitis. Can J Surg 39(2):142–146
26. Tedesco P, Lobo E, Fisichella PM, Way LW, Patti MG (2006) Laparoscopic fundoplication in elderly patients with gastroesophageal reflux disease. Arch Surg 141(3):289–292, discussion 292
27. Pilotto A, Franceschi M, Leandro G et al (2006) Clinical features of reflux esophagitis in older people: a study of 840 consecutive patients. J Am Geriatr Soc 54(10):1537–1542
28. Knutson JW, Slavin RG (1995) Sinusitis in the aged. Optimal management strategies. Drugs Aging 7(4):310–316
29. Norman DC, Toledo SD (1992) Infections in elderly persons. An altered clinical presentation. Clin Geriatr Med 8(4):713–719
30. Koch WM, Patel H, Brennan J, Boyle JO, Sidransky D (1995) Squamous cell carcinoma of the head and neck in the elderly. Arch Otolaryngol Head Neck Surg 121(3):262–265
31. Ehlinger P, Fossion E, Vrielinck L (1993) Carcinoma of the oral cavity in patients over 75 years of age. Int J Oral Maxillofac Surg 22(4):218–220
32. Chigot JP, Menegaux F, Achrafi H (1995) Should primary hyperparathyroidism be treated surgically in elderly patients older than 75 years? Surgery 117(4):397–401
33. Thomas PC, Grigg M (1996) Carotid artery surgery in the octogenarian. Aust N Z J Surg 66(4):231–234
34. Canto JG, Fincher C, Kiefe CI et al (2002) Atypical presentations among Medicare beneficiaries with unstable angina pectoris. Am J Cardiol 90(3):248–253
35. Hellmann DB (2003) Eurekapenia: a disease of medical residency training programs? Pharos Alpha Omega Alpha Honor Med Soc 66(2):24–26
36. Durso SC (2004) A bipolar disorder: eurekaphoria, then discouragement. Pharos Alpha Omega Alpha Honor Med Soc 67(3):49
37. Birim O, Zuydendorp HM, Maat AP, Kappetein AP, Eijkemans MJ, Bogers AJ (2003) Lung resection for non-small-cell lung cancer in patients older than 70: mortality, morbidity, and late survival compared with the general population. Ann Thorac Surg 76(6):1796–1801
38. Brock MV, Kim MP, Hooker CM et al (2004) Pulmonary resection in octogenarians with stage I nonsmall cell lung cancer: a 22-year experience. Ann Thorac Surg 77(1):271–277
39. Keagy BA, Pharr WF, Bowes DE, Wilcox BR (1984) A review of morbidity and mortality in elderly patients undergoing pulmonary resection. Am Surg 50(4):213–216
40. Au J, el-Oakley R, Cameron EW (1994) Pneumonectomy for bronchogenic carcinoma in the elderly. Eur J Cardiothorac Surg 8(5):247–250
41. Miller DL, Deschamps C, Jenkins GD, Bernard A, Allen MS, Pairolero PC (2002) Completion pneumonectomy: factors affecting operative mortality and cardiopulmonary morbidity. Ann Thorac Surg 74(3):876–883, discussion 883–874

42. Rostad H, Naalsund A, Strand TE, Jacobsen R, Talleraas O, Norstein J (2005) Results of pulmonary resection for lung cancer in Norway, patients older than 70 years. Eur J Cardiothorac Surg 27(2):325–328

43. Demmy TL, Plante AJ, Nwogu CE, Takita H, Anderson TM (2004) Discharge independence with minimally invasive lobectomy. Am J Surg 188(6):698–702

44. Jaklitsch MT, DeCamp MM Jr, Liptay MJ et al (1996) Video-assisted thoracic surgery in the elderly: a review of 307 cases. Chest 110(3):751–758

45. Nomori H, Horio H, Fuyuno G, Kobayashi R, Yashima H (1996) Respiratory muscle strength after lung resection with special reference to age and procedures of thoracotomy. Eur J Cardiothorac Surg 10(5):352–358

46. Yim AP (1996) Thoracoscopic surgery in the elderly population. Surg Endosc 10(9):880–882

47. Cattaneo SM, Park BJ, Wilton AS et al (2008) Use of video-assisted thoracic surgery for lobectomy in the elderly results in fewer complications. Ann Thorac Surg 85(1):231–235, discussion 235–236

48. Patel HJ, Williams DM, Upchurch GR Jr et al (2008) A comparison of open and endovascular descending thoracic aortic repair in patients older than 75 years of age. Ann Thorac Surg 85(5): 1597–1603, discussion 1603–1594

49. Bergus BO, Feng WC, Bert AA, Singh AK (1992) Aortic valve replacement (AVR): influence of age on operative morbidity and mortality. Eur J Cardiothorac Surg 6(3):118–121

50. Salomon NW, Page US, Bigelow JC, Krause AH, Okies JE, Metzdorff MT (1991) Coronary artery bypass grafting in elderly patients. Comparative results in a consecutive series of 469 patients older than 75 years. J Thorac Cardiovasc Surg 101(2):209–217, discussion 217–208

51. Lytle BW, Navia JL, Taylor PC et al (1997) Third coronary artery bypass operations: risks and costs. Ann Thorac Surg 64(5): 1287–1295

52. Elayda MA, Hall RJ, Reul RM et al (1993) Aortic valve replacement in patients 80 years and older. Operative risks and long-term results. Circulation 88(5 Pt 2):II11–II16

53. Fortner JG, Lincer RM (1990) Hepatic resection in the elderly. Ann Surg 211(2):141–145

54. Fong Y, Blumgart LH, Fortner JG, Brennan MF (1995) Pancreatic or liver resection for malignancy is safe and effective for the elderly. Ann Surg 222(4):426–434, discussion 434–427

55. Escarce JJ, Shea JA, Chen W, Qian Z, Schwartz JS (1995) Outcomes of open cholecystectomy in the elderly: a longitudinal analysis of 21,000 cases in the prelaparoscopic era. Surgery 117(2):156–164

56. Tsujitani S, Katano K, Oka A, Ikeguchi M, Maeta M, Kaibara N (1996) Limited operation for gastric cancer in the elderly. Br J Surg 83(6):836–839

57. Gretschel S, Estevez-Schwarz L, Hunerbein M, Schneider U, Schlag PM (2006) Gastric cancer surgery in elderly patients. World J Surg 30(8):1468–1474

58. Okada M, Koike T, Higashiyama M, Yamato Y, Kodama K, Tsubota N (2006) Radical sublobar resection for small-sized non-small cell lung cancer: a multicenter study. J Thorac Cardiovasc Surg 132(4):769–775

59. Mery CM, Pappas AN, Bueno R et al (2005) Similar long-term survival of elderly patients with non-small cell lung cancer treated with lobectomy or wedge resection within the surveillance, epidemiology, and end results database. Chest 128(1):237–245

60. Lawrence VA, Hazuda HP, Cornell JE et al (2004) Functional independence after major abdominal surgery in the elderly. J Am Coll Surg 199(5):762–772

61. Seymour DG, Vaz FG (1989) A prospective study of elderly general surgical patients: II Post-operative complications. Age Ageing 18(5):316–326

62. Dzankic S, Pastor D, Gonzalez C, Leung JM (2001) The prevalence and predictive value of abnormal preoperative laboratory tests in elderly surgical patients. Anesth Analg 93(2):301–308, 302nd contents page

63. Vaporciyan AA, Merriman KW, Ece F et al (2002) Incidence of major pulmonary morbidity after pneumonectomy: association with timing of smoking cessation. Ann Thorac Surg 73(2):420–425, discussion 425–426

64. Mizushima Y, Noto H, Sugiyama S et al (1997) Survival and prognosis after pneumonectomy for lung cancer in the elderly. Ann Thorac Surg 64(1):193–198

65. Reilly JJ (1997) Preparing for pulmonary resection: preoperative evaluation of patients. Chest 112(4 Suppl):206S–208S

66. Goldhaber SZ, Tapson VF (2004) A prospective registry of 5,451 patients with ultrasound-confirmed deep vein thrombosis. Am J Cardiol 93(2):259–262

67. Jacobs LG (2003) Prophylactic anticoagulation for venous thromboembolic disease in geriatric patients. J Am Geriatr Soc 51(10): 1472–1478

68. Berlauk JF, Abrams JH, Gilmour IJ, O'Connor SR, Knighton DR, Cerra FB (1991) Preoperative optimization of cardiovascular hemodynamics improves outcome in peripheral vascular surgery: a prospective, randomized clinical trial. Ann Surg 214(3):289–297, discussion 298–289

69. Bender JS, Smith-Meek MA, Jones CE (1997) Routine pulmonary artery catheterization does not reduce morbidity and mortality of elective vascular surgery: results of a prospective, randomized trial. Ann Surg 226(3):229–236, discussion 236–227

70. Ziegler DW, Wright JG, Choban PS, Flancbaum L (1997) A prospective randomized trial of preoperative "optimization" of cardiac function in patients undergoing elective peripheral vascular surgery. Surgery 122(3):584–592

71. Leppo JA (1995) Preoperative cardiac risk assessment for noncardiac surgery. Am J Cardiol 75(11):42D–51D

72. Biagini E, Elhendy A, Schinkel AF et al (2005) Long-term prediction of mortality in elderly persons by dobutamine stress echocardiography. J Gerontol A Biol Sci Med Sci 60(10):1333–1338

73. Pollock M, Roa J, Benditt J, Celli B (1993) Estimation of ventilatory reserve by stair climbing: a study in patients with chronic airflow obstruction. Chest 104(5):1378–1383

74. Brunelli A, Refai M, Xiume F et al (2008) Performance at symptom-limited stair-climbing test is associated with increased cardiopulmonary complications, mortality, and costs after major lung resection. Ann Thorac Surg 86(1):240–247, discussion 247–248

75. Win T, Jackson A, Groves AM, Sharples LD, Charman SC, Laroche CM (2006) Comparison of shuttle walk with measured peak oxygen consumption in patients with operable lung cancer. Thorax 61(1):57–60

76. Simonsick EM, Fan E, Fleg JL (2006) Estimating cardiorespiratory fitness in well-functioning older adults: treadmill validation of the long distance corridor walk. J Am Geriatr Soc 54(1): 127–132

77. Weinstein H, Bates AT, Spaltro BE, Thaler HT, Steingart RM (2007) Influence of preoperative exercise capacity on length of stay after thoracic cancer surgery. Ann Thorac Surg 84(1):197–202

78. Audisio RA, Pope D, Ramesh HS et al (2008) Shall we operate? Preoperative assessment in elderly cancer patients (PACE) can help. A SIOG surgical task force prospective study. Crit Rev Oncol Hematol 65(2):156–163

79. Internullo E, Moons J, Nafteux P et al (2008) Outcome after esophagectomy for cancer of the esophagus and GEJ in patients aged over 75 years. Eur J Cardiothorac Surg 33(6):1096–1104

80. Iwamoto K, Ichiyama S, Shimokata K, Nakashima N (1993) Postoperative pneumonia in elderly patients: incidence and mortality in comparison with younger patients. Intern Med 32(4):274–277

81. Kwon AH, Matsui Y (2006) Laparoscopic cholecystectomy in patients aged 80 years and over. World J Surg 30(7):1204–1210

82. Landau O, Kott I, Deutsch AA, Stelman E, Reiss R (1992) Multifactorial analysis of septic bile and septic complications in biliary surgery. World J Surg 16(5):962–964, discussion 964–965

83. Meijer WS, Schmitz PI, Jeekel J (1990) Meta-analysis of randomized, controlled clinical trials of antibiotic prophylaxis in biliary tract surgery. Br J Surg 77(3):283–290

84. Watters JM, Clancey SM, Moulton SB, Briere KM, Zhu JM (1993) Impaired recovery of strength in older patients after major abdominal surgery. Ann Surg 21(3):380–390, discussion 390–383

85. Kudsk KA, Tolley EA, DeWitt RC et al (2003) Preoperative albumin and surgical site identify surgical risk for major postoperative complications. JPEN J Parenter Enteral Nutr 27(1):1–9

86. Souba WW (1997) Nutritional support. N Engl J Med 336(1):41–48

87. Bittner R, Butters M, Ulrich M, Uppenbrink S, Beger HG (1996) Total gastrectomy. Updated operative mortality and long-term survival with particular reference to patients older than 70 years of age. Ann Surg 224(1):37–42

88. Myrdal G, Gustafsson G, Lambe M, Horte LG, Stahle E (2001) Outcome after lung cancer surgery. Factors predicting early mortality and major morbidity. Eur J Cardiothorac Surg 20(4):694–699

89. Allen MS, Darling GE, Pechet TT et al (2006) Morbidity and mortality of major pulmonary resections in patients with early-stage lung cancer: initial results of the randomized, prospective ACOSOG Z0030 trial. Ann Thorac Surg 81(3):1013–1019, discussion 1019–1020

90. Cerfolio RJ, Bryant AS (2006) Survival and outcomes of pulmonary resection for non-small cell lung cancer in the elderly: a nested case-control study. Ann Thorac Surg 82(2):424–429, discussion 429–430

91. Coyle KA, Smith RB 3rd, Salam AA, Dodson TF, Chaikof EL, Lumsden AB (1994) Carotid endarterectomy in the octogenarian. Ann Vasc Surg 8(5):417–420

92. Maehara Y, Oshiro T, Oiwa H et al (1995) Gastric carcinoma in patients over 70 years of age. Br J Surg 82(1):102–105

93. Jougon JB, Ballester M, Duffy J et al (1997) Esophagectomy for cancer in the patient aged 70 years and older. Ann Thorac Surg 63(5):1423–1427

94. de Perrot M, Licker M, Reymond MA, Robert J, Spiliopoulos A (1999) Influence of age on operative mortality and long-term survival after lung resection for bronchogenic carcinoma. Eur Respir J 14(2):419–422

95. Okada M, Nishio W, Sakamoto T, Harada H, Uchino K, Tsubota N (2003) Long-term survival and prognostic factors of five-year survivors with complete resection of non-small cell lung carcinoma. J Thorac Cardiovasc Surg 126(2):558–562

96. Thomas P, Sielezenff I, Rajni J, Giridicilli R, Fuentes P (1993) Is lung cancer resection justified in patients aged over 70 years? Eur J Cardiothorac Surg 7:246–251

97. Turrentine FE, Wang H, Simpson VB, Jones RS (2006) Surgical risk factors, morbidity, and mortality in elderly patients. J Am Coll Surg 203(6):865–877

98. Keller SM, Markovitz LJ, Wilder JR, Aufses AH Jr (1987) Emergency and elective surgery in patients over age 70. Am Surg 53(11):636–640

99. Bingener J, Richards ML, Schwesinger WH, Strodel WE, Sirinek KR (2003) Laparoscopic cholecystectomy for elderly patients: gold standard for golden years? Arch Surg 138(5):531–535, discussion 535–536

100. Tambyraja AL, Kumar S, Nixon SJ (2004) Outcome of laparoscopic cholecystectomy in patients 80 years and older. World J Surg 28(8):745–748

101. Tsai TP, Chaux A, Matloff JM et al (1994) Ten-year experience of cardiac surgery in patients aged 80 years and ove. Ann Thorac Surg 58(2):445–450, discussion 450–441

102. Tseng EE, Lee CA, Cameron DE et al (1997) Aortic valve replacement in the elderly. Risk factors and long-term results. Ann Surg 225(6):793–802, discussion 802–794

103. Bender JS, Magnuson TH, Zenilman ME et al (1996) Outcome following colon surgery in the octagenarian. Am Surg 62(4):276–279

104. Spivak H, Maele DV, Friedman I, Nussbaum M (1996) Colorectal surgery in octogenarians. J Am Coll Surg 183(1):46–50

105. Sisto D, Hoffman D, Frater RW (1993) Isolated coronary artery bypass grafting in one hundred octogenarian patients. J Thorac Cardiovasc Surg 106(5):940–942

106. Logeais Y, Langanay T, Roussin R et al (1994) Surgery for aortic stenosis in elderly patients. A study of surgical risk and predictive factors. Circulation 90(6):2891–2898

107. Maurice-Williams RS, Kitchen ND (1992) Intracranial tumours in the elderly: the effect of age on the outcome of first time surgery for meningiomas. Br J Neurosurg 6(2):131–137

108. Tan KY, Chen CM, Ng C, Tan SM, Tay KH (2006) Which octogenarians do poorly after major open abdominal surgery in our Asian population? World J Surg 30(4):547–552

109. Adam DJ, Craig SR, Sang CT, Cameron EW, Walker WS (1996) Esophagectomy for carcinoma in the octogenarian. Ann Thorac Surg 61(1):190–194

110. Mathisen DJ, Grillo HC, Wilkins EW Jr, Moncure AC, Hilgenberg AD (1988) Transthoracic esophagectomy: a safe approach to carcinoma of the esophagus. Ann Thorac Surg 45(2):137–143

111. Bandoh T, Isoyama T, Toyoshima H (1991) Total gastrectomy for gastric cancer in the elderly. Surgery 109(2):136–142

112. Katz NM, Chase GA (1997) Risks of cardiac operations for elderly patients: reduction of the age factor. Ann Thorac Surg 63(5):1309–1314

113. Bernstein EF, Dilley RB, Randolph HF 3rd (1988) The improving long-term outlook for patients over 70 years of age with abdominal aortic aneurysms. Ann Surg 207(3):318–322

114. Lo CY, van Heerden JA, Grant CS, Soreide JA, Warner MA, Ilstrup DM (1996) Adrenal surgery in the elderly: too risky? World J Surg 20(3):368–373, discussion 374

115. Giannice R, Foti E, Poerio A, Marana E, Mancuso S, Scambia G (2004) Perioperative morbidity and mortality in elderly gynecological oncological patients (≥70 years) by the American Society of Anesthesiologists Physical Status classes. Ann Surg Oncol 11(2):219–225

116. Social Security Online (2000) Period life table, 2000. Statistical tables. http://www.ssa.gov/OACT/STATS/table4c6.html. Actuarial Publications, Baltimore, MD. Accessed 8 Mar 2004

117. Minino AM, Heron MP, Smith BL (2006) Deaths: preliminary data for 2004. Natl Vital Stat Rep 54(19):1–49

118. Nugent WC, Edney MT, Hammerness PG, Dain BJ, Maurer LH, Rigas JR (1997) Non-small cell lung cancer at the extremes of age: impact on diagnosis and treatment. Ann Thorac Surg 63(1):193–197

119. Kuo CW, Chen YM, Chao JY, Tsai CM, Perng RP (2000) Non-small cell lung cancer in very young and very old patients. Chest 117(2):354–357

120. Fruh M, Rolland E, Pignon JP et al (2008) Pooled analysis of the effect of age on adjuvant cisplatin-based chemotherapy for completely resected non-small-cell lung cancer. J Clin Oncol 26(21):3573–3581

121. Cress RD, O'Malley CD, Leiserowitz GS, Campleman SL (2003) Patterns of chemotherapy use for women with ovarian cancer: a population-based study. J Clin Oncol 21(8):1530–1535

122. Moore DH (1994) Ovarian cancer in the elderly patient. Oncology (Huntingt) 8(12):21–25, discussion 25, 29–30

123. Edmonson JH, Su J, Krook JE (1993) Treatment of ovarian cancer in elderly women. Mayo Clinic-North Central Cancer Treatment Group studies. Cancer 71(2 Suppl):615–617

124. Singletary SE, Shallenberger R, Guinee VF (1993) Breast cancer in the elderly. Ann Surg 218(5):667–671

125. Wanebo HJ, Cole B, Chung M et al (1997) Is surgical management compromised in elderly patients with breast cancer? Ann Surg 225(5):579–586, discussion 586–579

126. Swanson RS, Sawicka J, Wood WC (1991) Treatment of carcinoma of the breast in the older geriatric patient. Surg Gynecol Obstet 173(6):465–469

127. van Dalsen AD, de Vries JE (1995) Treatment of breast cancer in elderly patients. J Surg Oncol 60(2):80–82

128. Guadagnoli E, Shapiro C, Gurwitz JH et al (1997) Age-related patterns of care: evidence against ageism in the treatment of early-stage breast cancer. J Clin Oncol 15(6):2338–2344

129. Hebert-Croteau N, Brisson J, Latreille J, Blanchette C, Deschenes L (1999) Compliance with consensus recommendations for the treatment of early stage breast carcinoma in elderly women. Cancer 85(5):1104–1113

130. Hurria A, Hurria A, Zuckerman E et al (2006) A prospective, longitudinal study of the functional status and quality of life of older patients with breast cancer receiving adjuvant chemotherapy. J Am Geriatr Soc 54(7):1119–1124

131. Silliman RA, Ganz PA (2006) Adjuvant chemotherapy use and outcomes in older women with breast cancer: what have we learned? J Clin Oncol 24(18):2697–2699

132. Bilimoria KY, Stewart AK, Palis BE, Bentrem DJ, Talamonti MS, Ko CY (2008) Adequacy and importance of lymph node evaluation for colon cancer in the elderly. J Am Coll Surg 206(2):247–254

133. Chalmers RT, Stonebridge PA, John TG, Murie JA (1993) Abdominal aortic aneurysm in the elderly. Br J Surg 80(9): 1122–1123

134. Blanche C, Matloff JM, Denton TA et al (1997) Cardiac operations in patients 90 years of age and older. Ann Thorac Surg 63(6):1685–1690

135. Finlayson E, Fan Z, Birkmeyer JD (2007) Outcomes in octogenarians undergoing high-risk cancer operation: a national study. J Am Coll Surg 205(6):729–734

136. Moskovitz AH, Rizk NP, Venkatraman E et al (2006) Mortality increases for octogenarians undergoing esophagogastrectomy for esophageal cancer. Ann Thorac Surg 82(6):2031–2036, discussion 2036

137. Ngaage DL, Cowen ME, Griffin S, Guvendik L, Cale AR (2008) Early neurological complications after coronary artery bypass grafting and valve surgery in octogenarians. Eur J Cardiothorac Surg 33(4):653–659

138. Leo F, Scanagatta P, Baglio P et al (2007) The risk of pneumonectomy over the age of 70. A case-control study. Eur J Cardiothorac Surg 31(5):780–782

139. Barnett SD, Halpin LS, Speir AM et al (2003) Postoperative complications among octogenarians after cardiovascular surgery. Ann Thorac Surg 76(3):726–731

140. Jarvinen O, Huhtala H, Laurikka J, Tarkka MR (2003) Higher age predicts adverse outcome and readmission after coronary artery bypass grafting. World J Surg 27(12):1317–1322

141. Lightner AM, Glasgow RE, Jordan TH et al (2004) Pancreatic resection in the elderly. J Am Coll Surg 198(5):697–706

142. Sosa JA, Mehta PJ, Wang TS, Boudourakis L, Roman SA (2008) A population-based study of outcomes from thyroidectomy in aging Americans: at what cost? J Am Coll Surg 206(3):1097–1105

143. Mamoun NF, Xu M, Sessler DI, Sabik JF, Bashour CA (2008) Propensity matched comparison of outcomes in older and younger patients after coronary artery bypass graft surgery. Ann Thorac Surg 85(6):1974–1979

144. Fraioli B, Pastore FS, Signoretti S, De Caro GM, Giuffre R (1999) The surgical treatment of pituitary adenomas in the eighth decade. Surg Neurol 51(3):261–266, discussion 266–267

145. Derks W, De Leeuw JR, Hordijk GJ, Winnubst JA (2003) Elderly patients with head and neck cancer: short-term effects of surgical treatment on quality of life. Clin Otolaryngol 28(5):399–405

146. Uruno T, Miyauchi A, Shimizu K et al (2005) Favorable surgical results in 433 elderly patients with papillary thyroid cancer. World J Surg 29(11):1497–1501, discussion 1502–1493

147. Salameh JR, Myers JL, Mukherjee D (200) Carotid endarterectomy in elderly patients: low complication rate with overnight stay. Arch Surg 137(11):1284–1287, discussion 1288

148. Durward QJ, Ragnarsson TS, Reeder RF, Case JL, Hughes CA (2005) Carotid endarterectomy in nonagenarians. Arch Surg 140(7):625–628, discussion 628

149. Beauford RB, Goldstein DJ, Sardari FF et al (2003) Multivessel off-pump revascularization in octogenarians: early and midterm outcomes. Ann Thorac Surg 76(1):12–17, discussion 17

150. Chiappini B, Camurri N, Loforte A, Di Marco L, Di Bartolomeo R, Marinelli G (2004) Outcome after aortic valve replacement in octogenarians. Ann Thorac Surg 78(1):85–89

151. Collart F, Feier H, Kerbaul F et al (2005) Valvular surgery in octogenarians: operative risks factors, evaluation of Euroscore and long term results. Eur J Cardiothorac Surg 27(2):276–280

152. Ferguson TB Jr, Hammill BG, Peterson ED, DeLong ER, Grover FL (2002) A decade of change–risk profiles and outcomes for isolated coronary artery bypass grafting procedures, 1990–1999: a report from the STS National Database Committee and the Duke Clinical Research Institute. Society of Thoracic Surgeons. Ann Thorac Surg 73(2):480–489, discussion 489–490

153. Huber CH, Goeber V, Berdat P, Carrel T, Eckstein F (2007) Benefits of cardiac surgery in octogenarians – a postoperative quality of life assessment. Eur J Cardiothorac Surg 31(6):1099–1105

154. Rice DC, Correa AM, Vaporciyan AA et al (2005) Preoperative chemoradiotherapy prior to esophagectomy in elderly patients is not associated with increased morbidity. Ann Thorac Surg 79(2):391–397, discussion 391–397

155. Ruol A, Portale G, Zaninotto G et al (2007) Results of esophagectomy for esophageal cancer in elderly patients: age has little influence on outcome and survival. J Thorac Cardiovasc Surg 133(5):1186–1192

156. Ruol A, Portale G, Castoro C et al (2007) Effects of neoadjuvant therapy on perioperative morbidity in elderly patients undergoing esophagectomy for esophageal cancer. Ann Surg Oncol 14(11):3243–3250

157. Poon RT, Law SY, Chu KM, Branicki FJ, Wong J (1998) Esophagectomy for carcinoma of the esophagus in the elderly: results of current surgical management. Ann Surg 227(3): 357–364

158. Kunisaki C, Akiyama H, Nomura M et al (2006) Comparison of surgical outcomes of gastric cancer in elderly and middle-aged patients. Am J Surg 191(2):216–224

159. Avital S, Kashtan H, Hadad R, Werbin N (1997) Survival of colorectal carcinoma in the elderly. A prospective study of colorectal carcinoma and a five-year follow-up. Dis Colon Rectum 40(5):523–529

160. Barrier A, Ferro L, Houry S, Lacaine F, Huguier M (2003) Rectal cancer surgery in patients more than 80 years of age. Am J Surg 185(1):54–57

161. Law WL, Choi HK, Ho JW, Lee YM, Seto CL (2006) Outcomes of surgery for mid and distal rectal cancer in the elderly. World J Surg 30(4):598–604

162. Aldrighetti L, Arru M, Caterini R et al (2003) Impact of advanced age on the outcome of liver resection. World J Surg 27(10):1149–1154

163. Cescon M, Grazi GL, Del Gaudio M et al (2003) Outcome of right hcpatectomies in patients older than 70 years. Arch Surg 138(5):547–552

164. Ferrero A, Vigano L, Polastri R et al (2005) Hepatectomy as treatment of choice for hepatocellular carcinoma in elderly cirrhotic patients. World J Surg 29(9):1101–1105

165. Menon KV, Al-Mukhtar A, Aldouri A, Prasad RK, Lodge PA, Toogood GJ (2006) Outcomes after major hepatectomy in elderly patients. J Am Coll Surg 203(5):677–683

166. Sohn TA, Yeo CJ, Cameron JL et al (1998) Should pancreaticoduodenectomy be performed in octogenarians? J Gastrointest Surg 2(3):207–216

167. Petrowsky H, Clavien PA (2005) Should we deny surgery for malignant hepato-pancreatico-biliary tumors to elderly patients? World J Surg 29(9):1093–1100

168. Geisler JP, Geisler HE (1994) Radical hysterectomy in patients 65 years of age and older. Gynecol Oncol 53(2):208–211

169. Anderson JG, Wixson RL, Tsai D, Stulberg SD, Chang RW (1996) Functional outcome and patient satisfaction in total knee patients over the age of 75. J Arthroplasty 11(7):831–840

170. Wurtz LD, Feinberg JR, Capello WN, Meldrum R, Kay PJ (2003) Elective primary total hip arthroplasty in octogenarians. J Gerontol A Biol Sci Med Sci 58(5):M468–M471

171. Hamel MB, Toth M, Legedza A, Rosen MP (2008) Joint replacement surgery in elderly patients with severe osteoarthritis of the hip or knee: decision making, postoperative recovery, and clinical outcomes. Arch Intern Med 168(13):1430–1440

172. Malata CM, Cooter RD, Batchelor AG, Simpson KH, Browning FS, Kay SP (1996) Microvascular free-tissue transfers in elderly patients: the leeds experience. Plast Reconstr Surg 98(7):1234–1241

173. Morgan JA, John R, Weinberg AD et al (2003) Long-term results of cardiac transplantation in patients 65 years of age and older: a comparative analysis. Ann Thorac Surg 76(6):1982–1987

174. Mahidhara R, Bastani S, Ross DJ et al (2008) Lung transplantation in older patients? J Thorac Cardiovasc Surg 135(2):412–420

175. Minor ME, Ellozy S, Carroccio A et al (2004) Endovascular aortic aneurysm repair in the octogenarian: is it worthwhile? Arch Surg 139(3):308–314

176. St Peter SD, Craft RO, Tiede JL, Swain JM (2005) Impact of advanced age on weight loss and health benefits after laparoscopic gastric bypass. Arch Surg 140(2):165–168

177. Chautard J, Alves A, Zalinski S, Bretagnol F, Valleur P, Panis Y (2008) Laparoscopic colorectal surgery in elderly patients: a matched case-control study in 178 patients. J Am Coll Surg 206(2):255–260

178. Gianetta E, de Cian F, Cuneo S et al (1997) Hernia repair in elderly patients. Br J Surg 84(7):983–985

179. Amemiya T, Oda K, Ando M et al (2007) Activities of daily living and quality of life of elderly patients after elective surgery for gastric and colorectal cancers. Ann Surg 246(2):222–228

180. Zierer A, Melby SJ, Lubahn JG, Sicard GA, Damiano RJ Jr, Moon MR (2006) Elective surgery for thoracic aortic aneurysms: late functional status and quality of life. Ann Thorac Surg 82(2):573–578

181. de Vincentiis C, Kunkl AB, Trimarchi S et al (2008) Aortic valve replacement in octogenarians: is biologic valve the unique solution? Ann Thorac Surg 85(4):1296–1301

182. Vicchio M, Della Corte A, De Santo LS et al (2008) Tissue versus mechanical prostheses: quality of life in octogenarians. Ann Thorac Surg 85(4):1290–1295

183. Dunlop WE, Rosenblood L, Lawrason L, Birdsall L, Rusnak CH (1993) Effects of age and severity of illness on outcome and length of stay in geriatric surgical patients. Am J Surg 165(5):577–580

184. Akoh JA, Mathew AM, Chalmers JW, Finlayson A, Auld GD (1994) Audit of major gastrointestinal surgery in patients aged 80 years or over. J R Coll Surg Edinb 39(4):208–213

185. Battafarano RJ, Piccirillo JF, Meyers BF et al (2002) Impact of comorbidity on survival after surgical resection in patients with stage I non-small cell lung cancer. J Thorac Cardiovasc Surg 123(2):280–287

186. Mehta RH, Eagle KA, Coombs LP et al (2002) Influence of age on outcomes in patients undergoing mitral valve replacement. Ann Thorac Surg 74(5):1459–1467

187. Muravchick S (2000) Anesthesia for the elderly. In: Miller RD (ed) Anesthesia, 5th edn. Churchill Livingston, Philadelphia, pp 2140–2156

188. Barzan L, Veronesi A, Caruso G et al (1990) Head and neck cancer and ageing: a retrospective study in 438 patients. J Laryngol Otol 104(8):634–640

189. Gupta R, Kawashima T, Ryu M, Okada T, Cho A, Takayama W (2004) Role of curative resection in octogenarians with malignancy. Am J Surg 188(3):282–287

190. Martin RC II, Jaques DP, Brennan MF, Karpeh M (2002) Extended local resection for advanced gastric cancer: increased survival versus increased morbidity. Ann Surg 236(2):159–165

191. Siegelmann-Danieli N, Khandelwal V, Wood GC et al (2006) Breast cancer in elderly women: outcome as affected by age, tumor features, comorbidities, and treatment approach. Clin Breast Cancer 7(1):59–66

192. Muravchick S (2000) Anesthesia for the elderly. In: Miller R (ed) Anesthesia, 5th edn. Churchill Livingstone, Philadelphia, pp 2140–2156

193. Lakatta EG (1994) Cardiovascular reserve capacity in healthy older humans. Aging (Milano) 6(4):213–223

194. Muravchick S (1997) Choosing an anesthetic for the elderly patient. Am Rev PAN 19:117–124

Chapter 21
Geriatric Models of Care

Elizabeth A. Capezuti, Marie Boltz, and Hongsoo Kim

Introduction

Models of care addressing the unique needs of older hospitalized patients can be traced to the comprehensive geriatric assessment (CGA) programs first developed in the 1970s [1]. CGA programs screen older patients at high risk for geriatric-specific problems, assess for modifiable risk factors, and implement evidence-based strategies consistent with the patient's treatment goals. Over the last 30 years changes in the health-care system, coupled with the increasing older adult population, has led to development of several geriatric models of care across all health-care settings. In general, the goals of these geriatric models of care in the hospital focus on (1) prevention of complications that occur more commonly in older adults and (2) address hospital factors that contribute to complications. This chapter provides a brief overview of complications that are more frequently found in older patients, care delivery issues that are addressed by geriatric models of care and a description of the most commonly employed hospital models.

Complications of Older Hospitalized Patients

Although patients aged 65 and over represent about 13% of the US population, they account for 40% of those undergoing surgical procedures in American hospitals [2]. In addition to the high proportion of older patients, the most troublesome finding is that older patients also represent a higher complication rate for certain conditions which subsequently lead to higher health-care costs. Age may be viewed as a proxy for multiple chronic diseases. Postoperative complications that are known determinants of short and long-term survival following major surgery such as

myocardial infarction and sepsis are associated with age due to the increased likelihood of co-morbidities such as cardiac disease [3].

Older adults are more likely to experience additional types of complications that, in addition to reducing survival, can result in loss of independence and lead to hospital readmission, increased usage of rehabilitation services, and new placement in a nursing home. Physical frailty and cognitive impairment [4–6] (either chronic dementia and/or delirium) can further compound an older person's vulnerability to complications during hospitalization [7, 8]. Frailty refers to "decreased reserves in multiple organ systems" [9] that is highly associated (after controlling for age, race, sex, and comorbid illness) with an increased risk for falls, cardiovascular disease, hypertension as well as reduced mobility, decreased functional status, institutionalization, and death (see Chap. 10) [10, 11].

Persons with dementia are more prone to negative outcomes related to disease management and hospitalization. Older patients with dementia hospitalized for exacerbation of a chronic disease have significantly longer lengths of hospital stays (LOS) as compared to older patients without dementia. For example, the LOS of older patient with COPD is 121 days/1,000 persons as compared to older patients with both COPD and dementia, who have a LOS of 361 days/1,000 persons [12]. For those who develop delirium (for both those with and without an underlying chronic dementia) during hospitalization, increased LOS and higher hospital costs is well documented [13]. The complex challenges of those adult patients with cognitive impairment are often not adequately addressed. Table 21.1 provides examples of common behaviors of cognitively impaired persons that can lead to complications.

Although geriatric models of care can improve the overall outcomes and experiences of hospitalization, in general, these programs are designed to target those adverse events that occur more commonly in older patients. Table 21.2 provides a summary of these complications and the clinical and cost outcomes associated with these complications. These complications are often referred to as "geriatric syndromes"

E.A. Capezuti (✉)
Hartford Institute for Geriatric Nursing, NYU College of Nursing,
726 Broadway, 10th Floor, New York, NY 10003, USA
e-mail: ec65@nyu.edu

R.A. Rosenthal et al. (eds.), *Principles and Practice of Geriatric Surgery*,
DOI 10.1007/978-1-4419-6999-6_21, © Springer Science+Business Media, LLC 2011

Table 21.1 Behaviors of cognitively impaired patients contributing to high complication rate

Behaviors	Example	Potential complication
Inability to follow directions	Does not use call bell to ask for assistance and gets out of bed without needed assistance	Fall-related injury
Removal of treatments	Pulls out central lines	Hemorrhage Infection Physical restraints and associated complications
Not able to communicate needs	In pain but not able to verbally communicate this to nurse	Functional decline
Wandering	Leaves unit and exits hospital in gown	Hypothermia Other injuries Use of physical and chemical restraints that increase likelihood of delirium, falls, fall-related injury, nutritional problems
Misinterprets visual and auditory cues	Resists staff attempts to assist the patient to get out of bed which is perceived as an assault and then hits staff	Agitation-related injury Overuse of psychoactive medication that increase likelihood of delirium, falls, and fall-related injury
Decreases inhibition of inappropriate behaviors	Removes clothing and walk down hallway nude	Agitation-related injury Overuse of psychoactive medication that increases likelihood of delirium, falls, and fall-related injury

Reference: Silverstein and Maslow [12]

which refer to "clinical conditions in older persons that do not fit into discrete disease categories." [14]

A US congressional mandate instituted on August 1, 2007 significantly changed the Inpatient Prospective Payment System that the Centers for Medicare & Medicaid Services (CMS) use to reimburse hospitals [15–17]. As of October 2008, hospitals will no longer receive payment for eight hospital-acquired conditions; three of these eight are complications that are known to occur most frequently in older inpatients and have been found to be reduced when geriatric models of care are employed [18]. These three complications (fall-related injury, pressure ulcer, and cathe-ter-associated urinary tract infection) are among the six adverse events or complications specifically associated with hospitalization of older adults. Although there are other geriatric syndromes (e.g., incontinence) and other potential complications associated with older inpatients (e.g., sleep deprivation, inadequate pain management, dehydration, adverse drug effects), many of these syndromes and compli-cations are either risk factors or outcomes of the following.

Functional Decline

Functional decline refers to the loss of the ability to perform basic activities of daily living (ADL). A systematic review of 30 studies examining correlates of functional decline found that between 15 and 76% of hospitalized elders experience dimin-ished performance in at least one ADL at discharge [19]. Of those with decline at discharge, only half will recover function at 3 months postdischarge, and, for many, this decline will result in permanent loss of independent living [20, 21]. Functional decline is considered a "profound marker of morbidity and mortality" [22, 23] resulting in longer lengths of stay, greater costs and increased rate of nursing home placement [24]. Among the ADLs, the ability to walk independently is considered the most critical in predicting health outcomes. Functional Mobility Decline, defined as new walking dependence, is associated with poor posthospitalization outcomes such as discharge to a nurs-ing home, continued impaired mobility and higher mortality rates [25]. The incidence of functional mobility decline occurs in 15–59% of hospitalized elders [26]. For older hip fracture patients, especially those with cognitive and affective disorders, there is a greater risk of functional decline and new nursing home placement [27, 28].

Fall-Related Injury

Roughly 2–5% of older adults fall during hospitalization [29]. The number of falls per 1,000 patient days is highest in hospi-tal units admitting mostly older adults such as geropsychiatry, rehabilitation, and geriatric medicine. Among hospitalized older adults, falls from bed account for approximately one-third of all falls. Almost one-third of all fall-related injuries occur among persons 85 years of age or older. Approximately 3–10% of falls happening in hospitals result in either serious or minor injuries [30]. Hip fractures, occurring in about 1–4% of hospital falls are particularly significant because older adults are more likely to suffer from a substantial decline in physical functioning and often require longer periods of active rehabilitation services as compared to younger persons [31].

Undernutrition/Malnutrition

Undernutrition and malnutrition are deficiency syndromes caused by inadequate intake or absorption of macronutrients. Malnutrition has long been associated with important adverse outcomes, such as increased morbidity and mortality and decreased quality of life. Weight loss and hypoalbuminemia are both strongly correlated with increased mortality in ill adults [32]. Body weight and body composition have important implications for physical functioning of older persons and the prevalence of malnutrition in older hospitalized patients has been estimated to be between 40 and 60% [33].

Pressure Ulcers

Pressure ulcers continue to present a major health problem for hospitalized adults with reported nosocomial incidence rates between 0.4 and 38% [34]. Pressure ulcers are highly correlated with age [35]. At least a fifth of pressure ulcers will progress to a more advanced stage of deterioration. Most ulcers develop in the sacrum and coccyx areas with rates higher in patients with mobility impairment. Pressure ulcers remain a major cause of morbidity and are associated with longer lengths of hospital stay. Nosocomial pressure ulcers and their progression in severity during hospitalization have been used as a quality care indicator [36].

Urinary Tract Infection

Approximately 4% of patients with urinary tract infection (UTIs) will develop bacteremia which is known to significantly increase in length of stay and is associated with higher mortality in older patients [37]. The major care-associated practice leading to UTI in older inpatients is the overuse of urinary catheters, defined as catheter use for longer than 2 days [38]. Catheter-associated urinary tract infection (CAUTI) is the most common nosocomial infection [39]. A study using a random sample of almost 36,000 Medicare patients undergoing major operations from 2,965 US hospitals reported that 86% had perioperative indwelling urinary catheters and among these 50% had catheters for longer than 2 days postoperatively. These patients' risk of developing a urinary tract infection was twice as likely compared to patients with catheterization [40]. Among another sample of approximately 39,000 Medicare patients undergoing major surgery who were discharged to a nursing home it was found that those patients discharged with catheters were at higher risk for rehospitalization for UTI and death within 30 days than patients who did not have catheters [41].

In addition to infection, catheter use is associated with immobility, delirium, and pain [42].

Delirium

Delirium, a transient state of cognitive impairment, may develop in both cognitively intact and impaired older adults. It is estimated that between 14 and 24% of older persons are admitted to the hospital with delirium, and an additional 6–56% of hospitalized elders will develop delirium during their hospitalization replace especially if they are admitted to an ICU [43]. Postoperative delirium is more likely to occur following hip fracture, cardiac, non-cardiac thoracic, aortic aneurysm, and abdominal surgery. Postoperative delirium is more likely in those deemed vulnerable. Patient vulnerability including presence of previous brain pathology, decreased ability to manage change, impaired sensory function, multiple co-morbidities and changes in pharmacodynamic responses to medications, are all suggested possible causes for delirium. In surgical patients both preoperative (use of narcotic analgesics, history of alcohol abuse and depression) and perioperative (greater intraoperative blood loss, more postoperative transfusions, postoperative hematocrit less than 30%, and severe postoperative pain) risk factors have been identified for delirium postoperatively [44]. Additionally, hospital practices that lead to iatrogenic events including use of physical restraints, malnutrition, more than three medications and urinary catheterization are also significantly associated with delirium [45]. There are no significant differences in incidence of postoperative delirium following general vs. epidural anesthesia.

Despite high incidence, most delirium goes undetected [46, 47] thus contributing to many negative consequences. Delirium is associated with poor hospital outcomes such as higher mortality rates, increased length of hospital stay, increased intensity of nursing care, greater health-care costs as well as increased risk of several adverse outcomes after discharge, including functional decline, persistent cognitive impairment, rehospitalization, and nursing home placement [48].

The occurrence of each of these complications leads to interventions that can often prolong the hospital stay. Following hospital discharge, they frequently contribute to death, institutionalization as well as disproportionately high rehospitalization rates, high emergency department usage, and increased need for rehabilitation therapy services. As illustrated in Table 21.2, the *interrelationships* among these various complications during hospitalization is obvious and also well documented [12]. The data supporting the importance of prevention, early detection, and treatment of these complications in older surgical patients is described in the ACOVE (Assessing Care of Vulnerable Elders) report, Quality Indicators for Hospitalization and Surgery in Vulnerable Elders [49].

TABLE 21.2 Complications in the older surgical patient[a]

Complication	Hospital factors[b]	Clinical outcome	Cost implications
Functional decline	• Immobility • Bed rest without medical/surgical indication • Physical restraint • Inappropriate medication prescribing • New psychoactive drug use • Obstacles in the hospital physical environment	• Reduced/loss of independence in function (activities of daily living) • Reduced/loss of ambulation • Pain • Increased rate of pressure ulcers, falls, fall-related injuries, and development of contractures	• Longer length of stay (LOS) • Increased rate of institutional or home-based rehabilitation • Nursing home placement
Fall-related injury	• Immobility • Physical restraint • Inappropriate medication prescribing • New psychoactive drug use • Obstacles in the hospital physical environment	• Pain • Fracture requiring surgical intervention • Reduced/loss of independence in function (activities of daily living) • Reduced/loss of ambulation	• Medicare will not pay for treatment[c] • Surgery • Longer LOS • Institutional or home-based rehabilitation • Nursing home placement
Under/malnutrition	• Immobility • Inattention to oral care • Lack of feeding assistance for those with physical or cognitive impairments	• Reduced wound healing • Discomfort due nasogastric tube placement • Percutaneous enteral access procedures (gastrostomy) • Delirium • Physical restraint to prevent tube removal • Aspiration • Functional decline	• Longer LOS • Surgery • Institutional or home-based enteral nutrition therapy
Pressure ulcer	• Immobility • Physical restraint • Under/malnutrition • Dehydration	• Immobility • Sleep deprivation • Pain • Sepsis • Septicemia • Surgical debridement • Surgical techniques (direct closure, flaps, and skin grafting)	• Medicare will not pay for treatment[b] • Longer LOS • Institutional or home-based skilled nursing treatment
Urinary tract infection (UTI: secondary to catheter use or CAUTI)	• Emergency room placement without indication • Incontinence treatment • No postsurgical monitoring of catheter use	• Immobility • Pain • Delirium • Acute pyelonephritis • Bacteremia • Sepsis • Prosthetic joint infection • Higher risk for death	• Medicare will not pay for treatment[b] • Longer LOS • Rehospitalization
Delirium	• Physical restraint • Inappropriate medication prescribing • New psychoactive drugs • Urinary catheterization • CAUTI • Immobility • Under/malnutrition • Dehydration	• Functional decline • Persistent cognitive impairment • Falls, injuries • Undetected infection • Sleep deprivation	• Longer LOS • Rehospitalization • Nursing home placement • Death

[a] Geriatric syndromes refer to "clinical conditions in older persons that do not fit into discrete disease categories." This may also include other conditions highly associated with aging such as frailty, sleep disorders, self-neglect. For the purpose of this review, these syndromes and potential complications are more narrowly defined

[b] Hospital factors. There is a myriad of patient and hospital factors that contribute to each complication, however, this list provides examples of those specific hospital practices that place the older adults at high risk and which are the focus of geriatric care model interventions

[c] As of October 2008, hospitals will no longer receive payment for 8 hospital-acquired conditions; 3 of these 8 indicated in the table are complications that are known to occur most frequently in older inpatients and have been found to be reduced when geriatric models of care are employed (fall-related injury, pressure ulcer, and catheter-associated urinary track infection)

Although patient characteristics, especially multiple co-morbidities, frailty, and cognitive impairment, may increase vulnerability of older inpatient to negative consequences, the hospital environment plays an independent and significant role in determining staff practice and subsequent patient outcomes such as iatrogenic complications. This has led to the development of geriatric models to address these hospital-based or institutional factors that are likely to contribute to complications among older patients. Effective resolution of these negative consequences is dependent on geriatric models that target both patient and environmental (institutional) risk factors.

Geriatric Care Model Objectives

Although geriatric models of care differ in their approach to prevent complications and address care delivery problems that can contribute to complications, all share a common set of general objectives. Although these objectives could be applied to any patient regardless of age, it is how geriatric care models apply these that are age-specific. Table 21.3 provides examples of processes and interventions to meet these six general objectives.

The six general objectives of geriatric care models are as follows.

TABLE 21.3 Geriatric care models: objectives, processes and interventions

Objective	Examples of processes	Examples of interventions
Educate health-care providers in core geriatric principles	• Resident training includes required geriatric rotation *or* mandatory geriatric rotation for residents • Institutional continuing education includes geriatric-specific training *or* Geriatric-specific interdisciplinary continuing education programs • Geriatric specialist responsible for geriatric training initiatives	• Hospital intranet includes geriatric programming • Journal club includes geriatric journals and/or articles focusing on geriatric outcomes • Medical, surgical, nursing, and interdisciplinary rounds includes geriatric case studies
Target risk factors for complications	• Policies, protocols, and documentation system includes assessment tools and practices that identify older adults at risk for complications • Assessment tools prompt providers to consult geriatric specialists for evaluation of high-risk problems • Geriatric specialist provides individual evaluation of risk factors	• Electronic medical record (EMR) provides alerts for medications prescribed that are known to increase fall risk • EMR prompts providers to document daily cognitive testing results • Hospital policy for daily cognitive assessment of at-risk patients • Cognitive assessment indicates delirium that leads to geriatric specialist consultation
Incorporate patient (family) choices and treatment goals	• Policies and protocols support and documentation system includes forms that elicit patient choices as well as family involvement in care • Geriatric nurses are prepared to coordinate an interdisciplinary evaluation and promote development of *informed* patient/family treatment goals and plan of care • Palliative care is consulted and provides informed choices to patients/families in situations of life-threatening illness	• Admission history includes evaluation of patient's preferences for postdischarge rehabilitation • Unlimited visiting hours and bedside recliners encourage family participation in recovery • Patient and family preferences for type and degree of family involvement is documented • Patient with Alzheimer's disease who is unable to verbally indicate needs is evaluated by palliative care specialist for pain evaluation/treatment
Employ evidence-based interventions	• Policies and protocols integrate geriatric specific implications • Education and training for all clinicians include core geriatric content	• Hospital protocol for urinary catheter removal within 2 days postsurgery • Unit-based mobility program • Physical environment reduces injury risk for nonambulatory patients with dementia such as low-height beds and bedside mats
Promote interdisciplinary communication	• Medical record facilitates patient information across disciplines • Processes in place to encourage face-to-face interaction among disciplines • Unit-based and hospital-wide committee includes geriatric specialist representation	• Interdisciplinary team rounds held bi-weekly • Programmatic initiatives include all applicable disciplines, e.g., physical and occupational therapy in unit-based mobility program • Co-manage patients across specialties such as geriatric oncology • Collaborate with other programs such as palliative care in providing symptom management
Emphasize discharge planning or transitional care	• Documentation system provides comprehensive hospital course information to primary care provider and other postdischarge providers (home care, nursing home, etc.) as well as elicits pertinent information *from* other providers	• Patient and caregiver receive comprehensive documentation of hospital treatment, changes in treatment plan, and postdischarge instructions • Understanding of instructions is evaluated before discharge • Phone follow-up postdischarge to evaluate patient condition and needs

Educate Health-Care Providers in Core Geriatric Principles

The complications most frequently encountered among older patients are often due to system-level problems. These include inadequate educational preparation of health-care providers to recognize age-specific factors that increase risk of complications. All geriatric care models require a coordinator or clinician with advanced geriatric education; however, the implementation of any model depends on direct care staff with the knowledge and competencies to deliver safe and evidence-based care to older patients. Thus, the coordinator or other geriatric clinician role includes teaching of other staff through rounds, journal clubs, conferences, and other internal institutional educational venues.

Target Risk Factors for Complications

Given the disproportion of certain complications or geriatric syndromes among hospitalized older adults, the clinical focus of all geriatric models is prevention via risk factor reduction and early detection of these problems. Some models may focus on a particular syndrome; however, the interrelationship of these complications and their shared risk factors often result in a reduction of the other geriatric syndromes. Targeting risk factors requires standardized assessment tools known to be valid and reliable for older adults. See the Hartford Institute's Try This and How to Try This series for examples of assessment instruments (http://www.hartfordign.org/trythis). Implementation of geriatric care models often include institutionalizing these practices such as incorporating these tools in the medical record as well as hospital policies, procedures, and protocols.

Incorporate Patient (Family) Choices and Treatment Goals

All health-care decisions should be guided by the patient's choices. Choices range from decisions about activity level and medication use to more complex issues including advance directives.

Decisions regarding life-sustaining treatment are often influenced by quality of life considerations balanced by the potential length of life. For family members acting in the best interests of patients who can no longer participate in decision-making, this can be a complicated dilemma. Life-sustaining treatments are often employed with very old patients who die in the course of hospitalization although most prefer comfort care. Geriatric models are meant to address this lack of congruence by supporting efforts to provide care that is more consistent with patients' preferences [50]. For this reason, many geriatric models work collaboratively or in conjunction with palliative care programs.

Employ Evidence-Based Interventions

Given that most physicians, nurses, and other health providers have received minimal content in their training regarding geriatrics, it is not surprising that there is a higher complication rate for older hospitalized patients. Advances in geriatric science, similar to other research-based approaches, are not readily employed in hospital care. Problems with polypharmacy, inappropriate medications (e.g., overuse of psychoactive), overuse of restraints, inadequate detection of delirium, depression, and undermanagement of pain are some of the many hospital factors that can contribute to poor outcomes. Thus, geriatric models promote the use of standardized evidence-based protocols.

Promote Interdisciplinary Communication

Since geriatric syndromes are not just medical problems but represent a complex interaction of medical, functional, psychological, and social issues, other disciplines such as nursing, pharmacy, social work, physical and occupational therapy are needed. Geriatric care models all include interdisciplinary teams, i.e., an approach that facilitates communication among disciplines.

Emphasize Discharge Planning (or Transitional Care)

Many older patients will require rehabilitation or skilled nursing services following hospitalization. Almost a quarter of older hospital patients are discharged to another institution such as a rehabilitation hospital or nursing home and more than 10% are discharged with home care [51]. Older adults are more likely to experience problems associated with discharge planning that can lead to delays in discharge and greater use of emergency service use and hospital readmission. Hospital readmission for older patients is most likely associated with medical errors in medication continuity [52, 53], diagnostic workup, or test follow-up [54]. These poor outcomes are attributed to a lack of coordination among health-care providers that can result in unresolved medical issues [55] and deficient preparation of patients and their caregivers to carry out discharge instructions [56]. One study found wide variations among providers in discharge planning effectiveness; the providers cited their lack of knowledge and experience when not making appropriate home-care referrals [57]. Thus, geriatric models not only focus on the inpatient experience but also the post-hospital care environment and the care transition following hospital discharge. Two of the six models consider the care transition a primary focus of their programs.

Geriatric Models

There are several types of geriatric models that are currently employed in hospitals throughout the USA. In addition to incorporating the original tenets central to comprehensive geriatric assessment (screen for those at high risk for geriatric-specific problems, assess for modifiable risk factors, and implement strategies consistent with the patients' treatment goals), all strive to deliver quality care for older adults in a cost-effective manner. Comprehensive geriatric assessment assumes that the systematic evaluation of a frail older person by a multidisciplinary health-care team will uncover actual or potential health problems. The considerable advances in geriatric health-care science over the last 30 years can then be applied to treating or preventing these conditions and thus result in better health outcomes.

Although the specific mode of intervening may differ among the models, they all address both common health problems and care delivery issues. The geriatric model may consider all geriatric syndromes or target specific ones such as delirium or functional decline. Similarly, the geriatric model may be employed as a hospital-wide approach, unit-based intervention, or focus on specific processes of hospitalization such as admission screening or discharge planning. Regardless of the structure of the geriatric model, all facilitate the general objectives listed in Table 21.3. Table 21.4 provides a summary of the clinical foci, unique features, coordination, and interventions for each of the six most commonly employed geriatric models of care.

Geriatric Consultation Service

Geriatric Consultation Service provides a geriatrician, a gero-psychiatrist, a geriatric clinical nurse specialist or an interdisciplinary team of geriatric health-care providers to conduct a comprehensive geriatric assessment or evaluate a specific condition (delirium), symptom (patient dislodges or removes treatment), or situation (adequacy of family support for discharge back to community setting). The consultation may be requested by another primary service for an individual patient or may be initiated by a hospital policy for all patients that are screened at high risk for geriatric-related complications or are admitted from a home-bound program or a nursing home [58].

Outside of academic medical centers, few hospitals have geriatric departments that can provide geriatricians or a geriatric consultation team. Although geriatric nurse specialists may be more prevalent in hospitals than geriatricians, many function without the benefit of a geriatric team or a geriatrician. Similar to geriatricians, it is difficult to evaluate their effectiveness when their practice is limited to a consultative role in which recommendations may not be followed or institutional resources are not adequately available for staff to implement [59].

Acute Care for the Elderly Units

Acute Care for the Elderly (ACE) Units are discrete geriatric care-focused units. Originally developed in the 1970s within Veterans Administration Hospitals, Geriatric Evaluation and Management (GEM) Units were meant to provide comprehensive geriatric assessment delivered by a multidisciplinary team with a focus on the rehabilitative needs of older patients. Multidisciplinary team rounds and patient-centered team conferences are considered the hallmarks of care. The core team includes a geriatrician, clinical nurse specialist, social worker as well as specialists from other disciplines providing consultation: occupational and physical therapy, nutrition, pharmacy, audiology, and psychology. GEM units usually have been redesigned to facilitate care of the older patient, which, in contrast to geriatric consultation services, have direct control over the implementation of team recommendations. Research conducted in the 1980s and 1990s have documented significant reductions in functional decline and suboptimal medication use as well as return to home postdischarge and, more recently, decreased rate of nursing home placement [60] among hospitalized veterans on GEMUs compared to general medical units.

Beginning in the 1990s, Acute Care of Elders (ACE) Units have been implemented in non-VA hospitals although they generally focus on more acutely ill patients than GEM units. These units utilize staff with geriatric expertise working collaboratively in an interdisciplinary team (fostered by care processes such as team rounds and family conferences) in a physical environment with adaptations to addresses age-related changes (e.g., flooring to reduce glare and low-height

Table 21.4 Core components of six geriatric care models

Model type	Clinical outcome focus[a]	Unique features	Program/team coordination	Interventions[b]
Geriatric Consultation	• Primary focus can vary depending on composition of consult team & may be specific to a surgical specialty or procedure	• Employed by primary provider request	• Individual consultant (geriatrician, gero-psychiatrist or geriatric nurse specialist) *or* • Interdisciplinary team that is coordinated by geriatric medicine or psychiatry fellow, geriatric nurse specialist or an administrative director	• Comprehensive geriatric assessment: medical, psychiatric, functional, and social • Recommends interventions based on consultant discipline (medicine, psychiatry, or team that includes nurses, social workers, and others) • Primary provider chooses which recommendation to employ
Acute Care for the Elderly (ACE)	• Functional decline	• Dedicated unit with explicit admission criteria • Requires interdisciplinary team • Redesign of physical environment to accommodate physical and cognitive needs	• Unit directed and/or team coordinated by geriatrician, geriatric nurse specialist, administrator or co-managed by clinician-manager	• Physical environment to promote patient mobility, orientation and staff observation • Interdisciplinary rounds facilitate care coordination and thus: 　○ Identify modifiable risk factors for geriatric syndromes and complications 　○ Prevent avoidable discharge delay 　○ Promote timely referrals to disciplines or specialists
NICHE: GRN/ACE	• Nursing processes related to all geriatric syndromes and potential complications such as avoiding restraint use, initiating urinary catheter removal	• Focus on improving nursing care of all geriatric syndromes • Prepares staff nurses to take active part in geriatric care management including coordinating or facilitating other geriatric models of care	• Program implementation by NICHE Coordinator (usually a geriatric nurse specialist) • Geriatric Resources Nurses (staff nurses with additional training) implement protocols • Depending on availability, other clinicians (geriatrician, hospitalist, social worker, etc.) work as interdisciplinary team	• Nurse-initiated protocols: 　○ Restraint and psychoactive drug reduction 　○ Functional mobility 　○ Fall/injury prevention 　○ Pressure ulcer assessment/treatment 　○ Prevention of UTI – early catheter removal 　○ Delirium assessment/treatment • Organizational strategies including measurement schema, performance improvement techniques, and management tools to promote implementation of above protocols
HELP	• Delirium prevention and early management	• Requires use of volunteers	• Elder Life Nurse Specialist or Elder Life Specialists coordinates interdisciplinary team (geriatrician, recreation therapy, physical therapy, etc.) and trained volunteers	• Delirium risk factor protocols: 　○ Mental orientation 　○ Therapeutic activities 　○ Early mobilization 　○ Vision and hearing adaptations 　○ Hydration and feeding assistance 　○ Sleep enhancement
APN Transitional Care Model	• Reducing complications specific during the transition from hospital to home	• Requires advanced practice nurse coordinator to follow patient in hospital and following discharge	• Advanced Practice Nurse (nurse practitioner or clinical nurse specialist)	• Protocols to assess/intervene with: 　○ Medication discrepancies and inappropriate medication usage 　○ Case management and APN surveillance across settings
The Care Transitions Intervention	• Reducing complications specific during the transition from hospital to home, such as preventing post-hospital medication discrepancies, increase likelihood of patient/caregiver detection of worsening condition	• Requires nurse transitions coach to follow patient in hospital and following discharge	• Transition Coach (nurse or advanced practice nurse) empowers patient and caregiver	• Personal Health Record includes data elements essential to promote productive patient–provider encounters across settings • Discharge Preparation Checklist to facilitate patient's knowledge of discharge instructions • Medication Discrepancy Tool used by transition coach to identify medication issues

[a]All programs are meant to address geriatric syndromes and potential complications. Geriatric syndromes refer to "clinical conditions in older persons that do not fit into discrete disease categories." This may also include other conditions highly associated with aging such as frailty, sleep disorders, self-neglect. For the purpose of this review, these syndromes and potential complications are more narrowly defined to 6 of the most common complications

[b]Interventions are guided by the use of standardized assessment tools known to be valid and reliable for older adults. See the Hartford Institute's Try This and How to Try This series for examples of assessment instruments (http://www.hartfordign.org/trythis)

beds to reduce fall-related injury), promote orientation (clocks and calendars) and facilitate staff observation (e.g., alarmed exit doors, windows inserted in walls and communal space for meals). The interdisciplinary team (led by geriatricians and/or geriatric nurse specialists) aims to facilitate care coordination and thus identify modifiable risk factors for geriatric syndromes and complications, prevent avoidable discharge delay, and promote timely referrals to disciplines/specialist.

Palmer et al. designed the first ACE unit at the University Hospitals of Cleveland [61]. A randomized controlled trial of Acute Care for Elders in an academic medical center reported improved functional status (ADL or activities of daily living, instrumental ADLs and ambulation) at discharge of patients hospitalized on the ACE unit compared to those on other units. Fewer patients from the ACE group were discharged to nursing homes. These beneficial effects were achieved without increasing in-hospital or postdischarge costs. There were no significant differences in mortality, length of stay, readmission, or hospital costs between the two groups [62]. In another randomized trial conducted in a community hospital, patients were randomly assigned to either ACE care or a regular care unit. Positive outcomes of the ACE intervention was demonstrated in several processes of care including a reduction in restraint use, days to discharge planning and use of high-risk medications. They also found benefit in a composite outcome of ADL improvement and nursing home placement but not in discharge ADL levels alone. There was no significant reduction in length of stay, hospital costs, or mortality in the ACE unit subjects compared to the regular unit subjects [63]. These savings are recognized in integrated health-care delivery systems such as the VA, Kaiser, and PACE (Program of All Inclusive Care of the Elderly); however, our current "silo-based" reimbursement system to individual hospitals does not provide incentives for postdischarge reductions in health services usage [64].

Since one unit cannot provide care for all older patients within a hospital, many hospitals use this unit for patients at highest risk for age-related complications. The unit is an excellent environment for training of all disciplines. ACE staff may also provide consultation throughout the hospital to export ACE principles throughout the health system.

Nurses Improving the Care of Health System Elders

Nurses Improving the Care of Health System Elders (NICHE; http://www.nicheprogram.org) is a national program aimed at system improvement to achieve positive outcomes for hospitalized older adults. NICHE has two main goals: improving the quality of care to patients and improving nurse competence. This is accomplished by "modifying the nurse practice environment with the infusion of geriatric-specific: (a) core values into the mission statement of the institution; (b) special equipment, supplies, and other resources; and (c) protocols and techniques that promote interdisciplinary collaboration." [65] NICHE includes several approaches, each of which facilitates transfusion of evidence-based geriatric best practices into hospital care. A geriatric nurse specialist as the NICHE Coordinator functions in both a "primary care" role (evaluating and managing patients directly) and in a leadership role (teaching and mentoring others and changing systems of care)." [66] Foundational to NICHE is the Geriatric Resource Nurse Model (GRN) which is an educational intervention model that prepares staff nurses as the clinical resource person on geriatric issues to other nurses on their unit. The GRN model provides staff nurses, via education and modeling by a NICHE coordinator, with specific content for improved knowledge of care management for geriatric syndromes. Clinical protocols and organizational strategies provide necessary tools to apply evidence-based practice. For example, in one NICHE orthopedic unit, GRNs received intensive education on the prevention and detection of delirium in a unit where the primary diagnoses were joint replacement and hip fracture repair. Utilizing a combination of standardized assessment of cognition and focused interventions to prevent post-op delirium, the unit realized a significant reduction in the incidence of delirium. Other systemic interventions utilized by the GRNs include a revised nursing database and delirium-specific order sets [67]. An evaluation of responses of 9,802 direct-care registered nurses from 75 acute care hospitals participating in NICHE found that a positive geriatric nurse practice environment was associated with positive geriatric care delivery. The independent contribution of all three aspects of the geriatric nurse practice environment (resource availability, institutional values, and capacity for collaboration) influences care delivery for hospitalized older adult patients. The study findings demonstrate that a nurse practice environment that provides adequate geriatric-specific resources (continuing education, education, specialty services), promotes interdisciplinary collaboration, and fosters patient, family, and nurse involvement in treatment-related decision-making is associated with quality geriatric care [64]. In single site studies, NICHE hospitals demonstrate improved clinical outcomes, rate of compliance with geriatric institutional protocols; cost-related outcomes; and nurse knowledge. In a study of eight hospitals, nurses reported higher quality of geriatric care following NICHE implementation [68].

NICHE also promotes a unit-based ACE model. The ACE model within NICHE emphasizes: (1) implementation of nurse-driven protocols, (2) geriatric training of all nursing staff, and (3) utilization of geriatric-specific units within a health system's overall geriatric care programming. Similar to other ACE studies, a NICHE-ACE unit in which the majority of the staff nurses were nationally certified in geriatric nursing reported lower fall and pressure ulcer rates, and lower length of stay when compared to overall hospital [69].

Since NICHE is a system-level approach it provides a structure for nurses to collaborate with other disciplines and to actively participate or coordinate other geriatric care models. For example, in hospitals with a geriatric department or consultation service, GRNs screen for appropriate referrals to these services and can effectively implement geriatric service recommendations with support from the NICHE coordinator. The models enhance NICHE program effectiveness by expanding the scope of geriatric programming within a health system.

The Hospital Elder Life Program

The Hospital Elder Life Program (HELP; http://elderlife. med.yale.edu/public/public-main.php) is a program designed to implement protocols that target six delirium risk factors: mental orientation, therapeutic activities, early mobilization, vision and hearing adaptations, hydration and feeding assistance, and sleep enhancement. These protocols were tested in several well-designed clinical trials and demonstrated significant reduction in the incidence of new delirium. Further, among those who did develop delirium, these protocols are associated with a significant reduction of total number of episodes and days with delirium, functional decline, costs of hospital services, and reduction in use of long-term nursing home services [70, 71].

HELP employs geriatric specialists of various disciplines (geriatrician, geriatric nurse specialist, recreation therapy, and physical therapy) working together as an interdisciplinary team with trained volunteers. The program is coordinated by Elder Life Specialists, typically an Elder Life Nurse Specialist who has advanced geriatric nursing education and is responsible for implementing nursing-related assessments and tracking of delirium risk factor protocol adherence. The latter depends on the involvement of well-trained and supervised volunteers in patient-care interventions [72]. The research-tested protocol was made available to hospitals in 2000. Implementation in many hospitals has been adapted based on hospital resources. This has led to wide variations in adherence to the intervention protocol. Although higher levels of adherence have been associated with lower rates of delirium, these adapted protocols continue to provide positive results [73].

Transitional Care Models

An American Geriatric Society Position Statement defines transitional care as a set of actions designed to ensure the coordination and continuity of health care as patients transfer between different locations or different levels of care within the same location [74]. Older adult patients with complex medical and social needs and their caregivers require assistance to effectively navigate the health-care system, including recovery from surgery and return to pre-morbid health and living arrangements. Two models have emerged that have demonstrated improved outcomes for older adults hospitalized for both medical and surgical interventions.

APN transitional care model utilizes advanced practice nurses (APNs) whose primary responsibility is to optimize the health of high-risk, cognitively intact older adults with a variety of medical and surgical conditions during hospitalization and for designing and overseeing the plan for follow-up care following discharge [75]. The APN work collaboratively with the older adult, family caregiver, physician, and other health team members and are guided by evidence-based protocols. The same nurse implements this plan after discharge by providing traditional home-care services and by phone availability 7 days a week. Three federally funded, randomized, controlled trials consistently demonstrated that this model of care improves older adults' satisfaction, reduces rehospitalizations, and decreases health-care costs [76–78].

Care transitions coaching or *care transitions intervention* (see http://www.caretransitions.org/index.asp) employs a nurse or "transitions coach" to encourage older patients and their family caregivers to assume more active roles during care transitions by facilitating self-management and direct communication between the patient/caregiver and primary care provider. The four content areas or "pillars" of the patient/caregiver intervention are as follows: (1) medication self-management, (2) a patient-centered record, (3) primary care and specialist follow-up, and (4) knowledge of "red flags" warning symptom or sign indicative of a worsening condition [79]. The Personal Health Record includes data elements essential to promote productive patient–provider encounters across settings such as an active health problem list; medications and allergies; a list of warning symptoms or signs that correspond to the patient's chronic illnesses; a checklist of activities that need to take place before and following discharge. This record is maintained by the patient and caregiver with assistance from the transition coach. The 4-week intervention begins in the hospital and continues through home visits and/or phone follow-up after discharge.

Several studies, including a randomized, controlled trial, found that patients who received this intervention had lower all-cause rehospitalization rates 30 and 90 days after discharge compared with control patients. Intervention patients also had lower rehospitalization rates for the same condition that they were admitted for in the index hospitalization at 90 and at 180 days than controls. Mean hospital costs were approximately $500 less for patients in the intervention group compared with controls [80].

New Specialty Models

In some hospitals, multiple geriatric models are employed. For example, a hospital may begin with NICHE. The NICHE coordinator, a geriatric nurse specialist, will then become an Elder Life Specialist to implement HELP hospital wide or within a discrete ACE unit. Often the core geriatric interdisciplinary team of any geriatric program screens patients for other related services such as palliative care, rehabilitative services, or pain management programs. Some have developed dual-function units such as merging an ACE unit with a palliative care unit [66]. Others have developed programs that merge geriatrics with other specialties. Examples include hip fracture, trauma, and oncology.

The American Academy of Orthopedic Surgeons recommends coordination of care and communication by providers as important aspects of quality care for hip fracture patients [81]. In response, several hospital programs that incorporate geriatric co-management of hip fracture patients have been developed. The expectation is that involvement of geriatricians in care management will avoid iatrogenic problems. For example, one program focuses on minimizing time to surgery and employment of standardized orders and protocols [82]. These programs have been shown to reduce delirium by over one-third, reduce severe delirium by over one-half, decrease predicted length of stay, readmission rates, complication rates, and mortality [83]. Others have developed a geriatric trauma team that include a geriatrician and geriatric advanced practice nurse who evaluate older trauma patients and share recommendations in weekly multidisciplinary rounds and performance improvement meetings of the trauma service. Most (91%) geriatric recommendations were followed and included: advanced care planning, disposition decisions to promote function, decreased inappropriate medications, and pain management [84].

Similarly, oncology programs have either developed geriatric – oncology consultation team or have developed geriatric – oncology units, some of which are part of an existing ACE unit [85, 86]. These programs report that older oncology patients have more complex medical and social needs than adult oncology patients and thus require input from both perspectives [87].

Conclusion

Although these models use different strategies, all share common goals of treatment. Each hospital or health system chooses a model based on the unique needs of that hospital's patient population, the resources available (geriatric specialists, bed capacity to support separate unit, volunteers, etc.) and especially senior administrator's commitment to geriatric programming. Since there is no direct reimbursement for many components of these models (interdisciplinary rounds, geriatric nurse specialist, volunteers, etc.) administrators seek external (grants, donor gifts) and internal funding (hospital foundation grants). They are motivated by the model's alignment to the hospitals strategic plan (e.g., excellence in senior care), the institution's mission, patient/family satisfaction, relationship with the community, and costs savings (i.e., reduction of complications). All of the models have demonstrated positive outcomes and each have been implemented in at least 50 hospitals; however, this still only represents a small proportion of American hospitals. Each model was originally developed with government and/or foundation support. Future survival of these models may depend on advancing the unique contributions of each within an integrated model that will enhance the hospital experience of the older patient.

Another problem influencing geriatric model implementation is availability of geriatric clinicians. Since significant geriatric medicine input is needed for many of these models, they generally are limited to academic medical centers, which only represent a small proportion of US hospitals. All of these models require providers with knowledge of core concepts in geriatrics; however, there is a significant shortage of fellowship-trained geriatricians, geriatric psychiatrists, master's prepared geriatric nurse specialists, as well as other disciplines [88]. In addition to efforts to increase the training of geriatric specialists, several initiatives are underway that involve specialty organizations, medical schools [89], and resident training programs [90, 91] to integrate principles of geriatric care into curriculums and practice. As more geriatrics is being integrated into undergraduate medical training and surgical resident training, knowledge of geriatric care principles and collaboration with geriatric models will enhance outcomes of the older surgical patients. The Council of the Section for Surgical and Related Medical Specialties in the American Geriatrics Society program provides the Geriatrics Syllabus for Specialists; a useful guide (lectures, PowerPoint presentations, etc.) geared toward providing vital information for surgeons caring for older patients as well as faculty leadership training to promote geriatric training and research within their disciplines. The initiative also enables surgical professional certifying bodies and societies to build the capacity of their members to provide better care of older adults [92].

Financial and administrative barriers deter the implementation of geriatric models. Medicare payment system focuses on provider-specific reimbursement and thus limits payment for organizational redesign, multidisciplinary teams or nurse-coordinators. The new CMS financial incentives that will not reimburse for nosocomial "never" events such as pressure ulcers, catheter-associated infections, and fall-related injury, may eventually encourage the use of these models [15]. A recent IOM report recommended that "payers should promote and reward the dissemination of those models of care for older adults that have been shown to be effective and efficient." [87] Incentives suggested included elimination of Medicare's co-payment disparity for mental health and enhanced payments for services under these models.

Finally, most of the research documenting complications of the older patient are based on studies combining both medical and surgical patients, thus future research should address the risk factors of these complications specific to surgical patients. Further, with the exception of hip fracture and cardiac surgery, additional studies should also identify complications within specific types of surgical procedures. This may provide important data to tailor models to specific surgical populations.

References

1. Rubenstein LZ (2008) Geriatric assessment programs. In: Capezuti EA, Siegler E, Mezey M (eds) The encyclopedia of elder care, 2nd edn. Springer, New York, NY, pp 346–349
2. Older patients: a growing concern for surgeons and related specialists, American Geriatrics Society – Geriatrics for Specialists. See http://www.americangeriatrics.org/specialists/involved.shtml. Assessed 3 February 2009
3. Khuri SF, Henderson WG, DePalma RG et al (2005) Determinants of long-term survival after major surgery and the adverse effect of postoperative complications. Ann Surg 242(3):326–341
4. Fortinsky RH, Covinsky KE, Palmer RM, Landefeld CS (1999) Effects of functional status changes before and during hospitalization on nursing home admission of older adults. J Gerontol A Biol Sci Med Sci 54(10):M521–M526
5. Gill TM, Williams CS, Tinetti ME (1999) The combined effects of baseline vulnerability and acute hospital events on the development of functional dependence among community-living older persons. J Gerontol A Biol Sci Med Sci 54(7):M377–M383
6. Gill TM, Williams CS, Richardson ED, Tinetti ME (1996) Impairments in physical performance and cognitive status as predisposing factors for functional dependence among nondisabled older persons. J Gerontol A Biol Sci Med Sci 51(6):M283–M288
7. Chodosh J, Sultzer DL, Lee ML et al (2007) Memory impairment among primary care veterans. Aging Ment Health 11(4):444–450
8. Naylor MD, Hirschman KB, Bowles KH, Bixby MB, Konick-McMahan J, Stephens C (2007) Care coordination for cognitively impaired older adults and their caregivers. Home Health Care Serv Q 26(4):57–78
9. Ahmed N, Mandel R, Fain MJ (2007) Frailty: an emerging geriatric syndrome. Am J Med 120(9):748–753
10. Walston J, Fried LP (1999) Frailty and the older man. Med Clin North Am 83:1173–1194
11. Fried LP, Tangen CM, Walston J et al (2001) Frailty in older adults: evidence for a phenotype. J Gerontol 56A:M146–M156
12. Maslow K (2006) How many people with dementia are hospitalized? In: Silverstein N, Maslow K (eds) Improving hospital care for persons with dementia. Springer, New York, NY, pp 3–22
13. Leslie DL, Marcantonio ER, Zhang Y, Leo-Summers L, Inouye SK (2008) One-year health care costs associated with delirium in the elderly population. Arch Intern Med 168(1):27–32
14. Inouye SK, Studenski S, Tinetti ME, Kuchel GA (2007) Geriatric syndromes: clinical, research, and policy implications of a core geriatric concept. J Am Geriatr Soc 55(5):780–791

15. Centers for Medicare & Medicaid Services (2007) Medicare program: changes to the hospital Inpatient Prospective Payment Systems and fiscal year 2008 rates. Fed Regist 72(162):47129–48175
16. Pronovost PJ, Goeschel CA, Wachter R (2008) The wisdom and justice of not paying for "preventable complications". JAMA 299(18):2197–2199
17. Wald HL, Kramer AM (2007) Nonpayment for harms resulting from medical care: catheter-associated urinary tract infections. JAMA 298(23):2782–2784
18. Flood KL, Rohlfing A, Le CV, Carr DB, Rich MW (2007) Geriatric syndromes in elderly patients admitted to an inpatient cardiology ward. J Hosp Med 2(6):394–400
19. McCusker J, Kakuma R, Abrahamowicz M (2002) Predictors of functional decline in hospitalized elderly patients: a systematic review. J Gerontol A Biol Sci Med Sci 57(9):M569–M771
20. Sager MA, Franke T, Inouye SK, Landefeld CS, Morgan TM, Rudberg MA et al (1996) Functional outcomes of acute medical illness and hospitalization in older persons. Arch Intern Med 156(6):645–652
21. Covinsky KE, Justice AC, Rosenthal GE, Palmer RM, Landefeld CS (1997) Measuring prognosis and case mix in hospitalized elders. The importance of functional status. J Gen Intern Med 12:203–208
22. Thomas DR (2002) Focus on functional decline in hospitalized older adults. J Gerontol A Biol Sci Med Sci 57(9):M567–M568
23. Walter LC, Brand RJ, Counsell SR et al (2001) Development and validation of a prognostic index for 1-year mortality in older adults after hospitalization. JAMA 285(23):2987–2994
24. Inouye SK, Wagner DR, Acampora D, Horwitz RI, Cooney LM, Tinetti ME (1993) A controlled trial of a nursing-centered intervention in hospitalized elderly patients: The Yale Geriatric Care Program. J Am Geriatr Soc 41:1353–1360
25. Mahoney JE, Sager MA, Jalaluddin M (1998) Use of an ambulation assistive device predicts functional decline associated with hospitalization. J Gerontol A Biol Sci Med Sci 54(2):M83–M88
26. Fox KM, Reuland M, Hawkes WG et al (1998) Accuracy of medical records in hip fracture. J Am Geriatr Soc 46(6):745–750
27. Coleman EA, Kramer AM, Kowalsky JC et al (2000) A comparison of functional outcomes after hip fracture in group/staff HMOs and fee-for-service systems. Eff Clin Pract 3(5):229–239
28. Givens JL, Sanft TB, Marcantonio ER (2008) Functional recovery after hip fracture: the combined effects of depressive symptoms, cognitive impairment, and delirium. J Am Geriatr Soc 56(6):1075–1079
29. Rubenstein LZ (2006) Falls in older people: epidemiology, risk factors and strategies for prevention. Age Ageing 35(Suppl 2):ii37–ii41
30. Rubenstein LZ, Josephson KR (2002) The epidemiology of falls and syncope. Clin Geriatr Med 18(2):141–158
31. Magaziner J, Hawkes W, Hebel JR et al (2000) Recovery from hip fracture in eight areas of function. J Gerontol A Biol Sci Med Sci 55(9):M498–M507
32. Sullivan DH, Bopp MM, Roberson PK (2002) Protein-energy undernutrition and life-threatening complications among the hospitalized elderly. J Gen Intern Med 17(12):923–932
33. Nutrition Screening Initiative. Nutrition state of principle, 2002. http://www.hospitalmedicine.org/geriresource/toolbox/determine.htm. Accessed 3 February 2009
34. Lyder CH (2003) Pressure ulcer prevention and management. JAMA 289(2):223–226
35. Whittington K, Patrick M, Roberts JL (2000) A national study of pressure ulcer prevalence and incidence in acute care hospitals. J Wound Ostomy Continence Nurs 27(4):209–215
36. Preston LCH, Grady JN J et al (2001) Quality of care for hospitalized medicare patients at risk for pressure ulcers. Arch Intern Med 161(12):1549–1554

37. Emori TG, Banerjee SN, Culver DH et al (1991) Nosocomial infections in elderly persons in the United States, 1986–1990: National Nosocomial Infections Surveillance System. Am J Med 91(3B):289S–293S

38. Kunin CM (2006) Urinary-catheter-associated infections in the elderly. Int J Antimicrob Agents 28(Suppl 1):S78–S81

39. Tambyah PA, Maki DG (2000) Catheter-associated urinary tract infection is rarely symptomatic: a prospective study of 1,497 catheterized patients. Arch Intern Med 160:678–682

40. Wald HL, Ma A, Bratzler DW, Kramer AM (2008) Indwelling urinary catheter use in the postoperative period: analysis of the national surgical infection prevention project data. Arch Surg 143(6):551–557

41. Wald HL, Epstein AM, Radcliff TA, Kramer AM (2008) Extended use of urinary catheters in older surgical patients: a patient safety problem? Infect Control Hosp Epidemiol 29(2):116–124

42. Saint S, Lipsky B, Goold S (2002) Urinary catheters: a one-point restraint? Ann Intern Med 137(2):125–127

43. Dubois MJ, Bergeron N, Dumont M et al (2001) Delirium in an intensive care unit. A study of risk factors. Intensive Care Med 27:1297–1304

44. Silverstein JH, Timberger M, Reich DL, Uysal S (2007) Central nervous system dysfunction after noncardiac surgery and anesthesia in the elderly. Anesthesiology 106(3):622–628

45. Inouye SK (2000) Prevention of delirium in hospitalized older patients: risk factors and targeted intervention strategies. Ann Med 32(4):257–263

46. Inouye SK, Schlesinger MJ, Lydon TJ (1999) Delirium: a symptom of how hospital care is failing older persons and a window to improve quality of hospital care. Am J Med 106(5):565–573

47. Inouye SK, Foreman MD, Mion LC, Katz KH, Cooney LM Jr (2001) Nurses' recognition of delirium and its symptoms: comparison of nurse and researcher ratings. Arch Intern Med 161(20):2467–2473

48. Inouye SK, Rushing JT, Foreman MD, Palmer RM, Pompei P (1998) Does delirium contribute to poor hospital outcomes? A three-site epidemiologic study. J Gen Intern Med 13(4):234–242

49. Arora VM, McGory ML, Fung CH (2007) Quality indicators for hospitalization and surgery in vulnerable elders. J Am Geriatr Soc 55(Suppl 2):S347–S358

50. Somogyi-Zalud E, Zhong Z, Hamel MB, Lynn J (2002) The use of life-sustaining treatments in hospitalized persons aged 80 and older. J Am Geriatr Soc 50(5):930–934

51. Coleman EA, Min SJ, Chomiak A, Kramer AM (2004) Posthospital care transitions: patterns, complications, and risk identification. Health Serv Res 39(5):1449–1465

52. Foust JB, Naylor MD, Boling PA, Cappuzzo KA (2005) Opportunities for improving post-hospital home medication management among older adults. Home Health Care Serv Q 24(1–2):101–122

53. Coleman EA, Smith JD, Raha D, Min SJ (2005) Posthospital medication discrepancies: prevalence and contributing factors. Arch Intern Med 165(16):1842–1847

54. Forster AJ, Murff HJ, Peterson JF, Gandhi TK, Bates DW (2003) The incidence and severity of adverse events affecting patients after discharge from the hospital. Ann Intern Med 138:161–167

55. Moore C, McGinn T, Halm E (2007) Tying up loose ends: discharging patients with unresolved medical issues. Arch Intern Med 167(12):1305–1311

56. Flacker J, Park W, Sims A (2007) Hospital discharge information and older patients: do they get what they need? J Hosp Med 2(5):291–296

57. Bowles KH, Naylor MD, Foust JB (2002) Patient characteristics at hospital discharge and a comparison of home care referral decisions. J Am Geriatr Soc 50(2):336–342

58. Agostini J, Baker D, Inouye S, Bogardus S (2001) Chapter 29: Multidisciplinary geriatric consultation services. Making health

care safer: a critical analysis of patient safety practices. AHRQ Publication No. 01-E058

59. Allen CM, Becker PM, McVey LJ, Saltz C, Feussner JR, Cohen HJ (1986) A randomized, controlled clinical trial of a geriatric consultation team. Compliance with recommendations. JAMA 255:2617–2621

60. Phibbs CS, Holty JE, Goldstein MK et al (2006) The effect of geriatrics evaluation and management on nursing home use and health care costs: results from a randomized trial. Med Care 44(1):91–95

61. Palmer RM, Landefeld CS, Kresevic DM, Kowal J (1994) A medical unit for the acute care of the elderly. J Am Geriatr Soc 42(5):54–55

62. Landefeld CS, Palmer RM, Kresevic DM, Fortinsky RH, Kowal J (1995) A randomized trial of care in a hospital medical unit especially designed to improve the functional outcomes of acutely ill older patients. N Engl J Med 332(20):1338–1344

63. Counsell SR, Holder CM, Liebenauer LL et al (2000) Effects of a multicomponent intervention on functional outcomes and processes of care in hospitalized older patients: a randomized controlled trial of acute care of elders (ACE) in a community hospital. J Am Geriatr Soc 48(12):1572–1581

64. Siu AL, Spragens LH, Inouye SK, Morrison RS, Leff B (2009) The ironic business case for chronic care in the acute care setting. Health Affairs 28(1):113–125

65. Boltz M, Capezuti E, Bowar-Ferres S et al (2008) Hospital nurses' perception of the geriatric nurse practice environment. J Nurs Scholarsh 40(3):282–289

66. Fletcher K, Hawkes P, Williams-Rosenthal S, Mariscal CS, Cox BA (2007) Using nurse practitioners to implement best practice care for the elderly during hospitalization: The NICHE journey at the University of Virginia medical center. Crit Care Nurs Clin North Am 19(3):321–337

67. Guthrie PF, Schumacher S, Edinger G (2006) A NICHE delirium prevention project for hospitalized elders. In: Silverstein N, Maslow K (eds) Improving hospital care for persons with dementia. Springer, New York, NY, pp 139–157

68. Boltz M, Capezuti E, Bowar-Ferres S et al (2008) Changes in the Geriatric Care Environment Associated with NICHE (Nurses Improving Care for HealthSystem Elders). Geriatr Nurs 29(3):176–185

69. LaReau R, Raphelson M (2005) The treatment of the hospitalized elderly patient in a specialized acute care of the elderly unit: A Southwest Michigan perspective. Southwest Mich Med J 2(3):21–27

70. Inouye SK, Bogardus ST, Charpentier PA et al (1999) A multicomponent intervention to prevent delirium in hospitalized older patients. N Engl J Med 1340(9):669–676

71. Inouye SK, Baker DI, Fugal P, Bradley EH, for the HELP Dissemination Project (2006) Dissemination of the hospital elder life program: implementation, adaptation, and successes. J Am Geriatr Soc 54(10):1492–1499

72. Bradley EH, Webster TR, Schlesinger M, Baker D, Inouye SK (2006) The roles of senior management in improving hospital experiences for frail older adults. J Healthc Manag 51(5):323–336

73. Inouye SK, Bogardus ST, Williams CS, Leo-Summers L, Agostini JV (2003) The role of adherence on the effectiveness of nonpharmacologic interventions: evidence from the delirium prevention trial. Arch Intern Med 163(8):958–964

74. Coleman EA, Boult C, American Geriatrics Society Health Care Systems Committee (2003) Improving the quality of transitional care for persons with complex care needs. J Am Geriatr Soc 51(4):556–557

75. Naylor M, Keating SA (2008) Transitional care. Am J Nurs 108(9 Suppl):58–63

76. Naylor M, Brooten D, Jones R, Lavizzo-Mourey R, Mezey M, Pauly M (1994) Comprehensive discharge planning for the

hospitalized elderly: a randomized clinical trial. Ann Intern Med 120:999–1006

77. Naylor MD, Brooten D, Campbell R et al (1999) Comprehensive discharge planning and home follow-up of hospitalized elders: a randomized clinical trial. JAMA 281(7):613–620

78. Naylor MD, Brooten DA, Campbell RL et al (2004) Transitional care of older adults hospitalized with heart failure: a randomized, controlled trial. J Am Geriatr Soc 52(5):675–684

79. Coleman EA, Smith JD, Frank JC, Min S, Parry C, Kramer AM (2004) Preparing patients and caregivers to participate in care delivered across settings: the care transitions intervention. J Am Geriatr Soc 52(11):1817–1825

80. Coleman EA, Parry C, Chalmers S, Min SJ (2006) The care transitions intervention: results of a randomized controlled trial. Arch Intern Med 166(17):1822–1828

81. Morris AH, Zuckerman JD, for the AAOS Council of Health Policy and Practice, American Academy of Orthopaedic Surgeons (2002) National Consensus Conference on improving the continuum of care for patients with hip fracture. J Bone Joint Surg Am 84-A(4):670–674

82. Friedman SM, Mendelson DA, Kates SL, McCann RM (2008) Geriatric co-management of proximal femur fractures: total quality management and protocol-driven care result in better outcomes for a frail patient population. J Am Geriatr Soc 56(7): 1349–1356

83. Marcantonio ER, Flacker JM, Wright RJ, Resnick NM (2001) Reducing delirium after hip fracture: a randomized trial. J Am Geriatr Soc 49(5):516–522

84. Fallon WF Jr, Rader E, Zyzanski S et al (2006) Geriatric outcomes are improved by a geriatric trauma consultation service. J Trauma 61(5):1040–1046

85. Flood KL, Carroll MB, Le CV, Ball L, Esker DA, Carr DB (2006) Geriatric syndromes in elderly patients admitted to an oncology-acute care for elders unit. J Clin Oncol 24(15):2298–2303

86. Retornaz F, Seux V, Pauly V, Soubeyrand J (2008) Geriatric assessment and care for older cancer inpatients admitted in acute care for elders unit. Crit Rev Oncol Hematol 68(2):165–171

87. Retornaz F, Seux V, Sourial N, Braud AC, Monette J, Bergman H, Soubeyrand J (2007) Comparison of the health and functional status between older inpatients with and without cancer admitted to a geriatric/internal medicine unit. J Gerontol A Biol Sci Med Sci 62(8):917–922

88. Committee on the Future Health Care Workforce for Older Americans, Institute of Medicine (2008) Retooling for an aging America: building the health care workforce. National Academies Press, Washington, DC

89. Wieland D, Eleazer GP, Bachman DL, Corbin D, Oldendick R, Boland R, Stewart T, Richeson N, Thornhill JT (2008) Does it stick? Effects of an integrated vertical undergraduate aging curriculum on medical and surgical residents. J Am Geriatr Soc 56(1):132–138

90. Burton PJF, Drach GW JR, Lundebjerg EJ, Solomon DH NE (2005) Geriatrics for residents in the surgical and medical specialties: implementation of curricula and training experiences. J Am Geriatr Soc 53(3):511–515

91. Burton PJF, Drach GW JR, Lundebjerg EJ, Solomon DH NE (2005) Geriatrics for residents in the surgical and medical specialties: implementation of curricula and training experiences. J Am Geriatr Soc 53(3):511–515

92. Council of the Section for Surgical and Related Medical Specialties in the American Geriatrics Society Program. http://www.american-geriatrics.org/specialists/default.shtml. Accessed 3 February 2009

Chapter 22
Preoperative Evaluation of the Older Surgical Patient

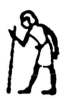

Lisa M. Walke and Ronnie A. Rosenthal

Simplified Assessment	Questions	Tests
Identify comorbidities	• Thorough history and review of systems	• Thorough physical examination
Medications	• Name all the prescription, herbal, and over-the-counter pills you take on a regular or as-needed basis	• Check medication lists or bottles
Function	• Can you walk up a flight of stairs carrying a bag of groceries?	• Timed Get Up and Go
Nutrition	• Have you lost ≥10 pounds in the last 6 months without trying to do so?	• Serum albumin • BMI
Cognition	• How is your memory? • Do you drink alcohol occasionally, with meals, or before going to bed? • In the past month, have you been sad, blue, down in the dumps or depressed? • In the past month, have you been a lot less interested in most things or unable to enjoy the things you used to enjoy?	• Three item recall • Clock drawing task • Geriatric depression scale

Introduction

Aging Epidemiology

Beginning in 2012, nearly 10,000 Americans will reach age 65, each day [1]. The number of older Americans is expected to increase from 35 million (12.4% of the total population) in 2000 to 71 million (19.6% of the total population) in 2030 [2]. As demonstrated in Fig. 22.1 [3], the proportion of adults who are ≥65 years of age is increasing, while the proportion of persons < age 55 is decreasing. In fact, individuals over age 85, dubbed the "oldest old," are the most rapidly growing segment of the population, and their number is expected to increase fivefold to almost 19 million by the year 2050 [2].

The aging of the American population has created the need to provide surgical care to an ever-increasing number of older persons. At present, 35% of all surgical procedures performed in the USA are on persons 65 years of age or older; the rate of surgical procedures performed per 10,000 is 4.4 in older patients compared with 1.5 in younger adults [4]. Approximately half of individuals over age 65 will have at least one major surgical procedure in the remainder of their lifetime [4]. Overall, workload varies considerably by specialty; persons of age 65 years and older represent 60% of the cases in general surgery and almost 90% of the cases in ophthalmology [5].

Over the past several decades, advances in surgical and anesthetic techniques have led to an overall decline in operative mortality in older patients [6]. The "risk" of surgery therefore has become somewhat less of a concern, whereas the need and ability to provide maximal disease management has increased. While age cannot be completely ignored, functional status and/or comorbid conditions usually contribute more to operative outcomes than age alone. However, there are physiological changes that occur with aging that warrant recognition in order to maximize perioperative outcomes. As the number of older surgical candidates continues to grow, it will become increasingly important for all surgeons to understand the special issues involved in the selection and evaluation of older patients for surgical care.

L.M. Walke (✉)
Department of Medicine, Yale University School of Medicine,
New Haven, CT, USA
and
Geriatrics Consult Service, Geriatrics & Extended Care Service,
VA Connecticut Healthcare System, New Haven, CT, USA
e-mail: lisa.walke@yale.edu

R.A. Rosenthal et al. (eds.), *Principles and Practice of Geriatric Surgery*,
DOI 10.1007/978-1-4419-6999-6_22, © Springer Science+Business Media, LLC 2011

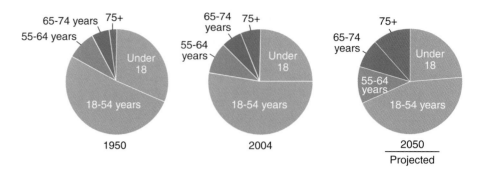

Figure 22.1 Population by age. Percent of population in five age groups: United States, 1950, 2004, and 2050 (from Centers for Disease Control and Prevention, National Center for Health Statistics, Health, United States, 2005).

Pattern of Surgical Disease in the Elderly

Before discussing the process of selecting and evaluating geriatric patients, it is important to note that the pattern of surgical disease in older patients is not always superimposable on the pattern seen in younger patients. The indication for surgery therefore may not be apparent until a complication has occurred. The absence of the classic signs and symptoms often leads to delays in treatment and errors in diagnosis. As a result, emergency surgical intervention is frequently necessary.

For example, older adults are twice as likely (33 vs. 16%) to have a right-sided colon cancer compared with younger adults [7]. As a result of this anatomical difference older adults may present more often with symptoms that are not initially associated with colorectal cancer, such as syncope and fatigue. Older adults with left-sided colon cancer often delay seeking medical care because they do not consider symptoms such as constipation to be abnormal. Thus, it is not surprising that up to 40% of older patients with colorectal cancer present for surgical intervention secondary to obstruction and/or perforation [7]. Further evidence of altered symptomatology in older persons is found in the pattern of presentation of biliary tract disease. The classic pattern of worsening biliary symptoms preceding the development of a complication is often absent in older adults. Consequently, up to two-thirds of the cholecystecomies in patients over the age of 65 are performed urgently or emergently compared with less than one-fifth in younger patients [8].

The high rate of emergency surgery in older adults is important because emergency surgery is associated with at least a threefold increase in mortality and morbidity. In one series of patients over the age of 70 years, emergency operations carried a mortality rate ten times greater than that for elective procedures [9]. Emergency surgery is also associated with a higher rate of long-term hospital stay (>30 days), more need for postoperative intensive care, larger decline in functional status, and increased need for postoperative nursing home placement [10].

Eliciting Patients' Preferences

Before the decision is made to proceed with elective surgery, a thorough discussion of the patient's goals of care and preferences is warranted. Items for consideration include the following:

- How clear is the indication for surgery, including the likelihood of progression of the disease?
- What is the likelihood of achieving equal or improved functional status?
- What degree of symptom improvement can be expected after the procedure?
- What quality of life can be expected with or without the surgery?
- Does the patient, and his or her family, understand the problem and the proposed solution?
- What is the risk of a negative outcome as determined by the nature of the procedure and the presence of comorbid conditions?

Fried et al. have shown that for older persons, the burden of treatment, the possible treatment outcomes (desirable vs. undesirable), and the likelihood of a particular outcome each influence treatment preferences [11]. Given various hypothetical situations, the majority of older patients (>70%) stated they would not want even a low-burden treatment if severe functional impairment or cognitive impairment was the expected outcome. As the likelihood of an adverse outcome increased, the number of patients who stated they would want treatment decreased. Thus, advance care planning that includes elucidation of patients' treatment preferences and designation of surrogate decision makers is one of the most important components of preoperative assessment for older surgical patients.

Objectives of Preoperative Assessment

Once these issues is addressed; the main thrust of the preoperative evaluation is to identify, and optimize, any coexisting disease processes or decline in physiologic reserve. With this information, an accurate risk/benefit determination can be made for each surgical intervention in each elderly patient. Although we refer to risk primarily as the chance of postoperative mortality and morbidity, risk in the elderly should also be assessed in terms of restoration of preoperative functional status and quality of life. For older patients, maintenance of independence, quality of life, and symptom resolution may be as important as, if not more so, than survival.

Efforts are currently underway to develop process-based quality indicators to improve perioperative care and subsequent outcomes for older patients undergoing ambulatory, major elective, or nonelective inpatient surgery [12]. Additional work is needed both to determine the feasibility of implementing quality indicators into routine care and to demonstrate improved patient outcomes secondary to their use.

General Evaluation

Affect of Age on Perioperative Outcomes

The general approach to the preoperative assessment is directed toward identifying those factors that place the patient at increased risk for postoperative complications or death. Although some of these factors are related to the surgical disease itself and to the type of operation required, the most important factors in the determination of risk are related to the overall health, function level, cognitive abilities, and nutritional status of the patient.

Many studies have demonstrated comparable outcomes among older and younger adult surgical patients. A retrospective analysis of cardiac surgery among octogenarians in Germany demonstrated that morality was associated with comorbid conditions (e.g., chronic obstructive pulmonary disease or heart failure), nonelective surgery, and male gender, but not with age [13]. Follow-up with these patients 3–5 years after surgery revealed that approximately 85% were clinically better than they were prior to surgery. Another German study examined outcomes for colorectal cancer patients who underwent surgery. While mortality rates were higher for patients ≥80 years than for patients <80 years (8.0 vs. 2.6%), specific morbidity related to the operation was not significantly different (20.5 vs. 19.9%) [14].

Yet, some evidence suggests that even after adjusting for comorbid conditions, age itself is associated with higher risk for adverse outcomes among patients undergoing noncardiac surgery [15, 16]. The reason for this increased risk is presently unclear. It is possible that confounders associated with aging exist but are unrecognized, and thus unadjusted for, in multivariate analyses. If true, the increased risk observed with increasing age would in fact be due to the confounders, not age itself. Nonetheless, many older adults tolerate surgery if it is well conducted and free of complications. However,

if complications arise, the additional stress associated with the complications exceeds the physiological reserves of many older adults.

Comorbidity

ASK the question	Do a thorough history including review of systems 2
DO the test	Do a complete physical exam

Over 80% of Americans aged ≥65 have at least one chronic condition and 50% have at least two [17]. The prevalence of comorbid diseases clearly rises with increasing age. The age-related increase in cardiac, pulmonary, renal, and hepatic comorbid conditions in a cohort of colon cancer patients over age 50 has previously been demonstrated [18]. The prevalence rates for some common chronic conditions experienced by older adults are depicted in Fig. 22.2 [1].

In a larger, more detailed review of comorbidity in elderly patients with colon cancer, Yancik et al. explored the increase in the number of additional conditions with age [19]. By age 75, patients with colon cancer had a mean of five disorders in addition to the primary cancer. For all adults, the influence of comorbid conditions on activity level increases substantially with age as demonstrated in Fig. 22.3 [3]. In addition, comorbid conditions more frequently contribute to the cancelation of surgery after hospital admission in older adults compared with younger adults [4].

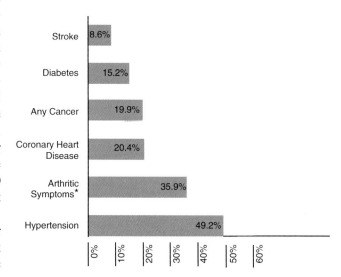

Figure 22.2 Prevalence of selected chronic conditions among adults age 65 and over, 2000–2001. *Asterisk* indicates a respondent was considered to have "arthritic symptoms" if s/he answered "yes" to the following questions: "During the past 12 months, have you had pain, aching, stiffness, or swelling in or around a joint?" and "Were these symptoms present on most days for at least one month?" (from Centers for Disease Control and Prevention, National Center for Health Statistics, National Health Interview Survey, 2000–2001).

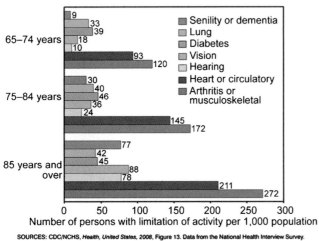

Activity limitation among older adults due to chronic conditions, 2005–2006

SOURCES: CDC/NCHS, *Health, United States, 2008*, Figure 13. Data from the National Health Interview Survey.

Figure 22.3 Limitation of activity caused by selected chronic health conditions among older adults, by age: United States, 2005–2006 (from [13]).

As the number of associated illnesses increases, so does the rate of perioperative complications. In a study on the effect of increasing comorbidity on outcome, Tiret and colleagues demonstrated a strong correlation between the number of conditions and the rate of perioperative complications. This effect was seen in all age groups but was most pronounced in the youngest and oldest patients [20]. Only a minimal increase in mortality and morbidity was seen in old patients who lacked coexisting disease. Such minimal increases were insignificant when compared with the three-fold increase associated with as few as two additional comorbidities. Other studies of outcome for both surgical and medical treatment demonstrate a similar correlation between comorbidity and poor treatment outcome [19, 21].

As is true for surgical disease itself, older adults often do not present with the "classical" signs and symptoms typically attributed to comorbid conditions. The search for comorbid conditions must therefore be diligent. In the Framingham heart study for example, myocardial infarction was unrecognized or silent in more than 40% of persons of age 75–84 compared with fewer than 20% of those of age 45–54 [22]. Thyroid dysfunction (either hyper or hypo), cognitive impairment, and malnutrition are among the many other coexisting disorders that may not be recognized during the initial history and physical examination. For example, one study of hospitalized medical patients over age of 75 years revealed that 63% of patients meeting criteria for cognitive impairment were not identified as impaired on their discharge summary [23]. Earlier studies demonstrate that 46% of moderate to severe nutritional deficits identified among patients during hospital admission had not been recognized by the primary caregiver in the community (Fig. 22.4) [24].

Frailty is another comorbid condition that is frequently not recognized by providers. But recent evidence suggests that frailty may be an important predictor of postoperative mortality in one study, patients who had four of the following

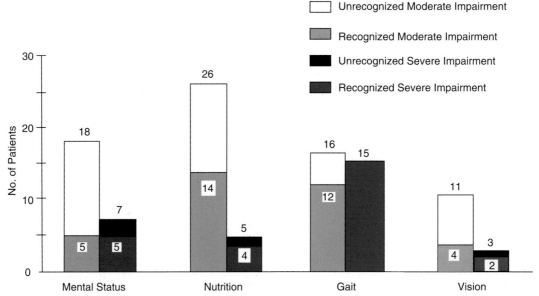

Prevalence and recognition by primary caregivers of functional impairment in 79 medical inpatients. Number at top of each bar represents total number of patients impaired in that functional area.

Figure 22.4 Patients found to have nutritional and mental status deficits during formal geriatric assessment at admission to the hospital compared to those identified by the primary caregiver in the community. *Lighter bars* indicate the results of formal assessment. It is seen that most of the nutritional deficits and a large percentage of mental status deficits were not recognized prior to admission to the hospital, indicating that these deficits are subtle and may not be appreciated without purposeful attempts to identify them (from Pinholt [24] with permission, Copyright © 1987 American Medical Association. All rights reserved).

TABLE 22.1 Herbal medicines and recommendations for discontinuation of use before surgery

Herb: common name(s)	Uses	Perioperative concerns	Preoperative discontinuation
Echinacea: purple coneflower root	Prophylaxis, treatment of viral, bacterial, fungal infections	Decreased effectiveness of immunosuppressants	No data
Ephedra: ma huang	Weight loss, increase energy	Tachycardia, hypertension	At least 24 h before surgery
Garlic: ajo	Lowers blood pressure, serum lipid and cholesterol level	May potentially increase risk of bleeding	At least 7 days before surgery
Ginkgo: duck foot tree, maidenhair tree, silver apricot	Cognitive disorders	Potential to increase risk of bleeding	At least 36 h before surgery
Ginseng: American ginseng, Asian ginseng, Chinese ginseng, Korean ginseng	Prevention of stress, restore homeostasis	Potential to increase risk of bleeding, hypoglycemia	At least 7 days before surgery
Kava: awa, intoxicating pepper, kawa	Anxiolytic sedative	Potential to increase sedative effect of anesthetics	At least 24 h before surgery
St. John's wort: amber, goat weed, hardhay, Hypericum, klamatheweed	Depression	Induction of cytochrome P450 enzymes, decreased serum digoxin levels	At least 5 days before surgery
Valerian: all heal, garden heliotrope, vandal root	Insomnia	Potential to increase sedative effect of anesthetics	No data

Source: Reprinted with permission from Ang-Lee et al. [27]. Copyright © 2001 American Medical Association. All rights reserved

six markers preoperatively had an increased risk of death within 6 months of their operation [25].

Mini_Cog score <4*
Albumin level <3.4 g/dL
≥1 fall within the prior 6 months
Hematocrit <35%
Katz disability score <6*
Charlson comorbidity score ≥3*

---

*For definition see below

Extensive testing for comorbidity in every organ system is neither cost-effective nor necessary for every patient. A thorough history and physical examination provide information that can direct further workup, if necessary. It is important, however, to adjust the history and physical examination to look for risk factors and signs and symptoms of the more common comorbid disorders. The addition of simple questions and simple tools for assessing functional, cognitive, and nutritional status significantly enhances understanding the individual elderly patient's true operative risk. When initial evaluation identifies specific disease or risk factors for disease, further workup may be indicated. Evaluation of specific organ systems is described later in the chapter.

Medication Assessment

ASK the question	Can you tell me all the prescription, herbal, and over-the-counter pills you take on a regular or as-needed basis
DO the test	Check medication lists or bottles

The vast majority of medications taken on a daily basis are consumed by adults over the age of 65 years. Thus, a comprehensive medication review is warranted for all older preoperative patients. Patients should specifically be queried regarding the use of herbal medications, given the potential for drug–herbal interaction and the low likelihood of self-report among patients. Education (≥12 years) and annual income (>$20,000) were found to be associated with herbal medication use in the multivariate logistic regression of one study [26]. A list of the most commonly taken herbal medicines, their uses, perioperative concerns, and recommended preoperative discontinuation time is found in Table 22.1 [27].

Geriatrics-Specific Evaluation

Functional Status Evaluation

ASK the question	"Can you carry a bag of groceries up a flight of steps without getting short of breath?"
DO the test	Timed Get Up and Go

Functional status can be measured in many different ways. Regardless of the methods, preoperative functional deficits have been shown to contribute to postoperative immobility, with associated complications such as atelectasis and pneumonia, multisystem deconditioning, increased length of stay, and increased mortality and morbidity. Individuals with poor preoperative function have longer hospitalizations, more surgical complications, and are more likely to die within 30 days of surgery when compared with individuals with good preoperative functional fitness [28]. Deconditioning is an important clinical entity that leads to further functional decline despite improvement in the acute illness [29]. The recovery period from deconditioning can be three or more times as long as the period of immobilization that led to the decline. Methods of measuring functional status are described below.

Measures of Functional Status

American Society of Anesthesiologists Classification

For decades, the American Society of Anesthesiologists (ASA) Physical Status Classification has been one of the most reliable and accurate predictors of surgical mortality. This simple classification ranks patients according to the functional limitations imposed by coexisting disease (see Table 25.4). Despite its subjective nature, ASA classification has repeatedly been shown to accurately predict postoperative outcomes. Curves for mortality versus ASA class in older patients are superimposable on those of younger patients, thus demonstrating that coexisting disease, rather than chronologic age, has the most profound impact on surgical outcome [30]. Even for patients over age 80, ASA classification has been shown to predict postoperative mortality accurately [31].

The value of the ASA classification is further demonstrated by the results of a large, multicenter Department of Veterans Affairs (VA) study begun in 1991, later referred to as the National Surgical Quality Improvement Project (NSQIP), in which surgical patients were assessed prospectively for operative risk. Risk-adjusted models were then created to allow comparison of the quality of surgical care among institutions [32]. Sixty-eight preoperative and intraoperative variables were collected, and nine models for mortality and morbidity (one for each subspecialty and one overall) were created [33, 34]. Serum albumin and ASA class were the top two risk factors for both mortality and morbidity. Disseminated cancer was ranked third for mortality while operation complexity was ranked for morbidity [35]. The ASA functional classification was the second most predictive factor for mortality and the most predictive for morbidity after serum albumin. A discussion of the predictive value of serum albumin is found below under "Nutritional Assessment."

Activities of Daily Living

Activities of daily living (ADLs) are physical tasks performed routinely, namely bathing, dressing, personal grooming, toileting, transferring, walking, and eating [36]. Instrumental activities of daily living (IADLs) are higher order tasks performed regularly such as telephone use, transportation, meal preparation, shopping, housework, medication management, and managing finances. Studies have demonstrated an association between ADLs or IADLs and operative outcomes. For example, the Preoperative Assessment of Cancer in the Elderly (PACE) study conducted

in the UK demonstrated that among older patients electively scheduled for cancer surgery, individuals with IADL dependence (RR 1.43), poor performance status (RR 1.52), and moderate/severe fatigue (RR 1.64) all had higher rates of postoperative complications [37]. Similar findings have also been demonstrated in less specific patient populations [38].

Exercise Capacity (in Metabolic Equivalents)

Exercise tolerance, as an indication of functional reserve, is the single most important predictor of cardiac and pulmonary complications following noncardiac surgery. In a study comparing Dripps Criteria (ASA), Goldman Clinical Criteria, pulmonary function tests, exercise tolerance, and several other variables, Gerson et al. demonstrated that the inability to raise the heart rate to 99 beats/min while doing 2 min of supine bicycle exercise was the most sensitive predictor of postoperative cardiac and pulmonary complications, and death [39, 40].

The physiologic basis for this finding has been further clarified by a study in which older patients performed supine ergometry while connected by mouthpiece to a metabolic cart [41]. The authors identified an anaerobic threshold – defined as the level of oxygen consumption above which circulatory supply could not meet metabolic demand – and correlated this threshold with surgical outcome. For those patients able to reach an anaerobic threshold of 11 ml/kg/min or more, the mortality was 0.8% compared with 18% for those unable to reach this threshold. Even in patients who experienced ischemia at the time of exercise testing, threshold levels were highly predictive of postoperative mortality (Table 22.2).

Formal exercise testing is neither readily available nor practical in a routine preoperative clinic. However, the metabolic requirements for many routine activities have already been determined and are quantified as metabolic equivalents (METs). The Duke's Activity Status Index is an example of a standardized self-assessment tool that quantifies METs [42]. One MET, defined as 3.5 ml/kg/min, represents the basal oxygen consumption of a 70-kg, 40-year-old man at rest. Estimated energy requirements for various activities are shown in Table 22.3 [43]. The inability to function above four METs has been associated with increased perioperative cardiac events and long-term risk. Functional capacity of the individual can be estimated by inquiring about the ability to perform these routine physical activities.

TABLE 22.2 Mortality in relation to anaerobic threshold

Anaerobic Threshold (ml/min/kg)	All patients		Patients with ischemia	
	No.	% Mortality	No.	% Mortality
<11	55	18	19	42
>11	132	0.8	25	4
	$p<0.001$		$p<0.01$	

Source: Reprinted with permission from Older et al. [41]

TABLE 22.3 Estimated energy requirements for various activities

	Can you...		Can you...
1 MET	Take care of yourself?	4 METs	Climb a flight of stairs or walk up a hill?
	Eat, dress, or use the toilet?		Walk on level ground at 4 mph (6.4 kph)?
	Walk indoors around the house?		Run a short distance?
	Walk a block or 2 on level ground at 2–3 mph (3.2–4.8 kph)?		Do heavy work around the house like scrubbing floors or lifting or moving heavy furniture?
4 METs	Do light work around the house like dusting or washing dishes?		Participate in moderate recreational activities like golf, bowling, dancing, doubles tennis, or throwing a baseball or football?
		Greater than 10 METs	Participate in strenuous sports like swimming, singles tennis, football, basketball, or skiing?

Source: Reprinted from Fleisher et al. [43], with permission from Elsevier

Tests of Functional Ability

Preoperative gait speed, balance, and upper extremity strength have been shown to correlate with postoperative recovery. Utilizing the Timed Get Up and Go, Hand Grip Strength, and Functional Reach Test as measures of physical status, Lawrence et al. have shown that older adults with intact preoperative physical status recover more quickly than persons with preoperative physical limitations [44]. Results from a study by Moriello et al. support the use of gait speed as a measure of postoperative recovery [45].

In addition, Lawrence et al. [44] demonstrated that recovery of various functions may not occur concurrently. While cognitive status recovery was relatively quick (3 weeks), gait speed (6 weeks), balance (6 weeks–3 months), and IADL abilities (3–6 months) took longer to return to preoperative levels [44]. Upper extremity strength measured by grip strength took the longest to recover and had not returned to baseline levels even after 6 months for some individuals. A description of the Timed Get Up and Go, Hand Grip Strength, and Functional Reach Tests is included below.

Timed Get Up and Go: For this test, participants are seated in a straight back chair. They are instructed to rise from the chair without using the armrests, ambulate 10 ft, turn around, walk back to the chair, and sit down. Completing the test in 10 s or less is a normal result.

Hand Grip Strength: This measure is calculated as the kilograms of pressure applied to a handheld dyanometer. Preoperative mean grip strength for the population of older patients examined by Lawrence et al. was 27 ± 11 kg [44].

Functional Reach Test: For this test, participants are asked to lean against the wall with their arm outstretched and their hand clenched in a fist. They are instructed to lean forward as far as possible without losing their balance. Persons who can reach 10 in. or more are at lowest risk for falling in the future.

Prehabilitation

It seems intuitive that improving exercise capacity preoperatively would result in better postoperative outcomes. However, to date, little data exist about the effectiveness of prehabilitation – exercise therapy conducted before surgery. However, what data do exist have shown postoperative benefits for some, but not all, patient groups. Orthopedic surgery patients engaged in prehabilitation did not show improvements in their health-related quality of life (HR-QOL) or recovery [28]. As reported by Carli, one study demonstrated that 275 elderly patients electively scheduled for abdominal or cardiac surgery, who participated in prehabilitation, had improved HR-QOL, fewer postoperative complications, shorter hospitalization, and lower levels of functional disability compared with a control group of sedentary patients [28]. More research in the area is clearly needed.

Nutritional Assessment

ASK the question	*"Have you lost 10 pounds or more in the last 6 months without trying to do so?"*
DO the test	*Height & weight (BMI), serum albumin*

Poor nutrition has been long recognized as a risk factor for pneumonia, poor wound healing, and other postoperative complications. Malnutrition, defined as a decrease in nutrient reserves, occurs in approximately 0–15% of community dwelling elderly persons, 35–65% of older patients in acute care hospitals, and 25–60% of institutionalized elderly [46] (see Chap. 6). Physiological changes that occur with aging, such as increased total body fat, loss of lean body mass, decreased bone density, and decreased total body water, may all affect nutritional requirements [47].

The assessment of nutritional status begins by understanding the risk factors for nutritional deficiency in older adults.

Factors that may lead to inadequate intake and utilization of nutrients include inability to access food (e.g., financial constraints, availability of food, limited mobility), lack of the desire to eat food (e.g., living alone, impaired mental status, chronic illness), inability to eat and/or absorb food (e.g., poor dentition, chronic gastrointestinal problems such as gastroesophageal reflux disease or diarrhea), and medications that interfere with appetite or nutrient metabolism.

Preoperative Serum Albumin

Serum albumin is a strong predictor of outcome in both non-surgical and surgical patients. Evidence demonstrates that low serum albumin in hospitalized elderly patients correlates with increased length of stay, increased rates of readmission, decreased rates of discharge to home, and increased all-cause mortality [48]. In surgical patients, low preoperative serum albumin has also been shown to correlate with postoperative morbidity and mortality [49]. Data from the NSQIP demonstrate an inverse relationship between serum albumin and 30-day morbidity and mortality (Fig. 22.5) [50].

Nutrition Screening Tests

Complicated markers of malnutrition exist [46] but are not necessary in the routine surgical setting. Subjective assessment by history and physical examination, in which risk factors and physical evidence of malnutrition are assessed, has been shown to be as effective as objective measures of nutritional status [51]. Additionally, there is evidence to support the use of a simple screening question "Have you lost 10 pounds or more in the last 6 months without trying to do so?" to diagnose malnutrition in older adults [52].

Body Mass Index (BMI) measured by weight in kilograms divided by height in meters squared, has been shown to correlate with surgical outcomes. Underweight and overweight persons have both been shown to have worse surgical outcomes compared with persons with normal weight [53, 54].

The Subjective Global Assessment (SGA) is one relatively simple reproducible tool for assessing nutritional status from the history and physical exam [55]. SGA ratings are most strongly influenced by loss of subcutaneous tissue, muscle wasting, and weight loss. In a study of patients undergoing elective gastrointestinal surgery, both SGA and serum albumin were predictive of postoperative nutrition-related complications [56].

The Mini Nutritional Assessment (MNA) is another instrument that is designed to identify older adults at risk for malnutrition [57]. A short form of the MNA has been developed and used preoperatively (Table 22.4) [58].

Preoperative Nutritional Supplementation

Data confirming that the reversal of nutritional defects, by using enteral or parenteral supplementation prior to surgery, improves outcomes are few and inconclusive. However, some initial studies suggest that improving preoperative nutrition may positively impact perioperative outcomes. In one such study, cardiac surgery patients who received a preoperative oral immune-enhancing nutritional supplement had lower rates of pneumonia compared with individuals who did not receive supplementation; rates of urinary tract and wound infections did not differ [59].

Information obtained during the preoperative nutritional assessment will be particularly useful for perioperative decisions regarding nutritional support. A flow diagram regarding which patients should be considered for nutritional support perioperatively is illustrated in Fig. 22.6 [47].

Cognitive Assessment

ASK the questions	*"Do you have problems with your memory?"* *"Do you drink alcohol during the day or before going to bed at night?"*
DO the test	*Mini-Cog*

The perioperative cognitive assessment tends to be undervalued and underapplied as a predictor of postoperative outcome. However, cognitive dysfunction as either a presurgical condition or postoperative complication can interfere with surgical treatment and postsurgical recovery. Patients with dementia and/or delirium have worse perioperative outcomes. Dementia, the clinical manifestation of chronic cognitive impairment, is *the* major risk factor for delirium, an acute

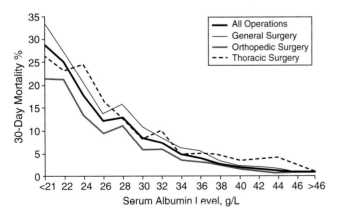

FIGURE 22.5 Relationship between albumin and 30 day mortality. Data from the National Surgical Quality Improvement Program showing 30-day operative mortality as a function of serum albumin for several different surgical specialties and for all specialties combined (reprinted with permission from [49]. Copyright © 1999 American Medical Association. All rights reserved).

TABLE 22.4 Mini-nutritional assessment-short form

Question	Score

A. Has food intake declined over the past three months due to loss of
   appetite, digestive problems, chewing or swallowing difficulties?
   0 = severe loss of appetite
   1 = moderate loss of appetite
   2 = no loss of appetite

B. Weight loss during last 3 months
   0 = weight loss greater than 3 kg (6.6 lbs)
   1 = does not know
   2 = weight loss between 1 and 3 kg (2.2 and 6.6 lbs)
   3 = no weight loss

C. Mobility
   0 = bed or chair bound
   1 = able to get out of bed/chair but does not go out
   2 = goes out

D. Has suffered psychological stress or acute disease in the past 3 months
   0 = yes
   2 = no

E. Neuropsychological problems
   0 = severe dementia or depression
   1 = mild dementia
   2 = no psychological problems

F. Body Mass Index (BMI) (weight in kilograms)/(height in meters)^2
   0 = BMI less than 19
   1 = BMI 19 to less than 21
   2 = BMI 21 to less than 23
   3 = BMI 23 or greater

Screening score (subtotal max. 14 points)
   12 points or greater: Normal – no need for further assessment
   11 points or below: Possible malnutrition – continue assessment

Source: Reprinted from Rubenstein et al. [58], with permission from the Oxford University Press

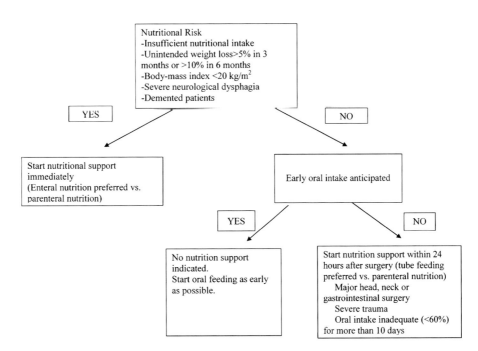

FIGURE 22.6 Decision flow chart for implementing perioperative nutrition support in geriatric patients (modified from Lugli [47], with permission from Elsevier).

reversible state of confusion, during hospitalization. As such, it is important to identify patients who have baseline cognitive impairment, even at mild levels, in the preoperative period.

Screening Tools for Dementia

There are several methods for evaluating baseline cognitive function in the elderly. Each of these instruments, although extremely informative, may take 5–10 min to administer which may not be practical in a busy preoperative clinic. The exception is the Mini-Cog, a quick and practical screening tool for dementia that can be completed in 2–4 min.

The Mini-Cog has sensitivity and specificity rates similar to the Folstein Mini Mental Status Examination (MMSE) and a standardized neuropsychological battery [60]. Participants are asked to recall three words and to draw a clock indicating an abstract time such as one forty five (1:45) or ten after 11 (11:10). The three item word recall assesses short-term memory, while the clock drawing task assesses for key features of executive function such as initiation, planning, and multistep processing. The instructions for the administration and scoring of the Mini-Cog can be found in Appendix 22.1.

The Folstein Mini Mental Status Examination (MMSE) has become widely accepted for its ease of administration and reliability [61]. The MMSE allocates a total of 30 points to five areas (1) orientation, (2) registration, (3) attention/calculation, (4) recall, and (5) language. MMSE scores are influenced by several factors including age and educational attainment. As such, MMSE scores should be interpreted according to population-based norms for age and educational level as shown in Table 22.5 [62].

The Telephone Interview for Cognitive Status (TICS) is a validated, reliable modification of the MMSE, which can be easily administered over the telephone [63]. The TICS has a maximum score of 38.

The St. Louis University Mental Status (SLUMS) Examination is a dementia screening instrument that allocates 30 points to four areas (1) orientation, (2) memory, (3) attention, and (4) executive function (Appendix 22.2) [64]. The sensitivity and specificity of the SLUMS has been shown to be similar to the MMSE; the SLUMS may be better able to detect mild cognitive impairment.

Delirium

Estimates of postoperative delirium rates vary significantly depending upon the type of surgery performed. Delirium is reported in <5% of older patients after cataract surgery, 35% of patients after vascular surgery, and 40–60% of older patients after hip fracture repair [65]. Delirious surgical patients have more major complications, longer hospitalizations, costlier hospital stays, higher rates of discharge to long-term care facilities, and higher rates of death compared with nondelirious patients [66]. In addition, postoperative delirium has been shown to persist for several months after surgery, up to three, in a significant percentage of older patients [67]. Thus, identifying preoperative patients at highest risk for delirium has the potential to significantly improve perioperative outcomes. Marcantonio et al. developed a clinical prediction rule for postoperative delirium from a large prospective study of major elective noncardiac surgery patients over age 50 years [66]. The independent correlates for postoperative delirium and the point system devised to quantify the risk of delirium are illustrated in Table 22.6. For additional information on delirium, please refer to Chap. 16.

Unrecognized alcohol abuse should always be included on the list of potential causes of delirium. Older adults may not report their intake of alcohol with meals or prior to bedtime. Forced abstinence as a result of hospitalization may present in a mild form such as evening agitation or

TABLE 22.5 Norms for the mini-mental state examination by age and education

Education	Age range							
	50–54	55–59	60–64	65–69	70–74	75–79	80–84	85+
0–4 years								
Mean	23	22	23	22	22	21	20	19
SD	2.6	2.7	1.9	1.7	2.0	2.2	2.9	2.3
5–8 years								
Mean	27	26	26	26	26	25	25	23
SD	2.4	2.9	2.3	1.7	1.8	2.1	1.9	3.3
9–12 years								
Mean	28	28	28	28	27	27	25	26
SD	2.2	2.2	1.7	1.4	1.6	1.5	2.3	2.0
13 or more years								
Mean	29	29	29	29	28	28	27	27
SD	1.9	1.5	1.3	1.0	1.6	1.6	0.9	1.3

TABLE 22.6 Clinical prediction rule for postoperative delirium

Risk factor	Points
Age ≥ 70 years	1
Alcohol abuse	1
TICS score < 30	1
SAS class IV	1
Markedly abnormal preoperative sodium, potassium, or glucose level	1
Aortic aneurysm surgery	2
Noncardiac thoracic surgery	1
Total points	Risk of delirium, %
0	2
1 or 2	11
≥3	50

"sundowning" or in a more severe form such as delirium tremors (DTs). Older patients should be specifically asked about mealtime and/or bedtime alcohol use. More comprehensive alcohol screening tools specifically designed for older adults, such as the Michigan Alcohol Screening Test-Geriatric Version [68] (see Appendix 22.3), are available.

Mental status changes in older surgical patients are often the earliest signs of a postoperative complication. If an older patient presents with an altered mental status in the perioperative period, knowledge of his or her preoperative cognitive status provides critical information for determining the extent and aggressiveness of intervention warranted.

Depressive Symptoms

Not all patients who perform poorly on screening examinations will have cognitive impairment. Patients with depressive symptoms may appear to have cognitive impairment as a result of providing little effort during testing. In addition, patients with depressed mood may exhibit less desire to participate in rehabilitation activities. Interestingly, one study [69] demonstrated an association between number of depressive symptoms reported by older adults on the Geriatric Depression Scale (GDS) and delirium. Persons who reported more depressive symptoms preoperatively had higher incidence rates, and more days, of delirium postoperatively.

The GDS [70] is a 15-item questionnaire that can be administered in person or over the telephone. Respondents provide a yes or no response to the questions posed. A score ≥5 indicates depression is a possibility. The GDS is reprinted in Appendix 22.4.

Specific Organ System Evaluations

Although cardiac and pulmonary complications are the most common postoperative events for older patients, physiological changes in the renal and hepatic systems also place older adults at risk. Complications due to specific organ system problems may prolong hospitalization and contribute to functional decline, necessitating the addition of rehabilitation services upon discharge. Thus, preoperative history or physical examination findings consistent with clinically significant cardiac, pulmonary, renal or hepatic disease warrant investigation, monitoring, and/or intervention.

Pulmonary Assessment

Comparatively much more attention has been paid to the preoperative evaluation and optimization of cardiac risk factors than pulmonary risk factors. However, there is evidence to support the assertion that pulmonary complications are equal determinants of postoperative morbidity, mortality, and length of stay for older surgical patients [71]. This assertion is supported by the findings of a large study in which the 30-day mortality rate for persons with postoperative pneumonia was 21 versus 2% for persons without postoperative pneumonia [72]. In the literature, pulmonary complications refer to a variety of conditions including pneumonia, respiratory insufficiency, respiratory failure, atelectasis, acute respiratory distress syndrome, and pleural effusions. It is important to remember that aspiration is one of the leading causes of these complications. While aspiration is possible in any age group, monitoring for aspiration is especially important in the elderly. As with all adverse surgical outcomes, pulmonary complications are more common following emergency operations. Given the high prevalence of emergency surgery in persons over the age of 65, this is of particular significance for older adults.

Risk Factors

Patient, procedure, and laboratory factors have all been implicated as increasing the odds of developing postoperative pulmonary complications. A recent systematic review examined the literature regarding risk factors and subsequent pulmonary complications [71]. The patient and procedure-related factors for which there was good or at least fair evidence to support the association between the risk factor and postoperative pulmonary complications are presented in Tables 22.7 and 22.8.

Patient-Related Risk Factors

Subtle nasopharyngeal dysfunction is frequently unrecognized in the elderly but is known to be a factor predisposing to aspiration pneumonia. Devices that traverse the oropharynx may further disrupt the normal swallowing process and

TABLE 22.7 Potential patient-related risk factors for postoperative pulmonary complications

Risk factor	Odds ratio
Advanced age	2.09–3.04
ASA class ≥ II	2.55–4.87
Heart failure	2.93
Functionally dependent	1.65–2.51
Chronic obstructive pulmonary disease	1.79
Weight loss	1.62
Impaired sensorium	1.39
Cigarette use	1.26
Alcohol use	1.21

Source: Modified from Smetana [71], with permission from the American College of Physicians

TABLE 22.8 Potential procedure-related risk factors for postoperative pulmonary complications

Risk factor	Odds ratio
Aortic aneurysm repair	6.90
Thoracic surgery	4.24
Abdominal surgery	3.01
Upper abdominal surgery	2.91
Neurosurgery	2.53
Prolonged surgery	2.26
Head and neck surgery	2.21
Emergency surgery	2.21
Vascular surgery	2.10
General anesthesia	1.83
Perioperative transfusion	1.47

Source: Modified from Smetana [71], with permission from the American College of Physicians

further increase the risk of aspiration. In one multivariate analysis, postoperative nasogastric intubation was the single most important variable associated with postoperative pulmonary complications [73]. In another study of cardiac surgery patients, the use of transesophageal echocardiography probes intraoperatively was significantly associated with the development of postoperative aspiration [74].

Several conditions, commonly found in older adults, increase the risk of aspiration. These include cognitive impairment, prior stroke, xerostomia (dry mouth), poor dentition, gastroesophageal reflux disease (GERD), and diabetes. Thus, aspiration precautions are particularly important in this population.

Several studies have examined the impact of age on postoperative pulmonary complications with equivocal results. Studies that were not controlled for the presence of comorbid conditions indicate 4–45% of persons over the age of 70 develop postoperative pulmonary complications. More recent reviews of the literature suggest that older age remains an independent predictor of postoperative pulmonary complications even after adjusting for comorbid conditions [71].

The ASA classification, a subjective assessment of overall functional and physical well-being (see above), has been shown to be an accurate predictor of postoperative cardiac and pulmonary status [75]. Similarly, functional dependence is an important determinant of postoperative pulmonary complications. Individuals who are either unable to complete any ADLs or require assistance from another person or device have been shown to have worse pulmonary outcomes compared with functionally independent persons [76].

The most commonly identified risk factor for postoperative pulmonary complications is chronic obstructive pulmonary disease. In multivariate analyses [72], the degree of obstructive disease (none to mild vs. moderate to severe) contributed to the degree of risk. Unintentional weight loss ≥10% in the prior 6 months, acute cognitive changes secondary to

delirium, cigarette smoking within the past 1 year, and consumption of >2 drinks/day in the past 2 weeks have all been shown to increase the risk of postoperative pulmonary complications [72]. Of note, individuals who discontinue smoking ≤8 weeks prior to surgery have higher rates of complications compared with individuals who were still actively smoking at the time of their operation.

Although obesity is widely thought to be associated with postoperative pulmonary complications, the incidence of pulmonary complications following surgery even for patients with morbid obesity is no higher than would be expected in a group of procedure-matched nonobese patients. In addition, there is little evidence that diabetes or well-controlled asthma affect postoperative pulmonary complication rates [71].

Procedure-Related Risk Factors

Procedure-related risk factors implicated in the development of postoperative pulmonary complications include the site of incision, type of anesthesia, duration of the procedure, amount of blood loss, type of repair (e.g., open vs. endovascular), and urgency of the operation (e.g., emergency vs. elective) [71].

The proximity of the surgical incision to the diaphragm has been long known to influence the rate of postoperative pulmonary complications. Upper abdominal incisions are accompanied by a 13–33% [77, 78] pulmonary complication rate, compared with a 0–16% [78, 79] rate for incisions in the lower abdomen. Rates as high as 40% are reported with thoracic incisions [79, 80]. Minimally invasive procedures, such as laparoscopic cholecystectomy, are associated with little risk of pulmonary complications. In several large series rates as low as 0.3–0.4% were reported [81, 82].

The importance of the type of anesthesia and the length of operation in terms of the incidence of postoperative pulmonary complications is less clear. Although most studies support the lower complication rate following regional anesthesia compared with general anesthesia, these results are not uniform. Duration of anesthesia of more than 3 h has been shown to be significant [73, 83].

In one retrospective analysis, intraoperative blood loss of more than 1,200 ml was an independent predictor of postoperative pneumonia [84]. This may be an indication of the complexity of the procedure or of underlying comorbidity. Although multiple transfusions are known to be immunosuppressive, the relation of transfusion to postoperative infection is not clear [85]. However, when combined with the declining immunologic competence associated with aging, a transfusion-related alteration in host defenses may facilitate the development of pneumonia in the elderly.

Pulmonary Assessment Tools

Tests for Aspiration Risk

Evaluation for aspiration is important for all older adults with conditions that place them at higher risk for aspiration, such as persons with a history of stroke, poor dentition, or GERD. The 3-ounce water swallow test is a time-efficient method to clinically screen individuals who are at risk for aspiration [86]. Individuals are asked to swallow 3 ounces (90 cc) of water without pausing. Persons who choke, cough, are unable to complete the task, or have a wet quality to their voice after completing the task are typically referred for fiberoptic endoscopic evaluation. One study of 3,000 individuals, 20% of whom were surgical patients, demonstrated that the water swallow test has high sensitivity and negative predictive value [86]. Thus, individuals who pass the swallow test have a high likelihood of passing a fiberoptic endoscopic evaluation. However, the swallow test had a high false positive rate such that half of the individuals who failed the swallow test did not demonstrate aspiration on a fiberoptic evaluation. Fiberoptic evaluation should, therefore, be reserved for those persons with known risk factors for aspiration. Aspiration precautions, however, should be observed for any patient with either a failed water swallow test or has a know risk factor for aspiration.

Laboratory/Radiology Tests

There is good evidence that an albumin level <35 g/L increases the odds of postoperative pulmonary complications by 2.53 [71]. The evidence that other laboratory tests, such as chest radiography, contribute to the predictions of postoperative risk, is less convincing. Even though chest radiographs are routinely ordered as part of a preoperative evaluation, it is rare that the radiograph illustrates issues that were not discovered during the history and physical examination [71]. Preoperative chest radiographs are arguably only beneficial for patients with established cardiopulmonary disease and/or adults over the age of 50 who will likely receive an incision close to the diaphragm [71].

Pulmonary Function Evaluation

Although previous guidelines for preoperative pulmonary function testing suggested that spirometry was indicated for every patient over the age of 70 years [87], more recent data refute that claim. The few studies that have compared clinical findings with spirometric measures do not uniformly support the use of spirometry over a comprehensive history and physical examination [71]. Abnormal chest findings on physical examination and chest radiography have been shown

Table 22.9 ACP guidelines for preoperative spirometry

Planned lung resection
Potential coronary artery bypass graft candidate
Known asthma
Known chronic obstructive pulmonary disease (COPD)
Probable undiagnosed COPD

Source: Data from Quaseem et al. [76]

to be highly associated with postoperative pulmonary complications; the data for spirometry is equivocal.

Present guidelines from the American College of Physicians for the use of preoperative pulmonary function tests are shown in Table 22.9 [76]. There is consensus that all patients undergoing lung resection should have pulmonary function tests. Individuals with uncharacterized pulmonary disease, known COPD or asthma, and questionable CABG candidacy should also be tested. However, those patients with normal physical examinations and good exercise tolerance do not benefit from additional studies.

A risk index has been developed to indentify the patients at highest risk for developing postoperative pneumonia [72]. Points are assigned depending upon the presence of various risk factors (Table 22.10); the maximum point value is 164. Individuals are classified into five risk classes: class I (0–15 points), class II (16–25 points), class III (26–40 points), class IV (41–55 points), or class V (>55 points). Persons in the lowest risk class have an average predicted probability of postoperative pneumonia of 0.24%; those in the highest class have a probability of 15.3%.

Cardiovascular Assessment

With the aging of America it is estimated that the annual number of noncardiac surgical procedures performed in older adults will increase from the present level of six million to approximately 12 million over the next 30 years [43]. Four procedures that constitute one-fourth of the surgeries performed in older adults, namely major intraabdominal, thoracic, vascular, and orthopedic procedures, have been associated with significant cardiovascular morbidity and mortality. Because cardiovascular events are a leading cause of perioperative complications and death, preoperative evaluation of cardiac risk has been studied extensively. The American College of Cardiology (ACC)/American Heart Association (AHA) Task Force on Practice Guidelines routinely publish guideline on perioperative cardiovascular evaluation and care for noncardiac surgery patients [43]. The recommendations provided in the guidelines are based upon the available scientific evidence as well as expert opinion; the objective is to improve patient care. Use of the guidelines is intended to clarify which patients would benefit from additional cardiac evaluation and what evaluation should be pursued, if any.

TABLE 22.10 Postoperative pneumonia risk index

Preoperative risk factor	Point value
Type of surgery	
Abdominal aortic aneurysm repair	15
Thoracic	14
Upper abdominal	10
Neck	8
Neurosurgery	8
Vascular	3
Age	
≥80 years	17
70–79 years	13
60–69 years	9
50–59 years	4
Functional status	
Totally dependent	10
Partially dependent	6
Weight loss > 10% in past 6 months	7
History of chronic obstructive pulmonary disease	5
General anesthesia	4
Impaired sensorium	4
History of cerebrovascular accident	4
Blood urea nitrogen level	
<2.86 mmol/L (<8 mg/dL)	4
7.85–10.7 mmol/L (22–30 mg/dL)	2
≥10.7 mmol/L (≥30 mg/dL)	3
Transfusion > 4 units	3
Emergency surgery	3
Steroid use for chronic condition	3
Current smoker within 1 year	3
Alcohol intake > 2 drinks/day in past 2 weeks	2

Source: Modified from Arozullah [72], with permission from the American College of Physicians

TABLE 22.11 Clinical predictors of increased perioperative cardiovascular risk

Active cardiac conditions

Unstable coronary syndromes
  Recent myocardial infarction (>7 days but <30 days) with evidence of important risk based on clinical symptoms or noninvasive study
  Unstable or severe angina (Canadian class III or IV) [58]
Decompensated heart failure
Significant arrhythmias
  High-grade atrioventricular block
  Symptomatic ventricular arrhythmias in the presence of underlying heart disease
  Supraventricular arrhythmias with uncontrolled ventricular rate
Severe valvular disease

Revised cardiac risk index

History of ischemic heart disease
History of cerebrovascular disease
History of compensated or prior heart failure
Diabetes mellitus
Renal insufficiency

Minor predictors

Advanced age (greater than 70 years)
Abnormal electrocardiographic findings
  Left ventricular hypertrophy
  Left bundle branch block
  ST-T abnormalities
Rhythm other than sinus
  Atrial fibrillation, for example
Uncontrolled systemic hypertension

Source: Reprinted from Fleisher et al. [43], with permission from Elsevier

Clinical Risk Factors

The previous terminology of major and intermediate risk factors has been replaced, respectively, with active cardiac conditions and Revised Cardiac Risk Index clinical risk factors. The terminology of minor clinical predictors remains the same. The clinical risk factors are listed in Table 22.11.

Perioperative Algorithm (Appendix 22.5)

Step 1: Determine the Urgency of Noncardiac Surgery

Preoperative cardiac evaluation is not necessary for emergency surgery. Patients should proceed directly to surgery; risk stratification and management can be performed perioperatively.

Step 2: Determine If Any Active Cardiac Conditions Exist

The presence of ≥1 active cardiac conditions warrants intervention and, unless deemed emergent, may result in a delay or cancelation of surgery. If no active cardiac conditions are present, proceed to the next step. Evidence suggests that cardiovascular intervention does not influence surgical outcomes in asymptomatic patients without active cardiac conditions. Therefore, preoperative cardiovascular screening is not necessary.

Step 3: Consider the Risk of the Planned Surgery

Cardiac risk stratification according to surgical procedure is listed in Table 22.12. If the proposed surgery is a low-risk procedure, stable patients may proceed to surgery without cardiovascular evaluation since the results of testing are unlikely to warrant a change of plans.

Step 4: Consider the Functional Capacity and Symptom Status of the Patient

Highly functional asymptomatic patients may proceed to surgery without cardiovascular evaluation, since the results of testing are unlikely to warrant a change of plans. As mentioned

TABLE 22.12 Cardiac risk stratification for noncardiac surgical procedures

Vascular (reported cardiac risk often more than 5%)

Aortic or other major vascular surgery

Peripheral vascular surgery

Intermediate (reported cardiac risk generally 1–5%)

Carotid endarterectomy

Head and neck surgery

Intraperitoneal and intrathoracic surgery

Orthopedic surgery

Prostate surgery

Low (reported cardiac risk generally less than 1%)

Endoscopic procedures

Superficial procedures

Cataract surgery

Breast surgery

Ambulatory surgery

Source: Reprinted from Fleisher et al. [43], with permission from Elsevier

Risk denotes combined incidence of cardiac death and nonfatal myocardial infarctions

above, questioning patients on their ability to perform certain activities for which the estimated MET values are known provides individual scoring of functional capacity (Table 22.3). Utilizing METs, functional capacity can be classified as excellent (>10), good (7–10), moderate (4–6), or poor (<4). Patients unable to meet a four-MET demand during most normal daily activities are at increased risk for perioperative cardiopulmonary and long-term complications.

Step 5: Determine If Clinical Risk Factors Are Present For Patients with Poor Functional Capacity or Symptoms

If no clinical risk factors are present, the patient may proceed to surgery without further evaluation. If ≥3 clinical risk factors are present, cardiac risk stratification (Table 22.12) must be considered.

Renal Assessment

Physiological Changes of the Aging Kidney

Renal insufficiency is often asymptomatic in older adults. Preoperative renal insufficiency is a strong predictor of perioperative cardiac and pulmonary morbidity [88]. Moreover, impaired preoperative kidney function increases the likelihood of perioperative kidney failure. Physiological changes that occur with aging, namely decreases in renal plasma flow and glomerular filtration rate (GFR), contribute to the increased rates of renal insufficiency among older adults.

Muscle mass also decreases with age. As a result, serum creatinine level may not accurately estimate renal function in older adults. (A complete discussion of changes in renal physiology can be found in Chap. 76.)

Glomerular Filtration Rate

Accurately assessing GFR is an essential component of the preoperative renal evaluation for older adults. GFR can be estimated via the Cockcroft–Gault equation for creatinine clearance (CrCl):

$$CrCl = (140 - age) \times \text{Ideal body weight} /$$
$$(\text{Serum creatinine} \times 72) (\times 0.85 \text{ for women})$$

$$\text{Ideal body weight} = 2.3 \text{ kg for every inch over 5 ft}$$
$$+ [50 \text{ kg (men) or } 45.5 \text{ kg (women)}]$$

More recent formulas, such as the Modification of Diet in Renal Disease (MDRD) equation, may also be used to calculate GFR and stage chronic kidney disease [89]. The MDRD equation takes into account serum creatinine level, age, race, and gender. A free online MDRD calculator can be accessed at http://www.mdrd.com.

In addition to calculating GFR, identifying patient medications that are cleared by the kidneys is warranted during a preoperative assessment. Medications that are cleared by the kidney may need to be administered at a lower dose, with a longer dosing interval, or avoided altogether in individuals with impaired GFR (<30 mg/dL). Avoiding dehydration preoperatively and perioperatively is a vitally important management issue. Older adults are predisposed to dehydration due to impairments with the thirst drive with increasing age. Thus, monitoring for appropriate hydration, especially in patients recently restarted on a diet after a period of nothing-by-mouth (NPO) status is warranted.

Hepatic Assessment

Liver failure is an important predictor of poor perioperative outcomes [88]. Physiological changes that occur with aging may increase the risk of hepatic dysfunction. Liver blood flow, size, and mass all decrease with increasing age, as does cytochrome P450 content. As a result, medications that undergo a first pass effect, such as nitrates, may have a higher serum concentration or higher bioavailability in older adults. Additionally, the metabolism of medications, in particular anesthetic agents, can be impaired in adults over the age of 65. Obtaining an accurate history of current and previous alcohol use should be incorporated into the preoperative hepatic assessment. Laboratory evaluation of liver function tests including albumin, and the coagulant profile are also recommended.

Processes of Care to Improve Outcomes

Preoperative Evaluation of Postoperative Needs

Once the decision to proceed with surgery has been made, planning for the postoperative period should begin. In particular, knowledge of the geriatric surgical patient's social support structure will help guide postoperative discharge decisions. A functionally independent individual living with involved family members, for example, requires far less ancillary support than a frail individual living alone. Preoperative patients who do not receive adequate support from family, friends, or paid professionals are unlikely to be discharged home postoperatively, when their needs are likely to be greater, unless additional support can be arranged. If a patient's needs exceed the level of assistance home services can provide, then short-term rehabilitation or long-term care placement may be indicated. Assistance with housework, laundry, and driving are just a few examples of needs that may originate during the postoperative period. If possible, patients should be encouraged to make arrangements for additional home support, prior to surgery. If informal assistance is not available, involving care coordination as early as possible may smooth the transition from hospital to home. Determining the level of additional support required and preparing for this support prior to surgery allows the patient to prepare for their entire recovery period and may positively affect compliance with follow-up care.

Surgery–Geriatrics Comanagement Models

As previously discussed, older adults have an increased risk of postoperative adverse outcomes including mortality, longer hospitalization, and new discharge to a long-term care facility. A combined surgery–geriatrics comanagement care model has been utilized in various hospitals outside of the USA for several years; some US hospitals have recently implemented similar models. Comprehensive Geriatric Assessment (CGA) is a common component of comanagement models instituted for patients scheduled for elective surgery. CGA typically includes preoperative cognitive, functional, and nutritional assessments; mood evaluation; and medication review. In one study, older patients who had CGA as part of a comanagement model had shorter hospitalizations (11.5 vs. 15.8 days) and fewer delayed discharges (24.1 vs. 70.4%) [90]. In another study, older hip fracture patients who were assessed by the geriatrics service within 24 h of admission and subsequently comanaged by geriatrics

and orthopedic surgery throughout the remainder of their hospitalization had lower rates of delirium (RR = 0.64) and severe delirium (RR = 0.4) compared with patients who received usual care [91]. A collaboration of surgeons and geriatricians in Japan has used the functional and cognitive components of CGA to predict which thoracic surgery patients are at highest risk for postoperative complications [92]. Additional studies are necessary in order to fully understand all the benefits afforded to older surgical patients who receive care via combined surgery–geriatrics comanagement programs. Perhaps comanagement programs will emerge as a low risk, cost-effective means to improve perioperative and postoperative outcomes for older surgical patients. Given the expected increase in the number of older adults in the next few decades, any intervention or model of care that improves outcomes for geriatric surgical patients would likely make a significant contribution to the overall US healthcare system.

Summary

Successful surgical care of the older patient requires a full understanding of the factors that will influence the postoperative recovery of each individual. Determining these factors need not take an excessive amount of time or require elaborate testing. A thorough history and physical examination will identify serious comorbidity that may direct additional specific testing. Assessment of the factors specific to the older patient can be done by asking these simple questions:

1. "Can you carry a bag of groceries up a flight of steps without getting short of breath?"
2. "Have you lost 10 pounds or more in the last 6 months without trying to do so?"
3. "Do you have problems with your memory?"
4. "Do you drink alcohol occasionally, with meals, or before going to bed?"

…and doing these three tests:

1. Timed Get Up and Go
2. Height, weight, BMI, serum albumin
3. Mini-Cog

The need for further testing or preoperative preparation will be guided by the results of these simple assessments.

Improving the care of the older surgical patient presents special challenges. However, these challenges may be overcome by developing patient-centered treatment plans that recognize individual preferences, geriatric-specific issues, and the physiological changes that occur with aging.

Appendix 22.1   Mini-Cog Screen for Dementia

Administration

1. Make sure you have the patient's attention. Instruct the patient to listen carefully to and remember three unrelated words and then to repeat the words back to you (to be sure the patient heard them)
2. Instruct the patient to draw the face of a clock, either on a blank sheet of paper, or on a sheet with the clock circle already drawn on the page. After the patient puts the numbers on the clock face, ask him or her to draw the hands of the clock to read a specific time (1:45 or 11:10 are commonly used). These instructions can be repeated, but no additional instructions should be given. If the patient cannot complete the clock-drawing test (CDT) in 3 min or less, move on to the next step
3. Ask the patient to repeat the three previously presented words

Scoring

Give 1 point for each recalled word after the CDT distractor. Score 0–3 for recall

Give 2 points for a normal CDT, and 0 points for an abnormal CDT. The CDT is considered normal if all numbers are depicted, once each, in the correct sequence and position, and the hands readably display the requested time. Add the recall and CDT scores together to get the Mini-Cog score

0–2 positive screen for dementia

3–5 negative screen for dementia

Source: Data from [60]

Appendix 22.2   St. Louis University Mental Status (SLUMS) Examination

1. What day of the week is it?	1 point	
2. What is the year?	1 point	
3. What state are we in?	1 point	
4. Please remember these five objects	I will ask you what they are later	
Apple Pen Tie House	Car	
5. You have \$100 and you go to the store and buy a dozen apples for \$3 and a tricycle for \$20		
How much did you spend?	1 point	
How much do you have left?	2 points	
6. Please name as many animals as you can in 1 min		
0–5 animals	0 points	
5–10 animals	1 point	
10–15 animals	2 points	
15+ animals	3 points	
7. What were the five objects I asked you to remember?	1 point for each one correct	
8. I am going to give you a series of numbers and I would like you to give them to me backwards. For example, if I say 42, you would say 24		
87	0 points	
649	1 point	
8,537	2 points	

9. This is a clock face. Please put in the hour markers and the time at 10 min to 11 o'clock

    Hour markers okay   2 points

    Time correct   2 points

10. Please place an X in the triangle

    Which of the above figures is the largest?

(continued)

Appendix 22.2 (continued)

11. I am going to tell you a story. Please listen carefully because afterwards, I'm going to ask you some questions about it

Jill was a very successful stockbroker. She made a lot of money on the stock market. She then met Jack, a devastatingly handsome man. She married him and had three children. They lived in Chicago. She then stopped work and stayed at home to bring up her children. When they were teenagers, she went back to work. She and Jack lived happily ever after

What was the female's name?	2 points
What work did she do?	2 points
When did she go back to work?	2 points
What state did she live in?	2 points

Scoring

High school education		Less than high school education
27–30	Normal	20–30
20–27	Mild cognitive impairment	14–19
1–19	Dementia	1–14

Source: Available at http://www.medschool.slu.edu/agingsuccessfully/pdfsurveys/slumsexam_05.pdf. (See also 64)

Appendix 22.3 Michigan Alcoholism Screening Test: Geriatric Version (MAST-G)

1.	After drinking have you ever noticed an increase in your heart rate or beating in your chest?	Yes	No
2.	When talking with others, do you ever underestimate how much you actually drink?	Yes	No
3.	Does alcohol make you sleepy so that you often fall asleep in your chair?	Yes	No
4.	After a few drinks, have you sometimes not eaten or been able to skip a meal because you didn't feel hungry?	Yes	No
5.	Does having a few drinks help decrease your shakiness or tremors?	Yes	No
6.	Does alcohol sometimes make it hard for you to remember parts of the day or night?	Yes	No
7.	Do you have rules for yourself that you won't drink before a certain time of the day?	Yes	No
8.	Have you lost interest in hobbies or activities you used to enjoy?	Yes	No
9.	When you wake up in the morning, do you ever have trouble remembering part of the night before?	Yes	No
10.	Does having a drink help you sleep?	Yes	No
11.	Do you hide your alcohol bottles from family members?	Yes	No
12.	After a social gathering, have you ever felt embarrassed because you drank too much?	Yes	No
13.	Have you ever been concerned that drinking might be harmful to your health?	Yes	No
14.	Do you like to end an evening with a nightcap?	Yes	No
15.	Did you find your drinking increased after someone close to you died?	Yes	No
16.	In general, would you prefer to have a few drinks at home rather than go out to social events?	Yes	No
17.	Are you drinking more now than in the past?	Yes	No
18.	Do you usually take a drink to relax or calm your nerves?	Yes	No
19.	Do you drink to take your mind off your problems?	Yes	No
20.	Have you ever increased your drinking after experiencing a loss in your life?	Yes	No
21.	Do you sometimes drive when you have had too much to drink?	Yes	No
22.	Has a doctor or nurse ever said they were worried or concerned about your drinking?	Yes	No
23.	Have you ever made rules to manage your drinking?	Yes	No
24.	When you feel lonely, does having a drink help?	Yes	No

Scoring: Five or more "Yes" responses are indicative of an alcohol problem
Source: from [67]

Appendix 22.4 The Geriatric Depression Scale (Short Form)
Choose the best answer for how you felt over the past week.

Date / /	Please tick ✔
1. Are you basically satisfied with your life?	Yes ☐ No ☐
2. Have you dropped many of your activities and interests?	**Yes** ☐ No ☐
3. Do you feel that your life is empty?	**Yes** ☐ No ☐
4. Do you often get bored?	**Yes** ☐ No ☐
5. Are you in good spirits most of the time?	Yes ☐ **No** ☐
6. Are you afraid that something bad is going to happen to you?	**Yes** ☐ No ☐
7. Do you feel happy most of the time?	Yes ☐ **No** ☐
8. Do you often feel helpless?	**Yes** ☐ No ☐
9. Do you prefer to stay at home, rather than going out and doing things?	**Yes** ☐ No ☐
10. Do you feel you have more problems with memory than most?	**Yes** ☐ No ☐
11. Do you think it is wonderful to be alive now?	Yes ☐ **No** ☐
12. Do you feel pretty worthless the way you are now?	**Yes** ☐ No ☐
13. Do you feel full of energy?	Yes ☐ **No** ☐
14. Do you feel that your situation is hopeless?	**Yes** ☐ No ☐
15. Do you think that most people are better off than you?	**Yes** ☐ No ☐
TOTAL SCORE	

Answers in **bold** indicate depression and receive one point. Scores greater than five suggest the presence of depression.

Source: material available at http://www.chcr.brown.edu/GDS_SHORT_FORM.PDF. See also Sheik and Yesavage [70]

Appendix 22.5   Cardiac Evaluation and Care Algorithm
Reprinted from Fleischer et al. [43]. Copyright 2007, with permission from Elsevier

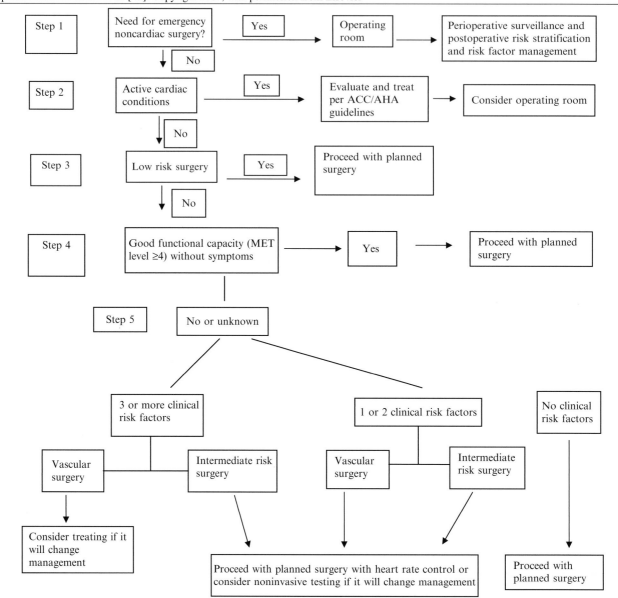

References

1. The State of Aging & Health in America (2004) http://www.cdc. gov/aging/pdf/State_of_Aging_and_Health. Accessed 21 Dec 2008
2. Centers for Disease Control & Prevention Public health & Aging (2003) Trends in aging – United States and Worldwide. MMWR 52(06):101–106
3. National Center for Health Statistics (2009) Health, United States, 2008, with chartbook. Hyattsville, MD (Figure 1)
4. Beliveau MM, Multach M (2003) Perioperative care for the elderly patient. Med Clin N Am 87:273–289
5. Owings MF, Kozak LJ (1998) Ambulatory and inpatient procedures in the United States, 1996. National Center for Health Statistics. Vital Health Stat 13(139). http://www.cdc.gov/nchs/data/series/ sr_13/sr13_139.pdf. Accessed 7 Oct 2008.

6. Thomas DR, Ritchie CS (1995) Preoperative assessment of older adults. J Am Geriatr Soc 43:811–821
7. Audisio RA et al (2004) The surgical management of elderly cancer patients: recommendations of the SIOG surgical task force. Eur J Cancer 40:926–938
8. Rosenthal RA, Andersen DK (1993) Surgery in the elderly: observations on the pathophysiology and treatment of cholelithiasis. Exp Gerontol 28:459
9. Keller SM et al (1987) Emergency and elective surgery in patients over age 70 years. Am Surg 53:636
10. Zenilman ME (1993) Considerations in surgery in the elderly. Advances in surgery in the elderly, vol 2, Master series in surgery. World Medical Press, New York
11. Fried TR, Bradley EH, Towle VR, Allore H (2003) Understanding the treatment preferences of seriously ill patients. N Engl J Med 346:1061–1066

12. McGory ML et al (2009) Developing quality indicators for elderly surgical patients. Ann Surg 250:338–347

13. Schmidtler FW et al (2008) Cardiac surgery for octogenarians – a suitable procedure? Twelve-year operative and post-hospital mortality in 641 patients over 80 years of age. Thorac Cardiovasc Surg 56(1):14–19

14. Marusch F, For the Working Group Colon/Rectum Cancer et al (2005) The impact of the risk factor "age" on the early postoperative results of surgery for colorectal carcinoma and its significance for perioperative management. World J Surg 29(8):1013–1021

15. Polanczyk CA et al (2001) Impact of age on perioperative complications and length of stay in patients undergoing noncardiac surgery. Ann Intern Med 134:637–643

16. Hamel MB, Henderson WG, Khuri SF, Daley J (2005) Surgical outcomes for patients aged 80 and older: morbidity and mortality from major noncardiac surgery. J Am Geriatr Soc 53:424–429

17. The State of Aging & Health in America (2007) http://www.cdc. gov/aging/pdf/saha_2007.pdf Accessed 12 Feb 2009

18. Boyd BJ et al (1980) Operative risk factors of colon resection in the elderly. Ann Surg 192:743

19. Yancik R et al (1998) Comorbidity and age as predictors of risk for early mortality of male and female colon carcinoma patients: a population based study. Cancer 82:2123–2134

20. Tiret L et al (1986) Complications associated with anaesthesia – a prospective survey in France. Can Anaesth Soc J 33:336–344

21. Escarce JJ et al (1995) Outcomes of open cholecystectomy in the elderly: a longitudinal analysis of 2,100 cases in the prelaparoscopic era. Surgery 117:156

22. Kannel WB, Dannenberg AV, Abbott RD (1985) Unrecognized myocardial infarction and hypertension: Framingham study. Am Heart J 109:581

23. Joray S, Wietlisbach V, Bula CJ (2004) Cognitive impairment in elderly medical inpatients: detection and associated six-month outcomes. Am J Geriatr Psychiatry 12:639–647

24. Pinholt EM et al (1987) Functional assessment of the elderly: a comparison of standard instruments with clinical judgement. Arch Intern Med 147:484

25. Robinson TN, Eiseman B, Wallace JI et al (2009) Redefining geriatric preoperative assessment, using frailty, disability and comorbidity. Ann Surg 250:449–455

26. Siddiqui U, Weinshel EH, Bini EJ (2005) Prevalence and predictors of herbal medication use in veterans with chronic Hepatitis C. J Clin Gastroenterol 39(4):344

27. Ang-Lee MK, Moss J, Yuan CS (2001) Herbal medicines and perioperative care. JAMA 286:208–216

28. Carli F, Zavorsky G (2005) Optimizing functional exercise capacity in the elderly surgical population. Curr Opin Clin Nutr Metab Care 8(1):23–32

29. Shahar A, Powers KA, Black JS (1996) The risk of postoperative deconditioning in older adults. J Am Geriatr Soc 44:471

30. Buxbaum JL, Schwartz AJ (1994) Perianesthetic considerations for the elderly patient. Surg Clin North Am 74:41–61

31. Djokovic JL, Hedley-White J (1979) Prediction of outcome of surgery and anesthesia in patients over 80. JAMA 242:2301

32. Khuri SF et al (1995) The National Veterans Administration Surgical Risk Study: risk adjustment for the comparative assessment of the quality of surgical care. J Am Coll Surg 180:519–531

33. Khuri SF et al (1997) Risk adjustment of the postoperative mortality rate for the comparative assessment of quality of surgical care: results of the National Veterans Affairs Surgical Risk Study. J Am Coll Surg 185:315–327

34. Daley J et al (1997) Risk adjustment of the postoperative morbidity rate for the comparative assessment of the quality of surgical care: results of the National Veterans Affairs Surgical Risk Study. J Am Coll Surg 185:341–351

35. Khuri SF et al (1998) The Department of Veterans Affairs' NSQIP. Ann Surg 228:491–507

36. Katz S, Ford AB, Moskowitz RW, Jackson BA, Jaffe MW (1963) Studies of illness in the aged; the index of activities of daily living: a standardized measure of biological and psychosocial function. JAMA 185:914–919

37. Audisio RA, For the PACE Participants et al (2008) Shall we operate? Preoperative assessment in elderly cancer patients (PACE) can help: a SIOG surgical task force prospective study. Crit Rev Oncol Hematol 65(2):156–163

38. Anderson DJ et al (2008) Poor functional status as a risk factor for surgical site infection due to methicillin-resistant *Staphylococcus aureus*. Infect Control Hosp Epidemiol 29:832–839

39. Gerson MC et al (1985) Cardiac prognosis in noncardiac geriatric surgery. Ann Intern Med 103:832

40. Gerson MC, Hurst JM, Hertzberg VS et al (1990) Prediction of cardiac and pulmonary complications related to elective abdominal and noncardiac thoracic surgery in geriatric patients. Am J Med 88:101–107

41. Older P et al (1993) Preoperative evaluation of cardiac function and ischemia in elderly patients by cardiopulmonary exercise testing. Chest 103:701

42. Hlatky MA et al (1989) A brief self-administered questionnaire to determine functional capacity (the Duke's Activity Status Index). Am J Cardiol 64:651

43. Fleischer LA et al (2007) ACC/AHA 2007 guidelines on perioperative cardiovascular evaluation and care for noncardiac surgery. JACC 50(17):e159–e241

44. Lawrence VA et al (2004) Functional independence after major abdominal surgery in the elderly. J Am Coll Surg 199:762–772

45. Moriello C, Mayo NE, Feldman L, Carli F (2008) Validating the six-minute walk test as a measure of recovery after elective colon resection surgery. Arch Phys Med Rehabil 89(6):1083–1089

46. Reuben DB, Greendale GA, Harrison GG (1995) Nutrition screening in older persons. J Am Geriatr Soc 43:415

47. Lugli AK, Wykes L, Carli F (2008) Strategies for perioperative nutrition support in obese, diabetic and geriatric patients. Clin Nutr 27:16–24

48. Corti M et al (1994) Serum albumin level and physical disability as predictors of mortality in older persons. JAMA 272:1036

49. Gibbs J, Cull W, Henderson W, Daley J, Hur K, Khuri SF (1999) Preoperative serum albumin level as a predictor of operative mortality and morbidity. Arch Surg 134:136

50. Rosenthal RA (2004) Nutritional concerns in the older surgical patient. J Am Coll Surg 199:785–791

51. Detsky AS et al (1987) What is subjective global assessment of nutritional status? JPEN J Parenter Enteral Nutr 11:8–13

52. National Guideline Clearinghouse. Unintentional weight loss in the elderly. http://www.guideline.gov/summary/summary. aspx?ss=15&doc_id=9435&nbr=5=56. Accessed 15 May 2009

53. Batsis JA et al (2009) Body mass index and risk of adverse cardiac events in elderly patients with hip fracture: a population-based study. J Am Geriatr Soc 57:419–426

54. Freedland SJ et al (2005) Obesity and capsular incision at the time of open retropubic radical prostatectomy. J Urol 174:1798–1801

55. Detsky AS et al (1987) Predicting nutrition-associated complications for patients undergoing gastrointestinal surgery. JPEN J Parenter Enteral Nutr 11:440–446

56. Souba WW (1997) Nutritional support. N Engl J Med 336:41

57. Guizog Y, Lauque S, Vellas BJ (2002) Identifying the elderly at risk for malnutrition: the mini nutritional assessment. Clin Geriatr Med 18:1–19

58. Rubenstein LZ, Harker JO, Salva A et al (2001) Screening for undernutrition in geriatric practice: developing the short form mini nutritional assessment (MNA-SF). J Gerontol A Biol Sci Med Sci 56A:M366–M372

59. Tepaske R, Velthuis H, Oudemans-van Straaten HM et al (2001) Effect of preoperative oral immune-enhancing nutritional supplement on patients at high risk of infection after cardiac surgery: a randomised placebo-controlled trial. Lancet 358:696–701

60. Borson S, Scanlan JM, Chen P, Ganguli M (2003) The mini-cog as a screen for dementia: validation in a population-based sample. J Am Geriatr Soc 51:1451–1454

61. Folstein MF, Folstein SE, McHugh PR (1975) The mini-mental state examination: a practical method for grading the cognitive state of patients for the clinician. J Psychiatr Res 12:189

62. Crum RM, Anthony JC, Bassett SS, Folstein MF (1993) Population-based norms for the mini-mental state examination by age and educational level. JAMA 269(18):2386–2391

63. Brandt J, Spencer M, Folstein MF (1988) The telephone interview for cognitive status. Neuropsychiatry Neuropsychol Behav Neurol 1:111

64. Tariq SH, Tumosa N, Chibnall JT, Perry MH, Morley JE (2006) Comparison of the Saint Louis University mental status examination and the mini-mental state examination for detecting dementia and mild neurocognitive disorder – a pilot study. Am J Geriatr Psychiatry 14:900–910

65. Amador LF, Goodwin JS (2005) Postoperative delirium in the older patient. J Am Coll Surg 200:767–773

66. Marcantonio ER, Goldman L, Mangione CM et al (1994) A clinical prediction rule for delirium after elective noncardiac surgery. JAMA 271:134

67. Moller JT, Cluitmans P, Rasmussen LS et al (1998) Long-term postoperative cognitive dysfunction in the elderly: ISPOCD1 study. Lancet 351:857

68. National Library of Medicine. Michigan alcoholism screening test-geriatric version (MAST-G). http://www.ncbi.nlm.nih.gov/books/bv.fcgi?rid=hstat5.table.49350. Accessed 8 Jun 2009

69. Leung JM, Sands LP (2005) Are preoperative depressive symptoms associated with postoperative delirium in geriatric surgical patients? J Gerontol A Biol Sci Med Sci 60A:1563–1568

70. Sheik JI, Yesavage JA (1986) Geriatric depression scale (GDS): recent evidence and development of a shorter version. Clin Gerontol 5:165–172

71. Smetana GW, Lawrence VA, Cornell JE (2006) Preoperative pulmonary risk stratification for noncardiothoracic surgery: systematic review for the American College of Physicians. Ann Intern Med 144:581–595

72. Arozullah AM, Khuri SF, Henderson WG, For the Participants in the National Veterans Affairs Surgical Quality Improvement Program (2001) Development and validation of a multifactorial risk index for predicting postoperative pneumonia after major noncardiac surgery. Ann Intern Med 135:847–857

73. Mitchell CK et al (1998) Multivariate analysis of factors associated with postoperative pulmonary complications following general elective surgery. Arch Surg 133:194–198

74. Hogue CW Jr et al (1995) Swallowing dysfunction after cardiac operations: associated adverse outcomes and risk factors including intraoperative transesophageal echocardiography. J Thorac Cardiovasc Surg 110:517–522

75. Hall JC et al (1991) A multivariate analysis of the risk of pulmonary complications after laparotomy. Chest 99:923–927

76. Qaseem A, For the Clinical Efficacy Assessment Subcommittee of the American College of Physicians et al (2006) Risk assessment for and strategies to reduce perioperative pulmonary complications for patients undergoing noncardiothoracic surgery: a guideline from the American College of Physicians. Ann Intern Med 144:575–580

77. Tarhan S et al (1973) Risk of anesthesia and surgery in patients with bronchitis and chronic obstructive pulmonary disease. Surgery 74:720–720

78. Pedersen T et al (1990) A prospective study of risk factors and cardiopulmonary complications associated with anaesthesia and surgery: risk indicators of cardiopulmonary morbidity. Acta Anaesthesiol Scand 34:144–155

79. Gracey DR et al (1979) Preoperative pulmonary preparation of patients with chronic obstructive pulmonary disease: a prospective study. Chest 76:123–129

80. Garibaldi RA et al (1981) Risk factors for postoperative pneumonia. Am J Med 70:677–680

81. Philips EH et al (1994) Comparison of laparoscopic cholecystectomy in obese and nonobese patients. Am Surg 60:316–321

82. Southern Surgical Club (1991) A prospective analysis of 1518 laparoscopic cholecystectomies. N Engl J Med 324:1073–1078

83. Smetana GW (1999) Current concepts: preoperative pulmonary evaluation. N Engl J Med 340:937–944

84. Fujita T, Sakurai K (1995) Multivariate analysis of risk factors for postoperative pneumonia. Am J Surg 169:304–307

85. Alexander JW (1991) Transfusion-induced immunomodulation and infection. Transfusion 31:195–196

86. Suiter DM, Leder SB (2008) Clinical utility of the 3-ounce water swallow test. Dysphagia 23:244–250

87. Tisi GM (1979) Preoperative evaluation of pulmonary function. Am Rev Respir Dis 119:293–310

88. Joehl RJ (2005) Preoperative evaluation: pulmonary, cardiac, renal dysfunction and comorbidities. Surg Clin N Am 85:1061–1073

89. Levey AS, For the Modification of Diet in Renal Disease Study Group et al (1999) A more accurate method to estimate glomerular filtration rate from serum creatinine: a new prediction equation. Ann Intern Med 130(16):461–470

90. Harari D et al (2007) Proactive care of older people undergoing surgery ('POPS'): designing, embedding, evaluating and funding a comprehensive geriatric assessment service for older elective surgical patients. Age Ageing 36:190–196

91. Marcantonio ER, Flacker JM, Wright RJ, Resnick NM (2001) Reducing delirium after hip fracture: a randomized trial. J Am Geriatr Soc 49:516–522

92. Fukuse T, Satoda N, Hijiya K, Fuinaga T (2005) Importance of a comprehensive geriatric assessment in prediction of complications following thoracic surgery in elderly patients. Chest 127:886–891

Chapter 23
Invited Commentary

Jerry G. Reves

Practice of surgery and anesthesiology has changed immensely over time. I can best comment on the field of anesthesiology from my vantage point as a cardiac anesthesiologist, but obviously, I have admired the progress and development of all anesthesiology during my professional time in the field since 1969.

I became a cardiac anesthesiologist because of my interest in the cardiovascular system and the ability to rapidly alter it with acute pharmacologic intervention during surgery. This preoccupation with cardiac surgery and anesthesia began in 1965 with my pharmacology research as a medical student and continues till today. Over this near half-century, we have witnessed great changes and improvements in the operative care of patients which merit commentary.

Of the many things that have changed over time, none is greater than patient selection and operative procedure. In early cardiac anesthesiology practice, virtually all patients had congenital heart disease or acquired valvular disease. The most morbid cardiovascular disease, coronary artery disease, was not amenable to the surgical approach until the latter half of the past century. At the same time, the age of the adult population with the disease has been steadily increasing. I recall the days when we were doing our initial investigations into the anesthetic effects of patients undergoing coronary bypass surgery and the average age was almost always 55 years. Today, the average age is much higher for patients undergoing coronary artery bypass surgery than in the past. Reasons for this include less smoking among patients, multiple available drugs such as statins that prevent cardiac events, and greater variety of nonsurgical medical interventions that delay surgery.

Older patients present a variety of problems to cardiac anesthesiologists. For example, as patients age, there is increased sensitivity to the central nervous system drugs that anesthesiologists use for sedation, sleep, analgesia, and anesthesia. Awareness of this is critical in prevention of "overdosing" the patients that results in unwanted hemodynamic problems and prolonged somnolence after surgery. There is no question that the tissue of older patients is not the same as younger patients, and this leads to surgical hemostasis issues that can be challenging for the anesthesiologist as well as surgeon. The entire coagulation system is also less functional as patients age, again raising management problems around coagulation for the anesthesiologist and surgeon. Although no organs function in the very old as they do in the young patient, the lungs and liver seem to be resilient to the aging process, and this is important in the all important areas of oxygenation and drug metabolism, respectively. However, renal function tends to decline, and some of the drugs administered by the anesthesiologist depend on good renal clearance including some muscle relaxants and some of the antiarrhythmic medications. Awareness of these potential problems can avoid postoperative complications.

The greatest organ of concern to the cardiac anesthesiologist caring for elderly patient is the brain. All central nervous system complications are increased with age. These complications vary in severity from temporary confusion to proven susceptibility to cognitive impairment that can prohibit patients from returning to preoperative functional levels. Stroke is the most profound and dreaded of the neurologic consequences of cardiac surgery. The causes of neurologic adverse events are still largely unknown but probably are a combination of compromised cerebral vascular perfusion, emboli from the aorta, air and other debris when the heart or aorta are opened, thrombi from the atria in patients with atrial fibrillation, and many other possible causes. It is devastating to anesthesiologist, surgeon, family, and patient when a surgery patient is never quite the same after the procedure, especially when the heart or aorta has been "fixed."

Despite the risks with cardiac surgery and the additional risk that age confers on these patients, the results over the years have steadily improved even as we have cared for older and more complicated patients. This is a result of many innovations and improvements. The first of these is the education

J.G. Reves (✉)
Department of Anesthesia and Perioperative Medicine,
Cell and Molecular Pharmacology & Experimental Therapeutic,
Medical University of South Carolina, Charleston, SC, USA
e-mail: revesj@musc.edu

R.A. Rosenthal et al. (eds.), *Principles and Practice of Geriatric Surgery*,
DOI 10.1007/978-1-4419-6999-6_23, © Springer Science+Business Media, LLC 2011

of the cardiac anesthesiologist. Many of the anesthesiologists today who practice cardiac anesthesia have had formal education and a fellowship. There are journals, textbooks, and a whole new field of cardiac anesthesiology that has emerged over the past 30 years. Evidence-based knowledge guides the cardiac anesthesiologist today. The many drugs used today by anesthesiologists are better than years ago, and the anesthesiologist has an array of compounds to tailor to the needs of the patient. Technology is vastly improved as well. Monitoring allows the anesthesiologist to assess the patient on virtually a beat-to-beat basis and to look at the heart's function with echocardiography. The anesthesiologist now is diagnostician of the heart's anatomy and physiology, as well as pharmacology. The development of better pump oxygenators and many other life-assist devices has made it possible to get through surgery for patients who would not have been able to in the past. Finally, a major development, in my experience, was the introduction of myocardial protection with cardioplegia in the 1970s. This permitted prolonged periods of safe heart stoppage to allow the surgeon to perform a more perfect operation. We are still searching for other organ protective strategies.

Cardiac surgery has vastly improved as has cardiac anesthesiology over the past half-century. The two disciplines are complementary approaches to improve patient outcomes even in the very old. The same is true for all of our many surgical fields. Neither the surgeon nor the anesthesiologist can justifiably claim to have improved surgery for the patient alone; it has been a marvelous team effort unmatched in all medicine.

Chapter 24
Physiologic Response to Anesthesia in the Elderly

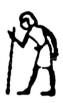

Aaron N. LacKamp and Frederick E. Sieber

Cardiovascular physiology: effects of anesthesia and aging

	Physiologic effects of anesthesia	Physiologic effects of aging	Combined effects of anesthesia and aging	Clinical implications
Venous	Slight dilation	Less compliant venous system	Decrease in preload	Greater fluctuation in preload for a given volume challenge
Arterial	Dilation	Decreased sympathetic response, stiffening of arterial system	Decreased systemic vascular resistance	Possible hypotension, increased vasopressor requirements
Heart	Decreased contractility	Diastolic dysfunction Left ventricular hypertrophy	Higher filling pressures needed to maintain cardiac output	Possible hypotension Susceptible to volume overload, dependant on late ventricular filling from atrial contribution
Baroreceptor	Response impaired	Response impaired	Response greatly impaired	Greater susceptibility to hypotension

Pulmonary physiology: effects of anesthesia and aging

	Physiologic effects of anesthesia	Physiologic effects of aging	Combined effects of anesthesia and aging and their clinical implications
Shunt	Hypoxic pulmonary vasoconstriction inhibited, atelectasis, V/Q̇ mismatching	V/Q̇ mismatching, increased closing capacity, increased PA pressures	Increased A-a gradient
Neuromodulation	Decreased response to hypoxia and hypercarbia	Decreased response to hypoxia and hypercarbia	Susceptible to hypercapnea Susceptible to hypoxemia Susceptible to residual anesthetic respiratory depressant effects
Mechanics	Decreased TV, $\dot{V}_E$, FRC (anesthetized and supine)	Decreased muscle mass, Loss of lung elasticity Decreased chest wall compliance	Increased work of breathing Increased dead space ventilation Susceptible to residual muscle relaxant
Protection	Impaired cough Impaired mucociliary clearance	Dysphagia, decreased cough reflex, decreased esophageal motility	Greater aspiration risk

Organ specific effects of anesthesia and aging

	Physiologic effects of anesthesia	Physiologic effects of aging	Clinical implications
Neurologic	Inhibition of neurotransmitter function	Decrease in neurotransmitters	Increased postoperative delirium and cognitive dysfunction
Renal	Decreased blood flow and glomerular filtration rate	Decreased renal mass	Decreased drug clearance; Susceptible to acute renal failure
Hepatic	Decreased blood flow		Decreased clearance of drugs with high hepatic extraction ratios
Endocrine	Impaired glucose tolerance	Impaired glucose tolerance	Hyperglycemia: Infection
Thermoregulation	Vasodilatation; decreased shivering threshold	Decreased muscle mass	Hypothermia: Infection Coagulopathy Intraoperative arrhythmia Postoperative myocardial infarction

A.N. LacKamp (✉)
Department of Anesthesiology and Critical Care Medicine, Johns
Hopkins Bayview Medical Center, Baltimore, MD, USA
e-mail: alackamp1@jhmi.edu

R.A. Rosenthal et al. (eds.), *Principles and Practice of Geriatric Surgery*,
DOI 10.1007/978-1-4419-6999-6_24, © Springer Science+Business Media, LLC 2011

Introduction

This chapter focuses on the physiologic components of aging and anesthesia that are likely to increase perioperative complications. The approach entails a separate description of anesthetic and aging physiology, followed by a discussion of how the two interact. Only the physiologic changes invoked by aging that provide important interactions with anesthesia are discussed. The reader is encouraged to consult relevant chapters contained in this textbook on preoperative assessment and specific organ systems for a more comprehensive discussion of the physiologic changes with aging.

Cardiovascular Implications of Anesthesia in the Elderly

Cardiovascular Effects of Anesthesia

Anesthetics decrease blood pressure by decreasing left ventricular contractility, decreasing systemic vascular resistance, and inhibiting baroreceptor function (Fig. 24.1).

Decreased ventricular contractility occurs with intravenous anesthetic agents. Propofol is the most common induction agent used today and is generally thought to be a direct

myocardial depressant. The negative inotropic effect of propofol is mediated by a decrease in intracellular Ca^{++} [1]. In fact, propofol is a greater myocardial depressant than the inhalational anesthetics [2]. Even ketamine, which produces a sympathetically mediated increased heart rate and blood pressure, causes some direct myocardial depressant effect [3, 4]. It appears that opioids have minimal effects on contractility [3]. It has been suggested that etomidate is the induction agent of choice in elderly patients with limited cardiovascular reserve [5]. In fact, hemodynamic stability after induction with this agent in severely compromised patients can be remarkable. Etomidate can cause transient adrenal depression [6,7], although the effect is of questionable significance.

In comparison to the intravenous agents, inhaled anesthetic agents are associated with less myocardial depression. Volatile anesthetics decrease inotropy by means of their effects on the L-type Ca^{++} channels, the sarcoplasmic reticulum, and the contractile apparatus [8]. Older drugs, such as halothane and enflurane, cause greater decreases in myocardial contractility than the modern agents isoflurane, sevoflurane, and desflurane [9–12]. Cardiac output is generally maintained under the modern agents because the myocardial depression is accompanied by afterload reduction [10, 13, 14].

Most anesthetic agents reduce afterload by decreasing arteriolar tone (Fig. 24.2). Propofol is a potent vasodilator [15]. Opioids are also vasodilators, though this effect is small when compared to propofol or the inhalational agents [16].

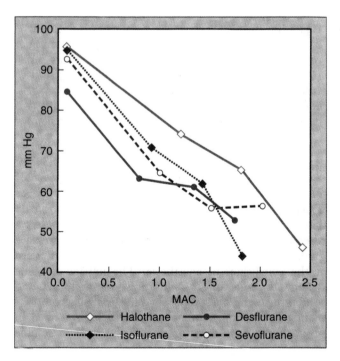

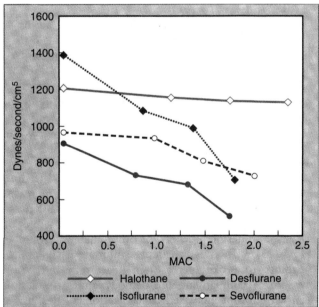

FIGURE 24.1 The effects of increasing concentrations (MAC) of halothane, isoflurane, desflurane, and sevoflurane on mean arterial pressure (mmHg) when administered to healthy volunteers. MAC is a means of defining dose of inhaled volatile anesthetics, higher MAC values representing higher anesthetic dose. One MAC equals the minimum alveolar concentration at which 50% of subjects aged 40 would not move in response to a surgical stimulus (used with permission from Calahan [121]).

FIGURE 24.2 The effects of increasing concentrations (MAC) of halothane, isoflurane, desflurane, and sevoflurane on systemic vascular resistance (dynes/s/cm⁵) when administered to healthy volunteers. MAC is a means of defining dose of inhaled volatile anesthetics, higher MAC values representing higher anesthetic dose. One MAC equals the minimum alveolar concentration at which 50% of subjects aged 40 would not move in response to a surgical stimulus (used with permission from Calahan [121]).

Anesthetic agents blunt baroreceptor function. The degree of inhibition depends on the anesthetic agents administered. As a result, tachycardia may not be observed in response to hypotension. Inhalational agents blunt baroreceptor function in a dose-dependent manner [17]. Although both opioids and propofol alter baroreceptor function, the effect is much less than observed with the inhalational agents [2]. Significant bradycardia can occur, however, because of the direct vagotonic effect of the opioids, especially fentanyl.

Anesthetic effects on venous pooling have been an area of intense investigation because of the possible causal relationship to deep vein thrombosis. However, the impact of general anesthetics on venous blood flow of the lower extremities is insignificant. Rather it seems that surgical stress is the primary mediator of perioperative decreases in venous blood flow [18].

Cardiovascular Changes with Aging That Effect Anesthetic Physiology

Cardiovascular aging is characterized by increased sympathetic tone, diminished β-adrenergic response, and stiffening of the left ventricle and venous and arterial systems. The increased sympathetic tone and arterial stiffening have several important long-term effects. Arterial stiffening causes hypertension late in systole, and this in turn causes an increased vascular load by means of increased pulse wave velocity and wave reflection [19]. This elevated vascular load is thought to be associated with the development of left ventricular hypertrophy [20].

With ventricular hypertrophy comes delayed relaxation and myocardial stiffening. Delayed relaxation impairs early diastolic filling [21]. This enhances the importance of late diastolic filling in maintaining cardiac output [22]. Late diastolic filling, however, must now overcome ventricular stiffness and that requires higher preload. The contribution of the atrial contraction to ventricular filling becomes critical and creates greater susceptibility to hypotension should atrial fibrillation occur. Thus, the combination of chronic hypertension and left ventricular hypertrophy contribute to a higher incidence of diastolic dysfunction in the elderly. To boost cardiac output in the setting of increased ventricular stiffness, elderly patients may depend on higher diastolic filling pressures. This impaired diastolic filling increases preload requirements. Elderly patients may be thereby predisposed to volume overload as they become increasingly reliant on preload to maintain cardiac output.

Another factor that affects diastolic filling of the ventricle is the relative time the heart spends in systole versus diastole. In the aging heart, length of diastole is shortened and systole is lengthened as a compensatory mechanism to maintain ejection fraction [23, 24]. Increased left ventricular filling does increase inotropy by means of the Starling forces, but the compensation for the systolic function is at the expense of higher diastolic pressures and greater time in systole [25–28]. Shortened diastolic time also affects coronary perfusion [27, 28].

Stiffening of the vessel walls occurs in the venous system with aging. Rigid veins fail to function as a preload buffer. The venous system normally contains 80% of blood volume, so low venous capacitance means that the aging venous system cannot accommodate excess volume or adapt to low volume states without a comparatively large change in filling pressure [29]. This loss of venous compliance may be associated with impairment in diastolic filling.

Conduction abnormalities occur in the elderly. Dilation and fibrotic change in the atria predispose the elderly to atrial fibrillation. Bradycardia is the second most common initiating rhythm after premature atrial contractions [30] and may increase the incidence of new onset atrial fibrillation. The high incidence of sinus bradycardia may be related to drop-out of sinus node pacemaker cells to as little as 10% of levels seen in young adults [23]. New onset atrial fibrillation during the perioperative period in the elderly frequently results in significant blood pressure changes. The cell populations in the aging AV node are maintained. AV conduction slows with aging, however, resulting in lengthened *P–R* interval [31, 32].

Cardiovascular responsiveness in the elderly is impaired. For instance, maximal heart rate decreases with aging, and can be estimated by the formula: maximum predicted heart rate = 220 – age [33]. As a consequence, the ability to increase cardiac output by means of an increase in heart rate is limited [20]. There is reduced adrenergic responsiveness [34], affecting both the β-adrenergic [5, 35] absolute heart rate [36] response and inotropy [37] and α-adrenergic mediated arteriolar tone [38].

Rapid response to hypotension is mediated by baroreceptor function. The stiffening of arterial walls in the elderly may contribute to the well-documented decrease in baroreceptor response. There is a decrease in baseline vagal tone [39] and consequently diminished carotid sinus baroreceptor response to hypotension in the elderly [40, 41].

The aging of the autonomic nervous system is characterized by progressively limited capacity to adapt to stress. A main concern of the anesthesia provider in evaluating the elderly patient is the response to acute hemodynamic challenges in which the autonomic nervous system and its effectors may play an important role. The preoperative history can provide some indication of the competence of the autonomic nervous system. The patient should be specifically questioned concerning signs and symptoms of exercise intolerance, orthostatic hypotension, temperature intolerance, and unusual patterns of sweating (especially increased upper body sweating). If the history suggests that autonomic nervous system responses are attenuated, one has good reason to suspect that blood pressure lability will occur perioperatively.

The Interplay of the Aging Cardiovascular System and the Effects of Anesthesia

Cardiovascular compensation occurs even in the healthy aging patient, and the significance of age-related change varies greatly on an individual basis. Physiologic limitations, however, may be unmasked by anesthesia.

The most frequent cardiovascular problem that occurs with anesthesia in the elderly is hemodynamic instability, which manifests itself primarily as hypotension. This effect is mediated through interactions with myocardium, preload, and afterload. Anesthesia causes sympatholysis which results in decreased afterload because the primary resistance vessels are sympathetic sensitive. However, the ability to augment cardiac output to maintain blood pressure in the face of decreased systemic vascular resistance is lessened. Anesthesia decreases contractility and inhibits baroreceptor responses. This makes the aging heart with diastolic dysfunction more dependent on adequate preload to maintain cardiac output. The margin of safety in administering an anesthetic decreases as the aging heart with diastolic dysfunction becomes increasingly preload dependant. Important clinical situations in which hypotension frequently occurs in the elderly in the setting of relative perioperative hypovolemia include causes such as chronic hypertension, prolonged NPO status, impaired renal salt conservation, and use of diuretics [5].

Most anesthetic drugs can be used safely without hemodynamic compromise in the elderly population if several principles are kept in mind. Anesthetic dose requirements of both intravenous induction agents and inhalational agents decrease with age. In addition, slower titration of medication as opposed to bolus administration may be warranted because changes in body composition alter the pharmacokinetics of intravenous agents. The loss of lean body mass, increase in percent body fat, and 20–30% decrease in blood volume observed with aging cause the initial drug bolus to be dispersed in a reduced volume of distribution. The so-called greater "sensitivity" of aged patients to the bolus administration of certain drugs has been related to a reduction in either the initial volume of distribution or the initial distribution clearance. In elderly patients compared to younger ones, the same bolus dose will generate a markedly higher plasma concentration and thus a greater pharmacologic effect.

The elderly are at increased risk of fluid overload during management of hypotension and correction of fluid deficits. The balance of euvolemia is more delicate in the elderly than in the younger patient, as the clinical range between hypovolemia and fluid overload is narrowed. Perioperative congestive heart failure in the elderly occurs in a bimodal type of time frame. It may first appear in the immediate recovery phase after anesthetic emergence. It is most likely to occur when sympathetic tone reappears and may be the result of pain or fluid shifts from the peripheral vasculature to the heart. It may next appear on postoperative day 2–3, and likely occurs with mobilization of extravascular fluid. Late postoperative congestive heart failure is exacerbated by underlying renal dysfunction, and its prevention requires physician attentiveness and diuresis.

Mode of ventilation during anesthesia can have significant cardiovascular effects in the elderly. Positive pressure ventilation decreases venous return via an increase in intrathoracic pressure. Similarly, hyperventilation can cause hypotension via impairment of venous return. An additional mechanism of hypotension is the decrease in sympathetic tone associated with hypocapnea [42–44]. Spontaneous ventilation is associated with less hypotension in the elderly patient with diminished cardiovascular reserve, because venous return is augmented during inspiration.

The prone position can be associated with a significant reduction in the cardiac index secondary to vena caval compression [45]. Both the sitting position and reverse Trendelenberg position decrease venous return and can worsen hypotension in severely preload-dependant elderly patients. Trendelenberg augments venous return. Lateral position is generally not associated with significant hemodynamic effects. Although right lateral decubitus has improved venous return over the supine and left lateral decubitus positions, the effect is probably minimal except in patients with congestive heart failure [46].

Laparoscopic insufflation causes decreased venous return. This, coupled with the depressant effect of anesthetic drugs, can result in hypotension. It is typical for $PaCO_2$ to slowly rise after 30 min of laparoscopy. This results from the increased CO_2 load and the decreased ability to eliminate CO_2 secondary to pneumoperitoneum. The hypercapnea and its associated increase in sympathetic tone [47] may cause hypertension and ectopy. Correction of hypercapnea requires ventilatory changes such as increased respiratory rate, tidal volume, and peak airway pressures, which may further impair venous return.

Elderly patients frequently take cardiovascular medications, which interact with anesthetics. For instance, bradycardias are apt to occur in anesthetized patients being treated with β-blockers and calcium channel blockers. Bradycardia may also be associated with anesthesia-specific medications such as high-dose narcotics, acetylcholinesterase inhibitors for reversal of neuromuscular junction blockade, and with a rare acetylcholine-like effect of succinylcholine (a short-acting neuromuscular relaxant). Under rare instances, heart block can occur; the risk increases with preexisting bundle branch block. Preoperative use of ACE inhibitors [48] and angiotensin receptor blockers [49] has been closely associated with increased risk of hypotension in anesthetized patients. It is controversial, however, whether discontinuing these medications preoperatively will decrease the incidence of perioperative hypotension.

Regional Anesthesia: Spinal and Epidural

Spinal and epidural anesthesia cause significant afterload reduction due to blockade of sympathetic fibers. Because the sympathetic fibers are small in diameter, they are highly susceptible to local anesthetic blockade. The sympathectomy associated with regional anesthesia has greater effects in the elderly because of limited ability to mount a compensatory response and possibly greater propensity to obtain a higher spinal anesthetic level [50]. With epidural anesthetics, the decreased compliance of the epidural space in the elderly is associated with achievement of a higher dermatome level of anesthesia with the same dose of local anesthetic in comparison to younger patients. A decrease in blood pressure with neuraxial blockade is nearly universal and often heralds the onset of motor and sensory blockade (Fig. 24.3). Preload reduction contributes to hypotension as well as afterload reduction. Tachycardia is the normal compensatory response but may be impaired in the elderly. With a very high sensory level (T1–T4), the cardioaccelerator fibers may be blocked, thus precluding the tachycardia response and predisposing the patient to severe hypotension and reduction in cardiac output. When hypotension occurs after administration of spinal anesthesia in the elderly, volume loading is generally insufficient to correct the hypotension, and vasopressors are generally required [51]. Furthermore, excessive volume loading can be associated with ventricular dysfunction [52].

It should be noted that the careless use of spinal anesthesia in a hypovolemic patient with limited cardiac reserve will likely result in cardiovascular collapse. These events are asso-

ciated with profound bradycardia resulting from activation of the Bezold–Jarisch reflex. When patients are hypovolemic and spinal anesthesia is to be used, it may be best to use a continuous catheter technique. This allows slow titration of drug so that hemodynamic changes have a slower onset and can be treated in a timely manner. Epidural anesthesia also can be administered slowly via a catheter so that the hemodynamic response can be gradual and controlled. Even with gradual administration, there is a risk of rapid hemodynamic changes if the patient is not closely monitored.

Spinal and epidural anesthesia can be desirable modes of anesthesia in the elderly in order to attenuate the stress response to surgery, avoid central nervous system depressants, avoid airway manipulation and its associated pulmonary complications, and to assist in postoperative pain management.

Pulmonary Implications of Anesthesia in the Elderly

Pulmonary Effects of Anesthesia

During spontaneous ventilation, the inhalational agents decrease tidal volume and minute ventilation [53–55]. This is associated with an increase in $PaCO_2$ and respiratory rate (Fig. 24.4). In the absence of opioids or other respiratory depressants, profound tachypnea can occur. Despite the increase in respiratory rate, however, the net effect on the alveoli is a decrease in ventilation. In the anesthetized state, spontaneous ventilation in the supine position results in decreased functional residual capacity due to cephalad displacement of the diaphragm and inward displacement of the ribcage [56]. The work of breathing [57] is increased because the weight of the abdominal contents must be displaced with inspiration. Decreased functional residual capacity means less oxygen reserve prior to any apneic interval.

Normal ventilatory drive depends on central and peripheral chemoreceptor response to hypercapnea, hydrogen ion concentration, and pH. The response to hypercapnea is independent and synergistic with the response to hypoxia. The carbon dioxide response curve is shifted to the right under anesthesia requiring higher CO_2 [58] for a given minute ventilation. Likewise, there is impaired response to hypoxia with even minimal residual inhalational anesthetic levels [59].

Ventilation–perfusion (V/Q) mismatching occurs during anesthesia and is caused largely by atelectasis [60] and impaired hypoxic pulmonary vasoconstriction. Atelectasis commonly forms in dependent regions of the lung shortly after induction of anesthesia and progresses as gas is absorbed from poorly ventilated regions [61]. Positive end-expiratory

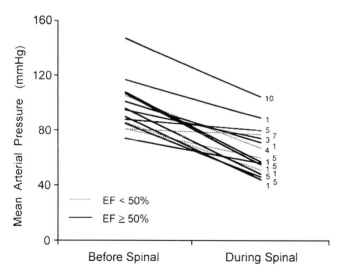

FIGURE 24.3 The effect of spinal anesthesia on mean arterial pressure is shown in 15 elderly men with cardiac disease. The thoracic block level is noted on the "during spinal" side of the graph. The four patients with a baseline ejection fraction (EF) less than 50% were no more or less likely to demonstrate significant decreases in mean arterial pressure than those with normal baseline ejection fraction (used with permission from Rooke et al. [122]).

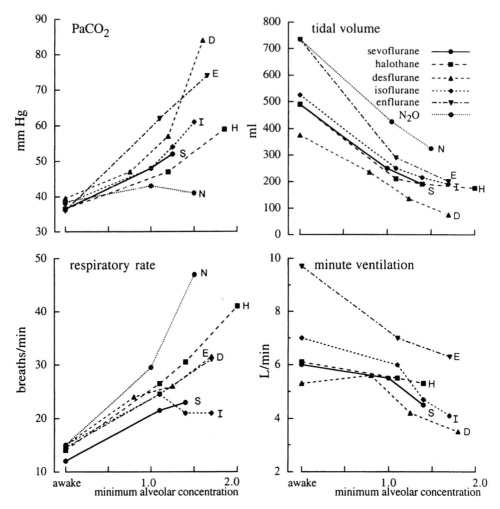

Figure 24.4 Comparison of mean changes in resting $PaCO_2$, tidal volume, respiratory rate, and minute ventilation in patients anesthetized with either halothane, isoflurane, enflurane, sevoflurane, desflurance, or nitrous oxide. Anesthetic-induced tachypnea compensates in part for the ventilatory depression caused by all volatile anesthetics (decrease in minute ventilation and tidal volume and concomitant increase in $PaCO_2$). Desflurane results in the greatest increase in $PaCO_2$ with corresponding reductions in tidal volume and minute ventilation. Isoflurane, like all other inhaled agents, increases respiratory rate, but does not result in dose-dependent tachypnea. MAC is a means of defining dose of inhaled volatile anesthetics, higher MAC values representing higher anesthetic dose. One MAC equals the minimum alveolar concentration at which 50% of subjects age 40d would not move in response to a surgical stimulus (used with permission from Barash et al. [123]).

pressure can reduce atelectasis formation, but large tidal volume recruitment maneuvers are generally necessary to reverse shunt [62]. Hypoxic pulmonary vasoconstriction reduces blood flow to underventilated regions, but this mechanism is partially inhibited by anesthetic agents [63].

Other anesthetic effects on the pulmonary system include impairment of bronchial mucociliary clearance in intubated patients [64, 65] and impairment of swallowing reflex from pharyngeal dysfunction and risk of aspiration at subhypnotic concentrations of anesthetic [66]. Decreased pharyngeal tone results in upper airway obstruction. The incidence of apnea due to upper airway obstruction is increased in obese individuals. Inhalational anesthetics are potent bronchial dilators in the face of bronchoconstriction [67], although bronchoconstriction can be induced during anesthesia by the stimulus of tracheal intubation [68] and by the inhalational agent desflurane [69].

Pulmonary Changes with Aging That Effect Anesthetic Physiology

The loss of muscle mass with aging does not spare the muscles of respiration. Decreased muscle strength in the intercostals and accessory muscles of respiration impairs the ability to perform maximal ventilatory maneuvers and impairs the ability to mount a strong cough. Clearance of secretions is in part dependent on the patient having sufficient strength to perform the maneuver. Elderly patients are less able to maintain adequate tidal volume and generate sufficient inspiratory or expiratory force. If the weakness is severe enough, it may interfere with extubation and weaning efforts.

Less efficient gas exchange is inherent in the aging lung. The incidence of overt chronic lung disease increases with age, a problem compounded by smoking. Normal structural changes account for some of the increased risk of respiratory compromise in the elderly. There is a loss of elasticity of the lung tissue, and the chest wall becomes less compliant. The result is increased residual volume of the lung. Total lung capacity remains unchanged or slightly decreases, but the increase in residual volume causes a decrease in vital capacity [70]. The effect is increased work of breathing for given level of gas exchange, and increased shunt and dead space. Functional residual capacity also increases along with residual volume, yet the geriatric patient is more susceptible to hypoxia stemming from the increased closing capacity of the small airways. As the aging lung loses elasticity, the smallest airways are no longer stented open by elastic tissue but instead rely on some minimal amount of lung inflation, or closing capacity, to maintain small airway patency. As lung volumes decrease with active expiration, there comes a point when the summation of intra-airway pressure and elastic forces stenting open distal air passages become insufficient to overcome the tendency of these distal airways to collapse. There is a general trend toward increased closing capacity with aging. By age 66, closing capacity exceeds FRC in the sitting position [71]. When closing capacity exceeds FRC, some portion of the lung will be ineffective in gas exchange during part of the respiratory cycle. This mechanism leads to increasing V/Q mismatch in the elderly and a gradual decrease in blood oxygenation. On average, the PaO_2 decreases 0.31 mmHg per year of age [70].

Other changes in the elderly that are of importance to anesthetic physiology include a blunting of the response to hypoxia and hypercarbia [72, 73]. In addition, aging leads to dysphagia, decreased esophageal motility, and decreased cough reflex.

The Interplay of the Aging Pulmonary System and the Effects of Anesthesia

Pulmonary complications are a major cause of postoperative morbidity in the elderly. Postoperative respiratory complications are associated with 40% of the perioperative deaths in patients older than 65 years of age [74]. The aging of the pulmonary system and anesthesia interact to increase the likelihood of these events. Increased A–a gradient is likely to occur under anesthesia. Impaired oxygenation is secondary to the anesthetic effects of decreased minute ventilation, increased atelectasis, and the aging effect of increased closing capacity. In addition, hypoxic pulmonary vasoconstriction is impeded by the aging effect on pulmonary vascular rigidity and by anesthetic inhibition. Ventilatory failure may occur secondary to the combined effects of anesthesia and aging to decrease minute

ventilation, depress hypoxic and hypercarbic respiratory drive, and increase the work of breathing in the face of decreased muscle mass. Many of the changes outlined act in concert with a less effective cough and impaired airway protective mechanisms to increase the risk of aspiration and pneumonia.

The pulmonary implications of residual anesthetic effects after emergence is a serious issue in the elderly. Of primary importance are the effects of muscle relaxants. Age-related pharmacokinetic and pharmacodynamic changes interact with the decrease in muscle mass to potentiate the effects of these drugs, thus increasing the risk of respiratory compromise in the early postoperative period [75–77]. The respiratory depressant effects of sedative agents, narcotics, and inhalational anesthetics are prolonged. As a special case, the inhaled anesthetics are eliminated primarily by the lung. Decreases in minute ventilation and cardiac output, as well as V/Q mismatch, will prolong the elimination of inhaled anesthetic agents [78, 79].

The insufflation pressure during laparoscopy displaces the diaphragm cephalad; this reduces tidal volumes toward that of the dead space volume. In this case, adequate ventilation is maintained either by increasing the airway pressure to maintain adequate tidal volume or by decreasing insufflation pressures. Under these conditions, atelectasis develops at an accelerated rate. Low levels of PEEP may be used in this setting as long as intrathoracic pressures do not impair venous return so as to cause hemodynamic compromise.

Regional Anesthesia and Pulmonary Implications

With spinal or epidural blockade of sufficient dermatomal height for abdominal procedures, the musculature of the thoracic cage will be anesthetized, eliminating the contribution of the intercostal muscles to respiration. Spontaneous ventilation is still possible, however, because the diaphragm is the major muscle of respiration. In these circumstances, loss of accessory muscle function may be an issue in patients with limited pulmonary reserve. Protective airway reflexes are maintained although cough may be impaired.

Spinal and epidural anesthesia have been advocated as a means of decreasing postoperative pulmonary complications, although there is little data to support this contention. Epidural anesthesia continued into the postoperative period may help in promoting early mobilization, cough, and deep breathing by relieving postoperative pain. In theory, spinal or epidural anesthesia helps to minimize the administration of central nervous system depressants during the perioperative period, thereby maintaining protective airway reflexes. It is common practice, however, for sedation to be administered during spinal and epidural anesthetics. Therefore, it is important to identify at risk patients, and verify recovery of protective reflexes in the elderly after an anesthetic, including sedation for spinal.

Physiologic Response to Anesthesia in the Aging Nervous System

Age-related decreases in central nervous system functional reserve lead to alterations in pharmacodynamics, and increased susceptibility to postoperative cognitive dysfunction and delirium.

Altered Pharmacodynamics

Brain sensitivity to most anesthetic agents increases with age. This necessitates decreasing the drug dose in the elderly (Fig. 24.5). Some components of the elderly drug response can be explained by pharmacokinetic changes associated with aging; these are specific to each drug. The underlying mechanism to explain altered brain pharmacodynamics is unclear at present. Altered brain pharmacodynamics may

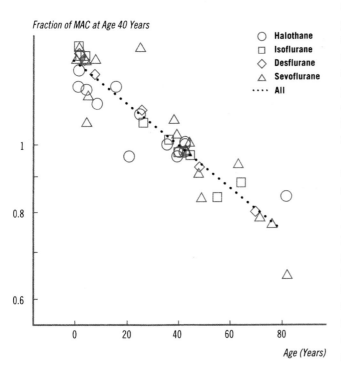

Figure 24.5 Aging influences MAC in humans for desflurane, isoflurane, halothane, and sevoflurane. MAC is at its peak in humans less than 1 year of age, decreasing by approximately 40% in older adults. MAC is a means of defining dose of inhaled volatile anesthetics, higher MAC values representing higher anesthetic dose. One MAC equals the minimum alveolar concentration at which 50% of subjects aged 40 would not move in response to a surgical stimulus (used with permission from Eger et al. [124]).

result from age-related changes in the receptors, signal transduction, or homeostatic mechanisms. Within the central nervous system, aging is associated with decreases in dopaminergic and cholinergic neurons and receptors as well as a decrease in the number of synapses. There are also alterations in brain phospholipid chemistry associated with changes in second messengers such as diacylglycerol [80]. A definitive association between these changes and age-related brain pharmacodynamics has yet to be established.

Increased Susceptibility to Postoperative Delirium and Cognitive Dysfunction

The incidence of postoperative delirium and postoperative cognitive dysfunction may exceed 50% in certain surgical populations [81]. The incidence of cognitive dysfunction in elderly patients after major surgery seems to be highest after cardiac surgery and hip fracture repair [82, 83]. Thus, postoperative delirium and postoperative cognitive dysfunction are two of the most common postoperative complications in the elderly, and their incidence may be higher than that of myocardial infarction or respiratory failure [81, 84, 85].

A wide variety of drugs are associated with delirium, many of which are used frequently in the perioperative period. These include benzodiazepines, anticholinergics, opioids, corticosteroids, anticonvulsants, antidopaminergic antiemetics, and H_2 antagonists [86]. Although a recent critical review of the literature concerning the relationship of psychoactive medications and delirium found that the evidence for an association is weak, the authors attributed this to methodological issues in the studies and concluded that a relationship may indeed exist [87].

The hypothesis that postoperative delirium is the result of age-associated central cholinergic deficiency has been the driving force behind studies examining the role of intraoperative management as it relates to postoperative delirium. Arguably, the most important decision concerning anesthetic management is whether patients should have a regional or general anesthetic. In theory, regional anesthetic techniques should be associated with a reduced incidence of postoperative delirium because these techniques minimize exposure to agents that influence central cholinergic activity and drugs that are associated with delirium in medical patients, such as opiates and benzodiazepines. Furthermore, regional anesthesia deeply suppresses the neuroendocrine stress response to surgery [88–90]. Unfortunately, studies to date have not demonstrated that regional anesthetic techniques reduce the incidence of postoperative delirium [91].

Postoperative pain increases the risk of postoperative delirium. Interestingly, maximum pain and pain with movement are not predictive of delirium. Only high levels of rest pain are associated with postoperative delirium [92]. As a class, opiates are not associated with postoperative delirium, except for meperidine [93]. This may be because of its atropine-like structure and influence on brain cholinergic activity. Postoperative use of benzodiazepines has also been associated with postoperative delirum [94].

It is important to recognize that postoperative delirium may be the presenting symptom of a number of complications, including sepsis, urinary tract infections, myocardial infarction, stroke, pneumonia, etc [95]. Thus, the first step in managing postoperative delirium is to identify and treat underlying medical and/or surgical causes.

Many surgeons are aware of patients who complain after surgery of difficulties performing cognitive tasks that they were previously able to do without difficulty. Postoperative cognitive dysfunction is the term used to describe this condition. It can consist of a variety of cognitive deficits. Unlike patients with postoperative delirium, however, those with postoperative cognitive dysfunction are generally alert and oriented.

In vitro and animal studies suggest that inhalational and intravenous anesthetic agents alter neuronal function after exposure [96–98]. Neurons exposed to volatile anesthetics in vitro have increased oligomerization and cytotoxicity of β-amyloid, the protein associated with Alzheimer disease [98]. In aged rats, exposure to anesthetic agents causes long-term declines in cognitive function [99–101]. The clinical relevance of these findings is unclear because studies examining the influence of regional versus general anesthesia on the incidence of postoperative cognitive dysfunction in humans have not found a difference between the two techniques [91, 102]. One reason may be that patients who received regional anesthesia in those studies also received intravenous sedatives. Another may be that postoperative management was not controlled. Stress plays a role in cognitive function [103]. Although regional anesthetic techniques attenuate the surgical stress response [88, 104], if these techniques were not continued into the postoperative period, any benefit may have been negated. Also, by not continuing regional analgesic techniques into the postoperative period, patients were exposed to higher doses of opiates, which may have influenced their cognitive outcomes. Interestingly, unlike the case with postoperative delirium, perioperative use of benzodiazepines is not associated with postoperative cognitive dysfunction [105, 106].

Though the exact mechanisms by which postoperative delirium and postoperative cognitive dysfunction occur are not well understood, the likely cause is an acute insult in a vulnerable patient. The degree of surgical or physiological insult required to precipitate postoperative delirium or postoperative cognitive dysfunction varies from patient to patient. In patients with a high degree of preoperative cognitive reserve, a substantial insult is required for postoperative delirium and/or postoperative cognitive dysfunction to occur. Conversely, in patients with a lower degree of cognitive reserve, a relatively minor stress is all that is necessary for postoperative delirium and/or postoperative cognitive dysfunction to develop [107].

Renal Implications of Anesthesia in the Elderly

Anesthesia decreases renal perfusion and glomerular filtration rate. When a patient receives an anesthetic, glomerular filtration rate may be acutely decreased by hypotension, redistribution of blood flow away from body core, or a specific pressure effect of laparoscopy. The potential for postoperative acute renal injury is greater with preexisting renal disease.

Drug excretion and metabolism by the kidney is proportionately decreased with aging. Many anesthetic drugs depend on renal elimination. Dose adjustment of most medications should be anticipated in the elderly. Of special note, many of the commonly used opioids and muscle relaxants have some component of renal elimination, and their effects are prolonged in the elderly. Fortunately, there are alternate drugs, with little or no dependence on renal elimination. Inhaled anesthetics are eliminated primarily by the respiratory route. Serum enzymes degrade certain drugs such as cisatracurium, remifentanil, and chloroprocaine. Due to the blood stream degradation of cisatracurium, this agent may be of special value in the elderly patient with renal impairment who requires muscle relaxation.

Hepatic Implications of Anesthesia in the Elderly

Hepatic functional reserve is fairly well maintained with healthy aging. As a result, anesthetic drug binding to serum proteins produced by the liver is not significantly affected. One potential effect of anesthesia is decreased hepatic blood flow. Hepatic blood flow parallels cardiac output and correlates with the rate of elimination of drugs with high hepatic extraction ratio [108, 109]. Commonly administered anesthetic agents with high hepatic extraction ratios include fentanyl, sufentanyl, lidocaine, meperidine, ketamine, and propofol. Drugs with lower hepatic extraction ratios are less impacted by hepatic blood flow.

Endocrine Implications of Anesthesia in the Elderly

Hyperglycemia is a frequent issue during surgery in the elderly patient. Inhalational anesthetics impair glucose tolerance. The mechanism is unclear but may be secondary to direct inhibition of insulin secretion [110]. Thus, hyperglycemia occurs in the anesthetized state with or without surgery. Insulin resistance and prevalence of diabetes is increased in the elderly. This effect is compounded in the face of obesity.

Thermoregulation

Normal human thermoregulation allows only small fluctuations in core temperature within the narrow interthreshold range of 0.2°C; this range can be extended to 2–4°C under the effects of anesthesia [111]. Multiple inputs from the core and periphery contribute to the detection of temperature variation. Peripheral sensation tends to contribute largely to behavioral aversion to unpleasant environments, while core sensing mechanisms have a relatively larger impact on autonomic responses [111]. The response to decreased temperature begins when the threshold of vasoconstriction is reached. Beyond the vasoconstriction threshold lays the threshold for the energy intensive shivering mechanism. Non-shivering thermogenesis, although important in neonates, is negligible in adults. The response to elevation in core temperature begins when the threshold for sweating is reached. With extremes of temperature elevation, active vasodilation can also occur [111].

During anesthesia, hypothermia is a common challenge as a consequence of several colluding factors. Preparations for surgery entail exposing large surfaces of the patient's skin. Operating rooms are traditionally kept very cool. Under anesthesia, vasodilation occurs as a direct anesthetic effect. This results in an immediate decrease in core body temperature from a redistribution of body heat from the core to the periphery, and eventually results in greater dissipation of heat to the environment. By central mechanisms, anesthesia decreases the threshold temperature for vasoconstriction and shivering, allowing drift of the core temperature.

The elderly are predisposed to hypothermia [70, 112] as a result of decreased muscle mass and neural and hormonal mechanisms. Thyroid function and overall metabolic rate decrease with aging. Decreased muscle mass leads to greater heat loss and less heat generation. The neural thermoregulatory mechanisms [112] are altered with a lowered threshold for vasoconstriction, decreased maximum vasoconstriction response, decreased α-adrenergic response [113, 114], and decreased thermal perception.

These changes with aging compound the tendency, present among all patients, to develop hypothermia during both general and spinal anesthesia. The effects occur across a wide spectrum of anesthetic techniques and agents [115].

Complications of hypothermia include possible coagulopathy [116, 117], increased risk of surgical wound infection [118], and increased cardiac risk [119, 120] secondary to hypermetabolism if shivering occurs after emergence from anesthesia. See the physiology table at the beginning of this chapter, which summarizes the interactions of anesthesia and aging in the brain, kidney, liver, endocrine system, and with thermoregulation.

Summary

Aging affects every body system, so the interplay between anesthesia and aging is necessarily complex. Because of decreases in hepatic and renal reserve, pharmacodynamic/pharmacokinetic changes must be taken into account when administering anesthetics. Other important considerations include the cardiopulmonary and neurologic systems. Labile hemodynamics and potential for diastolic heart failure are the important cardiovascular issues as compared to younger adults. The risks of postoperative ventilatory failure and pneumonia are increased in the elderly. Postoperative cognitive dysfunction is a common entity after all types of major surgery. At this time, it is difficult to define the optimal anesthetic for the elderly because both regional and general anesthesia affect many of these organ systems, and definitive data concerning the advantage of one anesthetic technique over another has yet to be established.

References

1. Kanaya N, Murray PA, Damron DS (1998) Propofol and ketamine only inhibit intracellular Ca2+ transients and contraction in rat ventricular myocytes at supraclinical concentrations. Anesthesiology 88(3):781–791
2. Nishikawa K, Kanaya N, Kawamata M, Namiki A (2004) Left ventricular mechanical performance in elderly patients after induction of anaesthesia. A comparison of inhalational induction with sevoflurane and intravenous induction with fentanyl and propofol. Anaesthesia 59(10):948–953
3. Kawakubo A, Fujigaki T, Uresino H, Zang S, Sumikawa K (1999) Comparative effects of etomidate, ketamine, propofol, and fentanyl on myocardial contractility in dogs. J Anesth 13(2):77–82
4. Gelissen HP, Epema AH, Henning RH, Krijnen HJ, Hennis PJ, den Hertog A (1996) Inotropic effects of propofol, thiopental, midazolam, etomidate, and ketamine on isolated human atrial muscle. Anesthesiology 84(2):397–403
5. Priebe HJ (2000) The aged cardiovascular risk patient. Br J Anaesth 85(5):763–778
6. Fragen RJ, Shanks CA, Molteni A, Avram MJ (1984) Effects of etomidate on hormonal responses to surgical stress. Anesthesiology 61(6):652–656
7. Wagner RL, White PF, Kan PB, Rosenthal MH, Feldman D (1984) Inhibition of adrenal steroidogenesis by the anesthetic etomidate. N Engl J Med 310(22):1415–1421
8. Hanley PJ, ter Keurs HE, Cannell MB (2004) Excitation-contraction coupling in the heart and the negative inotropic action of volatile anesthetics. Anesthesiology 101(4):999–1014

9. Weiskopf RB, Cahalan MK, Eger EI 2nd et al (1991) Cardiovascular actions of desflurane in normocarbic volunteers. Anesth Analg 73(2):143–156

10. Stevens WC, Cromwell TH, Halsey MJ, Eger EI 2nd, Shakespeare TF, Bahlman SH (1971) The cardiovascular effects of a new inhalation anesthetic, forane, in human volunteers at constant arterial carbon dioxide tension. Anesthesiology 35(1):8–16

11. Pagel PS, Kampine JP, Schmeling WT, Warltier DC (1991) Alteration of left ventricular diastolic function by desflurane, isoflurane, and halothane in the chronically instrumented dog with autonomic nervous system blockade. Anesthesiology 74(6):1103–1114

12. Malan TP Jr, DiNardo JA, Isner RJ et al (1995) Cardiovascular effects of sevoflurane compared with those of isoflurane in volunteers. Anesthesiology 83(5):918–928

13. Eger EI 2nd (1981) Isoflurane: a review. Anesthesiology 55(5):559–576

14. Bastard OG, Carter JG, Moyers JR, Bross BA (1984) Circulatory effects of isoflurane in patients with ischemic heart disease: a comparison with halothane. Anesth Analg 63(7):635–639

15. Rouby JJ, Andreev A, Leger P et al (1991) Peripheral vascular effects of thiopental and propofol in humans with artificial hearts. Anesthesiology 75(1):32–42

16. Moore PG, Quail AW, Cottee DB, McIlveen SA, White SW (2000) Effect of fentanyl on baroreflex control of circumflex coronary conductance. Clin Exp Pharmacol Physiol 27(12):1028–1033

17. Nagasaki G, Tanaka M, Nishikawa T (2001) The recovery profile of baroreflex control of heart rate after isoflurane or sevoflurane anesthesia in humans. Anesth Analg 93(5):1127–1131

18. Knaggs AL, Delis KT, Mason P, Macleod K (2005) Perioperative lower limb venous haemodynamics in patients under general anaesthesia. Br J Anaesth 94(3):292–295

19. Nichols WW, O'Rourke MF, Avolio AP et al (1985) Effects of age on ventricular-vascular coupling. Am J Cardiol 55(9):1179–1184

20. Levy D, Anderson KM, Savage DD, Kannel WB, Christiansen JC, Castelli WP (1988) Echocardiographically detected left ventricular hypertrophy: prevalence and risk factors. The Framingham heart study. Ann Intern Med 108(1):7–13

21. Schulman SP, Lakatta EG, Fleg JL, Lakatta L, Becker LC, Gerstenblith G (1992) Age-related decline in left ventricular filling at rest and exercise. Am J Physiol 263(6 Pt 2):H1932–H1938

22. Groban L (2005) Diastolic dysfunction in the older heart. J Cardiothorac Vasc Anesth 19(2):228–236

23. Rooke GA (2003) Cardiovascular aging and anesthetic implications. J Cardiothorac Vasc Anesth 17(4):512–523

24. O'Rourke MF (2007) Arterial aging: pathophysiological principles. Vasc Med 12(4):329–341

25. Plehn G, Vormbrock J, Perings C et al (2008) Loss of diastolic time as a mechanism of exercise-induced diastolic dysfunction in dilated cardiomyopathy. Am Heart J 155(6):1013–1019. doi:10.1016/j.ahj.2008.01.027

26. Siri FM, Malhotra A, Factor SM, Sonnenblick EH, Fein FS (1997) Prolonged ejection duration helps to maintain pump performance of the renal-hypertensive-diabetic rat heart: correlations between isolated papillary muscle function and ventricular performance in situ. Cardiovasc Res 34(1):230–240

27. Takehana K, Sugiura T, Nagahama Y, Hatada K, Okugawa S, Iwasaka T (2000) Cardiovascular response to combined static-dynamic exercise of patients with myocardial infarction. Coron Artery Dis 11(1):35–40

28. Arshad W, Duncan AM, Francis DP, O'Sullivan CA, Gibson DG, Henein MY (2004) Systole-diastole mismatch in hypertrophic cardiomyopathy is caused by stress induced left ventricular outflow tract obstruction. Am Heart J 148(5):903–909

29. Juneja R (2006) Anaesthesia for the elderly cardiac patient. Ann Card Anaesth 9(1):67–77

30. Hoffmann E, Sulke N, Edvardsson N et al (2006) New insights into the initiation of atrial fibrillation: a detailed intraindividual and interindividual analysis of the spontaneous onset of atrial fibrillation using new diagnostic pacemaker features. Circulation 113(16):1933–1941

31. Fleg JL, Das DN, Wright J, Lakatta EG (1990) Age-associated changes in the components of atrioventricular conduction in apparently healthy volunteers. J Gerontol 45(3):M95–M100

32. Erikssen J, Amlie JP, Thaulow E, Kjerkshus J (1982) PR interval in middle-aged men with overt and latent coronary heart disease compared to PR in angionegative and normal men of similar age. Clin Cardiol 5(6):353–359

33. Fleg JL, O'Connor F, Gerstenblith G et al (1995) Impact of age on the cardiovascular response to dynamic upright exercise in healthy men and women. J Appl Physiol 78(3):890–900

34. Bullington J, Mouton Perry SM, Rigby J et al (1989) The effect of advancing age on the sympathetic response to laryngoscopy and tracheal intubation. Anesth Analg 68(5):603–608

35. Folkow B, Svanborg A (1993) Physiology of cardiovascular aging. Physiol Rev 73(4):725–764

36. Poldermans D, Boersma E, Fioretti PM, van Urk H, Boomsma F, Man in't Veld AJ (1995) Cardiac chronotropic responsiveness to β-adrenoceptor stimulation is not reduced in the elderly. J Am Coll Cardiol 25(5):995–999

37. Hees PS, Fleg JL, Mirza ZA, Ahmed S, Siu CO, Shapiro EP (2006) Effects of normal aging on left ventricular lusitropic, inotropic, and chronotropic responses to dobutamine. J Am Coll Cardiol 47(7):1440–1447

38. Elliott HL, Sumner DJ, McLean K, Reid JL (1982) Effect of age on the responsiveness of vascular alpha-adrenoceptors in man. J Cardiovasc Pharmacol 4(3):388–392

39. Taylor JA, Hayano J, Seals DR (1995) Lesser vagal withdrawal during isometric exercise with age. J Appl Physiol 79(3):805–811

40. Laitinen T, Niskanen L, Geelen G, Lansimies E, Hartikainen J (2004) Age dependency of cardiovascular autonomic responses to head-up tilt in healthy subjects. J Appl Physiol 96(6):2333–2340. doi:10.1152/japplphysiol.00444.2003

41. Latson TW, Ashmore TH, Reinhart DJ, Klein KW, Giesecke AH (1994) Autonomic reflex dysfunction in patients presenting for elective surgery is associated with hypotension after anesthesia induction. Anesthesiology 80(2):326–337

42. Theye RA, Milde JH, Michenfelder JD (1966) Effect of hypocapnia on cardiac output during anesthesia. Anesthesiology 27(6):778–782

43. Markello R, Thweatt RC, Lauria JI, Baker JM, Schuder RJ (1969) Effect of hyperventilation on cardiac output during ether anesthesia. Anesth Analg 48(1):99–105

44. Hewitt PB, Chamberlain JH, Seed RF (1973) The effect of carbon dioxide on cardiac output in patients undergoing mechanical ventilation following open-heart surgery. Br J Anaesth 45(6):640–641

45. Sudheer PS, Logan SW, Ateleanu B, Hall JE (2006) Haemodynamic effects of the prone position: a comparison of propofol total intravenous and inhalation anaesthesia. Anaesthesia 61(2):138–141

46. Tanabe K, Ishibashi Y, Ohta T et al (1993) Effect of left and right lateral decubitus positions on mitral flow pattern by Doppler echocardiography in congestive heart failure. Am J Cardiol 71(8):751–753

47. Norman J, Atkinson SA (1970) The effect of cardiac sympathetic blockade on the relationship between cardiac output and carbon dioxide tension in the anaesthetized dog. Br J Anaesth 42(7):592–602

48. Licker M, Schweizer A, Hohn L, Farinelli C, Morel DR (2000) Cardiovascular responses to anesthetic induction in patients chronically treated with angiotensin-converting enzyme inhibitors. Can J Anaesth 47(5):433–440

49. Brabant SM, Bertrand M, Eyraud D, Darmon PL, Coriat P (1999) The hemodynamic effects of anesthetic induction in vascular surgical patients chronically treated with angiotensin II receptor antagonists. Anesth Analg 89(6):1388–1392

50. Simon MJ, Veering BT, Stienstra R, van Kleef JW, Burm AG (2002) The effects of age on neural blockade and hemodynamic changes after epidural anesthesia with ropivacaine. Anesth Analg 94(5):1325–1330, table of contents

51. Critchley LA, Stuart JC, Short TG, Gin T (1994) Haemodynamic effects of subarachnoid block in elderly patients. Br J Anaesth 73(4):464–470

52. Baron JF, Coriat P, Mundler O, Fauchet M, Bousseau D, Viars P (1987) Left ventricular global and regional function during lumbar epidural anesthesia in patients with and without angina pectoris. influence of volume loading. Anesthesiology 66(5):621–627

53. Fourcade HE, Stevens WC, Larson CP Jr et al (1971) The ventilatory effects of forane, a new inhaled anesthetic. Anesthesiology 35(1):26–31

54. Doi M, Ikeda K (1987) Respiratory effects of sevoflurane. Anesth Analg 66(3):241–244

55. Lockhart SH, Rampil IJ, Yasuda N, Eger EI 2nd, Weiskopf RB (1991) Depression of ventilation by desflurane in humans. Anesthesiology 74(3):484–488

56. Warner DO, Warner MA, Ritman EL (1995) Human chest wall function while awake and during halothane anesthesia. I. quiet breathing. Anesthesiology 82(1):6–19

57. Sprung J, Gajic O, Warner DO (2006) Review article: age related alterations in respiratory function - anesthetic considerations: [article de synthese: Les modifications de fonction respiratoire liees a l'age – considerations anesthesiques]. Can J Anaesth 53(12):1244–1257

58. Regan MJ, Eger EI 2nd (1966) Ventilatory responses to hypercapnia and hypoxia at normothermia and moderate hypothermia during constant-depth halothane anesthesia. Anesthesiology 27(5): 624–633

59. van den Elsen M, Sarton E, Teppema L, Berkenbosch A, Dahan A (1998) Influence of 0.1 minimum alveolar concentration of sevoflurane, desflurane and isoflurane on dynamic ventilatory response to hypercapnia in humans. Br J Anaesth 80(2):174–182

60. Tokics L, Hedenstierna G, Svensson L et al (1996) V/Q distribution and correlation to atelectasis in anesthetized paralyzed humans. J Appl Physiol 81(4):1822–1833

61. Gunnarsson L, Strandberg A, Brismar B, Tokics L, Lundquist H, Hedenstierna G (1989) Atelectasis and gas exchange impairment during enflurane/nitrous oxide anaesthesia. Acta Anaesthesiol Scand 33(8):629–637

62. Tokics L, Hedenstierna G, Strandberg A, Brismar B, Lundquist H (1987) Lung collapse and gas exchange during general anesthesia: effects of spontaneous breathing, muscle paralysis, and positive end-expiratory pressure. Anesthesiology 66(2):157–167

63. Pagel PS, Fu JL, Damask MC et al (1998) Desflurane and isoflurane produce similar alterations in systemic and pulmonary hemodynamics and arterial oxygenation in patients undergoing one-lung ventilation during thoracotomy. Anesth Analg 87(4):800–807

64. Forbes AR, Gamsu G (1979) Mucociliary clearance in the canine lung during and after general anesthesia. Anesthesiology 50(1):26–29

65. Keller C, Brimacombe J (1998) Bronchial mucus transport velocity in paralyzed anesthetized patients: a comparison of the laryngeal mask airway and cuffed tracheal tube. Anesth Analg 86(6):1280–1282

66. Sundman E, Witt H, Sandin R et al (2001) Pharyngeal function and airway protection during subhypnotic concentrations of propofol, isoflurane, and sevoflurane: volunteers examined by pharyngeal videoradiography and simultaneous manometry. Anesthesiology 95(5): 1125–1132

67. Rooke GA, Choi JH, Bishop MJ (1997) The effect of isoflurane, halothane, sevoflurane, and thiopental/nitrous oxide on respiratory system resistance after tracheal intubation. Anesthesiology 86(6):1294–1299

68. Hirshman CA, Bergman NA (1990) Factors influencing intrapulmonary airway calibre during anaesthesia. Br J Anaesth 65(1): 30–42

69. Goff MJ, Arain SR, Ficke DJ, Uhrich TD, Ebert TJ (2000) Absence of bronchodilation during desflurane anesthesia: a comparison to sevoflurane and thiopental. Anesthesiology 93(2):404–408

70. Tonner PH, Kampen J, Scholz J (2003) Pathophysiological changes in the elderly. Best Pract Res Clin Anaesthesiol 17(2):163–177

71. Leblanc P, Ruff F, Milic-Emili J (1970) Effects of age and body position on "airway closure" in man. J Appl Physiol 28(4):448–451

72. Kronenberg RS, Drage CW (1973) Attenuation of the ventilatory and heart rate responses to hypoxia and hypercapnia with aging in normal men. J Clin Invest 52(8):1812–1819

73. Wahba WM (1983) Influence of aging on lung function-clinical significance of changes from age twenty. Anesth Analg 62(8):764–776

74. Zaugg M, Lucchinetti E (2000) Respiratory function in the elderly. Anesthesiol Clin North America 18(1):47–58, vi

75. Murphy GS, Szokol JW, Marymont JH, Greenberg SB, Avram MJ, Vender JS (2008) Residual neuromuscular blockade and critical respiratory events in the postanesthesia care unit. Anesth Analg 107(1):130–137

76. Rose DK, Cohen MM, Wigglesworth DF, DeBoer DP (1994) Critical respiratory events in the postanesthesia care unit. patient, surgical, and anesthetic factors. Anesthesiology 81(2):410–418

77. Murphy GS, Szokol JW, Franklin M, Marymont JH, Avram MJ, Vender JS (2004) Postanesthesia care unit recovery times and neuromuscular blocking drugs: a prospective study of orthopedic surgical patients randomized to receive pancuronium or rocuronium. Anesth Analg 98(1):193–200, table of contents

78. Sprung J, Whalen FX, Comfere T et al (2009) Alveolar recruitment and arterial desflurane concentration during bariatric surgery. Anesth Analg 108(1):120–127

79. Lu CC, Tsai CS, Hu OY, Chen RM, Chen TL, Ho ST (2008) Pharmacokinetics of isoflurane in human blood. Pharmacology 81(4):344–349

80. Turnheim K (2003) When drug therapy gets old: pharmacokinetics and pharmacodynamics in the elderly. Exp Gerontol 38(8):843–853

81. Rasmussen LS, Moller JT (2000) Central nervous system dysfunction after anesthesia in the geriatric patient. Anesthesiol Clin North America 18(1):59–70, vi

82. Olofsson B, Lundstrom M, Borssen B, Nyberg L, Gustafson Y (2005) Delirium is associated with poor rehabilitation outcome in elderly patients treated for femoral neck fractures. Scand J Caring Sci 19(2):119–127

83. Newman MF, Kirchner JL, Phillips-Bute B et al (2001) Longitudinal assessment of neurocognitive function after coronary-artery bypass surgery. N Engl J Med 344(6):395–402

84. Lawrence VA, Hilsenbeck SG, Mulrow CD, Dhanda R, Sapp J, Page CP (1995) Incidence and hospital stay for cardiac and pulmonary complications after abdominal surgery. J Gen Intern Med 10(12):671–678

85. Ashton CM, Petersen NJ, Wray NP et al (1993) The incidence of perioperative myocardial infarction in men undergoing noncardiac surgery. Ann Intern Med 118(7):504–510

86. Alagiakrishnan K, Wiens CA (2004) An approach to drug induced delirium in the elderly. Postgrad Med J 80(945):388–393

87. Gaudreau JD, Gagnon P, Roy MA, Harel F, Tremblay A (2005) Association between psychoactive medications and delirium in hospitalized patients: a critical review. Psychosomatics 46(4): 302–316

88. Cosgrove DO, Jenkins JS (1974) The effects of epidural anaesthesia on the pituitary-adrenal response to surgery. Clin Sci Mol Med 46(3):403–407

89. Pflug AE, Halter JB (1981) Effect of spinal anesthesia on adrenergic tone and the neuroendocrine responses to surgical stress in humans. Anesthesiology 55(2):120–126

90. Seitz W, Luebbe N, Bechstein W, Fritz K, Kirchner E (1986) A comparison of two types of anaesthesia on the endocrine and

metabolic responses to anaesthesia and surgery. Eur J Anaesthesiol 3(4):283–294

91. Williams-Russo P, Sharrock NE, Mattis S, Szatrowski TP, Charlson ME (1995) Cognitive effects after epidural vs general anesthesia in older adults. A randomized trial. JAMA 274(1):44–50

92. Lynch EP, Lazor MA, Gellis JE, Orav J, Goldman L, Marcantonio ER (1998) The impact of postoperative pain on the development of postoperative delirium. Anesth Analg 86(4):781–785

93. Fong HK, Sands LP, Leung JM (2006) The role of postoperative analgesia in delirium and cognitive decline in elderly patients: a systematic review. Anesth Analg 102(4):1255–1266

94. Marcantonio ER, Juarez G, Goldman L et al (1994) The relationship of postoperative delirium with psychoactive medications. JAMA 272(19):1518–1522

95. Francis J, Martin D, Kapoor WN (1990) A prospective study of delirium in hospitalized elderly. JAMA 263(8):1097–1101

96. Hanning CD, Blokland A, Johnson M, Perry EK (2003) Effects of repeated anaesthesia on central cholinergic function in the rat cerebral cortex. Eur J Anaesthesiol 20(2):93–97

97. Jevtovic-Todorovic V, Todorovic SM, Mennerick S et al (1998) Nitrous oxide (laughing gas) is an NMDA antagonist, neuroprotectant and neurotoxin. Nat Med 4(4):460–463

98. Eckenhoff RG, Johansson JS, Wei H et al (2004) Inhaled anesthetic enhancement of amyloid-beta oligomerization and cytotoxicity. Anesthesiology 101(3):703–709

99. Blokland A, Honig W, Jolles J (2001) Long-term consequences of repeated pentobarbital anaesthesia on choice reaction time performance in ageing rats. Br J Anaesth 87(5):781–783

100. Culley DJ, Baxter M, Yukhananov R, Crosby G (2003) The memory effects of general anesthesia persist for weeks in young and aged rats. Anesth Analg 96(4):1004–1009, table of contents

101. Culley DJ, Baxter MG, Yukhananov R, Crosby G (2004) Long-term impairment of acquisition of a spatial memory task following isoflurane-nitrous oxide anesthesia in rats. Anesthesiology 100(2):309–314

102. Rasmussen LS, Johnson T, Kuipers HM et al (2003) Does anaesthesia cause postoperative cognitive dysfunction? A randomised study of regional versus general anaesthesia in 438 elderly patients. Acta Anaesthesiol Scand 47(3):260–266

103. Sapolsky RM (2000) Glucocorticoids and hippocampal atrophy in neuropsychiatric disorders. Arch Gen Psychiatry 57(10):925–935

104. Gordon NH, Scott DB, Percy Robb IW (1973) Modification of plasma corticosteroid concentrations during and after surgery by epidural blockade. Br Med J 1(5853):581–583

105. Moller JT, Cluitmans P, Rasmussen LS et al (1998) Long-term postoperative cognitive dysfunction in the elderly ISPOCD1 study. ISPOCD investigators. International study of post-operative cognitive dysfunction. Lancet 351(9106):857–861

106. Rasmussen LS, Steentoft A, Rasmussen H, Kristensen PA, Moller JT (1999) Benzodiazepines and postoperative cognitive dysfunction in the elderly. ISPOCD group. International study of postoperative cognitive dysfunction. Br J Anaesth 83(4):585–589

107. Inouye SK (2006) Delirium in older persons. N Engl J Med 354(11):1157–1165

108. Nies AS, Shand DG, Wilkinson GR (1976) Altered hepatic blood flow and drug disposition. Clin Pharmacokinet 1(2):135–155

109. Wilkinson GR, Shand DG (1975) Commentary: a physiological approach to hepatic drug clearance. Clin Pharmacol Ther 18(4):377–390

110. Tanaka T, Nabatame H, Tanifuji Y (2005) Insulin secretion and glucose utilization are impaired under general anesthesia with sevoflurane as well as isoflurane in a concentration-independent manner. J Anesth 19(4):277–281

111. Sessler DI (2005) Temperature monitoring. In: Miller RD (ed) Miller's anesthesia, 6th edn. Elsevier, Philadelphia, PA, p 1571

112. Frank SM, Raja SN, Bulcao C, Goldstein DS (2000) Age-related thermoregulatory differences during core cooling in humans. Am J Physiol Regul Integr Comp Physiol 279(1):R349–R354

113. Frank SM, Raja SN, Wu PK, el-Gamal N (1997) Alpha-adrenergic mechanisms of thermoregulation in humans. Ann N Y Acad Sci 813:101–110

114. Thompson CS, Holowatz LA, Kenney WL (2005) Attenuated noradrenergic sensitivity during local cooling in aged human skin. J Physiol 564(Pt 1):313–319

115. Ozaki M, Sessler DI, Suzuki H, Ozaki K, Atarashi K, Negishi C (1997) The threshold for thermoregulatory vasoconstriction during nitrous oxide/sevoflurane anesthesia is lower in elderly than in young patients. Ann N Y Acad Sci 813:789–791

116. Schmied H, Kurz A, Sessler DI, Kozek S, Reiter A (1996) Mild hypothermia increases blood loss and transfusion requirements during total hip arthroplasty. Lancet 347(8997):289–292

117. Winkler M, Akca O, Birkenberg B et al (2000) Aggressive warming reduces blood loss during hip arthroplasty. Anesth Analg 91(4):978–984

118. Polk HC Jr, Simpson CJ, Simmons BP, Alexander JW (1983) Guidelines for prevention of surgical wound infection. Arch Surg 118(10):1213–1217

119. Frank SM, Fleisher LA, Breslow MJ et al (1997) Perioperative maintenance of normothermia reduces the incidence of morbid cardiac events. A randomized clinical trial. JAMA 277(14):1127–1134

120. Frank SM, Beattie C, Christopherson R et al (1993) Unintentional hypothermia is associated with postoperative myocardial ischemia. the perioperative ischemia randomized anesthesia trial study group. Anesthesiology 78(3):468–476

121. Calahan MK (1996) Hemodynamic effects of inhaled anesthetics. Review courses. International Anesthesia Research Society, Cleveland, OH, pp 14–18

122. Rooke GA, Freund PR, Jacobson AF (1997) Hemodynamic response and change in organ blood volume during spinal anesthesia in elderly men with cardiac disease. Anesth Analg 85(1):99–105

123. Ebert TJ (2005) Inhalation anesthesia. In: Barash PG, Cullen BF, Stoelting RK (eds) Clinical anesthesia, 5th edn. Lippincott Williams & Wilkins, Philadelphia, PA, p 406

124. Eger EI, Weiskopf RB, Eisenkraft JB (eds) (2002) The pharmacology of inhaled anesthetics. Baxter Healthcare Corporation, New Providence, NJ, p 24

Chapter 25
Choosing the Best Anesthetic Regimen

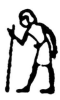

Sheila R. Barnett

Introduction

Why Is Anesthesia a Particular Concern in Elderly Patients?

The administration of anesthesia to a geriatric patient requires meticulous attention to detail and a clear understanding of the impact of aging on organ reserve and function. Older surgical patients present for surgery with complicated medical histories, limited physiologic reserve, and frequently unpredictable responses to anesthetic agents [1, 2]. In general, elderly frail patients with underlying chronic disease can be less tolerant of brief episodes of hemodynamic instability such as hypotension or desaturation that may not be preventable during the course of a surgery. While these events may be insignificant in a young patient and in the frail elder, they may lead to serious consequences, such as cardiac ischemia and arrhythmias [3, 4]. This chapter reviews the basic anesthetic concepts and discusses the impact of aging on the choice of anesthesia.

Choosing the Anesthetic Regimen

Regardless of the age of the patient, the choice of anesthesia is influenced by several factors: the patient's medical and psychological condition, the type and duration of the procedure or surgery, and the requirements of the surgery itself. The anesthesiologist is ultimately responsible to

S.R. Barnett (✉)
Department of Anesthesiology, Beth Israel Deaconess Medical Center, Harvard Medical School, Boston, MA, USA
e-mail: sbarnett@bidmc.harvard.edu

choose the regimen that is most appropriate for the patient and the surgeon. In many instances, the choice of the anesthesia is limited, for example, the elderly patient presenting with a perforated bowel and evidence of hemodynamic instability will require a general anesthesia with endotracheal intubation. In this example, there are no viable alternatives for the anesthetic type. However, even in this case and other similar cases in which the choice of anesthetic type is limited, the risks and benefits of the individual medications administered, the monitoring requirements, the positioning during the surgery, the duration of the surgery, and the post operative recovery plan will require thorough consideration [5]. For the older patient, the anesthesiologist must be prepared to tailor the anesthetic carefully to provide age appropriate care.

Using the case below, the challenges encountered by a "geriatric" anesthesiologist will be illustrated through a discussion of the case of Mr. Smith.

General Considerations for the Elderly Patient

Mortality and risk of an adverse event associated with surgery increase with advanced age [4, 6–9]. This is due to multiple factors including age related reductions in physiologic reserve, the increase in comorbid conditions, and the magnitude and type of the surgery itself. Complex emergency cases in the elderly carry the highest mortality with a suggested threefold increase in mortality. The risk of cardiac complications in geriatric patients following emergency surgery increases three to five times, and the chance of postoperative intubation and ventilation is five times that of a young patient undergoing a major emergency surgery. The magnitude and size of surgery are relevant: thoracotomy mortality in patients over the age of 70 years has been reported as high as 17% and emergency abdominal surgery in patients over the age of 80 years carries a mortality rate of 10–25%.

R.A. Rosenthal et al. (eds.), *Principles and Practice of Geriatric Surgery*,
DOI 10.1007/978-1-4419-6999-6_25, © Springer Science+Business Media, LLC 2011

CASE STUDY: PART 1

Mr. Smith is a 85-year-old male presenting with new right upper quadrant pain. He is scheduled for an upper endoscopy and ERCP with a possible biliary dilation. Past medical history includes known gallstones, chronic lower back pain, Parkinson's disease, and hypertension. Prior surgery includes brain surgery for his tremor 5 years ago, and a lumbar discectomy 15 years ago. He consults his primary care doctor regularly and a neurologist for his Parkinson's every 3 months. In the past 12 months, he has had an EKG, which showed left ventricular hypertrophy and nonspecific ST changes; he has not had any further cardiac testing. His medications include a beta blocker, levodopa, intermittent ibuprofen and he has a prescription for acetaminophen with codeine but as per his wife he rarely takes any pain medication. Mr. Smith lives with his wife, in the past 12 months he has had increasingly difficulty with ambulation and has fallen several times. His appearance and speech are consistent with severe Parkinson's. Depending on the results of the ERCP, he may or may not require either a laparoscopic cholecystectomy or a more extensive biliary surgery.

Mr. Smith has several medical issues that will challenge the anesthesiologist during each of the procedures proposed.

For the ERCP, sedation is routinely recommended. However, Mr. Smith's medical conditions will make sedation challenging and it is possible that a general anesthesia will ultimately be a safer choice.

For the potential follow-up procedures, either a laparoscopic cholecystectomy or an exploratory laparotomy, Mr. Smith will need a general anesthesia. Mr. Smith has a significant increased risk from delirium post operatively, and may need adjustment on his Parkinson's medication. Although a laparoscopic cholecystectomy is generally an ambulatory procedure, serious consideration will need to be given to admit Mr. Smith until it is clear that he is stable. A major exploratory laparotomy and biliary dissection carry a very high risk of mortality in his age group, especially in view of his overall apparent frailty. For the more extensive surgery, Mr. Smith will need a general anesthesia and invasive monitoring including an arterial line at a minimum and possibly a central venous line. Although he has no history of congestive heart failure, if significant blood loss is encountered, he may benefit from cardiac output monitoring to assist with volume resuscitation. Postoperatively recovery should include intensive care unit, possible ventilation, and appropriate pain control. Depending on his hemodynamic status, he could benefit from a postoperative thoracic epidural for the treatment of postoperative pain.

The occurrence of any complications appears to be a major factor influencing outcomes in the elderly surgical patient. Several studies have shown a significant increase in 30-day mortality in patients who experienced complications following noncardiac surgery. In addition, patients experiencing a cardiac or noncardiac complication had a threefold increase in length of stay. Thus avoiding complications, even minor ones, and conducting a careful review of the patients' physical and medical status prior to anesthesia must be a primary focus for all anesthesiologists taking care of older patients.

The increased morbidity experienced by older patients largely reflects the burden of disease encountered in this age group. In a study examining preoperative health status in elderly patients, over 84% of 544 patients had at least one comorbid condition [1]. Thirty percent of patients had three or more preoperative health conditions, 27% had two, and 28% had one preexisting disease. Hypertension (HTN) was the most commonly encountered comorbidity. Other common conditions included: diabetes mellitus, dysrhythmias, pulmonary

disease, neurologic disease, arthritis, and ischemic heart disease including congestive failure. Despite a long list of diseases, functional status and clinical evidence of congestive heart failure [1, 8] were the two most important predictors of adverse events postoperatively in this study. Functional status is particularly important and frequently impacted by the presence of a physical disability. In the oldest patients, over the age of 80 years, 74% have a disability and 35% of this group requires assistance with daily activities.

Anesthetic Choices

Aspiration

Regardless of the anesthetic regimen, protection of the airway is paramount. The geriatric patient is at increased risk of aspirating because of physiologic changes and common disease conditions [10]. A reduction in pharyngeal sensitivity has been demonstrated and common comorbidities such as a previous cerebrovascular accident, swallowing disorders, and diseases such as Parkinson lead to the increased possibility of aspiration. The development of aspiration pneumonia can be devastating in the older patient with reduced functional reserve. Thus, sedation should be administered cautiously in patients with an unprotected airway [11,12]. Pulmonary complications were among the most common in a study comparing young and elderly patients undergoing noncardiac surgery leading to both an increased length of stay and subsequent mortality [8].

General Anesthesia

The decision to use a general anesthesia is driven by the extent of the surgery, and the patient and surgeon preference [5]. A general endotracheal anesthesia with paralysis allows maximal exposure for abdominal surgery and is necessary for abdominal and laparoscopic surgeries. When paralysis is not required, provided the patient is fasting, not significantly obese with a low risk of aspiration and the surgery site, and positioning is appropriate, the laryngeal mask airway (LMA) has largely replaced the traditional mask anesthetic. For certain very brief surgeries a mask anesthetic is still desirable. Advantages of intubation compared with the LMA include the ability to protect the airway from aspiration, and possible reduction in the risk of development of intraoperative atelectasis through the use of positive pressure volume ventilation with or without additional positive pressure end-expiratory pressure. Mucociliary dysfunction occurs after using an LMA or an endotracheal tube, but it is worse following intubation.

In some instances, a patient will request to be asleep for a procedure and provided there is no additional risk, patient preferences should be followed. Dementia increases with age: in patients of 60–70 years old, the incidence ranges from 5 to 7%, while in those between 80 and 90 years old, the incidence ranges from 15 to 20%. Depending on the ability to cooperate, these patients may require a general anesthesia or deeper sedation than would normally be indicated by the procedure itself.

Regional Anesthesia

Regional anesthesia includes both neuraxial techniques such as spinal and epidural anesthesia and peripheral nerve blocks. Regional anesthesia may be administered as the primary anesthetic or as an adjuvant for pain relief during or after the surgery [13]. When utilized to treat postoperative pain, epidural analgesia and peripheral nerve blocks improve pain relief, functional outcomes, and have been shown to reduce hospital stay in selected patient groups. Advantages of a pure regional anesthesia include a reduction in the requirement for sedatives, preservation of spontaneous ventilation, the absence of airway instrumentation, and potential decrease the incidence of postoperative thrombosis and blood loss following orthopedic surgery [14].

The choice for a regional anesthesia vs. general anesthesia remains the subject of significant debate [14–17]. Despite increasing popularity of regional blocks such as intrascalene and femoral nerve blocks, there is no consistent data supporting a reduction in morbidity or mortality after general surgery.

Neuraxial Anesthesia

The spine undergoes significant age-related changes, including a gradual deterioration of the intervertebral disks, fibrosis of the intervertebral foramina, and a reduction in fat in the epidural space. In addition to making the placement of a spinal or epidural more challenging, these changes also result in a less compliant epidural space. When dosing the geriatric patient, enhanced local anesthetic spread can occur in the spinal column, and the dose of epidural medications should be reduced and given more slowly [18]. Similarly, local anesthetic administered through the spinal needle into the subarachnoid space can result in a variable and higher level of analgesia and sympathetic block in an older patient due to a decrease in the CSF and age-related changes in the pain fibers themselves [19, 20]. In addition to changes in the spread of local anesthetic agents, metabolism and clearance of these drugs are also delayed with advanced age. Lidocaine and other local anesthetic doses should be reduced for both neuraxial and peripheral nerve blocks. The enhanced cephalad spread of epidural and spinal local anesthetic agents also contributes to the increased hypotension observed in older patients from the consequent sympathectomy. Older patients are also more sensitive to the central effects of opioids and are at increased risk of apnea following neuraxial opioid administration.

Epidural analgesia can be employed postoperatively to improve pain control from large abdominal and thoracic incisions. Epidural analgesia includes several advantages over systemic narcotics including improved pain relief, less sedation, and improved respiratory mechanics. However, epidural anesthetics usually include low dose local anesthetic agents and this can be associated with a sympathetic blockade and subsequent potential vasodilatation and hypotension. The effects of the sympathectomy are often exaggerated in the elderly patient due to a combination of existing age-related declines in autonomic function and increased decline in vascular resistance. The increase in hypotension in older vs. younger patients can be a significant factor limiting the use of an epidural for postoperative analgesia or even a spinal for a procedure [3, 13, 20]. In general, fluid administration alone will not offset the impact of the sympathectomy and carries the risk of inducing congestive heart failure once the sympathectomy wears off and the fluid is returned to the central volume. Epidural- (or spinal) induced hypotension usually requires treatment with an alpha agonist such as phenylephrine [3, 13], and this may be undesirable in patients with tenuous blood supply or new vascular grafts. In general, if phenylephrine will be deemed unacceptable in the postoperative course then alternative postoperative pain management strategies to epidural anesthetics should be considered. Pure opioid analgesia through the epidural may be useful but significant complications with postoperative apnea have occurred and limited the use in elderly frail patients [21].

Absolute contraindications to neuraxial anesthesia include anticoagulation and antiplatelet medications. Other contraindications to neuraxial anesthetic include sepsis, bacteremia, and hypovolemia. Current recommendations suggest discontinuing warfarin for 3–5 days and allowing normalization of the INR to 1.5 or less prior to placing an epidural or spinal. Antiplatelet medications take several days or weeks to wear off and it is recommended that ticlopidine be stopped for 14 days and clopidogrel for 7 days at a minimum prior to a neuraxial anesthetic. Nonsteroidal anti-inflammatory drugs (NSAIDs) and aspirin can be continued. Twice daily low molecular heparin should be discontinued for 24 h, if only once per day then 12 h is sufficient [22].

In all patients in whom anticoagulation or antiplatelet medication is an issue, a serious discussion is needed regarding risks and benefits of discontinuing the medication and the plans for reinstituting the medications postoperatively. It is important that any plans to change a patient's anticoagulation medication involve a discussion with the patient's cardiologist or primary care physician.

Monitored Anesthesia Care

This is the most common type of anesthesia administered. A monitored anesthesia care (MAC) can range from the administration of minimal anxyiolysis to deep sedation. In older patients, continuous supplemental oxygen is recommended in all cases as physiological changes with aging result in a lower arterial oxygen tension on room air, even before the administration of sedation. In general, the medication administered by the anesthesia provider is supplemented by local anesthesia through infiltration or a field block administered by the surgeon. Patients undergoing an MAC need to be at least partially cooperative and able to lie still without significant pain; in the older patient with agitation, dementia, or chronic pain, this can be difficult and a lower threshold for recommending a general anesthesia may be needed. Similarly, an MAC may be unreasonable in patients with chronic cough or intractable tremors.

Minimum Requirements for Anesthesia

Regardless of the anesthetic technique chosen, there are certain minimum requirements that must be met for all patients undergoing an anesthesia. Patients must have a preoperative anesthetic evaluation, appropriate laboratory testing, pertinent consultations, and should receive instructions regarding NPO status and general information on "what to expect following their surgery and anesthesia." There are several options for the completion of the preanesthetic evaluation; the choice will depend on the patient, the surgeon, and the facility guidelines (Table 25.1).

When a preoperative testing clinic is utilized, the patient may meet with an anesthesiologist for a full discussion of anesthetic options. It is recommended that patients are not promised any particular anesthetic type in advance, the anesthesiologist assigned to the case should be free to make that decision. In general, older patients with complex medical

---

CASE STUDY: PART 2

Considering Mr. Smith, he has a high risk of aspiration due to his Parkinson's disease. In addition, it is not clear how cooperative he will be with only sedation. The plan for his ERCP should include the strong possibility of a general anesthesia with intubation. A general anesthesia will definitely be required for either his subsequent laparoscopic cholecystectomy or exploratory laparotomy and biliary dissection.

TABLE 25.1 Preoperative assessment alternatives and the elderly patient

	Advantages	Disadvantages
Preoperative assessment clinic	Reduction lab testing	Expensive
	Reduction consultations	Cost of administrative clerical staff
	Improved OR efficiency	Requires allocated hospital space and support
	Decrease in OR cancelations and delays	Primary MD maybe unaware of surgery
	Anesthesiology input	Second trip to hospital
	Specific NPO instructions	
Primary physician visit "clearance"	Patient known to MD	More laboratory testing
	Primary MD involved for postoperative care	No anesthesia discussion – especially detrimental in complex high risk cases
	No second hospital visit	No instructions for surgery
	Good for simple surgeries	Scheduling dependent on MD office availability
		Paperwork/clearance at remote site
Telephone interview	Convenient for patient	No anesthesia input
	Preoperative instructions including NPO	Difficult to reach patients at work
		Language barriers
		Advanced age usually an exclusion factor

Surveys

May be added to above visits/calls

Preoperative health survey	Simple	No instructions
	No extra visits	No anesthesia input
		No time to optimize medical conditions identified
		Mail return unreliable
Internet health quiz	Simple	No instructions
	Remote access to information	No anesthesia input
	Algorithm for laboratory testing	

histories are best seen prior to surgery to ensure that an appropriate work-up to optimize the patient's condition has been completed [23, 24].

Preoperative Assessment

The aims of the preoperative assessment are to prepare the patient for anesthesia, obtain consent for the anesthesia, and ensure that the patient is adequately prepared for their procedure. Chronological age may not accurately reflect a patient's physiological age, and a significant goal of the preoperative assessment is to estimate the patient's physiologic reserve function. The physiologic age reflects the combined impact of aging and comorbid conditions, and is more likely to be predictive of outcome than age in years alone (Table 25.2).

The assessment can begin with a general assessment of the geriatric patient: Does the patient look their age? Is there evidence of cognitive dysfunction or significant disability? Does the patient's caregiver answer all the questions? Patients with preexisting cognitive dysfunction are at higher risk from postoperative delirium and the anesthetic plan may need to

TABLE 25.2 The goals of the preoperative assessment

Obtain a thorough history and physical examination
Provide a risk assessment
Recognize high risk patients
Implement risk reduction strategies
Perform selected laboratory and cardiac testing
Improve control of perioperative diseases
Formulate and discuss the anesthetic plan
Obtain informed consent
Formulate a post operative plan
Reduce anxiety through education

Source: Data from [23]

be altered to accommodate the patient with cognitive or other disabilities.

Functional status should be assessed during the preoperative interview, and this is easily achieved using a simple scale as outlined in Table 25.3. Patients with reduced functional status (<4 METS) have an increased risk of cardiac morbidity and poor outcome following noncardiac surgery [25]. The anesthesiologist's physical examination should be focused including an airway examination and examination of the cardiopulmonary system and other relevant organs.

TABLE 25.3 Functional assessment scale

1 MET	Can you take care of yourself?
	Eat, dress, use the toilet?
	Walk indoors around the house
	Walk 1–2 blocks on level ground at 2–3 mph?
	Do light housework?
	Can you take care of yourself?
4 METS	Climb a flight of stairs? Carry groceries?
	Walk on level ground at 4 mph?
	Run a short distance
	Do heavy housework?
	Do moderate sports – golf, dance, doubles tennis?
	Climb a flight of stairs? Carry groceries?
10 METS	Play competitive sports? Singles tennis? Ski?

Source: Data from [25]

Laboratory and Other Testing

Large-scale preoperative laboratory testing in healthy individuals leads to an increase in false positive results and inappropriate work-ups [26, 27]. Several studies have demonstrated that preoperative screening laboratory testing rarely provides new information that would not otherwise have been obtained from a thorough history and physical examination [26, 28]. Anesthesiologists tend to order fewer laboratory tests compared with outside referral physicians and some have found financial benefit derived from anesthesiology-directed laboratory testing vs. other providers. Except for concurrence on the complete blood count, anesthesiologists generally order fewer tests compared with surgeons [29–31]. The data refers to laboratory testing that is being performed to allow safe administration of anesthesia, in all patients, there may be other reasons why additional laboratory testing is requested by a surgeon or primary care physician in the general course of a patient's disease work-up.

A Hemoglobin or hematocrit. It is indicated when the surgery is associated with significant blood loss potential or the patient has systemic disease and may be anemic. The American Society of Anesthesiologists (ASA) practice advisory on preoperative evaluation concluded that age alone was not an indication for a routine blood count before surgery [32]. However, anemia is more common in the elderly and may be poorly tolerated in patients with cardiac disease. In elderly patients undergoing significant surgery, it is not unreasonable to request a baseline hematocrit.

Coagulation studies. These studies are indicated in symptomatic patients with significant liver disease or known coagulopathic conditions. Baseline studies may also be valuable in patients who are undergoing major surgery with a high risk of blood loss that are likely to need blood products during the case. Patients on anticoagulants or those for whom postoperative anticoagulation is planned generally should have baseline studies. The other group of patients for whom coagulation profiles should be considered is those who will have an epidural or spinal placed [22].

Electrolytes and blood chemistry. Healthy elderly ambulatory patients or those with mild-to-moderate systemic disease such as hypertension do not need routine electrolyte levels drawn [29]. Patients scheduled for extensive procedures such as an exploratory laparotomy or a major vascular procedure should have baseline blood chemistries, as renal insufficiency occurs in advanced and hyponatremia is more common in geriatric patients. Although not routinely ordered, reduced albumin in frail older patients is a marker of increased risk of mortality and morbidity [33].

Electrocardiograms. An ECG should be done in patients with cardiac risk factors and a history of cardiac disease. Occult cardiac disease is extremely common in older patients and most institutions recommend age-related screening with ECGs. A common requirement is a preoperative ECG in males over the age of 45 years and females over 55 years. A prior ECG within 6 months of the surgery in the absence of ongoing symptoms or changes in cardiac status is frequently acceptable 32, 34, 35].

Consultations

Elderly patients have a very high incidence of cardiac conditions. Ischemic heart disease increases almost exponentially with age and is frequently under diagnosed. It is not surprising that cardiac complications are the most significant following surgery and anesthesia. However, the decision to obtain a cardiology work-up or consultation prior to surgery will depend on the severity of the patient's disease and the onset of symptoms. Scheduled surgery per se is not an indication for a cardiac work-up [24, 36].

Chest radiographs. These are not recommended preoperatively unless indicated by the history or dictated by the underlying diagnosis. Widespread routine chest X-rays led to significant morbidity in larger studies secondary to unnecessary follow-up on false positive examinations and unexpected findings were rare [27, 32, 37].

Institutionalized Patients

The preoperative assessment of institutionalized elderly patients can be especially challenging. It may be difficult or impractical to require these patients to come to a hospital or

---

CASE STUDY: PART 3

The preoperative assessment of Mr. Smith will provide critical information for the anesthesiologist. A visit to a preoperative clinic is advisable, and in addition to a general assessment for his Parkinson's disease, a brief cognitive assessment will be valuable to establish a baseline prior to any surgery. Mr. Smith has a very high risk of developing postoperative delirium and he and his family should be warned. In view of his potential for a more significant surgery following his ERCP, Mr. Smith should have baseline laboratory testing done including a blood count, electrolytes, and an ECG. From the current history, which does not indicate any new chest pain or shortness of breath, further cardiac testing is not warranted and a chest X-ray is not needed unless his chest exam reveals abnormalities. Mr. Smith's overall poor functional status is a significant concern if he is

required to ultimately undergo a major surgery. A baseline albumin may provide an indication of his nutritional status and if reduced, it may be associated with increased risk of mortality (see physical classification Table 25.4).

TABLE 25.4 ASA physical status classes

Class 1. A healthy patient (no physiologic, physical or psychological abnormalities)
Class 2. A patient with a mild systemic disease without limitation of daily activities
Class 3. A patient with severe systemic disease that limits activity but is not incapacitating
Class 4. A patient with incapacitating systemic disease that is a constant threat to life
Class 5. A moribund patient not expected to survive 24 h with or without the operation
Class 6. A brain dead patient whose organs are being removed for donor purposes
Add "E" to denote emergency surgery

---

faculty for a special preoperative visit. Frequently, a remote preoperative screen can be conducted. The facility physician can be asked to provide a brief history and physical and the results of any laboratory testing done recently. The preoperative examination can be completed the day of the surgery. Arrangements for consent from a legal guardian or family member should be made in advance to prevent delays on the day of surgery.

After the completion of the preoperative assessment the anesthesiologist assigns a physical status classification (ASA 1–6). The physical status classification reflects the patient's condition and underlying disease complexity, it is independent of the patient's age. A higher ASA classification carries independent diagnoses that lead to increased risk from surgery. In general, risk for anesthesia increases in patients with more advanced ASA classification. An E is added to the physical classification to designate a patient for whom a surgery is emergent. The ASA physical classification system is a useful way to communicate about patients and is used by many health care providers outside of anesthesia.

NPO Status (Table 25.5)

The ASA has published guidelines for liquid and solid foods prior to the administration of an anesthetic. For the older patient, it is important that these instructions are written and provided to both the caretaker and the patient when relevant.

TABLE 25.5 ASA guidelines for NPO status preoperatively

Substance	Minimum fasting period (h)
Clear liquids[a]	2
Breast milk	4
Infant formula	6
Non human milk	6
Light meal	6
Fried or fatty foods, meat	8

[a] *Clear liquids include*: water, fruit juices without pulp, clear tea, carbonated beverages, and black coffee

Medications

Elderly patients are on average taking three medications and patients must receive clear instructions on which medications should be held or continued on the day of surgery. In many instances, it is recommended that patients bring all their medications on the day of preoperative visit and/or provide a complete list of all medications in advance of the procedure.

As a general rule, most medications should be continued until the morning of surgery, especially cardiac and antihypertensive medications. Angiotension converting enzyme inhibitors (ACEIs) and angiotension receptor blockers (ARBs) have been associated with profound and prolonged hypotension following the induction of anesthesia and provided they are not being administered for congestive heart failure and these should be held prior to surgery. Similarly, diuretics can be continued in the presence of significant fluid

---

CASE STUDY: PART 4

Mr. Smith is an ASA 3 patient, his Parkinson's disease is significantly altering his daily life and appears progressive. His medication situation is particularly challenging to prevent acute worsening of his Parkinson's symptoms and he should be instructed to continue his Levo dopa until 3 h prior to surgery. He can take his other usual medications on the morning of surgery. He should be instructed to bring his medications with him to the holding area if his surgery is delayed; he should continue his scheduled anti-Parkinson's medication. Given his complex medications, all instructions should be clearly written for him (Table 25.6).

TABLE 25.6 Preoperative instructions

Instructions should be clearly written in simple language
Instructions should be specific avoiding vague or ambiguous terms such as "maybe"
Directions to exact location in the hospital
Recommendations on clothing and belongings
NPO recommendations – written down
Number to call with change in health

---

overload; however, for the most part thiazide diuretics can be held for patient convenience. As discussed above, anticoagulation and antiplatelet medications will restrict the anesthesia choices and the decision to hold anticoagulant and antiplatelet medications should be made by the surgeon. Whenever a change in these medications is planned, the patient's primary care physician should be informed and included in the decision. One-third of older patients have chronic pain and in these instances it is important to encourage patients to continue their analgesics until the day of surgery. The patient's tolerance to pain medication may require intraoperative adjustment of the anesthetic itself [38].

Special Considerations

Cardiac Adverse Events

In general, the risk of a cardiac event following a noncardiac surgery is 1–2%, and advanced age (over 65 years) is associated with an almost 2½-fold increase in risk of a significant event. Other risk factors described recently are consistent with those mentioned above: the presence of congestive heart failure (fourfold increase), emergency surgery (twofold), the need for a blood transfusion (almost threefold), and longer surgery (twofold increase). Past history of cardiac intervention, cerebrovascular, and hypertension disease was also significant (almost twofold increase) risk factors for an adverse event. The intraoperative hemodynamic course is probably relevant and this study suggested that episodes of hypotension and tachycardia increased chance of a postoperative event in high risk patients [3, 4, 6].

Pulmonary Disease

Five to fifteen percent of elderly patients undergoing surgery develop a postoperative pulmonary complication. The presence of chronic obstructive pulmonary disease (COPD) can increase the postoperative mortality rate by tenfold. Risk factors for postoperative pulmonary complications include severe COPD, advanced age, and undergoing high risk procedures, such as upper abdominal or intrathoracic surgery [8, 39]. The increased risk during surgery in the presence of COPD relates to a combination of factors related to the patient, the surgery, and the anesthesia. Patients may exhibit increased sensitivity to medications through alterations in central respiratory control and changes in sensitivity to hypoxemia and hypercapnia; in addition, changes in respiratory mechanics that occur during mechanical ventilation can persist postoperatively. These detrimental effects may be exaggerated by residual muscle paralysis and the development of atelectasis and consequent hypoxemia. The trauma induced by surgical incision can further limit optimal respiration and pulmonary mechanics. In these older patients, full reversal of muscle relaxant and adequate analgesia is particularly important to overcome the increased work of breathing associated with advanced age from stiffening of the chest wall and reduced elasticity of the lung tissues.

Elderly patient's exhibit reduced threshold for apnea following narcotic administration and a blunting of the responsiveness to rising carbon dioxide levels. These changes leave the geriatric patient susceptible to periods of apnea, desaturation, and respiratory arrest. Opioid sparing techniques using peripheral nerve blockade or alternate analgesic such as NSAIDs can be useful if they are compatible with the surgery [40].

Regional anesthesia may obviate the need to manipulate the airway and this may offer advantages in patients with severely reactive airways disease. However, caution is needed as COPD patients with significant disease may not tolerate the associated reduction in respiratory muscle function with a spinal or epidural anesthetic, especially if they are dependent on active expiration or have excessive secretions requiring frequent coughing [41]. These compromised patients may experience a significant respiratory depression with a neuraxial block. Intrascalene nerve blocks may be associated with diaphragmatic paralysis secondary to phrenic nerve paresis and should not be used in patients with significant lung disease.

Renal and Metabolic

Normal aging is associated with a steady decline in baseline renal function and the choice of anesthesia administered to a geriatric patient should take into account the potential reduction in baseline renal function. Postoperative renal failure is rare but associated with a high mortality rate, accounting for one-fifth of postoperative deaths in elderly patients [42]. Associated risk factors for acute postoperative renal failure include advanced age over 65 years, type 1 diabetes mellitus, preexisting renal insufficiency, major vascular surgery, and recent exposure to nephrotoxins including NSAIDS, radio contrast dye, and amino glycoside antibiotics. The postoperative renal failure is usually secondary to an ATN developing as a result of hypotension, hypovolemia, and/or dehydration.

Nervous System Assessment

In addition to predictable anatomical changes in the central nervous system, there is an increase in disorders of cognitive function with an increase in dementia, memory loss, and degenerative diseases such as Parkinson's disease. Anatomical changes include gradual atrophy of the brain, reduction in gray cells, and widening of the ventricles. Alterations in neurotransmitter levels and neuronal circuits lead to changes in memory and pharmacodynamic changes resulting in an increased sensitivity to certain medications such as midazolam and some of the opioids [43]. Alterations in pain perception result from age-related changes in the peripheral nervous system, such as a reduction in myelinated fibers. In general, elderly patient's exhibit increased pain thresholds, and this may contribute to the delay in presentation of painful conditions such as peritonitis.

Neurodegenerative disorders increase with age and may influence the administration of anesthesia. One of the most common is Parkinson's disease, which afflicts 3% of elderly persons over 65 years of age. Parkinson' disease results from a loss of dopaminergic cells in the ventrolateral aspect of the substantia nigra of the basal ganglia. Characteristic symptoms include resting tremor, bradykinesia, cogwheel rigidity, postural instability, and a shuffling gait. The disease is also associated with autonomic dysfunction and orthostatic hypotension is common and frequently exacerbated by medication such as L-DOPA and other treatments. Patients with Parkinson's disease have increased oral secretions and are at increased risk of aspiration and laryngospasm during anesthesia. Orthostatic hypotension may be profound and medications that induce vasodilatation such as propofol should be administered cautiously. Parkinson's medications should be continued until the time of surgery. L-DOPA (sinemet), the mainstay of treatment is only available orally with a relatively short half life of approximately 3 h. Unfortunately, Parkinson's patients have a very high incidence of postoperative confusion and delirium that may be difficult to treat. When possible, a regional anesthesia can be advantageous or a combined general regional technique that can lead to improved for postoperative pain control. When treating Parkinson's patients, it is important to avoid agents that may exacerbate the symptoms such as the phenothiazines and metoclopramide.

Postoperative Cognitive Disorders

Postoperative delirium and postoperative cognitive dysfunction (POCD) are common complications in the elderly population [43–45]. Delirium is an acute confusional state, usually appearing 1–3 days after surgery; it may persist for weeks to months in afflicted patients. The etiology is multifactorial including acute medical conditions such as sepsis, hypoxemia, urinary tract infections, and alcohol withdrawal. Certain medications including meperidine and medications with anticholinergic effects such as diphenhydramine and scopolamine are highly associated with delirium, and should be avoided in the elderly patient [46]. Patients with preexisting dementia, baseline cognitive difficulties and depression carry a high risk of developing delirium postoperatively. Delirium is associated with an increase in morbidity and mortality and also an increase in the length of stay and dependent living situations. When pharmacological intervention is required, low dose haloperidol starting at 0.25–0.5 mg intravenously may be administered for treatment for agitation. Midazolam has been associated with a paradoxical excitation in elderly patients with delirium and, in general, it is not recommended; similarly long acting benzodiazepines can accumulate in the older patient and should be avoided.

In contrast to delirium, POCD refers to a specific cognitive disorder generally recognized in the postoperative period and is ultimately diagnosed through neuropsychological testing. Studies have demonstrated that almost 10% of elderly patients receiving a general anesthesia had some cognitive dysfunction 3 months after surgery. The cause of POCD is unknown, and multiple studies have looked at the difference in prevalence between general and regional techniques [44, 47, 48]. To date there is no convincing evidence that regional anesthesia offers any cognitive advantages over general anesthesia.

The Intraoperative Course

Monitoring

Basic monitoring standards for all patients, including the elderly, undergoing anesthesia have been established by the ASA. The first standard requires the continuous presence of qualified anesthesia personnel in the operating room. The second standard requires a continuous assessment of the patient's oxygenation, ventilation, circulation, and temperature. Although these standards are not different for older patients, aging patients may have associated comorbid conditions that influence monitoring choices.

In most instances, oxygenation is continuously assessed using variable pitch pulse tone pulse oximetry. As a fall in oxygenation may actually be a late indicator of hypoventilation, ventilation should be monitored using end tidal carbon dioxide to provide early identification of hypoventilation and possible hypercapnia. In addition to continuous ECG monitoring, the ASA requires BP assessment at least every 5 min. The decision to use additional invasive monitoring depends on the patient and the procedure. In the older patient labile blood pressure is commonly encountered [49], and a low threshold for continuous arterial blood pressure monitoring should be maintained. An arterial line can assist in both the precise titration of medications and access for blood sampling during the case.

Aging cardiac changes render the older patient more susceptible to congestive heart failure in the event of excessive fluid administration or significant shifts in volume [3, 50]. Central monitoring of the central venous pressure or pulmonary artery catheter may be useful to manage the fluid administration during a case. Interpretation of the central pressure requires a careful consideration of the aging patients underlying physiologic condition. For instance, an older hypertensive patient with a "normal" CVP may actually be modestly hypovolemic. In general, elderly patients benefit from higher preloads and are very dependent on the atrial contraction during diastole. There is significant controversy over the utility of the PA catheter as a tool to measure volume status and guide fluid resuscitation and the role of the transesophageal echocardiogram is yet to be established.

The Surgery

Laparoscopic surgery carries significant advantages in the elderly patient including a more rapid recovery, less pain following surgery, and reduced fluid requirements [51–53]. Laparoscopic cholecystectomy has been associated with improved postoperative pulmonary function vs. open cholecystectomy, and that may be advantageous for the frail elder with reduced pulmonary reserve. General anesthesia with controlled ventilation is preferred to allow adequate abdominal insufflation. During the surgery absorption of CO_2 can result in hypercapnia and acidosis. The rise in intra-abdominal pressure accompanying the insufflation can lead to reduced venous return, increased peripheral resistance, and intrathoracic pressure leading to a diminished cardiac output and hypotension. In the frail elderly patient with reduced cardiac function these cardiovascular challenges can be significant, requiring increased monitoring, and adjustment of the anesthetic medications to optimize cardiac function.

Medications

A decrease in total body water and increase in adipose can lead to a change in distribution of medications. Specifically, the water soluble agents such as most induction agents are distributed in a smaller initial compartment, resulting in increased exposure of receptors and potentially augmented impact. In contrast, lipid soluble medications may be deposited in larger fat stores leading to prolonged and unpredictable recovery. Age-related hepatic changes and reduction in hepatic blood flow can result in a delay in the metabolism of certain drugs such as lidocaine [54]. Although albumin levels are usually preserved in health, they may be diminished in older patients with chronic disease, in general, the quality of protein binding may be reduced and these combined changes can lead to increased free fractions of tightly bound medication such as warfarin. For certain drugs such as the benzodiazepines and opioids, [55–57] age related increased sensitivity seems more related to changes in the pharmacodynamic and sensitivity of the receptors as opposed to an alteration in the distribution or clearance of the medications. In the next section, the impact of aging on individual agents will be considered [40].

Anxiolytics

Benzodiazepines provide anxiyiolyisis and amnesia. *Diazepam and lorazepam* are long acting anyxioltics compared with midazolam, and their administration has been associated with postoperative delirium. In general, these longer acting drugs should be avoided in frail geriatric patients, although lorazepam may be indicated in certain circumstances such as alcohol withdrawal [56, 58].

Midazolam is a water soluble benzodiazepine generally given intravenously as an anxiolytic prior to the induction of anesthesia or as an adjunct to sedation; it may even be used as the sole anesthetic agent for very brief procedures. It is metabolized via hepatic hydroxylation to its major metabolite 1-hydroxymidazolam that is subsequently conjugated and excreted. Pharmacodynamic changes with aging result in increased sensitivity to midazolam and the starting dose should be reduced to 0.5–1 mg, and increased slowly if needed [56]. There are very limited hemodynamic effects, although hypotension has been observed when midazolam is combined with fentanyl. In general, in older patients, it is advantageous to avoid midazolam altogether, and if needed in anxious patients the initial and subsequent doses should be reduced.

Induction Agents

Propofol or 2,6 di-isopropyl phenol is now the most commonly used intravenous anesthesia agent inside the operating room and also for procedures in remote locations. Propofol provides excellent hypnosis, a rapid recovery, and some protection against nausea and vomiting. Propofol also causes significant vasodilatation and potential hypotension that is exaggerated in older patients especially in the presence of hypovolemia. In general, older patients require less drug (20–60% reduction) to achieve the same level of anesthesia. The initial propofol dose in the older patient is distributed in a smaller central volume of distribution, and the peak concentration may be more pronounced and prolonged compared with a young patient in whom the redistribution occurs rapidly after the bolus dose. This translates to an increased sensitivity of older patients to smaller bolus doses and a delay to peak effect, including delayed peripheral vasodilatation. Thus in the elderly patients, it is important to reduce the bolus and increase the interval between repeated doses. Administration of even a small dose of propofol may result in respiratory arrest and for that reason it has been recommended that its use is limited to anesthesiologists or providers trained in basic airway management and resuscitation [40, 59].

Etomidate is another induction agent frequently used to induce anesthesia, especially in elderly patients, trauma victims, or emergency circumstances. In contrast to propofol, etomidate has almost no cardiovascular side effects and is preferred in the patient with unstable hemodynamics and poor cardiac reserve. In older patients with significant cardiac disease or unknown physiological reserve etomidate can be advantageous. In general, the induction dose should be reduced 25–50% in elderly patients.

Ketamine is a phencyclidine derivative, NMDA blocker that can produce dissociative anesthesia. Advantages of ketamine include absence of respiratory depression and analgesic properties. In the elderly patient, small doses of ketamine can reduce opioid requirements and offset the hypotensive effects of higher propofol doses during an MAC anesthetic. Its use has been associated with bad dreams and agitation in younger patients, but this may be less of a problem in the older patient when administered with low dose benzodiazepines or propofol. Preemptive low dose ketamine infusions in the postoperative period have been used to treat patients with significant pain that is resistant to traditional medications. The opioid sparing effects of ketamine can be very useful in the older compromised patient. At these lower doses, there has been no evidence of any increase in cognitive problems.

Opioids

Elderly patient's exhibit increased sensitivity to central respiratory effects of opioid medications, and this may lead to an increase in the risk of unrecognized postoperative hypoventilation and apnea. In general, all initial opioid doses should be reduced in older patients and careful monitoring of both oxygenation and ventilation is required [60, 61].

Fentanyl is a synthetic opioid, about 50-100 times as potent as morphine but not associated with histamine release. It is lipid soluble and has a rapid onset with little effect hemodynamically and relatively short duration. During induction of anesthesia, fentanyl has been shown to block the adverse hemodynamic effects of intubation [55, 62].

Remifentanil is another highly potent synthetic opioid that is becoming increasingly popular for short stimulating procedures and sedation, especially in elderly patients in whom significant perturbations of the cardiovascular system can be deleterious. Remifentanil is metabolized by rapid hydrolysis through esterases in blood and tissue, and is suitable for infusions. In older patients, the initial dose and infusion should be reduced by about 33%. When larger doses are administered bradycardia (that can be profound) and respiratory depression may occur and limit remifentnil's use [57].

Morphine is a popular opioid for postoperative pain [38, 61], frequently administered via a PCA [63]. Older patients show an increased sensitivity, decreased clearance, and in the presence of renal failure, the accumulation of metabolites can occur. Several studies have suggested that the initial postoperative requirements of morphine are similar in old and young patients but the maintenance doses should be reduced [64].

Meperidine is a short acting analgesic, which is *not* recommended in elderly patients. It has been associated with delirium and the accumulation of the metabolite normeperidine that can be neuroexcitatory and lead to seizures.

Neuromuscular Blocking Agents

Muscle relaxation during surgery is critical for exposure and to prevent patient movement, and is generally achieved through the administration of nondepolarizing drugs such as vecuronium and cisatracurium. These drugs are competitive antagonists of acetylcholine at the nicotinic receptor and act at the postjunctional membrane of the neuromuscular junction. The most important anesthetic concern for the elderly patients is the complete reversal of these agents at the end of the surgery. Even a small amount of residual drug effect could result in significant respiratory impairment in the recovery room. For this reason, the longer acting muscle relaxant pancuronium should be avoided altogether in older patients.

Inhalational Agents

General anesthesia usually includes the addition of a volatile anesthetic agent; the most popular agents include sevoflorane, desflorane, and isoflorane. It is well documented that older patients require less volatile anesthetic to attain a suitable depth of anesthesia. The amount of inhalational agent decreases linearly with aging so by age of 80 years a patient requires only about one-third that needed in a 20-year-old patient [65].

Other

Dexmetatomidine is an alpha 2 agonist, similar to clonidine, that is approved for sedation and has gained popularity as a sedative and anesthetic adjunct. Dexmetatomidine has powerful analgesic properties and can be used in small bolus or as a continuous infusion. In addition to providing sedation and analgesia, dexmetatomidine is also a hemodynamic depressant and its administration can cause significant hypotension and bradycardia. In general, the cardiovascular side effects limits the use in older patients with cardiac disease, but in certain cases such as plastics, the hypotensive effect may be valuable; offsetting the hypertensive effects of infiltration of local anesthesia that includes epinephrine [59]. The full extent of dexmetatomidine's role in postoperative analgesia has yet to be established.

Acetominophen is frequently overlooked as a useful opioid sparing analgesic in the immediate post-recovery phase. For the older patient without liver impairment, scheduled dosing is recommended and frequently combined with a multimodal approach that includes low doses of NSAIDs or opioids [66].

Ketorolac is a potent NSAID available for intravenous administration. It can be a useful adjunct for pain relief and result in significant opioid sparing. Ketorolac, like all NSAIDS, must be used cautiously in elderly patents, especially in patients with dehydration or renal failure, a history of gastrointestinal bleeding, or anticoagulant or antiplatelet therapy. Postoperatively ketorolac should be administered for a short duration less than 5 days, and in older patients the dose should be reduced 50% starting at 15 mg and not exceeding total 60 mg/24 h.

Gabapentin is an anticonvulsant that has strong analgesic effects [67]. The mechanism of action of gabapentin is not fully known, but probably involves the neurotransmitter gamma amino butyric acid (GABA) system. Single preoperative doses of gabapentin have been found to reduce pain intensity and opioid use in the first 24 h postoperatively. In addition, gabapentin administration is associated with a reduced incidence of postoperative nausea and vomiting, constipation, and urinary retention, although an increase in sedation has been noted, especially at higher doses.

Ambulatory Surgery

Older age is not a contraindication to ambulatory surgery. Indeed some studies have suggested elderly patients may be more able to be fast tracked through the recovery area and discharged, possibly due to a reduction in medications and a lighter level of sedation administered compared with young healthy patients [51]. In general, there is limited data on outcomes in older patients following surgery, however, there is the suggestion that intraoperative arrhythmias and hypertension are more common in older patients vs. younger and that the incidence of postoperative nausea may be diminished with age [7, 9]. Postoperative urinary retention

CASE STUDY: PART 5

After discussion among the anesthesiologist, the endoscopist, and the patient, a general anesthesia is agreed upon. Due to his high risk from aspiration and increased risk of significant complications in the event of an aspiration, the anesthesiologist proceeds with a general anesthesia and endotracheal intubation. The endoscopist is able to dilate his biliary duct at the time of the ERCP. During the procedure, Mr. Smith receives several boluses of phenylephrine for low blood pressure, but overall is hemodynamically stable and extubated at the end of the

case. Mr. Smith's Parkinson symptoms worsen temporarily and mobility is a significant problem. After reinstating his Parkinson medications, Mr. Smith is hospitalized for 4 days following the procedure. He is ultimately discharged home and his family notes that his memory appears slightly worse, for instance, he has more trouble with word finding, names, and dates than he did prior to the surgery, but he does not appear delirious. This appears to resolves over the next few months. His abdominal pain is better following the dilation and the patient and the family decline a laparoscopic cholecystectomy to remove remaining gall stones.

can lead to significant morbidity, for instance in older males following hernia repair. In general, urinary retention has been associated with the administration of opioids, regional anesthesia (spinal or epidural anesthetics), male sex, older age, and anticholinergic medications.

Temperature Control

In general, exposure of a nonanesthetized patient to a cold environment such as the operating room will result in activation of receptors peripherally and centrally that lead to vasoconstriction and an increase in heat production and basal metabolic rate. Usually the core temperature is maintained a few degrees higher than the peripheral tissues through tonic vasoconstriction. Unfortunately, normal aging results in the deterioration in thermoregulation both peripherally and centrally leading to an increased risk of hypothermia. The age-related physiologic changes blunt vasoconstriction and heat production, shivering is less effective and induced at lower temperatures compared with younger subjects. Furthermore, older patients have less lean body mass and lower basal metabolic rates at the outset, and they lose heat more quickly compared with younger patients.

The issues with temperature regulation are further exacerbated in the anesthetized elderly patient and the ability to withstand cold temperatures is inhibited in the presence of all anesthetic agents. Disordered temperature regulation has been observed following both general and regional anesthetics. The risks of hypothermia to an older patient are substantial and include myocardial ischemia, surgical infection, coagulopathy, bleeding, delayed drug metabolism, and arousal [68].

Since older patients may not respond appropriately to a drop in core temperature, the anesthetic plan should include the ability to actively warm older patients in and outside

of the operating room. Intraoperative heat loss may be minimized by prewarming surfaces and maintain room temperatures high until the patient is fully draped. Warmed forced air blankets have been associated with improved maintenance of temperature.

Summary

In summary, "choosing the best anesthetic" for the geriatric patient requires meticulous attention to detail, knowledge of the physiologic changes that can be expected to occur during aging and an understanding of common comorbidities found in the elderly population. The risk of anesthesia and surgery is increased in frail older patients and anesthetics should be designed to avoid side effects and eliminate the occurrence of even small complications.

References

1. Leung JM, Dzankic S (2001) Relative importance of preoperative health status versus intraoperative factors in predicting postoperative adverse outcomes in surgical patients. J Am Geriatr Soc 49:1080–1085
2. Hosking MP, Warner MA, Lobdel CM et al (1989) Outcomes of surgery in patients 90 years of age and older. JAMA 261:1909–1915
3. Rooke GA (2003) Cardiovascular aging and anesthetic implications. J Cardiothorac Vasc Anesth 17:512–523
4. Kheterpal S, O'Reilly M, Englesbe MJ, Rosenberg AL, Shamks AM, Zhang L, Rothman ED, Campbell DA, Tremper KK (2009) Preoperative and intraoperative predictors of cardiac adverse events after general, vascular and urological surgery. Anesthesiology 110:58–66
5. Cook DJ, Rooke GA (2003) Priorities in perioperative geriatrics. Anesth Analg 96:1823–1836
6. Turrentine FE, Wang H, Simpson VB, Jones RS (2006) Surgical risk factors, morbidity, and mortality in elderly patients. J Am Coll Surg 203:865–877

7. Pedersen T, Eliasen K, Henriksen E (1990) A prospective study of mortality associated with anaesthesia and surgery: risk indicators of mortality in hospital. Acta Anaesthesiol Scand 34(3):176–182

8. Manku K, Bacchetti P, Leung JM (2003) Prognostic significance of postoperative in-hospital complications in elderly patients. I. Long-term survival. Anesth Analg 96:583–589

9. Chung F, Mezei G, Tong D (1999) Adverse events in ambulatory surgery. A comparison between elderly and younger patients. Can J Anaesth 46(4):309–321

10. Marick PE, Kaplan DL (2003) Aspiration pneumonia and dyspghagia in the elderly. Chest 124:328–336

11. Wang CY, Ling LC, Cardosa MS, Wong AKH, Wong NW (2000) Hypoxia during upper gastrointestinal endoscopy with and without sedation and the effect of pre-oxygenation on oxygen saturation. Anaesthesia 55:654–658

12. Yano H, Iishi H, Tatsuta M et al (1998) Oxygen desaturation during sedation for colonoscopy in elderly patients. Hepatogastroenterology 45:2138–2141

13. Hang J (2007) The controversy of regional vs. general anesthesia in surgical outcomes. In: Seiber FE (ed) Geriatric anesthesia. McGraw Hill, Philadelphia, pp 253–266

14. Urwin SC, Parker MJ, Griffiths R (2000) General versus regional anaesthesia for hip fracture surgery: a meta-analysis of randomized trials. Br J Anaesth 84(4):450

15. Williams-Russo P, Sharrock NE, Mattis S et al (1995) Cognitive effects after epidural vs general anesthesia in older adults: a randomized trial. JAMA 274(1):44–50

16. Rasmussen LS, Johnson T, Kuipers HM et al (2003) Does anaesthesia cause postoperative cognitive dysfunction? A randomized study of regional versus general anaesthesia in 438 elderly patients. Acta Anaesthesiol Scand 47:260–266

17. Chung F, Meier R, Lautenschlager E et al (1987) General or spinal anesthesia: which is better in the elderly? Anesthesiology 67:422–427

18. Simon MJG, Veering BT, Stienstra R et al (2002) The effects of age on neural blockade and hemodynamic changes after epidural anesthesia with ropivicaine. Anesth Analg 94(5):1325–1330

19. Pitkanen M, Haapaniemi L, Tuominen M et al (1984) Influence of age on spinal anaesthesia with isobaric 0.5% bupivicaine. Br J Anaesth 56(3):279–284

20. Critchley LA (1996) Hypotension, subarachnoid block and the elderly patient. Anaesthesia 51(12):1139–1143

21. Gustafsson LL, Schildt B, Jacobsen K (1982) Adverse effects of extradural and intrathecal opiates: report of a nationwide survey in Sweden. Br J Anaesth 54(5):479–486

22. Conference C (2003) Reg Anesth Pain Med 28:172–197

23. Roizen MF (1989) Preoperative patient evaluation. Can J Anaesth 36:513–551

24. Fischer SP (1996) Development and effectiveness of an anesthesia preoperative evaluation clinic in a teaching hospital. Anesthesiology 85:196–206

25. Fleisher LA, Beckman JA, Brown KA et al (2007) AHA/ACC 2007 guidelines on perioperative cardiovascular evaluation and care for non cardiac surgery. J Am Coll Cardiol 50:1701–1732

26. Roizen MF (1998) The compelling rationale for less preoperative testing. Can J Anaesth 35:214–218

27. Bouillot JL et al (1996) Are routine preoperative chest radiographs useful in general surgery? Eur J Surg 162:597–604

28. Schein OD, Katz J, Bass EB et al (2000) The value of routine preoperative medical testing before cataract surgery. N Engl J Med 342:168–175

29. Narr BJ (1997) Outcomes of patients with no laboratory assessment before anesthesia and a surgical procedure. Mayo Clin Proc 72:505–509

30. Starsnic MA, Guarnieri DM, Norris MC (1997) Efficacy and financial benefit of an anesthesiologist-directed University Preadmission Evaluation Center. J Clin Anesth 9:299–305

31. Power LM, Thackray NM (1999) Reduction of preoperative investigations with the introduction of an anesthetist led preoperative assessment clinic. Anaesth Intensive Care 27:481–488

32. ASA Task Force (2002) Practice advisory for preanesthesia evaluation. A report by the ASA Task Force on preanesthesia evaluation. Anesthesiology 96:485–496

33. Gibb J, Cull W, Henderson W et al (1999) Preoperative serum albumin level as a predictor of operative mortality and morbidity. Arch Surg 134:36–42

34. Gold BS (1992) The utility of preoperative electrocardiograms in the ambulatory surgical patient. Arch Intern Med 152:301–305

35. Goldberger Al, OKonski M (1986) Utility of the routine electrocardiogram before surgery and on general hospital admission. Ann Intern Med 105:552

36. ACC/AHA Guidelines (2007) ACC/AHA 2007 on perioperative cardiovascular evaluation and care for noncardiac surgery. Circulation 116:e418–e500

37. Charpak Y et al (1998) Prospective assessment of a protocol for selective ordering of preoperative chest x-rays. Can J Anaesth 35:259–264

38. Kalso E, Edwards JE, Moore RA, McQuay HJ (2004) Opioids in chronic non-cancer pain: systematic review of efficacy and safety. Pain 112(3):372–380

39. Zaugg M, Lucchinetti E (2000) Respiratory function in the elderly. Anesthesiol Clin North America 18:47–58

40. Lortat-Jacob B, Sevrin F (2007) Pharmacology of intravenous drugs in the elderly. In: Seiber FE (ed) Geriatric anesthesia, Ch 8. McGraw Hill, New York, pp 91–105

41. Warner DO (2000) Preventing postoperative pulmonary complications. Anesthesiology 92:1467–1472

42. Novis BK et al (1994) Association of preoperative risk factors with postoperative acute renal failure. Anesth Analg 78:143–149

43. Silverstein JH, Timberger BA, Reich DL, Uysal S (2007) Central nervous system dysfunction after non cardiac surgery and anesthesia in the elderly. Anesthesiology 106:622–628

44. Moller JT et al (1998) Long-term postoperative cognitive dysfunction in the elderly: ISPOCD1 study. Lancet 351:857–861

45. Okeefe ST et al (1994) Postoperative delirium in the elderly. Br J Anaesth 73:673–687

46. Inouye SK (2006) Delirium in older persons. N Engl J Med 354(11):1157–1165

47. Williams-Russo P et al (1992) Post-operative delirium: predictors and prognosis in elderly orthopedic patients. J Am Geriatr Soc 40:759–767

48. Dasgupta M, Dumbrell AC (2006) Preoperative risk assessment for delirium after non cardiac surgery: a systematic review. J Am Geriatr Soc 54:1578–1589

49. Reich DL, Hossain S, Krol M et al (2005) Predictors of hypotension after induction of general anesthesia. Anesth Analg 101:622–628

50. Phillip B, Pastor D, Bellows W, Leung JM (2003) The prevalence of preoperative diastolic filling abnormalities in geriatric surgical patients. Anesth Analg 97:1214–1221

51. White PF, Kehlet H, Neal JM et al (2007) The role of the anesthesiologist in fast-track surgery: from multimodal analgesia to perioperative medical care. Anesth Analg 104:1380–1396

52. Hasuke S, Mesic D, Dizdarevic E, Keser D, Hadziselimovic S, Bazardzanovic M (2002) Pulmonary function after lapraroscopic and open cholecystectomy. Surg Endosc 16:163–165

53. Karayiannakis AJ, Makri GG, Mantzioka A, Karousos D, Karatzas G (1996) Posoperative pulmonary function after laparoscopic and open cholecystectomy. Br J Anaesth 77:448–452

54. Schucker DL (2005) Age related changes in liver structure and function: implications for disease? Exp Gerontol 40:650–659

55. Singleton MA, Rosen JI, Fisher DM (1988) Pharmacokinetics of fentanyl in the elderly. Br J Anaesth 60(6):619–622

56. Jacobs R et al (1995) Aging increases pharmacodynamic sensitivity to the hypnotic effects of midazolam. Anesth Analg 80: 143–148

57. Minto CF, Schnider T, Egan T et al (1997) Influence of age and gender on the pharmacokinetics and pharmacodynamics or remifentanil. Anesthesiology 86:10–23

58. Reidenberg MM, Levy M, Warner H et al (1978) Relationship between diazepam dose, plasma level, age, and central nervous system depression. Clin Pharmacol Ther 23:371–374

59. Arain SR, Ebert JE (2002) The efficacy, side effects, and recovery characteristics of dexmedetomidine versus propofol when used for intraoperative sedation. Anesth Analg 95:461–465

60. Cepeda MS, Farrar JT, Baumgarten M et al (2003) Side effects of opioids during short-term administration: effect of age, gender, and race. Clin Pharmacol Ther 74(2):102–112

61. Moore RA, McQuay HJ (2005) Prevalence of opioid adverse events in chronic non-malignant pain: systematic review of randomized trials of oral opioids. Arthritis Res Ther 7(5):R1046–R1051

62. Bentley JB, Borel JD, Nenad RE Jr et al (1987) Age and fentanyl pharmacokinetics. Anesth Analg 61(12):968–971

63. Sessler DI, Sessler DI (2008) Perioperative thermoregulation. In: Silverstein JH, Rooke GA, Reves JG, McLeskey CH (eds) Geriatric anesthesiology, 2nd edn, Springer, New York, pp 107–122

64. Aubrun F (2005) Management of postoperative analgesia in elderly patients. Reg Anesth Pain Med 30:363–379

65. Mapelson WW (1996) Effect of age on MAC in humans: a meta-analysis. Br J Anaesth 76:179–185

66. Remy C, Marret E, Bonnet F (2005) Effects of acetaminophen on morphine side-effects and consumption after major surgery: meta-analysis of randomized controlled trials. Br J Anaesth 94(4):505–513

67. Ho KY, Gan TJ, Habib AS (2006) Gabapentin and postoperative pain – a systematic review of randomized controlled trials. Pain 126(1–3):91–101

68. Gagliese L, Jackson M, Ritvo P, Wowk A, Katz J (2000) Age is not an impediment to effective use of patient-controlled analgesia by surgical patients. Anesthesiology 93(3):601–610

Chapter 26
Acute Postoperative Pain Management in Elderly Patients

Jack M. Berger

In their review article, Brennan, Carr, and Cousins conclude that "because pain management is the subject of many initiatives within the disciplines of medicine, ethics, and law, we are at an 'inflection point' in which unreasonable failure to treat pain is viewed worldwide as poor medicine, unethical practice, and an abrogation of a fundamental human right" [1]. In coming to this conclusion these authors review much of the medical ethics literature which taken together is summarized in their statement that "…a virtue ethics approach to bioethics would also yield a clear response to patient's pain. A virtuous doctor would place the recognition, monitoring, and treatment of pain as a high priority. To this end, a virtuous doctor would inquire regularly about pain, respond appropriately, and refer wisely if unable to control it" [1]. This of course became mandated by the Joint Commission for the Accreditation of Healthcare Organizations (JCAHO) in 2000–2002, and the declaration by the US Congress calling 2001–2010 the "Decade of Pain Control and Research" [1].

Brennan, Carr, and Cousins go on to state that "if there is a clear ethical duty to relieve suffering or to act virtuously by doing so, then one may argue that from that duty springs a *right*. The moral right to pain management emerges from, and is directly founded upon, the duty of the doctor to act ethically. Classically, the holder of a *right* has the capacity to enforce a duty in a person or institution. That 'other' has a duty to fulfill that *right*. Indeed, a basic tenet of the *philosophy of rights* is that a *right* can only exist if there is a preexisting obligation. If one accepts that a health professional has an obligation, where appropriate, *to manage pain*, then the patient has a concomitant *right*, where appropriate, to receive such care" [1].

It is clear that this right to receive adequate pain management is not more evident than in the postoperative surgical patient (of any age). Yet fear of uncontrolled postsurgical pain continues to be among the primary concerns of many patients about to undergo surgery [2]. This fear is not unfounded since, despite increasing research and clinical attention, many adult surgical patients continue to experience moderate to severe pain [3, 4]. Some improvement has been the result of the Joint Commission for the Accreditation of Healthcare Organizations (JAHCO) initiative for better pain management assessment and treatment as reported by Frasco et al., who demonstrated that there has been an increased use of morphine and prophylactic antiemetics in postanesthesia recovery rooms without a concomitant increase in length of stay in the recovery rooms [5].

The ill effects of inadequately treated pain in the acute postoperative period are summarized by Sinatra [6]. Acute pain leads to increased sympathetic activity which in turn leads to tachycardia and hypertension [6]. In elderly patients with coronary artery disease, the risk of myocardial infarction is therefore increased. Regional blood flow can be impaired which may increase the risk of postoperative infection. Fear and anxiety resulting from inadequate pain control can impair sleep and rehabilitation. Splinting and shallow breathing can lead to hypoxemia, atelectasis, and pneumonia [6] (Fig. 26.1).

Less well recognized is the fact that inadequate acute postsurgical pain management can lead to chronic pain syndromes [7, 8]. Without belaboring the point further, it is clear that these pathological effects of acute pain can lead to life threatening consequences and can also lead to chronic neuropathic pain states that can affect the future quality of the patient's life through a constellation of maladaptive physical, psychological, family, and social consequences. These chronic neuropathic pain states can be regarded as true disease entities leading to dependence on medication, reduced mobility, loss of strength, disturbances of sleep, and social consequences that can result in dissolution of family relations [9].

Ginsberg writing in Anesthesiology News, February 2002 commenting on a Canadian study of postoperative pain management states "Pain interferes with out-patients' activities, work, sleep, appetite, and concentration…Pain on the first day after surgery can be expected. But in the Canadian study, 7 days after surgery, 50% of patients had pain that interfered with activity or work, and 25% could not sleep because of

J.M. Berger (✉)
Department of Anesthesiology, Keck School of Medicine,
University of Southern California, LAC + USA Medical Center,
Los Angeles, CA, USA
e-mail: JMBerger@usc.edu

R.A. Rosenthal et al. (eds.), *Principles and Practice of Geriatric Surgery*,
DOI 10.1007/978-1-4419-6999-6_26, © Springer Science+Business Media, LLC 2011

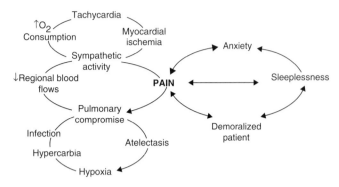

Figure 26.1 Harmful effects of unrelieved acute pain (reprinted from Sinatra [6], with permission from Elsevier).

pain" [10]. Ginsberg goes on to state that "Physicians as caregivers must take blame for inadequate pain treatment… in the Canadian study on day 1, 60% were given a mild opioid…by day 7, they only received tender loving care and chicken soup" [10].

These pathological consequences of uncontrolled pain may have greater consequences in the elderly population [11]. As the population ages, and surgical and anesthetic protocols become safer, the number of older patients undergoing surgery will grow [12]. By the year 2050, there will be a fourfold increase in the elderly population compared with only a 50% global population increase, and at that time 25% of the elderly will be over the age of 80 [13]. Elderly patients have surgery four times more frequently than the younger population [14].

However, there is little merit in considering the treatment of acute pain in the elderly population unless it differs from that provided to younger patients [13]. This begs the questions of whether elderly patients perceive pain differently from younger patients; are there changes in nociception that occur with aging, and do elderly patients process and respond to nociception differently?

Issues in treating pain in the elderly can therefore be broken down to:

- Sensitivity to painful stimuli – nociception
- Sensitivity of the central nervous system (CNS) (cognitive impairment)
- Pharmacodynamics/pharmacokinetics, organ function, and aging

    - Metabolism of drugs (liver function)
    - Excretion of drugs (renal function)

- Social concerns – addiction, pseudoaddiction, dependence, and tolerance
- Principles of titration of medications
- Role of interventional techniques and regional anesthetics

These issues will be addressed below.

Nociception Is Not Pain

Activity induced in the nociceptor and nociceptive pathways by a noxious stimulus is not "pain," which is always a psychological state. Although we appreciate that pain most often has a proximate physical cause, especially acute pain, activity in nociceptor systems is not equivalent to the "experience of pain" [15]. The recognition that pain serves an important biologic function related to survival raises the important question: to what extent do age-related changes in nociception impact on the capacity of the pain experience to fulfill an "enteroceptive" function such as thirst, hunger, and thermoception that constitute sensory indexes of the health of the body? [16]

Assessment and intervention for pain in the elderly should therefore begin with the assumption that all neurophysiologic processes subserving nociception are intact [17]. In fact Gagliese and Melzack demonstrated that age did not affect the rating of pain by postsurgical patients [18]. That is to say, tissue injury produces the same intensity of stimulus in an elderly person as in a young person.

There are data to suggest, however, that some impairment of $A\delta$ fibers occurs with aging, and therefore impedes the early warning of tissue injury [16]. There are also data that suggest that widespread and substantial changes in structure, neurochemistry, and function occur in the dorsal horn of the spinal cord and CNS with aging [16].

Multiple studies report reductions in the descending inhibitory modulating systems for nociception in the elderly [16, 19]. Gibson and Ferrell conclude that the reduced efficacy of endogenous analgesic systems might be expected to result in a more severe pain experience following prolonged noxious stimulation [16]. It is also possible that the documented decline in afferent transmission pathways could be offset by a commensurate reduction in the endogenous inhibitory mechanisms of older persons, with a net result of little or no change in the perceptual pain experience [16]. They further conclude that any deficit in endogenous analgesic response (which is stimulus intensity dependent) will become critical, thereby making it more difficult for persons of advanced age to cope with severe or persistent clinical pain conditions [16].

Gibson reviewed the literature on pain threshold and tolerance in elderly patients [20]. Evidence suggests that as age advances, pain threshold increases, but pain tolerance decreases. The net effect may be that elderly patients experience acute surgical pain in the same way as younger patients. It is clear that if a surgeon was to make a skin incision with a scalpel in an elderly unanesthetized patient, then the patient would most certainly scream with pain. Yet silent myocardial infarctions are more common in the elderly, and the bowel must be more distended before the elderly sense pain, often delaying the diagnosis of such conditions as a bowel obstruction [20, 21].

With respect to the heart, the complete absence of "the perception of pain" that can occur in the presence of myocardial ischemia, arteriolar occlusion, myocarditis, early acute endocarditis, valvular ulceration, etc. makes it difficult and yet extremely important to assess for pain in elderly patients recovering from surgery [22].

But while there is controversy over whether the number and integrity of nociceptors decreases with age, *the clinical position that age dulls the "sense of pain" is untenable* [16]. It is the processing of the nociceptive information that may be altered in the elderly, and the elderly may be more sensitive to the side effects of medications that are used to treat pain. These observations thereby give the impression that the elderly are less sensitive to pain. But no physiologic changes in pain perception in the elderly have been demonstrated according to a five-state study by Cleeland [21]. This is supported by the observation that age does not affect the success of traditional interventions for the treatment of pain [17].

Again one would not assume that a surgical incision in an elderly patient will "hurt" less and therefore does not need to be treated. Likewise, anyone who has observed an elderly patient with acute herpes zoster certainly can attest to the excruciating pain that these unfortunate patients report. If given adequate preoperative teaching, assessed preoperatively for any impediments to the use of patient-controlled analgesia (PCA), e.g., dementia, elderly patients were successfully started on PCA in the postanesthesia care unit after general anesthesia once they were awake and responsive enough to receive a loading dose of opioids titrated to comfort [17].

Postoperative Central Nervous System Dysfunction

Postoperative CNS dysfunction is a common complication in elderly surgical patients. Rohan and his associates reported that the incidence of postoperative cognitive dysfunction (POCD) in elderly patients on the first postoperative day after minor surgery performed under general anesthesia (either propofol or sevoflurane) was 47% compared with 7% for matched nonsurgical hospitalized patients [23]. The acute confusional state, postoperative delirium (POD), is also common and can occur in as many as 60% of patients depending on preoperative risk factors and the type of surgery [16]. Preoperative confusion has been found to be a predictor of POD [23]. Pain can lead to delirium which can complicate pain assessment [24]. At the same time, the effect of pain in patients who already have preexisting cognitive deficits or dementia with loss of communication skills, or even loss of basic reflexes (e.g., gag), may disturb the assessment of critical functions for the expression of pain [13].

Little is known of the neurophysiological relationships between pain- and age-related degenerative brain diseases. It has been reported that beginning at the age of 40 and continuing into late old age, there is reduced expression in the human brain of genes involved in learning and memory and neuronal survival [25]. But the ability for plasticity and new dendritic synapses (i.e., memory) is preserved even into old age [26].

It would appear that elderly patients are more susceptible to confusion and cognitive impairment, but retain some capacity to recover. It is not uncommon for elderly patients to go through a period of delirium postoperatively, and although recovery from the acute contusional state may be complete, POCD may persist for far longer. This is manifested by the complaint from the family that the elderly patient just never seemed "quite the same" again after the operation.

Pharmacodynamics/Pharmacokinetics, Organ Function, and Aging

Fine recently reviewed the issues of pharmacological management of persistent pain in older patients [27]. In general, the *pharmacodynamic* actions of drugs (what the drug does to the patient) are unaffected in the normal aging process. The molecular action of morphine is the same in all animals, although dose requirements to produce the same effect may change with age, and the therapeutic window between intended effect and side or adverse effects may be narrowed in the elderly [28, 29]. However, since centrally acting drugs may interact with a preexisting disease state, care must be taken when treating pain in patients with CNS disease such as Parkinsonism, Alzheimer dementia, or stroke.

The pharmacokinetic actions of drugs (what the patient does to the drug), on the other hand, are frequently affected by aging processes and disease states. Pharmacokinetic changes due to physical aging may complicate medication management [30]. Woodhouse and Mathur studied the 24-h cumulative PCA opioid administration as a function of age, and found that morphine and fentanyl both showed the expected reduction in dose by 50% in the elderly, but meperidine was more variable due to a more complex pharmacology [31]. This 50% reduction in PCA opioid analgesia requirement in elderly surgical patients compared with younger patients was confirmed by other investigators [17]. The patients in this study showed comparable levels of pain relief and satisfaction with this technology. Opioids have been shown to produce a greater incidence of respiratory depression in the elderly, but the elderly seem to be less sensitive with respect to nausea and vomiting [32].

The most important generalization from physiologic studies of aging is that although the basal function of the various organ systems may decline with aging *that the impact of this decline may not be functionally important at rest.* However, functional reserve and the ability to compensate for physiologic stress are reduced with aging [33]. With aging there is a decreased lean body mass and total body water and an increased proportion of body fat; these alter the volume of distribution and redistribution of drugs and alter their rates of clearance and elimination [33]. There is decreased liver mass and blood flow, which prolongs drug metabolism [34]. There is an age-related decrease in basal metabolic rate of the liver and a decline in albumin production of about 10% [35]. However, overall age-related changes in protein binding do not produce clinical difference in drug transport [36].

Drug biotransformation reactions can either lead to the inactivation of the parent compound, the conversion of an inactive compound to an active one, or result in metabolites that are even more active than the parent active drug [37]. Toxic metabolites are also produced that depend on rapid excretion to avoid harm to the organism. Drug biotransformation is usually an enzymatic process. Although most tissues have some enzymatic metabolism, most occurs in the liver. Patients with impaired liver function will therefore have altered metabolic capacity for drug elimination [37].

Renal blood flow is also compromised by aging; approximately 10% per decade of life after the age of 50 with a loss of renal parenchyma also [38]. Perioperative metabolic acidosis is relatively common in elderly patients who are less efficient in the renal excretion of acid [33]. Anesthetics, surgical stress, pain, sympathetic stimulation, and renal vasoconstrictive drugs may all compound subclinical renal insufficiency [33]. Cook and Rooke conclude that what is clear from a review of the physiologic changes with aging is that even the fit elderly patient's ability to compensate for perioperative stress is compromised. The cardiac, pulmonary, neurologic, and neuroendocrine changes that occur with aging make hypotension, low cardiac output, hypoxia, hypercarbia, and disordered fluid regulation more commonplace in the perioperative period. Furthermore, because baseline cardiac, pulmonary, renal, and neurologic function is typically adequate in the absence of acute challenges, it can be very difficult to predict the effect of perioperative stress on the older patient [33].

The kidney, lungs, GI tract, and skin all have some capacity to metabolize drugs. One of the major enzymatic systems for drug elimination with respect to analgesics and adjuvant analgesics is the cytochrome P450 system of enzymes. Drugs that are administered simultaneously and that are metabolized by the same enzyme system will compete for binding sites leading to altered blood levels [37].

The elderly have decreased renal function which increases the risk of nonsteroidal anti-inflammatory drug (NSAID) nephrotoxicity and accumulation of metabolites of drugs like meperidine. There is decreased plasma binding which increases blood levels of active drugs, opioids, and NSAIDs [even the specific cyclooxygenase 2 (COX-2) inhibitors, such as celecoxib (Celebrex®)]. [39]

To understand the cascade of renal effects of NSAIDs, it is necessary to look at the beneficial effects of the enzyme cyclooxygenase 1 (COX-1) on converting arachidonic acid to various prostaglandins. These prostaglandins are necessary for maintaining good renal blood flow, adequate glomerular filtration rate, and homeostasis of potassium and sodium retention through appropriate secretions of renin, aldosterone, and antidiuretic hormone (ADH). When the conversion of arachidonic acid to prostaglandins is inhibited by NSAID inhibition of COX-1, then the kidney comes under risk and losses its ability to regulate salt and water balance. This detrimental effect of NSAIDs on the kidney is potentiated by renal hypoperfusion states [40]. All NSAIDs can result in renal insufficiency; and with the exception of salicylsalicylic acid and choline magnesium trisalicylate, for which the risk is less, they can inhibit platelet aggregation and cause dyspepsia and gastric ulceration [41].

In a Canadian study of nearly 650,000 elderly patients being prescribed either traditional NSAIDs with or without a proton pump inhibitor (PPI), acetaminophen with or without a PPI, or NSAID and acetaminophen together with or without a PPI, it was found that when given together, an NSAID plus acetaminophen increased the risk of GI bleeding even with the addition of a PPI [42]. *Elderly patients must therefore be warned about the combined use of NSAIDs and acetaminophen that can be purchased over-the-counter.*

NASIDs have peripheral and central effects [43]. The "Constitutive" effects of the prostaglandins resulting from the actions of COX-1 also include protection of the stomach and intestinal lining, and preservation of platelet function [44]. The "Inducible" effects of COX-2 on conversion of arachidonic acid to prostaglandin E-2 leads to inflammation and pain. Blockade of the action of COX-2 reduces inflammation and pain without affecting the good effects of the prostaglandins that are COX-1 dependent [44, 45]. In the presence of inflammation, COX-2 can be found elevated in the CNS. This elevation is primarily due to upregulation of interleukin-1β. The action of COX-2 leads to increased levels of prostaglandin E2. *Antagonists of interleukin-1β or blocking COX-2 both lead to antinociception* [46]. The common NSAIDs are nonspecific because they have variable effects on blockade of COX-1 and COX-2. The most common oral NSAIDs used in clinical practice are shown in Table 26.1.

There is a ceiling dose effect to all of the NSAIDs, above which no further analgesia is obtained; and although the dose may vary it usually falls below the maximal recommended dose of the manufacturer [47]. In general, for elderly patients, agents with short half-lives (e.g., ibuprofen) are most appropriate; for patients with a history of dyspepsia, ulcer disease,

TABLE 26.1 Common oral NSAIDs by chemical class

Propionic acids	Salycilates	Fenamates	Oxicams	Acidic acids	Benzine-acidic acid
Ibuprofen (Motrin®)	Aspirin	Meclofenamate sodium (Meclomen®)	Piroxicam (Feldene®)	Tolmetin sodium (Tolectin®/DS)	Diclofenac sodium (Voltaren®) (Voltaren® XR)
Naproxen (Naprosyn®)	Diflunisal (Dolobid®)			Indomethacin (Indocin®) (Indocin® SR)	
Fenoprofen calcium (Nalfon®)	Salicylsalicylic acid (Disalcid®)			Sulindac (Clinoril®)	
Ketoprofen (Orudis®)	Choline magnesium trisalicylate (Trilisate®)				

Source: Data from Insel [60]

or bleeding diatheses, either salicylsalicylic acid or choline magnesium trisalicylate should be used if a traditional NSAID is indicated [41]. NSAIDs can be combined with opioids to enhance analgesia.

Parenteral NSAIDs

Parenteral NSAIDs (e.g., ketorolac) are being used increasingly for postoperative pain as sole analgesic agents and in conjunction with opioids as opioid-sparing agents [48]. The efficacy of ketorolac, currently the only available parenteral NSAID in the USA, has been well established with 30 mg being equianalgesic with 10 mg of parenteral morphine [48]. When used together, there was a significant reduction of adverse side effects of opioids due to a significant reduction in morphine requirements. Intravenous ketorolac has been shown to reduce opioid requirements for knee and hip replacement surgery by 35–44%, and by 50–75% for thoracotomy and upper abdominal surgery [49, 50]. While ketorolac can reduce opioid requirements, it is not potent enough to be used as a sole analgesic after major surgery such as intra-abdominal surgery [51].

Peak analgesia from ketorolac is typically seen 1–2 h after administration, and the half-life is approximately 6 h, although it may be prolonged in patients with reduced renal function or in the elderly. The manufacturer's recommended dose for elderly individuals or those with renal insufficiency is 15 mg every 6 h following a 30 mg loading dose, and doses as low as 7.5 mg q6h have been found to significantly reduce opioid requirements in such painful surgeries as spinal fusion [52].

Ketorolac has a side-effect profile similar to those of other NSAIDs. There appears to be a significantly increased risk of gastrointestinal bleeding in the elderly, particularly with high doses and with the duration of use of more than 5 days [53–55]. But when used in doses of 15 mg or less q6h for less than 3 days, toxicity seems to be minimal.

Parecoxib is a specific COX-2 inhibitor that is available in Europe for intravenous administration. In a study of parecoxib 40 mg IV administered on induction of general anesthesia, and then q12h for 24 h; improved postoperative analgesia without increased bleeding for total hip arthroplasty was observed. It is well known that COX-2 is responsible for the synthesis of prostaglandins, which sensitizes the nociceptor and acts as excitatory neuromediators in the CNS and in the periphery [45, 56].

In another study, parecoxib was found to be an effective analgesic in acute postoperative pain at 20 or 40 mg over placebo given either intravenously or intramuscularly. The number needed to treat (NNT) for parecoxib 20 mg IV for at least 50% pain relief over 6 h was 3.0 and for 40 mg was 2.2 [57]. This compares favorably with other analgesics, e.g., morphine 10 mg where the NNT was 3, ibuprofen 400 mg where the NNT was 2.7, and acetaminophen 1,000 mg where the NNT was 4.6 [58]. Ibuprofen was actually more effective than morphine at these doses. In direct comparison of 4 mg of intravenous morphine with 30 mg of intravenous ketorolac or 20 mg of intravenous paracoxib, the times to remedication were 3 h for morphine versus 5.5 h for both the ketorolac and paracoxib at the specified doses [59].

Symptomatic hepatic effects attributable to therapeutic use of most NSAIDs are extremely rare and usually mild except in over dosage of acetaminophen (not a true NSAID but used as a nonopiate analgesic) where fatal hepatic necrosis can occur. There is no clearly established explanation for why some compounds are more hepatotoxic than others. It is possible that some compounds undergo oxidation, probably to the phenylic ring structure, yielding highly reactive metabolites. Compounds that cause mild hepatic damage, such as diclofenac and bromfenac, may produce some reactive epoxides during biotransformation [60].

Impairment of wound healing has been attributed to the use of NSAIDs in the postoperative period. Studies have shown that there was no effect on epidermal wound healing with selective COX-2 and nonselective COX inhibitors in a mouse model. The authors propose that this was probably due to redundant mechanisms for wound repair, most of which are not influenced by the COX-2 inhibitors [61].

Power indicates in his review article that the data is conflicting with respect to bone healing and nonunion when these agents are used in orthopedic procedures [62]; but much of the adverse data come from animal studies which may not have clinical significance in humans [63, 64]. Short-term use of COX-2-specific inhibitors may play an important role in preventive analgesia for postoperative pain management [56, 65].

It is important to remember that COX-2-specific inhibitors do not affect platelet aggregation [45, 56] and therefore may pose a risk for myocardial infarction (MI) if the patient is taken off aspirin therapy. Since low-dose aspirin is increasingly being used for cardioprotection, it is important to note that coadministration of selective COX-2 inhibitors does not alter this protective effect [66]. It has recently been shown that celecoxib (Celebrex™) does not appear to be associated with an increased risk of serious cardiovascular thromboembolic events and it is the only remaining oral COX-2 inhibitor available in the USA [67]. It could therefore be used as a preoperative medication and continued postoperatively through healing (e.g., <10 days) as part of a multimodal preventive analgesic regimen, if the patient is able to take oral medications and does not have an allergy to sulfa-containing medications.

Opioids

Opioids are the closest drugs we currently have to an ideal analgesic. They exhibit no ceiling effect and can produce profound analgesia by progressive dose escalation. They are the most effective agents for the relief of any type of acute pain because of their predictable dose-dependent response.

Opioids have no significant long-term organ toxicity and can be used for years [68]. Addiction is negligible when opioids are used in the context of medical care [69].

It is clinically useful to classify opioids as weak or strong depending on their relative efficacy. Weak opioids are used for moderate or less severe pain, and their efficacy is limited by an increased incidence of side effects at higher doses (e.g., nausea and constipation with codeine, CNS with propoxyphene) [41].

Morley introduced a concept of "Broad Spectrum Opioids" versus "Narrow Spectrum Opioids" [70]. The narrow spectrum opioids have analgesic actions limited to the Mu, Kappa, and Delta opioid receptors. For purposes of acute postoperative pain management, we are primarily dealing with Mu opioid agonists. The broad spectrum opioids find more usefulness in chronic pain and neuropathic pain with their Mu opioid action enhanced by actions also as *N-methyl* d-*aspartate* (*NMDA*) receptor antagonists. In addition, some have central neuromodulating effects through inhibition of reuptake of serotonin and norepinephrine similar to many antidepressants. Some broad spectrum opioids have all three properties (e.g., methadone). These actions of the different opioids in common use are summarized in Table 26.2.

When opioids are used in a fixed oral dose mixed with a nonopioid analgesic, their efficacy is limited by the maximal safe dose for the acetaminophen, aspirin, or NSAID component. A list of the common combination oral opioids is shown in Table 26.3.

Strong opioids are used for more severe pain. They have a wide therapeutic window and no ceiling effect, with higher doses producing an increasing level of analgesia. They are the agents of choice for parenteral administration. Patients experiencing moderate pain should be started on a weak opioid. Patients whose pain is severe or whose pain persists, despite the use of a weak opioid, should be administered a strong opioid [41].

TABLE 26.2 Broad spectrum versus narrow spectrum opioid analgesics

Broad spectrum opioids with NMDA receptor blocking action	Broad spectrum opioids which inhibit reuptake of serotonin and norepinephrine	Narrow spectrum opioids with analgesic action limited as Mu opioid agonist
Methadone	Methadone	Morphine
Ketobemidone	Levorphanol	Hydromorphone
Dextroproxyphene	Dextromethorphan	Codeine
Dextromethorphan	D-Propoxyphene	Etorphine
Meperidine (pethidine)	Tramadol	Fentanyl
	Meperidine (Pethidine)	Sufentanil
		Oxycodone
		Hydrocodone
		Buprenorphine

Source: Data from Morley [70]

TABLE 26.3 Combination opioids available for oral administration

Trade name®	Opioid component	Dose of opioid (mg)	Adjuvant drug	Dose of adjuvant (mg)	Tabs/caps/day
Advil			Ibuprofen	200	12
E.S. Tylenol			Acetaminophen	500	8
Tylenol-3	Codeine	30	Acetaminophen	300	13
Tylenol-4	Codeine	60	Acetaminophen	300	13
Darvon	Propoxyphene	65			NL
Darvocet	Propoxyphene	65	Acetaminophen	325	13
Darvocet N-100	Propoxyphene	100	Acetaminophen	325	13
Vicodin	Hydrocodone	5	Acetaminophen	500	8
Vicodin ES	Hydrocodone	7.5	Acetaminophen	750	5
Lortab Elix	Hydrocodone	7.5	Acetaminophen	500	8
Lorcet 10/650	Hydrocodone	10	Acetaminophen	650	6
Norco	Hydrocodone	10	Acetaminophen	325	13
Vicoprofen	Hydrocodone	7.5	Ibuprofen	200	12
Percodan	Oxycodone	5	Aspirin	325	6
Percocet	Oxycodone	5	Acetaminophen	325	13
		10			
Tylox	Oxycodone	5	Acetaminophen	500	8
Oxycodone	Oxycodone	5			NL

The dose is limited by the adjuvant not by the opioid component. The maximum doses should be reduced in the elderly or in the presence of liver and renal insufficiency

Weak Opioid Agents

These are the most commonly prescribed opioids particularly in the elderly. They are available in various strengths and should be started in low doses in the elderly. Most are even scored so that half doses can be given.

Codeine, an alkaloid of opium, is the prototype "weak" analgesic. Although a parenteral preparation is available, it is nearly always given orally and often in a fixed mixture with a nonopioid analgesic. A 200 mg dose is equipotent to 30 mg of morphine. The half-life of codeine is 2.5–3.0 h [41]. Codeine is often combined with acetaminophen with or without caffeine in doses of 300 mg acetaminophen, 30 mg codeine, and 15 mg caffeine (e.g., Tylenol 3™).

Hydrocodone is a codeine derivative, available in the USA only in combination with acetaminophen, aspirin, or ibuprofen. It is more potent than codeine, although good data are lacking [41].

It should be remembered, however, that codeine (Tylenol™ 3 or 4), dihydrocodeine (Synalgos™ DC), and hydrocodone (Vicodin™, Lortab™, Norco™, etc.) do not have opioid action until they undergo metabolic conversion to morphine or hydromorphone by the action of the enzyme CYP2D6, one of the P450 group of enzymes [71]. Twenty percent of the population is reported to be deficient in this enzyme and therefore will have a poor response to these medications. In addition, there are a number of drugs which will depress the action of CYP2D6, such as: amiodarone (Cordarone®), fluoxetine (Prozac®), haloperidol (Haldol®), paroxetine (Paxil®), propafenone (Rythmol®), propoxyphene (Darvon®), quinidine, ritonavir (Norvir®), terbinafine (Lamisil®), thioridazine (Mellaril®), etc. [71].

Oxycodone is a semisynthetic derivative of the baine, an opium alkaloid. Because of its high bioavailability (>50%), it is suitable for oral administration and is 1.5 times more potent than morphine by this route and ten times more potent than codeine [72, 73]. When administered parenterally, its intensity and duration of analgesia are 25% less than those of morphine [73]. However, in the USA, oxycodone is exclusively an oral medication. Oxycodone given orally has a half-life of 2–3 h and duration of action of 4–5 h. It is metabolized like codeine: demethylated and conjugated in the liver and excreted in the urine [73]. Oxycodone has been considered a "weak" analgesic because of its use in a fixed combination with acetaminophen and aspirin, e.g., Percocet® (oxycodone 2.5, 5, or 10 mg with acetaminophen 325 mg) or Percodan® (oxycodone 5 mg with aspirin™ 325 mg) which limits its dose. When oxycodone is used alone, it has no ceiling effect for analgesia. It is more potent than morphine, and there are reports suggesting that it might have fewer side effects [74, 75]. Its availability in 5 mg tablets permits careful titration in patients with a narrow therapeutic margin. It is also available in extended-release preparations with doses of 10, 20, 40, and 80 mg without acetaminophen, which can be used for q12h dosing or occasionally q8h dosing.

Oxycodone is therefore a versatile and flexible oral medication that can be used to treat pain of any intensity requiring an opioid analgesic [41]. It is also interesting that patients who report poor analgesic effect from codeine- and hydrocodone-based opioids will report excellent analgesia from oxycodone-based analgesics. This is a result of enzymatic metabolism of oxycodone by CYP2D6. Therefore, the patients who are deficient in this enzyme cannot convert codeine or hydrocodone to morphine, but also will not metabolize oxycodone quickly and therefore have a prolonged effect from oxycodone [71]. The reverse would also be true in that those patients who genetically have high levels of CYP2D6 will get excellent analgesia from codeine or hydrocodone, but oxycodone although effective, will have a shortened duration and require more frequent dosing.

Propoxyphene (Darvon™ or Darvocet™, propoxyphene/acetaminophen) is a synthetic analgesic structurally related to methadone. It is approximately equipotent to codeine as an analgesic but lacks its antitussive properties. Its analgesic activity lasts 3–5 h, its half-life is 6–12 h, and its major metabolite is norpropoxyphene, which has a half-life of 30–36 h and may be responsible for some of the observed toxicity, particularly in the elderly [76]. Norpropoxyphene has local anesthetic effects similar to those of lidocaine, and high doses may cause arrhythmias. Seizures occur more often with propoxyphene intoxication than with other opioids. It is more difficult to manage and offers no advantage over other opioids, and therefore it is a poor choice of mild analgesic in the elderly [41].

Tramadol (Ultram®) is a weak opioid analgesic that also inhibits the reuptake of serotonin and norepinephrine. A tramadol dose of 50 mg appears to be equianalgesic with 60 mg of codeine [77]. Unlike other opioids, tramadol exhibits an analgesic ceiling, which limits its use for severe pain syndromes. Tramadol appears not to be associated with physical dependence but does have a relatively high incidence of associated nausea compared with that of other opioids [78]. Tramadol is also available as a combination drug with acetaminophen (Ultracet® 37.5 mg tramadol/325 mg acetaminophen) or as a sustained-release tramadol of 100 or 200 mg (Ultram® ER).

Strong Opioid Agents

As described by Morrison et al., *morphine* is the prototype strong opioid agonist [41, 79]. In the past, all other opioids were compared with morphine when determining their relative analgesic potency. But Shafer and Flood describe several concepts that must be considered when treating the elderly with opioids by bolus intravenous administration or by continuous infusions as is commonplace in the postoperative period [30].

They state that "the calculation of the equianalgesic dose is complicated by the relative intrinsic potency of the opioids, the different pharmacokinetic profiles, and the large differences in the rate of blood–brain equilibration." Further, because of these stated differences in the properties of the opioids, the equianalgesic dose also becomes a function of the time after the injection was made; and they give an example of fentanyl (50 μg), which has a rapid onset, will have the same effect at 10 min as 5 mg of morphine which has a slow onset time. However, at 60 min postinjection, 50 μg of fentanyl will have the same effect as 1 mg of morphine [30]. Thus, one must be careful in titrating morphine with frequent bolus doses since it may result in stacking the effect which may not become evident until 60 min later. It may be better to load a patient to comfort with fentanyl while starting a PCA with morphine or hydromorphone, in order to allow enough time for the longer acting and slower onset opioids to reach peak effect and steady state.

Like other "strong" opioids, there is no ceiling to the analgesic effect, although side effects, particularly sedation and confusion, may intervene before optimal analgesia. Morphine is metabolized in the liver, where it undergoes glucuronidation at the 3- and 6-positions. Morphine-3-glucuronide (M3G) and morphine-6-glucuronide (M6G) accumulate with chronic morphine administration [80]. M6G binds to Mu receptors with affinity similar to morphine but also binds to delta receptors, which may account for its higher analgesic potency [69, 81].

M6G appears to be 20 times more analgesic than morphine when administered directly in the periaqueductal gray, but only 0.077% of this metabolite crosses the intact blood–brain barrier following oral or parenteral administration [81, 82].

With single-dose morphine studies, the relative parenteral/oral potency ratio is 1:6 [83]. After chronic use, the ratio changes to 1:3 as a result of the accumulation of active metabolites [84]. There is experimental [85] and clinical [86] evidence that M3G, which has negligible affinity for opioid receptors and does not produce analgesia, has excitatory effects on neurons and can cause myoclonus and rarely a hyperalgesic state [81]. It is thought that the myoclonus and hyperalgesia precipitated by M3G are mediated by different receptor mechanisms [87].

The half-life of morphine is about 2 h but the onset time for analgesia from a bolus dose can be as long as 90 min [88]. Shafer and Flood comment that this slow onset of analgesia should make it difficult to titrate morphine [30] even though Auburn showed that titration of small morphine doses every 5 min was safe and effective in the elderly [28, 88].

Extended-release oral preparations of morphine have been available for many years in many different doses permitting q8h, q12h (MS Contin™), and once daily dosing (Kadian™ and Avinza™). Slow-release preparations should be used only after dose titration with morphine sulfate and only if the pain is expected to continue [41]. Morphine metabolites are eliminated by glomerular filtration and can accumulate in patients with renal insufficiency, leading to an increased incidence of side effects [89]. Morphine should be used with caution in the presence of renal failure; and if utilized, the dosing interval should be increased.

Hydromorphone (Dilaudid®) is a potent semisynthetic phenanthrene-derivative opioid agonist [22]. When single doses are administered parenterally, 2 mg of hydromorphone is equipotent to 10 mg of morphine. Hydromorphone is somewhat shorter acting than morphine but has a higher peak effect. Its bioavailability is 30–40% with an oral to parenteral ratio of 5:1 [90]. It has a half-life of 1.5–2.0 h, and active metabolites may accumulate during renal failure [91]. Because hydromorphone is highly water soluble, continuous subcutaneous infusion and intravenous infusions of hydromorphone result in similar analgesia and side effects [92].

Fentanyl is a synthetic phenylpiperidine-derivative opioid agonist that interacts primarily with Mu receptors [93]. It is 80–100 times more potent than morphine and highly lipophilic [30]. The onset time for analgesia when administered intravenously is 2–3 min making it an ideal agent for analgesic titration.

Fentanyl is also available in both a transdermal (Duragesic™) form and oral transmucosal (Actiq™) form. The transdermal form is not recommended, however, for the treatment of postoperative pain because the titration is lengthy and it lacks the flexibility, which is the cornerstone of treatment for acute and evolving pain. Oral transmucosal fentanyl is being used for severe breakthrough pain requiring rapid onset without intravenous access (e.g., at home). Its inherent safety is that the patient can discontinue administration with the onset of analgesia without having to use the entire dose.

Levorphanol (Levo-Dromoran™) is a synthetic opioid agonist structurally related to the phenanthrene-derivative opiates. It is a potent Mu agonist but also binds delta and kappa receptors [94]. When administered parenterally, 2 mg of levorphanol is equianalgesic to 10 mg of morphine [95]. Because it has a half-life of 12–30 h and duration of analgesia of 4–6 h, dose reduction may be required 2–4 days after starting the drug to avoid side effects resulting from drug accumulation. Levorphanol should not be used in patients with impaired renal function or encephalopathy because of the dangers of drug accumulation and the development of toxic serum levels. It should be used only for patients who cannot tolerate other opioids because of the combination of inadequate analgesia and intolerable side effects [96].

Because Levo-Dromoran™ is four to eight times as potent as morphine and has a longer half-life, the dosage in elderly patients with cancer or with other conditions for which chronic opioid therapy is indicated must be individualized. Because there is incomplete cross-tolerance among opioids, when converting a patient from morphine to Levo-Dromoran™, the total daily dose of oral Levo-Dromoran™ should begin at approximately 1/15 to 1/12 of the total daily dose of oral morphine that such patients had previously required and then the dose should be adjusted to the patient's clinical response not more frequently than every 72 h.

Methadone is a synthetic diphenylheptane-derivative opiate mu agonist. It is an inexpensive and effective analgesic, but its use is limited by the need for a carefully individualized dose and interval titration. When administered to opioid-naive patients, especially the elderly, the risk of overdose is high. It should therefore be used only for selected patients and only by individuals experienced with its use [97]. The oral bioavailability is high, ranging up to 100%, and it is rapidly absorbed from the gastrointestinal tract with measurable plasma concentrations within 30 min after oral administration [97, 98]. It has no active metabolites and its clearance is not affected by hepatic or renal disease [98].

When administered in single parenteral doses to opioid naïve patients, methadone is equipotent to morphine, with duration of analgesia of 4–6 h [99]. Its plasma level declines in a biexponential manner with a half-life of 2–3 h during the initial phase and 15–60 h during the terminal phase [100]. This biexponential decline accounts for the relatively short analgesic action and the tendency for drug accumulation with repeated dosing. A reduction in dose and interval frequency is often needed during the first few days of treatment to prevent side effects from overdosage [101]. The rare patient allergic to morphine and intolerant to fentanyl might benefit from methadone because of its different chemical structure. Furthermore, *since methadone is cleared almost exclusively by the liver, it can be a useful medication in patients with renal failure* [102].

Patients with neuropathic pain or opioid tolerance can often obtain relief when changed to methadone. However, methadone must be started at a much lower dose and increased slowly, with a frequency of not less than every 3 days. Breakthrough doses of the present opioid must be maintained during this transition period [103]. Another interesting recent finding concerning methadone is the report that it is a potent inducer of cell death in leukemia cells and inhibited proliferation of these cancer cells [104].

As stated previously, methadone also has antagonist action at the NMDA receptor site thus being effective in neuropathic pain states of tolerance, and has action on inhibiting reuptake of serotonin and norepinephrine effectively increasing the concentration of these antinociceptive hormones at the level of the spinal cord [103].

Meperidine (Demerol®), a synthetic phenylpiperidine-derivative mu agonist with anticholinergic properties, used to be the most commonly prescribed analgesic for acute pain and was widely used for chronic pain [41]. The reasons for this enthusiasm are unclear and irrational. Meperidine is reported to cause less biliary spasm than morphine [105].

This property, however, has not been shown to be clinically advantageous. The *CNS excitatory effects* that appear after chronic use, *particularly in the elderly*, and in patients with renal insufficiency are well substantiated, and the accumulation of its metabolite normeperidine causes multifocal myoclonus and grand mal seizure that are not reversed by naloxone [106, 107]. The half-life of meperidine is 3 h. Short-term treatment with meperidine has been associated with mild negative alterations in various elements of mood [107]. *Therefore, the physician order for 25 mg of Demerol® q4h i.m. PRN for pain in the elderly hip fracture patient should be discouraged.*

When administered to patients' receiving monoamine oxidase (MAO) inhibitors, severe respiratory depression or excitation, delirium, hyperpyrexia, and convulsions can occur [108]. The equianalgesic dose to 10 mg of parenteral morphine is 75–100 mg of meperidine. The oral/parenteral ratio is 1:4. Its use as an oral agent for long-term use is rare if ever justified because of its poor oral bioavailability and toxic metabolite (normeperidine); however, it still can be a useful agent for acute pain crisis in the emergency room or postanesthesia recovery room when patients have known neuropathic pain or acute opioid tolerance, or shivering [109, 110].

Principles of Dosing and Delivery Methods

Onset, peak, and duration of analgesia vary with the drug, route of administration, and individual patient. The recognition of this variability allows the appropriate choice of drug, route, and scheduling. The elderly exhibit a more pronounced pharmacologic effect after any weight-adjusted opioid dose. The analgesia is more intense, but the cognitive and respiratory effects and perhaps constipation are more severe. This enhanced effect is likely due to a lesser volume of distribution (approximately half that of younger patients), decreased clearance, and diminished target organ reserve (CNS, pulmonary function, and bowel function) [111, 112].

Other factors that influence opioid effects, but to a lesser degree than that of age, are body weight, severity of pain, abnormal renal function, nausea/vomiting, and cardiopulmonary insufficiency. After the initial dose determination, drugs are titrated based on the analgesic effect. For patients with severe acute pain, such as postoperative pain, parenteral morphine was usually the opioid of choice [41]. Today, at least in the well-monitored site of the postanesthesia recovery room, hydromorphone and fentanyl have become more common. Opioids should be titrated until one of the two endpoints is reached: adequate analgesia or the development of intolerable side effects [113].

Dose titration to comfort must be accomplished before beginning PCA. In this author's experience, one can utilize the total dose required to obtain comfort as a measure of the 3-h patient requirement in setting up a PCA. Basal infusion rates are not recommended for the elderly as accumulation of dose can occur during periods of sleep. But the lockout period must also be adjusted so that the patient has adequate time to experience the effect of the analgesic but short enough that the patient can "catch up" with his/her pain (see below).

PCA and Intravenous Infusions

PCA is a safe, effective modality for the delivery of opioids for pain that is expected to resolve (e.g., postoperative pain). The patient self-delivers fixed doses of an opioid by pressing a button. An overdose is infrequent because the patient must be alert to press the button and there is a lockout time between delivered doses during which pressing the button does not result in the delivery of medication. Family members must be cautioned not to press the button for their loved ones while the patient is sleeping in response to a groan or grimace. The usual PCA starting dose for morphine is 1 mg and for hydromorphone is 0.2 mg. The usual lockout time is 8, 10, or 15 min, although this should be adjusted for the individual patient depending on the severity of pain, the age of the patient, and whether there is a basal rate. Some advocate a low-dose basal infusion of opioid at night (e.g., morphine 0.5 mg/h or hydromorphone 0.1 mg/h) to avoid frequent awakenings because of pain, especially for the first 2–3 nights after surgery, although this may increase the daily morphine consumption [114]. Others feel that in the elderly it is better that the patients be allowed to awaken and press the PCA button on their own [115]. However, when PCA was compared with the more traditional "as-needed" administration of intramuscular opioids in a randomized trial involving postoperative pain control in elderly men, PCA using morphine without a basal rate was clearly found to result in better analgesia, fewer complications, less sedation, and higher patient satisfaction than intramuscular opioids [116].

For patients unable to operate PCA or in situations where PCA is not available, a continuous opioid infusion (e.g., morphine 0.5–1.0 mg/h or hydromorphone 0.10–0.25 mg/h) could be started and the patient observed for excessive sedation (reduce dose) or behavioral cues of pain (increase dose). This may be necessary for intubated patients or patients treated in end-of-life care. Frequent assessments focusing on face and body language that may indicate pain are essential, particularly during the first 24 h following surgery [41]. However, most hospitals might require an intensive care setting in order to provide a continuous infusion of opioid analgesia which the patient's condition may not warrant. It has also been shown that round the clock bolus dosing of intravenous opioids can provide good pain control if the patient is unable to use the PCA machine. This could be in the mode of "nurse-controlled analgesia," and would probably be safer than the continuous infusion.

For patients in whom pain is difficult to control, it has been shown that optimum pain control with minimal side effects could be obtained using PCA with a combination solution of 1 mg/ml morphine and 1 mg/ml ketamine, with a lockout period of 8 min [117]. This takes advantage of the ability of ketamine to block NMDA receptors and enhance the opioid analgesic effect of morphine.

When venous access is problematic, the subcutaneous route can be used. The infraclavicular area is generally the best site when a continuous infusion, PCA, or both are used. A 27-gage butterfly needle is well tolerated and can be maintained for 3–5 days, after which the site must be rotated. When intermittent dosing is required, an insulin syringe is used to minimize trauma. Doses for subcutaneous administration are equal to intravenous doses, and hydromorphone is the agent of choice because of its high potency and lipid insolubility. It is best to avoid the intramuscular route because of erratic absorption and pain from the injection [41]. One must remember, however, that the subcutaneous tissue site can only accommodate <2 ml volume per hour and so solutions must be concentrated. Hydromorphone being more soluble and more potent than morphine is suitable for concentrating.

Initial opioid doses are much higher for patients on chronic opioid therapy. For these patients, the presurgical opioid dose must be converted to a continuous infusion, and the as-needed PCA dose should be set equal to the hourly infusion dose. When converting oral opioids to parenteral opioids refer to an opioid conversion chart (Table 26.4). A patient receiving 180 mg of oral morphine every 24 h prior to surgery, for example, should be started postoperatively on 60 mg of morphine intravenously in 24 h (2.5 mg/h) and a PCA dose of 2.5 mg every 15 min. If the pain is severe, the continuous infusion rate should be increased. Patients on chronic opioid therapy have almost always developed tolerance to the respiratory suppressant and cognitive side effects of opioids, and so it is rare for these patients to develop these symptoms, even after receiving doses substantially higher than their baseline [41].

Oxycodone is not available for intravenous administration and so the oral dose must be converted to a morphine or hydromorphone equivalent to convert to an intravenous dose. Since oxycodone is about 1.5 times more potent than morphine, 120 mg/day of oxycodone (extended-release oxycodone) would be equivalent to 180 mg/day of oral morphine or 60 mg/day of intravenous morphine [41]. This equivalency can then be used to set up a PCA of morphine or hydromorphone (15 mg/day hydromorphone = 60 mg/day morphine).

When patients are being prepared for discharge from the hospital after surgery, it will usually be necessary to convert from their current pain control regimen to an oral medication regimen. This conversion should be made prior to discharge and it is recommended that at least 24 h of observation be allowed so that an adequate oral regimen can be established and tested prior to discharge.

For example, for conversion from intravenous or oral morphine to a fentanyl transdermal patch, one only needs to remember that 60 mg/day of intravenous morphine or 180 mg/day of oral morphine will equal a 100 µg/h transdermal fentanyl patch. As with all sustained-release opioids, this is for continuous pain that is opioid responsive. One still needs to consider breakthrough pain medications, fast onset, and short duration, for activity based pain. Since hydromorphone is about 4–5 times as potent as morphine, a similar conversion can be made from intravenous hydromorphone of 15 mg/day to a 100 µg/h transdermal fentanyl patch. Once patients have been receiving intravenous opioid medication for several days, the equianalgesic relationship between intravenous and oral doses changes from 1–6 (IV to oral) to closer to 1–3.

In the elderly, although there is increased CNS sensitivity to opioids leading to enhanced sedation, analgesia, and side effects including delirium, the experience of pain tends to counteract the sedative and respiratory effects of opioids as evidenced by the low rate of respiratory depression noted in postoperative patients receiving parenteral, PCA, or epidural opioids [118]. As stated earlier, pain itself can aggravate delirium.

Table 26.4 Equianalgesic doses of common intravenous and oral opioids

Drug	IV (mg)	Oral (mg)
Morphine	10	30
Hydromorphone (Dilaudid®)	1.5	7.5
Methadone[a]	10	12
Fentanyl	0.1 (100 µg)	N/A[b]
Meperidine (Demerol®)	100	300
Codeine	N/A	200
Oxycodone (Percodan®) (Percocet®)	N/A	20
Hydrocodone (Vicodin®) (Lorcet®)	N/A	30 (5 mg/tab Vicodin® with 500 mg acetaminophen)

Notice that the oral equivalent for 10 mg of intravenous morphine is 30 mg of oral hydrocodone. But when hydrocodone is combined with acetaminophen, the ratio is such that a toxic dose of acetaminophen would be taken with the hydrocodone. It is better to convert to a pure opioid agonist until such time that a reasonable dose of a combination medication can be given safely as shown in Table 26.3

[a] Not recommended for acute titration, ratio depends on the presence of prior opioid tolerance

[b] Oral transmucosal fentanyl is available in 200, 400, 800, and 1600 µg doses, and the transmucosal absorption depends on the duration of contact with the mucosa but will maximize at about 25% of the total dose with the remainder being swallowed and subject to a small degree of gastric absorption. An effervescent lozenge is also available in similar doses with a reported absorption of about 50%

Intraspinal Administration

Discovery of opioid receptors in the spinal cord provided a rationale for the administration of opioids into the epidural and subarachnoid spaces for the treatment of postoperative pain [119]. Reports have documented the efficacy and safety of this approach in a variety of patient populations [120–125]. The subarachnoid route is useful intraoperatively as part of a spinal anesthetic providing up to 24 h of postoperative analgesia after a single dose of morphine [126, 127]. For postoperative pain and acute pain in general, the epidural route is highly effective, especially if a combination of opioid plus local anesthetic is used [128]. When epidural analgesia was compared with parenteral opioid analgesia in a randomized study of high-risk surgical patients, epidural anesthesia was associated with significantly less postsurgical mortality and morbidity [128]. The epidural route is used for continuous infusion with or without patient-controlled epidural analgesia (PCEA). PCEA reduces analgesic requirements compared with continuous epidural infusion after major abdominal surgery [129].

When choosing the opioid for epidural infusion, it is important to consider the lipid solubility of the drug. Lipid-soluble drugs (fentanyl and sufentanil) are absorbed rapidly, resulting in a fast onset of analgesia [126, 127]. In addition, lipid-soluble agents concentrate at the spinal level where the tip of the epidural catheter is positioned. Thus, the tip of the catheter should be positioned, if possible, at the segmental level of the surgery.

Hydrophilic drugs (e.g., morphine) have a slower absorption rate and, upon entering the cerebrospinal fluid (CSF), have more rostral distribution. Morphine can cause more sedation and respiratory depression than fentanyl because of its ability to reach brain stem centers after penetrating the dura into the CSF [126, 127]. Fentanyl, on the other hand, tends to be sequestered in the fat tissue of the epidural space and absorbed rapidly by the vascular structures in the epidural space and reaches systemic plasma levels within 2 h of commencing an epidural infusion that would equal the same infusion rate given intravenously [130, 131]. Care must therefore be taken with fentanyl during the initial phases of the infusion, whereas the respiratory depressive effects of morphine or hydromorphone tend to be more delayed if they are to occur, and are the result of rostral spread of the opioid once it has diffused into the CSF rather than systemic absorption [126, 127].

For example, an epidural infusion of a solution containing 0.1 mg/ml of morphine at a rate of 10 ml/h would infuse a total of 2.4 mg of morphine in 24 h. Systemic absorption of this amount of morphine over 24 h would hardly produce respiratory depression in a postsurgical patient. Fentanyl on the other hand with a solution of 5 µg/ml infused epidurally at a rate of 10 ml/h, would provide 50 µg/h epidurally to be potentially absorbed systemically. Since fentanyl is 100 times more potent than morphine, this would be equivalent to 5 mg/h of intravenous morphine. This is a significant dose of morphine if given intravenously.

Various combinations of opioid and local anesthetic can be used to meet the needs of individual patients. Local anesthetic side effects include orthostatic hypotension, numbness/weakness, and urinary retention. Opioid side effects include sedation, urinary retention, and pruritis [132].

The local anesthetic/opioid ratio is adjusted based on the type and severity of side effects that develop. Complications of epidural infusions include accidental subarachnoid puncture with postdural puncture headache (generally benign and self-limiting), epidural hematoma, and epidural abscess. Side effects and complications are minimal if the catheters are inserted and monitored by those experienced with the technique [41].

For frail, elderly patients undergoing painful procedures (thoracotomy, extensive abdominal and pelvic surgery) and particularly for those with cognitive impairment, the epidural route is probably the best option for pain management because of its better analgesic efficacy/side effect profile (sedation/delirium, constipation, and postoperative complications) [133, 134].

Elderly patients undergo a high number of surgical interventions. The importance of adequate postoperative analgesia for reducing morbidity and mortality in the elderly is undisputed [33]. Epidural analgesia and I.V. PCA are both excellent postoperative techniques. Physicians are often reluctant to use PCA in older patients [135, 136]. However PCA was found to be effective in this population with the caveat that the patient is physically and mentally able to operate the machine [17].

Regional anesthetic techniques are excellent for the elderly. Although a fair amount of research has been published, data proving long-term benefit are lacking [33]. In a study of elderly patients following abdominal surgery, I.V. PCA versus PCEA, the I.V. PCA group had general anesthesia with sufentanil, isoflurane, nitrous oxide, and atracurium for muscle relaxation. Postoperative analgesic loading with 5 mg morphine intravenously was followed by morphine PCA of 1.5 mg, with a lockout of 8 min. The epidural group had a T7–T11 catheter placed, depending on surgery level, which was activated with 2% lidocaine with epinephrine 5 µg/ml, dosed to a T4 sensory level prior to the induction of general anesthesia. A solution of 0.25% bupivacaine plus 1 µg/ml sufentanil was infused continuously throughout the surgery and continued postoperatively with a solution of 0.125% bupivacaine plus 0.5 µg/ml sufcnta at 3–5 ml/h with 2–3 ml PCEA bolus and a lockout of 12 min [133]. The authors concluded that PCEA with local anesthetic and opioid provided better pain control, improved mental status, and better bowel function return than did traditional IV PCA morphine after general anesthesia. Orthostatic and mobility deficits were not a problem with the PCEA adjustments.

Carli et al. in a study of 64 patients for elective colon surgery randomized to an IV PCA group or epidural group found that epidural analgesia enhanced functional exercise capacity and health-related quality of life indicators after colonic surgery [134]. In this study, the PCA group had anesthetics consisting of 250 μg fentanyl, adjusted isoflurane, nitrous oxide, oxygen, and followed postoperatively with a PCA of morphine with no basal rate but a dose of 1–2 mg q5min. It was discontinued on day 3–4 if the verbal analog score was less than 3/10. The epidural group had T8–T9 catheters placed preoperatively and activated with 15–20 ml 0.5% bupivacaine to a sensory level of T4. General anesthesia was then induced and maintained with 100 μg fentanyl, maintenance 0.4% end tidal isoflurane, nitrous oxide, oxygen, and bolus doses of 5 ml 0.5% bupivacaine epidurally. Postoperatively, the epidural infusion was 4–15 ml/h of 0.1% bupivacaine and 2 μg/ml fentanyl and continued for 4 days.

The results indicated that the epidural group had improved outcomes for pain control, mobilization, gastrointestinal motility, and intake of protein and calories. This may be a function more of the local anesthetic, facilitating bowel function, thereby causing less nausea, and more willingness to eat. Decreased pain can also result in the same benefits, not just at rest but also with mobility, and less pain may ameliorate insulin sensitivity, hypercatabolism, and maintain muscle protein better. These benefits seemed to carry out to 6 weeks in the study of health-related quality of life indicators, leaving little doubt that epidural analgesia is even better than systemic opioids in the elderly [134].

Concomitant use of the epidural and parenteral routes is not recommended because (1) it makes titration of drugs overly complicated and (2) it becomes difficult to determine the origin of side effects if they develop. Generally, it is not advisable to maintain an epidural catheter for more than 8 days even if the site of insertion is without evidence of inflammation or infection. The source of epidural infection from continuous catheters is not well known but skin flora is considered the primary source [137]. If the epidural route is still needed, the catheter can be replaced with a new one at the segmental level above or below the insertion of the old catheter.

Pruritis is a common side effect of morphine administered either parenterally (intravenous or intramuscular) or spinally (intrathecal or epidural) [138]. However, the mechanisms and therefore effective treatments are different. Parenteral morphine results in histamine release in a dose-dependent manner and can be treated with antihistamines such as promethazine or dyhenhydramine. This pruritis is not ameliorated by naloxone and so is not Mu opioid receptor mediated [138].

Epidural or intrathecal morphine also produces pruritis which is through a central stimulating effect mediated through the mu opioid receptor. It is treated most effectively not with antihistamines but with a naloxone infusion at a low enough dose to ameliorate the pruritis without reversing the analgesic effect [138].

An additional benefit of spinal anesthesia has been suggested, although not yet proven. The perioperative period is characterized by a state of immunosuppression, which was shown in animal studies to underlie the promotion of tumor metastasis by surgery [139]. Bar-Yosef and his associates demonstrated that spinal anesthesia when added to general anesthesia reduced tumor recurrence in an animal model. They propone that as the immunosuppression of surgery is partly ascribed to the neuroendocrine stress response, it is hypothesized that spinal blockade, known to attenuate this response, may reduce the tumor-promoting effect of surgery. They therefore conclude that the addition of spinal block in their model had an advantage over the use of general anesthesia alone, and they suggest that it acts by reducing the neuroendocrine response to surgery [139].

These authors further state that since in clinical practice, an epidural block can be carried over into the postoperative period, it is reasonable to assume, but certainly proof is needed, that the favorable effect of prolonged epidural block on immune function and tumor metastasis will exceed the effect they found using short-term spinal block. This study provides the first experimental evidence that regional anesthesia may reduce postoperative metastatic development [139]. Controlled clinical studies are necessary to confirm this result in humans

Peripheral Nerve Block Analgesia

While epidural analgesia has been the gold standard for post-surgical analgesia for many years, the disadvantages of bilateral blockade when local anesthetics are employed, pruritis and nausea from spinal opioids, hypotension from local anesthetics, and the necessity for a Foley catheter have spurred interest and utilization of peripheral nerve blocks including continuous catheter techniques. With these techniques, unilateral blockade is possible using local anesthetic infusions without the addition of opioids to the infusions. However, patients will still need reduced doses of supplemental opioids as explained below.

With the interscalene technique, blockade of the shoulder is possible. The upper extremities below the shoulder are easily blocked with supraclavicular or infraclavicular techniques. And the lower extremities including the hips can be blocked with a combination of sciatic with lumbar plexus or the so-called 3-in-1 femoral block. The use of ultrasound needle guidance in addition to nerve stimulation techniques has made these procedures more accurate and less risky [140].

Thoracotomy pain can be blocked with paravertebral catheters, as can the pain from mastectomy surgery. Of significance is that in a recent report woman undergoing mastectomy for tumor removal had one-fourth the risk of metastatic recurrence when surgery was performed with a continuous paravertebral catheter. The catheter was placed at T2-3 through which a bolus of local anesthetic was given followed by a continuous infusion of local anesthetic. These patients also received general anesthesia with intravenous propofol. This group of patients was compared with a group that received general anesthesia alone [141]. The general anesthesia group had sevoflurane, fentanyl, and morphine with a postoperative morphine PCA. The paravertebral catheters were removed after 2 days.

Surgery and tissue injury cause the release of prostaglandins, histamine, potassium, hydrogen, oxygen radicals, bradykinins, substance P, and multiple cytokines involved in chemotaxis [141]. Vallejo also states that some opioids such as heroin inhibit the induction of nitric oxide, a molecule with a critical role in the regulation of immune response and resistance to infection challenges. Therefore, the above study supports that regional anesthesia may not only reduce the stress response associated with surgery, but also avoid anesthetic agents that may directly affect the immune response during the perioperative period, creating a friendlier cytokine environment. It is therefore important that regional anesthetic techniques be employed in a preemptive manor in tumor surgery instead of solely for postoperative pain management.

These blocks allow for unilateral analgesia, facilitating movement, and rehabilitation without the necessity of a Foley catheter. In addition, patients can safely be sent home with continuous catheters and infusions of local anesthetic, pulling the catheters out themselves when the disposable pumps are empty [142].

Just as postoperative epidural analgesia requires the participation of the anesthesiology department of the hospital, so does a peripheral nerve block service. Such a service is predicated upon the anesthesiology department having the expertise and personnel to oversee such a service.

Unfortunately, unlike epidural analgesia which can in fact provide complete analgesia without the need for supplemental intravenous or oral opioid analgesia (since opioids are administered spinally), peripheral nerve blockade cannot be used to completely eliminate the need for supplement opioid analgesics. In order to have complete analgesia, the local anesthetic dose would have to be high enough for a complete sensory blockade which is undesirable. The technique is designed instead to provide adequate analgesia that patients can be discharged from the same day of surgery to home, or remain in the hospital with the need for only oral opioid and anti-inflammatory analgesic supplementation. Decreasing the opioid analgesic requirements can result in reduced side effects such as nausea and constipation. Patient satisfaction is high with these techniques, and the incidence of complications is relatively low [143, 144].

In some orthopedic surgeries, bone graft may be harvested from the iliac crest. This can cause severe pain, which extends far out from the surgical procedure, and can become a chronic problem. It has been shown that the injection of morphine percutaneously into the prospective donor site can produce both immediate postoperative pain relief and long-term benefit [145, 146].

Although the mechanism of the long-term benefit of this technique is not known, there are at least three nerves that can be injured or entrapped in scar tissue at the donor site, the lateral femoral cutaneous nerve, the ilioinguinal nerve (retraction), or the superior cluneal nerves. It is possible that morphine inhibits sensitization of the nerve fibers. This author uses 10 ml of 1% ropivacaine with 2.5–3 mg of morphine injected by the surgeon along the iliac crest percutaneously prior to skin incision for the bone graft harvest.

Multimodal Techniques for Acute Postoperative Pain Management in the Elderly

Because patients rarely present with pure nociceptive pain (i.e., pain caused by activity in the neural pathways in response to damaging or potentially damaging stimuli) or neuropathic pain (i.e., pain initiated by a primary lesion or dysfunction in the nervous system), but rather, have a mixed pain syndrome (i.e., pain caused by a combination of both the primary injury and secondary effects), a rational polypharmacy approach that targets key peripheral and central pain mechanisms and modulating pathways may yield the best outcomes [147].

Oral Administration

Once pain is controlled and bowel function restored, analgesics should be changed to the oral route. Depending on individual variability and the type of surgery, this transition should occur 3–8 days after the surgery. Occasionally patients require parenteral or epidural opioids for a more prolonged period, usually because of intervening complications. Typically, patients require oral opioids for 5–10 days after parenteral or epidural opioids are discontinued. A certain percentage of patients, especially after more painful surgeries, require oral opioids for 2 weeks or longer [41].

Oral analgesics such as oxycodone or codeine are appropriate choices for a patient with mild-to-moderate pain [148].

Fixed combinations with nonopioid analgesics can be useful, but they sometimes limit the careful individualized titration that is the basis of therapeutic success. The oral transmucosal route may prove effective for rescue doses, but absorption is probably inadequate for more sustained relief. This latter statement also holds for the rectal route, which, additionally, is often uncomfortable for the patient and the caregiver.

One example of the difficulty with combination medications is conversion from intravenous PCA to oral. As seen in Table 26.4, the oral equivalent of hydrocodone to 10 mg of intravenous morphine is 30 mg. The usual combination of hydrocodone with acetaminophen is 5 and 500 mg, respectively. Therefore, six tablets of this combination drug would be necessary to equal 10 mg of intravenous morphine.

In patients suffering from continuous cancer pain, Foley recommended that the opioid analgesic should be administered regularly, including waking the patient from sleep at intervals based on the duration of analgesia for the given drug. This approach keeps the patient's pain at tolerable levels and often results in a reduction in the total amount of medication taken during a 24-h period [149]. In elderly patients with acute postsurgical pain, disrupting sleep to provide pain medication on a time contingent basis may be more detrimental than helpful. When the pain is present only during particular activities (e.g., physical therapy) or at particular times of the day, the opioid should be administered on an as-needed basis. It must be remembered that it takes approximately 1 h to reach peak serum levels after oral administration.

Special Circumstances

Some surgical procedures are associated with a higher risk of postoperative pain syndromes such as phantom limb pain syndrome after amputation. Regional anesthetic techniques offer the greatest protection; however, some patients either decline to have a regional blockade or the blocks are contraindicated for various reasons, and general anesthesia must be administered. General anesthetics alone do not protect the spinal cord from undergoing central sensitization leading to chronic neuropathic pain [150, 151]. But a polypharmaceutical approach, although not proven yet, seems to offer an advantage over traditional anesthetic and postoperative management techniques.

The following recommendations for the example of phantom limb pain prevention with amputation surgery are based on this author's experience, supported by the available evidenced-based medicine, which although limited in this regard, aims to target polypharmacy in such a way to help the brain modulate neuropathic pain [152]. The recommendations given below for this presented scenario of an amputation without the benefit of regional anesthesia is similar to the multimodal polypharmaceutical therapeutic recommendations of power, in which he reviews the uses of both opioid and nonopioid analgesics, anticonvulsants, and antidepressants in postoperative pain management [62].

As indicated above, in this author's experience, agents that have NMDA receptor blocking action like ketamine [153, 154], drugs with Mu opioid agonist action, tetrodotoxin resistance (TTXr) sodium channel blockers such as the local anesthetics, serotonin and norepinephrine reuptake inhibitors such as antidepressants [155–157], and neuronal calcium channel blockers such as the anticonvulsants gabapentin or pregabalin [158–163], and anti-inflammatory drugs if not contraindicated (see above), can all contribute to CNS protection. In such a case, preoperative oral gabapentin (Neurontin®) 300–1,200 mg [158–167] or pregabalin (Lyrica®) 75–150 mg, and if available a COX-2 inhibitor celecoxib (Celebrex®) 200 mg, can also be given orally which would alleviate the need for intraoperative ketorolac. It is true that COX-2 inhibitors are controversial with respect to patients at risk for stroke or myocardial infarction which makes up a large percentage of the elderly population. But there does not seem to be evidence that a single preoperative dose of 200 mg of celecoxib would pose a significant risk versus the benefit of preemptive analgesia [168].

Glucocorticoids given both preoperatively or postoperatively have been shown to reduce postoperative nausea and vomiting, and to decrease pain [169, 170]. Less than 8 mg of dexamethasone or 150 mg of methyprenisolone intravenously seem to be adequate.

Preoperative oral administration of clonidine, an α_2-agonist, reduces postoperative analgesic requirement as determined by IV morphine utilization via PCA after knee surgery [171], but not after major abdominal surgery [172]; whereas analgesia from intrathecally administered morphine was enhanced by oral clonidine premedication after total abdominal hysterectomy [173].

The recommended dose of gabapentin should be reduced from that given in the above references when dealing with the elderly population. Again this is an empiric decision of the author since the preoperative dose that would be appropriate in elderly patients has not been determined. But gabapentin and pregabalin have both been used in patients of all ages for the treatment of such conditions as postherpetic neuralgia [174]. Gabapentin in a dose of 600 mg preoperatively has also been found to decrease the incidence of nausea and vomiting and reduce the postoperative opioid requirements in a study of laparoscopic cholecystectomy patients [175].

Intraoperatively, the anesthesiologist (*again in this author's experience*) can administer several adjuvants that will also assist in protecting the spinal cord from excessive nociceptive input. Methadone would be a good choice for an opioid because of its NMDA receptor antagonist effect but it is often

TABLE 26.5 Antidepressants in clinical practice (Tricyclic antidepressants)

	Anticholinergic effects (sedation)	Dose range	Tolerability
Tricyclics			
Amitriptyline (Elavil®)	Least effect	10–25 mg qhs	
Desipramine (Norpramin®)	Least effect	10–25 mg qhs	Best
Doxipin (Sinequan®)	Most effect		Most sedating
Imipramine (Tofranil®)	Intermediate	10–25 mg/day	Best
Nortriptyline (Pamelor®)	Intermediate	10–25 mg/day	Best
Non-Tricyclics			
Venlafaxine (Effexor®)		≥150 mg/day	
Duloxetine (Cymbalta®)		30–120 mg/day	Best
Bupropion (Wellbutrin®SR)		150–300 mg/day	
Trazadone (Deseryl®)	Sleep aid in women	50–300 mg/day	Risk of priapism in men

Note: Dosages are low adjusted for the elderly patient. The antidepressants that are effective in pain management are those that have both serotonin and norepinephrine reuptake inhibition effects. The Tricyclic antidepressants all have these effects but their side effect profiles determine the tolerability of these drugs particularly by elderly patients, e.g., anticholinergic effects, sedation. The non-Tricyclic antidepressants that are effective in pain management tend to be less sedating and have a faster onset of effect with respect to decreasing neuropathic pain after initiation of therapy than the Tricyclic antidepressants that can require several weeks of treatment to become effective

unavailable and its slow onset of action is not suitable for intraoperative administration. Fentanyl would therefore be a logical choice since it is potent and more easily titrated due to its rapid onset of action when administered intravenously.

Although the data are not conclusive there is data to show that magnesium amplifies the analgesic effects of low-dose morphine in conditions of sustained pain [176]. Lysakowski et al., in a meta-analysis study of magnesium, concluded that the trials reviewed did not provide "convincing" evidence that perioperative magnesium has a favorable effect on postoperative pain intensity and analgesic requirements. Nevertheless, it may be worthwhile to further study the role of magnesium as a supplement to postoperative analgesia, since this molecule is inexpensive, relatively harmless, and the biological basis for its potential antinociceptive effect is promising [177]. There is a possibility that magnesium might have an additive or even synergistic effect with other NMDA antagonists, specifically ketamine although the optimum dose is not established [178, 179].

Considering the good tolerability of magnesium, these findings may have clinical application in neuropathic and persistent pain. Again the appropriate dose of magnesium is not known, but 30 mg/kg IV intraoperative administered prior to skin incision seems to be safe even in the elderly population. In combination with low-dose gabapentin, significant improvement in the effectiveness of morphine is observed in a rat model of nerve ligation neuropathic pain [166]. Referring to the above-stated preoperative dosing of gabapentin, the two should enhance the protective analgesic effect of the opioid used.

Low subanesthetic doses of ketamine (0.10–0.2 mg/kg IV intraoperative preincision) can be used for as part of the intravenous induction, and repeat doses q2h intraoperative can provide additional inhibition of activation of spinal cord NMDA receptors. Midazolam preinduction can reduce anxiety and also has an antagonist site on the NMDA receptor. As previously stated, if the patient is unable to take a COX-2 inhibitor (celecoxib), then ketorolac 7.5–15 mg should be given prior to amputation intraoperatively and continued q6h intravenously for 48 h. Lidocaine 1.5 mg/kg IV at the time of skin incision and repeated during the amputation as a general sodium channel blocker can all be helpful.

Postoperatively, the antineuropathic regimen should be continued until the wound (stump) has healed in terms of continued gabapentin or pregabalin (100–300 mg tid or 50 mg tid, respectively) along with an appropriate opioid, anti-inflammatory, and antidepressant (for serotonin and norepinephrine reuptake inhibition action).

Antidepressants that have been used in pain management are listed below (Table 26.5) along with starting doses and tolerability [147]. In summary, amitriptyline is probably the most studied in pain management and its efficacy is well established. Of the newest antidepressants that have been studied in pain management, duloxetine (a non-Tricyclic) is well tolerated with a fast onset of effect after the initiation of treatment [147].

Addiction, Dependence, Tolerance, and Pseudoaddiction

The fear of addiction or psychological dependence is one of the major barriers to the appropriate management of pain in the USA. Psychological dependence is the development of drug-seeking behavior that persists despite harm to the patient or others. Such drug-seeking behavior includes the hoarding of medication, use of medication for purposes other

TABLE 26.6 Choosing the best option for postoperative pain control in the elderly

Cognitively intact	Cognitively impaired
More painful procedures (e.g., thoracotomy, complex abdominal/pelvic surgery)	
Epidural: lipophilic opioid (e.g., fentanyl) plus local anesthetic as a continuous infusion with or without epidural PCA _or_	_Epidural_: opioid plus local anesthetic as a continuous infusion without PCA _or_
Intravenous: strong opioid as an intravenous infusion with intravenous PCA	_Intravenous_: strong opioid as a continuous infusion without PCA, or nurse administered "PCA" without a basal rate based on patient assessment
Less painful procedures (e.g., lower abdominal surgery, hip/knee replacement)	
Intravenous: strong opioid via PCA or given intravenously every 4–6 h	_Epidural_: opioid plus local anesthetic as a continuous infusion without PCA _or_
	Intravenous: strong opioid as a continuous infusion without PCA
If appropriate for the surgery, continuous peripheral nerve blocks with supplemental oral medications	If appropriate for the surgery, continuous peripheral nerve blocks with supplemental oral medications

Continuous epidural or peripheral nerve block techniques offer the best control of postoperative pain in the elderly patient but if not appropriate or contraindicated, then intravenous administration must be utilized. Transition to oral medications must be adequate to control pain prior to discharge. When intravenous access is not available and the oral route cannot be used, the subcutaneous route is better than the intramuscular route. When the subcutaneous route is used, the absorption is less erratic with hydromorphone (more lipid soluble) than with morphine. For intermittent dosing, it is best to use an insulin syringe. For continuous infusion, a 27-gage butterfly needle can be used. Postoperative orders for pain medication should be standing rather than PRN. The remarks "hold for excessive sedation" and "patient may refuse" add a safety valve to the order
PCA patient-controlled analgesia
Source: Data from Morrison et al. [41]

than control of pain, and obtaining opioids from multiple sources. It is important to distinguish true psychological dependence from "pseudoaddiction" [180], which can develop in patients who are undermedicated for their level of pain. Pseudoaddiction is drug-seeking behavior motivated by a need to obtain enough analgesia to control pain. When pain is appropriately managed and adequate analgesia provided, the behavior disappears. Although further research is needed, it appears that the incidence of psychological addiction in patients without a history of substance abuse and treated with opioids for control of pain is rare [69]. Fear of addiction should never limit the use of opioids for pain control in the elderly patient who has no history of substance abuse [41].

65 represent the most rapidly growing segment of the US population) and the increasing rates of surgery in this population. Until such research is completed, clinicians must continue to interpret the available data in the context of their knowledge of age-related physiologic changes, medication effects, side effect profiles, and clinical experience. This approach is summarized in Table 26.6 and results in appropriate pain management for most elderly surgical patients" [41]. The increased use of regional and peripheral nerve block techniques holds much promise for acute postsurgical pain management in the elderly population, as does our increasing knowledge of the pathophysiological mechanisms of pain translating into advances in the polypharmaceutical multimodal approach to pain management.

Conclusion

As aptly stated by Morrison, Carney, and Manfredi, in the first edition of this book, "good pain management in the elderly surgical patient is a complex, challenging undertaking of critical importance. Ensuring adequate analgesia requires an understanding of age-related changes in pharmacokinetics and pharmacodynamics, pain physiology, the appropriate use of analgesic agents, and knowledge of these agents' limitations and side effects. Unfortunately, few studies have focused on the assessment and treatment of pain in elderly individuals, and guidelines for analgesic therapy are often based on the experiences of young and middle-aged adults. Further research involving pain in the elderly is critically needed given the evolving changes in population demographics (persons over

References

1. Brennan F, Carr D, Cousins M (2007) Pain management: a fundamental human right. Anesth Analg 105:205–221
2. Rathmell JP, Wu CL, Sinatra RS et al (2006) Acute post-surgical pain Management critical appraisal of current practice. Reg Anesth Pain Med 31(4 Suppl 1):1–42
3. Gagliese L, Gauthier LR, Macpherson AK et al (2008) Correlates of postoperative pain and intravenous patient-controlled analgesia use in younger and older surgical patients. Pain Med 3:299–314
4. Apfelbaum JL, Chen C, Mehta SS, Gan TJ (2003) Postoperative pain experience: results from a national survey suggest postoperative pain continues to be undermanaged. Anesth Analg 97(2):534–540
5. Frasco PE, Sprung J, Trentman TL (2005) The impact of the Joint Commission for Accreditation of Healthcare Organizations pain initiative on perioperative opiate consumption and recovery room length of stay. Anesth Analg 100:162–168

6. Sinatra R (2002) Role of COX-2 inhibitors in the evolution of acute pain management. J Pain Symptom Manage 24(Suppl 1):S18–S27

7. Perkins F, Kehlet H et al (2000) Chronic pain as an outcome of surgery: a review of predictive factors. Anesthesiology 93(4): 1123–1133

8. Carr D, Goudas L (1999) Acute pain. Lancet 353:2052–2058

9. Siddall P, Cousins M (2004) Persistent pain as a disease entity: implications for clinical management. Anesth Analg 99:510–520

10. Beauregard L, Pomp A, Choiniere M (1998) Severity and impact of pain after day surgery. Can J Anesth 45:304–311

11. Chung F, Mezei G, Tong D (1999) Adverse events in ambulatory surgery: a comparison between elderly and younger patients. Can J Anesth 46(4):309–321

12. Ergina PL, Gold SL, Meakins JL (1993) Perioperative care of the elderly patient. World J Surg 17:192–198

13. McCleane G (2006) Pain and the elderly patient. In: McCleane G, Smith H (eds) Clinical management of the elderly patient in pain. The Haworth Medical Press, New York, Chapter 1

14. Rooke A, Reves J, Rosow C (2002) Anesthesiology and geriatric medicine: mutual needs and opportunities. Anesthesiology 96(1):2–4, Editorial

15. Sullivan M (2008) A biopsychomotor model of pain. Clin J Pain 24(4):281–290

16. Gibson S, Farrell M (2004) A review of age differences in the neurophysiology of nociception and the perceptual experience of pain. Clin J Pain 20(4):227–239

17. Gagliese L, Jackson M, Ritvo P et al (2000) Age is not an impediment to effective use of patient-controlled analgesia by surgical patients. Anesthesiology 93(3):601–610

18. Gagliese L, Melzack R (1997) The assessment of pain in the elderly. In: Lomrang J, Mostofsky D (eds) Handbook of pain and aging. New York, Plenum, pp 69–96

19. Shin S, Eisenach J (2004) Peripheral nerve injury sensitizes the response to visceral distension but not its inhibition by the antidepressant Milnacipran. Anesthesiology 100(3):671–675

20. Gibson SJ (2003) Pain and aging: the pain experiences over the adult lifespan. In: Proceedings of the 10th World Congress on Pain, IASP Press, Seattle, pp 767–790

21. Cleeland C (1998) Undertreatment of cancer pain in elderly patients. JAMA 279(23):1914–1915

22. Malliani A (1995) The conceptualization of cardiac pain as a nonspecific and unreliable alarm system. In: Gebhart G (ed) Visceral pain: progress in pain research and management, 5th edn. IASP Press, Seattle, pp 63–74, Chapter 4

23. Rohan D, Buggy D, Crowley S et al (2005) Increased incidence of postoperative cognitive dysfunction 24 hours after minor surgery in the elderly. Can J Anesth 52:137–142

24. Lynch EP, Lazor MH, Gellis JE et al (1998) The impact of postoperative pain on the development of postoperative delirium. Anesth Analg 86:781–785

25. Lu T, Pan Y, Kao S et al (2004) Gene regulation and DNA damage in the aging human brain. Nature 429(6994):883–891

26. Shors T, Miesegaes G, Beylin A et al (2001) Neurogenesis in the adult is involved in the formation of trace memories. Nature 410(6826):372–376

27. Fine P (2004) Pharmacological management of persistent pain in older patients. Clin J Pain 20(4):220–226

28. Auburn F, Monsel S, Langeron O et al (2002) Postoperative titration of intravenous Morphine in the elderly patient. Anesthesiology 96:17–23

29. Daykin A, Bowen D, Daunders D, Norman J (1986) Respiratory depression after morphine in the elderly. Anaesthesia 41:910–914

30. Shafer SL, Flood P (2008) The pharmacology of opioids. In: Silverstien JH, Rooke GA, Reves JG, McLeskey CH (eds) Geriatric anesthesiology, 2nd edn. Springer, New York, pp 209–228, Chapter 15

31. Woodhouse A, Mathur L (1997) The influence of age upon opioid analgesic use in the patient controlled analgesia environment. Anaesthesia 52:949–955

32. Cepeda M, Farrar J, Baumbarten M et al (2003) Side effects of opioids during short-term administration: effect of age, gender, and race. Clin Pharmacol Ther 74:102–112

33. Cook D, Rooke G (2003) Priorities in perioperative geriatrics. Anesth Analg 96:1823–1836

34. Silverstein J, Bloom H, Cassel C (1999) New challenges in anesthesia: new practice opportunities. Anesthesiol Clin North Am 17: 453–465

35. Henry C (2000) Mechanisms of changes in basal metabolism during aging. Eur J Clin Nutr 54:77–91

36. Grandison M, Boudinot F (2000) Age-related changes in protein binding of drugs: implications for therapy. Clin Pharmacokinet 38: 271–290

37. Benet L, Kroetz D, Sheiner L (1996) Pharmacokinetics: the dynamics of drug absorption, distribution, and elimination. In: Hardman J, Limbird L (eds) Goodman & Gilman's the pharmacological basis of therapeutics, 9th edn. McGraw-Hill, New York, pp 3–28, Chapter 1

38. Epstein M (1996) Aging and the kidney. J Am Soc Nephrol 7: 1106–1122

39. Lewis M (2008) Alterations in metabolic functions and electrolytes. In: Silverstein J, Rooke GA, Reves J, McLeskey C (eds) Geriatric anesthesiology, 2nd edn. Springer, New York, pp 97–106, Chapter 7

40. Miyoshi HR (2001) Systemic nonopioid analgesics. In: Loeser J, Butler S, Chapman C, Turk D (eds) Bonica's Management of Pain, 3rd edn. Lippincott Williams & Wilkins, Philadelphia, pp 1667–1681, Chapter 83

41. Morrison R, Carney M, Manfredi P (2001) Pain management. In: Rosenthal RA, Zenilman ME, Katlic MR (eds) Principles and practice of geriatric surgery. Springer, New York, Chapter 12

42. Rahme E, Barkam A, Nedjar H et al (2008) Hospitalizations for upper and lower GI events associated with traditional NSAIDs and acetaminophen among elderly in Quebec, Canada. Am J Gastroenterol 103(4):872–882

43. Ferreira S (1983) Prostaglandins: peripheral and central analgesia. In: Bonica J, Lindblom U, Iggo A (eds) Advances in pain research and therapy. Raven, New York

44. Gilron I, Milne B, Hong M (2003) Cyclooxygenase-2 inhibitors in postoperative pain management; Current evidence and future directions. Anesthesiology 99:1198–2008

45. Gajraj N (2003) Cyclooxygenase-2 inhibitors: review article. Anesth Analg 96:1720–1738

46. Samad T, Moore K, Sapirstein A et al (2001) Interleukin-1[beta]-mediated induction of Cox-2 in the CNS contributes to inflammatory pain hypersensitivity. Nature 410(6827):471–475

47. Jacox A, Carr DB, Payne R, et al (1994) Management of cancer pain. Clinical practice guideline no. 9. AHCPR Publication No. 94-0592. Agency for Health Care Policy and Research, U.S. Department of Health and Human Services, Rockville. Public Health Service, p 257

48. Cepeda M, Carr D, Miranda N et al (2005) Comparison of morphine, ketorolac, and their combination for postoperative pain, results from a large, randomized double-blind trial. Anesthesiology 103:1225–1232

49. Etches RC, Warriner CB, Badner N et al (1995) Continuous intravenous administration of ketorolac reduces pain and morphine consumption after total hip or knee arthroplasty. Anesth Analg 81:1175–1180

50. Stouten E, Armbuster S, Houmes R et al (1992) Comparison of ketorolac and morphine for postoperative pain after major surgery. Acta Anesthesiol Scand 336:716–721

51. Cepeda S, Vargas L, Ortegon G et al (1995) Comparative analgesic efficacy of patient-controlled analgesia with ketorolac versus morphine after elective intraabdominal operations. Anesth Analg 80:1150–1153

52. Reuben SS, Connelly N, Lurie S et al (1998) Dose-response of ketorolac as an adjunct to patient-controlled analgesia morphine in patients after spinal fusion surgery. Anesth Analg 87:98–102

53. Strom BL, Berlin JA, Kinman JL et al (1996) Parenteral ketorolac and risk of gastrointestinal and operative site bleeding: a postmarketing surveillance study. JAMA 275:376–382

54. Camu F, Lauwers MH, Vandersberghe C (1996) Side effects of NSAIDs and dosing recommendations for ketorolac. Acta Anaesthesiol Belg 47:143–149

55. Maliekal J, Elboim CM (1995) Gastrointestinal complications associated with intramuscular ketorolac tromethamine therapy in the elderly. Ann Pharmacother 29:698–701

56. Martinez V et al (2007) The influence of timing of administration on the analgesic efficacy of paracoxib in orthopedic surgery. Anesth Analg 104:1521–1527

57. Kranke P, Morin A, Roewer N, Leopold H (2004) Patients' global evaluation of analgesia and safety of injected parecoxib for postoperative pain: a quantitative systematic review. Anesth Analg 99:797–806

58. Hyllested M, Jones S, Pedersen J, Kehlet H (2002) Comparative effect of paracetamol, NSAIDs or their combination in postoperative pain management: a qualitative review. Br J Anesth 88:199–214

59. Barton S, Langeland F, Snabes M et al (2002) Efficacy and safety of intravenous parecoxib sodium in relieving acute postoperative pain following gynecologic laparotomy surgery. Anesthesiology 97:306–314

60. Insel P (1996) Analgesic-antipyretic and anti-inflammatory agents and drugs employed in the treatment of gout. In: Hardman J, Limbird L (eds) Goodman & Gilman's the pharmacological basis of therapeutics, 9th edn. McGraw-Hill, New York, pp 617–658, Chapter 27

61. Hardy MM et al (2003) Selective cyclooxygenase-2 inhibition does not alter keratinocyte wound responses in the mouse epidermis after abrasion. J Pharmacol Exp Ther 304:959–967

62. Power I (2005) Recent advances in postoperative pain therapy. Br J Anesth 95(1):43–51

63. Gerstenfeld L, Thiede M, Seibert K et al (2003) Differential inhibition of fracture healing by non-selective and cyclooxygenase-2 selective non steroidal anti-inflammatory drugs. J Orthop Res 21:670–675

64. Harder A, An Y (2003) The mechanism of the inhibitory effects of non steroidal anti-inflammatory drugs on bone healing: a concise review. J Clin Pharmacol 43:807–815

65. McCrory C, Lindahl S (2002) Cyclooxygenase inhibition for postoperative analgesia. Anesth Analg 95:169–176

66. Jones S, Power I (2005) Postoperative NSAIDs and COX-2 inhibitors: cardiovascular risks and benefits. Br J Anaesth 95:281–284, Editorial

67. White W, Faich G, Whelton A et al (2002) Comparison of thromboembolic events in patients treated with Celecoxib, a cyclooxygenase-2 specific inhibitor, versus ibuprofen or diclofenac. Am J Cardiol 89:425–430

68. Zuckerman L, Ferrante FM (1998) Nonopioid and opioid analgesics. In: Asburn M, Rice L (eds) The management of pain. Churchill Livingstone, New York, pp 111–140, Chapter 8

69. Fishbain D, Rosomoff H, Rosomoff R (1992) Drug abuse, dependence, and addiction in chronic pain patients. Clin J Pain 8:77–85

70. Morley J (1999) New perspectives in our use of opioids. Pain Forum 8(4):200–205

71. Supernaw J (2001) CYP2D6 enzyme and the efficacy of codeine and codeine-like drugs. Am J Pain Manag 11(1):30–31

72. Beaver W, Wallenstein S, Rogers A, Houde W (1978) Analgesic studies of codeine and oxycodone in patients with cancer. 1. Comparison of oral with intramuscular codeine and oral with intramuscular oxycodone. J Pharmacol Exp Ther 207:92–100

73. Beaver W, Wallenstein S, Rogers A, Houde R (1978) Analgesic studies of codeine and oxycodone in patients with cancer. 2. Comparison of intramuscular oxycodone with intramuscular morphine and codeine. J Pharmcol Exp Ther 207:101–108

74. Kantor T, Hopper M, Laska E (1981) Adverse effects of commonly ordered oral narcotics. J Clin Pharmacol 21:1–8

75. Kalso E, Vanio A (1987) Hallucinations during morphine but not during oxycodone treatment. Lancet 2:912

76. Chan G, Matzke G (1987) Effects of renal insufficiency on the pharmacokinetics and pharmacodynamics of opioid analgesics. Drug Intell Clin Pharm 21:773–783

77. Sunshine A (1994) New clinical experience with tramadol. Drugs 47:8–18

78. Moore R, McQuay H (1997) Single-patient data meta-analysis of 3453 postoperative patients: oral tramadol versus placebo, codeine, and combination analgesics. Pain 69:287–294

79. Hamilton G, Baskett TF (2000) In the arms of Morpheus: the development of morphine for postoperative pain relief: history of Anesthesia. Can J Anesth 47:367–374

80. Sawe J, Svensson J, Rane A (1983) Morphine metabolism in cancer patients on increasing oral doses – no evidence of autoinduction or dose-dependence. Br J Clin Pharmacol 16:85–93

81. Pasternak G, Bodnare R, Clarke J, Inturrisi C (1987) Morphine-6-glucuronide, a potent mu agonist. Life Sci 41:2845–2849

82. Portenoy R, Khan E, Layman M et al (1991) Chronic morphine therapy for cancer pain: plasma and cerebrospinal fluid morphine and morphine-6-glucuronide concentrations. Neurology 41:1457–1461

83. Houde R, Wallenstein S, Beaver W (1966) Evaluation of analgesics in patients with cancer pain. In: Lasagna L (ed) International encyclopedia of pharmacology and therapeutics. Pergamon, New York, pp 59–67

84. Twycross R (1975) The use of narcotic analgesics in terminal illness. J Med Ethics 1:10–17

85. Labella F, Pinsky C, Havlicek V (1979) Morphine derivatives with diminished opiate receptor potency show enhanced central excitatory activity. Brain Res 174:263–271

86. Morley J, Miles J, Wells J, Bowsher D (1992) Paradoxical pain. Lancet 340:1045

87. Smith M, Watt J, Cramond T (1990) Morphine-3-glucuronide: a potent antagonist of morphine analgesia. Life Sci 47:579–585

88. Skarke C, Darimont J, Schmidt H et al (2003) Analgesic effects of morphine and morphine-6-glucuronide in a transcutaneous electrical pain model in healthy volunteers. Clin Pharmacol Ther 73:303–311

89. Osborne R, Joel S, Slevin M (1986) Morphine intoxication in renal failure: the role of morphine-6-glucuronide. BMJ 292:1548–1549

90. Houde R (1986) Clinical analgesic studies of hydromorphone. Adv Pain Res Ther 8:129–135

91. Babul N, Darke A, Hagen N (1995) Hydromorphone metabolite accumulation in renal failure. J Pain Symptom Manage 10:184–186

92. Moulin D, Kreeft J, Murray-Parsons N, Bouquillon A (1991) Comparison of continuous subcutaneous and intravenous hydromorphone infusions for management of cancer pain. Lancet 337:465–468

93. Reisine T, Pasternak G, 9 (1996) Opioid analgesics and antagonists. In: Hardman J, Limbird L (eds) Goodman & Gillman's the pharmacological basis of therapeutics, 9th edn. McGraw-Hill, New York, pp 521–556, Chapter 23

94. Pasternak G (1993) Pharmacological mechanisms of opioid analgesia. Clin Neuropharmacol 16:1–18

95. Houde E, Wallenstein S, Beaver W (1975) Clinical measurement of pain. In: de Stevens G (ed) Analgesics. San Diego, Academic, pp 75–122

96. Dixon R, Crews T, Inturrisi C, Foley K (1983) Levorphanol pharmacokinetics and steady-state plasma concentrations in patients with pain. Res Commun Chem Pathol Pharmacol 41:3

97. Shir Y, Rosen G, Zeidin A, Davidson E (2001) Methadone is safe for treating hospitalized patients with severe pain. Can J Anesth 48:1109–1113

98. Faisinger R, Schoeller T, Bruera E (1993) Methadone in the management of chronic pain: a review. Pain 52:137–147

99. Beaver W, Wallenstein S, Houde R, Rogers A (1967) A clinical comparison of the analgesic effects of methadone and morphine administered intramuscularly and of oral and parenterally administered methadone. Clin Pharmacol Ther 8:415–426

100. Sawe J (1986) High dose morphine and methadone in cancer patients: clinical pharmacokinetic consideration of oral treatment. Clin Pharmacol 11:87–106

101. Morley J, Watt J, Wells J et al (1993) Methadone in pain uncontrolled by morphine. Lancet 342:1243

102. Kreek M, Schecter A, Gutjahr C, Hecht M (1980) Methadone use in patients with chronic renal disease. Drug Alcohol Depend 5:195–205

103. Mitra S, Sinatra R (2004) Perioperative management of acute pain in the opioid-dependant patient. Anesthesiology 101:212–227

104. Friesen C, Roscher A, Alt A, Miltner E (2008) Methadone, commonly used as maintenance medication for outpatient treatment of opioid dependence, kills leukemia cells and overcomes chemoresistance. Cancer Res 68(15):6059–6064

105. Radney P, Brodman E, Mankikar D, Duncalf D (1980) The effect of equi-analgesic doses of fentanyl, morphine, meperidine, and pentazocine on common bile duct pressure. Anaesthetist 29:26

106. Szeto H, Inturrisi C, Houde R et al (1977) Accumulation of normeperidine, an active metabolite of meperidine, in patients with renal failure and cancer. Ann Intern Med 86:738–740

107. Kaiko R, Foley K, Grabinski P et al (1983) Central nervous system excitatory effects of meperidine in cancer patients. Ann Neurol 13:180–185

108. Gillman P (2005) Monoamine oxidase inhibitors, opioid analgesics and serotonin toxicity: review Article. Br J Anaesth 95:434–441

109. Yamakura T, Sakimura K, Shimoji K (2000) N-Methyl-D-Aspartate receptor channel block by meperidine is dependent on extracellular pH. Anesth Analg 90:928–932

110. Kurz A, Ikeda T, Sessler D et al (1997) Meperidine decreases the shivering threshold twice as much as the vasoconstriction threshold. Anesthesiology 86:1046–1054

111. Klein U, Klein M, Sturm H et al (1976) The frequency of adverse drug reactions as dependent upon age, sex, and duration of hospitalization. Int J Clin Pharmacol Biopharm 13:187–1950

112. Crooks J (1983) Aging and drug disposition-pharmacodynamics. J Chronic Dis 36:85–90

113. Lasagna L, Beecher HK (1954) The analgesic effectiveness of nalorphine and nalorphine-morphine combinations in man. JAMA 112(3):356–363

114. Guler T, Unlugenc H, Gundogan Z (2004) A background infusion of morphine enhances patient controlled analgesia after cardiac surgery. Can J Anesth 51:718–722

115. Grass J (2005) Patient-controlled analgesia: review article. Anesth Analg 101:844–861

116. Egbert A, Parks L, Short L, Burnett M (1990) Randomized trial of postoperative patient-controlled analgesia vs intramuscular narcotics in frail elderly men. Arch Intern Med 150:1897–1903

117. Svedicic G, Gentilini A, Eichenberger U et al (2003) Combinations of morphine with Ketamine for patient-controlled analgesia: a new optimization method. Anesthesiology 98(5):1195–1205

118. Cashman J, Dolin S (2004) Respiratory and haemodynamic effects of acute postoperative pain management: evidence from published data. Br J Anaesth 93:212–223

119. Robertson DH, Lewerentz H, Holmes F (1978) Subarachnoid spinal analgesia. A comparative survey of current practice in Scotland and Sweden. Anaesthesia 33:913–923

120. Bernards C, Shen D, Sterling E et al (2003) Epidural, cerebrospinal fluid, and plasma pharmacokinetics of epidural opioids (part 1): differences among opioids. Anesthesiology 99:455–465

121. Bernards C, Shen D, Sterling E et al (2003) Epidural, cerebrospinal fluid, and plasma pharmacokinetics of epidural opioids (part 2): effect of epinephrine. Anesthesiology 99:466–475

122. Wang YK (1978) Soulagement de la douleur par injection intrathécale de sérotonine ou de morphine. Ann Anesth Fr 19:371–372

123. Bromage PR, Camporesi E, Chestnut D (1980) Epidural narcotics for postoperative analgesia. Anesth Analg 59:473–480

124. Reiz S, Ahlin J, Ahrenfeldt B et al (1981) Epidural morphine for postoperative pain relief. Acta Anaesthesiol Scand 25:111–114

125. Rawal N, Sjörstrand U, Dahlström B (1981) Postoperative pain relief by epidural morphine. Anesth Analg 60:726–731

126. Ummenhofer W, Arends R, Shen D, Bernards C (2000) Comparative spinal distribution and clearance kinetics of intrathecally administered morphine, fentanyl, alfentanil, and sufentanil. Anesthesiology 92:739–753

127. Angst M, Ramaswamy B, Riley E, Stanski D (2000) Lumbar epidural morphine in humans and supraspinal analgesia to experimental heat pain. Anesthesiology 92:312–324

128. Yeager M, Glass D, Neff R, Brinck-Johnsen T (1987) Epidural anesthesia and analgesia in high risk surgical patients. Anesthesiology 66:729–736

129. Standl T, Burmeister M-A, Ohnesorge H et al (2003) Can J Anesth 50:258–264

130. Coda B (1994) Pharmacology of epidural fentanyl, alfentanil, and sufentanil in volunteers. Anesthesiology 81:1149–1161

131. Loper KA, Ready LB, Downey M et al (1990) Epidural and intravenous fentanyl infusions are clinically equivalent after knee surgery. Anesth Analg 70:72–75

132. Gwirtz K, Young J, Byers R et al (1999) The safety and efficacy of intrathecal opioid analgesia for acute postoperative pain: seven years' experience with 5969 surgical patients at Indiana University Hospital. Anesth Analg 88:599–604

133. Mann C, Pouzeratte Y, Bocarra G et al (2000) Comparison of intravenous or epidural patient-controlled analgesia in the elderly after major abdominal surgery. Anesthesiology 92(2):433–441

134. Carli F, Phil M, Mayo N et al (2002) Epidural analgesia enhances functional exercise capacity and health related quality of life after colonic surgery. Results of a randomized trial. Anesthesiology 97(3):540–549

135. Dyer C, Ashton C (1995) Postoperative delirium: a review of 80 primary data-collection studies. Arch Intern Med 155(5):461–465

136. Gustafson Y, Berggren D, Brännström B et al (1988) Acute confusional states in elderly patients treated for femoral neck fracture. J Am Geriatr Soc 36:525–530

137. Sato S, Sakuragi T, Dan K (1996) Human skin flora as a potential source of epidural abscess. Anesthesiology 85:1276–1282

138. Twycross R, Greaves MW, Handwerker H et al (2003) Itch: scratching more than the surface. Q J Med 96:7–26

139. Bar-Yosef S, Melamed R, Page G et al (2001) Attenuation of the tumor-promoting effect of surgery by spinal blockade in rats. Anesthesiology 94:1066–1073

140. Marhofer P, Greher M, Kapral S (2005) Ultrasound guidance in regional anaesthesia: review Article. Br J Anaesth 94:7–17

141. Exadaktylos A, Buggy D, Donal J et al (2006) Can anesthetic technique for primary breast cancer surgery affect recurrence or metastasis? Anesthesiology 105:660–664

142. Swenson J, Bay N, Loose E et al (2006) Outpatient management of continuous peripheral nerve catheters placed using ultrasound guidance: an experience in 620 patients. Anesth Analg 103(6):1436–1443

143. Klein S (2005) Continuous peripheral nerve blocks, fewer excuses: editorial view. Anesthesiology 103:921–923

144. Liu S, Salinas F (2003) Continuous plexus and peripheral nerve blocks for postoperative analgesia: review article. Anesth Analg 96:263–272

145. Houghton A, Valdez J, Westland K (1998) Peripheral morphine administration blocks the development of hyperalgesia and allodynia after bone damage in the rat. Anesthesiology 89(1):190–201

146. Wilson P (1995) Pain relief following iliac crest bone harvesting. Br J Oral Maxillofac Surg 33:242–243

147. (2005) Management of chronic pain syndromes: issues and interventions. A CME program of the American Academy of Pain Medicine. Pain Med 6:S1–S21

148. World Health Organization (1990) Cancer pain relief and palliative care. WHO, Geneva

149. Foley KM (1985) The treatment of cancer pain. N Engl J Med 313:84–95

150. Woolf CJ, Chong MS (1993) Preemptive analgesia – treating postoperative pain by preventing the establishment of central sensitization. Anesth Analg 77:362–379

151. Abram SE, Yaksh TL (1993) Morphine, but not inhalational anesthesia, blocks post-injury facilitation. The role of preemptive suppression of afferent transmission. Anesthesiology 78:713–721

152. Giordano J (2005) The neurobiology of nociceptive and anti-nociceptive systems. Pain Physician 8(3):277–290

153. Zakine J, Samarcq D, Lorne E et al (2008) Postoperative ketamine administration decreases morphine consumption in major abdominal surgery: a prospective, randomized, double-blind, controlled study. Anesth Analg 106:1856–1861

154. Roytblat L, Korotkoruchko A, Katz J et al (1993) Postop pain: the effect of low-dose ketamine in addition to general anesthesia. Anesth Analg 77:1161–1165

155. Goldstein FJ (2002) Adjuncts to opioid therapy. J Am Osteopath Assoc 102(9 Suppl 3):S15–S20

156. Malseed RT, Goldstein FJ (1979) Enhancement of morphine analgesia by tricyclic antidepressants. Neuropharmacolgy 18:827–832

157. Ossipov MH, Malseed RT, Goldstein FJ (1994) Augmentation of central and peripheral morphine analgesia by desipramine. Arch Int Pharmacol 259:222–228

158. Dahl JB, Mathiesen O, Moniche S (2004) Protective premedication: an option with gabapentin and related drugs? A review of gabapentin and pregabalin in the treatment of post-operative pain. Acta Anaesthesiol Scand 48:1130–1136

159. Turan A, Kaya G, Karamanlioglu B, Pamukcu Z, Apfel CC (2006) Effect of oral gabapentin on postoperative epidural analgesia. Br J Anaesth 96:242–246

160. Saraswat V, Arora V (2008) Preemptive gabapentin vs pregabalin for acute postoperative pain after surgery under spinal Anaesthesia. Indian J Anaesth 52(6):829–834

161. Pandey CK, Singhal V, Kumar M et al (2005) Gabapentin provides effective postoperative analgesia whether administered pre-emptively or post-incision. Can J Anesth 52:827–831

162. Ménigaux C, Adam F, Guignard B et al (2005) Preoperative gabapentin decreases anxiety and improves early functional recovery from knee surgery. Anesth Analg 100:1394–1399

163. Gilron I (2007) Gabapentin and pregabalin for chronic neuropathic and early postsurgical pain: current evidence and future directions. Curr Opin Anaesthesiol 20:456–472

164. Dirks J, Fredensborg B, Christensen D et al (2002) A randomized study of the effects of single-dose gabapentin versus placebo on postoperative pain and morphine consumption after mastectomy. Anesthesiology 97(3):560–564

165. Gilron I (2002) Is gabapentin a "broad-spectrum" analgesic? Anesthesiology 97(3):537–538, Editorial

166. Matthews E, Dickerson A (2002) A combination of gabapentin and morphine mediates enhanced inhibitory effects on dorsal horn neuronal responses in a rat model of neuropathy. Anesthesiology 96(3):633–640

167. Hayashida K, Hideaki O, Kunie N, Eisenach J (2008) Gabapentin acts within the locus coeruleus to alleviate neuropathic pain. Anesthesiology 109(6):1077–1084

168. Clark DWJ, Layton D, Shakir SAW (2004) Do some inhibitors of COX-2 increase the risk of thromboembolic events? Linking pharmacology with pharmacoepidemiology. Drug Saf 27:427–456

169. Kardash K, Sarrazin F, Tessler M, Velly A (2008) Single-dose dexamethasone reduces dynamic pain after total hip arthroplasty. Pain Med 106(4):1253–1257

170. Romundstad L, Breivik H, Niemi G et al (2004) Methylprednisolone intravenously 1 day after surgery has sustained analgesic and opioid-sparing effects. Acta Anaesthesiol Scand 48:1223–1231

171. Park J, Forrest J, Kolesar R et al (1996) Oral clonidine reduces postoperative PCA morphine requirements. Can J Anaesth 43:900–906

172. Benhamou D, Narchi P, Hamza J et al (1994) Addition of oral clonidine to postoperative patient-controlled analgesia with i.v. morphine. Br J Anaesth 72:537–540

173. Goyagi T, Nishikawa T (1996) Oral clonidine premedication enhances the quality of postoperative analgesia by intrathecal morphine. Anesth Analg 82:1192–1196

174. Dirks J et al (2002) A randomized study of the effects of single-dose gabapentin versus placebo on postoperative pain and morphine consumption after mastectomy. Anesthesiology 97(3):560–564

175. Pandey CK, Priye S, Ambesh SP et al (2006) Prophylactic gabapentin for prevention of postoperative nausea and vomiting in patients undergoing laparoscopic cholecystectomy: a randomized, double-blind, placebo-controlled study. J Postgrad Med 552(2):97–100

176. Begon S, Pickering G, Eschalier A, Dubray C (2002) Magnesium increases morphine analgesic effect in different experimental models of pain. Anesthesiology 96(3):627–632

177. Lysakowski C, Dumont L, Czarnetzki C, Tramer M (2007) Magnesium as an adjuvant to postoperative analgesia: a systematic review of randomized trials. Anesth Analg 104:1532–1539

178. Begon S et al (2002) Magnesium increases morphine analgesic effect in different experimental models of pain. Anesthesiology 96(3):627–632

179. Hollman MW et al (2001) Modulation of NMDA receptor function by ketamine and magnesium. Part II: interactions with volatile anesthetics. Anesth Analg 92:1182–1191

180. Weissman D, Haddox J (1989) Opioid pseudoaddiction: an iatrogenic syndrome. Pain 36:363–366

Further Reading

181. NiChonchubhair A, Valacio R, Kelly J, O'keeffe S (1995) Use of the abbreviated mental test to detect delirium in elderly people. Br J Anaesth 75:481–482

182. Auburn F, Bunge D, Langeron O et al (2003) Postoperative morphine consumption in the elderly patient. Anesthesiology 99:160–165

183. Vallejo R (2009) In Anesthesia method during tumor surgery tied to cancer outcomes: new study from 2008 ASA buttresses previous findings favoring regional. Anesthesiology News January 35(1):1, 21

Chapter 27
Drug Usage in Surgical Patients: Preventing Medication-Related Problems

Richard A. Marottoli, Sean M. Jeffery, and Roshini C. Pinto-Powell

Examples of age-related physiologic changes affecting drug pharmacokinetics

Physiologic change	Direction of change	Drugs affected by this change	Result of change
Serum albumin	↓	Phenytoin, naproxen, valproate, and warfarin	Increased free (active) fraction of drug; increased effects
α_1-Acid glycoprotein	↑	Propranolol, antidepressants, lidocaine, methadone, and quinidine	Decreased free (active) fraction of drug; decreased effects
Body fat	↑	Fat-soluble drugs (e.g., benzodiazepines)	Increased volume of distribution; increased half-life and potential for accumulation
Lean muscle mass	↓	Digoxin	Decreased volume of distribution; increased concentration; lower loading dose is needed
Body water	↓	Water-soluble drugs (e.g., lithium)	Decreased volume of distribution; increased concentration and effects
Hepatic blood flow	↓	High-hepatic extraction ratio drugs (e.g., morphine, meperidine, lidocaine, and isosorbide)	Decreased first-pass metabolism; increased effects
Hepatic metabolism (phase 1: reduction, oxidation, hydroxylation, and demethylation)	↓	Diazepam, alprazolam, triazolam, theophylline, quinidine, propranolol, phenytoin, and imipramine	Decreased metabolism; increased half-life and concentration
Renal function	↓	Aminoglycosides, digoxin, ciprofloxacin, and allopurinol	Decreased clearance; increased effects, toxicity, or both

On January 1, 2011, the first of the Baby Boomers will turn 65 years old. And so will begin the largest increase in the number of older adults ever seen. To put this in perspective, in the entire history of mankind, two-thirds of all people who have ever lived to the age of 65 are alive today [1]. Advances in pharmacotherapy are partially responsible for this unprecedented increase in longevity and will play a central role in reducing morbidity and mortality in this aging cohort. However, when it comes to older adults, medications are often improperly dosed, overprescribed, and poorly monitored for signs of toxicity. Furthermore, changes in pharmacokinetics associated with aging leave little room for error. Surgeons operating on elderly patients should preoperatively identify potential medication-related problems (MRPs) that can result in postoperative complications. This chapter reviews some of the factors that contribute to MRPs in the elderly, general approaches to prescribing, signs and symptoms to monitor, and highlights of certain drug categories that are commonly used or have substantial potential to cause side effects in older adults.

Biology of Aging

After the age of 30, it is all downhill (Table 27.1). All organ systems decline in function to some extent with advancing age, but they decline at varying rates, and independent of each other. In the absence of disease, these declines are not sufficient to impair daily function [2, 3]. However, the overall reserve capacity of an organ system diminishes with age. Thus, the ability to withstand even a minor insult is decreased, and

R.A. Marottoli (✉)
Department of Internal Medicine (Geriatrics), Yale University School of Medicine, VA Connecticut Healthcare System, New Haven, CT 06510, USA
e-mail: richard.marottoli@ynhh.org

R.A. Rosenthal et al. (eds.), *Principles and Practice of Geriatric Surgery*,
DOI 10.1007/978-1-4419-6999-6_27, © Springer Science+Business Media, LLC 2011

TABLE 27.1 Pharmacokinetic changes with aging

Absorption	Extent not affected
	Rate is reduced or unaltered
	Increased gastric pH
	Unchanged passive diffusion
	Decreased active transport
	Decreased first-pass effect
	Decreased GI blood flow with certain diseases (e.g., HF)
Distribution	Decreased total body water
	Decreased lean body mass
	Decreased serum albumin
	Increased body fat
	Increased or decreased free fraction of highly plasma protein-bound drugs
	Higher concentration of water-soluble drugs
Metabolism	Decreased liver blood flow
	Decreased liver size
	Decreased enzymatic activity
	Variable decreased and increased $t_{1/2}$ for phase I oxidation drugs
	Decreased clearance and increased $t_{1/2}$ of drugs with high-extraction ratio
Excretion	Decreased GFR
	Decreased renal blood flow
	Decreased tubular function
	Decreased clearance and increased $t_{1/2}$ for drugs eliminated primarily by the kidneys

recovery may be delayed. Appreciating medication-related factors that affect an organ system's reserve capacity is an imperfect science. The principles of pharmacokinetics help frame an understanding of how physiologic changes with aging affect medications [4]. Understanding pharmacokinetic changes associated with aging can help surgeons better anticipate MRPs. Pharmacokinetics is defined as the delivery of a drug to its site of action. This includes drug absorption, distribution, metabolism, and excretion. These changes are reviewed here in general terms to provide a background for the discussion of individual drug classes [5].

Drug Absorption

The amount of oral drug absorption (bioavailability) is dependent on many factors not related to age, including the presence of food, drug ionization, and dosage formulation [6]. Absorption can occur anywhere along the gastrointestinal tract. Oral drug absorption can also include buccal absorption of orally disintegrating tablets (ODT) specifically designed for patients unable to swallow. Some formulations are specifically designed to release medication in response to changes in intestinal pH or osmolality. In general, older adults tend to have a slight increase in gastric pH. This increase is unlikely to result in altered drug absorption [6, 7]. Achlorhydria was once thought to be a consequence of aging. However, the

identification and treatment of indolent *Helicobacter pylori* infections has diminished achlorhydria as a concern.

Older adults tend to experience two alterations that can lead to clinically significant changes in the rate of oral drug absorption. First, changes in gastrointestinal blood flow may reduce portal circulation and delay gastric absorption. For example, these changes can be seen in some heart failure or cirrhosis patients with substantial hepatic congestion. And second, decreased gastric emptying, resulting from conditions such as Parkinson's disease or diabetes, may also delay the rate of absorption, but not the extent of drug absorbed [7, 8]. Unless therapeutic failure is observed, no changes in dosing are required to overcome delays in gastric absorption.

Oral bioavailability can be substantially altered in the presence of food, so called drug–food interactions. For example, patients who receive calcium supplementation while taking quinolones have a 50% reduction in the absorption of the quinolone due to chelation with calcium. The authors recommend discontinuing most calcium supplementation during the postoperative period to prevent potential chelation interactions with antibiotics. Bisphosphonate bioavailability is exceedingly low when taken with anything other than water. Levodopa absorption is substantially decreased when consumed with a high-protein meal [9]. In addition, certain foods can substantially alter drug levels and actions. Patients on warfarin who alter their intake of vitamin K-containing foods risk changes in their international normalized ratio (INR). Consumption of grapefruit irreversibly inhibits intestinal CYP-450 3A4 isoenzyme activity. This results in presystemic decreases in metabolism leading to increases in therapeutic concentrations that can last for up to 72 h. In summary, the rate of absorption may be delayed with aging, but the overall extent of absorption is unlikely to be altered.

Limited information is available about topical drug absorption changes as a result of aging. Topical administration is gaining popularity as a way to minimize first-pass metabolism, improve medication adherence, and provide more continuous therapeutic drug concentrations. For example, postoperative pain control may include the use of fentanyl or lidocaine patches. In general, decreases in skin thickness and integrity may alter drug absorption and subsequently peak concentrations. When comparing healthy young volunteers with healthy elderly volunteers receiving transdermal fentanyl patches, the older patients demonstrated higher systemic concentrations of fentanyl and correspondingly greater adverse effects resulting in drug discontinuation [10]. An additional concern when administering medications in patch form is the ability to safely remove the patch without damaging the underlying skin. Finally, all patches utilize adhesives that can cause localized skin irritation. The use of presurgical skin disinfectants and body preparations may contribute to heightened skin sensitivity to patch adhesives.

Distribution

The distribution of drugs is altered by the aging process. Total body and intracellular water decrease, as does muscle mass, whereas body fat increases [2, 3]. These changes have important implications for drug distribution that can affect both the half-life of a compound and the concentration of the drug in various tissues (e.g., lipophilic versus hydrophilic saturation). Water-soluble drugs tend to have an increased level per unit dose because of the decreased total body and intracellular water described above. Similarly, the volume of distribution for lipid-soluble drugs tends to be higher because of increased fat stores, resulting in prolonged and less predictable half-lives. Changes in protein binding can also alter receptor site activity. When medications exhibit substantial protein binding (generally >90%), the potential for protein-binding interactions due to changes in serum albumin becomes more pronounced. For example, in the case of low albumin levels, the relative proportion of free or unbound drug may be increased, enhancing the pharmacologic and toxic properties of the drug. To further illustrate this point, consider the highly protein bound drug phenytoin. By convention, when ordering phenytoin levels what is typically reported is the total drug level [11]. In the setting of low albumin, however, the free drug concentration may be high, resulting in toxicity despite a total level in the therapeutic range. In contrast, the carrier protein α_1-acid glycoprotein may increase with age, as it does with illness, so drugs that bind to this protein may have a lower proportion unbound; an example is propranolol [12]. Another caveat with drug levels is that normal ranges are often established on young persons, therefore targeting lower therapeutic drug levels may minimize the risk of toxicity. The important exception to this approach is for antibiotic therapy where specific minimum inhibitory concentrations (MIC) are specified. Finally, some evidence suggests that conformational changes in the ability of albumin to bind drugs increase as one ages [11]. Therefore, despite a normal albumin level, the affinity of albumin to bind to medications may be reduced.

Metabolism

First-pass metabolism and high-hepatic extraction ratio drugs, liver size, and blood flow tend to decrease with age by 20–30%. Drugs that depend on extensive first-pass metabolism may have higher therapeutic levels resulting from decreased hepatic metabolism [9, 13, 14]. Pertinent to a surgeon, it is estimated that morphine exhibits a 33% reduction in clearance in the elderly as a result of decreased first-pass metabolism [14]. Therefore, the effects of morphine may last longer in the elderly. However, this does not constitute a reason to avoid morphine in older patients. Drugs that have high-hepatic

extraction ratios also exhibit decreased metabolism and potentially increased therapeutic concentrations. Atorvastatin is a high-hepatic extraction ratio drug with increased serum concentration (40%) and area under the concentration curve (30%) [14]. Therefore, closer attention to liver function tests and potential dose reduction may be warranted. Similar findings occur with simvastatin and lovastatin.

Pharmacogenomics and the Cytochrome P450 Enzymes

Drug metabolism can be affected by diet, smoking, enzyme induction or inhibition, and alcohol intake [4, 14, 15]. Polymorphisms in the drug-metabolizing enzymes influence drug safety and efficacy. Pharmacogenomics refers to the influence of genes in determining drug metabolism, safety, and efficacy. As most drugs are metabolized by the liver and involve one or more enzymatic pathways, the ability to pre-screen a patient for potential genetic variants that affect drug response has clinical utility. Individualizing medication therapy based on a patient's specific metabolic genotype now exists for some medications. For example, the FDA approved genetic testing for warfarin in 2007. Completion of the Human Genome Project has helped accelerate the discovery of genetic variations affecting treatment response.

Appreciating potential changes in drug metabolism with aging and the influence of genetic factors that alter metabolic functions is central to the field of pharmacogenomics. For example, genetic polymorphism and changes in hepatic blood flow can explain interpatient variability to medications commonly used in the surgical intensive care unit [15]. The use of codeine in patients deficient in CYP2D6 results in poor conversion of codeine to morphine (the active metabolite) [14, 15]. Therefore, switching to an equianalgesic dose of morphine based on the failed codeine regimen can result in drug toxicity.

Conventional wisdom was that metabolism through the cytochrome (CYP) P450 system was impaired with aging. While some drugs metabolized via pathways involving microsomal oxidation are slowed with aging and may have active metabolites, broader probes for hepatic microsomal activity have shown inconsistent results [14–17]. For example, early studies of diazepam and chlordiazepoxide in the elderly demonstrated longer and less predictable half-lives. However, both these drugs are highly lipophilic and therefore have a larger volume of distribution given the increase in adipose tissue common in aging. Changes in drug distribution are now thought to account more for the prolonged and erratic half-life than decreases in metabolism [18, 19]. Regardless, neither agent is recommended for elderly patients.

Metabolism via glucuronide conjugation is minimally changed with advancing age, and metabolites tend to be

TABLE 27.2 Half-life of common benzodiazepines

Drug	Half-life in adults <65 years (h)	Half-life in adults ≥65 years (h)
Lorazepam	12.7	14.4
Alprazolam	11.7	15
Diazepam	M[a] 35.0–44.5	M 61.7–71.5
	F[b] 44.0–45.5	F 79.4–101
Chlordiazepoxide	10.1	18.2

Source: Data from [8, 18, 19]

[a] Male patients

[b] Female patients

inactive [14, 15]. Thus, drugs metabolized through these pathways, including benzodiazepines such as lorazepam, oxazepam, and temazepam, have shorter, more predictable half-lives and are therefore preferred for elderly patients (Table 27.2) [8, 18, 19]. Drug inhibition of enzymatic pathways typically occurs at a faster rate than induction of the same pathways. The ability to induce hepatic enzymes to the same extent as in younger individuals is unclear. Some agents commonly associated with enzyme induction include phenytoin, carbamezpine, phenobarbital, and chronic alcohol use. One potent inhibitor frequently used to control behavior in dementia patients is valproic acid.

Renal Elimination

The kidney is the main route of excretion for most drugs. On average, there are declines in glomerular filtration rate and renal blood flow with advancing age, although up to one-third of elderly persons have no substantial changes in renal function [20, 21]. Because of decreases in muscle mass and therefore creatinine production, serum creatinine levels may not accurately reflect renal function. Therefore, it is strongly recommended that creatinine clearance be calculated for every elderly patient. Even patients with seemingly normal serum creatinine levels may have a decreased creatinine clearance [22, 23]. Many formulas exist to estimate renal function [24–26]. It is important to recognize that all the available methods have limitations [27, 28]. The most widely used method is the Cockcroft and Gault equation:

$$\frac{[(140 - \text{Age}) \times (\text{Lean body weight in kilograms})]}{(72 \times \text{serum creatinine})} [\times 0.85 \text{ for women}]$$

This equation is valid when serum creatinine is at steady state. It is the authors' approach to use the resulting creatinine clearance to determine a range of possible renal function by adding and subtracting five points to the calculation. Many medications have specific dosing guidance based on creatinine clearance. Therefore, knowing the range of a patient's creatinine clearance allows for more conservative dosing if necessary and compensates for patient variability in

serum creatinine. When renal dose adjustments are necessary, surgeons should reduce the dosage or extend the dosing interval of primarily renally excreted drugs. This also applies to drugs with active metabolites that may have prolonged durations of action during renal insufficiency. One example of a medication commonly used in older adults is glyburide for type 2 diabetes. The dosing guidelines for glyburide recommend against using this product if the patient's creatinine clearance is <50 mL/min. The reason is an increased incidence of hypoglycemia secondary to reduced elimination of a renally active metabolite. Glipizide is the preferred sulfonylurea. To further emphasize the potential for hypoglycemia, the Veterans Health Administration (VHA) Pharmacy Benefits Management Services (PBM), Medical Advisory Panel (MAP), and Center for Medication Safety (VA Medsafe) issued a national bulletin advising providers to switch all patients with a calculated creatinine clearance of <50 mL/min to glipizide [29].

Medication-Related Problems in the Elderly

Polypharmacy and the Surgeon

Increases in the number of chronic conditions in the elderly generally result in increased medication use. Comorbidity is also associated with poor quality of life, physical disability, high health care use, and increased risk for adverse drug events and mortality [30–32]. Approximately 82% of older adults are treated for one or more conditions with 88% receiving a medication [33]. Prescription drug use is greatest in the elderly, with over one-third of all medications used annually [34]. Unfortunately, polypharmacy remains a significant problem for many older adults. Underuse, overuse, duplicate medication use, and ineffective medication use are by definition inappropriate medication use. Polypharmacy includes not only the number of medications a patient receives, but also potentially inappropriate medications that can lead to MRPs in older adults. In a nationally representative probability sample of community-dwelling adults aged 57–84 years old, Qato et al. found that more than half of older adults used five or more prescription medications, over-the-counter medications, or dietary supplements [35]. Almost one-third of this study population used five or more prescription medications and the prevalence of the use of five or more prescription medications increased steadily with age. Data from the Center for Medicare & Medicaid Services (CMS) estimate that 58% of community-dwelling elderly are taking three or more different acute and chronic medications in a year. CMS rates of medication use in long-term care are staggering with 67% of residents receiving nine or more different medications.

The increased emphasis on guideline-based medicine often results in patients receiving multiple agents for a condition in order to conform to "best practices." Patients with heart failure, hypertension, and diabetes can easily exceed six or more medications based on current clinical practice guidelines [36]. Medication management in elderly patients is more complex than in younger patients and each added medication increases the potential for interactions and adverse events. Medication errors and safety concerns in the elderly increase with each new prescription. For example, clinically significant drug interactions are more likely to occur when a patient takes five or more medications, and the likelihood for falls increases when an older adult takes four or more medications. Adding to the medication diaspora is the lack of coordination of prescribing in the elderly. Primary care physicians are unable to coordinate the multitude of specialists prescribing medications. Competitive pricing among major pharmacies often leads to patients filling prescriptions from multiple locations with no pharmacy holding a complete record of the patient's current medications. Collectively, there is a loss of control over ensuring medication safety and appropriateness.

It is unrealistic to expect surgeons to make substantive changes to a patient's chronic medications. Therefore, the issue of polypharmacy is more often a burden to the surgeon given the number of medications they must coordinate. While the absolute number of medications a geriatric surgery patient might receive may not change, the appropriateness of the prescribing should be optimized. When prescribing a new medication, attention to published lists of medications not to be used in the elderly (Beers criteria), avoidance of medications with known effects on cognition (anticholinergics and sedatives/hypnotics), and the judicious use of pain medication will help minimize the potential for polypharmacy-related complications [37–39]. In addition, particular attention should be given to any drugs with known narrow therapeutic windows to ensure proper monitoring for signs of toxicity. For example, warfarin is associated with five out of the top ten drug interactions in older adults (Table 27.3) [40]. Finally, any new symptom in an elderly patient should be considered a drug side effect until proven otherwise. During the course of treatment, the patient should be monitored closely and regularly for adverse effects. Regardless of age, 95% of all adverse drug reactions (ADRs) are predictable extensions of the pharmacology of the drug. Proper dosage adjustment based on renal and hepatic function can reduce the likelihood of experiencing an ADR. Once the desired effect is achieved and maintained, or the inciting event has passed, taper and discontinue the medication.

General Principles of Prescribing

The maxim of geriatric prescribing is to "start low, go slow, and sometimes say no." While perhaps overly simplistic and not applicable to all medications (i.e., antibiotics), the message is clear – medications are potentially dangerous in the elderly and should be used with caution [37–39]. Furthering the maxim, if starting low, it follows that you should also discontinue slow. Many drugs can be discontinued directly, but others (e.g., benzodiazepines and β-blockers) should be tapered to avoid adverse drug-withdrawal effects. With this background in mind, several underlying principles can help minimize the occurrence of MRPs and maximize adherence to prescribed drug regimens. Although they may seem rudimentary, they are nonetheless helpful to review (Table 27.4).

It is now required by the Joint Commission that all patients have their medications reconciled upon admission, discharge, or transfer within the hospital. Medication reconciliation can prevent MRPs resulting from forced adherence, a common occurrence resulting from a medication being restarted in a patient who stopped or changed their medication without notifying their primary provider. Elderly patients are often reluctant to admit they have stopped a medication or altered the dose. When reviewing medications, it is not enough to have the patient to recall their list of medications given the prevalence of cognitive impairment in older adults. The provider must also determine the dose and frequency of administration to assure accuracy when prescribing.

Table 27.3 Top ten drug interactions in the elderly

Warfarin – NSAIDs[a]
Warfarin – sulfa drugs
Warfarin – macrolides
Warfarin – quinolones[b]
Warfarin – phenytoin
ACE inhibitors – potassium supplements
ACE inhibitors – spironolactone
Digoxin – amiodarone
Digoxin – verapamil
Theophylline – quinolones[b]

Source: Reprinted with permission from the American Society of Consultant Pharmacists, Alexandria, VA. All rights reserved http://www.ascp.com [40]
[a] NSAID class does not include COX-2 inhibitors
[b] Quinolones that interact include: ciprofloxacin, enoxacin, norfloxacin, and ofloxacin

Table 27.4 Principles of safe geriatric prescribing

Take a detailed medication history (including over-the-counter and herbal/alternative preparations)
Establish clear, feasible therapeutic endpoints
Know the clinical pharmacology of drugs prescribed; use a few drugs well; balance safety with efficacy
Begin with a low dose of a drug and titrate up to achieve the desired response
Keep the regimen as simple as possible
Review medications regularly and discontinue those no longer needed
Remember that new symptoms (and illness) can be caused by a drug as well as by a new illness
Select the least costly alternative whenever possible
Encourage compliance. Utilize available pharmacy resources for counseling, written information, special packaging, and other reminder devices

When obtaining a full medication history, it is ideal to have the patient or a family member to bring all medications with them. The authors recommend instructing patients to bring all prescription and active nonprescription bottles to their presurgical screening visit. Actually examining the pill bottles can provide valuable information about the individual's medication management abilities. For example, you might be able to determine the number of providers following the patient, if they use only one pharmacy (important for drug interaction screening), if there is duplication of medications from multiple providers, the physical appearance of the bottles (recently filled prescription bottles that are filthy may be indicative of the individual's home environment), if the refills are on time, the pills are in the right bottles, pills are mixed together, and if the pill counts are accurate. Additional questions should probe for any new side effects or possible allergic reactions.

When assessing nonprescription medication usage, the authors advocate prompting patients with names of commonly used agents versus simply asking if they take any additional medications. The flow sheet in Table 27.5 is used by the authors to screen patients for OTC MRPs [41].

TABLE 27.5 Geriatric outpatient pharmacy interview

Name/Last 4: _____ Date:_____

Age:_____ Gender: M / F Race:_____ Confirm Allergies:_____

Last Visit:_____ Purpose of Visit: _____

Why does the patient think they are here?_____

General Appearance
- Y☐   N☐ cane/walker
- Y☐   N☐ glasses
- Y☐   N☐ hearing aids

Medication Management
- Y☐   N☐ Arrives with meds
- Y☐   N☐ Carries medication card
- Y☐   N☐ Medichest
- Y☐   N☐ Storagelocation_____
- Y☐   N☐ Medication assistance_____
- Y☐   N☐ Med reminders/alarms, etc

Social History
- Y☐   N☐ alcohol
- Y☐   N☐ tobacco

Medication ADL's
- Y☐   N☐ Young children at home
- Y☐   N☐ Can read label
- Y☐   N☐ Comprehends label instructions
- Y☐   N☐ Can open bottle
- Y☐   N☐ Pills in appropriate bottle
- Y☐   N☐ Other Pharmacy (location, meds):

Medication Adherence
Refill Method: ☐ phone ☐ mail
Refills on time: ☐ Yes   ☐ No

Missed dose:
☐daily ☐ weekly ☐monthly

What happens if you miss a dose:
- ☐ take when remember
- ☐ double next dose
- ☐ skip dose

Medication Reconciliation
(review prescription medications)

1. Medication Regimen Discrepancies
(i.e., changes in dose, frequency, product)

2. Non-VA OTC Meds (if so list)

Y☐   N☐ Vitamins

Y☐   N☐ Herbals/Natural Products

3. Other Medications

Side Effects?
If so, clarify ADR vs SE
How long?
What did they do when they had the SE?

Questions/Comments/Concerns?

Given that many drugs with potential toxicity and interactions are available without a prescription, every patient should also be asked about the use of OTC, herbal, or alternative medications. The pharmacist is a valuable resource for conducting the medication history/review. Pharmacist interventions with in-patients may decrease subsequent hospital and emergency visits and medication-related re-admissions [42, 43]. Inclusion of pharmacists on daily rounds in the intensive care units is encouraged to help improve overall prescribing [44]. Utilization of computerized provider order entry can further reduce medication errors [45]. When preparing discharge prescriptions, keep medication regimens simple. Once-daily dosing substantially improves adherence! If a complicated regimen is necessary, the hospital pharmacist may be able to arrange for the patient's community pharmacy to dispense the medication in a pill box or have them blister packed. These approaches may enhance adherence to the regimen. Providing the patients with a *legible* list of their medications with directions written in lay-terms is perhaps the single most important strategy to prevent MRPs. Many hospitals have pharmacists available for comprehensive medication counseling and to assist in streamlining regimens.

Specific Prescribing Issues

Delirium

Although seemingly a deviation from the topic, a discussion of delirium is warranted at this point because it is prevalent, potentially serious, potentially reversible, and because medications are leading contributors. This point is of particular importance in the hospital and during the perioperative period because a number of factors may contribute to the onset and propagation of delirium, including underlying cognitive impairment, change in environment, comorbid illnesses, the underlying illness prompting hospitalization or surgery, complications of that illness or procedures, anesthesia, the surgery itself, and a variety of medications, many of which are described below. The central focus in delirium is looking for and recognizing its appearance and then moving quickly to identify and correct the inciting factors.

Delirium is the acute or subacute development of an alteration in mental state that fluctuates during the course of the day. Standardized assessment instruments such as the confusion assessment method can be helpful for its detection [46]. Risk factors can be thought of as "predisposing factors," making one vulnerable to developing delirium, and "precipitating factors," which directly or indirectly lead to it. Among the predisposing factors are cognitive impairment, visual impairment, severe illness, and renal insufficiency [47]. Precipitating factors include the use of physical restraints,

malnutrition, bladder catheterization, iatrogenic events, and the number and type of medications [48]. Certain medications have been linked to a particular risk of postoperative delirium (e.g., meperidine and benzodiazepines) [49]. However, one study noted that the simultaneous addition of three or more medications to a drug regimen in the hospital was a significant contributing factor to delirium, suggesting that the sheer volume of new medications in certain hospitalized patients may be sufficient to overwhelm their reserve capacity (it should be noted that as the number of prescribed medications increased there was a greater likelihood of at least one of the medications being psychoactive) [48].

A number of strategies may be employed to try to decrease the risk of delirium, including attention to underlying illness and complications. The general prescribing principles outlined above may also be helpful along with specific examples detailed below when discussing individual drug categories. Another factor that is particularly problematic in the hospital setting is the scheduling of medications or treatments at night that require patients to be awakened, sometimes repeatedly. Although it may be necessary for acutely or severely ill patients or during the immediate postoperative period, it is helpful to attempt to minimize the occurrence later in the hospital course. Multifactorial interventions have been shown to reduce the incidence of delirium by 35–40% in medical and posthip fracture patients [50, 51].

Antipsychotics

Antipsychotics are used to treat hallucinations, delusions, paranoia, and extreme agitation or physical violence [52]. They tend to not be useful for pacing or wandering. Because of potential serious side effects, they should not be used to treat insomnia. It is important to look for delirium as the potential cause of a new-onset behavioral disturbance or thought disorder, so the underlying etiology can be determined and treatment of the primary process initiated.

Once a target sign or symptom is identified to gage the effectiveness of treatment, the choice of agent largely depends on the desired side effect. For the most part, neuroleptics are essentially equally effective, so the choice of agent depends on which side-effect profile fits the characteristics of the patient or is best tolerated by the patient. "Typical" agents, such as haloperidol (starting dose 0.25–0.5 mg, maximum daily dose 2.0 mg), are inexpensive and are available in oral, intramuscular, and intravenous preparations. The latter parenteral preparations may be particularly helpful in the setting of acute agitation or if the patient is unable to take oral medications. Haloperidol is more likely to produce extrapyramidal side effects, but less likely to cause sedation, orthostasis, and anticholinergic effects than lower potency agents. Among the extrapyramidal effects are parkinsonian features including tremor, bradykinesia, and masked fascies. Although these symptoms may fade over time, they have in the past also been treated with anticholinergic agents such as benztropine and trihexyphenidyl. This approach should be avoided because of the increased potential for delirium with concomitant therapy. A wiser approach might be to decrease the dose or switch to a different agent. Akathisia is manifested as motor restlessness, pacing, or disturbed sleep and may be reported as discomfort or anxiety. A danger is that these features may be misinterpreted as increasing psychosis, with the neuroleptic dose then being increased, resulting in worsened symptoms. As a result, it is often better to decrease the dose as an initial response to such symptoms to see if they are alleviated.

Tardive dyskinesia is a potential serious side effect of neuroleptic use and one of the reasons their use should be limited to the indications described above. Tardive dyskinesia starts as fine movement of the tongue, a facial tic, or lip smacking but may progress in the extreme to affect speech, eating, and breathing. Furthermore, it may be irreversible. Older adults and women are most likely to develop tardive dyskinesia, and it is more likely to be severe and less likely to be reversible in the older adults. It is less clear that treatment duration and type of agent are important contributors to risk [53, 54]. The primary treatment is to taper and discontinue the drug.

"Atypical" agents, such as risperidone (starting dose 0.25–0.5 mg, maximum daily dose 2.5 mg), have been touted as having fewer extrapyramidal side effects, although the risk does increase with increasing dosage. Olanzapine (starting dose 2.5–5 mg, maximum daily dose 20 mg) may be helpful in individuals who have insomnia or poor oral intake in addition to psychosis, although these effects may be problematic with longer-term use.

A number of precautions can be taken to minimize the risk or extent of side effects. Once the desired effect is achieved and the target symptom is alleviated, or the inciting event is resolved, the drug should be tapered and discontinued. Many of the problems with neuroleptic use result from patients being left on the drug long after the inciting event has resolved and after discharge from the hospital. If patients are discharged to a rehabilitation or long-term care facility, it is helpful to indicate a time limit to treatment with these agents, much as one would do with a course of antibiotics. If agents are prescribed on an as-needed, or pro re nata (PRN), basis, the indication for use and maximum daily dose should be clearly stated in the orders. The maximum daily doses provided for agents outlined above are guidelines; while they may be exceeded, this should be done cautiously and under close supervision because of the increased risk of side effects.

Of note, recent evidence has raised concern about the limited effectiveness of these agents in controlling behavioral symptoms and the potential risk of other serious adverse effects, such as cardiac and cerebrovascular events and death [55–57]. These effects have been noted in patients with dementia and with long-term use and higher doses, but they may affect the risk-benefit equation in a given patient. They also add to the importance of judiciously using these medications only for the appropriate indications (psychosis and agitation where the health and safety of the patient or caregivers is threatened) and at as low a dose and for as short a duration as is clinically necessary.

Antidepressants

The cardinal features of depression are the "vegetative" or depressive signs and symptoms, including increased or decreased sleep, decreased activity level, fatigue, decreased concentration, increased or decreased appetite or weight, motor slowing or agitation, guilt, suicidality, chronic somatic complaints, and pain [58]. Although standardized instruments, such as the Geriatric Depression Scale, can be useful adjuncts, diagnosis still often relies on the recognition of depressive signs and symptoms [59]. It is important to rule out underlying medical illnesses contributing to depression, such as stroke, myocardial infarction, congestive heart failure, thyroid disorders, uremia, and certain cancers. Medications may contribute as well, including central-acting antihypertensives and β-blockers, narcotics, neuroleptics, benzodiazepines, antihistamines, and sedative/hypnotics [60].

Once these contributing factors have been ruled out and target signs or symptoms identified, the choice of agent again depends in part on the characteristics or features of the patient and the desired side-effect profile [58, 61, 62]. There is currently a wide range of therapeutic options to treat depression. While early agents such as tricyclics can be effective, their side-effect profiles require much more caution when used in older patients. Tertiary amine tricyclics (e.g., amitriptyline, imipramine, and doxepin) were among the early agents used. Although still effective, their side effects are very poorly tolerated by elderly persons and they should be avoided. Their metabolites (secondary amine tricyclics such as nortriptyline and desipramine) are available and are preferred if a tricyclic is to be used. Like the low-potency neuroleptics, tricyclics also have potential side effects such as sedation, orthostasis, and anticholinergic effects. In addition, they have the potential to contribute to arrhythmias. While nortriptyline and desipramine have relatively low arrhythmogenicity, they should be used cautiously in persons with underlying conduction disorders, and PR and QRS intervals should be monitored periodically while on treatment. Desipramine is an activating agent and is preferable for persons who are apathetic, withdrawn, and anhedonic. Nortriptyline is a sedating agent and is preferred in individuals who are anxious or have sleep difficulties as well as depression. Blood levels are available for both agents and can be used to adjust doses depending on effect and side effects (nortriptyline has a therapeutic window – a level beyond the upper limit may lead to less effectiveness and more side effects) [63].

Because of their enhanced safety and tolerablility profiles, selective serotonin and norepinephine reuptake inhibitors (SSRI and SNRI) are the current preferred agents for treating depression in older patients [62, 64]. In general, citalopram/escitalopram, sertraline, and venlafaxine are safe, effective, and well-tolerated by older patients and are reasonable initial choices. For patients with certain associated features, other agents may be considered. For patients with poor sleep, poor intake, and anxiety as features of their depression, mirtazapine would be an option. For patients with pain and depression, duloxetine is an alternative. The latter options may minimize the number of medications by treating multiple symptoms with a single agent. Most agents take several weeks to have an effect on mood, but beneficial effects on sleep or appetite may be seen sooner. Potential side effects include gastrointestinal upset, change in sleep, headaches, dizziness, and sexual dysfunction.

Methylphenidate (starting dose 5 mg daily, maximum dose 10 mg twice a day, dosed early), which often exhibits an effect within 24–48 h, may be used as a bridging activating agent for particularly anhedonic or apathetic patients until other agents exert their effect, with its primary side effects being excessive arousal, gastrointestinal upset, and tachycardia [65]. Monoamine oxidase (MAO) inhibitors are used infrequently because of their potential serious interactions with certain medications and tyramine-containing foods. For life-threatening depression or patients refractory to medications, electroconvulsive therapy can be used safely and effectively in elderly persons [60].

Anxiolytics

Pharmacologic intervention for anxiety is warranted if symptoms are sufficiently severe to interfere with daily coping or enjoyment of life. In general, treatment should be short term: for a grief reaction or as an adjunct to supportive therapy to develop coping strategies. It is again important to rule out contributing disorders such as congestive heart failure and chronic obstructive pulmonary disease.

The mainstays of anxiolytic therapy are the benzodiazepines [52, 66]. Given the metabolic changes that occur with aging described above, short-acting agents such as lorazepam (starting dose 0.5 mg/day) and oxazepam (starting dose 7.5 mg/day) are preferred because of their more predictable half-lives and duration of action. All benzodiazepines share potential side effects, including sedation, dizziness, depression, confusion, agitation, and disinhibition. Dependence

can develop, and tolerance to their effects often occurs after 2–4 weeks of continuous use. Consequently, it is best to use these agents short term. Because a withdrawal reaction or "rebound" characterized by tremor and agitation can occur after abrupt withdrawal, benzodiazepines should be tapered prior to discontinuing. Buspirone (starting dose 5 mg twice a day) is a nonbenzodiazepine anxiolytic that is less likely to cause dependence, sedation, or psychomotor retardation. However, it has a delayed onset of action (several weeks) and lacks the soporific and muscle relaxant effects of benzodiazepines. Its primary side effects are dizziness and nausea. Barbiturates should be avoided because they are less effective and have greater addictive potential than other available agents [66, 67].

Sedative/Hypnotics

Disturbed sleep is a common complaint among older persons, particularly in the hospital [52, 68]. Part of this is due to changes that occur in sleep patterns with aging, including a phase shift (falling asleep and waking up earlier than in prior years) and more disruptions to sleep. Disturbed sleep may manifest as difficulty falling asleep, difficulty staying asleep, or early morning awakening. A variety of medical factors contribute to sleep difficulties, including anxiety, depression, pain, itching, nocturia, and congestive heart failure. Medications that may contribute include amphetamines, steroids, decongestants, caffeine, and alcohol. A number of other factors may play a role among hospitalized patients, including daytime naps, intravenous lines, catheters, traction, and frequent wakings for medications or treatments. After establishing by history if sleep is disturbed, the mainstay of treatment should be nonpharmacologic interventions directed at potential contributing factors.

If drug treatment is indicated, there are several potential choices that can be used safely and effectively short term (suggested maximum duration of use is 7–10 days). Among the benzodiazepines, short-acting agents are preferred because they are less likely to cause carryover sedation the following day. Temazepam (starting dose 7.5 mg) has a reasonable duration of action but a delayed onset of action and so must be given approximately 1–2 h before bedtime. Nonbenzodiazepine hypnotics, such as zolpidem, zaleplon, and eszopiclone, also appear relatively safe in older persons [69]. If the primary problem is difficulty falling asleep, ramelteon is another option. If persons are depressed and have sleep difficulties, treatment with a sedating antidepressant is preferable to separate treatment with two different medications. Similarly, if someone has a thought disorder and disturbed sleep, a sedating neuroleptic is preferred, but neuroleptics should not be used for sleep alone.

Pain Management

Pain is a common complaint among elderly persons and can have a substantial impact on affect and physical functioning. Adequate treatment is thus important, but caution must be exercised because of the strong potential for adverse effects with many of these agents. As such, it is helpful to follow the stepwise approach defined above for assessing the nature and extent of pain, determining its etiology, and starting with lower doses of less potent agents. A variety of instruments are available to help gage the current severity of pain and the effectiveness of treatment [70, 71].

The first line of therapy often consists of acetaminophen, aspirin, or nonsteroidal anti-inflammatory agents (NSAIDs) [71–73]. Although all three possess analgesic and antipyretic properties, acetaminophen lacks the anti-inflammatory properties of the other two classes. Acetaminophen is safe, effective, inexpensive, and well-tolerated by older persons. Caution should be exercised in the setting of liver disease or alcohol use, and there may be an increased risk of end-stage renal disease with high-dose long-term use [71, 74]. Caution must also be taken to ensure that patients avoid compound medications that include acetaminophen, which may contribute to their unknowingly exceeding recommended daily limits. Aspirin and the nonsteroidals can cause gastrointestinal bleeding or renal insufficiency and can interfere with platelet function. A variety of central nervous system (CNS) side effects may also be seen with nonsteroidals. Given that these three classes provide roughly equipotent analgesic effects, acetaminophen is a safer initial choice in the absence of inflammation. Of note, the most recent guidelines of the American Geriatrics Society recommend acetaminophen rather than nonsteroidals for the first line treatment of pain because of their side-effect profiles in older adults [73].

If pain is not controlled with these agents, opioid analgesics are the next line of treatment [71–73]. They are often characterized as mild or strong. Mild opioids, such as codeine and oxycodone, may provide relief alone or in conjunction with the nonopioid analgesics described above. Strong opioids, such as morphine, are used if pain remains unrelieved. All opioids have similar potential side effects, among which are respiratory depression, constipation, urinary retention, nausea and vomiting, delirium, and myoclonus. The patient should be monitored closely and appropriate dose adjustments made when these side effects appear. Prophylactic bowel regimens are often necessary and should be initiated when the narcotic is started. Tolerance to some of the effects may appear and may be facilitated by continuous, rather than as-needed, administration schedules. For respiratory depression, the opiate antagonist naloxone may be helpful. Meperidine should be avoided in the elderly, as it must be used with caution in patients with renal insufficiency and its metabolite, normeperidine, may cause seizures. Topical analgesics such as capsaicin may be helpful for conditions such as herpes zoster. Nonpharmacologic modalities such as heat, cold, massage, biofeedback, and transcutaneous electrical nerve stimulation (TENS) help in certain situations. Nerve blocks are another potential option for certain types of refractory pain. A recent trial of an interdisciplinary analgesic program in orthopedic patients found that intervention participants had less pain postoperatively and at 6 months and better physical performance [75].

Antihistamines

Histamine H_1 receptor blockers are commonly used for the treatment of allergies and allergic reactions; occasionally they are used as sedative/hypnotics. Because of their prominent anticholinergic properties, they should be used cautiously in the elderly. Newer agents with relatively low anticholinergic properties, such as loratadine, are preferred to treat allergy symptoms. Antihistamines such as diphenhydramine should not be used as sleep medications given the availability of safer agents.

Histamine H_2 receptor blockers, used to inhibit gastric acid secretion, can be safely used in elderly persons. All of these agents can cause alterations in mental status [76]. In general, the dose and duration of use should be kept to a minimum and always adjusted for renal function. If used prophylactically during the perioperative period, the dose should be decreased and ultimately discontinued as soon as possible.

Antibiotics

There are two major clinical categories of antibiotic usage among surgical inpatients: perioperative prophylaxis and the treatment of postoperative infections. Although this chapter does not deal with specific antibiotic recommendations, it addresses the general principles of antibiotic choice, dosing, and specific side effects in the geriatric patient.

As the population ages and as individuals live longer and productive lives through the benefits of advances in pharmacotherapy and medical technology, it has become important to consider technologic devices (grafts, stents, pacemakers, transplanted organs, and dialysis catheters) as important factors in the selection of antibiotics in the elderly surgical patient. Both the devices themselves, as well as the medications (immunosuppressive drugs and anticoagulants) that patients may be on as a result, need to be taken into consideration when choosing an antibiotic regimen. With the expansive antibiotic armamentarium currently available and new drugs being released with regular frequency, it is imperative that the proper choice of antibiotic be made by taking

TABLE 27.6 Selected antibiotics and their drug interactions

Antibiotic	Other drugs	Effect
Ampicillin	Anticoagulants	↑ Anticoagulation
Aminoglycosides	Amphotericin B	↑ Nephrotoxicity
	Cyclosporine	↑ Nephrotoxicity
	Loop diuretics	↑ Ototoxicity
	Neuromuscular blockers	↑ Respiratory paralysis
	NSAIDs	↑ Nephrotoxicity
	Vancomycin	↑ Nephrotoxicity
Cefoperazone, cefotetan	Anticoagulants	↑ Anticoagulation
Clindamycin	Muscle relaxants	↑ Frequency of respiratory paralysis
Ciprofloxacin	Antacids/sucralfate/ cations (vitamins and calcium supplements)	↓ Absorption of ciprofloxacin if taken within 2 h
	NSAIDs	↑ CNS stimulation/ seizures
	Anticoagulants	↑ Anticoagulation
Fluconazole	Tacrolimus	↑ Tacrolimus level with toxicity
	Cyclosporine	↑ Cyclosporine level, nephrotoxicity
	Ca channel blockers	↑ Ca channel blocker level
	Anticoagulants	↑ Anticoagulation
	Theophylline	↑ Theophylline level
Metronidazole	Alcohol	Disulfiram-like reaction
	Oral anticoagulants	↑ Anticoagulation
Imipenem cilastatin	Cyclosporine	↑ Cyclosporine level
Trimethoprim– sulfamethoxazole	Anticoagulants	↑Anticoagulation

Source: Data from [77]

into account possible drug interactions (Table 27.6), the side-effect profile of a particular drug, and the appropriate dose in a given patient [77].

The increasing antibiotic resistance noted in several strains of gram-positive bacteria has led to the development of new classes of antibiotics in an effort to combat this problem. All this has improved our ability to successfully care for and treat patients, but has also increased the risk of potential side effects and drug interactions to which patients are exposed. The advent of the electronic medical record, electronic prescribing systems, and electronic prescribing data bases have made the life of a busy clinician easier and have been shown to prevent adverse events [78].

While the maxim of geriatric prescribing, "start low, go slow" is true for most classes of drugs, this practice is not advisable with antibiotic use. This is especially true in the critically ill surgical patient and may in fact contribute to the problem of antimicrobial resistance. Understanding when pharmacokinetic changes in the elderly are important and

call for dose adjustments is imperative [79]. Proper dosing of antibiotics and other drugs in older adults reduces the incidence of ADRs. This point is especially important in light of the fact that the incidence of ADRs increases with advancing age and the effects are more serious in frail elderly patients than in their younger counterparts [80]. In general, improper dosing is a more frequent cause of error in therapy than is the use of an inappropriate drug [81].

Judicious clinical practice requires the prescribing physician to be aware of age-related changes in drug absorption, distribution, metabolism, and elimination. These have been described earlier in this chapter. Of these factors, the one with the most direct clinical relevance to antibiotic dosing is the decline in renal function. Many disease processes in the elderly, including most notably hypertension and diabetes, contribute to and accelerate this decline [80].

Most clinicians are aware of the need to decrease the dose of certain nephrotoxic antibiotics, such as aminoglycosides in the setting of frank renal insufficiency or decreased creatinine clearance. However, other commonly used drugs such as quinolones and most cephalosporins need to be dose-adjusted for a creatinine clearance of less than 30 ml/min [82]. Table 27.7 lists selected antibiotics whose dosages need to be adjusted [83, 84].

Although aminoglycosides remain important drugs for treating serious infections, alone or in combination with other drugs, the availability of newer agents (quinolones, monobactams, and carbapenems) with broad-spectrum coverage and less nephrotoxicity make the use of aminoglycosides less attractive in elderly persons. Risk factors for the development of aminoglycoside-induced nephrotoxicity include diabetes mellitus, dehydration, advanced age, and duration of treatment [85]. In addition to nephrotoxicity, aminoglycosides may also cause ototoxicity. This is more likely to occur in elderly patients especially if given in high dose or for prolonged periods because ototoxicity is cumulative. Furthermore, the risk of ototoxicity is greater in patients concomitantly taking a loop diuretic [86–88].

Evidence suggests that once-daily dosing of an aminoglycoside is at least as effective as, and less toxic than, conventional dosing regimens of multiple daily dosages as long as trough levels are monitored closely. Several analyses of pooled data from randomized controlled studies in adults found that once-daily aminoglycoside dosing may be associated with less nephrotoxicity and no greater ototoxicity than with conventional dosing [89–92]. Keep in mind, however, that once-daily aminoglycoside dosing is not appropriate for, or recommended in, any patient with a creatinine clearance <30 ml/min.

As mentioned above, although liver size and blood flow tend to decrease with age, in the absence of serious liver disease and subsequent hepatic dysfunction, antibiotic dosages do not need to be adjusted. Drug-induced hepatitis in patients treated with antituberculous agents, especially isoniazid,

TABLE 27.7 Selected antibiotics requiring dose adjustment during renal insufficiency

Antibiotic	Usual dose	Dose for CrCl 10–50 ml/min	Dose for CrCl <10 ml/min
Cefazolin	1–2 g q8 h	1–2 g q12 h	1–2 g q24–48 h
Cefuroxime	0.75–1.50 g q8 h	0.75–1.50 g q12 h	0.75–1.50 g q24 h
Ceftazidime	2 g q8 h	2 g q12–24 h	2 g q24–48 h
Cefotaxime	2 g q8 h	2 g q12–24 h	2 g q24 h
Penicillin G	0.5–4.0 million units q4 h	75% of dose	20–50% of dose
Ampicillin	1–2 g q6 h	1–2 g q6–12 h	1–2 g q12–24 h
Pipercillin tazobactam	3.375–4.5 g q6–8 h	2.25 g q6 h	2.25 g q8 h
Piperacillin	3–4 g q4–6 h	3–4 g q6–8 h	3–4 g q 8 h
Ticarcillin clavulanate	3.1 g q4 h	3.1 g q8–12 h	2 g q12 h
Aztreonam	2 g q8 h	50–75% of dose	25% of dose
Ertapenem	1 g q24 h	0.5 g q24 h	0.5 g q24 h
Imipenem cilastatin	0.5 g q6 h	0.25 g q6–12 h	0.125–0.25 g q12 h
Metronidazole	7.5 mg/kg q6 h	7.5 mg/kg q6 h	50% of dose
Vancomycin	1 g q12 h	1 g q 24–96 h	1 g q4–7 days
Gentamicin	1.7 mg/kg q8 h	1.7 mg/kg q12–24 h	1.7 mg/kg q48 h
Amikacin	7.5 mg/kg q12 h	7.5 mg/kg q24 h	7.5 mg/kg q48 h
Amphotericin B	0.4–1 mg/kg q24 h	0.4–1 mg/kg q24 h	0.4–1 mg/kg q24 h
Fluconazole	100–400 mg q24 h	50% of dose	50% of dose
Ciprofloxacin (IV)	400 mg q12 h	400 mg q12–24 h	400 mg q18–24 h

Source: Data from [84]

CrCl creatinine clearance

TABLE 27.8 Selected antibiotics requiring dose adjustment in the presence of severe hepatic dysfunction

Nafcillin

Cefoperazone

Clindamycin

Erythromycin

Ketoconazole

Isoniazid

Rifampin

increases in incidence from 2.8/1,000 in patients <35 years old to 7.7/1,000 in patients ≥55 years old [86, 93]. Therefore, liver function tests must be performed frequently prior to and during the course of antituberculous therapy. Antibiotics that require dose adjustments in patients with hepatic dysfunction include cefoperazone, clindamycin, erythromycin, isoniazid, ketoconazole, nafcillin, and rifampin (Table 27.8).

β-Lactam antibiotics (penicillins, cephalosporins, cephamycins, carbapenems, and monobactams) have varying characteristics of absorption, peak concentration, bioavailability, and metabolism. These topics are described in detail in standard texts and are not covered here. In general, bioavailability is relatively poor after oral administration, which has implications for the switch from intravenous to oral preparations, and pharmacokinetics are similar after intramuscular or intravenous administration [83].

Cephalosporins are relatively safe drugs to use in older persons. Dosages for certain cephalosporins need adjustment for renal insufficiency (Table 27.7). The broad spectrum of activity of ceftriaxone together with its convenient once-daily dosing make it an ideal drug for empiric use in a variety of clinical infections in the older adults [94, 95]. In addition, it has both renal and biliary excretion and as a result needs little adjustment for renal insufficiency. A lesser known side effect of ceftriaxone is the formation of biliary sludge with prolonged use [96].

Cefoperazone, a third-generation cephalosporin still in use especially for the treatment of intra-abdominal infections, has primarily biliary excretion and needs no adjustment for renal insufficiency; however, it can cause elevation of the prothrombin time [97]. This side effect is particularly important in the surgical patient. There are three proposed mechanisms of cephalosporin-associated hypoprothrombinemia, two of which involve the *N*-methylthiotetrazole (NMTT) moiety. The most plausible mechanism is NMTT inhibition of vitamin K epoxide reductase in the liver. Patients at increased risk for this adverse event include those with low vitamin K stores, specifically patients who are malnourished with low albumin concentrations and poor food intake. The elderly and patients with liver or renal dysfunction are examples of populations at potential risk. The manufacturer therefore recommends concomitant use of vitamin K once a week during cefoperazone administration, although epidemiologic studies suggest that bleeding complications with antibiotics in general may have more to do with other risk factors than the specific antibiotic [98–101]. It should also be noted that cefoperazone causes a mild disulfiram-like reaction when given within 72 h of alcohol ingestion.

Carbapenems (imipenem cilastatin, meropenem, and ertapenem) are a widely used class of drugs especially in the postoperative patient because of their broad spectrum of activity. Their pharmacokinetics are similar to that of cephalosporins, and they require dose adjustment for renal insufficiency because they are excreted renally. The cilastatin component of imipenem cilastatin has no antibacterial activity, but is used to inhibit renal tubular metabolism of imipenem, thereby increasing the urinary concentration of the active drug. Major adverse effects of the carbapenems, especially imipenem cilastatin, are related to the CNS, including seizures, somnolence, and confusion [102]. This is more likely to occur in the elderly with a history of a CNS lesion, prior seizure disorder, or renal failure.

Aztreonam is a monobactam that has only aerobic gram-negative bacterial coverage. Its pharmacokinetics are similar to that of the cephalosporins. It is frequently used in patients with renal insufficiency as a substitute for aminoglycosides, although it too needs dose adjustment in such patients. Its use in combination with β-lactam antibiotics for synergy (as with aminoglycosides for enterococcal or pseudomonal infections), however, has not been validated. It lacks cross-reactivity with other β-lactam antibiotics and can be used safely in patients with severe allergy to penicillin or cephalosporins [103, 104].

The fluorinated quinolones have gained wide usage during the past few decades. Compared with the older quinolones (norfloxacin and ciprofloxacin), the third- and fourth-generation quinolones (ofloxacin, levofloxacin, and moxifloxacin) have a broad spectrum of aerobic gram-positive and gram-negative bacterial activity along with the same excellent pharmacokinetic profile. The gram-positive coverage, especially in vitro activity against *Streptococcus pneumoniae*, of the earlier quinolones (ciprofloxacin) is not as good as that of the new generation of quinolones. In addition, they are active against intracellular organisms such as *Legionella*, *Mycoplasma*, *Chlamydia*, and *Mycobacteria*. They are well absorbed orally, with a high degree of bioavailability that makes them especially useful drugs in the transition from intravenous to oral dosing. They also have excellent tissue penetration. Care should be taken with the oral administration of these drugs to ensure that they are administered 2 h before or after antacids, sucralfate, or other multivalent metallic cations as their absorption can be severely impaired [105, 106]. Renally eliminated fluoroquinolones (ofloxacin and levofloxacin) need to be dose-adjusted when the creatinine clearance is <50 ml/min.

Along with the increased usage of this class of antibiotics, there have been reports of specific side effects when prescribing these drugs in older adults. Certain quinolones can cause QT interval prolongation. They should be avoided in patients with known prolongation of the QT interval, patients with uncorrected hypokalemia or hypomagnesemia, and patients receiving Class I or Class II antiarrhythmic drugs [107]. Elderly patients on corticosteroids, especially in the setting of chronic renal insufficiency, are also at risk for Achilles tendon rupture [108]. An important and well-documented drug interaction of quinolones with warfarin is particularly noteworthy in the postsurgical patient. The prothrombin time (PT) and INR need to be closely monitored to prevent bleeding complications [109, 110].

With the current escalating problem of antibiotic resistance and the increase in the numbers of resistant gram-positive infections (methicillin resistant *Staphylococcus aureus* and vancomycin resistant enterococci), several new antibiotics have been introduced in the past decade as an alternative to vancomycin. Linezolid and quinupristin dalfopristin are two such antibiotics. Linezolid, a fluorinated oxazolidinone active against gram-positive organisms, is a nonselective inhibitor of monoamine oxidase (MAOI). In the elderly patient with the potential for polypharmacy as discussed above, drug interactions need to be kept in mind when using this antibiotic. Linezolid is on the list of drugs with serotonergic activity that may cause serotonin syndrome – a potentially preventable complex of symptoms that may be fatal if not recognized early. The most common drug combinations associated with serotonin syndrome are MAOIs with selective serotonin reuptake inhibitors (SSRIs). Since SSRIs are frequently used for the treatment of depression, this is an important drug interaction to keep in mind [111–113].

No discussion of antibiotic use is complete without mention of *Clostridium difficile*-associated diarrhea (CDAD) – a challenge in the care of all hospitalized patients, particularly older ones. Surgical patients comprise 55–75% of all patients with CDAD [114]. Initial treatment regimens remain the same in this population and include oral metronidazole (cheap and effective) or oral vancomycin (expensive and concern for antibiotic resistance); however, there is an increased frequency of treatment failure and CDAD recurrence among elderly persons. Prolonged, tapering course of antibiotics, treatment with anion exchange resins, oral lactobacillus, or nonpathogenic yeast such as *Saccharomyces boulardii* and fecal transplants (enema with feces from healthy donors) or combinations of the above may need to be considered. None of these regimens has been proven superior to the others [115].

Summary

A number of factors can potentially influence the risk-benefit equation for drug use in an older population, including age-related physiologic changes in organ system function; increased likelihood of comorbid diseases affecting organ systems that are the intended site of drug action or are responsible for the metabolism or clearance of a drug; and increased likelihood of multiple chronic medications, which may increase the possibility of drug interactions. However, the vast majority of drugs can be used safely and effectively in older surgical patients if appropriate precautions are taken in the selection, dosing, and timing of drugs and in the active monitoring of effects and side effects.

References

1. Dychtwald K (1999) Age power. How the 21st century will be ruled by the new old. Penguin Putnam, New York, NY
2. Shock NW, Watkin DM, Yiengst MJ et al (1963) Age differences in the water content of the body as related to basal oxygen consumption in males. J Gerontol 18:1–8
3. Forbes GB, Reina JC (1970) Adult lean body mass declines with age: some longitudinal observations. Metabolism 19:653–663
4. Gilbaldi M (1992) Revisiting some factors contributing to variability. Ann Pharmacother 26(7–8):1002–1007
5. Hammerlein A, Derendorf H, Lowenthal D (1998) Pharmacokinetic and pharmacodynamic changes in the elderly. Clin Pharmacokinet 35:49–64
6. Pickering G (2004) Frail elderly, nutritional status and drugs. Arch Gerontol Geriatr 38:174–180
7. Hanlon JT, Ruby CM, Guay D, Artz M (2002) Geriatrics. In: DiPiro JT, Talbert RL, Yee GC et al (eds) Pharmacotherapy: a pathophysiologic approach, 5th edn. McGraw-Hill, New York, NY, pp 79–89
8. Turnheim K (1998) Drug dosage in the elderly: is it rational? Drugs Aging 13:357–359
9. Robertson DRC, Wood ND, Everest H et al (1989) The effect of age on the pharmacokinetics of levodopa administered alone and in the presence of carbidopa. Br J Clin Pharmacol 28:61–69
10. Holdsworth MT, Forman WB, Killilea TA et al (1994) Transdermal fentanyl disposition in elderly subjects. Gerontology 40(1):32–33
11. Tozer TN, Winter ME (2005) Phenytoin. In: Burton ME, Shaw LM, Schentag JJ, Evans WE (eds) Applied pharmacokinetics: principles of therapeutic drug monitoring, 4th edn. Lippincott Williams & Wilkins, Baltimore, pp 463–488
12. Paxton JW, Briant RH (1984) Alpha one-acid glycoprotein concentrations and propranolol binding in elderly patients with acute illness. Br J Clin Pharmacol 1:806–810
13. Castleden CM, George CF (1979) The effect of ageing on the hepatic clearance of propranolol. Br J Clin Pharmacol 7:49–54
14. Tanaka E (1998) In vivo age-related changes in hepatic drug-oxidizing capacity in humans. J Clin Pharm Ther 23:247–255
15. Herlinger C, Klotz U (2001) Drug metabolism and drug interactions in the elderly. Best Pract Res Clin Gastroenterol 15:897–918
16. Greenblatt DJ, Shader RI, Harmatz JS (1989) Implications of altered drug disposition in the elderly: studies of benzodiazepines. J Clin Pharmacol 29:866–872
17. Greenblatt DJ, Harmatz JS, Shader RI (1991) Clinical pharmacokinetics of anxiolytics and hypnotics in the elderly: therapeutic considerations. Part I. Clin Pharmacokinet 21:165–177
18. Divoll M, Greenblatt DJ, Ochs HR, Shader RI (1983) Absolute bioavailability of oral and intramuscular diazepam: effects of age and sex. Anesth Analg 62:1–8
19. Herman RJ, Wilkinson GR (1996) Disposition of diazepam in young and elderly subjects after acute and chronic dosing. Br J Clin Pharmacol 42:147–155
20. Rowe JW, Andres R, Tobin JD et al (1976) The effect of age on creatinine clearance in men: a cross-sectional and longitudinal study. J Gerontol 31:155–163
21. Lindeman RD, Tobin J, Shock NW (1985) Longitudinal studies on the rate of decline in renal function with age. J Am Geriatr Soc 33:278–285
22. Bertino JS Jr (1993) Measured versus estimated creatinine clearance in patients with low serum creatinine values. Ann Pharmacother 27:1439–1442
23. Smythe M, Hoffman J, Kizy K et al (1994) Estimating creatinine clearance in elderly patients with low serum creatinine concentrations. Am J Hosp Pharm 51:198–204
24. Cockcroft DW, Gault MH (1976) Prediction of creatinine clearance from serum creatinine. Nephron 16:31–41
25. Sanaka M, Takano K, Shimakura K et al (1996) Serum albumin for estimating creatinine clearance in elderly with muscle atrophy. Nephron 73:37–44
26. Levey AS, Bosch JP, Lewis JB et al (1999) A more accurate method to estimate glomerular filtration rate from serum creatinine: a new prediction equation. Ann Intern Med 130:461–470
27. Lamb EJ, Webb MC, Simpson DE et al (2003) Estimation of glomerular filtration rate in older patients with chronic renal insufficiency: is the modification of diet in renal disease formula an improvement? J Am Geriatr Soc 51:1012–1017
28. Reichley RM, Ritchie DJ, Bailey TC (1995) Analysis of various creatinine clearance formulas in predicting gentamicin elimination in patients with low serum creatinine. Pharmacotherapy 15:625–630
29. Anonymous (2009) Risk of severe hypoglycemia with glyburide use in elderly patients with renal insufficiency. Veterans Health Administration (VHA) Pharmacy Benefits Management Services (PBM), Medical Advisory Panel (MAP), & Center for Medication Safety (VA Medsafe), July 29
30. Gijsen R, Hoeymans N, Schellevis FG, Ruwaard D, Satariano WA, van den Bos GA (2001) Causes and consequences of comorbidity: a review. J Clin Epidemiol 54:661–674
31. Hoffman C, Rice D, Sung HY (1996) Persons with chronic conditions: their prevalence and costs. JAMA 276:1473–1479
32. Field TS, Gurwitz JH, Harrold LR et al (2004) Risk factors for adverse drug events among older adults in the ambulatory setting. J Am Geriatr Soc 52:1349–1354
33. Safran DG, Neuman P, Schoen C et al. (2002) Prescription drug coverage and seniors: how well are we closing the gap? Health Aff (suppl web exclusives):W253–W268. http://content.healthaffairs.org/cgi/reprint/hlthaff.w2.253v1.pdf. Accessed Feb 2009
34. Mojtabai R, Olfson M (2003) Medication costs, adherence, and health outcomes among Medicare beneficiaries. Health Aff 22:220–228
35. Qato DM, Alexander GC, Conti RM et al (2008) Use of prescription and over-the-counter medications and dietary supplements among older adults in the United States. JAMA 300(24):2867–2878
36. Boyd CM, Darer J, Boult C et al (2005) Clinical practice guidelines and quality of care for older patients with multiple comorbid diseases: implications for pay for performance. JAMA 294:716–724
37. Fick DM, Cooper JW, Wade WE et al (2003) Updating the Beers criteria for potentially inappropriate medication use in older adults: results of a US consensus panel of experts. Arch Intern Med 163(22):2716–2724
38. Beyth RJ, Shorr RI (2002) Principles of drug therapy in older patients: rational drug prescribing. Clin Geriatr Med 18:577–592
39. Sloan RW (1992) Principles of drug therapy in geriatric patients. Am Fam Physician 45:2709–2718
40. American Society of Consultant Pharmacists. Top ten dangerous drug interactions in long-term care. Available at http://www.scoup.net/M3Project/topten. Accessed Feb 2009
41. Jeffery SM (2009) Outpatient Geriatric Medication Reconciliation.
42. Hanlon JT, Weinberger M, Samsa GP et al (1996) A randomized, controlled trial of a clinical pharmacist intervention to improve prescribing in elderly outpatients with polypharmacy. Am J Med 100:428–437
43. Gillespie U, Alasaad A, Henrohn D et al (2009) A comprehensive pharmacist intervention to reduce morbidity in patients 80 years or older: a randomized controlled trial. Arch Intern Med 169:894–900
44. Richardson WC, Berwick DM, Bisgard JC et al (2000) The Institute of Medicine Report on Medical Errors: misunderstanding can do harm. Quality of Health Care in America Committee. MedGenMed 2(3):E42
45. Bates DW, Teich JM, Lee J et al (1999) The impact of computerized physician order entry on medication error prevention. J Am Med Inform Assoc 6(4):313–321

46. Inouye SK, van Dyck CH, Alessi CA et al (1990) Clarifying confusion: the confusion assessment method: a new method for detection of delirium. Ann Intern Med 113:941–948

47. Inouye SK, Viscoli CM, Horwitz RI et al (1993) A predictive model for delirium in hospitalized elderly medical patients based on admission characteristics. Ann Intern Med 119:474–481

48. Inouye SK, Charpentier PA (1996) Precipitating factors for delirium in hospitalized elderly persons: predictive model and interrelationship with baseline vulnerability. JAMA 275:852–857

49. Marcantonio ER, Juarez G, Goldman L et al (1994) The relationship of postoperative delirium with psychoactive medications. JAMA 272:1518–1522

50. Inouye SK, Bogardus ST, Charpentier PA et al (1999) Multicomponent intervention to prevent delirium in hospitalized older patients. N Engl J Med 340:669–676

51. Marcantonio ER, Flacker JM, Wright RJ, Resnick NM (2001) Reducing delirium after hip fracture. J Am Geriatr Soc 49: 516–522

52. Jenike MA (1988) Psychoactive drugs in the elderly: antipsychotics and anxiolytics. Geriatrics 43(9):53–65

53. Task Force on Late Neurological Effects of Antipsychotic Drugs (1980) Tardive dyskinesia: summary of a task force report of the American Psychiatric Association. Am J Psychiatry 137:1163–1172

54. Smith JM, Baldessarini RJ (1980) Changes in prevalence, severity, and recovery in tardive dyskinesia with age. Arch Gen Psychiatry 37:1368–1373

55. Schneider LS, Tariot PN, Dagerman KS et al (2006) Effectiveness of atypical antipsychotic drugs in patients with Alzheimer's disease. N Engl J Med 335:1525–1538

56. Ray WS, Chung CP, Murray KT et al (2009) Atypical antipsychotic drugs and the risk of sudden cardiac death. N Engl J Med 360: 225–235

57. Ballard C, Hanney ML, Theodoulou M et al (2009) The dementia antipsychotic withdrawal trial (DART-AD): long-term follow-up of a randomized placebo-controlled trial. Lancet Neurol 8:151–157

58. Jenike MA (1988) Psychoactive drugs in the elderly: antidepressants. Geriatrics 43(11):43–57

59. Yesavage JA, Brink TL, Rose TL et al (1983) Development and validation of a geriatric depression screening scale: a preliminary report. J Psychiatr Res 17:37–49

60. Stimmel GL, Gutierrez MA (1995) Psychiatric disorders. In: Delafuente JC, Stewart RB (eds) Therapeutics in the elderly, 2nd edn. Harvey Whitney Books, Cincinnati, pp 324–343

61. Tourigny-Rivard MF (1997) Pharmacotherapy of affective disorders in old age. Can J Psychiatry 42(suppl 1):10S–18S

62. Alexopoulos GS, Katz IR, Reynolds CF, et al (2001) The expert consensus guideline series: pharmacotherapy of depressive disorders in older patients. Postgrad Med (Special Report):1–86

63. Perry PJ, Pfohl BM, Holstad SG (1987) The relationship between antidepressant response and tricyclic antidepressant plasma concentrations: a retrospective analysis of the literature using logistic regression analysis. Clin Pharmacokinet 13:381–392

64. Mukai Y, Tampi RR (2009) Treatment of depression in the elderly: a review of the recent literature on the efficacy of single- versus dual-action antidepressants. Clin Ther 31:945–961

65. Wallace AE, Kofoed LL, West AN (1995) Double-blind, placebo-controlled trial of methylphenidate in older, depressed, medically ill patients. Am J Psychiatry 152:929–931

66. Schneider LS (1996) Overview of generalized anxiety disorder in the elderly. J Clin Psychiatry 57(suppl 7):34–45

67. Shuckit MA (1981) Current therapeutic options in the management of typical anxiety. J Clin Psychiatry 42(11, sect 2):15–26

68. Flamer HE (1995) Sleep problems. Med J Aust 162:603–607

69. Vaz Fragoso CA, Gill TM (2007) Sleep complaints in community-living older persons: a multifactorial geriatric syndrome. J Am Geriatr Soc 55:1853–1866

70. Herr KA, Mobily PR (1991) Pain assessment in the elderly: clinical considerations. J Gerontol Nurs 17(4):12–19

71. Ferrell BA (1991) Pain management in elderly people. J Am Geriatr Soc 39:64–73

72. Ferrell BA (1995) Pain evaluation and management in the nursing home. Ann Intern Med 123:681–687

73. American Geriatrics Society Panel (2009) Pharmacological management of persistent pain in older persons. J Am Geriatr Soc 57:1331–1346

74. Barrett BJ (1996) Acetaminophen and adverse chronic renal outcomes: an appraisal of the epidemiologic evidence. Am J Kidney Dis 28(suppl 1):S14–S19

75. Morrison RS, Flanagan S, Fischberg D et al (2009) A novel interdisciplinary analgesic program reduces pain and improves function in older patients after orthopedic surgery. J Am Geriatr Soc 57:1–10

76. Cantu TG, Korek JS (1991) Central nervous system reactions to histamine-2 receptor blockers. Ann Intern Med 114:1027–1034

77. Sanford JP, Gilbert DN, Moellering RC, Sande MA (eds). Anti-infective drug–drug interactions. In: The Sanford Guide to Antimicrobial Therapy; 27th edn. Vienna, VA: Antimicrobial Therapy, 1997:123–126.

78. Smith DH, Perrin N, Feldstein A et al (2006) The impact of prescribing safety alerts for elderly patients in an electronic medical record. Arch Intern Med 116:1098–1104

79. Bergman SJ, Speil C, Short M et al (2007) Pharmacokinetic and pharmacodynamic aspects of antibiotic use in high risk populations. Infect Dis Clin N Am 21:821–846

80. Gleckman RA (1995) Antibiotic concerns in the elderly. Infect Dis Clin North Am 9:575–590

81. Lesar TS, Lomaestro BM, Pohl H (1997) Medication-prescribing errors in a teaching hospital: a 9-year experience. Arch Intern Med 157:1569–1576

82. Gilbert DN, Bennett WM (1989) Use of antimicrobial agents in renal failure. Infect Dis Clin North Am 3:517–531

83. McCue JD (1992) Antimicrobial therapy. Clin Geriatr Med 8:925–945

84. Sanford JP, Gilbert DN, Moellering RC, Sande MA (eds) (1997) Dosage of antimicrobial drugs in adult patients with renal impairment. In: The Sanford Guide to antimicrobial therapy, 27th edn. Vienna, VA: Antimicrobial Therapy, pp 116–120

85. Mingeot-Leclercq MP, Tulkens PM (1999) Aminoglycosides: nephrotoxicity. Antimicrob Agents Chemother 43:100–112

86. Posner JD (1982) Particular problems of antibiotic use in the elderly. Geriatrics 37(8):49–54

87. Tablan OC, Reyes MP, Rintelmann WF et al (1984) Renal and auditory toxicity of high-dose, prolonged therapy with gentamicin and tobramycin in *Pseudomonas endocarditis*. J Infect Dis 149:257–263

88. Moore RD, Smith CR, Lietman PS (1984) Risk factors for the development of auditory toxicity in patients receiving aminoglycosides. J Infect Dis 149:23–30

89. Marra F, Partovi N, Jewesson P (1996) Aminoglycoside administration as a single daily dose. Drugs 52:344–370

90. Barza M, Ioannidis JPA, Cappelleri JC et al (1996) Single or multiple daily doses of aminoglycosides: a meta-analysis. BMJ 312:338–345

91. Hatala R, Dinh T, Cook DJ (1996) Once-daily aminoglycoside dosing in immunocompetent adults: a meta-analysis. Ann Intern Med 124:717–725

92. Raveh D, Kopyt M, Hite Y et al (2002) Risk factors for nephrotoxicity in elderly patients receiving once-daily aminoglycosides. Q J Med 95:291–297

93. Van den Brande P, van Steenbergen W, Vervoort G et al (1995) Aging and hepatotoxicity of isoniazid and rifampin in pulmonary tuberculosis. Am J Respir Crit Care Med 152:1705–1708

94. Mandell LA, Bergeron MG, Ronald AR et al (1989) Once-daily therapy with ceftriaxone compared with daily multiple-dose therapy with cefotaxime for serious bacterial infections: a randomized, double-blind study. J Infect Dis 160:433–441

95. Barriere SL, Flaherty JF (1984) Third-generation cephalosporins: a critical evaluation. Clin Pharm 3:351–373

96. Michielsen PP, Fierens H, Van Maercke YM (1992) Drug-induced gallbladder disease: incidence, etiology and management. Drug Saf 7:32–45

97. Brogden RN, Carmine A, Heel RC et al (1981) Cefoperazone: a review of its in vitro antimicrobial activity, pharmacological properties and therapeutic efficacy. Drugs 22:423–460

98. Rockoff SD, Blumenfrucht MJ, Irwin RJ et al (1992) Vitamin K supplementation during prophylactic use of cefoperazone in urologic surgery. Infection 20:146–148

99. Goss TF, Walawander CA, Grasela TH et al (1992) Prospective evaluation of risk factors for antibiotic-associated bleeding in critically ill patients. Pharmacotherapy 12:283–291

100. Grasela TH, Walawander CA, Welage LS et al (1989) Prospective surveillance of antibiotic-associated coagulopathy in 970 patients. Pharmacotherapy 9:158–164

101. Schentag JJ, Welage LS, Williams JS et al (1988) Kinetics and action of N-methylthiotetrazole in volunteers and patients: population-based clinical comparisons of antibiotics with and without this moiety. Am J Surg 155(5A):40–44

102. MacGregor RR, Gibson GA, Bland JA (1986) Imipenem pharmacokinetics and body fluid concentrations in patients receiving high-dose treatment for serious infections. Antimicrob Agents Chemother 29:188–192

103. Neu HC (1990) Aztreonam activity, pharmacology, and clinical uses. Am J Med 88(suppl 3C):2S–6S

104. Fillastre JP, Leroy A, Baudoin C et al (1985) Pharmacokinetics of aztreonam in patients with chronic renal failure. Clin Pharmacokinet 10:91–100

105. Davies BI, Maesen FPV (1989) Drug interactions with quinolones. Rev Infect Dis 11(suppl 5):S1083–S1090

106. Norrby SR, Ljungberg B (1989) Pharmacokinetics of fluorinated 4-quinolones in the aged. Rev Infect Dis 11(suppl 5):S1102–S1106

107. Stahlmann R, Lode H (2003) Fluoroquinolones in the elderly: safety considerations. Drugs Aging 20(4):289–302

108. van der Linden PD, Sturkenboom MC, Herings RM et al (2003) Increased risk of achilles tendon rupture with quinolone antibacterial use, especially in elderly patients taking oral corticosteroids. Arch Intern Med 163:1801–1807

109. Holbrook AM, Pereira JA, Labiris R et al (2005) Systematic overview of warfarin and its drug and food interactions. Arch Intern Med 165:1095–1106

110. Jones CB, Fugate SE (2002) Levofloxacin and warfarin interaction. Ann Pharmacother 36:1554–1557

111. Huang V, Gortney JS (2006) Risk of serotonin syndrome with concomitant administration of linezolid and serotonin agonists. Pharmacotherapy 26:1784–1793

112. Clark DB, Andrus MR, Byrd DC (2006) Drug interactions between linezolid and selective serotonin reuptake inhibitors: case report involving sertraline and review of the literature. Pharmacotherapy 26:269–276

113. Taylor JJ, Wilson JW, Estes LL (2006) Linezolid and serotonergic drug interactions: a retrospective survey. Clin Infect Dis 43:180–187

114. Jobe BA, Grasley A, Deveney KE et al (1995) *Clostridium difficile* colitis: an increasing hospital acquired illness. Am J Surg 169:480–483

115. Mylonakis E, Ryan ET, Calderwood SB (2001) *Clostridium difficile* – associated diarrhea. A review. Arch Intern Med 161:523–533

Chapter 28
Invited Commentary

Donald D. Trunkey

Injury in the elderly is increasing, and we now see a bimodal distribution of injury deaths. The first peak in death rates is in the 16 to 24 age group, and the second is after the age of 60. This increase in the number of elderly patients is due in no small part to the fact that they are more active, continue to drive, and remain involved in some risk-taking sports, such as skiing and driving motorcycles. One can ask, "When does 'old age' begin?" If one reviews the National Trauma Data Bank maintained by the American College of Surgeons, there appears to be an increase in deaths after the age of 45. I wish to emphasize the variability in the physiologic changes that occur in the aged. The most common comorbidities that I see are cirrhosis, smoking, heart disease, and chronic obstructive pulmonary disease.

There have been many recent changes in the management of shock and hemotherapy. One has to be careful in analyzing and applying some of these changes to the elderly. Data from Iraq and Afghanistan have confirmed what Cannon observed in World War I. It is important *not* to over-resuscitate the patient prior to surgical control of bleeding. The military studies show that minimal pre-hospital fluid should be given, corroborating Cannon's data in that keeping the blood pressure above 85 mm/Hg is optimal. However, this may not be applicable or should be modified in the case of elderly patients who have arterial sclerosis or congestive heart failure. One of the more dramatic changes shown recently by our military is in hemotherapy. During World War I, Cannon used whole blood. The component therapy data from Operation Enduring Freedom and Operation Iraqi Freedom have been modified to reflect a 1:1:1 ratio of packed red blood cells, fresh frozen plasma, and platelets and provide a statistically better outcome when compared to the earlier management of components. An even better outcome can be achieved with whole blood, which most surgeons believe to be the appropriate fluid to give for hypovolemic shock.

Another concept that is gaining credibility is the prevention and treatment of compartment syndromes. Compartment syndromes can occur in the cranial vault, hemithoraces, abdomen, pelvis, and the extremities. Neurosurgery has rightly pointed out the ravages of compartment syndrome within the cranial vault, and there has been aggressive management in the form of evacuation of hematomas, and even craniectomy. These problems are aggravated in the elderly because many of them come into the emergency room after major injury and are on Warfarin, Plavix, or aspirin. Although rapid reversal of these compounds is desirable, it is fraught with difficulties, particularly if one uses vitamin K, fresh frozen plasma, or platelets. These all take time to reverse. Some centers have used low-dose Factor VII with promising results, but there is the downside of increased thrombosis. Compartment syndromes, including air and blood within either hemithorax can usually be addressed once the patient arrives at the emergency department, but in some instances, can be relieved (tension) in the pre-hospital care. The compartment syndromes that develop in the abdomen and pelvis are partly preventable by prudent limitation of over-resuscitation, but in some instances will require leaving the abdomen open, packing the pelvis temporarily to gain hemostasis, and repeated damage control until the abdomen can be closed either primarily or at a later date after temporary closure with synthetic material.

A related issue is the triad of coagulopathy, hypothermia, and acidosis, which is often a complication of resuscitation. Oftentimes, this is preventable. Warming the patient should start in the prehospital setting, and acidosis can be partially ameliorated by use of balanced salt solutions. In the emergency room, this triad *must* be recognized early and aggressively addressed.

A particularly contentious issue in the elderly is futility of care in the emergency room and the ICU. This includes both quantitative and qualitative futility. Examples of quantitatively futile care would include full ventilatory support of a patient with documented brain death or an instance where there is no precedent for survival. Qualitative futility describes the nature of function following survival of a devastating insult. The descriptors of qualitative futility are dependent on

D.D. Trunkey (✉)
Department of Surgery, Oregon Health and Science University, Portland, OR 97239, USA
e-mail: trunkeyd@ohsu.edu

R.A. Rosenthal et al. (eds.), *Principles and Practice of Geriatric Surgery*,
DOI 10.1007/978-1-4419-6999-6_28, © Springer Science+Business Media, LLC 2011

personal preferences and are value-laden. For geriatric trauma patients, substantial erosion in the capability for independent living defines qualitative futility, with the range of individual preferences defining the specifics of the loss of function. For some elderly patients, becoming permanently dependent on the assistance of others for management of bodily function constitutes a qualitative futile outcome; while for others, coma and a requirement for mechanical ventilation would be the threshold for qualitative futility. Futilities are tough ethical issues that the surgeon and intensivist face almost on a daily basis. Unfortunately, when we studied this at our institution, our outcomes were mixed. Patients who were discharged to nursing homes, skilled nursing facilities, and rehabilitation centers had a higher death rate at 1 year than those discharged to their homes. Furthermore, those who had significant injury (ISS >15) were able to return immediately to independent living status in only 25% of instances. When discharged to secondary care institutions, many did not return to independent living status.

The elderly represent a heterogeneous group in the physiologic changes that occur during latter years. Comorbid factors described above also influence the elderly patient's response to injury and surgery. There are no simple rules in preventing futility, but the surgeon has to be aggressive in making decisions, working with the families, and trying to do what is best for the patient.

Chapter 29
Common Perioperative Complications in Older Patients

Sandhya A. Lagoo-Deenadayalan, Mark A. Newell, and Walter E. Pofahl

Introduction

As one of the fastest growing segments of the population, elderly patients account for an increasing percentage of operations in most practices. On the basis of the 2006 National Hospital Discharge Survey, patients aged 65 and older accounted for 35% of all procedures [1]. Elderly patients have a higher rate of postoperative complications. Two large studies found complication rates of 20–50% in patients aged 80 years and older [2, 3]. In contrast, younger patients had complication rates approximately half of that in the elderly patients. Table 29.1 outlines the relative frequency of specific complications in elderly patients undergoing a variety of noncardiac surgical procedures.

Elderly patients are similar to other patients in terms of the "typical" postoperative complications that can occur with an operation such as bleeding, infection, or technical errors. However, elderly patients are at risk for a group of unique complications owing to the physiologic changes of aging and the stress of the perioperative period. The underlying mechanisms for recognition, treatment, and prevention of these complications are the focus of this chapter.

There are some general principles for identifying, preventing, and treating postoperative complications in elderly patients. First and foremost, many postoperative complications in elderly patients have "atypical" presentations, making the recognition of postoperative complications difficult in this age group. For example, infectious complications do not necessarily present with fever and leukocytosis; delirium can be the sole clinical manifestation of an infectious complication.

The second principle is to actively search for and avoid complications. Every surgeon caring for elderly patients has had a case where a single, seemingly minor, postoperative complication spiraled into something more significant. This is because although elderly patients tolerate most elective operations, they have limited physiologic reserves to tolerate the increased physiologic stress of postoperative complications. After emergency operations, much of physiologic reserve is spent maintaining homeostasis, leaving even less reserve for complications. Therefore, it is imperative to avoid preventable complications such as those that result from a poor choice of medications.

The third principle is to perform an adequate preoperative risk assessment including functional status and cognitive assessment. In the elective setting, there is adequate time to fully evaluate the elderly patient for occult comorbidities and determine functional and cognitive status. Unfortunately, the same time is usually not available in the case of urgent or emergency operations. However, this information can often be obtained from caregivers and family. This has a direct impact on expected postoperative course, especially after emergency operations, and can help set expectations and goals of therapy.

Age-Related Complications

Delirium

Delirium is a relatively frequent complication following surgery in elderly patients. Table 29.2 outlines the rates of postoperative delirium for selected common procedures. The reported rates of postoperative delirium range from 15 to >50%. [4] The rate varies from <5% following cataract surgery to as high as 60% after hip replacement [5]. Elderly patients who develop delirium have longer postoperative hospital stays, are more likely to be discharged to a nursing home, less likely to regain full function, and have higher death rates at 30 days, 6 months, and 1 year [5–8].

W.E. Pofahl (✉)
Department of Surgery, Brody School of Medicine, East Carolina University, Pitt County Memorial Hospital, Greenville, NC, USA
e-mail: pofahlw@ecu.edu

R.A. Rosenthal et al. (eds.), *Principles and Practice of Geriatric Surgery*,
DOI 10.1007/978-1-4419-6999-6_29, © Springer Science+Business Media, LLC 2011

TABLE 29.1 Postoperative complications in elderly patients

Morbidity	Age	
	<80 ($n = 568,263$)	≥80 ($n = 26,648$)
	% Complication	
≥1 complication	12.1	20.0
Respiratory complications		
Pneumonia	2.3	5.6
>48 h on ventilator	2.1	3.5
Required reintubation	1.6	2.8
Pulmonary embolism	0.2	0.4
Urinary tract complications		
Urinary tract infection	2.2	5.6
Acute renal failure	0.4	0.6
Progressive renal failure	0.4	1.0
Cardiac complications		
Myocardial infarction	0.4	1.0
Pulmonary edema	0.6	1.0
Cardiac arrest	0.9	2.1
Wound complications		
Deep wound infection	1.4	1.3
Superficial wound infection	1.9	1.7
Wound dehiscence	0.9	0.9
Nervous system complications		
Cerebrovascular accident	0.3	0.7
Coma > 24 h	0.3	0.3
Peripheral nerve injury	0.3	0.3
Other complications		
Systemic sepsis	1.2	2.0
Bleeding requiring >4 units blood	1.0	1.5
Prolonged ileus	1.2	1.7
Deep-vein thrombosis	0.4	0.6
Graft or prosthesis failure	0.5	0.4

Source: Reprinted from Hamel et al. [2], with permission from Wiley Blackwell

TABLE 29.2 Rates of delirium following selected procedures

Procedure	Rate (%)
Cardiac surgery[a]	48
Aortic surgery[b]	30–50
Vascular bypass[b]	29
Cataract surgery[c]	<5
Hip surgery (elective)[b]	4–15
Hip surgery (emergency)[b]	19–44
Colorectal surgery[d]	38

[a] Data from Rudolph JL et al (2009) Circulation
[b] Data from Dasgupta and Dumbrell [12]
[c] Data from Milstein A et al (2002) Int Psychogeriatr
[d] Data from Beaussier M et al (2006) Reg Anesth Pain Med

Impact on Outcome

The development of postoperative delirium has a deleterious effect on postoperative outcomes. Specifically, postoperative delirium is associated with longer length of stay [6, 9], higher postoperative complication rates [9], higher probability of discharge to nursing home [6], poorer functional outcome [7, 10], and higher death rates at 6 [6] and 12 months [7]. This results in a greater financial burden of care for these patients. Robinson documented an average cost of hospitalization of $50,100 in patients who developed postoperative delirium [6]. In contrast, the average cost of hospitalization in patients who did not develop delirium was $31,600. Two studies of patients undergoing nonorthopedic operations documented a doubling of length of stay in patients with postoperative delirium when compared to patients who do not develop delirium [6, 9].

The development of delirium is also associated with higher rates of overall postoperative complications [9]. This is not unexpected as delirium is often the initial sign of a postoperative complication. However, a large study of patients who developed delirium after surgical treatment of hip fracture did not show an increased length of stay or increased postoperative complication rate when compared to patients who did not develop postoperative delirium [7].

There are also conflicting data on increased rates of discharge to nursing homes in patients who developed postoperative delirium. Robinson et al. [6] showed a significantly higher rate (33%) of postdischarge institutionalization in patients who developed delirium as compared to patients who did not (1%) following nonorthopedic procedures. In contrast, Edelstein et al. [7] did not find a significant increase in the rate of discharge to a skilled nursing facility for patients who developed delirium after hip fracture repair.

There is general agreement, however, that postoperative delirium is associated with worse functional recovery, as demonstrated by decline in basic activities of daily living at 1 [10] and 12 months [7] after treatment of hip fracture, and with a higher risk of death in the 6–12 months following operation [6, 7].

Etiology, Risk Factors, and Precipitating Factors

The underlying mechanisms of delirium are uncertain. However, it appears to represent an imbalance between central nervous system cholinergic and dopaminergic activity. The predominant theory is that underactivity of cholinergic system coupled with excessive dopaminergic activity can lead to delirium. This is supported by precipitation of delirium through use of anticholinergic or dopaminergic medications [11].

Delirium is the end result of a complex interaction between risk factors and precipitating events. Furthermore, in similar situations, similar patients may not necessarily develop delirium. A key component in preventing postoperative delirium is recognition of at-risk patients. The preoperative evaluation should include a detailed cataloging of the common risk factors noted in Table 29.3. The risk factor with the strongest association with development of postoperative delirium is preoperative cognitive impairment [12].

Table 29.3 Risk factors for and precipitating factors of delirium

Risk factors	Precipitating factors
Advanced age	Infection
Underlying cognitive impairment	Medications
Functional impairment	Hypoxemia
Coexisting medical comorbidities	Dehydration
Psychotropic medications	Sensory deprivation
Alcohol abuse	Electrolyte abnormalities
Sensory impairment	Unfamiliar environment
Immobility	Surgery
	Neurologic events
	Sleep deprivation/disruption
	Use of physical restraints
	Malnutrition
	Use of a bladder catheter

Table 29.4 Etiology of acute confusion in surgical patients

I	Infection
M	Metabolic
C	Cognitive, sensory
O	Oxygenation
N	Nutrition, swallowing
F	Function, pharmacy, Foley catheter
U	Unfamiliar environment
S	Stress, pain
E	Electrolytes/fluids
D	Dysfunction lung, liver, kidney, brain

Unfortunately, this and many of the other risk factors cannot be modified in the preoperative setting prior to elective operation. However, reduction in the severity of individual risk factors, such as visual and hearing impairment and immobility, has been shown to reduce the incidence of delirium [13]. In addition to risk factors noted in the table, the presence of preoperative pain is a risk factor for postoperative delirium [14]. This is a factor that can be mitigated prior to operation using an appropriate clinical strategy. Specifically, use of oral instead of intravenous analgesia is associated with lower rates of postoperative delirium in elderly patients.

During the perioperative period, the most important strategy to prevent delirium is to actively monitor, treat, and avoid the precipitating factors. Each precipitating factor is a marker for a risk factor, has the potential to increase the severity of risk factors, or can lead to development of complications for which delirium may be a sign. Use of physical restraints and bladder catheters both lead to immobilization. In addition, indwelling bladder catheters predispose to urinary tract infection, which can precipitate delirium. Factors that alter sensorium, such as sleep deprivation or disruption, medications, or neurologic events, can also precipitate delirium. It should be noted that neurologic events are an unusual, but often sought, cause of postoperative delirium.

Diagnosis

Delirium is distinguished from dementia by its acute onset and fluctuating course. Other components include inattention with the inability to focus, disorganized thinking, and altered level of consciousness. Although most clinicians are familiar with the agitated or hyperactive state of delirium, the condition can also present as somnolence. This can lead to misdiagnosis and attribution to other causes. The Confusion Assessment Method as proposed by Inouye [15] is a validated method to diagnose delirium. It requires the presence of acute onset with a fluctuating course and inattention. Either disorganized thinking or altered level of consciousness must

also be present to confirm the diagnosis. The presence or absence of each component is obtained by history or testing. Acute onset and fluctuating course are confirmed by direct observation or in the case of patients presenting with delirium through history from family and/or care providers. Inattention can be tested using simple tests such as counting backward (by threes or sevens) or naming months in reverse order. Disorganized thinking is noted on interviewing the patient. The patient will have rambling speech and/or illogical flow of ideas. He or she may switch between subjects of conversation unpredictably. Altered level of consciousness is defined as reduced clarity of surroundings – either lethargy/somnolence or hyperactivity/mania.

Evaluation and Treatment

Initial evaluation of patients with postoperative delirium is focused on assessing etiology and stabilizing the patient. Review of the preoperative history, including functional assessment and medications, is critical. The presence of risk factors as outlined should be determined. Possible precipitating factors should also be sought. A mnemonic for etiologies of acute confusion in surgical patients is shown in Table 29.4.

In those instances when postoperative delirium occurs, treatment is directed at identifying the underlying cause, providing supportive care and controlling symptoms (Fig. 29.1). Delirium is often a manifestation of other postoperative complications such as occult infection, anastomotic leak, hypoxia, hypovolemia, or electrolyte imbalance. A thorough investigation is indicated to evaluate and treat these possible etiologies. Unfortunately, a single, specific etiology is not identified in a significant number of cases. Supportive care includes many of the strategies used to prevent delirium and also includes measures to ensure airway protection, maintain adequate oxygenation, maintain fluid and electrolyte balance, and provide nutritional support. If possible, physical restraints should be avoided. Control of the patient's symptoms includes the prevention strategies previously discussed. Pharmacologic intervention should be reserved

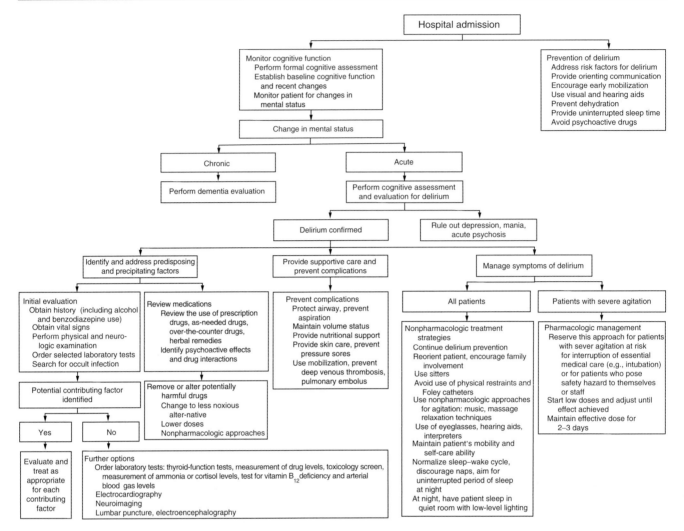

Figure 29.1 Prevention and management of delirium (reprinted from Inouye [11]. Copyright © Massachusetts Medical Society. All rights reserved).

for the most severe cases where patients are in danger of injuring themselves. Haloperidol (0.5–1 mg) is the preferred medication for pharmacologic intervention. Benzodiazepines – lorazepam is preferred – should only be used in cases of alcohol or benzodiazepine withdrawal.

Prevention

Strategies to prevent postoperative delirium are outlined in Table 29.5. Effective preventative measures involve multi-component interventions. An early trial demonstrated a reduction in the number and duration of episodes of delirium in medical patients [13]. The interventions to prevent cognitive impairment were orientation and therapeutic activities, prevention of sleep deprivation, early mobilization, communication methods and adaptive devices for hearing and visual impairment, and early intervention to treat dehydration. A subsequent randomized trial in patients with hip fracture found that geriatrics consultation with structured intervention

Table 29.5 Delirium prevention strategies

Orientation	Adequate oxygenation
Avoidance of restraints	Adequate pain management
Hearing aids	Medication review and avoidance
Eyeglasses	Adequate hydration
Family presence	
Bowel and bladder regimen	
Early mobilization	
Adaptive equipment	
Normal sleep/awake cycle	

reduced the rate of postoperative delirium when compared with standard care [16].

Studies on pharmacologic prevention of delirium have focused on several different medications. Randomized, placebo-controlled trials in surgical patients have evaluated the antipsychotic drug haloperidol [17], the cholinesterase inhibitor donepezil [18, 19], and the analgesic gabapentin [20]. Haloperidol prophylaxis was associated with reduced severity and duration of delirium in patients at intermediate or high risk for this complication following hip surgery. Hospital length of stay was also reduced; however, the incidence of delirium was unchanged [17]. The trials evaluating prophylactic treatment with donepezil also did not find a reduction in the incidence of delirium or a reduction in hospital length of stay [18, 19]. A single small study of gabapentin found reduced analgesic requirements and a reduced incidence of delirium in patients undergoing spine surgery when compared with placebo [20].

Falls

Greater than one third of persons 65 years of age and older fall each year [21]. Falls are common in the postoperative period although they are likely to be underreported as is the rate of functional disability. Various risk factors for falls have been identified including previous history of falls, dehydration, frequent toileting, cognitive dysfunction, gait disturbances, impaired balance and mobility, and conditions such as Alzheimer's disease. Sleep apnea is known to cause sleep fragmentation and daytime drowsiness, leading to a higher risk of falls [22, 23].

Behavioral disturbances occasionally require the use of restraints in older patients in the postoperative period. Restraints should be used only when clinically justified and with strict adherence to guidelines and required monitoring. Restraints do not reduce the incidence of falls. In a case control study, patients with restraints were more likely to fall than those without restraints [24].

Fall risk should be judged preoperatively by assessing the patient's ability to ambulate and by inquiring about any history of falls in the recent past, both from the patient and family. Those with a history of falls and difficulty ambulating can be referred for perioperative physical therapy. A history of problem alcohol drinking is also associated with increased fall risk [25].

The "Get Up and Go" test is an excellent method to evaluate mobility and balance. It requires a patient to get up from a chair, walk three meters, turn around, and sit down. The test is scored on a five-point scale with 1 = normal, 2 = very slightly abnormal, 3 = mildly abnormal, 4 = moderately abnormal, and 5 = severely abnormal. The patient is rated as a low fall risk (1) or a high fall risk (5) during the maneuver. If an elderly patient is able to accomplish the task in 20 s or less, they are likely to be independent in activities of daily living. Inability to complete the maneuver suggests a high risk of fall [26]. During a 6-month period following hip fracture surgery, 95% of subjects who fell had a test score of >24 s, while 93% of patients who did not fall had scores <24. The limitation of this study is that a moderate functional capacity is needed at the time of discharge to be able to perform in the test [27].

Another useful test for assessment of balance and mobility in frail older adults is the Hierarchical Assessment of Balance and Mobility [28]. The Hierarchical Assessment of Balance and Mobility is designed to be sensitive to changes in mobility of a patient in the postoperative period. A patient's mobility varies from being unable to move off pressure points to being able to grab the bed rail and roll and eventually being able to sit and ambulate. The assessment, therefore, measures mobility (unlimited, limited, limited with aid, one person hands on, one person stand-by, lying or sitting independently, positioning self in bed, in need of positioning), transfers (independent, one person standing by, one person minimal assist, one person assist, two person assist, or total lift), and ambulation (stable ambulation, stable dynamic standing, stable static standing, stable dynamic sitting, stable static sitting, impaired static sitting). Interventions that can prevent falls in the older hospitalized patient include medication review with removal of the offending medication, adequate hydration and monitoring of orthostatic blood pressure, management of postoperative delirium by identifying and treating the cause of delirium, balance and gait training, and adherence to a regular voiding schedule [29]. Problems with vision can lead to a higher incidence of falls in the postoperative period. Vision aids may have been taken away preoperatively, and it is critical that these are returned and made available to the patient in the postoperative period [13].

Functional Decline

Deconditioning is a complex process of physiological change following a period of inactivity, bed rest, or sedentary lifestyle. It results in functional losses in such areas as mental status, degree of continence, and ability to accomplish activities of daily living (Table 29.6). It is frequently associated with hospitalization and the postoperative period in the elderly. The most predictable effects of deconditioning are seen in the musculoskeletal system and include diminished muscle mass and decrease of muscle strength that can seriously limit mobility [30]. Deconditioning following surgery can be debilitating and impede functional recovery. Incontinence and constipation are consequences of deconditioning and can have a significant impact on functional recovery and restoration of Activities of Daily Living (ADL).

Prolonged bed rest following surgery is a risk factor for functional decline [31]. In a study of 223 patients older than 75 years of age who underwent elective surgery for gastric and colorectal cancers, 24% of patients showed a decrease in activities of daily living (ADL) at 1 month following surgery. However, only 3% of patients showed a decline at 6 months. This suggests that older patients are able to attain functional independence and also report better quality of life

TABLE 29.6 Immobility, deconditioning, and functional decline

Musculoskeletal	*Metabolic*
Atrophy	Negative nitrogen balance
Contractures	Impaired glucose tolerance
Bone loss (osteoporosis)	Altered drug pharmacokinetics
Cardiovascular	*Genitourinary*
Deconditioning	Infection
Decreased plasma volume	Retention
Orthostatic hypotension	Bladder stones
DVT and PE	Incontinence
Pulmonary	*Psychological*
Atrophy	Sensory deprivation
Contracture	Delirium/dementia
Bone loss	Depression
Gastrointestinal	*Skin*
Anorexia	Pressure ulcers
Constipation	
Impaction/incontinence	

after surgery [32]. Patients who show signs of functional decline in the early postoperative period benefit from early physical therapy consultation and discharge to a skilled nursing facility or to a nursing home until satisfactory recovery. A study conducted in patients in intensive care units and ranging from 40 to 70 years have shown that initiation of early physical therapy was safe in older adults, did not increase cost, and decreased length of stay in the intensive care unit as well as hospital length of stay [33]. Another study in patients between 36 and 69 years of age also showed that whole-body rehabilitation – consisting of interruption of sedation – and physical and occupational therapy in the earliest days following a critical illness resulted in better functional outcomes at hospital discharge [34].

Cognitive impairment has been shown to be associated with poor rehabilitation outcomes and increased surgical mortality [35], and dementia is also a predictor of functional disability [36]. Older patients with preexisting chronic renal disease are more likely to be frail and also have a higher risk of developing functional limitation and disability [37, 38]. This may be secondary to a heightened inflammatory state in chronic renal disease [39].

Other General Complications

Infection

Postoperative infections are an important cause of morbidity and mortality in elderly patients. Although little is known about specific decreases in immunologic competence, elderly patients may have diminished immune function, predisposing them to infection [40]. The most common sites of postoperative infection are the urinary tract, lungs, and surgical site [40].

Urinary tract infection (UTI) is typically due to prolonged bladder catheterization. Up to 25% of hospitalized patients have urinary catheters inserted; of these, 10–27% develop UTIs [41]. Eighty percent of nosocomial UTIs are associated with the use of urethral catheters [41] The need for catheterization is increased in elderly patients for several reasons including medication side effects, preexisting incontinence, prostatism, and decreased mobility, all of which hinder urination [40]. Symptoms of UTI in the elderly may be subtle. Postoperative confusion may be the first and only sign of a UTI [40].

As UTIs are associated with significant morbidity and excess hospital cost [42], methods to decrease this complication are warranted. Silver impregnated catheters have been shown to reduce the risk of asymptomatic bacteriuria in short-term catheterization and to provide a cost savings when compared to standard catheters [43]. Urethral catheters impregnated with antibiotics (minocycline, rifampicin, nitrofurazone) have also shown a reduction in asymptomatic bacteriuria for urethral catheterization of less than 1-week duration [43]. However, as the inappropriate use of urinary catheters in the elderly has been documented [44] and the risk of UTI increases with increasing duration of catheterization [45], avoidance of catheterization if possible and early removal of the catheter are important steps in preventing urinary tract infections postoperatively [40].

Nosocomial pneumonia (NP) is the second most frequent hospital-acquired infection and is common in patients undergoing general, noncardiac surgery [46, 47]. Ventilator-associated pneumonia (VAP) is an important subset of NP defined as pneumonia occurring 48–72 h after endotracheal intubation. NP is a leading cause of postoperative mortality in elderly patients [46]. Although NP in older patients does not have distinctive features or a different management approach when this illness arises in younger patients [48], certain risk factors including age and functional status render the elderly vulnerable for developing NP. Underlying comorbid conditions, malnutrition, and impaired immune function may increase the mortality associated with postoperative pneumonia in the elderly [40]. Nasogastric tubes, tracheal intubation, dementia, aspiration (see section "Pulmonary Complications"), recent chest or abdominal surgery, and immobility are additional risk factors [40, 46].

NP is diagnosed using clinical criteria such as fever, purulent sputum, leukocytosis, and the presence of new infiltrates on chest radiography combined with a quantitative lower respiratory tract specimen positive for organisms. The early and appropriate initiation of antibiotic therapy for the treatment of NP has been shown to decrease mortality [47].

Because inappropriate initial antibiotic therapy leads to worsened outcomes, broad-spectrum empiric antibiotics are used at first, and therapy is then tailored based upon final culture results and sensitivities. Strategies to reduce the risk of NP include standard precautions like hand washing and the use of personal protective equipment among health care providers; aspiration prevention methods (see section "Pulmonary Complications") including the use of endotracheal tubes with a dorsal lumen for drainage of tracheal secretions in the subglottic area; and early ambulation, deep breathing, and the use of incentive spirometry [49].

Surgical site infection (SSI) is a significant postoperative complication. SSI is the most common nosocomial infection in surgical patients, accounting for 38% of nosocomial infections in this patient population [50]. Not only is there substantial morbidity and mortality associated with SSI but the economic costs to the patient and health care delivery system are also high [51]. SSI is an infection that occurs somewhere in the operative field after a surgical intervention. Risks of developing SSI include those related to the operative procedure as well as patient-specific risks. Advanced age is considered a host-derived risk factor for surgical site infection [52]. In an analysis of deep incisional and organ/space surgical infections, elderly patients with these infections had longer hospitalizations, more frequent readmissions, and almost double the hospital charges as compared to elderly patients without postoperative infections. Most significantly, the elderly patients with these postoperative infections had a death rate that was more than three times that of the elderly patients without postoperative infections [53].

SSI is caused by organisms introduced into the surgical wound at the time of the operative procedure [51]. Most of these organisms originate from the patient's own flora, but exogenous sources of bacteria may also lead to infection. The implementation of proven surgical infection preventive practices such as appropriate antibiotic selection and administration, intraoperative maintenance of normothermia, the avoidance of shaving the surgical site until just prior to incising the skin, and ensuring perioperative euglycemia has been demonstrated to reduce the incidence of surgical site infection by 27% [52, 54]. Vigilant surveillance of surgical wounds postoperatively is necessary to ensure the early diagnosis and treatment of a wound infection, characterized by erythema at the wound edges and the presence of purulent drainage involving the wound or organ space. Treatment of SSI involves opening the incision and allowing adequate drainage. The use of antibiotics is discouraged unless there are systemic signs of infection. If antibiotics are to be used, the choice should be determined by the most likely pathogens for the operative procedure performed [51].

Complications of Specific Organ Systems

Cardiac Complications

Myocardial Ischemia and Infarction

Major cardiovascular complications following noncardiac surgery occur in over one million patients per year; many of these occur in elderly patients [55]. Cardiac events such as myocardial infarction or cardiac death occur in 1–5% of patients undergoing noncardiac surgery [56, 57]. Postoperative cardiovascular complications substantially increase the risk of other complications and death [58]. In one study, patients with cardiac complications were six times more likely to suffer a noncardiac complication than were those without cardiac complications [59]. At least 10% of all perioperative deaths result from myocardial complications [60].

The most common cardiac complications associated with surgery in elderly patients are myocardial ischemia and myocardial infarction [61]. In a study of 4,315 patients of 50 years of age and older who underwent nonemergent major noncardiac procedures, patients aged 70 years and older had a higher risk for cardiac complications including unstable angina and myocardial infarction, compared to patients younger than 60 years [62]. The elderly are also more likely to have heart failure associated with the myocardial infarction [63]. The mortality associated with perioperative myocardial infarction is approximately 30% [60].

Preexisting hypertension, diabetes mellitus, and history of cardiac or renal failure contribute to a higher incidence of perioperative myocardial infarction (5.1%), cardiac death (5.7%), or ischemia (12–17.7%) in elderly patients [61, 64]. Patients with coronary artery disease have a 4.1% incidence of perioperative myocardial infarction. The perioperative reinfarction rate in patients older than 65 years is 5.5% [61], compared to a 3.5–4.2% perioperative reinfarction rate in the general population. Additional risk factors in the elderly include the need for emergency surgery, major surgical procedures, American Society of Anesthesiologists (ASA) physical status III or IV, and poor nutritional status [61].

A large number of perioperative myocardial infarctions occur during the first 3 days after surgery, particularly on the 1st postoperative day [65, 66]. Although chest pain is the most common presenting symptom of myocardial ischemia in young patients, elderly patients may not experience chest pain. Myocardial ischemic events are silent in over 80% of elderly patients [66, 67]. Detecting episodes of ischemia during the postoperative period is often missed because of incisional pain, residual anesthetic effects, postoperative analgesia, and the lack of typical angina pain by elderly patients [66]. Atypical symptoms such as tachycardia, hypotension, dyspnea, respiratory failure, syncope, confusion, nausea, and excessive hyperglycemia in diabetics are more common presentations of myocardial ischemia in the elderly [60, 64, 66].

Monitoring for specific electrocardiographic changes, such as ST segment elevation and Q waves, accompanied by elevated CK, CK-MB isoenzyme, and troponin T and I levels enables the diagnosis of myocardial infarction [61]. Postoperative ST-segment changes more commonly demonstrate depression than elevation, and most myocardial infarctions are non-Q wave. This differs from what is seen in the nonsurgical setting, suggesting that perioperative myocardial infarctions are more often related to prolonged ischemia rather than acute thrombotic occlusion [66]. As such, EKGs should be obtained in the early postoperative period and between the 3rd and 5th postoperative days in high-risk patients [48].

Noncardiac surgery intensifies myocardial oxygen demand by raising catecholamine concentrations, resulting in an increased heart rate, blood pressure, and free fatty-acid concentrations. β-adrenergic blockers attenuate the effects of increased catecholamine levels and prevent perioperative cardiovascular complications [55]. In a large observational study, the perioperative administration of β-blockers was associated with clinically significant reductions in mortality among surgical patients considered at moderate or high risk for major cardiovascular complications based upon their Revised Cardiac Risk Index score. However, β-blockers were of no significant benefit – and were possibly harmful – in patients at low risk, suggesting that careful patient selection remains necessary [58].

β-blockade may have additional benefits in elderly patients. In one study, patients who received β-blockers were extubated sooner, had lower analgesic requirements, and were more alert sooner after surgery [57]. Prophylactic β-blocker therapy may attenuate the impact of myocardial infarction, resulting in lower in-hospital mortality rates [65].

Potential harmful effects from β-blockers include bradycardia, hypotension, bronchospasm, and congestive heart failure [38, 55, 57]. The use of perioperative β-blockade in patients who had not been receiving β-blockers long-term may also pose an additional risk in that withdrawal of β-blockers may lead to adrenergic hypersensitivity and possibly worsen outcomes [68].

Dysrhythmias

Dysrhythmias have been shown to increase postoperative cardiac morbidity in elderly patients [69]. Postoperative atrial arrhythmias are seen in 6.1% of elderly patients undergoing noncardiac surgery [70]. Electrolyte disturbances and/or increased sympathetic nervous system activity in the perioperative period may lead to cardiac dysrhythmias, although

myocardial ischemia or congestive heart failure must be considered [71].

To date, the only consistent preoperative risk factor for an increased incidence of atrial arrhythmias following surgery has been an age of 60 years or older [72]. In patients undergoing elective thoracic surgery, those aged 60 years or older were independently associated with development of atrial fibrillation [70]. Patients who developed postoperative pneumonia or acute respiratory failure were also at risk [70].

The timing of the onset of atrial arrhythmias is similar to that of postoperative myocardial ischemia and likely is related to autonomic nervous system imbalance [72]. These arrhythmias may also be precipitated by pulmonary disease such as pneumonia or pulmonary embolism, volume overload, hyperthyroidism, or sympathomimetic drugs. Atrial arrhythmia-onset peaks 2–3 days following surgery. Although usually well tolerated in younger patients, perioperative atrial arrhythmias can be associated with hemodynamic instability in elderly patients [72]. The complications of atrial fibrillation include stroke and congestive heart failure [73]. Atrial fibrillation is also associated with higher inpatient mortality when accompanied by myocardial infarction (25% vs. 16%) [73].

Management of atrial fibrillation consists of heart rhythm and rate control and prevention of thromboembolism. Although approximately 85% of atrial arrhythmias revert to sinus rhythm with rate-or rhythm-control strategies during hospitalization, recent data suggest that rhythm control by pharmacologic means or direct current electrical cardioversion offers little advantage to a rate-control strategy [72]. Atrial fibrillation responds well to intravenous rate control drugs such as β – and calcium-channel blockers [72]. β-blockers are preferred in patients who have ischemic heart disease but may be relatively contraindicated in patients with severe bronchospastic disease, congestive heart failure, severe sinus bradycardia, or high-degree atrioventricular block [72]. In patients who have Wolff–Parkinson–White syndrome with atrial fibrillation, amiodarone is recommended as first-line therapy [72]. Digoxin should be used as a first-line drug only in patients who have congestive heart failure because of its ineffectiveness in high-adrenergic states such as the perioperative period [72]. As it relates to thromboembolism, oral vitamin K antagonists and aspirin reduce the stroke risk by 68 and 21%, respectively [74]. In the perioperative period, the decision to use bridging anticoagulation with heparin and the timing of resuming anticoagulation postoperatively are dependent on risk of thromboembolism. Clinical prediction rules such as the Congestive Heart Failure-Hypertension-Age > 75-Diabetes-Stroke (CHADS$_2$) assist in risk stratification [75]. CHADS$_2$ estimates the risk of stroke by assigning one point for each of the five included conditions except stroke, which is assigned two points. The total score ranges from zero to six points; aspirin therapy is recommended for thromboembolism prevention for low-risk patients (<5% risk per year; CHADS$_2$ 0–2), whereas oral vitamin K antagonists are prescribed with higher risk patients (>5% risk per year; CHADS$_2$ 3–6) [76, 77].

Significant, sustained ventricular arrhythmias (ventricular tachycardia, ventricular fibrillation, torsade de point) occur less frequently than atrial arrhythmias perioperatively [70, 73]. In a study of patients undergoing major thoracic surgery with continuous postoperative electrocardiographic monitoring for 72 h, nonsustained ventricular tachycardia occurred in 15% of patients [76]. None of the patients required treatment for hemodynamic compromise. Postoperative atrial fibrillation was independently associated with ventricular tachycardia. This association between atrial and ventricular arrhythmias suggests that similar mechanisms may have a role in precipitating postoperative ventricular tachycardia [76].

Congestive Heart Failure

Congestive heart failure is present in 10% of individuals over 65 years of age and is a leading cause of postoperative morbidity and mortality following surgical procedures [69]. Preexisting congestive heart failure is associated with a two- to fourfold increase in postoperative cardiovascular complications, including myocardial infarction, supraventricular and ventricular dysrhythmias, hypotension or hypertension, and cardiac arrest [69, 78]. Heart failure can arise from any condition that compromises the contractility of the heart (systolic heart failure) or that interferes with the heart's ability to relax (diastolic heart failure) [79].

Risk factors for postoperative heart failure included preoperative symptomatic cardiac disease, male sex, and age ≥ 90 in one study of elderly patients with hip fracture undergoing operative repair [80]. Manifestations of postoperative heart failure usually occur within the initial 3 postoperative days [81]. Patients found to be in pulmonary edema postoperatively should be assessed for myocardial ischemia. This includes cardiac monitoring, electrocardiography, and serial cardiac enzyme measurements.

The treatment of postoperative heart failure with pulmonary edema, whether from systolic or diastolic dysfunction, differs little from the general management of heart failure. Angiotensin-converting enzyme inhibitors and diuretics are first-line therapy. In patients with acute decompensated heart failure, angiotensin-converting enzyme inhibitor therapy may need to be held, reduced, or discontinued if hypotension is a concern. In the presence of diuretic usage, electrolyte abnormalities (e.g., potassium, magnesium) should be diagnosed and corrected. β-blocker therapy can be used in heart failure secondary to myocardial ischemia unless hypotension precludes its usage. Digoxin is first-line therapy in heart failure associated with atrial fibrillation [78].

Pulmonary Complications

Pulmonary complications account for up to 40% of postoperative complications and 20% of potentially preventable deaths [82]. Postoperatively, pulmonary complications occur in 2.1–10.2% of elderly patients and include atelectasis, hypoxemia, hypoventilation, acute respiratory distress syndrome, and pneumonia. Development of these complications is associated with prolonged intensive care unit stay and increased mortality [61]. Increased age elevates the odds of developing a postoperative pulmonary complication nearly twofold [83]. Compared with patients younger than 60 years of age, patients of 70 years of age and above had a higher risk of respiratory complications including bacterial pneumonia, noncardiogenic pulmonary edema, and respiratory failure requiring intubation in one study [62].

Age-related alterations in pulmonary function combined with postoperative pulmonary pathophysiologic changes place the elderly patient at greater risk for complications [82]. The physiologic changes of aging lead to decreased lung volumes, expiratory flow rates, and oxygenation. Upper airway reflexes are also reduced, leading to loss of ability to clear secretions [82].

Clinical predictors of adverse pulmonary outcome include the site of surgery (chest, abdomen), duration and type of anesthesia, chronic obstructive pulmonary disease (COPD), asthma, preoperative hypersecretion of mucus, chest deformation, and perioperative nasogastric tube placement [61, 84]. In one multivariate analysis, postoperative nasogastric intubation was the single most important variable associated with postoperative pulmonary complications [85].

Aspiration

The process of deglutition involves a complex coordination of neuromuscular structures during its oral, pharyngeal, and esophageal phases [86]. Age-related changes affect each phase of the swallowing process, increasing the risk of aspiration in the elderly [86]. Aspiration, defined as the inhalation of oropharyngeal or gastric contents into the larynx and lower respiratory tract, is a prerequisite for aspiration pneumonia [86]. Other alterations with aging that contribute to aspiration pneumonia include a change of oropharyngeal colonization to pathogenic organisms, decreased immunity, and impaired pulmonary clearance [86].

The presence of other risk factors in the elderly make them particularly susceptible to oropharyngeal aspiration including dysphagia, poor oral hygiene, altered level of consciousness, and gastroesophageal reflux disease [60, 86] (see Table 29.7). As such, efforts to reduce postoperative aspiration in the elderly are indicated [87]. Elderly patients with signs and symptoms of dysphagia and recurrent pneumonia

TABLE 29.7 Risk factors for aspiration

Altered consciousness	Advanced age
Alcohol	Dysphagia
Substance abuse	Gastrointestinal motility disorders
Sedatives	Gastroesophageal reflux disease
Anesthesia	Recurrent emesis
Head trauma	Supine position
Seizures	Nasogastric tube
Other neurological disorders	Endotracheal intubation

require an assessment of swallowing function. Patients found on evaluation to be aspirating may require swallow therapy, modification of dietary consistency, upright positioning while feeding, and medications shown to improve dysphagia such as angiotensin-converting enzyme inhibitors, which prevent the breakdown of substance P, a neurotransmitter believed to play a role in the swallowing pathway [86, 88].

Respiratory Failure

Postoperative respiratory failure (PRF), the inability of the patient to be extubated within 48 h after surgery or the need for reintubation after postoperative extubation [89, 90], ranks first among the most serious postoperative pulmonary complications. The incidence of PRF in patients older than 65 years is estimated to be 3.85 per 1,000 elective surgery discharges compared to 1.41 per 1,000 elective surgery discharges in people aged 18–44 [91]. Risk factors for PRF include those that are patient-specific and operation-specific [89]. Age greater than 60 years, functional status, comorbidities, and severity of illness make up patient-specific risk factors. Operation-specific risk factors consist of the location of the incision in relation to the diaphragm, type of anesthesia administered, and the need for an emergent procedure [89]. Pneumonia, pulmonary edema, systemic sepsis, and cardiac arrest are postoperative pulmonary complications associated with PRF [89].

In patients with PRF, mechanical ventilation is used to improve gas exchange, to decrease work of breathing which can utilize as much as 50% of oxygen consumption, and to support fatigued respiratory muscles [91]. Different methods of ventilatory support are available to accomplish these goals. Positive end-expiratory pressure (PEEP) improves oxygenation by recruiting atelectatic areas of the lung. The use of PEEP leads to an increase in oxygenation by reducing intrapulmonary shunting [91].

Ultimately, an assessment has to be made to determine the timing of discontinuing ventilator support. This weaning process may be difficult in patients recovering from severe respiratory failure and prolonged mechanical ventilation. In a study to determine the major cause of planned extubation failure in critically ill elderly patients, inability to handle secretions was the most common airway cause of failure compared to upper airway obstruction in a younger group matched for severity of illness [92]. Traditional weaning parameters such as rapid shallow breathing index, negative inspiratory force, and minute ventilation were not predictive of elderly patients who ultimately failed extubation [92]. The in-hospital mortality for the elderly patients that failed extubation was 47% compared to 20% for the patients successfully extubated [92].

The need for early tracheostomy in elderly patients predicted to require prolonged intubation is controversial. Potential benefits of early (after 3–7 days of continuous ventilatory support) tracheostomy include improved patient comfort, decreased incidence of ventilator associated pneumonia (VAP), and decreased ICU and hospital lengths of stay. A recent retrospective cohort study of ventilated patients of 65 years or older was undertaken to compare outcomes in patients with more (late group) or less (early group) than 7 days of continuous ventilation who underwent tracheostomy [93]. The early tracheostomy group had shorter ICU and hospital admission time, decreased incidence of VAP, and a trend toward decreased mortality [93]. This study also demonstrated the ability to transfer elderly patients with tracheostomy to ventilator step-down units. Given the growing elderly population and need for ICU beds, early tracheostomy may permit more efficient usage of a valuable resource [93].

Prevention of Pulmonary Complications

Prevention of postoperative pulmonary complications in the elderly begins during the preoperative period. Assessing patients for sputum production is important as a productive cough correlates with respiratory failure [90]. Smoking cessation 8 weeks prior to the operation has been shown to improve mucociliary function and promote sputum clearance. The use of bronchodilators can aid expectoration. Providing instruction preoperatively on deep breathing exercises and the use of incentive spirometry facilitate the utilization of these maneuvers postoperatively when anesthesia and sedatives may decrease awareness and hinder education [90].

Postoperatively, an aggressive pulmonary toilet regimen is necessary to reduce pulmonary complications. Of utmost importance is adequate pain control. Splinting from inadequate pain control restricts lung expansion, limits cough to clear secretions, and leads to an increased risk for atelectasis, pneumonia, and hypoxia [69]. However, avoidance of excessive sedatives and narcotics is equally important. Appropriate analgesia will facilitate deep breathing and coughing, incentive spirometry, chest physiotherapy, and early ambulation [69, 82, 85].

Venous Thromboembolism

Venous thromboembolism (VTE) disproportionately affects the elderly [94]. Age is a well-accepted risk factor for VTE, with a mean age of approximately 60 years based on several studies. There is a linear increase in the prevalence of deep venous thrombosis and pulmonary embolism with age [95]. Ninety percent of all pulmonary emboli are estimated to occur in patients over age 50 [82]. The elderly are more likely to have prior recent hospitalization, atherosclerosis, heart failure, frailty, and immobility as factors responsible for their increased prevalence of VTE [94, 96].

For surgical patients, age over 60 years is associated with a high risk for postoperative VTE [94]. In these older patients not receiving prophylaxis, the incidence of proximal deep venous thrombosis is 4–8% and of PE is 2–4% [95]. These numbers are twice as high in high-risk categories that include cancer surgery, joint replacement, previous VTE, and trauma [94]. Because the elderly have a higher bleeding risk when treated with anticoagulants, a balance has to be achieved between optimal VTE prevention and the risk of bleeding complications [94, 97]. Care should be exercised with the use of anticoagulants in patients with creatinine clearance < 30 ml/min and serum creatinine > 2 mg/dl in that the pharmacokinetics of these medications may be affected, thereby increasing the bleeding risk [94].

Early ambulation can decrease the incidence of venous thrombosis with pulmonary embolus. Unfortunately, owing to comorbidity or deconditioning, elderly patients are frequently unable to accomplish this simple exercise [85]. Mechanical prophylactic measures to prevent VTE include graded compression stockings, intermittent pneumatic compression, and venous foot pumps. These devices are attractive in that they are efficacious and are void of bleeding risk. Compliance with these devices may not be optimal, however, because of patient discomfort [94]. Alternatively, the administration of pharmacologic prophylaxis can be verified in the medical record, and its use does not discourage ambulation [94]. Perioperative prophylaxis with unfractionated or low-molecular-weight heparin offers a cost-effective means of reducing the risk of VTE, thereby avoiding a number of postoperative deaths [82]. In high-risk bleeding patients, mechanical prophylactic measures may be all that is available.

Anemia

Preoperative anemia, characterized by less than the normal number of red blood cells (RBC), may be secondary to decreased production, increased destruction, or increased loss [98]. The World Health Organization has defined anemia as a hemoglobin count of less than 13 g/dl in adult men and less than 12 g/dl in nonpregnant women [98]. In elderly patients undergoing surgery, perioperative blood loss leading to or exacerbating anemia leads to increased morbidity and mortality, but the correction of anemia with RBC transfusions is fraught with debate [98–102].

RBC transfusions can be associated with transfusion complications, immunosuppression, and increased bacterial infections in hip fracture patients [98–101]. Conversely, perioperative anemia in the elderly may represent a further physiological insult due to increased cardiac demand and potential tissue hypoxia [100]. As such, the appropriate transfusion threshold in the elderly that would limit risk and optimize benefit would be advantageous.

Restrictive (transfusion for hemoglobin less than 7 g/dl) and liberal (transfusion for hemoglobin less than 10 g/dl) transfusion thresholds have been advocated in an attempt to balance the risks and potential benefits of RBC transfusion. In a randomized clinical trial comparing restrictive and liberal transfusion thresholds, critically ill patients in the restrictive group had similar mortality, and fewer patients developed myocardial infarction and congestive heart failure [98]. Caution should be exercised in extrapolating these results to an elderly population. In the elderly, anemia may impede functional mobility after hip surgery [100]; it may be associated with increased cardiovascular complications [101], mortality [101], and postoperative delirium [100] and may negatively impact quality of life [99]. Additional, well-designed randomized studies are needed to determine the optimal transfusion trigger in the elderly.

Urinary and Renal Dysfunction

Postoperative urinary retention is a frequent complication after surgery especially in elderly males. Although it is not a life-threatening complication, treatment with bladder catheterization puts patients at risk for urinary tract infection and its attendant complications. In one report, 69% of males undergoing hip arthroplasty required postoperative bladder catheterization [103]. Using logistic regression, the predicted probability of catheterization was 85% in males aged 70 years and older. In addition to age and male gender, intraoperative fluid requirement [104], operative duration, operation for rectal tumor, and postoperative pelvic infection [105] are associated with postoperative urinary retention. On the basis of the above noted studies, it would seem reasonable to recognize the risk factors for postoperative urinary retention and working to militate against those factors. Factors associated with postoperative urinary retention in elderly patients are outlined in Table 29.8.

Table 29.8 Factors associated with urinary retention in elderly patients

Age > 55 years
Intraoperative fluids > 750 cc
Operation duration > 4 h
Procedure for middle or lower rectal tumor
Presence of pelvic drain
Postoperative pelvic infection

Aging is associated with decreased renal cortical mass and a 30–50% decrease in the number of functioning glomeruli by the seventh decade [106]. This results in decreased creatinine clearance and decreased maximal urine concentrating capacity. Loss of muscle mass in the elderly patient can result in normal serum creatinine even in patients with decreased renal function. Creatinine clearance is a more accurate measure of renal function and estimated glomerular filtration rate based on the Cockcroft/Gault equation correlates well with creatinine clearance.

Chronic renal disease is prevalent in 11–25% of the elderly population and is an important comorbid condition in the perioperative period. In the general population, patients with chronic kidney disease are at higher risk for adverse outcomes such as death, cardiovascular disease, and hospitalizations [107]. Chronic renal disease is also associated with development of functional impairment [39]. Patients with chronic kidney disease have a higher incidence of hyperkalemia, infections, cardiac arrhythmia, and bleeding in the perioperative period [108].

Postoperative acute renal failure (ARF) is a significant etiology of renal failure, accounting for 25–50% of all cases [109–111]. However, ARF occurs infrequently after operation in elderly patients. In one study of cardiac surgery patients, 2.7% patients aged 70 years and older developed postoperative ARF [112]. In comparison, 1.9% patients younger than 70 years of age developed postoperative ARF. In contrast, another study of patients undergoing coronary artery bypass demonstrated a 3.2% rate of ARF in patients aged 80 and older; only 0.4% of patients younger than 80 years developed ARF. A study of elderly patients undergoing repair of femur fracture found that 24% developed postoperative kidney dysfunction, but none required renal replacement therapy [113].

Recovery of renal function is possible after developing ARF. Data on postoperative ARF are limited. A systematic review and meta-analysis found that approximately 30% of elderly patients do not recover renal function after ARF [114] as compared with 26% of younger patients. Despite failure to recover normal renal function, only 3–6% of elderly patients require long-term dialysis after ARF [115].

Acute renal failure in elderly patients in general and postoperative ARF specifically is associated with a high mortality rate. The mortality rate for patients with ARF (all causes) is 45–75% [115]. The mortality rate for postoperative ARF

in elderly patients in one study was 39%. In elderly patients undergoing cardiac surgery, postoperative renal failure was the most significant factor associated with postoperative death with an odds ratio of 4.4 [116]. In one study of patients undergoing cardiac surgery, the death rate in patients developing postoperative ARF was 56.1; however, there was no significant difference in mortality rates in the younger (61.9%) and older (50%) patient groups [112].

Gastrointestinal Complications

Postoperative Nausea and Vomiting

Postoperative nausea and vomiting (PONV) is a major concern in surgical patients, but less so in the elderly. Important risk factors for PONV include female gender, nonsmokers, history of PONV, and the use of postoperative opioids. Each risk factor can be accorded a point of 1. Total scores of 0, 1, 2, 3, or 4 are associated with a risk of PONV of 10, 20, 40, 60, and 80%, respectively [117]. Age is not an independent risk factor for PONV. There is >10% decreased risk of PONV for every decade of age in adults, starting at age 30 [118]. One of the factors that could be responsible for decreased PONV in older adults is the decrease in the doses of anesthetic agents administered. In a study involving 30,842 patients, fentanyl, propofol, midazolam, and isoflurane showed a 10, 8, 6, and 4% reduction in dose per decade of age, respectively [119]. Current consensus guidelines recommend use of regional anesthesia whenever possible as it is associated with a lower incidence of PONV in adults [120]. When general anesthesia is administered, use of propofol for induction and maintenance and avoidance of nitrous oxide can decrease the risk of PONV. Proper preoperative and intraoperative hydration are important in prevention of postoperative nausea and vomiting [121]. Metoclopramide should not be used in the elderly due to significant CNS side effects such as dyskinesia, drowsiness, and agitation. Prophylactic antiemetics should be used based on a risk score and are therefore not recommended in the elderly.

Dysphagia

There is an increased incidence of dysphagia in the elderly. ADL score has been shown to correlate with increased swallowing dysfunction [122]. Knowledge of preoperative nutritional habits is important so that appropriate foods can be offered in the postoperative period. Lack of dentures or offering solid foods in patients who are used to pureed/soft foods can result in inadequate intake and compromise postoperative recovery.

Impairment of swallowing is slow to resolve following extubation [122], especially after prolonged ventilation. This increases the risk of aspiration and subsequent aspiration pneumonia [123]. Aspiration precautions should be rigorously implemented in the postoperative period. These include elevation of the head end of the bed, seated position during meal intake, and specific food consistency.

Although it is not necessary to do a fiberoptic endoscopic evaluation of swallowing in all elderly patients, those with impaired preadmission functional status should be considered at high risk for aspiration and evaluated appropriately [124].

Gastroesophageal reflux disease (GERD) is common in elderly patients and prevalent in greater than 30% of the elderly population [125]. Unlike their younger counterparts, older patients with GERD may not complain of worsening symptoms. It is important to continue antireflux medications in the postoperative period. Proton pump inhibitors are more effective in elderly patients than H_2 blockers. Administration of proton pump inhibitors in the immediate postoperative period helps not only to control GERD but also serves as prophylaxis for bleeding from gastritis or peptic ulcer disease.

Postoperative Ileus

Surgical manipulation of the bowel can cause a prolonged postoperative ileus. Another factor in the development of ileus is the stimulation of opioid receptors. In a prospective study designed to compare surgical outcomes in patients greater or less than 80 years of age, the incidence of postoperative ileus was increased in the older patients [2]. Routine measures such as bowel rest, bowel decompression, and attention to nutrition (TPN) should be addressed.

Enhanced recovery after surgery (ERAS) is used in fast track surgery to reduce surgical stress response and support basic body functions by use of optimized analgesia, early mobilization, and early return to normal diet [126, 127]. This type of multidisciplinary intervention has been used effectively following colon surgery with significant success. It has led to a significant decrease in postoperative ileus and a decrease in hospital stay [128]. Prospective randomized trials are still needed to evaluate the effects of fast track surgery on older patients. While age should not be a contraindication to enroll patients in such a study, it will be critical to determine comorbidities in this group that would limit the benefits of such an intervention [129]. It is possible that while ERAS programs benefit those with significant comorbidities, the benefit may be most evident in vulnerable subgroups such as the elderly [130]. An upload antagonist such as ADL 8-2698 differs from other opioid-receptor antagonists in that it is potent, orally active, and poorly absorbed after oral administration. Once absorbed, the drug has a limited ability to cross the blood–brain barrier. Large doses of ADL 8-2698, thus, have the potential to antagonize gastrointestinal opioid receptors nearly completely without inhibiting the beneficial analgesic action of systemic opioids. These antagonists are able to counteract the effect of morphine on the GI tract [131]. Selective inhibition of GI opioid receptors by a peripherally restricted opioid antagonist can facilitate early recovery of bowel function, decreased hospital stay and still provide adequate pain relief [132].

Summary

As the number of elderly patients increase, they are accounting for a greater proportion of patients in most surgical practices. Therefore, surgeons, and all adult medical practitioners, must be aware of the unique complications associated with the surgical care of elderly patients. Because of their reduced physiologic reserve, elderly patients are less able to respond to and recover from postoperative complications. However, attempts to recognize, treat, and prevent these complications are complicated by atypical presentations.

Optimal care of elderly patients requires significant diligence. The presence of comorbidities and physiology of aging put this population at risk for "typical" complications such as cardiac dysrhythmias, myocardial infarction, pneumonia, and surgical site infection. Equally important, but often less appreciated, are the "atypical" complications that are more prevalent in elderly patients. Delirium is such a complication. It is much less common in younger patients. It is often misdiagnosed in elderly patients. The importance of this lies in the fact that postoperative delirium is often the initial sign of another postoperative complication.

The surgical care of elderly patients can be a gratifying part of surgical practice. By taking appropriate measures to prevent complications and by remaining vigilant, the perioperative experience for patient, surgeon, and the health care team has the opportunity to be rewarding.

References

1. DeFrances CJ, Lucas CA, Buie VC, Golosinskiy A (2006) National Hospital Discharge Survey. National Health Statistics Reports; no 5, National Center for Health Statistics 2008, Hyattsville, MD
2. Hamel MB, Henderson WG, Khuri SF, Daley J (2005) Surgical outcomes for patients aged 80 and older: morbidity and mortality from major noncardiac surgery. J Am Geriatr Soc 53:424–429
3. Turrentine FE, Wang H, Simpson VB, Jones RS (2006) Surgical risk factors, morbidity, and mortality in elderly patients. J Am Coll Surg 203:865–877
4. Agnosti JV, Inouye SK (2003) Delirium. In: Hazzard WR, Blass JP, Halter JP et al (eds) Principles of geriatric medicine and gerontology, 5th edn. McGraw-Hill, New York, NY, pp 1503–1515
5. Amador LF, Goodwin JS (2005) Postoperative delirium in the older patient. J Am Coll Surg 200:767–773

6. Robinson TN, Raeburn CD, Tran ZV, Angles EM, Brenner LA, Moss M (2009) Postoperative delirium in the elderly. Risk factors and outcomes. Ann Surg 249:173–178

7. Edelstein DM, Aharonoff GB, Karp A, Capla EL, Zuckerman JD, Koval KJ (2004) Effect of postoperative delirium on outcome after hip fracture. Clin Orthop Rel Res 422:195–200

8. McAvay GJ, Van Ness PH, Bogardus ST, Zhang Y, Leslie DL, Leo-Summers LS, Inouye SK (2006) Older adults discharged from the hospital with delirium: 1-year outcomes. J Am Geriatr Soc 54:1245–1250

9. Olin K, Eriksdotter-Jonhagen M, Jansson A, Herrington MK, Kristiansson M, Permert J (2005) Postoperative delirium in elderly patients after major abdominal surgery. Br J Surg 92:1559–1564

10. Marcantonio ER, Flacker JM, Michaels M, Resnick NM (2000) Delirium is independently associated with poor functional recovery after hip fracture. J Am Geriatr Soc 48:618–624

11. Inouye SK (2006) Delirium in older persons. N Engl J Med 354:1157–1165

12. Dasgupta M, Dumbrell AC (2006) Preoperative risk assessment for delirium after noncardiac surgery: a systematic review. J Am Geriatr Soc 54:1578–1589

13. Inouye SK, Bogardus ST, Charpentier PA, Leo-Summers L, Acampora D, Holford TR, Cooney LM (1999) A multicomponent intervention to prevent delirium in hospitalized older patients. N Engl J Med 340:669–676

14. Vaurio LE, Sands LP, Wang Y, Mullen EA, Leung JM (2006) Postoperative delirium: the importance of pain and pain management. Anesth Analg 102:1267–1273

15. Wei LA, Fearing MA, Sternberg EJ, Inouye SK (2008) The confusion assessment method: a systematic review of current usage. J Am Geriatr Soc 56:823–830

16. Marcantonio ER, Flacker JM, Wright RJ, Resnick NM (2001) Reducing delirium after hip fracture: a randomized trial. J Am Geriatr Soc 49:516–522

17. Kalisvaart KJ, de Jonghe JFM, Bogaards MJ, Vreeswijk R, Egberts TCG, Burger BJ, Eikelenboom P, van Gool WA (2005) Haloperidol prophylaxis for elderly hip-surgery patients at risk for delirium: a randomized placebo-controlled study. J Am Geriatr Soc 53:1658–1666

18. Liptzin B, Laki A, Garb JL, Fingeroth R, Krushell R (2005) Donepezil in the prevention and treatment of post-surgical delirium. Am J Geriatr Psychiatry 13:100–1106

19. Sampson EL, Raven PR, Ndhlovu PN et al (2007) A randomized, double-blind, placebo-controlled trial of donepezil hydrochloride (Aricept) for reducing the incidence of postoperative delirium after elective total hip replacement. Int J Geriatr Psychiatry 22:343–349

20. Leung JM, Sands LP, Rico M et al (2006) Pilot clinical trial of gabapentin to decrease postoperative delirium in older patients. Neurology 67:1251–1253

21. Tinetti ME (2003) Clinical practice: preventing falls in elderly persons. N Engl J Med 348:42–49

22. Sateia MJ (2003) Neuropsychological impairment and quality of life in obstructive sleep apnea. Clin Chest Med 24:249–259

23. Kaushik S, Wang JJ, Mitchell P (2007) Rise and fall of skeletal muscle size over the entire life span. J Am Geriatr Soc 55(7):1150

24. Tan KM, Austin B, Shaughnassy M et al (2005) Fall in an acute hospital and their relationship to restraint use. Ir J Med Sci 174(3):28–31

25. Cawthon PM, Harrison SL, Barrett-Connor E et al (2006) Alcohol intake and its relationship with bone mineral density, falls, and fracture risk in older men. J Am Geriatr Soc 54:1649–1657

26. Mathias S, Nayak US, Isaacs B (1986) Balance in elderly patients: the "get-up and go" test. Arch Phys Med Rehabil 67:387–389

27. Kristensen MT, Foss NB, Kehlet H (2007) Timed "up & go" test as a predictor of falls within 6 months after hip fracture surgery. Phys Ther 87:24–30

28. Rockwood K, Rockwood MR, Andrew M, Mitnitski A (2008) Reliability of the hierarchical assessment of balance and mobility in frail older adults. J Am Geriatr Soc 56:1213–1217

29. Amador LF, Loera JA (2007) Preventing postoperative falls in the older adult. J Am Coll Surg 204:447–453

30. Gillis A, MacDonald B (2005) Deconditioning in the hospitalized elderly. Can Nurse 101:16–20

31. Brown CJ, Friedkin RJ, Inouye SK (2004) Prevalence and outcomes of low mobility in hospitalized older patients. J Am Geriatr Soc 52:1263–1270

32. Amemiya T, Oda K, Ando M et al (2007) Activities of daily living and quality of life of elderly patients after elective surgery for gastric and colorectal cancers. Ann Surg 246:222–228

33. Morris PE, Goad A, Thompson C, Taylor K, Harry B, Passmore L, Ross A, Anderson L, Baker S, Sanchez M, Penley L, Howard A, Dixon L, Leach S, Small R, Hite RD, Haponik E (2008) Early intensive care unit mobility therapy in the treatment of acute respiratory failure. Crit Care Med 36:2238–2243

34. Schweickert WD, Pohlman MC, Pohlman AS, Nigos C, Pawlik AJ, Esbrook CL, Spears L, Miller M, Franczyk M, Deprizio D, Schmidt GA, Bowman A, Barr R, McCallister KE, Hall JB, Kress JP (2009) Early physical and occupational therapy in mechanically ventilated, critically ill patients: a randomised controlled trial. Lancet 373(9678):1874–1882

35. John AD, Sieber FE (2004) Age associated issues: geriatrics. Anesthesiol Clin North America 22:45–58

36. Sauvaget C, Yamada M, Fujiwara S et al (2002) Dementia as a predictor of functional disability. A four-year follow-up study. Gerontology 48(4):226–233

37. Shlipak MG, Stehman-Breen C, Fried LF et al (2004) The presence of frailty in elderly persons with chronic renal insufficiency. Am J Kidney Dis 43(5):861–867

38. Ferrucci L, Guralnik JM, Studenski S (2004) Designing randomized, controlled trials aimed at preventing or delaying functional decline and disability in frail, older persons: a consensus report. J Am Geriatr Soc 52(4):625–634

39. Fried LF, Lee JS, Shlipak M et al (2006) Chronic kidney disease and functional limitation in older people: health, aging and body composition study. J Am Geriatr Soc 54:750–756

40. Beliveau MM, Multach M (2003) Perioperative care for the elderly patient. Med Clin North Am 87:273–289

41. Cunha BA Urinary tract infections, males. eMedicine from WebMD. http://emedicine.medscape.com/article/231574-overview. Accessed 12 September 2009

42. Rupp ME, Fitzgerald T, Marion N et al (2004) Effect of silver-coated urinary catheters: efficacy, cost-effectiveness, and antimicrobial resistance. Am J Infect Control 32:445–450

43. Schumm K, Lam TB (2008) Types of urethral catheters for management of short-term voiding problems in hospitalized adults. Cochrane Database Syst Rev 16:CD004013

44. Hazelett SE, Tsai M, Gareri M et al (2006) The association between indwelling urinary catheter use in the elderly and urinary tract infection in acute care. BMC Geriatr 6:15

45. Foxman B (2002) Epidemiology of urinary tract infections: incidence, morbidity, and economic costs. Am J Med 113(Suppl 1A):5S–13S

46. Feldman C (2001) Pneumonia in the elderly. Med Clin North Am 85:1441–1459

47. Mehta RM, Niederman MS (2002) Nosocomial pneumonia. Curr Opin Infect Dis 15:387–394

48. Niederman MS, Brito V (2007) Pneumonia in the older patient. Clin Chest Med 28:751–771

49. Tablan OC, Anderson LJ, Besser R et al (2004) Guidelines for preventing health-care-associated pneumonia, 2003. MMWR Recomm Rep 53:1–36

50. Neumayer L, Hosowana P, Itani K et al (2007) Multivariable predictors of postoperative surgical site infection in general and vascular surgery: results from the patient safety in surgery study. J Am Coll Surg 204:1178–1187
51. Kirby JP, Mazuski JE (2009) Prevention of surgical site infection. Surg Clin North Am 89:365–389
52. Barie PS, Eachempati SR (2005) Surgical site infections. Surg Clin North Am 85:1115–1135
53. Kaye KS, Anderson DJ, Sloane R et al (2009) The effect of surgical site infection on older operative patients. J Am Geriatr Soc 57(1):45–54
54. Dellinger EP, Hausmann SM, Bratzler DW et al (2005) Hospitals collaborate to decrease surgical site infections. Am J Surg 190:9–15
55. Devereaux PJ, Yang H, Yusuf S, for the POISE Study Group et al (2008) Effects of extended-release metoprolol succinate in patients undergoing non-cardiac surgery (POISE trial): a randomized controlled trial. Lancet 371:1839–1847
56. McGory ML, Maggard MA, Ko CK (2005) A meta-analysis of perioperative beta blockade: what is the actual risk reduction? Surgery 138:171–179
57. Auerback AD, Goldman L (2002) Beta-blockers and reduction of cardiac events in noncardiac surgery. JAMA 287(11):1435–1444
58. Lindenauer PK, Pekow P, Wang K et al (2005) Perioperative beta-blocker therapy and mortality after major noncardiac surgery. N Engl J Med 353:349–361
59. Fleischmann KE, Goldman L, Young B et al (2003) Association between cardiac and noncardiac complications in patients undergoing noncardiac surgery: outcomes and effects on length of stay. Am J Med 115(7):515–520
60. Kulaylat MN, Dayton MT (2008) Surgical complications. In: Townsend CM Jr, Beauchamp RD, Evers BM, Mattox KL (eds) Sabiston textbook of surgery, 18th edn. Saunders Elsevier, Philadelphia, PA, pp 338–347
61. Jin F, Chung F (2001) Minimizing perioperative adverse events in the elderly. Br J Anaesth 87(4):608–624
62. Polanczyk CA, Marcantonio E, Goldman L et al (2001) Impact of age on perioperative complications and length of stay in patients undergoing noncardiac surgery. Ann Intern Med 134:637–643
63. Mehta RH, Rathore SS, Radford MJ et al (2001) Acute myocardial infarction in the elderly: differences by age. J Am Coll Cardiol 38:736
64. Woon VC, Lim KH (2003) Acute myocardial infarction in the elderly-differences compared with the young. Singapore Med J 44(8):414–418
65. Lindenauer PK, Fitzgerald J, Hoople N et al (2004) The potential preventability of postoperative myocardial infarction. Arch Intern Med 164:762–766
66. Ryder DL (2008) The use of beta-blockers to decrease adverse perioperative cardiac events. Dimens Crit Care Nurs 27(2):47–53
67. Badner NH, Knill RL, Brown JE et al (1998) Myocardial infarction after noncardiac surgery. Anesthesiology 88(3):572–578
68. Martinez EA, Pronovost P (2002) Perioperative beta-blockers in high-risk patients. J f Crit Care 17(2):105–113
69. Loran DB, Hyde BR, Zwischenberger JB (2005) Perioperative management of special populations: the geriatric patient. Surg Clin North Am 85:1259–1266
70. Amar D, Zhang H, Leung DHY et al (2002) Older age is the strongest predictor of postoperative atrial fibrillation. Anesthesiology 96:352–356
71. Ramsay JG (1999) Cardiac management in the ICU. Chest 115(5 Suppl):138S–144S
72. Amar D (2008) Prevention and management of perioperative arrhythmias in the thoracic surgical population. Anesthesiol Clin 26(2):325–335
73. Goodman S, Weiss Y, Weissman C (2008) Update on cardiac arrhythmias in the ICU. Curr Opin Crit Care 14(5):549–554
74. Fang MC, Chen J, Rich MW (2007) Atrial fibrillation in the elderly. Am J Med 120:481–487
75. Douketis JD, Berger PB, Dunn AS et al (2008) The perioperative management of antithrombotic therapy. Chest 133:299S–339S
76. Amar D, Zhang H, Roistacher N (2002) The incidence and outcome of ventricular arrhythmias after noncardiac thoracic surgery. Anesth Analg 95:537–543
77. Gage BF, Waterman AD, Shannon W et al (2001) Validation of clinical classification schemes for predicting stroke: results from the National Registry of Atrial Fibrillation. JAMA 285:2864–2870
78. Gilmore JC (2003) Heart failure and treatment: part II Perianesthesia management. J Perianesth Nurs 18:242–246
79. Gutierrez C, Blanchard DB (2004) Diastolic heart failure: challenges of diagnosis and treatment. Am Fam Physician 69:2609–2616
80. Roche JJW, Wenn RT, Sahota O et al (2005) Effect of comorbidities and postoperative complications on mortality after hip fracture in elderly people: prospective observational cohort study. BMJ 331:1374–1378
81. Hernandez AF, Newby LK, O'Connor CM (2004) Preoperative evaluation for major noncardiac surgery: focusing on heart failure. Arch Intern Med 164(13):1729–1736
82. Ergina PL, Gold SL, Meakins JL (1993) Perioperative care of the elderly patient. World J Surg 17:192–198
83. Brooks-Brunn JA (1997) Predictors of postoperative pulmonary complications following abdominal surgery. Chest 111:564–571
84. McAlister FA, Bertsch K, Man J et al (2005) Incidence of and risk factors for pulmonary complications after nonthoracic surgery. Am J Respir Crit Care Med 171(5):514–517
85. Gabeau D, Rosenthal RA (2001) Preoperative evaluation of the elderly surgical patient. In: Rosenthal RA, Zenilman ME, Katlic MR (eds) Principles and practice of geriatric surgery, 1st edn. Springer, New York, NY, pp 126–143
86. Kikawada M, Iwamoto T, Takasaki M (2005) Aspiration in the elderly. Drugs Aging 22:115–130
87. Cook DJ, Rooke GA (2003) Priorities in perioperative geriatrics. Anesth Analg 96:1823–1836
88. Marik PE, Kaplan D (2003) Aspiration pneumonia and dysphagia in the elderly. Chest 124:328–336
89. Arozullah AM, Daley J, Henderson WG et al (2000) Multifactorial risk index for predicting postoperative respiratory failure in men after major noncardiac surgery. Ann Surg 232:242–253
90. Gore DC (2007) Preoperative maneuvers to avert postoperative respiratory failure in elderly patients. Gerontology 53:438–444
91. Mendez-Tellez PA, Dorman T (2008) Postoperative respiratory failure. In: Cameron JL (ed) Current surgical therapy. Mosby, Baltimore, MD, pp 1196–1201
92. El Sohl AA, Bhat A, Gunen H et al (2004) Extubation failure in the elderly. Respir Med 98:661–668
93. Schneider GT, Christensen N, Doerr TD (2009) Early tracheotomy in elderly patients results in less ventilator-associated pneumonia. Otolaryngol Head Neck Surg 140:250–255
94. Jaffer AK, Brotman DJ (2006) Prevention of venous thromboembolism in the geriatric patient. Clin Geriatr Med 22(1):93–111
95. Kim V, Spandorfer J (2001) Epidemiology of venous thromboembolic disease. Emerg Med Clin North Am 19(4):839–859
96. Piazza G, Seddighzadeh A, Goldhaber SZ (2008) Deep-vein thrombosis in the elderly. Clin Appl Thromb Hemost 14:393–398
97. Di Minno G, Tifano A (2004) Challenges in the prevention of venous thromboembolism in the elderly. J Thromb Haemost 2:1292–1298
98. Kumar A, Carson JL (2008) Perioperative anemia in the elderly. Clin Geriatr Med 24:641–648
99. Conlon NP, Bale EP, Herbison GP et al (2008) Postoperative anemia and quality of life after primary hip arthroplasty in patients over 65 years old. Anesth Analg 106:1056–1061

100. Foss NB, Kristensen MT, Kehlet H (2008) Anaemia impedes functional mobility after hip fracture surgery. Age Aging 37:173–178

101. Foss NB, Kristensen MT, Jensen PS et al (2009) The effects of liberal versus restrictive transfusion thresholds on ambulation after hip fracture surgery. Transfusion 49:227–234

102. Wu W, Rathore SS, Wang Y et al (2001) Blood transfusion in elderly patients with acute myocardial infarction. N Engl J Med 345:1230–1236

103. Sarasin SM, Walton MJ, Singh HP, Clark DI (2006) Can a urinary tract symptom score predict the development of postoperative urinary retention in patients undergoing lower limb arthroplasty under spinal anaesthesia? A prospective study. Ann R Coll Surg Engl 88:394–398

104. Keita H, Diouf E, Tubach F, Brouwer T, Dahmani S, Mantz J, Desmonts J (2005) Predictive factors of early postoperative urinary retention in the postanesthesia care unit. Anesth Analg 101:592–596

105. Changchien CR, Yeh CY, Huang ST, Hsieh M, Chen J, Tang R (2007) Postoperative urinary retention after primary colorectal cancer resection via laparotomy: a prospective study of 2355 consecutive patients. Dis Colon Rectum 50:1688–1696

106. Frocht A, Fillit H (1984) Renal disease in the geriatric patient. J Am Geriatr Soc 32:28–39

107. Go AS, Chertow GM, Fan D, McCulloch CE, Hsu CY (2004) Chronic kidney disease and the risks of death, cardiovascular events, and hospitalization. N Engl J Med 351:1296–1305

108. Kellerman PS (1994) Perioperative care of the renal patient. Arch Intern Med 154:1674–1688

109. Kohli HS, Bhaskaran MC, Muthukumar T, Thennarasu K, Sud K, Jha V, Gupta KL, Sakhuja V (2000) Treatment-related acute renal failure in the elderly: a hospital-based prospective study. Nephrol Dial Transplant 15:212–217

110. Harmankaya O, Kaptanogullari H, Obek A (2002) Acute renal failure in the elderly: a five-year experience. Ren Fail 24:223–225

111. Sesso R, Roque A, Vicioso B, Stella S (2004) Prognosis of ARF in hospitalized elderly patients. Am J Kidney Dis 44:410–419

112. Noorgate NVD, Mouton V, Lamot C, Nooten GV, Dhondt A, Vanholder R, Afschrift M, Lameire N (2003) Outcome in a post-cardiac surgery population with acute renal failure requiring dialysis: does age make a difference? Nephrol Dial Transplant 18:732–736

113. Azevedo V, Silveira M, Santos J, Braz J, Braz L, Modolo N (2008) Postoperative renal function evaluation, through RIFLE criteria, of elderly patients who underwent femur fracture surgery under spinal anesthesia. Ren Fail 30:485–490

114. Schmitt R, Coca S, Kanbay M, Tinetti ME, Cantley LG, Parikh CR (2008) Recovery of kidney function after acute kidney injury in the elderly: a systematic review and meta-analysis. Am J Kidney Dis 52:262–271

115. Cheung CM, Ponnusamy A, Anderton JG (2008) Management of acute renal failure in the elderly patient: a clinician's guide. Drugs Aging 25:455–476

116. Bardacki H, Cheema FH, Topkara VK, Dang NC, Martens TP, Mercando ML, Forster CS, Benson AA, George I, Russo MJ, Oz MC, Esrig BC (2007) Discharge home rates are significantly lower for octogenarians undergoing coronary artery bypass surgery. Ann Thorac Surg 83:483–489

117. Apfel CC, Laara E, Koivuranta M et al (1999) A simplified risk score for predicting postoperative nausea and vomiting. Anesthesiology 91:693–700

118. Pierre S, Benais H, Pouymayou J (2002) Apfel's simplified score may favourably predict the risk of postoperative nausea and vomiting. Can J Anaesth 49:237–242

119. Martin G, Glass PS, Breslin DS et al (2003) A study of anesthetic drug utilization in different age groups. J Clin Anesth 15(3):194–200

120. Gan TJ, Meyer T, Apfel CC et al (2003) Consensus guidelines for managing postoperative nausea and vomiting. Anesth Analg 97:62–71

121. Adanir T, Aksun M, Ozgürböz U, Altin F, Sencan A (2008) Does preoperative hydration affect postoperative nausea and vomiting? A randomized, controlled trial. J Laparoendosc Adv Surg Tech A 18(1):1–4

122. El Solh A, Okada M, Bhat A, Pietrantoni C (2003) Swallowing disorders postorotracheal intubation in the elderly. Intensive Care Med 29:1451–1455

123. Marik PE (2001) Aspiration pneumonitis and aspiration pneumonia. N Engl J Med 344:665–671

124. Barquist E, Brown M, Cohn S et al (2001) Postextubation fiberoptic endoscopic evaluation of swallowing after prolonged endotracheal intubation: a randomized, prospective trial. Crit Care Med 29:1710–1713

125. Spechler SJ (1992) Epidemiology and natural history of gastro-oesophageal reflux disease. Digestion 51(Suppl 1):24–29, Review

126. Hendry PO, Hausel J, Nygren J, Lassen K, Dejong CH, Lungqvist O, Fearon KC (2009) Determinants of outcome after colorectal resection within an enhanced recovery programme. Enhanced Recovery After Surgery Study Group. Br J Surg 96:197–205

127. Raue W, Langelotz C, Neub H, Müller JM, Schwenk W (2000) "Fast-track" rehabilitation to enhance recovery after ileostomy closure – a prospective clinical trial. Zentralbl Chir 133(5):486–490

128. Chen HH, Wexner SD, Iroatulam AJ et al (2000) Laparoscopic colectomy compares favorably with colectomy by laparotomy for reduction of postoperative ileus. Dis Colon Rectum 43(1):61–65

129. Schlachta CM, Burpee SE, Fernandez C et al (2007) Optimizing recovery after laparoscopic colon surgery (ORAL-CS). Surg Endosc 21:2212–2219

130. Kehlet H, Wilmore DW (2002) Multimodal strategies to improve surgical outcome. Am J Surg 183:630–641

131. Taguchi A, Sharma N, Saleem RM, Sessler DI, Carpenter RL, Seyedsadr M, Kurz A (2001) Selective postoperative inhibition of gastrointestinal opioid receptors. N Engl J Med 345(13):935–940

132. Akca O, Doufas AG, Sessler DI (2002) Use of selective opiate receptor inhibitors to prevent postoperative ileus. Minerva Anestesiol 68(4):162–165

Chapter 30
Management and Outcomes of Intensive Care in the Geriatric Surgical Patient

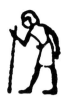

Gary T. Marshall and Scott R. Gunn

Introduction

Should we admit geriatric patients to the intensive care unit (ICU) at all? Of course, we believe the answer to this question is a qualified "yes"; otherwise, our chapter would be brief indeed. But, it is important to remember that rationing health care based upon age has been advocated as a strategy for limiting cost [1]. Refusal of ICU admission is common across many developed countries and has been reported to range between 24 and 46% of requested admissions [2–6]. In these studies, advanced age and previously poor functional status are the most common reasons for refusal to admit to the ICU. In 2004, Sinuf and coworkers systematically reviewed rationing of ICU resources and found that age and severity of illness were most strongly associated with a refusal to admit to the ICU [7]. Admission to the ICU carries with it a large commitment of health care resources. If we admit geriatric patients, how do we best allocate costly and limited ICU resources? At a time when the numbers of geriatric ICU patients [8] and the costs associated with ICU care are rapidly increasing, it becomes important to examine what outcomes can be expected if we are to provide ICU care to elderly patients.

Outcomes

Mortality

Mortality has traditionally been the primary outcome used to assess health care delivery. Mortality among elderly patients is substantial following hospital discharge. In a study of medical and surgical patients ≥70 years, 1-year survival was 56% in patients aged <85 years and 27% in those ≥85 years –

rates markedly lower than in a matched population (93%) [9]. Others have reported mortality rates in critically ill patients ≥85 years of 30% at ICU discharge, 43% at 30 days posthospital discharge, and 64% at 1 year [10]. In addition, age is an independent variable in many prognostic scoring systems such as Acute Physiology and Chronic Health Evaluation (APACHE) II [11], APACHE III [12], and the Simplified Acute Physiology Score (SAPS) II [13].

But, chronologic age alone is not the whole story. In one study, the impact of age on outcome weakened as the severity of the acute illness (or physiologic derangement) increased [14]. Margulies and coworkers found ICU mortality among surgical patients related to severity of illness (evaluated as SAPS) and did not differ significantly between nonagenarians and younger patients when stratified for SAPS [15]. In two reports of patients admitted to medical ICUs, old age no longer predicted mortality when acute severity of illness, diagnosis, and prior health were taken into account [16, 17]. As is clear from other chapters on physiologic changes associated with aging, the elderly are less able to maintain homeostasis in the face of pathologic stressors than are younger patients. It is to be expected, therefore, that they will have more marked derangements for any given "insult" (e.g., injury, infection, or surgical procedure) than the young. In other words, prognostic scoring systems which examine abnormal physiology such as the APACHE III or SAPS II should be expected to reflect increased mortality not only as a result of increased age but also – and perhaps more importantly – as a result of a decreased ability to maintain homeostasis.

Health-Related Quality of Life

While mortality remains an important metric for assessing health care, other outcomes such as quality-adjusted life years (QALYs), postdischarge placement status, and health-related quality of life (HR-QOL) are becoming increasingly relevant. To date, the largest review of HR-QOL literature in elderly patients after admission to the ICU was authored by

G.T. Marshall (✉)
Department of Trauma Surgery, University of Pittsburgh Medical Center, Pittsburgh, PA, USA
e-mail: marshallgt@upmc.edu

R.A. Rosenthal et al. (eds.), *Principles and Practice of Geriatric Surgery*,
DOI 10.1007/978-1-4419-6999-6_30, © Springer Science+Business Media, LLC 2011

Hennessy and colleagues in 2005 [18]. After an extensive MEDLINE review, they identified 16 studies that examined HR-QOL or functional status in geriatric patients after ICU admission. These studies included a total of 3,247 elderly survivors of critical care whose HR-QOL or functional status was assessed after ICU discharge. In their review, these investigators were limited in their ability to synthesize results across multiple studies results by study heterogeneity. For example, the authors found that most studies used varying assessments of severity of illness, chronic illness and prior functional status. They found a lack of consensus regarding definition of "elderly" and evaluation of outcomes using various methods and at various times. In addition, many studies suffer from a potential selection bias arising from criteria or policies for ICU admission [19]. Studies usually evaluate convenience samples of patients admitted to an ICU; information about potentially eligible patients who were not admitted is uncommon. Finally, most studies are ICU-based or institution-based rather than population-based and thus are limited by referral bias.

Despite limitations, these investigators found that the majority of published literature in this field (10 of 16 reviewed studies) supports the concept that aged ICU survivors maintain a good functional status and/or HR-QOL. There were some exceptions. For example, Vasquez Mata and coworkers found that their elderly cohort had the most reduction in HR-QOL as compared to a younger cohort [20]. Of note, Vasquez Mata used an assessment tool primarily focused on physical functioning without a subjective assessment of HR-QOL. While physical functioning plays a role in HR-QOL, other significant domains include social functioning, pain, fatigue, and ability to perform activities of daily living. It is possible that while physical function may decrease for geriatric ICU survivors, other domains may become more important in their overall assessment of HR-QOL. In another significant study, Montuclard and coworkers found that independence in activities of daily living was significantly decreased for elderly ICU survivors [21]. However, their unique inception cohort (subjects with an ICU length of stay >30 days) may limit this study's generalizability.

In the largest, single-center outcome study of geriatric patients who survive ICU admission (published after the review by Hennessy), Kaarlola and coinvestigators evaluated 883 elderly ICU survivors and 1,827 controls [22]. They found that cumulative 3-year mortality was higher among the aged (57% vs. 40% in the control group). Most (66%) elderly non-survivors died within 1 month of ICU discharge (Fig. 30.1).

In addition, geriatric patients had significantly fewer QALYs than age- and sex-matched controls. However, 97% of the geriatric survivors lived at home. 88% described their present state of health as good or satisfactory. In fact, 66% found it similar or better than 12 months prior, and 48% found it similar or better than before ICU admission.

Other Factors

The relation of age and severity of illness to mortality is further modified by specific diagnosis. In one study, patients admitted following trauma had the highest long-term survival compared to other diagnostic groups in a mixed ICU [23]. Age, severity of illness, and diagnosis were independent predictors of 1-year survival in a recent study of medical and surgical patients ≥70 years of age [9]. In a study in which many of the patients were admitted to the ICU following surgery or trauma, the survival of those who were alive 6 months following hospital discharge approached that of an age-, year-, and gender- matched general population [24]. The interaction of prior functional status and age may also influence mortality. In one study, patients ≥75 years of age who had functional limitations were six times more likely to die in hospital than those aged 50–64 years without limitations [25]. Among patients without functional limitation, there was no difference in mortality between the youngest and oldest groups. Physical activity status and quality of life prior to admission were significant predictors of survival in a mixed ICU population with large proportions of older and chronically ill patients [26].

Conclusions

As age increases and functional status declines, patients may become more willing to accept aggressive medical therapy. For example, Sage and coauthors found that increasing age was inversely related to patients' assessments of quality of life following discharge, but not to objective scores of physical and psychosocial disability [27]. These observations are consistent with the concept that individual and societal views of quality of life do not necessarily coincide in older patients, who may be more accepting of health-related limitations in life style than young patients [27, 28]. While more research is needed to accurately characterize the mortality and HR-QOL of elderly survivors of critical illness, currently, we believe that despite a higher mortality, aged patients with a reasonable preadmission functional status and severity of illness can likely be expected to benefit from ICU admission. It is probable that postdischarge functional status will be less than that of younger ICU survivors; however, elderly ICU survivors are likely to be satisfied with their postdischarge HR-QOL and may even rate it higher than preadmission. In the rest of this chapter, we examine common ICU-related problems as they relate to geriatric patients: respiratory failure, delirium, shock and hemodynamic monitoring, acute kidney injury and renal replacement therapy, nutrition, and finally care of the dying patient.

Self Evaluation of Health Status

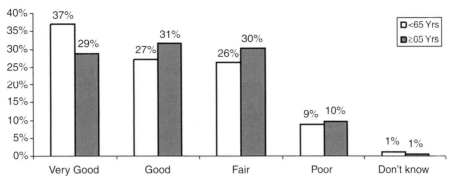

Satisfied with Present State of Health

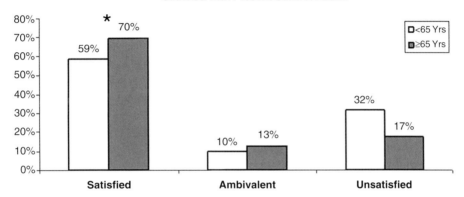

Figure 30.1 Health status and satisfaction among geriatric and younger ICU survivors. Rockwood and coworkers interviewed 143 geriatric (≥65 years) and 225 younger (<65 years) ICU survivors. They found no significant differences between the groups in self-evaluation of health status (*top figure*). However, they did find a statistically significant difference between groups (*asterisk*) in the number of respondents who were satisfied with their present state of health (data from Rockwood et al. [28]).

Respiratory Insufficiency and Failure

Changes in Pulmonary Function Associated with Aging

The aging process affects every aspect of respiratory physiology and oxygen transport, with important consequences for the geriatric patient with critical illness [29]. Pulmonary complications and adverse pulmonary events are common in elderly patient, following even elective surgical procedures [30–33]. The age-related changes that are most clinically relevant include declines in vital capacity, forced expiratory volume in 1 s, alveolar–arterial oxygen gradient, arterial oxygen tension, and maximal oxygen consumption. Ventilatory responses to hypoxia and hypercarbia are blunted [34, 35] Also relevant for the aged surgical patient is decreased sensitivity of the airways to noxious stimuli. Diminished airway sensitivity to stimuli such as refluxed gastric fluid in addition to impaired mucociliary transport and decreased cough strength renders the elderly patient at increased risk of silent pulmonary aspiration [36].

Outcomes

Outcomes of geriatric patients who require mechanical ventilation have been the focus of a number of conflicting reports. A hospital mortality of 52% and 1-year mortality of 63% have been identified in data compiled from multiple studies [19]. Age, severity of illness, comorbidity, and diagnosis are predictors of outcome in ventilated geriatric patients, as they are in elderly critically ill patients in general [19, 37]. In some studies, prolonged ventilation (defined as 15 days in one study and a total score of more than 100 for the number of days of ventilation plus age in years in another) has been accompanied by poor outcomes [37, 38], whereas in others, the duration of mechanical ventilation has not been significantly related to outcome [39, 40]. In a study of patients with acute respiratory distress syndrome (ARDS), age >60 was associated with a fivefold increase in mortality, presumably because of age-related impairments in cardiopulmonary regulatory mechanisms [29]. However other investigators have not found a statistically significant increase in mortality in elderly patients with ARDS [41]. In one of the largest studies on this question, Esteban and coauthors

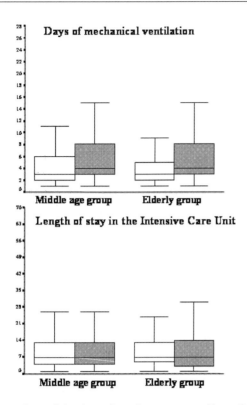

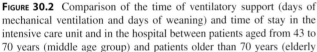

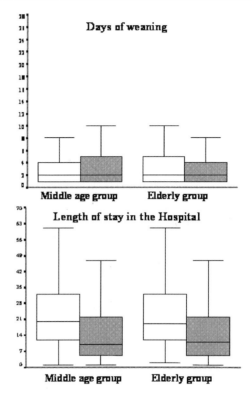

Figure 30.2 Comparison of the time of ventilatory support (days of mechanical ventilation and days of weaning) and time of stay in the intensive care unit and in the hospital between patients aged from 43 to 70 years (middle age group) and patients older than 70 years (elderly group). The *white boxes* correspond to patients who survive and the *gray boxes* to nonsurvivors. *Box plot* indicates the median and the interquantile range. *Bar* indicates the minimum and the maximum number of days (from Esteban et al. [43]. Reprinted with permission).

recently reviewed the database from the International Mechanical Ventilation Study [42] ($n = 5,183$) and found that patients >70 of age had similar intensity of care as compared to younger patients [43]. Their work supports conclusions of others that age alone is not a sufficient reason to withhold mechanical ventilation. They found that the most important risk factors for death in the elderly patient requiring mechanical ventilation were coexistent acute renal failure, shock, and limited functional status (Fig. 30.2).

Clinical Management

In our practice, we have found a number of techniques clinically useful on a daily basis. First, we avoid or minimize narcotics when at all possible in the aged. We have found regional techniques such as epidural analgesia or paravertebral blocks to be useful. Parenteral narcotics have been associated with more frequent respiratory disturbances following surgery, and regional techniques for pain management and nonnarcotic analgesics may therefore be particularly valuable in the geriatric patient [30]. It is also important to eliminate other medications, which might contribute to delirium in the aged patient, for example,

anticholinergics. Nonsteroidal pain relief would seem useful in this setting, but in practice, many elderly patients have absolute or relative contraindications to their use [44]. Second, we mobilize elderly patients as soon as possible. Assuming an upright position increases the functional residual capacity and should lessen the closure of small airways that is caused by the supine position. Oxygen consumption following thoracotomy is lower in the sitting than the supine position, suggesting that the work of breathing may be lessened when upright [45].

In the elderly, at-risk patient who is not mechanically ventilated, measures such as incentive spirometry (IS) and other lung recruitment maneuvers complement the basic measures of pain management and mobilization. We use a staged approach for managing pulmonary toileting in aged, compromised patients. First, we start with IS every 6 h. If patients are unable to attain volumes of at least 8–10 ml/kg ideal body weight on IS, then we add a noninvasive, lung expansion therapy: a single-use device attached to an oxygen flowmeter that provides positive airway pressure throughout the respiratory cycle. We continue to monitor IS volumes every 6 h while maintaining lung recruitment. Finally, if volumes are still below the desired 8–10 ml/kg, we initiate noninvasive pressure support ventilation while continuing to follow IS volumes when patients are off noninvasive ventilation.

While the techniques of mechanical ventilation and weaning may not differ in the elderly, they may require a longer period of support, given the impairments imposed by age, comorbidity, and acute illness. Caution should be exercised when liberating elderly patients from mechanical ventilation. Parameters used to predict successful weaning from mechanical ventilation in young patients appear less reliable in the elderly [46]. Even after successfully undergoing a trial of spontaneous breathing prior to extubation, elderly patients may not do as well as younger patients. The ARDSnet investigators examined age as a factor affecting outcome from acute lung injury and ARDS [47]. They found that although patients >70 years of age were able to breathe spontaneously for 2 h without ventilator assistance – a commonly accepted weaning parameter – at a similar time point to younger patients, the older patients had inferior outcomes, such as higher reintubation rates, longer ICU and hospital stays, and lower survival rates at 28 days.

Delirium

Definition, Assessment, and Incidence

Delirium is an acute state of confusion that develops over a short period of time and fluctuates over time. It is often the result of underlying organic derangements, such as infection, medical illness, and drug use or withdrawal. Delirium can be distinguished from dementia by its acute onset and fluctuating course. The assessment of acute changes in cognition is difficult in the ICU setting due to the severity of underlying disease and the frequent loss of verbal communication due to mechanical ventilation. One tool for assessment of delirium in the ICU, which was adapted from the Confusion Assessment Method (CAM), is the CAM-ICU [48]. It has been validated in several studies as being both highly sensitive and specific [48, 49]. Using CAM-ICU, delirium is diagnosed in two steps. First, a standardized sedation scale, such as the Richmond Agitation-Sedation Scale [50] is used to determine the level of consciousness. Any patient not determined to be comatose is then assessed for four features of delirium: (1) Acute onset of mental status changes or a fluctuating course, (2) inattention, (3) disorganized thinking, and (4) an altered level of consciousness. A diagnosis of delirium is made with the presence of both features (1) and (2) in addition to either feature (3) or (4) [48]. In a recent study of elderly patients admitted to the ICU, the rates of delirium were found to be >70% during their hospitalization. In the same study, the effect of dementia was also assessed. Patients with dementia had a 40% higher overall rate of delirium during hospitalization than those without dementia [51]. There is little doubt that as the elderly population ages, the prevalence and burden of delirium in the ICU will grow.

Predisposing Factors

Predisposing Factors for Delirium in the ICU

The risk factors for delirium are divided into host factors, which are present on admission to the ICU, and precipitating factors, which occur during the course of illness. It is this second group of factors that are potentially modifiable and therefore the target of therapeutic or prophylactic intervention [52, 53] (Table 30.1).

The use of sedative and analgesic medications deserves special attention. Nearly all patients in the ICU receive these medications. However, their use is not without detrimental effects. These effects include prolonged mechanical ventilation and an increased utilization of diagnostic studies for altered mental status when sedatives are used in a continuous, rather than intermittent, fashion. Daily interruption of sedation is one method used to avoid this complication [54]. Benzodiazepines and anticholinergics have been consistently linked to delirium in the elderly [55]. Pisani and coworkers recently published data showing that use of a benzodiazepine or opioid was associated with increased delirium duration, especially the first episode (relative risk of 1.64 with a 95% confidence interval of 1.27–2.10) [56]. Trials of newer agents have shown some promise. In a 2007 trial by Pandharipande et al., the use of dexmedetomidine (an alpha 2 agonist) was compared to lorazepam in mechanically ventilated patients. The use of dexmedetomidine was associated with more delirium-free days than lorazepam [57]. The data regarding the use of opioids is less clear. A study by Ouimet and coworkers demonstrated higher daily use of opioids in ICU patients without delirium [58]. Similarly, in a study of hip-fracture patients, Morrison and coauthors found that patients treated liberally with opioid analgesics were less likely to

TABLE 30.1   Predisposing factors for delirium in the ICU

Host factors	Critical illness related factors	Iatrogenic factors
Age	Acidosis	Immobilization
Alcoholism	Anemia	Catheters
Apolipoprotein E4	Fever/infection/sepsis	Medications
Polymorphism	Hypotension	Sleep disturbance
Cognitive impairment	Metabolic disturbances	
	Fever/hypothermia	
Depression	End organ dysfunction	
Hypertension	Respiratory disease/	
Smoking	hypoxia	
Vision or hearing loss	High severity of illness	

Source: Girard and Ely [53]

develop delirium than those who received less analgesia [59]. Meperidine is the exception, as it is consistently linked to the development of delirium, especially in the aged [60–62]. These findings point to the need for careful use of these agents with attention to providing adequate pain relief while avoiding oversedation.

Evaluation, Prevention, and Treatment

Once delirium is diagnosed, an underlying organic source must first be sought. A diminished level of consciousness may herald underlying infection or metabolic derangements, and these must be ruled out by careful history and physical examination. Within the ICU, risk factors more prevalent in the setting of critical illness must be addressed. These include infection, metabolic and electrolyte abnormalities, and medication exposure. If critical illness related factors are ruled out, other interventions may prove useful in reducing delirium such as repeated reorientation of the patient and activities designed to be cognitively stimulating; a nonpharmacologic sleep protocol; early mobilization and range of motion exercise; prompt removal of restraints and catheters; use of eyeglasses and hearing aids; and the early correction of dehydration [63]. These results were confirmed in patients after hip fracture [64] and in hospitalized geriatric patients [65] but have not yet been studied in the ICU.

After the use of nonpharmacologic strategies to minimize risk factors and addressing the metabolic derangements associated with critical care illness, consideration should be given to the use of pharmacologic agents to manage the symptoms of delirium. Currently, the clinical practice guideline from the Society of Critical Care Medicine recommends haloperidol as the drug of choice for treatment of delirium in the ICU [66]. This is also true for the geriatric patient [67]. Using intermittent intravenous injection, a 2-mg dose is recommended. Repeated doses are administered if symptoms are not controlled, doubling the previously administered dose every 15–20 min until agitation resolves. Once controlled, scheduled doses are given every 4–6 h and then tapered over several days. Side effects of haloperidol include QT interval prolongation, extrapyramidal symptoms, and neuroleptic malignant syndrome. Routine EKG monitoring is suggested to detect any QT prolongation [66]. Atypical antipsychotics, such as risperidone, ziprasidone, quetiapine, and olanzapine, may also have a role in the management of delirium. Although no placebo-controlled studies of these agents exist, early data suggests that these agents may be at least as effective as haloperidol and may have fewer side effects [68].

Outcomes

Among ICU patients, numerous adverse events have been associated with delirium. These include unplanned extubation, removal of catheters and drains, failed extubation, prolonged hospital stay, increased health care costs, and increased mortality. Milbrandt and colleagues studied patient charges in 275 consecutive, mechanically ventilated ICU patients and found the presence of delirium to be associated with 39% increased ICU cost (95% CI, 12–72%) and 31% higher hospital cost (95% CI, 1–70%) [69]. In addition to the acute adverse events associated with delirium in critically ill patients, multiple long-term detrimental effects have been noted. Ely and coworkers reported that delirium was associated with a threefold increase in the risk of death at 6 months [70]. Jackson and coauthors reviewed nine prospective studies a diverse group of hospitalized and critically ill patients and reported that delirium during hospitalization was associated with a cognitive decline over the following 1–3 years [71].

Shock and Hemodynamic Monitoring

Changes in the Cardiovascular System Associated with Aging

During the course of aging, there are structural and functional changes within the heart and vasculature which become important in the critical care of the geriatric patient. For example, there is a significant decrease in the compliance and distensibility of the aorta and vascular tree. This stiffening of the arteries results in an increase in afterload. The results of the increased afterload include left ventricular hypertrophy and decrease in diastolic compliance. Wall thickness increases of up to 30% have been documented. Diastolic compliance is also reduced, and when coupled with delayed diastolic filling observed in the elderly heart, results in nearly a 50% reduction in early diastolic ventricular filling. Ventricular filling becomes much more dependent on atrial contraction. Diastolic dysfunction and decreased left ventricular compliance means that the aging heart must achieve higher-end diastolic pressures to preserve preload and thus stroke volume. The clinical implications of these changes are that cardiac output is much more reliant on adequate preload and atrial systole. Hypovolemia must be avoided, and atrial arrhythmias must be controlled or addressed in the face of surgical stress and sepsis. In addition to normal age-related changes, clinicians must also take into account the effects of ischemic heart disease, which becomes increasingly prevalent with age. The Framingham Heart Study found that myocardial infarction was silent or unrecognized in over 40% of patients aged 75–84 years compared to under 20% in the group between age 45 and 54 years [72].

Monitoring and Management of Shock

Shock is best defined as a state of inadequate tissue perfusion. In the uncompensated state, it is easily recognized by tachycardia, oliguria, and hypotension. However, most critical care practitioners would prefer to recognize hypoperfusion before overt decompensation. The initial monitoring of the critically ill patient should include close attention to the physical exam, arterial blood pressure monitoring, and the urine output. We have found these parameters – and more importantly, their change over time – most useful in determining the response to resuscitative efforts, but they can fail to detect ongoing tissue hypoperfusion and hypoxia [73]. Even after hypotension has been corrected and urine output restored, a state of "compensated shock" may remain. In this condition, tissue hypoxia is ongoing, leading to multiple organ dysfunction and death. Hypoxia forces tissues to utilize anaerobic pathways, resulting in lactic acid production. Large amounts of H+ may then be produced. Base deficit, lactate level, and bicarbonate levels are frequently used to assess both the initial state of shock and to monitor the effects of ongoing resuscitation. Although no single end point is applicable to every scenario, it is important to repeatedly reexamine potentially "shocky" patients and follow them closely to determine the success or inadequacy of resuscitation.

The use of pulmonary artery catheters (PACs) is no longer de rigueur. There is currently no prospective evidence supporting their use. Friese and coworkers analyzed the National Trauma Data Bank and found higher mortality in trauma patients managed with a PAC. They did, however, find that those with severe injury who arrived in shock and older patients had a survival benefit when a PAC was used to guide management [74]. However, most evidence would contradict this. In a large meta-analysis, Shah and coworkers evaluated 13 randomized clinical trials. They concluded that in critically ill patients, the use of PACs neither increased mortality or hospital days nor did it confer benefit. The absence of benefit may have been the result of the lack of any clear or specific guidelines for treatment based on the data collected [75]. The PAC catheter was often used to drive "supranormal resuscitation," which sought to maximize cardiac index (>4.5 l/min/m^2) and oxygen delivery index (>600 ml/min/ m^2). Achieving these goals was associated with an increase in survival; however, there was no prospective evidence to suggest a benefit to attempting to attain these goals. Rather, the ability to achieve these goals appears to be a marker of the patient's physiologic reserve [76].

Mixed central venous oxygen saturation ($S_{cv}O_2$) may be a useful adjunct in determining the adequacy of oxygen delivery. A value of >70% is considered to be normal. Lower values are consistent with flow-dependent delivery of oxygen, and a variety of strategies have been published using $S_{cv}O_2$ as an end point for resuscitation. The most promising strategy was published by Rivers and coworkers in a group of patients with septic shock presenting to the emergency department. An early goal-directed resuscitation strategy aimed at achieving an $S_{cv}O_2$ of ≥70% resulted in a significant decrease in mortality (46.5% in the control group vs. 30.5% in the treatment group) [77]. Of interest, the mean age in the treatment group was 67.1 years (±17.4 SD).

Resuscitation with crystalloid, blood and the administration of vasopressors are all methods to improve tissue oxygen delivery [58]. Guidelines for the optimal use of these techniques are varied, and each approach is not without complications. Early restoration of circulating blood volume with blood products and crystalloid is crucial, especially in the elderly who are more dependent on effective ventricular filling to maximize cardiac output. In the early phase of resuscitation, fluids are probably superior to vasopressors for the maintenance of blood pressure [78]. Care, however, must be taken to avoid excessive amounts of crystalloid as this has been linked to cardiac and pulmonary complications, coagulopathy, and acid–base disturbances [79]. Transfusion of blood to restore adequate oxygen carrying capacity is vital in cases of frank anemia, but exact triggers for transfusion in the elderly are still debated. The Hebert study suggests a transfusion threshold value of <7 g/dl of hemoglobin, and this recommendation has been widely adopted. This study, however, excluded patients with chronic anemia, ischemic heart disease, or any patient in whom the attending physician was unwilling to tolerate a transfusion trigger of <7 g/dl [80]. In elderly patients with acute myocardial infarction, a lower 30-day mortality was associated with blood transfusion for hematocrit values <30% [81]. A hematocrit of <30% during operation is predictive of postoperative delirium [82]. Other studies have documented increased myocardial ischemia when intraoperative or postoperative hematocrit fell below 28% [83, 84]. Given the high incidence of ischemic cardiac disease – often silent in the elderly – care should be taken in setting a "one-size-fits-all" transfusion trigger in the geriatric population.

Once effective volume has been restored, inotropes may be required to augment oxygen delivery. The effects of aging can influence the choice of agents. In elderly patients, the response to β-agonists declines, with subsequent reduction in the inotropic, chronotropic, and vasodilatory effects of these medications. With these changes, nonadrenergic effects may be more pronounced. The stiffened aorta should also be taken into account, and the addition of afterload reducing agents may be useful [85]. With the geriatric patient, inotropic support may be required in atypical clinical settings such as septic shock. Viellard-Baron and coauthors found a high incidence of global left ventricular hypokinesia, defined as an ejection fraction of <45%, in a mixed group of patients presenting with septic shock (mean age 65 years). Hypokinesia was often present on initial evaluation. However, further cases were frequently unmasked after 24–48 h of therapy with norepinephrine, bringing the total incidence to about 60% [86]. This hypokinesia can be counteracted by the addition of inotropic agents such as dobutamine, the suggested inotrope for use in septic shock [87, 88]. After restoration of adequate circulating volume and the addition of inotropic support as needed to augment oxygen delivery, perfusion pressure should be maintained with vasopressors. In cases of severe sepsis, norepinephrine and dopamine are advocated as the initial vasopressors recommended in the Surviving Sepsis Guidelines, with a target mean arterial pressure of ≥65 mmHg [87, 88]. In summary, the clinician caring for the elderly patient with occult or overt shock must walk a fine line, using both fluids and inotropes, while paying close attention to detail. Frequent adjustments will be required as the clinical situation evolves.

Acute Kidney Injury and Renal Replacement Therapy

Changes in the Renal System Associated with Aging

The changes in renal function related to advancing age are significant in the management of critical illness. There are predictable declines in the glomerular filtration rate (GFR) and creatinine clearance. These declines, while significant, have little impact on the measured serum creatinine level, as there is a parallel reduction in the amount of creatinine produced. Fluid and electrolyte management deserves meticulous attention in the aged. With aging, homeostatic mechanisms become less capable of dealing with the fluid losses, acid–base disturbances, and electrolyte abnormalities often associated with surgery, trauma, and sepsis. Insensible losses are increased through surgery, wounds, and mechanical ventilation. The aging kidney is less able to concentrate urine and compensate for these losses. In addition, the normal thirst mechanism is often impaired in the geriatric patient. The net result is an increased propensity for hypovolemia, which can be particularly harmful in the elderly who rely on preload to maintain cardiac function. Compounding this

problem is the diminished capacity of the kidney to excrete acute salt and water loads, which can manifest as pulmonary insufficiency secondary to acute volume overload. Poor bicarbonate elimination also hampers renal compensation in acid–base disturbances. The key factors to successful management include meticulous attention to detail, frequent laboratory and physical assessment, and appropriate fluid administration to avoid any large or rapid changes in volume status, electrolytes, or acid–base loads.

Clinical Management

The incidence of acute kidney injury (AKI) increases with age and is 3.5 times more prevalent in those >70 years of age [89]. The etiology AKI is usually divided into three categories: prerenal, intrinsic, and postrenal. The elderly are especially vulnerable to prerenal AKI due to impaired autoregulation and high risk of hypovolemia. Prerenal causes include fluid losses, decreased intake and diuretic treatment, and reduced effective circulating blood volume secondary to impaired cardiac output, systemic vasodilatation, and renal artery stenosis. Acute tubular necrosis (ATN) accounts for up to 76% of cases of AKI in the ICU [90]. Although causes of AKI (hypovolemia, ATN, contrast induced nephropathy, NSAIDs, etc.) are no different in geriatric patients as compared younger ICU patients, age itself remains a major risk factor for the development of AKI in the ICU [91]. This may be due to the increased incidence of diabetes, hypertension, and underlying chronic kidney diseases in the elderly population.

The diagnostic approach to AKI should include a history and examination. A review of medications should focus on potential sources of kidney injury such as NSAIDs, intravenous contrast, diuretics, and angiotensin-converting enzyme inhibitors or angiotensin receptor blockers. Laboratory examination should include serum creatinine, urinalysis, urine electrolytes, urine creatinine, and osmolarity. These values can be used to determine the glomerular filtration rate and the fractional excretion of sodium. However, the fractional excretion of sodium is often confounded by diuretics in the elderly. Urine osmolarity, when <300 mOsm/kg, is indicative of intrinsic renal failure.

Management of AKI should first involve the treatment of life-threatening complications, such hyperkalemia, pulmonary edema, and metabolic acidosis. Second, all nephrotoxic agents should be discontinued. Finally, fluid and hemodynamic status should be optimized. Although still employed, there is no benefit to the use of "renal-dose" dopamine [92]. Furosemide may improve urine output, but it has no influence on return of renal function or survival, thus its utilization should be limited to maintaining fluid balance [93]. Mannitol has also been shown to have no efficacy in renal protection [93].

Outcomes: Renal Replacement Therapy

Renal replacement therapy (RRT) is required in approximately 85% of patients with oliguric renal failure and about 30% with nonoliguric renal failure [94]. Like tracheotomy, the initiation of RRT in the elderly is a significant decision point in the care of the elderly patient and should be approached with deliberation. Multiple recent studies have examined prognosis and outcomes following RRT during the course of critical illness. In a meta-analysis by Bagshaw, the mortality of ATN treated with RRT was reported at 46–74%. In studies confined to the critically ill, mortality was nearly 60% at 90 days. In the same analysis, quality of life was addressed, and studies consistently demonstrated lower global quality of life scores. However, survivors generally rated their quality of life acceptable [95]. In addition to survival, return of renal function, defined as freedom from RRT, is another important outcome measure. Schmitt and coworkers undertook a meta-analysis addressing recovery of kidney function after AKI in the elderly. They reported that 31.3% of the elderly did not recover function compared to 26% in younger patients (pooled RR, 1.28, 95% CI, 1.06–1.55). An interesting finding in their review was that the relative risk of nonrecovery was only slightly increased in the elderly when continuous RRT was used; however, this did not achieve statistical significance [96].

Nutrition

Body composition changes over the course of aging. Lean muscle mass is reduced up to 40% by the age of 80 with simultaneous increase in body fat. There is a corresponding decrease in muscle strength and decrease in resting energy expenditure by up to 15% [85]. As a result of this loss of muscle mass, the elderly patient may rapidly develop protein–energy malnutrition in the setting of acute illness and surgery. Ideally, nutritional support should be initiated within 24 h of admission to the ICU.

We routinely initiate "trickle feeds" as soon as vasopressor doses have stabilized and lactate levels are decreasing. Our preferred method of nutrition is the enteral route, with the choice of tube and position (gastric or postpyloric) determined by the clinical scenario. The use of early enteral nutrition in surgical patients has demonstrated reduced infection rates. No increase in the incidence of anastomotic failure has been documented, and there is a trend toward reduced mortality [97]. An audit of feeding practices by Taylor found that in patients greater than 64 years of age prolonged starvation (>5 days) resulted in higher mortality than those without nutrition 0–5 days, which was not found in younger patients. This suggested a greater susceptibility to starvation in the elderly [98]. Caloric requirements are reduced in the elderly; overfeeding

results in excess CO_2 production, mandating higher minute ventilation and should be avoided. Overfeeding will not decrease the amount of lean tissue loss, can increase fat synthesis, aggravated hyperglycemia, and can delay weaning from mechanical ventilation [99]. Deficiencies in micronutrients are common, and supplementation should be routine.

Impaired glucose tolerance increases with aging, and nearly 40% of the U.S. population over age 60 has either type 2 diabetes or impaired glucose tolerance. The mechanism of impaired glucose tolerance is a lifelong decline in insulin secretion by B-cells at a rate of 0.7% per year. No specific change in insulin sensitivity, as previously thought, has been identified [100]. Early evidence suggested that strict glycemic control may be beneficial for patients in the ICU with a decrease in mortality, especially when employed for more than 3 days [101, 102]. These initial findings generated controversy and concern over the risk of hypoglycemic events that occur during insulin therapy. The NICE-SUGAR study was undertaken to determine the best target for glycemic control in critical illness. In a study of over 6,000 ICU patients, subjects were randomized to intensive control or conventional control of blood sugar. The incidence of hypoglycemia was significantly greater in the intensive-control group (6.8% vs. 0.5%, $p < 0.001$). Mortality in this study was greater in the intensive-control group as well (27.5% vs. 24.9%, $p = 0.02$). The authors concluded that a blood glucose target of 180 mg/dl or less resulted in lower mortality than did a target of 81–108 mg/dl [103]. A growing problem faced by all clinicians is the epidemic of obesity. An increase in mortality has been documented with increase in BMI, and this trend continues in the elderly. Although not associated with an increase in mortality in the ICU, obesity is associated with increases in the duration of mechanical ventilation and ICU length of stay [104].

Caring for Dying Patients

Caring for dying patients is a natural part of working in the ICU, perhaps even more so with geriatric patients. A more complete discussion of palliative care and end-of-life decision making is presented in Chap. 18. However, this is such an integral part of caring for the geriatric ICU patient that it bears some repetition. Through experience, we have found that establishing consensus, providing open communication, and focusing on goals of therapy are effective tools in our daily practice.

Reaching Consensus

Before serious discussions with families, physicians need to have reached accord that curative therapy is not indicated. Of first importance in these discussions are an accurate diagnosis and an understanding of long-term outcomes. As we have outlined above, outcomes from critical illness in the elderly are influenced by prior health and functional status, the severity of the acute illness as manifested in the degree of physiologic derangement, and the specific diagnosis. We feel there is no justification for using chronologic age alone to predict the benefit to be obtained from intensive care or to exclude individuals from ICU care. In cases where a clear consensus cannot be obtained among physicians, we usually pursue curative care for a period of time, often 3–5 days. This is useful in the geriatric patient as it allows us to more accurately gauge their underlying physiologic reserve and response to treatment while allowing us to establish trust and rapport with the family.

Open Communication

When consensus among the health care team has been obtained, discussions with families regarding management must address the potential hazards during recovery from critical illness and thoughtful appraisal of the likely short-term and long-term outcomes. Other factors, such as expected life-span, HR-QOL, and potential pain and suffering associated with intensive care must be considered in the elderly. Although some patients may have an advanced directive or a "living will," we have found these documents are rarely helpful as they usually only apply to conditions that are unquestionably irreversible, such as persistent vegetative state. For example, an advance directive may not be helpful when treating a previously healthy and active septuagenarian who is now facing tracheotomy and possible long-term dialysis after surviving emergent repair of an abdominal aortic aneurysm.

End-of-life discussions are almost never concluded in a single setting and generally mature over time as the disease process and the patient's physiologic response becomes clear to both physician and family. It is helpful to have a single person in whom the family trusts lead the discussions. Trust from families is earned by being seen frequently at the patient's bedside. We have learned through sad experience that halls and patients' doorways are less than ideal locations for end-of-life discussions. Getting the setting right in a small conference room allows you to take control of the situation, provides an atmosphere where families and physicians can talk freely and gives at least the impression that you have the time sit and discuss the issues at length. We have found it important to avoid phrases such as "withdrawal of support" or "withdrawal of care." Instead, we emphasize with families that we alter our goal from cure to comfort – we provide a different kind of care. A comprehensive review of communicating "bad news" is beyond the scope of this chapter, but an excellent volume written by and for physicians has formed the foundation for our practice [105].

Goals of Therapy

Discussing goals of therapy and resolving conflicts can be problematic. Schneiderman and colleagues hypothesized that ethics consultations in the ICU reduce the use of life-sustaining treatments delivered to patients who ultimately do not survive to hospital discharge [106]. In a controlled trial, they randomized patients by site to early ethics consultation vs. standard care. The intervention involved ethics consultation in the ICU for conflicts and value disagreements either among the health-care team or between the team and patients or surrogates. Primary end points were ICU and hospital length of stay in patients who do not survive and patient/surrogate and health care provider satisfaction. The authors found that patients in the intervention group who died spent 3 fewer days in the hospital, 1.4 fewer days in the ICU, and 1.7 fewer days receiving mechanical ventilation than nonsurvivors in the control group. The authors concluded that ethics consultations reduced nonbeneficial care without increasing mortality. However, the intervention group had a slightly higher mortality rate (62.7% vs. 57.8%). Although this difference was not statistically significant, it may be meaningful. In a randomized trial, differences in outcomes that are not explained by differences in baseline characteristics or the concomitant interventions are usually attributed to the study intervention. It is not clear whether a higher mortality rate in this study would be good or bad.

In our own practice, we rarely have to resort to an ethics consultation to resolve conflicts regarding goals of therapy. We do not display a smorgasbord of options to patients and families and allow them to pick and choose a plateful of therapies. Instead, we present a therapeutic plan that is aimed at achieving a return to a quality of life that the patient would find acceptable. We are often forced to rely on heavily on information from family members and surrogates for our understanding of the patients' wishes regarding quality of life. We realize that understanding patients' wishes regarding quality of life and end-of-life decisions can be difficult. Cook and coworkers writing for the Canadian Critical Care Trials Group prospectively followed 851 patients with a mean age of 61.2 years who were receiving mechanical ventilation. Of these patients, 166 (19.5%) had mechanical ventilation withdrawn. Rather than age or the severity of the illness and organ dysfunction, the three strongest determinants of withdrawal of ventilation in critically ill patients were the physician's perception that the patient preferred not to use life support (hazard ratio, 4.19), the physician's prediction that the patient's likelihood of survival in the ICU was less than 10% (hazard ratio, 3.49), and a high likelihood of poor cognitive function (hazard ratio, 2.51) [107]. Surprisingly, Cook and coauthors did not find a significant relationship between withdrawal of ventilation and age, previous functional status, severity of illness, or severity of organ dysfunction. It should be concerning to all of us rendering care for elderly patients that the strongest determinate of withdrawal from mechanical ventilation was physicians' perception patients' wishes. Unfortunately, we know that patients' wishes regarding ICU admission or initiation of ventilation are frequently unknown at ICU admission [108]. In addition, patients' wishes may not correspond with the family members understanding of these wishes in elderly patients [109]. Finally, patients' assessments of their quality of life do not necessarily correlate with their wishes regarding life-sustaining therapy [83].

Despite these limitations, clinicians are daily called upon to make help families and surrogates navigate these waters with whatever information is available. When we feel that further critical care is unlikely to achieve a quality of life that would be acceptable – as previously defined in our discussions with patients when available or families and surrogates if not – we inform the patient or surrogates that we have done all that we can and that death or an unacceptable permanent debility is inevitable. For example, we would not broach renal replacement as a therapeutic option to the surrogates of nonagenarian with abdominal sepsis and multisystem organ failure. We admit that this approach may seem paternalistic, but we have found that families expect and appreciate this from physicians. The vast majority of families do not want to assume responsibility for a decision that they perceive as leading to the death of their patient, when in reality, it is often that the patient's disease process dictates the outcome. The decision surrogates are faced with is not whether death will occur, but how that death will happen. Occasionally, we are unable to reach a clear consensus with the family or surrogate decision makers. In these situations, we continue supportive therapy – usually with limitations about escalation – and reconvene the discussion in the near future. We have adopted this approach as it has been described by Cassell, a social anthropologist, who has studied extensively end-of-life decision making in the surgical ICU [110]. When employed properly, we have found this strategy effective in our daily practice without resort to ethics committees or outside intervention.

Process

For patients already in the ICU, the change in care from cure to comfort is best handled in the ICU. Patients and families are more at ease with staff they have come to know during their ICU stay. The challenge of titrating analgesia, removing invasive support, and managing family concerns are best met in the ICU. In this setting, our focus is on eliminating procedures, superfluous lines and tubes, and unnecessary medications while providing open visitation and effective analgesia [111]. Usually removing vasopressor therapy and reducing positive end-expiratory pressure to $0\ cmH_2O$ and the fraction of inspired oxygen to 25% will be all that is required. When weaning from mechanical ventilation, we typically switch to a pressure-targeted mode that delivers an adequate tidal volume and then titrate a short-acting narcotic infusion to a comfortable respiratory rate. We then decrease inspiratory pressures gradually while increasing the narcotics to keep a respiratory rate in the 14–20 breaths per minute range. Once inspiratory pressures are minimal, the patient can be extubated without concerns about distress or the bradypnea associated with bolus narcotic administration. This rapid, terminal weaning process is usually well tolerated by patients [112], avoids the gasping sometimes associated with terminal extubations done without a prior wean, and has been our practice at this institution since first described by Grenvik in 1983 [113]. We do not consider oxygen or feedings comfort measures. When mechanical ventilation has been removed and adequate analgesia obtained, a transfer out of the ICU to a more private atmosphere is usually in order. In conclusion, we have found that most of the difficulties regarding end-of-life care can be handled by assuring consensus among the health-care team prior to family discussions, establishing early, open, and honest communication between families and physicians and focusing on the overall goals of therapy while presenting a plan rather than multiple options.

Conclusion

Critical care of elderly patients both compares and contrasts with that of younger patients. It is different in that age has multifarious effects on all organ systems, and these age-related changes influence the way elderly patients respond to their critical illness and to treatment. It is similar in that the principles, procedures, techniques, and devices used to support organ system insufficiency or failure are the same and that with a comprehensive approach to care and close attention to detail many can survive their critical illness and resume a valued and enjoyable life.

References

1. Callahan D (1989) Old age and new policy. JAMA 261:905–906
2. Metcalfe MA, Sloggett A, McPherson K (1997) Mortality among appropriately referred patients refused admission to intensive-care units. Lancet 350:7–11

3. Azoulay E, Pochard F, Chevret S et al (2001) Compliance with triage to intensive care recommendations. Crit Care Med 29:2132–2136

4. Joynt GM, Gomersall CD, Tan P, Lee A, Cheng CA, Wong EL (2001) Prospective evaluation of patients refused admission to an intensive care unit: triage, futility and outcome. Intensive Care Med 27:1459–1465

5. Garrouste-Orgeas M, Montuclard L, Timsit JF, Misset B, Christias M, Carlet J (2003) Triaging patients to the ICU: a pilot study of factors influencing admission decisions and patient outcomes. Intensive Care Med 29:774–781

6. Garrouste-Orgeas M, Montuclard L, Timsit JF et al (2005) Predictors of intensive care unit refusal in French intensive care units: a multiple-center study. Crit Care Med 33:750–755

7. Sinuff T, Kahnamoui K, Cook DJ, Luce JM, Levy MM (2004) Rationing critical care beds: a systematic review. Crit Care Med 32:1588–1597

8. Angus DC, Kelley MA, Schmitz RJ, White A, Popovich J Jr (2000) Caring for the critically ill patient. Current and projected workforce requirements for care of the critically ill and patients with pulmonary disease: can we meet the requirements of an aging population? JAMA 284:2762–2770

9. Djaiani G, Ridley S (1997) Outcome of intensive care in the elderly. Anaesthesia 52:1130–1136

10. Kass JE, Castriotta RJ, Malakoff F (1992) Intensive care unit outcome in the very elderly. Crit Care Med 20:1666–1671

11. Knaus WA, Draper EA, Wagner DP, Zimmerman JE (1985) APACHE II: a severity of disease classification system. Crit Care Med 13:818–829

12. Knaus WA, Wagner DP, Draper EA et al (1991) The APACHE III prognostic system. Risk prediction of hospital mortality for critically ill hospitalized adults. Chest 100:1619–1636

13. Le Gall JR, Lemeshow S, Saulnier F (1993) A new Simplified Acute Physiology Score (SAPS II) based on a European/North American multicenter study. JAMA 270:2957–2963

14. Nicolas F, Le Gall JR, Alperovitch A, Loirat P, Villers D (1987) Influence of patients' age on survival, level of therapy and length of stay in intensive care units. Intensive Care Med 13:9–13

15. Margulies DR, Lekawa ME, Bjerke HS, Hiatt JR, Shabot MM (1993) Surgical intensive care in the nonagenarian. No basis for age discrimination. Arch Surg 128:753–756, discussion 6–8

16. Wu AW, Rubin HR, Rosen MJ (1990) Are elderly people less responsive to intensive care? J Am Geriatr Soc 38:621–627

17. McClish DK, Powell SH, Montenegro H, Nochomovitz M (1987) The impact of age on utilization of intensive care resources. J Am Geriatr Soc 35:983–988

18. Hennessy D, Juzwishin K, Yergens D, Noseworthy T, Doig C (2005) Outcomes of elderly survivors of intensive care: a review of the literature. Chest 127:1764–1774

19. Chelluri L, Grenvik A, Silverman M (1995) Intensive care for critically ill elderly: mortality, costs, and quality of life. Review of the literature. Arch Intern Med 155:1013–1022

20. Vazquez Mata G, Rivera Fernandez R, Gonzalez Carmona A et al (1992) Factors related to quality of life 12 months after discharge from an intensive care unit. Crit Care Med 20:1257–1262

21. Montuclard L, Garrouste-Orgeas M, Timsit JF, Misset B, De Jonghe B, Carlet J (2000) Outcome, functional autonomy, and quality of life of elderly patients with a long-term intensive care unit stay. Crit Care Med 28:3389–3395

22. Kaarlola A, Tallgren M, Pettila V (2006) Long-term survival, quality of life, and quality-adjusted life-years among critically ill elderly patients. Crit Care Med 34:2120–2126

23. Ridley S, Jackson R, Findlay J, Wallace P (1990) Long term survival after intensive care. BMJ 301:1127–1130

24. Zaren B, Bergstrom R (1989) Survival compared to the general population and changes in health status among intensive care patients. Acta Anaesthesiol Scand 33:6–12

25. Mayer-Oakes SA, Oye RK, Leake B (1991) Predictors of mortality in older patients following medical intensive care: the importance of functional status. J Am Geriatr Soc 39:862–868

26. Yinnon A, Zimran ARI, Hershko C (1989) Quality of life and survival following intensive medical care. QJM 71:347–357

27. Sage WM, Rosenthal MH, Silverman JF (1986) Is intensive care worth it? An assessment of input and outcome for the critically ill. Crit Care Med 14:777–782

28. Rockwood K, Noseworthy TW, Gibney RT et al (1993) One-year outcome of elderly and young patients admitted to intensive care units. Crit Care Med 21:687–691

29. Gee MH, Gottlieb JE, Albertine KH, Kubis JM, Peters SP, Fish JE (1990) Physiology of aging related to outcome in the adult respiratory distress syndrome. J Appl Physiol 69:822–829

30. Catley DM, Thornton C, Jordan C, Lehane JR, Royston D, Jones JG (1985) Pronounced, episodic oxygen desaturation in the postoperative period: its association with ventilatory pattern and analgesic regimen. Anesthesiology 63:20–28

31. Hall JC, Tarala RA, Hall JL, Mander J (1991) A multivariate analysis of the risk of pulmonary complications after laparotomy. Chest 99:923–927

32. Lawrence VA, Hilsenbeck SG, Mulrow CD, Dhanda R, Sapp J, Page CP (1995) Incidence and hospital stay for cardiac and pulmonary complications after abdominal surgery. J Gen Intern Med 10:671–678

33. Smetana GW (1999) Preoperative pulmonary evaluation. N Engl J Med 340:937–944

34. Kronenberg RS, Drage CW (1973) Attenuation of the ventilatory and heart rate responses to hypoxia and hypercapnia with aging in normal men. J Clin Invest 52:1812–1819

35. Peterson DD, Pack AI, Silage DA, Fishman AP (1981) Effects of aging on ventilatory and occlusion pressure responses to hypoxia and hypercapnia. Am Rev Respir Dis 124:387–391

36. Pontoppidan H, Beecher HK (1960) Progressive loss of protective reflexes in the airway with the advance of age. JAMA 174:2209–2213

37. Cohen IL, Lambrinos J (1995) Investigating the impact of age on outcome of mechanical ventilation using a population of 41,848 patients from a statewide database. Chest 107:1673–1680

38. Swinburne AJ, Fedullo AJ, Bixby K, Lee DK, Wahl GW (1993) Respiratory failure in the elderly. Analysis of outcome after treatment with mechanical ventilation. Arch Intern Med 153:1657–1662

39. Pesau B, Falger S, Berger E et al (1992) Influence of age on outcome of mechanically ventilated patients in an intensive care unit. Crit Care Med 20:489–492

40. Dardaine V, Constans T, Lasfargues G, Perrotin D, Ginies G (1995) Outcome of elderly patients requiring ventilatory support in intensive care. Aging (Milano) 7:221–227

41. Eachempati SR, Hydo LJ, Shou J, Barie PS (2007) Outcomes of acute respiratory distress syndrome (ARDS) in elderly patients. J Trauma 63:344–350

42. Esteban A, Anzueto A, Frutos F et al (2002) Characteristics and outcomes in adult patients receiving mechanical ventilation: a 28-day international study. JAMA 287:345–355

43. Esteban A, Anzueto A, Frutos-Vivar F et al (2004) Outcome of older patients receiving mechanical ventilation. Intensive Care Med 30:639–646

44. Visser LE, Graatsma HH, Stricker BH (2002) Contraindicated NSAIDs are frequently prescribed to elderly patients with peptic ulcer disease. Br J Clin Pharmacol 53:183–188

45. Brandi LS, Bertolini R, Janni A, Gioia A, Angeletti CA (1996) Energy metabolism of thoracic surgical patients in the early postoperative period. Effect of posture. Chest 109:630–637

46. Krieger BP, Ershowsky PF, Becker DA, Gazeroglu HB (1989) Evaluation of conventional criteria for predicting successful weaning

from mechanical ventilatory support in elderly patients. Crit Care Med 17:858–861

47. Ely EW, Wheeler AP, Thompson BT, Ancukiewicz M, Steinberg KP, Bernard GR (2002) Recovery rate and prognosis in older persons who develop acute lung injury and the acute respiratory distress syndrome. Ann Intern Med 136:25–36

48. Ely EW, Inouye SK, Bernard GR et al (2001) Delirium in mechanically ventilated patients: validity and reliability of the confusion assessment method for the intensive care unit (CAM-ICU). JAMA 286:2703–2710

49. Ely EW, Margolin R, Francis J et al (2001) Evaluation of delirium in critically ill patients: validation of the Confusion Assessment Method for the Intensive Care Unit (CAM-ICU). Crit Care Med 29:1370–1379

50. Sessler CN, Gosnell MS, Grap MJ et al (2002) The Richmond Agitation-Sedation Scale: validity and reliability in adult intensive care unit patients. Am J Respir Crit Care Med 166:1338–1344

51. McNicoll L, Pisani MA, Zhang Y, Ely EW, Siegel MD, Inouye SK (2003) Delirium in the intensive care unit: occurrence and clinical course in older patients. J Am Geriatr Soc 51:591–598

52. Ely EW, Siegel MD, Inouye SK (2001) Delirium in the intensive care unit: an under-recognized syndrome of organ dysfunction. Semin Respir Crit Care Med 22:115–126

53. Girard TD, Ely EW (2008) Delirium in the critically ill patient. Handb Clin Neurol 90:39–56

54. Kress JP, Pohlman AS, O'Connor MF, Hall JB (2000) Daily interruption of sedative infusions in critically ill patients undergoing mechanical ventilation. N Engl J Med 342:1471–1477

55. Tune LE, Bylsma FW (1991) Benzodiazepine-induced and anticholinergic-induced delirium in the elderly. Int Psychogeriatr 3:397–408

56. Pisani MA, Murphy TE, Araujo KL, Slattum P, Van Ness PH, Inouye SK (2009) Benzodiazepine and opioid use and the duration of intensive care unit delirium in an older population. Crit Care Med 37(1):177–183

57. Pandharipande PP, Pun BT, Herr DL et al (2007) Effect of sedation with dexmedetomidine vs lorazepam on acute brain dysfunction in mechanically ventilated patients: the MENDS randomized controlled trial. JAMA 298:2644–2653

58. Ouimet S, Kavanagh BP, Gottfried SB, Skrobik Y (2007) Incidence, risk factors and consequences of ICU delirium. Intensive Care Med 33:66–73

59. Morrison RS, Magaziner J, McLaughlin MA et al (2003) The impact of post-operative pain on outcomes following hip fracture. Pain 103:303–311

60. Eisendrath SJ, Goldman B, Douglas J, Dimatteo L, Van Dyke C (1987) Meperidine-induced delirium. Am J Psychiatry 144:1062–1065

61. Marcantonio ER, Juarez G, Goldman L et al (1994) The relationship of postoperative delirium with psychoactive medications. JAMA 272:1518–1522

62. Adunsky A, Levy R, Heim M, Mizrahi E, Arad M (2002) Meperidine analgesia and delirium in aged hip fracture patients. Arch Gerontol Geriatr 35:253–259

63. Inouye SK, Bogardus ST Jr, Charpentier PA et al (1999) A multicomponent intervention to prevent delirium in hospitalized older patients. N Engl J Med 340:669–676

64. Marcantonio ER, Flacker JM, Wright RJ, Resnick NM (2001) Reducing delirium after hip fracture: a randomized trial. J Am Geriatr Soc 49:516–522

65. Lundstrom M, Edlund A, Karlsson S, Brannstrom B, Bucht G, Gustafson Y (2005) A multifactorial intervention program reduces the duration of delirium, length of hospitalization, and mortality in delirious patients. J Am Geriatr Soc 53:622–628

66. Jacobi J, Fraser GL, Coursin DB et al (2002) Clinical practice guidelines for the sustained use of sedatives and analgesics in the critically ill adult. Crit Care Med 30:119–141

67. Leentjens AF, van der Mast RC (2005) Delirium in elderly people: an update. Curr Opin Psychiatry 18:325–330

68. Girard TD, Pandharipande PP, Ely EW (2008) Delirium in the intensive care unit. Crit Care 12(Suppl 3):S3

69. Milbrandt EB, Deppen S, Harrison PL et al (2004) Costs associated with delirium in mechanically ventilated patients. Crit Care Med 32:955–962

70. Ely EW, Shintani A, Truman B et al (2004) Delirium as a predictor of mortality in mechanically ventilated patients in the intensive care unit. JAMA 291:1753–1762

71. Jackson JC, Gordon SM, Hart RP, Hopkins RO, Ely EW (2004) The association between delirium and cognitive decline: a review of the empirical literature. Neuropsychol Rev 14:87–98

72. Kannel WB, Dannenberg AL, Abbott RD (1985) Unrecognized myocardial infarction and hypertension: the Framingham Study. Am Heart J 109:581–585

73. Abou-Khalil B, Scalea TM, Trooskin SZ, Henry SM, Hitchcock R (1994) Hemodynamic responses to shock in young trauma patients: need for invasive monitoring. Crit Care Med 22:633–639

74. Friese RS, Shafi S, Gentilello LM (2006) Pulmonary artery catheter use is associated with reduced mortality in severely injured patients: a National Trauma Data Bank analysis of 53,312 patients. Crit Care Med 34:1597–1601

75. Shah MR, Hasselblad V, Stevenson LW et al (2005) Impact of the pulmonary artery catheter in critically ill patients: meta-analysis of randomized clinical trials. JAMA 294:1664–1670

76. Velmahos GC, Demetriades D, Shoemaker WC et al (2000) Endpoints of resuscitation of critically injured patients: normal or supranormal? A prospective randomized trial. Ann Surg 232:409–418

77. Rivers E, Nguyen B, Havstad S et al (2001) Early goal-directed therapy in the treatment of severe sepsis and septic shock. N Engl J Med 345:1368–1377

78. Sperry JL, Minei JP, Frankel HL et al (2008) Early use of vasopressors after injury: caution before constriction. J Trauma 64:9–14

79. Cotton BA, Guy JS, Morris JA Jr, Abumrad NN (2006) The cellular, metabolic, and systemic consequences of aggressive fluid resuscitation strategies. Shock 26:115–121

80. Hebert PC, Wells G, Blajchman MA et al (1999) A multicenter, randomized, controlled clinical trial of transfusion requirements in critical care. Transfusion Requirements in Critical Care Investigators, Canadian Critical Care Trials Group. N Engl J Med 340:409–417

81. Wu WC, Rathore SS, Wang Y, Radford MJ, Krumholz HM (2001) Blood transfusion in elderly patients with acute myocardial infarction. N Engl J Med 345:1230–1236

82. Marcantonio ER, Goldman L, Mangione CM et al (1994) A clinical prediction rule for delirium after elective noncardiac surgery. JAMA 271:134–139

83. Nelson AH, Fleisher LA, Rosenbaum SH (1993) Relationship between postoperative anemia and cardiac morbidity in high-risk vascular patients in the intensive care unit. Crit Care Med 21:860–866

84. Hogue CW Jr, Goodnough LT, Monk TG (1998) Perioperative myocardial ischemic episodes are related to hematocrit level in patients undergoing radical prostatectomy. Transfusion 38:924–931

85. Rosenthal RA, Kavic SM (2004) Assessment and management of the geriatric patient. Crit Care Med 32:S92–S105

86. Vieillard-Baron A, Caille V, Charron C, Belliard G, Page B, Jardin F (2008) Actual incidence of global left ventricular hypokinesia in adult septic shock. Crit Care Med 36:1701–1706

87. Dellinger RP, Carlet JM, Masur H et al (2004) Surviving Sepsis Campaign guidelines for management of severe sepsis and septic shock. Crit Care Med 32:858–873

88. Dellinger RP, Levy MM, Carlet JM et al (2008) Surviving Sepsis Campaign: international guidelines for management of severe sepsis and septic shock: 2008. Crit Care Med 36:296–327

89. Pascual J, Orofino L, Liano F et al (1990) Incidence and prognosis of acute renal failure in older patients. J Am Geriatr Soc 38:25–30

90. Liano F, Junco E, Pascual J, Madero R, Verde E (1998) The spectrum of acute renal failure in the intensive care unit compared with that seen in other settings. The Madrid Acute Renal Failure Study Group. Kidney Int Suppl 66:S16–S24

91. de Mendonca A, Vincent JL, Suter PM et al (2000) Acute renal failure in the ICU: risk factors and outcome evaluated by the SOFA score. Intensive Care Med 26:915–921

92. Bellomo R, Chapman M, Finfer S, Hickling K, Myburgh J (2000) Low-dose dopamine in patients with early renal dysfunction: a placebo-controlled randomised trial. Australian and New Zealand Intensive Care Society (ANZICS) Clinical Trials Group. Lancet 356:2139–2143

93. Cheung CM, Ponnusamy A, Anderton JG (2008) Management of acute renal failure in the elderly patient: a clinician's guide. Drugs Aging 25:455–476

94. Star RA (1998) Treatment of acute renal failure. Kidney Int 54:1817–1831

95. Bagshaw SM (2006) The long-term outcome after acute renal failure. Curr Opin Crit Care 12:561–566

96. Schmitt R, Coca S, Kanbay M, Tinetti ME, Cantley LG, Parikh CR (2008) Recovery of kidney function after acute kidney injury in the elderly: a systematic review and meta-analysis. Am J Kidney Dis 52:262–271

97. Lewis SJ, Egger M, Sylvester PA, Thomas S (2001) Early enteral feeding versus "nil by mouth" after gastrointestinal surgery: systematic review and meta-analysis of controlled trials. BMJ 323:773–776

98. Taylor SJ (1993) Audit of nasogastric feeding practice at two acute hospitals: is early enteral feeding associated with reduced mortality and hospital stay? J Hum Nutr Diet 6:477–489

99. Reid C (2006) Frequency of under- and overfeeding in mechanically ventilated ICU patients: causes and possible consequences. J Hum Nutr Diet 19:13–22

100. Szoke E, Shrayyef MZ, Messing S et al (2008) Effect of aging on glucose homeostasis: accelerated deterioration of beta-cell function in individuals with impaired glucose tolerance. Diabetes Care 31:539–543

101. Van den Berghe G, Wouters P, Weekers F et al (2001) Intensive insulin therapy in the critically ill patients. N Engl J Med 345:1359–1367

102. Van den Berghe G, Wilmer A, Hermans G et al (2006) Intensive insulin therapy in the medical ICU. N Engl J Med 354:449–461

103. NICE-SUGAR Study Investigators (2009) Intensive versus conventional glucose control in critically ill patients. N Engl J Med 360(13):1283–1297

104. Akinnusi ME, Pineda LA, El Solh AA (2008) Effect of obesity on intensive care morbidity and mortality: a meta-analysis. Crit Care Med 36:151–158

105. Buckman R, Kason Y (1992) How to break bad news: a guide for health care professionals, 1st edn. John Hopkins University Press, Baltimore

106. Schneiderman LJ, Gilmer T, Teetzel HD et al (2003) Effect of ethics consultations on nonbeneficial life-sustaining treatments in the intensive care setting: a randomized controlled trial. JAMA 290:1166–1172

107. Cook D, Rocker G, Marshall J et al (2003) Withdrawal of mechanical ventilation in anticipation of death in the intensive care unit. N Engl J Med 349:1123–1132

108. Morrison RS, Olson E, Mertz KR, Meier DE (1995) The inaccessibility of advance directives on transfer from ambulatory to acute care settings. JAMA 274:478–482

109. Smucker WD, Houts RM, Danks JH, Ditto PH, Fagerlin A, Coppola KM (2000) Modal preferences predict elderly patients' life-sustaining treatment choices as well as patients' chosen surrogates do. Med Decis Making 20:271–280

110. Cassell J (2005) Life and death in intensive care, 1st edn. Temple University Press, Philadelphia

111. Brody H, Campbell ML, Faber-Langendoen K, Ogle KS (1997) Withdrawing intensive life-sustaining treatment – recommendations for compassionate clinical management. N Engl J Med 336:652–657

112. Campbell ML, Bizek KS, Thill M (1999) Patient responses during rapid terminal weaning from mechanical ventilation: a prospective study. Crit Care Med 27:73–77

113. Grenvik A (1983) "Terminal weaning"; discontinuance of life-support therapy in the terminally ill patient. Crit Care Med 11:394–395

Chapter 31
Care of the Injured Elderly

Jay Menaker and Thomas M. Scalea

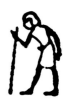

Injured Elderly

Trauma is the most common cause of death for those under the age of 44. Thus, some consider trauma to be exclusively a disease of the young [1]. However, as the population in the USA ages over the next several decades, the importance of falls and injuries in older patients will become more apparent. The elderly, defined as persons of age 65 or greater, [2–5] constitute one of the fastest growing segments of the US population. By the year 2030, the number of persons over age 65 will double relative to 2000, representing almost 20% of the nation's total population [6] (Fig. 31.1). This increase is the result of improvement in life expectancy and the aging baby boom generation. The Administration on Aging's Fiscal Year 2009 budget requested 1.381 billion dollars to assist in the long-term needs of these aging baby boomers [7].

In 2006, unintentional death was the fifth leading overall cause of death overall in the USA and the ninth for those over the age of 65 [8] (Table 31.1). Although the geriatric population in 2006 was approximately 12% of the total population [9], accidental deaths in this age group represented almost 31% of such deaths [8]. In 2006, the overall death rate from unintentional injury was 39.3 per 100,000 population [8]. However, in those between the ages of 65–74 years, it was 44 per 100,000, and for those over 74 years, it was 152.6 per 100,000. Decreased physical reserve, preexisting comorbidities, and a lack of provider understanding of the healthcare needs of older patients may all contribute to this finding [10].

Altered Physiology and Comorbidities

Aging causes changes in one's functional status and increases one's susceptibility to injury and mortality (Table 31.2). Progressive deterioration, which begins as subtle changes in the thirties, continues with increasing age. This rate of change varies from organ system to organ system and from individual to individual [11]. Advances in the treatment of debilitating medical conditions have enabled elders to live longer and healthier lives. This improvement in the quality of life allows them to remain physically active and mobile longer [12]. Ironically, an active life style has now been increasingly reported as a risk factor for injury in the elderly, including falls and motor vehicle crashes [13–15].

Preexisting medical conditions limit the ability of older persons to tolerate the increased physiologic demands associated with injury. "Resting organ function often is preserved, but the ability to augment performance in response to stress is greatly compromised" [16]. Comorbid conditions may also be the cause of the injury and, therefore, information must be carefully sought at the time of initial evaluation following the event. Treatment of the comorbid illness will likely be necessary in addition to that of the injury. Identifying the comorbidities may identify interventions to prevent recidivism.

By age 75, over two-thirds of injured patients have one or more chronic medical conditions [17] (Table 31.3). Bergeron et al. demonstrated that two-thirds of those over the age of 64 years had a comorbid disease [18]. In those who reached the age of 95 years, it was 81.5%. In another study, the incidence of having at least one preexisting medical condition was 29.4% for those between the age of 65 and 74 years, 34.7% for those between 75–84 years, and 37.3% for those over the age of 85 years [19]. These comorbidities are associated with decreased survival after trauma and independently predict mortality [15, 17, 18, 20–22]. Milzman et al. showed that mortality rose from 6.1% with one preexisting condition to 24.9% with three or more [17] (Table 31.4). Others have found similar results, demonstrating a two- to threefold

J. Menaker (✉)
Department of Surgery, University of Maryland Medical Center, R. Adams Cowley Shock Trauma Center, 22 S. Greene Street, Rm T1R60, Baltimore, MD 21201, USA
e-mail: jmenaker@umm.edu

R.A. Rosenthal et al. (eds.), *Principles and Practice of Geriatric Surgery*,
DOI 10.1007/978-1-4419-6999-6_31, © Springer Science+Business Media, LLC 2011

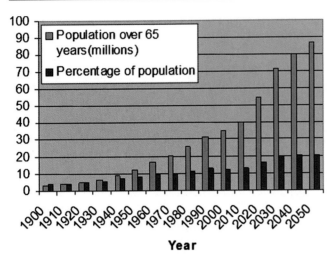

Figure 31.1 Population growth over time

Table 31.1 Causes of death

Leading causes of death (2006)	Leading causes of death, 65 years of age and older (2006)
Diseases of heart	Disease of heart
Malignant neoplasms	Malignant neoplasms
Cerebrovascular disease	Cerebrovascular disease
Chronic lower respiratory disease	Chronic lower respiratory disease
Accidents (unintentional injuries)	Alzheimer's disease
Alzheimer's disease	Diabetes mellitus
Diabetes mellitus	Influenza and pneumonia
Influenza and pneumonia	Nephritis, nephrotic syndrome
Nephritis, nephrotic syndrome	Accidents (unintentional)
Septicemia	Septicemia

Source: National Vital Statistics Reports, 11 June 2008

Table 31.2 Factors predisposing the elderly to injury

Reduced ability to react to environmental hazards
  Reduced hearing
  Presbyopia
  Significant degenerative joint disease
  Vertigo
Elderly placed in potentially dangerous situations
  Dementia
  Cardiovascular accident
  Coronary artery disease
    Dysrhythmias
    Myocardial infarction
    Postural hypotension
Increased consequences of injury
  Osteoporosis
  Cirrhosis
  Chronic obstructive pulmonary disease
  Coronary artery disease
  Disabling central nervous system disorders

The elderly may have chronic ailments that increase the likelihood and the consequences of injury

Table 31.3 Preexisting disease (PED) state vs. age

Age	15–24	25–34	35–44	45–54	55–64	65–74	>75
PED+	166	179	199	184	199	173	146
PED–	2,653	2,056	972	414	252	173	79
%PED+	5.8	8.0	17.0	30.8	44.1	50.0	64.9

Source: Reprinted with permission from Milzman et al. [17]

Table 31.4 Number of preexisting diseases and outcome

Number of PED	Survived	Died	Mortality (%)
0	6,341	211	3.2
1	868	56	6.1
2	197	36	15.5
≥3	67	22	24.9

Source: Reprinted with permission from Milzman et al. [17]

increase in hospital mortality rates for those older than 65 years as compared to younger counterparts [19, 23–25].

Once injured, the elderly may have an increased rate of complications from conditions such as cardiovascular or liver disease, diabetes, chronic obstructive pulmonary disease, and renal insufficiency. Smith and coworkers showed that complications occurred in 26% of their elderly population, the most common being infection (14.5%), followed by pulmonary (10.7%), cardiac (5.5%), and renal (3.7%) [26]. The authors also demonstrated that more than one complication following trauma was associated with a mortality of 30%. Bellemare et al. demonstrated that the elderly who developed pneumonia had significantly increased mortality compared to younger patients with pneumonia [27].

Influences of Senescence and Consequences of Comorbid Diseases

Senescence affects all organ systems but does so at varying degrees and at variable times during the aging process. Functional decline occurs in all organs. Increasing age may make it difficult to distinguish the impact of comorbid diseases on specific end-organ damage.

Central Nervous System

Subtle changes in cognition and memory are common in the elderly. Determining Glasgow Coma Scale (GCS) and distinguishing new neurologic findings from baseline can be problematic [28]. Dementia, hearing and visual difficulty, or fluctuation in an individual's baseline also make assessment of an elderly patient's mental status difficult. Family members will often be the best source of information to determine if an elderly patient is at baseline mental status. Once admitted to the hospital, the elderly patient may experience episodes of delirium, agitation, and confusion, even in the absence of injury. This can make it difficult to assess progression of brain injury.

Age-related brain atrophy between the 5th and 10th decade causes a reduction of approximately 15–20% of the cortical brain volume [28, 29]. A significant amount of blood can accumulate before neurologic symptoms appear [30]. Terry et al. demonstrated that the brain of an elderly person occupies only 82% of the skull, compared to 92% in younger individuals [31]. As the brain volume decreases, the dura remains adhered to the skull, causing an increase in the distance between the inner table of the skull and the outer surface of the brain. This lengthening causes the bridging veins to be pulled taut, thus rendering them more likely to sustain a shear-type injury during rotational stress, such as deceleration force in a motor-vehicle crash. Subdural hematomas are three times more common in the elderly. However, the risk of an epidural hematoma in the elderly is much lower because of the decrease in the epidural space [32].

Similarly, degenerative disease of the bony cervical spine narrows the central spinal canal and leads to an increased frequency of central cord syndrome, especially with extension-type forces [33]. Kato and colleagues demonstrated that degenerative changes and spinal stenosis represent important risk factors for cervical spine injuries [34]. In addition, degenerative changes can limit mobility and strength.

As the population ages, so does the portion of elderly persons who are "physically functional but cognitively impaired." For instance, patients with Alzheimer's disease have an additional 14–20% greater reduction in total cortical and forebrain brain volumes than expected during normal aging [28, 35]. One study documented 58.4 injuries per 100 person-years in patients with Alzheimer's disease [36]. More than 50% of those injured required treatment, and the likelihood of injury was associated with cognitive impairment and functional limitation.

Cardiovascular

With increasing age, myocardial contractility is depressed, and ventricular compliance falls for any given preload. The aged myocardium also fails to respond to heightened endogenous or exogenous catecholamines [37]. There is a fall in the maximum oxygen utilization, and maximum heart rate is reduced by about 30% between the age of 20 and 85 [38]. The incidence of dysrhythmia and subsequent syncope is increased, probably from conduction system ischemia [39]. Syncope may also be caused by medications, including β-blockers. Ventriculoarterial coupling is hampered by progressive arteriolar stiffening and loss of arterial elastance, leading to an increased frequency of orthostatic hypotension.

Cardiovascular disease is common in the elderly. Wilson described a 13.7% incidence of hypertension and 5.6% occurrence of symptomatic coronary artery disease (CAD) in a series of trauma patients over the age of 65. For those over 75 years of age, the incidence of symptomatic CAD was 12.9% [40]. More recently, Bochicchio et al. have demonstrated a 17% incidence of hypertension and a 9% incidence of CAD in a slightly younger (mean age of 43 years) cohort of critically ill trauma patients.[41].

Medications such as β-blockers, calcium channel blockers, or digoxin may blunt or inhibit tachycardia in response to acute intravascular volume loss and cloud the anticipated pattern of response to injury. In addition, CAD (especially right-sided coronary lesions) causes loss of autoregulation of coronary blood flow. Thus, as myocardial activity increases, the elderly can experience either occult or obvious cardiac ischemia with resultant pump failure [38]. In addition, some authors have reported as many as 78% of those over the age of 70 have amyloid deposits in the myocardium that can stiffen the heart and cause conduction defects and subsequent heart failure [11, 42].

The elderly cannot augment cardiac output and instead increase systemic vascular resistance [36]. This produces a falsely normal blood pressure and may very well correspond to profound shock. Scalea et al. have demonstrated that as many as 50% of those who had "normal" blood pressure in fact had evidence of occult cardiogenic shock and a subsequent poor outcome [16, 43].

Pulmonary

Elderly patients have a decreased respiratory reserve and decompensate quickly [44]. Decreases in respiratory function in the elderly result from changes in both the chest wall and the lungs [45, 46]. After the age of 30, a 4% per decade decrease in alveolar surface area results in a negative effect on gas exchange as well as forced expiratory flow [47]. Alveolar ducts enlarge, and the alveoli become flatter and shallower, reducing the area for gas exchange and leading to ventilation perfusion mismatch.

Decreases in chest wall compliance from anatomical changes such as kyphosis and a decline in respiratory muscle strength from muscle fiber atrophy lead to as much as 50% loss in maximal inspiratory and expiratory force [44]. Accessory muscles help to compensate for the decline in respiratory muscle atrophy. Lung elastance also progressively declines, causing a collapse of small airways and uneven alveolar ventilation. This results in increased closing volume of the lung.

Additionally, responses to hypoxia and hypercapnia are decreased by 50 and 40%, respectively [44]. The aging mucociliary function worsens, with fewer cilia per square centimeter. Secretion clearance is also impaired. This, in addition to poor dentition, increased oropharyngeal colonization, swallow dysfunction, and a decreased lower esophageal sphincter tone, predisposes the elderly to aspiration pneumonia and pulmonary infection [44]. Gram-negative organisms predominate in the oral flora, increasing the risk of pulmonary infection from aspiration [47].

Osteopenia of the thoracic cage may increase the rate of pulmonary contusions, rib fractures, and pneumo- and hemo-pneumothoraces as the bony thorax cannot absorb transmitted kinetic energy. Accordingly, flail chest in the elderly correlates with prolonged mechanical ventilation [48]. In those with a flail chest, age has been shown to be the strongest predictor of poor outcome and is directly proportional to mortality [49]. Elderly patients who sustain rib fractures have twice the mortality rate of younger patients with similar injuries [50]. The number of rib fractures increases, so does the incidence of pneumonia and death [50, 51]. Pain control is critical to allow deep breathing and prevent pulmonary complications.

Renal Disease

A number of structural changes occur in the kidney as one ages. Decrease in renal tubular length and thickening of basement membranes, as well as interstitial fibrosis and atherosclerosis of capillary beds, lead to ineffective secretion and resorption abilities of the aging kidney [32]. Between the age of 25 and 85, 40% of the nephrons become sclerotic. In addition, between the age of 30 and 85, there is a 20–25% decrease in renal mass, from renal cortical loss [52]. By age 80, the glomerular filtration rate (GFR) has decreased approximately 45%, but serum creatinine remains the same due to concomitant muscle mass loss [44]. Thus, serum creatinine for a given level of renal function is falsely low.

The lower GFR causes a diminished ability to concentrate urine in the aging kidney. A concomitant decrease in response to aldosterone and antidiuretic hormone further prevents the kidney from producing concentrated urine. Furthermore, diuretics prevent the aging kidney from concentrating the urine and make urine output a less reliable marker for renal perfusion in the elderly.

Once injured, the elderly who have renal insufficiency or failure may have additional problems. The platelet dysfunction commonly seen with renal failure may lead to prolonged bleeding even after minor trauma. Electrolyte disorders, most notably hyponatremia, hypo- or hyperkalemia, hypomagnesemia, and hypocalcemia may cause dysfunctional neural transmission, cardiac dysrhythmias, seizures, mental confusion, muscular weakness, or syncope.

Drugs used to evaluate and treat the older trauma victim may further impair renal function. Extensive imaging with iodinated contrast may damage already impaired renal parenchymal and tubular system and lead to contrast-mediated nephropathy. Nonsteroidal anti-inflammatory drugs (NSAIDs) are frequently used to treat pain and avoid the sedative effects of narcotics, but use of these agents is associated with a significant risk of interstitial nephritis. Life-threatening infections with gram-negative organisms may require aminoglycosides, but such therapy may induce renal dysfunction despite seemingly acceptable drug levels. Despite renal replacement therapies, acute renal failure in trauma patients results in a mortality rate of approximately 50%, regardless of cause [53–55].

Musculoskeletal

Degenerative joint disease is common in the elderly and results in limited range of motion around major axial joints and puts the individual at high risk of injury. Lean body mass decreases by 4% every 10 years after the age of 25 and 10% every 10 years after the age of 50 [32]. Osteoporosis, with loss of up to 60% of trabecular bone and 35% of cortical bone [30], has been cited as a major factor contributing to the high incidence of fractures seen in elderly trauma patients [56].

Aging also influences the site of cervical spine fractures. In younger patients, the lower cervical spine region is more mobile and is the location of many cervical spine injuries. However, in the elderly, the lower cervical spine is less mobile due to degenerative changes, and the more mobile region of C1 and C2 is more often the site of injuries in the elderly [57].

Gastrointestinal

There is decreased hepatic function in the elderly due to a 40% hepatic mass loss by the age of 80 [58, 59]. Preexisting liver dysfunction increases mortality after trauma [8, 20, 21]. Hepatic disease has the strongest effect on trauma mortality of all preexisting medical conditions and is associated with an increased mortality in elderly trauma patients with less severe injuries [8, 20]. Morris et al. demonstrated that cirrhosis, in trauma patients of any age, increased the risk of dying, with an odds ratio of 4.5 [21].

The elderly trauma patients are at an increased risk of intestinal infarction. Acute hemorrhage, neurogenic shock, or cardiac dysfunction from acute injury can all result in low flow states. In the elderly with underlying vascular calcification or mural thrombus, any decrease in flow can cause significant compromise to the bowel and result in intestinal ischemia. Additionally, geriatric patients often do not manifest peritoneal signs and tend not to localize pain, making the diagnosis difficult [32]. This lack of peritoneal irritation can be a result of decreased abdominal musculature. In addition, polypharmacy, dementia, or Alzheimer's can obscure the physical exam in the elderly, making the diagnosis of an intraabdominal injury more difficult.

Metabolic/Endocrine

By age 80, the elderly have lost almost 40% of their lean muscle mass [44]. During muscle breakdown for gluconeogenesis, critically ill patients lose a significant amount of muscle mass. As the elderly start with less muscle mass, the proportion of loss is greater [60]. Thus after injury, the elderly quickly become severely malnourished, and nutritional support should begin early. A 2005 Cochrane review on nutritional supplementation in the elderly suggested that early nutrition reduced unfavorable outcomes, long-term complications, and days spent in rehabilitation [61].

The most notable endocrinopathy of aging is glucose intolerance. This hyperglycemia is a result of both decreased secretion of insulin and increased resistance to insulin [11, 60, 62–64]. Increasing age is associated with an increase in serum glucose, but not an increase in insulin after mild or moderate trauma [63]. There is also a decrease in thyroid function and responsiveness to metabolic stress in the elderly. Aging cause fibrosis of the thyroid gland with a decrease in the amount of T3 released. This results in a lower basal metabolic rate [32]. The elderly also lose their natural responses to cold and are at a higher risk of hypothermia [65, 66]. Warming, therefore, should be implemented as quickly as possible after injury.

Epidemiology of Injury in the Elderly

Falls

Falls are the most common injury in the elderly. Most falls occur in or about the home, with the greatest number during winter [67]. Most tend to be ground-level falls, while falls from great heights are uncommon [30]. Between 30 and 40% of the population over 65 years of age who live in the community sustain a fall each year [68–73]. This is higher for persons living in long-term care facilities [69, 70, 72]. About 30–55% of falls in those over the age of 65 years cause minor injuries such as bruises and abrasions [73–75]. Fractures occur in 4–6%, 25% being hip fractures, while other major

injuries requiring hospitalization occur in an additional 2–10% [72, 76]. Elderly women are no more likely to fall, but sustain serious injury, usually fractures, more commonly than men [13, 77]. Men incur more CNS injuries and have higher mortality following falls [13]. This may be from higher risk-taking and underreporting of less severe fall injuries in men [13].

Inability to get up after a fall is common. In one study, 50% of the elderly could not get up without assistance from weakness or limited motion due to underlying musculoskeletal disabilities [77]. A large prospective study demonstrated that 14% of patients who fell were unable to get up after 5 min or more, and 3% of patients were down for longer than 20 min [73]. Another study showed that 41% of patients treated in an emergency room after a fall reported being unable to get up within 5 min, and 3% of patients lay on the floor for more than 3 h [78]. Prolonged down time can cause decubiti, dehydration, and even rhabdomyolysis.

Numerous studies [13, 76, 79, 80] have outlined the risk factors for falls among the elderly (Table 31.5). Debilitating chronic diseases such as parkinsonism, stroke, arthritis,

TABLE 31.5 Risk factors for falls and fall-related injuries

Chronic debilitating diseases
Parkinson's
Strokes
Arthritis
Anemia
Dementia
Neuromuscular disorders
Acute illnesses
Advanced age
Sensory impairments
Unsteady gait
Lower extremity weakness
Low body mass
Caucasian
Exercise[a]
Previous falls
Dependence for ADLs
Postural hypotension
Syncope
Dysrhythmias
Seizure
Carotid stenosis
Aortic stenosis
Medications
Benzodiazepines
Phenothiazines
Antidepressants
Diuretics
Laxatives
Diltiazem

ADLs activities of daily living
[a]Exercise has an inconsistent effect on the incidence of falls and fall-related injuries (see text)

dementia, and anemia are more prevalent in the population of elderly who sustain falls [81]. Among the other factors are older age, Caucasian race, history of previous falls, polypharmacy (especially psychotropic agents, diltiazem, laxatives, and diuretics), dependence for activities of daily living, low body mass and impaired mobility, muscle strength, gait, balance, vision, hearing, and cognition [73, 75, 76, 82]. These factors have all been correlated with an increased risk of falls and fall-related injury. The role of exercise as a risk factor is not clear. Exercise may lead to increased coordination and strength. While some studies have shown significant decreases in the incidence of falls, exercise also increases the exposure of the elderly to possible fall scenarios [81].

Falls amongst the elderly result from complex interactions of structural and physiologic disabilities. The consequences of a fall depend on such factors as the kinetic energy generated during the fall as well as the ability of the body structures to absorb and the fall surface to accept the energy. In addition, the protective responses, the garments of the faller, and the direction and body location of the impact will affect the outcome of the fall [77]. Functional consequences of the aging process along with an alteration in cognition may lead to increased risk-taking. Lack of realization of their limitations also predisposes the elderly to falls. Duthie suggested that approximately 25% of falls in the elderly were caused by an underlying medical problem [83]. Loss of muscle mass and changes in body composition result in decreased strength. Combined with a limited range of motion due to degenerative joint diseases, the elderly are less able to absorb the kinetic energy during a fall. Thus, many falls that are categorized as accidents are truly interactions between identifiable environmental hazards and increased individual susceptibility to those hazards from accumulated effects of age and disease [72]. Therefore, management of the elderly fall victim must include an investigation into the cause of the fall, which can frequently be determined from a thorough history.

Falls lead to life-altering consequences in the elderly. Approximately 8% of the elderly population seeks emergency care after a fall; 30–40% of older persons treated in the emergency department for a fall are hospitalized, with an average length of stay of 8–15 days [79, 84, 85]. In contrast to the younger patient seen in the ED after a fall, older patients usually do not die as a direct result of the fall. Instead, preexisting medical conditions and secondarily acquired complications are often the cause of death [21, 30]. As a result, complications from falls are the leading cause of death from injury in men and women over the age of 65 years [85].

The economic impact of falls in the elderly is huge. Numerous studies have attempted to estimate this financial impact; however, the wide variation on methodology makes it somewhat difficult to compare the results. Estimates range from $6.2 billion to $20 billion per year [86–89].

Motor Vehicle Collision

Motor vehicle collisions (MVC) are the second most common mechanism of injury in those 65 years of age and older. In 2005, over 177,000 elderly people suffered nonfatal injuries as a result of a MVC [90]. Injury pattern, however, is independent of age except for sternal fractures (11% elderly vs. 1.5% younger) [56]. Older drivers who are hospitalized after an MVC have significantly higher mortality rates, longer hospital stays, and are less likely to be discharged directly to their homes [91]. There is a greater frequency of intracranial hemorrhage and chest injury in the elder population that contribute to poor outcome as well. For similar injuries, older adults are five to six times more likely to die than their younger counterparts [30]. For those over 85 years of age, the fatality rate increases to seven to nine times that of younger drivers [92].

Elderly drivers appear to have lower crash rates compared with younger drivers, but they drive less often. When normalized for the number of miles driven, the >65 years group has the second highest crash rate after new drivers. The >85 years group has the highest per-mile-driven crash rate of all age groups. The elderly are more likely to be involved in vehicle–vehicle crashes, usually during daylight hours, close to home and frequently at intersections [93]. Cook et al. found that the elderly were no more likely to have a crash involving a right-hand turn but were more than twice likely to crash during a left-hand turn than younger drivers [94]. The elderly are also more likely to be found at fault by investigation officers [95].

Reduced vision or hearing, impaired judgment, and reduced reaction times are well recognized as factors leading to MVC in the elderly. Koepsell and coworkers showed that diabetes, especially when insulin-dependent, significantly increased the risk of a MVC with injury [96]. Rehm and Ross showed that elderly crash victims had a significantly higher incidence (74 vs. 14%) of underlying disease(s) such as cardiac, hypertension, diabetes, or neurologic diseases than did victims in the young cohort [95]. In addition, alcohol is less often involved in MVCs involving the elderly compared to younger drivers [95, 97].

Pedestrian–Motor Vehicle Collision

McCoy et al. showed the elderly were more likely to be involved in a pedestrian crash as a result of walking into oncoming vehicles, often due to confusion or impairment of visual or auditory acuity [56]. Reduced gait speed of the elderly pedestrian may be inadequate to complete the crosswalk at time-controlled traffic intersections, leaving the elder in the street exposed to inattentive drivers. In 1961, Haddon et al. demonstrated an increased risk of pedestrian crashes and fatalities with increasing age [98]. Others have corroborated this association [99, 100].

Burns

Deaths from burns are the fifth most common cause of unintentional injury death in the USA [101]. In 2005, there were approximately 3,200 fire/burn-related deaths in the USA. Of these, approximately one-third occurred in those over the age of 65 years [102], most of them sustained at home [103]. Diminished senses, impaired mentation, slower reaction time, reduced mobility, and bedridden states may decrease an elder's ability to identify fire and also to escape harm. This may result in a more severe injury and an increased likelihood of death [104].

Extensive burn in the elderly has a poor prognosis; however, the fatality rates from burns in this age group are variable. Lionelli et al. demonstrated an overall mortality of 47% in patients 75 years of age and older [105], while Covington et al. demonstrated a mortality of 60% in the same age group [106]. Lionelli also demonstrated a nearly 50% reduction in mortality when comparing rats in the 1970s to those in the 1980s and 1990s (77 vs. 41%). A study by McGill and colleagues demonstrated a 72% survival in the elderly burn victim when aggressive burn care was used [107].

The discharge of an elderly burn patient must be well thought out. For those with minor burns, returning to their home with some assistance will most likely be adequate. For those who have suffered more severe injury, rehabilitation will be required. Most importantly, for those who return home, an in-depth evaluation of home safety modification helps prevent recidivism.

Elder Abuse

The US National Academy of Sciences defines elder abuse as: "(a) intentional actions that cause harm or create a serious risk of harm to a vulnerable elder by a caregiver or other person who stands in a trust relationship to the elder or (b) failure by a caregiver to satisfy the elder's basic needs or to protect the elder from harm" [108]. The abuse includes physical, psychological, sexual, and financial, as well as neglect. Such injuries are considerably more subtle in their presentation than those from a physical assault.

Only 1 in 14 incidences of elder abuse come to the attention of the authorities [109]. Thomas estimated that the

TABLE 31.6 Risk factors for elder abuse

Increased frailty of the victim
Cognitive impairment of the victim
Mental illness of the abuser
Substance abuse by the abuser
Family history of violence or antisocial behavior
Victim and abuser live together
Isolation of the victim
Recent life stress

incidence of elder abuse ranges from 2 to 10% [110]. In a random-sample, community-based epidemiologic study, 3.2% of those surveyed reported to having been victims of either physical, or psychological abuse, or neglect since they turned 65 [109]. This number may underestimate the magnitude of the problem owing to the victim's reluctance to admit abuse for fear of loss of care, retribution from the abuser, or from being ashamed to be in an abusive relationship.

Risk factors should alert the healthcare provider to the diagnosis of abuse (Table 31.6) [111, 112]. Once suspicion is raised, the victim should be interviewed one-on-one to increase the likelihood of disclosure of the extent and details of the abuse. Victims may be embarrassed revealing such details to a group of health-care personnel. The details of the abuse should be documented completely in the medical record for the possibility of subsequent legal action. The physician who documents or suspects elder abuse is ethically obligated, and in most states legally bound, to report the case to an adult protective service agency.

The most important intervention is to protect the victim from danger. The victim may be reluctant to leave the care of their abuser because of ambivalence regardless of the perceived danger. Unless the victim lacks the cognitive skills to make informed decisions, individual liberty must not be compromised. The physician should interview the abuser in a nonconfrontational fashion to better understand the situation. The physician should acknowledge and empathize with the difficulty of shouldering the burden of elder care. Armed with this additional information, the physician is better prepared to intervene to break the abuse cycle.

Suicide

In 2004, suicide was the third leading cause of injury-related death for those 65 years of age and older [1]. Those over the age of 75 had the highest rate [113]. Only about 25% of the elderly who attempt suicide are actually successful [114]. Risk factors for suicide in the elderly population include psychiatric disorders, especially depression; medical conditions, especially cancer or chronic lung disease; moderate to heavy alcohol use; and social isolation. Changes in behavior such as altering a will, new preoccupation with religion, or giving away life possessions may be warning signs of impending suicide.

Management

Triage

Triage for the geriatric patient should provide the appropriate intensity of medical care, taking into account factors including severity of injury, cost, availability, prognosis for functional recovery, and patient desire. This process begins in the prehospital setting when decisions must be made regarding the appropriate facility [115]. In 2006, The American College of Surgery Committee on Trauma suggested that patients over the age of 55 years be triaged to a trauma center [116]. However, in reality, the elderly are the most undertriaged group and suffer increased morbidity and mortality as a result of underresuscitation [117].

Many of the physiologic and anatomic scores used in trauma correlate with outcomes in geriatric patients; however, these scores have little value in that they are not derivable at the time when triage decisions are made. The Trauma Score (TS), comprised of blood pressure, respiratory rate, respiratory effort, GCS, and capillary refill is readily obtainable and can be used to assist in triage. The minimal score is 0, and the maximal score is 16. The Revised Trauma Score (RTS) eliminates respiratory effort and capillary refill, resulting in a score range of 0–8. Osler et al. demonstrated that no patient with a TS<7 survived to reach the hospital and that no patient arriving at the hospital with a TS<9 survived the hospitalization [118]. Knudson and colleagues demonstrated a 100% mortality in those 65 years of age and older having a TS<7 [119]. This suggests that when geriatric patients have a TS<7, one must question the utility of aggressive treatment and resource allocation. A study of 374 patients over the age of 65 demonstrated an overall mortality of only 5% in those with a TS of 15 or 16, 25% in those with a TS of 12–14, and 65% in patients with a TS<12 [120]. These data suggest that appropriate triage and aggressive care, including admission to an ICU, for those with a TS of 7–14 may improve survival.

Initial Management and Resuscitation

The first few minutes of resuscitation of the elderly trauma victims differs very little from that of younger patients. Early intubation in the multi-injured elderly trauma patient should be considered as it reduces the work of breathing and may avoid progressive respiratory failure and cardiovascular collapse. As the elderly have limited cardiovascular reserve, they are vulnerable to hypotension from induction agents, and reduced doses should be used. In addition, limited pulmonary reserve may make preoxygenation difficult, causing rapid desaturation during intubation.

A normal blood pressure for a younger patient may be a relative hypotension for an elderly patient with history of hypertension. Geriatric patients are more likely to present in shock than younger patients matched for trauma and ISS [121]. In the Major Trauma Outcome Study (MTOS), Champion et al. showed that geriatric patients had four times the incidence of cardiovascular complications as the young cohort, supporting the importance of improving cardiovascular response of the elderly trauma patient to maximize survival potential [3].

Scalea and colleagues demonstrated that significant hemodynamic compromise occurs in elderly patients who were clinically stable after their initial evaluation for blunt trauma [43]. Over a 2-year period, all patients over the age of 65 who were hemodynamically stable after their initial resuscitation had pulmonary artery catheters (PACs) inserted. The authors defined patients to be in cardiogenic shock if they had a cardiac output (CO) of less than 3.5 L/M and/or a mixed venous saturation (MVO$_2$) of less than 50%. They demonstrated an increase in survival from 7 to 53% by early optimization of all patients with volume, inotropes, and afterload reduction. The authors concluded that emergent invasive monitoring identifies occult shock early and improves outcome. Schultz et al. performed a randomized trial of resuscitation in 70 patients with fractures of the hip [122]. The monitored group had a PAC placed, while the control group only had a central venous line placed. Despite numerous weaknesses in the study, the mortality for the monitored group was 2.9% and was 29% in the control group. In addition, DeMaria et al. concluded that aggressive treatment, including invasive monitoring, decreased mortality in trauma patients over 75 years of age [123]. To avoid potential complications associated with PACs, efforts have been made to develop alternative, less invasive techniques of cardiac output monitoring. Although initial studies have shown comparable accuracy and precision between the PAC and newer less invasive techniques, further studies are ongoing [124, 125].

Davis and Kaups showed that admission base deficit (BD) levels correlate with mortality in the geriatric population [126]. Although the authors used 55 years as their cutoff, a BD ≤−10 had an 80% mortality, −6 to −9 a 60% mortality, −3 to −5 a 23% mortality, and ≥−2 had an 18% mortality (Fig. 31.2). Other studies correlated the rate of serum lactate clearance after trauma with survival [127, 128]. Patients had a mortality rate over 75% if it took more than 48 h to normalize lactate.

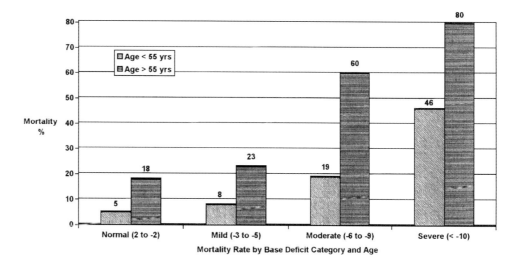

Figure 31.2 Mortality rate by base deficit category and age (reprinted with permission from Davis and Kaups [126]).

Management Considerations for Specific Injuries in the Elderly

Head Injuries

In persons 65 years of age and older, traumatic brain injury (TBI) is responsible for over 80,000 ED visits annually [129]. In 2006, over 2.8 billion dollars were spent on treating TBI in those older than 65 years [130]. Falls are the leading cause (51%), while MVCs are a distant second (9%) [129]. As many as 73% of elderly TBI patients may have at least one comorbid condition as compared to only 29% of younger patients [131]. Treatment of some of these chronic conditions includes the use of aspirin and warfarin, which increases the risk of TBI in the elderly. A study by Lavoie et al. found that 9% of the older patients with TBI were taking warfarin pre-injury and that it was associated with more severe TBI and a higher rate of mortality [132]. Older age has been well recognized as an independent predictor of worse outcome after TBI, even with relatively minor head injuries [133, 134] (Fig. 31.3). Older TBI patients also have been found to have longer length of stays, resulting in greater cost of care [135]. Significant TBI in the elderly can be caused by minimal trauma and may initially present with little or no neurologic deficits. In elderly patients with mild TBI (GCS 13–15), 14% of patients have a lesion on CT scan, four of which required neurosurgical intervention [136]. These authors recommended CT scan for patients over 65 years of age presenting with TBI. Due to the atrophy of the elderly brain, the distance traversed by the bridging veins is increased. This increased distance allows intracranial hemorrhages to have significant amount of room to expand prior to demonstrating any clinical signs. Thus, subdural hematomas are three times more common in the elderly [137].

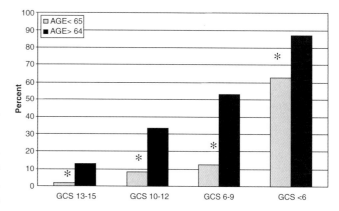

Figure 31.3 Percentage of elderly survivors and nonelderly survivors by GCS score (reprinted with permission from Susman et al. [134]).

Management of the head-injured elder is generally similar to that of the head-injured young patient: specifically rapid diagnosis of the specific neurologic injury using head CT scans and avoidance of secondary brain insult resulting from hypotension and hypoxia. Intracranial pressure (ICP) monitoring is paramount as is ensuring adequate cerebral perfusion pressure (CPP). A study by Czosnyka et al. demonstrated that ICPs decrease in the elderly, with a resultant increase in CPP [133]. The authors also demonstrated that there is a decrease in autoregulation in the elderly. Current guidelines for CPP management may not be appropriate for the elderly. Comorbidities may affect the responsiveness and perfusion needs of the cerebral vasculature in these patients.

Some studies have shown that preinjury warfarin use in the elderly had no effect on mortality in trauma patients [138, 139]. However, others have shown that it is, in fact, associated with increased frequency and severity of TBI, and a higher mortality [132, 140]. A study by Fortuna et al. demonstrated that those with a hemorrhagic brain injury on warfarin had a 34% mortality [141]. This was compared to those taking aspirin or clopidogrel, who had a mortality of 13 and 6%, respectively. All patients were similar in age and had similar ISS and head abbreviated injury score (AIS).

Any patient who has a traumatic hemorrhagic brain injury and an elevated INR should have the warfarin reversed. The risk of immediate mortality, related to the TBI, far outweigh risk for adverse thromboembolic events from the preexisting condition. Traditionally, fresh frozen plasma (FFP) has been used. Using a reversal protocol of 2 units of uncrossed FFP followed by an additional 2 U of matched FFP, Ivascu et al. demonstrated decreased reversal time from 4.3 to 1.9 h, with a subsequent improvement in mortality from 50 to 10% [142]. However, large volumes of FFP are often required to fully reverse warfarin. This can cause pulmonary edema and volume overload in the elderly patient with compromised cardiac and/or renal function. Alternatives to FFP do exist. Stein et al. demonstrated that a single dose on 1.2 mg of recombinant activated factor VIIa (rfVIIa) rapidly and effectively treats mild to moderate coagulopathy following injury [143]. In addition, they demonstrated that rfVIIa reduced the time to neurosurgical intervention (144 vs. 446 min) and decreased the use of blood products, without increasing the rate of thromboembolic complications [144]. In addition, despite having an increased pharmacy cost for those who have received rfVIIa, overall, the use of rfVIIa may actually decrease overall hospital charges [145]. Other alternatives include prothrombin complex concentrates (PCCs) as well as vitamin K and cryoprecipitate. Cartmill et al. demonstrated a more complete and quicker reversal time in patients on warfarin needing an emergent neurosurgical intervention using PCCs compared to FFP and vitamin K [146].

Elderly trauma patients on warfarin with TBI are particularly susceptible to clinical deterioration. In a recent study by Cohen et al., 56 of 77 patients with a GCS of 13–15 who were either discharged or admitted for observation had a clinical deterioration with a mortality rate greater that 80% [147]. As a result, any elderly patient on warfarin, with head trauma and a therapeutic INR, should be admitted and observed for a minimum of 12–24 h even if the initial head CT scan shows no injury [148]. A repeat CT scan should be done for any change in the patient's neurologic exam.

Spinal Injuries

Cervical fractures have a prevalence of 2.6–4.7% in patients older than 65 years [149, 150]. Low-energy falls are the most common mechanism among the elderly [151]. Injuries at the upper cervical region are associated with the longest hospital treatment. Golob et al. demonstrated a 22% in-hospital mortality in elderly patients with isolated cervical spine fractures [152].

Patients who are awake, alert, nonintoxicated, have no cervical tenderness, neurologic deficit, or distracting injury do not need any radiographic evaluation, regardless of age [153]. Although the three-view plain radiograph has been the traditional initial modality for cervical spine evaluation, many now use CT as the initial evaluation tool for cervical spine injury due to the high rate of missed injuries on plain films [154–159]. If a neurological deficit is present, then magnetic resonance (MR) should be used to evaluate ligamentous and/or spinal cord injury [160, 161].

Cervical stabilization is the primary end point, be it with a cervical collar, halo, or operation. A 1985 report by Pepin et al. stated that patients with odontoid fractures who were over the age of 75 years did not tolerate a halo and that surgical stabilization and an appropriate brace were superior [162]. Halo alone led to an increased rate of pneumonia and decubiti. In contrast, Malik et al. used a halo for ten patients over the age of 75 years, and most tolerated the halo relatively well [151]. Additionally, Weller et al. reported no complication with halo usage in patients over the age of 70 years [163]. The halo allows for mobilization in the early postinjury period, which is paramount in reducing complications.

Central cord syndrome (CCS), usually resulting from hyperextension, is more likely to occur in the elderly due to underlying cervical stenosis [93]. Patients usually present with upper extremity weakness that is greater than lower extremity weakness. A 1990 study by Penrod et al. demonstrated that at follow-up, 97% of younger patients with CCS were ambulatory, whereas only 41% of the elderly with CCS were able to walk. In addition, the younger patients with central cord syndrome achieved independence in self-care of bladder and bowel function more frequently than did the older group [164, 165]. DeVivo et al. demonstrated that the elderly, defined as those aged 61 years and older, had a 59% 2-year survival as compared to 95% in a younger cohort [166].

Thoracic Injuries

The elderly have a higher mortality from chest trauma as a result of the initial injury as well as secondary pulmonary insults [167, 168]. Routine use of cardiac enzymes, electrocardiogram (EKG), and echocardiography to identify cardiac injuries may be beneficial. Early intubation and mechanical ventilation should be considered for any elderly trauma patient that shows signs of respiratory compromise. Although intubation may increase pneumonia and the need for tracheostomy, the procedure may be lifesaving.

A number of studies have focused on rib fractures in the elderly and subsequent outcome. Cameron et al. demonstrated increased morbidity in the elderly with multiple fractures compared to younger patients [169]. In 2000, Bulger et al. retrospectively evaluated patients over the age of 65 years with rib fractures compared to those younger than 65 [50]. Despite similar ISS and chest abbreviated injury score (AIS), the elderly had fared significantly worse in all outcome measures (Table 31.7). Sharma and colleagues also demonstrated a twofold increase in mortality in the elderly with rib fractures [170]. Mortality increased as the number of rib fractures increased [50, 170] (Figs. 31.4 and 31.5).

Traumatic aortic injures (TAI) are often initially suspected by a widening of the mediastinum on a plain chest X-ray. Prior to the widespread use of CT scan, TAI was definitively diagnosed with the use of angiography. Over the last 10 years, there has been a significant change in the management of TAI from the traditional, standard operative repair (OR). A 1994 study by Camp et al. that compared OR in the young and the elderly demonstrated a 163-fold increased likelihood of mortality in the elderly [171]. In a 2006 study, Hirose et al. showed promise with nonoperative management in some high-risk elderly patients with small aortic tears [172].

Endovascular stent grafts (SG) were initially used for high-risk, multiply injured patients or those with comorbid disease, i.e., the elderly [173]. However, many centers now use them as their initial treatment of choice for TAI [174]. A 2008 multicenter American Association for the Surgery of Trauma (AAST) study compared 193 patients who had either an OR or endovascular SG for a TAI [174]. The study did not specifically breakdown outcome by age; however, using multivariable analysis, those over the age of 55 who received

TABLE 31.7 Outcome measures

Parameter	Age (years)		p Value
	≥65	18–64	
Mean ventilator days	4.3 ± 9.2	3.1 ± 9.2	=0.16
Mean ICU days	6.1 ± 10.0	4.0 ± 9.4	<0.05
Mean hospital days	15.2 ± 16.5	11.0 ± 13.1	<0.01
Mortality (%)	22	10	<0.001

Source: Reprinted from Bulger et al. [50] with permission from Wolters Kluwer Health
ICU intensive care unit

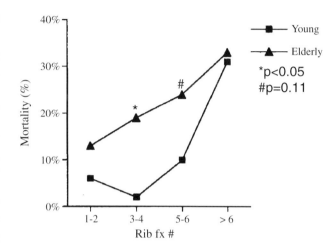

FIGURE 31.4 Relationship between mortality and number of rib fractures (reprinted with permission from Bulger et al. [50]).

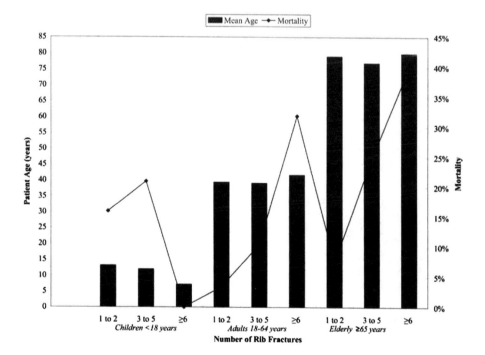

FIGURE 31.5 Mortality by number of rib fractures in all age groups (reprinted with permission from Sharma et al. [170]).

an endovascular SG had a significantly lower mortality. Unfortunately, the rates of long-term complications including delayed leak, migration, and thrombosis are currently unknown. It seems reasonable to assume an overall benefit for the elderly to have an SG placed as opposed to a thoracotomy performed.

Abdomen/Pelvis Injuries

Significant intraabdominal injury occurs in approximately one-third of elderly patients with multisystem trauma [175]. The clinical abdominal exam is less reliable in the elderly, and as such, liberal use of diagnostic studies is recommended [14, 175]. Ultrasound appears to be a reliable initial radiographic modality for evaluating an intraabdominal injury. Although free fluid on an ultrasound suggests an injury, it cannot differentiate between a solid organ injury and a hollow viscous injury. A study by Rozycki and colleagues demonstrated that ultrasound had an overall sensitivity of 83.3% and specificity of 99.7% [176]. In blunt trauma patients who were hypotensive (systolic blood pressure <90 mmHg), both sensitivity and specificity were 100%. Although the study did not evaluate the elderly per se, the oldest person in the study was 84 years old.

CT scan can be used to evaluate a hemodynamically stable patient to identify the presence of intraabdominal injuries. An IV contrast agent is typically used to better identify vascular injuries. This can often be problematic in the elderly for a number of reasons. Interactions with specific medication, such as metformin, can cause a lactic acidosis. In addition, contrast-induced nephropathy can be as high as 25% in patients with preexisting renal dysfunction, diabetes, advanced age, and concurrent usage of nephrotoxic drugs [177]. A meta-analysis suggested that pretreatment with N-acetylcysteine was most effective in preventing contrast-induced nephropathy [178]. However, most of the studies used pretreatment for 24 h, which is not feasible after injury. Merten et al. demonstrated that a protocol using pre- and posttreatment with bicarbonate was more effective than saline alone in preventing contrast nephropathy [179]. A 2006 review by Pannu et al. supports the use of hydration, bicarbonate, and low volumes of iso- or low-osmolar contrast in at-risk patients [180].

Nonoperative management of blunt splenic injuries has become standard of care. Early studies showed a high failure rate for those over the age of 55 years [181–183]. Recently, however, this has been challenged, and a number of studies have shown that age is not associated with increased failure rate [184–186]. Thus, age over 55 years is no longer considered a contraindication to nonoperative management of splenic injuries. Clinicians must monitor those with high-grade injuries and free pelvic fluid closely, as they have a higher failure rate.

Fractures

Hip fractures remain the most frequent cause of hospital admission after trauma in the elderly. Liberal use of CT scan or MR is wise in patients with high index of suspicion for fracture with negative plain radiographs [187]. Myers et al. showed that the mortality for men with hip fractures was 60% higher than for women [188]. In addition, factors associated with in-hospital death included sepsis, pneumonia, and gastrointestinal disorders. The risk of dying after hip fracture was doubled in patients with cardiac disease, cancer, or cerebrovascular disease. These authors concluded that the most important complication leading to in-hospital deaths after a hip fracture was sepsis.

Almost 30 years ago, Laskin et al. proposed a management scheme for intertrochanteric fractures in the elderly. This included early rigid fixation using compression hip screws to allow early mobilization and immediate weight bearing to assist with vigorous pulmonary toilet [189]. The longer the elderly remain bedridden, the more likely they are to have complications, including atelectasis, pneumonia, need for mechanical ventilation, venous thrombosis, muscle atrophy, and skin breakdown, all leading to longer hospital stay and increase in mortality. Thus, early orthopedic consultation, fracture fixation, and physical therapy are warranted.

Pelvic fractures are common in the elderly. A 2002 study by Henry et al. demonstrated that most elderly patients have lateral compression fractures, which are usually not associated with significant bleeding [190]. However, the authors found that the elderly are more likely to have fracture-associated hemorrhage and require angiography. In addition, the outcome for older patients with pelvic fractures was significantly worse than for younger patients. Recognizing these differences in fracture and bleeding patterns in the elderly identifies those at high risk and helps guide resuscitation.

Few studies have investigated management of other specific fractures in the elderly. Roumen et al. found that external fixation for unstable Colles' fractures was no more effective than nonoperative management in the elderly [191]. Ritchie et al. noted good limb salvage for open tibial fractures in patients over 60 years of age. Thus, age alone should not represent a contraindication to limb salvage in patients with severe open fractures and concomitant vascular injuries [192]. Helfet et al. reported that open reduction internal fixation (ORIF) of displaced acetabular fractures can yield good results in the elderly and obviate the need for a total hip replacement [193]. Bogner and colleagues demonstrated that a percutaneous reduction and internal fixation of the proximal humerus in patients over the age of 70 years provided a comfortable and mobile shoulder [194]. The authors state that this less invasive method provides a satisfactory alternative to replacement and traditional techniques of internal fixation.

Burns

Advances in burn care over the past 50 years have improved mortality rates across all age groups [195]. Although the elderly have a reduced rate of survival with less severe burns than their younger counterparts, the long-term outlook for those who do survive is somewhat optimistic. Manktelow et al. reported that 53% of those burned elders who survived did not have a more dependent living status on discharge [196]. Another 8% of patients achieved independent status within 5 years of the burn. Discharged patients did not have an accelerated death rate compared to that of the unburned population. In addition to the standard management of burn victims, the elderly present other challenges. The elderly burn victim may suffer hypoperfusion in the face of normal vital signs and adequate urine output. Bowser-Wallace et al. advocated hemodynamic monitoring for routine management of severe burns in the elderly [197]. They noted excellent survival in the elderly who were resuscitated with hypertonic lactated saline. Early wound closure has been viewed as a major advance in the management of young burn patients, resulting in decreased length of hospitalization and decreased mortality. Kara et al. demonstrated that early excision and grafting in the elderly yielded fewer episodes of infection, resulting in a reduction in hospital stay, but it did not improve survival [198]. Others have shown improvement in survival of elderly burn patients with early excision and grafting [199, 200].

Rehabilitation

The aim of rehabilitation is "to restore an individual to his/her former functional environmental status or, alternatively, to maintain or maximize remaining function" [201]. Unlike younger patients in whom rehabilitative outcomes are more apt to be dramatic, the geriatric patient is likely to make subtle progress. The degree of independence the patient is able to attain is dictated by these modest achievements and can mean the difference between living at home and living in a long-term care facility [201]. For many elders, independence is their ongoing reason to live. The physician caring for the injured elder must understand the importance of attaining or maintaining independence for their elderly patients and do whatever is necessary to achieve this. The elderly with chronic debilitating disease more frequently require rehabilitative services following trauma because of the limitations imposed by injury.

Long-Term Outcome

It is generally accepted that both short- and long-term outcomes after injury are considerably worse in the elderly than in younger patients. Despite this, The Eastern Association for the Surgery of Trauma (EAST) practice guidelines recommend that age should not be used as a criterion for limiting care as with aggressive initial management because as many as 85% return to independent living [117]. Others have demonstrated somewhat less promising outcomes of the injured elderly. A study of 38,000 patients over the age of 65 demonstrated that 50% went home and that 25% were discharged to a skilled nursing facility [202]. Taylor et al. demonstrated a nearly twofold increase in mortality risk in geriatric trauma patients even after controlling for comorbid diseases [5]. Inaba et al. reported in a study of injured elderly that, at long-term follow-up, only 68% of patients were living independently as compared to 98% before injury. Furthermore, an additional 20% required skilled home care [203].

Prevention

The first step toward prevention of injury is to recognize the individuals who are most likely to suffer injuries. Many of the factors that predispose the elderly to injury should be discovered on routine history-taking in the elderly patient. There are three injury-prevention approaches: (1) preevent strategies, focusing on increasing public awareness through education or influencing legislation, (2) event strategies, which involve interventions to reduce energy transfer during the injury, and (3) postevent strategies, which deal with efforts to improve resuscitation and reduce complications. In the elderly trauma population, the first two hold the most promise.

As an example, geriatric care groups have developed interventions such as home safety inspections, modifying medications known to affect balance adversely, gait training, and improving any correctable sensory deficits in an effort to reduce the incidence of falls. MVCs may potentially be avoided by identifying and reporting individuals who are unfit drivers. This includes persons with visual or hearing deficits, dementia, or disabling musculoskeletal disorders, and those using medications that decrease driving skills. In an effort to refresh skills and update traffic knowledge, driver education courses for adults over 55 years of age have been established by the American Association of Retired Persons (AARP) and the National Retired Teachers Association. Retting et al. showed that a pedestrian accident-prevention program significantly reduced the fatal and serious injury occurrence by 43 and 86%, respectively [204]. This program implemented prolongation of traffic-light times to accommodate the decreased gait of the elderly, modifications of road and crosswalk signs, tighter speed-limit enforcement, and safety-education presentations at senior centers.

End of Life/Withdrawal of Care

End-of-life and withdrawal-of-care discussions are often very difficult for families as well as the care providers. Although many elderly have advanced directives or living wills prior to getting injured, many do not. Despite good intention, the documents are often not helpful. It is then left to members of the patient's family to help guide the physician to provide the care the patient would want. It is often difficult to get the families to understand that they are to make decisions based on what their loved one would want, not what they would want.

The discussion regarding end of life and withdrawal of care is often a multistep process. The decision not to perform cardiopulmonary resuscitation or to intubate is often the first decision that families make. Often, it takes families some time to come to the reality that despite all medical advances, their loved will not survive. It is imperative to get as many family members as possible that want to be involved in the decision process together at one time. Although there is a hierarchy of legal decision makers, having all family members agree on the decision, can be critical. Utilizing pastoral care and or palliative care services often makes the process easier for all involved.

When the decision is made by the family to withdraw care, the physician must ensure a smooth process. Some families want to be present during the removal of life support, some do not. Adequate narcotics and sedatives help prevent any additional suffering. In addition, adequate medication can help minimize any visual discomfort, especially during removal from the ventilator. Turning off monitors and intravenous pumps and ensuring a quiet peaceful atmosphere for the patient and family enhances the family's experience.

CASE STUDY

AB, a 77-year-old female, with past medical history of atrial fibrillation, hypertension, and osteoporosis, was a restrained driver involved in a motor-vehicle collision. The patient was t-boned on the driver side by a car traveling at approximately 45 miles/h. On arrival, she denies any loss of consciousness, complains of some left-sided hip pain, which is worse with movement. In addition, she complains of left-sided chest pain, which is worse with deep inspiration. She denies any abdominal pain or back pain.

Past medical history: atrial fibrillation, hypertension, and osteoporosis

Past surgical history: appendectomy

Medications: warfarin, aspirin, metoprolol, alendronate, and multivitamin.

Allergies: none

Social history: denies alcohol, tobacco, or drug use

Family history: noncontributory

Physical Exam

Vital signs:

Height – 65 in.
Weight – 65 kg
Heart rate – 70 beats/min
Blood pressure – 105/60 mmHg

Respiratory rate – 30 breaths/min, shallow in nature
Oxygen saturation – 95% on 6 L by nasal cannula
EKG – rate-controlled atrial fibrillation

On exam, there is a left-sided scalp hematoma and small laceration that is not currently bleeding. The patient has significant left-sided rib tenderness on palpation; no subcutaneous soft tissue air is appreciated. She also has significant right hip and pelvis pain on palpation. The pelvis does not appear to be unstable. Distal extremities are cool to the touch. Pulse is intact. All other aspects of the physical exam are normal.

Lab work:

Sodium – 139 mmol/L	Chloride – 109 mmol/L
Potassium – 4.0 mmol/L	Bicarbonate – 19 mol/L — Glucose – 100 mg/dl
BUN – 35 mg/dl	Creatinine – 1.75 mg/dl
White blood cell count – 12 k/mcl	INR – 2.1
Hemoglobin – 10 g/dl	PTT – 30 s
Hematocrit – 32.0%	PT – 19.5 s
Platelets – 175 k/mcl	

Serial cardiac enzymes are normal
Lactic acid – 4.5 mmol/L

Arterial blood gas:

pH – 7.30
pCO_2 – 40 mmHg
pO_2 – 90 mmHg
O_2 Saturation – 95%
Base deficit – 6.5 mmol/L

(continued)

CASE STUDY (continued)

Radiographs:

Chest X-ray – multiple left-sided rib fractures, no pneumothorax, no hemothorax

CT scan

Head – scalp contusion, no intraparenchymal hemorrhage
Cervical spine – degenerative changes, no acute fractures or subluxations
Chest with IV contrast – left-sided rib fractures 5–10, no pneumothorax, small hemothorax, normal aorta
Abdomen/pelvis with IV contrast – left-sided inferior and superior rami fracture. Left-sided sacral fracture. Active extravasation in the pelvis. No solid or hollow viscous organ injury

Things to Consider

1. Early intubation in an elderly person with multiple rib fractures and labored breathing.
2. Insertion of an epidural catheter for administration of narcotics to assist with pulmonary toilet in setting of multiple rib fractures.
3. Mild hypotension and normal heart rate in setting of acute trauma may be related to medications patient is taking, i.e., beta blockers.
4. Administration of IV contrast for CT scan in the elderly patient with a decreased GFR and creatinine clearance.
5. The need for warfarin reversal in lieu of active bleeding in the pelvis.
6. The method by which warfarin can be reversed.
7. The need for invasive monitoring in the elderly trauma patient.

Hospital Course

AB received 2 U of fresh frozen plasma, which corrected her INR to 1.5. Her elevated INR and the fact that she has been on aspirin precluded her from getting an epidural catheter for pain management. However, she did receive a patient-controlled analgesia (PCA) pump to help with pain control and assist in pulmonary toilet.

Due to AB's signs of hypoperfusion including cold extremities, acidosis, and base deficit, a pulmonary artery catheter was placed. Initial cardiac index was 1.8 L/min/m^2, and mixed venous oxygen saturation was 55%. She was started on 2.5 mcg/kg/min of dobutamine, and a transthoracic echocardiogram was ordered.

Based on her abdominal and pelvic CT scan, it was felt that AB would best benefit from an interventional radiology consult, for possible embolization to stop her pelvic bleeding. At this time, AB was ordered a bicarbonate infusion as a strategy to help protect her renal function in the setting of an additional IV dye load. In addition, orthopedics was consulted regarding her pelvic fracture.

AB had successful angioembolization of pelvic bleeding; however, upon arrival at the intensive care unit, her work of breathing had increased. This was most likely multifactorial in nature, including volume from the fresh frozen plasma, volume from the bicarbonate infusion as well as supine posture for the angiographic procedure. AB was subsequently intubated for airway protection and maintenance of adequate oxygenation and ventilation.

The next day, AB had a repeat head CT to rule out delayed intraparenchymal hemorrhage, which was negative. The transthoracic echocardiogram demonstrated mildly depressed left ventricular function with an ejection fraction of 35% and no other abnormalities. Repeat lab values were significant for a decrease in hematocrit to 23% and a rise in the creatinine to 2.1 mg/dl; however, AB had adequate urine output. Because of the decreased hematocrit, she received 2 U of packed red blood cells. Following the transfusion, her cardiac index and mixed venous saturation were 2.9 L/min/m^2 and 68% respectively. Thus, AB was weaned off her dobutamine without incident.

Six days into her hospital course, AB was weaning from the ventilator, hemodynamically stable, and the pulmonary artery catheter had been removed. At this point, it was felt safe to place an epidural catheter for pain management to help facilitate extubation. AB was successfully extubated; however, approximately 36 h later, she was reintubated due to increased work of breathing and dropping oxygen saturation. After a discussion with her family as well as AB, it was determined that the safest thing for her was, as there was a likelihood of getting her successfully off the ventilator, to perform a tracheostomy. On day 9 of her hospital stay, AB had a tracheostomy performed and within 48 h, she was off the ventilator. She subsequently passed a swallow study and was able to eat on her own. Thirteen days after admission, AB was transferred to a rehabilitation center for further care.

References

1. CDC (2008) 10 Leading causes of death by age group, United States – 2004. National Center for Injury Prevention and Control, Office of Statistical Programming, Atlanta
2. Osler T, Baker SP, Long W (1997) A modification of the injury severity score that both improves accuracy and simplifies scoring. J Trauma 43:922–926
3. Champion HR, Copes WS, Buyer D et al (1989) Major trauma in geriatric patients. Am J Public Health 79:1278–1282
4. Grossman MD, Miller D, Scaff DW et al (2002) When is elder old? Effect of preexisting conditions on mortality in geriatric trauma. J Trauma 52:242–246
5. Taylor MD, Tracy JK, Meyer W et al (2002) Trauma in the elderly: intensive care unit resource use and outcome. J Trauma 53:407–414
6. US Census Bureau (2005) 65+ in the United States. US Census Bureau, Suitland
7. U.S. Administration on Aging, Department of Health and Human Services, Washington DC (2008) http://www.aoa.gov. Accessed 4 Nov 2008
8. Heron MP, Hoyert DL, Xu J, Scott C, Tejada-Vera B (2008) Death: preliminary data for 2006. Natl Vital Stat Rep 56:1–52
9. US Census Bureau (2007) Age data of the United States. Current Population Survey, Annual Social and Economic Supplement, Suitland, 2006
10. American College of Surgeons (2004) Advanced trauma life support for doctors, 7th edn. American College of Surgeons, Chicago, pp 263–274
11. Boss GR, Seegmiller JE (1981) Age-related physiological changes and their clinical significance. West J Med 135:434–440
12. Rosenbloom S (1988) The morbidity needs of the elderly. In: Transportation in an aging society. Special Report 218. Transportation Research Board, National Research Council, Washington, DC, p 21
13. Sattin RW, Lambert Huber DA, DeVito CA et al (1990) The incidence of fall injury events among the elderly in a defined population. Am J Epidemiol 131:1028–1037
14. Schwab CW, Kauder DR (1992) Trauma in the geriatric patient. Arch Surg 127:701–706
15. Viano DC, Culver CC, Evans L et al (1990) Involvement of older drivers in multi-vehicle side-impact crashes. Accid Anal Prev 22:177–188
16. Scalea TM (1996) Invited Commentary (for McMahon et al.: Co-morbidity and trauma in the elderly). World J Surg 20:116
17. Milzman DP, Boulanger BR, Rodriguez A et al (1992) Preexisting disease in trauma patients: a predictor of fate independent of age and ISS. J Trauma 32:236–243
18. Bergeron E, Rossignol M, Osler T et al (2004) Improving the TRISS methodology by restructuring age categories and adding com-morbidities. J Trauma 56:760–767
19. Hannan EL, Waller CH, Farrell LS et al (2004) Elderly trauma inpatients in New York state: 1994–1998. J Trauma 56:1297–1304
20. McGwin G Jr, MacLennan PA, Fife JB et al (2004) Preexisting conditions and mortality in older trauma patients. J Trauma 56:1291–1296
21. Morris JA Jr, MacKenzie EJ, Edelstein SL (1990) The effect of pre-existing conditions on mortality in trauma patients. JAMA 263:1942–1946
22. Mann NC, Cahn RM, Mullins RJ, Brand DM, Jurkovich GJ (2001) Survival among injured geriatric patients during construction of a statewide trauma system. J Trauma 50:1111–1116
23. Nagy KK, Smith RF, Roberts RR et al (2000) Prognosis of penetrating trauma in elderly patients: a comparison with younger patients. J Trauma 49:190–193
24. Perdue PW, Watts DD, Kaufmann CR, Trask AL (1998) Differences in mortality between elderly and younger adult trauma patients: geriatric status increases risk of delayed death. J Trauma 45:805–880
25. van der Sluis CK, Klasen HJ, Eisma WH et al (1996) Major trauma in young and old: what is the difference? J Trauma 40:78–82
26. Smith DP, Enderson BL, Maull KL et al (1990) Trauma in the elderly: determinants of outcome. South Med J 83:1717
27. Bellemare JF, Tepas JJ 3rd, Imani ER et al (1996) Complications of trauma care: risk analysis pneumonia in 10,001 adult trauma patients. Am Surg 62:207–211
28. Mouton PR, Martin LJ, Calhoun ME et al (1998) Cognitive decline strongly correlates with cortical atrophy in Alzheimer's dementia. Neurobiol Aging 19:371–377
29. Pakkenberg B, Gundersen HJ (1997) Neocortical neuron number in humans: effect of age and sex. J Comp Neurol 384:312–320
30. Mandavia D, Newton K (1998) Geriatric trauma. Emerg Med Clin North Am 16:257–274
31. Terry RD, DeTeresa R, Hansen LA (1987) Neocortical cell counts in normal human adult aging. Ann Neurol 21:530–539
32. Schulman CI, Alouidor R, McKenney MG (2008) Geriatric trauma. In: Feliciono DU, Mattex KL, Moore EE (eds.) Trauma, 6th edn. McGraw Hill, New York, pp 1003–1018
33. McGoldrick JM, Marx JA (1989) Traumatic central cord syndrome in a patient with os ondontoideum. Ann Emerg Med 18:1358–1361
34. Kato H, Kimura A, Sasaki R et al (2008) Cervical spinal cord injury without bony injury: a multicenter retrospective study of emergency and critical care centers in Japan. J Trauma 65(2):373–379
35. Regeur L, Jensen GB, Pakkenberg H et al (1994) No global neocorticol nerve cell loss in brains from patients with senile dementia of the Alzheimer's type. Neurobiol Aging 15:347–352
36. Oleske DM, Wilson RS, Bernard BA et al (1995) Epidemiology of injury in people with Alzheimer's disease. J Am Geriatr Soc 43:741–746
37. Lakatta EG (1980) Age-related alterations in the cardiovascular response to adrenergic mediated stress. Fed Proc 39:3173–3177
38. Lakatta EG, Levy D (2003) Arterial and cardiac aging: major share-holders in cardiovascular disease enterprises: Part II: the aging heart in health: links to heart disease. Circulation 107:346–354
39. Watters JM, McClaran JC (1991) The elderly surgical patient. In: The American college of surgeons: care of the surgical patient, vol 1. Scientific American, New York
40. Wilson RF (1994) Trauma in patients with pre-existing cardiac disease. Crit Care Clin 10:461–506
41. Bochicchio GV, Joshi M, Bochicchio K et al (2005) Incidence and impact of risk factors in critically ill trauma patients. World J Surg 30:114–118
42. Anous MM, Heimbach DM (1986) Causes of death and predictors in burned patients more than 60 years of age. J Trauma 26:135–139
43. Scalea TM, Simon HM, Duncan AO et al (1990) Geriatric blunt multiple trauma: improved survival with early invasive monitoring. J Trauma 30:129–134
44. Marik PE (2006) Management of the critically ill geriatric patient. Crit Care Med 34:176s–182s
45. DeLorey DS, Babb TG (1999) Progressive mechanical ventilatory constraints with aging. Am J Respir Crit Care Med 160:169–177
46. Zeleznik J (2003) Normative aging of the respiratory system. Clin Geriatr Med 19:1–18
47. Carpo RO (1998) Aging of the respiratory system. In: Fisherman AP (ed) Pulmonary diseases and disorders. McGraw Hill, New York, p 251
48. Allen JE, Schwab CW (1985) Blunt chest trauma in the elderly. Am Surg 51:697–700
49. Albaugh G, Kann B, Puc MM et al (2000) Age-adjusted outcomes in traumatic flail chest injuries in the elderly. Am Surg 66:978–981
50. Bulger E, Arneson MA, Mock CN et al (2000) Rib fractures in the elderly. J Trauma 48:1040–1047
51. Bergeron E, Lavoie A, Clas D et al (2003) Elderly trauma patients with rib fractures are at a greater risk for death and pneumonia. J Trauma 54:478–485
52. Beck LH (2000) The aging kidney. Defending a delicate balance of fluid and electrolytes. Geriatrics 55(26–28):31–32

53. Morris JA, Mucha P, Ross SE et al (1991) Acute post-traumatic renal failure: a multi-center perspective. J Trauma 31:1584–1590

54. Belzberg H, Cornwell EE, Berne TV (1996) The critical care of the severely injured patient II: pulmonary and renal support. Surg Clin North Am 76:971–983

55. Kunz A, Glinz W, Keusch G, Binswanger U (1984) Acute kidney failure in patients with multiple injuries. Schweiz Med Wochenschr 114:876–879

56. McCoy GF, Johnston BA, Duthie RB (1989) Injury to the elderly in road traffic accidents. J Trauma 29:494–497

57. Spivak JM, Weiss MA, Cotler JM et al (1994) Cervical spine injuries in patients 65 and older. Spine 19:2302–2306

58. Woodhouse KW, Mutch E, Williams FW et al (1984) The effect of aging on pathways of drug metabolism in human liver. Age Ageing 13:328–334

59. Kampmann JP, Sindinh J, Moller-Jorgensen I (1975) Effect of aging on liver function. Geriatrics 30:91–95

60. Robinson A (1995) Age, physical trauma and care. Can Med Assoc J 152:1453–1455

61. Avenell A, Handell HH (2005) Nutritional supplementation for hip fracture aftercare in older people. Cochrane Database Syst Rev 2:CD001880

62. Scheen AJ (2005) Diabetes mellitus in the elderly: insulin resistance and/or impaired insulin secretion? Diabetes Metab 31:5S27–5S34

63. Desai D, March R, Watters JM (1989) Hyperglycemia after trauma increases with age. J Trauma 28:719–723

64. Jeevanadam M, Petersen SR, Shamos RF (1993) Protein and glucose fuel kinetics and hormonal changes in elderly trauma patients. Metabolism 42:1255–1262

65. Wagner JA, Robinson S, Mariano RP (1974) Age and temperature regulation of humans in neutral and cold environments. Appl Physiol 37:562–565

66. Inoue Y, Nakao M, Araki T et al (1992) Thermoregulatory responses of young and older men to cold exposure. Eur J Appl Physiol Occup Physiol 65:492–498

67. Sjogren H, Bjornstig U (1991) Injuries to the elderly in the traffic environment. Accid Anal Prev 23:77–86

68. King MB, Tinetti ME (1996) A multifactorial approach to reducing injurious falls. Clin Geriatr Med 12:745–759

69. Thapa PB, Brockman KG, Gideon P et al (1996) Injurious falls in nonambulatory nursing home residents: a comparative study of circumstances, incidence, and risk factors. J Am Geriatr Soc 44:273

70. Tinetti ME, Liu W, Ginter SF (1992) Mechanical restraint use and fall-related injuries among residents of skilled nursing facilities. Ann Intern Med 116:369

71. Rubenstein LZ, Josephson KR (2002) The epidemiology of falls and syncope. Clin Geriatr Med 18:141

72. Rubenstein LZ (2006) Falls in older people: epidemiology, risk factors and strategies for prevention. Age Ageing 35:ii37–ii41

73. Nevitt MC, Cummings SR, Hudes ES (1991) Risk factors for injurious falls: a prospective study. J Gerontol Med Sci 46: M164–M170

74. Nevitt MC, Cummings SR, Kidd S et al (1989) Risk factors for recurrent nonsyncopal falls: a prospective study. JAMA 261:2663–2668

75. O'Loughlin JL, Robitaille Y, Boivin JF et al (1993) Incidence of and risk factors for falls and injurious falls among the community-dwelling elderly. Am J Epidemiol 137(3):342–354

76. Tinetti ME, Speechley M, Ginter SF (1988) Risk factors for falls among elderly persons lining in the community. N Engl J Med 319:1701–1707

77. Tinetti ME, Doucette J, Claus E (1995) Risk factors for serious injury during falls by older persons in the community. J Am Geriatr Soc 43:1214–1221

78. Tinetti ME, Liu W, Claus EB (1993) Predictors and prognosis of inability to get up after falls among elderly persons. JAMA 269:65–70

79. Grisso JA, Schwarz DF, Wolfson V et al (1992) The impact of falls in an inner-city elderly African-American population. J Am Geriatr Soc 40:673–678

80. Nelson RC, Amin MA (1990) Falls in the elderly. Emerg Med Clin North Am 8:309–324

81. Herndon JG, Helmick CG, Sattin RW et al (1997) Chronic medical conditions and risk of fall injury events at home in older adults. J Am Geriatr Soc 45:739–743

82. Kannus P, Parkkari J, Koskinen S et al (1999) Fall-induced injuries and deaths among older adults. JAMA 281:1895–1899

83. Duthie EH Jr (1989) Falls. Med Clin North Am 73:1321–1336

84. Sjogren H, Bjornstig U (1991) Injuries among the elderly in the hoke environment. J Aging Health 3:107–125

85. Sattin RW (1992) Falls among older persons: a public health perspective. Annu Rev Public Health 13:489–508

86. Englander F, Hodson TJ, Terregrossa RA (1996) Economic dimensions of slip and fall injuries. J Forensic Sci 41:733–746

87. Carroll NV, Slattum PW, Cox FM (2005) The cost of falls among the community dwelling elderly. J Manag Care Pharm 11: 307–316

88. Finkelstein E, Corso PS, Miller TR (2006) Incidence and economic burden of injuries in the United States. Oxford University Press, New York

89. Stevens JA, Corso PS, Finkelstein EA et al (2006) The costs of fatal and non-fatal falls among older adults. Inj Prev 12:290–295

90. Centers for Disease Control and Prevention (2006) Web-based injury statistics query and reporting system (WISQARS). National Center for Injury Prevention and Control, Centers for Disease Control and Prevention, Atlanta. http://www.cdc.gov/ncipc/wisqars. Accessed 16 Nov 2008

91. Bauza G, LaMorte WW, Burke PA et al (2008) High mortality in elderly drivers is associated with distinct injury pattern: analysis of 187m869 injured drivers. J Trauma 64:304–310

92. NHTSA (2008) Traffic safety facts 2007. Older populations. National Highway Traffic Safety Administration, Washington, DC. Accessed 16 Nov 2008

93. D'Andrea CC (2001) Geriatric trauma. In: Ferrera PC et al (eds) Trauma management: an emergency medicine approach. Mosby, St. Louis, MO, pp 533–545

94. Cook LJ, Knight S, Olson LM et al (2000) Motor vehicle crash characteristics and medical outcomes among older drivers in Utah, 1992-1995. Ann Emerg Med 35:585–591

95. Rehm CG, Ross SE (1995) Elderly drivers involved in road crashes: a profile. Am Surg 61:435–437

96. Koepsell TD, Wolf ME, McCloskey L et al (1994) Medical conditions and motor vehicle collision injuries in older adults. J Am Geriatr Soc 42:695–700

97. Quinlan KP, Brewer RD, Siegel P et al (2005) Alcohol-impaired driving among U.S. adults: 1993–2002. Am J Prev Med 28:346–350

98. Haddon W, Valien P, McCarroll J et al (1961) A controlled investigation of the characteristics of adult pedestrians fatally injured by motor vehicles in Manhattan. J Chronic Dis 14:655–678

99. Lane PL, McClafferty KJ, Nowak ES (1994) Pedestrians in real world collisions. J Trauma 36:231–236

100. Demetriades D, Murray J, Martin M et al (2004) Pedestrian injured by automobiles: relationship of age to injury type and severity. J Am Coll Surg 199:382–387

101. Centers for Disease Control and Prevention (2005) Web-based injury statistics query and reporting system (WISQARS). National Center for Injury Prevention and Control, Centers for Disease Control and Prevention, Atlanta. http://www.cdc.gov/ncipc/wisqars. Accessed 16 Nov 2008

102. Kung H-C, Hoyert DL, Xu J et al (2008) Deaths: final data for 2005. Natl Vital Stat Rep 56:1–121

103. Redlick F, Cooke A, Gomez M et al (2002) A survey of risk factors for burns in the elderly and prevention strategies. J Burn Care Rehabil 23:351–356

104. Barillo DJ, Goode R (1996) Fire fatality study: demographics of fire victims. Burns 22:85–88

105. Lionelli GT, Pickus EJ, Beckum OK et al (2005) A three decade analysis of factors affecting burn mortality in the elderly. Burns 31:958–963

106. Covington DS, Wainwright DJ, Parks DH (1996) Prognostic indicators in the elderly patient with burns. J Burn Care Rehabil 17:222–230

107. McGill V, Kowal-Vern A, Gamelli RL (2000) Outcome for older burn patients. Arch Surg 135:320–325

108. Bonnie RJ, Wallace RB (2003) Elder Mistreatment: abuse, neglect and exploitation in an aging America. National Academy Press, Washington, DC

109. Pillemer K, Finkelhor D (1988) The prevalence of elder abuse: random sample survey. Gerontologist 28:51–57

110. Thomas C (2002) First national study of elder abuse and neglect: contrast with results from other studies. J Elder Abuse Neglect 12:1–14

111. Lachs MS, Pillemer K (1995) Abuse and neglect of elderly persons: current concepts. N Engl J Med 332:437–443

112. Cammer Parris BE, Meier DE, Goldstein T et al (1995) Elder abuse and neglect: how to recognize warning signs and intervene. Geriatrics 50(4):47–51

113. Centers for Disease Control and Prevention (2005) Web-based injury statistics query and reporting system (WISQARS). National Center for Injury Prevention and Control, Centers for Disease Control and Prevention, Atlanta. http://www.cdc.gov/ncipc/wisqars. Accessed 24 Nov 2008

114. Goldsmith SK, Pellmar TC, Kleinman AM et al (2002) Reducing suicide: a national imperative. National Academy Press, Washington, DC

115. Jacobs DG, Plaisier BR, Barie PS et al (2003) Practice management guidelines for geriatric trauma: the EAST practice management guidelines work group. J Trauma 54:391–416

116. Committee on Trauma, American College of Surgeons (2006) Resources for the optimal care of the injured patient, 2006. American College of Surgeons, Chicago

117. Ma MH, MacKenzie EJ, Alcorta R et al (1999) Compliance with prehospital triage protocols for major trauma patients. J Trauma 46:168–175

118. Osler T, Hales K, Baack B et al (1988) Trauma in the elderly. Am J Surg 156:537–543

119. Knudson MM, Lieberman J, Morris JA Jr et al (1994) Mortality factors in geriatric blunt trauma patients. Arch Surg 129:448–453

120. Pellicane JV, Byrne K, DeMaria EJ (1992) Preventable complications and death from multiple organ failure among geriatric trauma victims. J Trauma 33:440–444

121. Clancy TV, Ramshaw DG, Maxwell JG et al (1997) Management outcomes in splenic injury: a statewide trauma center review. Ann Surg 226:17–24

122. Schultz RJ, Whitfield GF, LaMurra JJ et al (1985) The role of physiologic monitoring in patients with fractures of the hip. J Trauma 45:309–316

123. DeMaria EJ, Kenney PR, Merriam MA et al (1987) Survival after trauma in geriatric patients. Ann Surg 206:738–743

124. Goedje O, Hoeke K, Lichtwarck-Aschoff M et al (1999) Continuous cardiac output by femoral arterial thermodilution calibrated pulse contour analysis: comparison with pulmonary arterial thermodilution. Crit Care Med 27:2407–2412

125. Halvorsen PS, Espinoza A, Lundblad R et al (2006) Agreement between PiCCO pulse-contour analysis, pulmonary artery thermodilution and transthoracic thermodilution during off-pump coronary artery bypass surgery. Acta Anaesthesiol Scand 50:1050–1057

126. Davis JW, Kaups KL (1998) Base deficit in the elderly: a marker of severe injury and death. J Trauma 45:973–977

127. Abramson D, Scalea TM, Hitchcock R et al (1993) Lactate clearance and survival following injury. J Trauma 35:584–588

128. Rady MY, Rivers EP, Nowak RM (1996) Resuscitation of the critically ill in the ED: responses of blood pressure, heart rate, shock index, central venous oxygen saturation, and lactate. Am J Emerg Med 14:218–225

129. Langlois JA, Rutland-Brown W, Thomas KE (2004) Traumatic brain injury in the United States: Emergency department visits, hospitalizations and deaths. National Center for Injury Prevention and Control, Atlanta

130. Agency for Health Quality and Research (2008) Statistics on hospital stays. http://www.hcupnet.ahrq.gov. Accessed 26 Nov 2008

131. Mosenthal AC, Livingston DH, Lavery RF et al (2004) The effect of age on functional outcome in mild traumatic brain injury: 6-month report of a prospective multicenter trial. J Trauma 56:1042–1048

132. Lavoie A, Ratte S, Clas D et al (2004) Preinjury warfarin use among elderly patients with closed head injuries in a trauma center. J Trauma 56:802–807

133. Czosnyka M, Balestreri M, Steiner L et al (2005) Age, intracranial pressure, autoregulation, and outcome after brain trauma. J Neurosurg 102:450–454

134. Susman M, DiRusso SM, Sullivan T et al (2002) Traumatic brain injury in the elderly: increased mortality and worse functional outcome at discharge despite lower injury severity. J Trauma 53:219–224

135. Thompson HJ, McCormick WC, Kagan SH (2006) Traumatic brain injury in older adults: epidemiology, outcomes and future implications. J Am Geriatr Soc 54:1590–1595

136. Mack LR, Chan SB, Silva JC et al (2003) The use of head computed tomography in elderly patients sustaining minor head trauma. J Emerg Med 24:157–162

137. Demarest GB, Osler TM, Clevenger FW (1990) Injuries in the elderly: evaluation and initial response. Geriatrics 45:36–38

138. Wojcik R, Cipolle MD, Seislove E et al (2001) Preinjury warfarin does not impact outcome in trauma patients. J Trauma 51:1147–1152

139. Kennedy DM, Cipolle MD, Pasquale MD et al (2000) Impact of preinjury warfarin use in elderly trauma patients. J Trauma 48:451–453

140. Karni A, Holtzman R, Bass T et al (2001) Traumatic head injury in anticoagulated elderly patient: a lethal combination. Am Surg 67:1098–1100

141. Fortuna GR, Mueller EW, James LE et al (2008) The impact of preinjury antiplatelet and anticoagulant pharmacotherapy on outcomes in the elderly patients with hemorrhagic brain injury. Surgery 144:598–605

142. Ivascu FA, Janczyk RI, Junn FS et al (2006) Treatment of trauma patients with intracranial hemorrhage on preinjury warfarin. J Trauma 61:318–321

143. Stein DM, Dutton RP, Hess JR et al (2008) Low-dose recombinant factor VIIa for trauma patients with coagulopathy. Injury 39:1054–1061

144. Stein DM, Dutton RP, Kramer ME et al (2008) Recombinant factor VIIa: decreasing time to intervention in coagulopathic patients with severe traumatic brain injury. J Trauma 64:620–627

145. Stein DM, Dutton RP, Kramer ME, Scalea TM (2009) Reversal of coagulopathy in patients with traumatic brain injury: recombinant factor VIIa is more cost effective than plasma. J Trauma 66(1):63–72

146. Cartmill M, Dolan G, Byrne JL et al (2000) Prothrombin complex concentrate for oral anticoagulant reversal in neurosurgical emergencies. Br J Neurosurg 14:458–461

147. Cohen DB, Rinker C, Wilberger JE (2006) Traumatic brain injury in anticoagulated patients. J Trauma 60:553–557

148. Itshayek E, Rosenthal G, Fairfield S et al (2006) Delayed posttraumatic subdural hematoma in elderly patients on anticoagulation. Neurosurgery 58:851–856

149. Bub LD, Blackmore CC, Mann FA et al (2005) Cervical spine fractures in patients 65 years and older: a clinical prediction rule for blunt trauma. Radiology 234:143–149

150. Ngo B, Hoffman JR, Mower WR (2000) Cervical spine injury in the very elderly. Emerg Radiol 7:287–291

151. Malik SA, Murphy M, Connolly P et al (2008) Evaluation of morbidity, mortality and outcome following cervical spine injuries in elderly patients. Eur Spine J 17:585–591

152. Golob JF Jr, Claridge JA, Yowler CJ et al (2008) Isolated cervical spine fractures in the elderly: a deadly injury. J Trauma 64:311–315

153. Hoffman JR, Mower W, Wolfson AB et al (2000) Validity of a set of clinical criteria to rule out injury to the cervical spine in patients with blunt trauma. National emergency x-radiography utilization study group. N Engl J Med 343:94–99

154. Diaz JJ, Aulino JM, Collier B et al (2005) The early work-up for isolated ligamentous injury in the cervical spine: does computed tomography scan have a role? J Trauma 59.897–904

155. Besman A, Kaban J, Jacobs L et al (2003) False-negative plain cervical spine x-rays in blunt trauma. Am Surg 69:1010–1014

156. Woodring JJ, Lee C (1993) Limitations of cervical radiography in the evaluation of acute cervical trauma. J Trauma 34:32–39

157. Nunez DB Jr, Zuluaga A, Fuentes-Bernardo DA et al (1996) Cervical spine trauma: how much more do we learn by routinely using helical CT? Radiographics 16:1307–1321

158. Mower WR, Hoffman JR, Pollack CV et al (2001) Use of plain radiography to screen for cervical spine injuries. Ann Emerg Med 38:1–7

159. Barba CA, Taggert J, Morgan AS et al (2001) A new cervical spine clearance protocol using computed tomography. J Trauma 51:652–657

160. D'Alise MD, Benzel EC, Hart BL (1999) Magnetic resonance imaging evaluation of the cervical spine in the comatose or obtunded trauma patient. J Neurosurg 91:54–59

161. Benzel EC, Hart BL, Ball PA et al (1996) Magnetic resonance imaging for the evaluation of patients with occult cervical spine injury. J Neurosurg 85:824–829

162. Pepin JW, Bourne RB, Hawkins RJ (1985) Odontoid fractures, with special reference to the elderly patient. Clin Orthop 193:178–183

163. Weller SJ, Malek AM, Rossitch E (1997) Cervical spine fracture in the elderly. Surg Neurol 47:274–281

164. Penrod LE, Hegde SK, Ditunno JF Jr (1990) Age effect on prognosis for functional recovery in acute, traumatic central cord syndrome. Arch Phys Med Rehabil 71:963–968

165. Scivoletto G, Morganti B, Ditunno P et al (2003) Effects on age on spinal cord lesion patients' rehabilitation. Spinal Cord 41:457–464

166. DeVivo MJ, Kartus PL, Rutt RD et al (1990) The influence of age at time of spinal cord injury on rehabilitation outcome. Arch Neurol 47:687–691

167. Horst IIM, Obeid FN, Sorensen VJ et al (1986) Factors influencing survival of elderly trauma patients. Crit Care Med 14:681–684

168. Shorr RM, Rodriguez A, Indeck MC et al (1989) Blunt chest trauma in the elderly. J Trauma 29:234–237

169. Cameron P, Dziukas L, Hadj A et al (1996) Rib fractures in major trauma. Aust N Z Surg 66:530–534

170. Sharma OP, Oswanski MF, Jolly S (2008) Perils of rib fractures. Am Surg 74:310–314

171. Camp PC Jr, Rogers FB, Shackford SR et al (1994) Blunt traumatic thoracic aortic laceration in the elderly: an analysis of outcome. J Trauma 37:418–423

172. Hirose H, Gill IS, Malangoni NA (2006) Nonoperative management of traumatic aortic injury. J Trauma 60:547–601

173. Cook J, Salerno C, Krishnadasan B et al (2006) The effect of changing presentation and management on the outcome of blunt rupture of the thoracic aorta. J Thorac Cardiovasc Surg 131:594–600

174. Demetriades D, Velmahos GC, Scalea TM et al (2008) Operative repair or endovascular stent graft in blunt traumatic thoracic aortic injuries: results of an American Association for the Surgery of Trauma Multicenter Study. J Trauma 64:561–571

175. Levy DB, Hanlon DP, Townsend RN (1993) Geriatric trauma. Clin Geriatr Med 9:601–620

176. Rozycki GS, Ballard RB, Feliciano DV et al (1998) Surgeon-performed ultrasound for the assessment of truncal injuries: lessons learned from 1540 patients. Ann Surg 228:557–567

177. Morcos SK, Thomsen HS, Webb JA (1999) Contrast-media-induced nephrotoxicity: a consensus report. Contrast media safety committee, European Society of Urogenital Radiology (ESUR). Eur Radiol 9:1602–1613

178. Kelly AM, Dwamena B, Cronin P et al (2008) Meta-analysis of drugs for preventing contrast-induced nephropathy. Ann Int Med 148:284–294

179. Merten GJ, Burgess P, Gray LV et al (2004) Prevention of contrast-induced nephropathy with sodium bicarbonate. JAMA 291:2328–2334

180. Pannu N, Wiebe N, Tonelli M et al (2006) Prophylaxis strategies for contrast-induced nephropathy. JAMA 295:2765–2779

181. Smith JS, Cooney RN, Mucha P (1996) Nonoperative management of the ruptured spleen. A revalidation of criteria. Surgery 120:745–751

182. Smith JS, Wengrovitz MA, DeLong BS (1992) Prospective validation of criteria, including age, for safe, nonsurgical management of the ruptured spleen. J Trauma 33:363–369

183. Godley CD, Warren RL, Sheridan RL et al (1996) Nonoperative management of blunt splenic injury in adults: age over 55 years as a powerful indicator of failure. J Am Coll Surg 183:133–139

184. Krause KR, Howells GA, Bair HA et al (2000) Nonoperative management of blunt splenic injury in adults 55 years and older: a twenty-year experience. Am Surg 66:636–640

185. Albrecht RM, Schermer CR, Morris A (2002) Nonoperative management of blunt splenic injuries: factors influencing success in age >55 years. Am Surg 68:227–231

186. Haan JM, Biffl W, Knudson MM et al (2004) Splenic embolization revisited: a multicenter review. J Trauma 56:542–547

187. Grossheim LF (2007) Blunt trauma evaluation and management: pitfalls to avoid. Trauma Rep 8:1–12

188. Myers AH, Robinson EG, Van Natta ML et al (1991) Hip fractures among the elderly: factors associated with in-hospital mortality. Am J Epidemiol 134:1128–1137

189. Laskin RS, Gruber MA, Zimmerman AJ (1979) Intertrochanteric fractures of the hip in the elderly: a retrospective analysis of 236 cases. Clin Orthop Relat Res 141:188–195

190. Henry SM, Pollak AN, Jones AL et al (2002) Pelvic fracture in geriatric patients: a distinct clinical entity. J Trauma 53.15–20

191. Roumen RM, Hesp WL, Brüggink ED (1991) Unstable Colles' fractures in elderly patients. J Bone Joint Surg 73:307–311

192. Ritchie AJ, Small JO, Hart NB et al (1991) Type III tibial fractures in the elderly: results of 23 fractures in 20 patients. Injury 22:267–270

193. Helfet DL, Borrelli J Jr, DiPasquale T et al (1992) Stabilization of acetabular fractures in elderly patients. J Bone Joint Surg 74:753–765

194. Bogner R, Hübner C, Matis N et al (2008) Minimally invasive treatment of the three and four-part fractures of the proximal humerus in the elderly patients. J Bone Joint Surg Br 90:1602–1607

195. McGwin G Jr, Cross JM, Ford JW et al (2003) Long term trends in mortality according to age among adult burn patients. J Burn Care Rehabil 24:21–25

196. Manktelow A, Meyer AA, Herzog SR et al (1989) Analysis of life expectancy and living status of elderly patients surviving a burn injury. J Trauma 29:203–207

197. Bowser-Wallace BH, Cone JB, Caldwell FT Jr (1985) Hypertonic lactated saline resuscitation of severely burned patients over 60 years of age. J Trauma 25:22–26

198. Kara M, Peters WJ, Douglas LG et al (1990) An early surgical approach to burns in the elderly. J Trauma 30:430–432

199. Deitch EA, Clothier J (1983) Burns in the elderly: an early surgical approach. J Trauma 23:891–894
200. Scott-Conner CE, Love R, Wheeler W (1990) Does rapid wound closure improve survival in older patients with burns? Am Surg 56:57–60
201. Williams TK (1984) Rehabilitation in the aging: philosophy and approaches. In: Williams TK (ed) Rehabilitation in the aging. Raven, New York, p xiii
202. Richmond TS, Kauder D, Strumpf N et al (2002) Characteristics and outcomes of serious traumatic injury in older adults. J Am Geriatr Soc 50:215–222
203. Inaba K, Goecke M, Sharkey P et al (2003) Long term outcomes after injury in the elderly. J Trauma 54:486–491
204. Retting R, Schwartz SI, Kulewiicz M et al (1989) Queens Boulevard pedestrian safety project, New York City. MMWR Morb Mortal Wkly Rep 38:61

Chapter 32
Maximizing Postoperative Functional Recovery

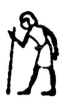

Leo M. Cooney

CASE STUDY

An 82-year-old man entered the hospital with fever and confusion. He had previously been living by himself in a small apartment, but had been going out of the apartment less and less over the past 6 months. His family noted that his memory had started to become impaired. They brought him to the Emergency Department because of acute confusion and a fever to 102°F. His evaluation revealed that he had acute cholecystitis with bacteremia. He was initially treated with antibiotics and a surgical drain. He then underwent a laparoscopic cholecystectomy.

During his hospitalization, he continued to be acutely confused. He required sedating medications and physical restraints, as he frequently tried to pull out his drains and intravenous lines. He developed a grade two pressure sore on his sacrum. He was initially treated with a Foley indwelling bladder catheter and later with an external catheter.

By the tenth hospital day, he had a normal white count, was afebrile, and his surgical wound had healed nicely. He was, however, unable to get out of bed by himself and unable to control his bladder and bowels and was still acutely confused. He required nursing home placement.

A higher and higher percentage of surgical procedures are now being done on patients 65 and older. The successful outcome of these procedures goes beyond traditional concerns about morbidity and mortality. For most patients, the most important result of these procedures is the ability to continue to live independently. Hospitalizations and surgical procedures often result in a decrease of older persons' ability to care for themselves, resulting in the need for daily care at home or nursing home placement. Surgeons must understand how to return their patients to the highest possible level of function, if they are going to provide them the best possible care.

Katz in 1963 outlined those functions that an individual must be able to do independently to live without the assistance of another individual. These "activities of daily living" include the ability to bathe, groom, dress, feed, and toilet oneself independently, as well as being able to transfer out of bed or chair and walk independently [1] (Table 32.1). "Instrumental activities of daily living" describe higher levels of activities needed to live independently in the community. These include preparing meals, shopping, using the telephone, cleaning one's home or apartment, driving or using public transportation, and managing one's own finances.

The ability to perform daily living activities is not only essential for the independence and life satisfaction of older adults, but also is the single most important predictor of mortality for older individuals. Virtually every study of prognosis has found that these seven daily living activities are more strongly associated with mortality than standard physiologic parameters. In many studies, the only condition that has a larger impact on mortality than function is metastatic cancer [2]. Difficulty with these daily living activities is also strongly predictive of nursing home placement.

Unfortunately, the process of hospitalization itself often causes a decline in function in older individuals; and 35–50% of patients over 65 experience a decline in function during hospitalization [3]. This decline is often unrelated to the reason for hospital admission and is associated with a prolonged hospital length of stay, increased need for nursing home placement, and increased mortality [4].

Older individuals are at a much higher risk for the complications of hospitalization and medical and surgical interventions than younger people [5]. The limited mental and physiologic reserve of older adults often contributes to these complications.

L.M. Cooney (✉)
Yale – New Haven Hospital, 20 York Street, Tomkins 17,
New Haven, CT 06504, USA
e-mail: leo.cooney@ynhh.org

R.A. Rosenthal et al. (eds.), *Principles and Practice of Geriatric Surgery*,
DOI 10.1007/978-1-4419-6999-6_32, © Springer Science+Business Media, LLC 2011

TABLE 32.1 Activities of daily living

Transfer
Walk
Bathe
Dress
Feed go to toilet
Continent of urine and stool

TABLE 32.2 Predictors of hospital decline

Altered mental status
Physical function prior to admission
Social function prior to admission
Frequency of going out of the home

Elderly patients have a high incidence of complications with therapy, including drug reactions, adverse effects of procedures, hospital-acquired infections, and other iatrogenic events [6].

When older patients are evaluated in acute hospitals, they often have significant functional problems. Warshaw found that 50% of patients over age 65 in a community hospital had mild or moderate confusion, 47% were incontinent of urine or catheterized, 65% could not ambulate independently, and 40% needed help with eating [7].

The most important contributor to loss of functional status during a hospitalization is altered mental status. The development of delirium, or acute confusional state, during a hospitalization has a major impact on a patient's function and long-term outcome. The major predisposing factor for the development of delirium is underlying dementia.

Delirium can now be easily diagnosed. Sharon Inouye's Confusion Assessment Method has become the international standard for the diagnosis of delirium. The four components of this instrument are (1) acute onset and fluctuating course, (2) inattention, (3) disorganized thinking, and (4) altered level of consciousness. The patient is classified as delirious if he/she exhibits 1 and 2 and either 3 or 4. Inattention is the key feature of delirium. Patients with inattention have difficulty focusing attention, are easily distractible, and have difficulty keeping track of what is being said [8].

The hospital environment itself can also precipitate delirium. There is a very high incidence of delirium in patients in intensive care units. The use of physical restraints can themselves produce delirium, and often severely complicate this condition. Lack of sleep caused by in-room intercoms, administration of medications, and the frequent measuring of vital signs often results in acute confusion.

Preoperative Assessment

The first step in promoting postoperative recovery is to assess the patient preoperatively for predictors of functional decline. The most important predictors of functional decline following surgery are patient's preexisting mental status, physical function, and social activities. Dementia is an extremely important predictor of outcome following surgical interventions. As noted above, dementia greatly increases the probability of a patient becoming delirious following surgery.

Dementia increases the mortality for hip fracture patients almost threefold [9]. Patients with dementia are two to three times as likely to die from pneumonia as patients without this condition [10].

Dementia is very common in older adults. The prevalence of this condition is roughly 1.5% between the ages of 65 and 70 and then doubles for each 5-year period after that. Thus, nearly 25% of individuals between 85 and 90 have some degree of dementia and almost 50% of those 90 and above have dementia [11]. Cognitive losses can be subtle. Many patients with mild-to-moderate dementia still have good social graces and do not appear, on casual observation, to have any major problems with their mental status. Although socially appropriate, patients with dementia are at very high risk for the development of delirium following a surgical procedure.

Memory loss is the most common feature of dementia. The best mental status screening test is the Folstein Mini Mental Status Test. This 30 point test takes only 5 min to administer. It has been studied and validated in populations throughout the world. The level of the patient's education must be considered in the interpretation of the results of this test. Patients with a high school education who scored 24 or less on this test should be evaluated for the presence of dementia. For individuals with an eighth grade education or less, a score of 19 is the level which requires a dementia evaluation.

It is important to determine how functional a patient is prior to hospital admission. Was that person able to get in and out of bed and walk independently, climb stairs, and walk good distances? Did that patient frequently fall?

Such measures of independence as how often one goes outside one's home or participates in outside social activities are excellent predictors of return of function following hip fracture surgery. Patients who are socially active have a much better outcome than individuals who stay in their own home or apartment and have limited social contacts.

The best screen for altered physical function is to observe the patient. The "get up and go" test observes the patient getting on and off a chair, walking a short distance, turning, and walking back to the chair. In addition, the surgeon should determine whether the patient can climb stairs, is still driving an automobile, does his/her own shopping, meal preparation, housekeeping, and other such activities. It is also extremely important to know patient's social support. Does that person have someone else living with him or her or other family members who can be available for assistance at home following hospital discharge? (Table 32.2).

Maintaining Function During Hospitalization

"Geriatric Vital Signs"

An older patient's physical, cognitive, and nutritional function is as vital to their assessment as blood pressure, pulse, and temperature. The geriatric vital signs are (1) Mental status (confused), (2) the ability to transfer in and out of bed and walk (immobility), (3) the patient's ability to take in adequate nutrition (poor nutrition), (4) continence of bowel and bladder (incontinence), and (5) the presence of any skin breakdown or pressure sores (skin breakdown) (Table 32.3).

Managing patients throughout their hospitalization is an essential step in returning patients to the highest possible level of function. In the first instance, patients who are at high risk for delirium and loss of physical function should be evaluated prior to surgery. Those patients at high risk should be monitored closely throughout their hospital stay. Patients with early or moderate dementia would benefit from close supervision on the part of families. Medications likely to produce delirium should be kept to a minimum.

Although dementia rarely has a medical cause, delirium is often caused by medical problems. The most common precipitants of delirium are an acute illness, being in an unfamiliar environment, and complications of medications [12]. The medications that are most likely to produce delirium are anticholinergic medications as well as sedatives and hypnotics. Long-acting sleep medications are particularly problematic. Medications such as diphenhydramine, often used for its sedating effects, are very apt to produce delirium because of strong anticholinergic qualities. Sedating medications such as benzodiazepines also frequently produce delirium. Long-acting pain medications can be another cause of confusion in elderly patients [13].

Any alteration in a patient's ability to follow the train of a conversation or follow the instructions of nurses or therapists should initiate an evaluation for delirium. The clinician should determine the presence of inattention, an acute onset and fluctuating course of the confusion, disorganized thinking, or altered level of consciousness. If these symptoms indicate that the patient is delirious, then the surgeon and nurse caring for that patient need to undertake a coordinated effort to control this condition. The surgeon should evaluate the patient for precipitants of delirium such as an acute illness, electrolyte or other physiologic abnormalities, or medications with anticholinergic, sedating, or hypnotic properties. The clinician should try and remove as many external devices as possible, such as indwelling bladder catheters, intravenous lines, and telemetry, and contact the patient's family to inform them about the nature and natural history of delirium. The nursing staff should place the patient under close observation, make sure that the patients have eyeglasses and hearing aids, provide continual orientation to the patient, and work with the patient's family to provide the patient with as much family assistance and supervision as possible. The use of physical restraints should be avoided, if at all possible. It is best to avoid medications in the management of delirium. If medications are necessary, most geriatric physicians suggest the use of low doses of antipsychotic agents such as haloperidol or risperidone if sedation is not needed, or quetiapine or olanzapine if the patient needs sedation in addition to control of agitation. Benzodiazepines, as noted above, should be avoided, as they often worsen delirium.

The very nature of nursing care can contribute to a loss of function for older hospitalized patients. Such activities as providing a bed pan, bathing, dressing, feeding, or administering medications may decrease the patient's ability to care for him or herself. Nurses prepare patients better for discharge if they assist them with various tasks and ensure that they can carry them out independently, rather than performing the tasks for the patient.

Continence of bowel and bladder is essential to an individual's independence. Indwelling bladder catheters should be removed as soon as possible after surgery. Transient urinary incontinence is common following surgery. Appropriate management of this problem can decrease the chances of permanent difficulties. If the nursing staff manages the incontinent patient with diapers and external catheters, it may be difficult to regain bladder control. Reassurance, frequent toileting of the patient, and assistance with mobility are likely to result in return of bladder control.

Physicians may also play a major role in the development of patient dependence. Sedatives and sleeping pills should be used with caution in older individuals. These medications often have a prolonged half life in the elderly and can cause lethargy and confusion. They are particularly problematic if the patient has any element of baseline dementia. The use of indwelling or external bladder catheters to monitor urine volume can result in at least temporary result of bladder control. The surgical approach to early postoperative ambulation has been well recognized for a number of years. Physicians and surgeons should realize, however, that the ability to transfer out of a bed or a chair is a more difficult task than walking and is more important to a patient's ability to live independently (Table 32.4).

TABLE 32.3 Geriatric vital signs

Confusion
Incontinence
Immobility
Skin breakdown
Poor nutrition

TABLE 32.4 Factors associated with hospital decline

Bed rest
Sedating or hypnotic drugs
Anticholinergic drugs
Prolonged use of bladder catheters
Use of physical restraints

Returning a patient to the highest level of function requires a concerted effort on the part of physicians, nursing staff, therapists, social workers, and discharge planners. The nursing staff and the patient's family are usually the best observers of the patient's mental status. A physician's major role is to listen. He/she should determine whether the patient has nighttime confusion, any problems recognizing family members, following commands, or attending to daily tasks. Although temporary confusion is common following anesthesia, any alterations in mental status that persists beyond 24 h after surgery, should be evaluated. Medications should be reviewed and a search undertaken to ensure that there are no acute medical problems causing the patient's delirium.

Patients who have significant care needs at the time of hospital discharge and insufficient help at home to provide these needs may be candidates for a short period of rehabilitation in a subacute or skilled nursing facility. It is essential that the patient's care be well coordinated between the physicians and staff at the acute-care hospital and the physician and staff at the subacute-care facility.

Posthospital Care

The final outcome of any surgical procedure is usually not clear until 4–6 weeks after the procedure. Posthospital rehabilitation and care play a major role in the success or failure of these procedures. It is the surgeon's responsibility to ensure that each patient receives the posthospital care most appropriate to his/her needs.

There are three options to posthospital care (1) acute rehabilitation units or hospitals, (2) subacute care in nursing homes or "skilled nursing facilities", and (3) home care.

Medicare has rather strict criteria for patients going to acute rehabilitation hospitals. Most of these patients have to fit into the small list of diagnostic categories including strokes, hips fractures, and other neurologic or orthopedic problems. To be eligible for this level of care, patients must need and receive at least 3 h per day of physical, occupational or speech therapy, and require a multidisciplinary approach from a team lead by physicians skilled in rehabilitation medicine. Most postoperative surgical patients are not eligible for this level of care, unless they have a complication such as a stroke.

Medicare does reimburse short-term rehabilitation care in skilled nursing facilities as long as the patient needs and receives restorative care or extensive nursing care that could not be provided at home. Although there is a 100-day maximum for this care, this care is covered only if the patient continues to make progress in his/her rehabilitation. In addition, there is a very substantial copayment required after the first 20 days of the nursing home stay. This copayment can make continued stay at these facilities difficult, if the patient does not have appropriate secondary insurance coverage.

Subacute Care

Medicare diagnosis-related group (DRG) reimbursement policies and the push to limit hospital lengths of stay have moved a great deal of the rehabilitation of older individuals into skilled nursing facilities. A number of these facilities have set up special units for "subacute care" [14].

A Swiss group has developed a predictive score to identify patients hospitalized on acute medical service risk of discharge to a postacute-care facility. These investigators found that data measured on the first hospital day was predictive of the need for posthospital care. The factors most predictive of discharge to a postacute-care facility were (1) the patient's partner's inability to provide home care, (2) inability to self-manage drug regimen, (3) number of active medical problems on admission, (4) dependency in bathing, and (5) dependency in transfers from bed to chair [15].

Although it may be logical and reasonable to use lower-acuity facilities for rehabilitation, use of these facilities without careful coordination of care between the acute and chronic care providers can lead to adverse outcomes. Fitzgerald et al. reported two important studies that demonstrated the problems associated with early transfers to skilled nursing facilities. These studies pointed out that the frequency of transfer of patients from acute hospitals to skilled nursing facilities for rehabilitation of a fractured hip more than doubled with introduction of the Medicare DRG-based reimbursement system [16, 17]. The greatest concern, however, was the increase of permanent nursing home placement from 13 to 39% after the introduction of prospective payment. These studies should caution the surgeon to ensure that temporary nursing home placements do not become permanent.

Bonar et al. studied the factors associated with permanent nursing home placement for patients transferred from hospitals to skilled nursing facilities for rehabilitation following hip fractures. She found that patients who were oriented, younger, could bathe independently, could transfer and walk independently, and had increased family involvement were more likely to be discharged from the nursing home to home. In addition, the number of physical therapy hours available in the nursing home predicted discharge home [18] (Table 32.5).

TABLE 32.5 Returning home from subacute facilities

Good mental status

Good daily living function

Integrated medical care

Intensity of rehabilitative services

Intensity of discharge planning

Good social support

Several studies have evaluated the outcome of older patients transferred from hospitals to rehabilitation hospitals, subacute nursing homes, and traditional nursing homes. Kramer et al. found that after adjusting for patients' admission cognitive and physical functions, stroke patients admitted to rehabilitation hospitals were more likely to return to the community and recover function in ADLs. For patients with fractured hips, however, there was no difference in outcome for patients admitted to rehabilitation hospitals, subacute nursing homes, or traditional nursing homes [19]. Kane et al. also found that stroke patients fared better when treated in rehabilitation hospitals and rehabilitative nursing homes. Although healthier hip fracture patients who received rehabilitative nursing home care fared better, the functional change for sicker hip fracture patients was not different between regular and rehabilitative nursing homes [20].

Fitzgerald et al., in their studies, found that one interesting fact about hip fracture patients who were able to return to their own home: patients followed by their own health maintenance physicians in the nursing home had a better chance of returning home than those who had a separate nursing home physician [17].

Although subacute-care facilities and traditional nursing homes may have a role in the rehabilitation of older surgical patients, it is important to ensure that the care given in these facilities is as coordinated as possible with the acute-care facility [21]. Surgeons should recognize that patients with altered mental status, substantial deficits in their ability to carry out ADLs, complex medical conditions, and limited social support at home are at substantial risk for permanent nursing home placement. The most complex aspect of returning an old person to his or her own home is the discharge planning process. The surgeon must ensure that the subacute-care facility has all the requisite resources and skills to carry out this complex process.

The integration of care between the acute-care and chronic-care facility requires, first and foremost, that the physicians caring for the patient in the nursing home setting be closely integrated with the acute-care physician. Communication between the acute-care providers must be complete and ongoing. Systems in which there is integrated physician coverage appear to have better rehabilitative outcomes and a higher frequency of patients returning home. An integrated system of care, in which the staff of the nursing home facility has complete access to the laboratory, diagnostic imaging, and other reports of the acute hospital, also increases the potential for improved care. The transition from an acute hospital to a skilled nursing facility requires very careful transmission of clinical information from the acute-care to the chronic-care providers. The most important information to transmit to the skilled nursing facility is the name of the responsible physician who has knowledge of the patient's hospital course, and how to readily reach that physician [22].

The discharge summary should give careful instructions for wound care [23], weight-bearing, diet, and medications. Medication lists should include the last doses given in the hospital. If medications are to be tapered or discontinued, a clear outline by date of the tapering course should be included. All recent significant laboratory tests should be listed within the discharge summary. Those tests that are still pending should be listed with appropriate follow-up outlined.

The goals of the subacute stay should be outlined. If the patient is on anticoagulation, the orders for anticoagulant should be listed with goal results for INRs, along with the most recent dose of anticoagulants and INR results.

Nutritional problems should be identified during the acute hospitalization and goals of nutritional therapy in the skilled nursing facility should be outlined. Nutritional supplements should be given at least 1 h before a meal. If parenteral feeding is used, instructions for these feedings should be clearly outlined [24].

The physician ultimately responsible for the patient's rehabilitation is the attending surgeon. He or she must ensure that those caring for the patient after hospitalization have a clear outline of the therapies indicated and should have easy access to that surgeon to answer any questions that they might have. Electronic access between the skilled nursing facility and discharging hospital is best, as this access could provide laboratory, diagnostic imaging, and operative and clinical information to the skilled nursing facility staff. In the final analysis, returning an individual to the highest possible level of function requires a concerted effort on the part of surgeons, physicians, nurses, physical therapists, discharge planners, and social workers to provide the patient with the highest possible level of function.

Patients who are confused or delirious at the time of hospital discharge do not do well in subacute-care facilities. The best management of delirious patients is to return them, as quickly as possible, into their own home environment. Another health care facility can often worsen patient's confusion. It is very difficult to rehabilitate a confused patient. If the patient's family cannot take the patient home in this condition, care must be coordinated very closely between the acute providers and physicians and nursing staff at the skilled nursing facility.

At the time of hospital discharge, the discharging surgeon must ensure (1) that the patient's mental status will allow continued rehabilitation at a subacute or home setting, (2) that the appropriate medical and rehabilitation care is well outlined to the subacute or home care providers, and (3) that those providing chronic care to the patient have immediate access to the responsible surgeon. Surgeons must recognize that this posthospital care is an important part of the recovery period from surgery and is the responsibility of the discharging surgeon.

References

1. Katz S, Ford A, Moskowitz R et al (1963) Studies of illness in the aged: the index of ADL; a standardized measure of biological and psychosocial function. JAMA 185:94–99
2. Walter LC, Brand RJ, Counsell SR et al (2001) Development and validation of a prognostic index for 1-year mortality in older adults after hospitalization. JAMA 285(23):2987–2994
3. Inouye SK, Wagner DR, Acampora D et al (1993) A predictive index for functional decline in hospitalized elderly medical patients. J Gen Intern Med 8:645–652
4. Hirsch CH, Sommers L, Olsen A et al (1990) The natural history of functional morbidity in hospitalized older patients. J Am Geriatr Soc 38:1296–1303
5. Creditor MC (1993) Hazards of hospitalization of the elderly. Ann Intern Med 11:219–223
6. Gillick MR, Serrell NA, Gillick LS (1982) Adverse consequences of hospitalization in the elderly. Soc Sci Med 16:1033–1038
7. Warshaw GA, Moore JT, Friedman SW et al (1982) Functional disability in the hospitalized elderly. JAMA 248:847–850
8. Inouye SK (1994) The dilemma of delirium: clinical and research controversies regarding delirium in hospitalized elderly medical patients. Am J Med 97:278–288
9. Miller CW (1978) Survival and ambulation following hip fracture. J Bone Joint Surg Am 60:930–933
10. Morrison RS, Siu AL (2000) Survival in end-stage dementia following acute illness. JAMA 284(1):47–52
11. Ferri CP, Prince M et al (2005) Global prevalence of dementia: a Delphi consensus study. Lancet 366:2112–2117
12. Inouye SK, Charpentier PA (1996) Precipitating factors for delirium in hospitalized elderly persons: predictive model and interrelationship with baseline vulnerability. JAMA 275:852–857
13. Pompei P, Foreman M, Rudberg M et al (1994) Delirium in hospitalized older persons: outcomes and predictors. J Am Geriatr Soc 42:809–815
14. Cotterill PG, Gage BJ (2002) Overview: medicare post-acute care since the Balanced Budget Act of 1997. Health Care Financ Rev 24(2):1–6
15. Simonet ML, Kossovsky MP, Chopard P, Sigaud P, Perneger TV, Gaspoz JM (2008) A predictive score to identify hospitalized patients' risk of discharge to a post-acute care facility. BMC Health Serv Res 8:154
16. Fitzgerald J, Fagan L, Tierney W et al (1987) Changing patterns of hip fracture care before and after implementation of the prospective payment system. JAMA 258:218–221
17. Fitzgerald J, Moore T, Dittus R (1988) The care of elderly patients with hip fracture: changes since implementation of the prospective payment system. N Engl J Med 319:1392–1397
18. Bonar S, Tinetti M, Speechley M et al (1990) Factors associated with short- versus long-term skilled nursing facility placement among community-living hip fracture patients. J Am Geriatr Soc 38:1139–1144
19. Kramer A, Steiner J, Schlenker R et al (1997) Outcomes and costs after hip fracture and stroke: a comparison of rehabilitation settings. JAMA 277:396–404
20. Kane R, Chen Q, Blewett L et al (1996) Do rehabilitative nursing homes improve the outcomes of care? J Am Geriatr Soc 44:545–554
21. Prvu Bettger JA, Stineman MG (2007) Effectiveness of multidisciplinary rehabilitation services in post-acute care: state-of-the-science. A review. Arch Phys Med Rehabil 88:1526–1534
22. Marcantonio ER, Yurkofsky M (2003) Subacute care. In: Hazzard WR, Blass JP, Halter JB, Ouslander JG, Tinetti M (eds) Principles of geriatric medicine and gerontology, 5th edn. McGraw Hill, New York, pp 181–196
23. Thomas DR, Kamel HK (2000) Wound management in postacute care. Clin Geriatr Med 16(4):783–803
24. Morley JE (2000) Management of nutritional problems in subacute care. Clin Geriatr Med 16(4):817–831

Section IV
Endocrine System/Breast

Chapter 33
Invited Commentary

Samuel A. Wells

Age-related alterations in endocrine function are important considerations in the surgical patient. Because the endocrine system is integrally related to virtually all bodily functions, it is unreasonable to think of the singular effects of a specific hormone deficiency. It is impossible to cover all aspects of the endocrinology of aging; however, we address some of the most significant.

Arguably, the most important endocrine change associated with aging arises in the pancreas and relates to the decreased availability of insulin. Forty percent of individuals aged 65–75 years have impaired glucose tolerance, the incidence of which increases with age. The abnormality goes undetected in many elderly patients, and they are at risk for developing vascular, ocular, and neurologic complications. In addition to decreased insulin secretion from the pancreatic beta cell, physical inactivity, poor diet, increased body weight, and decreased lean body mass contribute to glucose intolerance.

The incidence of thyroid abnormalities including autoimmune thyroiditis, the metabolic states of hypothyroidism and hyperthyroidism, thyroid nodules, and thyroid cancer also increases with age. The surgeon must be aware of the possibility of occult thyroid disease in the elderly. The failure to recognize the presence of occult hypothyroidism or hyperthyroidism in acutely ill surgical patients may result in increased operative and perioperative mortality.

There are significant decreases in cortical and trabecular bone as one ages. Loss of bone mineralization is particularly problematic in women, where trabecular bone loss accelerates at menopause and reaches a rate of 4% per year. Estrogen deficiency accounts for a 15–20% decrease in skeletal density, which is increased further in the presence of hyperparathyroidism, a disease that occurs primarily in postmenopausal women. Understandably, there is an increase in fracture rate in elderly patients not only due to decreased bone density but also because of a decrease in muscle strength and impaired coordination.

Menopause, one of the most dramatic age-related changes, is primarily associated with the loss of cyclic estradiol production. Menopause appears to be brought on by changes in both the ovarian follicles and the hypothalamus and pituitary. Long-term estrogen replacement therapy is beneficial for the skeleton, cardiovascular system, reproductive tract, skin, and central nervous system; however, estrogen replacement is associated with a modest but definitely increased incidence of breast cancer.

In aging men, there is a decline in serum testosterone levels and an accompanying reduction in the number of Leydig cells. Studies show that testosterone replacement in elderly men is associated with increased muscular strength, cognition, and red blood cell mass. However, testosterone administration has a stimulatory effect on the prostate, and the risk of enhancing the growth of an occult prostate cancer is a definite risk.

Hormonal changes also occur in the adrenal cortex, characterized by a decrease in circulating levels of dehydroepiandrosterone (DHEA), and in the pituitary gland, characterized by a reduction in growth hormone and insulin-like growth factor. There have been prospective randomized controlled trials in older adults, of DHEA administration compared to placebo. In subjects receiving DHEA, compared to those receiving placebo, circulating levels of DHEA and androgen were restored, and there was a sense of improved well-being. The risk of administering these agents relates to the direct or indirect stimulatory effect on the breast and prostate gland and perhaps other tissues. Similarly, growth hormone, administered in prospective randomized placebo-controlled trials, has been associated with increased muscle strength and bone mineral content. It has already been shown in patients with fractures or burns that administration of growth hormone has clear benefit in wound healing and return to independent living. As with DHEA, the question remains whether adverse effects will become evident with long-term administration of growth hormone. There is the possibility that administration of selected hormones would have a beneficial effect on the elderly surgical patient, as minimal adverse effects have been seen with their short-term administration.

S.A. Wells (✉)
Professor of Surgery, Department of Surgery,
Washington University Medical Center, St. Louis, MO, USA
e-mail: wellss@wudosis.wustl.edu

R.A. Rosenthal et al. (eds.), *Principles and Practice of Geriatric Surgery*,
DOI 10.1007/978-1-4419-6999-6_33, © Springer Science+Business Media, LLC 2011

The surgeon must understand that both profound and subtle changes occur in the endocrine system with aging and that these alterations influence the response of the older patient to surgical procedures. Replacement therapy for endocrine deficiencies is clearly indicated in the elderly patient whether in the emergent or the elective setting. However, much work remains to be done on the evaluation of hormonal administration in healthful elderly persons to clarify whether the benefits outweigh the risks. The question is important, as the results will influence how elderly patients respond to surgical treatment and to their underlying disease process.

Chapter 34
Surgical Disorders of the Thyroid in the Elderly

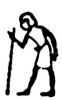

Leslie S. Wu, Julie Ann Sosa, and Robert Udelsman

CASE STUDY

JK is a 75-year-old woman with a right anterior neck mass identified on physical examination by her cardiologist. She described a globus sensation and dysphagia with solid foods, and had subjective hoarseness over the last year. She did not have a history of head or neck radiation, and there was no family history of glandular abnormalities. Her past medical history was significant for hypertension, hyperlipidemia, atrial fibrillation on chronic warfarin therapy, diabetes mellitus, osteopenia, and arthritis. Her past surgical history was notable for a cholecystectomy, hysterectomy for uterine fibroids, and left breast lumpectomy and radiation therapy for ductal carcinoma in situ. Family history is significant for "bad hearts." She was a former smoker. Her medications included warfarin, metoprolol, amlodipine, simvastatin, glucophage, glipizide, niacin, fish oil, calcium supplements with vitamin D, multivitamin, and acetaminophen as needed.

Physical examination revealed a well-developed woman in no acute distress. Her vital signs were within normal limits, and she appeared euthyroid. Focused exam was notable for a nontender 4-cm firm but mobile mass in the right anterior neck. The trachea was distracted slightly into the contralateral neck. The left thyroid lobe contained no palpable nodules. There was no cervical lymphadenopathy. Pemberton sign was absent, and there was no carotid bruit. The remainder of her physical exam was unremarkable.

On blood work, the patient was biochemically euthyroid with a thyroid-stimulating hormone (TSH) 2.5 mIU/L (normal 0.4–4.0 mIU/L). JK's geriatrician referred her to an endocrinologist, who, in turn, consulted a thyroid surgeon. JK underwent a dedicated neck ultrasound, which revealed a 60-g thyroid and a 4-cm nodule in the right lobe. It was hypoechoic with a small cystic component, microcalcifications, an irregular border, and possible extension into the overlying strap muscle. The left lobe contained two 4-mm nodules that were too small to characterize. Ultrasound-guided fine-needle aspiration (FNA) of the dominant right nodule was performed. Cytopathology was consistent with papillary thyroid cancer.

Introduction

The proportion of elderly people is growing steadily in Western societies as a consequence of increased life expectancy and reduced birth rates. Americans aged 80 years and older constituted 3.3% of the population in 2000; this is projected to increase to 7.7% in 2050 and 8.2% by 2070. In comparison, Americans 65–79 years of age constituted 9.3% of the population in 2000 and are projected to increase to 12.5% by 2050 and 12.9% by 2070 [1]. This phenomenon has generated numerous studies aimed at clarifying the physiologic and pathologic aspects of aging. Thyroid dysfunction can have profound clinical implications for elderly patients. Thyroid nodules are common, and the incidence of thyroid cancer increases with age.

Thyroid disease is common; 6.6% of the US population has thyroid disease, requires thyroid hormone supplementation, or both [2]. Based on results of autopsies performed on the general population, thyroid nodules have been found in up to 50% of asymptomatic patients [3]. The incidence of thyroid cancer has increased from 3.6 per 100,000 in 1973 to

J.A. Sosa (✉)
Department of Surgery, Maine Medical Center,
22 Bramhall St., Portland, ME, USA

R.A. Rosenthal et al. (eds.), *Principles and Practice of Geriatric Surgery*,
DOI 10.1007/978-1-4419-6999-6_34, © Springer Science+Business Media, LLC 2011

8.7 per 100,000 in 2002 – a 2.4-fold increase – with 87% of the increase due to the diagnosis of small differentiated thyroid cancers [4]. The association between increasing age and incidence of thyroid nodules makes diagnosis and treatment an important public health issue.

All thyroid diseases are encountered in the elderly; however, their prevalence and clinical expression differ from those observed in younger patients. Symptoms of aging can be confused easily with hypothyroidism. The clinical manifestations of thyroid dysfunction can be more vague, subtle, and hidden by a background of coexistent disease. Interpretation of thyroid function studies can be problematic in elderly patients, owing to difficulty in differentiating physiologic age-associated changes from alterations secondary to acute or chronic nonthyroidal illnesses [5]. And finally, the medical and surgical treatment of thyroid disease in the elderly is associated with an increased risk of complications attributed to the treatment itself [6].

Thyroid Function

The thyroid gland synthesizes the hormones thyroxine (T_4) and triiodothyronine (T_3), iodine-containing amino acids that regulate the body's metabolic rate. Adequate levels of thyroid hormone are necessary in infants for normal development of the central nervous system, in children for normal skeletal growth and maturation, and in adults for normal function of multiple organ systems [7]. Thyroid dysfunction is one of the most common endocrine disorders encountered in clinical practice. While abnormally high or low levels of thyroid hormones can be tolerated for long periods of time, usually there are symptoms and signs of thyroid dysfunction.

The effects of thyroid hormones are diffuse and important (Table 34.1). Thyroid hormones increase the activity of membrane-bound Na^+-K^+ adenosine triphosphate (ATP)-ase, increase heat production, and stimulate oxygen consumption ("calorigenesis"). Thyroid hormones also affect tissue growth

and maturation, help regulate lipid metabolism, increase cardiac contractility by stimulating the expression of myosin protein, and increase intestinal absorption of carbohydrates (Fig. 34.1) [8].

The usual biochemical measures of thyroid function, such as T_3, T_4, and thyroid-binding protein levels, change little with advancing age in the absence of systemic illness. Similarly, thyrotropin (TSH) levels and the production of

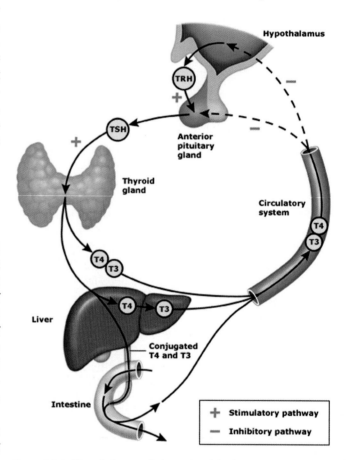

Figure 34.1 Hypothalamus–pituitary–thyroid axis with hormonal feedback mechanisms (reproduced with permission from Thyroid. In: Basow, DS, (Ed), Uptodate, Waltham, MA, 2010. Copyright © 2010 UpToDate, Inc. For more information, visit http://www.uptodate.com).

Table 34.1 Physiologic effects of thyroid hormones

Target tissue	Effect	Mechanism
Heart	Chronotropic	Increase number and affinity of beta-adrenergic receptors
	Inotropic	Enhance responses to circulating catecholamines
		Increase proportion of alpha myosin heavy chain (with higher ATPase activity)
Adipose tissue	Catabolic	Stimulate lipolysis
Muscle	Catabolic	Increase protein breakdown
Bone	Developmental and metabolic	Promote normal growth and skeletal development; accelerate bone turnover
Nervous system	Developmental	Promote normal brain development
Gut	Metabolic	Increase rate of carbohydrate absorption
Lipoprotein	Metabolic	Stimulate formation of LDL receptors
Other	Calorigenic	Stimulate oxygen consumption by metabolically active tissues (exceptions: adult brain, testes, uterus, lymph nodes, spleen, anterior pituitary)
		Increase metabolic rate

ATP adenosine triphosphate; *LDL* low-density lipoprotein

TSH in response to thyrotropin-releasing hormone (TRH) administration are relatively constant with increasing age [9]. In the past, hypothyroidism was considered an integral part of aging; however, more recent studies suggest that physiologic aging is associated with normal thyroid function [10]. The half-life of T_4 increases from 6.7 days in young adults to 9.3 days in those aged 80–90 years due to decreases in both fractional turnover rate and the distribution space of T_4. Peripheral conversion of T_4–T_3 is decreased, but the intrathyroidal conversion is increased, resulting in relatively stable T_3 levels in the elderly [11].

The Whickham survey documented the prevalence of thyroid disorders in a sample of 2,779 British adults, and the 20-year follow-up study was published in 1995 [12, 13]. The annual incidence of hypothyroidism was found to increase with age and correlate with the presence of thyroid autoantibodies or elevated TSH levels. Aging often is associated with an increased prevalence of antithyroid antibodies, but this age-dependent increase is observed commonly in unselected elderly subjects and not in healthy elderly populations selected for the absence of clinical or subclinical illnesses [14]. This suggests that thyroid autoimmune phenomena may not be the consequence of the aging process itself but, rather, an expression of age-associated disease.

Thyroid Dysfunction

Thyroid function can be evaluated by several biochemical measures, including total or free T_3 and T_4, and TSH [15]. The high incidence of comorbid illness in elderly people can confound assessment of thyroid function. Malnutrition, infection, sepsis, major surgery, poorly controlled diabetes mellitus, hepatic disease, renal failure, cerebrovascular disease, heart failure, malignancy, trauma, burns, and coma are all associated with alterations in thyroid function tests [16]. Depending on severity, stage, and drug effects, these nonthyroidal illnesses are associated with changes in the parameters of thyroid function that include low serum T_3, normal to low T_4, and normal to low or elevated TSH – the "euthyroid sick syndrome." Among acutely ill patients, 70% show a low T_3 state, and 30–50% of patients in intensive care units have low serum T_4 levels [17].

Findings in patients' personal and family histories indicate increased risk of developing thyroid dysfunction. Risk factors in personal history include goiter, surgery or radiotherapy affecting the thyroid gland, previous thyroid dysfunction, vitiligo, diabetes mellitus, pernicious anemia, leukotrichia, and medications, such as lithium carbonate and amiodarone, and iodine-containing compounds. Pertinent factors in family history are thyroid disease, pernicious anemia, diabetes mellitus, and primary adrenal insufficiency [18].

Measurement of serum TSH, a sensitive indicator of free thyroid hormone concentration in the presence of normal pituitary function, is often all that is required as a screening test for thyroid function. A decision analysis by Danese et al. reported that screening for thyroid disease by TSH measurement was particularly cost-effective in elderly female patients, as the clinical symptoms of thyroid dysfunction may be atypical in this age group [19]. Analyses of free hormone levels determine what is available for cellular metabolic regulation. In addition to thyroid function tests, diagnostic determination of thyroid autoantibodies can be useful. Antibodies to the TSH receptor are present in Graves' disease and also can be seen with other forms of autoimmune thyroid disease, such as Hashimoto's thyroiditis. Antithyroid peroxidase antibodies and antithyroglobulin antibodies are seen with all forms of autoimmune thyroid disease and may be present in patients with multinodular goiter. Assessment of the thyroid also should include imaging studies, such as ultrasound, nuclear medicine uptake scans, computed tomography (CT) scans, and magnetic resonance imaging (MRI).

Hypothyroidism

Epidemiology

The balance between central production and peripheral action of T_3 and T_4 is required for a euthyroid state. Clinical hypothyroidism usually is associated with decreased hormone production in the thyroid gland, although states of limited thyroid hormone activity in the periphery also can occur. In many underdeveloped countries or iodine-poor regions, lack of sufficient iodine intake explains a large percentage of hypothyroid conditions [20, 21]. In more developed countries, most cases of adult primary hypothyroidism (due to direct thyroid failure) are secondary to chronic autoimmune (Hashimoto's) thyroiditis, radioactive iodine (RAI) therapy, or surgery. Disorders of the pituitary or hypothalamus can cause diminished TSH secretion, producing hypothyroidism as a secondary or tertiary result. Finally, a host of medications, including the thioamide antithyroid drugs propylthiouracil (PTU) and methimazole (MMI), can produce hypothyroidism (Table 34.2).

There are two types of primary hypothyroidism. Clinical or overt primary hypothyroidism is characterized by elevated serum TSH and decreased serum T_3 and T_4 levels. Patients with subclinical primary hypothyroidism show mildly elevated serum TSH concentrations and normal serum thyroid hormone levels. Subclinical hypothyroidism is the most common thyroid dysfunction nationwide, with a markedly increased prevalence in the elderly, ranging from 4 to 15%

TABLE 34.2 Causes and pathogenetic mechanisms of hypothyroidism

Etiologic classification	Pathogenetic mechanism
Congenital	
	Aplasia or hypoplasia of thyroid gland
	Defects in hormone biosynthesis or action
Acquired	
Hashimoto's thyroiditis	Autoimmune destruction
Severe iodine deficiency	Diminished hormone synthesis, release
Thyroid ablation	Diminished hormone synthesis, release
Thyroid surgery	
[131]I radiation treatment of hyperthyroidism	
External beam radiation therapy for head and neck cancer	
	Diminished hormone synthesis,
Drugs	release
Iodine, inorganic	
Iodine, organic (amiodarone)	
Thioamides (propylthiouracil, methimazole)	
Potassium perchlorate	
Thiocyanate	
Lithium	
Hypopituitarism	Deficient TSH secretion
Hypothalamic disease	Deficient TRH secretion

TSH thyroid-stimulating hormone, *TRH* thyroid-release hormone
Source: Modified and reproduced from [94], with permission of The McGraw Hill Companies

for subclinical hypothyroidism and from 0.5 to 6% for overt hypothyroidism [22]. In the Whickham study, the risk of developing hypothyroidism was significantly increased in women between 75 and 80 years [12, 13].

Clinical and Diagnostic Evaluation

A comprehensive medical history should uncover symptoms that help establish the diagnosis, such as cold intolerance, weight gain, diminished appetite, constipation, and lethargy. On physical examination, a patient may exhibit hoarseness, bradycardia, periorbital or ankle edema, generalized muscle weakness, or delayed relaxation of deep tendon reflexes. The suspicion of hypothyroidism is raised by unexplained increases in serum cholesterol and creatine phosphokinase levels, severe constipation, congestive heart failure with restrictive cardiomyopathy, or macrocytic anemia [9].

Hypothyroidism is characterized by abnormally low serum T_4 and T_3 levels. Free thyroxine levels also are depressed. The serum TSH level is elevated in hypothyroidism, except in cases of pituitary or hypothalamic disease. TSH is the most sensitive test for early hypothyroidism, and

TABLE 34.3 Clinical findings in adult hypothyroidism

Symptoms

Slow thinking
Lethargy, decreased vigor
Dry skin, thickened hair, hair loss, broken nails
Diminished food intake, weight gain
Constipation
Menorrhagia, diminished libido
Cold intolerance

Signs

Round puffy face, slow speech, hoarseness
Hypokinesia, generalized muscle weakness, delayed deep tendon reflexes
Cold, dry, thick, scaling skin; dry, coarse, brittle hair; dry, ridged nails
Periorbital edema, ascites, pericardial effusion, ankle edema
Normal or faint cardiac impulse, indistinct heart sounds, bradycardia
Mental clouding, depression

Laboratory findings

Increased serum TSH
Decreased serum free thyroxine, total T_4 and T_3, resin T_4 or T_3 uptake, free thyroxine index
Decreased radioiodine uptake by thyroid gland
Diminished basal metabolic rate
Macrocytic anemia
Elevated serum cholesterol, creatine kinase
Decreased circulation time, low-voltage QRS complex on EKG

Source: Modified and reproduced from [95], with permission of The McGraw Hill Companies

marked elevations of serum TSH (>20 mU/L) are consistent with frank hypothyroidism. Modest TSH elevations (5–20 mU/L) may be found in euthyroid individuals with normal serum T_3 and T_4 levels and indicate impaired thyroid reserve and incipient hypothyroidism (Table 34.3) [23].

Many features of hypothyroidism are insidious and can be incorrectly attributed to aging. Hypothyroidism in elderly patients can be characterized by a paucity of specific signs and symptoms. Because of the high prevalence of hypothyroidism in women over 60 years, it is recommended that such individuals undergo annual screening with serum TSH measurement [24]. In addition, patients with other autoimmune diseases and those with unexplained depression or cognitive dysfunction should be screened with TSH measurements [25].

Treatment

The goal of therapy is to restore patients to a euthyroid state and normalize serum T_4 and TSH concentrations. Levothyroxine sodium, with its longer half-life and more stable serum concentration, is the treatment of choice for the routine management of hypothyroidism. Adults with hypothyroidism require approximately 1.7 mcg/kg of body weight per day for full replacement. For patients who are older than

50 years, a lower initial dosage is indicated, starting with 0.025–0.05 mg of levothyroxine daily, with clinical and biochemical reevaluations at 6- to 8-week intervals until serum TSH concentration is normalized [16]. In elderly patients with coexistent or suspected cardiac disease, levothyroxine therapy may precipitate angina or myocardial infarction. This is due to sensitivity to the hormone as a result of chronic depletion of catecholamines in the myocardium [10]. Monitoring serum TSH levels to ensure that they remain in the normal range will prevent the potential risk of overtreatment with levothyroxine.

Patients with subclinical hypothyroidism also can benefit from levothyroxine therapy. As many as 15% of elderly patients with subclinical hypothyroidism progress to overt hypothyroidism, particularly if the TSH concentration is greater than 10 mU/mL and thyroid autoantibodies are elevated [26]. Although early treatment prevents progression to frank hypothyroidism, hormone replacement therapy may exacerbate underlying cardiac disease. The decision whether to treat subclinical hypothyroidism should be made on an individual basis.

Hyperthyroidism

Epidemiology

The disease processes associated with increased thyroid secretion result in a hypermetabolic state. Increased thyroid secretion can be caused by primary alterations within the gland, most commonly due to Graves' disease in which TSH receptor autoantibodies stimulate thyroid follicular cells to produce excessive amounts of T_3 and T_4. Toxic adenoma (TA) and toxic multinodular goiter (TMNG, also known as Plummer's disease) are other common causes of hyperthyroidism, second in prevalence only to Graves' disease. They can appear at any age, although they most frequently occur in patients older than 40 years. Unlike Graves' disease, TA and TMNG are not believed to have an autoimmune etiology, since TSH receptor autoantibodies are absent. Less commonly, patients with multinodular goiter may become thyrotoxic without circulating antibodies if administered inorganic iodine compounds such as potassium iodide, or organic iodine compounds, such as the antiarrhythmic drug amiodarone. Patients from regions where goiter is endemic, so-called goiter belts, can develop thyrotoxicosis when given iodine supplementation (Jod-Basedow phenomenon) [20, 21]. Rarely, TSH-secreting pituitary adenomas (secondary hyperthyroidism) or TRH-secreting hypothalamic disorders (tertiary hyperthyroidism) may occur. Most hyperthyroid states result from thyroid gland dysfunction (Table 34.4). It is important to remember that thyrotoxicosis in the elderly can be caused easily by the administration of exogenous thyroid hormone.

TABLE 34.4 Causes and pathogenetic mechanisms of hyperthyroidism

Etiologic classification	Pathogenetic mechanism
Thyroid hormone overproduction	
Graves' disease	TSH-R-stimulating antibody
Toxic multinodular goiter	Autonomous hyperfunction
Follicular adenoma	Autonomous hyperfunction
Pituitary adenoma	TSH hypersecretion
Pituitary insensitivity	Resistance to thyroid hormone
Hypothalamic disease	Excess TRH production
Germ cell tumors	hCG stimulation
Struma ovarii	Functioning thyroid elements
Metastatic follicular thyroid cancer	Functioning metastases
Thyroid gland destruction	
Granulomatous thyroiditis	Release of stored hormone
Hashimoto's thyroiditis	Transient release of stored hormone
Other	
Thyrotoxicosis medicamentosa, thyrotoxicosis factitia	Ingestion of excessive exogenous thyroid hormone

TSH-R thyroid-stimulating hormone-receptor, *TRH* thyrotropin-releasing hormone, *hCG* human chorionic gonadotropin

Source: Modified and reproduced from [96], with permission of The McGraw Hill Companies

There are two types of primary hyperthyroidism based on thyroid function tests. Clinical primary hyperthyroidism is characterized by suppressed serum TSH and elevated serum total T_4 levels. Subclinical primary hyperthyroidism is defined by suppressed TSH and normal T_4 and T_3 levels. The prevalence of hyperthyroidism in the elderly ranges from 0.5 to 2.3% [27]. The Whickham survey demonstrated that hyperthyroidism did not increase in frequency with age or positive autoantibody status [12, 13]. Approximately 5% of elderly patients have subclinical hyperthyroidism [10].

Clinical and Diagnostic Evaluation

A detailed medical history will usually reveal sufficient clues to suggest the diagnosis of hyperthyroidism. Classic symptoms include heat intolerance, weight loss, increased appetite, palpitations, and emotional lability. Physical examination findings may include hyperkinesia, lid lag, periorbital edema, proptosis, proximal muscle weakness, and tachycardia (Table 34.5). Elderly hyperthyroid patients can display few signs and symptoms; this has been referred to as "apathetic hyperthyroidism." Orbital signs are often lacking with the exception of Graves' ophthalmopathy, which, if present, is usually worse than eye disease in the young (Fig. 34.2). Tachycardia in older patients is less common than that in younger patients, although it can be found in up to 50% of older patients. Congestive heart failure and angina are more frequent. Atrial fibrillation in thyrotoxic patients ranges from 9 to 22%, with a higher prevalence in elderly male patients [9]. Several studies also have demonstrated subtle abnormalities

TABLE 34.5 Clinical findings in adult hyperthyroidism

Symptoms

Alertness, emotional lability, nervousness, irritability

Poor concentration

Muscular weakness, fatigability

Palpitations

Voracious appetite, weight loss

Hyperdefecation

Heat intolerance

Signs

Hyperkinesia, rapid speech

Proximal muscle weakness, fine tremor

Fine, moist skin; fine, abundant hair; onycholysis

Lid lag, stare, chemosis, periorbital edema, proptosis

Accentuated first heart sound, tachycardia, atrial fibrillation, dyspnea

Laboratory findings

Suppressed serum TSH

Elevated serum free thyroxine, total T_4, resin T_3 or T_4 uptake, free thyroxine index

Increased radioiodine uptake by thyroid gland

Increased basal metabolic rate

Decreased serum cholesterol

TABLE 34.6 Adverse effects of major treatment modalities for hyperthyroidism

Treatment	Adverse effects
Antithyroid drugs (methimazole, propylthiouracil)	1–15% rash, arthralgias, fever, urticaria
	Rare: fulminant hepatitis, acute hepatic necrosis, glomerulonephritis, lupus-like syndrome, cholestatic hepatitis
	15–30%: elevated transaminases within first 2 months of therapy
	0.2–0.5%: agranulocytosis within first 3 months of therapy
Radioactive iodine	Transient or permanent hypothyroidism
	Recurrent or persistent hyperthyroidism
	Radiation thyroiditis
	Transient worsening of ophthalmopathy
	Hyperparathyroidism
	Thyrotoxic crisis
	Secondary gastrointestinal malignancy
	Radiation safety precautions
Surgery	Hypothyroidism
	Hypoparathyroidism
	Recurrent laryngeal nerve injury
	Hemorrhage
	Risk of anesthesia

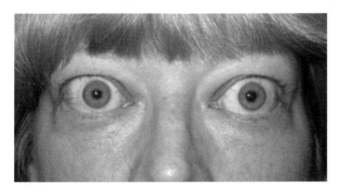

FIGURE 34.2 Exophthalmos in Graves' disease.

of cardiac contractility in individuals with subclinical hyperthyroidism, and one prospective study found that patients over age 65 years with TSH <0.1 mU/L had a threefold greater risk of developing atrial fibrillation than those with normal TSH levels [27]. Depression, lethargy, agitation, anxiety, dementia, and confusion have been reported as primary manifestations [26]. Because overt hyperthyroidism results in bone loss – through reduced absorption of dietary calcium, increased calcium excretion, increased bone turnover, and ultimately, decreased bone mineral density – the increased risk of osteoporosis and pathologic fracture is a pertinent feature of thyrotoxicosis in the elderly.

Treatment

Treatment of hyperthyroidism is directed toward lowering serum concentrations of thyroid hormones to reestablish a euthyroid state. There are three available modalities of treatment: antithyroid medications, radioactive iodine (^{131}I) therapy, and thyroid surgery. Each modality carries risks and benefits (Table 34.6).

Antithyroid Medication

Antithyroid medications interfere with one or more steps in the biosynthesis and secretion of thyroid hormone and include MMI and PTU. MMI is the preferred drug. Initial doses are MMI 10–40 mg three times daily and PTU 100–300 mg three times daily; these then can be reduced to once-daily dosing after the patient is rendered euthyroid. Rapidity of response is influenced by severity of the underlying disease, size of the gland, and dose and frequency of the agent used. In general, patients become euthyroid within 6–12 weeks of starting treatment [24].

Adverse reactions to both medications occur, including pruritus, arthralgias, and hepatic abnormalities. Hepatic necrosis caused by PTU and cholestatic jaundice associated with MMI are rare but recently have been the focus of attention. Agranulocytosis in response to either drug occurs in approximately 0.3% of patients, supporting routine monitoring of white blood cell counts [24]. In addition, Imseis and colleagues demonstrated that treatment with PTU reduced the efficacy of RAI therapy, an effect that was not found with MMI use [28]. This is of critical importance for patients who do not respond appropriately to antithyroid medications.

Long-term therapy can lead to remission, but as many as 40% of patients fail to remit after 2 years of treatment. The recurrence rate of disease is 60% after 6 months of therapy, with a latent period of 2–6 weeks. Because of this high failure rate, medical therapy with curative intent is primarily indicated in patients with small goiters, mildly elevated thyroid hormone levels, and who exhibit rapid remission with reduction of gland size [29].

In addition to preventing further synthesis of thyroid hormone, blockade of the catecholamine effects of thyroid hormone is especially important in elderly patients with underlying cardiac disease. The most useful adjuncts are beta-adrenergic blockers, which can provide symptomatic relief. Unfortunately, beta-blockers are contraindicated in patients with asthma or chronic obstructive pulmonary disease and those with heart block and congestive heart failure. In these patients, a calcium channel blocker such as diltiazem may be substituted [10, 24].

Radioactive Iodine Therapy

Radioactive iodine therapy (RAI) therapy is the standard treatment for thyrotoxicosis of Graves' disease in the USA. TMNG and toxic adenoma respond to ^{131}I, but surgery is more commonly employed. Advantages of RAI are avoidance of daily medications with the associated risk of noncompliance, symptoms of hyperthyroidism, and the risk of surgery. Thyrotoxic atrial fibrillation is likely to revert to sinus rhythm after a euthyroid state is established [10]. The overall risk of hypothyroidism with RAI necessitating lifelong replacement therapy is approximately 6% at 1 year and 82% at 25 years [30]. The insidious development of hypothyroidism is likely to occur following ^{131}I administration, and most patients eventually will require lifelong thyroid hormone replacement. Euthyroidism can take 4–6 months to achieve, and multiple doses may be required [29]. Because the effects of RAI may not be immediately evident, surgical resection in patients with antithyroid drug allergies, large goiters, more urgent cardiac issues, or coincident thyroid cancer may be more favorable.

In the USA, treatment of Graves' disease with RAI is the preferred therapy for most patients over the age of 21 years. Follow-up studies have not implicated RAI as a risk factor for development of secondary malignancies [31]. The main side effect of RAI is the development of hypothyroidism; most often, this occurs in patients with severe hyperthyroidism or very large goiters. Pretreatment with antithyroid medications before RAI reduces its effectiveness, primarily due to a radioactive-iodine-uptake (RAIU) independent effect [32]. This is particularly a problem with PTU, which can have a radioprotective effect [28]. However, in patients with severe hyperthyroidism, particularly in the presence of cardiac comorbidity, antithyroid medication pretreatment should

be performed for 4–8 weeks before RAI. Pretreatment reduces thyroid hormone secretion rapidly and thereby reduces the risk of thyrotoxic crisis soon after RAI [33].

The effect of RAI for Graves' hyperthyroidism associated with significant ophthalmopathy is controversial. In a prospective randomized study, Bartalena et al. evaluated the effects of RAI versus antithyroid medications and the effects of glucocorticoids in patients with or without Graves' ophthalmopathy. Among those treated with RAI, ophthalmopathy developed or worsened in 15% of patients 2–6 months after therapy. None of the patients with baseline ophthalmopathy in this group had improvement of eye disease. Among patients treated with a combination of RAI and glucocorticoids, 67% of patients with ophthalmopathy had improvement, and no patients had progression of eye disease [34].

RAI also provides effective treatment for TMNG and TA. Patients' characteristics that favor treatment with RAI include advanced age of patients, significant comorbidities, small goiters, adequate RAIU (>25%) as measured by thyroid uptake scans, prior surgery in the anterior neck, contraindications to surgery, and lack of access to a high-volume surgeon. Nygaard and colleagues reported a 52% rate of euthyroidism after a single ^{131}I treatment for TMNG, with an associated reduction in goiter volume by 40% at 24 months [35]. For TA, Nygaard et al. noted that 75% of patients were no longer hyperthyroid after their first RAI treatment, and that nodule volume showed a median reduction of 35% by 3 months and 45% by 24 months [36]. As demonstrated by Holm et al., hypothyroidism is the main side effect of RAI, with a higher incidence in patients who require more than one treatment to eliminate the hyperthyroid state [30].

Thyroid Surgery

Thyroid surgery should be considered if a patient has hyperthyroidism refractory to medical management, symptoms or signs of compression from goiter, coexisting hyperparathyroidism requiring surgery, large goiter, substernal or retrosternal goiter, insufficient RAIU (<25%), contraindications to RAI, thyroid nodule biopsy that is indeterminate or suspicious for thyroid cancer, or need for rapid correction of the thyrotoxic state [37]. Surgery for hyperthyroidism is advantageous because treatment is rapid, avoids the possible long-term risks of RAI and antithyroid medications, and it provides tissue for histologic examination. Risk of thyroid cancer in TMNG has been estimated to be 3%, although more recent data found an elevated risk of 21% [38, 39].

The operative complication rate is low when surgery is performed by high-volume thyroid surgeons [40]. In a recent cost-effectiveness analysis, surgery was more cost-effective than RAI unless patients had significant comorbidities that increased surgical mortality [41]. Near-total or total thyroidectomy should be performed for Graves' disease and TMNG, since subtotal thyroidectomy is associated with an attendant risk of persistent or recurrent disease. Ipsilateral thyroid lobectomy, not subtotal thyroid lobectomy or nodulectomy, is indicated for toxic adenomas [42, 43]. Hypothyroidism should be anticipated following near-total or total thyroidectomy [24, 41]. Following surgery, antithyroid medications should be stopped and beta-blockers weaned appropriately. Thyroid hormone replacement should be started at a dose appropriate for the patient's weight, with thyroid function levels monitored every 1–2 months until stable, and then at least annually. In the immediate postoperative period, serum calcium levels should be measured at 6 and 12 h after surgery, and oral calcium and vitamin D supplementation (rocaltrol) can be administered to reduce the likelihood of developing symptomatic hypocalcemia requiring readmission [44].

In the elderly, thyroidectomy has been shown to be associated with worser clinical and economic outcomes than in younger cohorts, as measured by length of hospital stay, mean total costs, immediate perioperative mortality, discharge status, and clinical complications (Table 34.7) [45]. Using the Charlson Comorbidity Index, the elderly (aged 65–79 years) and superelderly (aged >80 years) were stratified into healthy (none to two comorbidities) and sick (three or more comorbidities) subgroups. Their outcomes have been examined based on whether the procedure was performed by low-volume (1–29 thyroidectomies/year) versus high-volume (>30 thyroidectomies/year) surgeons. More experienced surgeons had better outcomes than their less experienced colleagues

(Fig. 34.3). A separate population-level study provided compelling evidence for a significant association between increased surgeon volume and improved patients' outcomes following surgical procedures for both benign and malignant thyroid disease [46]. The lowest-volume surgeons (1–9 thyroidectomies/year) operated on a substantially greater share of elderly patients, who, in turn, had less access to urban hospitals and teaching institutions [45]. For this older population, the surgical risks and benefits must be carefully weighed.

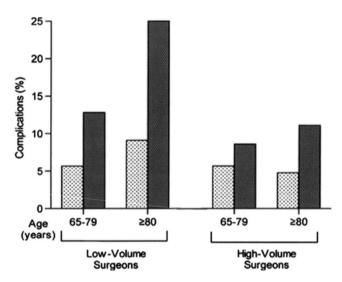

Figure 34.3 Complications of thyroidectomy for patients 65 years of age and older, by comorbidity and surgeon volume (reprinted with permission from [45] Copyright 2008, with permission of Elsevier).

Table 34.7 Unadjusted and adjusted clinical and economic outcomes from thyroidectomy, by patient age groups

Patient outcomes	Patient age groups (%)				
	18–44 years	45–64 years	65–79 years	80 years and older	p-Value
Unadjusted					
n (%)	8,053 (35.2)	9,959 (43.6)	4,092 (17.9)	744 (3.3)	
Mean total costs ($) (95% CI)	5,316 (5,174–5,459)	5,445 (5,343–5,547)	6,067 (5,850–6,285)	8,429 (7,339–9,519)	<0.001
Mean length of stay (days) (95% CI)	1.68 (1.63–1.73)	1.73 (1.68–1.77)	2.20 (2.11–2.30)	3.67 (3.19–4.15)	<0.001
In-hospital mortality (%)	2 (0)	7 (0.1)	8 (0.2)	6 (0.8)	<0.001
Patient discharge (%)					<0.001
Routine	7,998 (99.3)	9,827 (98.7)	3,907 (95.6)	621 (83.5)	
Home health care	26 (0.3)	75 (0.8)	104 (2.5)	50 (6.7)	
Transfer to intermediate care	2 (0)	11 (0.1)	2 (0)	3 (0.4)	
Other transfers	21 (0.3)	37 (0.4)	65 (1.6)	64 (8.6)	
Complications (%)	208 (2.6)	240 (3.4)	274 (6.7)	76 (10.2)	<0.001
Endocrine-specific complications[b] (%)	87 (1.1)	123 (1.2)	99 (2.4)	27 (3.6)	<0.001
Adjusted					
Mean total costs[c] ($) (95% CI)	4,905 (4,821–4,990)	5,263 (5,182–5,344)	5,917 (5,769–6,066)	7,084 (6,653–7,514)	<0.001
Mean length of stay[d] (days) (95% CI)	1.62 (1.58–1.66)	1.77 (1.73–1.81)	2.22 (2.15–2.30)	2.88 (2.67–3.10)	<0.001
Complications[e] (%)	6 (0.2)	15 (0.3)	41 (2.1)	19 (5.6)	<0.001

Source: Reproduced with permission from [45] Copyright 2008, with permission of Elsevier
[a] Significance was set at $\alpha = 0.05$
[b] Endocrine-specific complications include recurrent laryngeal nerve injury and hypoparathyroidism
[c] Adjusted for race, gender, hospital region, procedure, diagnosis, comorbidity, surgeon volume, household income, primary payor, and admission type
[d] Adjusted for race, gender, hospital region, procedure, diagnosis, comorbidity, surgeon volume, household income, primary payor, and admission type
[e] Adjusted for gender, region, procedure, diagnosis, comorbidity, surgeon volume, household income, primary expected payor, and admission type

Nodules

Epidemiology

Elderly patients frequently harbor thyroid nodules, and the incidence of thyroid nodules increases with age. Solitary palpable nodules occur in 4–7% of individuals and are approximately four times more prevalent in women than in men [47]. High-resolution ultrasound can detect thyroid nodules in 19–67% of randomly selected individuals, with higher frequencies in women and the elderly [48]. Exposure to radiation, particularly during childhood, is associated with an increased prevalence of thyroid nodules and papillary thyroid cancer. Iodine deficiency is associated with elevated risk of follicular thyroid cancer. Rapid growth, pain, and hoarseness are concerning for malignancy. Other risk factors for thyroid cancer include male gender, familial polyposis, Gardner's syndrome, Cowden's syndrome, familial papillary or medullary thyroid cancer, and multiple endocrine neoplasia (MEN) IIA or IIB syndrome. The clinical importance of thyroid nodules rests with the need to exclude thyroid cancer, which occurs in 5–10% of patients with thyroid nodules [47, 48].

Clinical and Diagnostic Evaluation

Following the discovery of a solitary thyroid nodule, subsequent management depends on the knowledge of a cost-effective workup. Most patients with a solitary thyroid nodule have a benign lesion; however, thyroid cancer is a consideration in all patients. Deciding between surveillance and nonoperative management or surgical therapy relies on careful analysis of the presentation and assessment with imaging modalities such as dedicated neck ultrasound and thyroid uptake scan, along with cytologic diagnosis provided by FNA biopsy (Fig. 34.4) [49].

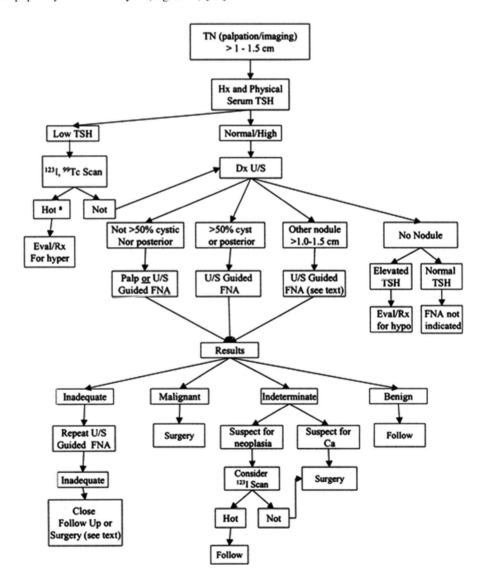

Figure 34.4 Algorithm for the evaluation of patients with one or more nodules (reprinted with permission from [5]).

The circumstances surrounding the onset and detection of the nodule and subsequent growth roughly correlate with malignant potential. Incidental subcentimeter nodules, identified during imaging procedures, have a very low probability of malignancy [50]. Slow growth over months to years can be seen with differentiated thyroid carcinomas or benign lesions. Rapid growth over days to weeks most commonly occurs with cyst formation in a goiter or hemorrhage into a preexisting cyst or nodule, but may rarely represent anaplastic thyroid carcinoma or primary thyroid lymphoma. Rapid onset of pain in a nodule often indicates hemorrhage into a goiter or benign adenoma. Slow onset of pain or hoarseness associated with a thyroid nodule is concerning for malignancy. Symptoms of hyperthyroidism are associated with an autonomous nodule (TA or "hot nodule") or TMNG.

With the discovery of a thyroid nodule, a complete history and physical examination focusing on the thyroid gland and adjacent cervical lymph nodes should be performed. Risk factors for thyroid cancer are a history of head and neck irradiation in childhood or adolescence (papillary thyroid cancer), family history of thyroid cancer in a first-degree relative (familial papillary or medullary thyroid cancer, MEN IIA or IIB), and total body irradiation for bone marrow transplantation. Physical examination findings suggestive of malignancy include vocal cord paresis or paralysis, fixation of the nodule to surrounding tissues, or cervical lymphadenopathy [50].

In general, use of a complete blood count or standard electrolyte evaluation is unhelpful in the evaluation of a patient with a thyroid nodule. Thyroid function tests, including measurement of T_3, T_4, and TSH levels, should be employed to identify patients with hyper- or hypothyroidism. In 2006, the American Thyroid Association (ATA) Guidelines Taskforce recommended that if serum TSH is subnormal for nodules greater than 1–1.5 cm in diameter, then a radionuclide thyroid scan should be performed to determine whether the nodule is functioning with tracer uptake greater than the surrounding normal thyroid tissue ("hot"), isofunctioning ("warm"), or nonfunctioning with tracer uptake less than the surrounding thyroid ("cold") (Fig. 34.5). In general, functional nodules rarely harbor malignancy [50]. However, a large series has shown that 16% of patients with cold nodules and 4% of patient with hot nodules had thyroid cancer documented by surgical resection [51]. It may be that the most useful current application for radionuclide scanning is in the setting of the workup for Graves' disease.

Based on the ATA Guidelines, the finding of a nodule that is 1–1.5 cm in size warrants consideration of ultrasound and biopsy. An exception can be made for an elderly patient with a growing hot nodule. The likelihood of a hot nodule causing clinical hyperthyroidism over time is a function of its size. If there is evidence of autonomous function, an elderly patient with a large nodule should be considered for either RAI or surgery to prevent the development of atrial fibrillation or other cardiac complications prevalent in this population [10, 41].

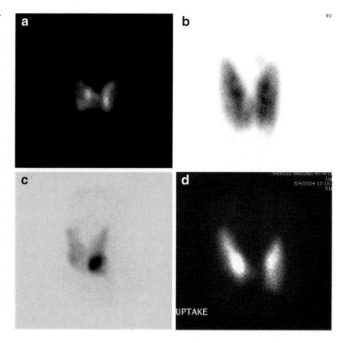

Figure 34.5 ^{123}I thyroid scintigraphy (thyroid "uptake" scans).

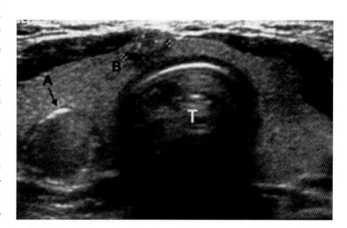

Figure 34.6 Transverse ultrasound image showing multifocal papillary thyroid carcinoma.

Ultrasonography of the thyroid is used as the initial imaging modality of a palpable nodule. It is helpful in determining volume and size, number of nodules, whether nodules are solid or cystic, and (with serial ultrasonography) whether there is interval growth. Use of ultrasound has expanded into the office setting and also is available for intraoperative evaluation. It is highly operator-dependent. Ultrasound cannot distinguish between benign and malignant pathologies [52]. Thyroid cancers are hypoechoic in almost 80% of cases; in 20% of cases, they appear as inhomogeneous lesions with solid hypoechoic and cystic changes. However, up to 1% of all carcinomas show a homogeneously hyperechoic echotexture. Papillary thyroid carcinomas often contain microcalcifications (Fig. 34.6), but these also can be seen within benign hyperplastic or regressive nodules [53, 54].

Subclinical, subcentimeter nodules in patients without personal or familial risk factors should undergo size assessment by ultrasound examination and follow-up studies at 6 and 12 months. FNA should be performed for nodules that are 1–1.5 cm in size, smaller nodules with irregular edges or rapid size progression, and in patients with risk factors for thyroid malignancy [55]. Ultrasound-guided FNA is the most accurate and cost-effective method for evaluating thyroid nodules and suspicious cervical lymph nodes. It can be readily performed by experienced clinicians in the outpatient setting. With the patient in a supine position and the neck extended, the skin overlying the nodule is cleansed. Infiltration of a local anesthetic agent is optional. A 23- to 25-gauge needle is inserted into the nodule. Ultrasound-guided FNA biopsy of a thyroid nodule has certain advantages, including the ability to biopsy small, nonpalpable nodules and to biopsy the solid component of a thyroid cyst. While maintaining gentle suction on the syringe, the needle is moved forward and backward through the nodule to draw tissue into the needle. Suction is released, and the needle is withdrawn. The aspirated fluid is spread on a microscope slide and air-dried or fixed according to the preferences of the examining cytopathologist [56, 57].

Assessment of FNA-acquired tissue by an experienced thyroid cytologist can identify reliably the characteristics of particular processes. The features of papillary thyroid carcinoma, such as nuclear grooves, intranuclear cytoplasmic inclusions, psammoma bodies, fine powdery chromatin, and papillary formations, may be seen. Bland follicular cells, mature lymphocytes, and hemosiderin-laden macrophages are typical of nodular goiter, Hashimoto's thyroiditis, or cystic degeneration of a benign nodule.

Traditionally, FNA biopsy results are divided into four categories: nondiagnostic, benign, indeterminate or suspicious for neoplasm, and malignant. Nondiagnostic aspirates are due to insufficient sampling and typically contain few follicular cells and scant colloid. Such results should prompt a repeat FNA biopsy [56]. If a nodule is benign on cytology, additional diagnostic studies or treatment are not routinely required. Indeterminate or suspicious cytology can be found in 15–30% of FNA specimens [37]. Follicular and Hürthle cell neoplasms fall into this category because malignancy is determined by histologic evidence of vascular or capsular invasion that only can be determined on histologic analysis. Specific molecular markers have been evaluated to improve diagnostic accuracy of cytology in the setting of these lesions. Recent ATA Guidelines do not advocate routine use of these markers; instead, ipsilateral thyroid lobectomy, or near-total or total thyroidectomy (if there are multiple or bilateral nodules) is recommended [50]. Finally, aspirates of malignant nodules have unequivocal cytopathologic features of malignancy. These specimens tend to be highly cellular and exhibit typical architechtural and cytologic features of primary thyroid carcinomas (papillary, medullary, or anaplastic),

lymphomas (primary or secondary), or metastatic tumors. Approximately 5% of aspirates fall into this category [58].

In the elderly population, primary thyroid lymphoma and anaplastic thyroid carcinoma are more common and present typically with a history of rapid nodule growth, often associated with subjective respiratory compromise and stridor. Prompt differential diagnosis is critical, as treatment options vary. Surgery, radiotherapy, and/or chemotherapy can be beneficial in the setting of primary thyroid lymphoma, while the treatment of anaplastic thyroid cancer is poorly effective and includes radiotherapy, palliative debulking, tracheostomy, and/or feeding tube placement.

Treatment

Patients with benign FNA results in the proper clinical setting should be followed-up periodically with focused physical examinations, as there is a false-negative rate of up to 5% with FNA [59]. Consideration should be given to ultrasound follow-up evaluation of nodule size and contour, and repeat FNA should be performed if the nodule increases in size or develops suspicious characteristics by ultrasound appearance or physical examination.

In the past, patients with benign nodules often were treated with thyrotropin-suppressive therapy with levothyroxine, which was thought to shrink some lesions and prevent enlargement of others. However, several studies indicate that only 20% of cytologically benign thyroid nodules undergo significant shrinkage with this therapy, and that 40–50% of these nodules shrink or disappear spontaneously. This may explain the apparent effectiveness of suppressive therapy reported in many uncontrolled clinical trials. Approximately 20% of cytologically benign thyroid nodules not treated with thyroid suppression enlarge over time, but only 5% of these nodules harbor malignancy [60, 61]. Given the potential long-term skeletal and cardiac effects of thyroid hormone, permanent suppressive therapy of presumed benign nodules is probably unwise in elderly women [10]. Furthermore, current ATA Guidelines do not recommend routine suppressive therapy of benign thyroid nodules [50].

Indications for surgical intervention include FNA findings of thyroid malignancy, suspicious for malignancy, or inconclusive neoplastic lesion; nodules with progressive growth in size; and, multiple thyroid nodules in the setting of prior ionizing radiation exposure [62]. In addition to resolving questions regarding malignancy, surgery can alleviate symptoms related to local mass effect on the upper aerodigestive tract. Patients can have dysphagia, chronic cough, or in the case of a substernal goiter, difficulty breathing. Substernal goiters are more common in the elderly [63, 64]. Often, elderly patients with long-standing goiter and respiratory complaints are diagnosed with asthma or chronic obstructive

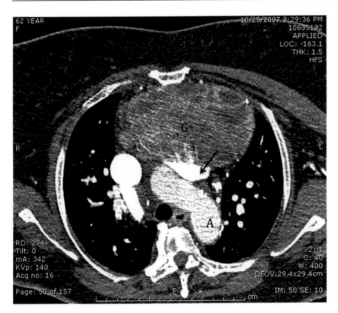

Figure 34.7 Computed tomography image of goiter with extensive substernal component.

pulmonary disease when the extent of airway compromise caused by the goiter is unrecognized. Routine chest radiograph, CT scan, or MRI can determine the extent of the goiter and status of the patient's airway (Fig. 34.7). In most cases, substernal goiters can be removed through a cervical Kocher incision, even in reoperative circumstances [63–65].

Neoplasia

Epidemiology

Thyroid cancer represents less than 1% of all malignancies in the USA, occurring in approximately 40 per one million people per year [1]. Six deaths per one million people occur annually. While the incidence of thyroid cancer in the USA more than doubled over the past 30 years, almost 90% of this increase was due to the diagnosis of differentiated thyroid cancers [4]. Ninety percent of thyroid malignancies are categorized as well-differentiated tumors arising from a follicular cell origin. These include papillary thyroid cancer, follicular thyroid cancer, and Hürthle cell cancer. Medullary thyroid cancer, which arises from thyroid parafollicular or C cells, accounts for about 6% of thyroid cancers, of which 20–30% are inherited in the form of familial medullary thyroid cancer or MEN types IIA and IIB. Anaplastic thyroid cancer, also derived from thyroid follicular cells, is an aggressive malignancy and is responsible for less than 1% of thyroid cancers, and 600 new cases per year. Approximately 1% of thyroid malignancies are primary thyroid lymphoma,

usually of the non-Hodgkin's B-cell type [66]. Metastatic disease to the thyroid is rare and most commonly originates from renal cell carcinomas, breast cancers, and lung cancers. Other tumors that have been shown to metastasize to the thyroid include melanoma and those from esophagus, stomach, pancreas, colon, rectum, uterus, and larynx [67, 68].

Clinical and Diagnostic Evaluation

Evaluation of a patient for thyroid cancer should begin with a thorough history and physical examination. This should be followed by ultrasonography with FNA, and occasionally, CT (usually without intravenous contrast in case it is a differentiated thyroid cancer that will necessitate adjuvant RAI therapy) or MRI. In addition to thyroid function tests, patients with medullary thyroid cancer require preoperative evaluation of calcitonin, carcinoembryonic antigen (CEA), and catecholamine levels (24-h urine measurement of epinephrine, norepinephrine, metanephrine, normetanephrine, vanillylmandelic acid, and dopamine levels), particularly if there is suspicion of MEN IIA or IIB syndrome. In addition, consideration should be given to genetic screening with a serum *RET* (rearranged during transfection) proto-oncogene screen for all patients with medullary thyroid cancer.

Papillary thyroid cancer is the most common form, representing 80% of thyroid cancers. Prognostically, it is the most favorable. This tumor tends to exhibit intra- and extraglandular lymphatic spread; unlike other malignancies, presence of lymphatic metastases generally does not adversely influence prognosis, especially in young patients under age 45 years. Recognized variants of papillary carcinoma include encapsulated, follicular, tall cell, columnar cell, clear cell, and diffuse sclerosing carcinomas. Follicular thyroid cancer is more aggressive. Malignant lesions exhibit vascular or capsular invasion, and they spread hematogeneously to lung and bone. Like follicular thyroid cancer, Hürthle cell cancer, an oncocytic tumor, is considered malignant if there is evidence of vascular or capsular invasion. Although considered well-differentiated, Hürthle cell carcinoma holds a significantly worse prognosis than its papillary or follicular counterparts, in part because only a minority of tumors demonstrate iodine avidity. While the mean age at presentation is 30–40 years for papillary carcinoma, mean age at presentation for follicular thyroid cancer is 50 years, and for Hürthle cell carcinoma, 60 years [69, 70].

Medullary thyroid cancer arises from the calcitonin-secreting parafollicular or C-cells, which are derived from neural crest cells during embryologic development. Sporadic medullary thyroid cancer represents 70% of all cases; it tends to be unilateral and occurs after 30 years of age. Inherited medullary thyroid cancer accounts for 20–30% of all cases; it is almost always bilateral, associated with C-cell hyperplasia, and usually occurs before 30 years of age. Familial medullary thyroid cancer can occur in the absence of associated endocrinopathy or as part of the MEN II syndromes. The pathologic features of medullary thyroid cancer include the presence of amyloid, a classic "salt-and-pepper" appearance of the cells, C-cell hyperplasia, and positive immunohistochemical staining for calcitonin and CEA. Patients present with a thyroid mass associated with cervical lymphadenopathy in up to 20% of cases. Symptoms are secondary to mass effect or to hypercalcitonism, as manifested by diarrhea and flushing. Hematogeneous metastases to the liver, lung, and bones occur with disease progression. Prognosis varies with extent of disease. Sporadic and MEN-IIB-associated medullary thyroid tumors are more aggressive, and they carry a worse prognosis than MEN IIA or familial forms of the disease [71].

With the reduction of iodine-deficiency-associated goiters in the USA, the incidence of anaplastic or undifferentiated carcinoma has decreased to less than 1% of thyroid cancers. It usually arises in a well-differentiated cancer and in patients older than 60 years. Patients may detail a history of rapid enlargement of a neck mass in conjunction with pain, hoarseness, dyspnea, and dysphagia. Physical examination often reveals a firm, fixed thyroid mass with palpable cervical lymph node metastases. On FNA, spindle cells, small cells, or giant cells suggest the diagnosis. In many cases, additional pathologic material will be required to obtain a histologic diagnosis. While anaplastic thyroid cancer is rare, it accounts for more than half of the 1,200 deaths attributed to thyroid cancer annually in the USA [72]. Given the overall aggressiveness of the disease as well as its late clinical presentation, prognosis is extremely poor, with a 90% mortality within a mean interval of 9 weeks [73, 74].

Primary thyroid lymphoma is usually of the non-Hodgkin's B-cell type. It tends to occur in elderly women who present with a rapidly growing, often painful, thyroid mass with compressive symptoms. The overall 5-year survival for lymphoma of the thyroid is 70%. Older age, single marital status, advanced stage (stages II–IV), and histologic subtype (large B-cell, follicular, or other non-Hodgkin's) are associated with worse survival [75]. Primary squamous cell carcinoma and metastatic disease is rare. The diagnosis is most often confirmed by FNA and rarely requires surgical intervention [73].

A number of clinical scoring systems have been developed to assess prognosis of differentiated thyroid cancer. These include AGES (age, grade, extent, size), AMES (age, metastasis, extent, size), and MACIS (metastasis, age, completeness of resection, invasion, size) [76,77]. For well-differentiated tumors, patients younger than 20 years, males older than 40 years, and females older than 50 years with cancers greater than 4 cm that have extended through the thyroid capsule and who have distant metastases are at higher risk of dying from the disease. In contrast, patients between ages 20 and 40 years with a tumor less than 4 cm confined to the thyroid are at low risk and have an excellent prognosis. The TMN staging system adopted by the American Joint Committee on Cancer

(AJCC), as well as the International Union Against Cancer (UICC), is universally accepted and is required by tumor boards for standardized reporting (Table 34.8) [50].

Treatment

The goals of initial therapy of differentiated thyroid cancer are to (1) remove the primary tumor, disease beyond the thyroid capsule, and involved cervical lymph nodes; (2) permit accurate staging of the disease; (3) minimize treatment-related morbidity; (4) facilitate postoperative treatment with RAI if appropriate; (5) allow for accurate long-term surveillance for recurrence; and (6) minimize risk of locoregional disease recurrence and metastatic spread [50].

Successful thyroid surgery requires an appreciation of the normal anatomic relations of the thyroid and parathyroids, the recurrent and superior laryngeal nerves, and the inferior thyroid arteries, as well as their common anatomic variations. Lo Gerfo and colleagues have shown that bilateral neck exploration under regional anesthesia can be performed safely in patients with thyroid disease [78, 79]. However, most surgeons prefer general endotracheal anesthesia. The relatively short duration of the procedure and lack of significant fluid shifts and hemodynamic changes allows it to be well-tolerated, even in older patients.

According to the ATA Guidelines, near-total or total thyroidectomy are acceptable operations for papillary thyroid cancer. They are followed by a 10-year survival rate in excess of 90%. Subtotal or partial lobectomy ("nodulectomy") is contraindicated. Total thyroidectomy is preferred over other operations because of the high incidence of multifocal disease, a clinical recurrence rate of 7% in the contralateral lobe if it is spared, and the ease of assessment for recurrence by serum thyroglobulin assay or radioiodine scan during follow-up exams. In addition, total thyroidectomy increases the efficacy of RAI therapy. Routine central compartment (level VI) neck dissection continues to be an area of great controversy. Although there are ample data that micrometastases to this level are not infrequent, central lymphadenectomy comes with increased attendant risk of recurrent laryngeal nerve injury and hypoparathyroidism. If there is palpable, biopsy-proven, or grossly apparent metastasis at the time of surgery, lymphadenectomy should be performed. However, if these conditions are not present and if postoperative RAI ablation is planned, dissection of nonpalpable central lymph nodes is debatable [80, 81]. A modified radical neck dissection (levels II–V), preserving the sternocleidomastoid muscle, spinal accessory nerve, and internal jugular vein, usually is indicated for patients with clinically palpable or biopsy-proven cervical adenopathy [82].

Patients with an FNA-diagnosis of follicular or Hürthle cell neoplasm should undergo ipsilateral thyroid lobectomy and isthmusectomy because approximately 20% of these

TABLE 34.8 American Joint Committee on Cancer (AJCC) pathologic-tumor-node metastasis (pTNM) system

Definition

Tx	Primary tumor cannot be assessed
T0	No evidence of primary tumor
T1	Tumor diameter 2 cm or less limited to the thyroid
T1a	Tumor diameter 1 cm or less limited to the thyroid
T1b	Tumor diameter 1–2 cm limited to the thyroid
T2	Primary tumor diameter >2–4 cm
T3	Primary tumor diameter >4 cm limited to thyroid or with minimal extrathyroidal extension
T4a	Tumor of any size extending beyond thyroid capsule to invade soft tissues, larynx, trachea, esophagus, recurrent laryngeal nerve (moderately advanced)
T4b	Tumor invades prevertebral fascia or encases carotid artery or mediastinal vessels (very advanced)
Nx	Regional lymph nodes cannot be assessed
N0	No regional lymph node metastasis
N1	Regional lymph node metastasis
N1a	Metastases to level VI (pretracheal, paratracheal, prelaryngeal/Delphian lymph nodes)
N1b	Metastases to unilateral, bilateral, contralateral cervical or superior mediastinal lymph nodes
Mx	Distant metastases not assessed
M0	No distant metastases
M1	Distant metastases

	Papillary or follicular		Medullary	Anaplastic
Stage	Age <45 years	Age >45 years	Any age	Any age
I	Any T, any N, M0	T1, N0, M0	T1, N0, M0	
II	Any T, any N, M1	T2, N0, M0	T2, N0, M0	
			T3, N0, M0	
III		T3, N0, M0	T1, N1a, M0	
		T1, N1a, M0	T2, N1a, M0	
		T2, N1a, M0	T3, N1a, M0	
		T3, N1a, M0		
IV				
A		T4a, N0, M0	T4a, N0, M0	T4a, any N, M0
		T4a, N1a, M0	T4a, N1a, M0	
		T1, N1b, M0	T1, N1b, M0	
		T2, N1b, M0	T2, N1b, M0	
		T3, N1b, M0	T3, N1b, M0	
		T4a, N1b, M0	T4a, N1b, M0	
B		T4b, any N, M0	T4b, any N, M0	T4b, any N, M0
C		Any T, any N, M1	Any T, any N, M1	Any T, any N, M1

Source: Used with permission of the American Joint Committee on Cancer (AJCC), Chicago, IL, The original source for this material is the AJCC Cancer Staging Manual, Seventh Edition (2010) published by Springer Science and Business Media, LLC, http://www.springerlink.com

lesions will prove to be carcinomas. The diagnosis of carcinoma is confirmed by the finding of capsular and vascular invasion on permanent histology. Detection of macroinvasion necessitates completion of thyroidectomy. Indications for total thyroidectomy include obvious extension of the lesion through the thyroid capsule, lesions greater than 4 cm (50–80% prove to be malignant), and contralateral nodularity or pathology. Follicular carcinoma is associated with a 10-year survival of 85% and 20-year survival of 70% [70]. Like papillary and follicular malignancies, Hürthle cell carcinomas produce thyroglobulin, a useful marker for postoperative surveillance. However, Hürthle cells are not iodine-avid; therefore, surgical resection is the mainstay of treatment.

In patients with papillary or follicular thyroid cancer, postoperative ablation with ^{131}I is used more frequently to eliminate residual thyroid tissue in order to decrease the risk of locoregional recurrence as well as to facilitate long-term surveillance with radioiodine scans. Several retrospective studies have demonstrated a significant reduction in the rates of disease recurrence and disease-associated mortality [70, 83]. In order to effectively administer postoperative RAI, the patient must be sufficiently hypothyroid as shown by elevated serum TSH levels. Levothyroxine is withheld or withdrawn for 4–6 weeks to maximize thyrotropin stimulation of the remaining thyroid tissue. The resulting hypothyroidism is tolerated poorly by some patients, and it may be attenuated by administration of liothyronine sodium to ensure a shorter duration of hypothyroidism. Recently, administration of recombinant human thyrotropin (rhTSH) has been used in lieu of traditional thyroid hormone withdrawal.

CASE STUDY RESOLUTION

JK's medical and surgical teams discussed the risks and benefits of total thyroidectomy with the patient, and the decision was made to proceed with surgery given the apparent aggressive nature of her cancer. Given her subjective hoarseness, indirect laryngoscopy was performed, and her vocal cord function was deemed to be intact; she had mild reflux. Appropriate medical and cardiologic clearance was obtained. The patient met with anesthesiology preoperatively. Her warfarin was stopped 5 days prior to surgery, as was her vitamin supplement. Total thyroidectomy with en bloc resection of the right strap muscle was performed, along with a right central lymph node dissection. The patient did well postoperatively; she had no evidence for change in voice or hypoparathyroidism. Her warfarin was restarted on postoperative day 1, and she was discharged home that day with follow-up with her cardiologist later in the week. Her final pathology revealed multifocal papillary thyroid cancer. The largest focus measured 4.1 cm in the right lobe, and an additional 5 mm focus was identified in the contralateral lobe. Lymphovascular invasion was seen, and there was extension of tumor into soft tissue, but surgical margins were negative. Three of ten lymph nodes were positive for metastatic disease, giving her an AJCC pT4aN1aMx, or stage IVA, papillary thyroid cancer. She met with endocrinology regarding adjuvant RAI therapy.

Successful remnant ablation with ^{131}I was equivalent after thyroxine withdrawal compared to rhTSH stimulation when the thyroxine therapy was stopped 1 day prior to the rhTSH injections and restarted the day following RAI [84–86].

Treatment for medullary thyroid cancer generally includes total thyroidectomy and central lymph node dissection. An ipsilateral or bilateral modified radical neck dissection is performed for lateral cervical lymph node disease. Tumor debulking may be helpful in alleviating diarrhea and flushing. Nutmeg oil, a combination of atropine sulfate and diphenoxylate hydrochloride, or subcutaneous somatostatin analogue has offered some relief from symptoms of metastatic disease [71]. Postoperatively, calcitonin remains a highly sensitive tumor marker and may remain elevated in patients who present with bulky disease. Preoperative basal calcitonin levels can individualize the extent of surgery and postoperative follow-up intervals. On multivariate analysis, preoperative basal serum calcitonin levels >500 pg/ml best predicted failure to achieve biochemical remission, followed by nodal metastasis and need for reoperation. Patients with nodal or distant metastases did not achieve biochemical remission when their preoperative basal calcitonin levels exceeded 3,000 pg/ml. Nodal metastasis emerged at basal calcitonin levels of 10–40 pg/ml, while distant metastases and extrathyroidal growth appeared with basal calcitonin levels of 150–400 pg/ml [87]. Despite this, some patients with medullary thyroid cancer survive for many years with minimal symptoms despite significant tumor burden. Chemotherapy is poorly effective in the management of locally advanced and metastatic medullary thyroid cancer, and the role of radiation therapy is questionable. The best results are achieved in familial medullary or MEN II kindreds where patients can be identified presymptomatically and appropriately treated [55, 71]. More recently, tyrosine kinase inhibitors have been shown to inhibit *RET* tyrosine kinase activity. Clinical studies are underway, but only preliminary results have been published [88, 89].

Anaplastic thyroid cancer most often is advanced at presentation, and it usually presents in the 6–7th decades of life. It is almost always unencapsulated and invades surrounding structures. Cervical lymphadenopathy and pulmonary metastases are common. It does not concentrate iodine or express thyroglobulin [90]. Although there is no satisfactory treatment for anaplastic cancer, local control can be attempted with palliative surgery, chemotherapy, or radiotherapy. Tumor debulking, tracheostomy, and feeding gastrostomy may be required for palliation [91]. In the rare instance of early anaplastic carcinoma localized to the thyroid, total thyroidectomy has resulted in long-term survival [92].

Primary non-Hodgkin's lymphoma of the thyroid is most common in elderly women, occurring most often in the background of autoimmune thyroid disease. Primary thyroid lymphoma usually is not a surgical disease, although surgeons often assist by obtaining adequate tissue to establish a diagnosis and determine tumor markers. Use of multimodality chemotherapy, particularly with anthracycline agents, and external radiotherapy results in dramatic tumor shrinkage and rapid resolution of airway compromise. The overall 5-year survival is approximately 70%, depending on stage and histologic type [71, 75, 93].

Conclusion

Thyroid disease is common in the elderly. In this population, the clinical manifestation of thyroid dysfunction can be subtle, often hidden by a background of coexistent disease. Hypo- and hyperthyroidism often are subclinical, and therapeutic decisions may be dictated by patients' preference and overall health status. The incidence of thyroid nodules increases with age, as does the risk of thyroid malignancy and the aggressiveness of the thyroid tumor. Surgery is the mainstay of treatment for thyroid cancer. Quality-of-life issues related to voice, swallowing, and calcium metabolism are especially salient in elderly patients. Thyroid surgery in this population is associated with increased attendant risk, but it can be performed safely, especially in the hands of high-volume thyroid surgeons. It is imperative that internists, geriatricians, endocrinologists, and thyroid surgeons work together as an interdisciplinary team to formulate and tailor treatment strategies.

References

1. United States Census Bureau (2008) Available at: http://www.census.gov/population/www/projections/natdet-d1a.html
2. Wu P (2000) Thyroid disease and diabetes. Clin Diabetes 18:1
3. Whitman ED, Norton JA (1994) Endocrine surgical diseases of elderly patients. Surg Clin North Am 74:127
4. Davies L, Welch HG (2006) Increasing incidence of thyroid cancer in the United States, 1973–2002. J Am Med Assoc 295:2164
5. Mariotti S et al (1995) The aging thyroid. Endocr Rev 16:686
6. Coburn MC, Wanebo HJ (1995) Age correlates with increased frequency of high risk factors in elderly patients with thyroid cancer. Am J Surg 170:471
7. Ganong WF (1991) The thyroid gland. In: Ganong WF (ed) Review of medical physiology. Appleton & Lange, Stamford, p 303
8. Goodman HM (2003) Thyroid gland. In: Johnson LR (ed) Essential medical physiology. Elsevier, San Diego, p 587
9. Mokshagundam S, Barzel US (1993) Thyroid disease in the elderly. J Am Geriatr Soc 41:1361
10. Chiovato L et al (1997) Thyroid diseases in the elderly. Ballieres Clin Endocrinol Metab 11(2):251
11. Gambert SR (1991) Environmental and physiologic variables. In: Braverman LE, Utiger RD (eds) The thyroid. Lippincott, Philadelphia, p 347
12. Tunbridge WMG et al (1977) The spectrum of thyroid disease in the community: the Whickham survey. Clin Endocrinol 7:481
13. Vanderpump MPJ et al (1995) The incidence of thyroid disorders in the community: a twenty-year follow-up of the Whickham survey. Clin Endocrinol 43:55
14. Pinchera A et al (1995) Thyroid autoimmunity and aging. Horm Res 43:64
15. Dayan CM (2001) Interpretation of thyroid function tests. Lancet 357:619
16. Surks MI et al (1990) American thyroid association guidelines for use of laboratory tests in thyroid disorders. JAMA 263:1529
17. Wong KT, Hershman JM (1992) Changes in thyroid function in nonthyroid illness. Trends Endocrinol Metab 3:8
18. Ladenson PW et al (2000) American thyroid association guidelines for detection of thyroid dysfunction. Arch Intern Med 160:1573
19. Danese MD et al (1996) Screening for mild thyroid failure at the periodic health examination: a decision and cost-effective analysis. J Am Med Assoc 276:2591
20. Laurberg P et al (1998) Iodine intake and the pattern of thyroid disorders: a comparative epidemiological study of thyroid abnormalities in the elderly in Iceland in Jutland, Denmark. J Clin Endocrinol Metab 83:765
21. Szabolcs I et al (1997) Comparative screening for thyroid disorders in old age in areas of iodine deficiency, long-term iodine prophylaxis, and abundant iodine intake. Clin Endocrinol 47:87
22. Cooper DS (2001) Subclinical hypothyroidism. N Engl J Med 345:260
23. Greenspan FS (2007) The thyroid gland. In: Garner D, Shoback D (eds) Basic and clinical endocrinology. McGraw, New York, p 209
24. Singer PA et al (1995) Treatment guidelines for patients with hyperthyroidism and hypothyroidism. JAMA 273:808
25. Surks MI et al (2004) Subclinical thyroid disease: scientific review and guidelines for diagnosis and management. JAMA 291:228
26. Roberts LM et al (2006) Is subclinical thyroid dysfunction in the elderly associated with depression or cognitive dysfunction? Ann Intern Med 145:573
27. Sawin CT et al (1994) Low serum thyrotropin concentrations as a risk factor for atrial fibrillation in older persons. N Engl J Med 331:1249
28. Imseis RE et al (1998) Pretreatment with propylthiouracil but not methimazole reduces the therapeutic efficacy of I-131 in hyperthyroidism. J Clin Endocrinol Metab 83:685
29. Boger MS, Perrier ND (2005) Graves' and Plummer's disease: medical and surgical management. In: Clark OH, Duh QY, Kebebew E (eds) Textbook of endocrine surgery. Elsevier, Philadelphia, p 54
30. Metso S et al (2004) Long-term follow-up study of radioiodine treatment of hyperthyroidism. Clin Endocrinol 61:641
31. Iagaru A, McDougall IR (2007) Treatment of thyrotoxicosis. J Nucl Med 48:379
32. Walter MA et al (2004) Radioiodine therapy in hyperthyroidism: inverse correlation of pretherapeutic iodine uptake level and post-therapeutic outcome. Eur J Clin Investig 34:365
33. Andrade V et al (2001) The effect of methimazole pretreatment on the efficacy of radioactive iodine treatment in Graves' hyperthyroidism: one-year follow-up of a prospective, randomized study. J Clin Endocrinol Metab 86:3488
34. Bartalena L et al (1998) Relation between therapy for hyperthyroidism and the course of Graves' ophthalmopathy. N Engl J Med 338:73
35. Nygaard B et al (1999) Radioiodine therapy for toxic multinodular goiter. Arch Intern Med 159:1364
36. Nygaard B et al (1999) Long term effect of radioactive iodine on thyroid function and size in patients with solitary autonomously functioning toxic thyroid nodules. Clin Endocrinol 50:191
37. Tuttle RM et al (1998) Clinical features associated with an increased risk of thyroid malignancy in patients with follicular neoplasia by fine-needle aspiration. Thyroid 8:377
38. Kang AS et al (2002) Current treatment of nodular goiter with hyperthyroidism (Plummer's disease): surgery versus radioiodine. Surgery 132:916
39. Pang H, Chen C (2007) Incidence of cancer in nodular goitres. Ann Acad Med Singapore 36:241
40. Andaker L et al (1992) Surgery for hyperthyroidism: hemithyrodectomy plus contralateral resection or bilateral resection: a prospective randomized study of postoperative complications and long-term results. World J Surg 16:765
41. Vidal-Trecan GM et al (2004) Radioiodine or surgery for toxic thyroid adenoma: dissecting an important decision. Thyroid 14:933
42. Reeve TS et al (1987) Total thyroidectomy: the preferred option for multinodular goiter. Ann Surg 203:782
43. Chao TC et al (1997) Reoperative thyroid surgery. World J Surg 21:644
44. Bellantone R et al (2002) Is routine supplementation therapy (calcium and vitamin D) useful after total thyroidectomy? Surgery 132:1109
45. Sosa JA et al (2008) A population-based study of outcomes from thyroidectomy in aging Americans: at what cost? J Am Coll Surg 206:1097
46. Sosa JA et al (1998) The importance of surgeon experience for clinical and economic outcomes from thyroidectomy. Ann Surg 228:320
47. Mazzaferri EL (1993) Management of a solitary thyroid nodule. N Engl J Med 328:553
48. Tan GH, Gharib H (1997) Thyroid incidentalomas: management approaches to nonpalpable nodules discovered incidentally on thyroid imaging. Ann Intern Med 126:226

49. Wong CKM, Wheeler MH (2000) Thyroid nodules: rational management. World J Surg 24:934
50. Cooper DS et al (2006) Management guidelines for patients with thyroid nodules and differentiated thyroid cancer. Thyroid 16(2):1
51. Shaha AR (2000) Controversies in the management of thyroid nodule. Laryngoscope 110:183
52. Boyd LA et al (1998) Preoperative evaluation and predictive value of fine-needle aspiration and frozen section of thyroid nodules. J Am Coll Surg 187:494
53. Hegedus L (2001) Tyroid ultrasound. Endocrinol Metab Clin North Am 30:339
54. Gritzmann N et al (2000) Sonography of the thyroid and parathyroid glands. Radiol Clin North Am 38:1131
55. Singer PA et al (1996) Treatment guidelines for patients with thyroid nodules and well-differentiated thyroid cancer. Arch Intern Med 156:2165
56. Gharib H (1994) Fine-needle aspiration biopsy of thyroid nodules: advantages, limitations, and effect. Mayo Clin Proc 69:44
57. Gharib H, Goelinci JR (1993) Fine-needle aspiration biopsy of the thyroid: an appraisal. Ann Intern Med 118:282
58. Gharib H et al (1993) Fine-needle aspiration cytology of the thyroid: a 12-year experience with 11,000 biopsies. Clin Lab Med 13:699
59. Ylagen LR et al (2004) Fine-needle aspiration of the thyroid: a cytohistologic correlation and study of discrepant cases. Thyroid 14:35
60. Cooper DS (1995) Thyroxine suppression therapy for benign thyroid nodular disease. J Clin Endocrinol Metab 80:331
61. Castro MR et al (2002) Effectiveness of thyroid hormone suppressive therapy in benign solitary thyroid nodules: a meta-analysis. J Clin Endocrinol Metab 87:4154
62. Kukora JS et al (2001) Thyroid nodule. In: Cameron JL (ed) Current surgical therapy. Mosby, St. Louis, p 636
63. Newman E, Shah A (1995) Substernal goiter. J Surg Oncol 60:207
64. Hsu B et al (1996) Recurrent substernal nodular goiter: incidence and management. Surgery 120:1072
65. Zeiger MA (2001) Nontoxic goiter. In: Cameron JL (ed) Current surgical therapy. Mosby, St. Louis, p 642
66. Samaan NA, Ordonez NG (1990) Uncommon types of thyroid cancer. Endocrinol Metab Clin North Am 19:637
67. Chen H et al (1999) Clinically significant, isolated metastatic disease to the thyroid gland. World J Surg 23:177
68. Wood K et al (2004) Metastases to the thyroid gland: the Royal Marsden experience. Eur J Surg Oncol 30:583
69. Schlumberger KJ (1998) Papillary and follicular thyroid carcinoma. N Engl J Med 338:297
70. Mazzaferri EL, Jhiang SM (1994) Long-term impact of initial surgical and medical therapy on papillary and follicular thyroid cancer. Am J Med 97:418
71. Moley JF (1995) Medullary thyroid cancer. Surg Clin North Am 75:405
72. Demeter JG et al (1991) Anaplastic thyroid carcinoma: risk factors and outcome. Surgery 110:956
73. Burman KD et al (1996) Unusual types of thyroid neoplasm's. Endocrinol Metab Clin North Am 25:49
74. Sugino K et al (2002) The important role of operations in the management of anaplastic thyroid carcinoma. Surgery 131:245
75. Graff-Baker A et al (2009) Prognosis of primary thyroid lymphoma: demographic, clinical and pathologic predictors of survival in 1408 cases. Surgery 146(6):1105–1115
76. Cady B, Rossi R (1988) An expanded view of risk-group definition in differentiated thyroid carcinoma. Surgery 104:948
77. Hay ID et al (1987) Ipsilateral lobectomy versus bilateral lobar resection in papillary thyroid carcinoma: a retrospective analysis of surgical outcome using a novel prognostic scoring system. Surgery 102:1088
78. Lo Gerfo P (1998) Local-regional anesthesia for thyroidectomy: evaluation as an outpatient procedure. Surgery 124:975
79. Lo Gerfo P (1999) Bilateral neck exploration for parathyroidectomy under local anesthesia: a viable technique for patients with coexisting thyroid disease with or without sestamibi scanning. Surgery 126:1011
80. Sosa JA, Udelsman R (2006) Papillary thyroid cancer. Surg Oncol Clin N Am 15:585
81. Dralle H, Machens A (2008) Surgical approaches in thyroid cancer and lymph-node metastases. Best Pract Res Clin Endocrinol Metab 22:971
82. Hay ID (1990) Papillary thyroid carcinoma. Endocrinol Metab Clin North Am 19:545
83. Samaan NA et al (1992) The results of various modalities of treatment of well-differentiated thyroid carcinomas: a retrospective review of 1599 patients. J Clin Endocrinol Metab 75:714
84. Pacini F et al (2002) Ablation of thyroid residues with 30 mCi (131) I: a comparison in thyroid cancer patients prepared with recombinant human TSH or thyroid hormone withdrawal. J Clin Endocrinol Metab 87:4063
85. Barbaro D et al (2003) Radioiodine treatment with 30 mCi after recombinant human thyrotropin stimulation in thyroid cancer: effectiveness for postsurgical remnants ablation and possible role of iodine content in L-thyroxine in the outcome of ablatin. J Clin Endocrinol Metab 88:4110
86. Ladenson PW et al (1997) Comparison of administration of recombinant human thyrotropin with withdrawal of thyroid hormone for radioactive iodine scanning patients with thyroid carcinoma. N Engl J Med 337:888
87. Machens A et al (2005) Prospects of remission in medullary thyroid carcinoma according to basal calcitonin level. J Clin Endocrinol Metab 90:2029
88. Cohen MS et al (2002) Inhibition of medullary thyroid carcinoma cell proliferation and RET phosphorylation by tyrosine kinase inhibitors. Surgery 132:960
89. Carlomagno F et al (2002) ZD6474, an orally available inhibitor of KDR tyrosine kinase activity, efficiently blocks oncogenic RET kinases. Cancer Res 62:7284
90. Chandrakanth A, Shaha AR (2006) Anaplastic thyroid cancer: biology, pathogenesis, prognostic factors, and treatment approaches. Ann Surg Oncol 13:453
91. Lang BH, Lo CY (2007) Surgical options in undifferentiated thyroid carcinoma. World J Surg 31:969
92. Brignardello E et al (2007) Anaplastic thyroid cancer: clinical outcome of 30 consecutive patients referred to a single institution in the past 5 years. Eur J Endocrinol 156:425
93. Matsuzuka F et al (1993) Clinical aspects of primary thyroid lymphoma: diagnosis and treatment based on our experience of 119 cases. Thyroid 3:93
94. McPhee SJ, Bauer DC (2000) Thyroid disease. In: McPhee SJ, Lingappa VR, Ganong WF, Lange JD (eds) Pathophysiology of disease. Lange, New York, p 491
95. McPhee SJ, Bauer DC (2000) Thyroid disease. In: McPhee SJ, Lingappa VR, Ganong WF, Lange JD (eds) Pathophysiology of disease. Lange, New York, p 493
96. McPhee SJ, Bauer DC (2000) Thyroid disease. In: McPhee SJ, Lingappa VR, Ganong WF, Lange JD (eds) Pathophysiology of disease. Lange, New York, p 487

Chapter 35
Parathyroid Disease in the Elderly

Leslie S. Wu, Sanziana A. Roman, and Robert Udelsman

CASE STUDY

An 82-year-old woman was brought to the Emergency Department with a 5-day history of worsening lethargy and confusion. From prior hospital records, her past medical history was notable for two episodes of nephrolithiasis, gastroesophageal reflux disease, and hypertension. Her medications included hydrochlorothiazide, metoprolol, omeprazole, and aspirin.

Physical examination revealed a frail-appearing woman, who was arousable to voice, and oriented only to person. She was afebrile and normotensive, but mildly tachycardic with a heart rate of 100 beats per minute. Neurologic exam was nonfocal. The remainder of her examination was significant only for poor skin turgor and dry mucous membranes.

Laboratory studies were notable for a normal white blood cell count, mild hemoconcentration, blood urea nitrogen (BUN) 25 mg/dL, serum creatinine 1.3 mg/dL, serum calcium 14.7 mg/dL, and albumin 4.3 g/dL. Urinalysis was negative.

The patient was admitted to the hospital with hypercalcemia. She was hydrated appropriately with intravenous crystalloid fluids, with subsequent improvement of her mental status and calcium level. Additional laboratory evaluation was obtained, revealing an intact parathyroid hormone (iPTH) level of 200 pg/ml. The patient was diagnosed with primary hyperparathyroidism.

Introduction

The primary function of the parathyroid glands is to maintain calcium homeostasis through the secretion of parathyroid hormone (PTH). This hormone is regulated by serum calcium through calcium-sensing receptors (CaSRs) on the parathyroid cell surface. In turn, most peripheral tissues, primarily kidney and bone, have PTH receptors which can affect varying functions. In the past, disturbances in this system were difficult to recognize until the development of clinically significant disease. With the development of better biochemical assays for serum PTH and calcium levels, subclinical derangements can be diagnosed before patients become symptomatic. The management of patients with the broad spectrum of metabolic calcium disturbances remains controversial.

Mineral Homeostasis

Plasma calcium exists in three phases: protein-bound, ionized, and complexed. Normally, approximately 1 g of inorganic calcium is absorbed daily in the proximal small intestine. About 45% of total blood calcium is protein-bound, predominantly to albumin, but also to globulins. A similar fraction is ionized. The rest is complexed to organic ions such as citrate, phosphate, and bicarbonate. Calcium is in constant flux between the extracellular and intracellular spaces, in bone, and in renal glomerular filtrate, which is reabsorbed by the normal kidney.

The ionized fraction of serum calcium controls vital cellular functions, such as neuromuscular transmission, muscle contraction, and blood clotting. Precise maintenance of calcium concentration within a very narrow range in extracelluar fluids is therefore critically important. The binding of calcium to albumin is pH-dependent, increasing with alkalosis, and decreasing with acidosis. Thus, if the ionized calcium is low, acidosis tends to protect an individual from manifesting the symptoms and signs of hypocalcemia; conversely, alkalosis predisposes a patient to symptomatic hypocalcemia.

L.S. Wu (✉)
Department of Surgery, Maine Medical Center, 887 Congress Str, Suite 400, Portland 04102, ME, USA
e-mail: miniwuwu@gmail.com

R.A. Rosenthal et al. (eds.), *Principles and Practice of Geriatric Surgery*,
DOI 10.1007/978-1-4419-6999-6_35, © Springer Science+Business Media, LLC 2011

FIGURE 35.1 Calcium metabolism.

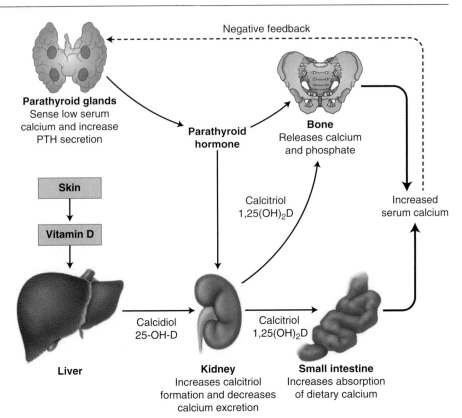

The adult body contains approximately 700 g of phosphate, primarily located in the teeth and bones. Plasma levels of calcium and phosphate are inversely related, and the primary agents responsible for calcium metabolism are PTH, vitamin D, and calcitonin (see Fig. 35.1) [1].

Parathyroid Hormone (PTH)

The chief cells of the parathyroid gland constantly monitor ionized calcium concentrations through their cell surface CaSR, thus allowing the circulating level of PTH to change within seconds after an alteration in serum calcium [2]. PTH secretory rates are related to serum ionized calcium and 1,25-dihydroxyvitamin D by an inverse sigmoidal relationship. Low ionized calcium concentrations maximally stimulate secretion, while increases in calcium suppress the production and release of PTH. PTH secretion is exquisitely sensitive to very small alterations in the calcium concentration, which have substantial effects on the rate of hormone synthesis and release.

PTH is synthesized within the parathyroid gland as a 115-amino-acid precursor molecule (preproPTH) that is successively cleaved within the cell to form the mature 84-amino-acid PTH. This form of the hormone is packaged into secretory granules and released into the circulation. Mature PTH is metabolized in the liver into the active N-terminal and inactive C-terminal fragments. The intact molecules and N-terminal fragments have half-lives of approximately 3–5 min, while the inactive C-terminal fragments have a half-life of hours. The C-terminal fragments are excreted by the kidneys, and usually accumulate to high levels in the serum of patients with renal failure.

PTH inhibits osteoblasts and stimulates osteoclasts. In the kidney, PTH causes a decrease in calcium clearance as well as increased renal excretion of phosphate by inhibiting its reabsorption in the tubules. In addition, PTH stimulates hydroxylation of 25-hydroxyvitamin D to 1,25-dihydroxyvitamin D, which allows for enhanced calcium absorption in the proximal intestine [3].

Vitamin D

The sterol 1,25-dihydroxyvitamin D, or calcitriol, is an essential mediator of calcium homeostasis. Calcitriol synthesis begins with ultraviolet activation of 7-dehydrocholesterol in the skin, generating cholecalciferol (vitamin D). In the liver, vitamin D is readily hydroxylated to 25-hydroxyvitamin D2, which in turn is hydroxylated to the potent calcitriol. This final step occurs in the kidney and is tightly regulated by PTH. In turn, calcitriol has a regulatory effect on PTH, by exerting a physiologic inhibition of the parathyroid glands [4].

Calcitonin

Parafollicular, or C cells, of the thyroid gland secrete the peptide hormone calcitonin. Calcitonin interacts with receptors in kidney and bone. The primary function of calcitonin is to lower serum calcium, and this hormone is released rapidly in response to hypercalcemia. It inhibits osteoclastic bone resorption and quickly blocks the release of calcium and phosphate from bone. Ultimately, this effect, along with the inhibition of resorption, leads to a fall in serum calcium and phosphate [3]. The physiologic effect of calcitonin in humans, however, is very modest.

Hypercalcemia

The most common reason for the finding of hypercalcemia in an elderly patient, in the oupatient setting, is primary hyperparathyroidism (HPTH), while hypercalcemia in the inpatient population often is secondary to malignancies. Diagnosing the correct etiology requires careful clinical evaluation of patients, as well as serologic and biochemical testing (Table 35.1) [5].

After a thorough history and physical examination, laboratory measurements of fasting serum calcium, PTH, creatinine, and vitamin D levels should be performed to determine if the hypercalcemia is parathyroid-mediated (in which serum PTH levels are elevated inappropriately) or non-parathyroid-mediated (in which serum PTH levels are suppressed appropriately). Normally, functioning parathyroid cells abruptly cease PTH release when the surrounding extracellular fluid calcium concentration is elevated. Therefore, in cases in which hypercalcemia results from a non-parathyroid-mediated condition, serum PTH levels will be suppressed [6].

Table 35.1 Differential diagnosis of hypercalcemia

Parathyroid-mediated	Non-parathyroid-mediated
Primary hyperparathyroidism	Malignancy-associated hypercalcemia
Parathyroid adenoma (85%)	Local osteolytic hypercalcemia
Parathyroid hyperplasia (15%)	Humoral hypercalcemia of malignancy (PTHrP and calcitriol)
Parathyroid carcinoma (<1%)	Granulomatous disease (sarcoidosis and tuberculosis)
Secondary/tertiary hyperparathyroidism	Endocrinopathies (hyperthyroidism and adrenal insufficiency)
Familial hypocalciuric hypocalemia	Drugs (thiazides, vitamin D and calcium)
Lithium therapy	Immobilization

Source: Modified and reproduced from [1]

Non-Parathyroid-Mediated Hypercalcemia

This category includes conditions in which patients have hypercalcemia and serum PTH levels that are suppressed appropriately; the parathyroid cells perceive excess extracellular calcium concentrations, and markedly reduce their hormonal release. Cancer is the most frequently diagnosed etiology of non-PTH-mediated hypercalcemia, particularly in the hospitalized population. This malignancy-associated hypercalcemia is classified into two primary forms, osteolytic and humoral.

The second form of malignancy-associated hypercalcemia is local osteolytic hypercalcemia, which occurs when a neoplasm directly invades the bony skeleton, resulting in localized destruction and calcium release. In contrast to malignant humoral hypercalcemia, local osteolytic hypercalcemia does not involve the elaboration of systemically active products. Rather, it appears to result from the production or local stimulation of bone-active cytokines as well as other osteoclast-activating factors. This form of pathologic hypercalcemia is most commonly associated with multiple myeloma; however, it has also been linked to adenocarcinoma of the breast and certain lymphomas [7].

Humoral hypercalcemia of malignancy results from the systemic effect of a circulating factor produced by the neoplasm. Most commonly, the factor involved is parathyroid hormone-related protein (PTHrP), a peptide that has been shown to recapitulate most of the metabolic effects of PTH, including stimulation of bone turnover and alteration in renal handling of both calcium and phosphate [7]. In humans, PTHrP serves as an important paracrine factor in may tissues, including skin, bone, breast, the central nervous system, and the vasculature. Neoplasms that elaborate PTHrP include squamous cell carcinomas (naso- and oro-pharynx, larynx, lung, esophagus, and cervix), adenocarcinoma of the breast and ovary, bladder transitional cell carcinoma, T-cell lymphomas, renal cell carcinoma, and carcinoid tumors. The other factor that may cause malignant humoral hypercalcemia is calcitriol, which is often associated with B-cell lymphomas [7, 8].

There are other benign, non-PTH-mediated causes of hypercalcemia encountered in the elderly. These include medications and supplements, such as thiazide diuretics and excess exogenous calcium, vitamin D, or vitamin A. Granulomatous diseases, such as sarcoidosis and tuberculosis, are associated with hypercalcemia through the direct production of calcitriol. In addition, several endocrinopathies are associated with hypercalcemia, including hyperthyroidism with augmented bone turnover, pheochromocytoma with PTHrP production, and adrenal insufficiency linked with decreased calcium clearance. Rarely, hypercalcemia may result from prolonged immobilization, particularly in settings in which bone turnover is already stimulated, such as recovery from fractures or surgery [3].

Parathyroid-Mediated Hypercalcemia

The differential diagnosis of parathyroid-mediated hypercalcemia includes HPTH, familial hypocalciuric hypocalcemia (FHH), and lithium therapy. The remainder of this chapter will focus primarily on the forms and treatment strategies of HPTH. However, FHH and lithium therapy briefly are discussed below, as the differences between these diagnoses are important.

FHH, also known as benign familial hypercalcemia, is an inherited autosomal dominant condition resulting from a deactivating mutation in the extracellular CaSR [9]. In this condition, the cell surface receptor is sub-normally activated by extracellular calcium. In the face of mild elevation of serum calcium, PTH levels are inappropriately normal or slightly elevated. However, urinary calcium excretion is reduced, due to the same defective CaSRs in the nephron, with subsequent increased urinary calcium reabsorption. Although FHH is classified as parathyroid-mediated, since PTH secretion is abnormal, it is a unique condition and distinct from the more common primary HPTH. Generally, it is diagnosed in younger patients with asymptomatic, mild hypercalcemia. The family history usually identifies affected relatives. It does not require surgical intervention, as parathyroidectomy will not cure the condition.

Chronic lithium therapy may increase serum calcium levels with inappropriately normal or mildly elevated PTH concentrations. Lithium appears to alter the sensitivity of the CaSR, thus increasing the set-point of extracellular calcium concentration. However, parathyroid adenomas and multigland hyperplasia have also been described in patients chronically treated with lithium [10]. Distinguishing those patients with drug-induced hypercalcemia from those with mild primary HPTH can be challenging.

Hyperparathyroidism

Hyperparathyroidism was first recognized during the 1920s and was thought to be a relatively uncommon condition, presenting usually as nephrolithiasis or as a complication of severe bony demineralization [5]. With the application of multiphasic blood testing revealing elevated serum calcium concentrations and the availability of accurate PTH determinations, HPTH now is recognized to be a more common disorder, particularly in the elderly population.

Primary Hyperparathyroidism

Primary hyperparathyroidism is the most common form of HPTH and is the most frequent explanation for hypercalcemia

in the outpatient setting. Population-based estimates reveal an overall incidence of approximately 25 per 100,000 in the general population with about 50,000 new cases occurring annually. The peak incidence is in the fifth to sixth decade of life, with a female to male ratio of about 3:2. Some studies estimate the overall prevalence of HPTH in the elderly at 2–3%, with approximately 200 cases/100,000 population [11].

The most common clinical presentation is that of asymptomatic, or minimally symptomatic, mild hypercalcemia. Primary HPTH generally is caused by a benign, solitary parathyroid adenoma in 80–85% of patients. In about 5% of patients, two distinct adenomas ("double adenoma") are found. Multigland parathyroid hyperplasia is present in 15–20%. In younger patients, this may be associated with familial syndromes, such as multiple endocrine neoplasia (MEN) types I and IIA. Patients with MEN-I have enlargement and hyperfunction of all parathyroid glands, whereas patients with MEN-IIA may have asymmetric parathyroid gland enlargement. The rare hyperparathyroidism-jaw tumor syndrome is another autosomal dominant inherited condition presenting with early-onset primary HPTH and fibro-osseous, cystic jaw neoplasms [12, 13]. Index cases of MEN syndromes are rare in the elderly patients, but certain mutations may manifest later in life, therefore in the appropriate clinical setting, MEN needs to be considered even in elderly patients.

Parathyroid carcinoma is a rare cause of primary HPTH, accounting for less than 1% of cases. In contrast to benign HPTH, it occurs equally in men and women. Patients with parathyroid carcinoma present most often in the fifth and sixth decades of life. Longstanding untreated primary HPTH may devolve into parathyroid carcinoma, which may then present in the elderly patients [14]. Although these tumors are slow-growing, they have a high propensity to recur locally, and recurrent disease is difficult to eradicate. Patients with recurrent and metastatic disease often suffer from severe, debilitating hypercalcemia, control of which may involve palliative surgical resection and the use of drugs, including bisphosphonates and calcimimetics, to lower the serum calcium level [15, 16].

Clinical and Diagnostic Evaluation

With the advent of routine serum calcium screening, the typical presentation of primary HPTH has changed from a severe, debilitating illness to a disease with subtle symptoms and physiologic derangements. Common signs include nephrolithiasis, nephrocalcinosis, osteopenia, and osteoporosis (Table 35.2) [17]. Hypertension is frequently present in patients with primary HPTH, and a variety of mechanisms have been proposed to explain this relationship. It appears to be most closely correlated with the degree of renal impairment seen in patients with hypercalcemia. However, one

TABLE 35.2 Symptoms and associated conditions in patients with primary hyperparathyroidism

Symptoms

Weakness, exhaustion, and fatigue

Bone pain, back pain, and joint pain

Polyuria, nocturia, and polydipsia

Loss of appetite, nausea, and dyspepsia

Memory loss and depression

Associated conditions

Weight loss

Bone fracture, joint swelling, and gout

Nephrolithiasis, hematuria from passage of renal calculus

Gastric ulcer, duodenal ulcer, and pancreatitis

Hypertension

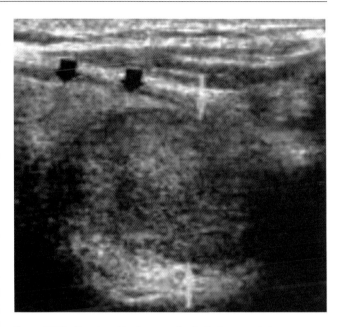

FIGURE 35.2 Parathyroid adenoma. Sagittal ultrasound shows a parathyroid adenoma (*white arrows*) behind the lower pole of the right thyroid lobe (*black arrows*).

study found that parathyroidectomy led to a substantial fall in both systolic and diastolic pressures in 54% of hypertensive subjects that appeared to be unrelated to improvement in renal function [18]. Most endocrine specialists do not believe that curative surgery in primary HPTH is associated with a significant improvement in hypertension.

There are many subtle abnormalities associated with primary HPTH, including decreased cognitive function, depression, lethargy, myalgias, arthralgias, constipation, and urinary symptoms, such as increased thirst and urinary frequency. Petersen performed psychiatric examinations on 54 patients with primary HPT and detected mental disturbances in more than 50% [19, 20]. However, it is often difficult to prove that these nonspecific findings result from primary HPTH because they are common in the elderly. In a general population cohort study of over 4,000 individuals, Schram et al. found that serum calcium levels that were at the upper range of normal or frankly elevated were associated with faster decline in cognitive function, particularly for patients over the age of 75 years [21].

The diagnosis of primary HPT typically is made by biochemical evidence of an elevated serum calcium concentration, usually in conjunction with an elevated serum intact PTH. Approximately half of patients with primary HPTH have hypophosphatemia. However, in the presence of significant renal impairment, serum phosphate levels may be elevated. Because of the effect of PTH on bicarbonate excretion in the kidney, patients with primary HPTH often have a hyperchloremic metabolic acidosis [13]. Approximately 10–40% of HPTH patients have elevated levels of alkaline phosphatase, which indicates some degree of increased bone turnover. Although osteitis fibrosa cystica, the classic form of parathyroid bone disease, is rarely seen today, even patients with mild disease can be seen to have biochemical or histologic evidence of bone involvement. Dual-energy X-ray absorption (DEXA) scanning of the lumbar spine, hip, and forearm has become the standard method for assessing bone density to diagnose osteoporosis in the setting of primary HPTH [22–24].

Patients with FHH must be distinguished from those with primary HPTH. This can be done with a 24-h urinary calcium excretion study, which is uniformly low in the setting of FHH. In contrast, patients with primary HPTH have a normal or elevated 24-h urinary excretion of calcium [9]. Postmenopausal women often have hypercalciuria for several years after the onset of menopause from estrogen decrease, therefore increased urinary calcium levels in this population may not always be due to hyperparathyroidism.

Although rare, parathyroid carcinoma should be suspected in patients who demonstrate a rapid and sustained rise in both their serum calcium and PTH levels. A palpable neck mass sometimes may be appreciated [25, 26]. A parathyroid adenoma is rarely, if ever, palpable on physical examination. Rather, this neck mass is more likely to represent a thyroid nodule.

There have been extensive discussions regarding the use and availability of preoperative imaging studies in patients with primary HPT. In the past, patients who had not undergone previous surgical exploration did not require any radiographic localization studies other than finding an experienced parathyroid surgeon. However, the increased use of minimally invasive parathyroidectomy techniques has mandated preoperative imaging.

Imaging studies can be sorted into noninvasive and invasive techniques. The noninvasive studies include the following: nuclear medicine scans, such as methoxyisobutylisonitrile (sestamibi) studies, which can be combined with single photon emission computed tomography (SPECT) imaging; ultrasound (Fig. 35.2); computed tomography (CT) scans; and magnetic resonance imaging (MRI). The noninvasive localization study of choice is a technetium (^{99m}Tc)-sestamibi scan with SPECT, which results in a three-dimensional reconstruction that can delineate the location of an enlarged parathyroid gland in 85% of cases (Fig. 35.3a, b).

Invasive techniques usually are reserved for re-operative cases, and include angiography and venous sampling for PTH gradients. Recently, the rapid PTH assay has been used in both the angiography suite as well as the operating room. It yields real-time feedback and has become invaluable in the development of minimally invasive techniques [27–29].

Most patients presenting with primary HPT are asymptomatic, or mildly, chronically ill with vague symptoms referable to the kidneys or the musculoskeleton. However, patients may become acutely and severely ill with acute hypercalcemia, or hyperparathyroid crisis. This disorder often can be seen in elderly patients, nursing home residents, or patients with cognitive deficits, such as dementia. Such patients often harbor mild to moderate hyperparathyroidism for years, but an inciting factor will cause acute worsening of the hypercalcemia. The most common etiology is simple dehydration from poor health, overuse of diuretic medications, gastroenteritis or viral illness. The onset is usually characterized by rapidly developing muscular weakness, nausea and vomiting, weight loss, drowsiness, fatigue, and confusion. The serum calcium concentration almost always is remarkably elevated (16–20 mg/dL). The offending parathyroid gland is usually large. The genesis of the condition involves uncontrolled PTH secretion followed by hypercalcemia, polyuria, dehydration, and reduced renal function, which worsens the hypercalcemia [10].

The management of severe hypercalcemia incorporates four primary aims: to correct dehydration; to enhance renal excretion of calcium; to inhibit bone resorption; and to treat the underlying disorder. Although the definitive therapy is resection of the hyperfunctioning parathyroid gland, it is unsafe to proceed with operative exploration until the serum calcium concentration is lowered. Resuscitation with 0.9% normal saline is instituted to maintain urinary output above 100 ml/h, and subsequent diuresis with loop diuretics increases the renal excretion of sodium and calcium. In the elderly patients, care must be taken to assess their cardiac function, so as to avoid overhydration and fluid overload. If the serum calcium level remains elevated, other agents that can lower the serum calcium concentration should be administered. These agents include bisphosphonates, calcitonin, and cinacalcet [10]. Often, multidisciplinary care is needed for these complex patients.

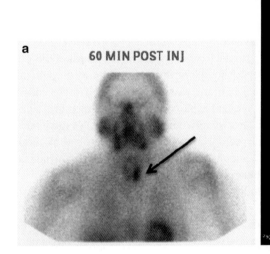

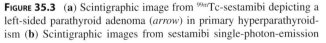

FIGURE 35.3 (**a**) Scintigraphic image from ^{99m}Tc-sestamibi depicting a left-sided parathyroid adenoma (*arrow*) in primary hyperparathyroidism (**b**) Scintigraphic images from sestamibi single-photon-emission tomography of the same patient presented in (**a**) depicting multiple rotational tomographic planes. The posterior location of the parathyroid adenoma (*arrow*) is consistent with a superior parathyroid gland.

Treatment

There has been considerable debate regarding the management of elderly patients with primary hyperparathyroidism. There is universal agreement that patients with clear symptoms and signs associated with hyperparathyroidism should undergo parathyroid surgery because parathyroidectomy is the only long-term effective treatment. However, controversy still exists about the management of patients with "asymptomatic" primary HPTH [30, 31]. Recent data suggest that these asymptomatic patients often have symptoms that are recognized in retrospect, once their HPTH has been cured. In addition, asymptomatic patients may suffer from neurocognitive deficits, depression, and anxiety, as well as progressive cardiovascular disease, and a suggestion of insulin resistance, which can result in premature death [32, 33].

In 1990 and 2002, the National Institutes of Health (NIH) convened consensus conferences to delineate the surgical indications in patients with both symptomatic and asymptomatic primary HPTH (Table 35.3) [34, 35]. In 2008, an international workshop on HPTH convened to review and update previous recommendations [36]. Guidelines also were created for the management of patients with asymptomatic primary HPTH who did not undergo surgery, including biannual serum calcium and annual serum creatinine measurements, as well as annual bone density measurements [35]. It has been suggested, however, that the NIH criteria for parathyroidectomy in asymptomatic patients are too limited and that all patients with primary HPTH should be referred for surgical therapy [37, 38].

There is no long-term effective pharmacologic treatment for primary HPTH. There are several pharmacologic agents that can transiently lower the serum calcium level (Table 35.4). These can limit further loss of bone by reducing the activation of new remodeling units in the skeleton. Estrogen replacement, salmon calcitonin, bisphosphonates, and more recently, calcimimetics (cinacalcet) have been used to treat primary HPTH in patients with complex comorbid medical conditions, either unwilling or considered unfit for surgery. In addition, glucocorticoids and calcimimetics can be employed during refractory hypercalcemia of metastatic parathyroid carcinoma [25, 27]. In the geriatric population, particularly in elderly postmenopausal women, it has been demonstrated that estrogen replacement therapy combined with either calcitriol or calcium supplements, appeared as effective as parathyroidectomy for the treatment of osteoporosis in the setting of primary HPTH [39–41]. In addition, the combination of calcitriol and calcium may be effective in reducing systolic hypertension associated with HPTH [42, 43]. However, these therapies are not definitive; with adequate preoperative parathyroid localization, experienced parathyroid surgeons may employ minimally invasive techniques with good outcomes in the elderly population [44].

Parathyroidectomy without preoperative localization studies has a high success rate (>95%) and a low complication rate. Complications associated with parathyroidectomy

TABLE 35.3 Surgical indications in patients with primary hyperparathyroidism

All symptomatic patients, including those with significant bone, renal, gastrointestinal, or neuromuscular symptoms typical of primary hyperparathyroidism

In otherwise asymptomatic patients:

Elevation of serum calcium by 1 mg/dl or more above the normal range (i.e., >11.5 mg/dl in most laboratories)

Marked elevation of 24-h urine calcium excretion (e.g., >400 mg)

Decreased creatinine clearance (e.g., reduced by >30% compared with age-matched normal person)

Significant reduction in bone density of more than 2.5 standard deviations below peak bone mass at any measured site (i.e., *T*-score <2.5)

Consistent follow-up is not possible or is undesirable because of coexisting medical conditions

Age younger than 50 years

Source: Modified from [30]. Copyright Elsevier (1994)

TABLE 35.4 Pharmacologic treatment for primary hyperparathyroidism

Pamidronate/bisphosphonates

Dosage	60–90 mg as a single dose
Adverse effects	Leukopenia, fever, and myalgia
Contraindications	Hypersensitivity
Special points	Onset 1–2 days with long half-life

Chronic oral sodium phosphates

Dosage	1–3 g daily
Adverse effects	Extraskeletal calcifications
Contraindications	Serum calcium >12 mg/dl, serum
Special points	phosphorus >3 mg/dl
	Not indicated in acute hypercalcemia

Calcitonin

Dosage	4–8 U/kg every 6–12 h
Adverse effects	Nausea, glucose intolerance
Contraindications	Allergic reactions
Special points	Effective within 2 h; can be used to lower serum calcium while awaiting effect of bisphosphonates

Furosemide

Dosage	20–40 mg up to three times daily
Adverse effects	Electrolyte imbalance
Contraindications	Anuria, hepatic coma, and
Special points	hypovolemia
	Hydration is essential

Cinacalcet*

Dosage	30–90 mg daily
Adverse effects	Nausea, vomiting, diarrhea
Contraindications	Hypersensitivity, and
Special points	hypocalcemia
	*Off-label use in primary HPTH except parathyroid carcinoma

include recurrent laryngeal nerve injury, transient or persistent hypocalcemia, postoperative hemorrhage, and pneumothorax [45]. Despite this, the specific operative approach has continued to evolve through the influence of a number of synergistic factors, including improvements in preoperative localization studies as mentioned above, rapid intraoperative PTH measurements, and adjunctive surgical technologies such as hand-held gamma detection probes and small videoscopic equipment. The net result has influenced patient selection so that the majority of parathyroid explorations are very well tolerated. However, difficult explorations remain difficult. Therefore, any surgeon performing parathyroidectomy must be facile and comfortable with standard four-gland parathyroid exploration. In fact, experienced parathyroid surgeons today achieve cure rates of up to 98% with both minimally invasive and conventional techniques [46].

The conventional technique for parathyroid exploration requires a bilateral cervical exploration. This operation is usually performed under general anesthesia, although it can be performed under bilateral regional superficial cervical block [47]. The goal is to identify all normal and abnormal parathyroid glands, thus distinguishing single-gland from multigland disease. Patients who have a single parathyroid adenoma undergo curative resection once the gland is removed. In the instance of multigland hyperplasia, a subtotal parathyroidectomy (leaving a remnant of one well-vascularized parathyroid gland in situ) is required. Total cervical parathyroidectomy with immediate heterotopic transplantation of parathyroid tissue is less desirable for patients with sporadic HPTH, but often is employed in the setting of familial HPTH, such as MEN-1.

The conventional approach has been challenged with increasing frequency in recent years, and minimally invasive parathyroid exploration is now performed routinely in several institutions. Three techniques have emerged: image-guided local exploration, most often in conjunction with intraoperative PTH assays; intraoperative gamma probe-guided exploration after sestamibi injection; and, image-guided video parathyroidectomy.

Image-guided local exploration has emerged as the most commonly employed minimally invasive technique. It is dependent on high-quality preoperative imaging, usually in the form of sestamibi scans, ultrasound studies, or, less commonly, CT scans. This technique is appropriate even for patients who have had multiple previous explorations, as long as the preoperative imaging is adequate [48, 49]. When performed by an experienced parathyroid surgeon well-versed in minimally invasive techniques, this surgical procedure can be performed on an outpatient basis and can avoid the risks of bilateral neck exploration and general anesthesia [50, 51]. This technique has become particularly more favorable for elderly patients with primary HPTH and additional comorbidities; these patients often are denied referral for parathyroidectomy because of the associated risks of general anesthesia and bilateral neck exploration.

Studies have shown that minimally invasive parathyroidectomy can be performed safely and can facilitate clinical care in these high-risk patients [52, 53].

Gamma probe exploration involves preoperative administration of $^{99\,m}$Tc-sestamibi to localize the abnormal parathyroid gland. The probe is then used in the operating room to find the area of increased radioactivity. In addition, the gamma probe can be used to measure radioactivity after tumor extraction to confirm the adequacy of resection. Although this technique has not gained widespread acceptance, the curative rates are comparable to the previously described technique [54].

Image-guided video parathyroidectomy has been employed by several investigators. Like the other minimally invasive techniques, preoperative imaging is required to locate the adenoma. The procedure usually requires general anesthesia with or without carbon dioxide insufflation to aid the dissection [55]. There may be very select patients in whom this technique is indicated. However, it is not a common procedure in elderly patients, as it offers no additional benefits for this specific patient population. This technique has not assumed a dominant role in parathyroid surgery in the US.

Clinical Outcomes

In the hands of an experienced parathyroid surgeon, it has been demonstrated that patients who underwent either conventional bilateral neck exploration or minimally invasive parathyroidectomy had equivalent cure rates. The rationale for parathyroidectomy is supported by evidence that in about 80% of patients, the clinical manifestations of primary HPTH improve after successful parathyroidectomy. Thus, fatigue, weakness, polydipsia, polyuria, bone and joint pain, constipation, nausea, and depression improve in most patients. This is also true for associated conditions – new renal stones usually stop forming, osteoporosis stabilizes or improves, pancreatitis becomes less likely, and peptic ulcer disease often resolves. In most patients, fracture risk and weakness also improve, and objective increase in muscular strength has been documented [56–60]. In addition, neurocognitive impairments, confusion, spatial learning deficits, and depression have been shown to improve after successful operative intervention. Patients can resume a regular diet with or without calcium supplementation, and hypercalcemia is not a concern when these patients are hospitalized for other medical conditions [61–65].

However, there is a natural reluctance to subject elderly patients to an operation when the advantages are less clear. Advances in parathyroid imaging resulting in a greater use of targeted or focused parathyroidectomy has opened the way for the inclusion of less fit patients into the potentially operable category. Chen et al. compared demographic and outcome data of elderly patients (>70 years of age) to those of younger patients (<70 years of age); and found that mental impairment, bone disease, and fatigue were more common in elderly patients, and nephrolithiasis was more frequent in younger patients. Elderly patients presented with more advanced disease, manifested by higher preoperative PTH levels. However, the cure rate, morbidity, and mortality in the elderly were indistinguishable from those of their younger cohorts [66]. Similarly, Bachar et al. found that there was no practical difference in perioperative management and surgical outcomes for patients over the age of 70 years, and concluded that surgeons should consider parathyroidectomy in primary HPTH patients regardless of age [67].

Several quality-of-life studies have been performed using standardized tools such as the SF-36 health survey in patients with primary HPTH, and have demonstrated that patients experience an improvement in health status and quality of life after operative correction [68, 69]. Furthermore, this benefit was independent of preoperative calcium levels [70]. Psychological distress, as measured by the General Health Questionnaire, has also been shown to be ameliorated by parathyroidectomy [71, 72]. The Parathyroid Assessment of Symptoms (PAS), a patient-based outcome tool, was developed specifically for patients with primary HPTH. A multicenter study using this questionnaire indicated that PAS is a reliable measure of the symptoms associated with HPTH, and that these symptoms improve after parathyroidectomy [73].

Both classic and more subtle clinical manifestations of primary HPTH warrant medical evaluation and, in most patients, parathyroidectomy. This especially is true when parathyroidectomy is performed by an experienced parathyroid surgeon, with a success rate greater than 97% and a very low complication rate. Furthermore, with the advent of minimally invasive techniques, these operations can often be done on an outpatient basis. Elderly patients are an especially vulnerable population, and should be referred to experienced parathyroid surgeons who have the knowledge, skill and available technology to perform these surgeries in minimally invasive fashion, with faster intraoperative times, less anesthetic requirements and low operative complications.

For patients with severe bone disease, often evidenced by markedly elevated preoperative blood alkaline phosphatase levels, subsequent "bone hunger" often necessitates postoperative treatment with calcium supplementation and calcitriol [56]. Normocalcemia generally is restored within the first 24 h after a successful parathyroidectomy, and this may be accompanied by mild paresthesia in the extremities. Symptoms may occur while the serum calcium level is within the normal range, reflecting the rapidity of change; however, this is usually transient and does not require treatment. Symptomatic hypocalcemia is more common in the elderly, in those with more severe preoperative HPTH, or in patients with evidence of high-turnover bone disease. Elderly patients may be magnesium deficient, and this may lead to a functional

hypoparathyroidism, which can be corrected by magnesium supplementation. Restoration of normocalcemia can be achieved with calcitriol in combination with supplemental calcium. It is sufficient to maintain the serum calcium within the lower part of the reference range in order to control symptoms. This also provides a greater margin of safety from hypercalcemia, which may be a particular risk in elderly patients with renal impairment [74].

Another and perhaps more important reason for recommending parathyroidectomy is that patients with primary HPTH appear to be at risk for premature death primarily because of cardiovascular disease and cancer, as documented by Palmer et al. and confirmed by Hedback et al. [75, 76] More importantly, the increased death rate, even in patients with mild primary HPTH, can be reversed by successful parathyroidectomy. Patients between the ages of 55 and 70 years seem to receive the greatest survival benefit.

Secondary and Tertiary Hyperparathyroidism

In contrast to the intrinsic feedback inhibition defect of primary HPTH, secondary HPTH is caused by chronic extrinsic overstimulation of otherwise normal parathyroid glands (Fig. 35.4a, b). Although it may result from malabsorption syndromes, celiac disease, or extreme dietary calcium or vitamin D deficiency, secondary HPTH occurs most commonly in the setting of chronic renal insufficiency associated with renal osteodystrophy. The stimulus for PTH hypersecretion is a reduced extracellular calcium concentration and reduced endogenous calcitriol production that is associated with reduced renal function [77, 78].

Tertiary hyperparathyroidism refers to the development, in the setting of longstanding secondary HPTH, of autonomous hypersecretion despite correction of the underlying case of PTH stimulation. This may be suspected when an individual with documented secondary HPTH develops refractory hypercalcemia, or after renal transplantation in a previously dialysis-dependent patient [79].

The distinction between secondary and tertiary HPTH is not critical when considering surgical intervention because refractoriness to medical therapy in secondary HPTH is functionally equivalent to the intrinsically refractory autonomy seen in tertiary HPTH. The indications and rationale for surgical therapy are the same. Elderly patients with renal disease are prone to severe bone loss, and seem to benefit from parathyroidectomy [78].

Clinical and Diagnostic Evaluation

Patients with chronic renal failure (CRF) have considerable morbidity and mortality. Classic clinical manifestations of worsening secondary HPTH are related to osteodystrophy

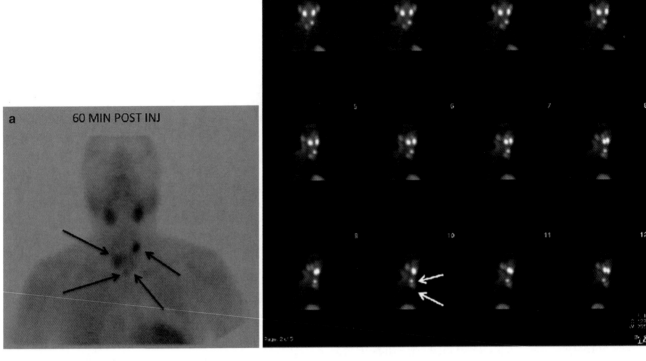

Figure 35.4 (**a**) Scintigraphic image from ^{99m}Tc-sestamibi depicting four-parathyroid-gland activity (*arrows*) in tertiary hyperparathyroidism. (**b**) Scintigraphic images from sestamibi single-photon-emission tomography of the same patient presented in Fig. 35.4a depicting multiple rotational tomographic planes. The right superior and inferior parathyroid glands (*arrows*) are visualized on sagittal view.

(pain, deformities, and fractures), extraskeletal calcifications, and the skin (pruritus and calciphylaxis).

Changes in bone structure due to secondary HPTH are common and begin early in the course of CRF. Renal osteodystrophy includes two major pathologies: osteitis fibrosa cystica and adynamic bone disease. In mixed osteodystrophy, features of both osteitis fibrosa and decreased mineralization coexist. The form and severity of the bone disease depend on the gender and age of the patient; the severity and duration of the CRF; metabolic acidosis; the characteristics of dialysis; calcitriol and PTH levels; dietary calcium and phosphate load; additional medications, particularly steroids; and associated endocrine diseases, such as diabetes mellitus. In addition, parathyroidectomy and renal transplantation can modify acutely the precarious balance of long-deranged mineral metabolism [80].

A disease of high bone turnover, osteitis fibrosa cystica is a consequence of elevated PTH secretion and is characterized by increased osteoclasts, osteoblasts, osteocytes, and fibroblasts. There is a correlation between the serum PTH level and the rate of bone turnover; and the probability of high-turnover bone disease increases with rising serum PTH concentrations. Serum PTH greater than 450 pg/ml is closely related to high-turnover bone disease in hemodialysis and peritoneal dialysis patients. It has become possible to suppress PTH secretion with the administration of calcium and vitamin D; therefore, the frequency of classic osteitis fibrosa

and mixed forms is decreasing, while the frequency of adynamic bone disease is increasing [81].

In contrast to osteitis fibrosa, adynamic bone disease is associated with low levels of serum PTH. This disease is characterized by unequal decreased numbers of both osteoclasts and osteoblasts, with a predominant deficiency of osteoblasts. Low bone formation rates lead to decreased bone mass [17, 81]. In the past, adynamic bone disease also was associated with high aluminum dialysis baths, but this has become less pronounced with modern dialysates.

There are three types of extraskeletal calcifications (systemic calcinosis): visceral, periarticular, and vascular. Visceral calcifications may involve the lungs, breast, myocardium, mitral valve, kidneys, and skeletal muscle. Patients often have hyperphosphatemia, an elevated calcium-phosphorus product, and increased PTH levels. Periarticular calcification or tumoral calcinosis results in calcific periarthritis and small-joint effusions; radiographically, calcifications can be seen around the joint. Vascular calcifications of both large and small vessels occur in 20% of patients with CRF, and may cause falsely elevated blood pressure measurements. Parathyroidectomy rarely affects vascular calcification, but usually diminishes nonvascular calcium deposits [82, 83].

The skin manifestations associated with secondary HPTH include pruritus and calciphylaxis. Pruritus affects up to 85% of hemodialysis patients. Although dramatic improvement of pruritus has been observed after parathyroidectomy, PTH does not seem to be directly involved in its pathogenesis. Rather, abnormal serum levels of phosphate, calcium, and magnesium may cause pruritus [84].

Calciphylaxis, or calcific uremic arteriolopathy, a rare syndrome of disseminated calcification, is a severe complication of secondary HPTH, and results in soft tissue calcification, vascular medial calcinosis, and arteriolar thrombosis leading to ischemic tissue necrosis. Patients present with painful, violaceous, mottled lesions that may progress to skin and subcutaneous tissue necrosis, nonhealing ulcers, and gangrene. Lesions are characteristically located in the hands and fingers, lower extremities, and occasionally lower abdomen. Patients usually have a high calcium-phosphate product, but not necessarily highly elevated PTH levels. The prognosis generally is poor, particularly in patients with truncal and proximal extremity lesions, with mortality approaching greater than 50%. When symptoms and signs of calciphylaxis are identified, the patient should be treated with phosphate binders and timely parathyroidectomy [85, 86]. Necrotic skin ulcers should be treated with standard wound care, debridement, and avoidance of superinfection. For large, non-healing ulcers, hyperbaric oxygen therapy has been employed with mixed results. Sodium thiosulfate has been shown to produce clinical improvement of calciphylaxis lesions. Bisphosphonates have been shown to be effective in animal models of calciphylaxis, and the mechanism of action is believed to be due to inhibition of macrophages and local proinflammatory cytokines as well as binding to calcified vascular smooth muscle cells to inhibit further arterial calcification. Cinacalcet is thought to decrease serum PTH levels and stabilize calcium and phosphate concentrations, and has been associated with improved pain control and ulcer healing. Calciphylaxis remains a poorly understood disease, as most of the data on these therapies consist of case reports [87].

Tertiary HPTH occurs most commonly following renal transplantation in a previously dialysis-dependent patient. Symptoms resemble those of primary HPTH and may include increased bone resorption, nephrolithiasis, and pancreatitis. Increased bone resorption is often exacerbated by preexisting osteodystrophy, and steroid-induced osteopenia. Tertiary HPTH is the main cause of nephrolithiasis in transplanted kidneys, presenting as painless hematuria in the grafted denervated kidney. Pancreatitis, which occurs in 2–6% of kidney transplant recipients, has a prevalence of 11% in those with hypercalcemia [88–90].

Treatment

The initial management of secondary and tertiary HPTH revolves around medical therapy with or without dialysis in order to maintain a stable mineral milieu. This therapy focuses on dietary phosphate restriction, vitamin D sterols, and calcimimetics [91].

Phosphate retention represents one of the major factors in the development of secondary HPTH. The first step to control serum phosphorus is to reduce phosphate intake. However, the extent of dietary phosphate restriction is limited by malnutrition associated with inadequate protein intake and often, poor patient compliance. Thus, the use of phosphate binders is required in almost all patients, particularly those who are dialysis-dependent. Phosphate binders can be calcium-based, aluminum-based, or neither calcium- or aluminum-based; the choice is dependent on the patient's calcium level [91].

After achieving the desired serum phosphorus levels with dietary restriction and the use of binders, secondary HPTH may often persist due to vitamin D deficiency. In this case, vitamin D should be substituted. Calcitriol is the most active metabolite of vitamin D; however, in the setting of CRF, there are potential adverse effects. Calcitriol promotes the intestinal absorption of calcium and phosphate, leading to hypercalcemia and hyperphosphatemia, with a subsequent rise in calcium-phosphate product, a known risk factor of mortality in CRF. In addition, oversuppression of PTH secretion can lead to adynamic bone disease and may, in turn, further aggravate hypercalcemia and hyperphosphatemia. Therefore, vitamin D should not be administered until the serum phosphorus is under adequate control. Several vitamin D analogs have been developed that retain a suppressive action on PTH and parathyroid gland growth with concomitantly less calcemic and phosphatemic activity. These include paricalcitol, doxercalciferol, and maxacalcitol [92].

The parathyroid CaSR regulates PTH secretion. In secondary HPTH there is underexpression of the CaSR, leading to partial loss of calcium-regulated PTH suppression. Calcimimetics allosterically modulate the CaSR, thereby sensitizing it to extracellular calcium ions. The reestablished calcium sensitivity leads to the suppression of PTH production. In contrast to vitamin D sterols, which show an effect on PTH levels in hours or days by inhibition of PTH synthesis, the modification of the CaSR and the resulting inhibition of PTH secretion leads to changes in serum PTH in minutes to a few hours. The advantage of calcimimetics, like cinacalcet hydrochloride, is the capacity to suppress PTH secretion with concomitant rise in serum calcium and phosphorus [93].

Parathyroidectomy is indicated when medical treatment fails to control progressive secondary HPTH. Clinical manifestations include persistence or worsening of skeletal symptoms, pruritus, and extraskeletal calcifications. Elevated intact PTH levels and a proven high-turnover bone disease are prerequisites for consideration of surgery. Calciphylaxis is an indication for immediate parathyroidectomy (Table 35.5) [86].

Indications for operative intervention in tertiary HPTH are similar to those of primary HPTH, namely, significant hypercalcemia, decline in creatinine clearance, nephrolithiasis,

TABLE 35.5 Indications for parathyroidectomy in secondary hyperparathyroidism

Appropriate medical treatment and elevated PTH levels and high-turnover bone disease with any of the following:
Bone pain that is disabling or dependent on continuous analgesic drugs
Pathologic fractures
Subperiosteal resorption documented on plain radiographic films
Hypercalcemia unresponsive to phosphate restriction and phosphate binding
Hyperphosphatemia unresponsive to phosphate restriction and binding
Severe pruritus
Extraskeletal nonvascular calcifications (systemic calcinosis)
Intractable anemia
Calciphylaxis

TABLE 35.6 Indications for parathyroidectomy after kidney transplantation

Subacute severe hypercalcemia
Persistent hypercalcemia and one of the following:
Deterioration of renal function
Nephrolithiasis
Progressive bone disease
Acute pancreatitis

acute pancreatitis, changes in mental status, or overt bone disease. Mild hypercalcemia alone does not appear to be a serious threat to the patient with a transplanted kidney, and its treatment remains controversial. However, impaired renal function in the presence of elevated PTH and hypercalcemia should be an indication for parathyroidectomy, especially in the elderly patients (Table 35.6) [88].

Preoperative preparation of dialysis patients includes control of hyperkalemia, hypomagnesemia, and hypervolemia with careful evaluation and treatment of hypertension and cardiovascular disease. Patients should receive oral calcitriol before surgery to avoid severe postoperative hypocalcemia. They should be dialyzed no longer than 1 day before parathyroidectomy and then again no later than 2 days after the operation. When parathyroidectomy is performed after kidney transplantation, immunosuppressive medications do not have to be interrupted in the perioperative period. However, replacement glucocorticoid doses should be administered [86–88].

The two accepted operative procedures for the management of secondary and tertiary HPTH are subtotal parathyroidectomy and total parathyroidectomy with immediate parathyroid autotransplantation [94]. The variability of the number of parathyroid glands is well known; in a report on 519 patients undergoing total parathyroidectomy with parathyroid forearm autotransplantation, supernumerary glands were found in 14.5% of patients. The most frequent location of supernumerary glands (39%) was the thymic tongue [95, 96]. Thus, transcervical thymectomy is performed routinely to decrease the risk of recurrent HPTH and to lower the rate of reoperations to the neck [97, 98].

Intraoperative PTH measurement is an established tool in determining the successful removal of parathyroid tissue in patients undergoing surgery for primary HPTH. Recent studies have provided evidence that intraoperative PTH monitoring also may be useful during surgery for secondary and tertiary HPTH. After subtotal or total parathyroidectomy, an appropriate and rapid decline of PTH levels is expected. A persistent elevated PTH, however, can result from non-identified supernumerary glands, and further identification and removal of additional parathyroid glands are indicated [99, 100].

Clinical Outcomes

The overall clinical result is considered good in 70–85% of patients who undergo successful parathyroidectomy. In a few days, bone pain improves in 60–80%, malaise in 75%, and joint pain in 85% of patients. Muscle weakness is alleviated in one third of the patients with improvement of radiologic signs in 95%. Pruritus decreases overnight in almost all patients and disappears in 60–80% [101].

Successful parathyroidectomy improves nonvisceral calcifications in 50–60% of patients. However, it does not change arterial calcification despite reduction in the calcium-phosphate product and PTH. Small peripheral arterial calcification may progress or even develop in approximately 56% of patients after operative intervention [101].

Conclusion

Hypercalcemia is a common finding in the elderly population. It appears to have widely encompassing effects on many aspects of geriatric health, from cognitive and psychiatric decline to diminished function of the cardiovascular, renal, bone, endocrine, and gastrointestinal systems. It may be associated with underlying malignancy, but concomitant intact PTH measurement usually is diagnostic. HPTH peaks in the fifth decade of life, but elderly patients are at increased risk to develop HPTH. Such patients should be evaluated carefully, and surgical interventions, when appropriate, should be undertaken by experienced parathyroid surgeons. With the advent of better imaging studies and minimally invasive operative techniques, elderly patients who may have been considered poor surgical candidates can now undergo safe and successful parathyroidectomy with improved health status, enhanced quality of life, and prolonged life expectancy.

CASE STUDY RESOLUTION

After appropriate medical management of acute hypercalcemia, including intravenous hydration, bisphosphate and furosemide therapy, the patient's serum calcium decreased to 10.8 mg/dL and her mental status returned to baseline. She underwent a sestamibi scan with SPECT, which revealed increased uptake in the right inferior anterior neck. After adequate medical evaluation, she underwent a minimally invasive parathyroidectomy with excision of a right inferior parathyroid adenoma. Intraoperative rapid PTH measurement documented adequate resection with a decline from her baseline 200 to 35 pg/ml at 10 min post-resection. The patient returned home the following day with a normal serum calcium level of 9.8 mg/dL, and a post-operative regimen of oral calcium supplementation. At 6 months post-operatively, she remained eucalcemic and did not have any further episodes of nephrolithasis.

References

1. Holt EH, Inzucchi SE (2007) Physiology and pathophysiology of the parathyroid glands and preoperative evaluation. In: Surgery of the thyroid and parathyroid glands. Springer, New York, p 235
2. Brown EM (1999) Physiology and pathophysiology of the extracellular calcium-sensing receptor. Am J Med 106:238
3. Bringhurst FR (1989) Calcium and phosphate distribution, turnover, and metabolic actions. In: DeGroot LJ (ed) Endocrinology. Saunders, Philadelphia, p 805
4. Norman AW et al (1982) The vitamin D endocrine system: steroid metabolism, hormone receptors and biologic response. Endocr Revi 3:331
5. Potts JT Jr (1996) Hyperparathyroidism and other hypercalcemic disorders. Adv Intern Med 41:165
6. Silverberg SJ et al (1999) Therapeutic controversies in primary hyperparathyroidism. J Clin Endocrinol Metab 84:2275
7. Rankin W et al (1997) Parathyroid hormone-related protein and hypercalcemia. Cancer 80:1564
8. Strewler GJ (2000) The physiology of parathyroid hormone-related protein. N Engl J Med 342:177
9. Brown EM (2000) Familial hypocalciuric hypercalcemia and other disorders with resistance to extracellular calcium. Endocrinol Metab Clin North Am 29:503
10. Ljunghall S et al (1991) Primary hyperparathyroidism: epidemiology, dianosis and clinical picture. World J Surg 15:681
11. Adami S et al (2002) Epidemiology of primary hyperparathyroidism in Europe. J Bone Miner Res 17(S2):N18
12. Bendz H et al (1996) Hyperparathyroidism and long-term lithium therapy: a cross-sectional study and the effect of lithium withdrawal. J Intern Med 240:357
13. Chen JD et al (2003) Hyperparathyroidism-jaw tumour syndrome. J Intern Med 253:634
14. Hundahl SA et al (1999) Two hundred eight-six cases of parathyroid carcinoma treated in the U.S. between 1985 and 1995: a National Cancer Data Base Report. The American College of Surgeons Commission on Cancer and the American Cancer Society. Cancer 86:538
15. Rodgers SE, Perrier ND (2006) Parathyroid carcinoma. Curr Opin Oncol 18:16
16. Koea JB, Shaw JH (1999) Parathyroid cancer: biology and management. Surg Oncol 8:155
17. Hruska KA, Teitelbaum SL (1995) Renal osteodystrophy. N Engl J Med 333:166
18. Diamond TW et al (1986) Parathyroid hypertension: a reversible disorder. Arch Intern Med 146:1709
19. Patten BM et al (1974) Neuromuscular disease and primary hyperparathyroidism. Ann Intern Med 80:182
20. Petersen P (1968) Psychiatric disorders in primary hyperparathyroidism. J Clin Endocrinol Metab 28:1491
21. Schram MT et al (2007) Serum calcium and cognitive function in old age. J Am Geriatr Soc 55:1786
22. Cummings SR et al (1995) Risk factors for hip fracture in white women: study of osteoporotic fractures research group. N Engl J Med 332:767
23. Dawson-Hughes B et al (1997) Effect of calcium and vitamin D supplementation on bone density in men and women 65 years of age or older. N Engl J Med 337:670
24. Eastell R (1998) Treatment of postmenopausal osteoporosis. N Engl J Med 339:736
25. Lang B, Lo CY (2006) Parathyroid cancer. Surg Oncol Clin N Am 15:573
26. Sandelin K et al (1992) Prognostic factors in parathyroid cancer: a review of 95 cases. World J Surg 16:724
27. Udelsman R (2001) Primary hyperparathyroidism. Curr Treat Options Oncol 2:365
28. Udelsman R (1996) Parathyroid imaging: the myth and the reality. Radiology 21:317
29. Udelsman R et al (2003) Rapid parathyroid hormone analysis during venous localization. Ann Surg 237:714
30. Clark OH (1994) "Asymptomatic" primary hyperparathyroidism: is parathyroidectomy indicated? Surgery 116:947
31. Clark OH et al (1991) Diagnosis and management of asymptomatic hyperparathyroidism: safety, efficacy, and deficiencies in our knowledge. J Bone Miner Res 6:S135
32. Uden P et al (1992) Primary hyperparathyroidism in younger and older patients: symptoms and outcome of surgery. World J Surg 16:791
33. Hedback G et al (1990) Premature death in patients operated on for primary hyperparathyroidism. World J Surg 14:829
34. NIH Consensus Development Conference Panel (1991) Diagnosis and management of asymptomatic primary hyperparathyroidism: consensus development state. Ann Intern Med 114:593
35. Bilezikian JP et al (2002) Summary statement from a workshop on aymptomatic primary hyperparathyroidism: a perspective for the 21st century. J Clin Endocrinol Metab 87:5353
36. Udelsman R et al (2009) Surgery for asymptomatic primary hyperparathyroidism: Proceedings of the Third International Workshop. J Clin Endocrinol Metab 94:366
37. Utiger RD (1999) Editorial: treatment of primary hyperparathyroidism. N Engl J Med 341:1301
38. Eigelberger MS et al (2004) The NIH criteria for parathyroidectomy in asymptomatic primary hyperparathyroidism: are they too limited? Ann Surg 239:528
39. Diamond T et al (1996) Estrogen replacement may be an alternative to parathyroid surgery for the treatment of osteoporosis in

elderly postmenopausal women presenting with primary hyperparathyroidism: a preliminary report. Osteoporos Int 6:329

40. Souberbielle JC et al (2001) Vitamin D status and redefining serum parathyroid hormone reference range in the elderly. J Clin Endocrinol Metab 86:3086

41. Quesada JM et al (1992) Influence of vitamin D on parathyroid function in the elderly. J Clin Endocrinol Metab 75:494

42. Pfeifer M et al (2001) Effects of a short-term vitamin D3 and calcium supplementation on blood pressure and parathyroid hormone levels in elderly women. J Clin Endocrinol Metab 86:1633

43. Tibblin S et al (1983) Hyperparathyroidism in the elderly. Ann Surg 197:135

44. Sosa JA et al (2008) A population-based study of outcomes from thyroidectomy in aging Americans: at what cost? J Am Coll Surg 206:1097

45. Guerrero MA et al (2007) Minimally invasive parathyroidectomy complicated by pneumothoraces: a report of 4 cases. J Surg Educ 64:101

46. Udelsman R (2002) Six hundred fifty-six consecutive explorations for primary hyperparathyroidism. Ann Surg 235:665

47. Lo Gerfo P (1999) Bilateral neck exploration for parathyroidectomy under local anesthesia: a viable technique for patients with coexisting thyroid disease with or without sestamibi scanning. Surgery 126:1011

48. Udelsman R, Donovan PI (2006) Remedial parathyroid surgery: changing trends in 130 consecutive cases. Ann Surg 244:471

49. Carty SE et al (1997) Concise parathyroidectomy: the impact of preoperative SPECT 99mTc sestamibi scanning and intraoperative quick parathyroid hormone assay. Surgery 122:1107

50. Chen H et al (1999) Outpatient minimally invasive parathyroidectomy: a combination of sestamibi-SPECT localization, cervical block anesthesia, and intraoperative parathyroid hormone assay. Surgery 126:1016

51. Irvin GL et al (1996) Ambulatory parathyroidectomy for primary hyperparathyroidism. Arch Surg 31:1074

52. Fang WL et al (2008) The management of high-risk patients with primary hyperparathyroidism—minimally invasive parathyroidectomy vs. medical treatment. Clin Endocrinol 68:520

53. Irvin GL III, Carneiro DM (2001) "Limited" parathyroidectomy in geriatric patients. Ann Surg 233:612

54. Chen H et al (2003) Radioguided parathyroidectomy is equally effective for both adenomatous and hyperplastic glands. Ann Surg 238:332

55. Miccoli P et al (1998) Endoscopic parathyroidectomy: report on an initial experience. Surgery 124:1077

56. Sheldon DG et al (2002) Surgical treatment of hyperparathyroidism improves health-related quality of life. Arch Surg 137:1022

57. Christiansen P et al (1999) Primary hyperparathyroidism: effect of parathyroidectomy on regional bone mineral density in Danish patients: a three-year follow-up study. Bone 25:589

58. Vestergaard P, Mosekilde L (2003) Cohort study on effects of parathyroid surgery on multiple outcomes in primary hyperparathyroidism. Br Med J 327:530

59. Chou FF et al (1995) Neuromuscular recovery after parathyroidectomy in primary hyperparathyroidism. Surgery 117:18

60. Tamura Y et al (2007) Remarkable increase in lumbar spine bone mineral density and amelioration in biochemical markers of bone turnover after parathyroidectomy in elderly patients with primary hyperparathyroidism: a 5-year follow-up study. J Bone Miner Metab 25:226

61. Burney RE et al (1998) Surgical correction of primary hyperparathyroidism improves quality of life. Surgery 124:987

62. Burney RE et al (1996) Assessment of patient outcomes after operation for primary hyperparathyroidism. Surgery 120:1013

63. Roman SA et al (2005) Parathyroidectomy improves neurocognitive deficits in patients with primary hyperparathyroidism. Surgery 138:1121

64. Roman SA, Sosa JA (2007) Psychiatric and cognitive aspects of primary hyperparathyroidism. Curr Opin Oncol 19:1

65. Papageorgiou SG et al (2008) Dementia as presenting symptom of primary hyperparathyroidism: favourable outcome after surgery. Clin Neurol Neurosurg 110:1038

66. Chen H et al (1998) Parathyroidectomy in the elderly: do the benefits outweigh the risks? World J Surg 22:531

67. Bachar G et al (2008) Comparison of perioperative management and outcome of parathyroidectomy between older and younger patients. Head Neck 30:1415

68. Talpos GB et al (2000) Randomized trial of parathyroidectomy in mild asymptomatic primary hyperparathyroidism: patient description and effects on the SF-36 health survey. Surgery 125:1013

69. Joborn C et al (1989) Self-rated psychiatric symptoms in patients operated on because of primary hyperparathyroidism and in patients with long-standing mild hypercalcemia. Surgery 105:72

70. Burney RE et al (1999) Health status improvement after surgical correct of primary hyperparathyroidism in patients with high and low preoperative calcium levels. Surgery 125:608

71. Okamoto T et al (2002) Outcome study of psychological distress and nonspecific symptoms in patients with mild primary hyperparathyroidism. Arch Surg 137:779

72. Solomon BL et al (1991) Psychologic symptoms before and after parathyroid surgery. Am J Med 96:101

73. Pasieka JL et al (2002) Patient-based surgical outcome tool demonstrating alleviation of symptoms following parathyroidectomy in patients with primary hyperparathyroidism. World J Surg 26:942

74. Sims R et al (2004) Hyperparathyroidism in the elderly patient. Drugs Aging 21:1013

75. Palmer M et al (1987) Survival and renal function in untreated hypercalcaemia: population-based cohort study with 14 years of follow-up. Lancet 1:59

76. Hedback G et al (1991) The influence of surgery on the risk of death in patients with primary hyperparathyroidism. World J Surg 15:399

77. Riggs BL et al (1978) A syndrome of osteoporosis, increased serum immunoreactive parathyroid hormone, and inappropriately low serum 1, 25-dihydroxyvitamin D. Mayo Clin Proc 53:701

78. Sitges-Serra A, Caralps-Riera A (1987) Hyperparathyroidism associated with renal disease: pathogenesis, natural history, and surgical treatment. Surg Clin North Am 67:359

79. Pietschmann P et al (1991) Bone metabolism in patients with functioning kidney grafts: increased serum levels of osteocalcin and parathyroid hormone despite normalization of kidney function. Nephron 59:533

80. Demeure MJ et al (1990) Results of surgical treatment for hyperparathyroidism associated with renal disease. Am J Surg 160:337

81. Qi Q et al (1995) Predictive value of serum parathyroid hormone levels for bone turnover in patients on chronic maintenance dialysis. Am J Kidney Dis 26:622

82. Coen G et al (2002) Renal osteodystrophy in predialysis and hemodialysis patients: comparison of histologic patterns and diagnostic predictivity of intact PTH. Nephron 91:103

83. Block GA et al (2004) Mineral metabolism, mortality, and morbidity in maintenance hemodialysis. J Am Soc Nephrol 15:2208

84. Massry SG et al (1968) Intractable pruritus as a manifestation of secondary hyperparathyroidism in uremia: disappearance of itching after subtotal parathyroidectomy. N Engl J Med 279:697

85. Roe SM et al (1994) Calciphylaxis: early recognition and management. Am J Surg 60:81

86. Duh QY et al (1991) Calciphylaxis in secondary hyperparathyroidism: diagnosis and parathyroidectomy. Arch Surg 126:1213

87. Raymond CB, Wazny LD (2008) Sodium thiosulfate, bisphosphonates, and cinacalcet for treatment of calciphylaxis. Am J Health-Syst Pharm 65:1419

88. D'Alessandro AM et al (1989) Tertiary hyperparathyroidism after renal transplantation: operative indications. Surgery 106:1049

89. David DS et al (1973) Hypercalcemia after renal transplantation: long-term follow-up data. N Engl J Med 289:398

90. Sitges-Serra A et al (1988) Pancreatitis and hyperparathyroidism. Br J Surg 75:158

91. Guller U, Mayr M (2007) Pathophysiology and treatment of secondary and tertiary hyperparathyroidism. In: Surgery of the thyroid and parathyroid glands. Springer, New York, p 293

92. Malluche HH et al (2002) Update on vitamin D and its newer analogues: actions and rationale for treatment in chronic renal failure. Kidney Int 62:367

93. Block GA et al (2004) Cinacalcet for secondary hyperparathyroidism in patients receiving hemodialysis. N Engl J Med 350(15):1516

94. Rothmund M et al (1991) Subtotal parathyroidectomy versus total parathyroidectomy and autotransplantation in secondary hyperparathyroidism: a randomized trial. World J Surg 15:745

95. Thompson NW et al (1982) The anatomy of primary hyperparathyroidism. Surgery 92:814

96. Akerstrom G et al (1984) Surgical anatomy of human parathyroid glands. Surgery 95:14

97. Numano M et al (1998) Surgical significance of supernumerary parathyroid glands in renal hyperparathyroidism. World J Surg 22:1098

98 Freeman JB et al (1976) Transcervical thymectomy: an integral part of neck exploration for hyperparathyroidism. Arch Surg 11:359

99. Clary BM et al (1997) Intraoperative parathyroid hormone monitoring during parathyroidectomy for secondary hyperparathyroidism. Surgery 122:1034

100. Chou FF et al (2002) Intraoperative parathyroid hormone measurement in patients with secondary hyperparathyroidism. Arch Surg 137:341

101. Pasieka JL, Parsons LL (2000) A prospective surgical outcome study assessing the impact of parathyroidectomy on symptoms in patients with secondary and tertiary hyperparathyroidism. Surgery 128:531

Chapter 36
Adrenal Tumors in Older Persons

Tobias Carling and Robert Udelsman

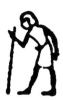

CASE STUDY

An 88-year-old male with a known left parotid gland tumor underwent a positron emission tomography/computed tomography (PET/CT) scan to rule out malignancy. The PET scan revealed uptake in the left retroperitoneal area, and the CT scan revealed a 4.0×3.0 cm mass of the left adrenal gland. The operation for his parotid gland tumor was postponed, and he underwent biochemical evaluation for endocrine hypersecretion. Twenty-four-hour urine collection revealed elevated levels of epinephrine, norepinephrine, and vanillylmandelic acid (VMA). Plasma levels of free metanephrine and normetanephrines were elevated, whereas serum cortisol, DHEA, potassium, calcitonin, plasma aldosterone concentration (PAC), renin activity (PRA), and 24-h urine collection of cortisol and aldosterone were all within normal limits. His past medical and surgical history are significant for a left parotid gland tumor, long-standing hypertension controlled with a β-blocker and an angiotensin-converting enzyme (ACE) inhibitor, atrial fibrillation, and benign prostatic hypertrophy (BPH). A recent echocardiogram revealed mild aortic stenosis and mitral valve prolapse with an ejection fraction of 55%. He had in the remote past undergone two intraabdominal operations: open cholecystectomy for acute cholecystitis and partial gastrectomy with vagotomy for a duodenal ulcer. His family history is negative for familial pheochromocytoma. He denies any chest pain, shortness of breath, palpitations, headache, pallor, diaphoresis, or any paroxysms (spells). The patient was started on α-blockade (doxazosin mesylate) and metyrosine and when adequately blocked underwent a laparoscopic left adrenalectomy. The operation was uneventful, although some adhesions were encountered from the prior gastrectomy. The patient remained hemodynamically stable during the operation but developed transient hypotension after ligation of the left adrenal vein. This was promptly controlled with volume expansion and intermittent norepinephrine by the dedicated pheochromocytoma anesthesia team. Postoperatively, the patient remained stable off antihypertensive medications. However, after removal of the Foley catheter, he was unable to void due to urinary retention. He was started on tamsulosin for BPH, discharged home on postoperative day 3, and returned for outpatient removal of his Foley catheter. Histopathological analysis revealed a 4.0×3.2×3.0 cm left adrenal pheochromocytoma. All margins were negative. However, marked cellular atypia and focal capsular invasion was identified, suggesting an aggressive phenotype. A definite diagnosis of malignant pheochromocytoma could not be made in the absence of invasive or metastatic disease. There is no evidence of recurrent disease based on biochemical and radiological surveillance for 3 years.

Introduction

Adrenal tumors are common, especially in older individuals. Numerous autopsy studies have examined the frequency of adrenal tumors, and in a review of 87,065 autopsies, adrenal lesions (>1 cm) were identified in 6% of patients [1]. Similarly, the prevalence of adrenal "incidentalomas" is 4% when detected by abdominal CT or magnetic resonance

T. Carling (✉)
Department of Surgery, Yale University School of Medicine, New Haven, CT, USA
e-mail: tobias.carling@yale.edu

imaging (MRI). The incidence of adrenal tumors increases with age. For instance, the likelihood of detecting an unsuspected adrenal lesion on an abdominal CT scan in individuals between 20 and 29 years of age is only 0.2% versus 7% in individuals over 70 years of age [1, 2]. The majority of adrenal tumors are clinically nonfunctioning, benign adrenocortical adenomas and usually do not require surgical intervention. However, surgeons also may encounter elderly patients with functioning benign adrenal tumors (cortisol-, aldosterone-, and catecholamine-producing) as well as malignant adrenal tumors (adrenocortical carcinoma; ACC, malignant pheochromocytoma, and metastasis to the adrenal). The management principles of adrenal tumors in older patients are similar to those in their younger counterparts. However, the diagnosis as well as the management may provide unique challenges in the elderly that are exemplified in the above case presentation: (1) the symptoms of hormone excess may be absent, subtle, atypical, and/or masked by medications, (2) the biochemical diagnosis of endocrine hypersecretion may be cumbersome due to drug interference, (3) the index of suspicion may be too low for an alternative diagnosis to essential hypertension, (4) laparoscopic surgery may be more difficult due to previous open abdominal procedures, (5) unanticipated complications may occur (e.g., urinary retention).

Anatomy and Pathophysiology

Anatomy

The adrenals are paired flat glands with a triangular shape, each weighing about 5 g. The medulla is of ectodermal origin and is derived from the neural crest. It contains homogeneous sheets of cells organized into nests. Cells have large varied nuclei and abundant cytoplasm packed with numerous secretory granules containing catecholamines and other substances specific to chromaffin cells. The cortex is of mesodermal origin and is derived from the adrenogenital ridge. The cortex is organized into three layers, each with a different function. The most superficial layer is the zona glomerulosa, responsible for aldosterone production. The middle zone is the zona fasciculata, containing radial columns of lipid-laden cells that primarily produce cortisol. The inner layer, zona reticularis, stores cholesterol for steroidogenesis and secretes sex hormones. The blood supply to the adrenal is threefold: via the superior adrenal arteries from the inferior phrenic arteries, the middle adrenal from the aorta, and the inferior adrenal artery from the renal arteries. Blood passes from the cortex to the medulla, and the gland is drained by a typically single central vein emptying into the vena cava on the right and the renal vein on the left.

Physiology

Steroid end products secreted by the adrenal cortex are metabolites of cholesterol. The common pathway is conversion of cholesterol to δ5-pregnenolone and then progesterone. In the zona glomerulosa, progesterone is converted through several steps to the mineralocorticoid aldosterone. In the other layers of the cortex, progesterone is converted first to 17-hydroxyprogesterone and then to either the 17-hydroxysteroid cortisol or the 17-ketosteroid sex hormones. Each day, the adrenal glands secrete 15–20 mg of cortisol, 25–30 mg of androgens, and 75–125 μg of aldosterone. The zona fasciculata and zona reticularis are responsible for glucocorticoid production. Secretion of cortisol is controlled via the hypothalamic–pituitary–adrenal (HPA) axis. Hypothalamic corticotropin-releasing hormone (CRH) causes release of adrenocorticotrophic hormone (ACTH) from the anterior pituitary gland, which stimulates the adrenal cortex to release cortisol. As cortisol concentration achieves the physiologic range of 15–20 μg/dl, it exerts a negative feedback on both hypothalamus and anterior pituitary secretion. ACTH has a plasma half-life of 25 min, and cortisol has a plasma half-life of 90 min [3]. ACTH and cortisol production are constant over life in normal, unstressed individuals. Adrenal androgen release is regulated by ACTH, whereas gonadal release of testosterone and estrogen are under a separate pathway of pituitary gonadotrophic control. Androgen production peaks at puberty and progressively declines with advancing age. The mineralocorticoid aldosterone is produced in the outermost layer of the adrenal cortex, the zona glomerulosa. Aldosterone secretion is primarily controlled through a renal pathway. Decreased arterial pressure or decreased serum sodium concentration is sensed by the juxtaglomerular apparatus and the macula densa, respectively. The result is production and release of renin, activating angiotensin I. Within the lung, angiotensin-converting enzyme (ACE) converts most of the angiotensin I to the angiotensin II. Circulating angiotensin II stimulates aldosterone secretion. To a lesser degree, aldosterone secretion is stimulated by direct effects of ACTH and elevated serum potassium. With aging, there is decreased production of aldosterone [4].

Stimulation of the adrenal medulla is via preganglionic sympathetic fibers, causing release of dopamine, norepinephrine, and epinephrine. Sympathetic neural outflow is increased by the fight-or-flight response, fear, emotional stress, upright posture, pain, cold, hypotension, hypoglycemia, and other stress. Norepinephrine exerts negative feedback at the preganglionic sympathetic receptors. With increasing age, there is no change in epinephrine levels, but norepinephrine and total plasma catecholamine are increased. However, this does not seem to be associated with hypertension in the elderly, which is probably due to an increased incidence and severity of atherosclerosis. This change in the cardiovascular system may also be responsible for the attenuated response to sympathetic stimuli seen in the elderly [4].

Molecular Pathology

Although familial adrenal tumors tend to have an age of onset earlier than their sporadic counterparts, the molecular genetics of such kindreds have contributed to the understanding of adrenal tumorigenesis (Table 36.1). Rare hereditary tumor syndromes predispose to adrenocortical tumor development. These include Li–Fraumeni's syndrome, Beckwith–Wiedemann syndrome, multiple endocrine neoplasia type 1 (MEN1), and the Carney Complex [5]. Li–Fraumeni's syndrome is a rare neoplasia syndrome caused by mutations of the tumor suppressor gene p53 that predispose patients to tumors of several origins (brain, breast, adrenal). Beckwith–Wiedemann syndrome is characterized by increased secretion of insulin-like growth factor 2 (IGF-2), resulting in hemihypertrophy, diabetes mellitus, and adrenocortical tumors in children. IGF-2 overproduction is mostly related to defects in genomic imprinting. Adrenocortical tumors arise in up to 40% of patients with MEN1. Mutations of the tumor suppressor gene *MEN1* on chromosome 11q13 are responsible for the development of MEN1 [6]. Studies of sporadic adrenocortical tumors suggest distinct molecular signatures between adrenal adenomas and ACC [7, 8]. However, detailed understanding of the molecular pathway leading to hormone-producing adrenal adenomas as well as ACC is lacking.

Pheochromocytomas occur either sporadically (80–90% of cases) or in four known familial syndromes – multiple endocrine neoplasia type 2 (MEN2), von Hippel–Lindau (VHL) disease, neurofibromatosis type 1 (NF 1), and succinate dehydrogenase (SDH) gene mutation [9]. The familial forms of pheochromocytoma are caused by the following genes: *RET* protooncogene, and the *VHL*, *NF1*, and *SDH* (*B*, *C*, and *D*) tumor suppressor genes, respectively. The age at presentation varies widely between the variants as well as between and within individual families. The underlying cause of sporadic pheochromocytoma is largely unknown, although genetic studies have identified several chromosomal loci with alterations in sporadic pheochromocytomas and abdominal paragangliomas. The most common chromosomal alteration is loss of the short arm of chromosome 1 [10].

Evaluation of the Adrenal Incidentaloma

In older persons, given the high and increasing prevalence of adrenal incidentalomas (defined as adrenal lesions >1 cm discovered serendipitously during radiological examination performed for reasons other than adrenal evaluation), a discussion about the management of such patients precedes the section about specific adrenal tumors. The overall goal is to identify patients who have functioning hormone-producing adrenal tumors (cortisol-, aldosterone-, or catecholamine-producing), or malignant adrenal tumors (ACC, malignant pheochromocytoma, or metastasis to the adrenal) [11]. Although all aspects of the evaluation of patients with adrenal incidentaloma have not been prospectively validated, an algorithm based on current clinical experience and data is shown (Fig. 36.1). A detailed history and physical exam is always of utmost importance, focusing on the signs and symptoms suggestive of adrenal hyperfunction or malignant disease (Table 36.2).

TABLE 36.1 Familial adrenal tumor disorders, genetic characteristics, adrenal and common nonadrenal manifestation

Disorder	Responsible gene	Chromosomal location	Adrenal manifestation	Associated manifestations
MEN1	*MEN1*	11q13	Adrenocortical adenomas	Tumors of the parathyroids, pituitary, endocrine pancreas
Li–Fraumeni	*p53*	17p13.1	Adrenocortical carcinoma	Sarcomas, breast cancer, brain tumors, leukemia
Beckwith–Wiedemann	*Genomic imprinting*	11p15.5	Adrenocortical adenomas and carcinomas	Congenital abnormalities, multiple tumors
Carney Complex	*PRKAR1A*	17q23-q24	Nodular, pigmented adrenal tumors	Multiple tumors, pigmented lesions of the skin and mucosae
MEN2A&B	*RET*	10q21	Pheochromocytoma, often bilateral	Medullary thyroid cancer, HPT in MEN2A. Marfanoid habitus and neuromas in MEN2B
von Hippel–Lindau	*VHL*	3p25-26	Pheochromocytoma	CNS hemangioblastoma, renal cell carcinoma, and pancreatic tumors
Familial Paraganglioma	*SDH B&D*	3q13-21, 11q23	Pheochromocytoma, paraganglioma	Leiomyomas and renal cancer
NF 1	*NF1*	17q11.2	Pheochromocytoma	Cafe-au-lait spots and fibromatous tumors, multiple tumors

MEN Multiple endocrine neoplasia; *NF* neurofibromatosis

Figure 36.1 Algorithm for evaluation of an older person with an adrenal incidentaloma. The algorithm should be individualized according to clinical circumstances, the imaging phenotype of the mass, the patient's age, comorbidities, and preferences.

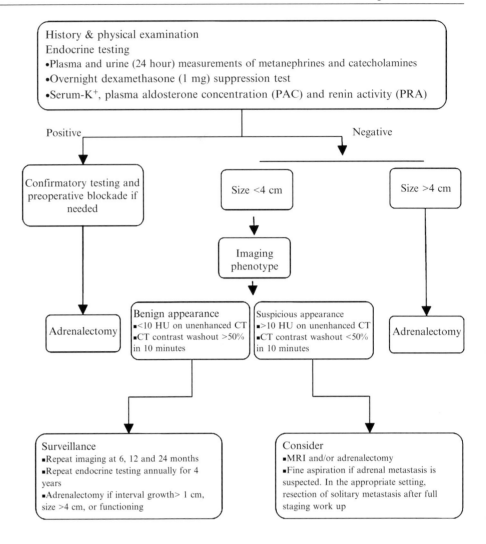

Clinically silent or overt pheochromocytoma occurs in 5% of adrenal incidentalomas. Only about 50% of such patients have hypertension, but clinically silent pheochromocytoma can be lethal [12]. The measurement of fractionated metanephrines and catecholamines in a 24-h urine specimen is recommended for all patients with adrenal incidentalomas (Table 36.2). The detection of elevated levels of fractionated metanephrines, catecholamines, or both has high sensitivity and specificity for pheochromocytoma (91–98%) [2]. The additional measurement of fractionated catecholamines in the 24-h urinary specimen increases the sensitivity of this approach by 5% and is especially helpful in diagnosing patients with dopamine-secreting neoplasms. In older individuals, the measurement of plasma-free metanephrines is less cumbersome than urine collections and has a higher sensitivity for pheochromocytoma (96–100%) [9]. However, the specificity is lower, especially in those older than 60 years of age (77%) [2]. The imaging characteristics of the adrenal mass can also be highly suggestive (but not diagnostic) of pheochromocytoma (Table 36.3 and Fig. 36.2). The findings consistent with pheochromocytoma is increased attenuation on an unenhanced CT scan, prominent vascularity, often

cystic changes, delayed clearance of contrast, and a high signal intensity on T2-weigthed MRI.

Clinical or subclinical (i.e., those lacking overt signs and symptoms of glucocorticoid excess) Cushing's syndrome is initially best evaluated with an overnight dexamethasone (1 mg) suppression test [2, 11, 13]. Although the optimal cut-off value is debated, the use of a cortisol level greater that 5 μg/dl is regarded as a reasonable criterion for clinically significant glucocorticoid secretory autonomy [11]. The specificity of the test is 91%, and if the result is abnormal, confirmatory testing should be performed (see section "Cortisol-Producing Adrenocortical Adenomas"). Approximately 5.3% of all patients with an adrenal incidentaloma have autonomous hypersecretion of cortisol (i.e., independent of a normal HPA axis) [2]. However, other studies have identified subclinical Cushing's syndrome in up to 20% of patients with incidentaloma [14–16].

At least 1% of adrenal incidentalomas have proven to be aldosterone-producing adenomas. Screening for hyperaldosteronism is routinely recommended for hypertensive patients who have an adrenal incidentaloma. Given that only a minority (9–37%) of patients with aldosterone-producing adenomas

TABLE 36.2 Symptoms and signs suggestive of adrenal hyperfunction or malignant disease, and suggested initial biochemical screening tests in older persons presenting with an adrenal incidentaloma

Disorder	Symptoms	Signs	Screening test
Pheochromocytoma	May be asymptomatic; Paroxysmal symptoms (spells) often extremely variable; may include palpitation, pallor, tremor, headache, and diaphoresis. Spells may be spontaneous or precipitated by postural change, anxiety, medications (e.g., metoclopramide, anesthetic agents), and maneuvers that increase intraabdominal pressure	Hypertension (paroxysmal or sustained), orthostatic hypotension, pallor, retinopathy, and fever	Plasma and urine (24 h collection) measurements of fractionated metanephrines and catecholamines. Imaging characteristics may be pathognomonic for pheochromocytoma
Cushing's syndrome	May be asymptomatic; symptoms may include weight gain with central obesity, facial rounding and plethora, supraclavicular and dorsocervical fat pads, easy bruising, thin skin, poor wound healing, purple striae, proximal muscle weakness, emotional and neurocognitive changes, opportunistic and fungal infections, acne, and hirsutism	Hypertension, osteopenia, osteoporosis, fasting hyperglycemia, diabetes mellitus, hypokalemia, hyperlipidemia, and leukocytosis	Overnight dexamethasone (1 mg) suppression test; serum cortisol >5 µg/dl is abnormal
Primary aldosteronism	Often asymptomatic. If hypokalemia is present, nocturia, polyuria, muscle cramps, and palpitations	Hypertension, mild or severe; occasionally hypokalemia and hypernatremia	Plasma aldosterone concentration (PAC) and plasma renin activity (PRA) [1]. PAC/PRA ratio ≥20 and a plasma aldosterone concentration of ≥15 ng/dl are positive results [2]
ACC	May include mass effect (e.g., abdominal pain) and symptoms related to adrenal hypersecretion of cortisol (Cushing's syndrome), androgens (hirsutism, acne, amenorrhea or oligomenorrhea, oily skin, and increased libido), estrogens (gynecomastia), or aldosterone (hypokalemia-related symptoms)	Hypertension, osteopenia, osteoporosis, fasting hyperglycemia, diabetes mellitus, hypokalemia, hyperlipidemia, and leukocytosis	Dependent on symptoms and index of suspicion
Metastatic cancer	History of extraadrenal cancer	Cancer specific signs	Dependent on history

ACC Adrenocortical carcinoma; (1) can be performed while the patient is receiving any antihypertensive drug except spironolactone, eplerenone, or high-dose amiloride; (2) may be laboratory-dependent
Source: Modified from Young [2]. Copyright © 2007 Massachusetts Medical Society. All rights reserved

demonstrate hypokalemia, the measurement of potassium levels alone is not reliable in screening for hyperaldosteronism [2, 11, 17]. The most reasonable screening test, especially in older individuals, is the ratio of the ambulatory morning plasma aldosterone concentration (PAC) to plasma renin activity (PRA) (Table 36.2). If this ratio is high (≥20), it is suggestive of hyperaldosteronism. However, the diagnosis of primary aldosteronism may need to be confirmed by an additional measurement of mineralocorticoid secretory autonomy (see section "Aldosterone-Producing Adrenocortical Adenomas").

A critical aspect of the evaluation of an adrenal incidentaloma is the assessment of malignant potential, which is based on size of the lesion and imaging characteristics. Overall, ACC is found in 4.7% and metastatic disease in 2.5% of adrenal incidentalomas. For patients who have a nonfunctioning mass, without a prior history of malignancy, the major determinant of whether to recommend surgical excision is the size of the lesion. Lesions smaller than 2 cm have an incidence of malignancy of less than 1%, lesions between 2 and 4 cm have an incidence of 3–5%, lesions between 4 and 6 cm have an incidence of 10–15%, and lesions over 6 cm have an incidence of 30–80%. The National Institutes of Health (NIH) state-of-the-science statement suggested that all lesions larger than 6 cm should have surgical excision and that those less than 4 cm may be observed with serial imaging, as outlined (Fig. 36.1). Some controversy exists whether all patients with lesions between 4 and 6 cm also should undergo adrenalectomy. The imaging characteristics may provide a guide in the management of these patients (Table 36.3). Additionally,

TABLE 36.3 Imaging characteristics of adrenal tumors

Feature	Adrenocortical adenoma	Adrenocortical carcinoma	Pheochromocytoma	Metastasis
Size	Small, usually <3 cm	Large, usually >4 cm, often >10 cm	Medium, usually 3–9 cm	Variable
Shape	Round or oval, smooth margins	Irregular, unclear margins	Round or oval, clear margins	Oval or irregular, unclear margins
Texture	Homogeneous	Heterogeneous, mixed densities	Heterogeneous, cystic areas	Heterogeneous, mixed densities
Laterality	Usually solitary, unilateral	Usually solitary, unilateral	Usually solitary, unilateral	Often bilateral
Unenhanced CT Attenuation	<10 HU	>10 HU (usually >25 HU)	>10 HU (usually >25 HU)	>10 HU (usually >25 HU)
Enhanced CT Vascularity	Not vascular	Usually vascular	Usually vascular	Usually vascular
Enhanced CT Rapidity of contrast washout	Fast	Slow	Slow	Slow
MRI – appearance on T2 weighted image	Isointense to liver	Hyperintense to liver	Markedly hyperintense to liver	Hyperintense to liver
Necrosis, hemorrhage, or calcifications	Rare	Common	Hemorrhage or cystic areas common	Occasional hemorrhage or cystic areas
Growth rate (per year)	Stable or slow (<1 cm)	Rapid (>2 cm)	Usually slow (0.5–1.0 cm)	Variable

HU Hounsfield units

Adrenal hemorrhage, myelolipomas, and cystic neoplasms are usually easily characterized based on their distinctive imaging characteristics [35, 38]. The presence of pure fat within an adrenal lesion on CT is consistent with myelolipoma

Source: Modified from Young [2].

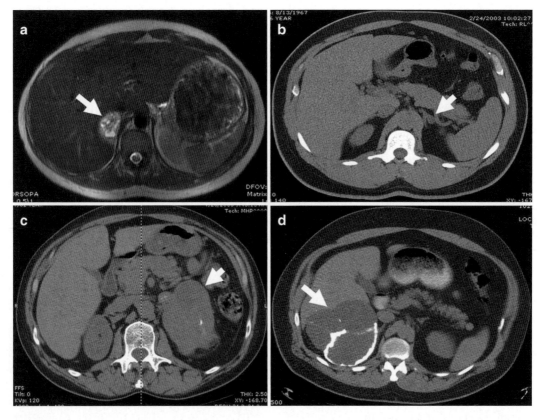

FIGURE 36.2 Representative image characteristics of older patients with adrenal tumors. (**a**) A 68-year-old female with a 4.9-cm right pheochromocytoma (*arrow*). T2-weighted image on MRI displays a partly cystic lesion markedly hyperintense compared to the liver. (**b**) A 72-year-old male with a 1.2-cm left adrenal incidentaloma (*arrow*). The unenhanced CT scan shows a small, round, homogeneous mass with low attenuation. Biochemical evaluation was consistent with primary hyperaldosteronism, and pathology revealed an adrenocortical adenoma. (**c**) A 69-year-old female with adrenocortical carcinoma arising from the left adrenal (*arrow*). The unenhanced CT scan shows a large (15 cm), heterogeneous tumor with irregular, unclear margins. There are multiple areas with mixed densities and necrosis and calcifications. (**d**) A 65-year-old male with a large (18 cm) cystic lymphangioma of the right adrenal gland. The unenhanced CT scan shows a heterogeneous cystic tumor but with regular smooth margins and a peripheral rim with calcifications.

factors such as age and presence of comorbid conditions may make surgery and anesthesia somewhat riskier. However, the vast majority of these patients can undergo a laparoscopic adrenalectomy, which is typically well tolerated.

Functioning Tumors

Cortisol-Producing Adrenocortical Adenomas

Cushing's syndrome is either ACTH-dependent (Cushing's disease, due to a cortisol-producing pituitary tumor; ectopic Cushing's syndrome, due to an ectopic ACTH-producing tumor) or ACTH-independent and adrenal in origin [18]. The signs and symptoms of Cushing's syndrome are summarized in Table 36.2. The biochemical evaluation is stepwise to first diagnose Cushing's syndrome and then to identify the origin of hypercortisolism (Fig. 36.3).

Patients with adrenal adenomas comprise 15–20% of all cases of Cushing's syndrome, and adrenal adenomas are the most common cause of ACTH-independent hypercortisolism, approximately 50–72% [16]. In one series of 85 elderly

patients, cortisol-secreting adenomas represented 37% of patients undergoing adrenalectomy for Cushing's syndrome and 8% of patients undergoing adrenalectomy for any reason [19]. The female/male ratio for adrenal Cushing's syndrome is as high as 9:1 [16], and the mean diameter of the adenomas is 3.9 cm [20]. However, the prevalence of cortisol-secreting adenomas may be higher than previously thought, and subclinical Cushing's syndrome has been reported in 5–20% of adrenal incidentalomas [14, 15]. It is unclear what percentage of patients with subclinical Cushing's syndrome will develop overt Cushing's syndrome over time. Given the morbidity of long-standing hypercortisolism, an aggressive surgical approach (unilateral adrenalectomy) has been advocated, but long-term health benefits remain to be clarified.

Prior to surgical intervention, careful radiological evaluation with CT and/or MRI is of paramount importance, to differentiate adrenal adenoma from ACC and bilateral adrenal hyperplasia. Bilateral adrenal hyperplasia may be ACTH-dependent, whereas the remaining bilateral lesions are due to ACTH-independent macronodular adrenal hyperplasia (AIMAH) and primary pigmented nodular adrenocortical disease (PPNAD).

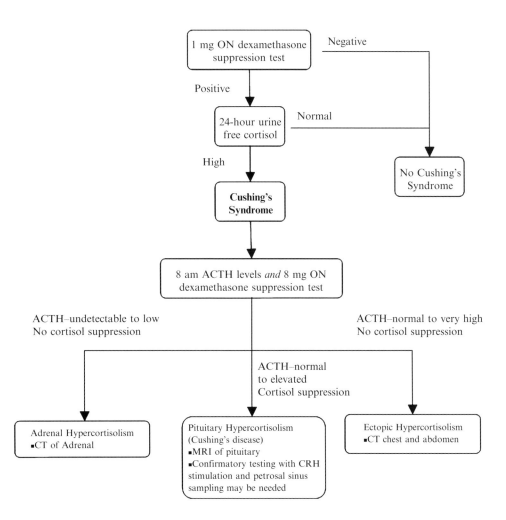

Figure 36.3 Algorithm for evaluation of elderly with suspected hypercortisolism. *ON* overnight; *ACTH* adrenocorticotrophic hormone; *CRH* corticotropin-releasing hormone.

The treatment of cortisol-producing adrenocortical adenomas is unilateral adrenalectomy, which can be performed laparoscopically, regardless of age, in the vast majority of cases [21]. Possible contraindications to the laparoscopic approach are a large tumor, suspicion of adrenocortical carcinoma, or the need for concurrent intraabdominal procedures. Tumor characteristics, not age, should determine the approach. Patients with hypercortisolism are at risk for increased morbidity and mortality due to thromboembolism, suppression of immune function, and delayed wound healing.

Elderly patients should not be excluded from surgery based on age alone, but the increased prevalence of associated medical problems during advanced age is associated with increased perioperative morbidity. In the rare cases of bilateral adenomas, AIMAH or PPNAD, bilateral adrenalectomy may be necessary [16]. Cortical-sparing bilateral adrenalectomy, when feasible, is attractive to preserve endogenous cortisol production in such patients [16]. For patients who have undergone unilateral adrenalectomy, replacement doses of glucocorticoids are given and tapered over time until return of function of the HPA axis is documented. The process, both physiologic and morphologic, may take weeks to months or beyond to complete.

Medical therapy for hypercortisolism, which include various steroidogenesis inhibitors, is limited to instances when surgery is not an option, or to briefly optimize a patient prior to definite surgical therapy [22].

Aldosterone-Producing Adrenocortical Adenomas

Conn's syndrome is due to excessive secretion of aldosterone, resulting in the signs and symptoms summarized in Table 36.2. Although it is a rare cause of hypertension (0.5–1.0%), in a series of elderly patients, an aldosterone-producing adrenocortical adenoma was the indication for 20% of adrenal resections (Table 36.4). As stated, all patients with an adrenal incidentaloma and hypertension should be screened for hyperaldosteronism, which is best performed with measurement of plasma aldosterone concentration (PAC) and plasma renin activity (PRA). A ratio of PAC/PRA ≥ 20 and a plasma aldosterone concentration of ≥ 15 ng/dl are consistent with the diagnosis. This test can be performed while the patient is receiving any antihypertensive drug except spironolactone, eplerenone, or high-dose amiloride. Hypokalemia is only present in 50% of patients with an aldosterone-producing adrenocortical tumor. Occasionally, confirmatory biochemical evaluation is needed with aldosterone suppression testing with either a saline infusion test or 24-h urinary aldosterone excretion test while the patient maintains a high-sodium diet [2]. Aldosterone-secreting

TABLE 36.4 Comparison of indications for adrenalectomy in all versus elderly patients

Diagnosis	% All patients	% >65 years of age
Pheochromocytoma	22–43	19
Adrenocortical carcinoma	18	8
Cushing's syndrome	17–18	22
Nonsecreting adenoma	16–18	31
Hyperaldosteronism	11–19	20
Virilizing/feminizing tumor	6	<1
Myelolipoma	4	<1
Cyst	2–5	<1
Metastasis	1	<1

Source: Data from refs. [19, 21, 47, 48]

adrenal adenomas account for 65–70% of primary aldosteronism, whereas the remaining is due to bilateral adrenal hyperplasia (BAH) and other rare causes.

Prior to surgical intervention, careful radiological evaluation with an adrenal CT is of paramount importance. Lateralization of the source of the excessive aldosterone secretion is critical to guide the management of primary aldosteronism. Distinguishing between unilateral and bilateral disease is important because unilateral adrenalectomy in patients with aldosterone-producing adenomas or unilateral adrenal hyperplasia results in normalization of hypokalemia; hypertension is improved in 100% and cured in 30–60% [17]. In BAH, unilateral or bilateral adrenalectomy seldom corrects the hypertension, and medical therapy is the treatment of choice. If the findings are unequivocal on CT, showing a >1 cm unilateral, attenuating lesion with a contralateral normal adrenal gland, no further evaluation is needed. However, if no tumor is found, or the tumor is less than 1 cm, or there are bilateral adrenal masses, further evaluation with adrenal venous sampling (AVS) for measurements of aldosterone and cortisol concentrations is warranted (Fig. 36.4). A ratio of aldosterone/cortisol fourfold greater than the contralateral side is indicative of a unilateral aldosterone-producing tumor, with a sensitivity of 95% and specificity of 100%. AVS is not a simple procedure and requires an experienced radiologist, especially with regard to catheterization of the short right adrenal vein.

Patients at all ages, with an acceptable operative risk and a lateralizing tumor (either by imaging and/or AVS), are candidates for adrenalectomy. Since the vast majority (>98%) of aldosterone-producing adenomas are small and benign, virtually all cases can be performed via a laparoscopic approach. As compared with open adrenalectomy, laparoscopic adrenalectomy is associated with shorter hospital stays and fewer complications. Hypertension is cured (defined as blood pressure <140/90 mmHg without the aid of antihypertensive drugs) in about 50% (range, 35–60%) of patients after unilateral adrenalectomy, with a cure rate as high as 56–77% when the cure threshold was blood pressure less than 160/95 mmHg [17]. Factors associated with resolution of hypertension

FIGURE 36.4 Algorithm for evaluation of an older patient with confirmed primary hyperaldosteronism.

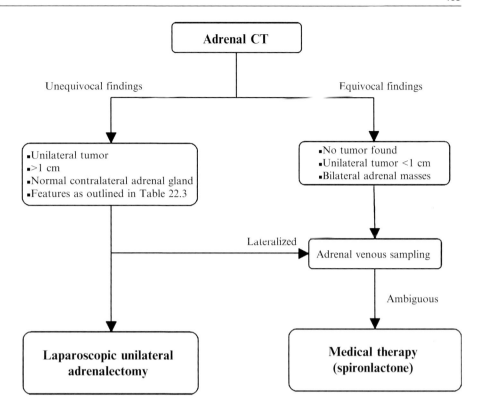

include preoperative use of two or fewer antihypertensive drugs, duration of hypertension less than 5 years, higher PAC to PRA ratio preoperatively, higher urinary aldosterone secretion, or positive preoperative response to spironolactone [17, 23, 24]. Advanced age and longer duration of hypertension have been suggested in some studies to be associated with a lower cure rate [17]

Medical management with spironolactone or amiloride is recommended for patients who do not undergo surgery [17]. Significant improvement can be achieved, but additional antihypertensive medications are needed in about 83% of cases. In the long term, adrenalectomy is more cost-effective than lifelong medical therapy [24].

Sex-Steroid Producing Adrenal Tumors

Androgen-secreting adrenal adenomas are rare. Virilization or feminization in the setting of an adrenal mass is most likely due to an adrenocortical carcinoma, especially in the elderly [25]. Androgens secreted by the adrenal cortex are dehydroepiandrosterone (DHEA) and androstenedione. They exert a direct effect and can also serve as precursors for testosterone and estrogen. Men can exhibit feminization, and women can experience hirsutism or virilization. Biochemical screening is performed when clinical signs are present. Signs of sex steroid excess are investigated in all such patients by measuring urinary 17-OH-progesterone. Urinary testosterone should be measured in women with virilization, as cases have been reported where testosterone but not 17-OH-progesterone was elevated. Estrogens are measured in men with feminization, as some patients with sex steroid-secreting adrenocortical carcinoma have had normal 17-OH-progesterone but elevated estrogens. When a tumor secreting androgens is detected, treatment is unilateral adrenalectomy, taking care to perform an adequate resection should the tumor prove to be a carcinoma (see section "Adrenocortical Carcinoma").

Adrenocortical Carcinoma

Adrenocortical carcinomas (ACC) are rare, with a yearly incidence of about 500 new cases in the United States, or about 0.5–2.0 cases per million inhabitants. Age at diagnosis ranges from 0 to 70 years (mean 46 years), and there is a bimodal distribution with peaks during the first and fifth decades. However, older persons do present with ACC and there is an increased incidence in the elderly of hormonally inactive tumors. The prevalence of ACC in cohorts of patients undergoing adrenalectomy is 8% in patients ≥64 years, 13% in those with incidentally diagnosed adrenal masses, and 18% in unselected patients. These findings are consistent with the Yale experience between 1997 and 2007, when 8.3% of patients operated on for ACC where above the age of 65 years (unpublished data). ACC is slightly more common in women, and tend to more often be hormonally active.

TABLE 36.5 Staging system for adrenocortical carcinoma (ACC), and percentage at diagnosis

Stage	TNM	(%) At diagnosis
I	T1 (Tumor≤5 cm), N0, M0	2.9
II	T2 (Tumor>5 cm), N0, M0	28.3
III	T3 (Tumor any size, local invasion), N0, M0 *or* T2, N1 (positive, mobile regional lymph node), M0	23.4
IV	T4 (Tumor any size, gross invasion of adjacent structures) *or* N2 (positive, fixed lymph node), *or* M1	45.4

Source: Data from Fraker [25]

The vast majority of patients present with stage III or IV and the overall prognosis is poor with a 5-year survival varying between 20 and 45% (Table 36.5) [25].

Earlier studies reported that about 50% of tumors were functional, but more recent series have noted hormone secretion in up to 79% of cases, most likely due to improvements in assay sensitivity [26]. Often, ACC may secrete multiple hormones and may change secretion according to size, growth rate, and differentiation. The biochemical workup depends on signs and symptoms of hormone excess (Table 36.2) and should also include DHEA-S, 17-OH-progesterone, androstenedione, testosterone, and 17β-estradiol (only in men and postmenopausal women) [27].

ACC tend to be large with imaging characteristics as outlined in Table 36.3 and exemplified in Fig. 36.2c. Local extension is present in 65% and metastasis in 25% of patients at diagnosis. Common sites of metastasis are lymph nodes, lung, liver, and bone; therefore, preoperative evaluation should include CT of the abdomen and chest. MRI and PET scan can be used to further establish the diagnosis preoperatively, as well as to identify metastatic disease. Fine needle aspiration is not helpful since it will not distinguish between a benign and malignant adrenocortical tumor [11].

The treatment of choice and the only chance for cure for ACC is complete surgical extirpation of the tumor and adrenal gland, en-bloc resection of invaded organs, and if necessary, periaortic/retroperitoneal lymphadenectomy. Noncurative surgical debulking is performed in approximately 20% of the cases, to ameliorate symptoms of endocrine hyperactivity. An open abdominal approach is advocated for ACC, to avoid tumor spillage, capsule rupture and to ensure adequate retroperitoneal resection and lymphadenectomy. Some authors suggest that a laparoscopic adrenalectomy can be considered for tumors that have no evidence of local invasion, extensive lymphadenopathy, or distant metastasis on preoperative imaging, thus ensuring clean resection margins, and are not too large to risk tumor spillage from manipulation. In patients with an aggressive surgical approach, the mean disease-free survival interval ranges from 12 to 22 months, although long-term survivors exist. Even in patients who underwent curative resection, up to 80% of patients developed locoregional recurrence or distant metastases [28].

Nonoperative management includes cytoreductive therapy with transarterial embolizations and radiofrequency ablation (RFA), which may ameliorate symptoms of endocrine hyperactivity [25]. The chemotherapeutic agent most commonly used in ACC is mitotane, which may also be used in the adjuvant setting [29]. The overall response rate has been reported to be between 14 and 36%, but most studies have shown no significant survival benefit [25, 29].

Pheochromocytoma and Abdominal Paraganglioma

Pheochromocytomas are rare catecholamine-producing tumors that derive from adrenomedullary tissue in about 80% of cases and from extraadrenal chromaffin tissue in about 20% of cases [30]. Pheochromocytomas arising in extraadrenal tissue are commonly called paragangliomas or (if in the region of the carotid body or aortic arch) chemodectomas. Regardless of location, pheochromocytomas share similar histopathological characteristics [9]. Pheochromocytomas can cause hypertension via exceptionally high circulating catecholamine levels, accounting for approximately 0.05–0.1% of cases of sustained hypertension. However, about 50% of patients with a pheochromocytoma have episodic or no hypertension [9]. The signs and symptoms associated with pheochromocytoma are summarized in Table 36.2. It has been estimated that in the United States, approximately 40,000 people have pheochromocytoma, with newly diagnosed pheochromocytoma averaging 800–1,600 cases per year in the general population [9]. Although the peak incidence occurs during the age of 30–50 years, older patients develop pheochromocytoma and may be asymptomatic or present with atypical symptoms, which may partly be masked by common medications such as β-blockers.

Measurement of plasma or urinary catecholamines and their metabolites, as well as serum chromogranin A, is the foundation of the biochemical diagnosis of pheochromocytoma. Urinary analysis of catecholamines and metanephrines should be performed in a 24-h urine sample collected in 6 M HCl, whereas plasma is collected in a fasting patient. Urinary metanephrine is the most specific diagnostic assay, whereas measurement of chromogranin A and plasma or urinary metanephrines are the most sensitive [31]. Measurement of urinary vanillylmandelic acid (VMA) has a false-negative rate of 41% in documenting catecholamine excess. In older individuals, the measurement of plasma-free metanephrines is less cumbersome than urine collections and has a higher sensitivity for pheochromocytoma (96–100%) [9]. However, the specificity is lower, especially in those older than 60 years (77%) [2].

The imaging characteristics of pheochromocytomas are summarized in Table 36.3 and exemplified in Fig. 36.2a. CT and/or MRI is sufficient in the vast majority of patients, but ^{131}I-metaiodobenzylguanidine scintigraphic scanning and PET scan may be useful, especially if there is a suspicion of bilateral, extraadrenal and/or malignant pheochromocytoma. PET imaging using 6-[^{18}F]-fluorodopamine, [^{18}F]-dihydroxyphenylalanine, [^{11}C]-hydroxyephedrine, or [^{11}C]-epinephrine are very promising, new, specific radionuclide localization techniques for pheochromocytoma [9]. Familial pheochromocytoma has increasingly been diagnosed due to advances in molecular and clinical genetics and likely represents a higher proportion than the classically quoted 10%. They tend to present at a younger age and more often with bilateral or extraadrenal lesions. Malignant pheochromocytoma occurs in 10–20% of cases and is three times as common in women. Extraadrenal lesions are two to three times likely to be malignant. Malignancy is proven by invasion of adjacent structures, nodal involvement, or metastasis. Sites of metastasis are bone, liver, lymph nodes, lungs, and brain. Histological differentiation between benign and malignant primary tumors remains unreliable.

Once a diagnosis of pheochromocytoma has been made, preoperative (1–2 weeks before surgery depending on response and level of catecholamine excess) α-blockade needs to be started. In older patients with significant cardiovascular comorbidities, this treatment may need to be performed in the inpatient setting [32]. There exist wide-ranging practices, international differences in available or approved therapies, and a scarcity of evidence-based studies comparing different therapies [32]. The overall principle, however, includes α-blockade for 1–2 weeks prior to surgery, with fluid replacement, and the addition of β-blockade if tachycardia is present. Metyrosine (Demser) is an analog of tyrosine that competitively inhibits tyrosine hydroxylase. Calcium channel blockers are also often used successfully either alone or as an adjunct. Phenoxybenzamine (Dibenzyline; irreversible, noncompetitive, α-adrenoceptor blocker) is most commonly used for preoperative blockade and is initially dosed at 10 mg twice a day with increments of 10–20 mg every 2–3 days [32].

The majority of pheochromocytomas and abdominal paragangliomas can be resected via a laparoscopic approach [33]. However, open exploration should be considered in cases of large tumors, known or suspected malignant disease, difficult-to-access periaortic paragangliomas, and when a pheochromocytoma has ruptured preoperatively. The key to safe surgery is effective preoperative blood pressure control, rigid intraoperative pressure management, and clear communication between surgeon and anesthesiologist. Elderly patients and patients with existing ischemic or congestive heart disease may require more meticulously regimented fluid administration, and a pulmonary artery catheter may be used to guide therapy. Recurrent and metastatic pheochromocytoma may be treated with surgical debulking and/or RFA or possibly [^{131}I]metaiodobenzylguanidine [34].

Nonfunctioning Tumors

Benign Adrenocortical Adenoma and Myelolipoma

Adrenal myelolipoma and nonfunctioning adrenocortical adenomas are the most common nonfunctioning tumors of the adrenal gland. The incidence increases with age, and as stated, adrenal lesions (>1 cm) are identified in 6% of autopsy studies [1]. The imaging characteristics of adrenocortical adenomas are summarized in Table 36.3, and the presence of pure fat within an adrenal lesion on CT is consistent with myelolipoma [35]. The workup of these lesions follow those of adrenal incidentaloma (see section "Evaluation of the Adrenal Incidentaloma").

Rare Adrenal Masses

A number of adrenal masses may be incidentally detected, and the differential diagnosis may include adrenolipoma, amyloidosis, ganglioneuroma, granuloma, hamartoma, hematoma, hemangioma, leiomyoma lipoma, neurofibroma, adrenal pseudocyst, lymphoma, and teratoma [36, 37]. Although rare in the United States, various infectious processes may cause an adrenal mass. These include fungal, tuberculosis, echinococcosis, and cryptococcosis [37]. Adrenal cysts can be infectious, lymphangiomatous, or angiomatous endothelial, cystic degenerative adenomas or embryonal retention cysts. Sometimes, the imaging characteristics of these particular lesions are suggestive [38, 39], as exemplified in Fig. 36.2d. Surgical resection may be needed due to mass effect or to prevent rupture, hemorrhage, or infection. Additionally, when malignancy cannot be excluded based on imaging, surgical resection is warranted. Again, the role for adrenal fine needle aspiration is limited to distinguishing adrenal tissue from metastatic tissue and less commonly infection.

Adrenal Metastasis

Metastasis to the adrenal gland occurs, with the most common sources being lung, breast, colon, kidney, and melanoma [40]. The imaging characteristics are variable as summarized in Table 36.2. Adrenal metastases are often bilateral. In select patients with isolated adrenal metastasis, after careful staging, improved survival for patients who underwent resection has been found in various tumor types [41–43]. If the patient elects to undergo resection, metastatic disease to the adrenal gland should be resected in any way that can give the most oncologic benefit to the patient. A laparoscopic approach may be used as long as oncologic principles are adhered to [42].

Surgical Management and Technique

Laparoscopic adrenalectomy has become the standard of care for the vast majority of adrenal masses. The benefits of minimally invasive techniques for the removal of the adrenal gland include decreased requirements for analgesics, improved patient satisfaction, and shorter hospital stay and recovery time when compared to open surgery [44]. The relative contraindications are size and malignancy, when there is a concern about adhering to oncologic principles. A variant of the minimally invasive approach is posterior retroperitoneoscopic adrenalectomy, which is especially useful in patients with previous open abdominal operations [45, 46]. Open adrenalectomy can be performed via a transperitoneal, retroperitoneal, or thoracoabdominal approach.

References

1. Kloos RT, Gross MD, Francis IR, Korobkin M, Shapiro B (1995) Incidentally discovered adrenal masses. Endocr Rev 16(4): 460–484
2. Young WF Jr (2007) Clinical practice. The incidentally discovered adrenal mass. N Engl J Med 356(6):601–610
3. Lindsay JR, Nieman LK (2005) The hypothalamic-pituitary-adrenal axis in pregnancy: challenges in disease detection and treatment. Endocr Rev 26(6):775–799
4. Ferrari M, Mantero F (2005) Male aging and hormones: the adrenal cortex. J Endocrinol Invest 28(11 Suppl Proceedings):92–95
5. Barlaskar FM, Hammer GD (2007) The molecular genetics of adrenocortical carcinoma. Rev Endocr Metab Disord 8(4):343–348
6. Carling T (2005) Multiple endocrine neoplasia syndrome: genetic basis for clinical management. Curr Opin Oncol 17(1):7–12
7. Else T, Giordano TJ, Hammer GD (2008) Evaluation of telomere length maintenance mechanisms in adrenocortical carcinoma. J Clin Endocrinol Metab 93(4):1442–1449
8. Giordano TJ (2006) Molecular pathology of adrenal cortical tumors: separating adenomas from carcinomas. Endocr Pathol 17(4):355–363
9. Pacak K, Eisenhofer G, Ahlman H et al (2007) Pheochromocytoma: recommendations for clinical practice from the First International Symposium. October 2005. Nat Clin Pract Endocrinol Metab 3(2):92–102
10. Carling T, Du Y, Fang W, Correa P, Huang S (2003) Intragenic allelic loss and promoter hypermethylation of the RIZ1 tumor suppressor gene in parathyroid tumors and pheochromocytomas. Surgery 134(6):932–939, discussion 939–940
11. NIH (2002) NIH state-of-the-science statement on management of the clinically inapparent adrenal mass ("incidentaloma"). NIH Consens State Sci Statements 19(2):1–25
12. Sutton MG, Sheps SG, Lie JT (1981) Prevalence of clinically unsuspected pheochromocytoma. Review of a 50-year autopsy series. Mayo Clin Proc 56(6):354–360
13. Emral R, Uysal AR, Asik M et al (2003) Prevalence of subclinical Cushing's syndrome in 70 patients with adrenal incidentaloma: clinical, biochemical and surgical outcomes. Endocr J 50(4): 399–408
14. Sippel RS, Chen H (2004) Subclinical Cushing's syndrome in adrenal incidentalomas. Surg Clin North Am 84(3):875–885
15. Terzolo M, Bovio S, Reimondo G et al (2005) Subclinical Cushing's syndrome in adrenal incidentalomas. Endocrinol Metab Clin North Am 34(2):423–439, x
16. Porterfield JR, Thompson GB, Young WF Jr et al (2008) Surgery for Cushing's syndrome: an historical review and recent ten-year experience. World J Surg 32(5):659–677
17. Funder JW, Carey RM, Fardella C et al (2008) Case detection, diagnosis, and treatment of patients with primary aldosteronism: an endocrine society clinical practice guideline. J Clin Endocrinol Metab 93(9):3266–3281
18. Stratakis CA (2008) Cushing syndrome caused by adrenocortical tumors and hyperplasias (corticotropin-independent Cushing syndrome). Endocr Dev 13:117–132
19. Lo CY, van Heerden JA, Grant CS, Soreide JA, Warner MA, Ilstrup DM (1996) Adrenal surgery in the elderly: too risky? World J Surg 20(3):368–373, discussion 374
20. van Heerden JA, Young WF Jr, Grant CS, Carpenter PC (1995) Adrenal surgery for hypercortisolism – surgical aspects. Surgery 117(4):466–472
21. Zeh HJ 3rd, Udelsman R (2003) One hundred laparoscopic adrenalectomies: a single surgeon's experience. Ann Surg Oncol 10(9): 1012–1017
22. Biller BM, Grossman AB, Stewart PM et al (2008) Treatment of adrenocorticotropin-dependent Cushing's syndrome: a consensus statement. J Clin Endocrinol Metab 93(7):2454–2462
23. Sawka AM, Young WF, Thompson GB et al (2001) Primary aldosteronism: factors associated with normalization of blood pressure after surgery. Ann Intern Med 135(4):258–261
24. Sywak M, Pasieka JL (2002) Long-term follow-up and cost benefit of adrenalectomy in patients with primary hyperaldosteronism. Br J Surg 89(12):1587–1593
25. Fraker D (2008) Adrenal tumors. In: DeVitaJr VT, Lawrence TS, Rosenberg SA (eds) Cancer: principles & practice of oncology, 8th edn. Lippincott-Raven, Philadelphia, pp 1690–1702
26. Tauchmanova L, Colao A, Marzano LA et al (2004) Andrenocortical carcinomas: twelve-year prospective experience. World J Surg 28(9):896–903
27. Allolio B, Fassnacht M (2006) Clinical review: adrenocortical carcinoma: clinical update. J Clin Endocrinol Metab 91(6): 2027–2037
28. Meyer A, Niemann U, Behrend M (2004) Experience with the surgical treatment of adrenal cortical carcinoma. Eur J Surg Oncol 30(4):444–449
29. Icard P, Goudet P, Charpenay C et al (2001) Adrenocortical carcinomas: surgical trends and results of a 253-patient series from the French Association of Endocrine Surgeons study group. World J Surg 25(7):891–897
30. Eisenhofer G, Siegert G, Kotzerke J, Bornstein SR, Pacak K (2008) Current progress and future challenges in the biochemical diagnosis and treatment of pheochromocytomas and paragangliomas. Horm Metab Res 40(5):329–337
31. Pacak K, Eisenhofer G (2007) An assessment of biochemical tests for the diagnosis of pheochromocytoma. Nat Clin Pract Endocrinol Metab 3(11):744–745
32. Pacak K (2007) Preoperative management of the pheochromocytoma patient. J Clin Endocrinol Metab 92(11):4069–4079
33. Ippolito G, Palazzo FF, Sebag F, Thakur A, Cherenko M, Henry JF (2008) Safety of laparoscopic adrenalectomy in patients with large pheochromocytomas: a single institution review. World J Surg 32(5):840–844, discussion 845–846

34. Lam MG, Lips CJ, Jager PL et al (2005) Repeated [131I] metaiodobenzylguanidine therapy in two patients with malignant pheochromocytoma. J Clin Endocrinol Metab 90(10):5888–5895

35. Udelsman R, Fishman EK (2000) Radiology of the adrenal. Endocrinol Metab Clin North Am 29(1):27–42, viii

36. Udelsman R, Dong H (2000) Case records of the Massachusetts General Hospital. Weekly clinicopathological exercises. Case 35-2000. An 82-year-old woman with bilateral adrenal masses and low-grade fever. N Engl J Med 343(20):1477–1483

37. Thompson GB, Young WF Jr (2003) Adrenal incidentaloma. Curr Opin Oncol 15(1):84–90

38. Guo YK, Yang ZG, Li Y et al (2007) Uncommon adrenal masses: CT and MRI features with histopathologic correlation. Eur J Radiol 62(3):359–370

39. Otal P, Escourrou G, Mazerolles C et al (1999) Imaging features of uncommon adrenal masses with histopathologic correlation. Radiographics 19(3):569–581

40. Gittens PR Jr, Solish AF, Trabulsi EJ (2008) Surgical management of metastatic disease to the adrenal gland. Semin Oncol 35(2):172–176

41. Mittendorf EA, Lim SJ, Schacherer CW et al (2008) Melanoma adrenal metastasis: natural history and surgical management. Am J Surg 195(3):363–368, discussion 368–369

42. Sebag F, Calzolari F, Harding J, Sierra M, Palazzo FF, Henry JF (2006) Isolated adrenal metastasis: the role of laparoscopic surgery. World J Surg 30(5):888–892

43. Saunders BD, Doherty GM (2004) Laparoscopic adrenalectomy for malignant disease. Lancet Oncol 5(12):718–726

44. Gumbs AA, Gagner M (2006) Laparoscopic adrenalectomy. Best Pract Res Clin Endocrinol Metab 20(3):483–499

45. Perrier ND, Kennamer DL, Bao R et al (2008) Posterior retroperi-toneoscopic adrenalectomy: preferred technique for removal of benign tumors and isolated metastases. Ann Surg 248(4): 666–674

46. Walz MK, Alesina PF, Wenger FA et al (2006) Posterior retroperitoneoscopic adrenalectomy – results of 560 procedures in 520 patients. Surgery 140(6):943–948, discussion 948–950

47. Linos DA, Stylopoulos N, Boukis M, Souvatzoglou A, Raptis S, Papadimitriou J (1997) Anterior, posterior, or laparoscopic approach for the management of adrenal diseases? Am J Surg 173(2): 120–125

48. Proye CA, Huart JY, Cuvillier XD, Assez NM, Gambardella B, Carnaille BM (1993) Safety of the posterior approach in adrenal surgery: experience in 105 cases. Surgery 114(6): 1126–1131

Chapter 37
Benign Breast Disease in Elderly Women and Men

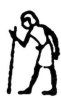

Kay O. Lovig and Barbara A. Ward

Physiologic Changes in the Breast

Familiarity with breast microanatomy and physiology aids in understanding benign breast physiology. The female breast is composed of ductal and lobular units. The main breast ducts arise from lactiferous sinuses in the nipple and divide several times to form small ducts and then the smallest ductal elements, or "ductules," which in fact form the lobular unit of the breast. The ductules also divide and terminate blindly with club-shaped endings. The ductules are sensitive to hormone stimulation; during pregnancy, they proliferate and form the alveolar components of the breast [1].

Ductal and lobular units of female breasts can be seen as early as during the neonatal period. Maternal estrogen, progesterone, mammotrophic peptides including prolactin, and human placental lactogen promote growth and development of fetal breasts. During the neonatal period, the ductal system shows evidence of secretory epithelium and surrounding myoepithelial cells, although these findings involute and a latent phase starts from childhood to puberty [2].

During puberty, hypothalamic synthesis of gonadotropin-releasing hormone (GnRH) begins. This hormone stimulates the release of follicle-stimulating hormone (FSH) and luteinizing hormone (LH) from the pituitary gland. The FSH then stimulates the ovaries, and estradiol synthesis begins. During the first few years of puberty, anovulatory cycles are common. Because of this, estradiol is the primary stimulant of the breast during this period. It promotes the elongation and branching of the ductal system and increases the volume of the breasts with fat deposition. When the luteal phase begins, progesterone stimulates dilatation of the ductal system and differentiates the alveolar cells to secretory cells.

The most dramatic alterations in the anatomy and physiology of the breast occur during pregnancy. Estrogen,

progesterone, prolactin, growth hormone (GH), cortisol, and insulin prepare the breast to lactate. Ductal and lobular units of the breast increase in size and complexity. Endings of the ductules become secretory alveoli during this period. Lactogenesis occurs throughout gestation, but lactopoiesis begins after delivery of the child. Estrogen and progesterone are believed to inhibit secretion of milk during gestation [3].

With aging, both men and women have significant fall in the production of most hormones when compared to young adults. The levels of growth hormone (GH) and insulin-like growth factor-1 (IGF-1) [4, 5], nocturnal melatonin [6], TSH [7], thyroid hormones [8], calcitonin [9], DHEA [10], aldosterone [11], estrogen [12, 13], and testosterone [14] progressively decrease with age in adult men and women. However, the only endocrine system for which there is a well-defined, abrupt, and universal change in function with age is the hypothalamic–pituitary–gonadal axis in women, seen in menopause. Menopause occurs at the mean age of 51 in normal women in the United States [15]. It is associated with a marked decline in the number of developing follicles, and with this, there is a parallel decrease in the concentration of inhibin B, a peptide that inhibits the production of follicular stimulating hormone (FSH), and thus a corresponding rise in FSH. During the earlier stages of menopause, there is preservation of estradiol secretion. However, in the later stage, ovarian secretion of estrogen and progesterone cease, subsequently resulting in breast involution. Lobules are mostly affected in this process. With the progression of involution, glandular epithelium is disrupted and phagocytized. Main ductal systems are least affected; they survive, but their number decreases and some develop cystic changes. Alterations occur in the elastic and collagen fibers, resulting in loss of supporting tissue, and fat deposition increases. The duration of involution of the breast is generally incomplete and variable. Although most of the lobular structures disappear, remnants and mature lobular structures can remain. Patient variability is significant [1, 16, 17].

In the aging male, there tends to be a gradual decrease in testosterone production by the aging testes and an increase in sex-hormone-binding-globulin (SHBG) levels, resulting

K.O. Lovig (✉)
Department of Internal Medicine, Greenwich Hospital,
Greenwich, CT, USA
e-mail: kayolovig@gmail.com

R.A. Rosenthal et al. (eds.), *Principles and Practice of Geriatric Surgery*,
DOI 10.1007/978-1-4419-6999-6_37, © Springer Science+Business Media, LLC 2011

in a fall in the free testosterone concentration with a reciprocal increase in the luteinizing hormone (LH) level. This rise in LH can result in enhanced Leydig cell stimulation and increased aromatization of testosterone to estradiol, thus increasing estradiol relative to testosterone in the aging male.

Gynecomastia

Gynecomastia is a benign proliferation of the glandular tissue of the male breast, which is caused by an increase in the ratio of estrogen to androgen activity. Gynecomastia occurring in middle-aged and elderly men has the highest prevalence at 50–80 years of age, with as many as 24–65% of men being affected [18]. True gynecomastia should be differentiated from both pseudogynecomastia as well as carcinoma, which is far less common. Pseudogynecomastia, which is often seen in obese men, is due to fat deposition without glandular proliferation and does not require further evaluation. Clinical features worrisome for breast carcinoma include a firm, eccentrically located asymmetric mass, often with fixation to the skin or underlying structures. Ulceration, axillary adenopathy, or a bloody nipple discharge may be present [19].

In true gynecomastia, a ridge of glandular tissue will be felt that is reasonably symmetrical to the overlying nipple–areolar complex.

Classification of Gynecomastia

Gynecomastia can be classified based on a number of different parameters, for example, pathogenesis, histopathology, and morphology, with the morphologic classification being based on subjective parameters. Cordova et al. proposed a scheme for morphological classification which can serve as a guide for the appropriate surgical technique once the diagnosis of benign gynecomastia has been confirmed [20]. These patients would have failed medical management as described below. Grade I and II are described as the nipple–areolar complex being above the inframammary fold. With these stages, ultrasound-assisted lipectomy and skin-sparing adenectomy are the procedure of choice. Once the nipple–areolar complex is at the same height as, or at most one centimeter below, the fold, the classification becomes Grade III. Here, it is necessary to remove the redundant skin by means of a periareolar removal of epidermis. Lastly, Grade IV was marked by ptosis, when the nipple–areolar complex is more than one centimeter below the fold. Stage IV requires reduction mammoplasty with upper repositioning of the nipple–areolar complex.

Etiology of Gynecomastia

The etiology of gynecomastia can be due to both physiologic as well as pathologic changes (see Table 37.1). Physiologic gynecomastia is more common is infants and adolescents boys and less so in adult men. However, aging is associated with an increase in the prevalence of hypogonadism. One previous study illustrated 20% of men older than 60 years of age and 50% of men older than 80 years of age were hypogonadal using total testosterone criteria (Table 37.1) [21, 22].

In addition to the increased prevalence of hypogonadism, there are multiple other hormonal changes occurring in the elderly man which likely account for "idiopathic" gynecomastia. First, aging is associated with an increase in body fat, and this adipose tissue is an active site of extraglandular aromatization of testosterone to estradiol and of androstenedione to estrone. In addition, gradual decreases in testosterone production results in a fall in free testosterone with a reciprocal increase in luteinizing hormone (LH). This rise in LH enhances Leydig cell stimulation, leading to increased aromatization of testosterone to estradiol.

Hypogonadism can also be due to pathological causes, which are broken down into primary and secondary hypogonadism. Primary hypogonadism can be due to a congenital abnormality such as Klinefelter's syndrome or due to testicular trauma, infection, infiltrative disorders, or vascular insufficiency. All of these etiologies of primary hypogonadism cause hormonal changes similar to those seen in the aging man, as described above. It is ultimately the reduction in testosterone production from the testes and a compensatory rise in LH that causes gynecomastia in these patients. Secondary hypogonadism is due to a hypothalamic or pituitary abnormality. Contrary to primary hypogonadism, these patients have a low production of LH, resulting in a low testosterone production rate and a low estradiol production from the testes. The adrenal cortex continues to produce estrogen precursors,

TABLE 37.1 Pathologic causes of gynecomastia

Pathologic etiology	Prevalence seen among men seeking help
Drugs	10–25%
Idiopathic	25%
Cirrhosis or malnutrition	8%
Male hypogonadism primary and secondary	Primary 8%, secondary 2%
Neoplasms	
Testicular-germ cell, Leydig cell Sertoli cell, sex cord	3%
Adrenal – adenoma or carcinoma	
Ectopic production of human chorionic gonadotropin	
Hyperthyroidism	1.5%
Renal disease and dialysis	1%

Source: Data from Braunstein [22]

which are aromatized in extraglandular tissue, thus causing gynecomastia.

One of the more prevalent causes of pathological gynecomastia is cirrhosis, which is a consequence of chronic liver disease characterized by replacement of liver tissue by fibrous scar tissue as well as regenerative nodules. Associated with these changes are an increased production rate of androstenedione to estrone and increased conversion of estrone to estradiol, all leading to gynecomastia [23].

Some of the less common causes of pathological gynecomastia are testicular tumors, hyperthyroidism, and chronic renal failure. Testicular tumors are associated with secretion of human chorionic gonadotropin (hCG). These high levels of hCG lead to Leydig cell dysfunction. In addition, hCG stimulates aromatase activity, which converts androgen precursors to estrone and estradiol, ultimately causing a relative increase in estradiol to testosterone production. Hyperthyroidism is often associated with elevated LH levels, again causing increased estradiol relative to testosterone production by Leydig cells.

Chronic renal failure is the progressive loss of renal function over a period of months to years. It is not entirely clear how dialysis and renal failure cause gynecomastia; however, there appears to be Leydig cell dysfunction in addition to decreased metabolic clearance of LH.

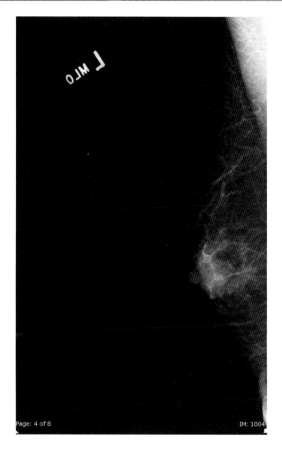

Figure 37.1 Mammogram showing typical gynecomastia.

Clinical Evaluation of Gynecomastia

When evaluating adult males for gynecomastia, it is important to take a thorough history including all possible medications that can cause gynecomastia, and perform a physical evaluation including a testicular exam. As discussed above, it is imperative to distinguish between gynecomastia and carcinoma, which typically appears as a firm asymmetric mass, possibly with ulceration, axillary adenopathy, or a bloody nipple discharge. If there is a suspicious lesion, mammography can accurately distinguish between malignant and benign male breast tissues and should be performed prior to a biopsy [24]. Gynecomastia is apparent as a triangular or a round area of increased density with flame-shaped margins (see Fig. 37.1). Male breast cancer presents as a well-defined mass eccentric to the nipple, with associated spiculation and calcification. Pseudogynecomastia is demonstrated as an extremely clear mammogram with no significant glandular tissue seen (see Fig. 37.2). There are no set guidelines with regard to mammography for patients who clinically appear to have true gynecomastia alone. Because some studies have found that mammography was able to identify cancer within what appeared to be purely gynecomastia, it is reasonable to include the exam [24]. Similarly, a breast ultrasound may be added when malignancy is suspected as this may also aid in

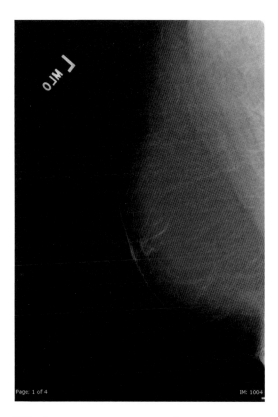

Figure 37.2 Clear mammogram documenting pseudogynecomastia.

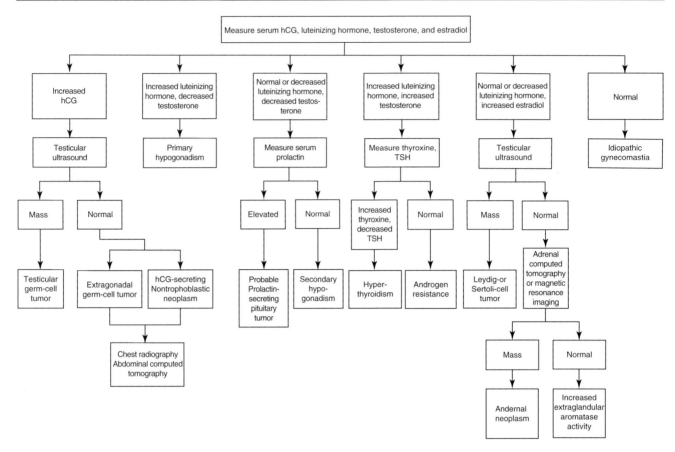

Figure 37.3 Algorithm for the laboratory evaluation of gynecomastia (reprinted with permission from Braunstein GD (2007) Gynecomastia. N Eng J Med 357:1229–1237. Copyright © 2007 Massachusetts Medical Society. All rights reserved).

targeting a core biopsy to confirm the diagnosis. The workup that is recommended for gynecomastia that is of recent onset or painful, without a clear etiology, is the following laboratory studies: hCG, LH, testosterone, and estradiol. Prolactin levels and thyroid function tests may be required as the algorithm suggests (see Fig. 37.3).

One last but significant cause of gynecomastia is medications and recreational drugs. Although a causal relation is well established with some drugs, the mechanism is unclear for most drugs (see Table 37.2) [25].

Treatment of Gynecomastia

While physiologic gynecomastia is more common among infants and adolescents, it is also possible in adults and the elderly. For this reason, it is recommended that men with gynecomastia initially be observed with a follow-up evaluation within 3 months. During these visits, it is important to identify possible medications or underlying treatable disorders as discussed above. For men in whom no cause can be identified, and the gynecomastia is tender and/or persists more than 3 months, it is recommended that the patient be started

Table 37.2 Medications and recreational drugs associated with gynecomastia

Antiandrogens/inhibitors of androgen	Drugs of abuse
Cyproterone acetate	Alcohol
Flutamide, bicalutamide, nilutamide	Amphetamines
Finasteride, dutasteride	Heroin
Spironolactone	Marijuana
Ketoconazole	Methadone
OTC herbal, i.e., Tea tree oil derivatives	*Hormones*
HAART therapy	Androgens
Antibiotics	Anabolic steroids
Ethionamide	Chorionic gonadotropin
Isoniazide	Estrogens
Ketoconazole	Growth hormone
Metronidazole	*Psychoactive drugs*
Antiulcer drugs	Diazepam
Cimetidine	Haloperidol
Ranitidine	Phenothiazines
Omeprazole	Tricyclic antidepressants
Cancer chemotherapeutic drugs	*Other*

Source: Data from Braunstein [22]

on a trial of medical therapy. It is important to note that medical therapy for gynecomastia is only effective in the early, active phase of gynecomastia, which is also when it is most symptomatic (0–12 months). The later phase of gynecomastia (greater than 12 months) is defined by fibrotic changes and disappearance of the inflammatory reaction. It is unlikely that any medical therapy will result in significant regression in the late fibrotic stage.

There are three types of medications that have been used for the early, inflammatory phase of gynecomastia. The first class is androgens (testosterone), which is only beneficial in hypogonadal men [26]. The second class of medications is selective estrogen receptor modulators (SERMS), such as tamoxifen and raloxifene. SERMS appear to decrease breast volume and significantly reduce breast tenderness. Complete breast regression is typically not achieved [27]. Lastly, aromatase inhibitors, which block estrogen biosynthesis, have been trialed to prevent gynecomastia. To date, clinical trials have not demonstrated an impressive benefit. Gynecomastia is common in men with prostate cancer undergoing androgen deprivation therapy. Medical therapy has limited benefit once gynecomastia is established in this patient population, and therefore, prevention of breast development is the goal. The two main strategies include pharmacologic therapy (antiestrogens or aromatase inhibitors) or radiotherapy [28].

If gynecomastia does not regress spontaneously or with medical therapy, is causing considerable discomfort or psychological distress, or is long-standing (greater than 12 months), then surgical therapy should be considered [29]. The extent of surgery depends on the severity of gynecomastia, but many patients are treated with a combination of direct surgical excision of glandular tissue and liposuction through a periareolar incision.

CASE STUDY

A 65-year-old retired fireman presents with a unilateral tender mass in the left retroareolar position. He is known through the diagnosis and treatment of his wife's early breast cancer, and she has done well. For the past several weeks, he has noted this mass and he is concerned, in part, given his wife's diagnosis. His past medical history is remarkable for hypertension and mild obesity. He has no issues with potency. His medications include atenolol and furosemide. Otherwise, he is healthy, and he reports moderate alcohol intake. He does not smoke.

On exam, the patient is a healthy-appearing male. His breasts are mildly asymmetric with the left being larger than the right. There are no other skin or nipple changes. There is a tender mass deep to the left nipple, located immediately behind the nipple. There is also a small amount of palpable breast tissue deep to the right nipple which is nontender. He has no palpable supraclavicular or axillary adenopathy. He refuses a testicular exam, but admits that everything is OK in that department.

Mammography demonstrates bilateral flame-shaped tissue in the retroareolar position which is concentric to the nipple. There is no suspicion of cancer.

The patient is offered a trial of observation and consideration for taking tamoxifen. He is not interested in tamoxifen as his wife had fairly significant hot flashes and some weight gain while taking it. After 3 months, he is still experiencing moderate tenderness, and he requests surgical excision. This is accomplished through a periareolar incision as an outpatient. Pathology demonstrates benign breast tissue. He does well but does require a postoperative aspiration of a small seroma in the office. At 3-month follow-up, he is happy with the cosmesis and remains pain-free. He returns a year later with the identical complaint on the right breast and again elects to undergo surgical excision with similar results.

Perimenopausal Benign Breast Disease

Although uncommon, we are faced more frequently with benign breast problems in an aging population. Benign breast disorders are exacerbated by menopause, however, and afterward their frequency sharply declines.

Mastalgia and Nodular Breasts

Mastalgia is a term applied to various conditions where pain is present in one or both breasts. Women commonly present with breast pain, and the etiology is typically puzzling. Although the clinician realizes that breast pain is rarely serious, patients are quite troubled by it and are usually worried that there may be an underlying malignancy. A thorough understanding of the classifications of breast pain, common etiologies, and treatment strategies is both helpful for the practitioner and reassuring to the patient.

Breast pain can be classified according to cyclic mastalgia, noncyclic mastalgia, and extramammary (nonbreast) pain [30]. Cyclic mastalgia refers to premenstrual breast pain experienced by most women and is accompanied by an increase in breast nodularity. This is accentuated when associated fibrocystic changes, including cysts, can cause focal severe pain, potentially relieved by cyst aspiration. This type of cyclic mastalgia usually resolves after menopause.

Noncyclic mastalgia generally starts in the fourth decade. In 50% of persons affected, it resolves after menopause, but in the other half, it persists [31]. Noncyclic mastalgia in the postmenopausal age group is less likely to respond to treatment but resolves spontaneously in up to 50% of cases [32]. Most patients assume that their pain is related to an underlying breast cancer. It is necessary to perform a thorough physical exam to rule out an underlying mass and to update the patient's mammogram and focal breast ultrasound as indicated. Tumyan et al. reported on 86 consecutive patients with focal breast pain in the absence of a breast mass. In their study, the negative predictive value of mammogram and ultrasound was 100% with a mean follow-up of 26.5 months [33]. This author has cared for two patients, however, who noted focal breast pain with normal imaging and developed very early cases of DCIS and invasive lobular carcinoma. Both had had contralateral breast cancers and had exhibited focal breast pain prior to that diagnosis as well. This should be considered extremely unusual, but as always, it is important to listen to the patient and respect their persistent concern. Additionally, it is reassuring for patients to understand that breast "tenderness" is normal. The breast is a highly sensitive organ, particularly involving the upper-outer quadrants and the nipple, and this sensitivity commonly persists in the elderly.

Prior to initiating therapy for mastalgia, sources of extramammary pain must be ruled out. Angina relating to coronary artery disease is the most critical possibility that must be considered in the elderly. More common, however, and poorly understood by most patients is costochondritis or "Tietze's Syndrome." This pain originates in the joint connecting the sternum to the upper seven ribs, although the second to fifth costochondral junctions are most commonly affected [34]. Chronic pain is described as a dull ache or pressure, but acute attacks are sharp and stabbing. Physical exam demonstrates a reproducible pain when pressure is applied to the area. It is worsened when moving the rib cage or taking a deep breath. Costochondritis can also be related to systemic arthritis, in which the treatment is dependent on the etiology. Otherwise, the mainstays of treatment are the nonsteroidal anti-inflammatories and avoidance of activities that provoke strain to this area. Steroids can also be injected into the specific costochondral junction, in severe, refractory cases. Khan et al. reported on the successful use of 1-ml 2% lignocaine and 1-ml 40-mg depomedrone injections in 104 women with an 83% success rate and no complications [35].

Other sources of extramammary pain include radiating pain from arthritic conditions or neural entrapment of the cervical and thoracic spine. Shingles should also be kept in mind as unilateral breast and back pain may precede the classical presentation with fever and skin blisters.

Mondor's disease is a less well-recognized condition of the breast which presents with a tender cord-like nodularity. This is a thrombophlebitis of the thoracoepigastric vein and most commonly is located superior and lateral to the nipple [36].

It can also be seen postoperatively when a superficial vein has been transected during the procedure. Trauma and radiation therapy can also contribute to this condition. There may be visible evidence of a vertically oriented nodularity as well as a palpable cord with tenderness. The tenderness may last 1–6 weeks although the cord may take longer to resolve. It can be treated with warm compresses and anti-inflammatories.

Hypothyroidism has been associated with breast pain. Although the exact mechanism is not understood, the breast has an affinity for thyroid hormone and iodine. The terminal part of the duct, the acini, and the ducts are lined with iodine-containing cells. When these levels are low, the breast becomes more sensitive to estrogen stimulation [37]. Given the frequency of thyroid disease in mature women, it is reasonable to include thyroid function testing and assessment of related symptoms of hypothyroidism in women with persistent mastalgia.

Once other sources of extramammary pain have been excluded, the patient and clinician can decide about the treatment, if any, for noncyclical breast pain. Caffeine and alcohol can contribute to mastalgia, so this should be mentioned. There are many medications that can contribute to breast pain and should also be assessed. Hormone replacement therapy (HRT) is known to increase breast pain, tenderness, and density. Macrocysts may persist on HRT postmenopausally and contribute to focal and global pain. Some patients are willing to tolerate these breast symptoms in light of the other benefits that HRT affords. Utilizing the lowest dose may reduce breast tenderness. Other medications such as antidepressants, cardiac drugs, and antihypertensives can cause breast pain, tenderness, and galactorrhea. Because these side effects may be uncommon, reviewing the side-effect profile of all newly introduced medications is prudent in an elderly patient with the recent onset of mastalgia.

Medical therapy for mastalgia has not been very simple or scientific in the past. Vitamin E, evening primrose Oil, and vitamin B6 have all been promoted, and for some patients, these remedies appear beneficial, particularly for cyclical mastalgia. Clinical trials, however, have not shown consistent results.

Rosolowich et al. reviewed the issue of mastalgia for The Society of Obstetricians and Gynecologists of Canada. They wanted to provide practice guidelines for Winnipeg Regional Health Authority Breast Health Centre. The results of their extensive review are as follows:

1. Education and reassurance is an integral part of mastalgia and should be the first-line treatment.
2. The use of a well-fitting bra that provides good support should be considered for the relief of cyclical and noncyclical mastalgia.
3. A change in dose, formulation, or scheduling should be considered for patients on HRT. HRT may be discontinued if appropriate.
4. Women with breast pain should not be advised to reduce caffeine intake.

5. Vitamin E should not be considered for the treatment of mastalgia.

6. There is presently insufficient evidence to recommend the use of evening primrose oil (EPO) in the treatment of breast pain.

7. Flaxseed should be considered as a first-line treatment for cyclical mastalgia.

8. Topical no steroidal anti-inflammatory (NSAID) gel, such as diclofenac 2% in pluronic lethicin organogel, should be considered for pain control for localized treatment of mastalgia.

9. Tamoxifen 10 mg daily or danazol 200 mg daily should be considered when first-line treatments are ineffective.

10. Mastectomy or partial mastectomy should not be considered an effective treatment for mastalgia [38].

Another study by Srivastava and colleagues examined randomized controlled trials comparing bromocryptine, danazol, EPO, and tamoxifen with placebo. While bromocryptine and danazol produced positive results, tamoxifen was associated with the fewest side effects and was considered the drug of first choice [39]. Other studies have confirmed the benefit of topical NSAIDs as a safe, effective, and rapid treatment modality [40, 41]. The use of toremifene has been controversial given its potential side effects, and lisuride maleate and iodine therapy are also mentioned in the literature.

Ductal Ectasia

Ductal ectasia, or dilatation of the ductal system, is frequently found in postmenopausal women. This can be found on clinical presentation with nipple discharge and nipple retraction or encountered when operating on the breast for other reasons. Grossly, the specimen consists of firm breast tissue with prominent ducts containing pasty or granular secretions. These secretions may be white, yellow, green, or brown. The walls of the ducts are firm as a result of periductal fibrosis, and sometimes calcium is noted in the ducts [42].

There may be spontaneous nipple discharge and nipple retraction, and the condition can be bilateral. The nipple retraction can appear slit-like in ductal ectasia, as opposed to the classic purse-string appearance with an underlying malignancy. This condition is also different from periductal mastitis, which is more common in young patients, associated with smoking, and results in granulomatous fistulization to the skin.

On imaging, ductal ectasia is typically symmetric with ultrasound demonstrating dilated ducts in a symmetrical fashion. Asymmetric and solitary ducts may be pathologic. Intraductal papilloma and carcinoma must be ruled out in these cases. If the patient has no palpable findings and a normal mammogram and ultrasound, it is highly unlikely that breast cancer is causing the nipple retraction. MRI can be done if further evaluation is warranted. Central excision of the retroareolar ducts can be performed to eliminate a persistent discharge and alleviate fear of malignancy.

Cystic Disease of the Breast

Breast cysts are common in women aged 40–50, particularly common around menopause. They can appear suddenly as a tender, palpable mass or discovered incidentally during radiologic screening.

There are two types of cysts, dependent on the cyst lining. One is lined with apocrine epithelium and the other with flattened epithelium. Simple cysts lined with flattened epithelium arise from dilatation of terminal portions of ductules and are generally small. Sometimes, they coalesce and form larger cysts, and they are regarded as physiologic changes of involution during menopause. Cysts that are palpable are generally apocrine cysts, and they may grow up to 4–5 cm in size. Apocrine cysts also originate from lobular units and also thought to be a physiologic change of the breast because they are common during the involutional phase of lactation and menopause. Cyst formation is further promoted by taking HRT following menopause [43].

Cysts surrounded by fatty tissue appear as round or oval, well-circumscribed masses on the mammogram. If they are surrounded by breast parenchyma, some of the contour may be obscured by dense breast tissue; generally, the posterior parts of the cysts are indistinct. Because some malignancies of the breast appear as smoothly contoured and round masses, it is recommended to undertake further diagnostic workup, especially in elderly patients. Ultrasound usually detects whether the lesion is cystic or solid. Simple cysts generally have smooth margins, and the contents of the cyst are anechoic. If echos are detected in the cyst, it can be the result of inflammation, intracystic papilloma, and extremely hypoechoic fibroadenoma, or a malignancy. Medullary carcinoma, in particular, must be considered first in the differential diagnosis. Aspiration biopsy aids in the diagnosis. If the fluid is green to brown and the lesion completely disappears after aspiration, it is consistent with a simple cyst and no further workup is necessary. Cyst fluid of this nature need not be sent for cytology. If a patient is postmenopausal and not on HRT, it is reasonable to analyze the fluid. A residual mass after cyst aspiration, rapid refilling of the cyst, solid papillary components in a cyst confirmed by ultrasonography, and atypical cells or papillary cells in a cyst aspirate are all reasons to perform an open biopsy to rule out malignancy [44]. Figure 37.4 depicts a complex cyst with atypical cells seen on aspiration. Excisional biopsy showed associated ductal carcinoma in situ (Fig. 37.4).

FIGURE 37.4 Complex cyst (ultrasound).

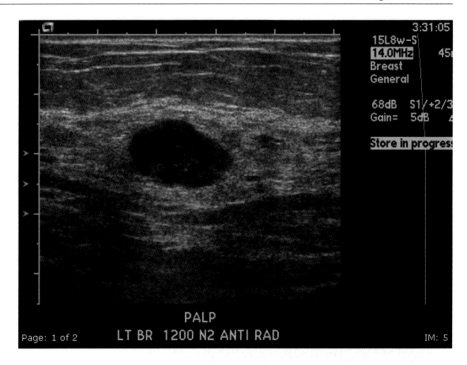

FIGURE 37.4 Complex cyst (ultrasound).

Fibroadenoma

Although fibroadenomas are commonly addressed in young patients, they rarely present issues in the elderly. They constitute approximately 12% of all breast masses in postmenopausal women. There are two classic structural types: intracanalicular or pericanalicular. Generally, the clinical examination, radiologic studies, and core biopsy confirm the diagnosis [45–47] Fibroadenomas involute after menopause and calcify. They are frequently seen on the mammogram associated with central heavy amorphous or peripheral course calcifications, sometimes referred to as "popcorn calcifications" (Fig. 37.5).

Fibroadenomas are considered an aberration of normal development. They do not arise from a single cell but from a single lobule and resemble hyperplastic lobules in the breast. They grow and lactate during pregnancy and degenerate during menopause, exhibiting their hormone dependence [47, 48]. In the elderly, fibroadenomas generally become less cellular and hyalinized, and sometimes, they become fibrotic or disappear in the breast without the influence of estrogen. Once the diagnosis is established, excision and observation are the two main options. Patients generally prefer excision, although the risk of their masses becoming malignant is no different from that of normal tissue. The problem, in general, is being certain of the diagnosis of a fibroadenoma, especially in the elderly where the suspicion of breast cancer is justifiably high [47]. Calcified, involuting fibroadenomas in the elderly do not deserve excision if they have been serially followed mammographically. Spiculation, architectural distortion, and fine and

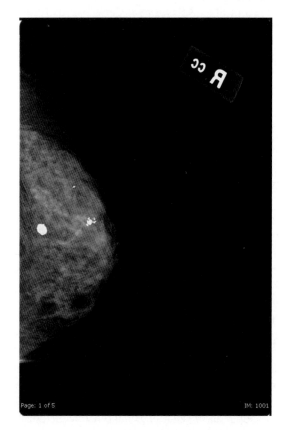

FIGURE 37.5 Mammogram demonstrating benign calcifications associated with fibroadenomas.

irregular calcifications are signs of coincidental cancer in a fibroadenoma, so further workup and treatment are needed in these patients [49].

Benign Breast Calcifications in the Elderly

Mammograms can demonstrate benign calcifications for many reasons, particularly in the elderly. Cysts can calcify, giving an "eggshell" appearance (see Fig. 37.6), and fibroadenomas may calcify as mentioned earlier. Calcifications may also be present secondary to fat necrosis, postsurgical scar, and suture calcification. Arteriosclerotic calcification is common in the elderly and is typically seen as long tubular structures that appear hollow.

Hormone Replacement Therapy and Mammographic Findings

In general, with the start of menopause, the overall density of the breast decreases owing to glandular atrophy and fatty replacement. The current standard for reporting breast density was established by the Breast Imaging Reporting and Data System (BIRADS). Category 1 describes a breast that is "almost entirely fat," while Category 2 shows "scattered fibroglandular" tissue. Category 3 reflects a "heterogeneously dense" breast, while Category 4 depicts "extremely dense" breast parenchyma.

Continuous HRT may increase mammographic densities in the elderly. Peck and Lowman first reported that HRT increases benign changes in the breast with involution after discontinuing treatment [50]. The mammographic changes attributed to HRT may be diffuse, symmetric, asymmetric, multifocal, or cystic densities. Roughly, it is accepted that one fourth of patients receiving HRT show evidence of increased breast density. Combination regimens with estrogen and progesterone are believed to produce this effect much more commonly than estrogen replacement alone [51, 52]. Tissue edema, proliferation of periductal connective tissue or ductal and lobular units may be responsible for the density. Patients who have lower baseline density percentages are more likely to develop breast densities with treatment. Generally, it takes months to years for these to develop. Persistence of breast densities in the elderly alters the sensitivity of the mammogram. In a large retrospective review of 8,779 postmenopausal women being screened in western Washington state, HRT was found to lower both the sensitivity and specificity of screening mammograms [53]. Invasive lobular carcinoma is of concern given that it is difficult to detect mammographically to begin with, and HRT may promote its development. Low-dose regimens may be helpful in patients with increased density of the breast, and discontinuation of HRT can be recommended.

Crandall et al. reviewed the association of breast discomfort with increases in breast density. In their study, postmenopausal women were randomly assigned to postmenopausal hormone therapy vs. placebo. New-onset breast discomfort was associated with an increase in mammographic breast density [54]. It has also been demonstrated that additional imaging is frequently required in women with either dense breast tissue or those on HRT [55]. Not surprisingly, it has also been shown that changes in density are dynamic, such that discontinuation of HRT will result in decreases in breast density [56].

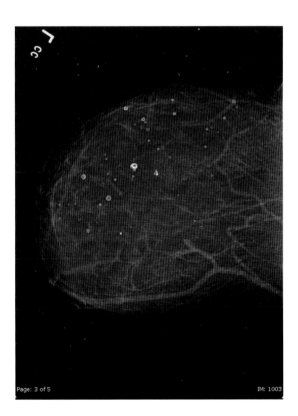

Figure 37.6 Mammogram demonstrating benign calcifying oil cysts.

References

1. Parks AG (1959) The microanatomy of the breast. Ann R Coll Surg 25:235–251
2. Anbazhagan R, Bartek J, Monaghan P, Gusteron BA (1991) Growth and development of the human infant breast. Am J Anat 192:407–417
3. Reyniak JV (1979) Endocrine physiology of the breast. J Reprod Med 22(6):303–309
4. Bando H et al (1991) Impaired secretion of growth hormone-releaseing hormone, growth hormone and IGF-1 in elderly men. Acta Endocrinol 124:31–33
5. Rudman D et al (1981) Impaired secretion of growth hormone secretion in the adult population: relation to age and adiposity. J Clin Invest 67:1361–1369
6. Waldhauser F, Kovacs J, Reiter E (1998) Age-related changes in melatonin levels in humans and its potential consequences for sleep disorders. Exp Gerontol 33:759–772
7. Weiner R, Utiger RD, Lew R, Emerson CH (1991) Age, sex and serum thyrotropin concentrations in primary hypothyroidism. Acta Endocrinol 124:364–369

8. Spaulding SW (1987) Age and the thyroid. Endocrinol Metab Clin North Am 16:1013–1025

9. Pedrazzoni M et al (1988) Calcitonin levels in normal women of various ages evaluated with a new sensitive radioimmunoassay. Horm Metab Res 20:118–119

10. Nafziger AN, Bowlin SJ, Jenkins PL, Pearson TA (1998) Longitudinal changes in dehydroepiandrosterone concentrations in men and women. J Lab Clin Med 131:316–323

11. Hegstad R et al (1983) Aging and aldosterone. Am J Med 74:442–448

12. Khosla S et al (1998) Relationship of serum sex steroid levels and bone turnover markers with bone mineral density in men and women: a key role for bioavailable estrogen. J Clin Endocrinol Metab 83:2266–2274

13. Sherman BM, West JH, Korenman SG (1976) The menopausal transition: analysis of LH, FSH, estradiol, and progesterone concentrations during menstrual cycles of older women. J Clin Endocrinol Metab 42:629–636

14. Deslypere JP, Vermeulen A (1984) Leydig cell function in normal men: effect of age, life-style, residence, diet and activity. J Clin Endocrinol Metab 59:955–962

15. McKinlay SM, Bifano NL, McKinlay JB (1985) Smoking and age at menopause in women. Ann Int Med 103:350

16. Vorherr H (1974) Menopausal mammary involution. In: Vorherr H (ed) The breast. Morphology, physiology, and lactation. Academic, San Diego, CA, pp 215–217

17. Tavossoli FA (1992) Postmenopausal involution (atrophy). In: Tavossoli FA (ed) Pathology of the breast. Elsevier, New York, NY, p 20

18. Lee PA (1975) The relationship of concentrations of serum hormones to pubertal gynecomastia. J Pediatr 86:212

19. Moore MP (1996) Male breast cancer. In: Harris JR, Lippman ME, Morrow M, Hellman CT (eds) Diseases of the breast, 2nd edn. Lippincott-Raven, Philadelphia, PA, p 859

20. Cordova A, Moschella F (2008) Algorithm for clinical evaluation and surgical treatment of gynaecomastia. J Plast Reconstr Aesthet Surg 61(1):41–49

21. Harman SM, Metter EJ, Robin JD et al (2001) Longitudinal effects of aging on serum total and free testosterone levels in healthy men. Baltimore Longitudinal Study of Aging. J Clin Endocrinol Metab 86:724–731

22. Braunstein GD (1993) Gynecomastia. N Engl J Med 328:490

23. Gordon GG, Olivo J, Fereidoon R et al (1975) Conversion of androgens to estrogen in cirrhosis of the liver. J Clin Endocrinol Metab 40:1018

24. Evans GF, Anthony T, Turnage RH et al (2001) The diagnostic accuracy of mammography in the evaluation of male breast disease. Am J Surg 181(2):96–100

25. DiLorenzo G, Perdona S, DePlacido S et al (2005) Gynecomastia and breast pain induced by adjuvant therapy with bicalutamide after radical prostatectomy in patients with prostate cancer: the role of tamoxifen and radiotherapy. J Urol 174(6):2197–2203

26. Kuhn J, Roca R, Laudat M et al (1983) Studies on the treatment of idiopathic gynecomastia with percutaneous dihydrotestosterone. Clin Endocrinol 19:513

27. Parker LN, Gray DR, Lai MK et al (1986) Treatment of gynecomastia with tamoxifen: a double-blind crossover study. Metabolism 35:705

28. Dicker AP (2003) The safety and tolerability of low dose irradiation for the management of gynecomastia caused by antiandrogen monotherapy. Lancet Oncol 4:30

29. Colombo-Benkmann M, Buse B, Stern J et al (1999) Indications for and results of surgical therapy for male gynecomastia. Am J Surg 178:60

30. Smith RL, Pruthi S, Fitzpatrick LA (2004) Evaluation and management of breast pain. Mayo Clin Proc 79(3):353–372

31. Fentiman I (2004) Management of breast pain. In: Harris JR, Lippman ME, Morrow M, Osborne CL (eds) Diseases of the breast, 3rd edn. Lippincott Williams and Wilkins, Philadelphia, PA, pp 57–61

32. Olawaiye A, Nithiam-Leitch M, Danakas G et al (2005) Mastalgia: a review of management. J Reprod Med 50(19):933–939

33. Tumhan L, Hoyt AC, Bassett LW (2005) Negative predictive value of sonography and mammography in patients with focal breast pain. Breast J 11(5):333–337

34. Kneece J (2003) Noncyclic pain. In: Kneece J (ed) Solving the mystery of breast pain, 2nd edn. Educare Publishing, Columbia, SC, pp 37–39

35. Khan HN, Rampaul R, Blabey RW (2004) Local anaesthetic and steroid combined injection therapy in the management of noncyclic mastalgia. Breast 13(2):129–132

36. Fentimen I (2004) Management of breast pain. In: Harris JR, Lippman ME, Morrow M, Osborne CL (eds) Diseases of the breast, 3rd edn. Lippincott Williams and Wilkins, Philadelphia, PA, pp 57–61

37. Kneece J (2003) Noncyclic pain. In: Kneece J (ed) Solving the mystery of breast pain, 2nd edn. Educare Publishing, Columbia, SC, p 40

38. Rosolowich V, Saettler E, Szuck B et al (2006) Mastalgia. J Obstet Gynaecol Can 28(1):49–74

39. Srivastava A, Mansel RE, Arvind N et al (2007) Evidence-based management of mastalgia: a meta-analysis of randomized trials. Breast 16(5):503–512

40. Quereshi S, Sultan N (2005) Topical nonsteroidal anti-inflammatory drugs versus oil of evening primrose in the treatment of mastalgia. J R Coll Surg Edinb Ireland 3(11):7–10

41. Colak T, Ipek T, Kanik A et al (2003) Efficacy of topical nonsteroidal anti-inflammatory drugs in mastalgia treatment. J Am Coll Surg 196(4):525–530

42. Rosen PP (1997) Mammary duct ectasia. In: Rosen PP (ed) Rosen's breast pathology. Lippincott-Raven, Philadelphia, PA, pp 29–32

43. Devitt JE (1996) Benign disorders of the breast in older women. Surg Gynecol Obstet 162:340–342

44. Heywang-Kobrunger SH, Scherer I, Dershaw DD (1997) Benign breast disorders. Thieme, Stuttgart, pp 141–165

45. Kern WH, Clark RW (1973) Retrogression of fibroadenomas of the breast. Am J Surg 126:56–59

46. Hunter TB, Roberts CC, Hunt R et al (1996) Occurrence of fibroadenomas in postmenopausal women referred for breast biopsy. J Am Geriatr Soc 44:61–64

47. Dixon JM (1991) Cystic disease and fibroadenoma of the breast: natural history and relation to breast cancer risk. Br Med Bull 47:258–271

48. Egan R (1988) Fibroadenoma. In: Egan R (ed) Breast imaging. Diagnosis and morphology of breast diseases. Saunders, Philadelphia, PA, pp 178–182

49. Kopans DB (1988) Benign and probably benign lesions. In: Kopans DB (ed) Breast imaging. Lippincott-Raven, Philadelphia, PA, pp 351–373

50. Peck DR, Lowman RM (1978) Estrogen and the postmenopausal breast: mammographic considerations. JAMA 240:1733–1735

51. Kaewrudee S, Anuwatnavin S, Kanpittaya J et al (2007) Effect of estrogen-progestin and estrogen on mammographic density. J Reprod Med 52(6):513–520

52. Aiello EJ, Buist DS, White E (2006) Do breast cancer risk factors modify the association between hormone therapy and mammographic density? Cancer Causes Control 17(10):1227–1235

53. Laya MB, Larson EB, Taplin SH et al (1996) Effect of estrogen replacement therapy on the specificity and sensitivity of screening mammography. J Natl Cancer Inst 88(10):643–649

54. Crandall CJ, Karlamangla A, Huang MH et al (2006) Association of new-onset breast discomfort with an increase in mammographic density during hormone therapy. Arch Int Med 166(15):1578–1584

55. Carney PA, Kasales CJ, Tosteson AN ct al (2004) Likelihood of additional work-up among women undergoing routine screening mammography: the impact of age, breast density, and hormone therapy use. Prev Med 39(1):48–55

56. Rutter CM, Mandelson MT, Laya MB et al (2001) Changes in breast density associated with initiation, discontinuation, and continuing use of hormone replacement therapy. JAMA 285(2):171–176

Chapter 38
Breast Cancer in Elderly Women

Monica Morrow and Lisa S. Wiechmann

CASE STUDY

An 80-year-old wheelchair-confined diabetic female is s/p right above the knee amputation after failed bypass grafting, and s/p two myocardial infarctions, most recently 3 years ago. She is not felt to be a candidate for revascularization. Her ejection fraction is 20%. She has occasional chest pain at rest. She also has an 80-packs-per-year smoking history, moderately severe arthritis, and mild dementia. She is managed by an endocrinologist, a cardiologist, her family doctor, and a rheumatologist. Her family doctor obtains a screening mammogram that demonstrates a 1.0-cm spiculated mass in the upper outer quadrant of the right breast. Breast exam is normal, and there is no adenopathy.

Management

This patient is highly unlikely to have her life prolonged by the detection of this cancer prior to the development of a palpable mass. Ideally, she would never have had a screening mammogram. Since she did, optimal management would include obtaining an ultrasound (US) to see if the mass is visible by US. If yes, a US-guided core biopsy would be far more comfortable for the patient than lying prone, with her breast in compression, for a stereotactic biopsy. The core biopsy demonstrates a Grade II, strongly estrogen receptor (ER)-positive and progesterone receptor (PR)-positive, HER-2-negative infiltrating ductal cancer. This patient is an appropriate candidate for primary endocrine therapy with tamoxifen or an aromatase inhibitor. Although removal of the primary tumor optimizes local control, in her case, this would entail needle localization prior to surgery, which would require her cooperation, as would a procedure done under local anesthesia. Her cardiopulmonary status places her at significant risk for general anesthesia. There is no indication for sentinel node biopsy since the identification of nodal metastases would not change her management. She should be followed with clinical breast exam. If a palpable mass develops in the breast, then surgical excision is warranted.

Breast cancer is the most common malignancy in American women aside from skin cancer, and the second leading cause of cancer death, exceeded only by lung cancer. It is estimated that there were 182,460 new breast cancer cases diagnosed in the United States in 2008, and 40,480 deaths. In addition to invasive breast cancer, carcinoma in situ (CIS), the earliest form of breast cancer, accounted for about 67,770 new cases in 2008 [1].

The incidence of breast cancer increases with age, and despite competing causes of mortality, breast cancer remains a significant cause of death in elderly women. Cancer is the leading cause of death in those 55–74 years of age and is second only to heart disease in the 75+ age group [2]. As life expectancy increases and the elderly population continues to grow, there will be an increasing number of elderly women diagnosed with breast cancer. Despite the high prevalence of this disease in the elderly, they largely have been excluded or discouraged from participating in clinical trials and often are not given the same therapeutic options as their younger counterparts [2, 3].

The goal of this chapter is to review the important issues related to the management of breast cancer in the elderly. These include age-specific issues regarding the value of mammographic screening, the selection of local surgical therapy, the need for adjuvant radiotherapy, the efficacy

M. Morrow (✉)
Breast Service, Department of Surgery, Memorial Sloan-Kettering
Cancer Center, New York, NY, USA
e-mail: morrowm@mskcc.org

and toxicity of systemic therapy, and the effect of mortality due to breast cancer in this population. Because there is no standard definition of "elderly," for the purposes of this chapter, an elderly patient is defined as one older than 70 years of age.

Epidemiology

Breast cancer incidence and mortality increase with age, with the greatest increase observed during the childbearing years. In Western countries, a continued increase in incidence is seen after menopause, whereas in Asian countries, the incidence decreases in elderly women [4, 5]. Approximately one half of the breast cancers in the United States are diagnosed in women aged 65 years and over. For women in this age group, an incidence rate of 322 cases per 100,000 population was noted in the SEER database [6], compared with 60 cases per 100,000 for women younger than age 65. The incidence rate for women aged 85 years or more rose to 375 cases per 100,000 population.

Although breast cancer incidence rates in the United States increased by 32% from 1980 to 1987 [7], a stabilization in female breast cancer incidence rates during 2001–2003 and a decrease in the number of breast cancer cases diagnosed in 2003 were observed [8]. Data from the National Program of Cancer Registries (NPCR) and the SEER registries [9] indicate that age-adjusted incidence rates for invasive breast cancer decreased significantly in women aged 50 years and older each year between 1999 and 2003, with the greatest decrease (6.1%) occurring from 2002 to 2003 (Fig. 38.1). The largest decreases were seen in women aged 55–59 years (11.3%), 60–64 years (10.6%), and 65–69 years (14.3%). Rates of in situ breast cancer also stabilized from 1999 to 2003 after increasing by more than 6.6% per year since 1981, with women aged 50–79 years experiencing a significant decrease in incidence during this period [10].

Over the past 25 years, the incidence of in situ carcinoma has increased in association with a decrease in regional disease and a stable metastatic disease rate [7]. Between 1987 and 1997, a decrease in breast cancer mortality was observed in the United States, with a 9% reduction in mortality for those aged 70–79 years. Approximately 50% of this mortality reduction is attributed to screening and 50% to improvements in therapy [11]. Despite the reported decreases in breast cancer mortality, it is important to keep in mind that breast cancer represents the underlying cause of death in 54.5, 37.1, and 30.7% of women aged 60–69, 70–79, and 80+ years, respectively, who are diagnosed with the disease [12].

As in young women, infiltrating ductal carcinoma is the most common histologic tumor type in the elderly, accounting for 77–85% of cases [6, 13]. The relatively favorable subtypes

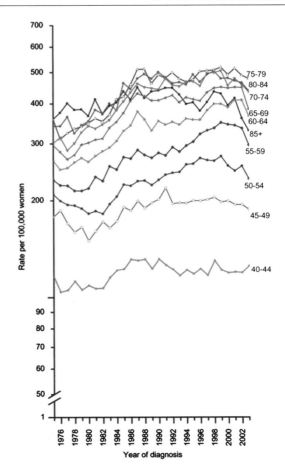

Figure 38.1 Age-adjusted breast cancer mortality rates for U.S. Caucasian women per 100,000 population. *Filled squares*, invasive; *diamonds*, localized; *triangles*, regional; *inverted triangles*, in situ; *open squares*, distant (from Chu et al. [7] Adapted with permission of the Oxford University Press).

of colloid and papillary carcinoma are observed more frequently in elderly women but still account for less than 10% of mammary carcinomas even in women aged 85 years or greater [6, 13, 14], whereas inflammatory and medullary carcinoma are seen less commonly in elderly women than in their younger counterparts [6, 14]. Breast cancers in elderly women are more likely to be moderately to well differentiated, contain estrogen receptors, and have a low thymidine labeling index [14].

Screening

Randomized studies have shown that screening for breast cancer with mammography reduces breast cancer mortality by approximately one third, especially for women aged 50–69 years at invitation to screening [15–17]. As life expectancy increases, attention has turned to determining an appropriate upper age limit for population-based mammography screening. Current guidelines are vague, indicating that chronological age alone should not be the reason for the cessation of regular screening. Theoretically, screening should be beneficial for women aged 70 years or greater, but evidence to support this statement is limited. To date, the only randomized screening trial that included women aged 70 years and greater was the Swedish Two-County trial [17]. In this study, 162,981 women aged 40–74 years were randomized to a screening or a control group. A 31% reduction in mortality from breast cancer and a 25% reduction in the rate of stage II or higher cancers were seen in the group invited to screening, and the benefit extended to patients aged 70–74 years.

Van Dijck et al. [18] reported the results of a nonrandomized trial of screening in 6,773 women aged 68–83 years, enrolled during 1977–1978 and followed through 1990. Women from the same birth cohort in a neighboring city without a screening program served as controls. Over the entire study period, the cumulative mortality rate ratio was 0.80 (95% CI, 0.53–1.22) for the screened women; at 9–13 years after the start of screening, it had decreased to 0.53 (95% CI, 0.27–1.04). A subsequent study by Jonsson et al. [19] attempted to evaluate the contribution of screening to decreasing breast cancer mortality in women aged 70–74 years. Breast cancer mortality for both the study (screened) and control (not screened) groups decreased during the study period, but with a mean screening interval of 22.8 months and a mean follow-up time of 10.1 years, a 24% reduction in breast cancer mortality was estimated in the screened group after adjusting for lead time bias.

In 2000, Smith-Bindman et al. in a study of 690,993 women aged 66–79 years reported that screening mammography was associated with a decreased risk of detecting metastatic breast cancer among elderly women [20]. Taplin et al. [21] retrospectively reviewed data from seven health-care plans dating from 1995 to 1999, comparing women aged 50 years or older who were diagnosed with late-stage (metastatic and/or tumor size≥3 cm; $n=1,347$) or early-stage (control subjects, $n=1,347$) breast cancers. The odds of having late-stage breast cancer were higher among women not undergoing screening (OR=2.17, 95% CI, 1.84–2.56; $p<0.001$); failure to screen was significantly associated with age>75 years (OR=2.77, 95% CI, 2.10–3.65), as well as lower socioeconomic status.

Mandelblatt et al. [22] used a decision analysis model to determine whether mammographic screening extends life for women aged 65 and greater in the presence and absence of comorbid conditions. Patients were stratified into age groups of 65–69, 70–74, 75–79, 80–84, and 85 years or greater. In each age category, women were further stratified into those with average health, those with mild diastolic hypertension, and women with symptomatic congestive heart failure, to determine the effect of comorbid conditions on screening benefit. Screening was found to save lives for

elderly women of all ages, although the magnitude of benefit decreased as the severity of the comorbidity increased. For a woman with breast cancer, screening prolonged life 617 days for the woman of average health aged 65–69 years, and 311 days for women in the same age group with congestive heart failure. The prolongations of survival for women older than 85 years in the same health groups were 178 and 126 days, respectively. The cost-effectiveness of annual screening ranged from $13,200 to $34,600 per year of life saved. In comparison, the cost per year of life saved by treating mild to moderate hypertension in the nonelderly is $16,000–$72,000 [22]. These estimates of cost are based on the use of annual screening mammograms. Moskowitz [23] calculated that owing to the longer lead times seen with breast cancer in older women, most of the benefits of screening could be obtained with a 2- to 3-year interval between studies.

Boer et al. [24] used a model incorporating the natural history of breast cancer and the known effect of screening to identify the optimum upper age limit for screening. Using a model in which preclinical duration of breast cancer was assumed not to increase after age 65, no upper limit for screening benefit was identified. If the duration of the preclinical phase was "pessimistically" assumed to increase in the elderly, screening up to age 80 was found to be of benefit. In a study of 2,067 million screening exams performed between 1998 and 2000, the overall breast cancer detection rates in the 50–69 and 70–75 age groups were, respectively, 4.2 and 14.2 per 1,000 initially screened women. The referral, biopsy, and detection rates were substantially higher in women aged 70–75 years than in their younger counterparts, and a significant trend toward a smaller tumor size distribution was observed [25]. These findings, summarized in Table 38.1, suggest that mammographic screening is a beneficial technique in the elderly.

The current United States Preventive Services Task Force guidelines recommend screening mammography for women aged 50–75 years [26]; however, a number of studies indicate that breast cancer screening in the elderly, whether by

TABLE 38.1 Outcomes of screening in older women

	Age group (years)	
	50–69	70–75
No. of screening exams	1,880,082	187,207
No. of women	18,902	3,429
% Additional imaging	33.9	24.9
% Biopsy	5.1	4.2
Screen detected cancers/1000	4.2	10.3
% In situ	14.8	11.6
% Node neg. (invasive only)	66.3	69.7
Positive predictive value of biopsy	70.0	79.0

Source: Data from Fracheboud et al. [25]

mammography or clinical breast examination, is underutilized. The National Cancer Institute Breast Cancer Screening Consortium [27] reported the results of 7 population-based surveys of women aged 50–74 years. In five of the seven studies, the rates of breast screening by mammography and breast examination in the 70–74 years age group were lower than those reported for other ages. This occurred despite the fact that more than 90% of women surveyed had a regular source of medical care.

Lack of awareness of breast cancer risk and screening procedures in elderly women contributes to the underutilization of these techniques. Leathar and Roberts [28] identified a lack of knowledge among elderly women about breast cancer, a pessimistic attitude toward disease outcome, and embarrassment about being examined as major barriers to screening. Fox et al. [29] conducted a telephone survey of 724 women aged 65 years and older to assess factors influencing the use of mammography. Only physician recommendation predicted a recent mammogram, with age, race, and health status found to be insignificant factors.

In 2001, data from the state-based Behavioral Risk Factor Surveillance System (BRFSS) and the National Health Interview Survey (NHIS) confirmed that the percentage of women who reported receiving mammography and clinical breast exam within 2 years was lower among older women (56.7% of women aged 70 years and older) compared with younger women (71.1% of women aged 50–69 years). Among both groups, those unable to perform a major activity of daily living were less likely to report receiving mammography within 2 years. Interestingly, most (62.7%) women aged 70 years and older reported having no activity limitation, and only 5.5% reported being unable to perform a major daily activity [30].

In 2007, Field et al. studied women aged 65 years or older when diagnosed with early-stage invasive breast cancer ($n = 1,762$). They assessed mammography use during 4 years of follow-up and found that the percentage of women having mammograms after treatment declined significantly during the studied time frame from 82% in the first year posttreatment to 68.5% in the 4th year of follow-up. Women at higher risk of recurrence (breast conservation without radiation therapy or higher stage) were less likely to have yearly mammograms, as were women without visits to breast cancer surgeons or oncologists, suggesting that underutilization of mammography is a problem for women at all levels of breast cancer risk [31].

Local Therapy of Breast Cancer

What constitutes appropriate local treatment for the elderly woman with breast cancer remains controversial. In the past, when mastectomy was the standard surgical therapy, the major debate in older women centered on dissection of the axillary nodes. The emergence of breast-conserving surgery and sentinel lymph node biopsy as accepted modalities for the local therapy of breast cancer, and the development of endocrine therapies such as tamoxifen and the aromatase inhibitors have increased the available options for local treatment in this population. When evaluating therapeutic options, it is important to consider not only the immediate morbidity and mortality of treatment but also the efficacy of the therapy in maintaining local control for the duration of the woman's life. Current options for the local management of breast carcinoma in the elderly include mastectomy, breast-conserving therapy consisting of excision and irradiation, or excision alone, and endocrine therapy.

Mastectomy

Mastectomy remains a common treatment in the elderly patient. A modified radical mastectomy includes removal of breast tissue, the underlying pectoralis fascia, and the axillary lymph nodes. In patients with clinically negative axillary lymph nodes, the modified radical mastectomy has been replaced by total (simple) mastectomy plus sentinel lymph node biopsy, an operative technique that is discussed later in this chapter. The 30-day operative mortality rate of any type of mastectomy is uniformly low, and the procedure is physically well tolerated. In a review of the SEER data from 1960 to 1973, Schneiderman and Axtell reported a 30-day operative mortality rate of 0.4% for the 37,745 patients treated during that period. For women aged 75 or older, the operative mortality was 0.8% during 1960–1966, and 0.9% during 1967–1973 [32]. Similar results have been noted in other studies, with mortality rates less than 4% commonly observed [33–36]. Davis et al. reported a 3% mortality rate for women aged 80 or older treated by mastectomy and a 7% incidence of major complications [33]. Hunt et al. in a study of 94 patients reported a complication rate of 20% in elderly patients, but the operative mortality was still only 1% [34]. Wound problems accounted for most of the complications in this series, while Kessler and Seton found cardiovascular and neurologic problems to be the most common cause of postoperative morbidity in their series [35]. Data on the morbidity and mortality of mastectomy in the elderly are summarized in Table 38.2. In patients with severe comorbidities, mastectomy has been performed using local anesthesia and regional nerve blocks [37]. Mastectomy under local anesthesia alone using the tumescent technique of infiltrating dilute lidocaine with epinephrine (25 ml of 1% lidocaine [250 mg] and 1 ml of 1:1,000 epinephrine [1 mg] in 1 L of Ringers lactate) via an infusion pump has also been reported [38]. Although

TABLE 38.2 Morbidity and mortality of mastectomy in the elderly

Study	Age (years)	No	Operative mortality (%)	Complications (%)
Hunt et al. [34]	>65	94	1.0	20
Schottenfield and Robbins [100]	>65	437	0.2	NS
Singletary et al. [36]	>69	157	1.9	24
Kesseler and Seton [35]	>70	82	1.2	11
Berg and Robbins [101]	>70	242	2.0	NS
Kraft and Block [102]	>75	75	4.5	NS
SEER 1967–1973 [32]	>75	NS	0.9	NS
Davis et al. [33]	>80	96	3.0	7

NS not stated

mastectomy is an excellent method for obtaining local control of breast cancer with a minimum number of outpatient visits, and although elderly women can undergo the procedure safely, these results are obtained at the expense of cosmesis.

Breast-Conserving Surgery in the Elderly

Since 1970, multiple prospective randomized trials have compared survival after breast conservation treatment to survival after mastectomy for stage I and II breast cancer. No survival advantage has been noted for mastectomy. Although most of these trials did not include women older than 70 years, the biologic rationale for breast preservation can be extrapolated to the elderly population. Several studies have suggested that elderly women may have a lower rate of breast recurrence after partial mastectomy and radiotherapy than their younger counterparts [39–41]. Fourquet et al. reported a 97% rate of control at 10 years for women older than 55 years compared to 85% for women aged 33–45 years and 71% for women aged 32 years or younger in a series of 518 patients [40]. Veronesi et al [41] and Clark et al. [39] have also reported a decreasing frequency of breast recurrence with increasing age. Some of these differences in local failure rates may be due to a higher incidence of adverse pathologic features, such as an extensive intraductal component or lymphatic invasion in young women, but older women appear to have lower local failure rates even after correction for pathologic features.

In addition, local recurrence rates can be affected by a number of treatment factors, such as the extent of surgical resection, the status of the surgical margin, and the use of adjuvant tamoxifen. In the National Surgical Adjuvant Breast Project (NSABP) B-14 trial, 2,644 axillary-node-negative patients, 38% of whom underwent breast-conserving therapy, were randomized to receive tamoxifen or placebo. After a median follow-up of 10 years, the rate of recurrence in the

TABLE 38.3 Contraindications to breast-conserving therapy with irradiation

Two or more primary tumors in separate quadrants of the breast

Diffuse malignant-appearing microcalcifications

Prior therapeutic irradiation to the breast region that requires retreatment to an excessively high total radiation dose

Persistent positive margins after reasonable surgical attempts

Source: American College of Radiology [43]

breast was 14.5% in the placebo arm compared to 3.4% in the tamoxifen group [42]. Thus, in women treated with breast-conserving therapy, including breast irradiation and tamoxifen, the incidence of local failure is low, and the small risk of a second surgery is not an appropriate reason to recommend that elderly women routinely undergo mastectomy. The standard contraindications to breast-conserving therapy (Table 38.3) used to determine the suitability of young women for breast-conserving therapy are applicable in older women as well [43].

High rates of mastectomy in the elderly have been attributed to patient choice. Some studies have indeed shown that BCT is chosen less frequently as age increases [44–46]. In contrast, Bleicher et al. [47] examined the role of age in the surgery decision-making process by surveying 1,279 patients aged 79 or younger from two SEER program registries. A majority of patients (80.3%) underwent BCT. There were no differences in patient preference for mastectomy on the basis of age, and in a logistic regression analysis, age and comorbidities were not significant predictors of mastectomy use.

The necessity for adjuvant radiotherapy in patients treated with breast conservation is a matter of particular interest in the elderly population. The Early Breast Cancer Trialists' Collaborative Group (EBCTCG) overview of randomized trials included ten trials of post-BCT radiotherapy with a total of 23,500 patients. The main analyses of local recurrence, breast cancer mortality, and overall mortality were stratified by age into five groups (<40, 40–49, 50–59, 60–69, and >70 years) [48]. The relative risk of recurrence, comparing those allocated to RT with those not, was about 0.3 in every trial, corresponding to a 5-year risk of local recurrence of 7% in the RT group versus 26% in the control. The absolute effects of post-BCS RT on local recurrence were greater in younger than in older women (5-year risk reductions of 22, 16, 12, and 11% for those aged <50, 50–59, 60–69, and >70 years, respectively). The proportional risk reduction for breast cancer mortality was less pronounced than that for local recurrence, with one breast cancer death averted at 15 years for every four local recurrences prevented in year 5. The lower absolute benefit of RT in older women coupled with the long follow-up period needed for mortality reductions to be observed makes it unlikely that RT will have a major impact upon survival in this population [48].

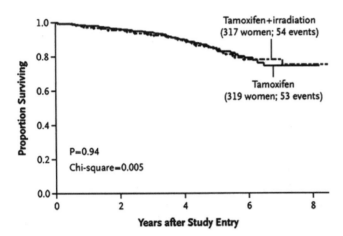

FIGURE 38.2 Overall survival in patients with ER-positive breast cancers 2 cm or less in size randomized to treatment with tamoxifen alone or tamoxifen plus irradiation. No survival difference between groups was observed (from Hughes et al. [50] Copyright © 2004 Massachusetts Medical Society. All rights reserved).

A similar age-related difference in the magnitude of benefit achieved with a boost dose of radiation was demonstrated in a randomized trial by Bartelink et al. [49] Although the use of a boost resulted in a statistically significant reduction in local recurrence in all age groups, the absolute benefit ranged from 10.4% at 10 years in women aged less than 40 years to approximately 3% in those older than 60 years [49].

Although the value of RT in the setting of BCS in the general population, and to some extent in elderly patients, has been demonstrated, the argument that older age may be associated with lower rates of recurrence, less aggressive tumor biology, and increased comorbidity has prompted investigation into the need for RT after breast-conserving surgery in this subgroup of patients. Hughes et al. [50] designed a prospective randomized trial that included 636 women aged 70 years or older who were randomly assigned to receive tamoxifen plus radiation therapy or tamoxifen alone to examine the benefit of RT in older women with small breast cancers. Eligibility criteria included ER-positive clinical stage I (tumor<2 cm, clinically node negative) breast carcinoma treated by lumpectomy. At a follow-up of 5 years, the locoregional recurrence rate was 1% in the tamoxifen + RT group versus 4% in the tamoxifen alone group ($p<0.001$). There were no significant differences in the rates of mastectomy, distant metastases, or overall survival between groups (Fig. 38.2). These findings suggest that lumpectomy plus adjuvant tamoxifen is a reasonable treatment choice for women aged 70 years or older with small, ER-positive breast cancers.

Practical issues, such as the difficulty in traveling to RT appointments daily for 6 weeks, play a significant role in the omission of RT in elderly women, and studies have examined the feasibility of alternative methods of radiation delivery. Kirova et al. [51] examined outcomes in a retrospective study of 367 women aged 70 years or greater treated with conventional RT (50 Gy, 25 fractions, 5 fractions weekly) or hypofractionated RT, which delivered a total dose of 32.5 Gy in five fractions of 6.5 Gy once weekly. At a median follow-up of 93 months, no differences in breast cancer deaths or local-recurrence-free survival were observed between the 50 patients receiving hypofractionated RT and those treated with conventional RT. The 5- and 7-year local-recurrence-free survival rates were 94% and 91% for the hypofractionated group. The Ontario Clinical Oncology Group reported one of the first trials of hypofractionation [52] in which 1,234 women with node-negative breast cancer and clear margins of excision after breast-conserving surgery and axillary dissection were randomized to accelerated hypofractionated whole-breast irradiation (AHWBI) of 42.5 Gy in 16 fractions over 22 days, or a more standard course of whole-breast irradiation (SWBI) of 50 Gy in 25 fractions over 35 days. The study was first reported in 2002 with a median follow-up of 5.8 years. The incidence of local recurrence at 5 years was 3.2% in the SWBI arm and 2.8% in the AHWBI arm, with no difference in cosmetic outcome. These results have been confirmed with additional follow-up, suggesting that this is an appropriate approach for older women who need to receive RT based on higher risk tumor characteristics [52]. In recent years, hypofractionation has also been used to deliver partial-breast irradiation (PBI). PBI is defined as the delivery of radiation to the surgical cavity plus a 1–2 cm margin after breast-conserving surgery. The rationale for PBI is that most local recurrences occur at the primary tumor site or immediately adjacent to it, rather than elsewhere in the breast. Numerous techniques have been developed, including interstitial brachytherapy, a single-source balloon catheter brachytherapy, three-dimensional conformal treatment with external beam, and intraoperative treatment (IORT). However, long-term outcomes are not yet available for any techniques of PBI. In addition, many of the patients selected for PBI are at very low risk for local recurrence in the absence of RT, raising questions as to whether the favorable outcomes reported in early nonrandomized studies are applicable to a wider spectrum of women with breast cancer. In spite of these concerns, the very brief period of time needed for treatment with PBI (5 days, or on the day of surgery in the case of IORT) make this an attractive approach for study in elderly women.

Overall, breast irradiation has been shown to be well tolerated in the elderly population. A tolerance study by Wyckoff et al. demonstrated that radiation dose, duration of therapy, number of treatment interruptions, and toxicities were no different in women older than 65 years compared to women aged less than 65 years [53]. When considering whether to omit breast irradiation after limited surgery, it is important to remember that most local failures occur within 6 years of surgery, leaving many elderly women at risk of this occurrence. Irradiation is well tolerated in the elderly population, and chronologic age alone is not an indication for its omission from breast-conserving therapy. In patients who do not undergo breast irradiation, a wider surgical resection (quadrantectomy) appears to decrease the risk of local recurrence.

Sentlnel Lymph Node Biopsy

The sentinel node is defined as the first lymph node/s to receive drainage from a particular cancer and can be identified by lymphatic mapping with a blue dye, a radioactive tracer, or both. Injection of the breast tissue around the tumor, the subareolar space, and the skin overlying the tumor have all successfully been utilized to identify a sentinel node. The success rate for identification of the sentinel node in prospective, multi-institutional studies is greater than 95% and improves with experience [54, 55]. When identified, the sentinel node is an accurate predictor of the status of the remaining nodes in the axilla in more than 90% of cases [54, 56, 57]. In the American College of Surgeons Oncology Group (ACOSOG) Z10 trial, increasing patient age was significantly associated with failure to identify a sentinel node [55], with the failure rate increasing from less than 1% in women aged less than 50 years to 2.7% for those aged 70 years and older ($p = 0.0004$). Others have reported excellent outcomes for SN biopsy in older patients. Gennari et al. reported a sentinel node identification rate of 100% in 241 consecutive patients aged 70 years or older who underwent sentinel node biopsy [58].

In the past, many elderly patients were not offered axillary staging because the complications associated with axillary lymph node dissection were felt to outweigh the potential benefits of the procedure. The sentinel lymph node biopsy technique allows patients with clinically node-negative breast cancer to undergo axillary staging with a significant decrease in morbidity. There are complications associated with the procedure, however. After 6 months of follow-up in the ACOSOG Z10 trial, decreased range of motion was observed in 4% of patients, axillary paresthesias in 9%, and lymphedema in 7%. Although paresthesias were more common in younger women, the incidence of lymphedema increased with age [59]. Thus, it is important to ensure that knowledge of nodal status is important for overall patient management prior to performing a sentinel node biopsy, since excellent outcomes have been reported after observation of the axilla in older women.

The International Breast Cancer Study Group conducted a prospective, randomized trial of axillary dissection versus observation in women aged 60 years and older [60]. The median patient age was 74 years, and all patients received tamoxifen. At a median follow-up of 6.6 years, axillary recurrence as a first event was observed in 2% of patients and did not differ between groups. This low rate of axillary failure is particularly noteworthy since most of the study participants did not receive radiotherapy. Differences in quality of life

TABLE 38.4 Comparison of the morbidity of SN biopsy and axillary dissection

Symptom	SN biopsy (%)	Axillary dissection (%)
Pain	8–14	23–72
Paresthesia	2–9	24 85
Decreased Range of Motion	0–6	18–27
Lymphedema	1–11	7–69

Source: Data from Lucci et al. [63], Veronesi et al. [65], and Schijven et al. [64]
SN Sentinel node

favoring no axillary surgery were present in the first 6–12 months postoperatively but were minimal with longer follow up. This study indicates that axillary observation is associated with a low risk of axillary recurrence but that when axillary dissection is necessary, it can be performed with a limited effect on quality of life. The impact of knowledge of axillary nodal status on treatment has been examined, with changes in planned therapy occurring in 14–38% of patients based on knowledge of nodal status [61, 62]. In aggregate, these studies suggest that when knowledge of axillary nodal status will not change therapy, axillary observation is a safe approach. When axillary staging is indicated, sentinel node biopsy is the procedure of choice, and axillary dissection can be safely carried out with acceptable morbidity in patients presenting with nodal involvement and those found to have metastases to the sentinel nodes. The morbidity of sentinel node biopsy and axillary dissection is compared in Table 38.4 [63–65].

Axillary dissection is an effective method for maintaining local control in the axilla with isolated axillary failures seen in only 1–2% of patients after the procedure [66, 67]. Major complications of axillary dissection, including injury or thrombosis of the axillary vein and injury to the motor nerves of the axilla, are uncommon, although significant short- and long-term morbidity are associated with the procedure (Table 38.4). Of the potential sequelae of the procedure, lymphedema of the arm is potentially associated with the greatest disability. The incidence of lymphedema following axillary dissection ranges from 1.5 to 62.5% [68–71] depending on the definition used, the length of follow-up, the method of detection employed, and the population studied. Several studies have suggested that older age is a risk factor for the development of lymphedema. Pezner et al. [71] noted lymphedema following breast-conserving treatment (including RT) in 25% of women aged 60 or older compared to 3 of 46 younger women (7%) ($p = 0.02$). Other studies have failed to identify an association between age and lymphedema [68–70]. Axillary dissection has also been shown to cause pain and decreased upper arm mobility [72], factors that can cause significant functional impairment in women with pre-existing limitations due to neurologic disease or arthritis. In patients with microscopic nodal involvement, axillary irradiation is an alternative to dissection to maintain local control [73], but in the presence of clinically evident, histologically confirmed nodal disease, axillary dissection remains the procedure of choice because failure rates after irradiation alone are higher than those seen with surgery in this clinical setting.

Primary Endocrine Therapy as an Alternative Local Therapy

Because of concerns regarding the morbidity and mortality of conventional surgical therapy for breast cancer in elderly women with comorbid conditions, considerable attention has been given to the use of tamoxifen as a primary treatment. In 2007, Hind et al. reviewed the evidence from randomized trials comparing primary endocrine therapy to surgery, with or without adjuvant endocrine therapy and/or radiation, in women aged 70 years or older [74]. Seven studies were included in the review, three reporting outcome data on surgery versus primary tamoxifen and four analyzing surgery plus endocrine therapy versus primary tamoxifen. Only one study selected patients on the basis of ER status. When comparing surgery alone to primary endocrine therapy, no significant difference in overall survival between interventions (HR 0.98, 95% CI, 0.74–1.30, $p=0.9$) was noted. One trial [75] reported adequate summary data to show a significant difference in progression-free survival (PFS) favoring surgery (HR 0.55, 95% CI, 0.39–0.77, $p=0.0006$). In the three trials comparing surgery plus adjuvant endocrine therapy to primary endocrine therapy [76–78], there was a nonsignificant trend in favor of surgery plus endocrine therapy (HR 0.86, 95% CI, 0.73–1.00, $p=0.06$). Only one trial [77] reported adequate data on PFS to calculate a significant difference favoring surgery plus endocrine therapy (HR 0.65, 95% CI, 0.53–0.81, $p=0.0001$), and two trials [76, 77] showed a significant decrease in local recurrence favoring surgery plus endocrine therapy (HR 0.28, 95% CI, 0.23–0.35, $p<0.00001$). These results are summarized in Table 38.5. The results of this review are based on a limited number of small studies of variable methodological quality, with significant heterogeneity among studies. Nonetheless, this review demonstrates that primary endocrine therapy is inferior to surgery plus endocrine therapy for the local control of breast cancer in ER-unselected, medically fit older women, independent of the type of surgery (mastectomy or wide excision alone). The meta-analysis showed no significant difference in overall survival between the two treatments, although one trial showed a small but significant survival advantage for surgery with adjuvant endocrine therapy where follow-up was extended to 13 years [76]. This review suggests that primary endocrine therapy should only be offered to women with ER-positive tumors who are not surgical candidates or who refuse surgery. In a cohort of women

Table 38.5 Primary endocrine therapy for breast cancer

Surgery vs. primary endocrine therapy

Trial	Median follow-up (years)	HR death (95% CI)
EORTC 10851	10	1.11 (0.75–1.65)
Nottingham 1	5	1.06 (0.59–1.92)
St. Georges	6	0.75 (0.44–1.26)

Surgery plus endocrine therapy vs. endocrine therapy

Trial	Median follow-up (years)	HR death (95% CI)	HR local failure (95% CI)
CRC	13	0.78 (0.63–0.96)	0.25 (0.19–0.32)
GRETA	7	0.98 (0.77–1.25)	0.38 (0.25–0.57)
Nottingham 2	5	0.80 (0.73–2.32)	Not available

HR hazard ratio; *EORTC* European Organization for Research and Treatment of Cancer; *CRC* Cancer Research Campaign; *GRETA* Italian Cooperative Group
Source: Data from Hind et al. [74]

with reduced life expectancy due to significant comorbid disease, primary endocrine therapy may be an appropriate treatment choice. The ESTEEM trial (Endocrine +/− Surgical Therapy for Elderly Women with Mammary Cancer), a national trial in the United Kingdom, will evaluate selection criteria for the use of primary endocrine therapy and hopefully clarify the indications for its use [74].

Systemic Therapy

Adjuvant therapy has come to play an increasingly large role in breast cancer management; however, its role in elderly women remains controversial. The value of adjuvant systemic therapy (endocrine therapy and chemotherapy) in the general population is best estimated from the meta-analysis of the Early Breast Cancer Trialists' Collaborative group which now includes 15 years of follow-up on more than 100,000 women entered on breast cancer clinical trials [79].

Tamoxifen is well established as an effective endocrine therapy for postmenopausal, ER-positive women with node-positive or node-negative breast cancer. The 2005 update of the meta-analysis by the Early Breast Cancer Trialists' Collaborative Group (EBCTCG) [79] demonstrated that only for ER-positive disease, adjuvant tamoxifen reduced the annual breast cancer death rate by 31% in all age groups (50, 50–69, and, >70 years) and that the absolute risk reduction after 5 years of tamoxifen was found to be similar for younger and older women [79].

Adjuvant therapy with tamoxifen for 5 years has been the standard of care for women with early-stage, endocrine-responsive breast cancer for many years [79]. However, the partial estrogen agonistic activity of tamoxifen and other selective ER modulators (SERMs) increases the risk of endometrial cancer and thromboembolic events [80]. Aromatase inhibitors (AIs) are an alternate form of endocrine therapy that profoundly reduce the already low-circulating endogenous levels of estrogens in postmenopausal women by blocking the synthesis of estrogens in nonovarian tissues, including breast tissue [81] AIs have been shown to be similar or superior to tamoxifen as first-line treatment for locally advanced and metastatic breast cancer [82], as well as in the adjuvant setting [82–84]. However, the side effect profiles of the AIs and tamoxifen differ, with AIs being associated with an increased risk of osteoporosis bone fractures and musculoskeletal complaints, and tamoxifen with an increased incidence of venous thrombosis, endometrial cancer, and cataracts. Crivellari et al. [85] have recently investigated whether the observed effects of letrozole compared to tamoxifen identified in the Breast International Group (BIG) 1-98 trial differed by age to determine whether treatment recommendations should be modified for elderly patients. In the elderly, letrozole significantly improved disease-free survival and was effective in reducing relapses, including distant metastases, when compared to tamoxifen; even though no convincing differences were observed in thromboembolic or cardiac events in the elderly group, data in the older (aged 64–75 years) cohort indicated that thromboembolic events appeared more common with tamoxifen and cardiac events with letrozole. Letrozole was also associated with a higher incidence of bone fractures, independent of age [85]. The choice between an AI and tamoxifen in the individual patient is often made on the basis of preexisting conditions, such as the presence of significant osteoporosis or a history of deep venous thrombosis, which would influence the risk/benefit ratio of one of the drugs.

There is considerable controversy regarding the use of adjuvant chemotherapy in elderly women. The EBCTCG overview [79] only included about 1,200 older women in trials of chemotherapy versus no chemotherapy, making it difficult to draw firm conclusions about efficacy, although the proportional reductions in recurrence and death were smaller in older women than in their younger counterparts. Chemotherapy is an appropriate treatment for many elderly patients with early breast cancer, but its use requires careful consideration of life expectancy, comorbidity, functional status, and other factors. Unlike endocrine therapy, toxicity can be substantial with a major effect on functional status. For healthy elderly women with hormone-receptor-negative tumors and life expectancies of at least 5 years, chemotherapy should be considered for node-positive patients and high-risk node-negative patients; the added value of chemotherapy to endocrine therapy can be estimated using the Adjuvant! program (www.adjuvantonline.com). A sample calculation from Adjuvant! is presented in Table 38.6.

Data indicate that women 65 years and older with node-positive breast cancer treated with newer state-of-the-art

Table 38.6 ER-positive tumors: 10-year mortality benefit of adjuvant treatment compared to no treatment by age and clinical characteristics in women of average health with grade 2 tumors (from www.adjuvantonline.com, version 7.0 – estimates only)

Size and node status	Treatment	Age in years		
		60	70	80
1.1–2.0 cm, node negative	Tamoxifen (%)	2.3	2	1.2
	T+CMF or AC (%)	2.7	2.2	1.5
	T+3rd Gen (%)	4.2	3.7	2.3
2.1–3.0 cm, node negative	Tamoxifen (%)	4.6	3.9	2.5
	T+CMF or AC (%)	5.4	4.6	2.9
	T+3rd Gen (%)	8.7	7.5	4.7
2.1–3.0 cm, 1–3 nodes	Tamoxifen (%)	8.7	7.4	4.6
	T+CMF or AC (%)	10 1	8.7	5.3
	T+3rd Gen (%)	16.9	14.5	9.0
2.1–3.0 cm, 10 plus nodes	Tamoxifen (%)	12.7	10.8	6.4
	T+CMF or AC (%)	15.2	12.8	7.6
	T+3rd Gen (%)	27.1	23	13.8

Source: Data from Muss [103]
CMF cyclophosphamide, methotrexate, 5-fluorouracil; *AC* doxorubicin, cyclophosphamide; *T* tamoxifen; *3rd Gen* third generation chemotherapy (i.e., AC plus a taxane)

chemotherapy regimens derive the same proportional benefits in relapse-free and overall survival as younger patients [86]; these benefits are more prominent in ER-negative, node-positive patients [87]. In comparing the efficacy in elderly patients (older than 65 years) of standard (CMF or AC) chemotherapeutic regimens versus capecitabine, an oral agent thought to be well suited for use in the elderly; Muss et al. have recently demonstrated that capecitabine was inferior to standard therapy [88].

Systemic therapy includes endocrine therapy, chemotherapy, and more recently, HER2-directed therapy. Trastuzumab combined with chemotherapy significantly improves survival in HER-2-positive patients compared to treatment with chemotherapy alone [89, 90]. Cardiac toxicity, reversible in most cases, is a major side effect of trastuzumab, and its incidence increases with age and anthracycline use. Elderly patients with HER-2-positive tumors at high risk for recurrence should be considered for nonanthracycline trastuzumab containing regimens such as docetaxel, carboplatin, and trastuzumab (TCH) if cardiac toxicity is a concern [91].

The decision to use adjuvant systemic therapy in elderly women must take into consideration coexisting morbidities and functional status; these may affect a woman's ability to tolerate breast cancer treatment and may decrease survival, regardless of age. The effects of comorbidity on survival can be reliably estimated from mathematical models that are publicly available [92]. This is important in view of the fact that nonbreast cancer causes of death are substantial in women aged 70 years and older, even in those with axillary nodal metastases [93] (Fig. 38.3).

Figure 38.3 Causes of death (breast cancer vs. nonbreast cancer) by stage at diagnosis in women aged 70 years and older at diagnosis (from Schairer et al. [93] Adapted with permission of the Oxford University Press).

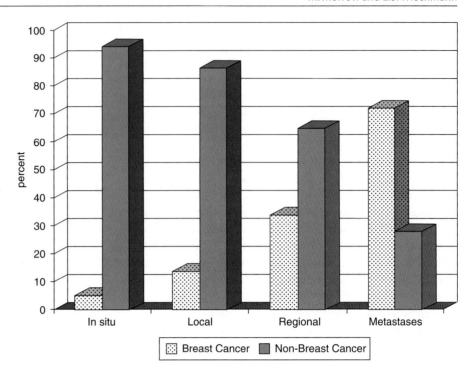

Patterns of Care in the Elderly

A number of studies suggest that age at breast cancer diagnosis is a major determinant of the type of therapy received. Outcome data concerning nonconventional breast cancer treatment in the elderly is conflicting, but studies have shown that a large portion of elderly patients do not receive conventional treatment for breast cancer. In 2001, Gadjos et al. retrospectively analyzed risk factors, presentation, pathologic findings, treatment, and outcomes of 206 women older than 70 years compared with those of 920 younger patients undergoing potentially curative operations for breast cancer between 1978 and 1998 [94]. Patients older than 70 years had fewer mastectomies, were less likely to undergo axillary node dissection, postoperative radiation, and chemotherapy, and received tamoxifen more frequently with no difference in rates of local and distant recurrence. In this series, undertreated elderly patients (54% of patients older than 70 years) were significantly older, but despite undertreatment by conventional criteria, the rates of local recurrence and distant metastasis were not increased in comparison with conventionally treated elderly patients. Enger et al. [95] also found that in their study of 1,859 women older than 65 years, women aged 75 years and older or with higher comorbidity indices were more likely to receive nonstandard primary

tumor therapy, to not receive axillary lymph node dissection, and to not receive radiation therapy after breast-conserving surgery.

More recently, Owusu et al. [96] have investigated whether the observed age-related disparities in breast cancer survival were related to differences in treatment received, by evaluating 659 women aged 65 years or older and treated for early breast cancer. In accordance with Enger et al., they found that women older than 75 years were less likely to receive axillary lymph node dissection, radiotherapy, definitive primary therapy, chemotherapy, and guideline therapy. This translated to a 7% absolute decrease in breast cancer-specific survival for women older than 75 years compared to those aged less than 75 years. Findings from this study indicated that as many as 66% of women aged greater than 75 years, and 45% of women aged 65–75 years received less than guideline therapy. These data are consistent with previous studies that demonstrate receipt of suboptimal therapy among elderly patients with early-stage breast cancer [97]. Owusu et al. showed that receipt of guideline therapy in the cohort of older women with early-stage breast cancer evaluated in their study was associated with improved outcomes, particularly among the very old.

Healthy vs. Frail Elderly Patients

Almost 30% of all invasive breast carcinomas occur in women older than 70 years [98]. By the year 2030, an even larger portion of breast cancer patients will be aged 65 years or older, and many will be affected by comorbid conditions. It is important to distinguish healthy from frail elderly patients and to develop clinical tools that guide clinicians when planning care. The following principles have been proposed for the management of *frail* elderly women. The benefit of screening mammography in these patients is questionable, and a clinical breast exam is likely to identify breast cancers that warrant intervention. Endocrine therapy may be a reasonable primary therapy in older, frail women with hormone-receptor-positive lesions. For ER-negative and PR-negative lesions, excision of the primary tumor may be adequate. Adjuvant endocrine therapy may be appropriate in frail elders with high-risk hormone-receptor-positive breast cancer; chemotherapy is rarely indicated regardless of tumor status. The majority of frail elders with metastases will have hormone-receptor-positive breast cancers, and endocrine therapy should be considered; those with receptor-negative tumors may be treated with single-agent chemotherapy or supportive care measures. Oncologists need to acquire the skills to appropriately identify frail elders so that they select appropriate therapies that will minimize toxicity and maintain quality of life.

Finally, when considering *healthy* elderly breast cancer patients, the data included above suggest that compliance with consensus recommendations for definitive locoregional treatment, usually defined as breast surgery with evaluation of the axillary lymph nodes and radiation therapy in patients undergoing breast-conserving procedures, is warranted. Standard guidelines for adjuvant systemic therapy, including chemotherapy, should also be utilized in this group [99].

Summary

- Screening mammography in healthy women up to age 75–80 years appears beneficial. It is not indicated in frail elders.
- Healthy elderly breast cancer patients should undergo surgery of the primary tumor (excision to negative margins or mastectomy) using standard selection criteria.
- Good local control is obtained with excision alone for T1-, ER-positive tumors. Radiotherapy should be given for others undergoing breast conserving therapy.
- Sentinel node biopsy is the axillary staging procedure of choice for clinically node-negative women if the finding of nodal metastases would alter treatment.
- Axillary dissection remains standard management for patients with macrometastases in the axilla.
- In frail elders, primary endocrine therapy (tamoxifen or an aromatase inhibitor) is the appropriate management of hormone-receptor-positive breast cancer.
- In the rare frail elderly patient with a hormone-receptor-negative tumor, excision alone may be the appropriate therapy.

References

1. American Cancer Society Cancer Statistics 2008. www.cancer. org. Accessed 16 February 2009
2. Bergman L, Dekker G, van Leeuwen FE, Huisman SJ, van Dam FS, van Dongen JA (1991) The effect of age on treatment choice and survival in elderly breast cancer patients. Cancer 67(9): 2227–2234
3. Trimble EL, Carter CL, Cain D, Freidlin B, Ungerleider RS, Friedman MA (1994) Representation of older patients in cancer treatment trials. Cancer 74(7 Suppl):2208–2214
4. MacMahon B, Cole P, Brown J (1973) Etiology of human breast cancer: a review. J Natl Cancer Inst 50(1):21–42
5. Waterhouse J, Muis C, Correa P (eds) (1976) Cancer incidence in 5 continents. Lyon International Agency for Research on Cancer, Lyon, AIRC Scientific Publications; No. 3
6. Yancik R, Ries LG, Yates JW (1989) Breast cancer in aging women. A population-based study of contrasts in stage, surgery, and survival. Cancer 63(5):976–981
7. Chu KC, Tarone RE, Kessler LG et al (1996) Recent trends in U.S. breast cancer incidence, survival, and mortality rates. J Natl Cancer Inst 88(21):1571–1579
8. Howe HL, Wu X, Ries LA et al (2006) Annual report to the nation on the status of cancer, 1975–2003, featuring cancer among U.S. Hispanic/Latino populations. Cancer 107(8):1711–1742
9. Ravdin PM, Cronin KA, Howlander N, Chelbowski RT, Berry DA (2006) A decrease in breast cancer incidence in the United States in 2003. In: 29th annual San Antonio breast cancer symposium, San Antonio, TX
10. Jemal A, Ward E, Thun MJ (2007) Recent trends in breast cancer incidence rates by age and tumor characteristics among U.S. women. Breast Cancer Res 9(3):R28
11. Berry DA, Cronin KA, Plevritis SK et al (2005) Effect of screening and adjuvant therapy on mortality from breast cancer. N Engl J Med 353(17):1784–1792
12. Du XL, Fox EE, Lai D (2008) Competing causes of death for women with breast cancer and change over time from 1975 to 2003. Am J Clin Oncol 31(2):105–116
13. Rosen PP, Lesser ML, Kinne DW (1985) Breast carcinoma at the extremes of age: a comparison of patients younger than 35 years and older than 75 years. J Surg Oncol 28(2):90–96
14. Schaefer G, Rosen PP, Lesser ML, Kinne DW, Beattie EJ Jr (1984) Breast carcinoma in elderly women: pathology, prognosis, and survival. Pathol Annu 19(Pt 1):195–219
15. Fletcher SW, Black W, Harris R, Rimer BK, Shapiro S (1993) Report of the International Workshop on Screening for Breast Cancer. J Natl Cancer Inst 85(20):1644–1656
16. Kerlikowske K, Grady D, Rubin SM, Sandrock C, Ernster VL (1995) Efficacy of screening mammography. A meta-analysis. JAMA 273(2):149–154
17. Tabar L, Fagerberg G, Duffy SW, Day NE (1989) The Swedish two county trial of mammographic screening for breast cancer: recent results and calculation of benefit. J Epidemiol Community Health 43(2):107–114
18. Van Dijck JA, Verbeek AL, Beex LV et al (1997) Breast-cancer mortality in a non-randomized trial on mammographic screening in women over age 65. Int J Cancer 70(2):164–168
19. Jonsson H, Tornberg S, Nystrom L, Lenner P (2003) Service screening with mammography of women aged 70–74 years in Sweden. Effects on breast cancer mortality. Cancer Detect Prev 27(5):360–369
20. Smith-Bindman R, Kerlikowske K, Gebretsadik T, Newman J (2000) Is screening mammography effective in elderly women? Am J Med 108(2):112–119
21. Taplin SH, Ichikawa L, Yood MU et al (2004) Reason for late-stage breast cancer: absence of screening or detection, or breakdown in follow-up? J Natl Cancer Inst 96(20):1518–1527

22. Mandelblatt JS, Wheat ME, Monane M, Moshief RD, Hollenberg JP, Tang J (1992) Breast cancer screening for elderly women with and without comorbid conditions. A decision analysis model. Ann Intern Med 116(9):722–730

23. Moskowitz M (1986) Breast cancer: age-specific growth rates and screening strategies. Radiology 161(1):37–41

24. Boer R, de Koning HJ, van Oortmarssen GJ, van der Maas PJ (1995) In search of the best upper age limit for breast cancer screening. Eur J Cancer 31A(12):2040–2043

25. Fracheboud J, Groenewoud JH, Boer R et al (2006) Seventy-five years is an appropriate upper age limit for population-based mammography screening. Int J Cancer 118(8):2020–2025

26. U.S. Preventative Services Task Force (1989) Guide to Clinical Preventative Services: an assessment of the effectiveness of 169 interventions. Williams & Wilkins, Baltimore

27. (1990) Screening mammography: a missed clinical opportunity? Results of the NCI Breast Cancer Screening Consortium and National Health Interview Survey Studies. JAMA 264(1):54–58

28. Leathar DS, Roberts MM (1985) Older women's attitudes towards breast disease, self examination, and screening facilities: implications for communication. Br Med J (Clin Res Ed) 290(6469):668–670

29. Fox SA, Siu AL, Stein JA (1994) The importance of physician communication on breast cancer screening of older women. Arch Intern Med 154(18):2058–2068

30. Caplan LS (2001) To screen or not to screen: the issue of breast cancer screening in older women. Public Health Rev 29(2–4):231–240

31. Field TS, Doubeni C, Fox MP et al (2008) Under utilization of surveillance mammography among older breast cancer survivors. J Gen Intern Med 23(2):158–163

32. Schneiderman MA, Axtell LM (1979) Deaths among female patients with carcinoma of the breast treated by a surgical procedure only. Surg Gynecol Obstet 148(2):193–195

33. Davis SJ, Karrer FW, Moor BJ, Rose SG, Eakins G (1985) Characteristics of breast cancer in women over 80 years of age. Am J Surg 150(6):655–658

34. Hunt KE, Fry DE, Bland KI (1980) Breast carcinoma in the elderly patient: an assessment of operative risk, morbidity and mortality. Am J Surg 140(3):339–342

35. Kesseler HJ, Seton JZ (1978) The treatment of operable breast cancer in the elderly female. Am J Surg 135(5):664–666

36. Singletary SE, Shallenberger R, Guinee VF (1993) Breast cancer in the elderly. Ann Surg 218(5):667–671

37. Oakley N, Dennison AR, Shorthouse AJ (1996) A prospective audit of simple mastectomy under local anaesthesia. Eur J Surg Oncol 22(2):134–136

38. Carlson GW (2005) Total mastectomy under local anesthesia: the tumescent technique. Breast J 11(2):100–102

39. Clark RM, Wilkinson RH, Miceli PN, MacDonald WD (1987) Breast cancer. Experiences with conservation therapy. Am J Clin Oncol 10(6):461–468

40. Fourquet A, Campana F, Zafrani B et al (1989) Prognostic factors of breast recurrence in the conservative management of early breast cancer: a 25-year follow-up. Int J Radiat Oncol Biol Phys 17(4):719–725

41. Veronesi U, Salvadori B, Luini A et al (1990) Conservative treatment of early breast cancer. Long-term results of 1232 cases treated with quadrantectomy, axillary dissection, and radiotherapy. Ann Surg 211(3):250–259

42. Fisher B, Dignam J, Bryant J et al (1996) Five versus more than five years of tamoxifen therapy for breast cancer patients with negative lymph nodes and estrogen receptor-positive tumors. J Natl Cancer Inst 88(21):1529–1542

43. American College of Radiology (2007) Practice guideline for the breast conservation therapy in the management of invasive breast carcinoma. J Am Coll Surg 205(2):362–376

44. Hiotis K, Ye W, Sposto R, Skinner KA (2005) Predictors of breast conservation therapy: size is not all that matters. Cancer 103(5):892–899

45. Mandelblatt JS, Hadley J, Kerner JF et al (2000) Patterns of breast carcinoma treatment in older women: patient preference and clinical and physical influences. Cancer 89(3):561–573

46. Wyld L, Garg DK, Kumar ID, Brown H, Reed MW (2004) Stage and treatment variation with age in postmenopausal women with breast cancer: compliance with guidelines. Br J Cancer 90(8):1486–1491

47. Bleicher RJ, Abrahamse P, Hawley ST, Katz SJ, Morrow M (2008) The influence of age on the breast surgery decision-making process. Ann Surg Oncol 15(3):854–862

48. Clarke M, Collins R, Darby S et al (2005) Effects of radiotherapy and of differences in the extent of surgery for early breast cancer on local recurrence and 15-year survival: an overview of the randomised trials. Lancet 366(9503):2087–2106

49. Bartelink H, Horiot JC, Poortmans PM et al (2007) Impact of a higher radiation dose on local control and survival in breast-conserving therapy of early breast cancer: 10-year results of the randomized boost versus no boost EORTC 22881-10882 trial. J Clin Oncol 25(22):3259–3265

50. Hughes KS, Schnaper LA, Berry D et al (2004) Lumpectomy plus tamoxifen with or without irradiation in women 70 years of age or older with early breast cancer. N Engl J Med 351(10):971–977

51. Kirova YM, Campana F, Savignoni A et al (2009) Breast-conserving treatment in the elderly: long-term results of adjuvant hypofractionated and normofractionated radiotherapy. Int J Radiat Oncol Biol Phys 75(1):76–81

52. Whelan T, Pignol JP, Julian J (2007) Long-term results of a randomized trial of accelerated hypofractionated whole breast irradiation following breast conserving surgery in women with node negative breast cancer. Breast Cancer 106:S6

53. Wyckoff J, Greenberg H, Sanderson R, Wallach P, Balducci L (1994) Breast irradiation in the older woman: a toxicity study. J Am Geriatr Soc 42(2):150–152

54. Krag DN, Anderson SJ, Julian TB et al (2007) Technical outcomes of sentinel-lymph-node resection and conventional axillary-lymph-node dissection in patients with clinically node-negative breast cancer: results from the NSABP B-32 randomised phase III trial. Lancet Oncol 8(10):881–888

55. Posther KE, McCall LM, Blumencranz PW et al (2005) Sentinel node skills verification and surgeon performance: data from a multicenter clinical trial for early-stage breast cancer. Ann Surg 242(4):593–599, discussion 599–602

56. Giuliano AE, Jones RC, Brennan M, Statman R (1997) Sentinel lymphadenectomy in breast cancer. J Clin Oncol 15(6):2345–2350

57. Veronesi U, Paganelli G, Galimberti V et al (1997) Sentinel-node biopsy to avoid axillary dissection in breast cancer with clinically negative lymph-nodes. Lancet 349(9069):1864–1867

58. Gennari R, Rotmensz N, Perego E, dos Santos G, Veronesi U (2004) Sentinel node biopsy in elderly breast cancer patients. Surg Oncol 13(4):193–196

59. Wilke LG, McCall LM, Posther KE et al (2006) Surgical complications associated with sentinel lymph node biopsy: results from a prospective international cooperative group trial. Ann Surg Oncol 13(4):491–500

60. Rudenstam CM, Zahrieh D, International Breast Cancer Study Group et al (2006) Randomized trial comparing axillary clearance versus no axillary clearance in older patients with breast cancer: first results of International Breast Cancer Study Group Trial 10-93. J Clin Oncol 24(3):337–344

61. DiFronzo LA, Hansen NM, Stern SL, Brennan MB, Giuliano AE (2000) Does sentinel lymphadenectomy improve staging and alter therapy in elderly women with breast cancer? Ann Surg Oncol 7(6):406–410

62. Hieken TJ, Nettnin S, Velasco JM (2004) The value of sentinel lymph node biopsy in elderly breast cancer patients. Am J Surg 188(4):440–442

63. Lucci A, McCall LM, Beitsch PD et al (2007) Surgical complications associated with sentinel lymph node dissection (SLND) plus axillary lymph node dissection compared with SLND alone in the American College of Surgeons Oncology Group Trial Z0011. J Clin Oncol 25(24):3657–3663

64. Schijven MP, Vingerhoets AJ, Rutten HJ et al (2003) Comparison of morbidity between axillary lymph node dissection and sentinel node biopsy. Eur J Surg Oncol 29(4):341–350

65. Veronesi U, Paganelli G, Viale G et al (2003) A randomized comparison of sentinel-node biopsy with routine axillary dissection in breast cancer. N Engl J Med 349(6):546–553

66. Fisher B, Redmond C, Fisher ER et al (1985) Ten-year results of a randomized clinical trial comparing radical mastectomy and total mastectomy with or without radiation. N Engl J Med 312(11):674–681

67. Halverson KJ, Taylor ME, Perez CA et al (1993) Regional nodal management and patterns of failure following conservative surgery and radiation therapy for stage I and II breast cancer. Int J Radiat Oncol Biol Phys 26(4):593–599

68. Britton RC, Nelson PA (1962) Causes and treatment of post-mastectomy lymphedema of the arm. Report of 114 cases. JAMA 180:95–102

69. Larson D, Weinstein M, Goldberg I et al (1986) Edema of the arm as a function of the extent of axillary surgery in patients with stage I-II carcinoma of the breast treated with primary radiotherapy. Int J Radiat Oncol Biol Phys 12(9):1575–1582

70. McLaughlin SA, Wright MJ, Morris KT et al (2008) Prevalence of lymphedema in women with breast cancer 5 years after sentinel lymph node biopsy or axillary dissection: objective measurements. J Clin Oncol 26(32):5213–5219

71. Pezner RD, Patterson MP, Hill LR et al (1986) Arm lymphedema in patients treated conservatively for breast cancer: relationship to patient age and axillary node dissection technique. Int J Radiat Oncol Biol Phys 12(12):2079–2083

72. Hladiuk M, Huchcroft S, Temple W, Schnurr BE (1992) Arm function after axillary dissection for breast cancer: a pilot study to provide parameter estimates. J Surg Oncol 50(1):47–52

73. Spruit PH, Siesling S, Elferink MA, Vonk EJ, Hoekstra CJ (2007) Regional radiotherapy versus an axillary lymph node dissection after lumpectomy: a safe alternative for an axillary lymph node dissection in a clinically uninvolved axilla in breast cancer. A case control study with 10 years follow up. Radiat Oncol 2:40

74. Hind D, Wyld L, Reed MW (2007) Surgery, with or without tamoxifen, vs tamoxifen alone for older women with operable breast cancer: cochrane review. Br J Cancer 96(7):1025–1029

75. Fentiman IS, Christiaens MR, Paridaens R et al (2003) Treatment of operable breast cancer in the elderly: a randomised clinical trial EORTC 10851 comparing tamoxifen alone with modified radical mastectomy. Eur J Cancer 39(3):309–316

76. Fennessy M, Bates T, MacRae K, Riley D, Houghton J, Baum M (2004) Late follow-up of a randomized trial of surgery plus tamoxifen versus tamoxifen alone in women aged over 70 years with operable breast cancer. Br J Surg 91(6):699–704

77. Mustacchi G, Ceccherini R, Milani S et al (2003) Tamoxifen alone versus adjuvant tamoxifen for operable breast cancer of the elderly: long-term results of the phase III randomized controlled multi-center GRETA trial. Ann Oncol 14(3):414–420

78. Willsher PC, Robertson JF, Chan SY, Jackson L, Blamey RW (1997) Locally advanced breast cancer: early results of a randomised trial of multimodal therapy versus initial hormone therapy. Eur J Cancer 33(1):45–49

79. Early Breast Cancer Trialists' Collaborative Group (2005) Effects of chemotherapy and hormonal therapy for early breast cancer on recurrence and 15-year survival: an overview of the randomised trials. Lancet 365(9472):1687–1717

80. McDonald CC, Alexander FE, Whyte BW, Forrest AP, Stewart HJ, The Scottish Cancer Trials Breast Group (1995) Cardiac and vascular morbidity in women receiving adjuvant tamoxifen for breast cancer in a randomized trial. Br Med J 311:977–980

81. Geisler J, Haynes B, Anker G, Dowsett M, Lonning PE (2002) Influence of letrozole and anastrozole on total body aromatization and plasma estrogen levels in postmenopausal breast cancer patients evaluated in a randomized, cross-over study. J Clin Oncol 20(3):751–757

82. Mouridsen H, Gershanovich M, Sun Y et al (2003) Phase III study of letrozole versus tamoxifen as first-line therapy of advanced breast cancer in postmenopausal women: analysis of survival and update of efficacy from the International Letrozole Breast Cancer Group. J Clin Oncol 21(11):2101–2109

83. Coates AS, Keshaviah A, Thurlimann B et al (2007) Five years of letrozole compared with tamoxifen as initial adjuvant therapy for postmenopausal women with endocrine-responsive early breast cancer: update of study BIG 1-98. J Clin Oncol 25(5):486–492

84. Forbes JF, Cuzick J, Arimidex, Tamoxifen, Alone or in Combination (ATAC) Trialists' Group et al (2008) Effect of anastrozole and tamoxifen as adjuvant treatment for early-stage breast cancer: 100-month analysis of the ATAC trial. Lancet Oncol 9(1):45–53

85. Crivellari D, Sun Z, Coates AS et al (2008) Letrozole compared with tamoxifen for elderly patients with endocrine-responsive early breast cancer: the BIG 1-98 trial. J Clin Oncol 26(12):1972–1979

86. Muss HB, Woolf S, Berry D et al (2005) Adjuvant chemotherapy in older and younger women with lymph node-positive breast cancer. JAMA 293(9):1073–1081

87. Giordano SH, Duan Z, Kuo YF, Hortobagyi GN, Goodwin JS (2006) Use and outcomes of adjuvant chemotherapy in older women with breast cancer. J Clin Oncol 24(18):2750–2756

88. Muss HB, Berry DL, Cirrincione C, Theodoulou M, Mauer A, Cohen H (2008) Standard chemotherapy (CMF or AC) versus capecitabine in early-stage breast cancer (BC) patients aged 65 and older: results of CALGB/CTSU 49907. 2008 ASCO Annual Meeting. J Clin Oncol 26(8 Supp):5–20, abstract 507

89. Piccart-Gebhart MJ, Procter M, Leyland-Jones B et al (2005) Trastuzumab after adjuvant chemotherapy in HER2-positive breast cancer. N Engl J Med 353(16):1659–1672

90. Romond EH, Perez EA, Bryant J et al (2005) Trastuzumab plus adjuvant chemotherapy for operable HER2-positive breast cancer. N Engl J Med 353(16):1673–1684

91. Slamon D, Eiermann W, Robert N, et al (2006) BCIRG 006: 2nd interim analysis phase III randomized trial comparing doxorubicin and cyclophosphamide followed by docetaxel (AC→T) with doxorubicin and cyclophosphamide followed by docetaxel and trastuzumab (AC→TH) with docetaxel, carboplatin and trastuzumab (TCH) in Her2neu positive early breast cancer patients (abstract 52). In: San Antonio breast cancer symposium, San Antonio, TX

92. Welch HG, Albertsen PC, Nease RF, Bubolz TA, Wasson JH (1996) Estimating treatment benefits for the elderly: the effect of competing risks. Ann Intern Med 124(6):577–584

93. Schairer C, Mink PJ, Carroll L, Devesa SS (2004) Probabilities of death from breast cancer and other causes among female breast cancer patients. J Natl Cancer Inst 96(17):1311–1321

94. Gajdos C, Tartter PI, Bleiweiss IJ, Lopchinsky RA, Bernstein JL (2001) The consequence of undertreating breast cancer in the elderly. J Am Coll Surg 192(6):698–707

95. Enger SM, Thwin SS, Buist DS et al (2006) Breast cancer treatment of older women in integrated health care settings. J Clin Oncol 24(27):4377–4383

96. Owusu C, Lash TL, Silliman RA (2007) Effectiveness of adjuvant tamoxifen therapy among older women with early stage breast cancer. Breast J 13(4):374–382

97. Du XL, Key CR, Osborne C, Mahnken JD, Goodwin JS (2003) Discrepancy between consensus recommendations and actual community use of adjuvant chemotherapy in women with breast cancer. Ann Intern Med 138(2):90–97

98. Landis SH, Murray T, Bolden S, Wingo PA (1998) Cancer statistics, 1998. CA Cancer J Clin 48(1):6–29

99. Allen C, Cox EB, Manton KG, Cohen HJ (1986) Breast cancer in the elderly. Current patterns of care. J Am Geriatr Soc 34(9):637–642

100. Schottenfeld D, Robbins GF (1971) Breast cancer in elderly women. Geriatrics 26(3):121–131

101. Berg JW, Robbins GF (1961) Modified mastectomy for older, poor risk patients. Surg Gynecol Obstet 113:631–634

102. Kraft RO, Block GE (1962) Mammary carcinoma in the aged patient. Ann Surg 156:981–985

103. Muss HB (2007) Adjuvant treatment of elderly breast cancer patients. Breast 16(Suppl 2):S159–S165. In: Proceedings of the 10th international conference on primary therapy of early breast cancer. St. Gallen, Switzerland, 14–17, March 2007

Chapter 39
Diabetes in the Elderly

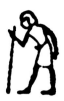

Klara Rosenquist and Kitt F. Petersen

Diabetes Mellitus

Diabetes mellitus is a metabolic disease characterized by hyperglycemia, resulting from a relative or absolute deficiency of insulin [1]. Type 2 diabetes is the most common chronic metabolic disease in the elderly, affecting ~30 million individuals 65 years of age or older in developed countries [2]. It is estimated that approximately 40% of people over the age of 65 have diabetes or impaired glucose tolerance (IGT) [3, 4] (Fig. 39.1).

The exact pathogenesis of the development of diabetes in the elderly remains unknown; however, epidemiological studies have shown that the transition from the normal state to overt type 2 diabetes in the elderly is typically characterized by deterioration in glucose tolerance [5, 6], which is due to relative or absolute insulinopenia. One current hypothesis holds that muscle insulin resistance develops with aging and leads to increased demand for insulin secretion by the beta cells in order to compensate for the insulin resistance. This continuous high demand for insulin secretion may over time cause beta-cell failure and thereby lead to overt type 2 diabetes. Several studies in the elderly have documented insulin resistance, independent on body weight, and found that insulin concentrations are two- to threefold increase in response to a standard oral glucose tolerance test (OGTT) [7]. The reason for muscle insulin resistance as a consequence of aging is still unclear. However, there is now strong cross-sectional evidence that insulin resistance in muscle can be attributed to accumulation of lipids (specific fatty acid metabolites such as diacylglycerol), which specifically blocks insulin signaling and thereby cause tissue-specific insulin resistance [8–12]. Application of magnetic resonance spectroscopy (MRS) studies to directly measure intramyocellular lipid content (IMCL) in muscle of healthy, normal

weight, sedentary older people has shown that the IMCL content is ~twofold higher in the older individuals when compared with young matched for body mass index and activity [7], suggesting a similar relation between increased IMCL and muscle insulin resistance in older as in young individuals [12]. This lipid accumulation in the muscle cells is likely caused by imbalance between delivery of fatty acids to the muscle call and the rate of oxidation within the cell. In support of this, MRS studies of mitochondrial ATP synthesis and basal rates of substrate oxidation via the tricarboxylic acid (TCA) cycle in vivo in young and elderly subjects have shown that both sides of mitochondrial function are reduced by ~40% in the elderly when compared with the young, suggesting that oxidation of lipids within the muscle is reduced in normal aging and thereby may be contributing to the build-up of lipids inside the muscle cell [7] (Fig. 39.2). Other factors may be involved in causing insulin resistance such as a systemic low-grade inflammation and the release of proinflammatory factors (adipocytokines) from adipose tissue such as adiponectin, IL-6, TNF-alpha, RBP-4, and other inflammatory factors, which are elevated in obesity and in type 2 diabetes [13]. These factors are not likely to be part of the early development of muscle-specific insulin resistance and no abnormalities in any of the adipocytokines have been found in healthy, normal weight, older individuals [7]. It seems likely that increases in adipose tissue mass in obesity and type 2 diabetes may contribute to chronic inflammation and proinflammatory states by increasing the recruitment of macrophages, which in turn, act in a feed forward mechanism to induce the release of proinflammatory cytokines that may contribute to systemic insulin resistance [14].

In this context, no signs of systemic inflammation or elevation of circulating adipocytokines have been consistently found in lean, young, healthy, insulin resistant offspring of parents with type 2 diabetes, a group that has muscle-specific insulin resistance [9, 15, 16], strongly suggesting that inflammation is not a primary factor in the early development of insulin resistance in muscle [15].

The link between muscle insulin resistance and the progression to overt type 2 diabetes is dependent on relative

K. Rosenquist (✉)
Department of Internal Medicine (Endocrinology),
Yale University School of Medicine, 333 Cedar Street,
P.O. Box 208020, New Haven, CT 06520-8020, USA
e-mail: klara.rosenquist@yale.edu

R.A. Rosenthal et al. (eds.), *Principles and Practice of Geriatric Surgery*,
DOI 10.1007/978-1-4419-6999-6_39, © Springer Science+Business Media, LLC 2011

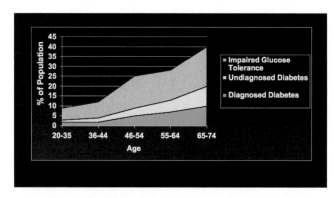

FIGURE 39.1 Prevalence of diabetes and glucose intolerance (reprinted with permission from Harris [4]).

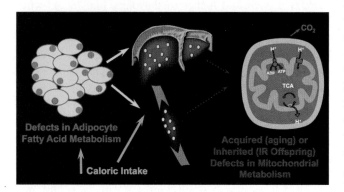

FIGURE 39.2 The road to insulin resistance.

TABLE 39.1 2003 American Diabetes Association diagnostic criteria for diabetes mellitus

Diabetes mellitus

A random serum glucose level ≥200 mg/dL plus classic diabetes symptoms

Fasting glucose level ≥126 mg/dL

Glucose level ≥200 mg/dL at 2 h during a standard OGTT

Impaired glucose tolerance (IGT)

Glucose level ≥140 mg/dL and <200 mg/dL at 2 h during a standard OGTT

Impaired fasting glucose (IFG)

Fasting glucose ≥110 and <126 mg/dL

or actual defects in pancreatic beta-cell function such that insulin secretion is insufficient for the appropriate lowering of postprandial blood glucose. Since pancreatic insulin secretion is a highly energy requiring process, it is currently speculated that reductions in beta-cell mitochondrial function could explain the development of defects in insulin secretion in the elderly and thus explain the high prevalence of diabetes in the elderly [7, 17].

The diagnosis of type 2 diabetes mellitus in young and elderly is similar as outlined by The Diabetes Expert Committee of the American Diabetes Association in 2003 (Table 39.1). The diagnosis is based on meeting one of three criteria: a random plasma glucose of ≥200 mg/dL confirmed on a subsequent day by a fasting plasma glucose (FPG) level

of ≥126 mg/dL, a 2 h plasma glucose of >200 mg/dL using the standardized OGTT (75 g of anhydrous glucose dissolved in water), or a random plasma glucose of ≥200 mg/dL with associated symptoms of polyuria, polydipsia, and unexplained weight loss [1]. The guidelines also distinguish a classification of altered glucose metabolism called impaired fasting glucose (IFG) and IGT to define a category of individuals that are at increased risk of developing diabetes over time. The diagnosis of IFG is made when an individual has FPG concentrations >110 mg/dL but <126 mg/dL, and IGT when 2-h plasma glucose values of the OGTT are ≥140 mg/dL but <200 mg/dL [1].

The ADA recommendations for glucose control are an FPG of 70–130 mg/dL and a hemoglobin$_{A1c}$ (Hb$_{A1c}$) level of <7.0% in adults [18]. According to past epidemiological studies, lowering Hb$_{A1c}$ into a normal range (i.e., <6%) is supposed to be associated with a decreased risk of diabetic complications. However, recently this has been questioned from data suggesting a potential increase in mortality with intense glucose lowering strategies in patients with type 2 diabetes and lowering of Hb$_{A1c}$ to <6% [19]. This study was terminated early given an increase in all causes of mortality of participants (mean age 62) in the intensive therapy group [19]. It is therefore prudent for the clinician to set individualized goals for elderly patients based on history of severe hypoglycemia, cognitive function, life expectancy, and comorbid conditions [18].

Therapeutic management options in elderly individuals are similar to those of younger individuals. As in younger individuals, dietary interventions and lifestyle modifications, including weight loss (medical nutrition therapy or MNT), are the cornerstone of diabetic management [18]. Dietary recommendations suggest weight loss diets for obese individuals, including either low carbohydrate (<130 g/day) or low fat for overall calorie restriction, a diet consisting of low saturated fat (<7% of total calories), a minimum of trans fats intake, and <130 g/day of carbohydrates for all diabetic individuals [18]. An exercise program may have beneficial effects on glucose intolerance, blood pressure control, weight control, lipid profile, and cardiovascular status [3]. Physical activity improves insulin sensitivity by stimulating noninsulin-dependent muscle glucose uptake and increasing substrate oxidation by increasing mitochondrial biogenesis [20, 21] as well as it improves glucose intolerance in diabetic subjects [22]; however, this too should be individualized in elderly patients based on functional status [18].

Medical management and therapeutic options are also similar to the options available in younger individuals. Currently, a number of oral medications are available for the management of older adults with diabetes (Table 39.2). Sulfonylurea drugs are the most widely used. They act initially by increasing pancreatic insulin secretion and later enhance insulin sensitivity, probably via a postreceptor mechanism [23]. Hypoglycemia is the main side effect associated with sulfonylurea drugs.

TABLE 39.2 Currently available oral hypoglycemic agents

Drug	Mechanism of action
Sulfonylureas	Enhances insulin secretion
Second generation	
Glimepiride	
Glipizide, sustained release	
Glyburide	
Glyburide, micronized	
Glimepiride	
α-Glucosidase inhibitor	Slows colonic carbohydrate absorption
Acarbose	
Miglitol	
Biguanide	Decreases hepatic glucose production; improves insulin sensitivity
Metformin	
Thiazolidenedione	Enhances muscle insulin sensitivity
Rosiglitazone	
Pioglitazone	
Nonsulfonylurea	Stimulates insulin secretion
Repaglinide	
Nateglinide	
DPP-4 inhibitor	Prolongs incretin activity
Sitagliptin	

Metformin works primarily by suppressing hepatic glucose production (by suppressing gluconeogenesis) and to a lesser extent by improving insulin sensitivity [24]. Metformin may result in loss of appetite and weight loss, a desirable side effect in obese diabetics. It should be avoided in persons over 80 years of age and should not be used in individuals with either renal insufficiency or heart failure.

The thiazolidinediones (TZDs) is the most recently introduced group of oral antidiabetic agents [25]. These agents function as ligands for nuclear receptor transcription factors (PPARgamma) that regulate genes involved in lipid metabolism and homeostasis. PPARgamma is preferentially expressed in adipose tissue. Activation of PPARgamma leads to adipocyte differentiation and improved insulin signaling of mature adipocytes. Although the main target for action of the TZDs is adipose tissue, their main effect in type 2 diabetes appears to be primarily by enhancing muscle insulin sensitivity [26]. This paradox may be explained by the mechanism of action of TZDs, which are fat cell proliferators and thus by creating more fat cells may act by redistribution of fat from the intramyocellular compartment into fat cells by providing extra storage depots [27]. Muscle insulin resistance in type 2 diabetes (and obesity) is likely caused by intramyocellular accumulation of lipids (certain fatty acids such as diacylglycerol and fatty acyl CoAs), which block intracellular insulin signaling and cause muscle insulin resistance [9, 10]. The TZDs (rosiglitazone and pioglitazone) may be used alone or in combination with other types of antidiabetic drugs such as metformin or sulfonylureas as

well as insulin. The combination of TZDs and metformin for the first time allows for direct targeting of the major pathological defects in type 2 diabetes, reducing hepatic glucose production and increasing muscle insulin sensitivity (stimulating postprandial muscle glucose uptake). The TZDs are generally well tolerated but can, however, cause fluid retention and are therefore contraindicated in patients with class III and IV heart failure [18]. A review of the studies of rosiglitazone led the FDA to conclude that this medication might increase the risk of heart attacks and angina [28], but left the association as inconclusive [29]. Additionally, there is not enough evidence that the risk of heart attack and angina is any greater with rosiglitazone than with other oral medicines used in the treatment of diabetes. Since troglitazone, the first generation of TZDs, was associated with liver injury, that liver enzymes must be measured before starting therapy and periodically thereafter [30].

As type 2 diabetes progresses in older persons adequate glycemic control is associated with an increased risk of adverse effects as a result of age-related changes in drug metabolism. Recently, incretin therapy has become available as novel oral antihyperglycemic treatment, which may prove significant in older persons [31, 32]. Incretins are gut hormones secreted from enteroendocrine cells into the blood within minutes after eating. The two main categories of incretin therapy currently available are: glucagon-like peptide-1 (GLP-1) analogs and inhibitors of GLP-1 degrading enzyme dipeptidyl peptidase-4 (DPP-4). DPP-4 inhibitors are orally active and they increase endogenous blood levels of active incretins, thus leading to prolonged incretin action. The elevated levels of GLP-1 are thought to be the mechanism underlying their blood glucose-lowering effects. There is accumulating evidence that use of incretin therapy, in particular the DPP-4 inhibitors, could offer significant advantages in older persons. Clinical evidence suggests that the DPP-4 inhibitors vildagliptin and sitagliptin are particularly suitable for frail and debilitated elderly patients because of their excellent tolerability profiles [33]. Importantly, these agents lack the gastrointestinal effects associated with metformin and alpha-glucosidase inhibitors taken alone and have a low risk of hypoglycemia. Specifically, sitagliptin has been approved by the US Food and Drug Administration (FDA) for use with diet and exercise to improve glycemic control in adult patients with type 2 diabetes. In randomized, placebo-controlled trials, sitagliptin provided a good treatment option for patients with type 2 diabetes as a monotherapy, or as an adjunct to metformin or a TZD when treatment with either drug alone provided inadequate glucose control [34]. It is also an alternative therapy for those patients who have contraindications or intolerability to other antidiabetic agents [34].

If oral agents are contraindicated or patients fail to respond, insulin is indicated. Physicians should not refrain from initiating insulin therapy in older diabetic patients simply because of age, however, insulin use requires that patients or caregivers have functional visual, motor, and cognitive skills. Most elderly diabetics do well on insulin injections [35], but physicians should regularly check the ability of their elderly patients to appropriately use the insulin syringe. As with all elderly diabetic patients the risk of hypoglycemia must be weighed against the benefits of tight glucose control and the realistic reduction of risk from microvascular complications. The short-term risk of hyperglycemia including poor wound healing, dehydration, and hyperglycemic hyperosmolar coma must also fit into this balance making this a decision that the clinician needs to consider carefully and on an individualized basis.

Substantial education and continuously monitoring for the degree of diabetic control and the development of chronic complications is key to the management of elderly diabetics. In addition to home glucose monitoring and regular assessments of glycosylated hemoglobin, ongoing care should include annual eye examinations, monitoring of renal function, and regular foot care [18].

References

1. Expert committee on the diagnosis and classification of diabetes mellitus (2003) Report of the expert committee on the diagnosis and classification of diabetes mellitus. Diabetes Care 26(Suppl 1): S5–S20
2. King H, Aubert RE, Herman WH (1998) Global burden of diabetes, 1995–2025: prevalence, numerical estimates, and projections. Diabetes Care 21(9):1414–1431
3. Singh I, Marshall MC Jr (1995) Diabetes mellitus in the elderly. Endocrinol Metab Clin North Am 24(2):255–272
4. Harris MI (1993) Undiagnosed NIDDM: clinical and public health issues. Diabetes Care 16(4):642–652
5. Sasaki A, Suzuki T, Horiuchi N (1982) Development of diabetes in Japanese subjects with impaired glucose tolerance: a seven year follow-up study. Diabetologia 22(3):154–157
6. Saad MF, Knowler WC, Pettitt DJ, Nelson RG, Mott DM, Bennett PH (1989) Sequential changes in serum insulin concentration during development of non-insulin-dependent diabetes. Lancet 1(8651):1356–1359
7. Petersen KF, Befroy D, Dufour S et al (2003) Mitochondrial dysfunction in the elderly: possible role in insulin resistance. Science 300(5622):1140–1142
8. Savage DB, Petersen KF, Shulman GI (2007) Disordered lipid metabolism and the pathogenesis of insulin resistance. Physiol Rev 87(2):507–520
9. Dresner A, Laurent D, Marcucci M et al (1999) Effects of free fatty acids on glucose transport and IRS-1-associated phosphatidylinositol 3-kinase activity. J Clin Invest 103(2):253–259
10. Yu C, Chen Y, Cline GW et al (2002) Mechanism by which fatty acids inhibit insulin activation of insulin receptor substrate-1 (IRS-1)-associated phosphatidylinositol 3-kinase activity in muscle. J Biol Chem 277(52):50230–50236
11. Savage DB, Petersen KF, Shulman GI (2005) Mechanisms of insulin resistance in humans and possible links with inflammation. Hypertension 45(5):828–833
12. Krssak M, Falk Petersen K, Dresner A et al (1999) Intramyocellular lipid concentrations are correlated with insulin sensitivity in humans: a 1H NMR spectroscopy study. Diabetologia 42(1):113–116
13. Petersen KF, Dufour S, Feng J et al (2006) Increased prevalence of insulin resistance and nonalcoholic fatty liver disease in Asian-Indian men. Proc Natl Acad Sci USA 103(48):18273–18277
14. Schenk S, Saberi M, Olefsky JM (2008) Insulin sensitivity: modulation by nutrients and inflammation. J Clin Invest 118(9): 2992–3002
15. Petersen KF, Dufour S, Befroy D, Garcia R, Shulman GI (2004) Impaired mitochondrial activity in the insulin-resistant offspring of patients with type 2 diabetes. N Engl J Med 350(7):664–671
16. Perseghin G, Price TB, Petersen KF et al (1996) Increased glucose transport-phosphorylation and muscle glycogen synthesis after exercise training in insulin-resistant subjects. N Engl J Med 335(18):1357–1362
17. Chang AM, Halter JB (2003) Aging and insulin secretion. Am J Physiol Endocrinol Metab 284(1):E7–E12
18. American Diabetes Association (2008) Standards of medical care in diabetes – 2008. Diabetes Care 31(Suppl 1):S12–S54
19. Gerstein HC, Miller ME, Byington RP et al (2008) Effects of intensive glucose lowering in type 2 diabetes. N Engl J Med 358(24):2545–2559
20. Conley KE, Marcinek DJ, Villarin J (2007) Mitochondrial dysfunction and age. Curr Opin Clin Nutr Metab Care 10(6):688–692
21. Hawley JA, Lessard SJ (2008) Exercise training-induced improvements in insulin action. Acta Physiol (Oxf) 192(1):127–135
22. LeBlanc J, Nadeau A, Richard D, Tremblay A (1981) Studies on the sparing effect of exercise on insulin requirements in human subjects. Metabolism 30(11):1119–1124
23. Gerich JE (1989) Oral hypoglycemic agents. N Engl J Med 321(18):1231–1245
24. Hundal RS, Krssak M, Dufour S et al (2000) Mechanism by which metformin reduces glucose production in type 2 diabetes. Diabetes 49(12):2063–2069
25. Fonseca VA, Valiquett TR, Huang SM, Ghazzi MN, Whitcomb RW (1998) Troglitazone monotherapy improves glycemic control in patients with type 2 diabetes mellitus: a randomized, controlled study. The Troglitazone Study Group. J Clin Endocrinol Metab 83(9):3169–3176
26. Petersen KF, Krssak M, Inzucchi S, Cline GW, Dufour S, Shulman GI (2000) Mechanism of troglitazone action in type 2 diabetes. Diabetes 49(5):827–831
27. Mayerson AB, Hundal RS, Dufour S et al (2002) The effects of rosiglitazone on insulin sensitivity, lipolysis, and hepatic and skeletal muscle triglyceride content in patients with type 2 diabetes. Diabetes 51(3):797–802
28. Nissen SE, Wolski K (2007) Effect of rosiglitazone on the risk of myocardial infarction and death from cardiovascular causes. N Engl J Med 356(24):2457–2471
29. Misbin RI (2007) Lessons from the Avandia controversy: a new paradigm for the development of drugs to treat type 2 diabetes. Diabetes Care 30(12):3141–3144
30. Faich GA, Moseley RH (2001) Troglitazone (Rezulin) and hepatic injury. Pharmacoepidemiol Drug Saf 10(6):537–547
31. Holst JJ, Vilsboll T, Deacon CF (2009) The incretin system and its role in type 2 diabetes mellitus. Mol Cell Endocrinol 297(1–2): 127–136
32. Kim W, Egan JM (2008) The role of incretins in glucose homeostasis and diabetes treatment. Pharmacol Rev 60(4):470–512
33. Abbatecola AM, Maggi S, Paolisso G (2008) New approaches to treating type 2 diabetes mellitus in the elderly: role of incretin therapies. Drugs Aging 25(11):913–925
34. Choy M, Lam S (2007) Sitagliptin: a novel drug for the treatment of type 2 diabetes. Cardiol Rev 15(5):264–271
35. Morley JE, Kaiser FE (1990) Unique aspects of diabetes mellitus in the elderly. Clin Geriatr Med 6(4):693–702

Section V
Oral Cavity, Eyes, Ears, Nose and Throat

Chapter 40
Invited Commentary

Frank E. Lucente

It is an honor to participate in this exciting venture by sharing some thoughts and reflections on the changing attitudes and approaches to the care of our elder patients who present with disorders or symptoms in the ear, nose, oral cavity, throat, and eye. Since the publication of the previous volume of this text in 2001, there have unquestionably been advances in the technical capabilities in all of these areas. However, with the population aged over 65 projected to increase from 39 million in 2009 to 70 million in 2020 and with the elderly currently comprising over 40% of medical specialty care, we have a mandate to include training in all medical and surgical aspects of geriatric care in our programs in undergraduate, graduate, and continuing medical education.

Disorders of the head and neck region are high on the list of geriatric impairments that threaten patients' viability and reduce their quality of life, including hearing loss, dizziness and vertigo, tinnitus, swallowing disorders, nasal respiratory disorders, loss of smell, loss of voice, reduction in vision, and neoplasms of this area. The authors of the following five chapters have done a superb job of discussing the substantive developments and advances in the provision of specialty care to the elderly and presenting many recommendations for care of specific medical issues in the head and neck region. I salute them for their achievements.

Looking back over my 40 year career in clinical otolaryngology, I am grateful for having had the opportunity to observe the advances in care of so many diseases that affect the elderly. In the area of head-and-neck cancer, we have seen the development of the multidisciplinary approach to tumor management with tremendous strides in surgery, radiation oncology, and medical oncology. The post-surgical rehabilitation of the cancer patient has also improved greatly through the introduction of reconstructive regional flaps and other techniques. In the area of otology, we have seen the development of cochlear implants and other devices and techniques that have restored hearing to thousands of elderly patients to whom we previously had little to offer. The development of functional endoscopic sinus surgery has brought relief to millions of elderly patients suffering from chronic rhinosinusitis. Finally, the incredible growth of the specialty of facial plastic and reconstructive surgery has enabled us to rejuvenate many elderly patients who have a strong desire for improved cosmetic appearance of the face and neck. Of course, these advances have not been without controversy as the profession attempts to balance its capabilities with the community's ability to afford them.

One of the most pressing challenges in this area is to assess the relevance of traditional ethical principles to the provision of compassionate and cost-effective care. We have generally been guided by three traditional ethical principles: *Beneficence*: Do only what is good for the patient but no harm. *Autonomy*: The patient has the right to decide what is best for her/himself. *Justice*: The rights of the individual need to be considered in the light of what is best for society as a whole.

In assessing the relationship between what is best for a single patient and what is best for society, a common challenge in the practice of many geriatric specialties, one confronts the issue of the so-called "technological imperative." This refers to the notion that "everything that can be done must be done." We frequently have to examine the use of procedures in patients with limited life expectancy as well as to assess screening programs that are used to identify diseases that are not likely to be treated because of the age of the patient.

As I look back over a 40-year period in training, practice, teaching, and administration as mentioned above, I am impressed with how our attitudes to care for the elderly have changed. As medical students in 1968, we studied and participated in the care of numerous geriatric patients but the focus was on their specific diseases, rather than on their geriatric status. In 1968, life expectancy for an American man was 67 years and for an American woman it was 74 years. In 2009, life expectancy for the man has increased to almost 76 years and for the woman to almost 81 years. Perhaps more

F.E. Lucente (✉)
Department of Otolaryngology, Downstate Medical Center, State University of New York, 450 Clarkson Avenue, Box 126, Brooklyn, NY 11203, USA
e-mail: Lucente@aol.com

importantly, US National Center for Health Statistics data show that the average number of years of life remaining for the current 75 year-old man is 11 and for the 75 year-old woman is 13. In other words, people are living significantly past the period in which they are contributing to the tax base that is supporting them and increased longevity has raised many financial and logistical issues.

One of the most critical ethical and socioeconomic challenges in this area relates to access for care for millions of elderly. Although the difficulties that confront physicians and surgeons in dealing with office and hospital costs are undeniable, it is discouraging to read numerous reports of denial of care to those unable to pay. While there are many wealthy elderly patients who can and should pay for their care, there are far more who struggle to pay more than Medicare covers. It is disheartening to hear so many reports of physicians closing their doors to these elderly patients. This is an ironic situation as these same physicians received their salary support from Medicare during their residency and without such support they would have had tremendous financial debts.

There is no easy resolution for this difficult situation. Physicians are bearing the burden of increasing costs of practice, including compliance with new regulations that appropriately focus on safe and expeditious patient care, as well as on HIPAA regulations that propose to protect patient confidentiality. However, at the same time, they are frequently seeing reductions in reimbursement for the best care that they can provide. Even the most well-intentioned and competent physician is stressed to provide cost-effective care to all patients who reach out to him/her.

As we confront the issue of access to care, we might note that even Hippocrates (466–377 B.C.) had some cogent observations. In "Precepts", Part 6 he wrote, "Sometimes give your services for nothing, calling to mind a previous benefactor or a present satisfaction. And if there be an opportunity of serving one who is a stranger in financial straits, give full assistance to all such. For where there is love of such, there is also love of art. For some patients, though conscious that their condition is perilous, recover their health simply through their contentment with the goodness of the physician" [1].

Another cogent guideline for addressing the ethical issues in geriatric care of the head-and-neck patients is found in the writings of the eighteenth century German philosopher, Immanuel Kant. His 1785 publication, Groundwork of the Metaphysics of Morals included his articulation of the "categorical imperative" in which he states, "Act only according to the maxim whereby you can at the same time will that it should become a universal law" [2]. If we were to follow his advice, we might view our work with our elderly patients in a different light and find it easier to cope with the challenges posed by the geriatric community.

References

1. Hippocrates (1868) Hippocrates: precepts, part 6. In: Jones WHS (ed) Hippocrates collected works I, Harvard University Press, Cambridge, p 236
2. Kant I Fundamental principles of the metaphysic of morals (http://philosophy.eserver.org/kant/metaphys-of-morals.txt)

Chapter 41
Changes in the Oral Cavity with Age

Susan Pugliese and Ajay R. Kashi

Alterations in oral motor functions in aging

Parameter	Changes with age
Lip posture	Drooling, angular cheilosis
Muscles of mastication	Efficiency of mastication
Tongue function	Speech, dysphagia, traumatic bite injury, snoring, sleep apnea
Swallowing	Dysphagia, regurgitation, choking
Taste	Dysgeusia, ageusia
Salivation	No significant changes in healthy older patients

Source: Reprinted with permission from Otomo-Corgel [7]. Copyright Elsevier (1996)

Introduction

Oral health and it's implications to one's overall health is often overlooked as insignificant or unimportant by the general population as well as the ever increasing geriatric population. The condition of the anatomical structures in the oral cavity (e.g., tongue, palate, teeth, and gums) can reflect the general health status of an individual. Although many pathologies alter the normal flora of the oral cavity in all age groups, older individuals typically present with certain changes in their oral cavity which are normal for their age [1]. Physicians and dental practitioners must be aware of pathologic findings versus normal findings in the oral cavity that are consistent with aging. Oral changes in the geriatric population have widespread implications ranging from the physical to the psychological and social well being of the individual.

It has been reported, for example, that the general prevalence of oral mucosal disease increases in the elderly population [2]. Pre-existing systemic conditions and changes in the oral cavity can influence surgical procedures and treatment outcomes in this age group. Elective surgical procedures typically require a thorough knowledge of the patients' current

medical status and the past medical history. The oral health status should be a vital part of the overall preoperative assessment of the geriatric general surgical patient. The inclusion of the oral status evaluation would in many cases prevent preoperative, intraoperative, and post operative delays and complications. This chapter discusses changes seen in the oral cavity of the geriatric sub-population. It is well documented that the geriatric population is growing in number. In the United States, people are living longer with and without chronic ailments requiring surgical intervention. In 1900, 3.1 million people or 4% of the population were 65 years or older; by 2005, this number had increased to 34.3 million people or 12.4% of the population, a tenfold increase in number [1]. In view of these statistics, this chapter is written to highlight and guide the general surgeon to some of the most common oral findings and their surgical implications in the geriatric population.

Changes Associated with Aging in the Oral Cavity

The advent of geriatric status in life is associated with changes in the oral cavity including xerostomia, worsening periodontal disease, and oral neoplasms. These changes affect the individual's physical, mental, and social status. For instance, the loss of teeth makes it difficult for communication, thus isolating the individual from his/her usual social environment. An altered motor performance is noticed in older individuals, for example, in lip posture, tongue function, swallowing and masticatory muscle function [3, 4]. Some of the consequences of altered tongue function in older individuals include difficulties in speech, dysphagia, traumatic bite injury, and nocturnal mouth breathing that can lead to a form of sleep apnea. Further, authors have previously reported that difficulty in swallowing can lead to laryngeal food penetration, regurgitation, and sometimes fatal choking [3]. These previously mentioned symptoms need to be taken into account before planning surgical procedures in the elderly.

A comprehensive oral examination performed prior to any surgical procedure(s) in geriatric patients can help to minimize

S. Pugliese (✉)
Department of Dentistry, University Hospital of Brooklyn, State University of New York, Downstate Medical Center, 450 Clarkson Ave., Brooklyn, NY 11203, USA
e-mail: susan.pugliese@downstate.edu

R.A. Rosenthal et al. (eds.), *Principles and Practice of Geriatric Surgery*,
DOI 10.1007/978-1-4419-6999-6_41, © Springer Science+Business Media, LLC 2011

complications during the surgery and the post-operative recovery period (this will also minimize the chances for aspiration, choking, hemorrhage, and regurgitation). In a study by Meurman et al. [5], it was reported that the majority of elderly individuals (~70% of 191; age range from 67 to 96 years) living at home before hospitalization showed dentogenic infection foci as evident from panoramic X-rays, although their infections did not correlate with infection parameters of blood. It was also noted from this study that the majority (96%) of dentate individuals had a poor periodontal condition, and edentulous individuals had positive yeast counts when compared to dentate individuals (84.4% vs. 66.1%, $P<0.05$) [5].

Tooth mobility, if left untreated, can lead to periodontal pocket formation between the tooth surface and gingival tissues. Further, this can lead to food accumulation and subsequent colonization by bacteria causing localized infection with the potential for wider systemic infections (e.g., cardiac valvular disease from oral bacterial colonization). The oral mucosa becomes more sensitive to mechanical damage as age progresses [6]. This may lead to easy bruising, either from minimal trauma (e.g., from sharp edges of denture margins) or nutritional deficiencies. Furthermore, it is also important to note that easy bruising of tissues can delay post-operative wound healing, thus emphasizing the need to take steps to minimize trauma during any surgical procedure. Missing teeth, dry mouth, and ill-fitting dentures can lead to a lack of social interaction in the elderly. If treatments to these underlying causes are not provided, it can lead to a severe lack of confidence and depression. Some of the common changes seen in the oral cavity of elderly patients are presented in the physiology table at the opening of this chapter [7].

Oral Manifestations of Systemic Disorders

Systemic diseases that most commonly affect older adults in the developed world are arthritis, cancer, chronic obstructive pulmonary diseases, diabetes, heart disease, hypertension, mental health conditions, osteoporosis, Parkinson's disease, and stroke [1]. Oral manifestations of systemic disorders and the drugs used to treat them can influence surgical treatments in the elderly. Further explanation of some of the commonly encountered systemic disorders and their consequences on treatment decisions is discussed.

Musculoskeletal Disorders: Osteoarthritis, Rheumatoid Arthritis, Osteoporosis

According to the World Health Organization, osteoarthritis will become the fourth leading cause of disability worldwide by 2020 [8]. Authors have reported that the strongest risk factor for osteoarthritis is age [9]. Some of the other risk factors include an increase in body weight, mechanical trauma, and laxity of the surrounding ligaments. It has been reported that almost half of the population older than 65 years of age suffers from arthritis [1]. One of the major reasons for the progression of osteoarthritis is the inability or decreased ability of the damaged cartilage to repair following injury. Secondary effects of osteoarthritis in the hands include difficulty in maintaining oral hygiene as a consequence of pain and impaired functional ability. This can lead to increased incidence of dental caries and periodontal disease in the elderly. Poor periodontal health is also known to contribute toward higher chances of systemic infections, thus having the potential for post-operative complications.

Presence of pain and lack of mobility can prevent people with osteoarthritis from visiting their dentist for routine oral healthcare. Most likely, a patient with arthritis or other musculoskeletal disorder will be consuming one or more medications to treat their illness. Typically, this can include pain killers, muscle relaxants, and drugs that prevent bone loss. Dental considerations in patients with musculoskeletal disorders range from the appropriate selection of drugs to helping patients with their oral hygiene needs. Simple steps including designing toothbrushes with large handles or encouraging patients to use electric toothbrushes can be beneficial in maintaining oral health. It has been reported that before invasive surgical procedures, corticosteroids and antibiotics need to be considered in elderly patients [1]. However, these drugs should be used with caution due to their systemic effects in the elderly.

Another important and common musculoskeletal disorder that affects the elderly includes osteoporosis. Dental considerations in osteoporosis include anecdotal reports of a side effect from the introduction of a recent class of drugs known as bisphosphonates to treat osteoporosis. These side effects include osteonecrosis of the lower jaw in some patients who are consuming this class of drugs and have undergone invasive dental procedures, although this clinical symptom has been reported to be more common in patients who are being treated for malignant diseases and who have received high-dose intravenous bisphosphonate therapy [10–12]. The exact mechanism that is responsible for the osteonecrosis seen in the jaws is yet to be ascertained and further clinical investigations and research needs to be carried out to better understand this important side effect. Before planning surgical procedures in elderly patients, it is important to consider the side effects and/or other drug interactions if patients are using this drug.

Cardiovascular Disease and Oral Health in the Elderly

Coronary heart disease was and remains the most likely cause of death in the geriatric population in the USA [1].

Oral health is correlated with initiation and/or progression of many cardiovascular pathologies (e.g., infective endocarditis), along with other factors. Poor periodontal health is one of the reasons for loss of teeth in the geriatric population, and for the colonization of oral pathogens on cardiac valves. Several etiologic factors including family history, lack of exercise, high cholesterol, smoking, and genetic factors contribute to cardiovascular disease. From a perspective of dentistry, people with fewer teeth generally prefer chewy foods including red meat and cakes, and avoid crunchy foods (e.g., carrots and dry breads) [13]. Further, high calorie, high fat foods can lead to higher chances of obesity and coronary heart disease in this population segment. Thus, it can be inferred that tooth loss, while not directly related to cardiovascular disease, has a significant secondary effect in terms of leading to cardiovascular disease (i.e., by choosing foods that are high in fat content). From a general surgical perspective, it is essential to be aware of the patient's general systemic health including their cardiac condition. Basic diagnostic tests including blood pressure, EKG recordings, and chest X-rays should be routine practice before invasive dental and surgical procedures are carried out in the elderly. Patients with certain cardiovascular conditions are typically required to take antibiotics prescribed by the American Heart Association and/or the American Dental Association before invasive dental procedures (e.g., deep scaling of roots, tooth extractions, periodontal/oral surgical procedures) [2, 3]. The complete list of medications including the recommended dosage and regime(s) is available from the published literature [14, 15]. Wilson et al. [15] advocate improved access to dental care and oral health in patients with underlying cardiac conditions that may be associated with increased risk of adverse outcomes from infective endocarditis (e.g., valvular heart disease). This will help to minimize the chance of infection in the surgical patient.

Diabetes and the Oral Cavity in the Elderly

There are more than 20 million individuals affected by diabetes mellitus in the USA [16]. The incidence of adult-onset (Type II) type of diabetes is more prevalent in people over the age of 50 years. The oral cavity is often reflective of signs suggestive of diabetes mellitus, some of which include multiple periodontal abscesses and slower wound healing following extractions or other oral surgical procedures. Full-mouth intra-oral periapical radiographs will usually reveal the presence of multiple periodontal abscesses in the diabetic patient. Furthermore, other soft tissue condition including candidiasis is more prevalent in the oral cavity of diabetics with poor glycemic control and denture use [16]. It is mandatory that blood sugar levels be determined before any invasive surgical procedure(s) in the elderly as it can

directly affect the duration of post-operative healing in addition to helping prevent complications (e.g., post-operative wound infections).

Mental Health Conditions and the Oral Cavity in the Elderly

Mental disorders constitute a range of serious illnesses. Among them, some of the important ones that warrant discussion include Alzheimer's and Parkinson's disease as these conditions mostly affect the elderly.

Alzheimer's Disease

Alzheimer's disease mostly affects the elderly population. It is the most common type of dementia and was first described by Alois Alzheimer in 1907. The incidence of Alzheimer's includes approximately 10% of older adults over 65 years of age and 45% over 85 years of age; the prevalence of this disease is expected to double by 2020 given the aging population in the USA [17, 18]. The cause of Alzheimer's remains unknown, although there are some reports implicating the loss of cholinergic neurons. Risk factors can include age, family history of dementia, and the presence of both ApoE4 alleles. Table 41.1 describes the signs and symptoms of Alzheimer's disease and the recommended dental management.

It has been reported that one-half of all patients with Alzheimer's need help with their personal care, and one third are eventually hospitalized [17]. Friedlander et al., mention that an inability to perform appropriate oral hygiene practices mainly results from impaired cognition, apraxia, and apathy in the middle stages of the disease. The authors also mention that there can be marked hyposalivation in these patients, especially localized to the submandibular salivary gland, and this can lead to symptoms of xerostomia [17]. The aim of dental treatment in Alzheimer's disease is to provide a realistic or meaningful solution to the patient's problems that can influence their quality of life positively. Simple procedures including taking care of sharp or jagged tooth/teeth and dentures can be more important initially than restoring carious teeth, as this might arouse intense anxiety in Alzheimer's patients. Complex dental procedures including tooth extractions and restorative dental procedures need to be carefully planned in such patients.

Several drugs that are routinely used in dentistry have been known to interact with drugs used to treat Alzheimer's. For instance, Alzheimer's drugs including Aricept (Donepezil), Razadyne (Galantamine), and Exelon (Rivastigmine) have been known to interact with non-steroidal anti-inflammatory drugs (NSAIDs) by increasing the chances for gastrointestinal

Table 41.1 Stages of Alzheimer's disease, signs, symptoms and dental considerations

Disease stage	Signs and symptoms	Dental findings	Dental management
Early stage	Reduced ability to follow instructions on the job, driving, shopping and housekeeping; require constant reminders	Changes in the oral cavity (e.g., coronal and root caries, plaque buildup) can be seen if the patient is unable to remember routine activities including maintenance of oral hygiene (i.e., brushing and flossing)	Routine dental treatment can be provided in most patients, aggressive preventive dentistry program (e.g., 3 month recall, oral examinations, prophylaxis, fluoride gel application, adjustment of prostheses)
Middle stage	Inability to work, easy to get confused, language impairment including comprehension and naming of objects, inability to do simple calculations, to tell time and loss of simple motor skills such as eating, dressing and solving simple puzzles; requires daily supervision	High incidence of xerostomia from antipsychotic medications, dry mouth, mucosal lesions, candidiasis, plaque and calculus buildup, periodontal disease, root caries, and high chances for aspiration pneumonia	Main focus of treatment should include maintaining dental status and minimizing deterioration, aggressive preventive dentistry program
Advanced stage	Patients may become rigid, incontinent, bedridden, present with generalized seizures; often require nursing care and supervision	High incidence of xerostomia from antipsychotic medications, dry mouth, mucosal lesions, candidiasis, plaque and calculus buildup, periodontal disease, root caries and high chances for aspiration pneumonia	Short appointments, non complex procedures; sedation (e.g., benzodiazepines) can be used for complex and tedious dental procedures, aggressive preventive dentistry program

(GI) bleeding and irritation. Other commonly used drugs in dentistry (e.g., Aspirin, Codeine, Clarithromycin, Erythromycin, and Opioid analgesics) have been reported to interact with drugs that are used to treat Alzheimer's disease [17]. It is best for the dentist to consult with the patient's physician to determine the level of cognition and ability to provide consent, to get information related to other underlying medical conditions (e.g., heart disease, diabetes, hypertension), and to complete a drug history before providing dental treatment and certifying that the patient is fit to undergo general surgical procedures.

Stroke

Stroke is the acute onset of neurological deficits persisting for at least 24 h. Two thirds of strokes occur in people over the age of 65 years and about 8% of the US population above 65 years of age has a history of stroke [1, 19]. Stroke or cerebrovascular accident is a serious medical condition that can have adverse effects on an individual's overall systemic health. The primary effects of these diseases might not be visible in the oral cavity, although they can have secondary effects in terms of deterioration of oral health status because of an inability to maintain oral health. This is mostly observed on the side of the face affected by stroke, as the individual lacks manual dexterity to maneuver the oral cleansing devices to clean their teeth. Some of the specific changes that can be seen in the oral cavity include halitosis, tooth decay, root caries, gingivitis, periodontal infections, and fungal infections (e.g., candidiasis). It is very important to emphasize that

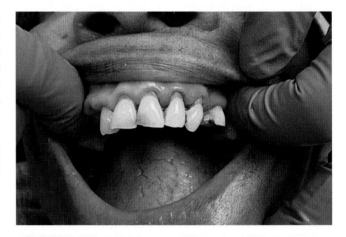

Figure 41.1 Root caries, partial edentulism, and gingival recession in an elderly patient.

patients with these diseases need special attention for their oral healthcare needs. MacDonald mentions that the incidence of root caries increases almost eightfold in patients with neurodegenerative disorders when compared to others living within the same community (Fig. 41.1) [20].

The dental professional will have to differentiate between a true deterioration of oral health (from a conscious lack of maintenance of oral health) and secondary oral health effects from an underlying illness (e.g., stroke, Alzheimer's). In the former scenario, patient education might work to reverse poor oral health, whereas the latter case will need special care in terms of assistance to care for an individual's oral health. During dental treatment, it is especially important in patients with stroke to ensure that foreign bodies are not aspirated into the pharynx as they might lack sensation on a particular side of their body and hence not have a normal gag reflex. Simple steps including talking to the patient slowly and not using complex language can be helpful. In addition, it is better to schedule dental appointments during the mid-morning in these patients [1]. It is important to note that elective and invasive dental procedures are generally deferred for a period of about 3 months following a stroke. This needs to be considered in a surgical treatment protocol, where the surgeon might need the patient to have dental treatment prior to a planned surgery.

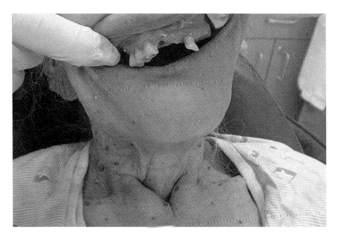

Figure 41.2 Oral cavity of a 78-year-old malnourished female patient. Note the poor periodontal condition of the teeth.

Nutritional Status and Dental Health in the Elderly

The nutritional status of elderly individuals is often compromised when compared to their younger counterparts due to a variety of reasons, including a higher incidence of systemic illnesses (e.g., diabetes) and medications that suppress the immune system. The overall nutritional status of an individual depends on a number of factors. For instance, it is known that gastrointestinal motility/health can be maintained with fiber in the diet and it has been reported that the presence of teeth will help with fiber intake [21]. However, it can be challenging for edentulous patients to chew fibrous foods, thus leading to higher chances of an imbalance in their general systemic health. Softening of foods (e.g., vegetables and fruits to assist with chewing in edentulous patients) can lead to denaturation of important nutrients including Vitamin C. In the long-term, this can lead to systemic illnesses including scurvy. Thus, Vitamin C deficiency can be correlated to the number of teeth present in the oral cavity. It has also been reported that Vitamin C remains one of the key nutrients that are missing in edentulous elderly individuals [21]. Figure 41.2 shows the oral cavity of a malnourished female patient, aged 78 years with a medical history of hypertension, dysphagia, diabetes mellitus, and psychiatric symptoms including depression and dementia. In addition to pain, she was unable to eat due to chronic periodontal disease and tooth mobility.

Edentulous conditions, when coupled with poor nutrition can have other consequences including bone resorption (more rapidly in the mandible when compared to the maxilla) (Fig. 41.3). This makes it difficult to fabricate stable mandibular dentures. Studies have shown that edentulous elderly patients generally consume less nutritious foods, particularly less protein, intrinsic and milk sugars, calcium, non-heme iron, niacin, and Vitamin C when compared to dentate people [21]. In order to improve wound healing following surgery, it is important to include nutritional supplements (e.g., multivitamin tablets, medications to improve the

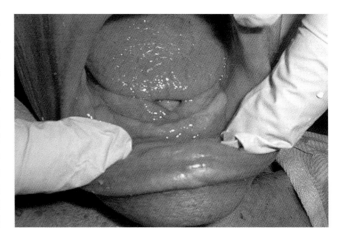

Figure 41.3 Complete edentulism of mandibular arch with resorption of the alveolar ridge in an elderly patient.

hemoglobin content of the blood) in the diets of the elderly. It must also be noted that a balanced diet tailored to elderly patients based on their chewing capability needs to be ensured post-operatively.

Aspiration Pneumonia

Aspiration pneumonia deserves special discussion because of the high chance of infection of the lungs from aspiration of oral contents and/or foreign objects in the geriatric population. This can occur as a result of higher incidence of dysphagia, stroke, and other neurological disorders in the geriatric surgical patient. Another important etiology for aspiration pneumonia includes accidental avulsion and aspiration of teeth from anesthetic intubation procedures during the pre-operative surgical preparation. Possible routes of entry for the avulsed teeth can include the trachea to enter the lungs or the esophagus to enter the stomach. Appropriate emergency measures including locating the tooth/teeth from chest or abdominal X-rays and their aspiration or surgical removal must be performed immediately. This is especially important in elderly patients to avoid pneumonia.

Aspiration pneumonia can lead to serious complications in elderly patients due to reduced ability to cope with illness from a higher likelihood of being immunocompromised. From a surgical perspective, it is important to note that aspiration pneumonia can lead to serious complications postoperatively (for instance, during the recovery period), and aspiration of oral contents including dried salivary debris has been known to cause infections and morbidity. One of the most common and often ignored changes (in the oral cavity) in older individuals is increased tooth mobility. Increased tooth mobility (usually associated with periodontal infections) in the elderly is associated with higher mortality as there is a greater chance for aspiration pneumonia.

The relationship between oral health and the mortality from pneumonia in an elderly Japanese population has been studied [22]. In this study, the authors evaluated 697 individuals (277 males and 420 females) who were 80 years old in 1997. The study results were documented between 1998 and 2002, during which 180 of the study patients died. According to their results, the adjusted mortality due to pneumonia was 3.9 times higher in persons with ten or more teeth with a probing depth exceeding 4 mm (periodontal pocket) than in those without periodontal pockets [22]. Some of the other findings reported from this study indicate that the number of Candida species on the lingual surface was much higher in those who died of pneumonia when compared to other participants [22]. This may be attributed to the possibility of an immunocompromised state in this age group, leading to resistance against virulent bacteria (mostly anaerobic gram-negative bacteria) and subsequent colonization by opportunistic pathogens including Candida.

Saliva

Diminished reserve capacity of individual organs (e.g., kidneys, gut, respiratory, and salivary glands) is an age-dependent phenomenon [23–25]. A loss of acinar cells of the salivary glands takes place with age although the salivary flow rate is maintained [23, 26, 27]. These findings might not have any adverse consequences during normal function, but they can become important in situations common to surgical patients: during physiologically stressful circumstances including surgery, with disease, and with intake of pharmacologic agents (e.g., anticholinergic drugs) that can compro-

mise the reserve capacity of salivary glands [23]. Reduced salivary volume can lead to a compromise of its rheological properties and consequent decrease in its ability to moisten the oral cavity and teeth. This can be a predisposing/contributing factor for rapid rise in the incidence of dental caries, infections and dry mouth.

Xerostomia

Xerostomia is also commonly known as "dry mouth." Although xerostomia can manifest at any age, it has been reported that this symptom is especially prevalent in the elderly population, particularly over the age of 65 years [28, 29]. Some authors suggest that approximately 25–30% of the population over the age of 65 years is affected by complaints of dry mouth [29, 30]. The sensation of dry mouth in the elderly is related to the use of drugs, radiotherapy, and autoimmune diseases including Sjogren's syndrome [27]. Among these previously mentioned causes for xerostomia, drugs are known to have significant effects when compared to the other two conditions. Clinicians have suggested causes for xerostomia [28], although the main etiologic factor remains idiopathic in nature. A reduction in the number of acini and an increase in the amount of fatty and fibrous tissues as age increases has been reported earlier by investigators [30]. However, Ship and Turner et al., have mentioned that healthy adults (i.e., without any complaints of systemic disease) remain relatively free from complaints of dry mouth [28, 29, 31].

Xerostomia needs be considered as a significant clinical complaint in the elderly because of its potential to affect an individual's daily activities. Thus, this clinical symptom needs to be given consideration in the overall treatment plan in the geriatric surgical patient. For instance, daily activities including wearing of dentures can be painful in patients with xerostomia. Furthermore, speaking and eating certain types of foods can also be a challenge in patients with xerostomia; this can also lead to psychological effects on the individual including a lack of social interaction [32].

Oral Mucosal Lesions in the Elderly

It is common to encounter mucosal lesions in the elderly, as the general immune response and healing capability of geriatric patients are poorer when compared to their younger counterparts. Aggressive treatment including patient education must be emphasized to treat and prevent oral mucosal lesions in the elderly, as this can also affect the general

TABLE 41.2   Oral mucous membrane lesions in the elderly

Problem	Cause	Treatment
Mucositis/glossitis	Systemic disease (e.g., diabetes, hematologic disease/anemia/leukemia, chronic mouth breathing) Nutritional deficiencies (especially Vit B complexes) Adverse drug reactions (e.g., aspirin, antibiotics, phenacetin)	Complete blood count and Vit B_{12} evaluation Rule out xerostomia Palliative mouthwash prescription, diphenhydramine (Benadryl)/kaolin (Kaopectate) in equal parts, 1-min rinse, then expectorate; or lidocaine (Xylocaine viscous) 2%
Infection from immunosuppression Candidiasis	Systemic disease (diabetes, leukemia) xerostomia Immunosuppression (prolonged steroid use) antibiotic or antineoplastic medications, ill-fitting prostheses	Improved oral hygiene Antifungal medications

Source: Reprinted with permission from Otomo-Corgel [7]. Copyright Elsevier (1996)

systemic health and surgical treatment decisions. A list of some of the commonly seen oral mucosal lesions in the elderly is shown in Table 41.2.

The incidence of oral neoplasms also increases with age. Some of the common etiological factors include a history of smoking, drinking, chewing tobacco, and genetic factors. It is important to note that many neoplasms are initially noticed in the oral cavity and can be an evidence of metastasis from other sites. Often, these tumors require dissection that can be disfiguring and alter oral function, thus affecting the general systemic health as well as the psychological state of the geriatric patient.

Opportunistic Infections

Opportunistic infections are quite common because of underlying factors including higher rates of systemic illnesses (e.g., diabetes) and a suppressed immune system in the geriatric population. Some of the commonly seen opportunistic infections in the oral cavity include candidiasis and oral manifestations of human immunodeficiency virus (HIV).

Candidiasis

In the United States, the three most common reasons for referrals by general dentists of older adults with oral mucosal lesions are suspected malignant lesions, inflammatory vesicular lesions and candidiasis [33, 34]. Candidal infection is an extremely common and often unnoticed condition in the geriatric general surgical patient (Fig. 41.4). Oral candidiasis is commonly encountered among denture wearers, in debilitation, diabetes, anemia, in those receiving chemotherapy or local irradiation, in patients consuming corticosteroids, or broad–spectrum antibiotics, and smoking [14, 35].

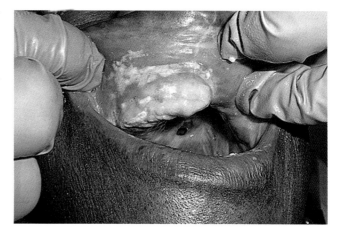

FIGURE 41.4   Oral candidiasis in a 58-year-old male operated for removal of squamous cell carcinoma of the palate. This patient was undergoing post-operative radiotherapy of the jaws along with chemotherapy.

It is also seen as a manifestation of other serious illnesses including HIV.

The fungus responsible for candidal infections is a normal part of the oral flora. It is overgrowth of these organisms (mostly due to a suppressed immune state) that leads to pathology which is often manifested by white, red, or white and red surface changes. It often appears under a denture as an acutely inflamed area in the exact shape of the denture or as white cheese like lesions that can be removed with a tongue blade. Candidiasis can be painful along with symptoms of halitosis and alterations in taste (dysgeusia). It occurs frequently due to improper denture use and maintenance, thus making it hard to diagnose and treat this condition effectively. There is a high likelihood that patients are unaware that they have this condition, although it can be long standing. In severe cases, it can be erosive and quite painful. Motor and cognitive skills are often diminished in the geriatric population, thus making it difficult to treat oral candidiasis as the treatments might require active participation on the patient's part.

CASE STUDY

A 58-year-old male patient that was referred to the dental clinic following surgery of the maxilla and palate for resection of squamous cell carcinoma is described. The tumor had invaded the left portion of the maxilla, hard and soft palates, left pterygomaxillary space, and the wall of the maxillary sinus. The patient's personal history included smoking for a period of 33 years and drinking, while his medical history included anemia and hypertension. He was operated for removal of the tumor mass, following which he was receiving radiation and chemotherapy. A communication between the palate and the maxillary sinus was present from the surgical procedure (Fig 41.4). This patient was referred to the dental clinic for an oral examination and rehabilitation of his oral cavity. During the oral examination, white patchy discoloration was observed, mainly on the upper borders of the maxillary arch and palatal regions (Fig. 41.4); a clinical diagnosis of candidal infection was made. Clinical diagnosis of candidal infection(s) can be confirmed with a smear or culture [34]. The clinical

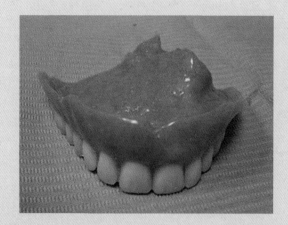

Figure 41.5 Maxillary denture incorporating the obturator to seal the communication between the oral cavity and orbit for speech and nutrition in a 58-year-old patient operated for removal of a tumor.

management of this patient included immediate and aggressive treatment of his candidal infection, fabrication of an obturator (Fig. 41.5) to close the communication between the oral cavity and the nasal cavity, educating the patient about denture care and the importance of maintaining oral hygiene.

Further, in patients with complicated medical/surgical histories, it is important to address systemic symptoms when providing treatment for the dental symptoms. For instance, radiation and chemotherapy will have the potential to further suppress the immune system in these patients, and hence, recurrent fungal infections including candidiasis are more prevalent in these individuals. Routine dental checkups are vital to ensure that the oral cavity is free from infection. The patient's physician should be part of the decision making team along with the dentist to provide the best available treatment.

It is important to note that the most common causes of a candidal overgrowth leading to infection are hyposalivation, high blood and salivary glucose, immune suppression, and the use of corticosteroids and antibiotics. Immunosuppressed patients are particularly predisposed to systemic, invasive infections of candidiasis. The gastrointestinal tract, trachea, lungs, liver, kidneys, and central nervous system are all potential sites for infection in disseminated systemic candidiasis and may result in septicemia, meningitis, hepatosplenic disease, and endocarditis [4]. It is important to identify the primary cause (whether it is denture related, drug related, or from an immunocompromised systemic state) and extent (local or systemic) of the infection before any treatment recommendations are made. In the case of localized infections, it is essential that the oral cavity be treated first to prevent recontamination of the tissues by the denture.

Treatment of oral candidiasis can be topical or systemic. The clinician might choose one mode over the other best treatment option based on the location and extent of the infection or immune status of the patient. Topical treatment generally includes Nystatin oral suspension: 100,000 U/ml, 5 cc swish and spit or swish and swallow (if pharyngeal involvement is suspected) for 14 days. This should be performed after meals and before going to bed. An alternative topical treatment for oral candidiasis is Clotrimazole troches, 10 mg, dissolved in the mouth five times a day for 14 days, taking care not to eat or drink for half an hour after ingestion. Systemic treatment for *Candida* includes either of the following antifungal medications: Nizoral (Ketoconazole) tablets, 200 mg, once daily with meal for 14 days, Diflucan (Fluconazole) tablets, 100 mg, two tablets stat followed by one tablet daily for 14 days, or Sporanox (Itraconazole) tablets, 100 mg, twice daily with meals for 14 days.

Oral hygiene and denture hygiene are essential to the resolution of the candidal infection. Simple steps including reminding patients never to sleep with dentures in their mouths (this gives the tissue in the oral cavity time for aeration) can be helpful in preventing future infections. The dentures should be thoroughly cleaned daily by soaking them in 1% sodium hypochlorite solution for 15 min followed by rinsing with running water for 2 min before sleeping [36]. It is prior to surgery that the geriatric patients may not be as capable cognitively and physiologically of responding to a fungal infection. Thus, it becomes essential that treatment be thorough and complete prior to surgery. This will prevent post operative complications and the possibility of an overwhelming systemic candidal infection.

Human Immunodeficiency Virus

The general surgeon will encounter a greater number of geriatric patients with HIV, either those newly infected or those with the virus as a chronic illness (the benefit of highly active antiretroviral therapy, or HAART). Furthermore, it has long been recognized that patients with HIV or AIDS will at some point in their disease progression or its chronic state exhibit one or more oral manifestations of the disease. It has been reported that as many as 90% of individuals with AIDS will eventually experience one or more oral lesions [37]. The presence of an oral lesion in the HIV patient can be an indicator of a high viral load or failing drug therapy that may need to be addressed prior to surgery. The surgeon should be aware of the more common oral manifestations of HIV/AIDS, as their presence may affect the general health of the patient and the surgical outcome of a procedure that the patient may be undergoing.

Some of the common oral manifestations of HIV/AIDS infection include oral candidiasis, hairy leukoplakia, angular cheilitis, recurrent aphthous ulcers, gingival disease, warts/condylomas, Kaposi's sarcoma, herpes, xerostomia, and salivary gland disease. Oral lesions can act as a conduit for the spread of infection and further compromise the immune function in AIDS patients, thus accelerating disease progression and death [38]. Thus, it is critical for the surgeon to look for these signs and symptoms, as they may affect his/her surgical treatment decision. The transmission of the virus seems to be somewhat different in the geriatric population when compared to the general population. The major etiologic factor for AIDS cases with advancing age include blood and blood product transfusion rather than homosexual contact and intravenous substance abuse [39].

HIV/AIDS in the geriatric population seems to take on new and challenging diagnostic and clinical characteristics, as many of the diseases or conditions associated with aging can lead to misdiagnosis and delay of appropriate treatment. Elderly patients are at an increased risk for contracting other infections when there is a diagnosis of HIV/AIDS already, thus highlighting its importance in surgical practice [40]. Ship and Wolff mention that the geriatric patient with HIV is at increased risk for developing other infections as the immune system declines in function as a result of the aging process [39].

The increasing prevalence of HIV infection in our general and geriatric population makes it important to include oral examination in the preoperative evaluation of patients. Often,

oral lesions are noted as the first indication of HIV/AIDS. In the initial stages of the disease, the viral count may be high and the CD4 count may be under 200, thus increasing the likelihood of the presence of one or more oral manifestations in an HIV infected individual. The presence of an oral lesion can raise the suspicion of the practitioner to investigate further to reach an accurate diagnosis and/or treatment of undiagnosed HIV infection. It is common to find HIV patients with altered hemoglobin B/hematocrit (HgB/HCT), white blood cell (WBC), absolute leukocyte count (ALC), absolute neutrophil count (ANC), and platelet counts. These findings can lead to higher incidence of intraoperative hemorrhage and postoperative infections [41]. Thus, an accurate diagnosis has a huge impact on intraoperative and post-operative surgical outcomes.

Elderly patients generally have declining social and cognitive skills and might often be incapable of reporting signs and symptoms that are a consequence of HIV/AIDS infections. This can lead to undiagnosed infections for long times and affect the health of the geriatric patient. It is vital for the physician/surgeon to be aware of the possibility of HIV infection in their patients and they must be trained to identify this disease and/or its symptoms prior to performing surgery. This process must include a review and evaluation of all the systems, including the oral cavity. The dentist and the general surgeon must consult with each other to make the preoperative evaluation of the geriatric patient accurate and complete to ensure acceptable surgical outcomes.

Surgical Considerations in the Geriatric Population

Normally, slower rates of wound healing and longer recovery times after surgical procedures can be expected to occur in the geriatric population. As mentioned previously, the oral mucosa becomes more sensitive to mechanical damage as age progresses [6]. Thus, it is important that surgical procedures be performed as non-invasively as possible in the elderly. In addition, other factors need to be carefully considered before embarking on surgical procedures in elderly patients. For instance, relying entirely on blood parameters of infection might not be sufficient to assume that the patient may not harbor a risk for a post-operative infection. The presence of dentogenic infection foci can be a positive finding regardless of a lack of infection parameters of blood. This might contribute to post-operative infections as the patients are generally under stress during the recovery phase of the surgery. Thus, it is highly recommended that physicians/surgeons refer geriatric patients for a complete oral health check-up before planned surgery. Oral sensorial complaints are more prevalent in elderly people who take

TABLE 41.3 Pre-operative dental evaluation in geriatric surgical patients

Structure	Examination	Findings	Surgical implications
Hard tissue(s)	Review of X-rays with probing of tooth surfaces	Carious lesions – thinning of enamel, tooth erosion	Pre and post-operative bacteremia
	Full mouth series	Narrowing of the pulp chamber	Avulsion of teeth during anesthetic administration
	Panorex baseline for relationship between mandible and maxilla	Neoplasms (e.g., cotton wool appearance)	Complicated post-operative course
		Bone cysts (traumatic and pathologic)	
		Osteonecrosis	
		Previous fractures	
		Pathological fractures	
	Documentation of carious lesions (both clinical and radiographic)	Deep lesions may penetrate the pulp chamber	Pre and post-operative infection
	Periodontal bone loss (vertical and horizontal); severity	Vertical and horizontal bone loss	Aspiration of loose teeth
		Bone spurs and bone lesions	
	Tooth mobility	Periodontal pockets and inflammation	Can affect intubation techniques and post-operative infections
	Abrasion, erosion, attrition		
Soft tissue(s)	Visual examination of hard and soft palate, oropharynx, tongue (dorsal, ventral, and lateral), lip, floor of mouth, vascularization of oral cavity	Thinning of oral mucosal tissues	Delicate mucosal tissues can be easily traumatized during intubation procedures leading to pain and difficulty when consuming foods
		Soft tissue lesions (benign and malignant)	Distant metastases
	Lymph nodes (intra-submandibular, and extraorally), anterior and posterior cervical nodes, subauricular, pre and post auricular	Can be palpated in inflammatory conditions and neoplasms as hard/indurated masses along the distribution of the lymphatic chain	Could delay surgical procedure(s) because of an active infection or neoplasm
	Gingival recession	Tooth root exposure	Higher chances for bacterial colonization on exposed tooth root surfaces, pre and post-operative complications

pharmaceutical drugs when compared to people who do not [29]. Surgical considerations in elderly patients include pre and post-operative side effects (i.e., Xerostomia, oral ulcers, and sensorial complaints) of drugs used during the surgical procedure in addition to the effects of other drugs that the patient consumes regularly. These side effects can also interfere with other daily activities such as eating, drinking, and talking. Table 41.3 provides a list of examination techniques that are used to determine if the oral tissues show signs of pathology and their surgical implications.

Summary

The components of successful aging are generally considered to be low probability of disease, avoidance of complications of chronic diseases, high functional capacity (both physical and cognitive), and active engagement with life, including interpersonal relationships and productive activity [42]. By the year 2030, the population of America is projected to be around 350 million, and one of every five or roughly 20% of these may be 65 years or older [43]. Lamster mentions that students currently enrolled in dental schools will be within their practice lives by the year 2030, which

highlights the need for emphasizing geriatric dental education in the present curriculum to address needs of this sub-group of people in the future [43]. It has been reported that the average dental practice would be expected to have about 260 or more patients 65 years of age or older [44], thus highlighting the need for dentists to be trained in diagnosing and treating symptoms of illness in the elderly.

Some medical needs of the geriatric sub-population will be different when compared to other sections of society. For example, comorbidities from some pairs of diseases (e.g., arthritis and heart disease), when occurring either alone or at the same time in the elderly can significantly increase the risk of disability. Diseases such as Alzheimer's which mostly affect the elderly might not have any direct effects on the oral cavity, although they can have secondary consequences related to the maintenance of optimum oral health. Psychiatric disorders including depression and medical conditions that interfere with motor skills and coordination (e.g., palsies, cerebrovascular events) can indirectly affect the maintenance of the oral health and general systemic health of elderly patients.

In summary, the clinician must be aware of the following points before surgically treating geriatric patients:

- The surgeon must not rely entirely on blood parameters of infection, but must be trained to look for other sources of infection including dental infection foci

- The surgeon must be aware of the most commonly occurring soft tissue lesions (i.e., oral neoplasms, vesiculoerosive disorders, and candidiasis) in the oral cavity of elderly patients
- It should be mandatory practice for the surgeon to include an oral examination of their patients pre-operatively to minimize post-operative complications
- The incidence of systemic illnesses and their oral manifestations is generally higher in the geriatric population when compared to their younger counterparts. Some of these symptoms include candidal infections from diabetes, immunosuppressed states, lymph node involvement from infections, oral neoplasms, and xerostomia from drug reactions and denture use.

References

1. Scully C, Ettinger RL (2007) The influence of systemic diseases on oral health care in older adults. J Am Dent Assoc 138:7S–14S
2. Scott J, Cheah SB (1989) The prevalence of oral mucosal lesions in the elderly in a surgical biopsy population: a retrospective analysis of 4042 cases. Gerodontology 8(3):73–78
3. Baum BJ, Bodner L (1983) Aging and oral motor function: evidence for altered performance among older persons. J Dent Res 62(1):2–6
4. Fucile S, Wright PM, Chan I, Yee S, Langlais M-E, Gisel EG (1998) Functional oral-motor skills: do they change with age? Dysphagia 13:195–201
5. Meurman JH, Pajukoski H, Snellman S, Zeiler S, Sulkava R (1997) Oral infections in home-living elderly patients admitted to an acute geriatric ward. J Dent Res 76(6):1271–1276
6. Avcu N, Ozbek M, Kurtoglu D, Kurtoglu E, Kansu O, Kansu H (2005) Oral findings and health status among hospitalized patients with physical disabilities, aged 60 or above. Arch Gerontol Geriatr 41:69–79
7. Otomo-Corgel J (1996) Periodontal treatment of geriatric patients. In: Carranza FA, Newman MG (eds) Clinical periodontology. W.B. Saunders, Philadelphia, pp 423–425
8. Woolf AD, Pfleger B (2003) Burden of major musculoskeletal conditions. Bull World Health Org 81(9):646–656
9. Kelsey JL, Lamster IB (2008) Influence of musculoskeletal conditions on oral health among older adults. Am J Public Health 98:1177–1183
10. Naveau A, Naveau B (2006) Osteonecrosis of the jaw in patients taking bisphosphonates. Joint Bone Spine 73:7–9
11. Ruggiero SL, Drew SJ (2007) Osteonecrosis of the jaws and bisphosphonate therapy. J Dent Res 11:1013–1021
12. Ruggiero SL, Fantasia J, Carlson E (2006) Bisphosphonate-related osteonecrosis of the jaw: background and guidelines for diagnosis, staging and management. Oral Surg Oral Med Oral Pathol Oral Radiol Endod 4:433–441
13. Hildebrandt GH, Loesche WJ, Lin C-F, Bretz WA (1995) Comparison of the number and type of dental functional units in geriatric populations with diverse medical backgrounds. J Prosthet Dent 3:253–261
14. Lockhart SR, Joly S, Vargas K, Swails-Wenger J, Enger L, Soll DR (1999) Natural defenses against *Candida* colonization breakdown in the oral cavities of the elderly. J Dent Res 78:857–868
15. Wilson W, Taubert KA, Gewitz M et al (2008) Prevention of infective endocarditis: guidelines from the American Heart Association: a guideline from the American Heart Association Rheumatic Fever, Endocarditis and Kawasaki Disease Committee, Council on Cardiovascular Disease in the Young, and the Council on Clinical Cardiology, Council on Cardiovascular Surgery and Anesthesia, and the Quality of Care and Outcomes Research Interdisciplinary Working Group. J Am Dent Assoc 139:3S–24S
16. Soell M, Hassan M, Miliauskaite A, Haikel Y, Selimovic D (2007) The oral cavity of elderly patients in diabetes. Diabetes Metab 33:S10–S18
17. Friedlander AH, Norman DC, Mahler ME, Norman KM, Yagiela JA (2006) Alzherimer's disease: psychopathology, medical management and dental implications. J Am Dent Assoc 137:1240–1251
18. Little JW, Flace DA, Miller CS, Rhodus NL (2007) Neurologic disorders. In: Dental management of the medically compromised patient, 7th edn. Mosby, St. Louis, MO, pp 464–487
19. Stroke: hope through research. http://www.ninds.nih.gov/disorders/stroke/detail_stroke.htm. Accessed 17 Dec 2008
20. MacDonald DE (2006) Principles of geriatric dentistry and their application to the older adult with a physical disability. Clin Geriatr Med 22:413–434
21. Sheiham A, Steele JG, Marcenes W, Lowe C, Finch S, Bates CJ, Prentice A, Walls AWG (2001) The relationship among dental status nutrient intake and nutritional status in older people. J Dent Res 80:408–413
22. Awano S, Ansai T, Takata Y, Soh I, Akifusa S, Hamasaki T, Yoshida A, Sonoki K, Fujisawa K, Takehara T (2008) Oral health and mortality risk from pneumonia in the elderly. J Dent Res 87:334–339
23. Ghezzi EM, Ship JA (2003) Aging and secretory reserve capacity of major salivary glands. J Dent Res 82:844–848
24. Janssens JP, Pache JC, Nicod LP (1999) Physiological changes in respiratory function associated with ageing. Eur Respir J 13:197–205
25. Epstein M (1996) Aging and the kidney. J Am Soc Nephrol 7:1106–1122
26. Tylenda CA, Ship JA, Fox PC, Baum BJ (1988) Evaluation of submandibular salivary flow rate in different age groups. J Dent Res 67:1225–1228
27. Vissink A, Spijkervet FKL, Amerongen AVN (1996) Aging and saliva: a review of the literature. Spec Care Dentist 16:95–103
28. Turner M, Jahangiri L, Ship JA (2008) Hyposalivation, xerostomia and the complete denture: a systematic review. J Am Dent Assoc 139:146–150
29. Turner MD, Ship JA (2007) Dry mouth and its effects on the oral health of elderly people. J Am Dent Assoc 138:15S–20S
30. Nagler RM, Hershkovich O (2005) Relationship between age, drugs, oral sensorial complaints and salivary profile. Arch Oral Biol 50:7–16
31. Ship JA, Pillemer SR, Baum BJ (2002) Xerostomia and the geriatric patient. J Am Geriatr Soc 50:535–543
32. Matear DW, Locker D, Stephens M, Lawrence HP (2006) Associations between xerostomia and health status indicators in the elderly. J R Soc Promot Health 126:79–85
33. Ettinger RL (2007) Oral health and the aging population. J Am Dent Assoc 138:5S–6S
34. Silverman S Jr (2007) Mucosal lesions in older adults. J Am Dent Assoc 138:41S–46S
35. Jackler RK, Kaplan MJ (1997) Ear, nose and throat. In: Tierney LM, Mcphee SJ, Papadakis MA (eds) Current medical diagnosis and treatment. Appleton and Lange, Stamford, pp 201–236
36. Oral candidiasis. http://www.dentalcare.com/soap/intermed/oral-can.htm. Accessed 17 Dec 2008
37. Silverman S Jr, Migliorati CA, Lozada-Nur F, Greenspan D, Conant MA (1986) Oral findings in people with or at high risk for AIDS: a study of 375 homosexual males. J Am Dent Assoc 112:187–192
38. Brown JB, Rosenstein D, Mullooly J, Rosetti MO, Robinson S (2002) Chiodo G impact of intensified dental care on outcomes in human immunodeficiency virus infection. AIDS Patient Care STDS 16:479–486

39. Ship JA, Wolff A (2006) AIDS and HIV-1 infection: clinical entities in geriatric dentistry. Gerodontology 8:27–32
40. Gardner ID (1980) The effect of aging on susceptibility to infection. Rev Infect Dis 2:801–810
41. Lauren LP (1999) Hematologic abnormalities among HIV-infected patients: associations of significance for dentistry. Oral Surg Oral Med Oral Pathol Oral Radiol Endod 88:561–567
42. Rowe JW, Kahn RL (1997) Successful aging. Gerontology 37:433–440
43. Lamster IB (2004) Oral health care services for older adults. Am J Public Health 94:699–702
44. Little JW, FD, Miller CS, Rhodus NL (2007) Dental management of older adults. In: Dental management of the medically compromised patient, 7th edn. Mosby, St. Louis, MO, pp 534–552

Chapter 42
Geriatric Ophthalmology

Andrew G. Lee and Hilary A. Beaver

CASE STUDY

An 87-year-old woman presents for a new patient exam with blurred vision in both eyes. She and her family feel that her vision has progressively worsened over the last few months, and she can no longer safely drive a car or perform her activities of daily living. They are worried about her ability to continue living alone without assistance. The patient complains that her glasses "don't seem to work anymore," and notes that she has had several unexplained falls over the past few weeks. She was last seen by an ophthalmologist 1 year ago. She missed multiple follow up appointments with that ophthalmologist because she "couldn't get a ride," She did not pursue therapy with them because they told her the problems were related to "old age," that she was "too old to have surgery," and that "nothing could be done" to improve her vision. Her prescription for eye drops has since expired. She feels depressed about her visual loss and anticipates a loss of independence. Her family believes there is a decline in her mental function, and that her dementia symptoms are worsening, and feel she is intermittently depressed.

She has a past medical history of poorly controlled diabetes mellitus, cataract, age-related macular degeneration (ARMD), and chronic open angle glaucoma. She is on insulin and topical timolol drops in both eyes. She smokes one pack of cigarettes per day and has done so for 50 years. Her family history is significant for diabetes, glaucoma, and macular degeneration.

On examination, her visual acuity is a slow 20/100 OD and 20/80 OS. Her external exam shows dermatochalasis, and her motility is normal. The pupils are normal without a relative afferent pupillary defect. The slit lamp examination shows bilateral nuclear sclerotic cataracts consistent with 20/70 visual acuity. The intraocular pressure is elevated in both eyes at 30 mm Hg, and she states she has not taken her eye drops since her prescription expired; the patient further observes that the drops make her "dizzy" and she is reluctant to restart therapy. The optic nerves show glaucomatous cupping to 0.8 cup to disc ratio bilaterally with an inferior vertical notch in both eyes. The macula shows multiple large macular drusen and mild eccentric geographic atrophy of the retinal pigment epithelium (RPE) consistent with the dry form of ARMD. She has a mild, scattered, dot and blot hemorrhages in the posterior pole consistent with mild non-proliferative diabetic retinopathy. Formal Humphrey Visual Field testing is unreliable OD, and the patient is not interested in completing the testing OS.

Significance of the Problem

The demographic shift towards an older population in the USA is well documented and has been discussed in other chapters in this text. The number of patients older than age 85 years (such as in our case vignette) is projected to double from 4.7 million in 2003 to 9.6 million in 2030, and by 2050 to 20.9 million. Ophthalmology as a specialty will be disproportionately affected by the demographic shift as the most common causes of chronic visual impairment all show an increased incidence and prevalence in the elderly population. The most common age-related visual problems with geriatric ophthalmic surgery implications are cataracts, glaucoma, diabetic retinopathy, and ARMD. The incidence of cataract dramatically increases with age and half of patients over the age of 75 will develop a visually significant cataract in one or both eyes. One quarter will have the non-exudative or "dry" form of ARMD, 5% will have the exudative or "wet"

A.G. Lee (✉)
Department of Ophthalmology, University of Iowa Hospitals and Clinics, 200 Hawkins Drive, PFP, Iowa City, IA 52242, USA
e-mail: andrew-lee@uiowa.edu

form of ARMD, and 2–10% will have glaucoma [1–5]. In addition, many other blinding disorders (e.g., giant cell arteritis, non-arteritic anterior ischemic optic neuropathy, cerebral stroke) are diseases primarily of the elderly.

Many of the blinding diseases of the elderly have vision preserving or vision saving surgical interventions. The Assessing Care of Vulnerable Elders (ACOVE) report shows that 40% of blindness among the elderly is either preventable or treatable [6]. The recognition and treatment of eye disease in the elderly has benefits beyond their visual improvement. One such example is falls, a common and significant cause of increased morbidity and mortality in the elderly. There is clear evidence that visual loss increases the risk of falling in older patients [7–10]. The loss of contrast sensitivity, depth perception, visual field, or visual acuity all increase the risk of falls and fractures [7–10]. The Beaver Dam Eye Study, a large epidemiologic study, showed that 943 of 2365 (11%) of elderly patients with impaired vision experienced a fall in the previous year compared to 4.4% in controls [2].

Visual loss may complicate other systemic comorbidities such as hearing loss, depression [11, 12] and anxiety, dementia, or delirium in the elderly patients [13, 14]. Population studies have shown that visual impairment affects overall health and functioning [15–17], self-esteem, the ability to drive, independent functioning, and activities of daily living in the elderly [18–23].

Major Ophthalmic Conditions in the Elderly

Age-Related Cataract

A cataract is an opacity that occurs in the native, crystalline lens that increases in incidence and prevalence with age. The crystalline lens is located behind the iris. The lens is composed of lens epithelial fibers contained by an anterior and posterior capsule. It is suspended from the ciliary body by zonules, which attach around the equator of the lens for 360°. Cataracts scatter and defocus the incoming light and thus can produce symptoms of loss of acuity, loss of detail, loss of contrast sensitivity, and increased glare. The clear or cataractous lens may be viewed through the pupil with a direct ophthalmoscope, but the best tool is a slit lamp biomicroscope. Examination by an eye care professional can document the severity, type, and progression of cataract. The different types of cataract are classified by type and location within the lens (e.g., anterior or posterior, cortical, nuclear, or subcapsular cataracts) (Fig. 42.1). The treatment for all visually significant and symptomatic cataracts is surgical extraction with placement of a synthetic or "pseudophakic" intraocular lens. The slit lamp appearance of the cataract and the quality

of the examiner's view of the fundus through the cataract may both be used to estimate a patient's likely visual potential after cataract surgery.

The American Academy of Ophthalmology (AAO) has developed written and specific guidelines in the form of a preferred practice pattern (PPP) for the evaluation, management, and surgical indications for cataracts. Although there are occasional exceptions, cataract surgery is considered an elective and outpatient procedure. In the elderly patient, the decision for cataract surgery is dependent upon the severity of the cataract, the functional status, the visual needs of the older patient, the individual patient's preferences, and the likelihood of improved visual and overall function after surgery [5]. The presence of a cataract alone is therefore not a sufficient indication for surgery. The potential functional impact on the activities of daily living must be considered in the decision making. Chronologic age alone is not a sufficient reason to elect to perform or to deny a patient cataract surgery; patients in their 90s can undergo successful cataract extraction, and frequently elect to proceed with subsequent fellow eye surgery.

Modern cataract surgery requires that the patient lie in a supine to slight reverse Trendelenburg position for up to an hour, though the surgical time is frequently shorter. The patient's face and torso are covered with a surgical drape with the surgical eye exposed. Anesthesia may be with topical agents, a retrobulbar injection, or general anesthesia based on patient factors such as anticoagulation, cooperation, and claustrophobia. Either a corneal or a scleral incision is used, with the surgeon viewing the field through an operating microscope. A continuous, circular opening or capsulorhexis is created in the anterior capsule, the lens removed, and the pseudophakic lens placed within the remaining anterior and posterior capsule. Phacoemulsification is currently the most common technique in the USA to remove the lens material. Ultrasound power is created by the vibration of a piezoelectric crystal located within the phacoemulsification handpiece, and is used to emulsify the lens. The lens fragments are aspirated from the eye through the same handpiece. Modern cataract surgery techniques are, in general, both well tolerated and efficient, and in the vast majority of cases produce an improvement in both visual and functional outcome with limited morbidity and mortality. Numerous studies have demonstrated the subjective and objective visual and functional benefit for cataract extraction in the overwhelming majority of patients (up to 92%) [24]. Local, and increasingly topical anesthesia techniques, allow for rapid surgical and recovery times, while minimizing the risk to the patient. The procedure itself has very low peri-operative and post-operative morbidity (e.g., bleeding, infection, increased intraocular pressure, retinal detachment, macular edema, need to remove intraocular lens) and exceedingly rare mortality. One relatively common post-operative event is posterior capsular opacification

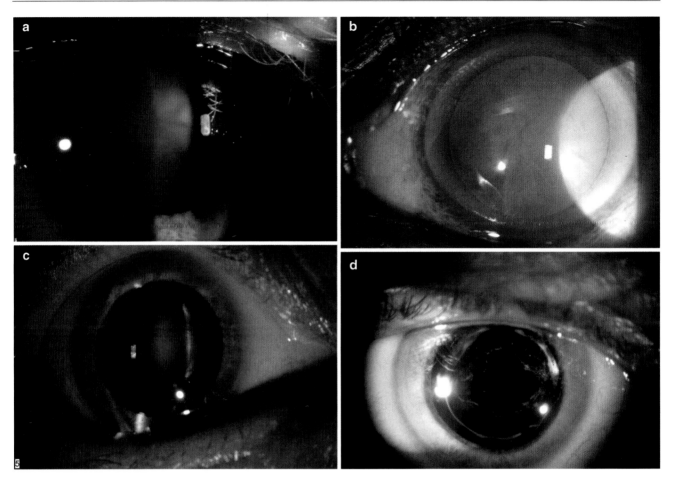

FIGURE 42.1   Cataracts. (**a**) Nuclear cataract. (**b**) Cortical cataract. (**c**) Posterior subcapsular cataract. (**d**) Posterior capsular opacity after YAG laser capsulotomy (photos courtesy of The University of Iowa Department of Opthalmology and Visual Sciences).

that may occur months to years after surgery. The capsule which surrounds the native lens preoperatively and now holds the replacement intraocular lens postoperatively may develop a secondary opacity (i.e., a posterior capsular opacification). This opacity may be treated using laser energy to produce a central opening in the capsule to clear the visual axis (i.e., YAG laser capsulotomy).

Age-Related Macular Degeneration

ARMD occurs most frequently in patients older than 50 years of age and increases in incidence and prevalence with increasing age. ARMD is a degenerative condition of the central portion of the retina called the macula, which is located temporal to the optic nerve and wreathed by the retinal vascular arcades. The receptive cells of the retina, the retinal photoreceptors, are supported by an underlying layer of retinal pigment epithelium (RPE). The RPE is in turn supplied by the underlying choroidal blood vessels. ARMD involves age-related damage to the photoreceptor and pigment epithelial layers of the retina.

ARMD is often classified into the "dry or wet" forms. The more common "dry form" presents with a loss of RPE, which may progress to geographic atrophy of the RPE within the macula, and may be associated with the formation of drusen. There is a secondary loss of the overlying photoreceptors and a resultant decrease in acuity. Patients with the "dry form" of ARMD may be asymptomatic (e.g., macular drusen) or may complain of unilateral or bilateral central visual loss. The visual loss may be static or slowly progressive and there is currently no effective treatment for the "dry form" of ARMD. Dry ARMD can be divided into three stages: (1) Early dry ARMD (i.e., small drusen or a few medium-sized drusen); (2) Intermediate dry ARMD (e.g., many medium-sized drusen or one or more large drusen); and (3) Advanced Dry ARMD with drusen and geographic atrophy of the RPE. The less common, but more visually disabling "wet form" of macular degeneration involves ingrowth of blood vessels from the choroid to the subretinal space (subretinal neovascularization) which leak serous fluid or hemorrhage. Patients present with distortion of their vision or sudden vision loss. Although age is the greatest risk factor for both forms of ARMD, other risk factors for ARMD include smoking,

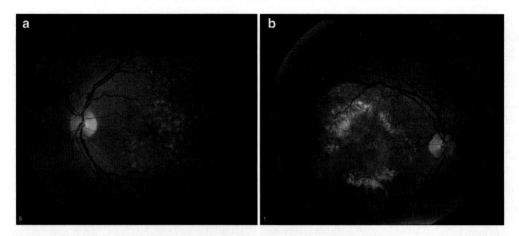

Figure 42.2 Age-related macular degeneration. (**a**) Dry form of ARMD characterized by drusen. (**b**) Wet form of ARMD with subretinal edema and exudate produced from an underlying choroidal neovascular membrane.

family history, blue eyes, obesity, white race, and female gender. The disease ophthalmoscopically is characterized by the following typical findings (Fig. 42.2) [25–30]:

1. Macular drusen (i.e., deposits of lipofuscin) under the retina forming visible yellow spots on ophthalmoscopic exam.
2. RPE hypopigmentation or hyperpigmentation.
3. Geographic atrophy of the RPE and underlying choriocapillaris.
4. Exudative neovascular maculopathy (i.e., the "wet form" of ARMD) with choroidal neovascularization, serous/hemorrhagic detachments of the sensory retina or RPE; hard exudates or hemorrhages, and subretinal or sub-RPE fibrovascular proliferation and eventually a disciform scar.

There remains no cure for ARMD, but newer preventive and therapeutic measures are being developed and tested [25–30]. Although a full description of the preventive dietary and lifestyle changes in ARMD is beyond the scope of this chapter, several studies have shown benefit in specific forms of ARMD. In the Age-Related Eye Disease Study (AREDS), a combination of antioxidants plus zinc (Table 42.1) was recommended for those patients with ARMD who are at high risk for developing advanced ARMD. These high risk individuals in this study were defined as those having (1) intermediate ARMD changes in one or both eyes characterized by the presence of either many medium-sized drusen or one or more large drusen or (2) advanced ARMD in one eye only characterized as either a breakdown of the light-sensitive cells and supporting tissue (RPE) in the macula (i.e., the advanced "dry form" of ARMD), or the development of the abnormal and fragile, leaky, new blood vessels under the retina (i.e., the "wet form" of ARMD). An eye care professional should examine the patient prior to instituting therapy as patients with early ARMD did not have benefit from treatment in the AREDS.

Table 42.1 AREDS multivitamin plus zinc formula [31]

500 mg of vitamin C
400 IU of vitamin E
15 mg of beta-carotene (often labeled as equivalent to 25,000 IU of vitamin A)
80 mg of zinc as zinc oxide
2 mg of copper as cupric oxide

The use of the AREDS supplements and other alternative and complementary therapies should be discussed with the patient and coordinated with their primary care provider. There are theoretic and real risks of side effects and drug interactions for all medications including vitamin and nutritional supplementation. The higher zinc concentration in the AREDS supplements can produce copper deficiency anemia, and copper was therefore included in the AREDS formulation. In addition, in the "antioxidants plus zinc" or "zinc alone" treatment arms there were genitourinary side effects, some of which required hospitalization (e.g., urinary tract infections, kidney stones, incontinence, and enlarged prostate) [31]. There is a risk of lung cancer in patients who smoke and who also take vitamin A. A "smoker's formula" of the AREDS multivitamins lacking the beta-carotene and substituting lutein is now commercially available; this formula was not available during the AREDS trial, and has not been clinically tested or found equivalent to the original AREDS formula.

As opposed to the "dry form" of ARMD, the "wet form" of ARMD is characterized by hemorrhage or exudate from new blood vessel formation under the retina (i.e., choroidal neovascular membrane). The wet form is considered advanced ARMD and therapy with the AREDS multivitamins should be instituted. Patients with subretinal neovascular membranes may be asymptomatic if the lesion is extrafoveal, or may be symptomatic with central or paracentral visual loss or visual distortion with subfoveal or juxtafoveal involvement. These patients often describe distortion of straight lines (i.e., metamorphopsia), or may have changes in image size (e.g., micropsia, macropsia) in addition to the loss of central acuity and a central scotoma ("blind spot") on visual field testing. The exudative "wet" form of ARMD in the past could sometimes be treated with laser therapy to eliminate the underlying subretinal neovascularization, but these membranes often recurred. Although the laser treatment destroys the fragile, leaky subretinal neovascularization, the laser is also destructive to the surrounding healthy retinal tissue and produced acute worsening of vision in centrally located (subfoveal) lesions. Only a small percentage of people with wet AMD can be successfully treated with laser because of the limitations based on total treatment size and on SRNVM characteristics. The laser is more effective for neovascularization that is adjacent to the fovea (juxtafoveal) rather than under the fovea (i.e., subfoveal). Recurrent membranes and the formation of new membranes are common in all locations, and repeated treatments are frequently necessary.

A subsequent adjunct to laser therapy is the use of a photosensitizing drug called verteporfin [32]. The laser light activates the drug within the membrane and enhances the laser's destructive effect on the fragile blood vessels of the SRNVM, allowing lower laser power use and producing less damage to the surrounding retina.

Modern therapy for "wet" ARMD has rapidly progressed and is now based on identified vascular endothelial growth factors (e.g., VEGF) that promote subretinal neovascularization. Anti-VEGF agents are now injected directly into the vitreous cavity, allowing for rapid regression of the neovascular membrane and stabilization or even return of vision. A series of multiple injections are frequently necessary. It is beyond the scope of this chapter to discuss the details of these agents, but early recognition and referral of treatable cases of ARMD is essential in both in the "dry" and "wet" forms [25–30]. We recommend that all patients with known ARMD be given information on the symptoms of ARMD progression (e.g., metamorphopsia) and a take home testing grid (i.e., Amsler grid), as well as regular monitoring by an eye care professional.

Glaucoma

Glaucoma is a common cause of visual loss in the elderly, affecting up to 2.5% of the population over the age of 40 years with an increasing incidence and prevalence with increasing age. Race influences the risk of developing glaucoma; glaucoma is present in up to 10% of elderly African Americans as compared with 2% of white patients. The etiology and

pathogenesis of glaucoma remain debated and are likely multifactorial. The disease is characterized pathologically by the loss of retinal ganglion cells beginning with those that pass through the superior and inferior poles of the optic nerve. The progressive loss of nerve fibers leads to a specific appearance of atrophy of the optic nerve, visible ophthalmoscopically as "cupping" of the optic disc (Fig. 42.3). The superior and inferior loss present with vertical elongation of the cup or even notching of the rim. The classification and description of the multiple types of glaucoma is beyond the scope of this text, but in general glaucoma is classified based upon the appearance of the draining apparatus (anterior angle) of the eye. The angle may be open (e.g., open angle glaucoma) or closed (i.e., angle closure glaucoma). Both forms of glaucoma may be primary or secondary (e.g., due to inflammation, trauma, neovascularization, mass effect, etc.). Primary open angle glaucoma (POAG) is the most common form in the elderly and will be the focus of the remainder of our discussion.

POAG is generally an adult disease with a bilateral, but often asymmetric presentation. The disease may initially be asymptomatic and is slowly progressive [33, 34]. Although increased intraocular pressure (IOP) above 21 mmHg is a risk factor for glaucoma, it is not the only factor, and some patients develop glaucomatous optic atrophy with "normal" pressures (i.e., normal tension glaucoma). Conversely, some patients with chronically elevated intraocular pressures may never develop glaucoma (ocular hypertension). The optic nerve damage of glaucoma produces painless, gradual, progressive visual field loss in a characteristic pattern. The peripheral

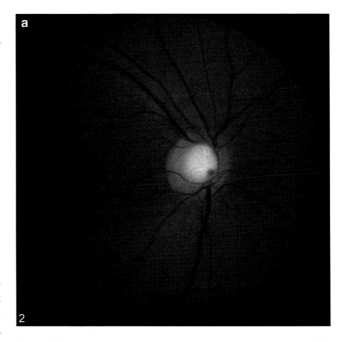

Figure 42.3 Glaucoma. (**a**) Glaucomatous cupping of the optic nerve OD.

b CENTRAL 30 - 2 THRESHOLD TEST

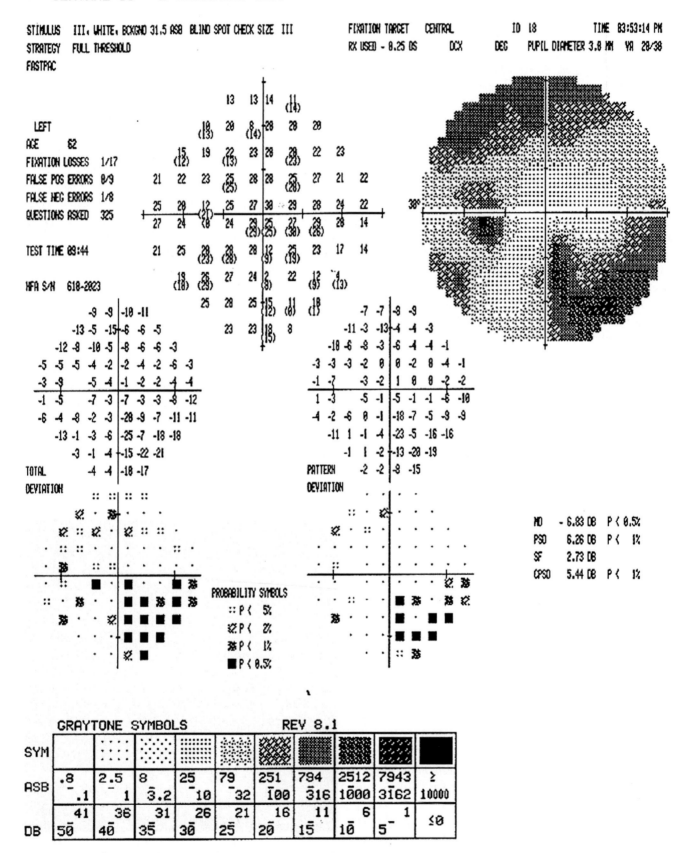

FIGURE 42.3 (continued) (b) Glaucomatous visual field loss as an inferior nasal step OS.

visual field is affected first, with the scotoma on formal visual field testing classically presenting in an arcuate pattern that is consistent with damage to the superior or inferior retinal nerve fiber layers. The appearance of atrophy of the optic nerve should match that expected based on the visual field. As opposed to ARMD where central visual loss is often the presenting symptom, the visual acuity and central vision tend to be preserved until late in the course of glaucoma.

Unfortunately, there is no cure for POAG. Medical treatments to lower the IOP with topical or less commonly systemic agents are the first line of therapy, and are used even in patients with borderline or normal IOP, but who have glaucomatous visual loss. The AAO has a PPP for POAG. In this PPP, the AAO recommended a 20% target reduction in IOP in POAG with progressive visual field loss and glaucomatous optic nerve damage. The management of POAG in the elderly is similar to that in younger patients, but there are some special considerations. Topical beta blockers, the previous "gold standard" of topical therapy, may not be the best first line choice in older patients with orthostatic hypotension as the beta blockade can cause or exacerbate hypotension, mask hypoglycemia in the diabetic, and exacerbate chronic obstructure pulmonary disease (COPD). Patients with severe degenerative arthritis may have difficulty administering their topical medications and might require assistance or special accommodations in this regard.

As stated above, glaucoma can occur despite normal IOP. In the Collaborative Normal Tension Glaucoma Study Group (a multicenter, randomized, and controlled trial), the treatment with IOP lowering agents produced a 20% reduction in rate of visual field loss at 3 years and a 40% reduction at 5 years if the IOP was reduced by 30% compared to untreated eyes [35, 36]. As with all treatment decisions, the AAO PPP recommends that the choice of treatment take into consideration the patient's quality of life, physical, visual, medical, psychological, and social circumstances [33].

POAG patients who have progression despite maximum tolerable medical therapy may require surgical treatment with either laser or incisional glaucoma surgery. As with medical treatment, the goal of laser or surgical therapy to lower the IOP to an acceptable target level is to prevent further loss of vision. With laser trabeculoplasty, the laser is applied to the trabecular meshwork in the angle of the eye to improve the outflow of aqueous fluid from the eye and lower IOP. Various types of incisional glaucoma surgery can also be performed (e.g., filtering surgery, tube shunts) to augment or bypass the eye's normal outflow system in the angle and lower IOP to a target level.

Diabetic Retinopathy

Diabetes occurs with increasing incidence with age, thus diabetic retinopathy is a common cause of visual loss in the elderly [37–41]. Both type I and type II diabetes may produce diabetic retinopathy, and because the incidence and severity of diabetic retinopathy increases with the duration of systemic disease, older patients are in general at higher risk for visual complications from diabetes. There are two types of diabetic retinopathy. The first type involves small vessel damage with hemorrhage and leakage, but is not associated with new blood vessel formation (i.e., non-proliferative diabetic retinopathy), and may or may not progress in an individual patient to new blood vessel formation (i.e., proliferative diabetic retinopathy). The non-proliferative form presents with retinal vascular changes, hemorrhages, and exudates (Fig. 42.4). Leakage of fluid from retinal microaneurysms into the central macula can produce retinal edema and visual loss (i.e., diabetic macular edema). Nonproliferative diabetic retinopathy without macular edema is usually asymptomatic, however. The type II diabetic is more likely to manifest diabetic macular edema, although it can occur in either form of diabetes. In contrast, proliferative diabetic retinopathy presents with new blood vessel formation (i.e., diabetic neovascularization) induced by vascular growth factors produced by the ischemic retina. These new blood vessels are often seen as net-like, friable fronds that can produce intraocular bleeding (i.e., vitreous hemorrhage) and secondary visual loss. Subsequent neovascular growth vertically into the vitreous scaffold or tangentially along the retina may produce a tractional retinal detachment. As the disease progresses, neovascularization may also develop on the iris or within the anterior chamber angle, leading to often intractable secondary neovascular glaucoma.

There is no medical cure for diabetic retinopathy. Tight control of blood glucose is recommended as the first line for the prevention and treatment of diabetic retinopathy. The Diabetes Control and Complications Trial (DCCT), is a randomized trial of patients with type I diabetes mellitus who were assigned either to intensive or to conventional glucose control. The aim of the intensive treatment arm was to achieve normal or near-normal blood glucose levels and target optimal glycosylated hemoglobin (hemoglobin A1c) levels. Four years after randomization, the proportion of diabetic patients with worsening diabetic retinopathy (e.g., proliferative retinopathy, macular edema, and the need for laser therapy) was lower in the intensive-therapy group compared with controls (odds reduction 72–87%, $P < 0.001$) [37]. Finally, hypertension and hyperlipidemia, often associated with diabetes, can both worsen diabetic retinopathy and should be optimally treated in patients with diabetic retinopathy.

Although there is no cure for diabetic retinopathy, that which reaches specific guidelines may be treated with laser therapy. Proliferative diabetic retinopathy may be treated with laser throughout the peripheral retina (i.e., panretinal photocoagulation) to destroy the ischemic retina and reduce the angiogenic stimulus for diabetic neovascularization. In contrast, patients with macular edema are treated with

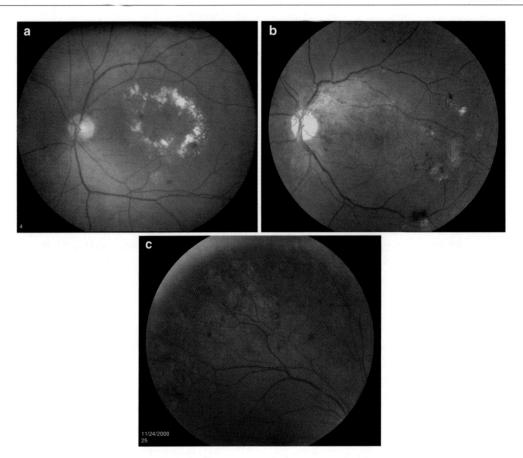

Figure 42.4 Diabetic retinopathy. (**a**) Non-proliferative diabetic retinopathy characterized by dot and blot retinal hemorrhages and macular edema with exudation. (**b**) Proliferative diabetic retinopathy characterized by neovascularization (new blood vessels) and retinal traction (courtesy of Thomas A. Weingeist, MD). (**c**) Periperal laser photocoagulation therapy for proliferative diabetic retinopathy.

focal laser treatments applied directly to the leaking microaneurysms or in a grid pattern to diffusely leaking macular tissue to reduce diabetic macular edema and improve the visual function. Multiple prior studies have demonstrated that laser treatment reduces the incidence and severity of visual loss and blindness due both to proliferative diabetic retinopathy and macular edema, and panretinal photocoagulation for proliferative diabetic retinopathy significantly reduced blindness [38–41]. Patients with diabetic tractional retinal detachments or non-resolving vitreous hemorrhages may also benefit from vitreoretinal surgery (e.g., vitrectomy with membrane peel).

Giant Cell Arteritis

Giant cell arteritis (GCA), also known as temporal arteritis, is a systemic inflammatory vasculitis affecting medium to large-sized arteries [42]. GCA is a disease of the elderly, especially older women. The dreaded complication of untreated GCA is permanent visual loss, typically due to arteritic anterior ischemic optic neuropathy. GCA is associated with systemic symptoms including new onset headache, scalp tenderness, ear or neck pain, pain with chewing (i.e., jaw claudication), and temporal artery pain or tenderness. The visual loss in GCA is often severe, and can be bilateral and simultaneous, or sequential. Although the visual loss is generally due to ischemia of the optic nerve (i.e., ischemic optic neuropathy), non-embolic central retinal artery, cilioretinal artery, or ophthalmic artery occlusions, as well as choroidal ischemia can occur (Fig. 42.5). Ischemic optic neuropathy typically occurs in the setting of swelling of the anterior portion of the optic disc that is visible within the eye (i.e., anterior ischemic optic neuropathy or AION), but in GCA the disc may appear normal (i.e., posterior ischemic optic neuropathy or PION) despite visual loss and evidenced by an optic neuropathy. Specialized testing (e.g., fluorescein angiography) may show choroidal perfusion delay in patients with GCA and visual loss due to AION or PION.

A stat erythrocyte sedimentation rate (ESR) and/or C-reactive protein (CRP) should be performed in patients suspected of having GCA, but normal laboratory testing does not exclude

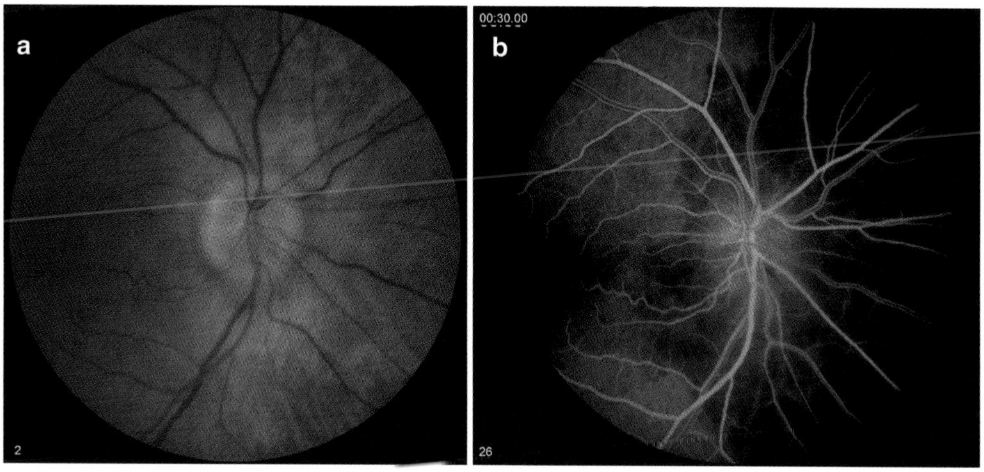

FIGURE 42.5 (a) Swollen optic nerve with disc hemorrhage in anterior ischemic optic neuropathy from giant cell arteritis. (b) Fluorescein angiogram demonstrating choroidal perfusion delay in choroidal distribution consistent with giant cell arteritis [(b), courtesy of The University of Iowa Department of Opthalmology and Visual Sciences].

GCA. Most patients with GCA have an elevated ESR (typically >50 mm/h), and the combination of the ESR and a CRP increases the sensitivity and specificity of either test alone.

In general, unless there are strong contraindications to treatment, patients suspected of having GCA should begin immediate corticosteroid therapy (e.g., oral prednisone at 1–1.5 mg/kg/day) and be scheduled for a confirmatory temporal artery biopsy with the next few weeks. It is highly recommended to confirm the diagnosis of GCA by temporal artery biopsy as the incidence of steroid related complications during treatment is high. When faced with steroid complications, a history of a positive biopsy reinforces the need to continue steroid or steroid sparing therapy for a full course of treatment. Although a unilateral temporal artery biopsy has a sensitivity of about 95% for the detection of GCA, if the clinical suspicion for the diagnosis remains high in the setting of a negative biopsy, then a contralateral biopsy should be considered [42]. Skip lesions, inadequate sample size, or inaccurate pathologic interpretation can produce false negative results in unilateral or even bilateral temporal artery biopsies.

Non-arteritic Anterior Ischemic Optic Neuropathy

In contrast to arteritic anterior ischemic optic neuropathy, patients can have ischemic optic neuropathy without GCA. The non-arteritic form of anterior ischemic optic neuropathy (NAION) is more common than the arteritic form, but the diagnosis of GCA should be considered in these patients. Like the arteritic form, NAION is characterized by acute unilateral visual loss, an ipsilateral relative afferent pupillary defect (RAPD), and a swollen optic nerve. NAION is typically associated with vasculopathic risk factors (e.g., hypertension, diabetes, smoking, and elevated cholesterol), but the precise etiology for NAION remains elusive. The major clinical consideration in AION in the elderly patient is excluding GCA (e.g., ESR/CRP and temporal artery biopsy). There is no proven effective treatment for NAION and management is typically directed against modifying the treatable vasculopathic risk factors and reducing the fellow eye risk for NAION.

CASE STUDY: RESOLUTION

We now return to our 87-year-old patient who presents with blurred vision in both eyes. The patient is brought in by her family for second opinion of progressive vision loss with declining activities of daily living and recent falls. This time the appropriate history and examination confirm that she had treatable cataracts, and reveal that part of her poor compliance with her glaucoma and dia-

betic regimens is because of her vision. Although she has a long standing history of poorly controlled diabetes mellitus, she now discloses that she is unable to check her blood glucose and administer her medications. She undergoes uncomplicated, sequential cataract extraction with intraocular lens placement under topical anesthesia. After the cataract extraction, her compliance with monitoring and treating her blood glucose improves. Her dizziness improves after her topical ocular anti-hypertensive therapy

(continued)

CASE STUDY (continued)

is switched from a beta blocker to a prostaglandin inhibitor. Her intraocular pressure measurements improve to normal and she proudly reports regular compliance. She has a 50 pack year tobacco history, but after realizing the improvement of her vision and reviewing the impact of tobacco on both glaucoma and macular degeneration she commences with smoking cessation treatment through her primary physician. The patient's diabetic retinopathy remained stable. Her vision improves to 20/20 in both eyes. She returns to driving and has not had a falling

episode since her last surgery. Although the cup to disc ratio remains 0.8 OU, she is better able to complete her formal visual field testing, which shows bilateral, but stable paracentral arcuate visual field loss. The drusen and geographic atrophy of the RPE are consistent with the dry form of severe age-related macular degeneration. She is started on AREDS formulation supplement therapy. Her family members feel that her mood and affect are improved after cataract surgery, and thank her new ophthalmologist for "not giving up on her" just because she is older.

TABLE 42.2 Visual loss in the elderly

Etiologies: Cataract, age-related macular degeneration (ARMD), glaucoma, diabetic retinopathy, ischemic optic neuropathy, giant cell arteritis

Worsens: Depression, dementia, fall risk and fractures, and hearing loss

Affects independence and daily activities

Prevention, therapy, and improvement with minimally invasive treatment

Summary

Non-ophthalmic care providers should be aware of the major age-related causes of visual loss in the elderly (e.g., cataract, ARMD, glaucoma, diabetic retinopathy, ischemic optic neuropathy, giant cell arteritis), should recognize the key features of each disorder, and should refer in a timely and appropriate manner to ophthalmology for evaluation and treatment. Visual loss has secondary impact on the elderly patient, including worsening of co-morbidities such as depression, dementia, fall risk, and hearing loss. Treating the visual loss might decrease the functional impact of these comorbidities (Table 42.2).

Acknowledgements This work was supported in part by an unrestricted grant from Research to Prevent Blindness, Inc., New York City, NY, the American Geriatrics Society, and the John A. Hartford Foundation.

References

1. U. S. Census Bureau (2005) 65+ in the United States: 2005. Current Population Reports, U.S. Department of Health and Human Services, National Institutes of Health, National Institute on Aging, U.S. Department of Commerce, Economics and Statistics, U. S. Census Bureau, Washington, DC
2. Klein R, Klein BE, Linton KL (1991) The beaver dam eye study: visual acuity. Ophthalmology 98:1013–1015
3. Tielsch JM, Javitt JC, Coleman A et al (1995) The prevalence of blindness and visual impairment among nursing home residents in Baltimore. N Engl J Med 332(18):1205–1209
4. Tielsch JM, Steinberg EP et al (1995) Preoperative functional expectations and post-operative outcomes among patients undergoing first eye cataract surgery. Arch Ophthalmol 113:1312–1318
5. American Academy of Ophthalmology (1996) Preferred practice patterns: cataract in the adult eye. American Academy of Ophthalmology, San Francisco, CA
6. Wenger NS, Shekelle PG (2001) Assessing care of vulnerable elders. ACOVE project overview. Ann Intern Med 135:642–646
7. Cummings SR, Nevitt MC, Browner WS, Stone K, Fox KM, Ensrud KE, Cauley J, Black D, Vogt TM (1995) Risk factors for hip fracture in white woman. Study of Osteoporotic Fractures Research Group. N Engl J Med 332(12):767–773
8. Kelsey JL, Browner WS, Seeley DG et al (1992) Risk factors for fractures of the distal forearm and proximal humerus. The Study of Osteoporotic Fractures Research Group. Am J Epidemiol 135(5): 477–489
9. Nevitt MC, Cummings SR, Kidd S, Black D (1989) Risk factors for recurrent nonsyncopal falls. A prospective study. JAMA 261(18): 2663–2668
10. Nevitt MC, Cummings SR, Hudes ES (1992) Risk factors for injurious falls: a prospective study. J Gerontol 46(5):M164–M170
11. Rovner BW, Zisselman PM, Shmuely-Dulitzki Y (1996) Depression and disability in older people with impaired vision: a follow-up study. J Am Geriatr Soc 44(2):181–184
12. Rovner BW, Ganguli M (1998) Depression and disability associated with impaired vision: the MoVies Project. J Am Geriatr Soc 46(5):617–619
13. Uhlmann RF, Larson EB, Koepsell TD et al (1992) Visual impairment and cognitive dysfunction in Alzheimer's disease. J Gen Intern Med 7(1):122
14. George J, Bleasdale S, Singleton SJ (1997) Causes and prognosis of delirium in elderly patients admitted to a district general hospital. Ageing 26(6):423–427
15. Salive ME, Guralnik J, Glynn RJ et al (1994) Association of visual impairment with mobility and physical function. J Am Geriatr Soc 42(3):287–292
16. West SK, Munoz B, Rubin GS (1997) Function and visual impairment in a population-based study of older adults. The SEE project. Invest Ophthalmol Vis Sci 38:72–82
17. Marx MS, Werner P, Cohen-Mansfield J, Feldman R (1992) The relationship between low vision and performance of activities of daily living in nursing home residents. J Am Geriatr Soc 40(10):1018–1020

18. Kosnik WD, Sekuler R, Kline DW (1990) Self-reported visual problems of older drivers. Hum Factors 32(5):597–608

19. Kline DW, Kline TJ, Fozard JL et al (1992) Vision, aging, and driving: the problems of older drivers. J Gerontol 47(1):P27–P34

20. Ball K, Owsley C, Stalvey B et al (1998) Driving avoidance and functional impairment in older drivers. Accid Anal Prev 30(3):313–322

21. McGwin G, Owsley C, Ball K (1998) Identifying crash involvement among older drivers: agreement between self-report and state records. Accid Anal Prev 30(6):781–791

22. Owsley C, Ball K, McGwin G et al (1998) Visual processing impairment and risk of motor vehicle crash among older adults. JAMA 279:1083–1088

23. Shipp MD, Penchansky R (1995) Vision testing and the elderly driver: is there a problem meriting policy change? J Am Optom Assoc 66(10):602

24. Javitt JC, Brenner MH, Curbow B, Legro MW, Street DA (1993) Outcomes of cataract surgery. Improvement in visual acuity and subjective visual function after surgery in the first, second, and both eyes. Arch Ophthalmol 111(5):686–691

25. American Academy of Ophthalmology (2001) Preferred practice patterns: age-related macular degeneration. http://www.ppp.org

26. Fine SL, Elman MJ, Ebert JE et al (1986) Earliest symptoms caused by neovascular membranes in the macula. Arch Ophthalmol 104:513–514

27. Fine SL (1985) Early detection of extra-foveal neovascular membranes by daily central visual field evaluation. Ophthalmology 92:603–609

28. Gelfand YA, Linn S, Miller B (1997) The application of the macular photocoagulation study eligibility criteria for laser treatments in age-related macular degeneration. Ophthalmic Surg Lasers 28:823–827

29. Klein ML, Jarizzo PA et al (1989) Growth features of choroidal neovascular membranes in age-related macular degeneration. Ophthalmology 96:1416–1421

30. Macular Photocoagulation Study Group (1994) Visual outcome after laser photocoagulation for subfoveal choroidal neovascularization secondary to age-related macular degeneration. The influence of initial lesion size and initial visual acuity. Arch Ophthalmol 112:480–488

31. Age-Related Eye Disease Study Research Group (2001) A randomized, placebo-controlled, clinical trial of high-dose supplementation with vitamins C and E, beta carotene, and zinc for age-related macular degeneration and vision loss: AREDS report no. 8. Arch Ophthalmol 119:1417–1436

32. Verteporfin Study Group (2001) Verteporfin therapy of subfoveal choroidal neovascularization in age-related macular degeneration: two-year results of a randomized clinical trial including lesions with occult with no classic choroidal neovascularization – verteporfin in photodynamic therapy report 2. Am J Ophthalmol 131(5):541–560

33. American Academy of Ophthalmology (2000) Preferred practice patterns. Primary open angle glaucoma. http://www.ppp.org

34. Hertzog LH, Albrecht KG, LaBree L, Lee PP (1996) Glaucoma care and conformance with preferred practice patterns. Ophthalmology 103:1009–1013

35. Collaborative Normal-Tension Glaucoma Study Group (1998) Comparison of glaucomatous progression between untreated patients with normal tension glaucoma and patients with therapeutically reduced intra-ocular pressures. Am J Ophthalmol 126: 487–497

36. Collaborative Normal-Tension Glaucoma Study Group (1998) The effectiveness of intra-ocular pressure reduction in the treatment of normal-tension glaucoma. Am J Ophthalmol 126:498–505

37. Diabetes Control and Complications Trial (2000) Retinopathy and nephropathy in patients with type 1 diabetes four years after a trial of intensive therapy. The Diabetes Control and Complications Trial/ Epidemiology of Diabetes Interventions and Complications Research Group. N Engl J Med 342(6):381–389

38. Diabetic Retinopathy Study Research Group (1987) Indications for photocoagulation treatment of diabetic retinopathy. DRS Study No. 14. Int Ophthalmol Clin 27:239–252

39. Diabetic Retinopathy Study Research Group (1981) Photocoagulation treatment of proliferative diabetic retinopathy: clinical applications of the DRS study findings. DRS report no. 8. Ophthalmology 88:583–600

40. Early Treatment Diabetic Retinopathy Study Research Group (1987) Photocoagulation for diabetic macular edema. ETDRS report number 4. Int Ophthalmol Clin 27:265–272

41. Early Treatment Diabetic Retinopathy Study Research Group (1991) Early photocoagulation for diabetic retinopathy. ETDRS report number 9. Ophthalmology 98:766–785

42. Lee AG, Brazis PW (1999) Temporal arteritis: a clinical approach. J Am Geriatr Soc 47:1364–1370

Chapter 43
Anatomic and Physiologic Changes in the Ears, Nose, and Throat

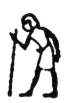

Ara A. Chalian and Sarah H. Kagan

Physiologic changes with age

Parameter	Change with age	Functional impact of change
The Ear		
Cartilage	Structural collapse	Potential cerumen impaction
Skin	Increased hair growth	Pruritus
	Increased cerumen	Potential cerumen impaction
		Limited hearing aide use
Ossicles	Increased rigidity	No known impact
Cochlea		Composite hearing loss
Organ of corti	Atrophy	Hair cell loss
Stria vascularis	Vascular changes	Neural fiber degeneration
		Decreased synapses
Auditory nerve	Decreased neurons	Hearing loss
	Decreased neuron size	
Central processing	Atherosclerosis	Hearing loss out of proportion with audiogram
Utricle and saccule	Decreased hair cells	Altered otoconia membrane
	Altered vestibular reflexes	
	Otoconial debris	Vertigo
		Falls/unsteadiness
The Nose		
Olfactory epithelium	Decreased neurogenesis	Composite change in olfaction
	Increased respiratory epithelium	Decreased olfactory sensation
		Danger – detecting noxious odors
		Altered nutrition
		Quality of life
	Decreased olfactory receptor neurons	
	Decreased olfactory cilia	
	Atrophy	Rhinitis
The Throat		
Laryngeal skeleton	Decreased elasticity	Contribution to voice changes
	Increased rigidity	Pitch
		Smoothness
		Projection
Mucosa/lamina propria	Increased vocal fold density	Vocal instability
		Rough phonation

A.A. Chalian (✉)
Department of Otorhinolaryngology: Head and Neck Surgery, Hospital of the University of Pennsylvania, 3400 Spruce Street, Philadelphia, PA 19104-4283, USA
e-mail: chaliana@uphs.upenn.edu

Introduction

Physiological and anatomical changes with age in the ear, nose, and throat have long been the subject of clinical interest; increasingly, they are the subject of basic and clinical investigations [1–7]. Nonetheless, the role of alterations in cells and tissues and distinctions among genetic, pathological, environmental, and interactive effects on cellular, tissue, and organ function are still emerging [3, 8–13]. Currently, presbycusis, presbystasis, presbyosmia, presbylarynx, and presbyphonia are the terms used to denote the functionally and clinically apparent manifestations of aging changes in the ear, nose, and throat [1, 2, 7, 14–18]. Presbyvertigo has also been proposed as a relevant term for matters of dizziness and falls in older adults though presbystasis is more commonly used [18]. Notably, presbypharynx is, while a parallel term to represent the manifestations of aging changes in the anatomy and physiology of the pharynx, not used in current literature. Instead, various uses of senescent swallowing and dysphagia predominate in the literature [19].

Research into conditions of the aging ears, nose, and throat offers a disparate and inconsistent body of evidence that connects aspects of the biology of aging, anatomy and histology, and functional changes. Related clinical literature has developed differentially, often relying on clinical observation and correlative science as well as treatment experience and case series reports. The magnitude of applicable science specific to the ears, nose, and throat varies by organ and senescent function. Similarly, the quality and quantity of translational science is inconsistent. Presbycusis is, for example, well studied with science that illuminates functional effects and clinical pearls [1, 20]. Conversely, presbyphonia and presbylarynx are only recently receiving significant attention in basic and clinical science [21]. Even with growing evidence of mechanisms, processes, and effects, direct translation of this evidence to care of the older surgical patient remains limited. Application thus requires careful review and interpretation.

This chapter describes important known anatomical and physiological changes with aging in the ear, nose, and throat. Each organ is addressed separately with focus on relevant changes in organ anatomy and physiology, and the chapter highlights alterations in function that result in presbycusis, presbystasis, presbyosmia, presbylarynx and presbyphonia, and senescent oropharyngeal anatomy and physiology, respectively. The sections detailing functional conditions of aging conclude with a brief summary of clinical surgical considerations. The chapter concludes with a summary of highlights.

The Aging Ear

Auditory Anatomy and Physiology

Targeted review of the anatomy and physiology of the ear predicates understanding presbycusis and presbystasis and their impact on function and implications for surgical care [1, 2, 7]. This section reviews in sequence the anatomy of the ear and aspects of physiology relevant to understanding presbycusis and presbystasis.

External Ear

The external ear, from pinna through ear canal to tympanic membrane, captures and intensifies sound in the 2–5 KHz range – frequencies in much of human speech – by acting as a resonator [15, 16, 22] (see Fig. 43.1). These external structures change with advancing age. Importantly, cartilage collapses, resulting in somewhat deceptive appearance of larger ears for many elders. Further, the tympanic membrane and the ossicular chain in the middle ear stiffen, though the functional impact is minor. The conductive aspects of hearing promoted by these structures do not change appreciably with age [9] (see Fig. 43.2). Instead, concerns that are cosmetic and mildly distressing emerge, including larger

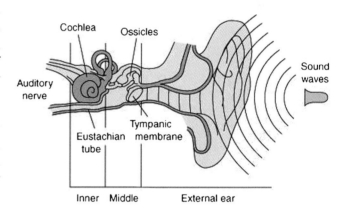

FIGURE 43.1 The ear and its divisions (reprinted from Lalwani AK. Current diagnosis and treatment of otolaryngology, head and neck surgery, 2nd edn, with permission from McGraw Hill Companies).

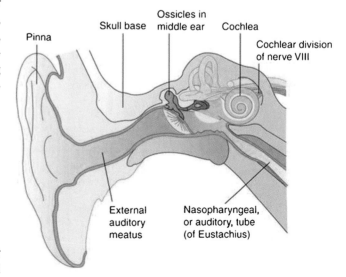

FIGURE 43.2 The ear (reprinted from Waxman SG. Clinical neuroanatomy, 26th edn, with permission from McGraw Hill Companies).

FIGURE **43.3** The middle ear
(reprinted from Lalwani AK.
Current diagnosis and treatment
of otolaryngology, head and neck
surgery, 2nd edn, with permission from McGraw Hill
Companies).

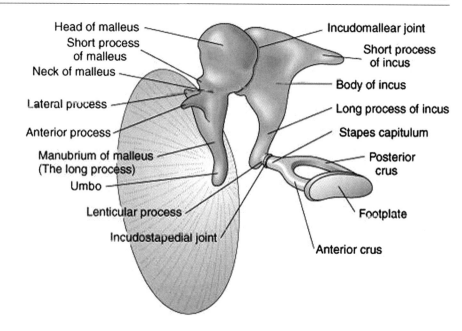

pinna size, more apparent cerumen production, and growth
of excessive hair in the pinna. Cerumen and hair growth
often result in complaints of pruritus. While these matters
may seem minor, they may influence acceptance and use of
hearing aides as well as prove distressing to some older
adults as they consider changes in appearance.

Middle Ear

Sound perception begins with vibration of the ossicular chain
[23, 24] (see Figs. 43.2 and 43.3). The tympanic membrane
and the ossicles (viz. malleus, incus, and stapes) are fairly
resistant to aging changes unlike larger skeletal bones. Thus,
age-related considerations and functional impact here are
minor if they are present at all [23].

Cochlea

The cochlea is the anterior portion of the inner ear, called the
bony labyrinth, which also contains the vestibule and the
semicircular canals [15] (see Fig. 43.4). This hollow bone
contains the neuroepithelium for auditory perception
(cochlea) and balance perception (vestibule and semicircular
canals) [16]. This section addresses aging changes in the
cochlea and the resultant condition of presbycusis. Alterations
in the vestibule and semicircular canals are discussed in a
following section to explicate presbystasis as a separate condition of aging in the ear.

A membranous canal, known as the cochlear duct, wraps
around a central bony core, the modiolus, for two and a half
to two and three-quarters turns through which the auditory
nerve fibers penetrate [9] (see Figs. 43.5 and 43.6). The
cochlear duct is divided into three compartments: the scala
tympani, scala media, and scala vestibule (see Fig. 43.7).
The scala media has a fluid composition (endolymph) different from that of the other two compartments (perilymph)
and contains the organ of Corti, which is the sensory organ
of hearing [9] (see Fig. 43.5). The organ of Corti rests on the
basilar membrane, which separates the scala media from the
scala tympani (see Fig. 43.6). The organ of Corti contains
afferent nerve endings (about 3,500 inner hair cells), affer-
ent/efferent nerve endings (approximately 12,000 outer hair
cells), and a variety of other supporting cells. The hair cells
communicate with the dendritic terminals of the bipolar
cochlear neurons whose cell bodies are located within the
modiolus. The hair cells serve as mechanoreceptors, converting the mechanical energy of basilar membrane displacement into an action potential to stimulate the ganglion
cells. The cochlea's capacity to analyze periodicity, syn-
chrony rate, phase, and spread of excitation of sound results
in specific ganglion cell population stimulation and ultimately the perception of sound frequency patterns in the
auditory cortex. The normal function of the cochlea occurs
as sound energy in the form of vibrations reaches the oval
window, the basilar membrane is set into motion and
vibrates. The stereocilia of the hair cells on the basement
membrane move and increase the permeability of the hair
cell to potassium that depolarizes the hair cell (see Fig. 43.8).

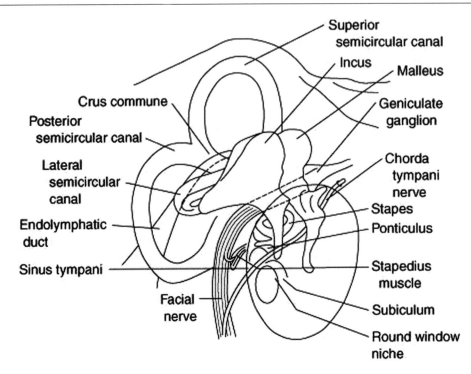

Figure 43.4 The inner ear in relation to the middle ear structures (reprinted from Lalwani AK. Current diagnosis and treatment of otolaryngology, head and neck surgery, 2nd edn, with permission from McGraw Hill Companies).

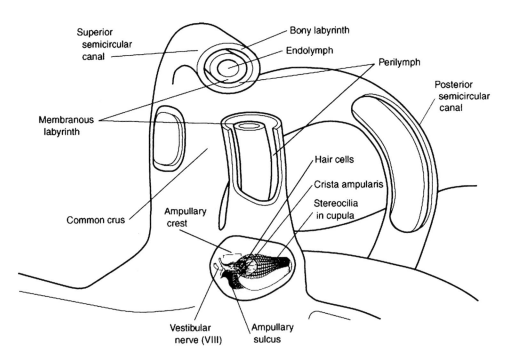

Figure 43.5 The semicircular canals (reprinted from Lalwani AK. Current diagnosis and treatment of otolaryngology, head and neck surgery, 2nd edn, with permission from McGraw Hill Companies).

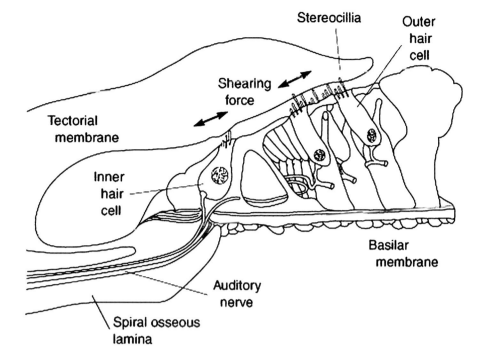

FIGURE 43.6 The organ of corti (reprinted from Lalwani AK. Current diagnosis and treatment of otolaryngology, head and neck surgery, with permission from McGraw Hill Companies).

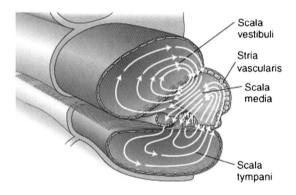

FIGURE 43.7 The cochlea, cross sectional view (reprinted from Lalwani AK. Current diagnosis and treatment of otolaryngology, head and neck surgery, with permission from McGraw Hill Companies).

A neurotransmitter is released by the hair cell onto the afferent ending of the cochlear nerve leading to a neurological signal [23].

Cochlear changes with advancing age result in presbycusis [15, 25]. Among the most significant alterations in anatomy and physiology include atrophy in the organ of Corti, vascular changes that affect the stria vascularis, and collapse of the cochlear duct [9, 26, 27]. These changes lead to hair cell loss, neural fiber degeneration, and reduction in number of synapses at the base of the hair cells [9, 25]. Accumulation of cochlear debris in the spiral bundles, abnormalities of the dendritic fibers and their sheaths in the osseous spiral lamina, and degenerative changes in the spiral ganglion cells and axons follow.

Auditory Nerve

The auditory nerve consists of about 30,000 afferent and 1,000 efferent bipolar neurons [9]. Ninety-five percent of the spiral ganglion is composed of myelinated (type 1) fibers that innervate only inner hair cells and nonmyelinated (type 2) fibers that innervate outer hair cells. The spiral ganglion is the densest at the mid and basal portions of the modiolus. The nerve fibers course in the nerve trunk in an orderly spatial arrangement (basal fibers located at the periphery and inferior portion of the nerve) through the temporal bone into the cerebellopontine angle into the pons to enter the cochlear nuclei [22].

Central Auditory Processing

Central auditory processing involves the cochlear nerve, the cochlear nuclei, and the auditory cerebral cortical regions [9, 28]. Through this process, the neuronal signal is appreciated as sound and interpreted by the cognitive regions of the brain to recognize content [16]. The process is bilateral. Three morphologically distinct auditory nuclei are appreciated within the pons. Upon entering the pons each fiber divides into an anterior branch, which terminates in the anterior part of the ventral cochlear nucleus, and a posterior branch, which again divides to terminate in the posterior part of the ventral cochlear nucleus and the dorsal cochlear nucleus.

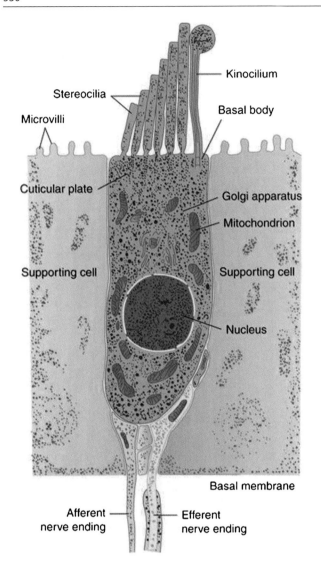

Microvilli **Stereocilia** **Kinocilium** **Basal body** **Cuticular plate** **Golgi apparatus** **Mitochondrion** **Supporting cell** **Supporting cell** **Nucleus** **Basal membrane** **Afferent nerve ending** **Efferent nerve ending**

Figure 43.8 A hair cell (reprinted from Waxman SG. Clinical neuroanatomy, 26th edn, with permission from McGraw Hill Companies).

aging on central auditory processing are a focus of dedicated current investigation [20, 30, 31].

Auditory Function

Changes in auditory function resulting in hearing impairment associated with aging is termed presbycusis, a prevalent and disabling condition [15]. Presbycusis results largely from aging changes in the inner ear and is a form of sensorineural hearing loss. Subtypes, however, can be detected on audiogram though the differences are likely to be functionally undetectable. They are sensory, neural, strial, and cochlear conductive presbycusis [15, 16]. Conductive hearing loss per se does not play a role in presbycusis. Early presbycusis effects high-frequency range, beyond the frequency characteristics of the human voice [15, 16]. Thus, early alterations in function are often imperceptible to older adults. With advancing age, hearing loss encroaches on the speech frequencies. Impairment then becomes consequential in daily activities. Despite the expectation of presbycusis, hearing loss among older adults is often multifactorial. The contribution of central auditory processing changes, along with the influence of genetics and family history of congenital hearing loss, cumulative environmental damage through occupational or leisure exposure, and use of ototoxic drugs should be considered [9, 10, 22]. Aminoglycosides and some chemotherapeutic agents are commonly identified as ototoxic medications. Additionally, other drug classes such as loop diuretics and beta blockers may damage auditory function, albeit in a manner that may be reversible [22].

Clinical Implications

Presbycusis, while seemingly peripherally related to surgical care, has direct impact on all processes of care from decision making through perioperative care to self-care after surgery. Gates and colleagues [32] suggest the simple screening question "Do you have a hearing problem now?" as the means to assess for impairment that results in disabling limitations in function. In elective surgeries, opportunity to refer for otolaryngologic assessment and clinical audiometric testing should result in improved interdisciplinary care. Emergent surgical care, conversely, requires anticipation of problems that require compensation including decision making, patient and family education, and postoperative care and the risk of reactions to the environment of care. Importantly, those older adults who wear hearing aides require additional support as their presbycusis may be inadequately corrected and central auditory processing problems unaddressed.

Cells from these nuclei send axons in a complex pattern from the contralateral superior and accessory olive areas to the lateral lemniscus, the inferior colliculus, and through the medial geniculate body to the auditory cortex in the temporal lobe [22].

Aging results in decrease in neurons in the cochlear nuclei and auditory centers [16]. Neurons decrease in size as well, thus altering their physiology. Diseases and injuries that alter brain anatomy and physiology – such as cerebral atherosclerosis and stroke or mild cognitive impairment and dementia – may further alter central auditory processing [16]. Changes in central auditory processing account for complaints in hearing that exceed that anticipated by the audiogram [29]. These changes are manifest in limited auditory comprehension in noisy environments and in failure of simple amplification through hearing aides to remedy complaints of dysfunction [29]. The effects of normal brain

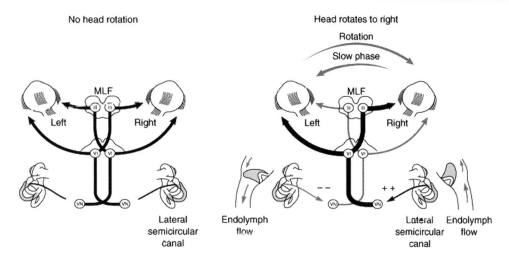

Figure 43.9 The vestibulo–ocular reflex (reprinted from Lalwani AK. Current diagnosis and treatment of otolaryngology, head and neck surgery, with permission from McGraw Hill Companies).

Vestibular Anatomy and Physiology

The vestibule is composed of three semicircular canals, the portions of the inner ear that are responsible for balance (see Fig. 43.5). The canals are posterior, superior, and horizontal, accounting for the dimensions in which the body is positioned in the physical environment of space [9, 10]. The otolithic organs are the utricle and the saccule; they are structured to respond to linear acceleration of the body in space [9, 10, 22]. The macula is the sensory portion of the utricle and the saccule. Type II hair cells are those that function in the vestibule (see Fig. 43.8). These cells are cylindrical with efferent and afferent synapses. Each type II hair cell contains approximately 50–100 stereocilia and one kinocilium. The kinocilium is located on one end of the hair cell, imparting anatomical polarization. Movement of the hair bundle toward the kinocilium causes an increase in the firing rate of the hair cell, while deflection away causes a decrease in the firing rate. In the lateral semicircular canal, the kinocilium is located near the utricle [9, 27]. The opposite is true in the superior and posterior semicircular canals (see Fig. 43.5). Cilia extend from hair cells to touch the statoconial membrane. It has a gelatinous consistency with calcareous particles embedded in that gelatinous layer. The surrounding endolymph has a lower specific gravity and, hence when the body accelerates, the hair cells of the macula are triggered. The central section of the statoconial membrane is called the striola. In the utricle, the hair cells are toward the striola. In the saccule, they are oriented away from the striola, again accounting for spatial dimension and direction of movement. The bipolar vestibular neurons create the inferior and superior vestibular neurons that merge when entering the brainstem [9, 27]. The vestibule is supplied by the labyrinthine artery.

The vestibular system senses linear and angular acceleration of the body. The semicircular canals sense angular acceleration while the otoliths sense linear acceleration. This system also coordinates eye–head movement. The vestibulo–ocular reflex enables focus on an object (see Fig. 43.9). The vestibule–spinal reflex accounts for postural placement of the body. Together, these physiological functions contribute to a sense of the body in space [33, 34]. Together with visual sensation and peripheral nervous system sensation in the feet, the vestibular reflexes create the complex sensory-perceptual system of proprioception [34]. Vestibular changes with age include alterations in the otoconia and in the hair cells [12, 18, 35, 36]. Atherosclerosis in the vascular supply and decline in the number of neurons in the vestibule further contribute to dysfunction and to altered vestibule–ocular and vestibule–spinal reflexes. Nevertheless, direct observation of the actual dysfunction is not possible given current assessment technology. Thus, clinical assessment relies on diagnosis by exclusion, employing means of inference including the caloric reflex test and other forms of electronystagmography [13, 18, 34]. These tests attribute vestibular function through manipulation of the vestibulo–ocular and the vestibulo–spinal reflexes and may create acute discomfort for patients [34].

Vestibular Function

Presbystasis is the condition in which age-related changes in the vestibular system result in altered balance and symptoms of dizziness and vertigo [2, 7, 18]. Vertigo and dizziness are common presenting complaints among older adults [10, 13, 37–39]. Nonetheless, presbystasis is a diagnosis of exclusion as vision and peripheral proprioception contribute to the sensation of dizziness and vertigo, which may culminate in a fall. Agrawal and colleagues [13] provide an elegant analysis of the prevalence of vestibular dysfunction among adults using a four-step test. The fourth step relies on standing on a foam-covered surface with an eye shield in place to isolate vestibular function. In their sample drawn of over 6,700 adults in the National Health and Nutrition Examination Survey, more than a third showed signs of vestibular dysfunction and could not remain standing without visual and proprioceptive cues. Prevalence was significantly associated with age. Almost half of those aged 60–69 and more than two-thirds of those aged 70–79, while the great majority of those over 80 years showed vestibular dysfunction [13]. Thus, the functional state of dizziness is likely to be presbystasis among the very old. However, aligned conditions such as benign paroxysmal positional vertigo (BPPV) and Meniere's disease must not be excluded [10, 37, 38]. BPPV is, in particular, a competing diagnosis that may create great distress from the periodic nature of its presentation. The mechanism of BPPV is suspected to be otoconial debris – which results from aging changes – moving in the semicircular canals and creating hypersensitivity to bodily movement [10, 38, 39]. Despite aging-related elements, BPPV is considered a separate, narrower condition than the breadth denoted by presbystasis.

Clinical Implications

Presbystasis is extremely common and thus an important clinical consideration throughout the surgical trajectory [13]. It creates risk of both minor and serious injury as well as discomforting sensations throughout the process of surgical care. Individuals affected by presbystasis then carry a clinically important risk of falling at some time during surgical treatment. Individualized plans of care should include attention to preoperative condition and reconditioning efforts as possible, as well as modification of the hospital environment and promotion of visual and proprioceptive cues [34]. Aspects of surgical care, including pharmacotherapy such as anesthetics, analgesics, and diuretics, may interact with altered balance and promote the potential to fall. As with presbycusis, elective surgery affords the opportunity for screening through preoperative history and physical assessment to generate appropriate referrals to otolaryngology and physical therapy [34]. These referrals aim for specialized assessment and discrete diagnosis along with treatment designed to mitigate the effects of presbystasis and promote visual and proprioceptive cues with spectacles, well-fitting footwear, and similar interventions. In emergency surgery, efforts to modify the hospital environment, provide compensatory support and supervision, use visual and ambulation aides, and integrate rehabilitative interventions for overall physical condition as well as vestibular accommodation are paramount.

The Aging Nose

Anatomy and Physiology

The nasal vault lies behind the external structures of the nose, through which air passes during respiration [40]. Inspired air enters through the nares. The nasal septum divides the vault in to two cavities, each of which contains three turbinates. Turbinates are rounded projections that extend the length of the cavity and labeled by position – superior, middle, and inferior. The space or valley below each turbinate is named for the turbinate above it. The paranasal sinuses drain into the meati. These sinuses, also labeled by location, are maxillary, frontal, ethmoid, and sphenoid. All the sinuses are lined with a specialized ciliated epithelium that secretes mucus and maintains mucosal flow with ciliary movement [41]. Together, the turbinates, mucus, and cilia insure humidification of inspired air and prevent gross and microscopic debris from entering the lower respiratory tract. The aging nose, like the external structures of the aging ear, is subject to cartilage collapse [40]. Few other changes in the nose are expressly linked to aging, though older adults may complain of more frequent rhinitis and sinusitis [42, 43]. Atrophic mucosa is a significant factor in these processes [41, 42]. The elderly may, as well, be more susceptible to nasal allergens and allergic rhinitis despite common clinical wisdom that allergen response declines with age [43].

The olfactory region is in the superior aspect of the nasal vault, a combination of olfactory and respiratory epithelial tissue [44–46] (see Figs. 43.10 and 43.11). Olfactory epithelium is organized into pseudostratified columnar shape with four cell types constituting this epithelium (viz. ciliated olfactory receptor neurons, sustentacular cells, microvillar cells of unknown function, and basal cells). Basal cells are the stem cell population responsible for differentiating and replacing lost olfactory receptor neurons [46]. Olfactory respiratory neurons transmit the signal from the odorant molecules to the central nervous system. Early in life, there is a balance between neurogenesis and the lifespan of the olfactory respiratory neurons. With aging, this process of neurogenesis degenerates and is no longer one of equilibrium in terms of maintenance of the type of the epithelium [44–46]. Additionally, there are increased patches of respiratory epithelium, representing a loss of the primary olfactory receptor neurons. The boundary between olfactory and respiratory epithelium becomes less well-defined with advancing age.

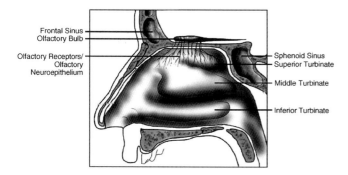

FIGURE 43.10   Olfactory neuroepithelium – sagittal view (reprinted from Wrobel BB, Leopold DA (2004) Smell and taste disorders. Facial Plast Surg Clin North Am 12(4):459–468, with permission from Elsevier).

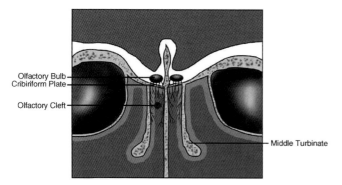

FIGURE 43.11   Olfactory neuroepithelium – coronal view (reprinted from Wrobel BB, Leopold DA. Smell and taste disorders (2004) Facial Plast Surg Clin North Am 12(4):459–468, with permission from Elsevier).

Thus, age-related changes in olfactory function are multifactorial and encompass interactions among the composition of olfactory epithelium, decline in specialized cell populations, and decline in olfactory cilia [44, 45].

Olfactory Function

Presbyosmia, loss of the sense of smell with aging, can significantly affect safety and quality of life [46]. Loss occurs on a continuum and is more correctly labeled by degree: anosmia (absent olfactory function), hyposmia (decline in olfactory function), and dysosmia (distorted olfactory function) [47]. Hyperosmia is less commonly noted in older adults. Well over half of adults aged 65–80 years of age have major olfactory disturbances [44–46]. The potential implications of olfactory loss are significant and range from inability to perceive noxious odors that present threats to environmental or food safety to depression and anhedonia [46]. Nonetheless, many patients are unaware of olfactory changes with age, will have no clinical response, and are unlikely to report changes to clinicians [46, 48].

Clinical Implications

The aging nose presents few clinical ramifications for surgical treatment. Cartilage collapse in the very old may challenge the utility of nasal intubation (endotracheal and nasogastric) and should be considered by the anesthesiologist and the surgeon. Effects of presbyosmia in surgical treatment are also limited. Clearly, attention to patients' complaints with otolaryngologic and neurological referrals is critical. Abrupt or distinct anosmia, rather than being a manifestation of aging changes, may be a sign of Alzheimer's disease as well as possibly being a harbinger of Parkinson's disease [46, 49–52]. Additionally, given the intersections of the senses of smell and taste, presbyosmic patients may report disabling dysgeusia rather than altered olfaction specifically [48]. Further, these patients may be malnourished as a result of this complex of conditions with commensurate risk of immune dysfunction and impaired postoperative wound healing. Thus, preoperative assessment of nutritional status and referrals to an otolaryngologist and to a registered dietician optimize care of patients in elective surgery. The same consultations are warranted as soon as possible after emergent surgery if presbyosmia, dysgeusia, or consequent or multifactorial malnutrition is suspected.

The Aging Throat

Anatomy and Physiology

The anatomy of the larynx, the central anatomical component of the throat, comprises a cartilaginous skeleton, internal and external muscles, and a mucosal lining [53] (see Figs. 43.12 and 43.13). The larynx and pharynx sit below the nasopharynx and the oropharynx to form, with the oral cavity and the nasal structures, the upper aerodigestive tract. The thyroid cartilage and the cricoid cartilage are visible anteriorly, with the cricoid forming the lower bound and the hyoid bone the upper bound of the organ (see Fig. 43.12). The two arytenoid cartilages are visible posterolaterally (see Fig. 43.12). These cartilaginous elements of the skeleton form two joints in the larynx. The cricoarytenoid joint is superior and the cricothyroid joint inferior at the posterior of the larynx. The vocal folds – or cords – attach to the arytenoids and form the glottis as their aperture (see Fig. 43.13). The cricothyroid muscles and the smaller vocalis muscle are responsible for tension and relaxation of the vocal folds. The posterior cricoarytenoid is the abductor of the vocal folds. The lateral cricoarytenoid, thyroarytenoid, and arytenoideus muscles adduct the vocal folds.

Branches of the inferior and superior thyroid arteries supply the larynx. Motor innervations arise from the cranial

Lateral section of the larynx

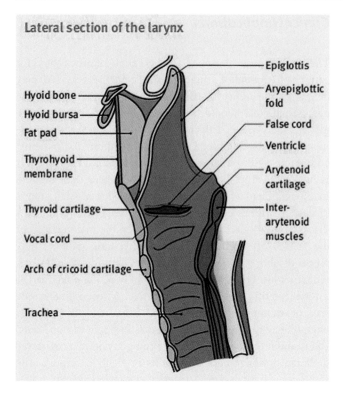

FIGURE 43.12 The larynx – lateral view (reprinted from Marchant W (2005) Anatomy of the larynx, trachea and bronchi. Anaesth Intensive Care Med 6(8):253–255, with permission from Elsevier).

Coronal section of the larynx

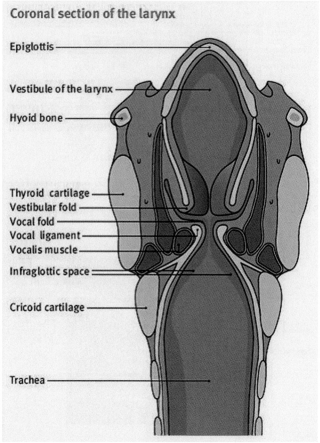

FIGURE 43.13 The larynx – coronal view. (reprinted from Marchant W (2005) Anatomy of the larynx, trachea and bronchi. Anaesth Intensive Care Med 6(8):253–255, with permission from Elsevier).

division of the accessory nerve, which travels with and therefore is clinically indistinguishable from the vagus nerve. The recurrent branch of the vagus nerve supplies almost all laryngeal muscles, save for the cricothyroid muscle that is innervated by the external laryngeal nerve. Sensory innervation is achieved through the internal laryngeal nerve above the vocal folds and the recurrent laryngeal nerve below them. These are branches of the vagus nerve that also supplies parasympathetic innervation.

The skeletal and muscular structures together create the form of the larynx [53]. In cross section, from the superior most aspect, the larynx begins with the aryepiglottic fold, the vestibule and the vestibular fold, the ventricle, the vocal fold, and the infraglottic cavity. The larynx is lined with mucosal tissue that maintains the humidity of inspired air during respiration and phonation, the central functions of the larynx. The mucosal lining also contributes to the pitch produced by the vibrating vocal folds when inspired air is drawn over them, creating phonation [53]. The epiglottis, which is critical to the laryngeal component in deglutition, sits behind the thyroid cartilage. The aryepiglotticus, thyroepiglotticus, and thyroarytenoid muscles close the larynx entirely, as during deglutition.

The pharynx begins behind the nasal structures, at the base of the skull, and extends to the cricoid cartilage [54] (see Fig. 43.14). At this point, the pharynx becomes the cervical

Sagittal view showing parts of the pharynx

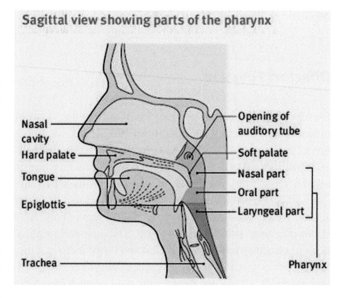

FIGURE 43.14 The oropharynx and pharynx – sagittal view (reprinted from Craven J (2005) Anatomy of the naso- and oropharynx. Anaesth Intensive Care Med 6(7):217–218, with permission from Elsevier.

portion of the esophagus. Unlike the complex larynx, the pharynx is a muscular tube. The outer anatomy of the pharynx is composed of three circular, skeletal muscle constrictors – superior, middle, and inferior. The inner muscular layer of the pharynx is composed of the stylopharyngeus, palatopharyngeus, and salpingopharyngeus muscles. Together these muscles support the successive contraction necessary to move a food bolus to the esophagus. In addition, the inferior constrictor maintains tone to function as a sphincter to limit air entering the digestive tract. Like the larynx, most motor innervation is supplied by branches of the accessory nerve. The stylopharyngeus muscle is the sole exception as it is innervated for motor and sensory function by the glossopharyngeal nerve. The glossopharyngeal nerve is the sensory supply for the pharynx, while the parasympathetic supply arises from branches of the vagus nerve. The functions of the pharynx and larynx require neuromuscular coordination and feedback for functional respiration, phonation, and deglutition, including protection of the respiratory and digestive tracts [54, 55].

The oral cavity is delimited anteriorly by the oral labia [54] (see Fig. 43.15). The muscles that control the lips and thus the oral cavity aperture are levator labii superioris, depressor anguli oris, and risorius. The cavity is lined with mucosal epithelium that covers the buccal surfaces and the hard palate. The transition to the soft palate marks the transition to the pharynx. Several muscles form the palatal aponeurosis: tensor veli palatini, levator veli palatini, palatopharyngeus, uvulus, and palatoglossus. German and Palmer [54] note that these muscles coordinate to open or close the airway during swallowing and to contribute to deglutition itself by altering the shape of the pharynx. The oral tongue and 32 permanent teeth are contained within the oral cavity. The muscles of the oral tongue include the extrinsic muscles – genioglossus, hyoglossus, styloglossus, and palatoglossus – which are innervated by hypoglossal and the vagus or accessory nerves and the intrinsic fibers – vertical, transverse, and longitudinal which are innervated by the hypoglossal nerve. The neuromuscular coordination of tongue movement is complex and involves the lingual nerve, branches of the glossopharyngeal nerve, and the internal laryngeal nerve in a minor capacity. The tongue, as well as aspects of adjacent structures like the soft palate, is covered with specialized papillae [56]. These papillae are found in fungiform, folliate, and vallate morphologies with a precise distribution over the tongue, creating the peripheral taste anatomy [48, 56]. Taste sensation is innervated by a branch of the facial nerve, the glossopharyngeal nerve, and the internal laryngeal nerve [48]. The muscles of the oral floor form the inferior boundary of the oral cavity and include digastric, mylohyoid, and geniohyoid muscles. Dentition arises from the maxilla and mandible, elements of the oral skeleton. The functions of the oral cavity are supported by adjacent structures without which mastication and transit of food are not possible. These components of oral function are the salivary glands, including the parotid, submandibular, sublingual, and minor salivary glands; the nasal structures, most importantly the olfactory epithelium with its direct contribution to chemosensation; and the muscles of mastication, temporalis, masseter, medial pterygoid, and lateral pterygoid [54].

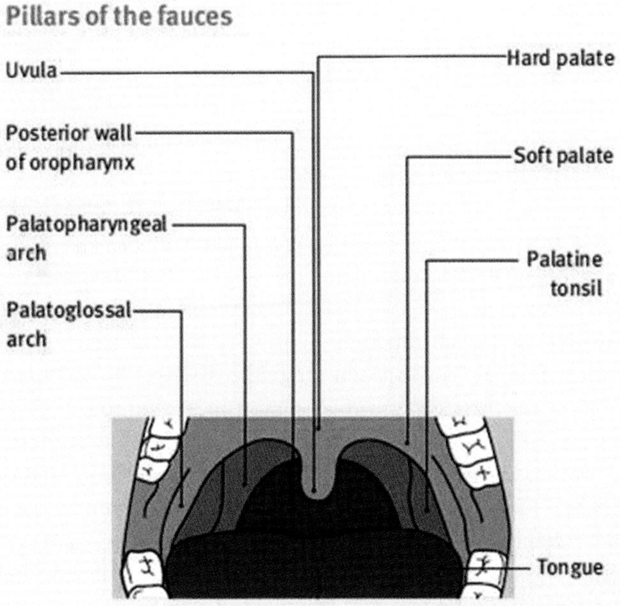

FIGURE 43.15 The oral cavity (reprinted from Craven J (2005) Anatomy of the naso- and oropharynx. Anaesth Intensive Care Med 6(7): 217–218, with permission from Elsevier).

Ageing Changes in Voice Function and Swallowing

Voice Function

Presbylarynx is the result of muscular atrophy and decreased elasticity in the muscular and skeletal components of the larynx [57, 58]. In fact, these changes begin early and are noted on examination as early as the fifth decade of life though functional effects are not noted by the individual potentially until the eighth or ninth decade of life if ever. Bowing of the vocal fold is the primary physical change. This bowing alters the aperture of the folds and results in incomplete closure causing a glottic gap. Other ligamentous and cartilaginous structures of the larynx are further altered with advancing age. The cartilaginous skeleton and joints ossify and the joints may become arthritic and dysfunctional. Microscopically, fibroblasts in the lamina propria may senesce and lose elasticity [17]. The lamina propria becomes denser as it produces less hyaluronic acid and more collagen. These changes alter the vibratory characteristics of the vocal folds [17, 53].

The voice changes experienced by older adults with advancing age are termed presbyphonia [17, 53]. The alterations in the laryngeal skeleton and function of the vocal folds include poor projection, shorter duration of phonation, and vocal roughness or instability. Importantly, presbyphonia is a diagnosis of exclusion [53]. It is the least common cause of vocal disturbance among older adults, accounting for approximately ten percent of voice complaints. More commonly, in order of incidence, older adults will suffer benign polyps, malignant vocal cord lesions, vocal cord paralysis, or functional dysphonia [53]. Neurodegenerative conditions, such as Parkinson's disease, also frequently create significant vocal dysfunction [53].

Oropharyngeal Function

Oropharyngeal function in later life is less a matter of tissue senescence [11, 54, 59, 60]. Dysfunction emerges more often as a product of "wear and tear" in the oral cavity with contributions of effects of local and systemic disease as well as treatment side effects of discrete functions like salivation [59]. Evidence points increasingly to decreased edentulism and increased functional dentition (i.e., 20 or more teeth) among older adults in both community and residential settings. Taste sensation likely remains relatively robust in the absence of pathology or significant presbyosmia [48]. Notably, as many as a third of all older adults experience xerostomia [60]. Nevertheless, age-related changes in salivary production are often indistinguishable from primary salivary disease and the contributions of medications with antihistamininergic and anticholingeric effects. Percival [61] notes that microbial flora of the oral cavity remain stable with age, all other factors being equal. However, conditions like xerostomia, changes in dentition and oral hygiene, and significant local disease, such as oral premalignant and malignant lesions, and systemic diseases including acute problems such as pneumonia and chronic concerns like Alzheimer's disease and Parkinson's disease may alter oral flora, salivary production, and functional capacity to perform hygiene [59–61]. As a result, oropharyngeal dysfunction among older adults is most often a complex and progressive cycle of direct and indirect functional changes [61]. Importantly, specific age-related alteration in taste is rarely noted, though Fukanaga and colleagues suggest that loss of taste perception may play a role in dysgeusia [62]. Dysguesia is more likely the result of presbyosmia or the effects of disease or its treatment that impairs olfaction, tastes, or both or effects contributory functions like salivation [11, 48, 54, 60]. Hall [11] notes that age-associated neuromuscular deconditioning or disease may result in oropharyngeal dyskinesia. There are resultant and often severe risks of dysphagia and aspiration, especially in stroke or with progressive neurodegenerative disease.

Clinical Implications

Presbylarynx and presbyphonia have circumscribed effects on surgical treatment. For patients who are distressed by presbyphonia, anxiety about being misunderstood or subjected to discrimination because of the "old" quality of their voices is likely real and thus a warranted concern. Attention to communication, discrete consideration of the basis for clinical decisions, and appropriate referrals to an otolaryngologist are important elements in addressing presbyphonia. Concerns about endotracheal intubation for surgery, given skeletal changes in the larynx, are probably theoretical and lack substantive evidence. However, rigidity in the cartilage and joints may offer some risk in the most affected elders, though the more clinical prominent issues of cervical spinal arthritis and kyphosis outweigh potential laryngeal rigidity. Skillful intubation with tacit recognition of laryngeal fragility is thus important in the absence of detailed and clinically relevant data. Nevertheless, postintubation voice changes may affect communication and comfort.

Oropharyngeal dysfunction among older adults poses significant risk and threats to surgical treatment. Such dysfunction may arise from aging changes in the anatomy and physiology of swallowing, dental pathology, comorbid disease that affects neuromuscular coordination, or any combination of these factors [8, 19, 63]. Side effects of intubation and anesthesia as well as postoperative healing, as it creates fatigue and saps functional reserves, may breach thresholds of functional compensation for dysphagia and aspiration. Elective surgery affords opportunity for integration of an interdisciplinary plan of care to assess and address for age-related and, more importantly, age-associated disease effects. Essential referrals include routine dental prophylaxis and treatment of dental caries and gingival disease that might affect tooth retention during the postoperative period as well as xerostomia; otolaryngologic and speech language assessment and intervention for diseases and dysfunction in deglutition, respiration, and phonation; and nutrition consultation and intervention to optimize visceral protein and overall nutritional status. These referrals are likely to be more successful given continuous collaboration with a particular patient's primary care provider. Comprehensive patient and family education further supports an effective plan of care and can be delivered by nurses on an outpatient basis before surgery, integrated into the inpatient care plan, and then reinforced during inpatient or outpatient rehabilitative postoperative follow-up.

Summary

Aspects of aging anatomy and physiology in the ears, nose, and throat have manifold and often consequential implications for surgical treatment of older adults. In the ears, presbycusis affects communication that results in possible problems in decision making and participation in perioperative care. Presbystasis is even more consequential as it is extremely common and results in significant risk of falls with the additive effects of anesthetics, analgesics, and diuretics, along with other postoperative interventions. Conversely, presbyosmia has little direct influence on surgical treatment save for implications of malnutrition when combined with the likelihood of dysgeusia and problems with food safety as a general concern. Presbyphonia conveys intermediate risk in surgical care for older adults. Older adults with noticeably affected voices may have difficulty in communication, both because of auditability and because of ageist discrimination for an "old" and infirm sounding voice. Finally, older adults with age-associated dental problems and acute or chronic disease that impinge upon neuromuscular coordination of the oropharynx are at significant risk for dysphagia and aspiration. The results of age-related functional changes in the anatomy and physiology of the ears, nose, and throat require thoughtfully integrated interdisciplinary surgical care. Knowledge of changes and functional implications is a rapidly evolving area of basic science and clinical investigation. Thus, surgeons can lead integration of a comprehensive plan of care that includes targeted referrals to specialists, preoperative preparation when possible, postoperative rehabilitation, and clear, consistent communication with patients, their family members, primary care providers, and other members of the interdisciplinary team. Modifications to the hospital environment that account for common sensory-perceptual and vocal changes, as well as ongoing patient and family education, further support successful care of the older surgical patient.

References

1. Belal A (1975) Presbycusis: physiological or pathological. J Laryngol Otol 89(10):1011–1025
2. Belal A, Glorig A (1986) Dysequilibrium of ageing (presbyastasis). J Laryngol Otol 100(09):1037–1041
3. Chen X, Thibeault SL (2008) Characteristics of age-related changes in cultured human vocal fold fibroblasts. Laryngoscope 118(9):1700–1704
4. Ju Z, Rudolph KL (2006) Telomeres and telomerase in cancer stem cells. Eur J Cancer 42(9):1197–1203
5. Thibeault SL, Glade RS, Li W (2006) Comparison of telomere length of vocal folds with different tissues: a physiological measurement of vocal senescence. J Voice 20(2):165–170
6. Walston J, Hadley EC, Ferrucci L et al (2006) Research agenda for frailty in older adults: toward a better understanding of physiology and etiology: summary from the American Geriatrics Society/National Institute on Aging Research Conference on Frailty in Older Adults. J Am Geriatr Soc 54(6):991–1001
7. Krmpotić-nemanić J (1969) Presbycusis, presbystasis and presbyosmia as consequences of the analogous biological process. Acta Otolaryngol 67(2–6):217–223
8. Robbins J, Hind J, Barczi S (2009) Disorders of swallowing. In: Halter J, Ouslander JG, Tinetti ME, Studenski S, High KP, Asthana S(eds) Hazzard's geriatric medicine and gerontology, 6th edn, Chap 41. McGraw-Hill, New York. http://www.accessmedicine.com/content.aspx?aID=5115738. Accessed 29 Dec 2009
9. Sha S-H, Talaska AE, Schacht J (2009) Age-related changes in the auditory system. In: Halter J, Ouslander JG, Tinetti ME, Studenski S, High KP, Asthana S (eds) Hazzard's geriatric medicine and gerontology, Chap 44. McGraw-Hill, New York. http://www.accessmedicine.com/content.aspx?aID=5116627. Accessed 29 Dec 2009
10. Nanda A, Besdine RW (2009) Dizziness. In: Halter J, Ouslander JG, Tinetti ME, Studenski S, High KP, Asthana S (eds) Hazzard's geriatric medicine and gerontology, 6th edn, Chap 56. McGraw-Hill, New York. http://www.accessmedicine.com/content.aspx?aID=5120291. Accessed 29 Dec 2009
11. Hall KE (2009) Effect of aging on gastrointestinal function. In: Halter J, Ouslander JG, Tinetti ME, Studenski S, High KP, Asthana S (eds) Hazzard's geriatric medicine and gerontology, 6th edn, Chap 89. McGraw-Hill, New York. http://www.accessmedicine.com/content.aspx?aID=5128150. Accessed 29 Jan 2009
12. Basta D, Todt I, Ernst A (2007) Characterization of age-related changes in vestibular evoked myogenic potentials. J Vestib Res 17(2–3):93–98
13. Agrawal Y, Carey JP, Della Santina CC, Schubert MC, Minor LB (2009) Disorders of balance and vestibular function in US adults: data from the National Health and Nutrition Examination Survey, 2001-2004. Arch Intern Med 169(10):938–944
14. Morsomme D, Jamart J, Boucquey D, Remade M (1997) Presbyphonia: voice differences between the sexes in the elderly. Comparison by maximum phonation time, phonation quotient and spectral analysis. Logoped Phoniatr Vocol 22(1):9–14
15. Gates GA, Mills JH (2005) Presbycusis. Lancet 366(9491):1111–1120
16. Busis SN (2006) Presbycusis. In: Calhoun KH, Eibling DE (eds) Geriatric otolaryngology. Taylor and Francis, New York, pp 77–90
17. Kendall K (2007) Presbyphonia: a review. Curr Opin Otolaryngol Head Neck Surg 15(3):137–140
18. Walther LE, Westhofen M (2007) Presbyvertigo-aging of otoconia and vestibular sensory cells. J Vestib Res 17(2–3):89–92
19. Ney DM, Weiss JM, Kind AJH, Robbins J (2009) Senescent swallowing: impact, strategies, and interventions. Nutr Clin Pract 24(3):395–413
20. Gates GA, Couropmitree NN, Myers RH (1999) Genetic associations in age-related hearing thresholds. Arch Otolaryngol Head Neck Surg 125(6):654–659
21. Kendall K (2007) Presbyphonia: a review. Curr Opin Otolaryngol Head Neck Surg 15(3):137–140
22. Howarth A, Shone GR (2006) Ageing and the auditory system. Postgrad Med J 82(965):166–171
23. Feeney MP, Sanford CA (2004) Age effects in the human middle ear: wideband acoustical measures. J Acoust Soc Am 116(6):3546–3558
24. Wiley TL, Nondahl DM, Cruickshanks KJ, Tweed TS (2005) Five-year changes in middle ear function for older adults. J Am Acad Audiol 16(3):129–139
25. Kusunoki T, Cureoglu S, Schachern PA, Baba K, Kariya S, Paparella MM (2004) Age-related histopathologic changes in the human cochlea: a temporal bone study. Otolaryngol Head Neck Surg 131(6):897–903

26. Suzuki T, Nomoto Y, Nakagawa T et al (2006) Age-dependent degeneration of the stria vascularis in human cochleae. Laryngoscope 116(10):1846–1850

27. Liu XZ, Yan D (2007) Ageing and hearing loss. J Pathol 211(2):188–197

28. Yilmaz ST, Sennaroglu G, Sennaroglu L, Kose SK (2007) Effect of age on speech recognition in noise and on contralateral transient evoked otoacoustic emission suppression. J Laryngol Otol 121(11):1029–1034

29. Tremblay K, Ross B (2007) Effects of age and age-related hearing loss on the brain. J Commun Disord 40(4):305–312

30. Gates GA, Mills D, B-h N, D'Agostino R, Rubel EW (2002) Effects of age on the distortion product otoacoustic emission growth functions. Hear Res 163(1–2):53–60

31. Caspary DM, Milbrandt JC, Helfert RH (1995) Central auditory aging: GABA changes in the inferior colliculus. Exp Gerontol 30(3–4):349–360

32. Gates GA, Murphy M, Rees TS, Fraher A (2003) Screening for handicapping hearing loss in the elderly. J Fam Pract 52(1):56–62

33. Deshpande N, Patla AE (2007) Visual-vestibular interaction during goal directed locomotion: effects of aging and blurring vision. Exp Brain Res 176(1):43–53

34. Whitney SL, Morris LO (2006) Multisensory Impairment in Older Adults: Evaluation and Intervention. In: Calhoun KH, Eibling DE (eds) Geriatric Otolaryngology. Taylor and Francis, New York, pp 109–123

35. Lee SK, Cha CI, Jung TS, Park DC, Yeo SG (2008) Age-related differences in parameters of vestibular evoked myogenic potentials. Acta Otolaryngol 128(1):66–72

36. Su H-C, Huang T-W, Young Y-H, Cheng P-W (2004) Aging effect on vestibular evoked myogenic potential. Otol Neurotol 25(6):977–980

37. Furman JM (2006) Benign Paroxysmal Positional Vertigo. In: Calhoun KH, Eibling DE (eds) Geriatric Otolaryngology. Taylor and Francis, New York, pp 155–163

38. Ekvall Hansson E, Mansson N-O, Hakansson A (2005) Benign paroxysmal positional vertigo among elderly patients in primary health care. Gerontology 51(6):386–389

39. Bhattacharyya N, Baugh RF, Orvidas L et al (2008) Clinical practice guideline: benign paroxysmal positional vertigo. Otolaryngol Head Neck Surg 139(5 Suppl 4):S47–S81

40. Moody M, Ross AT (2006) Rhinoplasty in the aging patient. Facial Plast Surg 22(2):112–119

41. Lindemann J, Sannwald D, Wiesmiller K (2008) Age-related changes in intranasal air conditioning in the elderly. Laryngoscope 118(8):1472–1475

42. Sahin-Yilmaz AA, Corey JP (2007) Rhinitis in the elderly. Clin Allergy Immunol 19:209–219

43. Chadwick SJ (2006) Allergic Rhinitis in the Elderly. In: Calhoun KH, Eibling DE (eds) Geriatric Otolaryngology. Taylor and Francis, New York, pp 213–224

44. Fong KL, Zacharek MA (2006) Olfaction and Aging. In: Calhoun KH, Eibling DE (eds) Geriatric otolaryngology. Taylor and Francis, New York, pp 173–180

45. Rawson NE (2006) Olfactory loss in aging. Sci Aging Knowledge Environ 2006(5):pe6

46. Lafreniere D, Mann N (2009) Anosmia: loss of smell in the elderly. Otolaryngol Clin North Am 42(1):123–131

47. Schiffman SS, Graham BG (2000) Taste and smell perception affect appetite and immunity in the elderly. Eur J Clin Nutr 54(6):S54

48. Mirza N (2006) Taste Changes in the Elderly. In: Calhoun KH, Eibling DE (eds) Geriatric Otolaryngology. Taylor and Francis, New York, pp 195–203

49. Wilson RS, Arnold SE, Schneider JA, Tang Y, Bennett DA (2007) The relationship between cerebral Alzheimer's disease pathology and odour identification in old age. J Neurol Neurosurg Psychiatry 78(1):30–35

50. Wilson RS, Schneider JA, Arnold SE, Tang Y, Boyle PA, Bennett DA (2007) Olfactory identification and incidence of mild cognitive impairment in older age. Arch Gen Psychiatry 64(7):802–808

51. Attems J, Lintner F, Jellinger KA (2005) Olfactory involvement in aging and Alzheimer's disease: an autopsy study. J Alzheimers Dis 7(2):149–157; discussion 173–180

52. Boesveldt S, de Muinck Keizer R, Wolters E, Berendse H (2009) Odor recognition memory is not independently impaired in Parkinson's disease. J Neural Transm 116(5):575–578

53. Sataloff RT, Linville SE (2006) The Effects of Age on Voice. In: Calhoun KH, Eibling DE (eds) Geratric Otolaryngology. Taylor and Francis, New York, pp 349–364

54. German RZ, Palmer JB (2006) Part 1 Oral cavity, pharynx and esophagus. In: Goyal R, Shaker R (eds) GI motility online. Nature Publishing, New York. http://www.nature.com/gimo/contents/pt1/full/gimo5.html#relatedcontent. Accessed 28 Dec 2009

55. Kawamura O, Easterling C, Aslam M, Rittmann T, Hofmann C, Shaker R (2004) Laryngo-upper esophageal sphincter contractile reflex in humans deteriorates with age. Gastroenterology 127(1):57–64

56. Gilbertson TA, Damak S, Margolskee RF (2000) The molecular physiology of taste transduction. Curr Opin Neurobiol 10(4):519–527

57. Kersing W, Jennekens FGI (2004) Age-related changes in human thyroarytenoid muscles: a histological and histochemical study. Eur Arch Otorhinolaryngol 261(7):386–392

58. Pontes P, Yamasaki R, Behlau M (2006) Morphological and functional aspects of the senile larynx. Folia Phoniatr Logop 58(3):151–158

59. Chalmers JM, Ettinger RL (2008) Public health issues in geriatric dentistry in the United States. Dent Clin North Am 52(2):423–446

60. Turner MD, Ship JA (2007) Dry mouth and its effects on the oral health of elderly people. J Am Dent Assoc 138(Suppl 1):15S–20S

61. Percival RS (2009) Changes in oral microflora and host defences with advanced age. http://www.springerlink.com/content/g3ul5987p4307264/about/. Microbiol Aging 131–152

62. Fukunaga A, Uematsu H, Sugimoto K (2005) Influences of aging on taste perception and oral somatic sensation. J Gerontol A Biol Sci Med Sci 60(1):109–113

63. Martin-Harris B, Brodsky MB, Michel Y, Ford CL, Walters B, Heffner J (2005) Breathing and swallowing dynamics across the adult lifespan. Arch Otolaryngol Head Neck Surg 131(9):762–770

Chapter 44
Geriatric Dysphagia

Neil N. Chheda, Gregory N. Postma, and Michael M. Johns

Introduction

Dysphagia, literally difficult or disordered eating, can refer to numerous difficulties with swallowing. The normal swallow consists of introduction of food into the oral cavity and its subsequent passage through the pharynx and esophagus into the stomach. Disorders of swallowing may be found along any point during this passage. A recent survey found that approximately one-third of independent, noninstitutionalized, elderly Americans reported a problem with swallowing [1]. In the year 2000, there were 35 million Americans over the age of 65 which represented 12.4% of the total population. By the year 2050, this population group is projected to number over 86 million and comprise over 20% of the total population [2]. With the "graying" of the American population, the prevalence of dysphagia is expected to increase.

Effects of dysphagia range from reduced enjoyment of meals to embarrassment at meals with resultant social isolation that can progress to depression. Life-threatening consequences include dehydration, weight loss, choking, airway obstruction, and aspiration pneumonia [3]. Pneumonia is currently the sixth leading cause of death. Aspiration pneumonia is the most common cause of death in patients with dysphagia secondary to a neurological condition [4].

After hospitalization, less than 2% of those under the age of 65 but over 20% of those over the age of 65 were discharged to a long-term care institution [5]. Analysis of this data showed that approximately 60% of nondysphagic stroke patients were discharged home compared with 21% of dysphagic stroke patients [6]. An estimated 60% of nursing home residents have dysphagia. Autopsy studies reveal that pneumonia is the cause of death in one-third to one-half of all deaths among nursing home residents [7].

Numerous etiologies exist for the increased incidence of dysphagia among the geriatric population. Studies have identified age-related changes to the normal swallow mechanism that result in a "slower" swallow with reduced sensation and less ability to compensate. Disease processes that affect swallowing, such as stroke and Parkinson's disease, are more prevalent in the geriatric population. In addition, social, psychological, and environmental changes occur, often in the setting of meal time activities.

Swallowing Physiology

The normal swallow process can be subdivided into three major phases: oral, pharyngeal, and esophageal. Of these, only the oral phase is under voluntary control. The oral phase is subdivided into an oral preparatory and oral transport phase where the food bolus is prepared into the proper consistency. During the pharyngeal phase, food is transported to the esophagus while the airway is protected from aspiration. The esophageal phase allows food to enter the remainder of the gastrointestinal system for digestion.

Prior to the swallowing process, the feeding process must occur – the voluntary delivery of food to the oral cavity. The individual requires the necessary cognition for food preparation and ability to schedule meal time. An intact extremity with proper coordination is needed to transport the food into the oral cavity. A functioning oral cavity is needed to receive the meal which requires the ability to open the mouth and coordinate the jaws and lips to receive the food.

The oral preparatory phase begins after the introduction of food into the mouth. The tone of the lips provided through the orbicularis oris musculature provides oral competency by preventing anterior spillage of the food bolus. Flavor and pleasure from eating are also derived during this phase. This phase can be voluntarily terminated if the taste, temperature, or consistency is not enjoyable. Through the coordination of the facial muscles such as the buccinator, the muscles of mastication (temporalis, medial and lateral ptygergoid, and masseter), the tongue, the soft palate, and the teeth, the food

M.M. Johns (✉)
Department of Otolaryngology, Emory University School of Medicine, Emory University Hospital, Emory Voice Center, Atlanta, GA, USA

R.A. Rosenthal et al. (eds.), *Principles and Practice of Geriatric Surgery*,
DOI 10.1007/978-1-4419-6999-6_44, © Springer Science+Business Media, LLC 2011

bolus is positioned and crushed into the appropriate texture and size for further handling. While the facial muscles are innervated by the facial nerve (cranial nerve VII), the muscles of mastication receive efferent signals from the trigeminal nerve (cranial nerve V). The tongue (cranial nerve XII) manipulates the bolus while the anterior movement of the soft palate (cranial nerve X) prevents premature passage of the food bolus while also opening the nasopharynx to increase the nasal airway.

After the food bolus has been adequately prepared by being chewed and mixed with saliva, as determined by various chemoreceptors and mechanoreceptors (cranial nerves V, IX, and X), the second part of the oral phase begins. Like the oral preparatory phase, the oral transport phase is under voluntary control. Through tongue manipulation, the food bolus is directed toward the oropharynx. After passing through the region of the faucal arches, branches of the glossopharyngeal and vagus nerve are stimulated and initiate the involuntary pharyngeal phase. Normal oral transport time ranges from 1 to 1.25 s regardless of viscosity [8].

While the nasopharynx is opened during the oral preparatory phase, actions of the velopharyngeal muscles during the pharyngeal phase close the nasopharynx to prevent nasal regurgitation. Posterior movement of the tongue and depression of the jaw direct the food bolus into the vallecula, the region between the base of tongue and epiglottis. Contraction of the suprahyoid muscles results in the superior and anterior movement of the larynx. By acting as a fulcrum, these actions invert the epiglottis and direct the movement of the food bolus from the vallecula into the two laterally located pyriform sinuses. The coordinate actions of the superior, middle, and inferior constrictor muscles result in an organized pharyngeal "squeeze" that moves the bolus in a superior to inferior direction through the pharynx. Mechanoreceptors, particularly of the tonsil pillars, stimulate the pharynx to continue to contract until the bolus has completely passed. The pharyngeal phase ends with passage of the food bolus through the upper esophageal sphincter (UES).

One of the primary objectives of the pharyngeal phase is the movement of food from the pharynx to the esophageal inlet while preventing passage of the bolus into the airway – aspiration. Mechanical defenses of the airway include the closure of both the true and false vocal folds, the inversion of the epiglottis over the laryngeal inlet, and the superior displacement of the larynx. Most frequently, respiration stops during the pharyngeal phase.

The UES is a manometrically defined region that is composed of the cricopharyngeus muscle, portions of the inferior pharyngeal constrictors, and the superior portion of the circular esophageal muscles. The cricopharyngeus is tonically active and in a "closed" state. Additional functions of the UES are the prevention of esophageal reflux and excessive air swallowing (aerophagia). The UES is opened through a five step process beginning with an inhibition of the tonic contraction. Elevation of the hyoid laryngeal complex results in passive opening. Passage of the food bolus distends the UES with a subsequent collapse when the bolus passes through. Finally, active contraction leads to closure of the UES.

Like the pharyngeal phase, the esophageal phase is under involuntary control. Two layers of muscle are present in the esophagus – an inner circular layer and an outer longitudinal layer. While skeletal muscle predominates in the proximal esophagus, in the distal esophagus smooth muscle is the main form. The lower esophageal sphincter marks the distal extent of the esophagus. Stimulation from bolus distension leads to lower esophageal sphincter opening through vagus nerve efferents. The food bolus normally passes through the esophagus into the stomach in 8–10 s.

Three primary patterns of esophageal peristalsis have been noted. Primary peristalsis is the peristaltic wave triggered by the brainstem swallowing center. Secondary peristaltic waves are induced by esophageal distension, retained food bolus, refluxate, or swallowed air. They serve to clear the esophagus of reflux or retained food bolus. Tertiary contractions are noncoordinated, dysfunctional contractions. These contractions are nonperistaltic and have no known physiologic role.

A complex system of neural coordination governs the swallow process. Areas of the cerebral cortex, particularly the precentral and inferior frontal gyrus, modulate the oral and pharyngeal phase. The brainstem provides primary coordination of swallowing and a normal swallow is possible in the absence of any cortical stimulation [9]. Though neural control centers and pathways are located in both sides of the cerebral cortex and brainstem, transcranial magnetic stimulation has shown asymmetrical cortical representation [10, 11]. Seventy-five percent of cases of oropharyngeal dysphagia have a neurological cause [12]. Esophageal contraction propagation receives input from both the brainstem as well as from local neural feedback through the myenteric plexus of Auerbach located within the wall of the esophagus. Primary peristalsis is from the vagal nucleus while secondary peristalsis is under esophageal control.

Age-Related Changes to Swallowing Mechanism

Globally with aging, there is decreased striated muscle fiber size, sarcopenia, with muscle tone decreasing between 20 and 25% [13]. In the alimentary system, changes in connective tissue result in decreased tensile strength that may lead to the development of diverticula. Particularly in the tongue, these changes are accompanied by an increase of fatty and connective tissue resulting in decreased strength and size. Osteoporosis and degenerative bony changes may alter cervical posture. For those patients who become edentulous, atrophy of the alveolar bone develops with reduced masticatory forces. Decreased salivary production affects bolus formation and manipulation. These changes in the oral phase do not often lead to significant difficulties as patients are able to modify their food intake to meet their needs (Table 44.1).

Bolus control is affected by the normal aging process. As a result of these age-related changes, there is decreased masticatory strength, reduced facial muscle strength with poor cup drinking, and reduced tongue strength and coordination [14, 15]. Compared with younger subjects, elderly patients tend to hold the bolus more posterior prior to the swallow [16]. Additional tongue movements were needed along with a slower swallow [17]. Yoshikawa evaluated the effect of age in comparing study participants who were all dentate and nonaspirators. The analysis found that the frequency of premature loss of liquid and increased oral and pharyngeal residue were greater in those over the age of 80 compared with younger control participants. In addition, oral transit time, pharyngeal delay time, and pharyngeal transit time in the dentate elderly group were found to be longer than in the younger group [18].

During the pharyngeal phase, age-related changes have more consequence compared with those of the oral phase. Manometry has shown that the amplitude, duration, and rate of pharyngeal pressure waves are not significantly changed in the elderly [19]. However, compared with younger individuals, the elderly have longer pharyngeal swallowing times and multiple swallows per bolus [20]. Aspiration is more likely as there is a three-time higher likelihood to inspire following swallowing rather than expire or breath hold. Aviv demonstrated a progressive increase in laryngeal sensory thresholds, believed to correlate with decreased laryngopharyngeal sensory discrimination that occurs with increasing age. The threshold values needed to stimulate the laryngeal adductor reflex for those greater than 61 years old were significantly greater than those between 20 and 40 years old and those between 41 and 60 years old [21].

Prior studies have suggested that reduced UES opening occurs with age [22]. More recent manometry studies, however, have shown no change or decreased resting tone of the UES [23]. Through primary peristalsis is often preserved, there is reduced secondary peristalsis causing decreased stripping of esophageal residue as well as an increase in the frequency of tertiary peristalsis [24]. Findings that manifest in the pharyngeal phase such as pooling of secretions in the pyriform sinuses may be due to changes in the esophageal phase, such as a stricture or poor motility.

Otherwise healthy individuals are usually able to compensate for the normal age-related swallowing changes without significant consequence. Certain disease processes with swallowing consequences, such as cerebrovascular accident and Parkinson's disease, occur with greater frequency in the elderly. Together, these normal age-related changes may put elderly individuals more at risk for dysphagia from other disease processes in a "two hit phenomenon." Medications, anatomical changes, and deconditioning may further contribute to the increased frequency of dysphagia seen in the elderly. The normal aging process often leads to a delay in bolus transit through the pharynx. Patients with COPD may be forced to inhale while the bolus is in the pharynx leading to aspiration. In addition, older patients may fatigue during eating and progress from a safe to an unsafe swallow.

TABLE 44.1 Common changes seen in the swallowing mechanism with aging

General
  Sarcopenia
  Connective tissue changes
  Osteoporosis
Oral phase
  Edentulous state
  Loss of tongue strength/coordination
  Reduced masticatory strength
  Reduced facial muscle tone
Pharyngeal phase
  Longer swallow time
  More swallows per bolus
  Reduced laryngopharyngeal sensation
  Reduced bolus control
  More likely to inspire during swallowing
Esophageal phase
  Possible reduced UES opening
  Decreased secondary peristalsis

Evaluation

History

Initial evaluation of dysphagia must include a careful history. In cases of a sudden onset, an etiology can often be identified such as stroke, acute illness, or intubation. However, there is often an insidious onset to dysphagia symptoms without a precise antecedent event. Questions should be asked about changes in diet, food consistency, number of meals consumed, and length of meals. A patient with feeding difficulties, which may be due to cognitive deficits, may eat frequent, irregularly spaced short meals, whereas patients with swallowing difficulty often have an increased meal time. Untreated dysphagia will ultimately lead to weight loss. However, in the initial period of recognized symptoms, some elderly patients may briefly experience a weight gain due to a change in food consistency such as consuming high caloric supplements. Three symptoms that have identified in an ambulatory geriatric population that are associated with a history of swallowing disorders are (1) taking a longer time to eat; (2) coughing, throat clearing, or choking, before, during, or after eating; and (3) a sensation of food stuck in the throat [1]. Querying the consistency of the food causing the most difficulty may aid in identification of the underlying etiology. Solid food dysphagia has traditionally been associated with an anatomic obstruction such as a stricture or web. Those reporting liquid dysphagia frequently have an underlying neurological dysfunction affecting coordination, sensation, or function. In cases of an insidious onset, patients may change their diet consistency to alleviate symptoms and may not readily recognize a difficulty with swallowing. Food avoidance may be an early indicator of dysphagia. Symptoms such as coughing with meals may indicate the presence of laryngeal penetration or aspiration. The regurgitation of undigested foods may suggest the presence of a diverticulum. Pain with swallowing, odynophagia, is an uncommon findings and may suggest an underlying malignancy.

Particularly for those with liquid dysphagia, a thorough neurological history should be ascertained. Specific signs to review include changes in gait, handwriting, and other fine motor skills that may reveal a global neurological condition. The responses from family and caregivers often provide accurate answers.

The past medical history should be queried for the presence of prior gastrointestinal conditions. Decreased pulmonary reserve, such as with advanced COPD, may also decrease swallow reserve. Recent endotracheal intubation should be identified as laryngeal sensation may be altered. Laryngeal function may also be affected by prior pulmonary, cardiac, cervical spine or neck (i.e., thyroid) procedures. In an ambulatory population, a history of esophageal reflux was identified as the most potent past medical history variable that identified in those with swallowing disorders.

Physical Examination

The physical examination should include an orderly, site-directed examination with particular attention to strength, fatigability, and coordination. Directed examination usually begins with the oral cavity. The lips are assessed for the ability to produce a complete seal, oral competency. Lip closure force has been found to correlate with markers of dysphagia such as weight loss, drooling, and food becoming "stuck" in the esophagus [25]. The presence and quality of the teeth may affect the ability to handle solids. Denture plates may block mechanoreceptors of the palate affecting afferent signals. Asymmetric palate elevation may indicate vagal

dysfunction. The tongue is assessed for the range of motion. Fasciculation of the tongue may indicate other neurological disease. The degree of laryngeal elevation with a dry swallow should be evaluated. The quality of the voice should be assessed. A thin or wet voice may suggest a laryngeal pathology. Dysarthria of the voice may indicate a central neurological disorder. Fixed neck adenopathy may indicate a neoplastic process.

Neurological assessment should include a basic level of arousal and orientation. A directed cranial nerve exam should be conducted. Those with dysfunction of the facial or hypoglossal nerve may have difficulty with bolus manipulation. The "gag reflex" tests sensory components of the glossopharyngeal nerve and motor function of the vagus nerve. The gag reflex, however, is not a normal component of swallowing. With the exception of an acute stroke, the presence or absence of the gag reflex has not been correlated with the risk of aspiration [26, 27]. Over one-third of healthy adults without dysphagia have an absent gag reflex.

Functional examination of swallow, particularly in inpatients, often begins with the bedside swallow assessment. Bedside evaluation begins with evaluation of patient's level of arousal, posture, voice quality, voluntary cough, and control of saliva. Patients are fed a small bolus and if successful are then given a larger and more complex bolus. Studies have demonstrated that bedside swallowing assessments may miss between one-third and one-half of significant aspiration seen on videofluoroscopy [28–30]. Leder and Espinosa found that while the sensitivity of the clinical bedside exam was 86%, its specificity was only 30%, and its false-positive rate was 70% [31]. The two most reliable signs from bedside swallow were reduced pharyngeal sensation and coughing with 50 cc water swallow [26].

Additional Studies

The barium swallow is a radiographic examination particularly useful for evaluating the mass occupying lesions of the pharynx and esophagus such as found with solid food dysphagia. The barium swallow aids in the identification of diverticulum as well as extrinsic compression such as from vascular structures. The density and consistency of the swallowed contrast material can be altered to aid in diagnosis.

The modified barium swallow (MBS) allows a dynamic evaluation of the swallow process (Fig. 44.1). This study is typically performed in a fluoroscopy suite with the collaboration of a speech-language pathologist and radiology personnel. Viewing of the fluoroscopic images allows for the evaluation of bolus movement and timing from the lips to passage through the LES. The MBS has traditionally been used as the gold standard for the evaluation of aspiration and

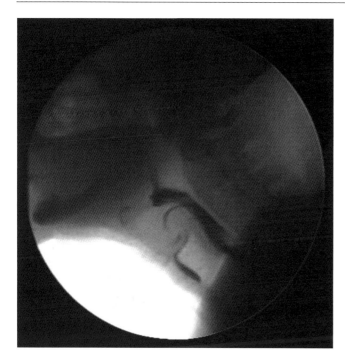

FIGURE 44.1 An image from a modified barium swallowing study demonstrating clear aspiration with barium entering the trachea.

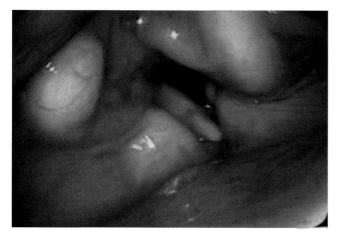

FIGURE 44.2 An image from a flexible endoscopic evaluation of swallowing. Note green colored material entering the larynx (penetration) and passing between the vocal folds (aspiration).

penetration. Compensatory maneuvers and rehabilitation strategies may be included at the time of examination.

Flexible endoscopic evaluation of swallow (FEES) is an ambulatory procedure that can also be used to evaluate the swallowing function and compensation technique [32, 33] (Fig. 44.2). In addition, the FEES examination can incorporate sensory testing for additional information (FEESST). Examination begins with an endoscopic examination of the pharynx and larynx. Important findings include the presence of secretions and the status of vocal fold mobility. The patient

is asked to produce a high pitched sound during which the pharyngeal walls are evaluated for symmetric contraction termed as the "pharyngeal squeeze."

After the endoscopic examination of anatomy is completed, the patient is fed various food consistencies, usually colored to enhance visualization. During the swallowing portion of the examination, a thickened fluid, such as applesauce, is used first as this is least likely to produce aspiration. After the swallow has been completed, endoscopy allows the assessment of bolus residue as well as laryngeal penetration (entry of food into the laryngeal inlet), regurgitation, or aspiration (entry of food below the level of the vocal folds). With an impaired swallow, food may accumulate in the hypopharynx, such as in the pyriform sinuses, and then overflow into the larynx in a delayed fashion. Food bolus that "clears" the UES but then re-enters the pharynx may be a sign of a Zenker's diverticulum, UES dysfunction, or poor esophageal motility.

In addition to its diagnostic value, the FEES examination can be used to guide compensatory maneuvers. For some patients, the visual feedback provided by endoscopy is easier to interpret than when seen on the MBS examination. One major disadvantage of the FEES examination is the "white-out" that occurs during the actual swallow as contraction of the pharyngeal walls and movement of the epiglottis temporarily obscure visualization.

Sensory testing can be incorporated into the FEES examination. During the FEESST examination, which was introduced in 1995 by Aviv, a calibrated air pulse is applied to the laryngeal mucosa at the junction of the arytenoid and aryepiglottic fold [34]. In the setting of normal physiology, a sufficient air pulse will stimulate the superior laryngeal nerve and activate the laryngeal adductor reflex resulting in glottic closure through the recurrent laryngeal nerve. This is an involuntary reflex arc and can be tested in those with cognitive deficits. Normative data for threshold pressures have been collected.

The MBS and FEES examination each possess relative advantages and should be used as complementary exams. Advantages of the MBS include the ability to evaluate the entire swallow including the esophageal phase which is not directly seen on FEES exam. Hyoid and laryngeal elevation, UES opening, and the degree of posterior movement of the tongue are better seen on MBS. Extrinsic compression is more easily identified. Disadvantages of the MBS include the need for radiation from the fluoroscopy equipment as well as the need to transport and position the patient in the fluoroscopy suite. A study found that in patients who had a MBS and FEES performed simultaneously, FEES examination graded the degree of dysphagia more severely [35]. A prospective, randomized study found no difference in pneumonia incidence whether MBS or FEESST was used to guide diet and swallow management [36].

The FEES exam allows for the diagnosis of subtle anatomic findings of the oropharynx, hypopharynx, and larynx. Native secretion can be easily identified and differentiated from ingested material. Examination can occur at bedside without the need for coordination with radiology personnel. Food bolus that pools in the pyriform sinus can accumulate and "spill" over into the laryngeal inlet. While both the FEES and MBS exam may be used to assess rehabilitative strategies, the biofeedback of the FEES examination may be more easily interpreted by the patient.

Esophagoscopy may be required during the workup of dysphagia. Traditionally, sedation has been required for the endoscopy. Adverse cardiopulmonary events related to sedation constitute a majority of the complications related to traditional esophagoscopy [37, 38]. Transnasal esophagoscopy (TNE) has emerged as a viable alternative. TNE can be safely and effectively performed with only local anesthesia and without the need for sedation. Endoscopic findings are diagnosed as accurately with TNE as EGD [39]. While the biopsy size is significantly smaller due to a smaller working channel, there was no difference in diagnostic ability between TNE and EGD [40, 41]. As the patient remains awake during the exam, the patient may be asked to swallow water or applesauce during exam such that a functional evaluation may also be incorporated into the examination. Direct examination of the mucosa allows for the detection of anatomic obstructions such as webs, rings, and strictures as well as the presence of esophagitis from causes including reflux and infection.

Quantitative assessment of peristalsis requires the use of manometry. Peristaltic pressure waves can be assessed for amplitude as well as timing and coordination. Conditions such as achalasia, ineffective esophageal motility, hypertonic UES, and diffuse esophageal spasm may be diagnosed through the use of manometry. Elderly patients with esophageal dysmotility tend to report different symptoms than younger patients.

Etiology

Cerebrovascular accident or stroke is the most common cause of dysphagia in the elderly. Forty-five to sixty-five percent of poststroke patients experience swallowing difficulties within the first 6 months after infarction [42, 43]. Approximately 25% of all patients die from aspiration pneumonia within 1 year of the stroke [44]. Results of the Paul Coverdall National Acute Stroke registry showed that only 45.5% of eligible stroke patients underwent dysphagia screening during their hospitalization [45]. Larger stroke infarctions have been associated with greater swallowing deficits with infarctions of the subcortical and periventricular regions associated with poor

Table 44.2 Common causes of geriatric dysphagia

Neurologic
Stroke
Parkinson
Other
Multiple sclerosis
ALS
Alzheimer's
Muscle disease
Myasthenia gravis
Muscular dystrophy
UES dysfunction
Structural UES
Functional UES
Zenker's diverticulum
Esophageal
Achalasia
Diffuse esophageal spasm
Esophagitis
Reflux
Infectious
Anatomic/structural
Neoplasm
Stricture
Web
Ring
Medication induced

tongue coordination and oral-phase dysphagia [46–48]. In addition to motor deficits, dysphagia may be secondary to lack of laryngopharyngeal sensory detection. Nearly one-half of patient recover to premorbid swallowing status within 1 week of the stroke and nearly 90% resume normal oral intake within 6 months after the event [49]. Swallow rehabilitation has been shown to improve the function though a temporary nonoral-feeding method may be required (Table 44.2).

Parkinson disease is the most common neuromuscular disease to cause dysphagia. The disease process affects the ability to initiate and coordinate complex motor tasks. An increase in oral pharyngeal transit time and decreased tongue movements have been noted [50]. Despite improvement of limb motor function with dopamine therapy, dysphagia may not improve. Swallow dysfunction is a late manifestation of Parkinson's disease typically diagnosed greater than 1 year after diagnosis [51].

In amyotrophic lateral sclerosis (ALS), initiation of the voluntary swallow is prolonged. Aspiration is a less common phenomenon as pharyngeal and laryngeal sensation remains intact. Swallow therapy has been beneficial though some may eventually progress to require nonoral-feeding methods [52]. Other neurological etiologies include traumatic brain injury, Alzheimer's disease, multiple sclerosis, brain malignancy, and Huntington's disease. Though rarely a presenting symptom, myasthenia gravis and muscular dystrophy may report dysphagia.

Medications may affect swallow function through several mechanisms. The most frequent mechanism is through xerostomia. Xerostomia is common with medications that have anticholinergic effects such as antihistamines, tricyclic antidepressants, neuroleptics, antiemetics, and antidiarrhea medications. Elderly patients in an inpatient setting who were given an antipsychotic medication were three times more likely to have swallowing dysfunction that an age-matched controls who were not taking an antipsychotic [53]. By affecting saliva production, xerostomia alters bolus formation and transport. Dehydration from diuretic use may worsen xerostomia.

Alteration of arousal level resulting in mental status changes may also affect swallowing and feeding function. Medications should be screened for sedative properties such as hypnotics, anxiolytics, muscle relaxants, and analgesics. Alcohol may compound sedative effect.

Medications may alter esophageal function. Particularly in those with xerostomia, this effect may be magnified as less saliva with its neutralizing sodium bicarbonate content is produced. Pill-induced esophagitis may cause odynophagia through four primary mechanisms [54]. Prolonged mucosal contact may result in a direct caustic effect such as is seen with clindamycin, potassium, alendronate, and quinidine. Esophageal pH may be altered through medications such as clindamycin, tetracycline, ascorbic acid, and iron resulting in an acid burn. Phenytoin may result in an alkaline burn. Doxycycline and nonsteroidal anti-inflammatory drugs may accumulate to toxic levels within the esophagus. Drugs such as calcium channel blockers, nitrates, and theophylline may result in relaxation of the lower esophageal sphincter and induce gastric reflux [55].

Pill-induced esophagitis may be diagnosed though esophagoscopy where a well demarcated ulcer may be seen surrounded by normal mucosa. The most common site of injury in the esophagus is the area posterior to the arch of the aorta which is a natural site of narrowing and an area of manometrically decreased peristalsis. Compensation strategies include taking medications with ample water, crushing pills or taking the medication in liquid form, avoiding a double swallow, and taking medications in an upright position [56].

Esophageal motility disorders may result in dysphagia symptoms. Manometry allows for a specific diagnosis. Achalasia refers to an aperistaltic esophageal body with elevated LES pressures. A characteristic "bird beak" pattern may be seen on barium esophagram. In contrast, patients with scleroderma will also have a nonperistaltic mid- and distal esophagus but with the absence of LES pressures waves. There are normal findings in the proximal esophagus. Diffuse esophageal spasm features at least 20% of uncoordinated, simultaneous contractions with some normal peristalsis. The mean pressures of the distal esophagus exceed 180 mmHg in "nutcracker" esophagus. Residual pressures

greater than 5 mmHg after swallowing suggest incomplete LES relaxation while LES pressures that do not exceed 10 mmHg indicate a hypotensive LES. Ribeiro et al. reported that when compared with younger patients, elderly patients were less likely to have normal esophageal motility and were more likely to have achalasia or diffuse esophageal spasm [57]. Among those with achalasia, as diagnosed by manometry, cough and dyspnea were more frequent complaints in the elderly than chest pain seen in younger patients [58]. A comparison of patients with known esophageal dysmotility found that elderly patients over 80 years old were more likely to report dysphagia as their main complaint and have significantly more complaints of dysphagia to solids and liquids than younger patients. Younger patients were more likely to report symptoms of heartburn [59].

The presence of an obstructing lesion should be suspected in those with solid food dysphagia. Esophageal webs have been found in the proximal esophagus, particularly in those with Plummer–Vinson syndrome (Fig. 44.3). Two forms of esophageal rings may be present. The less frequently seen Type A ring is a thick muscular ring found in the distal esophagus. These muscular rings do not respond well to dilation but may improve after botulism toxin injection. The Type B ring, also known as a Schatzki's ring, is found at the gastroesophageal junction. Rings with an opening diameter <13 mm tend to be symptomatic. The Type B ring responds to dilation or disruption.

Reflux esophagitis is a prevalent disease process found in the geriatric population [60]. Elderly patient were less likely to report classic gastroesophageal reflux symptoms such as heartburn or epigastric pain than younger patients. Instead, symptoms such as anorexia and dysphagia were more common [61]. The duration of reflux episodes, possibly secondary to

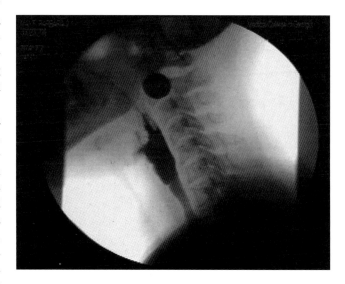

FIGURE 44.3 Fluoroscopic image of an anterior esophageal web at approximately the sixth cervical vertebra.

impaired esophageal motility, has been shown to be longer in the elderly [62]. Proton pump inhibitor therapy remains the primary therapeutic agent.

Candida albicans is the most frequent cause of infectious esophagitis. Risk factors for the development of a fungal esophagitis include immunodeficiency, diabetes, steroid use, and impaired esophageal motility. Candida colonies can also be seen among nonimmunosuppressed individuals as well. Treatment involves either a topical or systemic antifungal agent. Frank ulceration of the esophageal mucosa is uncommon and suggests a concurrent viral infection such as cytomegalovirus.

Cricopharyngeal (CP) dysfunction may contribute to dysphagia symptoms in the elderly. The dysfunction may be due to functional or structural reasons. Functional CP dysfunction refers to the failure of UES relaxation and has been associated with brainstem infarction, traumatic brain injury, and other neurological degenerative diseases. Figure 44.3 demonstrates the failure of CP relaxation with obstruction, commonly referred to as a cricopharyngeal bar. Structural CP dysfunction results in improper opening of the UES, despite relaxation of the UES musculature (Fig. 44.4). Structural CP dysfunction is commonly found in postradiation patients [63]. In addition, large cervical osteophytes in the region of the UES can lead to obstruction (Fig. 44.5).

Within the UES, manometric studies have demonstrated that the area superior to the horizontal fibers of the CP muscle is exposed to the highest pressures. This region, known as the Killian's dehiscence, has a low density of muscle fibers compared with the rest of the UES. Outpouching of the pharynx in this area, secondary to elevated CP pressures, may result in the development of a Zenker's diverticulum [64] (Fig. 44.6).

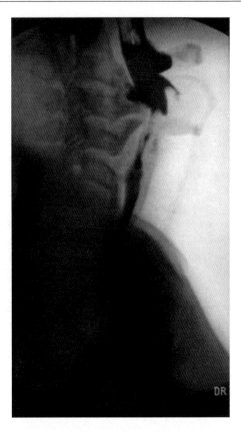

Figure 44.5 Large anterior cervical osteophytes at the level of the UES impairing the passage of food material into the esophagus.

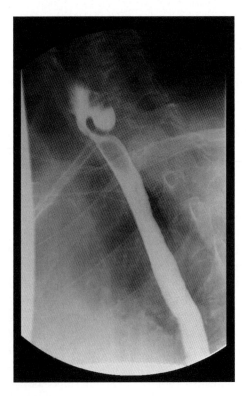

Figure 44.6 A large Zenker's diverticulum demonstrated as a pouch separate from the esophagus on barium swallow.

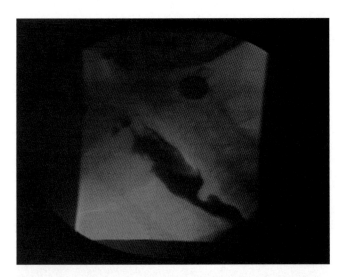

Figure 44.4 A cricopharyngeal bar, in this case, resulting from the failure of cricopharyngeal muscle relaxation despite excellent hyolaryngeal elevation during swallowing.

CASE STUDY

An 83-year-old man is accompanied by his 64-year-old daughter for a chief complaint of food "getting" stuck in his throat. He reports these symptoms have been present for years but have been getting worse. He states that recently at dinner, he felt like he was choking on a piece of chicken. His voice has gradually become softer over the years. He denies any weight loss or coughing with meal. His daughter, however, states that he coughs frequently after drinking his morning coffee. His past medical history is significant for a thyroidectemy 40 years ago, myocardial infarction at the age of 67, and COPD. He has a 50-pack-year history but quit smoking 5 years ago.

After a comprehensive physical examination, a laryngoscopy should be performed to evaluate the hypopharynx and laryngeal structures. Given his smoking history, the presence of a mucosal lesion would be concerning for a malignancy. The status of the vocal folds should be assessed in terms of mobility and "bulk" as "bowing" or atrophy of the vocal folds may be present. The pooling of secretions is highly suggestive of an obstruction or motility dysfunction.

Given his complaints of both solids and liquids, a FEES examination could be incorporated into the laryngoscopy. An alternative would be a MBS. Advantages of the FEES examination include the ability to perform without the need of a fluoroscopy suite and detailed views of the larynx. The MBS allows for the analysis of esophageal phase, particularly relevant given his solid food dysphagia. While both examinations allow for feedback, patient understanding of exam is usually greater with the FEES examination.

FEES examination demonstrated reduced pharyngeal muscular squeeze with retained secretions in the pyriform sinuses. Vocal fold mobility was normal and there were no masses present. Laryngeal sensation appeared reduced. MBS confirmed these observations and added the finding of mild esophageal dysmotility. There was no esophageal structures, diverticula, or masses noted on the esophagram.

The patient's dysphagia was attributed to age-related changes and a dietary and behavioral intervention program was initiated by the speech pathologist. He was counseled to chew foods well, take small bites, and alternate liquids and solids. These interventions controlled the patient's symptoms well.

Treatment

Two of the most important decisions that need to be made after the swallowing evaluation are whether the person is safe for oral swallowing and if so, with what consistencies and texture. Diets may be modified to exclude certain food consistencies. While diet modification may help prevent aspiration of ingested food, patients may remain at risk for aspiration of saliva or gastric refluxate. Swallow rehabilitation may include various methods to improve muscle function and coordination. These may include electrical stimulation, thermal stimulation, and muscle strength exercises. Additional strategies aim to optimize body posture and head position. Compensatory maneuvers, such as a supraglottic swallow, swallowing while breath holding, may improve function. Early intervention through swallow rehabilitation may allow a safe swallow and avoid or delay the need for nonoral feeding such as a gastrostomy tube.

In some patients, oral feeding may be considered unsafe and nonoral means of nutrition may be required. Two of the most common techniques are nutrition via a nasogastric tube or via a gastrostomy tube [65]. Nakajoh reported that the rate of aspiration pneumonia was significantly greater among dysphagic stroke patients who were fed orally versus those who had tube feedings, though the functional status of the orally fed group was higher [66]. No prospective, randomized trials

exist that compare oral versus PEG feeds in the advanced dementia population. However, analysis of the available data finds that among those with advanced dementia, tube feeds do not prevent aspiration pneumonia, prolonged survival, reduce the risk of pressure ulcers or infection, improved function, or provide palliation [67, 68].

Surgical Management

Because of the multifactorial nature of dysphagia in the older adult, surgery usually takes a secondary role to behavioral and dietary intervention. That being said, some specific problems can be well addressed with judicious use of surgery. The most common problems and the surgical techniques that can be utilized to treat them are summarized below.

Esophageal and Cricopharyngeal Narrowing

Strictures of the esophagus and cricopharyngeal segment are best initially managed with serial dilation in individuals who are able to tolerate anesthesia. The site of stricture can be visualized clearly on barium esophagram. Two important diagnostic considerations must be taken into account prior to dilation. Most importantly, the surgeon must identify the etiology of the narrowed segment with esophagoscopy and rule out carcinoma. Either rigid or flexible esophagoscopy can be utilized. Flexible endoscopic imaging, however, is favored because it can be easily performed under sedation or even awake, using TNE [69]. Stenotic segments at the cricopharyngeal segment need to be carefully evaluated in the geriatric patient. In many of these cases, the narrowing noted on barium swallow results from inadequate hyolaryngeal elevation and failure of cricopharyngeal opening, rather than true stenosis. Once the cricopharyngeal segment is identified as the true source of stenosis, the surgeon must differentiate whether the segment is stenotic or whether cricopharyngeal spasm is present. Stenotic segments respond to dilation (again after neoplasm is excluded).

Cricopharyngeal spasm is best treated with either botulinum toxin injection or cricopharyngeal myotomy. Cricopharyngeal myotomy has been traditionally performed with an external approach through the neck. Recently popularized endoscopic approaches offer a more minimally invasive approach, but long-term outcomes are pending [70].

With regard to dilation, serial dilation can be performed blindly with Maloney dilators or over a guide wire with Savary dilators. It can be performed under sedation or under general anesthesia. Caution should be used with rigid esophagoscopy due to reduced flexibility of the cervical spine and cervical osteophytes in older individuals, which make exposure difficult and increase the risk for esophageal perforation. Radial dilation using balloon dilators passed under flexible esophagoscopy has become more commonplace because of this risk.

Zenker's Diverticula

Zenker's diverticula occur at a natural muscular dehiscence between the cricopharyngeus muscle and the inferior constrictor (Killian's Triangle). They are easily visualized on barium swallow, but, because of their location by the esophageal inlet,

they are harder to identify on endoscopy. The flexible endoscope tends to fall into the pouch, and the natural esophageal opening can be difficult to find. Due to the more frail nature of the esophageal wall in elderly individuals, extra caution must be taken with any resistance to endoscope passage.

The decision to treat a Zenker's diverticulum depends on the severity of symptoms and the size of the pouch. Individuals with minimal dysphagia and a small pouch can be simply monitored. More severe symptoms warrant intervention. The treatment of Zenker's diverticula can be approached either through an external or an endoscopic approach. The familiar external approach involves cricopharyngeal myotomy (the most important step) plus diverticulectomy or diverticulopexy. Over the past decade, however, most patients are being treated with an endoscopic stapling or CO_2 laser division of the common wall between the cricopharyngeus and the pouch [71]. A cricopharyngeal myotomy is thereby also performed (Fig. 44.7a, b). This approach is less invasive, equally effective, has fewer complications, and in many areas has become the standard of care for initial treatment. Thus, in most situations, it is a more suitable initial approach in the geriatric patient.

Glottal Insufficiency

With age, the vocal folds become more atrophic, and individuals may have reduced glottal closure and protection of the airway during swallowing. Vocal fold paralysis also occurs more frequently in the elderly, usually arising iatrogenically from anterior cervical spine, thyroid, and thoracic surgery, or from carcinoma of the lung involving the recurrent laryngeal nerve. The resulting glottal insufficiency can vary in severity. Some patients have minimal symptoms limited to mild vocal difficulties and some have severe symptoms with near complete loss of voice and severe dysphagia. A careful assessment of the patient's voice and swallowing symptoms as well as a detailed laryngeal examination with in-office endoscopic laryngoscopy help direct treatment.

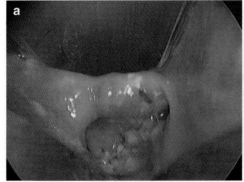 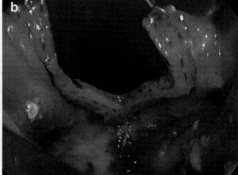

Figure 44.7 Endoscopic picture of a Zenker's diverticulum. (**a**) Note the pouch inferiorly containing food material and the party wall between the pouch and the esophagus anteriorly. (**b**) Endoscopic stapling of the pouch simultaneously divides the cricopharyngeus and opens the pouch into the native esophagus.

Glottal insufficiency can be treated with voice and swallowing therapy from a speech-language pathologist, vocal fold injection augmentation, and laryngeal framework surgery. An initial approach with therapy makes sense, particularly for dysphagia symptoms, as most swallowing symptoms are improved with behavioral strategies, such as chin-tuck swallowing and head-turn swallowing [72]. Surgical options are reserved for cases when therapy fails or is likely to fail due to the severity of disease.

While Teflon vocal fold injection has been largely abandoned due to granuloma formation, other injectables are well suited to augment the vocal folds and improve glottal insufficiency. Collagen, carboxymethylcellulose, and hyaluronic acid injectables offer temporary augmentation in situations where function is expected to return. Calcium hydroxylapatite can be used for more durable results. Vocal fold injection can be performed either under general anesthesia or awake in the office, endoscopy suite, or even at the bedside. Although less precise, awake injection offers the elderly patient significant advantage in avoiding general anesthesia.

Laryngeal framework surgery refers to two main procedures designed to reposition the vocal fold permanently: type-I thyroplasty and arytenoid adduction [73]. These procedures offer precise vocal fold medialization and are performed in the operating room under light sedation. Voice improvement has been clearly documented and although there is less evidence, swallowing improvement also occurs [74].

Other Procedures

Laryngectomy and laryngotracheal separation are uncommonly used for profound aspiration [75]. Laryngectomy separates the respiratory tract from the digestive tract and essentially eliminates aspiration. Patients experience significant loss of quality of life largely related the permanent tracheostoma and loss of laryngeal voice. Although voice can be restored through esophageal speech, tracheoesophageal puncture, and electrolaryngeal speech, laryngectomy is rarely performed for geriatric dysphagia. Laryngotracheal separation results in a similar effect as laryngectomy. Although theoretically reversible, voice rehabilitation is more difficult, and most patients can be managed with other techniques.

Tracheotomy is seldom performed for dysphagia alone, and should be considered a means for respiratory management. A tracheotomy does not prevent aspiration, and may, in fact, make aspiration worse [76]. However, patients with a tracheotomy have better pulmonary toilet and access to the respiratory system for suctioning and ventilator use. Because of these advantages, caution should be taken in decannulating patients with severe dysphagia.

Summary

Dysphagia is common in the geriatric patient causing significant functional and emotional quality-of-life impairment. Dysphagia in these patients is commonly multifactorial. Keen understanding of normal swallowing physiology and the common changes in the swallowing associated with aging are required in order to render an accurate diagnosis and therapeutic plan. MBS studies have been supplemented by flexible endoscopic evaluation of swallowing in the diagnostic armamentarium for these patients. Early involvement of speech-language pathology is critical in the assessment and intervention of geriatric dysphagia. Judicious use of surgery can positively impact dysphagia in select cases.

References

1. Roy N, Stemple J, Merrill RM, Thomas L (2007) Dysphagia in the elderly: preliminary evidence of prevalence, risk factors, and socioemotional effects. Ann Otol Rhinol Laryngol 116:858–865
2. US Census Bureau (2004) US interim projections by age, sex, race, and hispanic origin. http://www.census.gov/ipc/www/usinterimproj/
3. Leibovitz A, Baumoehl Y, Lubart E, Yaina A, Platinovitz N, Segal R (2007) Dehydration among long-term care elderly patients with oropharyngeal dysphagia. Gerontology 53:179–183
4. Ruiz M, Ewig S, Torres A, Arancibia F, Marco F, Mensa J, Sanchez M, Martinez JA (1999) Severe community-acquired pneumonia. Risk factors and follow-up epidemiology. Am J Respir Crit Care Med 160:923–929
5. Kozak LJ, DeFrances CJ, Hall MJ (2006) National Hospital Discharge Survey: 2004 annual summary with detailed diagnosis and procedure data. National Center for Health Statistics. Vital Health Stat 13:162
6. Altman KW, Schaefer SD, Yu GP, Hertegard S, Lundy DS, Blumin JH, Maronian NC, Heman-Ackah YD, Abitbol J, Casiano RR, Neurolaryngology Subcommittee of the American Academy of Otolaryngology – Head and Neck Surgery (2007) The voice and laryngeal dysfunction in stroke: a report from the Neurolaryngology Subcommittee of the American Academy of Otolaryngology – Head and Neck Surgery. Otolaryngol Head Neck Surg 136:873–881
7. Muder R (1998) Pneumonia in residents of long-term care facilities: epidemiology, etiology, management, and prevention. Am J Med 105:319–330
8. Schindler JS, Kelly JH (2002) Swallowing disorders in the elderly. Laryngoscope 112:589–602
9. Dray TG, Hillel AD, Miller RM (1998) Dysphagia caused by neurologic deficits. Otolaryngol Clin North Am 31:507–524
10. Singh S, Hamdy S (2006) Dysphagia in stroke patients. Postgrad Med J 82:383–391
11. Dziewas R, Warnecke T, Hamacher C, Oelenberg S, Teismann I, Kraemer C, Ritter M, Ringelstein EB, Schaebitz WR (2008) Do nasogastric tubes worsen dysphagia in patients with acute stroke? BMC Neurol 8:28
12. Ertekin C, Aydogdu I (2003) Neurophysiology of swallowing. Clin Neurophysiol 114:2226–2244
13. Forbes GB (1988) Body composition: influences of nutrition, disease, growth and aging. In: Shis ME, Young VR (eds) Modern nutrition in health and disease, 7th edn. Lea & Feibiger, Philadelphia

14. Jaradeh S (1994) Neurophysiology of swallowing in the aged. Dysphagia 9:218–220

15. Fucile S, Wright PM, Chan I, Yee S, Langlais ME, Gisel EG (1998) Functional oral-motor skills: do they change with age? Dysphagia 13:195–201

16. Stephen JR, Taves DH, Smith RC, Martin RE (2005) Bolus location at the initiation of the pharyngeal stage of swallowing in healthy older adults. Dysphagia 20:266–272

17. Bennett JW, van Lieshout PH, Steele CM (2007) Tongue control for speech and swallowing in healthy younger and older subjects. Int J Orofacial Myology 33:5–18

18. Yoshikawa M, Yoshida M, Nagasaki T, Tanimoto K, Tsuga K, Akagawa Y, Komatsu T (2005) Aspects of swallowing in healthy dentate elderly persons older than 80 years. J Gerontol A Biol Sci Med Sci 60:506–509

19. Robbins J, Hamilton JW, Lof GL, Kempster GB (1992) Oropharyngeal swallowing in normal adults of different ages. Gastroenterology 103:823–829

20. Nilsson H, Ekberg O, Olsson R, Hindfelt B (1996) Quantitative aspects of swallowing in an elderly nondysphagic population. Dysphagia 11:180–184

21. Aviv JE, Martin JH, Jones ME, Wee TA, Diamond B, Keen MS, Blitzer A (1994) Age-related changes in pharyngeal and supraglottic sensation. Ann Otol Rhinol Laryngol 103:749–752

22. Leonard R, Kendall K, McKenzie S (2004) UES opening and cricopharyngeal bar in nondysphagic elderly and nonelderly adults. Dysphagia 19:182–191

23. Shaker R, Ren J, Zamir Z, Sarna A, Liu J, Sui Z (1994) Effect of aging, position, and temperature on the threshold volume triggering pharyngeal swallows. Gastroenterology 107:396–402

24. Ren J, Shaker R, Kusano M, Podvrsan B, Metwally N, Dua KS, Sui Z (1995) Effect of aging on the secondary esophageal peristalsis: presbyesophagus revisited. Am J Physiol 268:G772–G779

25. Miura H, Kariyasu M, Sumi Y, Yamasaki K (2008) Labial closure force, activities of daily living, and cognitive function in frail elderly persons. Nippon Ronen Igakkai Zasshi 45:520–525

26. Martino R, Pron G, Diamant N (2000) Screening for oropharyngeal dysphagia in stroke: insufficient evidence for guidelines. Dysphagia 15:19–30

27. Leder SB (1996) Gag reflex and dysphagia. Head Neck 18:138–141

28. Marques CH, de Rosso AL, André C (2008) Bedside assessment of swallowing in stroke: water tests are not enough. Top Stroke Rehabil 15:378–383

29. Splaingard ML, Hutchins B, Sulton LD, Chaudhuri G (1988) Aspiration in rehabilitation patients: videofluoroscopy vs bedside clinical assessment. Arch Phys Med Rehabil 69:637–640

30. Smithard DG, O'Neill PA, England RE, Park CL, Wyatt R, Martin DF, Morris J (1997) The natural history of dysphagia following a stroke. Dysphagia 12:188–193

31. Leder SB, Espinosa JF (2002) Aspiration risk after acute stroke: comparison of clinical examination and fiberoptic endoscopic evaluation of swallowing. Dysphagia 17:214–218

32. Amin MR, Postma GN (2004) Office evaluation of swallowing. Ear Nose Throat J 83:13–16

33. Langmore SE, Schatz K, Olsen N (1988) Fiberoptic endoscopic examination of swallowing safety: a new procedure. Dysphagia 2:216–219

34. Aviv JE, Kim T, Sacco RL, Kaplan S, Goodhart K, Diamond B, Close LG (1998) FEESST: a new bedside endoscopic test of the motor and sensory components of swallowing. Ann Otol Rhinol Laryngol 107:378–387

35. Kelly AM, Drinnan MJ, Leslie P (2007) Assessing penetration and aspiration: how do videofluoroscopy and fiberoptic endoscopic evaluation of swallowing compare? Laryngoscope 117:1723–1727

36. Aviv JE (2000) Prospective, randomized outcome study of endoscopy versus modified barium swallow in patients with dysphagia. Laryngoscope 110:563–574

37. Waring JP, Baron TH, Hirota WK, Goldstein JL, Jacobson BC, Leighton JA, Mallery JS, Faigel DO, American Society for Gastrointestinal Endoscopy, Standards of Practice Committee (2003) Guidelines for conscious sedation and monitoring during gastrointestinal endoscopy. Gastrointest Endosc 58:317–322

38. Sharma VK, Nguyen CC, Crowell MD, Lieberman DA, de Garmo O, Fleisher DE (2007) A national study of cardiopulmonary unplanned events after GI endoscopy. Gastrointest Endosc 66:27–34

39. Postma GN, Bach KK, Belafsky PC, Koufman JA (2002) The role of transnasal esophagoscopy in head and neck oncology. Laryngoscope 112:2242–2243

40. Saeian K, Staff DM, Vasilopoulos S, Townsend WF, Almagro UA, Komorowski RA, Choi H, Shaker R (2002) Unsedated transnasal endoscopy accurately detects Barrett's metaplasia and dysplasia. Gastrointest Endosc 56:472–478

41. Jobe BA, Hunter JG, Chang EY, Kim CY, Eisen GM, Robinson JD, Diggs BS, O'Rourke RW, Rader AE, Schipper P, Sauer DA, Peters JH, Lieberman DA, Morris CD (2006) Office-based unsedated small-caliber endoscopy is equivalent to conventional sedated endoscopy in screening and surveillance for Barrett's esophagus: a randomized and blinded comparison. Am J Gastroenterol 101:2693–2703

42. Mann G, Hankey GJ, Cameron D (1999) Swallowing function after stroke: prognosis and prognostic factors at 6 months. Stroke 30:744–748

43. Gordon C, Hewer RL, Wade DT (1987) Dysphagia in acute stroke. Br Med J (Clin Res Ed) 295:411–414

44. Dray TG, Hillel AD, Miller RM (1998) Dysphagia caused by neurologic deficits. Otolaryngol Clin North Am 31:507–524

45. Reeves MJ, Broderick JP, Frankel M, LaBresh KA, Schwamm L, Moomaw CJ, Weiss P, Katzan I, Paul Coverdell Prototype Registries Writing Group, Arora S, Heinrich JP, Hickenbottom S, Karp H, Malarcher A, Mensah G, Reeves MJ (2006) The Paul Coverdell National Acute Stroke Registry: initial results from four prototypes. Am J Prev Med 31:S202–S209

46. Paciaroni M, Mazzotta G, Corea F, Caso V, Venti M, Milia P, Silvestrelli G, Palmerini F, Parnetti L, Gallai V (2004) Dysphagia following stroke. Eur Neurol 51:162–167

47. Brown M, Glassenberg M (1973) Mortality factors in patients with acute stroke. J Am Med Assoc 224:1493–1495

48. Daniels SK, Brailey K, Foundas AL (1999) Lingual discoordination and dysphagia following acute stroke: analyses of lesion localization. Dysphagia 14:85–92

49. Barer DH (1989) The natural history and functional consequences of dysphagia after hemispheric stroke. J Neurol Neurosurg Psychiatry 52:236–241

50. Nagaya M, Kachi T, Yamada T, Igata A (1998) Videofluorographic study of swallowing in Parkinson's disease. Dysphagia 13:95–100

51. Müller J, Wenning GK, Verny M, McKee A, Chaudhuri KR, Jellinger K, Poewe W, Litvan I (2001) Progression of dysarthria and dysphagia in postmortem-confirmed parkinsonian disorders. Arch Neurol 58:259–264

52. Grujic J, Coutaz M, Morisod J (2008) Amyotrophic lateral sclerosis also threatens the octogenarian. Rev Méd Suisse 4:1353–1357

53. Rudolph JL, Gardner KF, Gramigna GD, McGlinchey RE (2008) Antipsychotics and oropharyngeal dysphagia in hospitalized older patients. J Clin Psychopharmacol 28:532–535

54. Kikendall JW, Friedman AC, Oyewole MA, Fleischer D, Johnson LF (1983) Pill-induced esophageal injury. Case reports and review of the medical literature. Dig Dis Sci 28:174–182

55. Chami TN, Nikoomanesh P, Katz PO (1995) An unusual presentation of pill-induced esophagitis. Gastrointest Endosc 42:263–265

56. Misra SP, Dwivedi M (2002) Pill-induced esophagitis. Gastrointest Endosc 55:81
57. Ribeiro AC, Klingler PJ, Hinder RA, DeVault K (1998) Esophageal manometry: a comparison of findings in younger and older patients. Am J Gastroenterol 93:706–710
58. Kagansky N, Rimon E, Eliaz A, Levy S (2004) [Primary esophageal achalasia in octogenarians: does it really exist?]. Harefuah 143:775–778
59. Andrews JM, Fraser RJ, Heddle R, Hebbard G, Checklin H (2008) Is esophageal dysphagia in the extreme elderly (≥80 years) different to dysphagia younger adults? A clinical motility service audit. Dis Esophagus 21:656–659
60. Johnson DA (2004) Gastroesophageal reflux disease in the elderly – a prevalent and severe disease. Rev Gastroenterol Disord 4: S16–S24
61. Pilotto A, Franceschi M, Leandro G, Scarcelli C, D'Ambrosio LP, Seripa D, Perri F, Niro V, Paris F, Andriulli A, Di Mario F (2006) Clinical features of reflux esophagitis in older people: a study of 840 consecutive patients. J Am Geriatr Soc 54:1537–1542
62. Ferriolli E, Oliveira RB, Matsuda NM, Braga FJ, Dantas RO (1998) Aging, esophageal motility, and gastroesophageal reflux. J Am Geriatr Soc 46:1534–1537
63. Ekberg O, Nylander G (1982) Dysfunction of the cricopharyngeal muscle. A cineradiographic study of patients with dysphagia. Radiology 143:481–486
64. Cook IJ, Gabb M, Panagopoulos V, Jamieson GG, Dodds WJ, Dent J, Shearman DJ (1992) Pharyngeal (Zenker's) diverticulum is a disorder of upper esophageal sphincter opening. Gastroenterology 103:1229–1235
65. Nakajima M, Kimura K, Inatomi Y, Terasaki Y, Nagano K, Yonehara T, Uchino M, Minematsu K (2006) Intermittent oro-esophageal tube feeding in acute stroke patients – a pilot study. Acta Neurol Scand 113:36–39
66. Nakajoh K, Nakagawa T, Sekizawa K, Matsui T, Arai H, Sasaki H (2000) Relation between incidence of pneumonia and protective reflexes in post-stroke patients with oral or tube feeding. J Intern Med 247:39–42
67. Finucane TE, Christmas C, Leff BA (2007) Tube feeding in dementia: how incentives undermine health care quality and patient safety. J Am Med Dir Assoc 8:205–208
68. Cervo FA, Bryan L, Farber S (2006) To PEG or not to PEG: a review of evidence for placing feeding tubes in advanced dementia and the decision-making process. Geriatrics 61:30–35
69. Postma GN, Cohen JT, Belafsky PC, Halum SL, Gupta SK, Bach KK, Koufman JA (2005) Transnasal esophagoscopy: revisited (over 700 consecutive cases). Laryngoscope 115(2):321–323
70. Pitman M, Weissbrod P (2009) Endoscopic CO2 laser cricopharyngeal myotomy. Laryngoscope 119(1):45–53
71. Hillel AT, Flint PW (2009) Evolution of endoscopic surgical therapy for Zenker's diverticulum. Laryngoscope 119(1):39–44
72. Robbins J, Butler SG, Daniels SK, Diez Gross R, Langmore S, Lazarus CL, Martin-Harris B, McCabe D, Musson N, Rosenbek J (2008) Swallowing and dysphagia rehabilitation: translating principles of neural plasticity into clinically oriented evidence. J Speech Lang Hear Res 51(1):S276–S300
73. Mahieu HF (2006) Practical applications of laryngeal framework surgery. Otolaryngol Clin North Am 39(1):55–75
74. McCulloch TM, Hoffman HT, Andrews BT et al (2000) Arytenoid adduction combined with GoreTex medialization thyroplasty. Laryngoscope 110:1306–1311
75. Eibling DE, Snyderman CH, Eibling C (1995) Laryngotracheal separation for intractable aspiration: a retrospective review of 34 patients. Laryngoscope 105:83–85
76. Sharma OP, Oswanski MF, Singer D et al (2007) Swallowing disorders in trauma patients: impact of tracheostomy. Am Surg 73:1117–1121

Chapter 45
Head and Neck Cancer in the Elderly

Babak Givi and Ashok R. Shaha

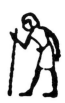

The head and neck region harbors a wide variety of malignancies. While the majority are easily treatable skin cancers, the bulk of mortality and morbidity comes from squamous cell carcinomas of the upper aerodigestive tract. Head and neck cancers account for approximately 3–5% of all cancers in the US. In 2007, more than 33,000 people were suffering from oral cavity, pharynx and laryngeal cancers in the US [1]. Moreover, head and neck cancers afflict the elderly population disproportionately.

The management of head and neck cancers has undergone major changes with the advent of new modalities such as organ preservation, partial resection, and microvascular free tissue transfers. In addition, new advances in chemotherapy and radiotherapy have offered new hope for patients. Few other areas of the body harbor as many critical organs as the head and neck. Consequently, diseases and treatments can cause significant morbidity and loss of critical function for the patient. While the results of surgery have improved quite significantly through the years, there are still major challenges in this field. One of the main problems is control of locoregional recurrence where there are few therapeutic options and treatment modalities can cause significant morbidity. Another important treatment aspect for head and neck cancers is the importance of multidisciplinary involvement. The roles of speech therapists, nutritionists, pain management, and maxillofacial prosthodontists can be as important as those of head and neck surgeons, medical oncologists, and radiation therapists. In spite of higher prevalence of head and neck cancers in the elderly population, there is paucity of data on the management and outcome of this group. Many myths and beliefs have prevented elderly patients from receiving standard therapies [2]. Traditionally, surgeons are reluctant to endeavor more aggressive surgical resections on this population. Furthermore, more recent trials of combined modality treatments such as concurrent chemoradiation, often have excluded elderly candidates [3]. This lack of data adds

to the challenges of head and neck cancer practitioner in planning optimal management of elderly patients. There is not always specific data or recommendations in management of different subsites of head and neck cancer in elderly. Based on evidence, these differences will be discussed in each section.

Clinical Anatomy of the Head and Neck

A basic understanding of anatomy is essential for all practitioners involved in the care of head and neck cancer patients. The upper aerodigestive tract is divided into the nose and paranasal sinuses, oral cavity, pharynx, and larynx (Fig. 45.1). Salivary gland anatomy will be discussed later in this chapter.

The nasal cavity consists of the space between the vestibule of the nose anteriorly and nasopharynx posteriorly. The lateral walls are bounded by turbinates and the nasal septum stands medially. The cribriform plate superiorly and hard palate inferiorly form the other two boundaries. The openings of frontal, maxillary, and ethmoid sinuses lie in the middle meatus between the middle and inferior turbinates. Tumor blockage of these openings can cause symptoms of sinusitis and opacification of sinuses on radiologic studies. The maxillary sinus is the most common site for paranasal sinus tumors. The maxillary sinus is divided by an imaginary plane (Ohngren's line) that runs between the medial canthus of the eye and the angle of mandible into the anteroinferior and superoposterior sections. Tumors of superoposterior section are more challenging, since treatment often requires management of orbital floor and skull base. Up to 15% of patients with maxillary sinus tumors will present with metastases to cervical node levels I and II. Sphenoid and frontal sinus tumors are quite uncommon.

The oral cavity is defined as the space between the vermilion of the lips and the junction of the hard and soft palate superiorly, and circumvallate papillae inferiorly. It is further divided into the vestibule (the space between the cheek and the teeth) and the oral cavity proper. Further subsites of

A.R. Shaha (✉)
Department of Surgery, Memorial Sloan Kettering Cancer Center,
1275 York Avenue, New York, NY 10065, USA
e-mail: givib@mskcc.org

R.A. Rosenthal et al. (eds.), *Principles and Practice of Geriatric Surgery*,
DOI 10.1007/978-1-4419-6999-6_45, © Springer Science+Business Media, LLC 2011

Figure 45.1 Sagittal section of the upper aerodigestive tract (From N Eng J med 328: 184–194, 1993).

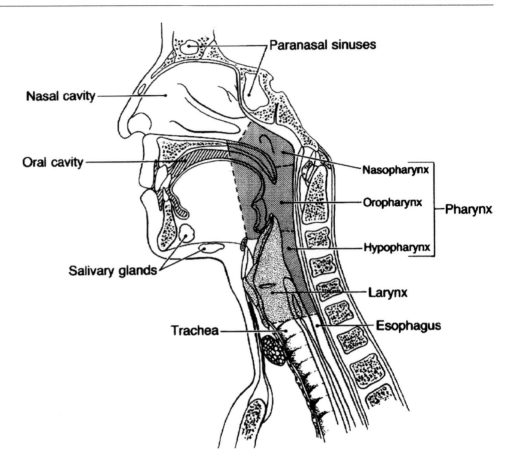

mouth include the lips, buccal mucosa, lower and upper alveolar ridges, retromolar trigone, floor of the mouth, hard palate, and anterior two-thirds of the tongue (oral tongue). Tumors of the oral cavity usually metastasize first to level I, then to level II and III of the cervical lymph nodes.

The pharynx is a muscular tube that communicates with the nasal, oral, and laryngeal cavities. It is divided into the nasopharynx superiorly, the oropharynx in the middle, and the hypopharynx inferiorly. The region between the skull base and the junction of the hard and soft palate is the nasopharynx. The oropharynx includes the base of tongue, vallecula, soft palate, tonsil, tonsillar fossa, and posterior pharyngeal wall. The hypopharynx consists of three areas: the pyriform sinus, the posterior pharyngeal wall between vallecula and cricoarytenoid joints, and the postcricoid area from the arytenoid cartilage to the inferior border of cricoid cartilage. Lymphatic drainage depends on the location of the lesion. While the nasopharynx drains into the upper part of the posterior triangle, the oropharynx drains to level II, and hypopharynx drains to levels II, III, and IV nodes. Base of the tongue lesion and those close to the midline have a propensity to metastasize bilaterally.

The larynx is divided into three parts. The supraglottic larynx extends from the hypopharynx to a horizontal plane passing through laryngeal ventricle. The epiglottis, aryepiglottic folds, arytenoid and false vocal cords make up the supraglottic larynx. This area has rich lymphatic drainage and lesions tend to metastasize early and bilaterally to the jugular chain. The glottic larynx, on the other hand, has very few lymphatic channels. This phenomenon, in addition to early symptoms due to hoarseness resulting from true vocal cord lesions, makes glottic cancer the most favorable of laryngeal cancers in terms of prognosis. Subglottic tumors are extremely rare. Most commonly, a glottic tumor extends to the subglottic area. Tumors involving the subglottic area tend to metastasize to the jugular chain and tracheoesophageal nodes.

A thorough knowledge of the anatomy and classification of lymphatic structure of the head and neck is of utmost importance to all practitioners of head and neck cancers. Cervical lymph nodes are the most common site of metastases from different head and neck cancers and also a common locus of recurrence. The most commonly used method for classification of cervical lymph nodes is the one originally devised by the Head and Neck Service at Memorial Sloan-Kettering Cancer Center almost half a century ago and later adopted by American Head and Neck Society. The most recent revision was published in 2002 [4]. Since then minor refinements have been added to this classification [5]. In this system, the lymphatics of the neck are divided into six levels (Fig. 45.2). Level I is submandibular triangle lymph nodes; level II is upper jugular; level III is mid jugular; level IV is lower jugular; level V is posterior triangle lymph nodes; and level VI is anterior compartment, prelaryngeal, and paratracheal lymph nodes. Nodes in the superior mediastinum below suprasternal notch and above innominate artery are considered level VII. Levels I, II, and V are further subdivided into A and B sublevels. Level IA is submental lymph nodes; IB is submandibular; IIA is upper jugular lymph nodes below the spinal accessory nerve; IIB is upper jugular lymph nodes above the spinal accessory nerve; VA is spinal accessory nodes; and VB is transverse cervical and supraclavicular nodes. Over much of the past century, management of cervical lymph nodes revolved around extensive radical operations (radical neck dissection) with emphasis on removal of all the lymph nodes and non-critical structures. Although this approach was effective in controlling the disease, it carried significant morbidity, the most well known being "shoulder syndrome" [6]. With improved understanding of the natural course of the disease and patterns of metastatic spread, this operation has evolved into a more selective and specific procedure (modified radical neck dissection and selective neck dissection) that removes only the most at risk lymphatic basins and tries to preserve the non-involved structures such as the internal jugular vein, accessory nerve, and sternocleidomastoid muscle. The details of lymphatic spread will be discussed later with each individual site.

Epidemiology and Risk Factors

Worldwide, head and neck cancers are among the ten most frequent cancers in men. More recent data analysis subdivides head and neck cancers into oral cavity and pharynx in one group and larynx in another group. Based on most recent global data from 2002, the 5 year prevalence of head and neck cancers is estimated at more than one million people for oral cavity and pharynx, and more than 450,000 for larynx cancer [7]. The prevalence of head and neck cancer was 1.4 times higher in less developed countries than developed regions of the world, which underscores the importance of developing and improving healthcare systems in these regions [8]. Globally, the highest rates of tongue and mouth cancer are reported from South Karachi, Pakistan for both men and women. Oropharynx and tonsil cancers were highest in Loire, France. Larynx cancer was highest in Basque, Spain and Sao Paolo, Brazil [8]. In the US, cancers of head and neck comprise about 3.3% of new cancer cases and 2% of all mortality from cancer, based on 2008 data [1]. Oral cavity and pharynx cancers are currently the eighth most common cancer in men in the United States. Head and neck cancers were 2.7 times more common in men than women.

In general, the incidence of head and neck cancers in US is declining; however, there is an observed increase in certain subpopulations. While the annual percentage change over a 30 year period among African American women was minus 1.38%, analysis of the 5 year period between 2000 and 2004 showed an increase of 3.18% [9]. Worldwide, the picture is heterogeneous. In eastern and northern Europe, oral cavity and tongue cancers are increasing in incidence, while declining for men in France and Italy. The incidence of head and neck cancers is increasing amongst women in Germany, France, and the UK, and for both men and women in Spain. China and India show decreases in incidence for both men and women, while Japan shows an increase in both. In Latin America, pharynx cancer incidence is on the rise everywhere except in Costa Rica. The incidence of larynx cancer is

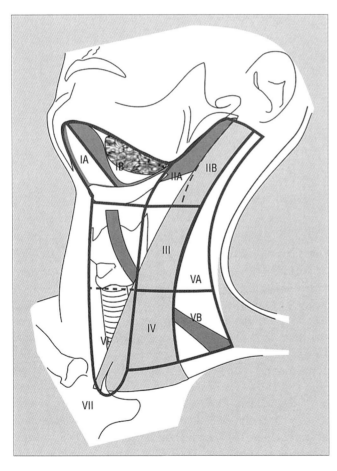

FIGURE 45.2 Anatomic boundaries of six levels and sublevels of neck (From Archives of Ottolaryngology Head and Neck Surgery. 2008 May;134(5):536–538).

mostly stable or decreasing worldwide, except in those few countries such as Japan, Denmark, Norway, and Spain (only in women) which show increases [10].

Head and neck cancers are much more common in the elderly. The median age of diagnosis for oral cavity and pharynx cancers is 62 and for larynx cancer is 64 years old [11]. As the population grows older, an increase in the number of patients with head and neck cancers is expected.

The most well known and well studied risk factors for head and neck cancers are cigarette smoking and alcohol consumption. At least 75% of head and neck cancers diagnosed in industrialized countries can be attributed to the combination of these two risk factors. Based on a meta-analysis of multiple studies worldwide, current cigarette smokers have a relative risk of 6.98 for developing larynx cancer, 6.76 for pharynx, and 3.43 for oral cavity cancers [12]. Former smokers are still at risk, although the risk is reduced depending on the years of abstinence. Smoking cessation around the age of 50 can reduce the risk by 50%, however, cessation at about 30 years of age brings down the risk by up to 90% [13]. Other forms of tobacco use have all been shown to be associated with an increased risk of head and neck cancer. Chewing tobacco is shown to be a risk factor for hypopharyngeal cancer in never-smokers in a study from India [14]. Passive (involuntary or secondhand) smoking at home or work is also associated with increased risk [15].

Alcohol seems to have a synergistic effect on the carcinogenic potential of tobacco. In addition, it has now been determined to be an independent risk factor for developing oropharynx, hypopharynx, and larynx cancers in never-smokers [16]. There are no meaningful differences in consumption of different types of alcohol and the risk is closely associated with frequency of alcohol consumption.

Viruses are known to be linked to the development of head and neck cancers. The most well known is Epstein-Barr Virus (EBV) and its association with nasopharyngeal cancer [17]. One of the more recently identified viruses is Human Papilloma Virus (HPV). HPV 16, a sexually transmitted virus, is now considered an etiologic factor for cancers of oropharynx. HPV has been attributed to the increase in incidence of oropharyngeal cancers in men between 40–59 years old and among non-smokers and non-drinkers. Currently, it is estimated that 20–25% of head and neck cancers are associated with HPV [18]. Cancers associated with HPV infection in general carry a better prognosis [19].

Other studied risk factors for developing head and neck cancers are oral carcinogens such as chewing betel nut with lime and catechu (in a quid of betel leaf called paan); dietary factors – there is an inverse ratio between consumption of fruits and vegetables and development of head and neck cancers [20, 21]; tooth loss [22], and even socioeconomic status [23]. Plummer–Vinson syndrome is associated with a high incidence of postcricoid carcinoma in Europe, but this condition is quite rare in the US. There are a few occupations that are associated with a higher risk for head and neck cancer. Nickel refining is associated with laryngeal cancer, woodworking with cancers of nasal cavity and paranasal sinuses, and steel and textile workers with oral cancers. Genetically inherited syndromes such as Li-Fraumeni and Bloom can cause an increase in risk of head and neck cancers through increased susceptibility to environmental carcinogens. The significance of heavy exposure to carcinogens is less pronounced in cancers developing after seventh decade of life, as well as genetic mutations such as p53 [24].

Prevention

A large number of head and neck cancers can be prevented by modifications in lifestyle. Smoking cessation and limiting alcohol use show the greatest proven benefit. Limiting exposure to known toxins and maintaining dental hygiene are of potential benefit and feasible with minimal cost. Early intervention in documented premalignant lesions or second primary tumors after treatment may reduce the risk of further progression of disease. Vitamin A analogs and cis-retinoic acid were initially implicated with beneficial effects in preventing second primary tumors, but subsequent trials did not show any benefit [25, 26]. Because of the role of HPV in developing oropharyngeal cancers, vaccination against this virus might eventually become an accepted method of prevention.

Natural History of the Disease

Although diagnosis of most head and neck cancers is relatively easier than cancers of internal organs, only one-third of patients with oral cavity and pharynx cancers are diagnosed while the disease is still localized. About 44% of patients are diagnosed with regional disease and 14% with distant metastasis. Head and neck cancers in most cases follow an orderly pattern of progression. Squamous cell carcinomas arise from expansion of a genetically altered population of epithelial cells. Cell populations that have the potential of invasion will produce a number of proteases and also recruit local fibroblasts and macrophages to actively destroy the epithelial basal membrane [27]. After destruction of basal membrane there is the potential of regional and distant spread of tumor.

Based on a series of studies at Memorial-Sloan Kettering Cancer Center by Shah and colleagues [28–31], there is a

TABLE 45.1 Percentage of metastatic lymph nodes involved in elective (*E*) and therapeutic (*T*) radical neck dissections

Level of nodes	Primary site							
	Oral cavity		Oropharynx		Hypopharynx		Larynx	
	E (%)	T (%)	E (%)	T (%)	E (%)	T (%)	E (%)	T (%)
I	58	61	7	17	0	10	14	8
II	51	57	80	85	75	78	52	68
III	26	44	60	50	75	75	55	70
IV	9	20	27	33	0	47	24	35
V	2	4	7	11	0	11	7	5

Source: Reprinted from Shah JP (1990) Patterns of cervical lymph node metastasis from squamous carcinomas of the upper aerodigestive tract. Am J Surg 160(4):405–409

better understanding of patterns of lymphatic spread in head and neck cancers. Lymphatic spread happens in an orderly fashion in the majority of cases based on the location of tumor (Table 45.1). These patterns will be discussed separately for individual tumors. A number of characteristics are predictors of high probability of distant metastasis. Location of the primary tumor, initial T and N stage of the neoplasm, and the presence or absence of locoregional control above the clavicle are the most important ones [32]. Primary tumors of hypopharynx, oropharynx, and oral cavity of high T stage are associated with the highest incidence of distant metastasis. Patients with advanced nodal disease also have a high risk of distant metastasis, especially if the jugular vein is invaded or if soft tissues of the neck are extensively involved by the disease. The lungs are the most common site of distant metastasis and account for approximately 66% of cases [32]. Multiple pulmonary nodules are a very suspicious sign of distant metastasis in head and neck cancers; however, a solitary pulmonary nodule might make it quite difficult to distinguish a second primary in the lung from a metastatic lesion. Other sites include bone (22%), liver (10%), skin, mediastinum, and bone marrow.

Other less frequent patterns of spread might happen in selected subpopulations of patients. Tumors may spread along the nerves. This is particularly important in treatment planning for tumors that involve the mandible and might invade the inferior alveolar nerve. Direct invasion of other nerves in the neck, such as the hypoglossal, lingual, vagus and the sympathetic chain, may also occur by tumors in their vicinity. High grade tumors of parotid glands are well known to involve the facial nerve, especially when they are large and bulky. Benign tumors almost never cause paralysis even when they are of substantial size. Another route is aberrant metastatic spread. This is more common in patients who have undergone previous treatment for head and neck cancer. Patients after radiotherapy or radical neck dissection are at risk for developing aberrant metastases to the neck, and subcutaneous and cutaneous sites.

Second Primary Tumors

Head and neck cancer patients are at risk of harboring (synchronous) or developing (metachronous) a second primary tumor. Carcinogens such as tobacco and alcohol will affect the entire mucosal surface (field cancerization) [33] and the potential for malignant transformation remains even after removal of the noxious agent. These tumors can be a "true second primary tumor" with a different genetic fingerprint from the index lesion, or can be similar to the index tumor and arise from the premalignant lesions in the affected field (second field tumor) [34]. The annual incidence of second primary tumors is estimated to be approximately 4% [35–37]. Overall incidence can be as high as 27% in some reports [35] and as low as 9% in others [38]. These tumors are more common in younger patients [38] and the median time to presentation is around 3 years [38]. The prognosis of second primary tumors is not favorable [39]. This phenomenon necessitates the continued and long term close follow-up of the head and neck cancer patients.

Clinical Presentation

Many cancers of head and neck can be easily detected by patients or on routine examination. A chronic ulcer, new or persistent lump in the neck (Fig. 45.3), or new onset of hoarseness or dysphagia are such examples. In spite of these obvious alarming symptoms, two out of three head and neck cancer patients will be diagnosed in an advanced stage. This is in part due to patients' negligence, but also reflects a component of delayed diagnosis in some cases [40, 41]. It is wise to consider the possibility of cancer in high risk patients with the new onset of symptoms, even when they are non-specific and vague. Symptoms and signs of head and neck cancer can be divided into two groups: local symptoms and generalized symptoms. The most common generalized symptom in head

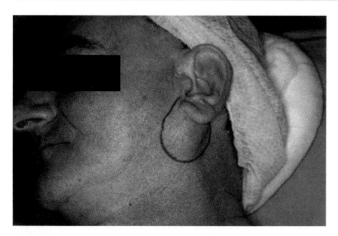

Figure 45.3 Left neck mass. Slowly growing asymptomatic mass in an otherwise healthy elderly man. Final diagnosis was pleomorphic adenoma of left parotid gland.

and neck cancer is unexplained weight loss and usually happens late in the course of disease, or when it is related to difficulties in swallowing (dysphagia). Local symptoms depend on the location of tumor. Some tumors can be symptomatic at a very early stage. True vocal cord tumors are such an example. On the other hand, tumors of nasopharynx or hypopharynx can go undetected for long periods of time.

Nasal cavity and paranasal sinus tumors can remain undetected for extended periods of time. Most of the early symptoms such as nasal obstruction, rhinorrhea, and sinus congestion are quite similar to benign processes of sinusitis and allergic rhinitis. Late symptoms can include recurrent epistaxis, malar swelling, and diplopia that may happen in advanced stages of maxillary sinus tumors. Oral cavity tumors usually manifest with painful ulcerations, slurred speech, bleeding or an exophytic mass. Nasopharyngeal cancers may present in early stages with unilateral otitis media. Oropharynx and hypopharyngeal tumors can cause odynophagia, dysphagia, change of voice and, occasionally, airway obstruction. Laryngeal tumors can become symptomatic very early if they are located on vocal cords with changes in voice. Supraglottic and subglottic cancers can be relatively asymptomatic for long periods and show up later with dysphagia, odynophagia, and throat pain, or airway compromise.

Pain is not commonly associated with early head and neck cancers. Most commonly the pain is mediated by branches of the trigeminal, or glossopharyngeal and vagus nerves. Pharyngeal and laryngeal tumors can cause referred pain in ear through the glossopharyngeal and vagus nerves. Hypopharyngeal and base of tongue tumors also can cause ear pain through the nerve of Arnold (auricular branch of facial nerve). In advanced cases, patients may present with involvement of skin of the face and neck, mandibular involvement and loss of teeth, severe pain, and dysphagia, or

airway distress. Oral cavity tumors can erode through the subcutaneous tissue and skin and cause an orocutaneous fistula in advanced, neglected cases.

Diagnostic Workup

A complete history and physical exam is the first step in assessing any patient with suspicion for head and neck cancer. In obtaining the history, attention to symptoms and signs more related to head and neck tumors such as non-healing ulcers, sore throat, hoarseness or any voice changes is of obvious importance. In addition, asking about symptoms of otalgia, odynophagia, malar swelling, etc. that patients might not relate to their problem can reveal valuable information. General symptoms of malaise, fatigue, and weight loss should not be overlooked either. A complete exam of head and neck region involves several steps. Examination starts with a detailed survey of the region visually and continues by palpation of thyroid gland, neck, and bimanual examination of the floor of the mouth and base of the tongue. Mirror examination of the larynx and rigid or fiberoptic nasopharyngolaryngoscopy should be considered part of a routine head and neck exam. Certain areas are prone to be overlooked. The examiner should pay attention to the scalp, the nape of the neck, and the gingivolabial and gingivobuccal sulci. Most head and neck surgeons perform fine needle aspiration (FNA) of suspicious neck masses or thyroid nodules and salivary gland tumors as an office procedure, or they may be performed with ultrasound for better localization of the mass.

Imaging

Conventional X-rays, except for a Panorex of the mandible, are of very limited value in evaluating head and neck cancers and are not being used. A panoramic view of the mandible, however, is still valuable in assessing the possibility of mandibular invasion and also in preoperative evaluation for mandibular reconstruction with tissue transfer. A routine chest X-ray is performed in all head and neck cancer patients to rule out possible lung metastasis. Ultrasound is quite helpful in assessing neck masses, thyroid nodules, and in directing FNA of suspected lesions. The CT scan has become the mainstay of imaging in head and neck cancers. This modality provides excellent detail in deep tumors, relation of tumors with adjacent structures, and also in assessing the lymphatics of the head and neck (Fig. 45.4). The CT scan has superior resolution to MRI in assessing bony structures and should be obtained if there is any suspicion of bony involvement. MRI is commonly used and provides superior resolution in assessing

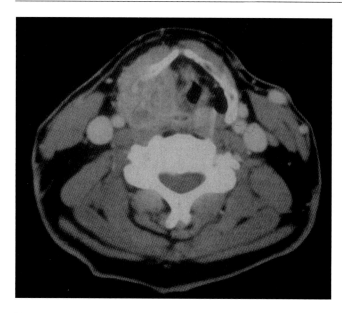

FIGURE 45.4 CT Scan image of advanced hypopharyngeal tumor. The image provides excellent details in extent of local invasion to adjacent structures. Note destruction of thyroid cartilage and invasion of larynx by tumor.

soft tissue, blood vessels, and nerves. It is not uncommon now to obtain both CT and MRI in assessing some head and neck tumors such as parapharyngeal space masses. Functional imaging using fluorodeoxyglucose-positron emission tomography (FDG-PET) is being used more commonly, especially for initial evaluation and follow-up of patients with malignant neoplasms. This modality is quite sensitive in detecting nodal spread or distant metastasis or both [42]. The Combined PET and CT provides more accurate results than each modality alone and is being utilized more often [43]. PET is especially helpful in the follow-up of patients and surveillance for recurrent disease.

Examination Under Anesthesia

Examination under anesthesia (EUA) is an important diagnostic and staging tool for the head and neck surgeon. This modality can be used in examining patients with oral cavity tumors with trismus, and patients with pharyngeal and laryngeal cancers. Rigid esophagoscopy is probably not needed in all patients, but in patients with hypopharyngeal tumors, a thorough examination of the esophagus is mandatory to determine the extent of the lesion. Bronchoscopy is also performed in select cases based on the judgment of the treating physician and the nature of the disease, such as subglottic tumors.

Similar to all areas of oncology an accurate tissue diagnosis is the cornerstone of the management. The role of head and neck surgeon in obtaining adequate and appropriate tissue is

as important as the pathologist that interprets the specimen. A few techniques are commonly used: punch biopsy, excisional biopsy, curettage, core-needle biopsy, and FNA. Each of these techniques is valuable in assessing certain types of lesions.

Punch biopsy is used quite commonly in mucosal lesions of head and neck. The preferred place is in the periphery of the lesion and the forceps commonly used is a cup forceps. A small sample usually is adequate to make a diagnosis. If a lesion is necrotic or appears to be infected, then the tissue should be obtained from a fleshy non-ulcerated section of the lesion. Small oral cavity lesions can be easily excised as a whole and submitted as an excisional biopsy with satisfactory margins. In cases of diffuse leukoplakia or erythroplakia, using vital dyes such as toluidine blue can be quite helpful to guide the surgeon to the most suspicious area. Incisional biopsy is used in lesions of the skin and soft tissue, and submucosal masses of the oral cavity and pharynx. Sampling irradiated tissue can be challenging since there can be edema or late radiation changes such as scarring and fibrosis. Asking for frozen samples to ascertain adequacy of tissue can be quite helpful in expediting the diagnostic process and avoiding extra procedures.

Fine needle aspiration was first described by Hayes Martin in 1930 [44]; however, out of fear of tumor implantation in the needle tract, it was not utilized extensively until the 1970s. Currently, FNA is the method of choice for evaluating most head and neck masses and is especially useful in assessing cervical lymphadenopathy [45], thyroid nodule, and salivary gland masses [46]. All practitioners dealing with head and neck cancer should be quite proficient in this technique. FNA biopsy interpretation requires a pathologist experienced in cytology.

The results of FNA biopsy can be interpreted as adequate or inadequate. If the sample is adequate, it can be metastatic squamous cell carcinoma, metastatic adenocarcinoma, metastatic thyroid carcinoma, or suspicious for lymphoma. An algorithm can be used in patients presenting with malignant features (Fig. 45.5). As valuable as FNA biopsy is in diagnosis, there are possible pitfalls and the clinician should interpret the results in the context of the all the available information. Further investigation, such as open biopsy, should be pursued if there are discrepancies between the results of FNA and the clinical picture.

Molecular Genetics and Pathogenesis

Over the past few decades major advances in understanding the genetic basis of development of squamous cell carcinomas of head and neck has occurred. The prevailing theories at this time propose a model of progressive genetic and

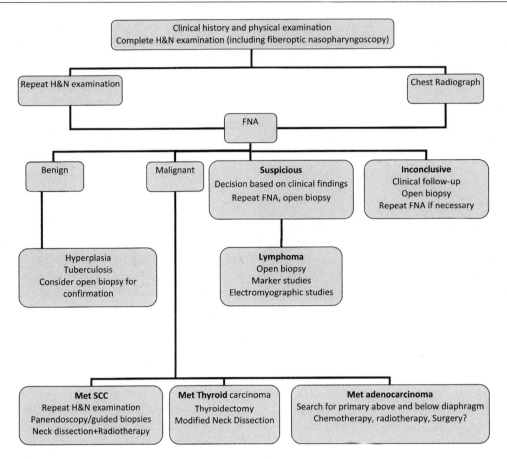

Figure 45.5 Algorithm for the management of cervical lymphade-nopathy. (*H&N*) Head and Neck, (*FNA*) Fine Needle Aspiration, (*Met*) Metastatic, (*SCC*) Squamous cell carcinoma (Reprinted from Shaha A et al (1986) Fine-needle aspiration in the diagnosis of cervical lymphadenopathy. Am J Surg 152(4):420–423).

phenotypic changes from normal mucosa to hyperplasia to premalignant lesion, carcinoma in situ and finally invasive cancer [47–49]. The genetic alterations in general cause activation of proto-oncogenes and inactivation of tumor suppressor genes. This can happen through deletion, point mutation, promoter methylation, or gene amplification. The most common genetic abnormality in premalignant lesions and head and neck SCCs is loss of heterozygosity in chromosomal region 9p21 [50, 51]. This abnormality is seen in 70–80% of cases. Loss of chromosomal heterozygosity (LOH) in 3p, 17p, 11q, and 13q are also seen in premalignant lesions and head and neck cancers with decreasing frequency [52–55]. LOH in chromosome 17p and p53 gene mutation are seen in 50% of head and neck cancers [56, 57]. Loss of 9p21 is considered an early event in progression of squamous neoplasia. This abnormality is seen in up to 30% of squamous hyperplasia [50, 51, 58]. On the other hand, abnormalities such as 17p loss and p53 deletion happen later in the process [59, 60]. Other abnormalities are associated with different tumor behavior. Amplification of 11q13 is associated with increased rate of lymph node metastases and overall poor prognosis [61–63]. Deletion of

the p53 gene has been associated with reduced survival after surgical treatment of head and neck cancers [64]. Interestingly this mutation is less common in head and cancer occurring after 70 years old [24].

Another relatively recent discovery is the role of Epidermal Growth Factor Receptor (EGFR) in head and neck cancers. EGFR belongs to the family of tyrosine kinase receptors. Binding of ligands results in activation of many downstream cascades that regulate cell proliferation, apoptosis, metastatic potential, and angiogenesis. EGFR can also be activated by other factors such as platelet derived growth factor and insulin-like growth factor. EGFR protein expression is seen in 90% or more of head and neck cancers [65] and many retrospective studies have shown that tumors that overexpress EGFR have a poor prognosis [66]. New medications (Cetuximab) have now been developed to target this receptor with successful results [67]. Angiogenesis is considered a fundamental process in the progression of malignant tumors. There are many proangiogenic and antiangiogenic factors that regulate this process. Vascular endothelial growth factor (VEGF) and its receptors have been extensively studied and their role in other solid tumors is established [68]. VEGF also can be upregulated in head and neck cancers with prognostic significance [69]. Antiangiogenesis drugs are currently under investigation for use against head and neck SCCs.

Pathologic Classification

The majority of the upper aerodigestive tract is covered with squamous epithelial cells and therefore the majority of tumors in this area arise from these cells (squamous cell carcinoma). Other well known, but less frequent tumors can occur. Adenocarcinomas, melanomas, minor salivary gland tumors, sarcomas, and lymphomas have all been described to arise from this region.

In the spectrum of squamous cell malignancies, there are a few terms to describe premalignant and different varieties of malignant neoplasms. Oral epithelial dysplasia manifests itself in two dominant forms. Leukoplakia is defined as a predominantly white lesion that cannot be wiped away and cannot be characterized as any other specific disease entity on the basis of clinical features. Erythroplakia is defined as a red, velvety surface lesion. Lesions consisting of mixed white and red lesions are called "erythroleukoplakia" or "speckled leukoplakia". In general, the risk of cancer arising from erythroplakia is considered higher than leukoplakia and in mixed lesions the red areas are more prone to transform to malignancy. Under the microscope these lesions show a range of histologic changes from nondysplastic epithelial hyperplasia to nuclear pleomorphism, increased mitoses, and architectural disturbances. The risk of developing malignancy in leukoplakic and erythroplakic lesions is dependent on the degree of dysplasia and other histologic factors. In lesions where dysplasia is present the risk can range from 11 to 36% depending on the length of follow-up [70–72]. Proliferative verrucous leukoplakia has been reported to have a malignant transformation rate as high as 70% [73].

Verrucous carcinoma is a rare and low grade variant of squamous cell carcinoma. It is more common in older men with a long standing history of smokeless tobacco abuse and comprises only 3% of oral cavity cancers in the US [74]. The appearance is quite unique and characteristic. It occurs most commonly in the buccal mucosa, the mandibular or maxillary vestibule, or the alveolar ridge and corresponds with the site of tobacco placement. The tumor usually appears as white, diffuse, thickened plaque with a distinct warty or papillary surface. Verrucous carcinoma is considered a low grade squamous cell carcinoma. It generally has a better prognosis due to its exophytic and slow growth pattern and highly differentiated nature. It can undergo dedifferentiation to more aggressive forms [75, 76]. The treatment is generally surgical excision, but primary radiotherapy has

also been successfully used. Sarcomatoid and basaloid varieties of squamous cell carcinoma on the other hand are more aggressive and have a higher rate of lymph node metastases. Basaloid carcinoma also has a high rate of distant metastases [77].

Other subtypes of squamous cell carcinoma in the head and neck are exophytic, ulcerating, and infiltrating. Infiltrating tumors usually have a worse prognosis. Tumors with lymphoid stroma are classified as lymphoepithelial carcinomas or lymphoepitheliomas. These are usually poorly differentiated tumors that most commonly occur in the nasopharynx and tonsil. They are quite radiosensitive.

A few other pathologic factors have been mentioned as determinants of prognosis. Presence of lymphatic, vascular, or perineural invasions are among those. Depth of invasion has been shown to predict a higher likelihood of cervical lymph node involvement [78].

Staging

Accurate staging of head and neck cancers is extremely important in determining the prognosis, treatment plans, and expected outcomes. It is recommended that all the information be gathered accurately and entered in the medical record as primary data. The staging systems have changed multiple times through history and without doubt will undergo more modifications. The advantage of retaining primary data lies in the fact that even when the classification systems change, one can accurately stage the patient in the correct group.

The staging system currently used for head and neck cancers is based on the sixth edition of AJCC-UICC TNM system [79]. The last modification was introduced in 2003 and significant changes were implemented [80]. This system is based on the characteristics of primary tumor (T), extent of nodal involvement (N), and status of distant metastasis (M). The T stage is primarily based on size and is site specific in head and neck cancer. One of the major changes in the new edition was subdivision of stage T4 to T4a and T4b, to differentiate between locally advanced tumors that are surgically resectable (T4a) and those that are not (T4b) (Tables 45.2–45.6).

The N stage is uniform for all head and neck cancers except tumors of nasopharynx and thyroid (Tables 45.7 and 45.8). M stage is based on absence (M0) or presence (M1) of distant metastasis (Table 45.9). The overall stage of the tumor consists of stages I–IV. Stage IV is now subdivided into three categories (IVa, IVb, and IVc) mostly based on the reorganization of T stage category. Stage I and II are considered early disease and prognosis in general is more favorable than advanced (III and IV) cancers (Tables 45.10 and 45.11).

TABLE 45.2 T staging for tumors of the lip and oral cavity

TX	Primary tumor cannot be assessed
T0	No evidence of primary tumor
Tis	Carcinoma in situ
T1	Tumor 2 cm or less in greatest dimension
T2	Tumor more than 2 cm but not more than 4 cm in greatest dimension
T3	Tumor more than 4 cm in greatest dimension
T4a	Moderately advanced local disease
Lip	Tumor invades through cortical bone, inferior alveolar nerve, floor of mouth, or skin of face, that is, chin or nose
Oral cavity	Tumor invades adjacent structures only (e.g., through cortical bone [mandible or maxilla] into deep [extrinsic] muscle of tongue [genioglossus, hyoglossus, palatoglossus, and styloglossus], maxillary sinus, skin of face)
T4b	Very advanced local disease
	Tumor involves masticator space, pterygoid plates, or skull base and/or encases internal carotid artery

Source: Used with permission of the American Joint Committee on Cancer (AJCC®), Chicago, Illinois. The original source for this material is the AJCC Cancer Staging Handbook, Seventh Edition (2009) Page 55, published by Springer Science and Business Media, LLC, www.springerlink.com

Principles of Treatment

Treatment of head and neck cancers is truly a multimodality, comprehensive, and team-based discipline. A multidisciplinary approach is the basic foundation of management of head and neck cancers. It requires considering many factors as diverse as tumor characteristics and patient's overall health to availability of resources and expertise. The most sensible treatment regimen is the one that is tailored to the patient's specific needs and circumstances. The treatment regimen will differ based on tumor site, depth of invasion, pathology, and clinical behavior. On the patient side, age, co-morbidities, risk factors, and patient cooperation and preferences are all very important factors. The availability of resources and expertise and the practicality of the treatment regimen are also significant determinants of the ultimate plan. Only a comprehensive approach involving all practitioners along with the active participation of the patient and their support group will maximize the chances of optimal treatment. While the majority of principles of treatment are the same for the elderly population, there exist notable

TABLE 45.3 T staging for tumors of the pharynx

TX	Primary tumor cannot be assessed
T0	No evidence of primary tumor
Tis	Carcinoma in situ
Nasopharynx	
T1	Tumor confined to the nasopharynx, or tumor extends to oropharynx and/or nasal cavity without parapharyngeal extension[a]
T2	Tumor with parapharyngeal extension[a]
T3	Tumor involves bony structures of skull base and/or paranasal sinuses
T4	Tumor with intracranial extension and/or involvement of cranial nerves, hypopharynx, orbit or with extension to the infratemporal fossa/masticator space
Oropharynx	
T1	Tumor 2 cm or less in greatest dimension
T2	Tumor more than 2 cm but not more than 4 cm in greatest dimension
T3	Tumor more than 4 cm in greatest dimension
T4a	Moderately advanced local disease
	Tumor invades the larynx, extrinsic muscle of tongue, medial pterygoid, hard palate, or mandible[b]
T4b	Very advanced local disease
	Tumor invades lateral pterygoid muscle, pterygoid plates, lateral nasopharynx, or skull base or encases carotid artery
Hypopharynx	
T1	Tumor limited to 1 subsite of hypopharynx and/or 2 cm or less in greatest dimension
T2	Tumor invades more than 1 subsite of hypopharynx or an adjacent site, or measures more than 2 cm, but not more than 4 cm in greatest diameter without fixation of hemilarynx
T3	Tumor measures more than 4 cm in greatest dimension or with fixation of hemilarynx or extension to esophagus
T4a	Moderately advanced local disease
	Tumor invades thyroid/cricoid cartilage, hyoid bone, thyroid gland, or central compartment soft tissue[c]
T4b	Very advanced local disease
	Tumor invades prevertebral fascia, encases carotid artery, or involves mediastinal structures

Source: Used with permission of the American Joint Committee on Cancer (AJCC®), Chicago, Illinois. The original source for this material is the AJCC Cancer Staging Handbook, Seventh Edition (2009) Page 69, published by Springer Science and Business Media, LLC, www.springerlink.com
[a] Note: Parapharyngeal extension denotes posterolateral infiltration of tumor
[b] Note: Mucosal extension to lingual surface of epiglottis from primary tumor of the base of the tongue and vallecula does not constitute invasion of larynx
[c] Note: Central compartment soft tissue includes prelaryngeal strap muscles and subcutaneous fat

TABLE 45.4 T staging for tumors of the larynx

TX	Primary tumor cannot be assessed
T0	No evidence of primary tumor
Tis	Carcinoma in situ

Supraglottis

T1	Tumor limited to one subsite of supraglottis with normal vocal cord mobility
T2	Tumor invades mucosa of more than one adjacent subsite of supraglottis, or glottis, or region outside the supraglottis (e.g., mucosa of base of tongue, vallecula, medial wall of pyriform sinus) without fixation of the larynx
T3	Tumor limited to larynx with vocal cord fixation and/or invades any of the following: postcricoid area, preepiglottic space, paraglottic space, and/or inner cortex of thyroid cartilage erosion
T4a	Moderately advanced local disease
	Tumor invades through the thyroid cartilage and/or invades tissues beyond the larynx (e.g., trachea, soft tissues of neck including deep extrinsic muscle of the tongue, strap muscles, thyroid, or esophagus)
T4b	Very advanced local disease
	Tumor invades prevertebral space, encases carotid artery, or invades mediastinal structures

Glottis

T1	Tumor limited to the vocal cord(s) (may involve anterior or posterior commissure) with normal mobility
T1a	Tumor limited to one vocal cord
T1b	Tumor involves both vocal cords
T2	Tumor extends to supraglottis and/or subglottis and/or with impaired vocal cord mobility
T3	Tumor limited to larynx with vocal cord fixation and/or invasion of paraglottic space, and/or inner cortex of the thyroid cartilage
T4a	Moderately advanced local disease
	Tumor invades through the outer cortex of the thyroid cartilage and/or invades tissues beyond the larynx (e.g., trachea, soft tissues of neck including deep extrinsic muscles of the tongue, strap muscles, thyroid, or esophagus)
T4b	Very advanced local disease
	Tumor invades prevertebral space, encases carotid artery or invades mediastinal structures

Subglottis

T1	Tumor limited to the subglottis
T2	Tumor extends to vocal cord(s) with normal or impaired mobility
T3	Tumor limited to larynx with vocal cord fixation
T4a	Moderately advanced local disease
	Tumor invades cricoid or thyroid cartilage and/or invades tissues beyond the larynx (e.g., trachea, soft tissues of neck including deep extrinsic muscles of the tongue, strap muscles, thyroid, or esophagus)
T4b	Very advanced local disease
	Tumor invades prevertebral space, encases carotid artery, or involves mediastinal structures

Source: Used with permission of the American Joint Committee on Cancer (AJCC®), Chicago, Illinois. The original source for this material is the AJCC Cancer Staging Handbook, Seventh Edition (2009) pp: 84–85, published by Springer Science and Business Media, LLC, www.springerlink.com

differences. These differences will be discussed in each modality and for each subsite. Similar to other areas of geriatric medicine, comprehensive geriatric assessment [81, 82] is an essential part of approach to the treatment of head and neck cancer in elderly.

The three pillars of treatment in head and neck cancers are surgery, radiotherapy, and chemotherapy. Chemotherapy is the most recently adopted modality, but in recent years noteworthy evidence has made it a mainstream component of head and neck cancer treatment, especially in the form of multimodality treatments.

Surgery continues to be the standard and most established treatment for the majority of head and neck cancers. Although the principles of surgical treatment have been established for more than a hundred years, new techniques, technologies,

and concepts continue to propel the field into new frontiers. The emphasis is now on minimizing the sequela of surgery and maximizing the preservation of form and function. A few major advances have revolutionized surgical treatment of head and neck cancer. The first one is the acceptance of selective, more precise, and more limited resections based on the knowledge of the anatomy and clinical behavior of the tumor. Laser microsurgery of laryngeal tumors and transoral resection of pharyngeal tumors, without the need for mandibulotomy, and widespread use of selective neck dissection, are prominent examples. By far the most significant improvement is the introduction and subsequent refinements of free tissue transfer for reconstruction of surgical defects. This technique allows for extensive surgical resection of advanced tumors and reconstructing the resultant defect with

TABLE 45.5 T staging for tumors of the nasal cavity and paranasal sinuses

TX	Primary tumor cannot be assessed
T0	No evidence of primary tumor
Tis	Carcinoma in situ

Maxillary sinus

T1	Tumor limited to the maxillary sinus mucosa with no erosion or destruction of bone
T2	Tumor causing bone erosion or destruction including extension into the hard palate and/or middle nasal meatus, except extension to posterior wall of maxillary sinus and pterygoid plates
T3	Tumor invades any of the following: bone of the posterior wall of maxillary sinus, subcutaneous tissues, floor or medial wall of orbit, pterygoid fossa, and ethmoid sinuses
T4a	Moderately advanced local disease
	Tumor invades anterior orbital contents, skin of cheek, pterygoid plates, infratemporal fossa, cribriform plate, sphenoid or frontal sinuses
T4b	Very advanced local disease
	Tumor invades any of the following: orbital apex, dura, brain, middle cranial fossa, cranial nerves other than maxillary division of trigeminal nerve (V2), nasopharynx, or clivus

Nasal cavity and ethmoid sinus

T1	Tumor restricted to any one subsite, with or without bony invasion
T2	Tumor invading two subsites in a single region or extending to involve an adjacent region within the nasoethmoidal complex, with or without bony invasion
T3	Tumor extends to invade the medial wall or floor of the orbit, maxillary sinus, palate, or cribriform plate
T4a	Moderately advanced local disease
	Tumor invades any of the following: anterior orbital contents, skin of nose or cheek, minimal extension to anterior cranial fossa, pterygoid plates, sphenoid or frontal sinuses
T4b	Very advanced local disease
	Tumor invades any of the following: orbital apex, brain, middle cranial fossa, cranial nerves other than V_2, nasopharynx, or clivus

Source: Used with permission of the American Joint Committee on Cancer (AJCC®), Chicago, Illinois. The original source for this material is the AJCC Cancer Staging Handbook, Seventh Edition (2009), page 98, published by Springer Science and Business Media, LLC, www.springerlink.com

TABLE 45.6 T staging for tumors of the major salivary glands

TX	Primary tumor cannot be assessed
T0	No evidence of primary tumor
T1	Tumor 2 cm or less in greatest dimension without extraparenchymal extension[a]
T2	Tumor more than 2 cm but not more than 4 cm in greatest dimension without extraparenchymal extension[a]
T3	Tumor more than 4 cm and/or tumor having extraparenchymal extension[a]
T4a	Moderately advanced local disease
	Tumor invades skin, mandible, ear canal, and/or facial nerve
T4b	Very advanced local disease
	Tumor invades skull base and/or pterygoid plates and/or encases carotid artery

Source: Used with permission of the American Joint Committee on Cancer (AJCC®), Chicago, Illinois. The original source for this material is the AJCC Cancer Staging Handbook, Seventh Edition (2009) Page 105, published by Springer Science and Business Media, LLC, www.springerlink.com

[a] Note: Extraparenchymal extension is clinical or macroscopic evidence of invasion of soft tissues. Microscopic evidence alone does not constitute extraparenchymal extension for classification purposes

autologous tissue with excellent functional and cosmetic results and long term durability. More recently, robotic surgery has been explored by a few select institutions in treatment of early tonsil and oropharyngeal cancers as well as skull base tumors [83–87]. The initial results are promising; however, the eventual benefits and advantages of this technique over current standards will need further investigation.

Surgical excision also provides the clinician with the most accurate data on the pathology of the tumor, extent of invasion, and status of regional lymph nodes. It's not uncommon to upstage tumors based on the findings of the surgical specimen and final pathology report. This information is quite valuable in tailoring further courses of therapy and determining the need for adjuvant radiotherapy. Currently there are no uniform unresectability criteria; however, most surgeons consider invasion of carotid artery, base of skull, and prevertebral musculature as unresectable disease.

Assessing elderly patients for the most suitable surgical therapy continues to be a dilemma for head and neck

TABLE 45.7 N staging for all head and neck sites except the nasopharynx and thyroid

NX	Regional lymph nodes cannot be assessed
N0	No regional lymph node metastasis
N1*	Metastasis in a single ipsilateral lymph node, 3 cm or less in greatest dimension
N2*	Metastasis in a single ipsilateral lymph node, more than 3 cm but not more than 6 cm in greatest dimension; or in multiple ipsilateral lymph nodes, none more than 6 cm in greatest dimension; or in bilateral or contralateral lymph nodes, none more than 6 cm in greatest dimension
N2a	Metastasis in a single ipsilateral lymph node more than 3 cm but not more than 6 cm in greatest dimension
N2b*	Metastasis in multiple ipsilateral lymph nodes, none more than 6 cm in greatest dimension
N2c	Metastasis in bilateral or contralateral lymph nodes, none more than 6 cm in greatest dimension
N3*	Metastasis in a lymph more than 6 cm in greatest dimension

Source: Used with permission of the American Joint Committee on Cancer (AJCC®), Chicago, Illinois. The original source for this material is the AJCC Cancer Staging Handbook, Seventh Edition (2009), page 45, published by Springer Science and Business Media, LLC, www.springerlink.com
*Note: A designation of "U" or "L" may be used for any N stage to indicate metastasis above the lower border of the cricoid (U) or below the lower border of the cricoid (L). Similarly, clinical/radiological ECS should be recorded as E– or E+, and histopathologic ECS should be designated En, Em, or Eg

TABLE 45.8 N staging for tumors of the nasopharynx

NX	Regional lymph nodes cannot be assessed
N0	No regional lymph node metastasis
N1	Unilateral metastasis in lymph node(s), 6 cm or less in greatest dimension, above the supraclavicular fossa, and/or unilateral or bilateral, retropharyngeal lymph nodes, 6 cm or less, in greatest dimension[a]
N2	Bilateral metastasis in lymph node(s), 6 cm or less in greatest dimension, above the supraclavicular fossa[a]
N3	Metastasis in a lymph node(s) >6 cm and/or to supra-clavicular fossa
N3a	Greater than 6 cm in dimension
N3b	Extension to the supraclavicular fossa[b]

Source: Used with permission of the American Joint Committee on Cancer (AJCC®), Chicago, Illinois. The original source for this material is the AJCC Cancer Staging Handbook, Seventh Edition (2009), page 70, published by Springer Science and Business Media, LLC, www.springerlink.com
[a] Note: Midline nodes are considered ipsilateral nodes
[b] Note: Supraclavicular zone or fossa is relevant to the staging of nasopharyngeal carcinoma and is the triangular region originally described by Ho. It is defined by three points: (1) the superior margin of the sternal end of the clavicle, (2) the superior margin of the lateral end of the clavicle, (3) the point where the neck meets the shoulder. Note that this would include caudal portions of levels IV and VB. All cases with lymph nodes (whole or part) in the fossa are considered N3b

TABLE 45.9 M staging for head and neck tumors

M0	No distant metastasis
M1	Distant metastasis

Source: Used with permission of the American Joint Committee on Cancer (AJCC®), Chicago, Illinois. The original source for this material is the AJCC Cancer Staging Handbook, Seventh Edition (2009), page 45, published by Springer Science and Business Media, LLC, www.springerlink.com

TABLE 45.10 Stage grouping for all head and neck sites except the nasopharynx and thyroid

Stage group	T stage	N stage	M stage
0	Tis	N0	M0
I	T1	N0	M0
II	T2	N0	M0
III	T3	N0	M0
	T1	N1	M0
	T2	N1	M0
	T3	N1	M0
IVA	T4a	N0	M0
	T4a	N1	M0
	T1	N2	M0
	T2	N2	M0
	T3	N2	M0
	T4a	N2	M0
IVB	Any T	N3	M0
	T4b	Any N	M0
IVC	Any T	Any N	M1

Source: Used with permission of the American Joint Committee on Cancer (AJCC®), Chicago, Illinois. The original source for this material is the AJCC Cancer Staging Handbook, Seventh Edition (2009), page 49, published by Springer Science and Business Media, LLC, www.springerlink.com

TABLE 45.11 Stage grouping for tumors of the nasopharynx

Stage group	T stage	N stage	M stage
0	Tis	N0	M0
I	T1	N0	M0
II	T1	N1	M0
	T2	N0	M0
	T2	N1	M0
III	T1	N2	M0
	T2	N2	M0
	T3	N0	M0
	T3	N1	M0
	T3	N2	M0
IVA	T4	N0	M0
	T4	N1	M0
	T4	N2	M0
IVB	Any T	N3	M0
IVC	Any T	Any N	M1

Source: Used with permission of the American Joint Committee on Cancer (AJCC®), Chicago, Illinois. The original source for this material is the AJCC Cancer Staging Handbook, Seventh Edition (2009), page 63, published by Springer Science and Business Media, LLC, www.springerlink.com

surgeons. Many patients have other comorbidities that can affect the outcome of surgery negatively. Age, per se, is not a contraindication to surgical therapy as shown in multiple studies [88–91]. Comorbidities, on the other hand, consistently have been cited as an independent negative prognostic factor [88, 92]. The outcome of surgery is similar to younger patient groups. Furthermore, perioperative complication rate and quality of life after surgery is quite comparable with younger patients [93, 94]. A few specific areas deserve special attention. Microvascular free tissue transfer while possible and successful in elderly, requires careful assessment and selection of suitable patients. This technique can be utilized safely; however, there may be a higher complication rate and that is, again, related to accompanying comorbidities [95–97]. Time under anesthesia is another significant predictor of morbidity [88]. This factor has to be considered when recommending procedures that involve free tissue transfer, since this technique adds a significant time to the duration of operation. A number of procedures, such as supraglottic laryngectomy are generally tolerated worse in elderly due to increased risk of aspiration. It's advisable to avoid such procedures or carefully assess the candidate's biologic age and status to assure desirable outcome [98].

Radiotherapy is used as the primary treatment for tumors of nasopharynx, early stage glottic larynx, tonsil, and base of tongue, as well as adjuvant therapy for most other head and neck cancers in advanced stages. Postoperative radiation has been shown to improve local control and survival better than surgery alone [99]. New techniques and concepts such as "Intensity Modulated Radiation Therapy" (IMRT), hyperfractionation, and accelerated fractionation have brought better efficacy and less toxicity.

Advanced tumors are commonly treated with multimodality therapy consisting of surgery and adjuvant radiotherapy. The advantages of radiotherapy in a postoperative setting are reduced wound complications, reduction in target tumor volume, and clear definition of the extent of tumor. Adjuvant radiotherapy should be considered in all locally advanced cancers and also in patients with early cancers with sinister pathologic features. These features are listed in Table 45.12 [100].

There are multiple methods and techniques to deliver ionizing energy to the tissues. In general, the methods are divided into teletherapy (external beam radiation) and brachytherapy. In teletherapy, the source of ionizing beam is away from the patient. The energy can be in the form of ionizing rays such as photons, X-rays, or gamma rays; or in the form of high energy particles such as electrons, neutrons, or proton beams. In brachytherapy the source of radiation is implanted in the patient. Each technique has its own advantages and applications. Electron beams are superficially penetrating and are used as a boost to superficial areas (e.g., posterior neck nodes). On the other hand, photon beam radiation spares the skin relatively and affects the deeper tissues

TABLE 45.12 Indications for postoperative radiotherapy

Primary tumor features
Advanced T stage (bulky tumor; involvement of bone, nerves, skin)
High histologic grade
Positive surgical margins
Lymphovascular invasion
Perineural spread

Lymphatic spread features
Involvement of more than two nodes
Involvement of more than one level of the neck
Lymph node >3 cm (N2, N3 disease)
Extracapsular spread
Microscopic or gross residual disease in the neck
Involvement of critical level of neck nodes (Levels IV and V)

Source: Reprinted with permission from Shaha AR et al (2001) Head and neck cancer. In: Osteen RT, Gansler TS, Lenhard RE (eds) Clinical oncology. American Cancer Society, Atlanta, GA, pp 297–329

more specifically. For lesions of nasopharynx, oral cavity, and oropharynx, brachytherapy in form of radioisotope implants (Iodine, Iridium, Radium, or Gold) can be quite useful. The methods of delivery have undergone significant improvement in the past few decades. For IMRT, a computer-controlled machine is used to produce a three-dimensional model in which many radiation beams are used to optimize the dose in the target area, while sparing normal tissues. More recently tomotherapy, which integrates CT or PET-CT technology into a linear accelerator, has been introduced and is being used more frequently. Cyberknife or stereotactic radiosurgery is another new development that is currently being explored for head and neck cancers. These methods, although quite exciting, have not been validated in prospective controlled trials yet [101, 102].

The typical radiotherapy regimen for head and neck cancers consists of daily fractions of 1.8 c–2.0 cGy, 5 days a week to a maximum dose of 70 Gy over 7 weeks. For most adjuvant treatments a total dose of 60–66 Gy is administered. When extracapsular extension is present, increasing the dose to 63 Gy improves locoregional control [103]. The toxicity of radiation escalates exponentially and becomes quite significant, especially in doses above 70 Gy.

In general, it is preferable to start postoperative radiotherapy within 6 weeks after surgery. Long term delays or interruptions in treatment are not desirable, theoretically due to repopulation of cancer cells. Cancer cells in general cannot repair the radiation damage as fast as normal tissue. In order to take advantage of this phenomenon, two techniques have been introduced: hyperfractionation and accelerated fractionation. In hyperfractionation, two to three reduced dose fractions are delivered every day (1.1–1.25 Gy/fraction). This method achieves a higher total dose without increasing the chronic toxic effects of a standard dose. Accelerated fractionation uses fractions of 1.6–1.8 Gy more than once a day and the goal is to achieve 10 Gy per week in a reduced time compared to standard fractionation. So far most studies have shown modest improvement in locoregional control and marginal improvement in survival [104, 105]. The combination of altered fractionation and chemotherapy has been more promising [106–108].

Radiotherapy has been used extensively in treatment and palliation of elderly head and neck cancer patients. Strong evidence supports both safety and efficacy of this modality and clearly shows that age is not a limiting factor in utilization of radiotherapy [109–111]. Radiotherapy in general has similar efficacy and side effect profile in elderly patients and general population [112, 113]. It has even been used successfully in patients older than 90 years old [114]. Although traditionally elderly patients have been treated with lower doses of radiation, there is no evidence that this is necessary. All studies have shown that elderly patients can tolerate and benefit from the standard regimens of radiation without increased morbidity and mortality. Newer modalities of radiotherapy such as altered fractionation and IMRT has been used in elderly patients. Since these modalities have been introduced more recently specific data on elderly population is scant. There is suggestion of reduced benefit of hyperfractionation in elderly patients and those with poor performance status [115]. IMRT is also used widely in treatment of different head and neck cancers, but more evidence needs to be acquired to determine if there are differences in treatment and complication profiles of this technique in elderly patients. In general early and late toxicities of radiotherapy occur with similar frequency in elderly and general population. The management of toxicities such as xerostomia and mucositis is the same as in younger patients. Elderly patients might need to be monitored more carefully during the treatment, since they are more susceptible to loss of fluids and electrolytes [116].

Chemotherapy has evolved quite significantly in recent history from a palliative option to a central component of treatment of locally advanced tumors. Cisplatin is considered a standard agent in combination with radiation and other agents. Carboplatin, the other platinum agent, is less toxic, but also less active against squamous cell cancers. They both are comparable radiosensitizing agents. Taxane-based agents are quite active and have been used in induction regimens for locally advanced tumors. One of the more significant advances is the use of EGFR inhibitors. Cetuximab is the first agent that has successfully been used in treating head and neck cancers [67, 117]. Other novel therapies that are being investigated include monoclonal antibodies or multiselective tyrosine kinase inhibitors against EGFR or other dysregulated pathways in head and neck cancer, and antiangiogenesis agents. The combination of these novel therapies with chemotherapy and radiation is actively being pursued. At present time there is no specific data in use of cetuximab in elderly patients; however, ongoing studies at this time are recruiting elderly patients.

Only about one-third of patients with head and neck cancer will present in early stages (I and II). In early stage disease, the tendency is to use one modality that offers the best chance for cure and minimizes morbidity. The preferred method of treatment in oral cavity cancers is surgery for the primary tumor with elective neck dissection based on the probability of lymph node metastases [118]. This method offers the best functional outcome and most accurate staging. It also avoids the late toxic effects of radiotherapy. In addition, in case of recurrence, radiotherapy can be used as a salvage option. For early stage laryngeal tumors, either organ preserving surgery or radiotherapy are acceptable and will produce comparable functional results and cure rates [119–121]. The choice depends on tumor location, local expertise, and patient's preferences. For early laryngeal lesions, laser excision is the preferred modality. In early-stage tumors of the oropharynx and hypopharynx, radiotherapy is usually recommended as the first choice. It produces similar cure rates to surgery with less morbidity [122, 123].

Treatment of locally advanced disease uses a multimodality approach based on surgery, radiation and chemotherapy. One of the major advances of treating this category is the introduction of chemoradiotherapy, which concurrently uses chemotherapy and radiation. Many trials have shown the superiority of chemoradiotherapy in comparison to radiotherapy alone with regard to locoregional control, disease free survival, and in some studies overall survival [124, 125]. In postoperative settings adding chemotherapy to radiation showed benefit, especially in the presence of extracapsular spread or positive margins [126]. In general, the same principles are used for advanced disease with the addition of chemoradiation or radiation to surgery. In oral cavity cancers, advanced tumors are treated with surgery followed by radiation or chemoradiation. Advanced oropharyngeal tumors are treated with primary chemoradiation that offers good efficacy and functional results. In cases of advanced laryngeal cancer, many experts still advocate primary surgery, since preserving an already dysfunctional organ does not add much to the quality of life and the failure rate of chemoradiotherapy is high in these situations.

Management of the neck is an integral part of the treatment of advanced head and neck cancers. Patients exhibiting positive margins, multiple positive nodes, or extranodal spread are generally considered candidates for postoperative chemoradiotherapy. However, use of this aggressive adjuvant therapy needs to be balanced against possible complications such as severe mucositis, neutropenia, and pharyngeal stricture.

The standard chemotherapy regimen is platinum based. Cetuximab plus radiation has been successfully used and should be strongly considered in patients who cannot tolerate standard chemotherapy. Induction chemotherapy has the potential to reduce the incidence of distant metastases.

Although platinum based regimens produce high response rates initially and result in good locoregional control, most of the trials have failed to show any survival benefit [127]. Introduction of taxane-based agents has improved survival or organ preservation [128–130]. Concurrent chemotherapy has been shown in a series of meta-analyses to be the most effective method and has the potential of becoming the standard of care. The most recent data indicates a 6.5% survival benefit at 5 years with this method [3].

Unlike radiation, which is fairly well tolerated and there is overwhelming evidence in its benefits in elderly population, not enough data exists for chemotherapy regimens. In addition, quite a few studies have shown higher complication and toxicity rate in elderly populations [131]. The benefits of chemotherapy also seem to be more pronounced in younger patients. This preliminary evidence should not discourage practitioners in considering elderly patients for chemotherapy. Certain elderly patients can benefit from these new regimens by careful assessment and attention to overall status of the patient and the disease.

Unknown Primary Tumors

A solitary lateral neck mass in adults is always suspicious for malignancy. Primary malignancies of the neck are extremely rare and these masses are most commonly a metastatic lymph node. If the source of malignancy is not found after a thorough history, physical exam, endoscopy and imaging, then it is classified as an "unknown primary tumor". The most common sites for lymph node involvement are upper jugular lymph nodes (level II) (Fig. 45.6) followed by middle and lower jugular nodes (level III and IV). The location of lymphadenopathy usually correlates with the origin of the tumor. In general, two-thirds of all primaries arise from supraclavicular sources. These primaries are located in nasopharynx and oropharynx in one-third of cases; tonsil and base of tongue in another third, and the rest come from different locations. A few can arise in the hypopharynx. Most metastases from infraclavicular sources (two-thirds of cases) will involve supraclavicular lymph nodes (level IV). Generally, 50% of the primaries are found in the lungs. Breasts, stomach, pancreas, and ovaries contribute to the rest of cases.

The clinician who encounters a patient with an isolated neck mass should resist the temptation to perform an excisional biopsy as a first step. Multiple studies have shown that such an intervention will increase the incidence of wound complications, local recurrences, and distant metastases [132–135]. The approach should be systematic and stepwise, preferably by a practitioner well versed in management of head and neck cancers and capable of performing different diagnostic and therapeutic procedures that might be required in the course of work-up and treatment. The first step is a thorough history and physical exam including nasopharyngoscopy and fiberoptic laryngoscopy. FNA of the suspicious lymph node should be the next step. If FNA results confirm malignancy or is suspicious then further work-up is necessary. Even if the results are inconclusive or benign, in high risk patients it is advisable to proceed with a thorough work-up. Imaging, preferably by CT and MRI, are necessary to find the possible primary and better delineate the extent of disease in the neck. T2 weighted MRI images are superior in characterizing submucosal lesions [136]. EBV antibody titers may be helpful in directing a diagnosis toward nasopharyngeal primaries. Examination under anesthesia is the next step. A panendoscopy should be performed to inspect the nasopharynx, larynx, pharynx, esophagus, and lungs very carefully. While blind biopsies do not offer high yield, directed biopsies of suspicious areas in endoscopy can be quite helpful. Directed biopsies should be based on the findings of the endoscopy, the patterns of lymphatic spread and the location of the metastatic lymph nodes. Some references have advocated ipsilateral tonsillectomy at the time of panendoscopy, especially if the involved lymph node is at level II (upper jugular) [137].

If after all these interventions a source is still not found or the FNA findings are highly suspicious for lymphoma, then performing an open biopsy is prudent. Before attempting the biopsy, the patient should be informed of the possible need for a formal neck dissection based on intraoperative findings. If the practitioner or the patient would rather wait for the permanent pathology specimen, it is extremely important to plan the incision in a way that can be excised if a definitive operation becomes necessary.

The standard treatment for metastatic squamous cell carcinoma of the neck with an unknown primary is neck dissection plus postoperative radiotherapy. Patients with N1 and

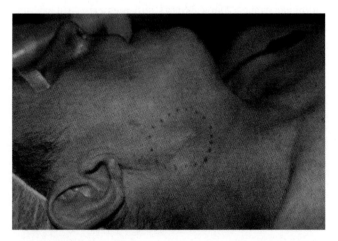

Figure 45.6 Right neck mass. Metastatic cutaneous squamous cell carcinoma to level II (upper jugular) lymph nodes. Primary source was unknown at the time of presentation.

extracapsular spread, or N2 and N3 disease will benefit the most from postoperative radiation to the neck. In cases of N1 disease without extracapsular spread there are different opinions. Some advocate surgery alone, some recommend excision of the node only with postoperative radiation and others press for neck dissection plus postoperative radiation. The practice and extent of prophylactic radiotherapy is a matter of controversy [138]. Irradiation of the involved side of the neck plus the contralateral side, nasopharynx, ipsilateral tonsil, and base of tongue has been advocated. The benefit of this approach been questioned and several adverse effects have been raised. Prophylactic radiation can induce later mucosal tumors. It causes significant morbidity in the form of xerostomia, dysphagia, and dental problems. Lastly, if the primary tumor is an excised skin cancer, or from an infraclavicular source, the patient will not benefit from radiation. In cases of positive EBV antibody it is recommended to include the nasopharynx in the radiation field. The rate of manifestation of primary tumors post radiation is 4–16%, which is the same as the rate of second primaries.

In general, patients with unknown primaries should be under close surveillance after treatment whether or not they receive postoperative radiation. Recurrence rates after treatment range from 11 to 14% for mucosal malignancies. The prognosis of recurrence is dependent on pathologic features of the tumor such as grade and presence of extracapsular spread. Patients whose primary tumor was never found have the best prognosis.

In cases of adenocarcinoma metastatic to the cervical lymph nodes, the majority of patients have other areas of distal metastases and the overall outcome is not dependent on the treatment of the neck. The primary tumor is usually infraclavicular and occasionally can be found in salivary glands [139]. Metastatic adenocarcinoma in the upper part of the neck is generally from the major or minor salivary glands and is commonly considered a surgical problem, while metastatic adenocarcinoma in the lower part of the neck is most likely from the lung or abdominal organs and considered to be a systemic disease and not a surgical problem.

Treatment of the Neck

Cervical lymph nodes are the most common site of metastases from head and neck cancers. Adequate and effective treatment of the neck is of utmost importance in management of head and neck cancer patients. The principles of treatment have been established for more than 100 years now and continue to evolve. Cervical lymphadenectomy was introduced by Butlin and was expanded to radical neck dissection by Crile. This operation was subsequently popularized by Hayes Martin. Radical neck dissection, although an effective cancer operation, carried a significant burden of morbidity. In this operation, all the lymphatic tissues of the neck from level I to level V are removed in addition to the sternocleidomastoid muscle, internal jugular vein, and spinal accessory nerve. A long list of morbidities accompanied this operation. The most significant is "shoulder syndrome" due to sacrifice of the spinal accessory nerve. A detailed list can be found in Table 45.13. Suarez from Argentina and later Bocca from Italy introduced the concept of functional neck dissection which was subsequently transformed to modified radical neck dissection. In this modification, the structures that were not directly involved with cancer were spared. Many studies have shown that the efficacy of RND and MRND are comparable and they both offer equivalent oncologic results. MRND, especially when all three structures are preserved, is a much less morbid operation than RND. Later, based on works by Lindberg and then Shah, the patterns of

TABLE 45.13 Complications of radical neck dissection

Timing and nature of complication	Sequelae
Intraoperative	
Injury to nerves	
Marginal mandibular nerve	Deformity of angle of mouth
Hypoglossal nerve	Difficulty in moving the tongue
Vagus nerve	Hoarseness, aspiration
Sympathetic chain	Horner's syndrome
Phrenic nerve	Paralyzed ipsilateral diaphragm
Brachial plexus	Weakness or paralysis of limb muscles
Injury to thoracic or major lymphatic duct	Chyle leak
Injury to dome of pleura	Pneumothorax (tension)
Injury to pharynx or esophagus	Salivary fistula
Other complications	
Stimulation of carotid bulb	Bradycardia
Injury to internal carotid artery	Stroke
Air embolism through major venous injury	Hypotension, death
Early and Intermediate postoperative	
Reactionary or secondary hemorrhage	Hematoma
Carotid artery exposure and rupture	Stroke, Death
Physiologic consequences	
Spinal accessory nerve	Shoulder dysfunction
Other nerves	Anesthesia of skin flaps, ear lobe, and cheek
Internal jugular vein ligation (bilateral)	Cerebral edema, airway obstruction, blindness, edema of face and neck

Source: Reprinted with permission from Shaha AR et al (2001) Head and neck cancer. In: Osteen RT, Gansler TS, Lenhard RE (eds) Clinical oncology. American Cancer Society, Atlanta, GA, pp 297–329

TABLE 45.14 Classification of neck dissection

1991 Classification	2002 Classification
Radical neck dissection	Radical neck dissection
Modified radical neck dissection	Modified radical neck dissection
Selective neck dissection	Selective neck dissection
Supraomohyoid	Each variation is depicted by
Lateral	"SND" and the use of
Posterolateral	parentheses to denote the
Anterior	levels or sublevels
	removed
Extended neck dissection	Extended neck dissection

Source: Robbins KT et al (2002) Neck dissection classification update: revisions proposed by the American Head and Neck Society and the American Academy of Otolaryngology-Head and Neck Surgery. Arch Otolaryngol Head Neck Surg 128(7): 751–758

lymphatic spread for different sites of head and neck cancers were defined. This knowledge led to the introduction of selective node dissection in which only the nodal groups at highest risk of metastases are removed, which spares the patient from the morbidity associated with comprehensive neck dissection. All of these modifications caused significant cluttering of the nomenclature. In an effort to standardize the vocabulary, the American Academy of Otolaryngology-Head and Neck Surgery convened a special task force in 1991. This task force published a report for standardizing different variations of neck dissection. The report was then updated in 2002. Currently, most head and neck surgeons use this classification when addressing the different variations of neck dissection. The 1991 and 2001 classifications are compared in Table 45.14.

In general, cervical lymph nodes are addressed in three different settings. First is management of the neck in clinically N0 disease, where there is no evidence of metastases in clinical examination and imaging. There is still controversy on the necessity and extent of dissection. A few guidelines are generally accepted. The need for elective neck dissection is justified if the probability of occult metastases is about 15–20%. The neck can be addressed either by radiotherapy or by neck dissection, but the tendency is to perform selective neck dissection. This will minimize the morbidity and avoid long term consequences of radiation. When the risk of metastases is less than 15%, it is not justified to subject the other 85% without disease to treatment. An exception is when addressing the primary tumor will require access through the neck. In these cases, selective neck dissection can be added to the procedure without significantly increasing the morbidity.

In terms of the extent of lymphadenectomy in elective neck dissection, there is now good evidence to guide clinicians. This evidence is mostly based on works of Shah et al., who established the patterns of lymphatic spread in head and neck cancers. Based on his work and other investigators such

as Byers et al., selective node dissection is widely accepted as adequate treatment in elective neck dissection. In general, for tumors of the oral cavity, dissection of levels I–III is performed. Levels II through IV are dissected in oropharyngeal tumors; however, quite often surgical access requires dissection of level I nodes and in this case levels I–IV are dissected. For hypopharynx and laryngeal tumors, levels II through IV are removed.

If there is evidence of disease in the neck, the traditional treatment was to perform radical neck dissection. Interestingly, even in presence of clinical evidence for lymph node metastases, disease will be found in approximately 80–85% of specimens. Nowadays, based on many prior studies, the tendency is to preserve the organs that are not directly involved with the disease. There are studies that show preservation of the spinal accessory nerve or jugular vein will not jeopardize the efficacy of the operation. Based on this evidence, it is generally accepted that modified radical neck dissection is equivalent to radical neck dissection as long as the preserved organs are not directly involved with the tumor. The next leap of faith was applying the principles of selective neck dissection to the node positive patient. There is quite a bit of controversy on this topic. An important principle is to treat the neck with radiation after neck dissection in all cases of node positive disease, except for a few special cases. Postoperative radiation improves local control from 30 to 50% for surgery alone to 70% even in cases of N2 and N3 disease. There are quite a few studies demonstrating that selective node dissection can be comparable to modified radical neck dissection as long as postoperative radiotherapy is used. While it can be said that the standard is still to perform modified radical neck dissection for node positive disease, there is an ever growing application of selective neck dissection in this group. The levels of dissection are as described for elective neck dissection. If there is evidence of disease in the specimen, the majority of practitioners will recommend postoperative adjuvant radiotherapy. In the N3 neck and when the extent of disease is beyond the first and second echelon of nodal drainage, the tendency is to perform comprehensive neck dissection and adjuvant radiotherapy, instead of selective neck dissection.

The last application of neck dissection is planned neck dissection or in cases of recurrence after definitive chemoradiation. Performing neck dissection is fraught with complications in this setting. There are not that many studies that provide evidence as to the effectiveness of the operation. In general, it is recommended to perform planned neck dissection in N2 and N3 disease after chemoradiation regardless of evidence of residual disease. However this approach was recently modified with the routine use of PET scans in the follow-up of patients receiving chemoRT. Patients with PET negative results are generally observed. In cases of N1 disease where there is no evidence of disease, most will observe the patient.

As to the extent of operation, most agree on comprehensive neck dissection with preservation of the spinal accessory nerve if possible. With widespread use of PET scans and other biologic studies and markers, these recommendations will probably change and more tailored approaches based on the biology of the tumor will be adopted.

The use of radiotherapy to address disease in the neck is quite established now. Radiotherapy can be used alone in treating disease in the neck. A dose of 60 Gy results in sterilization of 90% of pathologically involved nodes that are less than 2 cm. As the disease bulk increases, it takes higher doses of radiation to control the disease and at the same time, the rate of control decreases. For nodes larger than 3 cm, doses of 70 Gy can achieve control in approximately 80% of cases. Except for nasopharyngeal and tonsillar cancers that are very radiosensitive, nodes significantly larger than 3 cm rarely disappear with radiation alone. Based on these facts, N2 and N3 disease are treated with a combination of surgery and radiation. In preoperative settings, doses of 50–60 Gy are administered to the involved node. In postoperative settings, the dose is around 66 Gy. Another important factor is to avoid delay between therapies. On average, it is desirable to proceed with the next modality in 4–6 weeks. Further delays might cause repopulation of cancer cells and also increases morbidity.

Nasal Cavity and Paranasal Sinuses

Tumors arising from the paranasal sinuses are rare. They only comprise 3% of head and neck cancers. The most common malignant tumor is squamous cell carcinoma (80%) followed by adenoid cystic carcinoma and adenocarcinoma (10%), and numerous other tumors such as neuroendocrine tumors, malignant melanoma, sarcomas, and hematopoietic and lymphatic tumors. The most common site for squamous cell carcinoma is the maxillary sinus followed by the ethmoid sinus. Most symptoms are quite similar to benign processes of the sinuses (nasal obstruction, rhinorrhea, and congestion) and therefore most are diagnosed later in their course. Advanced symptoms include facial pain, diplopia, proptosis, or symptoms of intracranial invasion like headache, neuropathies, and frontal lobe syndrome. CT scanning and especially MRI are preferred imaging methods.

Since most tumors are found in advanced stages, treatment usually includes surgery and radiation. Depending on the size and location of tumor, different surgical techniques are used. External ethmoidectomy is the most limited operation and is used for benign tumors of the ethmoid region or biopsy of sphenoethmoidal region tumors. For small tumors of the lateral nasal wall, medial maxillectomy through a lateral rhinotomy approach is the procedure of choice. Partial maxillectomy can be used in treating infrastructure maxillary tumors. This operation is technically easier and cosmetic results are quite good. Local control with this approach is quite acceptable. Suprastructure lesions on the other hand are more challenging. They usually require total maxillectomy with reconstruction of the orbital floor. Orbital exenteration might become necessary depending on the extent of orbital invasion by tumor. The most extensive surgeries require craniofacial resection with an intracranial approach by a neurosurgeon and facial approach by a head and neck surgeon for tumors that involve the base of the skull. Endoscopic approaches have become quite popular recently and a few select centers resect malignant tumors by this technique. This approach, however, is mainly used for benign and intermediate tumors [140]. More recently reports of using surgical robots in skull base tumors in preclinical stages have emerged [83]. Appropriate rehabilitation after surgery is very important in this group of patients. This goal is achieved by involvement of a prosthodontist for smaller defects and use of microvascular free tissue transfers for larger and more complex ones. Small defects usually can be covered with a split thickness skin graft and then a temporary prosthesis placed in the defect. After the defect has stabilized a final prosthesis is fashioned.

Most cases will require adjuvant radiotherapy. The delivery of radiation is more complicated because of the proximity of the brain, spinal cord, and orbit. The complication profile of radiotherapy has been reduced by the advent of IMRT techniques, which reduces the dose to sensitive and noninvolved organs [141]. The 5-year survival rate of maxillary tumors treated with surgery and radiation is 46–67% [141–143]. Cervical lymph node metastasis occurs in approximately 15–25% of cases and is usually a bad prognostic feature [144]. More recently, reports of chemoradiotherapy have shown more promise in controlling these tumors. A report from Japan has shown impressive results with use of radiation and concurrent arterial infusion of 5-FU, tumor reduction surgery, and immunotherapy. They improved 5-year survival by more than 20% from 20 to 54% [145]. Other reports also have shown benefit by using concurrent cisplatin and split course radiotherapy in advanced cases [146].

Adenocarcinomas harbor equally poor outcome (5 year survival of only 20% in poorly differentiated tumors). They are more common in professions related to woodworking, furniture making, and leather-work [147]. They are quite aggressive locally and the best chance is en bloc resection if possible. Adenoid cystic carcinomas have a favorable 5-year survival of 75% but the 15-year survival declines to 20% [148]. These tumors can spread along nerve sheath structures and have a tendency toward distant metastases rather than regional metastases [148]. In spite of this fact, the most common cause of death is invasion of the skull base. Treatment is surgical with added adjuvant radiation if margins are suspicious.

Nasopharynx

Nasopharyngeal carcinoma (NPC) is a relatively rare disease outside parts of southern China, Hong Kong, and Singapore. It is more common in the Chinese population of these areas and the risk of cancer goes down with emigration, but is still much higher than other ethnicities [149]. It is more common in men than women (2.5:1). A multifactorial pathogenesis has been proposed based on patterns of distribution. Genetic susceptibility, latent EBV infection, dietary habits, and smoking are all well known factors. EBV infection plays a crucial role in progression to severe dysplasia. Diets high in preserved food, salted fish and deficient in carotene, fresh fruit and fiber have also been implicated [150].

The World Health Organization (WHO) has divided NPC into three subtypes [151]. WHO type I is keratinizing squamous cell carcinoma. This subtype is relatively more common among cases in the US (20–30%), but is rare in Asia (1–3%). WHO type II is non-keratinizing carcinoma. WHO type III is undifferentiated carcinoma or lymphoepithelioma. Types II and III are more radiosensitive and achieve better local control but have higher rates of distant metastases [152, 153].

NPC patients are relatively younger than the rest of head and neck cancer patients. Incidence starts to increase in second decade of life and peaks in fourth and fifth decade. The most common presenting symptom is cervical lymphadenopathy. Lymphadenopathy starts at the jugulodigastric nodes (level II) and continues to progress downward to levels III and IV. Other symptoms include nasal obstruction, epistaxis, otitis media, and referred pain to the ears. Multiple cranial nerve palsy can be seen (cranial nerves VI, IV, and V, and in case of extension to jugular foramen cranial nerves IX, X, and XI). Five percent of patients will present with distant metastases, most commonly to bones followed by the lungs and liver [154].

Diagnostic work-up includes a detailed history and physical including nasopharyngoscopy. The most common sites of origin are the Rosenmuller fossa and nasopharyngeal roof. Biopsies should be taken for histologies. If biopsy of a cervical lymph node is required, FNA is the preferred method and open biopsies should be avoided. EBV DNA titers have prognostic value and should be checked. In case of suspicious disease, high titers of EBV antibody are very sensitive and specific. Liver function tests may be helpful in ruling out liver metastases. The preferred imaging modality is MRI, which provides excellent soft tissue details. A chest X-ray should be obtained to rule out metastases. Staging is based on the sixth edition of AJCC-UICC TNM system and is detailed in Tables 45.3, 45.8 and 45.11.

The primary treatment for nasopharyngeal cancer is radiotherapy. NPC is extremely radiosensitive and even bulky lymphadenopathy responds well to radiotherapy. In addition, these tumors are difficult to access surgically and the morbidity of surgery can be quite high. External beam radiation is the most commonly used method, although there is a role for brachytherapy in selected cases when the disease volume is not very large. Fields of radiation include the primary tumor, retropharyngeal nodes, and bilateral neck and supraclavicular nodes. Doses of 70–76 Gy are administered to the diseased areas. Prophylactic doses of 50–60 Gy are administered to at risk areas in the neck. With the advent of new radiotherapy techniques such as three-dimensional conformal, IMRT, and altered fractionation, the morbidity of treatment is reduced, and the incidence of "geographic miss" is lower. Radiation boost in the form of brachytherapy can be used in T1 and T2 lesions to improve local control. Overall survival for use of radiation therapy alone is in the range of 50–76%. Results are excellent in early stage disease. For locally advanced disease, addition of chemotherapy in the forms of induction, concurrent and adjuvant chemotherapy has added improved survival and local control rates. The two most commonly used drugs are cisplatin and 5-FU. The role of surgery is limited to treating residual or recurrent disease. Neck dissection after radiotherapy for residual disease can be performed. In cases of brachytherapy, the surgeon can play a role in inserting brachytherapy catheters.

Recurrent disease can be treated with radiotherapy or surgical excision. If detected early, there is a potential for control and these patients need to be treated aggressively. Follow-up of the patients should include careful physical exam, radiologic imaging, and laboratory tests to monitor potential treatment-related side effects including pituitary dysfunction should be considered.

Oral Cavity

Oral cavity cancers have the chance of being detected relatively earlier than other head and neck cancers. However, common manifestations with benign oral disease make delays in diagnosis quite possible as well. Oral cavity cancers, including lip cancers, account for about 13% of head and neck cancers [155]. It is slightly more common in men. A majority of cases are squamous cell carcinoma with adenocarcinoma, verrucous carcinoma, lymphoma, and Kaposi's sarcoma constituting the rest.

The most common presenting symptom is a nonhealing ulcer (Fig. 45.7). The most common sites are the tongue and floor of the mouth. The most recent staging is described in Tables 45.2 and 45.10. The treatment plan is based on the location, stage, relation to the mandible, and incidence of occult or gross nodal metastases. Early stage lesions can be treated effectively with one modality (surgery or radiation). More advanced lesions usually require a combination of different modalities.

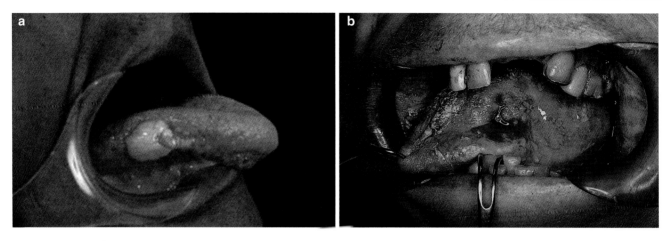

Figure 45.7 (a) Early tongue cancer (b) Advanced tongue cancer presenting as nonhealing ulcer. Note poor dental hygiene.

Most lip lesions occur in the lower lip and men are afflicted more commonly than women. Most malignancies of the lower lip are squamous cell carcinomas, while the upper lip harbors more basal cell carcinomas. Risk factors include prolonged sun exposure, fair skin complexion, immunosuppression, and tobacco abuse.

Choice of treatment depends on the size and location of the tumor. For small lesions, V-shaped resection with primary closure or a local flap is quite adequate. Excision of lesions up to one-third of lip length by this method results in acceptable functional and cosmetic outcome. For lesions between one-third and two-thirds of lip length usually involve a lip switch flap (Abbe-Estlander). For larger lesions and those which involve the commissure, options are a Gilles fan flap, bilateral advancement flap, and Karapandzic flap or radial forearm free flap [156]. Surgical excision can cause microstomia and oral incompetence, which are more common after removal of large lesions. Cervical metastases are rare (10%) and prophylactic neck dissection is not recommended. In cases of clinically positive lymph nodes, therapeutic neck dissection is indicated. Positive margins, perineural invasion, and positive cervical nodes, among others, are indications for adjuvant radiotherapy. Five-year survival for T1 and T2 lesions is excellent (90%). For larger lesions (T3 and T4) survival is decreased to 75%. Presence of cervical metastases lowers survival to almost 50%.

Cancers of the oral tongue are more common on the posterolateral aspect (75%) than on the anterolateral and ventral surfaces (20%). These tumors arise in the epithelium and invade deeper tissues. Patterns of invasion can be varied. The tumor can spread to the midline and contralateral side, posteriorly to base of the tongue or inferiorly to the floor of the mouth. In extreme cases they can involve the mandible. Perineural invasion can happen and will cause numbness, fasciculation, and atrophy of the tongue. Most lesions (75%) are diagnosed in an early stage (T1, T2). Partial glossectomy with negative margins provides good oncologic and functional

results. Resection of one-fourth to one-third of the oral tongue can be tolerated quite well with minimal adverse functional effects. The defect can be left open to heal with secondary intention or covered with a split thickness skin graft. If excision of the tumor requires removal of half of the tongue, the best strategy is to repair the defect with a fasciocutaneous free flap (radial forearm or anterolateral thigh). If a significant portion of the floor of the mouth are to be removed, again free flap reconstruction provides the best outcome. Tongue tumors are distinct in that depth of invasion is a better predictor of presence of cervical node metastases than T stage [78]. Based on a meta-analysis of multiple studies, for tumors with depth of invasion more than 4 mm, prophylactic neck dissection is recommended, since the probability of neck metastases is around 16%. Another phenomenon is the possibility of skip metastases. Tongue lesions can skip level I and II neck nodes and present in levels III and IV in almost 16% of cases. Based on this observation, some authorities advocate removal of neck nodes from level I to IV instead of performing a supraomohyoid neck dissection (level I–III) [157]. Lesions close to the midline may require bilateral neck dissection. Advanced lesions (III or IV) and those with positive or close surgical margins, neck nodes metastases will require adjuvant radiation which will improve locoregional control. The 5-year survival for early stage tumors is 75% and for advanced cancers (III and IV) is almost 50%.

Floor of mouth lesions are more common in men and usually present in the sixth decade of life. For small lesions, transoral excision is adequate and provides excellent results. The defect can be left open to be closed by secondary intention or with a split thickness skin graft. For larger lesions, immediate reconstruction with a free flap or local flaps is usually necessary. If the lesion is close to submandibular salivary glands, excision of the gland becomes necessary in a majority of cases. More extensive lesions may require different forms of mandibulectomy. Cervical metastases are common and can be found in up to 50% of cases. Lesions in the anterior floor of the mouth can metastasize bilaterally. Submandibular lymph nodes are most commonly affected. Survival for floor of mouth cancers are 90% for stage I disease, 80% for stage II, 65% for stage III, and 30% for stage IV [158, 159].

Buccal lesions are most common in users of smokeless tobacco and are usually located in the region of the third mandibular molar. Surgery and radiation have equal success in treating these cancers. However, surgery is preferred for most lesions since the rate of complications is lower. Primary radiotherapy is considered for patients who are not appropriate candidates for surgery and immediate reconstruction. Small lesions can be excised transorally. Larger lesions with involvement of the oral commissure, full thickness of cheek, skin or mandible will require composite resection and immediate reconstruction with free flap tissue transfer. For advanced lesions adjuvant radiation therapy is indicated. The incidence of lymph node metastases is relatively low and neck dissection is reserved for advanced cases or clinically positive nodes. Five-year survival is around 75% for stage I, 65% for stage II, 30–60% for stage III, and 20–50% for stage IV [160, 161].

Alveolar ridge tumors are relatively uncommon and account for approximately 10% of oral cavity cancers. Mandibular lesions are more common than maxillary gingival tumors. Close proximity to bone makes osseous invasion more common in these tumors. Management of the mandible will be discussed in detail later. Overall incidence of lymph node metastases is quite high (25%). This fact makes prophylactic and therapeutic neck dissection much more common in management of alveolar ridge tumors. Treatment is surgical excision and, in advanced tumors, adjuvant radiotherapy. Primary radiotherapy is not recommended in tumors with bony invasion. For early stage disease the 5-year survival is as good as 85%. In patients with metastatic spread, survival ranges from 35 to 59% [162, 163].

Retromolar trigone tumors usually present in advanced stages. Mandible involvement is common and invasion of the tonsillar fossa, faucial arch, and base of tongue happen often. Surgical treatment followed by radiation is the preferred method of treatment. Because of proximity to bone, surgical excision usually involves marginal or segmental mandibulectomy for more advanced tumors. Most of these tumors have metastasized to neck nodes at diagnosis and neck dissection is commonly performed at the time of surgical therapy. Survival ranges from 76% for T1 to 54% for T4 lesions at 5 years. Patients without nodal involvement have an overall survival of 69%. This rate falls down to 56% for N1 and 26% for N2 disease. Patients who have undergone surgery and adjuvant radiotherapy have better survival than primary radiation (44% vs. 23%) [164].

Hard palate tumors are mostly squamous cell carcinoma; however minor salivary gland tumors, mucosal melanoma and Kaposi's sarcoma can occur in this location. Treatment is mainly surgical and depends on the stage and extent of tumor requiring different degrees of maxillectomy (infrastructure in earlier lesion and total maxillectomy for more advanced tumors). The rate of metastases is low and prophylactic neck dissection is not routinely performed. The 5-year survival is reported from 40 to 60% [165, 166].

Oropharynx

The most common sites are the tonsil and base of tongue for cancers of oropharynx. Cancers of the soft palate and pharyngeal wall do occur, but are less common. Oropharyngeal cancers are on the rise especially in non-smokers and younger men. In general these tumors tend to be diagnosed late and there is a high incidence of lymphatic spread at the time of diagnosis. Radiation is used as primary treatment for oropharyngeal cancers much more commonly than oral cavity tumors due to the high morbidity of surgical excision in this region. Similar to oral cavity, advanced tumors require a combination of surgical and radiation therapies.

Tonsils are the most common site and account for almost 75% of oropharyngeal cancers. Most early cancers are asymptomatic. It is not uncommon to find cervical lymphadenopathy as the presenting symptom of tonsillar cancer (Fig. 45.8). The incidence of positive lymph nodes at presentation is as high as 40–76% in different reports. The most common site of lymph node metastases is level II nodes; however, retropharyngeal and parapharyngeal nodes can also

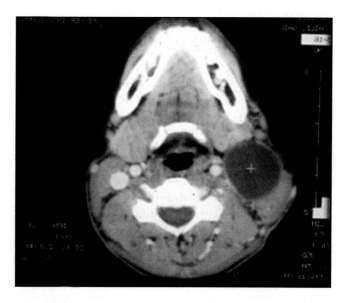

FIGURE 45.8 CT scan of neck. Metastatic tonsillar cancer to left level II lymph node. Note cystic appearance of lymph node. This is one of the characteristic features of tonsillar metastases and can be mistaken with bronchial cleft cyst.

be afflicted. These tumors tend to invade the base of tongue in most advanced cases. For early tonsillar tumors, surgery and radiation yield equal results. Surgical treatment is composed of radical tonsillectomy plus neck dissection. In current practice, majority of cases are treated with radiation primarily. Radiation fields include the primary site and ipsilateral neck, including retropharyngeal nodes. It is important to spare the contralateral parotid gland to reduce the complication of xerostomia. Radiation alone results in local control of 70–90%. Salvage surgery is also successful in two-thirds of patients. This combination results in ultimate local control of 90% in early stages. In advanced lesions (T3–T4), the combination of surgery and radiotherapy is standard practice. Resection of large lesions through the mouth is difficult and many patients will require a lower lip splitting incision with mandibulotomy. More recently, interest in using a surgical robot to resect these tumors without mandibulotomy has arisen in multiple centers [167, 168]. Comprehensive neck dissection is an integral part of surgery. Adjuvant radiation improves local control quite significantly. Surgery plus adjuvant radiation results in overall 5-year survival of 75% versus 48% for surgery alone [169, 170]. T-stage specific survival of tonsillar cancer is 89%, 55%, 49%, and 30% for T1 through T4 lesions respectively.

Base of tongue tumors are usually quite a challenge for the head and neck cancer practitioner. These tumors remain asymptomatic for a long time, usually present in advanced stages, have regional lymph node involvement (>60%), and have a tendency to metastasize to both sides of the neck (20%) (Fig. 45.9). Most of these tumors require a multidisciplinary approach and treatment. In early tumors it might be possible to resect the tumor transorally combined with neck dissection. Nearly 50% of the tongue base can be removed with very good functional results. Resection can be done using surgical laser or a more conventional method. Very good survival (52% at 5 years) and excellent functional results (92% could tolerate a normal diet and 88% had understandable speech) can be expected using this method [171]. For larger tumors, resection often involves other approaches such as transhyoid, lateral pharyngotomy or mandibular swing. The need for postoperative radiation depends on characteristics of the tumor, margins, and degree of involvement of lymph nodes. In general 5-year disease specific survival for tongue base tumors using surgery is reported as 65% [169]. This is quite comparable to primary radiotherapy [172].

Due to significant morbidity of surgery in most tumors, primary radiotherapy has become the method of choice in most cases. A combination of external beam radiation and brachytherapy has been an effective treatment both in maintaining function and offering comparable survival to other methods [173]. In general, more advanced tumors are treated with radiation to primary sites, neck nodes including retropharyngeal nodes, and in case of positive nodes, planned neck dissection after radiotherapy. Adding chemotherapy to radiation has shown an added benefit in local control and survival. The most effective method consists of concurrent chemotherapy and the most effective agents are platinum based chemotherapeutics [3, 174]. Primary surgical therapy is not used as often nowadays to treat advanced tumors. Treatment usually requires mandibulotomy to gain access and may involve total glossectomy, supraglottic, or even total laryngectomy and the need for free flap tissue transfer. Neck dissection is performed at the time of resection almost routinely. A significant number of patients will require adjuvant radiation to cervical lymph node beds. As it is apparent from the extent of surgery, functional consequences are quite devastating and patients will have significant difficulty in speech and swallowing. It has to be noted also that primary radiation and chemotherapy is not without complication and a number of patients will be afflicted with xerostomia, loss of taste, temporary and permanent dysphagia, pharyngeal or esophageal stenosis, osteoradionecrosis, and radiation induced malignancies. These issues show clearly the burden of this disease and its treatments on patients and the practitioners. The most recent data shows disease specific survival of 65%, 54%, 44%, and 30% for stages I–IV respectively [175].

Management of Mandible

Management of the mandible is necessary in a few scenarios. The mandible can be directly involved with the tumor, or it may limit the access to the tumor. Because of these issues, a comprehensive and careful pretreatment evaluation of the mandible is necessary in all oral cavity and oropharynx tumors. Careful physical exam remains one of the best

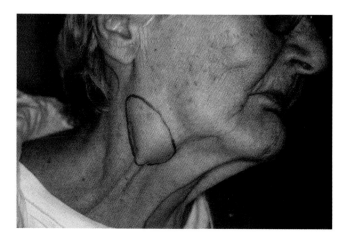

Figure 45.9 Right neck mass. Primary tumor was asymptomatic base of tongue cancer that was found during exam under anesthesia in an otherwise asymptomatic elderly woman.

Figure 45.10 Various types of marginal mandibulectomies: vertical, horizontal, and oblique cuts (Reprinted with permission from Shaha AR (1992) Marginal mandibulectomy for carcinoma of the floor of the mouth. J Surg Oncol 49:116–119).

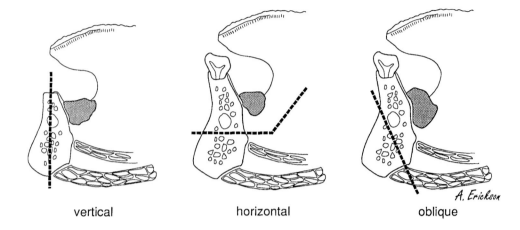

vertical   horizontal   oblique

methods for assessment of mandibular involvement [176]. A Panorex view of the mandible, although not accurate in determining the extent of disease, is still helpful in delineating the extent of resection and surgical planning. In recent years tremendous improvements in CT and MRI imaging techniques have been made. There is still controversy as to which modality is the best. In general, CT is quite specific, but might miss subtle invasions (false negative). MRI on the other hand, is very sensitive, but will overstate mandibular invasion. One strategy is to obtain the MRI first and if there is no evidence of invasion, the practitioner can be reassured the possibility is quite low. If there is still doubt, it might be necessary to proceed with CT scanning. On the other hand, most surgeons will obtain the CT as first modality because of its easy interpretation, great bone details, and lower cost. This is an ongoing debate and cases should be decided on their own specific characteristics [177]. The CT interpretation for the mandible may be difficult due to artifacts from dental fillings. Dentascan is another great technique for mandible evaluation. PET/CT in recent years has been commonly utilized. Its role in finding mandibular invasion has not yet been well determined. SPECT imaging is used in some centers, mostly in Europe as an accurate modality to find mandibular invasion [178]. This modality is not being commonly used in the US.

The mode of tumor spread to the mandible has been studied extensively and our understanding of this process has evolved through the years. It was first believed that tumors spread to cervical lymph nodes through the lymphatic channels that perforate the periosteum and bony structure of mandible. Nowadays we know that tumors invade the mandible directly. There are two patterns, erosive and infiltrative. The infiltrative pattern happens in more advanced cases and has a much worse prognosis. Tumors travel in the mucosa and submucosa until they reach the periosteum. In dentate patients tumor cells migrate through dental sockets into the mandible. In edentulous patients tumors enter the mandible by moving to the occlusal surface first and then through the dental pits [179].

There is always debate regarding the extent of mandibulectomy. Traditionally, most bony invasions were treated by segmental mandibulectomy. Many studies have shown that as long as negative margins are acquired, marginal mandibulectomy is as effective as segmental mandibulectomy [179–182]. Marginal mandibulectomy can be achieved via a horizontal, vertical, or oblique cut (Fig. 45.10). The oblique cut has a few advantages. Retention of a strong mandible remnant and better tumor clearance are among those. The defect can usually be closed by advancement of adjacent mucosa or split thickness skin graft if necessary. Very small defects can be left open to heal by secondary intention or use of Alloderm and larger defects might need a free tissue transfer flap for optimal functional results.

If obtaining negative margins necessitates segmental mandibulectomy, the defect is routinely filled with bone containing a free tissue transfer. The most commonly used donor sites are the fibula, iliac crest, and scapula. These microvascular flaps tolerate radiotherapy quite well and cosmetic and functional results are quite good [183]. There is also possibility of dental implants after completion of therapy. Fibula free flap is the most commonly used technique and osseointegration works very well with the fibula. Many studies have shown similar success rate for free tissue transfer in elderly population. Most important risk factors are medical comorbidities and ASA class of patient [184, 185].

When there is a need to perform mandibulotomy to gain access to tumors of the oral cavity or oropharynx, the preferred sites are midline or paramedian. Lateral mandibulotomy is not recommended since it cuts the mandibular nerve and artery. A paramedian site is better than midline since the inferior alveolar nerve and artery can be preserved, genial muscles can be spared, the osteotomy site can be placed in the natural space between canine and incisor teeth and avoid dental extraction, the osteotomy site is outside the radiation field and finally the segments can be fixed adequately with plates or wires. After the osteotomy is done, a mandibular swing is performed and the mucosa of the floor of the mouth is incised along the medial aspect of the mandible toward the tumor. This approach gives good exposure to parapharyngeal tumors including the deep lobe of the parotid. The cosmetic and functional results are quite good in experienced hands [186]. Segmental mandibulectomy is not recommended solely to gain access.

Osteoradionecrosis is one of the devastating complications of radiotherapy. Treatment is usually difficult, lengthy, and less than satisfactory. Prophylactic measures such as careful dental evaluation and extraction of unhealthy teeth before treatment, fluoride treatment, and regular follow-up during radiotherapy are quite important. Sometimes it is difficult to distinguish between recurrent tumor and osteoradionecrosis. More recently, PET scanning is used as a helpful modality to distinguish between these two [187]. Early limited osteoradionecrosis may respond to debridement, long term antibiotics, extensive oral irrigation, and hyperbaric oxygen. For more extensive cases, surgical excision and immediate reconstruction with free tissue transfer might be the only option [188].

Hypopharynx

Tumors arising from the hypopharynx are rare. The most common subsite is the pyriform sinus followed by the posterior pharyngeal wall and post-cricoid region. These tumors can remain asymptomatic for extended periods of time and the majority are diagnosed in advanced stages. Almost two-thirds of patients already have cervical lymph node involvement at diagnosis. It is also not uncommon for these tumors to metastasize bilaterally, since the hypopharynx has a rich lymphatic plexus. Because of these characteristics, most of these patients will require multimodality treatments. If surgery is used as primary treatment, depending on the extent of disease, there are several options. For early stage, small tumors (T1 and T2), partial pharyngectomy with either primary closure or myocutaneous flap or free flap is possible. Based on size and location of the lesion it might become necessary to perform partial laryngopharyngectomy or supracricoid hemilaryngectomy. For larger lesions, total laryngopharyngectomy is used. If the tumor has spread to the cervical esophagus, total laryngopharyngoesophagectomy is performed. Reconstruction of such defects is achieved by free jejunal flap in laryngopharyngectomy and gastric pull-up and pharyngogastrostomy in laryngopharyngoesophagectomy cases. In all surgical methods, neck dissection is performed from level II to IV. Many patients will still require adjuvant radiotherapy, which will improve locoregional control and survival. Because of obvious morbidity of surgical treatments, it is quite common to treat these tumors primarily by radiotherapy or chemoradiotherapy. The results of these approaches are not as good as radiotherapy for laryngeal cancers [189, 190]. Surgery with postoperative radiation offers similar locoregional control and survival rates to definitive chemoradiation; however, the rate of larynx preservation is higher in the chemoradiation group. Unfortunately the retained organ is not always functional and a significant number of patients will suffer from dysphagia and laryngeal dysfunction [190]. The overall prognosis for hypopharyngeal tumors is quite poor. The 5-year survival for N0–N1 disease is around 28–57% and for N2–N3 disease is 0–20%. These numbers are similar between different treatment modalities. Hypopharynx cancers remain a challenging topic for head and neck cancer practitioners and these patients should be considered for clinical trials of new modalities if possible.

Larynx

Laryngeal cancers are divided into three groups. Most common are glottic (51%), followed by supraglottic (32%), and subglottic (2%). The remainder of cases are either overlapping the two regions of the larynx (4%), or arise from the epiglottis (1%), or laryngeal cartilage (1%) [191].

In recent years significant improvements and changes have occurred in the management of laryngeal cancers due to seminal studies and introduction of new surgical techniques. In general, laryngeal cancer is divided into early and advanced stage for management purposes. In early laryngeal cancer, the emphasis is on using one modality and preserving maximal function without jeopardizing the oncologic principles of treatment. In advanced cases, multimodality treatment is used and the patient is given the best chance of preserving function and long term survival by a combination of chemotherapy, radiation, and surgery.

Glottic cancer has the best chance of being detected early. Lesions in this region become symptomatic at an early stage (hoarseness). This feature, combined with the fact that vocal cords have sparse lymphatic plexus and lymph node spread is not common, gives this group the best prognosis. Surgery and radiation are equally effective in treating T1 and T2 glottic tumors. Surgical treatments include endoscopic CO_2 laser excision in small tumors, and partial laryngectomy or hemilaryngectomy in larger lesions. The voice quality and cure rates after these procedures are excellent. Using transoral excision the 5-year local control rate is in range of 83–93% for T1 lesions and 73–89% for T2 lesions. These favorable results translate into disease specific survival rates of 96–99% for T1 lesions and 83–97% for T2 lesions [192]. Voice quality is best with endoscopic laser excision. Definitive radiotherapy is equally effective in treating early glottic cancer. There is no need to radiate the lymphatic basins of the neck since the incidence of lymph node metastases is extremely low. The voice quality is better than partial laryngectomy procedures. The results are extremely good. Five-year regional control is 85–94% for T1 and 68–80% for T2 lesions. Disease specific survival again is in the range of 93–98% for T1 lesions and 70–88% for T2 lesions. In cases of radiation failure, salvage surgery with either partial or total laryngectomy is successful 60–97% of the time [193, 194]. It is important to pay careful attention to anatomic details of the tumor before choosing one modality over another. The most suitable tumors are the ones in the middle third of the vocal cords. Hypomobility of cords, suspicion of deeper involvement, and involvement of the anterior commissure are considered adverse factors for primary radiation therapy. Some histologic types are also relatively resistant to radiation (verrucous, adenocarcinoma, and sarcoma) and therefore should be treated surgically.

Early supraglottic cancers on the other hand have an increased risk of lymphatic spread and cervical lymph nodes are routinely addressed at the time of treatment of the primary tumor. The tendency is to use one modality to treat both primary sites and lymphatic basins. Definitive radiotherapy can be used to treat early supraglottic cancer. Different series have reported excellent success rates of 80–100% in T1 lesions and 70–85% for T2 lesions [195, 196]. The best results are achieved in small superficial tumors. Primary surgical treatment is also quite effective in treating early supraglottic cancer. Transoral laser excision is used with excellent results (90–95% for T1 and 70–80% for T2 lesions) [197, 198]. Elderly patients tolerate this procedure quite well and the incidence of complications is not higher than general population [199]. This modality can be used in conjunction with neck dissection or postoperative adjuvant radiotherapy [200]. In one series, use of adjuvant radiotherapy in T2 lesions resulted in 97% control of the primary site [198]. Another mode of surgical treatment is open partial laryngectomy. This modality has been studied extensively and the results are consistently good [195]. In this procedure the entire supraglottic unit including the epiglottis and the aryepiglottic folds down to the false vocal cords with the overlying thyroid cartilage and the intervening preepiglottic space are removed. Similar to transoral excision, it is important to address lymphatics by bilateral neck dissection from levels II to IV. The quality of voice is quite good. Not all patients are good candidates for this procedure though, since there is a risk of postoperative aspiration and swallowing problems. Unfortunately incidence of aspiration is higher in older patients and this fact makes selection of suitable patients more complicated [201]. Early subglottic cancer is seen extremely rarely and there is not much evidence in outcomes of treatment.

Advanced laryngeal cancer is one of the areas of head and neck cancer that has undergone revolutionary changes in management. Traditionally, advanced tumors (T3 and T4) were treated by total laryngectomy and adjuvant radiation.

Tumors with evidence of cartilage involvement are not good candidates for definitive radiation therapy since the recurrence rate is quite high. In 1991, a study by the Department of Veterans Affairs compared induction chemotherapy with 5-fluorouracil and cisplatinum, and radiation to surgery and adjuvant radiation in previously untreated stage III and IV laryngeal cancer [202]. In this study two-thirds of patients responded well to chemotherapy and larynges were preserved. Survival was similar to the laryngectomy and radiation group. Later on, another study showed that concurrent chemotherapy is better than induction chemotherapy in larynx preservation (88% vs. 75%) and locoregional control (78% vs. 61%); however, there was no difference in survival and concurrent chemotherapy had more toxicity [203]. On the basis of these studies, it is a common practice now to treat advanced laryngeal cancer with concurrent chemoradiation. A few notes of caution should be considered before adopting organ preservation protocols. These protocols are not as effective in treating T4 tumors. Toxicity is quite high and in most cases they offer only modest survival advantage (4–6% only in concurrent protocols) [3]. Concurrent chemotherapy is also not as effective in older patients [3]. Detecting recurrent tumors in cases of chemoradiotherapy can be difficult since there are radiation changes that can mimic recurrence. The most commonly used modality is PET scanning and the results are encouraging. The sensitivity of FDG-PET is 84–100% and specificity is 61–93% for detecting recurrent cancer [204]. Salvage total laryngectomy and adjuvant radiation is used to treat organ preservation failures. In general up to 40% of patients in organ preservation protocols eventually require salvage surgery. Surgery is technically more difficult and the rate of complications in this setting is quite high (30–60% for wound problems and pharyngocutaneous fistulas). The 5-year survival is usually around 35% after salvage surgery [205–208]. A pectoralis muscle flap may be used to buttress the suture line.

Recurrent and Metastatic Cancer

A significant number of patients with locally advanced head and neck cancer will develop locoregional or distant relapses (Fig. 45.11). This usually occurs in first 2 years after treatment. Salvage surgery is an option for those who have resectable locoregional disease [208]. Resection of a recurrent tumor should encompass the entire initial extent of the primary tumor rather than the localized recurrent nidus. Recurrent tumors in the skull base or the ones invading prevertebral fascia or adhere to vertebral bodies are usually considered non-resectable. Re-irradiation with or without chemotherapy has also been investigated [209] and has shown

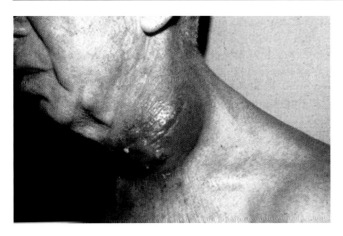

Figure 45.11 Advanced recurrent metastatic cancer in the neck after primary treatment. Note extensive involvement of skin.

better results than observation after salvage surgery. By far the most common method of treatment is chemotherapy, however. The goal is to extend survival and provide symptom palliation. Many agents such as methotrexate, bleomycin, carboplatin, and fluorouracil have been used as single agents in recurrent and metastatic disease [210]. Most trials are small and gains are modest. Two drug combinations improve response rates, but there is no gain in survival [210]. Fluorouracil plus cisplatin is the most commonly used combination. Taxanes plus cisplatin also shows equal results in recurrent cases but not superior to fluorouracil plus cisplatin [211]. Currently there is no standard second-line regimen for recurrent head and neck cancer. Addition of cetuximab to cisplatin and fluorouracil has shown promise [212]. Cetuximab has been also effective in platinum resistant tumors [213]. Gefitinib (EGFR-tyrosin kinase inhibitor) has also been used in clinical trials, but did not show any survival benefit over intravenous methotrexate [214].

Salivary Gland Tumors

The salivary glands are divided into major and minor. Major glands are the parotid, submandibular, and sublingual. Minor salivary glands are distributed throughout the mucosa of the upper aerodigestive tract. The highest concentration is in the hard and soft palate [215]. The majority of parotid tumors are benign (75%), while almost half of other submandibular salivary gland tumors are malignant. In contrast, a majority of minor salivary gland tumors are malignant (80%) [215]. Salivary gland tumors are relatively rare and there is no specific consideration in management of elderly patients. The general principles of treatments are the same in this population.

Patients with malignant tumors or tumors of minor salivary gland tend to be slightly older than patients with benign tumors or those of parotid gland [216].

The parotid gland is the largest major salivary gland. It is also the most common site of salivary gland tumors (65% of all salivary gland tumors). The gland is between the dermis laterally and the masseter muscle and sternocleidomastoid muscle medially. The lateral parapharyngeal space is medial to the parotid gland. The facial nerve divides the gland into two artificial lobes. The bulk of the gland is superficial to the nerve and most tumors arise from this portion. Thorough knowledge of facial nerve anatomy and its course is crucial to successful parotid surgery. The facial nerve exits the skull through the stylomastoid foramen and passes lateral to the styloid process. The main trunk lies at the junction of three anatomic structures: the posterior belly of digastric muscle, the bony auditory canal, and the tip of mastoid process. The nerve then enters the parotid gland and divides into the upper zygomaticotemporal and lower cervicomandibular divisions. By the time the nerve exits the gland it has been divided into five branches: temporal, zygomaticoorbital, buccal, mandibular, and cervical. Two branches are of critical functional importance – the orbital branch innervating the eyelid, and the mandibular branch innervating the lip. Injury to these two branches causes considerable cosmetic and functional disability. The parotid duct (Stensen) exits the gland anteriorly over the masseter muscle and then pierces the buccinator muscle to enter the oral cavity opposite the second maxillary molar on the buccal mucosa.

The submandibular gland is the second largest major salivary gland. It lies in the submandibular triangle on the hyoglossus muscle. Each gland is divided into two lobes by the posterior edge of the mylohyoid muscle. Wharton's duct runs from the deeper portion of the gland anteriorly under the mylohyoid muscle and drains into the floor of the mouth just lateral to the frenulum of the tongue. Three nerves are in proximity to the submandibular glands: lingual, hypoglossal, and ramus mandibularis. It is important to pay close attention to function of these nerves in the management of submandibular tumors.

Sublingual glands are the smallest of the three. They are located under the mucosa of the floor of the mouth above the mylohyoid muscle. The borders are the mandible laterally, the genioglossus medially, and the submandibular gland posteriorly. There are many minor sublingual ducts that open into the oral cavity (ducts of Rivinus). Some of these ducts join each other to form the major ducts of Bartholin. The ducts of Bartholin join the submandibular duct. The lingual nerve comes down laterally to the anterior end of the sublingual gland and runs along its inferior border. It then runs parallel to the submandibular duct until ascending into the tongue.

Diagnostic Work-up

A physical examination can give valuable information on most major salivary gland tumors, especially in the parotid. A hard fixed mass in the parotid gland is always suspicious for malignancy. Paresis or paralysis of the facial nerve is almost always an indicator of malignancy since benign processes do not easily cause paralysis even when they become quite large.

The most commonly used imaging modalities are CT scan and MRI. CT scan is available and quicker to perform. It is better in delineating bone destruction and invasion. MRI in general is superior to CT. It provides better anatomical detail and superior soft tissue differentiation. MRI is particularly helpful in deep lobe parotid tumors, minor salivary gland tumors, and vascular and neurogenic tumors [217]. PET scanning is usually not used in initial evaluation of salivary gland tumors.

FNA of salivary gland tumors can be quite helpful. Overall sensitivity of FNA ranges from 85 to 99% and the overall specificity is from 96 to 100% [46, 218–220]. FNA is more accurate for benign lesions than malignant ones. It is also very good in distinguishing between salivary and non salivary processes (lymphoma). Occasionally, a benign lesion such as mixed tumor can be interpreted as adenoid cystic carcinoma. Usefulness of FNA is highly dependent on the experience of cytopathologist. In general, FNA is a simple, easy to perform technique that can provide valuable information to better manage the lesion. FNA results can change the management of major salivary gland tumors in almost 35% of cases [221].

Staging of major salivary gland tumors is described in Tables 45.6, 45.7, 45.9, and 45.10. Minor salivary gland tumors are staged similar to squamous cell carcinomas.

Benign Tumors

Most benign tumors occur in the parotid gland. The most common are mixed tumor followed by Whartin's tumors. Oncocytoma, benign lymphoepithelial, and myoepithelial lesions are rarely seen. Almost 80% of parotid tumors are benign mixed tumors. These are called mixed since they show morphologic diversity with epithelial and connective tissue components such as myxoid, chondroid, and fibroid. They grow slowly in general, but occasionally rapid growth is observed in some patients with longstanding tumors. This might be due to development of carcinoma in a benign mixed tumor (carcinoma ex-pleomorphic adenoma). This situation can occur in 1–7% of cases [222]. The majority of these tumors are located in the superficial lobe of the parotid gland. They can also occur in minor salivary glands of the palate and upper lip. Many other sites have also been reported as origins of mixed tumors (buccal mucosa, base of tongue, parapharyngeal space, and nasal cavity). Pleomorphic adenoma is also the most common benign tumor of the lacrimal gland.

The most appropriate treatment is superficial parotidectomy with preservation of the facial nerve. In cases of deep lobe tumors, facial nerve function can be preserved and surgery usually involves enucleation of the tumor. On occasion, a very large deep lobe tumor might require a lower lip split incision and mandibulotomy for access. The principle is to remove the tumor with negative margins to avoid recurrence. Tumors that are enucleated or incompletely removed are at risk for recurrence. Any mass in the parotid area should be considered a parotid tumor and adequate treatment consisting of superficial parotidectomy and facial nerve identification and preservation should be performed.

Papillary cystadenoma lymphomatosum or Whartin's tumor is the second most common benign salivary gland tumor and consists of 10–15% of parotid tumors. These tumors are found exclusively in the parotid gland and are believed to originate from periparotid or intra parotid lymph nodes. Whartin's tumors are more common in men and are associated with cigarette smoking. Bilateral tumors can occur in 10% of cases. The risk of malignant transformation is extremely low. FNA is quite accurate in diagnosing Whartin's tumors. Treatment is superficial parotidectomy with facial nerve preservation.

Oncocytomas are rare tumors of the parotid gland (1%). They are fleshy, slow growing tumors. In the parotid they are usually well circumscribed and encapsulated but not in minor salivary glands. These tumors can show high uptake of technetium-99m and will be enhanced in radionuclide scans. Surgical excision with negative margins is the treatment of choice. Oncocytomas are resistant to radiation.

Myoepitheliomas are quite rare (less than 1%). They can occur in major and minor salivary glands. The tumor consists of myoepithelial cells exclusively. Sometimes it is difficult to distinguish myoepitheliomas from mixed tumors clinically since they present a slow growing painless mass. They should be differentiated from plasmacytomas and other tumors with spindle cells (neurilemoma, fibroma, meningioma, and leiomyoma). They usually occur in the third to sixth decade of life and there is no gender predilection. Treatment is surgical excision.

Malignant Salivary Tumors

Malignant salivary tumors are rare. They consist of 6% of head and neck cancers and 13% of salivary gland tumors. The most common type is mucoepidermoid carcinoma followed by adenoid cystic carcinoma and adenocarcinoma.

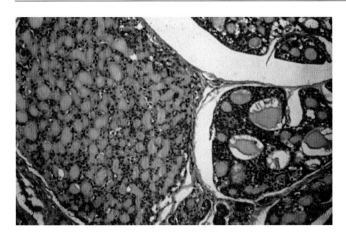

FIGURE 45.12 Hematoxylin-Eosin staining of adenoid cystic carcinoma. This slide shows cribriform pattern of tumor that is associated with lower grade and better prognosis.

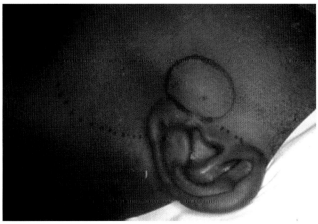

FIGURE 45.13 Large left parotid tumor. The marking shows the incision for standard superficial parotidectomy (modified Blair's incision).

Mucoepidermoid carcinomas originate in the salivary duct epithelium and comprise 44% of parotid malignancies. They are classified as low, intermediate, and high grade histologically. Low grade tumors act more like benign mixed tumors with slow growth, low recurrence rates, and rare distant metastases. Superficial parotidectomy with preservation of the facial nerve is the adequate treatment and 5-year survival is as good as 95% [223]. High grade tumors on the other hand show local invasion, facial nerve involvement, and lymph node metastases as high as 50% at presentation. The prognosis for this group is dismal [223].

Adenoid cystic carcinoma constitutes the most common malignancy of the minor salivary gland and submandibular gland and 10–15% of malignant parotid tumors. They show three distinct histologic patterns: cribriform, tubular, and solid. Cribriform pattern has the best prognosis and solid, the worst (Fig. 45.12). Adenoid cystic carcinoma can show unpredictable behavior. It is usually characterized by slow growth, neurotropism, local recurrence, and distant metastases. Cervical metastases are infrequent, but late distant metastases are common [216]. Treatment is surgical excision and postoperative radiation. Cervical lymph node dissection is usually not performed.

The malignant mixed tumor is a category consisting of carcinoma ex-pleomorphic adenoma, carcinosarcoma, and metastasizing mixed tumor. These are similar but distinct malignancies. The malignant mixed tumor category accounts for 5–12% of salivary gland malignancies. Carcinoma ex-pleomorphic adenoma is a carcinoma arising from a longstanding benign mixed tumor. True malignant mixed tumors show elements of carcinoma and sarcoma simultaneously. They are usually grouped with carcinoma ex-pleomorphic adenomas. Metastasizing mixed tumors are characterized by primary tumor and metastases that appear completely benign under the microscope. Cervical metastases are present in 15% of this category at presentation. Treatment is surgical excision including cervical lymphadenectomy and postoperative radiation.

Treatment of Salivary Tumors

Surgery

Surgical excision is the mainstay of treatment for malignant and benign salivary tumors. The minimal operation for parotid lesions is superficial parotidectomy with identification and preservation of the facial nerve (Fig. 45.13). Enucleation is not recommended uniformly. Most tumors of the superficial parotid can be addressed with this modality. Deep lobe tumors are more challenging. Total parotidectomy might be necessary to remove the tumor in its entirety. Every effort should be made to preserve a functioning facial nerve. Most of the time with careful dissection, a deep lobe parotid tumor can be removed without injury to the facial nerve branches. If the bulk of the tumor is in the parapharyngeal space and adjacent to the pharyngeal wall, a mandibulotomy approach might be a more suitable choice for exposure and excision of the mass. If the nerve is adherent to the tumor but functional, it can be peeled off carefully. In these cases, postoperative radiotherapy is indicated. If the nerve has already been invaded or paralyzed, or in rare cases a functioning nerve has to be sacrificed, immediate nerve grafting using cable interposition grafts from the greater auricular nerve, or cervical plexus, or sural nerve should be attempted. In order to protect eye function and closure, a gold weight can be implanted in cases of nerve sacrifice or paralysis due to tumor invasion.

Excision of submandibular gland tumors requires removal of the entire contents of the submandibular triangle. This becomes complicated due to the presence of three important nerves in this area, the ramus mandibularis, hypoglossal, and lingual nerves. If the tumor is close or attached to mandible, removal of the periosteum or even a segment of mandible is necessary. As part of the procedure, supraomohyoid neck dissection might be performed.

Minor salivary gland tumors are treated by wide local excision. This might require full thickness excision or infrastructure partial maxillectomy in hard palate tumors. The resultant defect should be covered with a dental obturator.

Palpable nodes at presentation should be addressed with modified or radical neck dissection. Elective neck dissection from level I to III is recommended for tumors >4 cm, high grade mucoepidermoid carcinoma, squamous cell carcinoma, adenocarcinoma, and undifferentiated carcinoma. For other patients if a transcervical approach is used, elective neck dissection should be included. If suspicious lymph nodes are encountered at the time of surgery, it is recommended that a comprehensive neck dissection be performed.

Radiation

Radiation is being used frequently nowadays in treatment of salivary gland tumors. It improves locoregional control and overall survival [224]. Indications for postoperative radiotherapy include advanced inoperable cancer, high-grade, high-stage primary tumor, positive margins, deep lobe malignant tumors, lymph node metastases, and tumor spillage at the time of surgery. Also in high-stage adenoid cystic carcinomas, due to the high recurrence rate, postoperative radiotherapy is recommended. Neutron therapy has shown improved locoregional control in adenoid cystic carcinoma in comparison to traditional photon irradiation (56% vs. 17%). It also improved 5-year survival for patients with adenoid cystic carcinoma and acinic cell carcinoma. However, 5% of patients experienced severe toxicity [225]. Neutron therapy is available only in a few centers in the US and is generally used for inoperable salivary tumors.

Chemotherapy

There is scant experience with chemotherapy in the treatment of salivary gland tumors. Fluorouracil, cisplatin, doxorubicin, and cyclophosphamide have been used in few patients [226]. The initial response is usually around 50%, but only lasts for 7–10 months [227]. In patients with complete response, survival was >19 months [228]. Overall success of chemotherapy has been disappointing. Concomitant use of radiation and chemotherapy might show some improvement in survival over radiation alone [229]. Immunotherapy with EGFR blockers might also become an option for treating salivary gland tumors [230].

Prognosis

Tumor stage is the most important prognostic factor [216, 231]. The overall 10-year survival rates for stages I–III are approximately 90%, 65%, and 22%. Grade is also important. Low grade tumors have 10 year survival as high as 90%, while high grade tumors survival rates are only around 25%. Adenocarcinoma, malignant mixed tumor, adenoid cystic, and squamous cell carcinomas have worse prognosis than acinic or low grade mucoepidermoid tumors. Submandibular and minor salivary gland tumors are more aggressive than parotid tumors in general. Gross nerve involvement, and bone and skin invasion have also been implicated as adverse prognostic factors [231, 232].

Follow-up of Head and Neck Cancer Patients

Patients treated for head and neck cancer need close and regular follow-up. The standard regimen consists of visits every 6–8 weeks in the first year followed by 2–3 month visits in the second year, 3–4 month visits in the third year, and biannual or annual visits thereafter for life. The extent of investigation in each visit is a matter of debate. Each patient should be evaluated individually with a program tailored to his or her particular needs. Some patients with deep tumors might require CT scanning while others will be adequately followed by physical exam. Chest radiographs are usually adequate to monitor for pulmonary metastases. The radiographs should be interpreted carefully and compared to previous studies. Routine endoscopy of the aerodigestive tract is not of proven value and should be performed in select cases or when symptoms suggesting problems in the lungs or esophagus arise. Patients treated with an organ preservation approach by chemoradiotherapy are best followed with careful physical examination along with PET scan. PET scan and specially PET CT is being used more often as a sensitive tool for follow up of patients [204]. Negative results are usually quite reassuring; however, positive changes have to be interpreted carefully to rule out other causes such as inflammation or infection.

References

1. Jemal A, Siegel R, Ward E, Hao Y, Xu J, Murray T et al (2008) Cancer statistics, 2008. CA Cancer J Clin 58(2):71–96
2. Kusaba R, Sakamoto K, Mori K, Umeno T, Nakashima T (2001) Laboratory data and treatment outcomes of head and neck tumor patients in the elderly. Auris Nasus Larynx 28(2):161–168

3. Pignon JP, le Maitre A, Maillard E, Bourhis J (2009) Meta-analysis of chemotherapy in head and neck cancer (MACH-NC): an update on 93 randomised trials and 17,346 patients. Radiother Oncol 92(1):4–14

4. Robbins KT, Clayman G, Levine PA, Medina J, Sessions R, Shaha A et al (2002) Neck dissection classification update: revisions proposed by the American Head and Neck Society and the American Academy of Otolaryngology-Head and Neck Surgery. Arch Otolaryngol Head Neck Surg 128(7):751–758

5. Robbins KT, Shaha AR, Medina JE, Califano JA, Wolf GT, Ferlito A et al (2008) Consensus statement on the classification and terminology of neck dissection. Arch Otolaryngol Head Neck Surg 134(5):536–538

6. Nahum AM, Mullally W, Marmor L (1961) A syndrome resulting from radical neck dissection. Arch Otolaryngol 74:424–428

7. Parkin DM, Bray F, Ferlay J, Pisani P (2005) Global cancer statistics, 2002. CA Cancer J Clin 55(2):74–108

8. Curado MP, Hashibe M (2009) Recent changes in the epidemiology of head and neck cancer. Curr Opin Oncol 21(3):194–200

9. Kingsley K, O'Malley S, Ditmyer M, Chino M (2008) Analysis of oral cancer epidemiology in the US reveals state-specific trends: implications for oral cancer prevention. BMC Public Health 8:87

10. Parkin DM, Whelan SL, Ferlay J, Storm H (2005) Cancer incidence in five continents. IARC CancerBase, IARC, Lyon France

11. Hayat MJ, Howlader N, Reichman ME, Edwards BK (2007) Cancer statistics, trends, and multiple primary cancer analyses from the Surveillance, Epidemiology, and End Results (SEER) Program. Oncologist 12(1):20–37

12. Gandini S, Botteri E, Iodice S, Boniol M, Lowenfels AB, Maisonneuve P et al (2008) Tobacco smoking and cancer: a meta-analysis. Int J Cancer 122(1):155–164

13. Bosetti C, Gallus S, Peto R, Negri E, Talamini R, Tavani A et al (2008) Tobacco smoking, smoking cessation, and cumulative risk of upper aerodigestive tract cancers. Am J Epidemiol 167(4):468–473

14. Sapkota A, Gajalakshmi V, Jetly DH, Roychowdhury S, Dikshit RP, Brennan P et al (2007) Smokeless tobacco and increased risk of hypopharyngeal and laryngeal cancers: a multicentric case-control study from India. Int J Cancer 121(8):1793–1798

15. Lee YC, Boffetta P, Sturgis EM, Wei Q, Zhang ZF, Muscat J et al (2008) Involuntary smoking and head and neck cancer risk: pooled analysis in the International Head and Neck Cancer Epidemiology Consortium. Cancer Epidemiol Biomarkers Prev 17(8):1974–1981

16. Hashibe M, Brennan P, Benhamou S, Castellsague X, Chen C, Curado MP et al (2007) Alcohol drinking in never users of tobacco, cigarette smoking in never drinkers, and the risk of head and neck cancer: pooled analysis in the International Head and Neck Cancer Epidemiology Consortium. J Natl Cancer Inst 99(10):777–789

17. Raab-Traub N (2002) Epstein-Barr virus in the pathogenesis of NPC. Semin Cancer Biol 12(6):431–441

18. Kreimer AR, Clifford GM, Boyle P, Franceschi S (2005) Human papillomavirus types in head and neck squamous cell carcinomas worldwide: a systematic review. Cancer Epidemiol Biomarkers Prev 14(2):467–475

19. Ragin CC, Taioli E (2007) Survival of squamous cell carcinoma of the head and neck in relation to human papillomavirus infection: review and meta-analysis. Int J Cancer 121(8):1813–1820

20. De Stefani E, Boffetta P, Ronco AL, Deneo-Pellegrini H, Acosta G, Mendilaharsu M (2007) Dietary patterns and risk of laryngeal cancer: an exploratory factor analysis in Uruguayan men. Int J Cancer 121(5):1086–1091

21. Freedman ND, Park Y, Subar AF, Hollenbeck AR, Leitzmann MF, Schatzkin A et al (2008) Fruit and vegetable intake and head and neck cancer risk in a large United States prospective cohort study. Int J Cancer 122(10):2330–2336

22. Hiraki A, Matsuo K, Suzuki T, Kawase T, Tajima K (2008) Teeth loss and risk of cancer at 14 common sites in Japanese. Cancer Epidemiol Biomarkers Prev 17(5):1222–1227

23. Conway DI, Petticrew M, Marlborough H, Berthiller J, Hashibe M, Macpherson LM (2008) Socioeconomic inequalities and oral cancer risk: a systematic review and meta-analysis of case-control studies. Int J Cancer 122(12):2811–2819

24. Koch WM, Patel H, Brennan J, Boyle JO, Sidransky D (1995) Squamous cell carcinoma of the head and neck in the elderly. Arch Otolaryngol Head Neck Surg 121(3):262–265

25. Lippman SM, Lee JJ, Karp DD, Vokes EE, Benner SE, Goodman GE et al (2001) Randomized phase III intergroup trial of isotretinoin to prevent second primary tumors in stage I non-small-cell lung cancer. J Natl Cancer Inst 93(8):605–618

26. Khuri FR, Lee JJ, Lippman SM, Kim ES, Cooper JS, Benner SE et al (2006) Randomized phase III trial of low-dose isotretinoin for prevention of second primary tumors in stage I and II head and neck cancer patients. J Natl Cancer Inst 98(7):441–450

27. Joyce JA, Pollard JW (2009) Microenvironmental regulation of metastasis. Nat Rev Cancer 9(4):239–252

28. Shah JP (1990) Patterns of cervical lymph node metastasis from squamous carcinomas of the upper aerodigestive tract. Am J Surg 160(4):405–409

29. Shah JP, Candela FC, Poddar AK (1990) The patterns of cervical lymph node metastases from squamous carcinoma of the oral cavity. Cancer 66(1):109–113

30. Candela FC, Kothari K, Shah JP (1990) Patterns of cervical node metastases from squamous carcinoma of the oropharynx and hypopharynx. Head Neck 12(3):197–203

31. Candela FC, Shah J, Jaques DP, Shah JP (1990) Patterns of cervical node metastases from squamous carcinoma of the larynx. Arch Otolaryngol Head Neck Surg 116(4):432–435

32. Ferlito A, Shaha AR, Silver CE, Rinaldo A, Mondin V (2001) Incidence and sites of distant metastases from head and neck cancer. ORL J Otorhinolaryngol Relat Spec 63(4):202–207

33. Slaughter DP, Southwick HW, Smejkal W (1953) Field cancerization in oral stratified squamous epithelium; clinical implications of multicentric origin. Cancer 6(5):963–968

34. Braakhuis BJ, Tabor MP, Leemans CR, van der Waal I, Snow GB, Brakenhoff RH (2002) Second primary tumors and field cancerization in oral and oropharyngeal cancer: molecular techniques provide new insights and definitions. Head Neck 24(2):198–206

35. Tepperman BS, Fitzpatrick PJ (1981) Second respiratory and upper digestive tract cancers after oral cancer. Lancet 2(8246):547–549

36. Leon X, Quer M, Diez S, Orus C, Lopez Pousa A, Burgues J (1999) Second neoplasm in patients with head and neck cancer. Head Neck 21(3):204–210

37. Boysen M, Loven JO (1993) Second malignant neoplasms in patients with head and neck squamous cell carcinomas. Acta Oncol 32(3):283–288

38. Jones AS, Morar P, Phillips DE, Field JK, Husband D, Helliwell TR (1995) Second primary tumors in patients with head and neck squamous cell carcinoma. Cancer 75(6):1343–1353

39. Rennemo E, Zatterstrom U, Boysen M (2008) Impact of second primary tumors on survival in head and neck cancer: an analysis of 2,063 cases. Laryngoscope 118(8):1350–1356

40. McGurk M, Chan C, Jones J, O'Regan E, Sherriff M (2005) Delay in diagnosis and its effect on outcome in head and neck cancer. Br J Oral Maxillofac Surg 43(4):281–284

41. Teppo H, Alho OP (2008) Relative importance of diagnostic delays in different head and neck cancers. Clin Otolaryngol 33(4):325–330

42. Ng SH, Yen TC, Chang JT, Chan SC, Ko SF, Wang HM et al (2006) Prospective study of [18F]fluorodeoxyglucose positron emission tomography and computed tomography and magnetic

resonance imaging in oral cavity squamous cell carcinoma with palpably negative neck. J Clin Oncol 24(27):4371–4376

43. Branstetter BF IV, Blodgett TM, Zimmer LA, Snyderman CH, Johnson JT, Raman S et al (2005) Head and neck malignancy: is PET/CT more accurate than PET or CT alone? Radiology 235(2):580–586

44. Martin HE, Ellis EB (1930) Biopsy by needle puncture and aspiration. Ann Surg 92(2):169–181

45. Shaha A, Webber C, Marti J (1986) Fine-needle aspiration in the diagnosis of cervical lymphadenopathy. Am J Surg 152(4):420–423

46. Shaha AR, Webber C, DiMaio T, Jaffe BM (1990) Needle aspiration biopsy in salivary gland lesions. Am J Surg 160(4):373–376

47. Califano J, van der Riet P, Westra W, Nawroz H, Clayman G, Piantadosi S et al (1996) Genetic progression model for head and neck cancer: implications for field cancerization. Cancer Res 56(11):2488–2492

48. Ha PK, Califano JA (2006) Promoter methylation and inactivation of tumour-suppressor genes in oral squamous-cell carcinoma. Lancet Oncol 7(1):77–82

49. Perez-Ordonez B, Beauchemin M, Jordan RC (2006) Molecular biology of squamous cell carcinoma of the head and neck. J Clin Pathol 59(5):445–453

50. van der Riet P, Nawroz H, Hruban RH, Corio R, Tokino K, Koch W et al (1994) Frequent loss of chromosome 9p21-22 early in head and neck cancer progression. Cancer Res 54(5):1156–1158

51. Mao L, Lee JS, Fan YH, Ro JY, Batsakis JG, Lippman S et al (1996) Frequent microsatellite alterations at chromosomes 9p21 and 3p14 in oral premalignant lesions and their value in cancer risk assessment. Nat Med 2(6):682–685

52. Garnis C, Baldwin C, Zhang L, Rosin MP, Lam WL (2003) Use of complete coverage array comparative genomic hybridization to define copy number alterations on chromosome 3p in oral squamous cell carcinomas. Cancer Res 63(24):8582–8585

53. Hogg RP, Honorio S, Martinez A, Agathanggelou A, Dallol A, Fullwood P et al (2002) Frequent 3p allele loss and epigenetic inactivation of the RASSF1A tumour suppressor gene from region 3p21.3 in head and neck squamous cell carcinoma. Eur J Cancer 38(12):1585–1592

54. Rowley H, Jones A, Spandidos D, Field J (1996) Definition of a tumor suppressor gene locus on the short arm of chromosome 3 in squamous cell carcinoma of the head and neck by means of microsatellite markers. Arch Otolaryngol Head Neck Surg 122(5):497–501

55. Masayesva BG, Ha P, Garrett-Mayer E, Pilkington T, Mao R, Pevsner J et al (2004) Gene expression alterations over large chromosomal regions in cancers include multiple genes unrelated to malignant progression. Proc Natl Acad Sci USA 101(23):8715–8720

56. Nawroz H, van der Riet P, Hruban RH, Koch W, Ruppert JM, Sidransky D (1994) Allelotype of head and neck squamous cell carcinoma. Cancer Res 54(5):1152–1155

57. van Houten VM, Tabor MP, van den Brekel MW, Kummer JA, Denkers F, Dijkstra J et al (2002) Mutated p53 as a molecular marker for the diagnosis of head and neck cancer. J Pathol 198(4):476–486

58. Rosin MP, Cheng X, Poh C, Lam WL, Huang Y, Lovas J et al (2000) Use of allelic loss to predict malignant risk for low-grade oral epithelial dysplasia. Clin Cancer Res 6(2):357–362

59. Boyle JO, Hakim J, Koch W, van der Riet P, Hruban RH, Roa RA et al (1993) The incidence of p53 mutations increases with progression of head and neck cancer. Cancer Res 53(19):4477–4480

60. Shahnavaz SA, Regezi JA, Bradley G, Dube ID, Jordan RC (2000) p53 gene mutations in sequential oral epithelial dysplasias and squamous cell carcinomas. J Pathol 190(4):417–422

61. Meredith SD, Levine PA, Burns JA, Gaffey MJ, Boyd JC, Weiss LM et al (1995) Chromosome 11q13 amplification in head and neck squamous cell carcinoma. Association with poor prognosis. Arch Otolaryngol Head Neck Surg 121(7):790–794

62. Michalides R, van Veelen N, Hart A, Loftus B, Wientjens E, Balm A (1995) Overexpression of cyclin D1 correlates with recurrence in a group of forty-seven operable squamous cell carcinomas of the head and neck. Cancer Res 55(5):975–978

63. Maruya S, Issa JP, Weber RS, Rosenthal DI, Haviland JC, Lotan R et al (2004) Differential methylation status of tumor-associated genes in head and neck squamous carcinoma: incidence and potential implications. Clin Cancer Res 10(11):3825–3830

64. Poeta ML, Manola J, Goldwasser MA, Forastiere A, Benoit N, Califano JA et al (2007) TP53 mutations and survival in squamous-cell carcinoma of the head and neck. N Engl J Med 357(25):2552–2561

65. Grandis JR, Tweardy DJ (1993) Elevated levels of transforming growth factor alpha and epidermal growth factor receptor messenger RNA are early markers of carcinogenesis in head and neck cancer. Cancer Res 53(15):3579–3584

66. Rubin Grandis J, Melhem MF, Gooding WE, Day R, Holst VA, Wagener MM et al (1998) Levels of TGF-alpha and EGFR protein in head and neck squamous cell carcinoma and patient survival. J Natl Cancer Inst 90(11):824–832

67. Karamouzis MV, Grandis JR, Argiris A (2007) Therapies directed against epidermal growth factor receptor in aerodigestive carcinomas. JAMA 298(1):70–82

68. Ferrara N (2005) VEGF as a therapeutic target in cancer. Oncology 69(Suppl 3):11–16

69. Smith BD, Smith GL, Carter D, Sasaki CT, Haffty BG (2000) Prognostic significance of vascular endothelial growth factor protein levels in oral and oropharyngeal squamous cell carcinoma. J Clin Oncol 18(10):2046–2052

70. Silverman S, American Cancer Society (1990) Oral cancer, 3rd edn. American Cancer Society, Atlantic

71. Silverman S Jr, Gorsky M, Lozada F (1984) Oral leukoplakia and malignant transformation. A follow-up study of 257 patients. Cancer 53(3):563–568

72. Bouquot JE, Gorlin RJ (1986) Leukoplakia, lichen planus, and other oral keratoses in 23, 616 white Americans over the age of 35 years. Oral Surg Oral Med Oral Pathol 61(4):373–381

73. Silverman S Jr, Gorsky M (1997) Proliferative verrucous leukoplakia: a follow-up study of 54 cases. Oral Surg Oral Med Oral Pathol Oral Radiol Endod 84(2):154–157

74. Bouquot JE (1998) Oral verrucous carcinoma. Incidence in two US populations. Oral Surg Oral Med Oral Pathol Oral Radiol Endod 86(3):318–324

75. Ackerman LV (1948) Verrucous carcinoma of the oral cavity. Surgery 23(4):670–678

76. Hansen LS, Olson JA, Silverman S Jr (1985) Proliferative verrucous leukoplakia. A long-term study of thirty patients. Oral Surg Oral Med Oral Pathol 60(3):285–298

77. Banks ER, Frierson HF Jr, Mills SE, George E, Zarbo RJ, Swanson PE (1992) Basaloid squamous cell carcinoma of the head and neck. A clinicopathologic and immunohistochemical study of 40 cases. Am J Surg Pathol 16(10):939–946

78. Huang SH, Hwang D, Lockwood G, Goldstein DP, O'Sullivan B (2009) Predictive value of tumor thickness for cervical lymph-node involvement in squamous cell carcinoma of the oral cavity: a meta-analysis of reported studies. Cancer 115(7):1489–1497

79. Greene FL, American Joint Committee on Cancer, American Cancer Society (2002) AJCC cancer staging manual, 6th edn. Springer, New York

80. Patel SG, Shah JP (2005) TNM staging of cancers of the head and neck: striving for uniformity among diversity. CA Cancer J Clin 55(4):242–258, quiz 61–2, 64

81. Cohen HJ, Feussner JR, Weinberger M, Carnes M, Hamdy RC, Hsieh F et al (2002) A controlled trial of inpatient and outpatient geriatric evaluation and management. N Engl J Med 346(12):905–912

82. Kuo HK, Scandrett KG, Dave J, Mitchell SL (2004) The influence of outpatient comprehensive geriatric assessment on survival: a meta-analysis. Arch Gerontol Geriatr 39(3):245–254

83. Hanna EY, Holsinger C, DeMonte F, Kupferman M (2007) Robotic endoscopic surgery of the skull base: a novel surgical approach. Arch Otolaryngol Head Neck Surg 133(12):1209–1214

84. O'Malley BW Jr, Weinstein GS (2007) Robotic skull base surgery: preclinical investigations to human clinical application. Arch Otolaryngol Head Neck Surg 133(12):1215–1219

85. Weinstein GS, O'Malley BW Jr, Snyder W, Sherman E, Quon H (2007) Transoral robotic surgery: radical tonsillectomy. Arch Otolaryngol Head Neck Surg 133(12):1220–1226

86. Genden EM, Desai S, Sung CK (2009) Transoral robotic surgery for the management of head and neck cancer: a preliminary experience. Head Neck 31(3):283–289

87. Boudreaux BA, Rosenthal EL, Magnuson JS, Newman JR, Desmond RA, Clemons L et al (2009) Robot-assisted surgery for upper aerodigestive tract neoplasms. Arch Otolaryngol Head Neck Surg 135(4):397–401

88. Boruk M, Chernobilsky B, Rosenfeld RM, Har-El G (2005) Age as a prognostic factor for complications of major head and neck surgery. Arch Otolaryngol Head Neck Surg 131(7):605–609

89. Clayman GL, Eicher SA, Sicard MW, Razmpa E, Goepfert H (1998) Surgical outcomes in head and neck cancer patients 80 years of age and older. Head Neck 20(3):216–223

90. McGuirt WF, Davis SP III (1995) Demographic portrayal and outcome analysis of head and neck cancer surgery in the elderly. Arch Otolaryngol Head Neck Surg 121(2):150–154

91. McGuirt WF, Loevy S, McCabe BF, Krause CJ (1977) The risks of major head and neck surgery in the aged population. Laryngoscope 87(8):1378–1382

92. Sanabria A, Carvalho AL, Melo RL, Magrin J, Ikeda MK, Vartanian JG et al (2008) Predictive factors for complications in elderly patients who underwent head and neck oncologic surgery. Head Neck 30(2):170–177

93. Zabrodsky M, Calabrese L, Tosoni A, Ansarin M, Giugliano G, Bruschini R et al (2004) Major surgery in elderly head and neck cancer patients: immediate and long-term surgical results and complication rates. Surg Oncol 13(4):249–255

94. Derks W, De Leeuw JR, Hordijk GJ, Winnubst JA (2003) Elderly patients with head and neck cancer: short-term effects of surgical treatment on quality of life. Clin Otolaryngol Allied Sci 28(5):399–405

95. Shestak KC, Jones NF, Wu W, Johnson JT, Myers EN (1992) Effect of advanced age and medical disease on the outcome of microvascular reconstruction for head and neck defects. Head Neck 14(1):14–18

96. Singh B, Cordeiro PG, Santamaria E, Shaha AR, Pfister DG, Shah JP (1999) Factors associated with complications in microvascular reconstruction of head and neck defects. Plast Reconstr Surg 103(2):403–411

97. Suh JD, Sercarz JA, Abemayor E, Calcaterra TC, Rawnsley JD, Alam D et al (2004) Analysis of outcome and complications in 400 cases of microvascular head and neck reconstruction. Arch Otolaryngol Head Neck Surg 130(8):962–966

98. Laccourreye O, Brasnu D, Perie S, Muscatello L, Menard M, Weinstein G (1998) Supracricoid partial laryngectomies in the elderly: mortality, complications, and functional outcome. Laryngoscope 108(2):237–242

99. Vikram B, Strong EW, Shah JP, Spiro R (1984) Failure at the primary site following multimodality treatment in advanced head and neck cancer. Head Neck Surg 6(3):720–723

100. Shaha AR, Patel SG, Shasha D, Harrison LB (2001) Head and neck cancer. In: Lenhard RE, Osteen RT, Gansler TS, American Cancer Society (eds) Clinical oncology, 1st edn. American Cancer Society, Atlanta, GA, pp 297–329

101. Ding M, Newman F, Raben D (2005) New radiation therapy techniques for the treatment of head and neck cancer. Otolaryngol Clin North Am 38(2):371–395, vii–viii

102. Voynov G, Heron DE, Burton S, Grandis J, Quinn A, Ferris R et al (2006) Frameless stereotactic radiosurgery for recurrent head and neck carcinoma. Technol Cancer Res Treat 5(5):529–535

103. Peters LJ, Goepfert H, Ang KK, Byers RM, Maor MH, Guillamondegui O et al (1993) Evaluation of the dose for postoperative radiation therapy of head and neck cancer: first report of a prospective randomized trial. Int J Radiat Oncol Biol Phys 26(1):3–11

104. Nguyen LN, Ang KK (2002) Radiotherapy for cancer of the head and neck: altered fractionation regimens. Lancet Oncol 3(11):693–701

105. Fu KK, Pajak TF, Trotti A, Jones CU, Spencer SA, Phillips TL, et al (2000) A Radiation Therapy Oncology Group (RTOG) phase III randomized study to compare hyperfractionation and two variants of accelerated fractionation to standard fractionation radiotherapy for head and neck squamous cell carcinomas: first report of RTOG 9003. Int J Radiat Oncol Biol Phys 48(1):7–16

106. Semrau R, Mueller RP, Stuetzer H, Staar S, Schroeder U, Guntinas-Lichius O et al (2006) Efficacy of intensified hyperfractionated and accelerated radiotherapy and concurrent chemotherapy with carboplatin and 5-fluorouracil: updated results of a randomized multicentric trial in advanced head-and-neck cancer. Int J Radiat Oncol Biol Phys 64(5):1308–1316

107. Brizel DM, Albers ME, Fisher SR, Scher RL, Richtsmeier WJ, Hars V et al (1998) Hyperfractionated irradiation with or without concurrent chemotherapy for locally advanced head and neck cancer. N Engl J Med 338(25):1798–1804

108. Jeremic B, Shibamoto Y, Milicic B, Nikolic N, Dagovic A, Aleksandrovic J et al (2000) Hyperfractionated radiation therapy with or without concurrent low-dose daily cisplatin in locally advanced squamous cell carcinoma of the head and neck: a prospective randomized trial. J Clin Oncol 18(7):1458–1464

109. Pignon T, Horiot JC, Van den Bogaert W, Van Glabbeke M, Scalliet P (1996) No age limit for radical radiotherapy in head and neck tumours. Eur J Cancer 32A(12):2075–2081

110. Zachariah B, Balducci L, Venkattaramanabalaji GV, Casey L, Greenberg HM, DelRegato JA (1997) Radiotherapy for cancer patients aged 80 and older: a study of effectiveness and side effects. Int J Radiat Oncol Biol Phys 39(5):1125–1129

111. Schilcher B, Curschmann J (1995) Clinical results of radiotherapy in 140 elderly patients treated at Basel University Hospital between 1980 and 1985. Int J Radiat Oncol Biol Phys 33(3):774

112. Lusinchi A, Bourhis J, Wibault P, Le Ridant AM, Eschwege F (1990) Radiation therapy for head and neck cancers in the elderly. Int J Radiat Oncol Biol Phys 18(4):819–823

113. Huguenin P, Sauer M, Glanzmann C, Lutolf UM (1996) Radiotherapy for carcinomas of the head and neck in elderly patients. Strahlenther Onkol 172(9):485–488

114. Oguchi M, Ikeda H, Watanabe T, Shikama N, Ohata T, Okazaki Y et al (1998) Experiences of 23 patients > or = 90 years of age treated with radiation therapy. Int J Radiat Oncol Biol Phys 41(2):407–413

115. Bourhis J, Overgaard J, Audry H, Ang KK, Saunders M, Bernier J et al (2006) Hyperfractionated or accelerated radiotherapy in head and neck cancer: a meta-analysis. Lancet 368(9538):843–854

116. Geinitz H, Zimmermann FB, Molls M (1999) Radiotherapy of the elderly patient. Radiotherapy tolerance and results in older patients. Strahlenther Onkol 175(3):119–127

117. Bonner JA, Harari PM, Giralt J, Azarnia N, Shin DM, Cohen RB et al (2006) Radiotherapy plus cetuximab for squamous-cell carcinoma of the head and neck. N Engl J Med 354(6):567–578

118. Duvvuri U, Simental AA Jr, D'Angelo G, Johnson JT, Ferris RL, Gooding W et al (2004) Elective neck dissection and survival in

patients with squamous cell carcinoma of the oral cavity and oropharynx. Laryngoscope 114(12):2228–2234

119. Dey P, Arnold D, Wight R, MacKenzie K, Kelly C, Wilson J (2002) Radiotherapy versus open surgery versus endolaryngeal surgery (with or without laser) for early laryngeal squamous cell cancer. Cochrane Database Syst Rev (2):CD002027

120. Jones AS, Fish B, Fenton JE, Husband DJ (2004) The treatment of early laryngeal cancers (T1-T2 N0): surgery or irradiation? Head Neck 26(2):127–135

121. Mendenhall WM, Werning JW, Hinerman RW, Amdur RJ, Villaret DB (2004) Management of T1-T2 glottic carcinomas. Cancer 100(9):1786–1792

122. Mendenhall WM, Morris CG, Amdur RJ, Hinerman RW, Malyapa RS, Werning JW et al (2006) Definitive radiotherapy for tonsillar squamous cell carcinoma. Am J Clin Oncol 29(3):290–297

123. Nakamura K, Shioyama Y, Kawashima M, Saito Y, Nakamura N, Nakata K et al (2006) Multi-institutional analysis of early squamous cell carcinoma of the hypopharynx treated with radical radiotherapy. Int J Radiat Oncol Biol Phys 65(4): 1045–1050

124. Pignon JP, Bourhis J, Domenge C, Designe L (2000) Chemotherapy added to locoregional treatment for head and neck squamous-cell carcinoma: three meta-analyses of updated individual data. MACH-NC Collaborative Group. Meta-Analysis of Chemotherapy on Head and Neck Cancer. Lancet 355(9208):949–955

125. Pignon JP, le Maitre A, Bourhis J (2007) Meta-Analyses of Chemotherapy in Head and Neck Cancer (MACH-NC): an update. Int J Radiat Oncol Biol Phys 69(2 Suppl):S112–S114

126. Bernier J, Cooper JS, Pajak TF, van Glabbeke M, Bourhis J, Forastiere A et al (2005) Defining risk levels in locally advanced head and neck cancers: a comparative analysis of concurrent post-operative radiation plus chemotherapy trials of the EORTC (#22931) and RTOG (# 9501). Head Neck 27(10):843–850

127. Argiris A (2005) Induction chemotherapy for head and neck cancer: will history repeat itself? J Natl Compr Canc Netw 3(3):393–403

128. Hitt R, Lopez-Pousa A, Martinez-Trufero J, Escrig V, Carles J, Rizo A et al (2005) Phase III study comparing cisplatin plus fluorouracil to paclitaxel, cisplatin, and fluorouracil induction chemotherapy followed by chemoradiotherapy in locally advanced head and neck cancer. J Clin Oncol 23(34):8636–8645

129. Posner MR, Hershock DM, Blajman CR, Mickiewicz E, Winquist E, Gorbounova V et al (2007) Cisplatin and fluorouracil alone or with docetaxel in head and neck cancer. N Engl J Med 357(17):1705–1715

130. Pointreau Y, Garaud P, Chapet S, Sire C, Tuchais C, Tortochaux J et al (2009) Randomized trial of induction chemotherapy with cisplatin and 5-fluorouracil with or without docetaxel for larynx preservation. J Natl Cancer Inst 101(7):498–506

131. Argiris A, Li Y, Murphy BA, Langer CJ, Forastiere AA (2004) Outcome of elderly patients with recurrent or metastatic head and neck cancer treated with cisplatin-based chemotherapy. J Clin Oncol 22(2):262–268

132. McGuirt WF, McCabe BF (1978) Significance of node biopsy before definitive treatment of cervical metastatic carcinoma. Laryngoscope 88(4):594–597

133. Gooder P, Palmer M (1984) Cervical lymph node biopsy – a study of its morbidity. J Laryngol Otol 98(10):1031–1040

134. Birchall MA, Stafford ND, Walsh-Waring GP (1991) Malignant neck lumps: a measured approach. Ann R Coll Surg Engl 73(2):91–95

135. Jones AS, Cook JA, Phillips DE, Roland NR (1993) Squamous carcinoma presenting as an enlarged cervical lymph node. Cancer 72(5):1756–1761

136. Underhill T, McGuirt WF, Williams DW (2000) Advances in imaging in head and neck tumors. Curr Opin Otolaryngol Head Neck Surg 8:91–97

137. Righi PD, Sofferman RA (1995) Screening unilateral tonsillectomy in the unknown primary. Laryngoscope 105(5 Pt 1):548–550

138. Freeman D, Mendenhall WM, Parsons JT, Million RR (1992) Unknown primary squamous cell carcinoma of the head and neck: is mucosal irradiation necessary? Int J Radiat Oncol Biol Phys 23(4):889–890

139. Lee NK, Byers RM, Abbruzzese JL, Wolf P (1991) Metastatic adenocarcinoma to the neck from an unknown primary source. Am J Surg 162(4):306–309

140. Reh DD, Lane AP (2009) The role of endoscopic sinus surgery in the management of sinonasal inverted papilloma. Curr Opin Otolaryngol Head Neck Surg 17(1):6–10

141. Hoppe BS, Stegman LD, Zelefsky MJ, Rosenzweig KE, Wolden SL, Patel SG et al (2007) Treatment of nasal cavity and paranasal sinus cancer with modern radiotherapy techniques in the postoperative setting – the MSKCC experience. Int J Radiat Oncol Biol Phys 67(3):691–702

142. Dulguerov P, Jacobsen MS, Allal AS, Lehmann W, Calcaterra T (2001) Nasal and paranasal sinus carcinoma: are we making progress? A series of 220 patients and a systematic review. Cancer 92(12):3012–3029

143. Hoppe BS, Wolden SL, Zelefsky MJ, Mechalakos JG, Shah JP, Kraus DH et al (2008) Postoperative intensity-modulated radiation therapy for cancers of the paranasal sinuses, nasal cavity, and lacrimal glands: technique, early outcomes, and toxicity. Head Neck 30(7):925–932

144. Le QT, Fu KK, Kaplan MJ, Terris DJ, Fee WE, Goffinet DR (2000) Lymph node metastasis in maxillary sinus carcinoma. Int J Radiat Oncol Biol Phys 46(3):541–549

145. Hayashi T, Nonaka S, Bandoh N, Kobayashi Y, Imada M, Harabuchi Y (2001) Treatment outcome of maxillary sinus squamous cell carcinoma. Cancer 92(6):1495–1503

146. Choi KN, Rotman M, Aziz H, Sohn CK, Schulsinger A, Torres C et al (1997) Concomitant infusion cisplatin and hyperfractionated radiotherapy for locally advanced nasopharyngeal and paranasal sinus tumors. Int J Radiat Oncol Biol Phys 39(4):823–829

147. Klintenberg C, Olofsson J, Hellquist H, Sokjer H (1984) Adenocarcinoma of the ethmoid sinuses. A review of 28 cases with special reference to wood dust exposure. Cancer 54(3):482–488

148. Hyams V (1984) Pathology of the nose and paranasal sinuses. In: English G (ed) Otolaryngology. Harper & Row, New York

149. Dickson RI (1981) Nasopharyngeal carcinoma: an evaluation of 209 patients. Laryngoscope 91(3):333–354

150. Yuan JM, Wang XL, Xiang YB, Gao YT, Ross RK, Yu MC (2000) Preserved foods in relation to risk of nasopharyngeal carcinoma in Shanghai, China. Int J Cancer 85(3):358–363

151. Shanmugaratnam K, Sobin LH (1978) Nasopharyngeal carcinoma. In: Shanmugaratnam K, Sobin LH (eds) International histological classification of tumors. World Health Organization, Geneva

152. Marks JE, Phillips JL, Menck HR (1998) The National Cancer Data Base report on the relationship of race and national origin to the histology of nasopharyngeal carcinoma. Cancer 83(3): 582–588

153. Reddy SP, Raslan WF, Gooneratne S, Kathuria S, Marks JE (1995) Prognostic significance of keratinization in nasopharyngeal carcinoma. Am J Otolaryngol 16(2):103–108

154. Sham JS, Cheung YK, Chan FL, Choy D (1990) Nasopharyngeal carcinoma: pattern of skeletal metastases. Br J Radiol 63(747): 202–205

155. Cooper JS, Porter K, Mallin K, Hoffman IIT, Weber RS, Ang KK et al (2009) National Cancer Database report on cancer of the head and neck: 10-year update. Head Neck 31(6):748–758

156. Langstein HN, Robb GL (2005) Lip and perioral reconstruction. Clin Plast Surg 32(3):431–445, viii

157. Byers RM, Weber RS, Andrews T, McGill D, Kare R, Wolf P (1997) Frequency and therapeutic implications of "skip metastases"

in the neck from squamous carcinoma of the oral tongue. Head Neck 19(1):14–19

158. Shaha AR, Spiro RH, Shah JP, Strong EW (1984) Squamous carcinoma of the floor of the mouth. Am J Surg 148(4):455–459

159. Rodgers LW Jr, Stringer SP, Mendenhall WM, Parsons JT, Cassisi NJ, Million RR (1993) Management of squamous cell carcinoma of the floor of mouth. Head Neck 15(1):16–19

160. Bloom ND, Spiro RH (1980) Carcinoma of the cheek mucosa. A retrospective analysis. Am J Surg 140(4):556–559

161. Diaz EM Jr, Holsinger FC, Zuniga ER, Roberts DB, Sorensen DM (2003) Squamous cell carcinoma of the buccal mucosa: one institution's experience with 119 previously untreated patients. Head Neck 25(4):267–273

162. Soo KC, Spiro RH, King W, Harvey W, Strong EW (1988) Squamous carcinoma of the gums. Am J Surg 156(4):281–285

163. Byers RM, Newman R, Russell N, Yue A (1981) Results of treatment for squamous carcinoma of the lower gum. Cancer 47(9):2236–2238

164. Huang CJ, Chao KS, Tsai J, Simpson JR, Haughey B, Spector GJ et al (2001) Cancer of retromolar trigone: long-term radiation therapy outcome. Head Neck 23(9):758–763

165. Evans JF, Shah JP (1981) Epidermoid carcinoma of the palate. Am J Surg 142(4):451–455

166. Konrad HR, Canalis RF, Calcaterra TC (1978) Epidermoid carcinoma of the palate. Arch Otolaryngol 104(4):208–212

167. Holsinger FC, McWhorter AJ, Menard M, Garcia D, Laccourreye O (2005) Transoral lateral oropharyngectomy for squamous cell carcinoma of the tonsillar region: I. Technique, complications, and functional results. Arch Otolaryngol Head Neck Surg 131(7):583–591

168. O'Malley BW Jr, Weinstein GS, Hockstein NG (2006) Transoral robotic surgery (TORS): glottic microsurgery in a canine model. J Voice 20(2):263–268

169. Foote RL, Schild SE, Thompson WM, Buskirk SJ, Olsen KD, Stanley RJ et al (1994) Tonsil cancer. Patterns of failure after surgery alone and surgery combined with postoperative radiation therapy. Cancer 73(10):2638–2647

170. Osborne RF, Brown JJ (2004) Carcinoma of the oral pharynx: an analysis of subsite treatment heterogeneity. Surg Oncol Clin N Am 13(1):71–80

171. Steiner W, Fierek O, Ambrosch P, Hommerich CP, Kron M (2003) Transoral laser microsurgery for squamous cell carcinoma of the base of the tongue. Arch Otolaryngol Head Neck Surg 129(1):36–43

172. Weber RS, Gidley P, Morrison WH, Peters LJ, Hankins P, Wolf P et al (1990) Treatment selection for carcinoma of the base of the tongue. Am J Surg 160(4):415–419

173. Harrison LB, Zelefsky MJ, Sessions RB, Fass DE, Armstrong JG, Pfister DG et al (1992) Base-of-tongue cancer treated with external beam irradiation plus brachytherapy: oncologic and functional outcome. Radiology 184(1):267–270

174. Denis F, Garaud P, Bardet E, Alfonsi M, Sire C, Germain T et al (2004) Final results of the 94-01 French Head and Neck Oncology and Radiotherapy Group randomized trial comparing radiotherapy alone with concomitant radiochemotherapy in advanced-stage oropharynx carcinoma. J Clin Oncol 22(1):69–76

175. Zhen W, Karnell LH, Hoffman HT, Funk GF, Buatti JM, Menck HR (2004) The National Cancer Data Base report on squamous cell carcinoma of the base of tongue. Head Neck 26(8):660–674

176. Shaha AR (1991) Preoperative evaluation of the mandible in patients with carcinoma of the floor of mouth. Head Neck 13(5):398–402

177. Ahmad A, Branstetter BF IV (2008) CT versus MR: still a tough decision. Otolaryngol Clin North Am 41(1):1–22, v

178. Van Cann EM, Koole R, Oyen WJ, de Rooy JW, de Wilde PC, Slootweg PJ et al (2008) Assessment of mandibular invasion of squamous cell carcinoma by various modes of imaging: constructing a diagnostic algorithm. Int J Oral Maxillofac Surg 37(6):535–541

179. Genden EM, Rinaldo A, Jacobson A, Shaha AR, Suarez C, Lowry J et al (2005) Management of mandibular invasion: when is a marginal mandibulectomy appropriate? Oral Oncol 41(8):776–782

180. O'Brien CJ, Adams JR, McNeil EB, Taylor P, Laniewski P, Clifford A et al (2003) Influence of bone invasion and extent of mandibular resection on local control of cancers of the oral cavity and oropharynx. Int J Oral Maxillofac Surg 32(5):492–497

181. Munoz Guerra MF, Naval Gias L, Campo FR, Perez JS (2003) Marginal and segmental mandibulectomy in patients with oral cancer: a statistical analysis of 106 cases. J Oral Maxillofac Surg 61(11):1289–1296

182. Patel RS, Dirven R, Clark JR, Swinson BD, Gao K, O'Brien CJ (2008) The prognostic impact of extent of bone invasion and extent of bone resection in oral carcinoma. Laryngoscope 118(5):780–785

183. Urken ML, Buchbinder D, Costantino PD, Sinha U, Okay D, Lawson W et al (1998) Oromandibular reconstruction using microvascular composite flaps: report of 210 cases. Arch Otolaryngol Head Neck Surg 124(1):46–55

184. Jones NF, Jarrahy R, Song JI, Kaufman MR, Markowitz B (2007) Postoperative medical complications – not microsurgical complications – negatively influence the morbidity, mortality, and true costs after microsurgical reconstruction for head and neck cancer. Plast Reconstr Surg 119(7):2053–2060

185. Howard MA, Cordeiro PG, Disa J, Samson W, Gonen M, Schoelle RN et al (2005) Free tissue transfer in the elderly: incidence of perioperative complications following microsurgical reconstruction of 197 septuagenarians and octogenarians. Plast Reconstr Surg 116(6):1659–1668, discussion 69–71

186. Spiro RH, Gerold FP, Shah JP, Sessions RB, Strong EW (1985) Mandibulotomy approach to oropharyngeal tumors. Am J Surg 150(4):466–469

187. Menda Y, Graham MM (2005) Update on 18F-fluorodeoxyglucose/positron emission tomography and positron emission tomography/computed tomography imaging of squamous head and neck cancers. Semin Nucl Med 35(4):214–219

188. Shaha AR, Cordeiro PG, Hidalgo DA, Spiro RH, Strong EW, Zlotolow I et al (1997) Resection and immediate microvascular reconstruction in the management of osteoradionecrosis of the mandible. Head Neck 19(5):406–411

189. Kraus DH, Pfister DG, Harrison LB, Shah JP, Spiro RH, Armstrong JG et al (1994) Larynx preservation with combined chemotherapy and radiation therapy in advanced hypopharynx cancer. Otolaryngol Head Neck Surg 111(1):31–37

190. Gourin CG, Terris DJ (2004) Carcinoma of the hypopharynx. Surg Oncol Clin N Am 13(1):81–98

191. Hoffman HT, Porter K, Karnell LH, Cooper JS, Weber RS, Langer CJ et al (2006) Laryngeal cancer in the United States: changes in demographics, patterns of care, and survival. Laryngoscope 116(9 Pt 2 Suppl 111):1–13

192. Back G, Sood S (2005) The management of early laryngeal cancer: options for patients and therapists. Curr Opin Otolaryngol Head Neck Surg 13(2):85–91

193. Biller HF, Lawson W (1986) Partial laryngectomy for vocal cord cancer with marked limitation or fixation of the vocal cord. Laryngoscope 96(1):61–64

194. Ganly I, Patel SG, Matsuo J, Singh B, Kraus DH, Boyle JO et al (2006) Results of surgical salvage after failure of definitive radiation therapy for early-stage squamous cell carcinoma of the glottic larynx. Arch Otolaryngol Head Neck Surg 132(1):59–66

195. Orus C, Leon X, Vega M, Quer M (2000) Initial treatment of the early stages (I, II) of supraglottic squamous cell carcinoma: partial laryngectomy versus radiotherapy. Eur Arch Otorhinolaryngol 257(9):512–516

196. Hinerman RW, Mendenhall WM, Amdur RJ, Stringer SP, Villaret DB, Robbins KT (2002) Carcinoma of the supraglottic larynx: treatment results with radiotherapy alone or with planned neck dissection. Head Neck 24(5):456–467

197. Ambrosch P, Kron M, Steiner W (1998) Carbon dioxide laser microsurgery for early supraglottic carcinoma. Ann Otol Rhinol Laryngol 107(8):680–688

198. Davis RK, Kriskovich MD, Galloway EB III, Buntin CS, Jepsen MC (2004) Endoscopic supraglottic laryngectomy with postoperative irradiation. Ann Otol Rhinol Laryngol 113(2):132–138

199. Sesterhenn AM, Dunne AA, Werner JA (2006) Complications after CO(2) laser surgery of laryngeal cancer in the elderly. Acta Otolaryngol 126(5):530–535

200. Agrawal A, Moon J, Davis RK, Sakr WA, Giri SP, Valentino J et al (2007) Transoral carbon dioxide laser supraglottic laryngectomy and irradiation in stage I, II, and III squamous cell carcinoma of the supraglottic larynx: report of Southwest Oncology Group Phase 2 Trial S9709. Arch Otolaryngol Head Neck Surg 133(10):1044–1050

201. Cabanillas R, Rodrigo JP, Llorente JL, Suarez V, Ortega P, Suarez C (2004) Functional outcomes of transoral laser surgery of supraglottic carcinoma compared with a transcervical approach. Head Neck 26(8):653–659

202. (1991) Induction chemotherapy plus radiation compared with surgery plus radiation in patients with advanced laryngeal cancer. The Department of Veterans Affairs Laryngeal Cancer Study Group. N Engl J Med 324(24):1685–1690

203. Forastiere AA, Goepfert H, Maor M, Pajak TF, Weber R, Morrison W et al (2003) Concurrent chemotherapy and radiotherapy for organ preservation in advanced laryngeal cancer. N Engl J Med 349(22):2091–2098

204. Wong RJ (2008) Current status of FDG-PET for head and neck cancer. J Surg Oncol 97(8):649–652

205. Davidson J, Briant D, Gullane P, Keane T, Rawlinson E (1994) The role of surgery following radiotherapy failure for advanced laryngopharyngeal cancer. A prospective study. Arch Otolaryngol Head Neck Surg 120(3):269–276

206. Sassler AM, Esclamado RM, Wolf GT (1995) Surgery after organ preservation therapy. Analysis of wound complications. Arch Otolaryngol Head Neck Surg 121(2):162–165

207. Panje WR, Namon AJ, Vokes E, Haraf DJ, Weichselbaum RR (1995) Surgical management of the head and neck cancer patient following concomitant multimodality therapy. Laryngoscope 105(1):97–101

208. Weber RS, Berkey BA, Forastiere A, Cooper J, Maor M, Goepfert H et al (2003) Outcome of salvage total laryngectomy following organ preservation therapy: the Radiation Therapy Oncology Group trial 91-11. Arch Otolaryngol Head Neck Surg 129(1):44–49

209. Janot F, de Raucourt D, Benhamou E, Ferron C, Dolivet G, Bensadoun RJ et al (2008) Randomized trial of postoperative reirradiation combined with chemotherapy after salvage surgery compared with salvage surgery alone in head and neck carcinoma. J Clin Oncol 26(34):5518–5523

210. Colevas AD (2006) Chemotherapy options for patients with metastatic or recurrent squamous cell carcinoma of the head and neck. J Clin Oncol 24(17):2644–2652

211. Gibson MK, Li Y, Murphy B, Hussain MH, DeConti RC, Ensley J et al (2005) Randomized phase III evaluation of cisplatin plus fluorouracil versus cisplatin plus paclitaxel in advanced head and neck cancer (E1395): an intergroup trial of the Eastern Cooperative Oncology Group. J Clin Oncol 23(15):3562–3567

212. Pfister DG, Su YB, Kraus DH, Wolden SL, Lis E, Aliff TB et al (2006) Concurrent cetuximab, cisplatin, and concomitant boost radiotherapy for locoregionally advanced, squamous cell head and neck cancer: a pilot phase II study of a new combined-modality paradigm. J Clin Oncol 24(7):1072–1078

213. Vermorken JB, Trigo J, Hitt R, Koralewski P, Diaz-Rubio E, Rolland F et al (2007) Open-label, uncontrolled, multicenter phase II study to evaluate the efficacy and toxicity of cetuximab as a single agent in patients with recurrent and/or metastatic squamous cell carcinoma of the head and neck who failed to respond to platinum-based therapy. J Clin Oncol 25(16):2171–2177

214. Stewart JS, Cohen EE, Licitra L, Van Herpen CM, Khorprasert C, Soulieres D et al (2009) Phase III study of gefitinib 250 compared with intravenous methotrexate for recurrent squamous cell carcinoma of the head and neck. J Clin Oncol 27(11):1864–1871

215. Shah JP, Ihde JK (1990) Salivary gland tumors. Curr Probl Surg 27(12):775–883

216. Spiro RH (1986) Salivary neoplasms: overview of a 35-year experience with 2,807 patients. Head Neck Surg 8(3):177–184

217. Rabinov JD (2000) Imaging of salivary gland pathology. Radiol Clin North Am 38(5):1047–1057, x–xi

218. Al-Khafaji BM, Afify AM (2001) Salivary gland fine needle aspiration using the ThinPrep technique: diagnostic accuracy, cytologic artifacts and pitfalls. Acta Cytol 45(4):567–574

219. Michael CW, Hunter B (2000) Interpretation of fine-needle aspirates processed by the ThinPrep technique: cytologic artifacts and diagnostic pitfalls. Diagn Cytopathol 23(1):6–13

220. Stewart CJ, MacKenzie K, McGarry GW, Mowat A (2000) Fine-needle aspiration cytology of salivary gland: a review of 341 cases. Diagn Cytopathol 22(3):139–146

221. Heller KS, Dubner S, Chess Q, Attie JN (1992) Value of fine needle aspiration biopsy of salivary gland masses in clinical decision-making. Am J Surg 164(6):667–670

222. Seifert G (1992) Histopathology of malignant salivary gland tumours. Eur J Cancer B Oral Oncol 28B(1):49–56

223. Nascimento AG, Amaral LP, Prado LA, Kligerman J, Silveira TR (1986) Mucoepidermoid carcinoma of salivary glands: a clinicopathologic study of 46 cases. Head Neck Surg 8(6):409–417

224. Spiro RH, Armstrong J, Harrison L, Geller NL, Lin SY, Strong EW (1989) Carcinoma of major salivary glands. Recent trends. Arch Otolaryngol Head Neck Surg 115(3):316–321

225. Douglas JG, Lee S, Laramore GE, Austin-Seymour M, Koh W, Griffin TW (1999) Neutron radiotherapy for the treatment of locally advanced major salivary gland tumors. Head Neck 21(3):255–263

226. Kaplan MJ, Johns ME, Cantrell RW (1986) Chemotherapy for salivary gland cancer. Otolaryngol Head Neck Surg 95(2):165–170

227. Airoldi M, Pedani F, Succo G, Gabriele AM, Ragona R, Marchionatti S et al (2001) Phase II randomized trial comparing vinorelbine versus vinorelbine plus cisplatin in patients with recurrent salivary gland malignancies. Cancer 91(3):541–547

228. Ruzich JC, Ciesla MC, Clark JI (2002) Response to paclitaxel and carboplatin in metastatic salivary gland cancer: a case report. Head Neck 24(4):406–410

229. Hocwald E, Korkmaz H, Yoo GH, Adsay V, Shibuya TY, Abrams J et al (2001) Prognostic factors in major salivary gland cancer. Laryngoscope 111(8):1434–1439

230. Hamakawa H, Nakashiro K, Sumida T, Shintani S, Myers JN, Takes RP et al (2008) Basic evidence of molecular targeted therapy for oral cancer and salivary gland cancer. Head Neck 30(6):800–809

231. Gomez DR, Hoppe BS, Wolden SL, Zhung JE, Patel SG, Kraus DH et al (2008) Outcomes and prognostic variables in adenoid cystic carcinoma of the head and neck: a recent experience. Int J Radiat Oncol Biol Phys 70(5):1365–1372

232. Terhaard CH, Lubsen H, Van der Tweel I, Hilgers FJ, Eijkenboom WM, Marres HA et al (2004) Salivary gland carcinoma: independent prognostic factors for locoregional control, distant metastases, and overall survival: results of the Dutch head and neck oncology cooperative group. Head Neck 26(8):681–692, discussion 92–3

Section VI
Respiratory System

Chapter 46
Invited Commentary

Earle W. Wilkins Jr.

A life span of 90 years provides an opportunity to look at the past, to compare surgery of the chest today and what it was like 25 or more years ago. Such a review should tell us what we have learned and what we do need to learn yet.

Early History

Certain mileposts stand out. The principles of one-stage lobectomy with individual ligature technique were formulated by Harold Brunn of San Francisco in 1929 [1]. Evarts Graham of St. Louis performed the first successful pneumonectomy for bronchogenic carcinoma in 1933 [2]. Edward Churchill of Boston, in collaboration with his fellow Ronald Belsey, defined the technique of segmental lobectomy in 1938 [3]. In the related field of esophageal surgery, William Adams and Dallas Phemister of Chicago had successfully carried out a resection of a carcinoma of the distal esophagus with intrathoracic esophagogastric anastomosis, also in 1938 [4]. Further historical details in the evolving story of surgery of the respiratory tract are provided in "General Thoracic Surgery: History and Development," Chap. 1 in Pearson's *Thoracic Surgery*, 2nd ed. (2002).

The Past: 1944–1985

By the beginning of my days in surgery, pulmonary resection had become an established and safe technical procedure. These decades saw improvements in the fields of diagnosis, technical details of surgery including instrumentation, advances in anesthesiology, the introduction of antibiotics, and particularly in the postoperative care of the patient.

E.W. Wilkins Jr. (✉)
Department of Surgery, Massachusetts General Hospital,
Boston, MA, USA
e-mail: ewwilki@roadrunner.com

1. *Extent of surgical resection*: Until 1950, Graham's pneumonectomy was the standard operation for lung cancer. A somewhat revolutionary and initially disputed report from Churchill and Richard Sweet (1950) [5] demonstrated that lobectomy, when technically possible, was an adequate and potentially curative procedure. Both of these men, my mentors, were true pioneers in the field of thoracic surgery; both became president of the American Association for Thoracic Surgery. A later president, Leo Eloesser, commented "the attempt to eradicate cancer by progressively increasing the anatomic limits of operation is not the right road to follow." Thus, lobectomy became the operation of choice.

2. *Staging*: As it became clear that invasion of lymphatics and lymph node metastases were determinants in the possibility of cure for bronchogenic carcinoma, the concept of preoperative staging was developed. An early technique, popularized by Griffith Pearson of Toronto, was mediastinoscopy [6]. This permitted direct visualization and biopsy of mediastinal and bronchial lymph nodes. Computed tomographic (CT) scanning provided a noninvasive method of assessing the mediastinum for the presence of enlarged nodes, but without pathologic tissue diagnosis. A more recent scanning technique, positron emission tomography (PET) is particularly helpful in assessing mediastinal node involvement. Precise information provided by these studies guided the decision of surgery vs. radiation or other nonoperative therapy.

3. *Postoperative care*: The era saw an evolution of postoperative care from the early recovery room to the intensive care unit (ICU). The original ICU established in 1958 at the Massachusetts General Hospital was planned for the care of postthymectomy patients with myasthenia gravis. It proved invaluable in the care of patients with pulmonary resections, especially those undergoing pneumonectomy. Respiratory physical therapy for the pulmonary patient, both pre- and postoperatively, became an integral component of care. A whole spectrum of new antibiotics became available for prophylactic use.

4. *Anesthesia*: Not to be forgotten in the progress of managing surgery for the respiratory patient was the role of the

R.A. Rosenthal et al. (eds.), *Principles and Practice of Geriatric Surgery*,
DOI 10.1007/978-1-4419-6999-6_46, © Springer Science+Business Media, LLC 2011

anesthesiologist. Measurement of arterial blood gases became routine. The use of pulse oximetry and continuous observation of arterial blood pressure and electrocardiographic tracing became regular monitoring techniques. The depth of necessary analgesia could be managed by a host of newer pharmacologic agents. The employment of the double-lumen endotracheal tube allowed the thoracic surgeon better technical access to mediastinal structures in his intraoperative dissections.

5. *The endotracheal tube* underwent a major modification. An unfortunate increase in the incidence of postintubation tracheal strictures proved to be the result of pressure ischemia of the tracheal wall resulting from tubes with the noncompliant inflatable cuff. Grillo and Cooper developed the large volume, low-pressure cuff, the so-called "floppy" cuff, which not only avoided the early postintubation stricture but also permitted longer term ventilatory mechanical assistance without serious damage to the trachea [7].

6. The *key* for developments in this period is encompassed in the word *Safety*: a safe conduct of the operated patient via safer selection, safer extent of operation, safe anesthesia, and safe postoperative care.

The Present Day: 1986 Onward

This is a term used since my departure from the chest operating scene. Happily, surgical care of the respiratory patient marches steadily forward. This includes in particular the geriatric patient.

1. *Video-assisted thoracoscopic surgery* (*VATS*). This technique is certainly the striking advance in the field of general thoracic surgery in recent decades. It makes possible an entirely different access to surgery within the thoracic cavities, perhaps as big a change as in all the preceding half century. The utilization of multiple mini-incisions, remarkable magnifying fiber-optic visualization, and an impressive array of specially devised instrumentation make for a more comfortable postoperative patient and a shorter stay in the hospital. It is a strangely new technique for the older surgeon, requiring looking horizontally at a monitoring screen rather than downward at the patient's chest.

   In general, VATS resections may be preferred for lobectomies, segmental, and other nonanatomic excisions, and for an excellent approach to thymectomy for myasthenia and for most thymic tumors. It is not a technique for large pulmonary tumors, for sleeve or other extended resections, such as the approach and access to superior sulcus tumors. Many skilled VATS surgeons object to pneumonectomy through this approach. The surgeon must always be prepared to convert to open thoracotomy for cases with difficult anatomy, extent of tumor, or unexpected event such as major hemorrhage.

2. *Induction chemotherapy*: It has long been a policy to irradiate the mediastinum of patients in whom positive lymph nodes were found at time of resection (stage III). Although this adjuvant (postoperative) therapy has enhanced local control, it has not resulted in improved long-term survival. Similarly, adjuvant chemotherapy alone has not proved beneficial in stage III patients. The result has been a shift to the use of induction (preoperative) chemotherapy in an effort to improve length of survival. Chemotherapy, either adjuvant or induction, with or without irradiation, has not proved curative in the absence of resection.

   An encouraging development has been the increasing role of the surgeon in the study and analysis of results in the use of induction chemotherapy. He has become his own oncologist. Numerous current randomized trials with varying drug combinations, with and without irradiation, remain in the evaluation phase of study. The General Thoracic Surgical Club has taken on such evaluating reviews at its annual meetings. It is difficult for this "noncombatant" to comprehend clearly the results thus far. There is an apparent survival benefit in the use of adjuvant chemotherapy in resected patients with N1–N2 disease, and it is reasonably clear that patients resected for stage IIA disease derive survival benefit from induction chemotherapy or chemoradiation.

   Again, thus far, it is difficult to anticipate cures. Its role in elderly patients is certainly far from clear. One must balance the often distressing side effects with survival time gained.

3. *Advances in surgical techniques*: By 1986, most surgical techniques dealing with lung cancer had become standard. Yet, there has been refinement in techniques in the recent era. The surgical management of superior sulcus tumors is one example. Operability, the likelihood of en bloc total removal of the tumor, improved with the use of induction chemoradiation and with the ease of resection facilitated by choosing the incisional approach. Depending upon the location of the primary tumor, the two commonly used approaches are the anterior cervicothoracic and the posterior.

   Familiarity with the technique of sleeve bronchial resections has led to greater use of these parenchyma sparing procedures. They constitute another advance in the goal of avoiding pneumonectomy. This is especially desirable in the elderly patient avoiding higher rates of complications and limitations in life style. Bronchoplasty has become a standard procedure for the accomplished thoracic surgeon. The potential addition of carinal resection for so-called T4 tumors has been added to the surgeon's skills. It usually is accomplished with a right pneumonectomy and anastomosis of the distal trachea to the left main stem bronchus. It is a procedure used only when every other patient factor is favorable and only by the most skilled operator and anesthesiologist. It has limited use in the geriatric patient. The *key* summary for this era is a combination of improved patient comfort and ongoing efforts with combination therapies to increase lengths of survival. The question remains: what is the role for and the details of chemotherapy?

Personal Commentary

1. The *geriatric patient*, already self-selected by virtue of mere survival, is a reasonable candidate for lobectomy for cancer of the lung. This is especially true with the VATS technique. Pneumonectomy should be undertaken with urgent caution. Left pneumonectomy is certainly better tolerated than the right.
2. Preoperative staging, by scanning techniques and/or mediastinoscopy, is essential. The finding of N2 disease should raise an alert as to whether surgical resection is indicated in the elderly patient.
3. Preservation of as much lung parenchyma as possible is the sine qua non in resections in the geriatric patient. Where possible, segmental resection or nonanatomic wedge resection is acceptable.
4. The use of inductive or adjuvant therapy with resections of the lung is a debatable consideration in the elderly. It should be an individual, not a routine, decision based on physiologic and life-style considerations.
5. Contraindications to pulmonary resections arise from physiologic, not chronologic, age. Particular attention in evaluation of candidacy for operation must be directed to cardiovascular status, pulmonary function, and the presence of metabolic or other malignant disease.
6. Personal experience: In a review of 426 pulmonary resections (unpublished data), there were *four* hospital deaths in 81 pneumonectomies (*4.9%*), while in lobectomies, the mortality was *1.6%*. Once again, where technically possible, lobectomy is the preferred operation. Special attention must be paid to the right pneumonectomy patient, whether geriatric or younger. Two of the mentioned mortalities resulted from bronchial stump leakage. Closure had been accomplished by the interrupted suture technique in patients who had accompanying mediastinal node dissections. Interruption of the arterial blood supply to the stump, related to the thorough mediastinal lymph node dissection, may have been a contributing factor in nonhealing.
7. Carcinoma of the lung remains the greatest cause of cancer deaths in patients of both genders. With maximal surgical therapy, no more than *20% of all* such patients are being cured. The establishment of the optimum inductive or adjuvant therapy, chemotherapy and/or radiation remains a difficult goal. Promising new approaches are on the horizon. At the Massachusetts General Hospital, biopsies of lung cancers are being scanned for genetic mutations (*tumor genotyping*), information from which may guide the oncologist in selecting specific chemotherapeutic drugs (*targeted therapy*) for specific tumors.
8. The surgeon remains a key, perhaps *the* key figure in the curative management of lung cancer. He should not forget the words of Emily Dickinson:

Surgeons must be very careful
When they take the knife,
Underneath their fine incisions
Lies the culprit – Life!

References

1. Brunn H (1929) Surgical principles underlying one-stage lobectomy. Arch Surg 18:490
2. Graham EA, Singer JJ (1933) Successful removal of an entire lung for carcinoma of the bronchus. JAMA 101:1371
3. Churchill ED, Belsey R (1939) Segmental pneumonectomy in bronchiectasis: lingula segment of left upper lobe. Ann Surg 109:481
4. Adams W, Phemister DB (1938) Carcinoma of the lower esophagus: report of a successful resection and esophagogastrostomy. J Thorac Surg 7:621
5. Churchill ED, Sweet RH, Soutter L, Scannell JG (1950) The surgical management of carcinoma of the lung. J Thorac Surg 20:349
6. Pearson FG (1965) Mediastinoscopy: a method of biopsy in the superior mediastinum. J Thorac Cardiovasc Surg 49:11
7. Grillo HC, Cooper JD, Geffin B et al (1971) A low pressure cuff for tracheostomy tubes to minimize tracheal injury: a comparative clinical trial. J Thorac Cardiovasc Surg 62:898

Chapter 47
Physiologic Changes in Respiratory Function

Edward J. Campbell

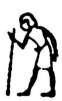

Physiologic changes with age: pulmonary

Parameter	Change with age	Functional impact of change
Chest shape	↑ AP diameter	No significant impact
	Mild-mod kyphosis	
Conducting airways	Calcification	Insignificant ↑ deadspace
	Mild ↑ size	
	Mucus gland hypertrophy	Minimal significance
Lung parenchyma	Enlarged alveolar ducts	Similar to mild emphysema
	V/Q mismatch	**Decreased reserve**
	↓ Elastic recoil	
Bellows apparatus	↑ Chest wall rigidity	Increased work of breathing
	↓ Respiratory muscle strength	Highly individual
Ventilatory control	↓↓ **Response to hypercapnia and hypoxemia**	Impaired homeostasis under stress
		Signs of distress subtle

Most important messages in bold
AP anteroposterior; *V/Q*: ventilation/perfusion

A substantial proportion of the excess operative risk among elderly patients is attributable to respiratory complications. The excess risk is explained in part by structural and functional changes in the respiratory system associated with aging. These changes are progressive even in individuals who enjoy apparently good health and are most marked beyond 60 years of age.

In youth, healthy individuals have a physiologic reserve (a marked excess of functional capacity over the amount needed to meet metabolic needs at rest or with stress). The respiratory system draws on this reserve as its function declines with age. Aged individuals thus become vulnerable to the stress, disease, and injuries that are weathered much more easily by the young.

The routine activities of healthy elderly persons are not limited by this decreasing respiratory system function. Thus, the effects of age may not be apparent until they need to draw on their physiologic reserves during stress, such as postoperative recovery or complications. An awareness of the inevitable, but possibly hidden, age-related changes in the respiratory system helps the surgeon anticipate and treat respiratory complications in elderly patients.

The purely age-related changes in the respiratory system are complicated by other accompaniments of aging. The lungs are exposed to a lifetime of environmental stresses, including tobacco smoke, respiratory infections, air pollutants, and occupational exposures to dusts and fumes. Elderly individuals also often have increasingly sedentary lifestyles and decreasing fitness.

As an introduction to the topics to be reviewed in this chapter, the various components of the respiratory system are shown in Table 47.1. Table 47.1 also contains introductory comments about structural and functional changes with age.

Airways and Lung Parenchyma Lung Shape

The lungs are closely applied to the chest wall, and their overall shape is determined by the chest wall shape. The increases in anteroposterior diameter of the lungs with age and the more rounded shape that results are presumably due to

E.J. Campbell (✉)
Department of Internal Medicine, University of Utah Health Sciences Center, 5505 East Pioneer Fork Road, Salt Lake City, UT 84108, USA
e-mail: ecampbell@aatdetection.com

R.A. Rosenthal et al. (eds.), *Principles and Practice of Geriatric Surgery*,
DOI 10.1007/978-1-4419-6999-6_47, © Springer Science+Business Media, LLC 2011

Table 47.1 Respiratory system and changes with aging

Functional division	Components	Function	Change(s) with aging
Conducting airways	Airways not involved in gas exchange	Transport gas to and from lung parenchyma	Calcification and other minor changes
Lung parenchyma	Respiratory bronchioles through alveoli and supporting structures	Exchanges gas between alveoli and pulmonary capillaries	Enlarged alveolar ducts; ventilation–perfusion mismatching
Bellows apparatus	Chest wall and respiratory muscles	Provides support for lung structure and applies force to lung	Increased rigidity of chest wall, some decrease in respiratory muscle strength
Ventilatory control	Respiratory control center; carotid and aortic bodies	Alters ventilation to match metabolic needs	Markedly decreased responses to hypoxemia and hypercapnia

changes in the shape of the surrounding thoracic cage. These changes are not thought to have functional consequences.

Conducting Airways

The conducting airways consist of the air passages from the mouth to the level of the respiratory bronchioles. The volume of the conducting airways determines the anatomic dead space. Their size, shape, and branching pattern are the major determinants of airway resistance. The large cartilaginous airways show a modest increase in size with age, resulting in slight but probably functionally insignificant increases in anatomic dead space [1]. Calcification of cartilage in the walls of the central airways and hypertrophy of bronchial mucous glands are seen during advanced age, but these and other changes in the extraparenchymal conducting airways appear to have little or no physiologic significance.

Lung Parenchyma

The respiratory bronchioles and alveolar ducts undergo progressive enlargement with age, beginning as early as age 30 or 40 but observable most prominently after the age of 60 (Fig. 47.1). The proportion of the lung made up of alveolar ducts increases, and alveolar septa become shortened, leading to a flattened appearance of the alveoli. The proportion of alveolar air decreases as the volume of air in alveolar ducts increases [2]. The distance between alveolar walls (the mean linear intercept, or MLI) increases, whereas the surface/volume ratio of the lung decreases. As a result of these changes, the alveolar surface area decreases by approximately 15% by age 70.

Superficially, the morphologic changes in the lung with aging are similar to those observed with mild pulmonary emphysema. To be classified as emphysema, however, the anatomic changes must consist of airspace enlargement in

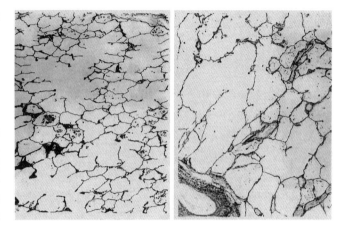

Figure 47.1 Histologic changes in the aging lung. Normal lung of a 36-year-old woman (*left*). Lung of a 93-year-old woman (*right*). Alveolar ducts are dilated, and shortening of interalveolar septa is observed (photomicrographs courtesy of Charles Kuhn III, MD, with permission of the Mayo Foundation).

the gas-exchanging zone of the lung (distal to the terminal bronchioles) and must show evidence that the airspace enlargement is due to alveolar wall destruction, with fusion of adjacent airspaces [3]. For a time, there was considerable debate as to the cause and classification of the airspace enlargement seen with advanced age. Debate centered on whether the airspace enlargement was a "senile" form of emphysema.

Pump [4] and several early authors thought they could identify "emphysematous" lesions in aged lungs. However, Pump studied only two lungs (from 78- to 80-year-old men), one of whom had been a heavy smoker. Ryan and colleagues resisted the term "emphysema" and called the age-related structural changes "ductectasia" because of the prominent finding of enlarged alveolar ducts [5]. Significant alveolar wall destruction as a cause of emphysema appears to be unlikely, as Thurlbeck and Angus have shown that the number of alveoli per unit area remains constant in mature lungs [2]. The latter authors considered the changes to be a "rearrangement of the geometry of the lung." A National Heart, Lung, and Blood Institute Workshop on the definition of emphysema weighed the available evidence and decided not to include age-related changes in the lung parenchyma under the definition of emphysema [3]. To avoid confusion and to simplify the nomenclature, they recommended use of the term "aging lung" to apply to the uniform airspace enlargement that develops with increasing age.

Mechanical Properties of the Lungs

The lungs exert an inward force in the intact thoracic cage. The retractile force of the lungs, or "elastic recoil," can be measured during life by estimating the pleural pressure with an esophageal balloon. Measurements are taken at progressively decreasing lung volumes from total lung capacity (TLC) to functional residual capacity (FRC), when the airways are open and there is no airflow. The negative pleural pressure is generated by the lungs' elastic recoil forces.

Figure 47.2 compares the elastic recoil pressures of a young man, a normal elderly adult, and a patient with emphysema. The normal elderly individual and the patient with

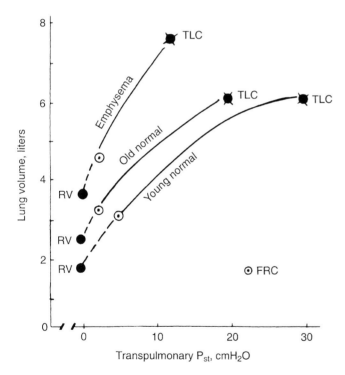

Figure 47.2 Static pressure–volume curves of the lungs illustrating elastic recoil forces and compliance. To generate these data, transpulmonary pressure (which reflects lung elastic recoil) is measured at various lung volumes with an esophageal balloon. At any lung volume, the recoil pressure is less in the aged than in the young individual. This results in a pressure–volume relation that is shifted upward and to the left. A curve for a patient with emphysema is shown for comparison. With emphysema, recoil pressures are much less than in normal elderly individuals, and lung compliance (the slope of the curve) is markedly abnormal (from Pride [6], with permission).

emphysema have a greater decrease in elastic recoil pressure than does a young person. This is reflected in the leftward shift of their pressure–volume curves [7, 8]. Emphysema produces a much greater loss of elastic recoil than is caused by aging alone.

There has been some disagreement as to whether aging changes lung compliance (the slope of the curve in Fig. 47.2) or, alternatively, is accompanied by a parallel leftward shift of the pressure–volume curve with aging (no change in compliance). There is general agreement if small changes in lung compliance do occur, they are not physiologically significant.

Changes in Lung Recoil Due to Surface Forces

The loss of surface area with age reduces the area of gas–liquid interface, resulting in a decrease in the surface tension forces. This ultimately causes a decrease in the lung elastic recoil. This change has important effects on lung function (especially on the function of small airways and expiratory flow).

Changes in Structural Macromolecules

Elastic fibers consist in large part of an extremely hydrophobic, highly cross-linked, and highly elastic macromolecule (elastin). They form a continuous skeleton that follows the airways and pulmonary vessels and extends to a fine meshwork in the alveolar septa [9]. These fibers are thought to contribute substantially to lung elasticity. The amount of elastin in the lungs has been studied in an attempt to determine the cause of decreasing lung elastic recoil with age. Analysis of whole lungs has revealed that the elastin content actually increases (rather than decreases) with age [10]. More recent evidence indicates that the increase in lung elastin with age is accounted for by an increase in pleural elastin; parenchymal elastin does not change [9].

Careful studies of the elastic fibers in the lung parenchyma by two independent methods have shown that they are remarkably stable following postnatal lung growth. Modeling of radiocarbon data [11] indicates that the "mean carbon residence time" in elastin is 74 years (Fig. 47.3). It is correct to consider that lung parenchymal elastin is stable over the human life span. These elastic fibers probably provide a metabolically inert scaffold for the structure of the lung. Thus, there are no age-related changes in lung elastin that provide an explanation for the decrease in elastic recoil forces observed in the elderly.

Although human studies have not been done, studies in rodents and birds suggest that lung collagen fibers, like elastic

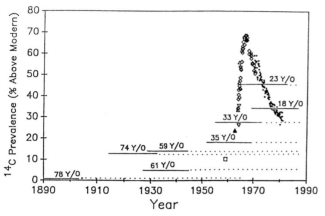

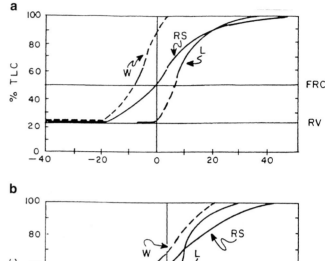

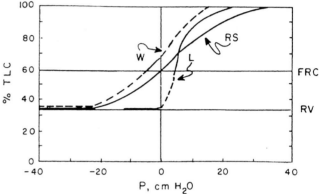

Figure 47.3 Turnover of elastic fibers in human lung parenchyma. Radiocarbon (^{14}C) prevalence in lung elastin is shown on the ordinate, with zero being the level before atmospheric nuclear weapons testing began. Levels above zero reflect protein synthesis that has occurred since the 1960s (% Above Modern). The symbols are data from human tissues that exhibit rapid turnover, sampled during the years shown [11]. Each horizontal line represents an analysis of human lung parenchymal elastin from a single individual. The age at time of death is shown for each subject. The lengths and positioning of the solid portions of the lines correspond to timing and duration of fetal and postnatal lung growth, and the interrupted portions of the lines represent the remainder of the individuals' life spans. The vertical position of each line represents the ^{14}C prevalence measured in that sample. Note that the ^{14}C prevalence measured in the elastin samples reflects the ^{14}C prevalence in the biosphere during the period of lung growth. Individuals whose lungs had ceased growing before the nuclear weapons age had little nuclear weapons-related ^{14}C in their lung elastin, demonstrating that minimal lung elastin turnover occurred during adulthood (from Shapiro et al. [11], with permission).

Figure 47.4 Static compliance relations of the components of the respiratory system. *L* lungs, *W* chest wall, *RS* total respiratory system, *TLC* total lung capacity, *FRC* functional reserve capacity, *RV* residual volume, *P* pressure gradient, (**a**) A 20-year-old man; (**b**) A 60-year-old man. Note that the static compliance of the chest wall is substantially decreased (reduced slope) in the older individual, whereas FRC (resting volume of the respiratory system, or the point at which the pressure gradient across the respiratory system is zero) increases somewhat. Note again (compare with Fig. 35.2) that the static recoil pressure of the lungs is reduced in the older subject.

fibers, are long-lived. Finally, although some qualitative changes in collagen during aging have been described (decreases in solubility and increases in intermolecular cross-links), they appear to have no relation to changes in lung elastic recoil.

Chest Wall

The chest wall becomes more rigid with advancing age [8, 12]. As can be seen in Fig. 47.4, the static pressure–volume curve of the chest wall is shifted to the right and is less steep (indicating decreased compliance) with increasing age [13]. It is known that the articulations of the ribs with the sternum and the spinal column may become calcified, and the compliance of the rib articulations decreases with age. The changes in rib articulations may be compounded by the development of kyphosis due to osteoporosis. The decreasing compliance of the chest wall demands more work from the respiratory muscles. For example, in a 70-year-old person, approximately 70% of the total elastic work of breathing is expended on the chest wall, whereas this value is 40% in a 20-year-old.

Muscles of Respiration

Age-related changes in nonrespiratory skeletal muscle include decreased work capacity owing to alterations in the efficiency of muscle energy metabolism, atrophy of motor units, and electromyographic abnormalities. Based on lessons learned with other skeletal muscles, it, at first, appeared likely that age-related abnormalities in respiratory muscles would also be found.

An early study by Black and Hyatt [14] appeared to confirm age-related decrements in respiratory muscle function by measuring maximal inspiratory pressure (PI_{max}) and maximal expiratory pressure (PE_{max}) in 120 normal individuals (both smokers and nonsmokers) between the ages 20 and 70. Maximal respiratory pressures in women were 65–70% of those in men. No significant age-related changes were observed in individuals under the age of 55. Trends toward reduced maximal respiratory pressure with age were seen for both sexes and with both PI_{max} and $PE_{max.}$ With the numbers of men studied, the change with age in PI_{max} was not statistically significant for the male gender.

More recently, McElvaney and coworkers [15] have come to a different conclusion in a similar study of 104 healthy individuals over the age of 55. They found large variation in maximal respiratory pressures from individual to individual (as had Black and Hyatt) but no significant correlation with age. In contrast, in a third population of 160 healthy individuals who ranged in age from 16 to 75 years, Chen and Kuo found significant gender differences in maximal respiratory pressures as well as trends toward decrements with age for both PI_{max} and PE_{max} in both genders [16]. The age-related change in PE_{max} in the male subjects was not statistically significant with the sample size studied. When the 40 individuals of both genders in the youngest age group (16–30 years) were compared with the 40 individuals in the oldest group (61–75 years), the decrement in PI_{max} was 32–36%, and the decrement in P^emax was 13–23%. Representative findings for maximal respiratory pressures in women are illustrated in Fig. 47.5.

Chen and Kuo measured inspiratory muscle endurance against a resistive load and found significant decrements with age [16]. Physically active men had greater inspiratory muscle endurance than sedentary men.

In summary, it appears that when populations of healthy individuals of widely differing ages are studied, moderate

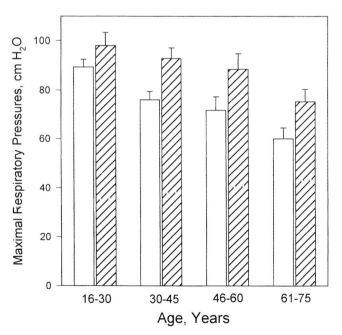

FIGURE 47.5 Representative variations in maximal respiratory pressure with age among women. Inspiratory and expiratory measurements were made at residual volume and total lung capacity, respectively. *Open bars*, maximal inspiratory pressure; *hatched bars*, maximal expiratory pressure. *Error bars* are standard errors of the mean. The variations with age were statistically significant but were small in magnitude (from Chen and Kuo [16], with permission).

age-related decrements in respiratory muscle strength and endurance can be found. These studies usually define "healthy" only by the absence of disease and do not control for physical activity. They are complicated by marked interindividual variability, and longitudinal studies have not been reported. Respiratory muscle function may be better preserved with age than that of other skeletal muscles because of a straining effect of the continuous respiratory muscle activity. Finally, physical activity may have an additional straining effect that enhances inspiratory muscle endurance in all age groups.

Control of Breathing

Stanley and colleagues have found that elderly subjects (mean age 69 years) have a slower, more variable respiratory rate than a young control group [17, 18]. It is doubtful that this isolated observation has any functional significance, but it did suggest that ventilatory control changes with aging.

More important is that ventilation becomes much less responsive to stress in elderly individuals. It is well known that in young individuals sensitive ventilatory control mechanisms match minute ventilation closely to metabolic demands. As a result, arterial blood-gas values remain stable throughout a wide range of activities from rest to strenuous exertion, whereas oxygen consumption and carbon dioxide production vary widely. Similarly, when the efficiency of gas exchange is diminished by a variety of lung problems (e.g., atelectasis and pneumonia) or congestive heart failure, appropriate increases in minute ventilation minimize the potential for resulting hypercapnia or hypoxemia in healthy young individuals.

To compare old and young individuals, ventilatory control mechanisms have typically been tested by inducing either hypoxemia or hypercapnia while monitoring ventilatory parameters. Such tests have shown striking differences between young and elderly individuals in ventilatory and cardiac responses [19–22].

Diminished Ventilatory Response to Hypercapnia

Kronenberg and Drage [21] compared the ventilatory responses to hypercapnia while $PACO_2$ was allowed to rise to 65 mmHg. The elderly individuals had a significantly diminished ventilatory response to hypercapnia, measured as the slope of the relation between ventilation and $PACO_2$.

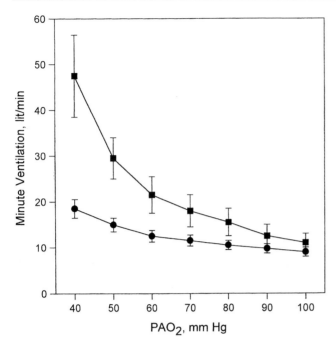

Figure 47.6 Variations in ventilatory responses to hypoxia, with age. Eight normal men aged 64–73 years (mean 69.6 years) (*circles*) were compared to young controls aged 22–30 years (mean 25.6 years) (*squares*). Ventilation was measured while the subjects were exposed to isocapnic progressive hypoxia by a rebreathing method. Values are means ± SEM. Note that the ventilatory responses were strikingly attenuated in the older individuals (from Kronenberg and Drage [21], with permission).

Diminished Ventilatory Response to Hypoxia

When these same authors [21] measured the ventilatory response to hypoxia, the contrasts between young and aged individuals were even more dramatic (Fig. 47.6). The ventilatory response to PAO_2 40 mmHg was uniformly smaller in the old subjects, and there was no overlap between the groups. The mean minute ventilation values at PAO_2 40 mmHg were 40.1 and 10.2 L/min in the young and old groups, respectively.

Diminished Occlusion Pressure Responses

Peterson and Fishman [23] showed that the differences in responses of elderly subjects to both hypercapnia and hypoxia are due to a lesser increase in tidal volume during stress, whereas the ventilatory rate increases normally. These authors also measured airway occlusion pressures, which are valuable indices of respiratory drive that are not affected by either respiratory muscle strength or respiratory mechanics. The measurements, called P_{100}, are the negative pressures at the mouth when measured 100 ms after the start of inspiration

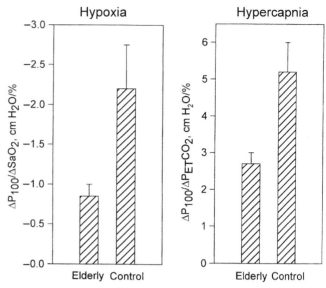

Figure 47.7 Variations in occlusion pressure responses to hypoxia and hypercapnia, with age. Data are slopes of the relations between occlusion pressure responses and either SaO_2 or end-tidal PCO_2; *error bars* are the SEM. Occlusion pressure responses are an indicator of ventilatory drive independent of chest wall compliance and respiratory muscle strength. The elderly individuals showed significantly and strikingly diminished ventilatory drives in response to both hypoxia and hypercapnia (from Peterson and Fishman [23], with permission).

against an occluded airway. The occlusion pressure responses to both hypoxia and hypercapnia (Fig. 47.7) were significantly reduced in ten elderly subjects (mean age 73.3 years) when compared to those of nine young control subjects (mean age 24.4 years) [22].

In summary, the compensatory change in tidal volume in response to either hypoxemia or hypercapnia is reduced (often strikingly) with age. The less-effective homeostasis is apparently due to reduced responsiveness of either the ventilatory drive or the neural output from the respiratory center. It has not been determined whether the diminished ventilatory drive results from altered chemoreceptor function or altered function of the respiratory center. Kronenberg and Drage favored altered receptor function based on their observation that elderly subjects responded to an alveolar oxygen tension of 40 mmHg with only an 11% increase in heart rate, whereas the young subjects responded with a 45% increase [21].

Respiratory Load Compensation and Dyspnea

Normally, when there is a change in the mechanical workload of the respiratory system (e.g., with lung disease, changes in posture, or mouth versus nose breathing), there is a reflex compensation that maintains the ventilation constant. To study the effects of aging, Akiyama and colleagues [24] measured responses to inspiratory flow-resistive loading in young and elderly individuals. In the young control group, inspiratory loading resulted in an increase in P_{100} at each level of induced hypercapnia, such that inspiratory loading did not change the ventilatory response to hypercapnia. In marked contrast, the P_{100} in the elderly group did not change when an inspiratory load was applied. Thus, ventilatory responses to hypercapnia were reduced during inspiratory loading in the elderly group.

At each level of PCO_2, the intensity of perceived dyspnea in response to inspiratory loading was higher in the elderly than in the control group. Thus, the sensation of dyspnea was intact or enhanced in the elderly subjects, while their compensatory responses were reduced.

Pulmonary Circulation

Pulmonary artery catheterization studies have typically been biased in that only subsets of patients have been reported. The reported studies were performed on individuals who had signs and symptoms that led to referral for heart catheterization. These individuals are probably not representative of "healthy" young and old cohorts. Furthermore, age-related changes in the pulmonary circulation are difficult or impossible to distinguish from changes due to heart disease or age-related changes in cardiac function. Even if they are real, the minor increases in pulmonary vascular resistance and age-related increases in pulmonary artery wedge pressure are probably not physiologically significant.

Pulmonary Function Tests

Several measurements of lung function and exercise capacity decline with age. However, descriptions of "normal" age-related changes are confounded by an increasing prevalence of disease, chronic illness, medication use, and an increasingly sedentary lifestyle. The influences of all of these factors are difficult to distinguish from each other. Superficially, it appears that longitudinal studies would provide the optimal design for distinguishing the effects of age from other influences. Longitudinal studies, however, have methodological problems and biases of their own, the most obvious being that the healthy elderly represent a healthy survival population. Regardless, it does seem that age alone has potentially important effects on lung function.

Lung Volumes

Figure 47.8 illustrates typical lung volume changes with aging based on cross-sectional studies. TLC, the volume of air in the lungs at the end of a maximal inspiration, is marked by the point at which the recoil pressure exerted by the respiratory system is exactly counterbalanced by the PI_{max} generated by the respiratory muscles. Cross-sectional studies of TLC summarized by the European Coal and Steel Community [25, 26], when combined, demonstrated no significant age coefficients for either men or women [25, 26].

Both slow and forced vital capacity (FVC) decline with age more rapidly in men than women. Average decrements in vital capacity per year vary considerably; in cross-sectional studies, declines range from 21 to 33 ml/year in men and 18 to 29 ml/year in women. Ware and colleagues [27], in a study containing both longitudinal and cross-sectional computations, found cross-sectional decreases in FVC for men and women to be −34 and −27.8 ml/year, respectively. Cross-sectional studies of residual volume (RV) and the RV/TLC ratio consistently show increases with age. In the young, RV (the volume of air in the lungs at the end of a maximal expiration) is the volume at which the outward static recoil pressure of the respiratory system is counterbalanced by the maximal pressure exerted by the expiratory muscles. In old subjects, the expiratory flow never completely reaches zero, and RV is determined in part by the length of time an individual can

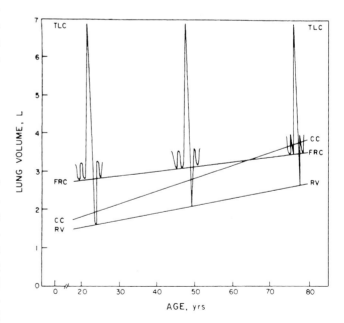

Figure 47.8 Lung volume changes with age. *TLC* total lung capacity, *CC* closing capacity, *FRC* functional residual capacity, *RV* residual volume. Although not labeled, the vital capacity is TLC minus RV. The most consistent age-related changes are an increase in RV and a decrease in ventilatory capacity (from Peterson and Fishman [23], with permission).

maintain the expiratory effort. Other factors leading to an increased RV with aging include loss of lung recoil, decreased chest wall compliance, decreased expiratory muscle force, and increased small airway closure (air trapping) in dependent lung zones [6].

FRC is also determined by the balance of the elastic recoil forces of the lung and chest wall, but in this instance, the equilibrium occurs at the end of a quiet (unforced) exhalation. Because lung recoil decreases and the chest wall stiffens with age, one would expect the FRC to increase. Cross-sectional studies, however, show inconsistent results, with most showing no change in FRC with aging. Studies that do find an increase in FRC with aging show a small positive age coefficient on the order of 7–16 ml/year. McClaran et al.'s longitudinal study found the FRC to increase 40 ml/year, but again the change was not significant [28]. Despite the conflicting data, it is generally believed that FRC increases somewhat with aging.

Loss of lung recoil also changes the volume at which airway closure occurs. When adults exhale fully, small airways close in the region of the terminal bronchioles in dependent lung zones. The lung volume at which this closure begins is measured as the closing volume or, if it is added to the residual volume, closing capacity. Closing volume increases linearly with age from about 5–10% of TLC at age 20 to about 30% of TLC at age 70. The loss of lung elastic recoil, a possible decrease in the recoil of the intrapulmonary airways, and decreases in small airway diameter probably explain most of the change in closing volume.

On average, closing volume encroaches on tidal volume by about age 44 when subjects are supine and at about age 65 when they are seated (Fig. 47.8). Airway closure during tidal breathing explains part of the decrease in arterial oxygen tension observed with aging.

Airflow

Although essentially all expiratory flows measured during a maximum expiratory maneuver decrease with age, the declines are most evident at low lung volumes (Fig. 47.9). Nunn and Dregg [29], in a study of 225 male and 228 healthy female nonsmokers, reported a modest decrease in peak expiratory flow (PEF) with aging. The rate of decline in FVC and forced expiratory volume at 1 s (FEV_1) with age tends to be more in (1) men, (2) tall individuals, (3) individuals with large baseline values, and (4) individuals with increased airway reactivity. Total airway resistance, measured at FRC, does not change with aging.

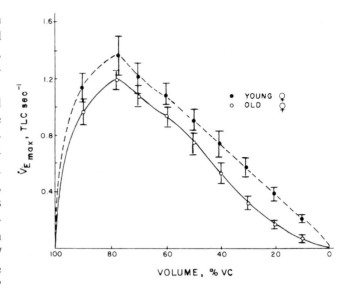

Figure 47.9 Maximal flow-volume curves, showing the changes in expiratory flow rates with age. Data are for elderly women (mean age 63 years) and control young women (mean age 25 years). Although all flows tend to be reduced with aging, the reduction in flow is most evident at lower lung volumes, where the flow-volume curve is concave in regard to the volume axis (from Peterson and Fishman [23], with permission).

Gas Exchange

The carbon monoxide diffusing capacity (DL_{CO}) declines with age. Early cross-sectional studies reported a linear decline in DL_{CO} of about −0.1 ml CO/min/mmHg/year for men and −0.15 ml/min/mmHg/year for women [30, 31]. These declines are roughly 0.5% per year. In a large representative sample of US adult men, Neas and Schwartz [32] found an almost identical linear fall in DL_{CO}. In women, however, they found a nonlinear, quadratic decline in DL_{CO} with age. After age 47, the nonlinear component was not significant, and the decline in DL_{CO} was identical to that in the earlier studies. The decline in DL_{CO} with age did not vary with race.

The decline in DL_{CO} with age is not explained by increased nonhomogeneity of gas distribution. Measured DL_{CO} decreases as the alveolar PO_2 increases and the venous hemoglobin concentration falls. Neither alveolar PO_2 nor hemoglobin concentration varies enough with age to explain the aging-related decline in DL_{CO}. The magnitude of the decline in DL_{CO} corresponds fairly well to the magnitude of the known aging-related decrease in the internal surface area of the lung.

Although alveolar oxygen pressure (PAO_2) remains constant with age, arterial PO_2 decreases, and the alveolar–arterial oxygen tension gradient ($PA-aO_2$) increases with

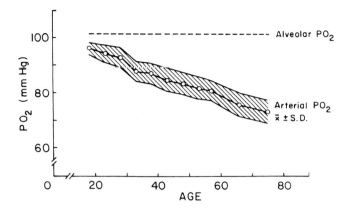

Figure 47.10 Decreasing arterial oxygen tension (PO_2) with age. The lack of change in alveolar oxygen tension is also shown for comparison with PaO_2. The widening alveolar–arterial partial pressure difference for oxygen results from the development of basilar areas of low ventilation/perfusion ratios due to airway closure in the elderly (modified from Sorbini et al. [33], with permission).

aging (Fig. 47.10). The decline in PaO_2 with aging is more pronounced when subjects are studied in a recumbent as contrasted with an upright position. The most likely explanation for the decline in PaO_2 with aging is increased mismatching of ventilation to blood flow ($\dot{V}/\dot{Q}$) as airway closure begins to occur during tidal breathing.

Summary and Implications for Geriatric Surgery

Aging is accompanied by readily measurable changes in respiratory system mechanics, gas exchange, ventilatory control, and respiratory muscle strength. Despite these changes, the activities of normal elderly individuals are not limited because they have substantial functional reserve of the respiratory system early in their lives. When anticipating operative morbidity and potential operative complications, however, the surgeon must be aware that elderly patients have lost much, or all, of their respiratory reserve. Operative stresses, pain, and bed rest are always less well tolerated by the respiratory system of elderly patients.

Changes in ventilatory control among geriatric patients deserve special attention. Because of changes in chemoreceptor function and respiratory center function, elderly individuals respond differently to hypoxemia and hypercapnia than their younger counterparts. Thus, an elderly patient who is developing respiratory failure may appear comfortable and may not be tachypneic or tachycardic. Vigilance and awareness on the part of the health-care team allow detection of respiratory complications early, through measurement of oxygen saturation and arterial blood gases. Such vigilance allows appropriate *nonemergent* interventions.

Acknowledgment Supported in part by U.S. Public Health Service grant 46440.

References

1. Gibellino F, Osmanliev DP, Watson A, Pride NB (1985) Increase in tracheal size with age: implications for maximal expiratory flow. Am Rev Respir Dis 132:784–787
2. Thurlbeck WM, Angus GE (1975) Growth and aging of the normal human lung. Chest 67:3S–7S
3. Snider GL, Kleinerman J, Thurlbeck WM, Bengali ZH (1985) The definition of emphysema: Report of a National Heart, Lung, and Blood Institute, Division of Lung Diseases workshop. Am Rev Respir Dis 132:182–185
4. Pump KK (1971) The aged lung. Chest 60:571–577
5. Ryan SF, Vincent TN, Mitchell RS, Filley GF, Dart G (1965) Ductectasia: an asymptomatic pulmonary change related to age. Med Thorac 22:181–187
6. Pride NB (1974) Pulmonary distensibility in age and disease. Bull Eur Physiopathol Respir 124:103–108
7. Knudson RJ, Clark DF, Kennedy TC, Knudson DE (1977) Effect of aging alone on mechanical properties of the normal adult human lung. J Appl Physiol 43:1054–1062
8. Turner JM, Mead J, Wohl ME (1968) Elasticity of human lungs in relation to age. J Appl Physiol 25:664–671
9. Pierce JA, Ebert RV (1965) Fibrous network of the lung and its change with age. Thorax 20:469–476
10. Pierce JA, Hocott JB, Ebert RV (1961) The collagen and elastin content of the lung in emphysema. Ann Intern Med 55:210–222
11. Shapiro SD, Pierce JA, Endicott SK, Campbell EJ (1991) Marked longevity of human lung parenchymal elastic fibers deduced from prevalence of d-aspartate and nuclear weapons-related radiocarbon. J Clin Invest 87:1828–1834
12. Mittman C, Edelman NH, Norris AH, Shock NW (1965) Relationship between chest wall and pulmonary compliance and age. J Appl Physiol 20:1211–1216
13. Crapo RO, Campbell EJ (1998) Aging of the respiratory system. In: Fishman AP, Elias JA, Fishman JA, Grippi MA, Kaiser LR, Senior RM (eds) Fishman's pulmonary diseases and disorders. McGraw-Hill, New York, pp 251–264
14. Black LF, Hyatt RE (1969) Maximal respiratory pressures: normal values and relationship to age and sex. Am Rev Respir Dis 99:696–702
15. McElvaney GL, Blackie S, Morrison NJ, Wilcox PG, Fairbarn MS, Pardy RL (1995) Maximal static respiratory pressures in the normal elderly. Am Rev Respir Dis 139:277–281
16. Chen H-S, Kuo C-S (1989) Relationship between respiratory muscle function and age, sex, and other factors. J Appl Physiol 56:1143–1150
17. Stanley G, Verotta D, Craft N, Siegel RA, Schwartz JB (1996) Age and autonomic effects on interrelationships between lung volume and heart rate. Am J Physiol 270:H1833–H1840
18. Stanley G, Verotta D, Craft N, Siegel RA, Schwartz JB (1997) Age effects on interrelationships between lung volume and heart rate during standing. Am J Physiol 273:H2128–H2134
19. Brichetto MJ, Millman RP, Peterson DD, Silage DA, Pack AI (1984) Effect of aging on ventilatory response to exercise and CO_2. J Appl Physiol 56:1143–1150
20. Chapman KR, Cherniack NS (1987) Aging effects on the interaction of hypercapnia and hypoxia as ventilatory stimuli. J Gerontol 42:202–209
21. Kronenberg RS, Drage CW (1973) Attenuation of the ventilatory and heart rate responses to hypoxia and hypercapnia with aging in normal men. J Clin Invest 53:1812–1819

22. Peterson DD, Pack AI, Silage DA, Fishman AP (1981) Effects of aging on the ventilatory and occlusion pressure responses to hypoxia and hypercapnia. Am Rev Respir Dis 124:387–391

23. Peterson DD, Fishman AP (1992) Aging of the respiratory system. In: Fishman AP (ed) Update: pulmonary diseases and disorders. McGraw-Hill, New York, pp 1–17

24. Akiyama Y, Nishimura M, Kobayashi S, Yamamoto M, Miyamoto K, Kawakami Y (1993) Effects of aging on respiratory load compensation and dyspnea sensation. Am Rev Respir Dis 148:1586–1591

25. Quanjer PH (1983) Standardized lung function. Bull Eur Physiopathol Respir 19:45–51

26. Quanjer PH (1983) Standardized lung function. Bull Eur Physiopathol Respir 19:66–92

27. Ware JH, Dockery DW, Louis TA et al (1990) Longitudinal and cross-sectional estimates of pulmonary function decline in never-smoking adults. Am J Epidemiol 131:685–700

28. McClaran SR, Babcock MA, Pegelow DF, Reddan WG, Dempsey JA (1995) Longitudinal effects of aging on lung function at rest and exercise in healthy active fit elderly adults. J Appl Physiol 78:1957–1958

29. Nunn AJ, Gregg I (1989) New regression equations for predicting peak expiratory flow in adults. Br Med J 298:1068–1070

30. Crapo RO, Gardner RM (1987) Single breath carbon monoxide diffusing capacity (transfer factor): recommendations for a standard technique. Am Rev Respir Dis 136:1299–1307

31. Stam H, Hrachovina V, Stijnen T, Versprille A (1994) Diffusing capacity dependent on lung volume and age in normal subjects. J Appl Physiol 76:2356–2363

32. Neas LM, Schwartz J (1966) The determinants of pulmonary diffusing capacity in a national sample of U.S. adults. Am J Respir Crit Care Med 153:656–664

33. Sorbini CA, Grassi V, Solinas E, Muiesan G (1968) Arterial oxygen tension in relation to age in healthy subjects. Respiration 25:3–13

Chapter 48
Pulmonary Surgery for Malignant Disease in the Elderly

Sarah E. Billmeier and Michael T. Jaklitsch

CASE STUDY

Ms. Jones is an 82-year-old F who was in her usual state of good health when she developed a fever and cough. A chest X-ray revealed left upper lobe pneumonia and she was successfully treated with a course of antibiotics. Three months later her pneumonia recurred, and at that time a chest CT showed a left upper lobe nodule. A biopsy of the nodule was consistent with adenocarcinoma, and she was referred for thoracic surgery evaluation.

On evaluation Ms. Jones is found to be healthy and active, despite recent flares of arthritis in her hands. Her family refers to her as "well preserved." She walks daily for a quarter mile with her family, shops for her own groceries and enjoys gardening. She carries a basket of laundry up two flights of stairs every day, and carries two bags of groceries at a time into the kitchen

from her car. She had a myocardial infarction 17 years ago and 2 years ago had a cardiac stent placed. She has a history of reflux disease which seems to be worsening over the past year. She has osteoarthritis and the kyphosis in her back has become quite obvious. She has a distant 27-pack year smoking history. She has extensive social supports and is viewed as the matriarch of a family that includes 6 children and 21 grandchildren. Her first great grandchild is expected this fall. She is active in her church and volunteers at a shelter serving meals once a month.

Pulmonary function tests are notable for good lung function with an FEV1 of 1.8 L (81% predicted) and an FVC of 2.6 L (88% predicted). She is able to walk 1,400 feet in 6 min without hypoxia. She is able to climb two flights of stairs without difficulty. A brain MRI, bronchoscopy, and mediastinoscopy are all negative. How does Ms. Jones advanced age affect her management?

Introduction

With the aging of the baby boomer population, the number of people in the USA over 65 is expected to nearly double by 2040. Currently 12.5% of the US population is over the age of 65, and this percentage is projected to increase to 20% by the year 2050. The average life expectancy in the USA is 77.8 and projected to increase to over 80 by 2050 [1–4].

Older patients increasingly present for consideration of thoracic surgery, and determining the optimal management for this group of patients will be a more frequent challenge in the future. While elderly patients present with a spectrum of thoracic disease, both benign and malignant, patients with

cancer comprise the largest and most studied subset of this population.

Lung cancer is a disease of the elderly. The median age of diagnosis for lung cancer in the USA is 71 years and over 65% of patients are diagnosed after age 65. National Cancer Institute statistics indicate that lung cancer is the leading cause of cancer mortality in men and women [5, 6]. In 2008 an estimated 215,020 Americans will be diagnosed and 161,840 people will die of lung cancer. Over 100,000 lung cancer deaths will be in patients over the age of 65 [7].

Non-small cell lung cancer (NSCLC) comprises 80–85% of primary lung tumors, small cell lung cancer (SCLC) makes up 15–20% and 1–2% are pulmonary carcinoid [8–10]. SCLC is usually widely metastatic at time of diagnosis, and rarely under the purview of the surgeon; however, the percentage of lung cancer patients with SCLC histology falls with age [10]. Surgical resection of NSCLC and pulmonary carcinoid offers the best chance for oncologic cure. Additionally, retrospective

---

S.E. Billmeier (✉)
General Surgery, Brigham and Women's Hospital, Boston, MA, USA
e-mail: sbillmeier@partners.org

R.A. Rosenthal et al. (eds.), *Principles and Practice of Geriatric Surgery*,
DOI 10.1007/978-1-4419-6999-6_48, © Springer Science+Business Media, LLC 2011

evidence suggests that resection of isolated metastases to the lung may improve survival.

The decision to undergo surgical resection for malignant disease should not be based on age alone. An understanding of the unique qualities of this patient population has lead to improved surgical outcomes for the elderly over the last several decades. Patient evaluation, selection, and peri-operative management must all be adapted to provide best possible care for the increasing numbers of aged patients undergoing surgery for cancer. Management of an elderly lung cancer patient requires a global consideration of the characteristics of aging, differences in tumor presentation and histology, and co-morbidities that tend to accumulate over time. The initial interview with a patient and family members is used to elucidate important variables that may impact operative risk and expectations of the recovery process. These questions should elucidate the current independent status of the patient, social supports, mood, and signs of reduced activity or physical limitations. After all, the elderly population is a heterogeneous group of patients ranging in functional reserve from the surprisingly well preserved to the wheelchair bound.

Physiologic Changes of Age

Physiologic changes of the respiratory system associated with aging include reduced chest wall compliance with stiffening of calcified costal cartilages and narrowing of the intervertebral disc space. A progressively restricted ribcage is accompanied by decreased diaphragmatic excursion. Postoperative weakness of the hemi-diaphragm in this group can lead to otherwise unexplained respiratory failure. There is a reduction of lung elastic recoil with loss of alveolar architecture producing a decreased alveolar gas exchange surface. The loss of lung elastic recoil and decreased lung compliance diminishes negative intrapleural pressure, which then prevents reopening of the small airways, resulting in air trapping and inadequate ventilation. Functionally this manifests in a gradual decline of vital capacity and partial pressure of oxygen (Po_2), with an increase in residual volume. Progressive atrophy creates weakness of the respiratory musculature. Decline in motor power of the accessory muscles and a stiffening of the chest wall also result in a declining forced expiratory volume in 1 s (FEV1). Changes in lung compliance are not uniformly distributed. Higher respiratory rates therefore increase ventilation–perfusion mismatch. Additionally, there is a decrease in central nervous system responsiveness. The elderly exhibit a blunted ventilatory response to both hypoxic and hypercapneic insults [11, 12].

Physiologic changes in lung mechanics make elderly patients particularly sensitive to narcotics and muscle relaxants, as well as to supine positioning. Elderly patients are also at increased risk for respiratory tract infections, due to waning immune responses [13]. Smoking in particular has been shown to cause bronchial mucociliary dysfunction [14]. which has been associated with increased susceptibility to infection [15]. Finally, elderly patients with marked kyphosis and accompanying paraesophageal diaphragmatic hernias are at particular risk for postoperative aspiration.

Increasing age is associated with declines in other organ systems as well. There is a decline in glomerular filtration rate, an increasing incidence of heart disease, and an increasing incidence of cognitive dysfunction. Changes in body composition decrease the volume of distribution of water-soluble drugs [16]. Additionally, elderly patients take more medications than younger patients and are vulnerable to adverse drug effects.

Preoperative Evaluation

Elderly patients are at increased risk for preoperative morbidity and mortality due to both decreased ability to recover physiologic homeostasis after surgical stress and co-morbid conditions. Older patients represent a heterogeneous population, and should be offered surgery based on physiologic rather than chronological age. A thorough preoperative assessment is imperative to determine whether a patient is an appropriate surgical candidate and to predict and avoid postoperative complications. Numerous risk assessment tools have been created to define preoperative variables that correlate with poor outcomes; however, an easy to use, strongly predictive tool, has been elusive. Geriatric assessment tools aimed at predicting outcomes in the specific elderly surgical population remain under study.

All patients in consideration for lung cancer resection surgery require a complete history and physical exam with particular attention to characterization of symptoms, smoking history, and weight loss. At a minimum, patients should undergo a chest X-ray, electrocardiogram, a room air arterial blood gas, pulmonary function tests for patients undergoing lung resection, basic laboratory work, and a complete staging evaluation. Further workup can be determined based on symptoms or the status of co-morbid conditions.

Accurate diagnosis and staging is of utmost importance to ensure that patients are appropriately chosen for operative resection. Elderly patients should have radiographic and surgical staging of suspected lung cancers in the same manner as younger counterparts. Only after the exact stage is known can rational treatment decisions be made. Therefore, elderly patients should have chest CT scans to image suspected lung nodules, PET scans to look for metastatic disease, brain scans to look for occult metastases and, if indicated, cervical mediastinoscopy to stage mediastinal nodes. Elderly patients with suspected lung nodules should not be denied this standard workup unless their functional status is so impaired that treatment is not possible.

Cardiac Risk Assessment

The American Heart Association (AHA) and American College of Cardiology (ACC) developed consensus practice guideline for peri-operative cardiovascular evaluation for non-cardiac surgery that provides a template for assessing patients of all ages [17]. The AHA/ACC guidelines describe a step-wise approach to preoperative surgery with risk stratification and further imaging determined by utilizing symptoms, clinical predictors, and functional capacity. Clinical history should focus on assessment for coronary risk factors and physical capacity including the ability to climb two flights of stairs or walk one block. In general, patients with poor functional status, or patients with a history of angina or claudication should undergo noninvasive testing. In thoracic surgery patients it may be difficult to determine if symptom etiology is the result of cardiac or pulmonary pathology, thus it is appropriate to have a low threshold for additional cardiac imaging and assessment by a cardiologist to assist with risk stratification.

Supraventricular tachycardias are very common after thoracic surgery, with increased risk for older patients or those with a faster preoperative heart rate [18]. The risk of postoperative atrial fibrillation is 19% in patients undergoing lung resection for cancer [19]. Randomized trials of thoracic surgery patients have determined that calcium channel blockers or beta-blockers can reduce the incidence of postoperative atrial fibrillation by 50–60%; however, beta-blockers were associated with an increased risk of pulmonary edema. Neither class of medication reduced mortality. Three trials showed that digitalis increased the risk of atrial arrhythmias [20]. Beta-blockers and calcium channel blockers will both reduce postoperative atrial fibrillation; however, beta-blockers are preferred by some due to their broader benefits of cardiac risk reduction. On the other hand, up to half the doses of postoperative beta-blocker may have to be held due to transient hypotension or bradycardia, leading others to recommend the use of calcium channel blockers.

Pulmonary Risk Assessment

All patients under consideration for lung resection surgery should have pulmonary function tests performed. FEV1 by spirometry is the most common measured value used to determine a patient's suitability for surgery. In the 1970s, data obtained from over 2,000 patients showed a <5% mortality rate for patients with an FEV1 >1.5 L for lobectomy and >2 L for pneumonectomy [21, 22]. Absolute values for FEV1 may create a bias against older people; however, a value of >80% of predicted has been quoted by some as sufficient for a patient to undergo pneumonectomy without further pulmonary testing [23]. In reviewing more recent spirometry studies performed from NSCLC patients in 1994–2000, Datta and

Lahiri concluded that increased postoperative morbidity and mortality were predicted by an FEV1 of <2 L or <60% predicted for pneumonectomy, an FEV1 of <1.6 L for lobectomy, and <0.6 L for wedge or segmentectomy [24].

Lung resections have been undertaken in patients with much poorer lung function. In 2005, Linden et al. published data from a series of 100 consecutive patients with preoperative FEV1 of <35% predicted undergoing lung tumor resection. In this series, there was a 1% mortality rate (single case of perforated colonic diverticulum) and a 36% complication rate. Morbidity was dominated by 22% of patients with prolonged air leaks. Eleven patients were discharged with a new oxygen requirement, and four patients developed pneumonia. Only one patient was discharged on a ventilator and three other patients required intubation for >48 h [25].

In a study of 237 patients, Ferguson et al. found preoperative diffusion capacity for carbon monoxide (DLCO) to be more predictive of postoperative mortality than FEV1. In this study, a DLCO of <60% predicted was associated with increased mortality and a DLCO of <80% predicted was predictive of increased pulmonary complications [26]. Other studies, however, have not found this parameter to be a significant predictor of postoperative complications [27, 28]. DLCO and spirometry may be used as complimentary tests, particularly in patients with diffuse parenchymal disease or dyspnea that is out of proportion to the FEV1, with a low DLCO prompting further evaluation [22].

Formal and simple exercise testing evaluates the cardiopulmonary system under induced physiological stress and also has been found to be predictive of postoperative complications. Girish et al. prospectively studied symptom-limited stair climbing in thoracic and upper abdominal surgery patients. No complications occurred in patients who could climb seven flights of stairs, while 89% of patients unable to climb one flight of stairs had complications. Inability to climb two flights of stairs had a positive predictive value of 80%. The ability of patients to climb stairs was found to be inversely related to the length of postoperative hospital stay [29]. The 6-min walk test (6MWT) measures the distanced walked over a period of 6 min. A normal patient is able to cover at least 1,400 feet in 6 min. In a qualitative review, Solway concluded that the 6MWT was easy to administer and more reflective of activities of daily living than other walk tests [30]. While stair climbing and 6MWT are easy to perform, their use in elderly patients may be limited by orthopedic impairments, peripheral vascular insufficiency or neurological impairments.

As published previously [31], a recommended preoperative pulmonary evaluation for an elderly patient should consist of spirometry, pulmonary diffusion capacity of the lung for carbon monoxide (DLCO), room air ABG, and exercise tolerance tests including stair climbing and 6-min walk. Patients with an FEV1 >1 L and no major abnormality of other tests (FEV1/FVC >50%, DLCO >50% predicted, ABG paO_2 >45 mm Hg, tolerance of exercise tests) may

Figure 48.1 Recommended pulmonary evaluation for patients undergoing lung resection surgery. *DLCO* diffusion capacity for carbon monoxide, *ABG* arterial blood gas, *FEV1* forced expiratory volume in 1 s, *FVC* forced vital capacity, *VO₂ Max* maximal oxygen consumption, *PPO* predicted postoperative.

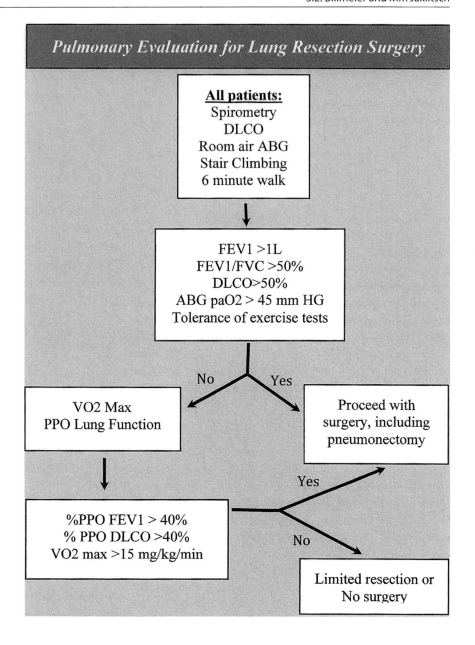

safely proceed with surgery, including pneumonectomy (Fig. 48.1).

Further evaluation for patients who fall outside these criteria include ventilation/perfusion scans to calculate predicted postoperative (PPO) lung function and VO₂ max testing. A PPO FEV1 threshold of 0.8 L [32] or 0.7 L [33] has been suggested as a lower limit value for proceeding with lung resection. Absolute values of PPO FEV1 can underestimate postoperative lung function in people with small stature or the elderly, and can thus be converted into percent-predicted postoperative (% PPO) lung function. Multiple studies have suggested that morbidity increases at a threshold % PPO FEV1 of <40%, or a % PPO DLCO of <40% [26, 34–37].

Measurement of maximal oxygen consumption (VO₂ max) by formal cardiopulmonary exercise testing is helpful to further risk stratify patients with borderline lung function. A VO₂ max of <10 ml/kg/min had a very high operative morbidity (26% total in combined data) in several small case series. VO₂ max values of 10–15 ml/kg/min had an intermediate peri-operative morbidity (8.3% total) whereas patients with >15 mg/kg/min can proceed with lung resection surgery with an acceptable mortality rate [22].

Cognitive Assessment

The likelihood of returning to baseline physical and mental function after surgery is one of the most important outcomes for an elderly patient. While patients and their families accept that there will be a postoperative recovery time in the hospital or rehabilitation setting, it is difficult to assess the magnitude of this functional decline and predict the risk of permanent loss of independence. There is a paucity of data assessing changes in quality of life after thoracic surgery in the elderly, and few studies that assess whether surgery triggers postoperative loss of independence, or change in need for assistance or living requirements. A study of 68 octogenarians undergoing pulmonary resections at Johns Hopkins Medical Institutions showed that 80% of patients were discharged directly to home from the hospital rather than to rehab, offering some proxy information regarding immediate postoperative return to function [38]. Moller et al. published a study in 1998 that showed a 25% rate of cognitive dysfunction at 1 week postop from major noncardiac surgery in elderly patients (average age 68), with continued dysfunction in 9% at 3 months [39]. Data from many studies verify a high incidence of postoperative cognitive dysfunction in the first week after surgery, and dysfunction does tend to increase with age. Only one other study has substantiated long-term declines over controls, and some have suggested that declines found in these studies may be due to random variation [40, 41]. Karneko et al. determined that preoperative dementia was a risk factor for postoperative delirium [42]. Furthermore, Fukuse et al. found that thoracic surgery patients with preoperative dementia, as estimated by the mini-mental status exam (MMS), were fourfold more likely to have postoperative complications [43].

Geriatric Assessments

There are multiple assessment indices that have been applied to elderly patients to link preoperative function with risk for poor outcome. Functional status describes the ability to perform self-care, self-maintenance, and physical activities. Traditional measures used to assess functional status are activities of daily living (ADLs) and instrumental activities of daily living (IADLs). ADLs are six basic self-care skills, including the ability to bathe, dress, go to the toilet, transfer from a bed to chair, maintain continence, and feed one's self. IADLs include higher functioning skills that are used to maintain independence in the community. This scale assesses ability to use the telephone, go shopping, prepare food, perform housekeeping and laundry, use various modes of transportation, assume responsibility for medications, and

the ability to handle finances. Need for assistance in these tasks has been predictive of prolonged hospital stay, nursing home placement and home-care requirements [44, 45]. Poor nutritional status, defined as a BMI <22 kg/m^2 has been associated with increased need for assistance with ADLs and a decreased 1-year survival [46]. A lower ADL score is associated with postoperative complications [47]. The information source reporting a patient's functional status biases the results, with self-reported scores rating higher than scores reported by a significant other or nurse [48].

Performance status is a standardized scale designed to measure the ability of a cancer patient to perform ordinary tasks. There are two scales, the Karnofsky performance scale, which ranges from 0 (dead) to 100 (normal) and the ECOG scale that ranges from 0 (asymptomatic) to 5 (dead). Comparisons of the two scales have been validated with a large sample of patients [49]. Performance status has been used to select patients for entry into chemotherapy trials; however, it is also well accepted to be associated with postoperative morbidity [50–52].

Postoperative Care

Postoperative management must be optimized specifically for the elderly population. Narcotic use should be minimized whenever possible to prevent delirium, and appropriate elderly patients should be assessed for preoperative placement of a thoracic epidural catheter for analgesia. Benzodiazapines and medications for sleep should also be minimized. Excellent pulmonary hygiene must be maintained with frequent chest physiotherapy and early ambulation. At our institution, thoracic ambulation carts, as shown in Fig. 48.2, are used to facilitate walking patients who require oxygen, and are otherwise tethered with multiple lines and catheters. Forearms are supported by pads while hands wrap around a handbrake. Oxygen tanks and ambulatory saturation monitors are stored along the sides. Pleural drainage systems can be suspended from the side rails. A cloth strap is used to secure the patient to the cart during ambulation.

Non-small Cell Lung Cancer

Stage at Presentation

Elderly patients more frequently have early-stage disease, compared to younger patients with lung cancer. O'Rourke et al. used a database of 22,874 patients to demonstrate that percentage of patients with surgically resectable disease at

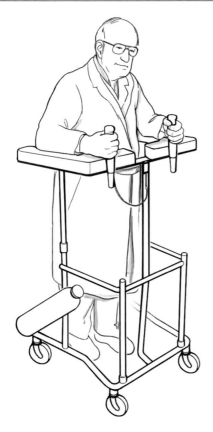

Figure 48.2 Thoracic ambulation cart used to facilitate early postoperative ambulation (artwork by Marcia Williams).

diagnosis increases with age. The percent of lung cancer patients with local stage NSCLC increased from 15.3% of those aged 54 years or younger, to 19.2% of those aged 55–64 years, to 21.9% of those aged 65–74 years, and to 25.4% of those aged 75 years or older [53]. Data published from the Surveillance, epidemiology, and end results (SEER) database in 2005 analyzing a cohort of 14,555 patients with early-stage NSCLC showed that the frequency of stage I disease increased from 79% in patients <65 to 87% in patients age 75 or greater [54]. Thus, although the elderly are at higher risk of developing lung cancer, a higher proportion present with potentially curable disease.

Histology

Elderly patients are more likely to be diagnosed with squamous cell carcinoma (SCC) over other histology types [10, 55, 56]. Mery et al.'s analysis of the SEER database showed that the frequency of SCC increased from 27% in patients <65 years old, to 38% in patients 75 and older, with parallel decreases in frequency of adenocarcinoma from 61 to 50% in corresponding age groups [54]. SCCs are associated with a higher incidence of local disease [53], tend to

have lower recurrence rates and may have longer survival times than non-squamous cell cancers [57–59]. Squamous cell tumors are more likely to be centrally located however, and thus are more likely to require pneumonectomy for curative resection.

Extent of Resection

Surgical resection for NSCLC offers the best chance for cure. The extent of NSCLC resection in elderly patients has been extensively debated, with advocates for limited resections for the aged. Lobectomy, removal of one of the five lobes of the lung and associated lymph nodes within a single pleural membrane, is considered standard of care for surgical resection of early-stage NSCLC [60]. Unfortunately there are multiple studies that substantiate age as a risk factor for death after thoracotomy. Using data from the 1960s and 1970s, several small single institution studies published operative mortality rates of 14–27% for the elderly depending on age and type of surgery [61–64]. These findings were confirmed by a multiinstitution study by the Lung Cancer Study Group in 1983. Ginsberg et al. reviewed 2,200 cases of lung resection for cancer and found that operative mortality increased proportionally with age. Patients with age <60 had a 1.3% 30-day mortality rate, with increasing rates of 4.1, 7.0, and 8.1% mortality rates for the 60–69, 70–79, and 80 or greater age groups, respectively [65].

More recently, Mery et al. determined a 30-day postoperative mortality rate of 14,555 patients who had undergone curative resections for treating stage I or II NSCLC over the period of 1992–1997. In an analysis of patients undergoing all types of surgery, there was a 0.45% mortality rate for those under age 65 years old, 0.6% for ages 65–74, and 1.2% for patients age 75 or older ($p = 0.001$). Mortality differences were found to be primarily due to differences in survival of patient undergoing lobectomy, with 0.3, 0.5, and 1.5% mortality, respectively, for these corresponding age groups ($p = 0.0001$). The difference in peri-operative mortality was statistically similar for patients undergoing limited resection [66]. Prior published reports likewise did not identify a difference in expected operative mortality after thoracotomy if lung-sparing operations were performed [67–69].

The American College of Surgeons Oncology Group (ACOSOG) Z0030 Study published morbidity and mortality data in 2006 for 1,023 clinically resectable T1 or T2, N0 or non-hilar N1 NSCLC patients randomized over a period from 1999 to 2004 to undergo pulmonary resection with lymph node sampling vs. mediastinal lymph node dissection. Their age-stratified morbidity and mortality data is shown in Table 48.1. Notably, overall mortality was 1.4%, improved from Ginsberg's reported 3.8%, and was not statistically associated with age [70]. Ninety percent of patients in

TABLE 48.1 ACOSOG Z0030 Study age-stratified morbidity and mortality after resection for clinically resectable T1 or T2, N0 or non-hilar N1 NSCLC

Event	Age <50 ($n=35$)	50–59 ($n=171$)	60–69 ($n=386$)	70–79 ($n=361$)	80+ ($n=70$)
One or more complications	8 (23%)	50 (29%)	136 (35%)	162 (45%)	34 (49%)
Air leak >7 days	1 (3%)	14 (8%)	24 (6%)	33 (9%)	6 (9%)
Chest tube drainage >7 days	0	14 (8%)	42 (11%)	53 (15%)	9 (13%)
Chylothorax	1 (3%)	3 (2%)	3 (1%)	5 (1%)	1 (1%)
Hemorrhage	1 (3%)	3 (2%)	10 (3%)	16 (4%)	4 (6%)
Recurrent nerve injury	0	0	5 (1%)	2 (<1%)	0
Atrial arrhythmia	1 (3%)	13 (8%)	53 (14%)	68 (19%)	12 (17%)
Respiratory	4 (12%)	8 (5%)	30 (8%)	29 (8%)	3 (4%)
Death	1 (2.6%)	0	3 (0.8%)	8 (2.2%)	2 (2.9%)

Source: Reprinted with permission from [70] Copyright Elsevier 2005

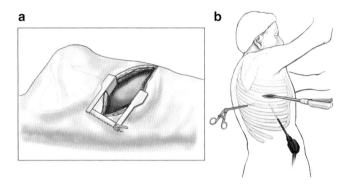

FIGURE 48.3 Lung resection surgery via (**a**) posteriolateral thoracotomy (**b**) video-assisted thoracoscopic surgery (artwork by Marcia Williams).

the ACOSOG Z0030 study underwent resection via a thoracotomy, with the remaining procedures performed as video-assisted thoracic surgery (VATS) or VATS-assisted resections. Operative mortality reported by Ginsberg for pneumonectomy and lobectomy was 6.2 and 2.9%, respectively, compared with 0 and 1.3%, in the ACOSOG study. Notably the pneumonectomy rate of the earlier study was 25.6 vs. 4% in ACOSOG, likely partially explaining the higher mortality rate of the earlier study. The complication rate did rise as age increased, with 49% of patients in the 80 and over age group experiencing one or more complication.

The operative risk of death after pulmonary resections is largely attributable to two anatomical disruptions. First there is the loss of functional lung tissue, and secondly there is the morbidity and mortality introduced by the access thoracotomy. Operative strategies particular to the elderly population addresses both of these fronts, with use of video-assisted thoracoscopic surgery (VATS) to minimize the chest wall disruption of a thoracotomy and by consideration of limited resections for the most elderly. Figure 48.3 illustrates the difference in the disruption of chest wall musculature between thoracotomy and VATS approaches.

VATS is defined as surgery performed through two or three incisions that are 2 cm in length. A utility incision <10 cm long may be used, without spreading of the ribs.

VATS procedures in the elderly have been shown to have lower morbidity, lower rates of postoperative delirium and result in earlier ambulation, a lower narcotic requirement, and a quicker recovery time [71–75].

Limited resections, consisting of either a sementectomy or wedge resection, remove less lung tissue and are usually performed via VATS. These operations are associated with less peri-operative morbidity and mortality; however, do not completely remove draining lymphatics and may be associated with poorer oncologic outcomes. A randomized trial by the Lung Cancer Study Group of limited resection vs. lobectomy for T1 N0 disease revealed a tripling of locoregional recurrence with limited resection, and a trend toward improved survival in the lobectomy group [76]. Divergence of the survival curves between lobectomy and limited resection did not occur until 3 years after surgery, however, indicating a potential role for limited resection in patients with a shorter expected life span. Additional studies have concluded that limited resection remains a "compromise" treatment for elderly patients or those with limited cardiopulmonary reserve [77]. An age-stratified analysis of 14,555 patients in the SEER database, showed no benefit for lobectomy over limited resection in patients over age 71 [54]. Figure 48.4 shows a schematic of the range of lung resections. The decision to perform a limited resection vs. a lobectomy must take into account the patient's ability to tolerate a larger surgery and potential associated complications vs. a smaller resection with less durable oncologic outcomes.

Pulmonary Carcinoid

Pulmonary carcinoids represent 1–2% of lung tumors. They consist of a spectrum of neuroendocrine tumors that are divided into those with typical (TC) or atypical (AC) histological features. While carcinoids tend to present in younger patients, atypical tumors are often diagnosed about 10 years later than typical carcinoid, occurring in the sixth decade.

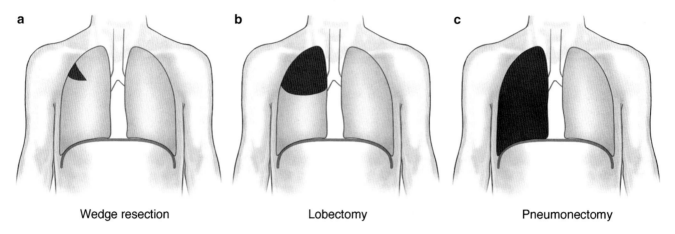

Figure 48.4 Extent of resection, (**a**) wedge resection, (**b**) lobectomy, (**c**) and pneumonectomy (artwork by Marcia Williams).

Atypical carcinoids tend to be larger, are usually localized to the peripheral lung fields, and are more aggressive than typical carcinoids. The 5-year survival is 40–60 vs. 90% for indolent typical carcinoids [78]. Limited resection with wedge or segmentectomy is the preferred treatment for localized carcinoids. More extensive resection has been advocated for atypical carcinoids, with extent of resection mirroring recommendations for NSCLC [79, 80].

Surgical Resection for Pulmonary Metastases

Metastasis to the lungs is a common oncologic problem. Pulmonary metastases tend to be an indicator of widely metastatic disease; however, in some patients metastases to the lungs may occur in isolation. Retrospective evidence suggests that highly selected patients may have improved survival after resection of pulmonary metastases. Indications for the procedure include (1) control of the primary site, (2) metastatic disease isolated to the thorax, (3) resectable disease, and (4) sufficient cardiopulmonary reserve for the operation [81]. Most studies have found that age does not have a prognostic influence on overall survival [82–87].

The largest evaluation of outcomes after lung metastasectomy comes from the International Registry of Lung Metastases. Established in 1990, the registry enrolls all patients who have undergone resection of lung metastases with curative intent. Of the 5,206 patients enrolled between 1991 and 1995, 43% of lung metastases were epithelial in origin, 42% were sarcomas, 7% were germ cell tumors, 6% were melanomas, and 2% were other types. Single metastases accounted for 46% and multiple metastases 52%. Germ cell tumors had the best survival and melanoma the poorest survival at 5 and 10 years (68% at 5 years and 63% at 10 years vs. 21 and 14%, respectively). The survival rates for epithelial

tumors and sarcomas did not differ significantly (37% at 5 years and 21% at 10 years vs. 31 and 26%, respectively). Rates of recurrence also varied by histology type, with 64% for sarcomas and melanoma, 46% for epithelial and 26% for germ cell tumors with a median time to recurrence of 10 months. In a multivariate analysis, disease-free interval (DFI), number of metastases and tumor type were highly prognostic of long-term survival. Based on these findings, Pastorino et al. proposed four prognostic groupings to provide a framework for management. Group I consisted of patients with resectable metastases, a DFI ≥ 36 months and a single metastasis. Group II patients had resectable metastases, and a DFI of <36 months or multiple metastases. Group III again had resectable lesions and both a DFI of <36 months and multiple metastases. Patients with unresectable metastases made up group IV. Median survival for these four groups were 61, 34, 24, and 14 months for groups I–IV, respectively [87].

The use of VATS over thoracotomy for lung metastasectomy is controversial, as the surgeon is not able to palpate the lung for additional lesions. In 1994, Collie et al. reported that conventional CT missed up to 50% of pulmonary metastases found at surgery [88]. Furthermore, McCormack et al. found additional malignant lesions at thoracotomy in 56% of patients after initial VATS exploration, and thus concluded that thoracotomy with manual palpation was the gold standard for metastasectomy [89]. Preoperative evaluation with PET has a reported sensitivity of up to 94% for lesions 1.1–1.9 cm; however, it has limited ability to detect smaller lesions [90]. Other investigators, however, found no difference in rates of recurrence or survival between VATS and thoracotomy [91, 92]. As advances in imaging technology increase the ability to detect smaller lesions, it is likely that the use of VATS will become more commonplace, particularly in older patients. Elderly patients with isolated pulmonary metastases and adequate cardiopulmonary reserve should be considered for surgical resection.

CASE STUDY UPDATE

Given Ms. Jones' relatively good health and performance status, her expected life expectancy was felt to be at least 5 years, and that this would be shortened without resection of her cancer. As an octogenarian, a limited VATS resection was chosen over thoracotomy to reduce perioperative morbidity and mortality. She underwent a VATS left upper lobe wedge resection and mediastinal nodal sampling without event, and was discharged home on postoperative day 4. Her pathology returned as T1 N0 Mx bronchioalveolar carcinoma (BAC). Ms. Jones continued to do well until 18 months after her surgery when a new contralateral right upper lobe spiculated mass was detected on follow-up chest CT scan. Interval follow-up CT showed slow growth of this nodule and a lack of

lymphadenopathy. A bone scan and head CT was negative for metastatic disease. Diagnostically, it was unclear if this was a metastasis, a new primary tumor, or a benign nodule. She otherwise remained in good health and elected to proceed with VATS wedge resection of this second nodule. Pathology from this resection again proved to be BAC.

Two years after her second resection her chest CT showed evidence of recurrence of BAC, now in the left lower lobe, and she developed a left pulmonary effusion. She began to have progressive shortness of breath and was started on gefitinib. This stabilized her disease and her symptoms for another 12 months. She eventually succumbed to her disease, 5 years after her initial diagnosis. Her functional status remained excellent for four and a half of those years.

Treatment Patterns of Elderly Cancer Patients

There are multiple studies that point to the under-treatment of cancer in the elderly, for both lung cancer and other diseases [93]. Published data from the SEER database showed that the frequency of limited resections increased with age, with a decline of pneumonectomies and lobectomies with age. Approximately, 30% of the most elderly patients in the database were denied surgery or were offered only palliative surgery, in contrast with only 8% of the youngest patients [54]. Age is associated with declines in functional reserve and organ function, and optimal treatment is often affected by co-morbid conditions. Adding to the complexity involved in treatment, the elderly have often not participated in clinical trials, often forcing clinicians to rely primarily on retrospective data for treatment decisions [94].

Using 2004 data, the life expectancy of an 80-year-old in the USA is 9.1 years (8.2 years for males, 9.8 years for females), whereas the median survival for elderly patients with untreated early-stage lung cancer is only 14 months [95]. This suggests that life limitation for an 80-year-old with lung cancer is likely to be cancer related [96]. Table 48.2 [97] shows life table data from 2004 for patients older than 65.

Summary Recommendations

Resection of pulmonary malignancies has been shown to be safe in selected elderly patients. Age alone should not be a contraindication to a therapy that offers the best chance for cure for early-stage cancer patients. A thorough preoperative assessment can help individualize the morbidity and mortality risk of surgery for each patient, and thus provide both surgeon and patient with the information needed for operative decision-making. Operative interventions in the elderly require coordinated attention to the specific requirements of the aged. Efforts must be made to balance complete oncologic resection with the elderly's limited tolerance for homeostatic insult. Specialized multidisciplinary care provided by primary-care physicians, geriatric specialists, cardiologists, oncologists, surgeons, anesthesia, nursing, physical therapy, and nutrition optimize care for the elderly thoracic surgery patient.

TABLE 48.2 Life expectancy by age, USA, 2004

Age	Total	Male	Female
65	18.7	17.1	20.0
70	15.1	13.7	16.2
75	11.9	10.7	12.8
80	9.1	8.2	9.8
85	6.8	6.1	7.2
90	5.0	4.4	5.2

Source: Data from [97]

References

1. Kung HC, Hoyery DL, Xu J (2008) Deaths: final data for 2005. Center for Disease Control. Natl Vital Stat Rep 56(10):1–124

2. US Census Bureau, Population Division (2008) Table 2. Projections of the population by selected age groups and sex for the United States: 2010 to 2050 (NP2008-T2). Release Date 14 Aug 2008

3. US Census Bureau, Population Division (2008) Table 3. Percent distribution of the projected population by selected age groups and sex for the United States: 2010 to 2050 (NP2008-T3). Release Date 14 Aug 2008

4. National Projections Program, Population Division (2000) NP-T7-B projected life expectancy at birth by race and Hispanic origin, 1999–2100. U.S. Census Bureau, Washington, DC

5. American Cancer Society, Cancer Facts & Figures (2008) Age-adjusted cancer death rates, males by site. http://www.cancer.org/docroot/MED/content/MED_1_1_Most_Requested_Graphs_and_Figures_2008.asp

6. American Cancer Society, Cancer Facts & Figures (2008) Age-adjusted cancer death rates, females by site. http://www.cancer.org/docroot/MED/content/MED_1_1_Most_Requested_Graphs_and_Figures_2008.asp

7. Ries LAG, Melbert D, Krapcho M et al (2008) SEER cancer statistics review, 1975–2005. National Cancer Institute, Bethesda, MD, http://seer.cancer.gov/csr/1975_2005/, based on November 2007 SEER data submission, posted to the SEER web site

8. Gridelli C, Langer C, Maione P, Rossi A, Schild SE (2007) Lung cancer in the elderly. J Clin Oncol 25(14):1898–1907

9. Hage R, de la Riviere AB, Seldenrijk C, van den Bosch JM (2003) Update in pulmonary carcinoid tumors: a review article. Ann Surg Oncol 10(6):697–704

10. Teeter SM, Holmes FF, McFarlane MJ (1987) Lung carcinoma in the elderly population. Influence of histology on the inverse relationship of stage to age. Cancer 60(6):1331–1336

11. Rossi A, Ganassini A, Tantucci C et al (1996) Aging and the respiratory system. Aging (Milano) 8(3):143–161

12. Janssens JP, Pache JC, Nicod LP (1999) Physiological changes in respiratory function associated with ageing. Eur Respir J 13:197–205

13. Meyer KC (2004) Lung infections and aging. Ageing Res Rev 3(1):55–67

14. Verra F, Escudier E, Lebargy F et al (1995) Ciliary abnormalities in bronchial epithelium of smokers, ex-smokers, and nonsmokers. Am J Respir Crit Care Med 151(3):630–634

15. Salathe M, O'Riordan TG, Wanner A (1996) Treatment of mucociliary dysfunction. Chest 110:1048–1057

16. McLesky CH (1992) Anesthesia for the geriatric patient. In: Barash PG, Cullen BF, Staelting RK (eds) Clinical anasthesia, 2nd edn. JB Lippincott, Philadelphia, pp 1353–1383

17. Eagle KA, Berger PB, Calkins H et al (2002) ACC/AHA guideline update for perioperative cardiovascular evauation for noncardiac surgery. Circulation 105:1257–1267

18. Passman RS, Gingold DS, Amar D et al (2005) Prediction rule for atrial fibrillation after major noncardiac thoracic surgery. Ann Thorac Surg 79:1698–1703

19. Roselli EE, Murthy SC, Rice TW et al (2005) Atrial fibrillation complicating lung cancer resection. J Thorac Cardiovasc Surg 130:438–444

20. Sedrakyan A, Treasure T, Browne J et al (2005) Pharmacologic prophylaxis for postoperative atrial tachyarrhythmia in general thoracic surgery: evidence from randomized clinical trials. J Thorac Cardiovasc Surg 129:997–1005

21. British Thoracic Sociert (2001) Society of cardiothoracic surgeons of Great Britain and Ireland working party. Guidelines on the selection of patients with lung cancer for surgery. Thorax 56:89–108

22. Colice GL, Shafazand S, Griffin JP et al (2007) Physiologic evaluation of the patient with lung cancer being considered for resectional surgery: ACCP evidence-based clinical practice guidelines (2nd ed). Chest 132:161–177

23. Wyser C, Stulz P, Soler M et al (1999) Prospective evaluation of an algorithm for the functional assessment of lung resection candidates. Am J Respir Crit Care Med 159:1450–1456

24. Datta D, Lahiri B (2003) Preoperative evaluation of patients undergoing lung resection surgery. Chest 123:2096–2103

25. Linden PA, Bueno R, Colson YL et al (2005) Lung resection in patients with preoperative FEV1 < 35% predicted. Chest 127: 1984–1990

26. Ferguson MK, Little L, Rizzo L et al (1988) Diffusing capacity predicts morbidity and mortality after pulmonary resection. J Thorac Cardiovasc Surg 96:894–900

27. Stephan F, Boucheseiche S, Hollande J et al (2000) Pulmonary complications following lung resection: a comprehensive analysis of incidence and possible risk factors. Chest 118:1263–1270

28. Botsen PC, Block AJ, Moulder PC (1981) Relationship between preoperative pulmonary function tests and complications after thoracotomy. Surg Gynecol Obstet 52:813–815

29. Girish M, Trayner E, Dammann O et al (2001) Symptom-limited stair climbing as a predictor of postoperative cardiopulmonary complications after high risk surgery. Chest 120:1147–1151

30. Solway S, Brooks D, Lacasses Y et al (2001) A qualitative systematic overview of the measurement properties of functional walk tests used in the cardiorespiratory domain. Chest 119(1):256–270

31. Jaklitsch MT, Mery CM, Audisio RA (2003) The use of surgery to treat lung cancer in elderly patients. Lancet Oncol 4:463–471

32. Olsen GN, Block AJ, Tobias JA (1974) Prediction of postpnemonectomy pulmonary function using quantitative macroaggregate lung scanning. Chest 66:13–16

33. Pate P, Tenholder MF, Griffin JP et al (1996) Preoperative assessment of the high-risk patient for lung resection. Ann Thorac Surg 61:1494–1500

34. Markos J, Mullan BP, Hillman DR et al (1989) Preoperative assessment as a predictor of mortality and morbidity after lung resection. Am Rev Respir Dis 139:902–910

35. Bolliger CT, Wyser C, Boser H et al (1995) Lung scanning and exercise testing for the prediction of postoperative peformance in lung resection candidates at increased risk of complications. Chest 108:341–348

36. Holden DA, Rice TW, Stefmach K et al (1992) Exercise testing, 6-min walk, and stair climb in the evaluation of patients at high risk for pulmonary resection. Chest 102:1774–1779

37. Wahi R, McMurtry MJ, DeCaro LF et al (1989) Determinants of perioperative morbidity and mortality after pneumonectomy. Ann Thorac Surg 48:33–37

38. Brock MV, Kim MP, Hooker CM et al (2004) Pulmonary resection in octogenarians with stage I nonsmall cell lung cancer: a 22-year experience. Ann Thorac Surg 77:271–277

39. Moller JT, Cluitmans P, Rasmussen LS et al (1998) Long-term postoperative cognitive dysfunction in the elderly: ISPOCD1 study. Lancet 351:857–861

40. Rasmussen LS, Siersma VD (2004) ISPOCD Group: postoperative cognitive dysfunction: true deterioration versus random variation. Acta Anaesthesiol Scand 48:1137–1143

41. Newman S, Stygall J, Shaefi S et al (2007) Postoperative cognitive dysfunction after noncardiac surgery. Anesthesiology 106:572–590

42. Kaneko T, Takahashi S, Naka T et al (1997) Postoperative delirium following gastrointestinal surgery in elderly patients. Surg Today 27:107–111

43. Fukuse T, Satoda N, Hijiya K et al (2005) Importance of a comprehensive geriatric assessment in prediction of complications following thoracic surgery in elderly patients. Chest 127:886–891

44. Narian O, Rubenstein L et al (1988) Predictors of immediate and 6 month outcomes in hospitalized elderly patients. The importance of functional status. J Am Geriatr Society 36:775–783

45. Reuben D, Rubenstein L et al (1992) Value of functional staus as a predictor of mortality: results of a prospective study. Am J Med 93(6):663–669

46. Landi F, Giuseppe G et al (1999) Body mass index and mortality among older people living in the community. J Am Geriatr Soc 47:1072

47. Audisio RA, Ramesh H, Longo W et al (2005) Preoperative assessment of surgical risk in oncogeriatric patients. Oncologist 10:262–268

48. Rubenstein LZ, Schairer C, Wieland GD, Kane R (1984) Systematic biases in functional status assessment of elderly adults: effects of different data sources. J Gerontol 39(6):686–691

49. Buccheri G, Ferrigno D, Tamburini M (1996) Karnofsky and ECOG performance status scoring in lung cancer: a prospective, longitudinal study of 536 patients from a single institution. Eur J Cancer 32A(7):1135–1141

50. Harpole DH Jr, Herndon JF 2nd, Young WG Jr et al (1995) Stage I nonsmall cell lung cancer: a multivariate analysis of treatment methods and patterns of recurrence. Cancer 76:787–796

51. Stamatis G, Djuric D, Eberhardt W et al (2002) Postoperative morbidity and mortality after induction chemoradiotherapy for locally advancer lung cancer: an analysis of 350 operated patients. Eur J Cardiothorac Surg 22:292–297

52. Ferguson MK, Vigneswaran WT (2008) Diffusing capacity predicts morbidity after lung resection in patients without obstructive lung disease. Ann Thorac Surg 85(4):1158–1164

53. O'Rourke MA, Feussner JR, Feigl P et al (1987) Age trends of lung cancer stage at diagnosis: implications for lung cancer screening in the elderly. JAMA 258:921–926

54. Mery CM, Pappas AN, Bueno R et al (2005) Similar long-term survival of elderly patients with non-small cell lung cancer treated with lobectomy or wedge resection within the Surveillance, Epidemiology, and End Results database. Chest 128:237–245

55. Weinmann M, Jeremie B, Toomes H et al (2003) Treatment of lung cancer in the elderly. Part I. Non-small cell lung cancer. Lung Cancer 39:233–253

56. Morandi U, Stefani A, Golinelli M et al (1997) Results of surgical resection in patients over the age of 70 years with non small-cell lung cancer. Eur J Cardiothorac Surg 11:432–439

57. Gail MH, Eagan RT, Feld R et al (1984) Prognostic factors in patients with resected state I non-small cell lung cancer: a report from the Lung Cancer Study Group. Cancer 54:1802–1813

58. Mountain CF, Lukeman JM, Hammar SP et al (1987) Lung cancer classification: the relationship of disease extent and cell type to survival in a clinical trials population. J Surg Oncol 35:147–156

59. Deslauriers J, Gregoire J (2000) Surgical therapy of early non-small cell lung cancer. Chest 117(suppl):104S–109S

60. Faulkner SL (2000) Is lobectomy the "gold standard" for stage I lung cancer in year 2000? Chest 118(suppl):119S

61. Bates M (1970) Results of surgery for bronchial carcinoma in patients aged 70 and over. Thorax 25:77–78

62. Evans EW (1973) Resection of bronchial carcinoma in the elderly. Thorax 28:86–88

63. Kirsh MM, Rotman H, Bove E et al (1976) Major pulmonary resection for bronchial carcinoma in the elderly. Ann Thorac Surg 22:369–373

64. Harviel JD, McNamara JJ, Straehley CJ (1978) Surgical treatment of lung cancer in patients over the age of 70 years. J Thorac Cardiovasc Surg 75:802–805

65. Ginsberg RJ, Hill LD, Eagan RT et al (1983) Modern thirty-day operative mortality for surgical resections in lung cancer. J Thorac Cardiovasc Surg 86:654–658

66. Mery CM, Jaklitch MT (2006) Lung resection in the elderly, correspondence. Chest 129:496–497

67. Albano WA (1977) Should elderly patients undergo surgery for cancer. Geriatrics 32:105–108

68. Breyer RH, Zippe C, Pharr WF et al (1981) Thoracotomy in patients over age seventy years: ten-year experience. J Thorac Cardiovasc Surg 81:187–193

69. Zapatero J, Madrigal L, Lago J et al (1990) Thoracic surgery in the elderly: review of 100 cases. Acta Chir Hung 31:227–234

70. Allen MS, Darling GE, Pechet TT et al (2006) ACOSOG Z0030 Study Group. Morbidity and mortality of major pulmonary resections in patients with early-stage lung cancer: initial results of the randomized, prospective ACOSOG Z0030 trial. Ann Thorac Surg 81(3):1013–1019

71. Decamp MM Jr, Jaklitsch MT, Mentzer SJ et al (1995) The safety and versatility of video-thoracoscopy: a prospective analysis of 895 cases. J Am Coll Surg 181:113–120

72. McKenna R (1994) Thoracoscopic lobectomy with mediastinal sampling in 80 year-old patients. Chest 106:1902–1904

73. Landreneau RL, Sugarbaker DJ, Mack MJ et al (1993) Postoperative pain-related morbidity: video-assisted thoracic surgery versus thoracotomy. Ann Thorac Surg 56:1285–1289

74. Jaklitsch MT, Bueno R, Swanson SJ et al (1996) Video-assisted thoracic surgery in the elderly: a review of 307 cases. Chest 110:751–758

75. Cattaneo SM, Park BJ, Wilton AS et al (2008) Use of video-assisted thoracic surgery for lobectomy in the elderly results in fewer complications. Ann Thorac Surg 85:231–236

76. Ginsberg RJ, Rubinstein LV (1995) Randomized trial of lobectomy versus limited resection for T1 N0 non-small cell lung cancer. Lung Cancer Study Group. Ann Thorac Surg 60(3):615–622, discussion 622–623

77. Landreneau RJ, Sugarbaker DJ, Mack MJ et al (1997) Wedge resection versus lobectomy for stage I (T1 N0 M0) non-small-cell lung cancer. J Thorac Cardiovasc Surg 113(4):691–700

78. Kulke MH, Mayer RJ (1999) Carcinoid tumors. N Engl J Med 340(11):858–868

79. Marty-Ane C, Costes V, Pujol J et al (1995) Carcinoid tumors of the lung: do atypical features require aggressive management? Ann Thorac Surg 59(1):78–83

80. Mezzetti M, Raveglia F, Panigalli T et al (2003) Assessment of outcomes in typical and atypical carcinoids according to latest WHO classification. Ann Thorac Surg 76(6):1838–1842

81. Jaklitsch MT, Mery CM, Lukanich JM et al (2001) Sequential thoracic metastasectomy prolongs survival by re-establishing local control within the chest. J Thorac Cardiovasc Surg 121(4):657–667

82. Inoue M, Ohta M, Iuchi K et al (2004) Benefits of surgery for patients with pulmonary metastases from colorectal carcinoma. Ann Thorac Surg 78(1):238–244

83. Weiser MR, Downey RJ, Leung DH, Brennan MF (2000) Repeat resection of pulmonary metastases in patients with soft-tissue sarcoma. J Am Coll Surg 191(2):184–190, discussion 190–191

84. Saito Y, Omiya H, Kohno K et al (2002) Pulmonary metastasectomy for 165 patients with colorectal carcinoma: A prognostic assessment. J Thorac Cardiovasc Surg 124(5):1007–1013

85. Pfannschmidt J (2003) Prognostic factors and survival after complete resection of pulmonary metastases from colorectal carcinoma: experiences in 167 patients. J Thorac Cardiovasc Surg 126(3):732–739

86. Carballo M, Maish M, Jaroszewski D, Holmes C (2009) Video-assisted thoracic surgery (VATS) as a safe alternative for the resection of pulmonary metastases: a retrospective cohort study. J Cardiothorac Surg 4(1):13

87. The International Registry of Lung Metastases, Writing Committee, Pastorino U et al (1997) Long-term results of lung metastasectomy: prognostic analyses based on 5206 cases. J Thorac Cardiovasc Surg 113(1):37–49

88. Collie DA, Wright AR, Williams JR et al (1994) Comparison of spiral-acquisition computed tomography and conventional computed tomography in the assessment of pulmonary metastatic disease. Br J Radiol 67(797):436–444

89. McCormack PM, Bains MS, Begg CB et al (1996) Role of video-assisted thoracic surgery in the treatment of pulmonary metastases: results of a prospective trial. Ann Thorac Surg 62(1): 213–216

90. Reinhardt M, Wiethoelter N, Matthies A et al (2006) PET recognition of pulmonary metastases on PET/CT imaging: impact of attenuation-corrected and non-attenuation-corrected PET images. Eur J Nucl Med Mol Imaging 33(2):134–139

91. Nakajima J, Takamoto S, Tanaka M et al (2001) Thoracoscopic surgery and conventional open thoracotomy in metastatic lung cancer. Surg Endosc 15(8):849–853

92. Mutsaerts E, Zoetmulder F, Meijer S et al (2002) Long term survival of thoracoscopic metastasectomy vs metastasectomy by thoracotomy in patients with a solitary pulmonary lesion. Eur J Surg Oncol 28(8):864–868

93. Samet J, Hunt WC, Key C et al (1986) Choice of cancer therapy varies with age of patient. JAMA 255:3385–3390

94. Gridelli C, Langer C, Maione P et al (2007) Lung cancer in the elderly. J Clin Oncol 25(14):1898–1907

95. McGarry RC, Song G, des Rosiers P et al (2002) Observation-only management of early stage, medically inoperable lung cancer: poor outcome. Chest 121:1155–1158

96. Yellin A, Brenfield JR (1985) Surgery for bronchogenic carcinoma in the elderly. Am Rev Respir Dis 131:197

97. Arias E (2007) United States life tables, 2004. Natl Vital Stat Rep 56(9):1–39.

Section VII
Cardiovascular System

Chapter 49
Invited Commentary

Timothy J. Gardner

Cardiovascular illnesses in the elderly are, in many respects, a natural consequence of aging. The aging process is associated with degeneration of organs and their functions, including the brain, heart, musculoskeletal system, and vascular system. Cardiovascular illnesses, such as ischemic heart disease, peripheral vascular disease, and congestive heart failure can be expected to occur in some form or other as we age; and nearly everyone who survives into their eighties has evidence of cardiovascular pathology. It is interesting that when questioned about their preferred mode of demise, many older people indicate that they would choose to sustain a sudden fatal cardiac event over such unpleasant terminal illnesses as cancer, stroke, dementia, or other afflictions of the elderly.

Many of the dramatic advances in the management of cardiovascular diseases during the past 30 years have been directed toward premature or "unnatural" cardiovascular conditions such as ischemic heart disease in young people, cardiomyopathies causing heart failure in young adults, valvular heart conditions creating disability in middle-aged people, and the like. Coronary bypass grafting and percutaneous coronary angioplasty were offered initially only to young patients with disabling angina. Heart transplantation was undertaken initially only in patients 50 years or younger. Even today, cardiac transplantation is considered inappropriate for people in their late fifties and older.

Along with the survival improvement and increased longevity for young people with heart disease that has occurred over the past two to three decades, the general population, especially in prosperous and developed countries, has been blessed with increasing longevity, as many preventable causes of early deaths are being dealt with successfully. With the enhanced life expectancy, has come changing expectations among our aging fellow citizens. Retirement is no longer viewed as the end of one's useful lifetime, but rather, as a period of enrichment during which the rewards of a productive life can be realized and enjoyed. One's ability to function successfully as an elderly member of society – that is, being able to remain independent and to participate in a variety of important social, physical, and intellectual activities – ends up defining one's quality of life. If an elderly individual develops a cancer that is unfavorable for successful treatment, that patient and his or her family usually accept the inevitability of death and attempt to deal with the pain and suffering associated with the disease and the need to prepare for dying. The prevailing attitude toward many cardiovascular conditions in the elderly, however, is often different. We often do not accept as readily the inevitability of continued deterioration and death from cardiovascular illnesses, even when such problems occur in older individuals.

What, then, should be the proper approach to cardiovascular disease in the elderly? Because heart and vascular diseases are a natural consequence of aging, should we develop limits indicating at what age one should cease and desist from treating the cardiovascular condition invasively and let "nature takes its course?" Should a patient's age of 75 or 80 become the cutoff for such advanced cardiovascular therapies as angioplasty, coronary bypass grafting, or placement of internal cardiac defibrillators? On the other hand, in view of our observation that most elderly people want to live as long as possible with a suitable quality of life, should we offer aortic valve replacement to the octogenarian who is functionally intact except for heart-related episodes of syncope from isolated critical aortic valve stenosis? Should we broaden the criteria for eligibility for heart transplantation to old patients who may, in fact, have an extended life expectancy if the current disabling heart failure is adequately managed by cardiac transplantation? There are no easy answers to these and similar questions. They involve a host of considerations beyond the scope of whether an operation can be done safely on a given patient or if there are identifiable preoperative patient characteristics that allow accurate risk factor analysis.

What must be acknowledged by all who are concerned with health care for the elderly is that there will be a continuing and

T.J. Gardner (✉)
Center for Heart and Vascular Health, Christiana Health Care System, 4755 Ogletown-Stanton Road, Newark, DE 19718, USA
e-mail: tgardner@christianacare.org

R.A. Rosenthal et al. (eds.), *Principles and Practice of Geriatric Surgery*,
DOI 10.1007/978-1-4419-6999-6_49, © Springer Science+Business Media, LLC 2011

dramatic increase in the percent of elderly in the population and a notable increase in the number of those surviving beyond 80 years of age. Because of the nature of cardiovascular illnesses, it is likely that such conditions will predominate among our aging population, and that illnesses such as unstable angina in an 80-year-old woman who is living alone successfully will mandate interventional treatment even though the risk of death or complications with angioplasty or surgery is increased. Likewise, the 85-year-old man who is living comfortably in a retirement home, but develops an acute myocardial infarction should be given the opportunity to receive intravenous thrombolytic therapy despite his age and despite the increased risk of adverse bleeding events.

The challenge that must be faced when considering the expanded application of advanced or invasive therapies for cardiovascular disease in the elderly is that of defining and predicting the expected outcomes of various treatments in terms of immediate and long-term survival along with complications, morbidities, and the restoration of one's quality of life. Epidemiologic methods and techniques should be used in an attempt to account for survival differences among elderly patients with specific cardiovascular conditions. Using such information, risk profiles that are based on the individual's health characteristics and are predictive of treatment success or failure can be developed and discussed before undertaking advanced treatments.

In addition, it is mandatory to recognize differences between elderly patients and younger individuals with cardiovascular illnesses. Even such simple concepts as variations in pharmacokinetics in an old patient compared to that in the young, "general population" in whom most clinical trials have been performed becomes an important challenge. For example, despite the fact that there may be statistically validated efficacy associated with the use of a β-blocker for certain cardiovascular conditions, such a medication when used in an elderly patient may result in disabling complications, such as syncope or heart block. Percutaneous coronary angioplasty or intraarterial stenting from the usual femoral artery approach may be precluded in the elderly patient with severe peripheral vascular disease. Coronary artery bypass grafting, which has negligible mortality risks in otherwise healthy young patients, is much riskier even in the "healthy" elderly patient, with a substantially higher likelihood of death or disabling stroke.

Treatments for cardiovascular illness that, when successful, prolong life and enhance the quality of that life should not be withheld from an elderly patient simply based on that individual's age. On the other hand, we must recognize that invasive therapies, including catheter interventions and especially major surgical procedures, are likely to be less successful and more often associated with complications because of age-related comorbidities and other degenerative conditions. To determine accurately the risk–benefit relation of a suggested treatment, we must be able to stratify the risks according to the patient's individual characteristics including his or her advanced age. Successful treatment of the elderly individual with cardiovascular disease requires also the committed interest and attention of specialists who are willing and able to view their elderly patients with the same discrimination that pediatric specialists are called upon to utilize when caring for young children.

Finally, a commitment to preserve and sustain the useful life of our elderly patients must be supported by a societal commitment to support advanced medical therapies for these individuals. In virtually every developed country of the world, health care for the elderly is provided through government support for medical care. Each society must continuously renew its commitment to supporting and caring in the most appropriate way for its elderly citizens. The challenge and responsibility for those in medicine is to provide advanced medical care to elderly patients only when it is appropriate, that is, when it can be expected to sustain useful life for that patient. The challenges of the aging society, which we will face for the foreseeable future, are immense. It is predictable that much of the focus in medical care will remain on management of cardiovascular illnesses in the elderly.

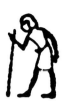

Chapter 50
Physiologic Changes in Cardiac Function with Aging

Wilbert S. Aronow and William H. Frishman

Age-related changes in the cardiovascular system, overt and occult cardiovascular disease, and decreased physical activity affect cardiovascular function in older persons. With aging, there is a loss of myocytes in both the left and right ventricles with a progressive increase in myocyte cell volume per nucleus in both ventricles [1]. There is also a progressive decrease in the number of pacemaker cells in the sinus node, with only 10% of the number of cells present at age 20 remaining at age 75 [2].

Gonzalez et al. [3] have shown in an animal model that chronologic age also leads to telomeric shortening in cardiac progenitor cells. Aging affects the growth and differential potential of cardiac stem cells, interfering not only with their ability to sustain physiologic cell turnover but also with their capacity to adapt to increases in pressure and volume loads [4, 5].

Afterload

Resistance to the ejection of blood by the left ventricle (LV) is termed afterload. There are two components to afterload: peripheral vascular resistance (PVR) and characteristic aortic impedance. PVR is the steady-state component and provides opposition to steady blood flow. Characteristic aortic impedance is the dynamic component and opposes pulsatile blood flow. PVR is calculated by dividing the mean arterial pressure by the cardiac output; it is inversely proportional to the cross-sectional area of the PV beds. Characteristic aortic impedance is measured as the time variation in mean arterial pressure/flow through the aorta; it is inversely proportional to the arterial compliance (the distensibility of the arterial wall). An indirect measurement of afterload is the pulse wave velocity, which measures the propagation speed of pressure

waves traveling from proximal to distal arterial segments; it increases as arteries become less compliant.

With aging, the large elastic arteries become dilated with a decrease in compliance [6]. Progressive thickening of the aortic media and intima are associated with aortic enlargement [7]. There is an age-associated increase in arterial stiffness resulting from changes in the arterial media, such as thickening of the smooth muscle layers, increased fragmentation of elastin, an increase in the amount and characteristics of collagen, and increased calcification [8]. These structural changes are associated with a decrease in aortic distensibility due to increased aortic stiffness with an increase in pulse wave velocity [9]. The structural changes in the arterial wall are independent of coexisting atherosclerosis. Avolio et al. [9] showed an increase in pulse wave velocity with age in farmers from Guanzhou Province in southern China despite a low prevalence of atherosclerosis in this population. The age-associated increase in stiffness and decrease in distensibility of large elastic arteries is not found in distal arteries [10].

Impedance spectral patterns have demonstrated an age-related increase in characteristic aortic impedance and PVR [11]. The decrease in arterial PV vascular beds [11]. PVR was not age-related in healthy persons screened for occult coronary artery disease (CAD) in the Baltimore Longitudinal Study of Aging [12], but increased with age in persons not screened for occult CAD [13]. Arterial stiffening appearing as an increase in pulse wave velocity is associated with degeneration of the vascular media independent of atherosclerosis. Arterial stiffening causes earlier occurrence of wave reflection from peripheral sites to the ascending aorta during LV ejection. Therefore, aortic and carotid phasic pressures increase to a greater magnitude at a later time during LV ejection, causing an increase in systolic and pulse pressures and a delayed peak in the aortic pressure pulse contour.

Circulating levels of catecholamines increase with age, especially with stress, although β-adrenergic vasodilation of vascular smooth muscle decreases [14]. α-Adrenergic vasoconstriction of vascular smooth muscle does not change with age [15]. The impaired vasodilator response to β-adrenergic

W.S. Aronow (✉)
Cardiology Division, New York Medical College,
Macy Pavilion, Room 138, Valhalla, NY 10595, USA
e-mail: wsaronow@aol.com

R.A. Rosenthal et al. (eds.), *Principles and Practice of Geriatric Surgery*,
DOI 10.1007/978-1-4419-6999-6_50, © Springer Science+Business Media, LLC 2011

stimulation with age is most important during exercise and contributes to the increased afterload associated with aging.

Increased afterload results in an increase in blood pressure. With aging, there is an increase in systolic blood pressure (SBP) and a widened pulse pressure. A slight reduction in diastolic blood pressure occurs after the sixth decade [16]. The increase in SBP is due to interactions of aging, cardiovascular disease, and lifestyle factors, such as dietary sodium intake, body weight, and level of physical activity. An age-associated increase in the index of aortic stiffening was not found in normotensive persons on a low sodium chloride diet [17]. The increase in carotid augmentation index (an index of aortic stiffening) in highly trained elderly men was half of that expected on the basis of age alone [18]. The prevalence of abnormal aortic stiffness increases steeply in the community with advancing age, especially in the presence of diabetes mellitus and obesity [19].

As aortic compliance decreases with aging, the transfer of kinetic energy from the blood ejected during LV systole to potential energy stored in the elasticity of the aortic wall is reduced. Consequently, return of the potential energy stored in the elasticity of the aortic wall back to the kinetic energy of blood flow during diastole also is reduced. Therefore, the LV must eject its stroke volume into a less compliant aorta with greater pressure and force to achieve adequate cardiac output. The increased pulse wave velocity also causes the pressure in the aorta to increase and peak later during systole, contributing to the increased SBP and widened pulse pressure.

Posterior LV wall thickness increased with increasing age in normotensive men and women screened for occult CAD in the Baltimore Longitudinal Study of Aging [20]. Data from persons in this study suggested that the increase in LV wall thickness associated with aging is mediated by an increase in SBP. Aging is also associated with an increase in the prevalence of hypertension and cardiovascular disease and, therefore, with the LV hypertrophy (LVH) seen by echocardiography.

Age-associated LVH is caused by an increase in the volume but not in the number of cardiac myocytes. Fibroblasts undergo hyperplasia, and collagen is deposited in the myocardial interstitium. Increased afterload results in increased LV systolic stress, and the addition of sarcomeres, in parallel, causes increased LV wall thickness with a normal or reduced LV chamber size and an increased relative wall thickness.

In the Framingham Heart Study, echocardiographic LVH was observed in 33% of men and 49% of women older than 70 years [21]. In our elderly population, echocardiographic LVH was found in 226 of 554 men (41%) with a mean age of 80 years and in 539 of 1,243 women (43%) with a mean age of 82 years [22].

In our elderly population, systolic or diastolic hypertension was present in 255 of 664 men (38%) with a mean age of 80 years and in 651 of 1,488 women (44%) with a mean

age of 82 years [23]. In another study of our elderly population, systolic or diastolic hypertension occurred in 108 of 215 Blacks (50%) with a mean age of 81 years, in 411 of 1,140 Whites (36%) with a mean age of 82 years, and in 19 of 54 Hispanics (35%) with a mean age 81 years [24]. Echocardiographically diagnosed LVH occurred in 66 of 92 hypertensive Blacks (72%), in 194 of 346 hypertensive Whites (56%), and in 8 of 15 hypertensive Hispanics (53%) [24]. However, it was observed in only 2 of our 88 elderly persons (2%) without hypertension or overt cardiac disease [25].

Regular aerobic endurance exercise attenuates age-related decreases in central arterial compliance and restores levels in previously sedentary healthy middle-aged and elderly men [26]. Regular aerobic endurance exercise also can prevent the age-associated loss in endothelium-dependent vasodilation and restore levels in previously sedentary middle-aged and elderly healthy men [27]. These are mechanisms by which regular aerobic endurance exercise contributes to a reduced risk of cardiovascular disease in the elderly [26, 27].

Preload

Preload is the filling volume of the LV. Preload is determined by many factors that influence blood return to the heart and by the mechanical properties of the heart during diastolic filling of the LV.

Resting LV end-diastolic volume, measured by radionuclide ventriculography using multiple gated pool acquisition imaging or by echocardiography, is not age-related in healthy persons, indicating that the resting preload does not change with age [6, 12, 28]. Although resting preload does not change with age, LV early diastolic filling decreases with age.

Passive filling of the LV occurs during the rapid filling and diastasis phases of early diastole. With age, LV stiffness is increased, LV compliance reduced, LV wall thickness increased, LV relaxation impaired, and LV early diastolic filling reduced. This may result in hypotension if preload is reduced. An age-related increase in SBP also decreases LV early diastolic filling, leading to hypotension if preload is decreased. LV filling during early diastole is reduced 50% from age 20 to 80 [6, 29, 30].

Despite the decrease in early diastolic filling of the LV with age, preload is maintained because left atrial contraction becomes more vigorous to increase late diastolic filling of the LV [6, 28–34]. Augmentation of late diastolic filling of the LV prevents a reduction in LV end-diastolic volume. The ratio of late diastolic Doppler peak transmitral velocity (peak atrial, or A wave, velocity) to early diastolic Doppler peak transmitral velocity (peak rapid filling, or E wave, velocity) increases from approximately 0.6 at 30 years of age to 1.2 at 70 years of age [35]. A reduction in the E/A wave ratio with age reflects a decrease in LV compliance. An age-related increase in left atrial size resulting from increased wall stress due to increased left atrial pressure counteracts the effects of reduced LV compliance with age. In our older population, 619 of 1,797 older persons (34%) had echocardiographic left atrial enlargement [22].

Age was the most powerful independent variable LV filling in healthy persons in the Framingham Heart Study [36]. Age was inversely associated with the E wave (peak early diastolic filling velocity) and was directly associated with the A wave (peak late diastolic filling velocity). Other independent variables that contributed to a lesser degree to LV filling were heart rate, PR interval measured from the electrocardiogram (ECG), gender, LV systolic function, and SBP. Increasing the heart rate decreases peak early diastolic filling and increases peak late diastolic filling velocity. The PR interval on the ECG is inversely associated with peak early diastolic filling velocity. Women have slightly higher peak early diastolic filling velocities than men. LV systolic function is directly associated with peak early diastolic filling velocity. Increasing the SBP increases the peak late diastolic filling velocity [36, 37]. Age-associated abnormalities in Doppler measures of myocardial filling and relaxation are only partially minimized by lifelong endurance training [38].

A decrease in preload is not well tolerated in older persons. Decreased intravascular volume, reduced venous return to the heart, vasodilation by drugs or disease states, and use of drugs such as nitrates or diuretics decrease preload and may cause reduced cardiac output and hypotension in older persons. Reduced compliance of the LV and decreased cardiac and vascular responsiveness to β-adrenergic stimulation [39] cause elderly persons to be highly dependent on the Frank–Starling mechanism to increase cardiac output. Older persons are more susceptible to developing orthostatic hypotension [40–42]. Impaired baroreceptor reflex sensitivity [43], reduced cardiac responsiveness to β-adrenergic stimulation [36], loss of arterial compliance, reduced venous return due to increased venous distensibility, impaired compensatory mechanisms for maintenance of fluid volume and electrolyte balance, increased incidence of common precipitating diseases and disorders, and the use of multiple drugs contribute to orthostatic hypotension. Older persons are also more susceptible to developing postprandial hypotension [43–46].

Marked decreases in postprandial SBP in the elderly may predispose them to symptomatic hypotension and to falls, syncope, angina pectoris, and transient cerebral ischemic attacks [44–48]. At 29-month follow-up, a marked reduction in postprandial SBP in older persons was associated with an increased incidence of falls, syncope, new coronary events, new stroke, and total mortality [48]. Whether therapeutic interventions to prevent a marked decrease in postprandial SBP in elderly persons can reduce the incidence of these outcomes at long-term follow-up must be investigated.

Because left atrial contraction can contribute up to 50% of LV filling in a poorly compliant LV, the development of atrial fibrillation may result in a marked decrease in cardiac output because of loss of the left atrial contribution to LV late diastolic filling. A rapid ventricular rate associated with atrial fibrillation also decreases the time for diastolic filling of the LV, resulting in a marked reduction in cardiac output.

The incidence of chronic atrial fibrillation also is increased with age [49, 50]. In 2,101 elderly persons in a nursing home, the prevalence of chronic atrial fibrillation was 5% in persons aged 60–70 years, 13–14% in persons aged 71–90 years, and 22% in persons aged 91 years and older [50]. Atrial fibrillation in old persons is associated with an increased incidence of new thromboembolic stroke [49, 50] and new coronary events [51, 52].

Cardiac output increases during exercise in healthy old persons owing to an increase in venous return to the heart, increasing the diastolic filling of the LV and allowing an increased stroke volume to be ejected during exercise (Frank–Starling mechanism) [53]. The maximal heart rate response to exercise decreased with age in healthy subjects in the Baltimore Longitudinal Study of Aging [12], whereas exercise stroke volume increased with age to maintain the exercise cardiac output. The increase in exercise stroke volume resulted from an increase in LV end-diastolic volume (preload) via the Frank–Starling mechanism. In contrast, healthy nonelderly persons achieved an increase in exercise cardiac output primarily by an increase in heart rate. Exercise stroke volume increased in nonelderly healthy persons owing to a slight increase in the LV end-diastolic volume and a large reduction in the LV end-systolic volume. The exercise-induced increase in heart rate and decrease in LV end-systolic volume in nonelderly persons is probably mediated by β-adrenergic stimulation. The increase in LV end-diastolic volume during exercise in healthy older persons suggests that the age-associated decrease in resting early diastolic filling of the LV does not persist during exercise.

Contractility

The intrinsic ability of the heart to generate force does not change with age in healthy persons, although the duration of contraction and relaxation is prolonged in senescent animals [54, 55]. Prolongation of the LV ejection time [56] and the pre-ejection period [57] with age in healthy persons indicates that prolongation of contraction occurs with age. Prolongation of the duration of contraction in senescent animals is associated with increased muscle stiffness and prolongation of the action potential duration [58]. These age-related changes are associated with cellular changes in the excitation-contraction coupling mechanism [59] and are an adaptive response to preserve contractile function in response to an age-induced increase in afterload.

There is no decrease in resting LV ejection fraction (LVEF) or circumferential fiber shortening in old persons with no evidence of heart disease [6, 12, 28, 60, 61]. However, systolic function with exercise decreases with age. In the Baltimore Longitudinal Study of Aging, old persons showed less exercise-induced increase in LVEF than did younger persons because of an age-related increase in LV end-systolic volume [12]. However, the absolute values of LVEF at maximal exercise LV ventricular contractility in healthy old persons during maximal exercise are manifestations of reduced β-adrenergic responsiveness, with aging partially offset by exercise-induced dilation of the LV [62].

Diastolic Function

Aging is associated with prolongation of the isovolumic relaxation time, decreased early diastolic filling of the LV, and augmented late diastolic filling of the LV [29, 32, 35]. Normal aging changes that affect the LV diastolic function include increased SBP, increased LV wall thickness, reduced LV early diastolic filling, prolonged LV diastolic relaxation, increased left atrial size, and increased LV late diastolic filling [63].

With age occurs slowing of the rate at which calcium is sequestered by the sarcoplasmic reticulum following myocardial excitation, which causes decreased relaxation of the LV [59, 64, 65]. Accumulation of calcium at the onset of diastole may decrease LV diastolic relaxation and early diastolic filling [64]. Decreased oxidative phosphorylation and cumulative mitochondrial peroxidation occurring with age may also decrease the LV diastolic function [66, 67].

Increased LV stiffness with age due to increased interstitial fibrosis and cross-linking of collagen in the heart impairs LV diastolic relaxation and filling [1, 68–70]. Myocardial ischemia in the absence of CAD caused by decreases in capillary density and coronary reserve with age may further reduce LV diastolic function in old persons [1, 71].

In addition to a decrease in LV diastolic relaxation and early diastolic filling caused by age, old persons are more likely to have LV diastolic dysfunction because they have an increased prevalence of hypertension, myocardial ischemia due to CAD, and LVH due to hypertension, CAD, valvular aortic stenosis, hypertrophic cardiomyopathy, and other cardiac disorders. The increased stiffness of the LV and prolonged LV relaxation time reduce LV early diastolic filling and cause higher LV end-diastolic pressures at rest and during exercise in old persons [72, 73].

In patients with congestive heart failure (CHF) associated with LV systolic dysfunction, the LVEF <50%. Amount of

myocardial fiber shortening is reduced, the stroke volume is decreased, the LV is dilated, and the patient is symptomatic.

With CHF, due to LV diastolic dysfunction with normal LV systolic function, the LVEF is normal. Kitzman et al. [74] showed that during exercise, persons with CHF and normal LV systolic function but abnormal LV diastolic function were unable to increase stroke volume normally, even in the presence of increased LV filling pressure. Myocardial hypertrophy, ischemia, or fibrosis causes slow or incomplete LV filling at normal left atrial pressures. The left atrial pressure increases to augment left ventricular filling, resulting in pulmonary and systemic venous congestion. The development of atrial fibrillation may also cause a decrease in cardiac output and the development of pulmonary and systemic venous congestion because of loss of the left atrial contribution to LV late diastolic filling and reduced diastolic filling time due to a rapid ventricular rate.

In a prospective study of 2,535 persons older than 60 years (mean 82 years), CHF developed in 677 persons (27%) [75]. In a prospective study of 1,160 men and 2,464 women older than 60 years, mean age 81 years, CHF developed in 29% of older men and in 26% of older women [76]. Elderly persons are more likely than nonelderly persons to develop CHF because of abnormal LV diastolic dysfunction with normal LV systolic function. Table 50.1 shows that the prevalence of normal LVEF in older persons with CHF ranges from 34 to 52% [75, 77–82]. The prevalence of normal LVEF with CHF is also higher in old women than in old men [75, 78–82].

A normal LVEF was present in older persons with CHF in 44% of 55 African-American men versus 58% of 110 African-American women, in 46% of 24 Hispanic men versus 56% of 34 Hispanic women, in 35% of 148 white men versus 57% of 303 white women, and in 38% of 227 older men versus 57% of 447 older women [82]. Table 50.2 shows the prevalence of a normal LVEF in 572 older persons with CHF in men and women of different age groups [75]. In the

Table 50.1 Prevalence of normal left ventricular ejection fraction (LVEF) in older persons with congestive heart failure (CHF)

Study	Results for patients with CHF and normal LVEF
Wong [77]	41% of 54 persons, mean age 80 years
Aronow [78]	47% of 247 persons, mean age 82 years
Cardiovascular Health Study [79]	59% of 186 persons, mean age 73 years
Framingham Heart Study [80]	51% of 73 persons, mean age 73 years
Pernenkil [81]	34% of 501 persons, mean age 81 years
Aronow [75]	50% of 572 persons, mean age 82 years
Aronow [82]	51% of 674 persons, mean age 81 years

TABLE 50.2 Association of congestive heart failure with normal left ventricular ejection fraction with gender and age in 572 older persons

Age (years)	Normal left ventricular ejection fraction
60–69	22% of 18 men and 37% of 38 women
70–79	33% of 54 men and 44% of 79 women
80–89	41% of 86 men and 59% of 219 women
≥90	47% of 19 men and 73% of 59 women
All ages	37% of 177 men and 56% of 395 women with congestive heart failure

Source: Adapted from Aronow et al. [75]

community, advancing age and female gender are associated with increases in vascular and ventricular systolic and diastolic stiffness even in the absence of cardiovascular disease [83] This contributes to the increased prevalence of CHF with a normal LVEF in elderly persons, especially in elderly women.

LVEF should be measured in all patients with CHF in order that appropriate therapy may be given [84–88]. For example, digoxin should not be used to treat persons with CHF and normal LVEF if sinus rhythm is present [63, 89–93]. By increasing contractility through increasing intracellular calcium ion concentration, digoxin may increase LV stiffness, increasing left ventricular filling pressure, and adversely affecting CHF due to LV diastolic dysfunction. Patients with CHF due to abnormal LVEF tolerate higher doses of diuretics than do patients with CHF and normal LVEF. Patients with CHF due to LV diastolic dysfunction with normal LVEF need high LV filling pressures to maintain an adequate stroke volume and cardiac output and cannot tolerate intravascular depletion. These patients should be treated with a low-salt diet with cautious use of diuretics, rather than with large doses of diuretics. Patients with abnormal LVEF should not be treated with calcium channel blockers [94, 95].

Cardiovascular Response to Exercise

The maximal oxygen consumption (VO_{2max}) is the best overall measurement of cardiovascular fitness [96]. VO_{2max} is the product of cardiac output and systemic arteriovenous oxygen difference at peak exercise. Maximal cardiac output – the heart rate multiplied by the stroke volume at peak exercise – is a more direct measurement of cardiovascular reserve than is VO_{2max} [96]. VO_{2max} is reduced with age [97, 98]. The degree of reduction of VO_{2max} with age is affected by physical conditioning, subclinical CAD, smoking, and body weight. Table 50.3 lists the cardiovascular responses to exercise in healthy old persons.

In the Baltimore Longitudinal Study of Aging, older male athletes had a higher peak exercise VO_{2max} than older sedentary men [99]. The greater peak exercise VO_{2max} in older male athletes than in older sedentary men was achieved by a higher

cardiac index and a greater systemic arteriovenous oxygen difference. The higher peak exercise cardiac index in older male athletes than in older sedentary men was due to a higher stroke volume index with similar maximal heart rates. Long-term endurance training also is associated with enhanced ventricular diastolic filling indices [100]. Older age is associated with a reduced exercise efficiency and an increase in the oxygen cost of exercise, which contributes to a reduced exercise capacity. These age-related changes are reversed with exercise training [101].

A reduction in maximal systemic arteriovenous oxygen difference occurs with age [102]. The decrease in muscle mass with age may play a major role in the decrease in systemic arteriovenous oxygen difference at peak exercise and in VO_{2max} [103].

Fleg et al. [104] also investigated the effect of age on peak upright cycle exercise in healthy sedentary men and women aged 22–86 years in the Baltimore Longitudinal Study of Aging. Peak cycle work rate was reduced with age in both men and women but was greater in men than in women at any age. Both men and women had peak exercise reductions in heart rate, cardiac index, and LVEF and increases in the LV end-diastolic volume index and end-systolic volume index with age. Peak exercise stroke volume index did not vary with age in men or women. The exercise-induced decrease in LV end-systolic volume index and the increases in cardiac index, stroke volume index, and LVEF from rest were greater in older men than in older women.

Age-Related Changes in Cardiovascular Function

Table 50.3 lists some age-related changes in cardiovascular function in healthy old persons. Contractility at rest does not change with age, but the duration of LV contraction and relaxation is prolonged. Age-associated reductions in maximal heart rate and in LV contractility during maximal exercise are manifestations of reduced β-adrenergic responsiveness with age partially offset by exercise-induced dilation of the LV.

Reduced arterial compliance contributes more to the age-related increase in afterload than does the loss of peripheral vascular beds. The impaired vasodilator response to β-adrenergic stimulation with age is most important during exercise and contributes to the increased afterload associated with age. Resting preload does not change with age. LV early diastolic filling is reduced with age. Augmentation of late diastolic filling of the LV prevents a reduction in LV end-diastolic volume with age. The maximal heart rate response to exercise is reduced with age. Exercise stroke volume is increased with age to maintain

TABLE 50.3 Cardiovascular responses to exercise in healthy old persons

Maximal heart rate is reduced with age

Exercise stroke volume is increased with age to maintain cardiac output

Increased exercise stroke volume with age results primarily from increase in LV end-diastolic volume by Frank–Starling mechanism

Reduction in muscle mass with age plays role in age-associated decreases in systemic arteriovenous oxygen difference and in VO_{2max} at peak exercise

LV end-diastolic and end-systolic volumes are increased during peak exercise with age

Peak exercise LV ejection fraction is reduced with age

Exercise-induced decrease in the LV end-systolic volume index and increases in the cardiac index, stroke volume index, and LV ejection fraction from rest are greater in old men than in old women

Contractility at rest does not change with age

Duration of LV contraction and relaxation is prolonged with age

Reduction in arterial compliance contributes more to age-related increase in afterload than does loss of peripheral vascular beds

Resting preload does not change with age

LV early diastolic filling is reduced with age

Augmentation of late diastolic filling of the LV prevents a reduction in LV end-diastolic volume with age

Age-associated reductions in maximal heart rate and LV contractility during maximal exercise are manifestations of reduced β-adrenergic responsiveness with age partially offset by exercise-induced dilation of the LV

Aging selectively impairs endothelium-dependent function

LV left ventricle, left ventricular

the exercise cardiac output, resulting from an increase in preload by the Frank–Starling mechanism. VO_{2max} and the systemic arteriovenous oxygen difference at peak exercise are reduced with age. Aging also selectively impairs endothelium-dependent function [105].

In addition to age-related changes in cardiovascular function and deconditioning due to a sedentary lifestyle, old persons also have a higher prevalence and incidence of cardiovascular disorders that impair cardiovascular performance than do nonelderly persons. Old persons are more likely than nonelderly persons to develop CHF secondary to abnormal LV diastolic dysfunction with normal LV systolic function.

Treatment of Congestive Heart Failure

The LVEF should be measured in all persons with CHF so appropriate therapy may be given [84–88]. For example, digoxin should not be used to treat persons with CHF and

normal LVEF if a sinus rhythm is present [63, 89–93]. Large doses of diuretics and nitrates should also be used cautiously in persons with CHF and a normal LVEF [95].

Calcium channel blockers such as diltiazem, nifedipine, and verapamil exacerbate CHF associated with abnormal LVEF [106]. Diltiazem increased mortality in patients with pulmonary congestion associated with abnormal LVEF after myocardial infarction [107]. The Multicenter Diltiazem Postinfarction Trial showed, in persons with a LVEF less than 40%, that late CHF at follow-up was increased in patients randomized to diltiazem (21%) versus those randomized to placebo (12%) [108]. Prospective studies have found that the vasoselective calcium channel blockers amlodipine [109] and felodipine [110] did not significantly affect survival compared with placebo in patients with CHF associated with abnormal LVEF. There was a significantly higher incidence of pulmonary edema in the persons treated with amlodipine (15%) than in persons treated with placebo (10%) [109]. The American College of Cardiology (ACC)/American Heart Association (AHA) guidelines recommend that calcium channel blockers should not be given to persons with CHF associated with abnormal LVEF [94].

Abnormal Left Ventricular Ejection Fraction

Table 50.4 shows the ACC/AHA Class I recommendations for treating patients with current or prior symptoms of CHF with reduced LVEF [94]. Older persons with CHF associated with abnormal LVEF should be treated with a low sodium diet and with diuretics plus an angiotensin-converting enzyme (ACE) inhibitor [111, 112] plus a β-blocker such as metoprolol CR/XL [113], carvedilol [114], bisoprolol [115], or nebivolol [116]. An angiotensin receptor blocker should be used if the patient is intolerant to an ACE inhibitor because of cough or angioneurotic edema [117]. Regular physical activity such as walking should be encouraged in patients with mild to moderate HF to improve functional status and to decrease symptoms. Patients with CHF who are dyspneic at rest at a low work level may benefit from a formal cardiac rehabilitation program [118].

An implant cardioverter defibrillator and cardiac resynchronization therapy should be used according to ACC/AHA guidelines [94, 119–121]. An aldosterone antagonist such as spironolactone [122] or eplerenone [123] should be used according to ACC/AHA guidelines [94].

Table 50.5 shows the ACC/AHA Class IIa recommendations for treating patients with current or prior symptoms of CHF with reduced LVEF [94]. Isosorbide dinitrate plus hydralazine was very effective in treating Blacks with CHF

TABLE 50.4 Class I recommendations for treating persons with current or prior symptoms of heart failure with decreased left ventricular ejection fraction

Treat underlying and precipitating causes of heart failure

Use diuretics and salt restriction in persons with fluid retention

Use ACE inhibitors

Use β-blockers

Use angiotensin II receptor blockers if intolerant to ACE inhibitors because of cough or angioneurotic edema

Avoid or withdraw nonsteroidal anti-inflammatory drugs, most antiarrhythmic drugs, and calcium channel blockers

Recommend exercise training

Implant cardioverter-defibrillator in persons with a history of cardiac arrest, ventricular fibrillation, or hemodynamically unstable ventricular tachycardia

Implant cardioverter-defibrillator in persons with ischemic heart disease ≥40 days postmyocardial infarction or nonischemic cardiomyopathy, a LVEF ≤30%, NYHA Class II or III symptoms on optimal medical therapy, and an expectation of survival of ≥1 year

Use cardiac resynchronization therapy in persons with a LVEH ≤35%, NYHA Class III or IV symptoms despite optimal therapy, and a QRS duration >120 ms

Add an aldosterone antagonist in selected patients with moderately severe to severe symptoms of heart failure who can be carefully monitored for renal function and potassium concentration (serum creatinine should be ≤2.5 mg/dl in men and ≤2.0 mg/dl in women; serum potassium should be <5.0 mEq/l)

Source: Adapted from Hunt et al. [94]

ACE angiotensin converting enzyme, *LVEF* left ventricular ejection fraction, *NYHA* New York Heart Association

TABLE 50.5 Class IIa recommendations for treating persons with current or prior symptoms of heart failure with decreased left ventricular ejection fraction

Angiotensin II receptor blockers may be used instead of ACE inhibitors if patients are already taking them for other reasons

Add hydralazine plus a nitrate to patients with persistent symptoms

Implant cardioverter-defibrillator in patients with LVEF of 30–35% from any origin with NYHA Class II or III symptoms on optimal medical therapy with a life expectancy of >1 year

Digoxin can be used in patients with persistent symptoms to reduce hospitalization for heart failure

Source: Adapted from Hunt et al. [94]

ACE angiotensin converting enzyme, *LVEF* left ventricular ejection fraction, *NYHA* New York Heart Association

TABLE 50.6 Therapy of patients with heart failure and normal left ventricular ejection fraction

Treat underlying and precipitating causes of heart failure

Avoid use of inappropriate drugs such as nonsteroidal anti-inflammatory drugs

Treat hypertension, especially systolic hypertension, hyperlipidemia, myocardial ischemia, and anemia

Treat with cautious use of diuretics

Treat with β-blockers

Treat with angiotensin-converting enzyme (ACE) inhibitor or angiotensin receptor blocker if patient cannot tolerate ACE inhibitor because of cough, angioneurotic edema, rash, or altered taste sensation

Add isosorbide dinitrate plus hydralazine if heart failure persists

Avoid digoxin if sinus rhythm is present

Exercise training as an adjunctive approach to improve clinical status in ambulatory patients

Source: Data from Hunt et al. [94]

and rejuvenation in vitro [3, 5, 128]. Cardiac stem cell therapy may become perhaps a novel strategy for the devastating problem of heart failure in the old population.

Normal Left Ventricular Ejection Fraction

Table 50.6 shows the therapy for older persons with CHF associated with a normal LVEF. β-Blockers [116, 129], ACE inhibitors [130, 131], and angiotensin receptor blockers [132] are efficacious in the treatment of these patients.

In older persons with CHF associated with a normal LVEF, pulmonary congestion is reduced by a low sodium diet, diuretics, and nitrates. Sinus rhythm is maintained to increase the LV filling time. The ventricular rate is slowed below 90 beats per minute by a β-blocker to increase LV filling time. Myocardial ischemia should be decreased and is best achieved by giving a β-blocker. Elevated SBP is decreased by diuretics and an ACE inhibitor. The LV mass is reduced by an ACE inhibitor. LV relaxation should be improved by ACE inhibitors or β-blockers.

Cardiovascular Disease

In addition to age-related changes in cardiovascular function and deconditioning due to a sedentary lifestyle, old persons also have a higher prevalence and incidence of cardiovascular disorders, which impair cardiovascular performance, than nonelderly persons. Table 50.7 lists the prevalence of some cardiovascular disorders in an elderly population in a long-term health care facility [76, 133, 134].

in the African-American Heart failure trial [124, 125]. The serum digoxin level should be maintained between 0.5 and 0.8 ng/ml to avoid an increase in mortality [95, 126, 127].

In experimental studies, the recognition of factors enhancing the activation of the cardiac stem cell pool, their mobilization and translocation, however, suggest that the detrimental effects of aging on the heart might be prevented in the future by local stimulation of cardiac stem cells or the intramyocardial delivery of cardiac stem cells following their expansion

TABLE 50.7 Prevalence of cardiovascular disorders in older persons in a long-term health-care facility

Cardiovascular disorder	Mean age (years)	Prevalence Number	%
Coronary artery disease [76]	81	1,521/3,624	42
Thromboembolic stroke [76]	81	1,131/3,624	31
Peripheral arterial disease [76]	81	1,011/3,624	28
40–100% Extracranial carotid arterial disease [133]	81	281/1,846	19
Congestive heart failure [76]	81	978/3,624	27
Hypertension [76]	81	2,136/3,624	59
Aortic stenosis [134]	81	463/2,805	17
Mitral annular calcium [134]	81	1,321/2,805	47
≥1+Mitral regurgitation [134]	81	928/2,805	33
≥1+Aortic regurgitation [134]	81	824/2,805	29
Rheumatic mitral stenosis [134]	81	37/2,805	1
Hypertrophic cardiomyopathy [134]	81	108/2,805	4
Idiopathic dilated cardiomyopathy [134]	81	29/2,805	1
Atrial fibrillation [76]	81	495/3,624	14
Pacemaker rhythm [76]	81	186/3,624	5
Abnormal left ventricular ejection fraction [134]	81	687/2,805	24
Left ventricular hypertrophy [134]	81	1,224/2,805	44
Left atrial enlargement [134]	81	987/2,805	35

Aortic Valve Disease

Valvular aortic stenosis in old persons is usually due to stiffening, scarring, and calcification of aortic valve leaflets. Calcific deposits in the aortic valve are common and may lead to valvular aortic stenosis [22, 135–137]. Calcific deposits in the aortic valve were present in 22 of 40 necropsied patients (55%) aged 90–103 years [136]. Aortic cuspal calcium was present in 295 of 752 men (36%), mean age 80 years, and in 672 of 1,663 women (40%), mean age 82 years [137].

Calcific valvular aortic stenosis was present at autopsy in 18% of 366 octogenarians [138]. Valvular aortic stenosis was diagnosed by continuous-wave Doppler echocardiography in 463 of 2,805 old persons (17%) with a mean age 81 years [76]. Severe aortic stenosis was present in 2% of these 2,805 old persons [76]. Severe aortic stenosis was also diagnosed in 3% of 501 persons aged 75–86 years in the Helsinki Ageing Study [139].

Aortic valve calcium, mitral annular calcium, and coronary artery disease in older persons have similar predisposing factors for atherosclerosis [137, 139–145]. Older patients with extracranial carotid arterial disease [140] and with peripheral arterial disease [141] have an increased prevalence of aortic stenosis. Older patients with aortic stenosis [146–148] and with valvular aortic sclerosis [148, 149] have an increased incidence of new coronary events.

The prevalence of aortic regurgitation also increases with age [22, 150, 151]. Aortic regurgitation was diagnosed by pulsed Doppler recordings of the aortic valve in 526 of 1,797 old persons (29%) with a mean age of 81 years [76]. Severe or moderate aortic regurgitation was diagnosed by pulsed Doppler recordings of the aortic valve in 74 of 450 old patients with a mean age of 82 years [152]. Margonato et al.

[150] linked the increased prevalence of aortic regurgitation with age to aortic valve thickening.

Mitral Valvular Disease

Two degenerative aging processes – mitral annular calcification and mucoid (or myxomatous) degeneration of the mitral valve leaflets and chordae tendineae – can cause significant mitral valvular dysfunction [153–155]. Mitral annular calcification was diagnosed by two-dimensional echocardiography in 36% of 924 elderly men and in 52% of 1,881 elderly women, mean age 81 years [76]. Mitral annular calcium was present in 11 of 57 persons (19%) 62–70 years of age, in 53 of 158 persons (34%) 71–80 years of age, in 190 of 301 persons (63%) 81–90 years of age, in 75 of 85 persons (88%) 91–100 years of age, and in 3 of 3 persons (100%) 101–103 years of age [156].

Breakdown of lipid deposits on the ventricular surface of the posterior mitral leaflet at or below the mitral annulus and on the aortic surfaces of the aortic valve cusps is probably responsible for the calcification [157]. Elderly men and women with mitral annular calcium have a higher prevalence of CAD [158–160], of peripheral arterial disease [160, 161], of extracranial carotid arterial disease [160, 162, 163], and of aortic atherosclerotic disease [160] than elderly men and women without mitral annular calcium.

Conduction Defects

The increased prevalence of conduction defects in old persons is due to age-related degeneration of the conduction system and to the development of cardiovascular disease.

TABLE 50.8 Prevalence of conduction defects in 1,153 old persons

Defect	Prevalence (%)
First-degree atrioventricular block	6
Left anterior fascicular block	8
Right bundle branch block	10
Left bundle branch block	4
Intraventricular conduction defect	3
Second-degree atrioventricular block	1
Pacemaker rhythm	4

Source: Adapted from Aronow [165]

Aging is associated with regional conduction slowing, anatomically determined conduction delay at the crista, and structural changes including areas of low voltage [164]. Impairment of sinus node function and an increase in atrial refractoriness occur with aging, predisposing to atrial fibrillation [164]. Table 50.8 lists the prevalence of conduction defects in 1,153 old persons, mean age 82 years [165]. At a 45-month follow-up, old persons with second-degree atrioventricular block, left bundle branch block, intraventricular conduction defect, and pacer rhythm had an increased incidence of new coronary events [165]. At the 45-month follow-up, old persons with first-degree atrioventricular block, left anterior fascicular block, or right bundle branch block did not have an increased incidence of new coronary events [165].

Conclusions

Cardiovascular function in elderly persons is significantly affected by the aging process itself and by those acquired diseases of the cardiovascular system that are more prevalent with age. These physiologic and pathologic changes of the aging cardiovascular system must be taken into consideration during the clinical assessment and management of elderly patients who need to undergo surgical procedures and general anesthesia.

References

1. Olivetti G, Melissari M, Capasso JM et al (1991) Cardiomyopathy of the aging human heart: myocyte loss and reactive cellular hypertrophy. Circ Res 68:1560–1568
2. Davies MJ (1988) The pathological basis of arrhythmias. Geriatr Cardiovasc Med 1:181–183
3. Gonzalez A, Rota M, Nurzynska D et al (2008) Activation of cardiac progenitor cells reverses the failing heart senescent phenotype and prolongs lifespan. Circ Res 102:597–606
4. Anversa P (2005) Aging and longevity. The IGF-1 enigma. Circ Res 97:411–414
5. Anversa P, Rota M, Urbanek K et al (2005) Myocardial aging – a stem cell problem. Basic Res Cardiol 100:482–493
6. Gerstenblith G, Fredericksen J, Yin FCP et al (1977) Echocardiographic assessment of a normal adult aging population. Circulation 56:273–278
7. Safar M (1990) Aging and its effects on the cardiovascular system. Drugs 39(suppl 1):1–8
8. Yin FCP (1980) The aging vasculature and its effects on the heart. In: Weisfeldt ML (ed) The aging heart: its function and response to stress. Raven, New York, pp 137–214
9. Avolio AP, Fa-Quan D, Wei-Qiang L et al (1985) Effects of aging on arterial distensibility in populations with high and low prevalence of hypertension: comparison between urban and rural communities in China. Circulation 71:202–210
10. Boutouyrie P, Laurent S, Benetos A et al (1992) Opposing effects of ageing on distal and proximal large arteries in hypertensives. J Hypertens 10:587–591
11. Nichols WW, O'Rourke MF, Avolio AP et al (1985) Effects of age on ventricular-vascular coupling. Am J Cardiol 55:1179–1184
12. Rodeheffer RJ, Gerstenblith G, Becker LC et al (1984) Exercise cardiac output is maintained with advancing age in healthy human subjects: cardiac dilatation and increased stroke volume compensate for a diminished heart rate. Circulation 69:203–213
13. Brandfonbrener M, Landowne M, Shock NW (1955) Changes in cardiac output with age. Circulation 12:557–566
14. Pan HY, Hoffman BB, Pershe RA et al (1986) Decline in beta-adrenergic receptor-mediated vascular relaxation with aging in man. J Pharmacol Exp Ther 239:802–807
15. Buhler F, Kowski W, Van Brumeler P (1980) Plasma catecholamines and cardiac, renal and peripheral vascular adrenoceptor mediated response in different age groups in normal and hypertensive subjects. Clin Exp Hypertens 2:409–426
16. Landahl S, Bengtsson C, Sigurdsson JA et al (1986) Age-related change in blood pressure. Hypertension 8:1044–1049
17. Avolio AP, Clyde KM, Beard TC et al (1986) Improved arterial distensibility in normotensive subjects on a low salt diet. Arteriosclerosis 6:166–169
18. Vaitkevicius PV, Fleg JL, Engel JH et al (1993) Effects of age and aerobic capacity on arterial stiffness in healthy adults. Circulation 88:1456–1462
19. Mitchell GF, Guo C-Y, Benjamin EJ et al (2007) Cross-sectional correlates of increased aortic stiffness in the community. The Framingham Heart Study. Circulation 115:2628–2636
20. Lima JAC, Gerstenblith G, Weiss JL et al (1988) Systolic blood pressure, not age mediates the age-related increase in left ventricular wall thickness within a normotensive population (abstract). J Am Coll Cardiol 11:81A
21. Levy D, Anderson KM, Savage DD et al (1988) Echocardiographically detected left ventricular hypertrophy: prevalence and risk factors: the Framingham heart study. Ann Intern Med 108:7–13
22. Aronow WS, Ahn C, Kronzon I (1997) Prevalence of echocardiographic findings in 554 men and in 1243 women aged >60 years in a long-term health care facility. Am J Cardiol 79:379–380
23. Aronow WS, Ahn C (1996) Risk factors for new coronary events in a large cohort of very elderly patients with and without coronary artery disease. Am J Cardiol 77:864–866
24. Aronow WS, Kronzon I (1991) Prevalence of coronary risk factors in elderly Blacks and Whites. J Am Geriatr Soc 39:567–570
25. Aronow WS, Koenigsberg M, Schwartz KS (1988) Usefulness of echocardiographic left ventricular hypertrophy in predicting new coronary events and atherothrombotic brain infarction in patients over 62 years of age. Am J Cardiol 61:1130–1132
26. Tanaka H, Dinenno FA, Monahan KD et al (2000) Aging, habitual exercise, and dynamic arterial compliance. Circulation 102:1270–1275
27. DeSouza CA, Shapiro LF, Clevenger CM et al (2000) Regular aerobic exercise prevents and restores age-related declines in endothelium-dependent vasodilation in healthy men. Circulation 102:1351–1357
28. Gardin JM, Henry WL, Savage DD et al (1979) Echocardiographic measurements in normal subjects: evaluation of an adult population without clinically apparent heart disease. J Clin Ultrasound 7:439–447

29. Bryg RJ, Williams GA, Labovitz AJ (1987) Effect of aging on left ventricular diastolic filling in normal subjects. Am J Cardiol 59:971–974

30. Iskandrian AS, Aakki A (1986) Age related changes in left ventricular diastolic performance. Am Heart J 112:75–78

31. Spirito P, Maron BJ (1988) Influence of aging on Doppler echocardiographic indices of left ventricular diastolic function. Br Heart J 59:672–679

32. Miyatake K, Okamoto J, Kinoshita N et al (1984) Augmentation of atrial contribution to left ventricular flow with aging as assessed by intracardiac Doppler flowmetry. Am J Cardiol 53:587–589

33. Sartori MP, Quinones MA, Kuo LC (1987) Relation of Doppler-derived left ventricular filling parameters to age and radius/thickness ratio in normal and pathologic states. Am J Cardiol 59:1179–1182

34. Fleg JL, Shapiro EP, O'Connor F et al (1995) Left ventricular diastolic filling performance in older male athletes. JAMA 273:1371–1375

35. Gardin JM, Rohan MK, Davidson DM et al (1987) Doppler transmitral flow velocity parameters: relationship between age, body surface area, blood pressure and gender in normal subjects. Am J Noninvasive Cardiol 1:3–10

36. Benjamin EG, Levy D, Anderson KM et al (1992) Determination of Doppler indexes of left ventricular diastolic function in normal subjects (the Framingham heart study). Am J Cardiol 70:508–515

37. Villari B, Hess OM, Kaufmann P et al (1992) Effect of aortic valve stenosis (pressure overload) and regurgitation (volume overload) on left ventricular systolic and diastolic function. Am J Cardiol 69:927–934

38. Prasad A, Popovic ZB, Arbab-Zadeh A et al (2007) The effects of aging and physical activity on Doppler measures of diastolic function. Am J Cardiol 99:1629–1636

39. Lakatta EG (1980) Age-related alterations in the cardiovascular response to adrenergic mediated stress. Fed Proc 39:3173–3177

40. Robbins AS, Rubenstein LZ (1984) Postural hypotension in the elderly. J Am Geriatr Soc 32:769–774

41. Aronow WS, Lee NH, Sales FF et al (1988) Prevalence of postural hypotension in elderly patients in a long-term health care facility. Am J Cardiol 62:336

42. Lipsitz LA, Jonsson PV, Marks BL et al (1990) Reduced supine cardiac volumes and diastolic filling rates in elderly patients with chronic medical conditions: implications for postural blood pressure homeostasis. J Am Geriatr Soc 38:103–107

43. Gribbin B, Pickering TG, Sleight P et al (1971) Effect of age and high blood pressure on baroreflex sensitivity in man. Circ Res 29:424–431

44. Lipsitz LA, Nyquist RP Jr, Wei JY et al (1983) Postprandial reduction in blood pressure in the elderly. N Engl J Med 309:81–83

45. Vaitkevicius PV, Esserwein DM, Maynard AK et al (1991) Frequency and importance of postprandial blood pressure reduction of elderly nursing-home patients. Ann Intern Med 115:865–870

46. Aronow WS, Ahn C (1994) Postprandial hypotension in 499 elderly persons in a long-term health care facility. J Am Geriatr Soc 42:930–932

47. Kamata T, Yokota T, Furukawa T et al (1994) Cerebral ischemic attack caused by postprandial hypotension. Stroke 25:511–513

48. Aronow WS, Ahn C (1997) Association of postprandial hypotension with incidence of falls, syncope, coronary events, stroke, and total mortality at 29-month follow-up in 499 older nursing home residents. J Am Geriatr Soc 45:1051–1053

49. Wolf PA, Abbott RD, Kannel WB (1991) Atrial fibrillation as an independent risk factor for stroke: the Framingham study. Stroke 22:983–988

50. Aronow WS, Ahn C, Gutstein H (1996) Prevalence of atrial fibrillation and association of atrial fibrillation with prior and new thromboembolic stroke in elderly patients. J Am Geriatr Soc 44:521–523

51. Kannel WB, Abbott RD, Savage DD et al (1982) Epidemiologic features of chronic atrial fibrillation: the Framingham study. N Engl J Med 306:1018–1022

52. Aronow WS, Ahn C, Mercando AD et al (1995) Correlation of atrial fibrillation, paroxysmal supraventricular tachycardia, and sinus rhythm with incidences of new coronary events in 1359 patients, mean age 81 years, with heart disease. Am J Cardiol 75:182–184

53. Poliner LR, Dehmer GJ, Lewis SE et al (1980) Left ventricular performance in normal subjects: a comparison of the responses to exercise in the upright and supine positions. Circulation 62:528–534

54. Fraticelli A, Josephson R, Danziger R et al (1989) Morphological and contractile characteristics of rat cardiac myocytes from maturation to senescence. Am J Physiol 257:H259–H265

55. Capasso JM, Malhotra A, Remly RM (1983) Effects of age on mechanical and electrical performance of rat myocardium. Am J Physiol 245:H72–H81

56. Willems JL, Roelandt H, DeGeest H et al (1970) The left ventricular ejection time in elderly subjects. Circulation 42:37–42

57. Shaw DJ, Rothbaum DA, Angell CS et al (1973) The effect of age and blood pressure upon the systolic time intervals in males aged 20–89 years. J Gerontol 28:133–139

58. Lakatta EG (1987) Do hypertension and aging have similar effects on the myocardium? Circulation 75(suppl 1):69–77

59. Lakatta EG, Yin FCP (1982) Myocardial aging: functional alterations and related cellular mechanisms. Am J Physiol 242: H927–H941

60. Port S, Cobb FR, Coleman RE et al (1980) Effect of age on the response of the left ventricular ejection fraction to exercise. N Engl J Med 303:1133–1137

61. Aronow WS, Stein PD, Sabbah HN et al (1989) Resting left ventricular ejection fraction in elderly patients without evidence of heart disease. Am J Cardiol 63:368–369

62. Fleg JL, Schulman S, O'Connor F et al (1994) Effect of acute β-adrenergic receptor blockade on age-associated changes in cardiovascular performance during dynamic exercise. Circulation 90:2333–2341

63. Tresch DD, McGough MF (1995) Heart failure with normal systolic function: a common disorder in older people. J Am Geriatr Soc 43:1035–1042

64. Wei JY, Spurgeon HA, Lakatta EG (1984) Excitation-contraction in rat myocardium: alterations with adult aging. Am J Physiol 246:H784–H791

65. Morgan JP, Morgan KG (1984) Calcium and cardiovascular function: intracellular calcium levels during contraction and relaxation of mammalian cardiac and vascular smooth muscle as detected with aequorin. Am J Med 77(suppl 5A):33–46

66. Bandy B, Davison AJ (1990) Mitochondrial mutations may increase oxidative stress: implications for carcinogenesis and aging? Free Radic Biol Med 8:523–539

67. Corral-Debrinski M, Stepien G, Shoffner JM et al (1991) Hypoxemia is associated with mitochondrial DNA damage and gene induction: implications for cardiac disease. JAMA 266:1812–1816

68. Lie JT, Hammond PI (1988) Pathology of the senescent heart: anatomic observations on 237 autopsy studies of patients 90 to 105 years old. Mayo Clin Proc 63:552–564

69. Schaub MC (1964) The aging of collagen in the heart muscle. Gerontologia 10:38–41

70. Verzar F (1969) The stages and consequences of aging collagen. Gerontologia 15:233–239

71. Hachamovitch R, Wicker P, Capasso JM et al (1989) Alterations of coronary blood flow and reserve with aging in Fischer 344 rats. Am J Physiol 256:H66–H73

72. Ogawa T, Spina R, Martin WH III et al (1992) Effects of aging, sex and physical training on cardiovascular responses to exercise. Circulation 86:494–503

73. Manning WJ, Shannon RP, Santinga JA et al (1989) Reversal of changes in left ventricular diastolic filling associated with normal aging using diltiazem. Am J Cardiol 67:894–896

74. Kitzman DW, Higginbotham MB, Cobb FR et al (1991) Exercise intolerance in patients with heart failure and preserved left ventricular systolic function: failure of the Frank–Starling mechanism. J Am Coll Cardiol 17:1065–1072

75. Aronow WS, Ahn C, Kronzon I (1998) Normal left ventricular ejection fraction in older persons with congestive heart failure. Chest 113:867–869

76. Aronow WS, Ahn C, Gutstein H (2002) Prevalence and incidence of cardiovascular disease in 1160 older men and 2464 older women in a long-term health care facility. J Gerontol A Biol Med Sci 57:M45–M46

77. Wong WF, Gold S, Fukuyama O et al (1989) Diastolic dysfunction in elderly patients with congestive heart failure. Am J Cardiol 63:1526–1528

78. Aronow WS, Ahn C, Kronzon I (1990) Prognosis of congestive heart failure in elderly patients with normal versus abnormal left ventricular systolic function associated with coronary artery disease. Am J Cardiol 66:1257–1259

79. Kitzman DW, Gardin JM, Arnold A et al (1996) Heart failure with preserved systolic LV function in the elderly: clinical and echocardiographic correlates from the Cardiovascular Health Study (abstract). Circulation 94(suppl 1):I433

80. Vasan RS, Benjamin EJ, Evans JC et al (1995) Prevalence and clinical correlates of diastolic heart failure: Framingham heart study (abstract). Circulation 92(suppl 1):666

81. Pernenkil R, Vinson JM, Shah AS et al (1997) Course and prognosis in patients ≥70 years of age with congestive heart failure and normal versus abnormal left ventricular ejection fraction. Am J Cardiol 79:216–219

82. Aronow WS, Ahn C, Kronzon I (1999) Comparison of incidences of congestive heart failure in older African-Americans, Hispanics, and whites. Am J Cardiol 84:611–612

83. Redfield MM, Jacobsen SJ, Borlaug BA et al (2005) Age-and gender-related ventricular-vascular stiffening. A community-based study. Circulation 112:2254–2262

84. Konstam MA, Dracup K, Baker DW et al (1994) Heart failure: management of patients with left-ventricular systolic dysfunction. Quick Reference Guide for Clinicians, No. 11, AHCPR Publication No. 94-0613. Agency for Health Care Policy and Research, Rockville, MD, June 1994, pp 1–21

85. Aronow WS (1994) Echocardiography should be performed in all elderly patients with congestive heart failure. J Am Geriatr Soc 42:1300–1302

86. Williams JF Jr, Bristow MR, Fowler MB et al (1995) Guidelines for the evaluation and management of heart failure. Report of the American College of Cardiology/American Heart Association Task Force on Practice Guidelines (Committee on Evaluation and Management of Heart Failure). J Am Coll Cardiol 26:1376–1398

87. American Medical Directors Association (1996) Heart failure. Clinical practice guideline. American Medical Directors Association, Columbia, MD, pp 1–8

88. Aronow WS (1998) Commentary on American Geriatrics Society Clinical Practice Guidelines from AHCPR Guidelines on Heart Failure: Evaluation and Treatment of Patients with Left Ventricular Systolic Dysfunction. J Am Geriatr Soc 46:525–529

89. Aronow WS (1991) Digoxin or angiotensin converting enzyme inhibitors for congestive heart failure in geriatric patients: which is the preferred treatment? Drugs Aging 1:98–103

90. Rich MW, McSherry F, Williford WO et al (2001) Effect of age on mortality, hospitalizations and response to digoxin in patients with heart failure: the DIG study. J Am Coll Cardiol 38:806–813

91. Ahmed A, Aronow WS, Fleg JL (2006) Predictors of mortality and hospitalization in women with heart failure in the Digitalis Investigation Group trial. Am J Ther 13:325–331

92. Ahmed A, Rich MW, Fleg JL et al (2006) Effects of digoxin on morbidity and mortality in diastolic heart failure. The Ancillary Digitalis Investigation Group trial. Circulation 114:397–403

93. Ahmed A, Zile MR, Rich MW et al (2007) Hospitalizations due to unstable angina pectoris in diastolic and systolic heart failure. Am J Cardiol 99:460–464

94. Hunt SA, Abraham WT, Feldman AM et al (2005) ACC/AHA 2005 guideline update for the diagnosis and management of chronic heart failure in the adult – summary article. A report of the American College of Cardiology/American Heart Association Task Force on Practice Guidelines (Writing Committee to Update the 2001 Guidelines for the Evaluation and Management of Heart Failure). Developed in collaboration with the American College of Chest Physicians and the International Society for Heart and Lung Transplantation. Endorsed by the Heart Rhythm Society. J Am Coll Cardiol 46:1116–1143

95. Aronow WS (2006) Epidemiology, pathophysiology, prognosis, and treatment of systolic and diastolic heart failure. Cardiol Rev 14:108–124

96. Fleg JL (1986) Alterations in cardiovascular structure and function with advancing age. Am J Cardiol 57:33C–44C

97. Dehn MM, Bruce RA (1972) Longitudinal variations in maximal oxygen intake with age and activity. J Appl Physiol 33:805–807

98. Heath GW, Hagberg JM, Ehsani AA (1981) A physiological comparison of young and older endurance athletes. J Appl Physiol 51:634–640

99. Fleg JL, Schulman SP, O'Connor FC et al (1994) Cardiovascular responses to exhaustive upright cycle exercise in highly trained older men. J Appl Physiol 77:1500–1506

100. Forman DE, Manning WJ, Hauser R et al (1992) Enhanced left ventricular diastolic filling associated with long-term endurance training. J Gerontol 47:M56–M58

101. Woo JS, Derleth C, Stratton JR, Levy WC (2006) The influence of age, gender, and training on exercise efficiency. J Am Coll Cardiol 47:1049–1057

102. Julius S, Amery A, Whitlock LS et al (1967) Influence of age on the hemodynamic response to exercise. Circulation 36:222–230

103. Fleg JL, Lakatta EG (1988) Role of muscle loss in the age-associated reduction in VO_{2max}. J Appl Physiol 65:1147–1151

104. Fleg JL, O'Connor F, Gerstenblith G et al (1995) Impact of age on the cardiovascular response to dynamic upright exercise in healthy men and women. J Appl Physiol 78:890–900

105. Chauhan A, More RS, Mullins PA et al (1996) Aging-associated endothelial dysfunction in humans is reversed by l-arginine. J Am Coll Cardiol 28:1796–1804

106. Elkayam U, Amin J, Mehra A et al (1990) A prospective, randomized, double-blind, crossover study to compare the efficacy and safety of chronic nifedipine therapy with that of isosorbide dinitrate and their combination in the treatment of chronic congestive heart failure. Circulation 82:1954–1961

107. Multicenter Diltiazem Postinfarction Trial Research Group (1988) The effect of diltiazem on mortality and reinfarction after myocardial infarction. N Engl J Med 319:385–392

108. Goldstein RE, Boccuzzi SJ, Cruess D et al (1991) Diltiazem increases late-onset congestive heart failure in postinfarction patients with early reduction in ejection fraction. Circulation 83:52–60

109. Packer M, O'Connor CM, Ghali JK et al (1996) Effect of amlodipine on morbidity and mortality in severe chronic heart failure. N Engl J Med 335:1107–1114

110. Cohn JN, Ziesche SM, Loss LE et al (1997) Effect of the calcium antagonist felodipine as supplementary vasodilator therapy in patients with chronic heart failure treated with enalapril. V-HeFT III. Circulation 96:856–863

111. Garg R, Yusuf S (1995) Collaborative Group on ACE Inhibitor Trials. Overview of randomized trials of angiotensin-converting

enzyme inhibitory on mortality and morbidity in patients with heart failure. JAMA 273:1450–1456

112. Pitt B, Segal R, Martinez FA et al (1997) Randomised trial of losartan versus captopril in patients over 65 with heart failure (Evaluation of Losartan in the Elderly Study, ELITE). Lancet 349:747–752

113. MERIT-HF Study Group (1999) Effect of metoprolol CR/XL in chronic heart failure: Metoprolol CR/XL Randomised Intervention Trial in Congestive Heart Failure (MERIT-HF). Lancet 353:2001–2007

114. Packer M, Coats AJS, Fowler MB et al (2001) Effect of carvedilol on survival in chronic heart failure. N Engl J Med 344:651–658

115. CIBIS-II Investigators and Committees (1999) The Cardiac Insufficiency Bisoprolol Study II (CIBIS-II): a randomised trial. Lancet 353:9–13

116. Flather MD, Shibata MC, Coats AJS et al (2005) Randomized trial to determine the effect of nebivolol on mortality and cardiovascular hospital admission in elderly patients with heart failure (SENIORS). Eur Heart J 26:215–225

117. Granger CB, McMurray JJV, Yusuf S et al (2003) Effects of candesartan in patients with chronic heart failure and reduced left-ventricular systolic function intolerant to angiotensin-converting-enzyme inhibitors: the CHARM-Alternative trial. Lancet 362:772–776

118. Aronow WS (2001) Exercise therapy for older persons with cardiovascular disease. Am J Geriatr Cardiol 10:245–252

119. Bardy GH, Lee KL, Mark DB et al (2005) Amiodarone or an implantable cardioverter-defibrillator for congestive heart failure. N Eng J Med 352:225–237

120. Aronow WS (2005) CRT plus ICD in congestive heart failure. Use of cardiac resynchronization therapy and an implantable cardioverter-defibrillator in heart failure patients with abnormal left ventricular dysfunction. Geriatrics 60(2):24–28

121. Cleland JGF, Daubert J-C, Erdmann E et al (2005) The effect of cardiac resynchronization on morbidity and mortality in heart failure. N Engl J Med 352:1539–1549

122. Pitt B, Zannad F, Remme WJ et al (1999) The effect of spironolactone on morbidity and mortality in patients with severe heart failure. N Engl J Med 341:709–717

123. Pitt B, Remme W, Zannad F et al (2003) Eplerenone, a selective aldosterone blocker, in patients with left ventricular dysfunction after myocardial infarction. N Engl J Med 348:1309–1321

124. Taylor AL, Ziesche S, Yancy C et al (2004) Combination of isosorbide dinitrate and hydralazine in blacks with heart failure. N Engl J Med 351:2049–2057

125. Aronow WS (2005) Race, drugs, and heart failure. Geriatrics 60(7):8–9

126. Rathore SS, Curtis JP, Wang Y et al (2003) Association of serum digoxin concentration and outcomes in patients with heart failure. JAMA 289:871–878

127. Ahmed A, Aban IB, Weaver MT et al (2006) Serum digoxin concentration and outcomes in women with heart failure: a bi-directional effect and a possible effect modification by ejection fraction. Eur J Heart Fail 8:409–441

128. Bolli R, Anversa P (2007) Stem cells and cardiac aging. In: Leri A, Anversa P, Frishman WH (eds) Cardiovascular regeneration and stem cell therapy. Blackwell Futura, Malden, MA, pp 171–181

129. Aronow WS, Ahn C, Kronzon I (1997) Effect of propranolol versus no propranolol on total mortality plus nonfatal myocardial infarction in older patients with prior myocardial infarction, congestive heart failure, and left ventricular ejection fraction ≥40% treated with diuretics plus angiotensin-converting-enzyme inhibitors. Am J Cardiol 80:207–209

130. Aronow WS, Kronzon I (1993) Effect of enalapril on congestive heart failure treated with diuretics in elderly patients with prior myocardial infarction and normal left ventricular ejection fraction. Am J Cardiol 71:602–604

131. Cleland JG, Tendera M, Adamus J et al (2006) The perindopril in elderly people with chronic heart failure (PEP-CHF) study. Eur Heart J 27:2257–2259

132. Yusuf S, Pfeffer MA, Swedberg K et al (2003) Effects of candesartan in patients with chronic heart failure and preserved left-ventricular ejection fraction: the CHARM-Preserved trial. Lancet 362:777–781

133. Aronow WS, Ahn C, Schoenfeld MR, Gutstein H (1999) Association of extracranial carotid arterial disease and chronic atrial fibrillation with the incidence of new thromboembolic stroke in 1,846 older persons. Am J Cardiol 83:1403–1404

134. Aronow WS, Ahn C, Kronzon I (2001) Comparison of echocardiographic abnormalities in African-American, Hispanic, and white men and women aged >60 years. Am J Cardiol 87:1131–1133

135. Roberts WC, Perloff JK, Constantino T (1971) Severe valvular aortic stenosis in patients over 65 years of age. Am J Cardiol 27:497–506

136. Waller BF, Roberts WC (1983) Cardiovascular disease in the very elderly: an analysis of 40 necropsy patients aged 90 years or over. Am J Cardiol 51:403–421

137. Aronow WS, Schwartz KS, Koenigsberg M (1987) Correlation of serum lipids, calcium, and phosphorus, diabetes mellitus and history of systemic hypertension with presence or absence of calcified or thickened aortic cusps or root in elderly patients. Am J Cardiol 59:998–999

138. Shirani J, Yousefi J, Roberts WC (1995) Major cardiac findings at necropsy in 366 American octogenarians. Am J Cardiol 75:151–156

139. Lindroos M, Kupari M, Heikkila J et al (1993) Prevalence of aortic valve abnormalities in the elderly: an echocardiographic study of a random population sample. J Am Coll Cardiol 21:1220–1225

140. Aronow WS, Kronzon I, Schoenfeld MR (1995) Prevalence of extracranial carotid arterial disease and of valvular aortic stenosis and their association in the elderly. Am J Cardiol 75:304–305

141. Aronow WS, Ahn C, Kronzon I (2001) Association of valvular aortic stenosis with symptomatic peripheral arterial disease in older persons. Am J Cardiol 88:1046–1047

142. Nassimiha D, Aronow WS, Ahn C, Goldman ME (2001) Rate of progression of valvular aortic stenosis in persons ≥60 years. Am J Cardiol 87:807–809

143. Nassimiha D, Aronow WS, Ahn C, Goldman ME (2001) Association of coronary risk factors with progression of valvular aortic stenosis in older persons. Am J Cardiol 87:1313–1314

144. Palta S, Pai AM, Gill KS, Pai RG (2000) New insights into the progression of aortic stenosis. Implications for secondary prevention. Circulation 101:2497–2502

145. Aronow WS, Schwartz KS, Koenigsberg M (1987) Correlation of serum lipids, calcium and phosphorus, diabetes mellitus, aortic valve stenosis and history of systemic hypertension with presence or absence of mitral anular calcium in persons older than 62 years in a long-term health care facility. Am J Cardiol 59:381–382

146. Aronow WS, Ahn C, Shirani J, Kronzon I (1998) Comparison of frequency of new coronary events in older persons with mild, moderate, and severe valvular aortic stenosis with those without aortic stenosis. Am J Cardiol 81:647–649

147. Livanainen AM, Lindroos M, Tilvis R et al (1996) Natural history of aortic valve stenosis of varying severity in the elderly. Am J Cardiol 78:97–101

148. Otto CM, Lind BK, Kitzman DW et al (1999) Association of aortic-valve sclerosis with cardiovascular mortality and morbidity in the elderly. N Engl J Med 341:142–147

149. Aronow WS (1999) Shirani J, Kronzon I. Comparison of frequency of new coronary events in older subjects with and without valvular aortic sclerosis. Am J Cardiol 83:599–600

150. Margonato A, Cianflone D, Carlino M et al (1989) Frequence and significance of aortic valve thickening in older asymptomatic patients and its relation to aortic regurgitation. Am J Cardiol 64:1061–1062

151. Akasaka T, Yoshikawa J, Yoshida K et al (1987) Age-related valvular regurgitation: a study by pulsed Doppler echocardiography. Circulation 76:262–265

152. Aronow WS, Kronzon I (1989) Correlation of prevalence and severity of aortic regurgitation detected by pulsed Doppler echocardiography with the murmur of aortic regurgitation in elderly patients in a long-term health care facility. Am J Cardiol 63:128–129

153. Sell S, Scully RE (1965) Aging changes in the aortic and mitral valves. Am J Pathol 46:345–365

154. Pomerance A, Darby AJ, Hodkinson HM (1978) Valvular calcification in the elderly: possible pathogenic factors. J Gerontol 33:672–676

155. Roberts WC (1986) The senile cardiac calcification syndrome. Am J Cardiol 58:572–574

156. Aronow WS, Schwartz KS, Koenigsberg M (1987) Correlation of atrial fibrillation with presence of absence of mitral annular calcium in 604 persons older than 60 years. Am J Cardiol 59:1213–1214

157. Roberts WC, Perloff JK (1972) Mitral valvular disease: a clinicopathologic survey of the conditions causing the mitral valve to function abnormally. Ann Intern Med 77:939–975

158. Aronow WS, Ahm C, Kronzon I (1999) Association of mitral annular calcium and of aortic cuspal calcium with coronary artery disease in older patients. Am J Cardiol 84:1084–1085

159. Adler Y, Herz I, Vaturi M et al (1998) Mitral annular calcium detected by transthoracic echocardiography is a marker for high prevalence and severity of coronary artery disease in patients undergoing coronary angiography. Am J Cardiol 82:1183–1186

160. Tolstrup K, Roldan CA, Qualls CR, Crawford MH (2002) Aortic valve sclerosis, mitral annular calcium, and aortic root sclerosis as markers of atherosclerosis in men. Am J Cardiol 89:1030–1034

161. Aronow WS, Ahn C, Kronzon I (2001) Association of mitral annular calcium with symptomatic peripheral arterial disease in older persons. Am J Cardiol 88:333–334

162. Antonini-Canterin F, Capanna M, Manfroni A, Brieda M, Grandis U, Sbaraglia F, Cervesato E, Pavan D, Nicolosi GL (2001) Association between mitral annular calcium and carotid artery stenosis and role of age and gender. Am J Cardiol 88:581–583

163. Seo Y, Ishimitsu T, Ishizu T et al (2005) Relationship between mitral annular calcification and severity of carotid atherosclerosis in patients with symptomatic ischemic cerebrovascular disease. J Cardiol 46:17–24

164. Kistler PM, Sanders P, Fynn SP et al (2004) Electrophysiologic and electroanatomic changes in the human atrium associated with aging. J Am Coll Cardiol 44:109–116

165. Aronow WS (1991) Correlation of arrhythmias and conduction defects on the resting electrocardiogram with new cardiac events in 1,153 elderly patients. Am J Noninvasive Cardiol 75:182–184

Chapter 51
Risk Factors for Atherosclerosis in the Elderly

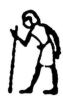

Wilbert S. Aronow and William H. Frishman

Coronary artery disease (CAD), peripheral arterial disease (PAD), atherothrombotic brain infarction (ABI), and extracranial carotid arterial disease (ECAD) are more common in old individuals than in middle-aged ones. CAD is the leading cause of death in old persons, especially those with PAD, ABI, or ECAD. This chapter discusses risk factors for CAD, PAD, ABI, and ECAD in old persons.

Cigarette Smoking

Coronary Artery Disease

The Chicago Stroke Study demonstrated that current cigarette smokers, age 65–74, had a 52% higher mortality from CAD than nonsmokers, ex-smokers, and pipe and cigar smokers [1]. Ex-smokers who had stopped smoking for 1–5 years had similar mortality from CAD as nonsmokers. The Systolic Hypertension in the Elderly Program pilot project found that smoking was a predictor of a first cardiovascular event and myocardial infarction (MI)/sudden death [2]. During a 30-year follow-up of subjects 65 years of age and older in the Framingham Heart Study, cigarette smoking was not associated with the incidence of CAD but was associated with mortality from CAD [3].

During a 12-year follow-up of men aged 65–74 in the Honolulu Heart Program, cigarette smoking was an independent risk factor for nonfatal MI and fatal CAD [4]. The absolute excess risk associated with cigarette smoking was 1.9 times higher in old men than in middle-aged men. At 5-year follow-up of old subjects (age ≥ 65) in three communities, cigarette smokers were shown to have a higher incidence of cardiovascular mortality than nonsmokers [5]. The relative risk for cardiovascular mortality was 2.0 in male smokers

and 1.6 in female smokers. The incidence of cardiovascular death in former smokers was similar to those who had never smoked [5].

At 40-month follow-up of 664 old men (mean age 80 years) and 48-month follow-up of 1,488 old women (mean age 82 years), cigarette smoking was demonstrated by multivariate analysis to increase the relative risk of new coronary events 2.2 and 2.0 times, respectively (Table 51.1) [6]. During a 42-month mean follow-up of 410 old Blacks and Whites with hypertension (mean age 81), the odds ratio for developing new coronary events was 2.0 in cigarette smokers [7]. It has also been observed that cigarette smoking aggravates angina pectoris and precipitates silent myocardial ischemia in old persons with CAD.

In the Coronary Artery Surgery Study (CASS) Registry, subjects over the age of 65 who continued smoking had an increased risk of developing MI or sudden death compared with those who stopped smoking during the year before enrolling in the study [8]. Furthermore, increasing age did not decrease the beneficial effects of smoking cessation.

In the Bronx Longitudinal Aging Study (BAS), whose cohort consisted of subjects 75–85 years of age at study onset, 10% of the cohort were smoking at study onset, and 46% reported having smoked in the past [8]. In the various BAS multivariate analyses, cigarette smoking history was shown to be an independent predictor of both cardiovascular morbidity and mortality and the development of MI.

Peripheral Arterial Disease

Numerous studies have shown that cigarette smoking is a risk factor for PAD in men and women [9–17]. In a study of 1,911 old subjects (mean age 81 years), current cigarette smoking was shown to increase the prevalence of symptomatic PAD 2.6 and 4.6 times in old men and women, respectively (Table 51.1) [9]. At 43-month follow-up of 291 old subjects (mean age 82 years) with PAD, multivariate analysis demonstrated that cigarette smoking was an independent predictor of new coronary events, with a relative risk of 1.6 [18].

W.S. Aronow (✉)
Cardiology Division, New York Medical College, Macy Pavilion, Room 138, Valhalla, NY, 10595, USA
e-mail: wsaronow@aol.com

R.A. Rosenthal et al. (eds.), *Principles and Practice of Geriatric Surgery*,
DOI 10.1007/978-1-4419-6999-6_51, © Springer Science+Business Media, LLC 2011

TABLE 51.1 Association of cigarette smoking with new coronary events, peripheral arterial disease, new atherothrombotic brain infarction, and extracranial carotid arterial disease in elderly men and women

Study	Elderly men			Elderly women		
	No. of patients	Mean follow-up (months)	Relative risk	No. of patients	Mean follow-up (months)	Relative risk
Incidence of new coronary events [6]	664	40	2.2	1,488	48	2.0
Prevalence of PAD [9]	467	–	2.6	1,444	–	4.6
Incidence of new ABI [23]	664	42	1.5	1,488	48	1.9
Prevalence of 40–100% ECAD in 1,063 men and women [24]			4.0			

PAD peripheral arterial disease, *ABI* atherothrombotic brain infarction, *ECAD* extracranial carotid arterial disease

Atherothrombotic Brain Infarction

A meta-analysis of 32 studies showed that cigarette smoking is a risk factor for ABI in men and women and carries a relative risk of 1.9 [19]. In the Medical Research Council (MRC) Trial, the incidence of strokes was 2.3 times higher in smokers than in nonsmokers [20]. Moreover, nonsmokers who received propranolol as antihypertensive therapy had a reduction in the incidence of stroke that cigarette smokers did not have. In the Framingham Heart Study, during a 26-year follow-up, cigarette smoking increased the incidence of new ABI 1.6 and 1.9 times in men and women, respectively [21]. Furthermore, the incidence of stroke in smokers who used >40 cigarettes daily was twice as high as in those who used <10 cigarettes daily. The impact of cigarette smoking did not diminish with increasing age. The risk of stroke was substantially decreased within 2 years of quitting smoking, with the incidence of stroke returning to the level of nonsmokers 5 years after smoking cessation. Although elderly individuals who quit smoking have higher cerebral perfusion levels than old persons who continue to smoke, their cerebral perfusion levels are lower than those who have never smoked [22].

At 42-month follow-up of 664 old men (mean age 80) and 48-month follow-up of 1,488 old women (mean age 82), cigarette smoking was demonstrated by multivariate analysis to increase the relative risk for ABI 1.5 and 1.9 times in men and women, respectively (Table 51.1) [23].

Extracranial Carotid Arterial Disease

Numerous studies have demonstrated that cigarette smoking is a strong risk factor for ECAD [24–29]. In a study of 1,063 old subjects (mean age 81 years), cigarette smoking was found by multivariate analysis to increase the prevalence of 40–100% ECAD 4.2 times (Table 51.1) [24].

On the basis of the available data, old men and women who smoke should be strongly encouraged to stop. In these individuals, cigarette smoking is a risk factor for CAD, PAD, ABI, and ECAD, as well as for other disorders including pulmonary disease and lung cancer. Smoking cessation should reduce mortality due to CAD, stroke, and other cardiovascular diseases and all-cause mortality in elderly persons.

Approaches to smoking cessation include the use of nicotine patches or nicotine polacrilex gum, which are available over the counter [30]. If this therapy is unsuccessful, nicotine nasal spray or treatment with the antidepressant buproprion and/or varenicline should be considered [30–32]. A nicotine inhaler may also be used [32]. The dosage and duration of treatment of each of these pharmacotherapies are discussed in detail elsewhere [32]. Concomitant behavioral therapy may also be needed [33]. Repeated physician advice is very important in the treatment of smoking addiction.

Hypertension

Coronary Artery Disease

Increased peripheral vascular resistance is the cause of systolic and diastolic hypertension in old persons. *Systolic hypertension* is diagnosed if the systolic blood pressure is 140 mmHg or higher on three occasions, and *diastolic hypertension* is diagnosed if the diastolic blood pressure is 90 mmHg or higher on three occasions [34]. *Isolated systolic hypertension* is diagnosed when the systolic blood pressure is 140 mmHg or higher on three occasions but diastolic blood pressure is normal [34].

In 1,414 old subjects (mean age 82 years), the prevalence of systolic or diastolic hypertension was higher in Blacks than in Hispanics or Whites [35]. In a study of 1,051 old individuals with hypertension, isolated systolic hypertension occurred in two-thirds of the persons [36]. Although both diastolic and isolated systolic hypertension are associated with increased cardiovascular morbidity and mortality in old individuals, increased systolic blood pressure is the greater risk factor [37].

The higher the systolic or diastolic blood pressure, the greater the morbidity/mortality from CAD in old men and women. During a 30-year follow-up of subjects 65 years and older in the Framingham Heart Study, systolic hypertension correlated with the incidence of CAD in men and women [3]. Diastolic hypertension correlated with CAD in old men but not in old women. At 40-month follow-up of 664 old men and 48 month follow-up of 1,488 old women, systolic or diastolic hypertension was demonstrated by multivariate analysis to increase the relative risk of new coronary events 2.0 and 1.6 times, respectively (Table 51.2) [6].

In the BAS [38], no relation was found between hypertension and the development of fatal MI, but a relation did exist for the development of clinically unrecognized MI, especially among hypertensives not on medication. Antihypertensive drugs have been shown to reduce new coronary events in the elderly hypertensive population [39–44]. The Joint National Committee on Detection, Evaluation, and Treatment of High Blood Pressure recommends diuretics or β-blockers as initial drug therapy because these drugs have been demonstrated to reduce cardiovascular morbidity and mortality in controlled clinical trials [35]. The particular antihypertensive agent selected as monotherapy should depend on the associated medical conditions. For example, old individuals with hypertension who have had an MI or who have angina pectoris, myocardial ischemia, or complex ventricular arrhythmias should be treated initially with a β-blocker [44]. Old hypertensive persons with congestive heart failure associated with abnormal or normal left ventricular ejection fraction should receive a diuretic, an angiotensin-converting enzyme (ACE) inhibitor, and a β-blocker [45–53]. Old persons with hypertension who have diabetes mellitus or left ventricular hypertrophy (LVH) should initially be treated with an ACE inhibitor [35, 54].

Old persons with hypertension and a prior MI should be treated with both β-blockers and ACE inhibitors [35, 55–58].

Peripheral Arterial Disease

Numerous studies have demonstrated that hypertension is a risk factor for PAD [10–12, 14–18]. In a study of 1,911 old persons (mean age 81 years), systolic or diastolic hypertension was observed to increase the prevalence of PAD 2.2 times in men and 2.8 times in women (Table 51.2) [10]. At 43-month follow-up of 291 old subjects with PAD (mean age 82), new coronary events developed in 165 patients (57%) [19].

Hypertension should be adequately controlled to decrease cardiovascular mortality and morbidity in persons with PAD. The blood pressure should be reduced to <140/90 mmHg and to <130/80 mmHg in patients with diabetes mellitus or chronic renal insufficiency, respectively [35, 55]. Among persons with PAD in the Appropriate Blood Pressure Control in Diabetes Trial, the incidence of cardiovascular events in persons treated with antihypertensive drug therapy with enalapril or nisoldipine was 13.6% if the mean blood pressure was reduced to 128/75 mmHg versus 38.7% if the mean blood pressure was reduced to 137/81 mmHg [59].

Atherothrombotic Brain Infarction

Numerous studies have documented that both systolic and diastolic hypertension increase the incidence of stroke in old persons [24, 39–43, 60–62]. Indeed, the higher the systolic or diastolic blood pressure, the greater the incidence of stroke. During a 30-year follow-up of men and women of age 65–94 years in the Framingham Heart Study, systolic blood pressure was the single risk factor most strongly correlated with ABI or transient cerebral ischemic attack [63]. At 42-month follow-up of 664 old men and 48-month follow-up of 1,488 old women, systolic or diastolic hypertension was demonstrated by multivariate analysis to increase the relative risk of ABI 2.2 times in men and 2.4 times in women (Table 51.2) [24].

In the BAS, subjects with measured hypertension had a significantly increased incidence of stroke (1.9/100 person-years) compared with that in controls (0.6/100 person-years) [9]. Previous studies have used a definition of hypertension as systolic blood pressure >160 mmHg, diastolic blood pressure >95 mmHg, or both to show an increased risk of stroke [24, 39–43, 60–62]. The findings in the BAS extended the risk of stroke to this oldest-old age group; [9] and considering the strict study values used, it suggested that the risk exists even

TABLE 51.2 Association of systolic or diastolic hypertension with new coronary events, peripheral arterial disease, and new atherothrombotic brain infarction in elderly men and women

Study	Elderly men			Elderly women		
	No. of patients	Mean follow-up (months)	Relative risk	No. of patients	Mean follow-up (months)	Relative risk
Incidence of new coronary events [6]	664	40	2.0	1,488	48	1.6
Prevalence of PAD [9]	467	–	2.2	1,444	–	2.8
Incidence of new ABI [23]	664	42	2.2	1,488	48	2.4

at levels of blood pressure not previously uniformly considered to be elevated by others. The BAS also showed an association between blood pressure elevation and the risk of vascular dementia [9], suggesting that some dementias could be prevented by blood pressure lowering [64].

Antihypertensive drug therapy has been shown to reduce the incidence of new ABI in old individuals [39–43, 61]. A systolic blood pressure of 140–160 mmHg causes an increased risk for cardiovascular disease that is equivalent to a diastolic blood pressure of 95–105 mmHg [38]. Consequently, the clinician should consider the treatment of old persons with systolic blood pressures in this range. Although nonpharmacologic interventions are indicated [65], there are currently no data showing that drug therapy for systolic blood pressures of 140–160 mmHg reduces the incidence of stroke in old persons. Nevertheless, the presence of LVH, target organ damage, and other risk factors for stroke would cause the authors to treat these individuals with antihypertensive drug therapy [66, 67].

Extracranial Carotid Arterial Disease

Numerous studies have demonstrated by univariate analysis that hypertension is a risk factor for ECAD [25–27, 29, 68]. According to multivariate analysis, however, hypertension is a risk factor in some studies [26, 68] but not in others [25, 26]. In a study of 1,283 old subjects (mean age 81), LVH was more prevalent in those with systolic or diastolic hypertension and ECAD than in those with systolic or diastolic hypertension alone [69].

Left Ventricular Hypertrophy

Coronary Events

LVH caused by hypertension or other cardiovascular disease is not only a marker of but also a contributor to cardiovascular morbidity and mortality in the elderly population. Indeed, old persons with electrocardiographic (ECG) and echocardiographic evidence of LVH have an increased risk of developing new coronary events [7, 70–75].

During a 4-year follow-up of 406 old men and 735 old women in the Framingham Heart Study, echocardiographic LVH was 15.3 times more sensitive for predicting new coronary events in men and 4.3 times more sensitive in women than ECG LVH [73]. The relative risk for new coronary events per 50 g/m increases in LV mass/height was 1.67 and 1.60 for old men and women, respectively [73].

At a 37-month follow-up of 360 old subjects (mean age 82 years) with hypertension or CAD, echocardiographic LVH was 4.3 times more sensitive for predicting new coronary events than ECG LVH [71]. Multivariate analysis of 472 old hypertensive subjects followed for 45 months showed that echocardiographic LVH was an independent risk factor for new coronary events, with a relative risk of 3.2 [75].

In the BAS a multivariate analysis showed that baseline ECG LVH is an independent predictor of MI and overall mortality. Those subjects who developed new LVH on ECG during follow-up had a 3.4 times higher total death rate and a 6.6-fold greater relative risk of cardiovascular death [9].

Atherothrombotic Brain Infarction

Elderly persons with ECG [7, 70–72] and echocardiographic [7, 71, 74–77] LVH have an increased risk of developing a new ABI. During an 8-year follow-up of 447 old men and 783 old women in the Framingham Heart Study, the hazard ratio for new cerebrovascular events was 1.45 for each quartile increase in the LV mass/height ratio after adjustments were made for age, sex, and cardiovascular disease [76]. At the 37-month follow-up of 360 old persons with hypertension and CAD, echocardiographic LVH was 4.0 times more sensitive for predicting a new ABI than ECG LVH [71]. Multivariate analysis of 472 old subjects with hypertension followed for 45 months revealed that echocardiographic LVH was an independent risk factor for a new ABI, with a relative risk of 2.9 [75]. Among 1,482 old persons (mean age 82 years) followed for 45 months, multivariate analysis also showed that echocardiographic LVH was an independent risk factor for a new ABI, with a risk ratio of 2.3 [77].

Physicians should try to prevent LVH from developing or progressing in persons with hypertension or other cardiovascular disease. The effect of various antihypertensive drugs on reducing LV mass is discussed elsewhere [78, 79]. A meta-analysis of 109 treatment studies showed that ACE inhibitors are more effective than other antihypertensive drugs in decreasing LV mass [79].

Reduction of LV mass with antihypertensive agents does not cause deterioration of LV systolic function and may improve LV diastolic function. Data from the Framingham Heart Study have shown a decrease of cardiovascular events in patients with the regression of LVH [80]. In patients with uncomplicated hypertension followed for 10.2 years, the Cornell group found that the development of LVH increases and the regression of LVH decreases the incidence of new cardiovascular events [81]. Regression of ECG LVH by antihypertensive treatment was associated with a 30% significant reduction in sudden cardiac death independently of treatment modality, blood pressure reduction, prevalent CAD, and other cardiovascular risk factors in hypertensive patients with LVH [82]. In addition, the BAS demonstrated that old subjects who developed new ECG LVH had a higher incidence of cardiovascular morbidity and mortality than old persons without ECG LVH [72] based on a 10-year follow-up. Old persons in whom the ECG pattern of LVH disappeared over time had a lower incidence of cardiovascular morbidity and mortality than old persons with persistent LVH [72].

Dyslipidemia

Serum Total Cholesterol and Coronary Artery Disease

Serum total cholesterol was an independent risk factor for CAD in old men and women in the Framingham Heart Study [83]. Among subjects with prior MI in this study, serum total cholesterol was most strongly related to death from CAD and to all-cause mortality in persons of age ≥65 years [84]. Many other studies have demonstrated that a higher serum total cholesterol level is a risk factor for new coronary events in old men and women [2, 6, 85, 86].

During a 9-year follow-up of 350 men and women with a mean age of 79 years, the BAS demonstrated that a consistently elevated low-density lipoprotein (LDL) cholesterol was associated with the development of MI in women [87]. In the Established Populations for Epidemiologic Studies of the Elderly study, serum total cholesterol was a risk factor for CAD-associated mortality in old women but not in old men [88]. At 40-month follow-up of 664 old men and 48-month follow-up of 1,488 old women, there was a 1.12 times higher probability of developing new coronary events in men and women for each 10 mg/dl increase in serum total cholesterol (Table 51.3) [6].

During a 5.4-year median follow-up of 1,021 old men and women with CAD and hypercholesterolemia in the Scandinavian Simvastatin Survival Study (4S), patients treated with simvastatin had a 34% reduction in mortality, a 43% reduction in CAD mortality, a 34% reduction in major coronary events, a 33% reduction in nonfatal MI, a 33% reduction in any acute CAD-related event, a 34% reduction in any atherosclerosis-related endpoint, and a 41% reduction in coronary revascularization [89]. The absolute risk reduction for both all-cause mortality and CAD mortality was approximately twice as great in older persons as in those younger than 65 years of age.

In the Cholesterol and Recurrent Events (CARE) Trial, 4,159 men and women with MI, serum total cholesterol levels

TABLE 51.3 Association of abnormal serum lipids with new coronary events and with new atherothrombotic brain infarction in 664 old men and 1,488 old women

	New coronary events		New antithrombotic brain infarction	
	Relative risk			
	Men	Women	Men	Women
Serum total cholesterol	1.12[a]	1.12[a]	NS	1.06[a]
Serum HDL cholesterol	1.70[b]	1.95[b]	NS	1.14[b]
Serum triglycerides	NS	1.02[c]	NS	NS

HDL high-density lipoprotein, NS nonsignificant
Source: Adapted from Aronow et al. [6, 23], with permission from Elsevier
[a]For an increment of 10 mg/dl of serum total cholesterol
[b]For a decrement of 10 mg/dl of serum HDL cholesterol
[c]For an increment of 10 mg/dl of serum triglycerides

<240 mg/dl, and serum LDL cholesterol ≥115 mg/dl were followed over a 5-year period [90]. The trial showed a 27% reduction in major coronary events in subjects 60–75 years of age who were randomized to pravastatin at study event; a 20% reduction in major coronary events was observed in subjects <60 years of age who were randomized to pravastatin. Furthermore, the reduction in coronary events was greater in women (46%) than in men (20%). On the basis of these data, old men and women with CAD and elevated total or LDL cholesterol should be treated with a statin drug.

At 6.1-year mean follow-up of 9,014 men and women (3,514 of whom were aged 65–75 years) with MI (64%) or unstable angina pectoris (36%) and serum total cholesterol levels of 155–271 mg/dl in the Long-Term Intervention With Pravastatin in Ischemic Disease Study (LIPID), compared with placebo, pravastatin 40 mg daily significantly reduced all-cause mortality by 22%, death from CAD by 24%, fatal and nonfatal MI by 29%, death from cardiovascular disease by 25%, need for coronary artery bypass surgery by 22%, need for coronary angioplasty by 19%, hospitalization for unstable angina pectoris by 12%, and stroke by 19% [91]. The absolute benefits of treatment with pravastatin were greater in groups of persons at higher absolute risk for a major coronary event such as older persons, those with a higher serum LDL-cholesterol level, those with a lower serum high-density lipoprotein (HDL)-cholesterol level, and those with a history of diabetes mellitus or smoking.

At 5-year follow-up of 20,536 British men and women (10,697 of whom were aged 65–80 years) with either CAD, occlusive arterial disease of non-coronary arteries, diabetes mellitus or treated hypertension and no serum lipid requirement in the Heart Protection Study, compared with placebo, simvastatin 40 mg daily significantly reduced all-cause mortality by 13%, any vascular mortality by 17%, major coronary events by 27%, any stroke by 25%, any revascularization procedure by 24%, and any major vascular event by 24% [92]. In the 1,263 persons aged 75–80 years at study entry and 80–85 years at follow-up, any major vascular event was significantly reduced 28% by simvastatin. Lowering serum LDL cholesterol from <116 to <77 mg/dl by simvastatin caused a 25% significant reduction in vascular events.

In the Heart Protection Study, 3,500 persons had initial serum LDL-cholesterol levels <100 mg/dl [92]. Decrease of serum LDL cholesterol from 97 to 65 mg/dl by simvastatin in these persons caused a similar decrease in risk as did treating patients with higher serum LDL-cholesterol levels. The Heart Protection Study Investigators recommended treating persons at high risk for cardiovascular events with statins, regardless of the initial levels of serum lipids, age, or gender [92].

On the basis of these data and other data [92–96], the American College of Cardiology/American Heart Association (ACC/AHA) guidelines [55] and the updated National Cholesterol Education Program III guidelines [97] state that in very high-risk persons, targeting a serum LDL-cholesterol level of <70 mg/dl is a reasonable clinical strategy. When a high-risk person has hypertriglyceridemia or low HDL cholesterol, consideration can be given to combining a fibrate or nicotinic acid with an LDL cholesterol-lowering drug [55, 97].

Serum HDL Cholesterol and Coronary Artery Disease

A low level of serum HDL cholesterol is a risk factor for new coronary events in old men and women [2, 6, 83, 87, 88, 98, 99]. In the Framingham Heart Study [83] and in the Established Populations for Epidemiologic Studies of the Elderly study [88], a low serum HDL was a more powerful predictor of new coronary events than was the total cholesterol.

During a 9-year follow-up of 350 men and women in the BAS, a consistently low HDL-cholesterol level was independently associated with the development of MI, cardiovascular disease, or death in men [87]. At a 40-month follow-up of 664 old men and 48-month follow-up of 1,488 old women, multivariate analysis showed that there was a 1.7 times higher probability of developing new coronary events in men and 1.95 times higher probability in women for each 10 mg/dl decrement in serum HDL cholesterol (Table 51.3) [6].

Serum Triglycerides and Coronary Artery Disease

High-serum triglycerides have been reported to be a risk factor for new coronary events in old women but not in old men [6, 83]. At a 40-month follow-up of 664 old men and 48-month follow-up of 1,488 old women, multivariate analysis showed that serum triglyceride levels were not a risk factor for new coronary events in the men and were a weak risk factor in the women (Table 51.3) [6].

Serum Lipids and Peripheral Arterial Disease

Some studies have shown an association between increased serum total cholesterol and PAD [10, 11, 14–18, 100, 101] but other studies have not [102]. A low serum HDL-cholesterol level, however, has been shown to be associated with PAD [10, 11, 14–18, 100, 101]. In a study of 559 old men and 1,275 old women (mean age 81 years), an inverse association was found between serum HDL cholesterol and PAD [101]. Multivariate analysis demonstrated a 1.24 times higher probability of having PAD for each 10 mg/dl decrement of serum HDL cholesterol.

Increased serum triglycerides have been associated with PAD in some studies [13, 14] but not in others [10, 11, 100, 101]. In a study of 559 old men and 1,275 old women, serum triglycerides were associated with PAD in both men and women according to univariate analysis but not according to multivariate analysis [101].

Treatment of hypercholesterolemia with statins has been demonstrated to reduce the incidence of cardiovascular events and mortality in older persons with PAD [92, 103]. Three double-blind, randomized, placebo-controlled studies have also demonstrated that statins improve walking performance in persons with PAD [104–106].

Serum Lipids and Atherothrombotic Brain Infarction

The Framingham Study found that serum total and HDL-cholesterol levels were not associated with new ABIs in old men or women [107]. However, the serum total cholesterol HDL-cholesterol ratio was associated with new ABIs in the women but not in the men. Very low-density lipoprotein (VLDL) levels were not associated with new ABIs in older men or women [107].

The Multiple Risk Factor Intervention Trial revealed an association between serum total cholesterol and death from nonhemorrhagic stroke in men [108]. Bihari-Varga et al. [109] demonstrated an inverse relation between serum HDL cholesterol and ABIs in men and women. At 42-month follow-up of 664 old men and 48-month follow-up of 1,488 older women, multivariate analysis showed no association between serum lipids and new ABIs in the men. There was an association between serum total cholesterol and an inverse association between HDL cholesterol and new ABIs in the women (Table 51.3) [24]. In this population, there was a 1.06 times higher probability of developing a new ABI for each 10 mg/dl increment in serum total cholesterol. Likewise, there was a 1.14 times higher probability of developing a new ABI for each 10 mg/dl decrement in serum HDL cholesterol.

In the Scandinavian Simvastatin Survival Study, patients treated with simvastatin had a 27% reduction in new ABIs [89]. In the Cholesterol and Recurrent Events Trial, patients treated with pravastatin had a 31% reduction in new ABIs [90]. A meta-analysis of four primary prevention trials and eight secondary prevention trials of CAD that used simvastatin, pravastatin, or lovastatin to reduce serum total cholesterol levels demonstrated a 27% reduction in new ABIs [110]. Many other studies reported since then have also demonstrated a significant reduction in ischemic stroke in patients treated with statins [91, 92, 111–114].

At 3-year follow-up of 1,410 patients, mean age 81 years, with prior MI and a serum LDL cholesterol of 125 mg/dl or higher, use of statins significantly reduced stroke by 60% [112]. Decreasing serum LDL cholesterol to less than 90 mg/dl was associated with a 7% incidence of new stroke, whereas decreasing serum LDL cholesterol to 90–99 mg/dl was associated with a 16% incidence of new stroke. The lower the serum LDL cholesterol in elderly persons treated with statins, the greater was the reduction in new stroke [112] and in new coronary events [95]. In 4,731 patients, mean age 63 years, with stroke or transient ischemic attack, reduction of serum LDL cholesterol at least 50% by atorvastatin caused a significant reduction in stroke of 31% and in major coronary events of 37% at 4.9-year follow-up [114]. These data support the use of statins to reduce elevated serum total and LDL-cholesterol levels in old men and women to prevent new thrombotic and/or embolic strokes and new coronary events.

A meta-analysis by our group has shown an increased risk of cerebral hemorrhage in patients receiving statins compared with those individuals not receiving statins. The mechanism for this finding is not known, and the data would suggest that patients with a history of cerebral hemorrhage or those individuals with a cerebral hemorrhage on a statin did not receive this therapy for cholesterol lowering [115].

Serum Lipids and Extracranial Carotid Arterial Disease

Elevated serum total cholesterol [25, 116, 117] and decreased serum HDL cholesterol [25, 27, 29, 32, 116, 117] are risk factors for ECAD. In 1,189 persons of age 66–93 years in the Framingham study, there was a strong association between the severity of ECAD and the serum total cholesterol, as measured 8 years before the carotid studies [116]. In women, but not in men, there was a strong inverse association between the severity of ECAD and the serum HDL cholesterol level measured 8 years before the carotid studies and concurrently [116].

In a study of 1,063 old persons, increased total cholesterol and decreased HDL cholesterol, but not serum triglycerides, were found to be risk factors for ECAD [25]. There was a 1.17 times higher probability of having 40–100% ECAD for each 10 mg/dl increment of serum total cholesterol and a 1.66 times higher probability of having 40–100% ECAD for each 10 mg/dl decrement of serum HDL cholesterol. Many studies have demonstrated the beneficial effects of lipid-lowering drug therapy on carotid atherosclerosis and on coronary events [118–121]. At 21-month follow-up of 449 patients with severe carotid arterial disease who did not undergo revascularization, use of statins caused a 87% significant reduction in the incidence of new stroke or new MI or death [121].

Diabetes Mellitus

Coronary Artery Disease

Diabetes mellitus is a risk factor for new coronary events in old men and women [6, 122]. At a 40-month follow-up of 664 old men and 48-month follow-up of 1,488 old women, diabetes mellitus was shown by multivariate analysis to increase the relative risk of new coronary events 1.9 and 1.8 times in men and women, respectively (Table 51.4) [6]. In the BAS diabetes mellitus, by history or a fasting blood glucose level

TABLE 51.4   Association of diabetes mellitus with new coronary events, peripheral arterial disease, new atherothrombotic brain infarction, and new extracranial carotid arterial disease in old men and women

Study	Older men			Older women		
	No. of patients	Mean follow-up (months)	Relative risk	No. of patients	Mean follow-up (months)	Relative risk
Incidence of new coronary events [6]	664	40	1.9	1,488	48	1.8
Prevalence of PAD [9]	467	–	2.4	1,444	–	3.0
Incidence of new ABI [23]	664	42	1.5	1,488	48	1.5
Prevalence of 40–100% ECAD in 1,063 men and women [24]			1.7			

PAD peripheral arterial disease, *ABI* atherothrombotic brain infarction, *ECAD* extracranial carotid arterial disease

of >140 mg/dl was associated with an increased incidence risk of all-cause mortality and cardiovascular disease [9].

Diabetic patients are more often obese and have higher serum LDL- and VLDL-cholesterol levels and lower serum HDL-cholesterol levels than do nondiabetics. Diabetics also have a higher prevalence of hypertension and LVH. These risk factors contribute to their higher incidence of new coronary events and new ABIs and the higher prevalence of PAD and ECAD. The drug of choice for treating hypertension in diabetics is an ACE inhibitor or angiotensin receptor blocker [35, 54]. The blood pressure should be lowered to <130/80 mmHg. The serum LDL cholesterol should be reduced to <70 mg/dl by a statin in diabetics [55, 97].

Diabetics with microalbuminuria have more severe angiographic CAD than diabetics without microalbuminuria [123]. Diabetics also have a significant increasing trend of hemoglobin A_{1c} levels over the increasing number of vessels with CAD [124]. Diabetics have a higher prevalence of unrecognized MI and a higher prevalence of silent myocardial ischemia without a history of angina pectoris than nondiabetics [125]. The hemoglobin A_{1c} level should be reduced to <7% in patients with diabetes mellitus [55].

Peripheral Arterial Disease

Diabetes mellitus is a risk factor for PAD in men and women [10–18]. In a study of 467 old men and 1,444 old women, diabetes mellitus was found to increase the prevalence of PAD 2.4 times in men and 3.0 times in women (Table 51.4) [10]. The higher the hemoglobin A_{1c} levels in diabetics with PAD, the higher the prevalence of severe PAD [126].

Atherothrombotic Brain Infarction

Diabetes mellitus is a risk factor for new ABIs in old men and women [23, 107, 127]. At a 42-month follow-up of 664 old men and a 48-month follow-up of 1,488 old women, diabetes was found by multivariate analysis to increase the relative risk for new ABIs 1.5 times in both men and women (Table 51.4) [24].

Extracranial Carotid Arterial Disease

Some studies [25, 128] have shown an association between diabetes mellitus and ECAD, whereas other studies [27] have not. In a study of 1,063 old men and women, diabetes mellitus was demonstrated by multivariate analysis to increase the prevalence of 40–100% ECAD 1.7 times [25].

Obesity

In the Framingham Heart Study, obesity was demonstrated to be a risk factor for new coronary events in old men and women [122]. A disproportionate distribution of fat to the abdomen, as assessed by the waist/hip circumference ratio, has also been shown to be a risk factor for cardiovascular disease, mortality due to CAD, and total mortality [129, 130]. At a 40-month follow-up of 664 old men and a 48-month follow-up of 1,488 old women, obesity was shown to be a risk factor for new coronary events in both men and women by univariate but not multivariate analysis [6].

In the BAS, body surface area was also not predictive. There were no subjects with major obesity problems [9]. In elderly subjects, maintenance of weight and appetite is a sign of health. Indeed, when old subjects lose weight and have reductions in their cholesterol, it may signify starvation, an occult malignancy, or a major cognitive problem.

The Framingham Heart Study showed that relative weight, according to Metropolitan Life Insurance criteria, was not associated with intermittent claudication in women but was inversely associated with intermittent claudication in men [63]. In a study of 244 old men and 625 old women, obesity did not significantly increase the prevalence of PAD in the men, but it did increase the prevalence of PAD 1.8 times in the women [11].

The Framingham Heart Study showed that relative weight was not a risk factor for new ABIs in old men but was a weak risk factor in old women [107]. Barrett-Connor and Khaw [127] observed no association between body mass index and new ABIs in old men and women. At a 42-month follow-up of 664 old men, obesity was not a risk factor for new ABIs [24]. At a 48-month follow-up of 1,488 old women, obesity was a risk factor for new ABIs by univariate analysis but not multivariate analysis [24]. Obesity is not a risk factor for ECAD [23, 27].

Physical Inactivity

Physical inactivity is associated with obesity, hypertension, dyslipidemia, and hyperglycemia. Paffenbarger et al. [131] found that individuals of age 65–79 years with a physical activity index >2,000 kcal/week have a better survival rate than those with an index <2,000 kcal/week. Wenger [132] discussed physiologic bases for the decrease in habitual physical activity with age and noted studies suggesting that physical activity is beneficial in preventing CAD. The relation of physical inactivity to ABI is unclear [107, 133].

Moderate exercise programs suitable for old persons include walking, climbing stairs, swimming, and bicycling.

TABLE 51.5 Association of gender with incidence of new coronary events, prevalence of peripheral arterial disease, incidence of new thromboembolic stroke, and prevalence of 40–100% extracranial carotid arterial disease in old men and women

Study	Old men			Old women		
	No. of patients	Mean follow-up (months)	Incidence or prevalence (%)	No. of patients	Mean follow-up (months)	Incidence or prevalence (%)
Incidence of new coronary events [135]	1,160	46	46	2,464	46	44
Prevalence of peripheral arterial disease [135]	1,160	–	32*	2,464	–	26
Incidence of new thromboembolic stroke [135]	644	46	23	2,464	46	21
Prevalence of 40–100% ECAD [24]	435	–	18	1,057	–	15

ECAD extracranial carotid arterial disease
*$p=0.0001$

Exercise training programs are not only beneficial for preventing CAD [132], but have also been demonstrated to improve endurance and functional capacity in old men with CAD [134].

Age

The incidence of new coronary events increases with age in old men and women [6, 122]. The incidence of PAD [10, 63] and ABI [24, 107] also increased with age. In the BAS, age was the strongest independent predictor of total mortality, cardiovascular mortality, MI, stroke, and dementia [9].

Gender

At a 46-month follow-up of 1,160 old men (mean age 80 years) and of 2,464 old women (mean age 81 years), the incidence of new coronary events was not significantly different in the men (46%) and the women (44%) (Table 51.5) [135]. The prevalence of PAD in the old men (32%) was higher than in the old women (26%) ($p=0.0001$) (Table 51.5). The incidence of new thromboembolic stroke was not significantly different between the men (23%) than in the women (21%) (Table 51.5) [135]. The prevalence of 40–100% ECAD was not significantly different for 435 old men (18%) and 1,057 old women (15%) with a mean age of 82 years. In the BAS, the incidence of MI was higher in women than in men [9].

Race

Black men are 2.5 times more likely to die of stroke than white men, and black women are 2.4 times more likely to die of stroke than white women [136]. Table 51.6 shows the prevalence of CAD, PAD, and ABI in 268 elderly Blacks (mean age 81), 71 elderly Hispanics (mean age 81), and 1,310 elderly Whites (mean age 82) [137]. The prevalence of CAD was not significantly different among the Blacks, Hispanics, and Whites. However, the prevalence of PAD was significantly higher in the Blacks than in Whites. Likewise, the prevalence of ABI was significantly higher in the Blacks than in either Hispanics or Whites.

Prior Coronary Artery Disease, Peripheral Arterial Disease, and Atherothrombotic Brain Infarction

At a 40-month follow-up of 664 old men and a 48-month follow-up of 1,488 old women, prior CAD was shown by multivariate analysis to increase the relative risk of new coronary events 1.7 times in men and 1.9 times in women [6]. At a 43-month follow-up of 291 old persons (mean age 82) with PAD, prior CAD was shown to be an independent risk factor for new coronary events, with a relative risk of 2.7 [19].

In the BAS, over an average range of 5–8 years of follow-up, the incidences of cardiovascular disease and mortality in subjects with evidence of infarct at baseline were 8.8 and 5.9 per 100 person-years versus 4.7 and 3.9 per 100 person-years in controls, respectively. The rates of development of unrecognized MI (Q-wave) were 2.4 and 3.2 per 100 person-years, respectively, for recognized MI. The rate of development of either a recognized or unrecognized MI was three times more likely in those with a history of a prior infarct [9].

Old persons with prior ABI or transient cerebral ischemic attacks have a higher incidence of ABI [7, 24, 138]. At a 42-month follow-up of 664 old men and a 48-month follow-up of 1,488 old women, multivariate analysis showed that a prior ABI increased the relative risk of a new ABI 2.6 times in men and 2.9 times in women [24].

Table 51.6 Prevalence of coronary artery disease, peripheral arterial disease, and atherothrombotic brain infarction in elderly Blacks, Hispanics, and Whites

Disorder	Prevalence (%)		
	Blacks ($n=268$)	Hispanics ($n=71$)	Whites ($n=1,310$)
CAD	46	34	41
PAD	29*	24	23
ABI	47**	31	22

Source: Adapted from Aronow [137]
*$p<0.05$ comparing Blacks with Whites
**$p<0.001$ comparing Blacks with Whites and <0.02 comparing Blacks with Hispanics

Table 51.7 Prevalence of coexistence of coronary artery disease, peripheral arterial disease, and atherothrombotic brain infarction in 1,886 elderly persons

Condition	Prevalence (%)		
	CAD	PAD	ABI
ABI present	53	33	–
PAD present	58	–	34
CAD present	–	33	32

Source: Adapted from Aronow and Ahn [148], with permission from Elsevier

Table 51.8 Prevalence of coexistence of coronary artery disease, peripheral arterial disease, and ischemic stroke in 1,802 older persons in an academic geriatrics practice

Condition	Prevalence (%)		
	CAD	PAD	ABI
Stroke present	56	28	–
PAD present	68	–	42
CAD present	–	26	32

Source: Adapted from Ness and Aronow [149], with permission from John Wiley & Sons, Inc.

Coexistence of Coronary Artery Disease, Peripheral Arterial Disease, and Atherothrombotic Brain Infarction

Persons with PAD [15, 19, 139–143] or cerebrovascular disease [144–146] are at increased risk for developing new coronary events. The Framingham Heart Study demonstrated that the age-adjusted incidence of stroke was more than doubled in patients with CAD [107]. In a study of 110 old persons (mean age 82) with chronic atrial fibrillation, logistic regression analysis revealed that a prior MI was an independent predictor of thromboembolic stroke, with an odds ratio of 4.8 [147].

Table 51.7 shows the prevalence of coexistence of CAD, PAD, and ABI in a study of 1,886 old persons (580 men and 1,306 women) whose mean age was 81 years [148]. If CAD was present, 33% had coexistent PAD and 32% had coexistent ABI. If PAD was present, 58% had coexistent CAD and 34% had coexistent ABI. If ABI was present, 53% had coexistent CAD and 33% had coexistent PAD.

Table 51.8 shows the prevalence of coexistence of CAD, PAD, and ischemic stroke in a study of 1,802 old persons (474 men and 1,328 women) whose mean age was 80 years [149]. If CAD was present, 26% had coexistent PAD and 32% had coexistent ischemic stroke. If PAD was present, 68% had coexistent CAD and 42% had coexistent ischemic stroke. If ischemic stroke was present, 56% had coexistent CAD and 28% had coexistent PAD.

Table 51.9 Factors associated with increased independent risk of incident morbidity or cardiovascular disease in the oldest old[a]: Bronx Longitudinal Aging Study

Age

Smoking history

Diabetes mellitus

History of past MI (clinically apparent or silent) documented on ECG

LVH by ECG (including new onset)

Cardiomegaly by chest radiography (including new onset)

Nonsustained ventricular tachycardia on 24-h Holter ECG

Persistent HDL cholesterol ≤30 mg/dl in men; persistent LDL cholesterol ≥171 mg/dl in women

Hypertension, both combined systolic and diastolic and isolated systolic

Prolongation of the RR interval on resting ECG

Nonspecific ST and T-wave abnormalities on resting ECG (unrelated to LV or past MI)

Digoxin use

Unfavorable baseline self-rated health assessment

Development of dementia

High vitamin B$_{12}$ level

MI myocardial infarction, *ECG* electrocardiography, *LVH* left ventricular hypertrophy
Source: Reprinted from Frishman et al. [38], with permission from Elsevier
[a]Age: 75–85 years

Conclusion

Many of the risk factors and markers for atherosclerosis complicated by CAD, cerebrovascular disease, and PAD seen during middle age continue to be operative in the elderly (Table 51.9) [9].

References

1. Jajich CL, Ostfield AM, Freeman DH Jr (1984) Smoking and coronary heart disease mortality in the elderly. JAMA 252:2831–2834
2. Siegel D, Kuller L, Lazarus NB et al (1987) Predictors of cardiovascular events and mortality in the systolic hypertension in the elderly program pilot project. Am J Epidemiol 126:385–399
3. Kannel WB, Vokonas PS (1986) Primary risk factors for coronary heart disease in the elderly: the Framingham study. In: Wenger

NK, Furberg CD, Pitt B (eds) coronary heart disease in the elderly. Elsevier, New York, pp 60–92

4. Benfante R, Reed D, Frank J (1991) Does cigarette smoking have an independent effect on coronary heart disease incidence in the elderly? Am J Public Health 81:897–899

5. LaCroix AZ, Lang J, Scherr P et al (1991) Smoking and mortality among older men and women in three communities. N Engl J Med 324:1619–1625

6. Aronow WS, Ahn C (1996) Risk factors for coronary events in a large cohort of very elderly patients with and without coronary artery disease. Am J Cardiol 77:864–866

7. Aronow WS, Ahn C, Kronzon I et al (1991) Congestive heart failure, coronary events and atherothrombotic brain infarction in elderly blacks and whites with systemic hypertension and with and without echocardiographic and electrocardiographic evidence of left ventricular hypertrophy. Am J Cardiol 67: 295 299

8. Hermanson B, Omenn GS, Kronmal RA et al (1988) Beneficial six-year outcome of smoking cessation in older men and women with coronary artery disease: results from the CASS registry. N Engl J Med 319:1365–1369

9. Ness J, Aronow WS, Ahn C (2000) Risk factors for peripheral arterial disease in an academic hospital-based geriatrics practice. J Am Geriatr Soc 48:312–314

10. Aronow WS, Sales FF, Etienne F et al (1988) Prevalence of peripheral arterial disease and its correlation with risk factors for peripheral arterial disease in elderly patients in a long-term health care facility. Am J Cardiol 62:644–646

11. Kannel WB, McGee DL (1985) Update on some epidemiologic features of intermittent claudication: the Framingham study. J Am Geriatr Soc 33:13–18

12. Pomrehn P, Duncan B, Weissfeld L et al (1986) The association of dyslipoproteinemia with symptoms and signs of peripheral arterial disease: the Lipid Research Clinics Program Prevalence Study. Circulation 73(Suppl I):100–107

13. Beach KW, Brunzell JD, Strandness DE Jr (1982) Prevalence of severe arteriosclerosis obliterans in patients with diabetes mellitus: relation to smoking and form of therapy. Arteriosclerosis 2:275–280

14. Reunanen A, Takkunen H, Aromaa A (1982) Prevalence of intermittent claudication and its effect on mortality. Acta Med Scand 211:249–256

15. Ness J, Aronow WS, Newkirk E, McDanel D (2005) Prevalence of symptomatic peripheral arterial disease, modifiable risk factors, and appropriate use of drugs in the treatment of peripheral arterial disease in older persons seen in a university general medicine clinic. J Gerontol Med Sci 60A:M255–M257

16. Murabito JM, Evans JC, Nieto K et al (2002) Prevalence and clinical correlates of peripheral arterial disease in the Framingham Offspring Study. Am Heart J 143:961–965

17. Sukhija R, Yalamanchili K, Aronow WS (2003) Prevalence of left main coronary artery disease, of 3-vessel or 4-vessel coronary artery disease, and of obstructive coronary artery disease in patients with and without peripheral arterial disease undergoing coronary angiography for suspected coronary artery disease. Am J Cardiol 92:304–305

18. Aronow WS, Ahn C, Mercando AD et al (1992) Prognostic significance of silent ischemia in elderly patients with peripheral arterial disease with and without previous myocardial infarction. Am J Cardiol 69:137–139

19. Shinton R, Beevers G (1989) Meta-analysis of relation between cigarette smoking and stroke. Br Med J 298:789–794

20. Medical Research Council Working Party (1985) MRC trial of treatment of mild hypertension: principal results. Br Med J Clin Res 291:97–104

21. Wolf PA, D'Agostino PS, Kannel WB et al (1988) Cigarette smoking as a risk factor for stroke: the Framingham study. JAMA 259:1025–1029

22. Rodgers RL, Meyer JS, Judd BW et al (1985) Abstention from cigarette smoking improves cerebral perfusion among elderly chronic smokers. JAMA 253:2970–2974

23. Aronow WS, Ahn C, Gutstein H (1996) Risk factors for new atherothrombotic brain infarction in 664 older men and 1488 older women. Am J Cardiol 77:1380–1383

24. Aronow WS, Ahn C, Schoenfeld MR (1993) Risk factors for extracranial internal or common carotid arterial disease in elderly patients. Am J Cardiol 71:1479–1481

25. Candelise L, Bianchi F, Galligoni F et al (1984) Italian multicenter study on reversible cerebral ischemic attacks. III. Influence of age and risk factors on cerebrovascular atherosclerosis. Stroke 15:379–382

26. Crouse JR III, Toole JF, McKinney WM (1987) Risk factors for extracranial carotid artery atherosclerosis. Stroke 18:990–996

27. Tell GS, Howard G, McKinney WM et al (1989) Cigarette smoking cessation and extracranial carotid atherosclerosis. JAMA 261:1178–1180

28. Bots ML, Breslau BJ, Briet E et al (1992) Cardiovascular determinants of carotid artery disease: the Rotterdam Elderly Study. Hypertension 19:717–720

29. Tell GS, Polak JF, Ward BJ et al (1994) Relation of smoking with carotid artery wall thickness and stenosis in older adults: the Cardiovascular Health Study. Circulation 90:2905–2908

30. Benowitz NL (1997) Treating tobacco addiction: nicotine or no nicotine. N Eng J Med 337:1230–1231

31. Hurt RD, Sachs DPL, Glover ED et al (1997) A comparison of sustained-release buproprion and placebo for smoking cessation. N Eng J Med 337:1195–1202

32. Frishman WH, Mitta W, Kupersmith A, Ky T (2006) Nicotine and non-nicotine smoking cessation pharmacotherapies. Cardiol in Rev 14:57–73

33. Tonnesen P, Fryd V, Hansen M et al (1988) Effect of nicotine chewing gum in combination with group counseling on the cessation of smoking. N Eng J Med 318:15–18

34. Chobanian AV, Bakris GL, Black HR, Joint National Committee et al (2003) The Seventh Report of the Joint National Committee on Prevention, Detection, Evaluation, and Treatment of High Blood Pressure: the JNC 7 report. JAMA 289:2560–2572

35. Aronow WS, Kronzon I (1991) Prevalence of coronary risk factors in elderly blacks and whites. J Am Geriatr Soc 39:567–570

36. Ness MG, JN AWS (1999) Drug treatment of hypertension in older persons in an academic hospital-based geriatrics practice. J Am Geriatr Soc 47:597–599

37. Applegate WB, Rutan GH (1992) Advances in management of hypertension in older persons. J Am Geriatr Soc 40:1164–1174

38. Frishman WH, Sokol S, Aronson M et al (1998) Risk factors for cardiovascular and cerebrovascular diseases and dementia in the elderly: findings from the Bronx Longitudinal Aging Study. Curr Probl Cardiol 23:1–68

39. Amery A, Birkenhager W, Brixko P et al (1985) Mortality and morbidity results from the European Working Party on Hypertension in Elderly Trial. Lancet 1:1349–1354

40. Dahlof B, Lindholm LH, Hansson L et al (1991) Morbidity and mortality in the Swedish Trial in Old Patients with Hypertension (STOP Hypertension). Lancet 338:1281–1285

41. SHEP Cooperative Research Group (1991) Prevention of stroke by antihypertensive drug treatment in older persons with isolated systolic hypertension: final results of the Systolic Hypertension in the Elderly Program (SHEP). JAMA 265:3255–3264

42. MRC Working Party (1992) Medical Research Council Trial on treatment of hypertension in older adults: principal results. Br Med J 304:405–412

43. Staessen JA, Fagard R, Thijs L et al (1997) Randomised double-blind comparison of placebo and active treatment for older patients with isolated systolic hypertension. Lancet 350:757–764

44. Aronow WS, Ahn C, Mercando AD et al (1994) Effect of propranolol versus no antiarrhythmic drug on sudden cardiac death, total cardiac death, and total death in patients ≥62 years of age with heart disease, complex ventricular arrhythmias, and left ventricular ejection fraction ≥40%. Am J Cardiol 74:267–270

45. Hunt SA, Abraham WT, Chin MH et al (2005) ACC/AHA 2005 guideline update for the diagnosis and management of chronic heart failure in the adult-summary article. A report of the American College of Cardiology/American Heart Association Task Force on Practice Guidelines (Writing Committee to Update the 2001 Guidelines for the Evaluation and Management of Heart Failure). Developed in collaboration with the American College of Chest Physicians and the International Society for Heart and Lung Transplantation. Endorsed by the Heart Rhythm Society. Circulation 112:e154–e235

46. Aronow WS (2006) Epidemiology, pathophysiology, prognosis, and treatment of systolic and diastolic heart failure. Cardiol Rev 14:108–124

47. Cleland JG, Tendera M, Adamus J et al (2006) The perindopril in elderly people with chronic heart failure (PEP-CHF) study. Eur Heart J 27:2257–2259

48. Yusuf S, Pfeffer MA, Swedberg K et al (2003) Effects of candesartan in patients with chronic heart failure and preserved left-ventricular ejection fraction: the CHARM-Preserved trial. Lancet 362:777–781

49. Aronow WS, Kronzon I (1993) Effect of enalapril on congestive heart failure treated with diuretics in elderly patients with prior myocardial infarction and normal left ventricular ejection fraction. Am J Cardiol 71:602–604

50. MERIT-HF Study Group (1999) Effect of metoprolol CR/XL in chronic heart failure: Metoprolol CR/XL Randomised Intervention Trial in Congestive Heart Failure (MERIT-HF). Lancet 353:2001–2007

51. Packer M, Coats AJS, Fowler MB et al (2001) Effect of carvedilol on survival in chronic heart failure. N Engl J Med 344:651–658

52. Flather MD, Shibata MC, Coats AJS et al (2005) Randomized trial to determine the effect of nebivolol on mortality and cardiovascular hospital admission in elderly patients with heart failure (SENIORS). Eur Heart J 26:215–225

53. Aronow WS, Ahn C, Kronzon I (1997) Effect of propranolol versus no propranolol on total mortality plus nonfatal myocardial infarction in older patients with prior myocardial infarction, congestive heart failure, and left ventricular ejection fraction ≥40% treated with diuretics plus angiotensin-converting-enzyme inhibitors. Am J Cardiol 80:207–209

54. American Diabetes Association (2003) Treatment of hypertension of adults with diabetes. Diabetes Care 26(Suppl 1):580–582

55. Smith SC Jr, Allen J, Blair SN et al (2006) ACC/AHA guidelines for secondary prevention for patients with coronary and other atherosclerotic vascular disease: 2006 update: endorsed by the National Heart, Lung, and Blood Institute. Circulation 113:2363–2372

56. HOPE (Heart Outcomes Prevention Evaluation) Study Investigators (2000) Effects of an angiotensin-converting-enzyme inhibitor, ramipril, on cardiovascular events in high-risk patients. N Engl J Med 342:145–153

57. Aronow WS, Ahn C, Kronzon I (2001) Effect of beta blockers alone, of angiotensin-converting enzyme inhibitors alone, and of beta blockers plus angiotensin-converting enzyme inhibitors on new coronary events and on congestive heart failure in older persons with healed myocardial infarcts and asymptomatic left ventricular systolic dysfunction. Am J Cardiol 88:1298–1300

58. Aronow WS, Ahn C (2002) Incidence of new coronary events in older persons with prior myocardial infarction and systemic hypertension treated with beta blockers, angiotensin-converting enzyme inhibitors, diuretics, calcium antagonists, and alpha blockers. Am J Cardiol 89:1207–1209

59. Mehler PS, Coll JR, Estacio R et al (2003) Intensive blood pressure control reduces the risk of cardiovascular events in patients with peripheral arterial disease and type 2 diabetes. Circulation 107:753–756

60. Garland C, Barrett-Connor E, Suarez L et al (1983) Isolated systolic hypertension and mortality after age 60 years: a prospective population-based study. Am J Epidemiol 118:365–376

61. Coope J, Warrender TS (1986) Randomised trial of treatment of hypertension in elderly patients in primary care. Br Med J 293:1145–1151

62. Beckett NS, Peters R, Fletcher AE et al (2008) Treatment of hypertension in patients 80 years of age or older. N Engl J Med 358:1887–1898

63. Stokes J III, Kannel WB, Wolf PA et al (1987) The relative importance of selected risk factors for various manifestations of cardiovascular disease among men and women from 35 to 64 years old: 30 years of follow-up in the Framingham study. Circulation 75(Suppl V):V65–V73

64. Aronow WS, Frishman WH (2006) Effects of antihypertensive drug treatment on cognitive function and the risk of dementia. Clin Geriatr 114:25–28

65. Applegate WB, Miller ST, Elam JT et al (1992) Nonpharmacologic intervention to reduce blood pressure in older patients with mild hypertension. Arch Intern Med 152:1162–1166

66. Aronow WS, Frishman WH (2004) Treatment of hypertension and prevention of ischemic stroke. Curr Cardiol Rep 6:124–129

67. Lavie CJ, Ventura HO, Messerli FH (1994) Left ventricular hypertrophy in the elderly. Cardiol Elder 2:362–369

68. Ruben S, Espeland MA, Ryu J et al (1988) Individual variation in susceptibility to extracranial carotid atherosclerosis. Arteriosclerosis 8:389–397

69. Aronow WS, Kronzon I, Schoenfeld MR (1995) Left ventricular hypertrophy is more prevalent in patients with systemic hypertension with extracranial carotid arterial disease than in patients with systemic hypertension without extracranial carotid arterial disease. Am J Cardiol 76:192–193

70. Kannel WB, Dannenberg AL, Levy D (1987) Population implications of electrocardiographic left ventricular hypertrophy. Am J Cardiol 60:85I–93I

71. Aronow WS, Koenigsberg M, Schwartz KS (1989) Usefulness of echocardiographic and electrocardiographic left ventricular hypertrophy in predicting new cardiac events and atherothrombotic brain infarction in elderly patients with systemic hypertension or coronary artery disease. Am J Noninvasive Cardiol 3:367–370

72. Kahn S, Frishman WH, Weissman S et al (1996) Left ventricular hypertrophy on electrocardiogram: prognostic implications from a 10 year cohort study of older subjects: a report from the Bronx Longitudinal Aging Study. J Am Geriatr Soc 44:524–529

73. Levy D, Garrison RJ, Savage DD et al (1989) Left ventricular mass and incidence of coronary heart disease in an elderly cohort: the Framingham Heart Study. Ann Intern Med 110:101–107

74. Aronow WS, Koenigsberg M, Schwartz KS (1988) Usefulness of echocardiographic left ventricular hypertrophy in predicting new coronary events and atherothrombotic brain infarction in patients over 62 years of age. Am J Cardiol 61:1130–1132

75. Aronow WS, Ahn C, Kronzon I et al (1997) Association of plasma renin activity and echocardiographic left ventricular hypertrophy with frequency of new coronary events and new atherothrombotic brain infarction in older persons with systemic hypertension. Am J Cardiol 79:1543–1545

76. Bikkina M, Levy D, Evans JC et al (1994) Left ventricular mass and risk of stroke in an elderly cohort: the Framingham Heart Study. JAMA 272:33–36

77. Aronow WS, Ahn C, Kronzon I et al (1997) Association of extracranial carotid arterial disease, prior atherothrombotic brain infarction, systemic hypertension, and left ventricular hypertrophy with the incidence of new atherothrombotic brain infarction at 45 month follow-up of 1482 older patients. Am J Cardiol 79:991–993

78. Aronow WS (1992) Left ventricular hypertrophy. J Am Geriatr Soc 40:71–80

79. Dahlof B, Pennert K, Hansson L (1992) Reversal of left ventricular hypertrophy in hypertensive patients: a meta-analysis of 109 treatment studies. Am J Hypertens 5:95–110

80. Levy D, Solomon M, D'Agostino RB et al (1994) Prognostic implications of baseline electro-cardiographic features and their serial changes in subjects with left ventricular hypertrophy. Circulation 90:1786–1793

81. Koren MJ, Devereux RB, Casale PN et al (1991) Relation of left ventricular mass and geometry to morbidity and mortality in uncomplicated essential hypertension. Ann Intern Med 114:345–352

82. Wachtell K, Okin PM, Olsen MH et al (2007) Regression of electrocardiographic left ventricular hypertrophy during antihypertensive therapy and reduction in sudden cardiac death. The LIFE Study. Circulation 116:700–705

83. Castelli SP, Wilson PWF, Levy D, Anderson K (1989) Cardiovascular risk factors in the elderly. Am J Cardiol 63:12H–19H

84. Wong ND, Wilson PWF, Kannel WB (1991) Serum cholesterol as a prognostic factor after myocardial infarction: the Framingham study. Ann Intern Med 115:687–693

85. Benfante R, Reed D (1990) Is elevated serum cholesterol level a factor for coronary heart disease in the elderly? JAMA 263:393–396

86. Rubin SM, Sidney S, Black DM et al (1990) High blood cholesterol in elderly men and the excess risk for coronary heart disease. Ann Intern Med 113:916–920

87. Zimetbaum P, Frishman WH, Ooi WL et al (1992) Plasma lipids and lipoproteins and the incidence of cardiovascular disease in the very elderly: the Bronx Aging Study. Arterioscler Thromb 12:416–423

88. Corti M-C, Guralnik JM, Salive ME et al (1995) HDL cholesterol predicts coronary heart disease mortality in older persons. JAMA 274:539–544

89. Miettinen TA, Pyorala K, Olsson AG et al (1997) Cholesterol-lowering therapy in women and elderly patients with myocardial infarction or angina pectoris. Findings from the Scandinavian Simvastatin Survival Study (4S). Circulation 96:4211–4218

90. Sacks FM, Pfefer MA, Moye LA et al (1996) The effect of pravastatin on coronary events after myocardial infarction in patients with average cholesterol levels. N Engl J Med 335:1001–1009

91. The Long-Term Intervention with Pravastatin in Ischaemic Disease (LIPID) Study Group (1998) Prevention of cardiovascular events and death with pravastatin in patients with coronary heart disease and a broad range of initial cholesterol levels. N Engl J Med 339:1349–1357

92. Heart Protection Study Collaborative Group (2002) MRC/BHF Heart Protection Study of cholesterol lowering with simvastatin in 20, 536 high-risk individuals: a randomised placebo-controlled trial. Lancet 360:7–22

93. Cannon CP, Braunwald E, McCabe CH et al (2004) Comparison of intensive and moderate lipid lowering with statins after acute coronary syndromes. N Engl J Med 350:1495–1504

94. LaRosa JC, Grundy SM, Waters DD et al (2005) Intensive lipid lowering with atorvastatin in patients with stable coronary disease. N Eng J Med 352:1425–1435

95. Aronow WS, Ahn C (2002) Incidence of new coronary events in older persons with prior myocardial infarction and serum low-density lipoprotein cholesterol ≥125 mg/dL treated with statins versus no lipid-lowering drug. Am J Cardiol 89:67–69

96. Nissen SE, Tuzcu EM, Schoenhagen P et al (2004) Effect of intensive compared with moderate lipid-lowering therapy on progression of coronary atherosclerosis. A randomized controlled trial. JAMA 291:1071–1080

97. Grundy SM, Cleeman JI, Merz CN et al (2004) Implications of recent clinical trials for the National Cholesterol Education Program Adult Treatment Panel III guidelines. Circulation 110:227–239

98. Aronow WS, Ahn C (1994) Correlation of serum lipids with the presence or absence of coronary artery disease in 1793 men and women aged ≥62 years. Am J Cardiol 73:702–703

99. Lavie CJ, Milani RV (1991) National Cholesterol Education Program's recommendations and implications of "missing" high-density lipoprotein cholesterol in cardiac rehabilitation programs. Am J Cardiol 68:1087–1088

100. Fowkes FGR, Housley E, Riemersma RA et al (1992) Smoking, lipids, glucose intolerance, and blood pressure as risk factors for peripheral atherosclerosis compared with ischemic heart disease in the Edinburgh Artery Study. Am J Epidemiol 135:331–340

101. Aronow WS, Ahn C (1994) Correlation of serum lipids with the presence or absence of atherothrombotic brain infarction and peripheral arterial disease in 1834 men and women aged ≥62 years. Am J Cardiol 73:995–997

102. Criqui MH, Browner D, Fronek A et al (1989) Peripheral arterial disease in large vessels is epidemiologically distinct from small vessel disease: an analysis of risk factors. Am J Epidemiol 129:1110–1119

103. Aronow WS, Ahn C (2002) Frequency of new coronary events in older persons with peripheral arterial disease and serum low-density lipoprotein cholesterol ≥125 mg/dl treated with statins versus no lipid-lowering drug. Am J Cardiol 90:789–791

104. Aronow WS, Nayak D, Woodworth S, Ahn C (2003) Effect of simvastatin versus placebo on treadmill exercise time until the onset of intermittent claudication in older patients with peripheral arterial disease at 6 months and at 1 year after treatment. Am J Cardiol 92:711–712

105. Mohler ER III, Hiatt WR, Creager MA (2003) Cholesterol reduction with atorvastatin improves walking distance in patients with peripheral arterial disease. Circulation 108:1481–1486

106. Mondillo S, Ballo P, Barbati R et al (2003) Effects of simvastatin on walking performance and symptoms of intermittent claudication in hypercholesterolemic patients with peripheral vascular disease. Am J Med 114:359–364

107. Wolf PA (1999) Cerebrovascular disease in the elderly. In: Tresch DD, Aronow WS (eds) Cardiovascular disease in the elderly patient. Marcel Dekker, New York, pp 125–147

108. Iso H, Jacobs DR Jr, Wentworth D et al (1989) Serum cholesterol levels and six year mortality from stroke in 350, 977 men screened for the Multiple Risk Factor Intervention trial. N Engl J Med 320:904–910

109. Bihari-Varga M, Szekely J, Gruber E (1981) Plasma high density lipoproteins in coronary, cerebral and peripheral vascular disease: the influence of various risk factors. Atherosclerosis 40:337–345

110. Crouse JR III, Byington RP, Hoen HM et al (1997) Reductase inhibitor monotherapy and stroke prevention. Arch Intern Med 157:1305–1310

111. Sever PS, Dahlof B, Poulter NR et al (2003) Prevention of coronary and stroke events with atorvastatin in hypertensive patients who have average or lower-than-average cholesterol concentrations, in the Anglo-Scandinavian Cardiac Outcomes Trial – Lipid Lowering Arm (ASCOT-LLA): a multicentre randomised controlled trial. Lancet 361:1149–1158

112. Aronow WS, Ahn C, Gutstein H (2002) Incidence of new atherothrombotic brain infarction in older persons with prior myocardial infarction and serum low-density lipoprotein cholesterol ≥125 mg/dL treated with statins versus no lipid-lowering drug. J Gerontol Med Sci 57A:M333–M335

113. Aronow WS, Ahn C, Gutstein H (2002) Reduction of new coronary events and of new atherothrombotic brain infarction in older persons with diabetes mellitus, prior myocardial infarction, and serum low-density lipoprotein cholesterol ≥125 mg/dL treated with statins. J Gerontol Med Sci 57A:M747–M750

114. Amarenco P, Goldstein LB, Szarek M et al (2007) Effects of intense low-density lipoprotein cholesterol reduction in patients with stroke or transient ischemic attack. The Stroke Prevention by Aggressive Reduction in Cholesterol Levels (SPARCL) Trial. Stroke 38:3198–3204

115. Warshafsky S, Packard D, Marks SJ et al (1999) Efficacy of 3-hydroxy-3-methylglutaryl coenzyme A reductase inhibitors for prevention of stroke. J Gen Intern Med 14:763–774

116. O'Leary DH, Anderson KM, Wolf PA et al (1992) Cholesterol and carotid atherosclerosis in older persons: the Framingham study. Ann Epidemiol 2:147–153

117. Salonen R, Seppanen K, Raurmaa R et al (1988) Prevalence of carotid atherosclerosis and serum cholesterol levels in eastern Finland. Arteriosclerosis 8:788–792

118. Blankenhorn DH, Selzer RH, Crawford DW et al (1993) Beneficial effects of colestipol-niacin therapy on the common carotid artery: two and four year reduction of intima-media thickness measured by ultrasound. Circulation 88:20–28

119. Furberg CD, Adams HP, Applegate WB et al (1994) Effect of lovastatin on early carotid atherosclerosis and cardiovascular events. Circulation 90:1679–1687

120. Crouse JR III, Byington RP, Bond MG et al (1995) Pravastatin, lipids and atherosclerosis in the carotid arteries (PLAC-II). Am J Cardiol 75:455–459

121. Ravipati G, Aronow WS, Ahn C et al (2006) Incidence of new stroke or new myocardial infarction or death in patients with severe carotid arterial disease treated with and without statins. Am J Cardiol 98:1170–1171

122. Vokonas PS, Kannel WB (2008) Epidemiology of coronary heart disease in the elderly. In: Aronow WS, Fleg JL, Rich MW (eds) Cardiovascular disease in the elderly, 4th edn. Informa Healthcare, New York, pp 215–241

123. Sukhija R, Aronow WS, Kakar P et al (2006) Relation of microalbuminuria and coronary artery disease in patients with and without diabetes mellitus. Am J Cardiol 98:279–281

124. Ravipati G, Aronow WS, Ahn C et al (2006) Association of hemoglobin A_{1c} level with the severity of coronary artery disease in patients with diabetes mellitus. Am J Cardiol 97:968–969

125. DeLuca AJ, Kaplan S, Aronow WS et al (2006) Comparison of prevalence of unrecognized myocardial infarction and of silent myocardial ischemia detected by a treadmill exercise sestamibi stress test in patients with versus without diabetes mellitus. Am J Cardiol 98:1045–1046

126. Aronow WS, Ahn C, Weiss MB, Babu S (2007) Relation of increased hemoglobin A_{1c} levels to severity of peripheral arterial disease in patients with diabetes mellitus. Am J Cardiol 99:1468–1469

127. Barrett-Connor E, Khaw K-T (1988) Diabetes mellitus: an independent risk factor for stroke. Am J Epidemiol 128:116–123

128. Bogousslavsky J, Regli F, Van Melle G (1985) Risk factors and concomitants of internal carotid arterial occlusion or stenosis: a controlled study of 159 cases. Arch Neurol 42:864–867

129. Kannel WB, Cupples LA, Ramaswami R et al (1991) Regional obesity and risk of cardiovascular disease. J Clin Epidemiol 44:183–190

130. Folsom AR, Kaye SA, Sellers TA et al (1993) Body fat distribution and 5 year risk of death in older women. JAMA 269:483–487

131. Paffenbarger RS Jr, Hyde RT, Wing AL et al (1986) Physical activity, all-cause mortality, and longevity of college alumni. N Engl J Med 314:605–613

132. Wenger NK (1994) Physical inactivity as a risk factor for coronary heart disease in the elderly. Cardiol Elder 2:375–379

133. Paffenbarger RS Jr, Wing AL (1967) Characteristics in youth predisposing to fatal stroke in later years. Lancet 1:753–754

134. Williams MA, Maresh CM, Aronow WS et al (1984) The value of early outpatient cardiac exercise programs for the elderly in comparison with other selected age groups. Eur Heart J 5(Suppl E):113–115

135. Aronow WS, Ahn C, Gutstein H (2002) Prevalence and incidence of cardiovascular disease in 1160 older men and 2464 older women in a long-term health care facility. J Gerontol Med Sci 57A:M45–M46

136. Gillum RF (1988) Stroke in blacks. Stroke 19:1–9

137. Aronow WS (1992) Prevalence of atherothrombotic brain infarction, coronary artery disease and peripheral arterial disease in elderly blacks, Hispanics and whites. Am J Cardiol 70:1212–1213

138. Aronow WS, Ahn C, Schoenfeld M et al (1992) Extracranial carotid arterial disease: a prognostic factor for atherothrombotic brain infarction and cerebral transient ischemic attack. N Y State J Med 92:424–425

139. Hertzer NR, Beven EG, Young JR et al (1984) Coronary artery disease in peripheral vascular patients: a classification of 1000 coronary angiograms and results of surgical management. Ann Surg 199:223–233

140. Smith GD, Shipley MJ, Rose G (1990) Intermittent claudication, heart disease risk factors and mortality: the Whitehall study. Circulation 82:1925–1931

141. Criqui MH, Langer RD, Fronek A et al (1992) Mortality over a period of 10 years in patients with peripheral arterial disease. N Engl J Med 326:381–386

142. Vogt MT, Cauley JA, Newman AB et al (1993) Decreased ankle/arm blood pressure index and mortality in elderly women. JAMA 270:465–469

143. Newman AB, Tyrrell KS, Kuller LH (1997) Mortality over four years in SHEP participants with a low ankle-arm index. J Am Geriatr Soc 45:1472–1478

144. Chimowitz MI, Mancini GBJ (1992) Asymptomatic coronary artery disease in patients with stroke: prevalence, prognosis, diagnosis and treatment. Stroke 23:433–436

145. Aronow WS, Ahn C, Schoenfeld MR et al (1993) Prognostic significance of silent myocardial ischemia in patients >61 years of age with extracranial internal or common carotid arterial disease with and without previous myocardial infarction. Am J Cardiol 71:115–117

146. Aronow WS, Schoenfeld MR (1992) Forty-five month follow-up of extracranial carotid arterial disease for new coronary events in elderly patients. Coron Artery Dis 3:249–251

147. Aronow WS, Gutstein H, Hsieh FY (1989) Risk factors for thromboembolic stroke in elderly patients with chronic atrial fibrillation. Am J Cardiol 63:366–367

148. Aronow WS, Ahn C (1994) Prevalence of coexistence of coronary artery disease, peripheral arterial disease, and atherothrombotic brain infarction in men and women ≥62 years of age. Am J Cardiol 74:64–65

149. Ness J, Aronow WS (1999) Prevalence of coexistence of coronary artery disease, ischemic stroke, and peripheral arterial disease in older persons, mean age 80 years, in an academic hospital-based geriatrics practice. J Am Geriatr Soc 47:1255–1256

Chapter 52
Cardiac Surgery in the Elderly

Margarita T. Camacho and Pooja R. Raval

As the elderly population steadily rises each year, so does the number of patients referred for cardiac surgical procedures. The U.S. Census Bureau predicted that there would be approximately 7.4 million people over the age of 80 by 2008, as compared to 6.2 million in 2000 [1]. Recent data reported that elderly patients over the age of 70 with no functional limitations could expect to live 14.3 years longer, compared with 11.6 years for those with limitation in at least one activity of daily living [2]. A formidable challenge facing cardiologists and cardiac surgeons is the appropriate treatment of the 40% of a growing elderly population that suffers from symptomatic cardiovascular disease [3]. The morbidity and mortality associated with cardiac surgical procedures in the elderly has substantially decreased since the late 1980s [4], although it is still higher than that of younger counterparts less than 70 years of age [5]. Reports of acceptable mortality rates and improved long-term quality of life justify cardiac operations in most symptomatic elderly patients. Only recently large studies have focused on risk analyses and outcomes in an effort to provide the clinician with as much evidence-based literature as possible to make the most appropriate decisions for many of these complex elderly patients.

Characteristics of the Elderly Cardiac Surgery Population

Despite the lack of consensus regarding the definition of "elderly," the perioperative cardiac surgery mortality rates rise significantly in patients older than 75 years of age [6]. An individual older than age 80 has more than three times the risk of death after coronary artery bypass than does a similar 50-year-old patient [7]. The increased risks of death and major complications are due not only to the natural processes of aging that result in associated comorbidities, but also to the fact that cardiovascular disease, the major cause of death and disability among elderly patients, is diagnosed at a more advanced state in this old population.

The aging process is influenced by a variety of genetic and environmental factors and occurs at somewhat different rates in every individual. The older the patient, the more likely is the presence of multiple chronic noncardiac diseases, increased tissue fragility, and limited organ reserves for stressful events [7]. Postoperative complications such as pneumonia, renal failure, stroke, and dementia are more prevalent and contribute significantly to perioperative morbidity and mortality. More than 50% of elderly individuals have at least one or more chronic medical conditions [8]. In addition to the routine preoperative assessment, other issues that must be evaluated include the degree of cognitive, neurologic, renal, respiratory, and immune impairment and the presence of other noncoronary atherosclerosis. Approximately one in three patients older than age 80 has some degree of cognitive dysfunction [9], and it is important to establish a baseline level of performance prior to surgical intervention [10]. Tests with age-specific normative standards include the Wechsler Adult Intelligence Scale, the Controlled Oral Word Association, and the Multilingual Aphasia Examination [11]. Patients with previously compromised cognitive function are at highest risk for such postoperative complications as delirium and progressive cognitive dysfunction. Depression is a common problem in patients of all ages and has been reported to follow cardiac surgery. It is clearly more pronounced in the elderly patient who may live alone and have few social support systems.

By age 80, there is a 25% decrease in kidney mass and 40% reduction in glomerular filtration rate (GFR) [10]. Due to the decrease in lean muscle mass, a decrease in GFR may not be reflected by an increase in serum creatinine concentration, and therefore a "normal" creatinine level in an octogenarian may be misleading. A more useful assessment of renal

M.T. Camacho (✉)
Department of Cardiothoracic Surgery, Newark Beth Israel Medical Center, Newark, NJ, USA
e-mail: mcamacho@sbhcs.com

R.A. Rosenthal et al. (eds.), *Principles and Practice of Geriatric Surgery*,
DOI 10.1007/978-1-4419-6999-6_52, © Springer Science+Business Media, LLC 2011

function in the elderly patient is the age-related creatinine clearance (Ccr)

$$Ccr\ (ml/min) = \frac{(140 - Age) \times (Ideal\ body\ weight\ in\ kilograms)}{72 \times Serum\ creatinine},$$

where normal is 75–125 ml/min. Renal function should be evaluated both before and after cardiac catheterization, and the amount of renally excreted dye used during angiography should be kept to an absolute minimum, employing nonionic contrast materials. The transient episodes of hypotension that inevitably occur during cardiopulmonary bypass may worsen any preexisting renal dysfunction; in this age group, perioperative renal insufficiency is a strong positive predictor of postoperative mortality [6, 12–14].

Old patients have declining cellular immunity and are therefore more predisposed to developing invasive bacterial and viral infections [10]. In addition to the bacterial colonization of the respiratory, urinary, and gastrointestinal tracts, there is a risk of infection from other monitoring lines and catheters used during cardiac surgery, such as central lines, Swan–Ganz catheters, and mediastinal drainage tubes. Leukocytosis is frequently absent or depressed in an elderly patient, who otherwise commonly exhibits atypical signs of infection such as hypothermia or confusion. Although most cardiac surgery patients are not cachexic or nutritionally depleted owing to their cardiac disease, it is important to assess the preoperative nutritional status of an elderly individual whose other organ reserves are already limited. Adequate nutrition is vital for wound healing and for avoiding infection and ventilatory dependence. Ideally, the serum albumin concentration should be >3.5 mg/dl, and there should be no history of recent significant (>5%) weight loss.

Numerous physiologic changes affect the cardiovascular system with advancing age. There is a decrease in vascular elasticity: The aorta and large arteries become much less compliant, resulting in an increase in peripheral vascular resistance. Left ventricular stiffness is increased [15], as is the ventricular septal thickness [16], and may require higher filling pressures to maintain adequate forward flow. During exercise there is a decrease in peak heart rate and ejection fraction, likely due to reduced responsiveness to circulating catecholamines [17–19]. Autopsy studies of octogenarians revealed that atherosclerotic heart disease with more than 75% narrowing in at least one major coronary vessel was the most common abnormality (present in 60% of patients). In fact, coronary disease was the most common single cause of death, with the most frequent manifestation being acute myocardial infarction [16]. Finally, compared with younger age groups, the heart of the elderly individual has smaller ventricular cavities and tortuous coronary arteries [20–22].

In light of these morphologic findings, it is not surprising that by age 80 at least 20% of this population have an established clinical diagnosis of coronary artery disease, and that eventually 67% of elderly patients die from this disease.

Elderly patients tend to have more advanced coronary artery disease than their younger counterparts by the time they are referred for cardiac surgery. Compared with the Coronary Artery Surgery Study (CASS) with a patient population of mean age 68 years [23], octogenarians were found to have a higher incidence of three-vessel coronary disease (87% vs. 61%; $p < 0.05$), left main or left main-equivalent disease (50% vs. 3%, $p < 0.0001$), and significant left ventricular dysfunction (19% vs. 4% had an ejection fraction <35%, $p < 0.01$) [24]. Older patients are more symptomatic on presentation; many series report that more than 90% of octogenarians are New York Heart Association (NYHA) functional class III–IV preoperatively [13, 25–31]. When compared with younger patients, a significantly higher percentage of elderly patients are referred for more urgent or emergent procedures, which carry substantially increased risks of major morbidity and mortality [7, 13, 24, 29, 31–34]. This underscores the need to prevent emergent and urgent surgical interventions.

A common finding in elderly patients is calcification and intimal disease of the aorta, which can crack and embolize when the ascending aorta is clamped or manipulated during cardiac operations. Such embolization to cerebral vessels is the principal cause of perioperative stroke in this age group [35]. Other causes of surgery-related neurologic deficits include transient episodes of systemic hypotension during cardiopulmonary bypass and air embolism from procedures that necessitate opening cardiac chambers or great vessels, such as aortic or mitral valve operations. Although aortic valve calcification is present in more than 55% of patients over the age of 90, only 5% eventually develop significant hemodynamic valvular stenosis [36]. One important difference between aortic and mitral valve disorders in the elderly is that aortic valve disease is usually associated with preserved left ventricular function, whereas mitral valve disease in the elderly is often ischemic in nature and is associated with significant ventricular dysfunction. Davis et al. [37] noted that only 29% of elderly patients with significant aortic valve disease had concomitant disease of two or more coronary vessels, compared with 46% of patients with significant mitral valve disease.

Predictors of Perioperative Morbidity and Mortality

As experience with the surgical treatment of cardiac disease in septuagenarians has grown, the literature has focused on the surgical outcome in octogenarians (Table 52.1). Many of these studies have reported predictors of perioperative morbidity

TABLE 52.1 Cardiac surgical procedures in the octogenarian: results and average length of hospital stay

Study	Year	No.	Procedure	Mortality (%)	Complication rate (%)	Mean postoperative LOS	% Survival (years)
Deiwick et al. [34]	1997	101	Mixed	8	73		88 (1)
							73 (5)
Gehlot et al. [38]	1996	322	AVR mixed	14	53	11.0	83 (1)
							60 (5)
Sahar et al. [39]	1996	42	Mixed	7	24		
Logeais et al. [40]	1995	200	Mixed	12	35	12.7	82 (1)
							75 (2)
							57 (5)
Cane et al. [12]	1995	121	Mixed	9	49		
Klima et al. [41]	1994	75	Mixed	8	21		
Yashar et al. [42]	1993	43	Mixed	9	38		
Glower et al. [26]	1992	86	CABG	14	29	10.0	64 (3)
Freeman et al. [31]	1991	191	Mixed	20	30	16.4	92 (1)
							87 (2)
							82 (3)
							78 (4)
Tsai et al. [43]	1991	157	CABG	7	20		85 (1)
							62 (5)
Ko et al. [28]	1991	100	CABG	12	24		
Mullany et al. [44]	1990	159	CABG	11	73		84 (1)
							71 (5)
Naunheim et al. [33]	1990	103	Mixed	17	71		90 (1)
Kowalchuk et al. [45]	1990	53	Mixed	11	38		81 (2)
Fiore et al. [46]	1989	25	Mixed	20	72	18.0	79 (1)
				Valve			69 (2)
Naunheim et al. [24]	1987	23	Mixed	22	67	14.3	94 (1)
							82 (2)
Rich et al. [47]	1985	25	Mixed	4	92	19.5	84 (2)

Mixed series includes valve and coronary bypass procedures and/or valve+coronary bypass procedures; *AVR* aortic valve replacement, *CABG* coronary artery bypass grafting, *LOS* length of stay in hospital

and mortality based on extensive univariate and multivariate analyses. This information has proved vital in identifying specific factors that may be optimized preoperatively and has provided physicians and patients with the ability to make timely treatment decisions based on expected short-term and long-term outcomes.

Several studies have shown that a decreased ejection fraction is a significant predictor of hospital mortality following cardiac surgery. This is even more predictive of an adverse outcome in octogenarians. A number of series have reported hospital mortality rates of 3–6, 5–13, and 24–43% in patients with normal, moderately impaired, and severely impaired (ejection fraction < 0.30) left ventricular function, respectively [48–50]. In a multivariate analysis of factors involving 159 octogenarians who underwent isolated coronary artery bypass, Mullaney et al. [44] found that an ejection fraction less than 0.50% was the most important predictor of adverse survival ($p < 0.01$). Ko and coworkers, who analyzed 100 consecutive octogenarians undergoing isolated coronary artery bypass, also found a decreased ejection fraction to be the most significant predictor of perioperative mortality ($p < 0.002$). In fact, an ejection fraction less than 30% was associated with a mortality rate of 43% [28].

High NYHA functional cardiac class was highly predictive of hospital mortality in numerous studies [13, 16, 19, 22, 25, 26, 31, 45] In their series of 76 octogenarians undergoing a variety of cardiac surgery procedures, Tsai et al. [48] found that 94% of the hospital deaths were in patients who presented in NYHA functional class IV. In a study of 24,461 patients 80 years and older who underwent isolated coronary artery bypass, measures of more acute coronary disease, such as acute myocardial infarction (MI) before bypass surgery, predicted higher procedural and long-term mortality rates [49]. This relation with acute coronary artery disease has been borne out by numerous other authors [24, 26, 28].

Combined coronary surgery procedures and mitral valve replacement (MVR) have been shown to carry significantly higher hospital mortality rates in the elderly population [19, 27, 32, 36, 37, 39, 42, 45]. In the early 1990s, Davis and coworkers reported operative mortality rates of 5.3% for aortic valve replacement (AVR), 20.4% for MVR, and 5.8% for isolated coronary artery bypass [37]. Several years earlier, Naunheim et al. reported even higher hospital mortality rates of 50% for MVR, 9% for AVR, and 67% for double valve replacement combined with coronary revascularization [33]. More recent outcomes for those aged 75

Table 52.2 Comparison of mortality rates by procedure status (elective vs. urgent vs. emergent)

Study	Year	No.	Procedure	Mortality (%)			
				Overall	Elective	Urgent	Emergency
Diewick et al. [34]	1997	101	Mixed	7.9	4.7		23.5
Williams et al. [13]	1995	300	CABG	11.0	9.6	11.0	33.3
Diegeler et al. [29]	1995	54	Mixed	9.2	6.1		40.0
Freeman et al. [31]	1991	191	Mixed	18.8			35.9
Ko et al. [28]	1991	100	CABG	12.0	2.8	13.5	33.3
Naunheim et al. [32]	1990	103	Mixed	16.5		10.0	29.0
Naunheim et al. [24]	1987	23	Mixed	22.0	11.0		75.0

See Table 52.1 for explanation of abbreviations

and above at Newark Beth Israel Medical Center, a participant in The Society of Thoracic Surgeons 2004–2008 database, reveal mortality rates of only 4.8% for isolated AVR, 0% for isolated MVR, and 3.0% for isolated CABG (personal communication).

The outcome after valve replacement in elderly patients is primarily a function of the myocardial performance, which decreases as the severity of any associated coronary artery disease increases. Old patients undergoing AVR tend to have a well-functioning ventricle; the degree of coronary artery disease tends to be less than that in patients undergoing MVR. Patients requiring mitral valve surgery tend to have more serious ischemic disease, which can irreversibly damage the myocardium and result in higher perioperative mortality [20–22, 27]. Furthermore, combined procedures require longer cardiopulmonary bypass times and longer ischemic cross-clamp times, two factors that are predictors of operative mortality as well [19, 24, 26, 28].

In addition to presenting with more advanced disease than their younger counterparts, a higher percentage of octogenarians are referred for urgent or emergent surgical intervention. As noted in Table 52.2, urgent and emergent operations are associated with extremely high mortality rates, particularly if a mitral valve procedure is performed independently or in combination with other procedures. These increased mortality rates reflect the progression and severity of the cardiac disease and the lack of functional reserve for stressful events in this older population. Another related factor, preoperative hemodynamic instability, was described by several authors as the need for an intra-aortic balloon pump (IABP) [15, 19, 24, 25, 33, 39], preoperative admission to the coronary care unit [34, 38, 44], and preoperative use of inotropes and vasoactive medications [33, 50]. Each was found to be a significant predictor of hospital mortality. Multivariate analyses by Williams and coworkers, who studied a group of 300 octogenarians who underwent isolated coronary artery bypass, revealed that preoperative renal dysfunction (creatinine > 2.0 mg/dl), pulmonary insufficiency, and postoperative sternal wound infection were strong predictors of hospital mortality [13]. Tsai and coworkers found that 67% of the elderly patients with postoperative mediastinal bleeding necessitating reoperation ultimately died [48].

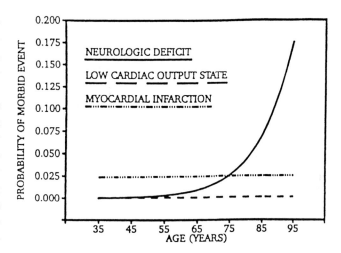

Figure 52.1 Effect of advanced age on the predicted probability of neurologic and cardiac morbidity (from Tuman et al. [51], with permission).

In a prospective study of 2,000 patients undergoing coronary artery bypass, Tuman et al. [51] studied the effect of age on neurologic outcome. The rate of neurologic complications rose significantly with age; patients <65 years old had a 0.9% stroke rate, whereas those aged 65–74 and >75 had rates of 3.6 and 8.9%, respectively ($p = 0.0005$). Suspected causes of serious neurologic events (in patients unresponsive for more than 10 days) include atheromatous emboli from the ascending aorta, hypotension or low-flow state during cardiopulmonary bypass, and preexisting critical extracranial or intracranial cerebrovascular disease. The mortality rate in this group of patients who sustained significant strokes was 74% (Fig. 52.1) [51]. Perioperative mortality associated with perioperative stroke in younger patients, although still formidable, was less than half of this frequency (24–26%).

Quality of Life

Although the short-term and intermediate-term survival for elderly patients undergoing cardiac surgery is somewhat less than their younger cohorts, the long-term survival for octogenarians after open heart surgery compares favorably with survival for the general US population of similar age. In a series of 600 consecutive patients 80 years or older undergoing various open heart procedures, the 5-year actuarial survival, including hospital mortality, was $63 \pm 2\%$. Survival in this group was identical to that for the simultaneous general US octogenarian population [14]. Excellent long-term results have been achieved by several groups in octogenarians after mitral valve surgery, aortic valve surgery, and coronary artery bypass surgery [40, 52, 53].

Of as great importance to the elderly as survival is the associated quality of life. Several authors have shown that most (81–93%) of the octogenarians who survive open heart surgery "feel" as good and frequently better than before their operations [14, 29, 40, 53]. An equally high percentage (75–84%) of octogenarians believed in retrospect that having decided to have a cardiac surgical procedure after age 80 had been a good choice [14, 54]. The precise and objective measurements of quality of life may be difficult to quantify. Based on well-studied populations, it has been possible to construct instruments that reliably assess the various domains of daily living, thereby producing a meaningful reproducible measurement of quality of life [55–57].

The NYHA angina functional class and cardiac failure functional class reflect symptom-free living with regard to chest pain and dyspnea. Octogenarians have consistently demonstrated substantial improvement in their NYHA angina functional class and cardiac failure functional class after open heart surgery. In several reports, most (68–92%) of the octogenarians who survived open heart surgery were in NYHA functional class I or II during long-term follow-up. This improvement was seen after isolated coronary artery bypass operations, valve operations, and combined operations (Table 52.3). When a well-validated health care index, the SF-36, was employed to study prospectively a cohort of elderly and nonelderly patients, those over 75 years of age enjoyed an identical long-term improvement in each of the seven domains of the SF-36. Indeed, as many of the elderly patients had low quality of life SF-36 scores preoperatively as their younger cohorts, their improvements were even greater, as both populations ended up with statistically identical SF 36 scores 6 months following surgery. Any neurologic injury associated with the diagnostic and surgical process dramatically affected their quality of life adversely when compared with those old patients who did not suffer any neurologic injury.

Many octogenarian patients live alone and consequently have impaired ability to carry out activities of daily living, which places them at a significant disadvantage. Karnofsky dependency category (KDC) and social support index (SSI) reflect the degree of help needed by patients. Glower and coworkers, using the KDC, showed that the median performance status in a group of octogenarians undergoing isolated coronary artery bypass

TABLE 52.3 Change in functional class after cardiac surgical procedures

				Functional class change (%)	
				Preoperative	Postoperative
Study	Year	No	Procedure	FC III–IV	FC I–II
Deiwick et al. [34]	1997	101	Mixed	88	83
Morris et al. [25]	1996	474	CABG	93	92
Gehlot et al. [38]	1996	322	Mixed	86	82
Sahar et al. [39]	1996	42	Mixed	87	90
Williams et al. [13]	1995	300	CABG	98	98
Logeais et al. [40]	1995	200	Mixed	74	99
Cane et al. [12]	1995	121	Mixed	69	84
Diegeler et al. [29]	1995	54	Mixed	100	92
Adkins et al. [58]	1995	42	Mixed	64	97
Tsai et al. [27]	1994	528	Mixed	99	70
Yashar et al. [42]	1993	43	Mixed	98	79
Tsai et al. [43]	1991	157	CABG	96	73
Ko et al. [28]	1991	100	CABG	100	94
McGrath et al. [30]	1991	54	Mixed	96	94
Mullaney et al. [44]	1990	159	CABG	97	89
Merrill et al. [59]	1990	40	Mixed	100	100
Edmunds et al. [60]	1988	100	Mixed	90	98
Naunheim et al. [24]	1987	23	Mixed	94	83

FC functional class

grafting improved from 20% preoperatively to 70% at hospital discharge, with 89% of survivors being discharged home [26]. Kumar et al. showed that when there was a significant decrease in the level of social support needed by octogenarians after open heart surgery, the mean KDC and mean SSI decreased significantly at the short-term follow-up (less than 2 years) [54]. These improvements were also present but significantly less evident at the long-term follow-up (more than 5 years). It is likely that significant comorbid conditions limit the ability of octogenarians to live independently long term, although they remain symptom-free from a cardiac point of view and do well in the short term.

As mentioned above, the subjective indicators of quality of life for octogenarians after open heart surgery are complex and involve a number of modalities relating to various domains of life. In the study by Kumar et al., indices for satisfaction with marriage, children, and overall life, feelings about the present life, and general affect were assessed. In the short term, the indices for satisfaction with overall life and eight bipolar items assessing general affect showed significant improvements, although all these improvements became less evident at long-term follow-up [54]. Perhaps the symptomatic benefits and the value of cardiac surgery as seen subjectively by the patients lie in the question, "Would you choose to undergo cardiac surgery again?" Virtually all the current studies in the literature have shown that most octogenarians would have made the same decision to undergo open heart surgery retrospectively.

Possible Strategies to Decrease Operative Risk

Improvements in surgical techniques and anesthesia have increased the confidence of cardiac surgeons performing operations on an elderly population with increased perioperative risk. Awareness of the problems unique to this growing population of elderly patients, along with recent statistical data highlighting the impact of these problems on morbidity and mortality, can help the medical team recommend the most appropriate treatment choice and timing of intervention in each individual case.

The two principal causes of perioperative cerebrovascular accidents (CVAs) in elderly patients undergoing cardiac surgery are embolization (air, atheroma, and calcific debris) and hypotension resulting in inadequate perfusion of the central nervous system. Preoperative evaluation of the ascending aorta and carotid arteries and intraoperative assessment of the proximal aorta using transesophageal or epiaortic echocardiography may alter the conduct of the procedure, minimize intraoperative manipulation, and thereby significantly reduce the incidence of stroke [34, 35, 39, 51, 61]. Such information enables the surgeon to avoid cannulation or direct manipulation of heavily diseased portions of the aorta where atheromas may dislodge or where plaque disruption may cause aortic dissection. The presence of extensive atheromatous or calcific disease, which precludes safe manipulation of the ascending aorta in patients with advanced coronary disease, leaves the surgeon with several choices.

1. Abandon the surgical procedure and consider nonoperative or nonbypass revascularization, such as angioplasty, transmyocardial revascularization, or angiogenesis.
2. Perform surgical revascularization on a beating heart, using one or both internal thoracic arteries or nonaortic-based grafts.
3. Establish cardiopulmonary bypass via the femoral, axillary, or other systemic nondiseased artery and perform graft replacement or endarterectomy of the ascending

aorta [34, 35]. The latter alternative is an aggressive, complex procedure and in the elderly population it should be reserved for the very good risk patient with no significant comorbidities.

Diffuse systemic atherosclerosis is more prevalent in the elderly than in younger patients; as such, special precautions should be taken to ensure adequate cerebral and renal perfusion perioperatively. Maintaining high perfusion pressures while on cardiopulmonary bypass can help decrease the incidence of ischemic stroke [62, 63]. Control of atrial arrhythmias and avoidance of episodes of sustained arterial hypotension due to hypovolemia or medications are important during the immediate postoperative period. Although there is still controversy regarding the management of asymptomatic carotid disease, it is believed that known carotid disease in the elderly population is a risk factor for postoperative CVA [14, 34, 44, 51]. Morris et al. [25] recommended routine preoperative assessment of carotid artery disease in octogenarians and advocated carotid endarterectomy if significant disease is found. If symptomatic carotid artery disease is diagnosed prior to cardiac surgical intervention, consideration should be given to performing a staged or a combined procedure. If asymptomatic significant carotid disease is discovered by Doppler preoperatively (>75% stenosis bilaterally or lesser degrees of unilateral stenosis in the presence of an occluded contralateral artery), concomitant carotid endarterectomy may decrease the risk of perioperative stroke [61].

Because of the significant increase in mortality associated with urgent or emergent operative procedures (Table 52.2), all possible measures must be taken to optimize the elderly patient preoperatively and possibly convert an urgent or emergent situation to a more elective one. Careful selection of elderly patients in this setting is critical, and one must evaluate the patient's mental status and existing comorbidities when determining the potential for meaningful survival before recommending operation. Aggressive preoperative medical management includes the use, when necessary, of intravenous nitroglycerin or heparin (or both), inotropic and ventilatory support, and if absolutely necessary, the IABP. Although numerous studies have reported that preoperative use of the IABP is a significant predictor of perioperative mortality [12, 14, 33, 50], it likely reflects the severity of the elderly patient's underlying cardiac disease, rather than any inherent risk in using the device. Sisto et al. [64] reported that in 25 consecutive octogenarians requiring IABP insertion, there were no significant complications related to device insertion; and of 20 patients who eventually underwent surgery after IABP, only two patients (10%) died in hospital. This operative mortality rate is significantly better than that reported by others for urgent/emergent cases (Table 52.2).

There is a strong association between early postoperative death and prolonged ventilatory dependence [60], which can develop quickly in the elderly patient. As soon as the patient awakens from general anesthesia, respiratory muscles must be exercised. Pulmonary hygiene and physiotherapy must be aggressive with early and progressive ambulation. Unlike their younger counterparts, elderly patients have much less functional reserve, and therefore a successful first attempt at extubation and mobilization ensures the best outcome. Intraoperatively, exquisite care must be taken to avoid injury to the phrenic nerve during harvesting of the internal thoracic artery, and use of bilateral internal thoracic arteries should generally be avoided [65].

Nephrotoxic drugs should be avoided; or, if necessary, doses should be adjusted in light of the decreased renal function in elderly patients. Intravenous renal dosage dopamine hydrochloride (1–2 μg/kg/min) may have benefit when used for any patient with preexisting renal insufficiency. Because of the high mortality associated with perioperative renal failure in this population [13, 38, 43, 66, 67], an aggressive approach to optimize preoperative renal function is essential. Although rigorous studies demonstrating the benefit of "renal dopamine" are inconclusive, many centers use this drug to enhance urine flow during and immediately after cardiac surgery.

Cognitive function is one of the most important factors affecting overall outcome and is one of the most difficult neurologic outcome parameters to measure and assess. Delirium and confusion are common in the postoperative elderly individual and can hinder important initial attempts to extubate and mobilize a patient. Encephalopathy changes are seen in as many as 30% of all bypass patients and 50% of elderly patients. Sensory deficits such as those due to hearing or vision impairments can be addressed as soon as the patient awakens by providing hearing aids and eyeglasses. Invasive lines and monitoring equipment should be removed as soon as the patient is medically possible to facilitate mobilization. Transfer out of an intensive care unit (ICU) setting, when possible, helps restore the sleep–wake cycle. Family members should stay with confused patients to offer reassurance and encouragement. Long-acting benzodiazepines should be avoided or other sedative/hypnotic medications altered to prevent excessive sedation, confusion, and respiratory depression. Haloperidol is a more appropriate drug for the management of delirium in this patient population because of its short-acting effect and safety margin in the postoperative cardiothoracic patient. Small doses are usually effective, and the patient can be rapidly weaned in conjunction with professional and family encouragement.

Octogenarians are more likely to develop sternal dehiscence due to osteoporosis of the sternum. The use of bilateral internal thoracic arteries should be avoided. Sternal wound infection has been shown to be a positive predictor of mortality in this group of patients [13].

Aggressive management is essential and includes early institution of intravenous antibiotics, timely debridement, and either primary reconstruction or secondary closure with a wound vacuum device. Adequate nutrition and pulmonary physiotherapy are critical to success. Staged closures are to be avoided in this population, other than for the most advanced infections, which should then undergo coverage and secondary closure as rapidly as possible.

Utley and Leyland described a highly selected group of 25 patients over the age of 80 who underwent coronary artery bypass with no hospital deaths [68]. Patients were selected on the basis of their ability to achieve acceptable functional recovery after operation. All patients were living at home alone or with relatives preoperatively, and they were ambulatory and capable of caring for their own personal needs. They were counseled preoperatively regarding the importance of early ambulation and self-care postoperatively. Four patients were rejected for surgery based on mental or physical senility, previous debilitating strokes, or a history of long-term institutional care. Anesthetic management included the use of short-acting agents and minimal use of postoperative sedation. Patients were extubated within 9–48 h postoperatively, and many were ambulatory and eating on the first postoperative day. Although this restrictive degree of patient selection is not appropriate in most cases, it illustrates how outcome can be strongly influenced by preexisting functional status and meticulous perioperative care.

Nonsurgical Alternatives

During the current era of health care reform, there is considerable interest in providing the most appropriate care for patients more than 80 years of age at an "acceptable" cost [69]. As coronary bypass surgery is the most common major operation performed in the USA (more than 300,000 done annually), the use of coronary bypass in the very elderly is an important issue in the present cost-conscious environment. Medicare data from 1987 to 1990 indicated that the use of this operation in patients more than 80 years of age increased by 67% during that time period [49]. The projected rise in the number of coronary bypass procedures to be done in these patients and associated costs is impressive (Fig. 52.2) [49]. Numerous studies have shown a considerable increase in length of stay (3–4 days longer) and hospital costs ($3,000–$6,000 more) in patients over 80 years old versus their younger counterparts. Failure to provide this service, however, often results in repeated and prolonged hospitalization, the need for multidrug therapy, and poorer quality of life, not to mention the emotional impact on patients and their families [7, 49].

In one series of octogenarians, when coronary surgery was compared with medical therapy, the overall cost, annual reinterventions, coronary disease-associated readmissions, and mortality were favored in the surgical group. Several studies have attempted to compare the treatment results of less expensive alternatives to coronary bypass surgery. In elderly patients, percutaneous transluminal coronary angioplasty (PTCA) has the advantages of shorter hospital stay, less immobilization, and lower cost compared with coronary artery bypass; however, coronary bypass confers greater and more durable freedom from angina, less need for future repeat interventional measures, and overall improved quality of life [36, 70, 71]. Although Mick et al. [72] reported that the procedural complication rates in matched groups of patients undergoing coronary bypass versus PTCA were similar, Braunstein et al. [70] observed that PTCA in the setting of unstable angina was associated with high initial morbidity but long-term survival roughly equivalent to that after coronary bypass surgery. As mentioned above, compared with medical noninterventional therapy, coronary artery bypass provides a significant survival advantage and improved quality of life. Ko et al. [71] compared 36 octogenarians who underwent coronary artery bypass with 29 octogenarians who continued medical noninterventional therapy and found that the functional class did not change in the latter group but improved significantly in the former group (NYHA functional class decreased from 3.4 to 1.2, $p < 0.01$). The 3-year survival rate of 77% for the surgical group was similar to the survival of octogenarians in the general US population and was significantly better than that of 55% for the medical group. In summary, coronary bypass surgery provided improved long-term survival and functional benefit compared with medical therapy and improved the quality of life compared with PTCA.

The New Era of Mechanical Circulatory Assist

In the mid-1980s, implantable mechanical circulatory assist devices were introduced in FDA clinical trials for patients with severe left ventricular dysfunction who were awaiting transplant and would otherwise not survive without such support. The most popular device in this early era, the HeartMate pneumatic left ventricular assist device (LVAD), enabled patients to ambulate and exercise on treadmills while in-hospital. The advantages of LVAD therapy for the often debilitated, deconditioned patients were significant and resulted in improved outcomes for heart transplant recipients who were able to optimize their physical and physiologic conditions prior to transplant. Since then the LVADs have become smaller (Figs. 52.3 and 52.4), more durable, and associated with increased survival rates when compared with the earlier models [73]. The smaller size and decreased postoperative complications have enabled this technology to be offered to the elderly population with acceptable perioperative risk.

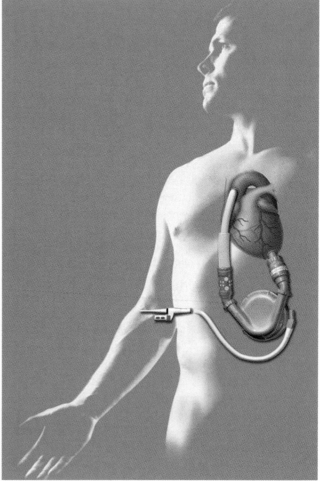

FIGURE 52.3 HeartMate II LVAD (reprinted with permission of Thoratec Corporation).

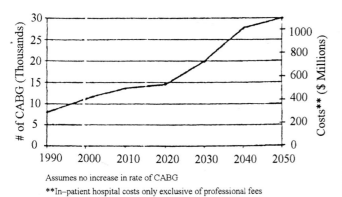

Assumes no increase in rate of CABG

**In-patient hospital costs only exclusive of professional fees

FIGURE 52.2 Projected number of bypass surgery (CABG) procedures performed per year in octogenarians (*left axis*) and the corresponding projected costs for these procedures (in 1990 dollars) (*right axis*) (from Peterson et al. [49], with permission).

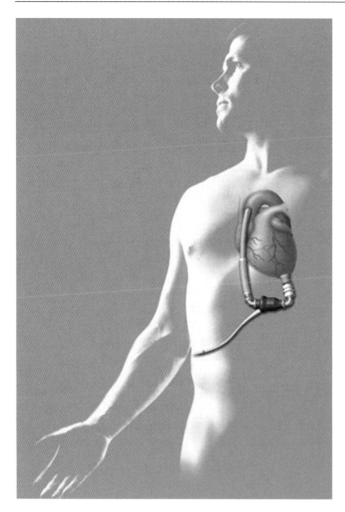

FIGURE 52.4 Mechanical circulatory support device placement (reprinted with permission of Thoratec Corporation).

The oldest patients with these smaller LVADs are octogenarians who, like their younger counterparts, are leading productive lives outside the hospital.

For a selective group of elderly but active patients who suffer hemodynamic compromise due to severe cardiac dysfunction, a temporary mechanical assist device can be implanted if there is hope of cardiac recovery, such as after a large myocardial infarction. Newer devices in this category, such as the Thoratec CentriMag, have been associated with fewer complications and improved survival (personal communication).

Guidelines for Therapy in the Elderly Cardiac Surgery Patient

During the process of deciding whether to offer cardiac surgical intervention to elderly patients, the relief of symptoms and improvement in quality of life should assume more

importance than the issue of increased life expectancy. When surgical revascularization is considered in this patient population, numerous social, ethical, and clinical issues arise. Comorbidities, quality of life, and concerns raised by the patient's family should be acknowledged and factored into the decision-making process. It is important to integrate the patient's and family's wishes, but one must focus the therapeutic decisions on the patient's advance directives. Emergency cases in these patients may be associated with more than 70% mortality risk, and therefore nonoperative treatment must be strongly considered. Asymptomatic patients should continue medical treatment unless there is critical (>70%) left main coronary artery stenosis, which is associated with significantly reduced life expectancy. Numerous groups (Table 52.2) have observed significantly increased mortality when combined procedures were performed. One study, comparing the operative mortalities for isolated AVR and isolated coronary artery bypass to combined AVR + coronary bypass, demonstrated five- to sixfold increased operative mortality in the combined procedure group [48]. In situations where two or three disease processes exist, the surgical plan should be modified to avoid such increased risks. For example, in an elderly patient with angina, severe coronary artery disease, and noncritical aortic stenosis, coronary revascularization alone may be the best option. Such patients are usually not at risk for a serious morbid event due to their aortic stenosis [36]. Conversely, in a patient with critical aortic stenosis, congestive heart failure, preserved or mildly impaired left ventricular function, and noncritical coronary lesions (<70–80% stenosis), valve replacement alone may be the best alternative. Fiore et al. [46] noted that of the early deaths of patients undergoing combined AVR + coronary bypass, 60% were due to low cardiac output; the patients who had died had little or no angina preoperatively, but each had considerable congestive heart failure and may have been better served by valve replacement alone.

Definitive treatment of isolated aortic stenosis is surgical replacement of the valve, preferably with a bioprosthesis that prevents a lifelong requirement for anticoagulation. The tissue valves have demonstrated impressive freedom from structural deterioration and reoperation at 10 or even 15 years in patients older than 65 years of age. Stentless bioprostheses may have some advantage in elderly small aortic root patients, but long-term benefit and durability remain unproven. Percutaneous balloon valvuloplasty may offer effective initial palliation, but medium- and long-term durability results have been disappointing. Symptoms recurred within 1 year in most patients and necessitated subsequent surgery [74, 75].

Chronic aortic regurgitation may be well tolerated for several decades before congestive heart failure occurs. Once symptoms appear and ventricular dilatation begins, AVR

CASE STUDY: CROSSING THE FRONTIER

Stanley M., an active male in his late 1970s, presented to a local hospital near his home in New Jersey after suffering a large myocardial infarction. Due to hemodynamic instability, he received an IABP, was intubated and transferred to Newark Beth Israel Medical Center for further treatment. Despite high-dose inotropes, he was not able to be weaned from the IABP and remained intubated. He received an implantable LVAD, the newer and smaller HeartMate II, as part of a clinical trial. He was able to be extubated and weaned from the IABP, and was discharged home to lead an active life that includes travel and caring for his brother. Had this technology not been available to Stanley, he would have expired in the hospital [77].

---

should be offered before chronic volume overload results in symptomatic irreversible myocardial and pulmonary damage. The most appropriate time to replace the valve is soon after left ventricular dilatation begins.

Surgery is usually recommended for mitral stenosis patients with NYHA functional class II–III heart failure and a calculated mitral valve area less than 1.0 cm^2. Percutaneous balloon mitral valvuloplasty, unlike the similar treatment for stenotic aortic valves, may be useful when only the mitral valve leaflets are impaired and there is no significant calcification or regurgitation. The subvalvular apparatus should be functional and not destroyed, as can happen with advanced rheumatic valve disease [76]. Mitral valve balloon valvuloplasty usually provides relatively long-term relief of dyspnea but is frequently not possible in elderly patients with advanced disease and heavily calcified mitral valves. MVR, although the definitive treatment for mitral valve stenosis, carries significantly increased procedural mortality either alone or combined with other procedures in the elderly. Naunheim et al. [33] observed operative risks of 42% for either MVR alone or MVR + coronary bypass. Combined MVR + AVR was associated with a 67% risk of surgical mortality, further suggesting a limited role for MVR in this elderly population. These procedures require prolonged periods of cardiopulmonary bypass and global cardiac ischemia, both of which are poorly tolerated by such patients with limited cardiac and other organ reserve. For these reasons, Fiore et al. [46] recommended that every effort be made to keep such operations simple and expeditious.

In patients with advanced coronary artery disease who may be at high risk for complications arising from cardiopulmonary bypass, such as those with severe calcific disease of the ascending aorta (precluding safe insertion of cannulas), a history of stroke, or end-stage pulmonary or renal failure, an alternate option is surgical revascularization on a beating heart. Technologic advances in pericardial retraction systems and stabilization devices have enabled the surgeon to perform anastomoses on a beating heart with the use of newer surgical techniques. However, there is a significant learning curve, as the surgical field is not nearly as optimal as that produced by cardiopulmonary bypass and ischemic arrest. Recent reports have observed a failure rate of 10% even in experienced hands. Although a reasonable alternative for patients who would otherwise have no interventional options, the increased risk of technical failure must be kept in mind and discussed with the patient and family.

Finally, for elderly patients in previously good physical and mental condition who suffer from acute or chronic severe ventricular dysfunction, both short-term and long-term mechanical circulatory assist devices are available at an acceptable operative risk, compared with their earlier counterparts.

Conclusions

As the elderly population has grown, so have the number of elderly patients being referred for cardiac surgery and their disease complexity. For the most part, these patients can be offered conventional surgical procedures with acceptable mortality, morbidity, and long-term quality of life expectations. Indeed, the perioperative complications are somewhat more numerous than for younger patients even when they are compared for procedure and matched for other risk factors.

This incremental morbidity and mortality is seen across the entire population but is most pronounced in emergently operated patients. With the availability of new and different techniques to accomplish myocardial revascularization and valvular repair and replacement, and the recent availability of mechanical assist devices, the range of procedures available for elderly patients with hemodynamically important heart disease is increasing at a rate almost faster than the population itself has grown. It is therefore critical that the health care professionals caring for these older patients are aware of ongoing developments in these areas and carefully stratify the preoperative risk factors to best select the least morbid and most effective procedure that is currently available.

Acknowledgments The authors wish to acknowledge the invaluable assistance of Melissa L. Wong and Gladys Madrid RN for the creation of this manuscript.

References

1. Table 1: Annual Estimates of the Resident Population by Sex and Five-year Age Groups for the United States: April 1, 2000 to July 1, 2008 (NC-EST2008-01). Source: Population Division, US Census Bureau; Release Date May 14, 2009 and Table 4: Annual Estimates of the Resident Population for the United States April 1, 2000 to July 1, 2008 (NST-EST 2008-01). Source: Population Division, US Census BUREAU; Release date December 22, 2008

2. Lubitz J, Kiming C, Kramarow E et al (2003) Health, life expectancy and health care spending among the elderly. N Engl J Med 349:1048–1055

3. Horvath KA, DiSesa VJ, Peigh PS et al (1990) Favorable results of coronary artery bypass grafting in patients older than 75 years. J Thorac Cardiovasc Surg 99:92–96

4. Maganti M, Rao V, Brister S et al (2009) Decreasing mortality for coronary artery bypass surgery in octogenarians. Can J Cardiol 25(2):e32–e35

5. Canver C, Nichols R, Cooler S et al (1996) Influence of increasing age on long-term survival after coronary artery bypass grafting. Ann Thorac Surg 62:1123–1127

6. Srinivasan A, Oo A, Grayson A et al (2004) Mid-term survival after cardiac surgery in elderly patients: analysis of predictors for increased mortality. Interact Cardiovasc Thorac Surg 3:289–293

7. Alexander KP, Peterson ED (1997) Coronary artery bypass grafting in the elderly. Am Heart J 134:856–864

8. Kern LS (1991) The elderly heart surgery patient. Crit Care Nurs Clin North Am 3:749–756

9. Mezey MD, Rauckhorst LH, Stokes SA (1993) Health assessment of the older individual, 2nd edn. Springer, New York

10. Smith Rossi M (1995) The octogenarian cardiac surgery patient. J Cardiovasc Nurs 9(4):75–95

11. Sweet J, Finnin E, Wolfe P et al (2008) Absence of cognitive decline one year after coronary bypass surgery: comparison to non-surgical and healthy controls. Ann Thorac Surg 85:1571–1578

12. Cane ME, Chen C, Bailey BM et al (1995) CABG in octogenarians: early and late events and actuarial survival in comparison with a matched population. Ann Thorac Surg 60:1033–1037

13. Williams DB, Carrillo RG, Traad EA et al (1995) Determinants of operative mortality in octogenarians undergoing coronary bypass. Ann Thorac Surg 60:1038–1043

14. Akins CW, Daggett WM, Vlahakes GJ et al (1997) Cardiac operations in patients 80 years old and older. Ann Thorac Surg 64:606–615

15. Iskandrian AS, Segal BL (1991) Should cardiac surgery be performed in octogenarians? J Am Coll Cardiol 18:36–37

16. Shirani J, Yousefi J, Roberts WC (1995) Major cardiac findings at necropsy in 366 American octogenarians. Am J Cardiol 75:151–156

17. Iskandrian AS, Hakki AH (1985) The effects of aging after coronary artery bypass grafting on the regulation of cardiac output during upright exercise. Int J Cardiol 7:347–360

18. Hakki AH, DePace NL, Iskandrian AS (1983) Effect of age on left ventricular function during exercise in patients with coronary artery disease. J Am Coll Cardiol 2(4):645–651

19. Iskandrian AS, Hakki AH (1986) Age-related changes in left ventricular diastolic performance. Am Heart J 112:75–78

20. Roberts WC (1993) Ninety three hearts ≥90 years of age. Am J Cardiol 71:599–602

21. Waller BF, Roberts WC (1983) Cardiovascular disease in the very elderly: analysis of 40 necropsy patients aged 90 years or older. Am J Cardiol 51:403–421

22. Roberts WC (1988) The aging heart. Mayo Clin Proc 63:205–206

23. Gersh BJ, Kronmal RA, Schaff HV et al (1983) Long-term (5 year) results of coronary bypass surgery in patients 65 years or older: a report from the Coronary Artery Surgery Study. Circulation 66(Suppl II):190–199

24. Naunheim KS, Kern MJ, McBride LR et al (1987) Coronary artery bypass surgery in patients aged 80 years or older. Am J Cardiol 59:804–807

25. Morris RJ, Strong MD, Grunewald KE et al (1996) Internal thoracic artery for coronary artery grafting in octogenarians. Ann Thorac Surg 62:16–22

26. Glower DD, Christopher TD, Milano CA et al (1992) Performance status and outcome after coronary artery bypass grafting in persons aged 80 to 93 years. Am J Cardiol 70:567–571

27. Tsai T, Chaux A, Matloff JM et al (1994) Ten-year experience of cardiac surgery in patients aged 80 years and over. Ann Thorac Surg 58:445–451

28. Ko W, Krieger KH, Lazenby WD et al (1991) Isolated coronary artery bypass grafting in one hundred consecutive octogenarian patients. J Thorac Cardiovasc Surg 102:532–538

29. Diegeler A, Autschbach R, Falk V et al (1995) Open heart surgery in the octogenarians: a study on long-term survival and quality of life. Thorac Cardiovasc Surg 43:265–270

30. McGrath LB, Adkins MS, Chen C et al (1991) Actuarial survival and other events following valve surgery in octogenarians: comparison with age-, sex-, and race-matched population. Eur J Cardiothorac Surg 5:319–325

31. Freeman WK, Schaff HV, O'Brien PC et al (1991) Cardiac surgery in the octogenarian: perioperative outcome and clinical follow-up. J Am Coll Cardiol 18:29–35

32. Bashour TT, Hanna ES, Myler RK et al (1990) Cardiac surgery in patients over the age of 80 years. Clin Cardiol 13:267–270

33. Naunheim KS, Dean PA, Fiore AC et al (1990) Cardiac surgery in the octogenarian. Eur J Cardiothorac Surg 4:130–135

34. Deiwick M, Tandler R, Mollhoff TH et al (1997) Heart surgery in patients aged eight years and above: determinants of morbidity and mortality. Thorac Cardiovasc Surg 45:119–126

35. Wareing TH, Davila-Roman VG, Barzilai B et al (1992) Management of the severely atherosclerotic ascending aorta during cardiac operations: a strategy for detection and treatment. J Thorac Cardiovasc Surg 103:453–462

36. Cannon LA, Marshall JM (1993) Cardiac disease in the elderly population. Clin Geriatr Med 9:499–525

37. Davis EA, Gardner TJ, Gillinov AM et al (1993) Valvular disease in the elderly: influence on surgical results. Ann Thorac Surg 55:333–338

38. Gehlot A, Mullany CJ, Ilstrup D et al (1996) Aortic valve replacement in patients aged eighty years and older: early and long-term results. J Thorac Cardiovasc Surg 111:1026–1036

39. Sahar G, Raanani E, Sagie A et al (1996) Surgical results in cardiac patients over the age of 80 years. Isr J Med Sci 32:1322–1325

40. Logeais Y, Roussin R, Langanay T et al (1995) Aortic valve replacement for aortic stenosis in 200 consecutive octogenarians. J Heart Valve Dis 4(Suppl 1):S64–S71

41. Klima U, Wimmer-Greinecker G, Mair R et al (1994) The octogenarians: a new challenge in cardiac surgery? Thorac Cardiovasc Surg 42:212–217

42. Yashar JJ, Yashar AG, Torres D, Hittner K (1993) Favorable results of coronary artery bypass and/or valve replacement in octogenarians. Cardiovasc Surg 1:68–71

43. Tsai T, Nessim S, Kass RM et al (1991) Morbidity and mortality after coronary artery bypass in octogenarians. Ann Thorac Surg 51:983–986

44. Mullany CJ, Darling GE, Pluth JR et al (1990) Early and late results after isolated coronary artery bypass surgery in 159 patients aged 80 years and older. Circulation 82(Suppl IV):229–236

45. Kowalchuk GJ, Siu SC, McAuliffe LS et al (1990) Coronary artery bypass in octogenarians: early and late results. J Am Coll Cardiol 15:35A

46. Fiore AC, Naunheim KS, Barner HB et al (1989) Valve replacement in the octogenarian. Ann Thorac Surg 48:104–108

47. Rich MW, Sandza JG, Kleiger RE et al (1985) Cardiac operations in patients over 80 years of age. J Thorac Cardiovasc Surg 90:56–60

48. Tsai TP, Matloff JM, Gray RJ et al (1986) Cardiac surgery in the octogenarian. J Thorac Cardiovasc Surg 91:924–928

49. Peterson ED, Cowper PA, Jollis JG et al (1995) Outcomes of coronary artery bypass graft surgery in 24,461 patients aged 80 years or older. Circulation 92(Suppl II):85–91

50. Curtis JJ, Walls JT, Boley TM et al (1994) Coronary revascularization in the elderly: determinants of operative mortality. Ann Thorac Surg 58:1069–1072

51. Tuman KJ, McCarthy RJ, Najafi H et al (1992) Differential effects of advanced age on neurologic and cardiac risks of coronary artery operations. J Thorac Cardiovasc Surg 104:1510–1517

52. Lee EM, Porter JN, Shapiro LM et al (1997) Mitral valve surgery in the elderly. Heart Valve Dis 6:22–31

53. Culliford AT, Galloway AC, Colvin SB et al (1991) Aortic valve replacement for aortic stenosis in persons aged 80 years and over. Am J Cardiol 67:1256–1260

54. Kumar P, Zehr KJ, Cameron DE et al (1995) Quality of life in octogenarians after open heart surgery. Chest 108:919–926

55. Remington M, Tyrer PJ, Newson-Smith J et al (1979) Comparative reliability of categorical and analogue rating scales in the assessment of psychiatric symptomatology. Psychol Med 9:765–770

56. Campbell A, Converse PE, Ridgers WL (1976) The quality of American life. Russell Sage, New York, pp 1–583

57. Bradburn NM (1969) The structure of psychological well-being. Aldine, Chicago, pp 214–215

58. Adkins M, Amalfitano D, Harnum NA et al (1995) Efficacy of combined coronary revascularization and valve procedures in octogenarians. Chest 108:927–931

59. Merrill WH, Steward JR, Frist WH et al (1990) Cardiac surgery in patients age 80 years or older. Ann Surg 211:772–776

60. Edmunds LH, Stephenson LW, Edie RN et al (1988) Open-heart surgery in octogenarians. N Engl J Med 319:131–136

61. Berens ES, Kouchoukos NT, Murphy SF et al (1992) Preoperative carotid artery screening in elderly patients undergoing cardiac surgery. J Vasc Surg 15:313–323

62. Grawlee GP, Cordell AR, Graham JE et al (1985) Coronary revascularization in patients with bilateral internal carotid occlusion. J Thorac Cardiovasc Surg 90:921–925

63. Brener BJ, Bried DK, Alpert J et al (1987) The risk of stroke in patients with asymptomatic carotid stenosis undergoing cardiac surgery: a follow-up study. J Vasc Surg 5:269–279

64. Sisto DA, Hoffman DM, Fernandes S, Frater RWM (1992) Is use of the intraaortic balloon pump in octogenarians justified? Ann Thorac Surg 54:507–511

65. He GW, Acuff TE, Ryan WH et al (1994) Determinants of operative mortality in elderly patients undergoing coronary artery bypass grafting. J Thorac Cardiovasc Surg 108:73–81

66. Ennabli K, Pelletier LC (1986) Morbidity and mortality of coronary artery surgery after the age of 70 years. Ann Thorac Surg 42:197–200

67. Higgins TL, Estafanous FG, Loop FD et al (1992) Stratification of morbidity and mortality outcome by pre-operative risk factors in coronary artery bypass patients: a clinical severity score. JAMA 267:2344–2348

68. Utley JR, Leyland SA (1991) Coronary artery bypass grafting in the octogenarian. J Thorac Cardiovasc Surg 101:866–870

69. Weintraub WS (1995) Coronary operations in octogenarians: can we select the patients? Ann Thorac Surg 60:875–876

70. Braunstein EM, Bajwa TK, Andrei L et al (1991) Early and late outcome of revascularization for unstable angina in octogenarians. J Am Coll Cardiol 17:151A

71. Ko W, Gold JP, Lazzaro R et al (1992) Survival analysis of octogenarian patients with coronary artery disease managed by elective coronary artery bypass surgery versus conventional medical treatment. Circulation 86(Suppl II):191–197

72. Mick MJ, Simpfendorfer C, Arnold AZ et al (1991) Early and late results of coronary angioplasty and bypass in octogenarians. Am J Cardiol 68:1316–1320

73. Camacho M, Baran D, Martin A et al (2009) Improved survival in high-risk patients with smaller implantable LVAD's: single-center experience over 3 years. J Heart Lung Transplant 28(2):S274

74. Dancy M (1989) Dawkins, Ward D. Balloon dilatation of the aortic valve; limited success and early restenosis. Br Heart J 60:236–239

75. Litvack F, Jakubowski AT, Buchbinder NA et al (1988) Lack of sustained clinical improvement in an elderly population after percutaneous aortic valvuloplasty. Am J Cardiol 62:270–275

76. Palacios I, Block PC, Brandi S et al (1987) Percutaneous balloon valvotomy for patients with severe mitral stenosis. Circulation 75:778–786

77. Health Care Today: post-acute care. Producer: Paula Levine. January 2008

Chapter 53
Invited Commentary

Frank J. Veith

The diseases of the vascular system discussed on this section comprise, in the elderly, primarily different manifestations of arteriosclerosis.

Occlusive arterial disease is the result of extensive plaque formation which can itself produce flow reducing arterial stenoses or occlusions. Plaque rupture and associated thrombosis or embolization can worsen the occlusive process.

Several generalities apply to arteriosclerotic occlusive disease. First, although most elderly patients have many arteriosclerotic plaques or lesions, most of these do not need to be treated. There is considerable reserve in the arterial system, so that the occlusive process must be extensive before symptoms occur. Although a single occlusive lesion can cause intermittent claudication, such single lesions in the elderly are often asymptomatic. Furthermore, all invasive treatments, with open surgical or endovascular techniques, are imperfect with frequent early and late failures. Therefore, most patients with occlusive lesions, certainly those who are asymptomatic or have mild symptoms, should not be treated invasively. Conservative treatment with reassurance that their limbs will probably not be threatened is usually best.

Second, more advanced limb threatening ischemia or so called critical limb ischemia (CLI) usually only occurs in patients who have multilevel occlusive disease. Only when this is associated with gangrene, a non-healing ulcer or true ischemic rest pain is aggressive interventional or surgical treatment justified. Such treatment may involve procedures which deal with small crural arteries below the knee, and may be difficult even for highly skilled specialists. Nevertheless, as we have shown for many decades, such aggressive efforts to save threatened limbs are almost always worthwhile even in elderly patients and those with diabetes [1, 2].

Third, patients with critical lower limb ischemia have a limited life expectancy with half of such patients dying within the first 5 years of their first revascularization procedure [1, 2]. Nevertheless many of these patients will have a failure of their revascularization with a renewed threat to their limb. Redo procedures, either surgical or interventional, usually can salvage the extremity, and have been shown to be worthwhile [1, 2]. Although such procedures can require considerable skill, they are an important part of the care of CLI patients.

Fourth, although surgical bypasses supplemented by catheter based treatments such as balloon angioplasty constituted the mainstay of treatment for arteriosclerotic occlusive disease for many decades, in the last 10–15 years there has been a paradigm shift in the treatment of this entity. Catheter based treatments are becoming the first therapeutic option for most patients requiring treatment for lower limb ischemia. Nevertheless 20–35% of these patients will require an open surgical procedure at some time in the course of their disease [3].

Extracranial cerebrovascular disease is primarily arteriosclerotic disease at the bifurcation of the common carotid artery into its internal and external branches in the neck. Plaques at this location can produce cerebral emboli, which can lead to strokes or transient neurological motor, sensory, or visual symptoms. When such symptoms occur in the absence of other pathology, the plaque is considered symptomatic. Over the last 50 years, carotid endarterectomy (CEA) has become the standard of care for such symptomatic plaques and also for high grade stenotic plaques that have not yet produced symptoms (asymptomatic plaques). More recently carotid artery angioplasty and stenting (CAS) has emerged as an alternate treatment for symptomatic and asymptomatic carotid plaques, and is being promoted and performed more commonly, particularly by interventional cardiologists.

There are three important facts to consider in this area. First, to date, all randomized trials comparing CEA to CAS for symptomatic carotid disease have shown CAS to be inferior to CEA. Second, CAS in elderly patients over 75 years of age has repeatedly been shown to be excessively risky. Although these facts may change as the technology improves, CEA should remain the treatment of choice for symptomatic carotid stenosis patients, particularly the elderly, unless there

F.J. Veith (✉)
Department of Surgery, New York University, 4455 Douglas Ave, Bronx, NY 10471, USA
e-mail: fjvmd@msn.com

R.A. Rosenthal et al. (eds.), *Principles and Practice of Geriatric Surgery*,
DOI 10.1007/978-1-4419-6999-6_53, © Springer Science+Business Media, LLC 2011

are compelling contraindications to a surgical procedure in the neck (radiation, scarring, a tracheostomy, or a high lesion).

Third, medical treatment for asymptomatic carotid stenosis has made dramatic advances in the last decade. Treatment with statins, antiplatelet agents, ACE inhibitors, and better control of blood pressure and diabetes has been shown to alter plaque pathology and behavior, and to dramatically reduce the risk of stroke in arterioclerotic patients. It is therefore likely that few if any asymptomatic patients with carotid stenosis will benefit from either CEA or CAS, although level I evidence to prove this is not available.

Treatment of aneurysms. Although aneurysms can occur anywhere in the arterial tree, this commentary will deal only with those of the abdominal and thoracic aorta (AAA and TAA). Since 1992 and continuing to the present, there has been a paradigm shift in the way.

AAAs and TAAs are being treated. Before 1992, the standard of care for the treatment of AAAs and TAAs that had reached a size that required treatment (5–5.5 cm for AAAs and >6 cm for TAAs) was open surgical exclusion of the aneurysm with a prosthetic polyester graft. Increasingly, over the last 17 years, the standard of care has been shifting to endovascular repair with an endovascular graft or stent-graft. This shift has already occurred for most elective AAAs although a proportion still require open repair for anatomical reasons. This proportion is shrinking as better technology, particularly branched endografts, becomes available. The shift to endovascular repair is also occurring for many TAAs and most ruptured AAAs [4].

Unlike CEA versus CAS where the differences in morbidity between the open and endovascular procedures are minimal, the differences between open and endovascular repair of abdominal and thoracic aneurysms are substantial. Because of this morbidity differential, it is likely that endovascular procedures will ultimately replace most open repairs of abdominal and thoracic aneurysms. However, this replacement evolution is still ongoing and in some cases is still controversial. Thus, currently there is still a need for open surgical repair in some patients with aortic aneurysm disease.

References

1. Veith FJ, Gupta SK, Samson RH et al (1981) Progress in limb salvage by reconstructive arterial surgery combined with new or improved adjunctive procedures. Ann Surg 194:386–401
2. Veith FJ, Gupta SK, Wengerter KR et al (1990) Changing arteriosclerotic disease patterns and management strategies in lower limb threatening ischemia. Ann Surg 212:402–414
3. Veith FJ, Cayne NS, Gargiulo NJ, Ascher E, Lipsitz EC (2009) Surgical options for critical limb ischemia. In: Bosiers M, Schneider PA (eds) Critical limb ischemia. Informa Healthcare USA, New York, pp 195–208
4. Veith FJ, Lachat M, Mayer D et al (2009) Collected world and single center experience with endovascular treatment of ruptured abdominal aortic aneurysms. Ann Surg 250(5):818–824

Chapter 54
Surgical Treatment of Vascular Occlusive Disease

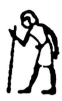

Amanda Feigel and Alan Dardik

Peripheral arterial disease (PAD) describes the spectrum of disease, from asymptomatic to severe, of diminished or absent arterial blood flow to the lower extremities or abdominal viscera. PAD is usually distinguished from extracranial and intracranial carotid disease, as well as coronary disease, although all of these entities are usually and most commonly caused by atherosclerosis. Symptoms of PAD can be present either acutely, caused by plaque rupture releasing distal emboli, or chronically, caused by the progressive intimal thickening leading to decreased luminal diameter and subsequent reduced distal blood flow. As atherosclerotic intimal thickening is typically indolent, slowly accumulating plaque reducing blood flow over many years, the elderly population is commonly affected with PAD. This chapter focuses on the impact of PAD in the lower extremity and visceral circulations in elderly patients. Recent advances in minimally invasive technologies, particularly endovascular treatments, have increased options for treatment of PAD in the elderly patient. However, the evidence for the efficacy of these newer technologies is rarely established in the elderly population.

CASE STUDY

An 85-year-old man presents for a second opinion regarding a right great toe ulcer that was ischemic, but not infected. He had a history of claudication treated with exercise approximately 10 years prior to presentation. He also had a history of coronary artery disease treated by coronary artery bypass approximately 8 years ago. There is a history of hypertension and type II diabetes but no recent smoking. He takes aspirin and a statin.

The physical exam is remarkable for his vascular exam. Femoral pulses are 2+ bilaterally, but there are no palpable popliteal, dorsalis pedis, or posterior pulses bilaterally. The ankle-brachial index is 0.3 on the right and 0.5 on the left. The right great toe has an ulcer that is clearly ischemic, painful to the point that motion is reduced; there is no cellulitis or exudate. There is no gangrene. The contralateral foot has trophic changes but is not frankly ischemic.

The patient claims to be able to perform his basic activities of daily living, but exam shows that he is probably chronically malnourished and mildly dehydrated, although there are no signs of dementia. He lives alone, having been recently widowed. The patient has already had an opinion from a general surgeon recommending primary amputation for his severe vascular disease; your office confirms these records and notes that the surgeon's opinion was based both on the patient's age as well as a computed tomogram (CT) angiogram. The patient is particularly concerned as he believes that an amputation will prevent him from returning home, forcing him to move permanently to a nursing home.

Incidence and Epidemiology

The incidence of PAD is typically noted to range from 3 to 10% in the general population, but the incidence increases to 15–20% in patients older than 70 years [1]. The prevalence of PAD increases dramatically with age (Fig. 54.1). For

A. Dardik (✉)
Department of Surgery, Yale University School of Medicine, New Haven, CT, USA
e-mail: alan.dardik@yale.edu

R.A. Rosenthal et al. (eds.), *Principles and Practice of Geriatric Surgery*,
DOI 10.1007/978-1-4419-6999-6_54, © Springer Science+Business Media, LLC 2011

Prevalence of Symptomatic PAD

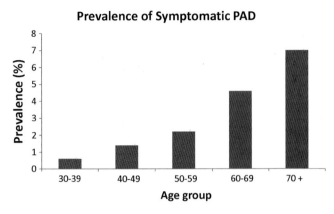

FIGURE 54.1 Increasing prevalence of PAD with age.

example, the PARTNERS study found that PAD was present in 29% of patients either ≥70 or 50–69 with a risk factor for PAD [2]. Additional risk factors independent of age include non-White ethnicity, male gender, smoking history, diabetes, hypertension, and dyslipidemia.

The increased incidence and prevalence of PAD in the elderly is especially significant since presence of PAD, even if only asymptomatic, increases the risk of coronary and cerebral arterial disease [2]. Patients with either claudication or critical limb ischemia have reduced long-term survival compared to age-matched control patients; for example, 10-year survival is reduced from 90 to 50% in patients with claudication and to 10% in patients with critical limb ischemia [1].

Patient Assessment

The initial evaluation of elderly patients with arterial occlusive disease is critical. Atherosclerotic disease of the aortoiliac segment is often asymptomatic in many elderly patients secondary to their sedentary life style. Few elderly patients present with lower extremity or buttock claudication secondary to either isolated infrainguinal or aortoiliac disease. Instead, they more commonly present with limb-threatening lower extremity ischemia (rest pain, ischemic ulceration, gangrene) secondary to multilevel arterial occlusive disease. The combined burden of aortoiliac and infrainguinal arterial occlusive disease can be more difficult to assess and treat in this patient population. After a complete physical examination that includes a careful pulse examination, noninvasive studies are helpful for evaluating the patient's arterial disease. The vascular laboratory may aid in the evaluation and selection of patients for single or multilevel revascularization. If an intervention is indicated, further invasive studies may be performed to define the best intervention for the individual patient, although recent technological advances may limit the need for invasive purely diagnostic studies.

The ankle-brachial index (ABI) is determined by dividing the ankle pressure in each lower limb by the higher of the two brachial pressures. Patients with normal circulation have an ABI in the range of 1.0–1.2, those with claudication have reduced ABIs in the range of 0.40–0.90, and those with limb-threatening ischemia have ABIs in the range of 0–0.5. An important limitation of measuring lower extremity pressure occurs in patients with heavily calcified vessels, mostly diabetics and patients with end-stage renal disease. In these patients, the ABI is falsely elevated owing to the higher pressure required to occlude calcified vessels, and in some cases, the vessels are not occluded even with pressures higher than 300 mmHg. However, all-cause mortality is increased both in patients with reduced ABI as well as in patients with elevated and incompressible ABI [3].

Pulse volume recordings (PVR) are obtained using a calibrated air plethysmograph. A PVR waveform is generated for different levels of the lower extremity using standard blood pressure cuffs. The increase in pressure within the cuff resulting from the volume increase during systole is recorded as a pulse wave. The tracings are characterized as normal when there is a brisk rise during systole and a dicrotic notch, as moderately abnormal when there is loss of the notch and a more prolonged downslope, and as severely abnormal when there is a flattened wave. The absolute amplitudes are not comparable from patient to patient, but serial PVRs have been shown to be highly reproducible, making them useful for following the course of patients with severe peripheral vascular disease. In addition, this test cannot easily differentiate proximal femoral disease from iliac occlusive disease. Figure 54.2 shows a typical PVR tracing demonstrating both thigh (superficial femoral artery) and tibial disease on the right.

Duplex scanning can be a useful noninvasive technique for assessing the aortoiliac and infrainguinal arterial system. A variety of studies have evaluated the ability of this technique to predict iliac artery stenoses. Kohler et al. initially suggested that duplex scanning had excellent sensitivity (89%) and specificity (90%) when used to predict an iliac stenosis of 50% or more [4]. Three subsequent studies by Langsfeld et al. [5], Moneta et al. [6], and Legemate et al. [7] corroborated these findings with sensitivities ranging from 81 to 89% and specificities ranging from 88 to 99%. These noninvasive evaluations may be useful for evaluating the elderly prior to invasive procedures such as angiography and angioplasty.

Until recently, computed tomography angiography (CTA) has had limited use in the evaluation of aortoiliac occlusive disease other than simple identification of severely calcified arteries or lesions. However, faster, new generation spiral CT scanners have the capability of three-dimensional reconstructions and provide significantly improved images (Fig. 54.3). The outstanding resolution of the newer generation of these studies has led to their routine use to evaluate patients with PAD in many centers. A distinct advantage of these new CTA

FIGURE 54.2 Typical PVR tracing demonstrating both thigh (superficial femoral artery) and tibial disease on the right.

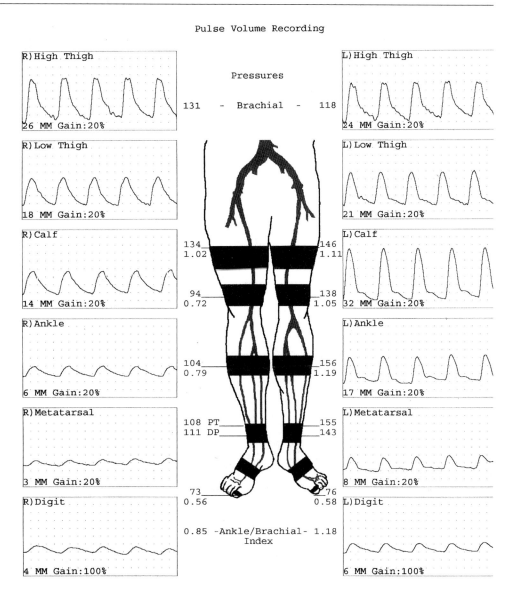

is the ability to simultaneously identify coronary artery disease, and thus perform risk stratification [8]. However, approximately 150 cc of intravenous contrast dye is required for most CTA, limiting the use to patients with essentially normal renal function. As the newer generations of CT scanners become faster, they have increased ability to accurately image elderly patients who, due to comorbidities such as congestive heart failure, may have limited tolerance to lie still for the duration of the study. As such, CTA is becoming more popular as a diagnostic tool in elderly patients.

Magnetic resonance angiography (MRA) is noninvasive, does not require contrast agents, and allows good arterial imaging. Owens et al. [9] and Carpenter et al. [10] showed that MRA may be more sensitive than arteriography when imaging distal lower extremity runoff vessels. Carpenter et al. [11] also reported that MRA had a 100% positive predicted value (PPV) and a 98.6% negative predicted value (NPV)

when compared to contrast angiography for evaluating patients with aortoiliac occlusive disease. These findings have not been widely reproduced, but this noninvasive modality has the potential to replace contrast arteriography in the evaluation of these patients. Current images are generally inadequate for therapeutic planning in most centers, but as the associated hardware and software improve, and interest by dedicated MR radiologists increases, the role of MRA in the assessment of occlusive disease of the aortoiliac segments will increase [12].

Intraarterial contrast angiography is considered the gold standard for evaluating patients with arterial occlusive disease. This modality provides the diagnostic information necessary to plan the treatment of most vascular patients with arterial occlusive disease. Complete evaluation of the existing arterial disease from the aorta to the pedal vessels is typically necessary for elderly patients as they commonly have

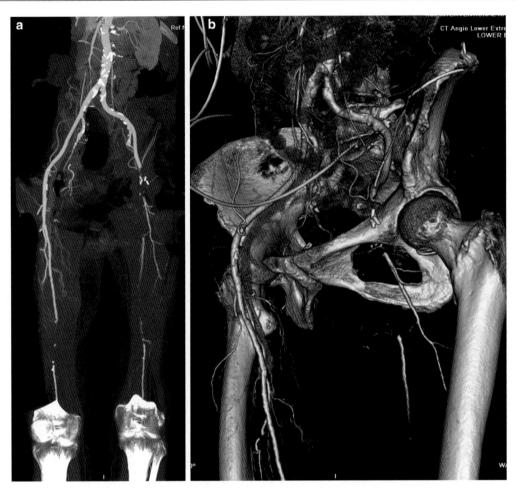

Figure 54.3 Utility of CTA in diagnosis of PAD. CTA shows occlusion of left common femoral artery and superficial artery. (**a**) Two-dimensional coronal reconstruction. (**b**) Three-dimensional reconstruction.

multilevel occlusive disease. The addition of intraarterial pressure measurements at the time of arteriography improves the accuracy of detecting clinically significant stenosis. Pressure measurements after intraarterial injection of a vasodilatory drug such as papaverine are used to evaluate the significance of aortoiliac stenoses under conditions of stress that require increased blood flow through these vessels. A systolic pressure gradient across the lesion of more than 15 mmHg is considered hemodynamically significant.

The complication rate of arteriography in the general population is only 1.7–3.3% [13]. Elderly patients with severe aortoiliac or infrainguinal disease must be carefully evaluated before the procedure, as local and systemic complications are more likely than in the general population. The transfemoral approach is the safest, but other options (e.g., translumbar, transbrachial, or transaxillary approach) may have to be used for patients with weak or nonpalpable femoral pulses. These alternative approaches have higher local complication rates. Complications include hematomas, pseudoaneurysms, dissections, thrombosis, and embolization.

Renal insufficiency is an important complication of angiography. Renal impairment associated with contrast agents occurs in 6.5–8.2% of patients who undergo arteriography [14, 15]. Patients with preexisting azotemia and a baseline serum creatinine level >2.0 mg/dl are at the highest risk of renal complications after angiography. Elderly patients have a low creatinine clearance rate for a given serum creatinine level, so they should always be considered at high risk for nephrotoxicity. All possible precautions must be taken to limit the renal insult. The use of low osmolar contrast agents has been shown by some to decrease the incidence of renal impairment [16, 17], but these findings are not universal [18]. Adequate hydration prior to arteriography is an effective maneuver to diminish the risk of contrast nephropathy. Mannitol is used for its osmotic diuretic effect to help prevent contrast toxicity. Vasodilators such as dopamine have also been used because the nephrotoxic effect of contrast agents is considered to be partly due to intrarenal vasoconstriction. Dopamine has been shown to be better than mannitol for preventing contrast-related renal insufficiency [19]. Unfortunately, many elderly patients have moderate to severe cardiac disease, and aggressive hydration may lead to congestive heart failure, cardiac ischemia, and arrhythmias. In addition, the use of dopamine may lead to cardiac complications. Careful hydration and judicious use of mannitol, dopamine, and contrast agents can decrease the incidence of renal impairment associated with arteriography.

TABLE 54.1	Signs of acute arterial ischemia
Pain	
Paralysis	
Pallor	
Paresthesia	
Pulselessness	
Poikilothermia	

Therapeutic Management

Medical management of PAD focuses on lifestyle modification to reduce risk factors for progression of atherosclerotic disease. These include smoking cessation, addition of a lipid lowering agent such as a statin, antiplatelet therapy, and increased daily exercise, as well as supervised exercise classes. Conservative management is invariant for all patients regardless of age. When it has become evident that medical therapy has failed, surgical and/or interventional approaches become the mainstay of treatment.

Elderly patients with mainly aortoiliac occlusive disease rarely require an intervention. Patients with claudication should be treated initially by maximizing the management of the known risk factors for the development of atherosclerosis, an exercise or walking program, and the use of potentially helpful oral agents such as pentoxifylline. The small group of patients with severe, debilitating claudication that has failed the initial treatment protocol generally request an intervention. In addition, patients who present with limb-threatening ischemia secondary to multilevel occlusive disease should be considered for intervention.

Acute Thromboembolic Disease

Severe forms of acute ischemia typically result from embolic occlusion of a previously patent vessel. Sources of embolism are typically of a cardiac nature but can also originate from aneurysms and proximal arteries. Occlusion of a vessel from progressive growth of a thrombus is more gradual and allows for development of collateral vessels. Therefore, chronic occlusive disease typically results in less severe ischemia and pain compared to acute disease.

Acute arterial ischemia presents similarly in elderly and younger patients with early neurological signs including pain, weakness, pallor, paresthesias, and lastly pulselessness in affected extremities (Table 54.1). Pain is the most common complaint, and numbness of the web space between the first and second toes is the earliest neurologic sign of ischemia. Extremities are relatively resilient to ischemic conditions for up to 5–6 h, after which irreversible damage may

occur. However, elderly patients may be reticent to complain and as such may present at a later stage of disease.

Systemic anticoagulation with intravenous heparin will prevent propagation of either the embolus or thrombus distal to the site of occlusion resulting from stagnant flow. A traditional angiogram or a CT angiogram can be performed to determine the area of occlusion. Once the location is known, early revascularization is often indicated to salvage the extremity. This can be accomplished by either surgical intervention and placement of a bypass graft, such as femoral-popliteal bypass, or through endovascular techniques for patients who may not be operative candidates or otherwise have amenable anatomy.

Chronic Occlusive Disease

Claudication rarely indicates a risk for limb loss and typically responds to lifestyle modifications. Conversely, rest pain represents critical ischemic disease in which blood flow is insufficient even for basal metabolism. Rest pain occurs in the dorsum of the foot and is increased in intensity when the limb is elevated and resolves with dangling the affected limb, allowing gravitational forces to assist perfusion. Additional signs of markedly decreased blood flow include loss of hair, thinning skin, and muscle wasting. Rest pain represents the presence of critical ischemia, similar to gangrene and non-healing ulcers; thus, the patient with rest pain should be evaluated for revascularization expeditiously.

PAD: Surgical Intervention

Femoral-popliteal bypass is usually performed for limb-threatening ischemia or severe, lifestyle-limiting claudication. Numerous reports have documented that elderly patients more frequently require surgery for limb-threatening ischemia, with operative urgency, than for claudication alone. Autologous saphenous vein remains the conduit of choice, with polytetrafluoroethylene (PTFE), dacron, and human umbilical vein being the most common prosthetics used when autologous vein is not available.

TABLE 54.2 Outcome of femoral-popliteal bypass grafts in elderly patients

Trial (Reference)	Year	Level of evidence	Randomized patients (n)	Intervention/ design	Median follow-up	Minor end point	Major end point	Age	Interpretations/ comments
[20]	2000	1b	240	Randomized multicenter	21 Months	Graft thrombosis	Death	≥65	5-year patency 55%
[21]	2001	2b	349	Retrospective cohort series	3 Years	Limb salvage	Graft patency	>70	5-year patency 82%
[22]	1986	4	168	Case series	–	Graft thrombosis	Death	≥80	3-year patency 62%
[23]	1987	4	46	Case series	41 Months	Graft thrombosis	Death	≥80	83-year patency 78%
[24]	1989	4	50	Case series	–	Graft thrombosis, limb salvage	Death	≥80	3-year limb salvage 80%

Outcomes of femoral-popliteal bypass graft placement in elderly patients are reviewed in Table 54.2. Two studies provide good evidence that elderly patients undergo femoral-popliteal bypass with patency at least equivalent to, and possibly even better than, that achievable in younger patients. In a multicenter, randomized trial comparing prosthetic grafts used in above-knee bypass, Green et al. reported that the type of prosthetic graft has little effect on outcome, but patients over 65 years old had significantly greater 5-year graft patency compared with younger patients (55% vs. 36%) [20]. Similarly, Lau et al. reported improved 5-year vein graft patency in patients over 70 years of age compared with patients less than 70 years of age (82% vs. 72%) [21]. All studies reported excellent limb salvage in elderly patients [20–24].

Outcome after more distal infrageniculate bypass surgery is similarly favorable in the elderly. Hearn et al. reported in a retrospective cohort series that patients ≥70 years of age had 5-year primary and secondary graft patency rates of 61 and 74%, respectively, which was similar to patients under the age of 70 years who had rates of 76 and 79%, respectively [25]. Similarly, excellent results of case series have been reported [26, 27].

We believe that if an elderly patient faced with a need for limb salvage can tolerate the perioperative mortality and morbidity risk of the cardiovascular stress of the procedure, the limited evidence available favors an aggressive approach to bypass surgery. However, the minimally invasive nature of endovascular procedures and their overall efficacy in short-term reports have led many authors to advocate for this therapy primarily in elderly patients.

Endovascular

The use of percutaneous transluminal balloon angioplasty (PTA) for the treatment of aortoiliac occlusive disease and superficial femoral arterial disease, with or without the use of intravascular stents, has flourished over the past decade. Multiple series in the literature have described a variety of factors that can affect the long-term results of iliac angioplasty

TABLE 54.3 Predictors of success after balloon angioplasty

Larger artery
Shorter lesion
Less severe clinical indication (claudication vs. critical limb ischemia)
Less severe degree of stenosis (stenosis vs. occlusion)
Excellent runoff distal to lesion (excellent vs. compromised)

and are now known to be applicable to balloon angioplasty in general (Table 54.3). Predictors of a long-term successful outcome after balloon angioplasty include the location of the lesion (common iliac lesions respond better than external iliac artery lesions), indication for therapy (patients with claudication respond better than those with limb-threatening ischemia), severity of the lesion (arterial stenoses respond better than arterial occlusions), and arterial runoff distal to the lesion (lesions with good runoff respond better than those with poor runoff).

A recent Italian study has reported the results of 37 elderly patients aged 80–89 with critical limb ischemia at high risk for surgery; 102 lesions were treated with PTA [28]. The overall technical success was 84%; however, 85% of patients had reocclusion within 1 year. Despite this high rate of restenosis and reocclusion, complete or partial wound healing was achieved in 80%, and rest pain was improved in 57% of patients, achieving a total limb salvage rate of 74% [28]. The authors suggest that even temporary vascular patency after PTA enables adequate wound healing in elderly patients, recommending a primary endovascular approach. Similar results were found in an Israeli study [29]. Most recent series similarly report excellent limb salvage despite low primary patency as assisted primary and secondary patency rates are excellent [30].

Early reports on the results of angioplasty supported the use of stents after angioplasty failures, dissections, or more complex lesions to improve the results of iliac artery interventions. The role of stenting after angioplasty remains controversial, with some authors recommending primary stenting and others advocating a more selective approach. We have found that high-risk patients, including elderly patients, have excellent results after stent placement in the superficial femoral artery [31].

Numerous additional variations on the basic angioplasty theme are currently being evaluated in patients with PAD, including elderly patients. Some of these options include: (1) subintimal angioplasty, in which the wire is intentionally placed in a dissection plane in the arterial media, to assist crossing of otherwise difficult lesions; (2) remote endarterectomy/plaque excision, in which the plaque is shaved off layers at a time; (3) laser atherectomy, in which a laser is used to destroy the plaque; (4) orbital atherectomy, in which a diamond-coated crown rotates to "sand away" plaque; (5) cryoplasty, the use of liquid nitrogen to inflate the angioplasty balloon, simultaneously freezing the plaque; (6) cutting balloon, in which fine microtomes are placed on the balloon to limit dissection and promote expansion of calcified plaques; (7) resorbable stents, in which a stent is placed that is absorbable with time; (8) covered stents, in which a totally endovascular endoluminal "bypass" can be performed; and (9) drug-eluting stents, in which pharmacological agents that prevent restenosis are delivered from the stent. None of these adjunctive therapies has been convincingly found to have long-term benefits at this time, in any group of patients, let alone elderly patients. It is likely that additional technologies will be developed and evaluated in the future, and the continued proliferation of these advances, coupled with the desire to treat patients with the latest advances, will continue to prevent timely randomized prospective studies of these endovascular technologies.

The Columbia group recently has reported its results of plaque excision using the Silverhawk atherectomy device [32]. 579 lesions in 275 patients, with a mean age of 70 years, were treated; 37% were claudicants, and 63% had critical limb ischemia. The authors reported 18-month primary patency of 53%, and secondary patency of 75%; limb salvage was 92% [32]. These excellent results require confirmation from additional groups, as results in younger cohort groups are not so optimistic.

Similarly, the Below-the-Knee Chill Study reported its initial experience with Cryoplasty (cold balloon angioplasty). 108 patients with a mean age of 73 years, presenting with critical limb ischemia, were treated and followed for 6 months; there were six major amputations (6.6%) and five deaths; amputation-free survival was 89% [33]. However, in a group of 64 patients with a mean age of 81 years, Samson reported only 38% freedom from restenosis at 24 months and an extra $1,700 cost per procedure for cryoplasty, suggesting that this therapeutic modality is not cost-effective [34].

We believe that a balanced approach is needed when infrapopliteal angioplasty is required. Restenosis, reintervention, and amputation are high after tibial angioplasty performed for critical limb ischemia, although an attempt at PTA is often indicated; excellent limb salvage rates may be obtained with careful follow-up and reintervention when necessary, including surgical bypass [35].

Stem Cell Therapy

The use of autologous stem cells for patients with unreconstructable ischemia is being explored. Initial results have described both bone marrow-derived as well as circulating peripheral blood-derived stem cell isolation; these stem cells are then reinjected into the ischemic leg to promote angiogenesis and arteriogenesis, resulting in relief of rest pain, healing of ulcers, and limb salvage [36, 37]. However, randomized trials have yet to confirm these exciting reports, preventing widespread usage of this technology to date. The use of stem cell therapy in elderly patients is not intuitive, as elderly patients may have reduced stem cell numbers, function, quality, and ability to isolate these cells from the marrow or circulation, compared to younger patients. Nonetheless, stem cell therapy may be an exciting alternative therapy for patients without other options, and its minimally invasive nature is especially appealing to elderly patients.

Chronic Visceral Ischemia

Progressive atherosclerotic stenosis and occlusion of the visceral arteries is often asymptomatic but ultimately can result in end organ damage to either the kidneys or the bowel. Renal artery stenosis is a relatively less common location for atherosclerotic lesions compared to the usual peripheral and cardiac locations; a renal artery stenosis greater than 60% may stimulate the kidney to release renin into the bloodstream, resulting in brittle hypertension. This affects 6.8% of patients older than 65 years [38]. Renovascular hypertension, however, is associated with increased risk of adverse coronary events in these patients [38]. If medical management fails, traditional surgical revascularization has excellent results; Benjamin et al. reported that age ≥60 was not a risk factor for mortality after renal artery bypass [39]. However, percutaneous angioplasty with placement of endoluminal stents is currently the most common procedure performed. Success rates of 65–80% and restenosis rates of 11–17% have been reported for the general population [40–42]. A French group found renal artery angioplasty to reduce by 60% the number of patients requiring two or more medications for blood pressure control [43]. However, this study excluded patients over the age of 75, and its findings have not been verified in the elderly population. The Wake Forest group reported its results of

110 renal artery angioplasty/stent placements in 99 patients, with a mean age of 69 years; the glomerular filtration rate was improved in only 28%, and the number of antihypertensive agents decreased modestly (3.3 ± 1.2 versus 3.1 ± 1.3 postintervention, $P = 0.009$) [42].

Asymptomatic celiac trunk or mesenteric artery stenosis is common, present in 17.5% of the population over 70 years of age, but was not associated with increased mortality [44]. Chronic mesenteric ischemia, resulting in intestinal angina, is thought to be associated with progression of disease beyond a single vessel and/or loss of collaterals. Acute occlusion of blood flow to the bowel by an embolic source can be a catastrophic event to the elderly patient and is associated with high mortality. Nonocclusive acute occlusion typically occurs in the critically ill and elderly who have low cardiac output states combined with diffuse mesenteric vasoconstriction.

Options for surgical correction of mesenteric stenoses or emboli include percutaneous angioplasty, stent placement, endarterectomy, and bypass procedures, all with limited success. Mesenteric artery endarterectomy and bypass is generally reported to be a safe and durable surgical procedure in patients with good surgical risk; operative mortality is typically <5% in elective cases. However, increased mortality is associated with age as well as renal insufficiency, suggesting a role for minimally invasive therapy in elderly patients [45].

Brown et al. [46] retrospectively analyzed 14 patients with a mean age of 73 years, having undergone mesenteric angioplasty and stent placement. This group reported a high early restenosis rate resulting in 53% of patients requiring reintervention within the 13-month follow-up period. However, 93% of patients remained symptom-free at the conclusion of the study [46]. Similarly, high symptom-free rates have been reported with mesenteric artery reconstruction, 80% at 5 years and 60% at 10 years [47]. Given these excellent functional results, mesenteric artery angioplasty with stent placement can be reasonably recommended for patients with limited life expectancy; however, surgical artery reconstruction remains the treatment of choice for patients with average life expectancy.

Summary

Vascular surgery is stressful in all patients and certainly in the elderly. Larger operations such as aortobifemoral bypass have increased perioperative morbidity and mortality that all patients with extensive comorbidities, such as many elderly patients, have difficulty tolerating with ease. For these physiologically elderly patients, minimally invasive approaches such as PTA, without or with stent placement, may be beneficial; long-term results may or may not be beneficial in this group of patients with limited life expectancy. On the other hand, the technically proficient conduct of most high-risk vascular surgical procedures, with aggressive pre-, intra-, and postoperative medical optimization, allows safe application to elderly patients [48]. Operations that are more limited in

---

CASE STUDY

An angiogram that you perform shows mild disease in the superficial femoral artery as well as severe proximal tibial disease; the dominant runoff vessel to the foot is the anterior tibial artery (Fig. 54.4). The patient's cardiologist believes that he is at moderate risk for procedures, but if beta-blockers are given perioperatively, no additional preoperative testing needs to be performed.

The patient is taken to the operating room where the superficial artery disease (Fig. 54.5a) is treated with both cryoplasty (Fig. 54.5b, c) as well as a 5 mm × 30 mm stent (Fig. 54.5d, e). The outflow disease is treated by an SFA-anterior tibial bypass using the ipsilateral vein.

After a 1-week postoperative recovery, the patient was able to be discharged to home, with a visiting nurse to monitor the healing toe. Follow-up at 3 months showed that the toe ulcer healed completely, and the patient was able to resume independent living.

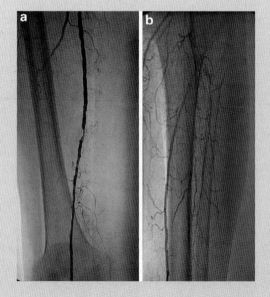

Figure 54.4 Angiogram showing: (**a**) mild superficial femoral disease, (**b**) severe proximal tibial disease.

(continued)

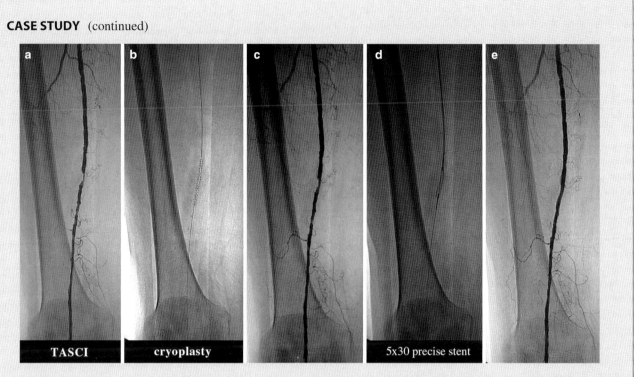

CASE STUDY (continued)

FIGURE 54.5 Angiogram showing endovascular treatment of the superficial femoral artery disease. (**a**) Primary lesion at the distal SFA; (**b**) cryoplasty of the lesion; (**c**) postcryoplasty appearance; (**d**) stent placement; (**e**) final appearance of the treated lesion.

scope, producing less physiological disturbance, are usually well tolerated by elderly patients. For example, carotid endarterectomy provides stroke-free survival benefit, and peripheral bypass surgery provides limb salvage; these procedures should not be denied to patients on the basis of age alone.

References

1. Norgren L, Hiatt WR, Dormandy JA, Nehler MR, Harris KA, Fowkes FG (2007) Inter-Society Consensus for the Management of Peripheral Arterial Disease (TASC II). J Vasc Surg 45(Suppl S):S5–S67
2. Hirsch A, Criqui M, Treat Jacobson D, Regensteiner J, Creager M, Olin J et al (2001) Peripheral arterial disease detection, awareness, and treatment in primary care. JAMA 286(11):1317–1324
3. Resnick HE et al (2004) Relationship of high and low ankle brachial index to all-cause and cardiovascular disease mortality: the Strong Heart Study. Circulation 109(6):733–739
4. Kohler TR, Nance DR, Cramer MM et al (1987) Duplex scanning for diagnosis of aortoiliac and femoropopliteal disease: a prospective study. Circulation 76:1074–1080
5. Langsfeld M, Nupute J, Hershey FB et al (1988) The use of deep duplex scanning to predict hemodynamically significant aortoiliac stenoses. J Vasc Surg 7:395–399
6. Moneta GL, Yeager RA, Antonovic R et al (1992) Accuracy of lower extremity arterial duplex mapping. J Vasc Surg 15:275–284
7. Legemate DA, Teeuwen C, Hoenveld H et al (1991) Value of duplex scanning compared with angiography and pressure measurement in the assessment of aortoiliac lesions. Br J Surg 78:1003–1008
8. Schlösser FJ, Mojibian HR, Dardik A, Verhagen HJ, Moll FL, Muhs BE (2008) Simultaneous sizing and preoperative risk stratification for thoracic endovascular aneurysm repair: role of gated computed tomography. J Vasc Surg 48(3):561–570
9. Owens RS, Carpenter JP, Baum RA et al (1992) Magnetic resonance imaging of angiographically occult runoff vessels in peripheral arterial occlusive disease. N Engl J Med 326:1577–1581
10. Carpenter JP, Owens RS, Baum RA et al (1992) Magnetic resonance angiography of peripheral runoff vessels. J Vasc Surg 16:807–815
11. Carpenter JP, Owens RS, Holland GA et al (1994) Magnetic resonance angiography of the aorta, iliac, and femoral arteries. Surgery 116:17–23
12. Arlart IP, Guhl L, Edleman RR (1992) Magnetic resonance angiography of the abdominal aorta. Cardiovasc Intervent Radiol 15:43
13. Hessel SJ, Adams DF, Abrams HL (1981) Complications of angiography. Radiology 138:273–281
14. Gomes AS, Baker JD, Martin-Paredero V et al (1985) Acute renal dysfunction after major arteriography. AJR Am J Roentgenol 145:1249–1253
15. Martin-Paredero V, Dixon SM, Baker JD et al (1983) Risk of renal failure after major angiography. Arch Surg 118:1417–1420
16. Nikonoff T, Skau T, Berglund J et al (1993) Effects of femoral arteriography and low osmolar contrast agents on renal function. Acta Radiol 34:88–91
17. Katholi RE, Taylor GJ, Woods WT et al (1993) Nephrotoxicity of nonionic low-osmolality versus ionic high-osmolality contrast media: a prospective double-blind randomized comparison in human beings. Radiology 186:183–187
18. Lautin EM, Freeman NJ, Schoenfeld AH et al (1991) Radiocontrast-associated renal dysfunction: a comparison of lower-osmolality and conventional high-osmolality contrast media. AJR Am J Roentgenol 157:59–65

19. Hall KA, Wong RW, Hunger GC et al (1992) Contrast-induced nephrotoxicity: the effects of vasodilator therapy. J Surg Res 53:317–320

20. Green RM et al (2000) Prosthetic above-knee femoropopliteal bypass grafting: five-year results of a randomized trial. J Vasc Surg 31:417–425

21. Lau H, Cheng SWK (2001) Long-term prognosis of femoropopliteal bypass: an analysis of 349 consecutive revascularizations. ANZ J Surg 71:335–340

22. Scher LA et al (1986) Limb salvage in octogenarians and nonagenarians. Surgery 99:160–165

23. Cogbill TH et al (1987) Late results of peripheral vascular surgery in patients 80 years of age and older. Arch Surg 122:581–586

24. Friedman SG et al (1989) Limb salvage in elderly patients. Is aggressive surgical therapy warranted? J. Cardiovasc Surg 30:848–851

25. Hearn AT et al (1996) Analysis of autogenous vein femoral-infrapopliteal bypass for limb salvage in the elderly. Cardiovasc Surg 4:105–109

26. O'Mara CS et al (1987) Distal bypass for limb salvage in very elderly patients. Am Surg 53(2):66–70

27. Illuminati G et al (2000) Distal polytetrafluoroethylene bypass in patients older than 75 years. Arch Surg 135:780–784

28. Amato B, Iuliano GP, Markabauoi AK et al (2005) Endovascular procedures in critical leg ischemia of elderly patients. Acta Biomed 76(Suppl 1):11–15

29. Atar E, Siegel Y, Avrahami R, Bartal G, Bachar GN, Belenky A (2005) Balloon angioplasty of popliteal and crural arteries in elderly with critical chronic limb ischemia. Eur J Radiol 53(2):287–292

30. Kudo T, Chandra FA, Ahn SS (2005) The effectiveness of percutaneous transluminal angioplasty for the treatment of critical limb ischemia: a 10-year experience. J Vasc Surg 41(3):423–435

31. Nishibe T, Kondo Y, Nishibe M, Muto A, Dardik A (2009) Stent placement for superficial femoral arterial occlusive disease in high-risk patients: preliminary results. Surg Today 39(1):21–26

32. McKinsey JF, Goldstein L, Khan HU, Graham A, Rezeyat C, Morrissey NJ, Sambol E, Kent KC (2008) Novel treatment of patients with lower extremity ischemia: use of percutaneous atherectomy in 579 lesions. Ann Surg 248(4):519–528

33. Das T, McNamara T, Gray B, Sedillo GJ, Turley BR, Kollmeyer K, Rogoff M, Aruny JE (2007) Cryoplasty therapy for limb salvage in patients with critical limb ischemia. J Endovasc Ther 14(6):753–762

34. Samson RH, Showalter DP, Lepore M Jr, Nair DG, Merigliano K (2008) CryoPlasty therapy of the superficial femoral and popliteal arteries: a reappraisal after 44 months' experience. J Vasc Surg 48(3):634–637

35. Giles KA, Pomposelli FB, Hamdan AD, Blattman SB, Panossian H, Schermerhorn ML (2008) Infrapopliteal angioplasty for critical limb ischemia: relation of TransAtlantic InterSociety Consensus class to outcome in 176 limbs. J Vasc Surg 48(1):128–136

36. Tateishi-Yuyama E, Matsubara H, Murohara T, Ikeda U, Shintani S, Masaki H, Amano K, Kishimoto Y, Yoshimoto K, Akashi H, Shimada K, Iwasaka T, Imaizumi T, Therapeutic Angiogenesis using Cell Transplantation (TACT) Study Investigators (2002) Therapeutic angiogenesis for patients with limb ischaemia by autologous transplantation of bone-marrow cells: a pilot study and a randomised controlled trial. Lancet 360(9331):427–435

37. Ishida A, Ohya Y, Sakuda H, Ohshiro K, Higashiuesato Y, Nakaema M, Matsubara S, Yakabi S, Kakihana A, Ueda M, Miyagi C, Yamane N, Koja K, Komori K, Takishita S (2005) Autologous peripheral blood mononuclear cell implantation for patients with peripheral arterial disease improves limb ischemia. Circ J 69(10):1260–1265

38. Edwards MS, Craven TE, Burke GL, Dean RH, Hansen KJ (2005) Renovascular disease and the risk of adverse coronary events in the elderly: a prospective, population-based study. Arch Intern Med 165(2):207–213

39. Benjamin ME, Hansen KJ, Craven TE, Keith DR, Plonk GW, Geary RL, Dean RH (1996) Combined aortic and renal artery surgery. A contemporary experience. Ann Surg 223(5):555–565

40. Burket MW, Cooper CJ, Kennedy DJ et al (2000) Renal artery angioplasty and stent placement: predictors of a favorable outcome. Am Heart J 139(1 Pt 1):64–71

41. Rocha-Singh K, Jaff MR, Rosenfield K (2005) Evaluation of the safety and effectiveness of renal artery stenting after unsuccessful balloon angioplasty: the ASPIRE-2 study. J Am Coll Cardiol 46(5):776–783

42. Corriere MA, Pearce JD, Edwards MS, Stafford JM, Hansen KJ (2008) Endovascular management of atherosclerotic renovascular disease: early results following primary intervention. J Vasc Surg 48(3):580–587

43. Plouin PF, Chatellier G, Darne B, Raynaud A (1998) Blood pressure outcome of angioplasty in atherosclerotic renal artery stenosis: a randomized trial. Essai Multicentrique Medicaments vs Angioplastie (EMMA) Study Group. Hypertension 31(3):823–829

44. Hansen KJ, Wilson DB, Craven TE, Pearce JD, English WP, Edwards MS, Ayerdi J, Burke GL (2004) Mesenteric artery disease in the elderly. J Vasc Surg 40(1):45–52

45. Mell MW, Acher CW, Hoch JR, Tefera G, Turnipseed WD (2008) Outcomes after endarterectomy for chronic mesenteric ischemia. J Vasc Surg 48(5):1132–1138

46. Brown DJ, Schermerhorn ML, Powell RJ et al (2005) Mesenteric stenting for chronic mesenteric ischemia. J Vasc Surg 42(2):268–274

47. Cho JS, Carr JA, Jacobsen G, Shepard AD, Nypaver TJ, Reddy DJ (2002) Long-term outcome after mesenteric artery reconstruction: a 37-year experience. J Vasc Surg 35(3):453–460

48. Barkhordarian S, Dardik A (2004) Preoperative assessment and management to prevent complications during high-risk vascular surgery. Crit Care Med 32(Suppl 4):S174–S185

Chapter 55
Natural History and Treatment of Extracranial Cerebrovascular Disease in the Elderly

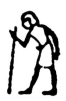

George H. Meier and Carlos Rosales

Cerebrovascular disease, specifically stroke, continues to increase despite improvements in the treatment and outcomes of cardiovascular disease in general. Many believe that the development of cerebrovascular atherosclerosis is simply a normal consequence of aging, as the incidence of stroke increases with age, rising almost sevenfold between the ages of 55 and 85 [1]. Despite a better understanding and advances in medical management, cerebrovascular disease remains the third leading cause of death in the United States [2]. It is therefore not surprising that carotid endarterectomy remains one of the most common peripheral vascular operations done in the United States [3]. Current estimates suggest that the population over the age of 65 will more than double by the year 2050 [4], by which time the likely increase in cerebrovascular disease will result in a marked impact on medical care. The correct and cost-effective management of cerebrovascular disease is therefore increasingly important as the population ages.

Cerebral infarction can be caused by intracerebral hemorrhage or embolic disorders. Although hemodynamic flow limitations can occur, flow-related cerebral ischemia is rare. Previous studies have suggested that about 60% of cerebrovascular events originate with atherosclerotic disease outside the heart [5]. Thus, most embolic strokes should be preventable if the extracranial vascular disease can be diagnosed and treated prior to an irreversible cerebrovascular event. This intervention may be as simple as limiting plaque growth with medical management once carotid disease is discovered, or it may require complex reopening of the arterial supply with surgical or endovascular techniques. Stroke prevention requires not only modification of risk factors for atherosclerosis but also appropriate selection of patients for intervention prior to the occurrence of a limiting cerebrovascular event.

Risk factor modification in those with atherosclerosis is an area of intense, ongoing investigation and review.

Traditional risk factors for atherosclerotic disease such as smoking [6], hypertension [7], and diabetes [8] remain significant for patients with extracranial atherosclerosis. Research suggests that other risk factors such as elevated homocysteine [9] and low-density lipoprotein (LDL) cholesterol [10–12] may be important in lowering the ultimate risk of stroke. Elevated homocysteine levels in the bloodstream have been implicated in numerous atherosclerotic disease processes [13, 14]. Whereas homozygous individuals with a deficiency of enzymes to metabolize homocysteine often die at a young age secondary to coronary disease [15], heterozygous individuals maintain function but appear to have an increased tendency to develop atherosclerosis. The management of these elevations is relatively simple, as three inducible enzyme systems allow breakdown of homocysteine into safer metabolites. These inducible systems increase their activity in response to folate, vitamin B_6, and vitamin B_{12}, respectively. While it remains simple to replace these vitamins, multiple studies have shown no benefit in cardiovascular disease prevention [16, 17].

The cholesterol saga has been a fundamental issue with respect to coronary disease for years. Cholesterol has traditionally been linked to coronary atherosclerosis [18] but has also been implicated strongly in cerebrovascular disease [19]. Whereas atherosclerotic plaque initiation is little influenced by cholesterol levels, progression of plaque already in place is clearly accelerated by elevated cholesterol levels. Evidence suggests that the reduction of cholesterol using 3-hydroxy-3-methylglutaryl coenzyme A (HMG-CoA) reductase inhibitors, even in individuals with normal levels, may lower the risk of subsequent cardiac events [20]. The CARE trial demonstrated a 31% reduced incidence of stroke with the use of pravastatin in patients with previous myocardial infarction [21]. The largest trial thus far is the Heart Protection Study, which showed a significant reduction in stroke/TIA on patients taking simvastatin versus placebo. When evaluating all cardiovascular end points, a relative risk reduction of 23.6% was achieved [22]. The SPARCL trial took patients with recent stroke or TIA and randomized them to atorvastatin or placebo. The stroke rate for the

G.H. Meier (✉)
Department of Vascular Surgery, University Hospital of Cincinnati, Cincinnati, OH, USA
e-mail: george.meier@uc.edu

placebo group was 13.1% versus 11.2% for the treatment group (RRR 2.2%). The absolute risk reduction for major cardiovascular events was 3.5%. When examining the subset of patients with carotid stenosis in the SPARCL trial, atorvastatin was associated with a 33% reduction in the risk of any stroke, and the need for carotid revascularization was reduced by 56% [23, 24]. These and multiple other studies have proven that statins are clearly beneficial in stroke prevention and should be used in all patients with carotid disease.

Antiplatelet therapy is another very important tool when managing cerebrovascular disease. Multiple trials have shown the benefit of aspirin in stroke prevention. The International Stroke Trial showed a reduction of reinfarction rate within 2 weeks of an ischemic stroke in patients treated with aspirin [25]. In the CAST study, those patients treated with aspirin had a 12% RRR for stroke and death in the 4 weeks following acute stroke [26]. Several recent studies have evaluated the role of clopidogrel in stroke prevention. The Clopidogrel Versus Aspirin in Patients at Risk of Ischemic Events Trial (CAPRIE) concluded that clopidogrel was slightly superior to aspirin in stroke prevention on patients with generalized atherosclerosis (8.7% RRR) [27–29]. This risk reduction is even higher (22.7%) in patients with disease in multiple vascular beds. The effects of aspirin alone versus aspirin and clopidogrel were evaluated in the CHARISMA trial [30, 31]. CHARISMA randomized patients with cardiovascular disease or multiple risk factors to either aspirin or aspirin and clopidogrel and looked at myocardial infarction, stroke, or death as the primary end point. The risk of future ischemic events in the aspirin group was 7.3% versus 6.8% for the dual therapy group. The relative risk reduction of 0.93 was not statistically significant. The RRR for symptomatic patients was statistically significant at 12% ($p=0.046$). Antiplatelet agents are proven of benefit to patients with proven stroke and should therefore be prescribed to all patients with carotid artery disease. Aspirin at either low or high dose is adequate for most patients, but clopidogrel should be considered in some situations, particularly in those patients with atherosclerotic disease in multiple vascular beds.

Early prospective randomized trials evaluating carotid treatments relied on a "Best Medical Management" arm for comparison to surgical treatment. While the standards of medical management at the time of these trials were quite different than today, best medical management today includes the use of statin therapy, antiplatelet agents, and other medical agents that were not available for routine use during previous trials. Clearly, physicians have become much better at slowing the progression of atherosclerotic disease with many new modalities not previously available. As a result, many observers question the comparisons previously used; current best medical therapy may be significantly better than that used for the trials and therefore raise questions as to whether or not the conclusions of the trials

remain valid in the current era. For this reason, historical controls are probably insufficient to determine outcomes for care. Newer trials have included new medical management arms whenever possible. Eventually, medical management should be effective at preventing progression of atherosclerotic disease; until that time, the medical management standard will be slowly drifting toward overall better outcomes.

Pathophysiology

Atherosclerotic disease begins early in life as plaque initiation starts in areas at risk for atherosclerotic degeneration [32, 33]. Most atherosclerosis is well explained by this mechanism, although some fundamental contradictions remain. If atherosclerosis is a progressive degenerative disease, it would be reasonably expected that its incidence would continue to increase with increasing age. Indeed, this appears to be true for cerebrovascular disease, but it is distinctly contrary to existing data relative to both coronary [34] and iliac [35] disease. In those distributions, a plateau occurs in the incidence of atherosclerosis, with decreasing incidence of disease once a certain age is reached. The explanation for this discrepancy is complex, and whether there is a real plateau in disease progression in these anatomic areas or whether a selection bias exists remains unclear. What data are available suggest that no such plateau exists for cerebrovascular disease, with the incidence of disease increasing with increasing age [35, 36]. Additionally, the increased incidence of cerebrovascular disease further explains the resultant increased incidence of stroke with increasing age [37].

The atherosclerotic plaque of cerebrovascular disease is no different from that associated with coronary or peripheral vascular disease. The initiating event appears to be the development of a lesion on the intimal surface of the artery, particularly in areas of low shear stress [38]. The carotid bifurcation has been studied extensively, as plaque formation in this distribution is more anatomically consistent than that seen in most other locations. Essentially, the bifurcation of the carotid artery generates an area of high velocity (and therefore high shear stress) at the septum between the external and internal carotid arteries and an area of low shear stress at the bulb of the internal carotid artery opposite the bifurcation. In fact, with the advent of color flow duplex ultrasonography, this area of flow separation and reversal can be easily defined in normal individuals. The flow phantom models of shear-related atherosclerosis have been best defined in this anatomic location. These models clearly demonstrate the areas of flow separation and resultant flow reversal opposite the bifurcation, where atherosclerosis is found consistently. Therefore, flow patterns at the carotid bifurcation appear to be important in the initiation and progression of atherosclerotic plaque in the cerebrovascular system.

A second issue associated with atherosclerotic plaque progression is the concept of intraplaque hemorrhage (Fig. 55.1). With coronary artery disease, intraplaque hemorrhage is a well-accepted mechanism of sudden plaque progression associated with an acute myocardial event. Similarly, carotid atherosclerosis has been studied extensively relative to plaque morphology and intraplaque hemorrhage. The small blood vessels that traverse the complex intimal plaque of mature atherosclerosis are subject to significant hemodynamic effects, resulting in an increased risk of vessel rupture, with attendant intraplaque hemorrhage. Recently, new techniques in high-resolution ultrasound using intravenous ultrasound contrast have demonstrated this neovascularization of the plaque, suggesting that these images may predict which plaques are vulnerable [39–41]. The concept of plaque vulnerability becomes important when trying to predict which lesions are likely to progress and potentially cause symptoms. The association of intraplaque hemorrhage with increasing stenosis has been well documented [42]. Additionally, there has been a significant association of intraplaque hemorrhage with symptomatic carotid stenosis [43–46]. In this instance, the presence of subintimal hemorrhage results in intimal ulceration and embolization of residual intraplaque clot and debris, producing the characteristic microemboli associated with transient ischemic attacks (TIAs) [47]. Thus, intraplaque hemorrhage is associated with the severity of stenosis as well as the symptoms, suggesting that intraplaque hemorrhage may be the link between degree of stenosis and the incidence of symptoms. As a result, prediction of which plaques have an increased risk of intraplaque hemorrhage becomes important for both surveillance and asymptomatic intervention.

The origin of symptoms related to carotid atherosclerosis has not always been well defined. According to the hemodynamic theory, the symptoms associated with carotid stenosis were related to flow limitations and resultant cortical ischemia. In contrast, the embolic theory held that degeneration of the atherosclerotic plaque resulted in microemboli, and clot

formation caused macroemboli and stroke. The stumbling block for the embolic theory was the recurrent nature of similar symptoms with repeated episodes of transient ischemia. If a second TIA occurred, it was often with the same symptoms as seen during the previous attacks. How embolic debris could produce such repetitive symptoms was unclear. Two landmark studies served to resolve the conflict. First, the hemodynamics was evaluated by Kendall and Marshall [48]. In this study, patients with TIAs were subjected to pharmacologically induced hypotension. As the blood pressure was decreased, the patients were monitored for neurologic changes. None of these patients developed symptoms when their mean blood pressure was decreased significantly. Therefore, hemodynamic causes of transient ischemia seemed less likely [49].

The second study that ended the hemodynamic embolic controversy was performed by Millikin at the Mayo Clinic [50]. In this study, baboons were anesthetized, and needles were inserted into the carotid flow. Small metallic beads were injected via these needles, and the brains were evaluated for the ultimate location of the beads. In a classic illustration from that study, the brain of one of the baboons was seen to have six beads lined up in the middle cerebral artery (Fig. 55.2). The insertion of the beads at a specific point in the flow resulted in emboli at a specific destination determined by the laminar flow patterns in the artery. In other words, the origin of the embolus determined its ultimate resting point. Thus, in one clear demonstration, the issue of recurrent symptoms resulting from multiple embolic events was resolved, confirming the embolic theory to be the best explanation for both TIAs and strokes [51, 52].

Given this evolution, the issue of hemodynamics has become a secondary issue in symptomatic cerebrovascular disease. Nonetheless, although certain patients clearly have flow compromise as an etiology for symptoms, their definition

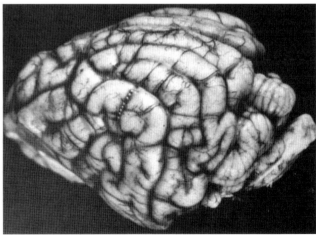

Figure 55.2 Experimental demonstration of repetitive embolizations. In this baboon brain, embolization of metal spheres lodged in the same arterial segment with each sequential injection.

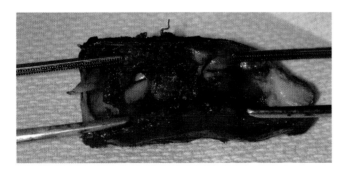

Figure 55.1 Intraplaque hemorrhage associated with high-grade carotid stenosis.

remains difficult. Anatomic studies have demonstrated that the circle of Willis, the traditional anatomic structure responsible for flow redistribution at the base of the brain, is incomplete in at least 25% of patients [53, 54]. With an incomplete circle of Willis, blood flow may be limited in its redistribution, resulting in areas of potential underperfusion. With additional atherosclerotic obstruction of the cerebral vessels, collateral flow may be compromised because of one of these congenital abnormalities in the circle of Willis. With a complete circle of Willis, normal anterior (carotid) circulation equates with normal posterior perfusion, even in the absence of native vertebral flow. In contrast, if one or both posterior communicating arteries are absent, vertebral or basilar artery disease may result in posterior circulation symptoms with completely normal anterior circulation. Given the frequency of abnormalities in the circle of Willis, maldistribution of flow is certainly possible in the setting of severe carotid or vertebral artery stenosis or occlusion.

Hemodynamic issues remain important when discussing watershed ischemia. Watershed ischemia occurs when perfusion to a segment of the brain is limited hemodynamically to a level below the blood flow necessary to maintain cell integrity. Infarctions then occur at the junction between two blood supplies, the so-called watershed zones. Watershed ischemia remains a topic of some controversy, but its occurrence remains ill-defined and sporadic. The classic scenario for watershed infarction due to underlying hemodynamic compromise occurs most commonly with open heart surgery using cardiopulmonary bypass. If a critical stenosis or occlusion is present, the diminished perfusion associated with the nonpulsatile, limited pressure flow of the heart–lung machine can produce watershed infarction in an area at risk. Carotid endarterectomy or carotid stenting prior to or simultaneous with coronary artery bypass surgery is done in an attempt to prevent these watershed infarctions [55–57].

The possibility of hemodynamic flow disturbance is reinforced by the occurrence of reperfusion syndromes after correction of severe carotid stenoses. In this scenario, the severe upstream stenosis results in the loss of autoregulation in the downstream cerebrovascular bed, with localized brain edema and risk of intracerebral hemorrhage resulting from reperfusion [58, 59]. Clearly, this loss of autoregulation represents a flow-limited response to a hemodynamically significant stenosis [60]. The difficulty is that flow-related ischemia is diffuse rather than focal, and evaluation of flow limitation is difficult with conventional intracranial imaging. Nonetheless, positron emission tomography has provided a window into overall brain blood flow and metabolism [61] and provides experimental insights into the frequency of flow limitation in the clinical setting. For the present, however, the basis for diagnosis and treatment of cerebrovascular disease focuses on the presence of a potential embolic focus, rather than on any potential for cerebrovascular flow limitation.

Diagnosis

Diagnostic testing in patients with cerebrovascular disease is essentially limited to two major areas: extracranial arterial imaging and intracranial arterial imaging. Each plays a fundamental role in the assessment of patients for carotid intervention. Because cerebral revascularization is focused on the extracranial carotid and vertebral arteries, arterial imaging is most important in these locations. Intracranial arterial imaging remains important, but its role continues to evolve as new modalities and technologies become available.

Anatomic definition in extracranial cerebrovascular disease is limited to two fundamental testing modalities: color duplex ultrasonography and arteriography. Each of these modalities has significant advantages and disadvantages, requiring more complete definition of their utility. Color duplex ultrasonography is a noninvasive technique for evaluating blood flow in any location accessible to an ultrasound beam (Fig. 55.3). The carotid and vertebral circulations were the initial focus of vascular ultrasonography development and remain the test bed for ongoing research in ultrasonographic diagnosis. Consistent visualization can be achieved in this location, resulting in reproducible diagnostic assessment of the severity and pattern of stenosis. Estimation of the degree of stenosis is based on several criteria, including peak systolic velocity, internal carotid/common carotid velocity ratios, and end-diastolic velocity. The most widely used criteria remain those of Strandness [62]. These criteria were developed to define percentage narrowing of the carotid bulb and have been verified in studies involving both angiographic and pathologic correlates [63]. Today, most carotid interventions are performed based on the data gathered from duplex ultrasound. It is also the standard to follow asymptomatic carotid stenosis with duplex ultrasound alone.

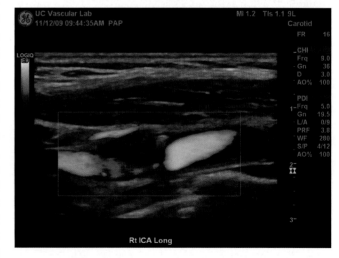

Figure 55.3 Duplex assessment of carotid using power Doppler.

The arteriographic assessment of cerebrovascular disease has remained essentially unchanged since the first cerebral angiogram by Moniz in 1927 [64]. Angiography results from injection of a radiopaque tracer intraluminally followed by exposure of an X-ray film or with use of a digital image intensifier. The choice of tracer today is usually a newer low osmolar nonionic contrast that has both lower incidence of allergic reactions and lower direct tissue toxicity. While traditional angiography involved X-ray film, currently, digital image processing techniques are used which not only lower radiation dose and contrast load but also provide archival images for digital storage (Fig. 55.4). While some institutions routinely use angiography for the diagnosis of cerebrovascular disease, many institutions have evolved to intervention based on ultrasound alone. As a result, angiographic diagnosis of cerebrovascular disease has faded, only to be somewhat revived by its use as a basis for carotid stenting. No specific combination of techniques dominates the arteriographic diagnosis of cerebrovascular disease, and institutional experience is more important than perceived advantages of one technique over another.

The diagnosis of atherosclerosis by arteriography requires documentation of intraluminal narrowing of the involved artery viewed in two planes. Because angiography is fundamentally a two-dimensional technique and atherosclerosis is three-dimensional, the assessment of luminal narrowing requires perpendicular perspectives to state the degree of narrowing accurately. Measurement of internal carotid narrowing has traditionally been a calculation of the minimum residual lumen relative to an estimated arterial diameter in the carotid bulb. This estimation of the carotid bulb diameter is subject to interpretation and often results in overestimation of the degree of luminal narrowing. Fundamentally, the significance of any carotid stenosis resides in the degree of luminal encroachment relative to the outflow arterial diameter. This approach was first applied to the assessment of arteriographic diameter reduction in the NASCET trial [65] and subsequently was used for the Asymptomatic Carotid Atherosclerosis Study (ACAS) [66] as well. Currently, minimum residual lumen is compared to outflow arterial diameter for calculating the degree of stenosis. This technique is utilized both in ultrasound as well as an angiographic imaging. Angiography today is generally not necessary before surgery; it is most commonly used before a carotid stent or if the duplex ultrasound findings are unclear.

The earliest form of evaluation for intracranial pathology was the use of computed tomography without intravenous contrast [67]. While this new technology was revolutionary in its days, it was limited by the lack of vascular definition, ultimately necessitating IV contrast to define the limits of the vessels within the cerebral circulation. The addition of intravenous contrast to conventional CT imaging of the head and neck allowed not only the definition of intracranial parenchymal pathology but also the potential for vascular anatomic definition (Fig. 55.5). It only remained for high-resolution scanning techniques to be developed to allow angiographic equivalence using spiral CT technology.

Currently, CT angiography is used as a preliminary step in imaging in many patients with symptomatic carotid disease; evaluation for intracranial pathology can be coupled with surface mapping of the arteries to define three-dimensional anatomy for both the intracranial and extracranial vessels. What are the limitations of CT angiography? Primarily, the limitations center on differentiating the presence of intravenous contrast from that of the calcific vessel [68–70]. Calcium appears as a bright tissue on CT imaging and when it is confluent with the IV contrast, the interface between the two cannot be easily differentiated. As a result, calcified atherosclerosis, a common component of advanced extracranial carotid plaque, can be a confounding factor that limits the interpretation of luminal stenosis relative to the plaque associated with the stenosis. Nonetheless, as a screening tool, computed tomographic angiography is a useful adjunct prior to planning procedures, particularly when contrast angiography will be employed at the time of treatment such as with carotid stenting. In the setting, intracranial pathology is ruled out, and an estimate of anatomic disease is achieved. When coupled with duplex ultrasonography of

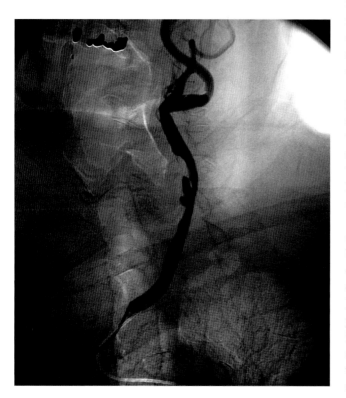

Figure 55.4 Arteriographic image of left common carotid stenosis with ulceration.

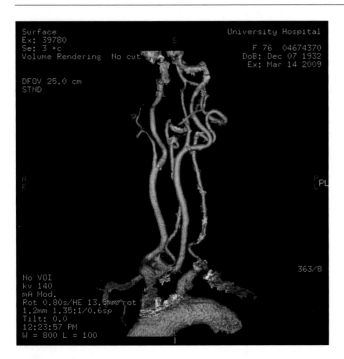

FIGURE 55.5 Surface mapping of CTA image showing normal carotid anatomy.

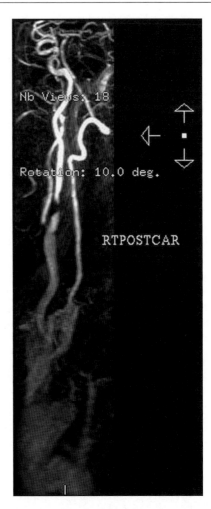

FIGURE 55.6 Magnetic resonance angiogram demonstrating signal dropout associated with stenosis.

the carotid bifurcation, a highly accurate assessment of the degree of vascular disease in the extracranial carotid circulation can be achieved.

The most promising technology for intracranial and vascular imaging has been magnetic resonance imaging. With advances in magnetic resonance techniques, the possibility of a noninvasive technique for arterial imaging becomes more likely [71]. The difficulty with magnetic resonance angiography (MRA) lies in differentiating stenosis from occlusion. Any significant stenosis results in downstream turbulence. As a result, turbulence mixes once-aligned magnetic dipoles, resulting in signal dropout. Similarly, an absence of magnetic dipoles as is seen with arterial occlusion can also lead to signal dropout. Therefore, conventional time-of-flight MRA techniques overestimate arterial stenoses (Fig. 55.6), making diagnosis of stenosis versus occlusion reliant on other imaging techniques. Many studies have evaluated this issue. In high-grade stenosis, the correlation with ultrasound is high. Unfortunately, it is in the patient with moderate degrees of stenosis where the correlations fall off: MRA often overcalls the degree of stenosis in moderate or lesser levels of carotid disease [72]. Nonetheless, the combination of arterial imaging with intracranial parenchymal imaging makes MRA attractive in symptomatic patients. If intervention is contemplated, however, carotid evaluation with duplex ultrasonography or angiography is necessary.

Treatment

Management of the Symptomatic Patient

Over the past few years, management of symptomatic carotid disease has progressed from an algorithm based on anecdotal reports to one based on significant scientific data owing primarily to publication of the NASCET study [73]. The prognosis of surgical versus medical management is clearly defined for the symptomatic population. More recently carotid stenting has been used in the symptomatic patient and is currently approved for "high-risk" patients with symptomatic disease. Despite the data that exist, numerous questions arise specific to an elderly population.

The NASCET trial for patients with symptomatic carotid disease enrolled only patients less than 80 years of age for a randomized study of surgery versus medical therapy.

Therefore, although the conclusions remain important, the results of necessity must be extrapolated to the elderly population over 79 years of age. The NASCET trial was terminated early in the high-grade stenosis group because of the significant benefit of surgery relative to medical therapy in patients with more than 70% stenosis by NASCET criteria. These results have been extended to the patient population with 49–70% stenosis demonstrating similar (though more limited) benefits to surgical management [74]. Although these data remain the cornerstone of treatment decisions for symptomatic patients, many assumptions are necessary for applying these data to the elderly population.

In the NASCET severe stenosis (>70%) group, a statistically beneficial result from surgical treatment was seen at the 3-month follow-up. Therefore, patients with symptomatic carotid disease would be expected to benefit from surgery if their operative risk was acceptable and their life expectancy was at least 3 months. Obviously, most patients treated surgically would be expected to have a life expectancy of at least 3 months. Therefore, the main issue of the decision to treat elderly symptomatic patients rests in the estimation of operative risk.

The operative risk associated with carotid disease centers on two factors: stroke risk and cardiac risk. Either factor may result in morbidity or mortality, but most studies report their results as a combined risk of stroke or death after endarterectomy. American Heart Association (AHA) guidelines [75] suggest that the upper limits for an acceptable stroke/death rate after carotid endarterectomy for TIAs should be 5%. In the NASCET trial, it was in fact 5.8% overall. Monitoring surgeon-specific and institution-specific stroke/death rates after carotid endarterectomy is a basic requirement for recommending surgical revascularization. Many investigators have studied the stroke/death rates after carotid endarterectomy in elderly patients [76–95]. There does not appear to be dramatically increased operative risks due to age alone, as most studies support the use of surgical endarterectomy in the elderly. Nonetheless, all surgical series suffer from an inherent selection bias: patients at too high risk or who are too ill may simply never be offered the procedure, skewing the results further in favor of operative intervention. In the NASCET trial, this bias was applied equally to both groups, as the randomization occurred between medical and surgical therapy only after patient entry. Therefore, all candidates in this study were appropriate for surgical management. In retrospective studies concerning the safety of carotid endarterectomy in the elderly, these controls do not exist, resulting in potential selection bias. These data demonstrate that the stroke/death rate after carotid endarterectomy in the elderly is not significantly increased over that of a more traditional patient population.

The risk of anesthesia for carotid endarterectomy has been a topic of debate for many years. Although general anesthesia is a safe, effective technique for operations on the carotid artery, proponents of local or regional anesthesia argue that the intensive care unit (ICU) stay [96] and overall length of stay [97] are both reduced, thus decreasing cost. The basic philosophy is inextricably bound to that of shunt usage: Surgeons who routinely shunt intraoperatively are more likely to use general anesthesia, as neurologic monitoring is optional. If selective shunting is employed, the decision to shunt rests on the detection of neurologic changes suggestive of cerebral ischemia. In the patient under general anesthesia, this can be provided by continuous electroencephalographic (EEG) monitoring using either a formal 16-lead EEG or compressed spectral array EEG. In the patient under regional anesthesia, neurologic monitoring is more direct, resulting from changes in the patient's neurologic examination while undergoing surgery. No evidence exists to support one anesthetic or shunting technique over another in the elderly patient undergoing carotid endarterectomy.

In the past 10 years, many studies have been undertaken to evaluate the role of carotid stenting in the treatment of carotid artery disease (Fig. 55.7). One of the early studies, the Carotid and Vertebral Artery Transluminal Angioplasty Study (CAVATAS) randomized 504 patients to be treated with angioplasty, angioplasty plus stenting, or carotid endarterectomy [98]. In this study, the 30-day stroke and death rate were similar in the endovascular and surgical groups. A common criticism of the CAVATAS study is the high rate of surgical morbidity and mortality: in this group of primarily symptomatic patients, the stroke morbidity and death rate was 9.9% in the surgical group. Additionally, the surgical group suffered cranial nerve injury in 8.7%, with no cranial nerve issues seen in the endovascular group. The overall conclusion from this early paper was that major outcomes were similar for both carotid artery stenting and carotid endarterectomy; nonetheless, increased minor complications were seen in the carotid endarterectomy patients.

The next major step in understanding carotid artery stenting occurred with publication of the SAPPHIRE trial in 2005 [99]. In this study, 334 patients with asymptomatic carotid stenosis greater than 50% or and a cinematic carotid stenosis of greater than 80% and who were considered high-risk surgical candidates were randomized to either carotid stenting or carotid endarterectomy. While no statistically significant difference was seen in the rate of stroke and death in these two populations, when myocardial infarction within 30 days after the procedure was included as an end point, the results developed statistical significance. While the inclusion of myocardial infarction within 30 days was a nuance that had not been used in previous studies, its addition to the SAPPHIRE outcomes resulted in a trend toward clear benefit to carotid stenting in high-risk patients. The study remains the cornerstone upon which carotid artery stenting was founded.

Figure 55.7 Carotid stent placement. Preintervention carotid stenosis (*left*), stent across stenosis (*center*), and final appearance after deployment (*right*).

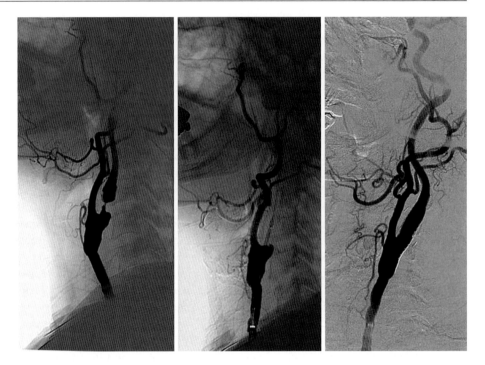

A Cochrane review in 2004 evaluated the available data from five randomized trials involving 1,269 patients [100]. The conclusion from this study was that 30-day and 1-year safety data showed no significant difference between carotid artery stenting and carotid endarterectomy. Additionally, the increased rates of cranial nerve injury and minor complications were once again noted in the surgical group compared to the stent group.

Based on the data at this point, the FDA conditionally approved carotid artery stenting in high-risk patients with greater than 70% symptomatic stenosis. These criteria were then endorsed by the Centers for Medicare and Medicaid Services as accepted indications for reimbursement for carotid artery stenting [101] (Table 55.1).

Of note, since the early use of carotid artery stenting, there has been an apparent increase in the risk of stroke in those patients greater than 80 years of age. An extensive body of data access to confirm the fact that patients greater than 80 years of age are at high risk for stroke after carotid artery stenting. The reasons for this are not clear; carotid endarterectomy patients do not appear to have the same increase in risk associated with advanced age. One of the more promising explanations has to do with the amount of aortic arch calcification: those patients greater than 80 years of age typically have an increased amount of aortic arch calcification involving the great vessels [102]. Negotiation of the aortic arch with a long sheath in these patients presumably results in an increased risk of atheroembolism from the calcium that collects with advanced age. While definitive data remains elusive, many studies have confirmed the statistical association of an increased stroke risk with an age greater than 80 years.

Table 55.1 Medicare requirements for carotid stenting reimbursement

CMS requirements for reimbursement for carotid stent placement

Stenosis > 70% using NASCET methodology

Use of both an FDA-approved embolic protection device and stent

High risk

- Congestive heart failure (CHF) class III/IV
- Left ventricular ejection fraction (LVEF) < 30%
- Unstable angina
- Contralateral carotid occlusion
- Recent myocardial infraction (MI)
- Previous CEA with recurrent stenosis
- Prior radiation treatment to the neck
- Other conditions that were used to determine patients at high risk for CEA in the prior carotid artery stenting trials and studies

In summary, any patient who is symptomatic because of extracranial carotid atherosclerosis and is of acceptable procedural risk should be offered intervention. The benefits of surgical revascularization are clear-cut, with improved outcome at both short-term and long-term follow-up; in high surgical risk patients, carotid stent placement using embolic protection appears to be an equivalent treatment. The selection of patients for carotid surgery versus carotid stenting will remain in evolution for the foreseeable future.

Management of the Asymptomatic Patient

With the publication of the ACAS trial [66], many questions related to the management of asymptomatic extracranial vascular disease were answered, but many more were raised.

Although a statistically significant decrease in stroke rate was achieved in male patients with at least 60% stenosis of the internal carotid artery, this protocol was limited to a population less than 79 years old. Therefore, extrapolation is necessary to apply these data to the very elderly population. In the ACAS trial, the patient group who most significantly benefited from prophylactic carotid endarterectomy was men, with a 79% risk reduction at the 5-year follow-up. Nonetheless, in this group, the absolute risk reduction at 5 years was only 8%, yielding a yearly risk reduction of only 1.6%. Given this modest risk reduction, the procedure-related stroke/death rate of 2.3% becomes an important determinant of the overall benefit. If the operative morbidity and mortality of carotid endarterectomy are excessive, the benefit is reduced further, and the overall efficacy reduced. Once again, the surgeon-specific and institution-specific risks must be accurately defined prior to recommending intervention. Similarly, the risk of operation in any given patient must be considered carefully, as any increase in operative stroke or death risk tempers the benefits seen. The stroke/death risk of cerebral angiography in the ACAS trial was surprisingly high at 1.2%. Therefore, the routine use of angiography further elevates the morbidity and mortality, potentially compromising the benefit of endarterectomy. Currently, many centers have adopted new strategies to lower the risk of carotid intervention in asymptomatic individuals. Foremost in this strategy is the elimination of routine arteriography prior to carotid surgery. Angiography is reserved for patients in whom unexplained findings are present on preoperative duplex ultrasonography. Using this strategy of selective angiography, preoperative arteriography can be avoided in up to 85% of the patients, lowering the risk of angiography (by extrapolation of ACAS data) to less than 0.2%. The loss of routine preoperative angiography in carotid surgery has two risks: failure to diagnose tandem intracranial or proximal lesions and failure to diagnose the high carotid bifurcation preoperatively. The risk of tandem lesions resides in the limitations to flow imposed across a fresh endarterectomy by a proximal or downstream lesion. Nonetheless, the risk of stroke following endarterectomy has not been documented to be higher in patients with tandem lesions [103, 104]. Similarly, tandem lesions do not seem to impose an increased stroke risk after successful extracranial carotid endarterectomy [105, 106]. Therefore, the risk of surgery and the risk of subsequent stroke are not significantly increased by the presence of tandem lesions. It appears that tandem carotid and intracranial stenosis occur in less than 10–15% of patients with carotid stenosis [107], implying that angiography contributes little to the management of most of these patients [108, 109].

The relative risk imposed by a high carotid bifurcation is much more difficult to define. Although numerous strategies have been developed to assist the surgical approach to the high carotid lesion, none has been without complications. The incremental benefit of knowing preoperatively that the bifurcation is higher than usual resides in the ability to change the surgical approach to compensate for the anatomic variation and improve the ease of operation. Because there does not appear to be a widely accepted alternative to the conventional approach, the preoperative diagnosis of a high carotid bifurcation serves only to provide a psychological advantage to the surgeon rather than a physical one. No data exist to justify the use of preoperative angiography or duplex ultrasound to define the high carotid bifurcation.

Although operation for asymptomatic carotid stenosis is an accepted technique, particularly in the male patient, there clearly are questions about who should undergo this treatment option. Foremost in this regard is the estimation of the patient's life expectancy. If an annual benefit of 1.2% stroke reduction is to be realized with surgery compared to medical management, the longer the patient survives after endarterectomy, the greater the benefit of operation. Similarly, as discussed above, if the patient is at high risk during surgery (for any reason), the annual benefit of surgery decreases. Therefore, patient selection for asymptomatic carotid endarterectomy requires consideration of the patient's risk during operation and the patient's overall health and life expectancy. If for any reason the patient's risk during operation is increased, medical management should be considered. Likewise, if the patient's health is so fragile that reliable long-term life expectancy cannot be assumed, medical management may be the best option.

In an in-depth cost analysis of carotid endarterectomy for asymptomatic disease, Cronenwett and colleagues estimated the cost-effectiveness of carotid endarterectomy with advancing age [110]. Although the cost-effectiveness of carotid endarterectomy under age 72 seemed conclusive, the costs increased exponentially to age 79 where the cost-effectiveness was marginal. By this algorithm, carotid endarterectomy for asymptomatic disease would not be considered cost-effective at age 80 or above. This is a theoretic issue related to an "average" elderly population. Obviously, some elderly patients have sufficient long-term survival to warrant carotid endarterectomy. Others just as obviously are medical candidates only. The difficulty remains in those in-between cases where selection criteria and operative risk are not clear-cut. In these situations, an in-depth analysis of risk and benefit is probably secondary to a truly informed consent discussion with the patient and family. In this way, the ultimate decision is left to the individual most directly involved, with the surgeon providing guidance where appropriate.

The treatment of asymptomatic patients with carotid stenting is significantly more controversial. While the use of carotid stenting in high-risk symptomatic patients is accepted, its use in high-risk asymptomatic patients is problematic. Traditionally, the surgical treatment of asymptomatic carotid disease has been limited to good-risk patients with an acceptable 5-year life expectancy based on the results of the ACAS trial. Given the limitations to treatment of good-risk asymptomatic patients, defining a high-risk group has been controversial. Nonetheless, there are probably some groups worthy of consideration for treatment in high-risk asymptomatic patients. Specifically, high risk based on anatomic criteria such as neck irradiation or previous neck surgery will define a population that may have an acceptable long-term life expectancy but has increased risk of local complications with surgery. Less well defined are the high-risk anatomic criteria associated with surgical intervention such as the presence of a high carotid bifurcation or the presence of a contralateral carotid occlusion. At the present, treatment of asymptomatic carotid stenosis is restricted to carotid endarterectomy except as part of an approved clinical trial.

Special Issues Related to Aging

Although carotid disease in general increases with increasing age, certain issues arise with aging that require further discussion. All of these problems can occur at any age, but the increased incidence in the elderly population requires explanation and elaboration.

Tortuosity of the Carotid Arteries

The coiling and kinking of the carotid arteries can be severe, resulting in stenosis or even complete vascular loops. The first references to carotid artery tortuosity appeared in relation to tonsillectomy, where the tortuous artery proved to be at risk for inadvertent injury [111]. The first recognition of neurologic symptoms referable to carotid artery tortuosity was during the early 1950s, with recommendations for arteriopexy of the artery to the sternocleidomastoid muscle [112]. During the late 1950s, cases of cortical stroke associated with carotid kinks were reported, with successful treatment in all cases by arterial resection [113]. From this point forward, the standard treatment of carotid coils has been resection or advancement of the redundant artery, which continues to be the treatment of choice today.

For a number of reasons, the exact incidence of extreme tortuosity of the extracranial carotid arteries is difficult to determine. Many patients are asymptomatic and may never come to medical attention. This situation is further confused by the lack of standard definitions as to what constitutes a kink, a coil, or a tortuosity. Tortuosity has been defined as excessive length of an artery (Fig. 55.8). This is a relative judgment, and the lengthening of the arterial tree is limited by fixation at branch points. Therefore, elongation often results in tortuosity moving away from bifurcations. If the elongation occurs between two points of fixation, kinks or coils can occur. Kinks are defined as an abrupt change in the direction of the artery, reducing the diameter of the arterial lumen (Fig. 55.9). Coils are redundant loops of artery without

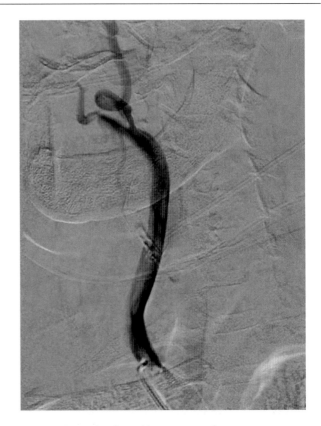

FIGURE 55.8 Example of carotid artery tortuosity.

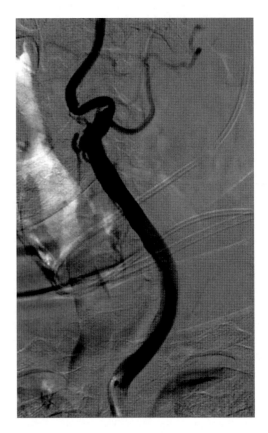

FIGURE 55.9 Example of carotid artery kink.

luminal encroachment, lacking the acute change in direction. Both kinks and coils are subsets of the vessels exhibiting tortuosity, all of which can lead to boundary layer separation with an associated increased risk of cerebrovascular events.

Angiographic studies suggest that tortuosity is common in the carotid circulation, occurring in 31% of 1,438 consecutive carotid arteriograms in one study [114]. In the same series, coils were seen in 7% and kinks in 5%. An additional study of 1,000 consecutive arteriograms suggested a 16% incidence of kinks [115]. The incidence of kinks has been associated with female sex, advanced age, hypertension, kyphosis, and obesity [116]. Estimates have suggested that fewer than 5% of patients with carotid atherosclerosis who come to operative intervention have clinically significant associated carotid tortuosity.

As previously outlined, the main therapy for carotid tortuosity or kinking is resection and advancement of the redundant segment, often in the form of an eversion carotid endarterectomy. A detailed discussion of the techniques of resection and reanastomosis is beyond the scope of this chapter, but segmental resection of either the internal or common carotid artery, with or without carotid endarterectomy, is the standard treatment. Using this technique, successful outcomes with low-stroke rates are the norm [117]. Of note, carotid stenting is significantly more difficult in a tortuous carotid artery due to the difficulties of landing the stent within a relatively straight segment of the artery.

"Dizziness" and Other Global Symptoms

The incidence of dizziness, vertigo, and syncope in the elderly population is epidemic, affecting an estimated 50% of the population over 65 years of age [118]. The causes of these symptoms are myriad, including inner ear problems, vision problems, loss of sympathetic tone, and cerebrovascular disease. Of all the symptoms related to cerebrovascular disease, this one remains unlikely to be related to cerebral blood flow. Because dizziness is a global rather than cortical symptom, the extent of cerebrovascular disease must be extreme if the symptoms are to arise from atherosclerotic disease.

Typical "drop" attacks associated with posterior circulation disease relate to loss of motor function due to cerebellar ischemia, often without loss of consciousness (cortical perfusion). These episodes are rare in the absence of combined system disease; if posterior circulation vascular disease is the only atherosclerosis present, no symptoms occur. Only when posterior disease is combined with circle of Willis or carotid disease do symptoms typically occur. If only 15% of the population over age 65 have carotid disease, a substantially smaller population of these individuals would be expected to have significant posterior circulation

disease in addition. No matter how the calculations are derived, most dizziness cannot be accounted for byatherosclerotic obstruction.

Assessment for Generalized Atherosclerosis Using the Carotid System

The most readily accessible site for assessment of early atherosclerosis remains the carotid bifurcation [119]. The presence of significant systemic vascular disease can be predicted with reasonable accuracy using duplex ultrasonography to measure intimal thickness [120–127]. Therefore, as a screening tool for atherosclerosis, carotid duplex ultrasonography may play an increasing role in the future.

To measure the carotid intimal–medial thickness (CIMT), a scan of the common carotid artery is performed, being careful to avoid segments of the artery with significant disease [128, 129]. Usually, far-wall CIMT is measured and is currently the standard rather than near-wall IMT (Fig. 55.10). The distance from the intimal reflection to the medial reflection is the measurement used, and an average is generated manually or automatically over a variable distance. There are many issues with this measurement, notably that many labs have undertaken this without validation. Since many software packages are available to perform this measurement automatically, there is some reliance on this technology to yield accuracy and reproducibility yet validation studies remain lacking. For the foreseeable future, CIMT will remain an experimental tool, to be used as part of a research protocol rather than a clinically appropriate generalized screening methodology. Currently, many commercial ventures are offering atherosclerotic screening using CIMT; its current utility remains controversial, and it remains for larger studies to better define the populations that could potentially benefit from such screening.

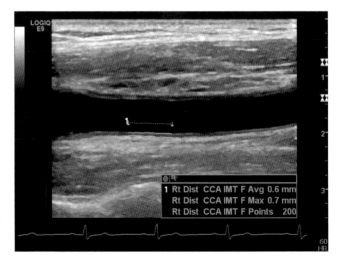

Figure 55.10 Measurement of carotid intimal–medial thickness (CIMT).

Conclusions

Carotid disease is a continuing issue in the care of the elderly. The incidence of cerebrovascular disease is increasing as the population ages, resulting in an ever-greater focus on the appropriateness of vascular care in this population. Although future studies may refine the overall management of cerebrovascular disease in the elderly, the need for intervention in symptomatic and asymptomatic patients with significant carotid disease has been better defined for this form of vascular disease than in virtually any other arterial distribution. No other area of vascular disease has been subjected to the multiple large, prospective, randomized trials as has been done with carotid disease; nonetheless, more is needed. Therefore, while the utility of carotid interventions has been uniquely studied as few other procedures have, a better understanding continues to evolve. The future direction for carotid intervention clearly includes carotid angioplasty and stent placement. Nonetheless, the exact role of endarterectomy and stenting and the appropriate patient selection remains to be defined.

References

1. Robins M, Baum HM (1981) National survey of stroke incidence. Stroke 12(Suppl 1):45–57
2. Matsumoto N, Whisnant JP, Kurland LT et al (1973) Natural history of stroke in Rochester, Minnesota, 1955 through 1969: an extension of a previous study, 1945 through 1954. Stroke 4:20–29
3. Pokras R, Dyken ML (1988) Dramatic changes in the performance of endarterectomy for diseases of the extracranial arteries in the head. Stroke 19:1289–1296
4. Day J (2008) Population projections of the United States by age, sex, race, and Hispanic origin: 2008 to 2050. U.S. Bureau of the Census, Current Population Reports. Government Printing Office, Washington, DC
5. Wolf PA, Kannel WB, Dawber TR (1978) Prospective investigation: the Framingham study and the epidemiology of stroke. Adv Neurol 19:107–120
6. Tell GS, Polak JF, Ward BJ et al (1994) Relation of smoking with carotid artery wall thickness and stenosis in older adults: the Cardiovascular Health Study; the Cardiovascular Health Study (CHS) Collaborative Research Group. Circulation 90:2905–2908
7. Glagov S, Rowley DA, Kohut R (1961) Atherosclerosis of human aorta and its coronary and renal arteries. Arch Pathol Lab Med 72:558–562
8. Bell ET (1957) Atherosclerotic gangrene of the lower extremities in diabetic and nondiabetic persons. Am J Clin Pathol 28:27–35
9. Selhub J, Jacques PF, Bostom AG et al (1995) Association between plasma homocysteine concentrations and extra-cranial carotid-artery stenosis. N Engl J Med 332:286–291
10. Kannel WB, Castelli WP, Gordon T et al (1971) Serum cholesterol, lipoprotein, and the risk of coronary heart disease: the Framingham study. Ann Intern Med 74:1–12
11. Lipids Research Clinics Program (1984) The Lipids Research Clinics Primary Prevention Trials results. II. The relationship of reduction and incidence of coronary heart disease to cholesterol lowering. JAMA 251:365–374
12. Multiple Risk Factor Intervention Trial Research Group (1982) Multiple risk factor intervention trial: risk factor changes and mortality rates. JAMA 248:1465–1477
13. Kang SS, Wong PW, Malinow MR (1992) Hyperhomocyst(e)inemia as a risk factor for occlusive vascular disease. Annu Rev Nutr 12:279–298
14. Ueland PM, Refsum H, Brattström L (1992) Plasma homocysteine and cardiac disease. In: Francis RB (ed) Atherosclerotic cardiovascular disease, hemostasis, and endothelial function. Marcel Dekker, New York, pp 183–236
15. Nygård O, Nordrehaug JE, Refsum H et al (1997) Plasma homo cysteine levels and mortality in patients with coronary artery disease. N Engl J Med 337:230–236
16. Albert CM, Cook NR et al (2008) Effect of folic acid and B vitamins on risk of cardiovascular events and total mortality among women at high risk for cardiovascular disease: a randomized trial. JAMA 299(17):2027–2036
17. Bazzano LA, Reynolds K et al (2006) Effect of folic acid supplementation on risk of cardiovascular diseases: a meta-analysis of randomized controlled trials. JAMA 296(22):2720–2726
18. Cornfeld J (1962) Joint dependence of risk of coronary heart disease on serum cholesterol and systolic blood pressure. Fed Proc 21(Suppl 2):58
19. O'Leary DH, Anderson KM, Wolf PA et al (1992) Cholesterol and carotid atherosclerosis in older persons: the Framingham study. Ann Epidemiol 2:147–153
20. Sacks FM, Pfeffer MA, Moye LA et al (1996) The effect of pravastatin on coronary events after myocardial infarction in patients with average cholesterol levels. N Engl J Med 335:1001–1009
21. Flaker GC et al (1999) Pravastatin prevents clinical events in revascularized patients with average cholesterol concentrations. Cholesterol and Recurrent Events CARE Investigators. J Am Coll Cardiol 34(1):106–112
22. Collins R et al (2004) Effects of cholesterol-lowering with simvastatin on stroke and other major vascular events in 20536 people with cerebrovascular disease or other high-risk conditions. Lancet 363(9411):757–767
23. Sillesen H et al (2008) Atorvastatin reduces the risk of cardiovascular events in patients with carotid atherosclerosis: a secondary analysis of the Stroke Prevention by Aggressive Reduction in Cholesterol Levels (SPARCL) trial. Stroke 39(12):3297–3302
24. Amarenco P et al (2006) High-dose atorvastatin after stroke or transient ischemic attack. N Engl J Med 355(6):549–559
25. (1997) The International Stroke Trial (IST): a randomised trial of aspirin, subcutaneous heparin, both, or neither among 19435 patients with acute ischaemic stroke. International Stroke Trial Collaborative Group. Lancet 349(9065):1569–1581
26. (1997) CAST: randomised placebo-controlled trial of early aspirin use in 20,000 patients with acute ischaemic stroke. CAST (Chinese Acute Stroke Trial) Collaborative Group. Lancet 349(9066): 1641–1649
27. Dippel DW (1998) The results of CAPRIE, IST and CAST. Clopidogrel vs. Aspirin in Patients at Risk of Ischaemic Events. International Stroke Trial. Chinese Acute Stroke Trial. Thromb Res 92(1 Suppl 1):S13–S16
28. Creager MA (1998) Results of the CAPRIE trial: efficacy and safety of clopidogrel. Clopidogrel versus aspirin in patients at risk of ischaemic events. Vasc Med 3(3):257–260
29. (1996) A randomised, blinded, trial of clopidogrel versus aspirin in patients at risk of ischaemic events (CAPRIE). CAPRIE Steering Committee. Lancet 348(9038):1329–1339
30. Bhatt DL et al (2006) Clopidogrel and aspirin versus aspirin alone for the prevention of atherothrombotic events. N Engl J Med 354(16):1706–1717
31. Bhatt DL, Topol EJ (2004) Clopidogrel added to aspirin versus aspirin alone in secondary prevention and high-risk primary

prevention: rationale and design of the Clopidogrel for High Atherothrombotic Risk and Ischemic Stabilization, Management, and Avoidance (CHARISMA) trial. Am Heart J 148(2):263–268

32. Ross R (1986) The pathogenesis of atherosclerosis: an update. N Engl J Med 14:488–500

33. Ross R (1999) Atherosclerosis: an inflammatory disease. N Engl J Med 340:115–126

34. Bild DE, Fitzpatrick A, Fried LP et al (1993) Age-related trends in cardiovascular morbidity and physical functioning in the elderly: the cardiovascular health study. J Am Geriatr Soc 41:1047–1056

35. Weber G, Bianciardi G, Bussani R et al (1988) Atherosclerosis and aging: a morphometric study on arterial lesions of elderly and very elderly necropsy subjects. Arch Pathol Lab Med 112:1066–1070

36. Homma S, Ishida H, Hasegawa H et al (1997) Carotid intima-medial thickness and the occurrence of plaque in centenarians: data from the Tokyo Centenarian Study. Jpn J Geriatr 34:139–146

37. Shuaib A, Boyle C (1994) Stroke in the elderly. Curr Opin Neurol 7:41–47

38. Zarins CK, Giddens DP, Bharadvaj BK et al (1983) Carotid bifurcation atherosclerosis: quantitative correlation of plaque localization with flow velocity profiles and wall shear stress. Circ Res 53:502–514

39. Granada JF, Feinstein SB (2008) Imaging of the vasa vasorum. Nat Clin Pract Cardiovasc Med 5(Suppl 2):S18–S25

40. Shah F et al (2007) Contrast-enhanced ultrasound imaging of atherosclerotic carotid plaque neovascularization: a new surrogate marker of atherosclerosis? Vasc Med 12(4):291–297

41. Feinstein SB (2006) Contrast ultrasound imaging of the carotid artery vasa vasorum and atherosclerotic plaque neovascularization. J Am Coll Cardiol 48(2):236–243

42. Theile BL, Strandness DE (1993) Distribution of intracranial and extracranial arterial lesions in patients with symptomatic cerebrovascular disease. In: Bernstein EF (ed) Vascular diagnosis, 4th edn. Mosby, St. Louis, pp 302–307

43. Imparato AM, Riles TS, Mintzer R et al (1983) The importance of hemorrhage in the relationship between gross morphologic characteristics and cerebral symptoms in 376 carotid artery plaques. Ann Surg 197:195–203

44. Lusby RJ, Ferrell LD, Ehrenfeld WK et al (1982) Carotid plaque hemorrhage: its role in production of cerebral ischemia. Arch Surg 117:1479–1488

45. Fryer JA, Myers PC, Appleberg M (1987) Carotid intraplaque hemorrhage: the significance of neovascularity. J Vasc Surg 6:341–349

46. Persson AV, Robichaux WT, Silverman M (1983) The natural history of carotid plaque development. Arch Surg 118:1048–1052

47. Polak JF, O'Leary DH, Kronmal RA et al (1993) Sonographic evaluation of carotid artery atherosclerosis in the elderly: relationship of disease severity to stroke and transient ischemic attack. Radiology 188:363–370

48. Kendall RE, Marshall J (1963) Role of hypotension in the genesis of transient focal cerebral ischemic attacks. Br Med J 2:344–348

49. Fazekas JF, Alman RW (1964) The role of hypotension in transitory focal cerebral ischemia. Am J Med Sci 248:567–570

50. Millikin CH (1965) The pathogenesis of transient focal cerebral ischemia. Circulation 32:438–448

51. Brass LM, Fayad PB, Levine SR (1992) Transient ischemic attacks in the elderly: diagnosis and treatment. Geriatrics 47:36–53

52. Perez-Burkhardt JL, Gonzalez-Fajardo JA, Rodriguez E, Mateo AM (1994) Amaurosis fugax as a symptom of carotid artery stenosis: its relationship with ulcerated plaque. J Cardiovasc Surg (Torino) 35:15–18

53. Alpers BJ, Berry RG, Paddison RM (1959) Anatomical studies of the circle of Willis in normal brain. Arch Neurol Psychiatry 81:409–422

54. Powers WJ, Press GW, Grubb RL et al (1987) The effect of hemodynamically significant carotid artery disease on the hemodynamic status of the cerebral circulation. Ann Intern Med 106:27–35

55. Berens ES, Kouchoukos NT, Murphy SF, Wareing TH (1992) Preoperative carotid artery screening in elderly patients undergoing cardiac surgery. J Vasc Surg 15:313–321

56. Halpin DP, Riggins S, Carmichael JD et al (1994) Management of coexistent carotid and coronary artery disease. South Med J 87:187–189

57. Sayers RD, Thompson MM, Underwood MJ et al (1993) Early results of combined carotid endarterectomy and coronary artery bypass grafting in patients with severe coronary and carotid artery disease. J R Coll Surg Edinb 38:340–343

58. Reigel MM, Hollier LH, Sundt TM et al (1987) Cerebral hyperperfusion syndrome: a cause of neurologic dysfunction after carotid endarterectomy. J Vasc Surg 5:628–634

59. Powers AD, Smith RR (1990) Hyperperfusion syndrome after carotid endarterectomy: a transcranial Doppler evaluation. Neurosurgery 26:56–60

60. Naylor AR, Merrick MV, Gillespie I et al (1994) Prevalence of impaired cerebrovascular reserve in patients with symptomatic carotid artery disease. Br J Surg 81:45–48

61. Syrota A, Castaing M, Rougemont D et al (1983) Tissue acid-base balance and oxygen metabolism in human cerebral infarction studied with positron emission tomography. Ann Neurol 14:419–428

62. Zierler RE, Phillips DJ, Beach KW et al (1987) Noninvasive assessment of normal carotid bifurcation hemodynamics with color-flow ultrasound imaging. Ultrasound Med Biol 13:471–476

63. Zierler RE, Kohler TR, Strandness DE (1990) Duplex scanning of normal or minimally diseased carotid arteries: correlation with arteriography and clinical outcome. J Vasc Surg 12:447–454

64. Moniz E (1927) L'encéphalographie artérielle, son importance dans la localisation des tumeurs cérébrales. Rev Neurol 2:72

65. Eliasziw M, Smith RF, Singh N et al (1994) Further comments on the measurement of carotid stenosis from angiograms. Stroke 25:2445–2449

66. Executive Committee for the Asymptomatic Carotid Atherosclerosis Study (1995) Endarterectomy for asymptomatic carotid artery stenosis. JAMA 273:1421–1428

67. Larson EB, Omenn GS, Loop JW (1978) Computed tomography in patients with cerebrovascular disease: impact of a new technology on patient care. AJR Am J Roentgenol 131(1):35–40

68. Uwatoko T et al (2007) Carotid artery calcification on multislice detector-row computed tomography. Cerebrovasc Dis 24(1):20–26

69. Koelemay MJ et al (2004) Systematic review of computed tomographic angiography for assessment of carotid artery disease. Stroke 35(10):2306–2312

70. Patel SG et al (2002) Outcome, observer reliability, and patient preferences if CTA, MRA, or Doppler ultrasound were used, individually or together, instead of digital subtraction angiography before carotid endarterectomy. J Neurol Neurosurg Psychiatry 73(1):21–28

71. Mittl RL Jr, Broderick M, Carpenter JP et al (1994) Blinded-reader comparison of magnetic resonance angiography and duplex ultrasonography for carotid artery bifurcation stenosis. Stroke 25:4–10

72. Debrey SM et al (2008) Diagnostic accuracy of magnetic resonance angiography for internal carotid artery disease: a systematic review and meta-analysis. Stroke 39(8):2237–2248

73. North American Symptomatic Carotid Endarterectomy Trial Collaborators (1991) Beneficial effects of carotid endarterectomy in symptomatic patients with high-grade carotid stenosis. N Engl J Med 325:445–453

74. Barnett HJM, Taylor DW, Eliasziw M et al (1998) Benefit of carotid endarterectomy in patients with symptomatic moderate or severe stenosis. N Engl J Med 339:1415–1425

75. Moore WS, Barnett HJ, Beebe HG et al (1995) Guidelines for carotid endarterectomy: a multidisciplinary consensus statement from the Ad Hoc Committee, American Heart Association. Circulation 91:566–579

76. Treiman RL, Wagner WH, Foran RF et al (1992) Carotid endarterectomy in the elderly. Ann Vasc Surg 6:321–324

77. Nunnelee JD, Kurgan A, Auer AI (1995) Carotid endarterectomy in elderly vascular patients: experience in a community hospital. Geriatr Nurs 16:121–123

78. Perler BA, Dardik A, Burleyson GP et al (1998) Influence of age and hospital volume on the results of carotid endarterectomy: a statewide analysis of 9918 cases. J Vasc Surg 27:25–33

79. Fisher ES, Malenka DJ, Solomon NA et al (1989) Risk of carotid endarterectomy in the elderly. Am J Public Health 79:1617–1620

80. Schultz RD, Feldhaus RJ (1988) Carotid endarterectomy in octogenarians and nonagenarians. Surg Gynecol Obstet 166:245–251

81. Kerdiles Y, Lucas A, Podeur L et al (1997) Results of carotid surgery in elderly patients. J Cardiovasc Surg (Torino) 38:327–334

82. Van Damme H, Lacroix H, Desiron Q et al (1996) Carotid surgery in octogenarians: is it worthwhile? Acta Chir Belg 96:71–77

83. Thomas PC, Grigg M (1996) Carotid artery surgery in the octogenarian. Aust NZ J Surg 66:231–234

84. Favre JP, Guy JM, Frering V et al (1994) Carotid surgery in the octogenarian. Ann Vasc Surg 8:421–426

85. Coyle KA, Smith RB, Salam AA et al (1994) Carotid endarterectomy in the octogenarian. Ann Vasc Surg 8:417–420

86. Perler BA, Williams GM (1994) Carotid endarterectomy in the very elderly: is it worthwhile? Surgery 116:479–483

87. Meyer FB, Meissner I, Fode NC et al (1991) Carotid endarterectomy in elderly patients. Mayo Clin Proc 66:464–469

88. Brooks RH, Park RE, Chassin MR et al (1990) Carotid endarterectomy for elderly patients: predicting complications. Ann Intern Med 113:747–753

89. Pinkerton JA, Gholkar VR (1990) Should patient age be a consideration in carotid endarterectomy? J Vasc Surg 11:650–658

90. Kastrup A, Groschel K (2007) Carotid endarterectomy versus carotid stenting: an updated review of randomized trials and subgroup analyses. Acta Chir Belg 107(2):119–128

91. Grego F et al (2005) Is carotid endarterectomy in octogenarians more dangerous than in younger patients? J Cardiovasc Surg (Torino) 46(5):477–483

92. Hingorani A et al (2004) Carotid endarterectomy in octogenarians and nonagenarians: is it worth the effort? Acta Chir Belg 104(4):384–387

93. Metz R et al (2002) Carotid endarterectomy in octogenarians with symptomatic high-grade internal carotid artery stenosis: long-term clinical and duplex follow-up. Vasc Endovascular Surg 36(6):409–414

94. Ballotta E et al (1999) Carotid endarterectomy in symptomatic and asymptomatic patients aged 75 years or more: perioperative mortality and stroke risk rates. Ann Vasc Surg 13(2):158–163

95. Roques XF, Baudet EM, Clerc F (1991) Results of carotid endarterectomy in patients 75 years of age and older. J Cardiovasc Surg (Torino) 32:726–731

96. Back MR, Harward TR, Huber TS et al (1997) Improving the cost-effectiveness of carotid endarterectomy. J Vasc Surg 26:456–462

97. Allen BT, Anderson CB, Rubin BG et al (1994) The influence of anesthetic technique on perioperative complications after carotid endarterectomy. J Vasc Surg 19:834–843

98. (2001) Endovascular versus surgical treatment in patients with carotid stenosis in the Carotid and Vertebral Artery Transluminal Angioplasty Study (CAVATAS): a randomised trial. Lancet 357(9270):1729–1737

99. Yadav JS et al (2004) Protected carotid-artery stenting versus endarterectomy in high-risk patients. N Engl J Med 351(15):1493–1501

100. Coward LJ, Featherstone RL, Brown MM (2004) Percutaneous transluminal angioplasty and stenting for carotid artery stenosis. Cochrane Database Syst Rev (2):CD000515

101. CMS Manual System, Pub 100-03 Medicare National Coverage Determinations. Department of Health & Human Services (DHHS), Centers for Medicare & Medicaid Services (CMS). 24 December 2008

102. Bazan HA et al (2007) Increased aortic arch calcification in patients older than 75 years: implications for carotid artery stenting in elderly patients. J Vasc Surg 46(5):841–845

103. Moore WS (1988) Does tandem lesion mean tandem risk in patients with carotid artery disease? J Vasc Surg 7:454–455

104. Lord RS, Raj TB, Graham AR (1987) Carotid endarterectomy, siphon stenosis, collateral hemispheric pressure and perioperative cerebral infarction. J Vasc Surg 6:391–397

105. Schuler JJ, Flanigan DP, Lim LT et al (1982) The effect of carotid siphon stenosis on stroke rate, death, and relief of symptoms following elective carotid endarterectomy. Surgery 92:1058–1067

106. Borozean PG, Schuler JJ, LaRosa MP et al (1984) The natural history of isolated carotid siphon stenosis. J Vasc Surg 1:744–749

107. Akers DL, Bell WH, Kerstein MD (1988) Does intracranial dye study contribute to evaluation of carotid disease? Am J Surg 156:87–90

108. Ricotta JJ, Holen J, Schenk E et al (1984) Is routine angiography necessary prior to carotid endarterectomy? J Vasc Surg 1:96–102

109. Moore WS, Ziomek S, Quiñones-Baldrich WJ et al (1988) Can clinical evaluation and noninvasive testing substitute for arteriography in the evaluation of carotid artery disease? Ann Surg 298:91–94

110. Cronenwett JL, Birkmeyer JD, Nackman GB et al (1997) Cost-effectiveness of carotid endarterectomy in asymptomatic patients. J Vasc Surg 25:298–311

111. Kelly AB (1891) Pulsating vessels in the pharynx. Glasgow Med J 49:28–30

112. Riser MM, Geraud J, Ducoudray J et al (1951) Dolicho-carotide interne avec syndrome vertigineux. Rev Neurol 85:10–12

113. Quattlebaum JK, Upson ET, Neville RL (1959) Stroke associated with elongation and kinking of the internal carotid artery. Ann Surg 150:824–832

114. Weibel J, Fields WS (1965) Tortuosity, coiling and kinking of the internal carotid artery. I. Etiology and radiographic anatomy. Neurology 15:7–11

115. Metz H, Murray-Leslie RM, Bannister RG et al (1961) Kinking of the internal carotid artery. Lancet 1:424–426

116. Bauer R, Sheehan S, Meyer JS (1961) Arteriographic study of cerebrovascular disease. II. Cerebral symptoms due to kinking, tortuosity, and compression of carotid and vertebral arteries in the neck. Arch Neurol 4:119

117. Mascoli F, Mari C, Liboni A et al (1987) The elongation of the internal carotid artery: diagnosis and surgical treatment. J Cardiovasc Surg 28:9–11

118. Yardley L, Owen N, Nazareth I, Luxon L (1998) Prevalence and presentation of dizziness in a general practice community sample of working age people. Br J Gen Pract 48:1131–1135

119. Niskanen L, Rauramaa R, Miettinen H et al (1996) Carotid artery intima-media thickness in elderly patients with NIDDM and in nondiabetic subjects. Stroke 27:1986–1992

120. Bots ML et al (1997) Common carotid intima-media thickness and risk of stroke and myocardial infarction: the Rotterdam Study. Circulation 96(5):1432–1437

121. Allan PL et al (1997) Relationship between carotid intima-media thickness and symptomatic and asymptomatic peripheral arterial disease. The Edinburgh Artery Study. Stroke 28(2): 348–353

122. Hodis HN, Mack WJ, Barth J (1996) Carotid intima-media thickness as a surrogate end point for coronary artery disease. Circulation 94(9):2311–2312

123. Sharma K et al (2009) Clinical and research applications of carotid intima-media thickness. Am J Cardiol 103(9):1316–1320

124. Espeland MA et al (2005) Carotid intimal-media thickness as a surrogate for cardiovascular disease events in trials of HMG-CoA reductase inhibitors. Curr Control Trials Cardiovasc Med 6(1):3

125. Basu AK et al (2005) Carotid intima media thickness: an independent marker for assessment of macrovascular risk in diabetic patients. J Indian Med Assoc 103(4):234–236

126. Stein JH et al (2004) Vascular age: integrating carotid intima-media thickness measurements with global coronary risk assessment. Clin Cardiol 27(7):388–392

127. Kablak-Ziembicka A et al (2004) Association of increased carotid intima-media thickness with the extent of coronary artery disease. Heart 90(11):1286–1290

128. Coll B, Feinstein SB (2008) Carotid intima-media thickness measurements: techniques and clinical relevance. Curr Atheroscler Rep 10(5):444–450

129. Stein JH et al (2008) Use of carotid ultrasound to identify subclinical vascular disease and evaluate cardiovascular disease risk: a consensus statement from the American Society of Echocardiography Carotid Intima-Media Thickness Task Force. Endorsed by the Society for Vascular Medicine. J Am Soc Echocardiogr 21(2):93–111, quiz 189–190

Chapter 56
Natural History and Treatment of Aneurysms

Michael Wilderman and Gregorio A. Sicard

Introduction and Historical Review

Any standard medical dictionary will describe an aneurysm as a localized abnormal enlarging or ballooning of a particular segment of an artery, greater than 50% of the normal caliber, commonly related to weakness in the wall of the blood vessel [1]. The most common location of an extracranial aneurysm is the infrarenal abdominal aorta. Using the above definition, an aorta with a diameter greater than 3 cm can therefore be considered aneurysmal, although normal aortic diameters vary with age, sex, and body habitus. Histologically, an abdominal aortic aneurysm (AAA) is characterized by macrophage degradation of the medial elastin lamellar architecture by metalloproteinases [2–5].

Aneurysms have been documented for thousands of years; in fact the Ebers Papyrus in 2000 BC discusses traumatic aneurysms of the peripheral arteries [6]. Antyllus, a Greek surgeon living in Rome, described the first elective procedure to treat an aneurysm using a method of proximal and distal ligation of the artery feeding the aneurysm, along with opening the sac and evacuation of its contents [7]. In the sixteenth century, a Flemish anatomist named Andreas Versalias wrote about an abdominal aortic aneurysm in his work *De humani corporis fabrica (On the Workings of the Human Body)* [8]. It was not until 1923 when Rudolph Matas performed the successful technical ligation of a ruptured syphilitic infrarenal AAA that anyone had deviated from Antyllus's technique [9]. Since Matas's technique carried a very high mortality, other surgeons attempted various alternative therapies such as wrapping the aneurysmal wall with various materials such as fascia lata, skin grafts, polyvinyl sponge, and even cellophane, in an attempt to prevent aneurysmal rupture, along with attempting to induce aneurysm thrombosis with wires [10–13]. Unfortunately, the morbidity and mortality of these procedures remained high and none of their results were all that good.

Alexis Carrel, the 1912 Nobel Laureate, initially reported on the contemporary technique for an open AAA repair, perfected in animals, consisting of replacing a segment of aorta with a segment from another artery or vein [14–17]. In 1951, Charles DuBost details a more successful approach using a thoraco-retroperitoneal incision to replace the aneurysmal infrarenal aorta with a thoracic-aortic homograft in a technique mimicking Carrel's [18]. In Houston in 1953, Denton Cooley and Michael DeBakey wrote of their success using an analogous technique [19]. The use of homografts was relatively short lived due to graft degeneration and subsequent graft rupture. When Voorhees et al. (1952) used a new material for vascular conduit, Vinyon-N, marked the next major breakthrough [20]. Around the same time, Blakemore placed the first Vinyon-N graft in a patient with a ruptured AAA. Sadly, this patient expired, but the graft was patent at autopsy [21]. In 1954, Voorhees and Blakemore described their results in 16 patients with AAA repaired using Vinyon-N grafts and nine patients (56%) survived [22, 23]. These advances forced companies to evaluate various types of potential arterial conduits. In 1958, Michael DeBakey's group in Houston wrote about a significant group of patients undergoing AAA repairs with knitted Dacron grafts [24]. In 1966, Creech and colleagues continued to refine the surgical procedure by introducing an endoaneurysmorrhaphy with intraluminal graft placement, the standard open technique used today [25]. Over the next 20 years, many series were reported with operative mortalities in the 10–15% range, using polyester grafts.

Prevalence, Incidence, and Risk Factors

Elderly white males are the most common patients to present with AAA. Moreover, it is age related with increasing frequency in men 60 years or older. AAA is two to six times more common in men than women, and two to three times more common in white men than African-American men.

M. Wilderman (✉)
Division of Vascular Surgery, Barnes Jewish Hospital, Washington University, St. Louis, MO 63110, USA
e-mail: wildermanm@wudosis.wustl.edu

R.A. Rosenthal et al. (eds.), *Principles and Practice of Geriatric Surgery*,
DOI 10.1007/978-1-4419-6999-6_56, © Springer Science+Business Media, LLC 2011

In men, aneurysms are first diagnosed around age 50 and reach a peak incidence at age 80. In women, they tend to present around age 60, with a steady increase after that [26–28]. The incidence of developing an AAA has varied from 3 to 117 per 100,000 person years [29–32]. Lederle et al. [33] reported that 2.6% of screened patients with a normal ultrasound 4 years prior now had AAAs. They also reported an incidence of AAA of 6.5 per thousand person years. While AAAs do not demonstrate a clear genetic transmission pattern, many papers suggest that 15–20% of first-order relatives of patients with AAAs will have one themselves [34–36].

AAA tend to be related to the process of atherosclerosis. Patients who develop AAA tend to show signs and symptoms of atherosclerosis in other arterial beds, such as their coronary carotid or peripheral arteries. Thus, patients who tend to have risk factors for atherosclerosis, such as smoking, hypertension, and hypercholesterolemia, may develop AAA [37–40].

Rupture of an AAA is the tenth leading cause of death in elderly males. Although this is the case, the majority of AAAs are found accidentally and only rarely will they be symptomatic Therefore, a ruptured AAA may be the patient's first knowledge or presentation of his aneurysm. Ruptured AAAs have an extremely high mortality (greater than 90% overall). Even patients who make to a hospital alive will have 40–50% mortality. Thus, the chief focus of AAA therapy is to treat in advance so to avoid rupture. Treatment of ruptured AAAs is very costly to the healthcare industry. Breckwoldt et al. found that emergent interventions for patients with ruptured AAAs led to hospital losses of $24,655 [41]. A report of Great Britain demonstrated that about 2,000 lives and nearly $50 million could be saved if AAAs were repaired prior to rupture [42]. Another study from the UK found that the total costs of emergency AAA repair were 96,700.69 pounds sterling, with a cost per life saved of 24,175.17 pounds sterling. The total cost of elective AAA repair was 76,583.22, with a cost per life saved of 5,470.23 pounds sterling. Emergency intervention was found to cost five times more than an elective procedure, per life saved, per year [43].

Clinical Presentation, Diagnosis of AAA, and What to Do About It?

The most likely presentation of AAA is as an incidental finding by the patient or treating physician on physical examination, diagnostic imaging for another reason, or in the operating room at the time of laparotomy for other reasons. The most dreaded presentation of AAA is that of hemodynamic instability and rupture. Free rupture into the peritoneal cavity is usually a fatal event, but thankfully, most patients who rupture do so into their retroperitoneum which will somewhat contain the rupture. It is this condition that is sometimes termed "a leaking" AAA. These patients may present with signs or symptoms of back, abdominal, or flank pain from the rupture or pressure or compressive symptoms relating to the hematoma compressing adjacent structures. On physical examination, the patient may have a tender pulsatile mass. Back pain can be due to erosion of the AAA into an adjacent lumber body, although it is most often due to the presence of hematoma from the AAA [44]. Flank pain is usually due to pressure and can radiate to the left groin because of pressure on the ureter. It has been well documented that a patient can present with a contained leak without hemodynamic changes and be discharged without a thorough workup only to represent in shock, so heightened awareness is required and an elderly patient presenting with abdominal or back pain must have AAA included in any differential diagnosis.

If an aneurysm ruptures, it does not always rupture into the retroperitoneum or peritoneal cavity. AAA can rupture into the duodenum. The typical presentation of this aortoduodenal fistula is a "herald" or small upper gastrointestinal (GI) tract bleed, followed by massive exsanguinating GI hemorrhage. The classic location for this is in the third portion of the duodenum and must be evaluated in any patient presenting with a GI bleed. Other GI symptoms, such as bowel obstruction, are also possible due to a large AAA compressing the GI tract, although this is rare. AAA can also rupture into the inferior vena cava. The classic presentation of this is high output congestive heart failure associated with venous hypertension, a widened pulse pressure, a continuous harsh abdominal bruit, and lower extremity swelling.

Another, although rare, presentation is due to an inflammatory or infectious AAA. These AAA are noted to have an intense desmoplastic reaction around the infrarenal aorta that involves adjacent structures. These AAA will produce local and systemic symptoms such as malaise, fever, vague abdominal, or back pain, along with weight loss and anorexia. These patients typically have an elevated white blood cell (WBC) count and the erythrocyte sedimentation rate (ESR) will be elevated in nearly 75% of the patients. The involved adjacent structures are the duodenum (90%), the inferior vena cava (50%), and the ureters (25%) [45].

One other presentation is that of thromboembolic symptoms. Since most AAA are lined with mural thrombus, pieces can break off and travel downstream, leading to ischemia. Therefore, patients presenting with embolic type symptoms must be evaluated for the presence of an aneurysm.

Most patients with AAA are asymptomatic and with the risk, morbidity, mortality, and cost if a patient presents with a ruptured AAA, targeted screening of high-risk population has become a vital. Schermerhorn et al. report that ultrasound screening for AAA was cost effective and beneficial for men 65–74 years of age with known risk factors such as coronary artery disease (CAD), smoking, or a family history of AAA [46]. Another study Derubertis et al. established that while women have a lower incidence of AAA than men, those over 65, with a history of smoking or heart disease are at a higher risk and should also be considered for screening [47]. Most screening programs have been developed outside of the USA [48–56]. Kim et al. published the UK results for a large randomized trial which demonstrated an early mortality benefit of screening ultrasonography for AAA which is sustained long term and that the cost effectiveness of screening improves over time [57]. Beginning on January 1, 2007, Medicare started to offer a free, one-time, ultrasound screening benefit to check for AAA's in qualified seniors. To qualify for this program, men had to have smoked at least 100 cigarettes in their lifetime. In addition, family history of AAA was an inclusion criterion for this program. Medicare linked this pared screening ultrasound to their "Welcome to Medicare Physical Exam," also known as the "Initial Preventive Physical Exam (IPPE)." This benefit became a law on February 8, 2006 as the Screening Abdominal Aortic Aneurysms Very Efficiently Act, (SAAAVE) a provision of S.1932, the Deficit Reduction Act of 2005. The ultrasound can occur anytime, but patients must have had their IPPE within 6 months of their 65th birthday. Today, many national medical societies as well as industry supporters are attempting to influence Medicare into expanding the screening test for *ALL* Medicare patients. 70,495 men age 65–74 participated in the Multicentre Aneurysm Screening Study (MASS) and were randomized to receiving either ultrasound screening or no screening for AAA. Of the 33,839 patients randomized to ultrasound screening, 80% actually underwent an ultrasound and 5% of the men had AAAs greater than 3 cm. Four years into the trial, 65 AAA-related deaths occurred in the screened group compared with 113 AAA-related deaths in the nonscreened control group. Although neither this trial nor any other will be able to show a significant reduction in all-cause mortality, MASS did show a 32% reduction in AAA-related mortality in the group who received ultrasound screening [56]. Given these findings regarding screening for AAA, most physicians, including vascular surgeons will screen male patients greater than 60–65 years of age, who currently smoke or have smoked in the past, along with those with a known family history of AAA. Currently, the most common manner in which patients learn that they have AAA is when AAAs are found incidentally when they are imaged, either with ultrasound, CT scan, or MRI for other diseases or symptomatology.

Once a diagnosis of AAA has been made, the question is: What is the best treatment strategy? One attempt to answer this was made by a group led by Lederle. They reported on the Department of Veterans Affairs Aneurysm Detection and Management (ADAM) Study. This multicenter randomized clinical trial was intended to compare long-term AAA survival from two treatment modalities, immediate open surgical repair for managing all AAAs less than 5.5 cm versus observation and surveillance and open surgical treatment when aneurysm reached 5.5 cm. A total of 1,136 patients were enrolled at 16 VA medical centers. The mean follow-up time was 4.8 years. This study noted that there was no significant difference between either group in terms of long-term mortality. They concluded that there was no long-term survival advantage with early surgical intervention in patients with AAA smaller than 5.5 cm even when the operative mortality is very low. They thus recommended surveillance of small AAAs and deferring open repair until the AAA has enlarged to 5.5 cm [58].

A similar study conducted in the UK found similar results. Powell et al. reported in 2007 on the long-term follow-up of 1,090 patients enrolled in the UK Small Aneurysm Trial between 1991 and 1995 and followed for 10 years. They found no long-term survival benefit of early elective open repair of small, 4–5.4 cm, AAAs. Even after successful repair, the mortality among these patients was higher than the general population [59].

Once the adequate aortic conduit to replace the aorta was confirmed surgeons began to pay closer attention to the overall medical condition of the patient with the AAA and ways to improve the intraoperative and postoperative care in order to significantly improve perioperative and in-hospital mortality. In the last 20 years, this approach of preoperatively maximizing the health status of the patient prior to AAA open repair has significantly impacted mortality with recent series reporting <5%, 30-day mortality consistently (Table 56.1) [60–71].

TABLE 56.1 Operative mortality following elective infrarenal AAA [60–71]

Authors	n	30-Day mortality (%)
Heller et al. (2000)	358,521	5.6
Huber et al. (2001)	16,450	4.2
Hertzer et al. (2002)	1,135	1.2
Lee et al. (2004)	4,607	3.8
Greenhalgh et al. (2004) (randomized)	539	4.7
Akkersdijk et al. (2004)	16,466	7.3
Anderson et al. (2005)	783 (2002)	4.21 (2002)
	1,043 (2001)	3.55 (2001)
	1,238 (2000)	4.12 (2000)
Lifeline registry of SVS 2005	334	1.4
Blankensteijn et al. (2005) (randomized)	178	4.6
Hua et al. (2005)	582	3.95
Sicard et al. (2006)	61 (high risk)	5.1
Bush et al. (2007)	1,580 (high risk)	5.2

While mortality has declined over the years, especially in centers with high volumes, not everyone with AAA needs an operation right away. The question is who needs an operation and who can be observed? It has been documented that the risk of rupture of a known AAA is based on its maximal diameter. Aneurysms between 3 and 5 cm have less than 1% per year chance of rupturing. Aneurysms with diameters between 5½ and 6 cm have between 5 and 10% chance of rupturing in a given year. Those between 6 and 7 cm rupture at a rate of 10–20%. Those between 7 and 8 cm have a 20–30% chance of rupturing in that year. Aneurysms found to be greater than 8 cm rupture at a rate anywhere between 30 and 50% per year. One other vital factor is rapid expansion. Those aneurysms that have enlarged by more than 0.5 cm in a given 6 months also have a higher likelihood of rupturing. Therefore, it is generally accepted that aneurysms less than 5½ cm, given the low likelihood of rupturing, can be safely followed with at least yearly ultrasound, recognizing that the growth pattern of AAA is that of discontinuous. Some studies have suggested that women with AAAs should have their aneurysms fixed at a slightly smaller diameter (between 5.0 and 5.5 cm) as compared to men. Most aneurysms, especially smaller ones, tend to grow at a rate of 0.3–0.5 cm per year [72–74]. Table 56.2 lists the rate of rupture of AAA for a given size.

If a patient has symptoms of abdominal or back pain of the patient's AAA has demonstrated rapid growth, they should probably be fixed more expeditiously, even if they do not meet absolute size criteria. Other factors that have been associated with increased expansion or rupture rate are advanced age, severe CAD, chronic obstructive pulmonary disease (COPD), female, uncontrolled hypertension, or the presence of a large volume of luminal thrombus.

A group from Dartmouth led by Mark Fillinger looked at mechanical wall stress and concluded that it is a key predictor of rupture risk for AAA. A mathematical analysis of AAA geometry, known as finite element analysis, has been suggested to be a theoretically better way to estimate wall stress and the risk of rupture. It was first performed in two dimensional shapes, then later in three dimensional shapes, and most recently actual AAA shapes obtained from CT scan data [75]. Using this model, Fillinger's group looked at three groups of patients: those who presented with a ruptured AAA, those who were symptomatic and required

urgent surgery, and those who underwent elective AAA repairs. They found that peak wall stress was significantly higher in ruptured AAA and symptomatic groups compared with that of the elective repair group comparing diameter-matched subjects. The group also realized that the location of maximal wall stress in their series was not at the site of maximal AAA diameter but rather in the posterolateral location, the site where most ruptures occur. Fillinger et al. thus concluded that peak wall stress calculated with computer modeling appears to assess risk rupture more accurately than AAA diameter alone. Fillinger et al. [76] later report that for AAAs under observation, elevated wall stress associated with rupture is not simply an acute event near the time of rupture. While these studies have been very exciting, a drawback to its widespread use is the cost and time required to make these models. Another limitation to its widespread use is that most physicians are not used to stress values. Fillinger's group has thought about creating "severe or critical" stress values similar to velocity thresholds for carotid duplex scanning. While Fillinger's colleagues do not advocate stress modeling in all patients, it can certainly add more information, especially in patients at the highest risk for surgery.

Preoperative Risk Stratification and Decision Making

The goal of therapy for AAA is to prevent aneurysmal rupture. Currently, there are two effective treatment modalities to treat AAA, and thus exclude the AAA from pressurized blood flow. The first is an endoluminally placed covered stent graft (EVAR) that can be inserted either via the femoral or iliac artery. The second is an open surgical exclusion of the AAA, along with an interposition synthetic graft. Both techniques have advantages and disadvantages, and therefore each case must be evaluated separately, based on a patient's age, comorbidities, and aortic anatomy.

If a patient is found to have a symptomatic AAA (i.e., back or abdominal pain or hypotension), urgent surgical intervention is the only true chance for survival. Stable patients can undergo cross-sectional imaging to assess their potential for an endoluminal approach, along with laboratory tests. If the patient is unstable, then the patient should be taken directly to the operating room for an open repair.

Current recommendations are to repair asymptomatic male patients with aneurysms greater than 5.5 cm or asymptomatic female patients with aneurysms greater than 5.0 cm. A vascular surgeon will determine the most appropriate treatment option by taking into account preoperative evaluations such as aneurysmal anatomy, along with the patient's age and other commodities. In 1995, a group led by Steyerberg created six independent risk factors for operative mortality

TABLE 56.2 Rate of rupture based on size of AAA

Size of AAA (cm)	Annual rupture risk (%)
≤4.0	0.3
4–4.9	1.5
5–5.9	6.5
6–7	20
7–8	30

after elective AAA repair, along with their relative risks. The most important risk factors from most important to least important were renal dysfunction and a creatinine greater than 1.8, congestive heart failure with cardiogenic pulmonary edema, jugular venous distention, the presence of ischemic changes (ST depression greater than 2 mm) on a preoperative ECG, history of a prior myocardial infarction, pulmonary dysfunction including COPD, dyspnea on exertion or prior lung surgery, older age, and female gender. Based on their findings, they report that a standard elective open AAA has a operative mortality of 5%, which could rise as high as 40% if many of the aforementioned risk factors were present, and decline to less than 3% if none were present [77]. Since that time, other studies have validated this. In 2001, Hallin et al. found between a four- and ninefold increase in mortality risk in patients with renal failure alone. They also found that CAD only had between two and a half and fivefold increase in mortality risk [78].

Another important aspect is the specific surgeon and hospital. This variability is directly proportional to the number of AAA operations that are performed by the given surgeon or center per year. Larger hospital performing more AAA operations have much better outcomes than less experienced surgeons or smaller centers [79]. In 2003, a group led by Dimick concluded that high-volume hospitals that perform more than 35 open AAA per year have a 30-day mortality of 3%, as compared to low-volume centers that have a 30-day mortality of 5.5%. They also reported that high-volume surgeons with specialty training in vascular surgery, working at high-volume hospitals have the best outcomes [80].

The first critical move in evaluating a patient with an asymptomatic AAA is a thorough personal and family history and careful physical examination. Family history is a key component of the patient's preoperative assessment. If a patient has a family history of AAA, earlier repair is warranted, regardless of the method, because their risk of rupture is higher when matched with comparable sized AAA in patients without a family history [81–83]. In addition, some basic laboratory data should be collected. These first steps should help a vascular surgeon decide what kind if any operation can or should be performed to fix this AAA. In addition, any of the preoperative risks, such as any cardiopulmonary troubles, should be optimized prior to surgery. Another key fact to think about is whether the patient's current life expectancy is long enough and their quality of life is good enough to justify an intervention.

Age has been one key variable that has shown to be statistically significant when comparing mortality among groups of patients being treated with AAA. Hertzer et al. reported on a large series of patients treated with open AAA from the Cleveland Clinic. They found that age greater than 74 years significantly affected outcomes. They found a risk ratio of 2.2 in their series in these patients [63, 84]. Others have reported

similar findings of higher incidence of adverse outcomes in patients greater than 75 or 80 years of age who underwent open AAA repairs [85–87]. Based on these results, older patients, especially octogenarians, may benefit from EVAR. Sicard et al. reported that when comparing EVAR to a conventional open repair of AAA in octogenarians, the mortality, the complication rate, and extent and gravity of these complications were higher in the octogenarian group [86]. Dardik et al. reported an in-hospital mortality of patients undergoing elective AAA repair of 3.5%. However, in his series, the death rate for patients in their sixth decade was 2.2% compared with 7.3% in octogenarians [79]. These findings may sway a vascular surgeon to treat an octogenarian via EVAR if possible.

To decrease overall operative mortality, perioperative cardiac optimization is vital, especially since CAD is the main cause of early and late mortality after AAA [88]. The American College of Cardiology (ACC) has standardized preoperative cardiac evaluation for noncardiac surgery, based on their best long-term data and created categories for the risk of the procedure and the clinical risk to the patient. Patients with unstable coronary syndromes such as acute or recent MI (less than 30 days) or unstable angina, decompensated CHF, significant arrhythmias such as high-grade AV block or symptomatic ventricular arrhythmias, or severe valvular disease are considered to have major cardiac risks. Those patients with intermediate risks would have symptoms such as mild angina, prior MI by history or the presence of Q waves on an ECG, compensated CHF, insulin-dependent diabetes mellitus, or renal insufficiency. Those patients with minor risk factors include those who are of advanced age, have an abnormal ECG (left ventricular hypertrophy and left bundle branch block), have a history of a prior stroke, or have uncontrolled hypertension [89].

Van Damme et al. from Europe reported on 156 patients prospectively, assessing cardiac risk before vascular surgery. They found that in patients without clinical markers of CAD, noninvasive cardiac testing did not predict cardiac complications. In patients with definite clinical of ECG evidence of CAD, a dobutamine stress test provided additional information and optimized risk stratification. Moreover, they found that a negative stress test had a high negative predictive value [90]. In 2006, Poldermans et al. reported for intermediate risk patients, cardiac testing can be safely omitted, provided that patients are treated with beta-blockers to keep their heart rates until tight control [91]. Recently, the coronary artery revascularization prophylaxis (CARP) trial in patients with CAD and stable cardiac complaints compared preoperative coronary revascularization with either coronary artery bypass grafting (CABG) or percutaneous coronary intervention versus no coronary revascularization in preparation for major vascular surgery [92]. Five hundred and ten patients were randomized and 258 were assigned to a strategy of preoperative coronary revascularization, while 252 received no revascularization procedure. Coronary revascularization prior to elective vascular surgery did not improve long-term survival. In addition, there did not appear to be any reduction in postoperative myocardial infarctions (MI) or deaths in the revascularized group. One other report from Kertai et al. looking at 570 patients found that statin therapy lowered the incidence of the composite endpoint of MI or death from 11 to 3.7% [93].

Fleisher et al. reported on the latest ACC/American Heart Association (AHA) Guidelines on perioperative cardiovascular evaluation and care for noncardiac surgery. They determined that successful evaluation and management requires teamwork and communication. The group felt that indications for cardiac testing and treatments are the same as in the nonoperative setting, but the timing of such evaluations is dependent upon the urgency of the surgery, patient risk factors, and surgery specific considerations. The use of testing, both invasive and noninvasive should be limited to those that affect patient management. In addition, they concluded that the preoperative evaluation was their first cardiac risk stratification, both short and long term, and treatment strategies could be implemented to reduce a patient's long-term risk [89]. This study has also concluded that perioperative beta blockade is crucial for pre-, peri-, and postoperative cardiac protection.

Even though CAD and cardiac risk stratification are the number one risk for aortic surgery, other conditions need to be evaluated, too. Patients who smoke should be encouraged to stop smoking before surgery. Patients with a history of pulmonary insufficiency require preoperative pulmonary function testing. Some patients with severe bronchospastic pulmonary disease may even need to be optimized with bronchodilator therapy or steroids prior to open AAA repair. If a patient requires persistent continuous oxygen therapy, he may not be a suitable candidate for an open surgical repair.

If a patient has a history of having a stroke or transient ischemic attack (TIA) or if a carotid bruit is present on physical exam, a carotid duplex scan should be performed. If a high-grade stenosis is found in the internal carotid artery, carotid revascularization should precede elective AAA repair.

Some centers routinely perform arteriography on patients with AAA to better determine certain anatomic factors prior to deciding which technique to perform to treat the AAA. In patients with hypertension and chronic renal insufficiency where renovascular disease may be present, better renal artery anatomy needs to be known. Also, patients with claudication may need some anatomic evaluation to assess the level or levels of disease. In addition, if there is some history of mesenteric ischemia or the AAA is in close proximity to the renal arteries, better visceral vessel anatomy is required for preoperative planning. Today, depending on the center, some of today's high-quality CT scanners or MRI machines can be as useful as traditional arteriography.

Surgical Techniques

The principal aim of surgical intervention is to eliminate aneurysmal flow and wall tension, thus preventing future dilatation and rupture [94]. There are two basic approaches to treating AAA, the older more traditional open surgical repair and endovascular repair of abdominal aortic aneurysms (EVAR). To date, open repairs have proven to be more durable long term and require less follow-up than endoluminal repairs, as long as patients can tolerate the open surgery. Conrad et al. reported in 2007 on a large series of AAA from Massachusetts General Hospital and found that open AAA repairs are safe and durable with an excellent 10-year survival in patients less than 75 years. In addition, the freedom from graft-related reintervention is superior to EVAR [95]. A large series published by Hertzer et al. also showed a low 30-day mortality and excellent long-term survival with open AAA repair [63]. One issue for today's younger vascular surgeons and current vascular surgery residents (VSR) is the fact that with newer and better endovascular devices, fewer open infrarenal AAAs are being performed each year. From 2001 to 2005, the mean volume of elective open infrarenal AAA repairs declined by 27%. During that same period, EVAR procedures for the VSR have increased by 212%.

A model was created by Barnes et al. to predict outcomes for EVAR using the following preoperative variables: age, aneurysm size, ASA class, gender, preoperative creatinine, aortic neck angle, infrarenal neck diameter, and infrarenal neck length [96].

Endovascular Repair of Abdominal Aortic Aneurysms

Over the past 15 years, EVAR has become widely accepted as a means of treating aneurysms located in the infrarenal portion of the aorta. In addition, as more endovascular grafts with broader applications become commercially available, the number of EVARs performed worldwide continues to increase. A group led by Parodi et al. reported of the first endoluminal repair of AAA in 1991 [97]. Since that time, numerous devices have come to market and numerous clinical trials have been published [61, 65, 67–71, 98–100]. Endoluminal methods allow the surgeon to access the arterial system from the femoral arteries, rather than requiring a

Figure 56.1 (**a** and **b**) This two CT scans demonstrate a completed EVAR with the graft in proper position.

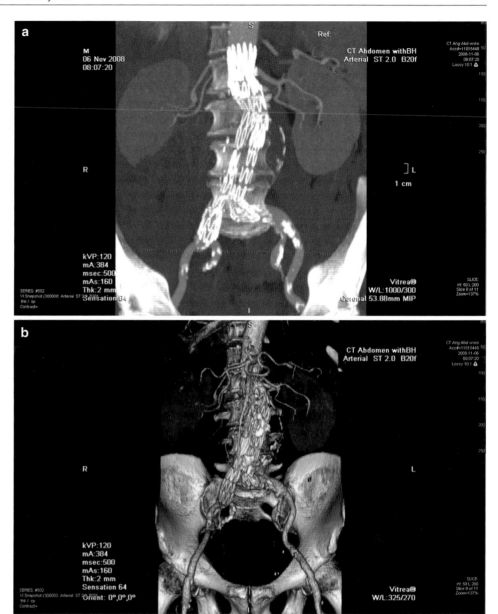

deep and extensive pelvic dissection, with its associated potential complications. This approach is even more useful in patients who are at high-operative risk due to significant medical comorbidities, prior abdominal or pelvic surgery, abdominal or pelvic radiation, lower abdominal stomas, or morbid obesity [101]. Endovascular repairs have been shown to reduce operative morbidity, mortality, length of hospital stay, and postprocedure disability [102]. The basic technical procedure involves placing an endovascular graft across the AAA below the renal arteries and above the hypogastric arteries and exclude it from arterial blood flow and systemic arterial pressure (Fig. 56.1a, b). This type of repair requires at least a 2 cm landing or attachment zone of normal infrarenal aorta above the graft and enough common iliac distal to

the aneurysm to achieve an adequate seal. Two randomized trials, EVAR-1 and DREAM trials, demonstrated a significantly lower mortality for EVAR when compared with open repair, but a higher reintervention requirement for EVAR [68, 69]. Both trials still support treating even low-risk surgical candidates with EVAR. Another report by Sicard et al. looked at EVAR as a long-term solution for patients at high risk for open surgery. The group found the EVAR for large AAA using FDA approved devices is safe and provides long lasting protection from AAA-related mortality and is certainly comparable to open repair at 4 years after the procedure [70]. Table 56.3 lists the results from the pivotal trials for each of the five current commercially available devices [103–107].

TABLE 56.3 Results from pivotal trials of long-term follow-up of each of the commercially available devices

	AneuRx (medtronic) (%)	Excluder (WL gore) (%)	Zenith (cook) (%)	Powerlink (endologix) (%)	Talent (medtronic) (%)
Freedom from rupture (at 5 years)	96.8	99.8	100	100	98.2
Freedom from conversion (at 5 years)	92.2	97	98.2	97.9	99.1
Freedom from aneurysm-related death (at 5 years)	96	98.2	97.8	97.9	96.5
Migration (at 5 years)	6.4	0.5	0.4	4.3	0.8% at 1 year not followed any longer
Probability of survival (at 5 years)	60.1	70	83	78.1	71.1

Open Technical Considerations

Once a patient and physician have agreed on an open repair, and the patient has been deemed medically suitable for open surgery, the specific approach and operation is individualized and based on a few factors. CT scan imaging provides the best method to assess the anatomical factors that will influence the open repair. The most critical is the shape and configuration of the aneurysm. The neck, the portion of the aorta immediately below the renal arteries, along with the iliac arteries must be assessed. If the iliac arteries have significant occlusive disease, the graft may have to be sewn to the femoral arteries. Another factor is the patient's pulmonary status because some approaches may be better if the patient has severe COPD. Finally, has the patient had other surgeries in the past, and if so, what types of surgery. These factors, along with operator comfort, will determine which approach is utilized. The two most frequently used incisions are a left retroperitoneal incision and a midline incision from the patient's xiphoid to his pubis. A transverse incision has also been described, especially for patients with multiple upper abdominal surgeries.

When AAA is repaired via the transabdominal approach, the patient is placed in a supine position. After entering the abdominal cavity, a full exploration of the abdominal contents should occur to rule out other intra-abdominal pathology that might have not been visible in the CT scan. If an unexpected lesion is discovered, it must be evaluated and a surgeon must make a judgment as to how best to proceed. Our group and others strongly discourages combining a sterile vascular case with a potentially contaminated gastrointestinal case.

The next step is to superiorly retract the transverse colon and greater omentum. The small bowel is the eviscerated to the right side of the abdomen, thus exposing the base of the mesenteries of the left colon and the small intestine. The posterior peritoneum is then incised from the ligament of Treitz to the aortic bifurcation, thus exposing the infrarenal aorta (Fig. 56.2). To identify the neck of the AAA, the peritoneum should be incised until at least the level of the left renal vein crossing. In rare occasions of juxtarenal aneurysm, the left renal vein can

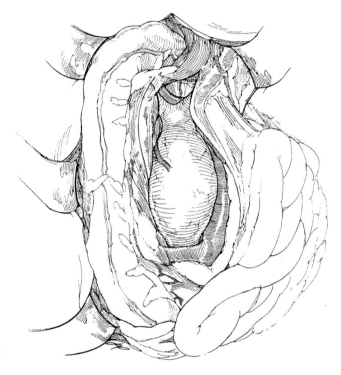

FIGURE 56.2 This drawing depicts the view of AAA via a transabdominal approach. The small intestines are mobilized to the patient's *right* and the left colon is reflected to the patient's *left*. The retroperitoneum has been opened, exposing the AAA.

be divided close to the IVC and/or reanastomosed if indicated. If the left renal vein is divided, it is important to preserve the left gonadal and adrenal vein to preserve left renal function. Once an adequate area proximally is exposed to cross clamp, the iliac arteries must also be exposed for cross-clamping. If the aneurysm involves one or more than one iliac, the dissection must be extended to the bifurcation of the common iliac(s) assuring identification of ureters and parasympathetic pudendal fibers. Usually circumferential aortic or iliac dissection is not necessary and may avoid venous injuries. One other key is constant communication between the surgical and the anesthesia teams to aid in proper intraoperative management.

Once clamps are applied, the aneurysm sac is then opened longitudinally and the mural thrombus should be removed. AAA with an adequate infrarenal neck to apply a clamp to

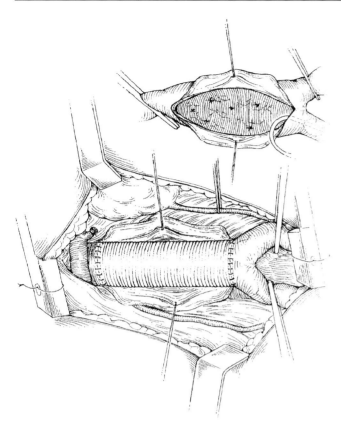

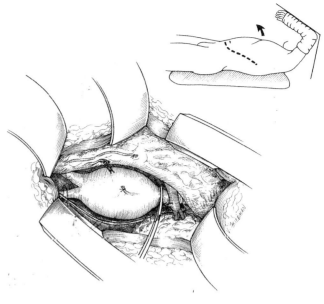

FIGURE 56.4 This drawing depicts the exposure and incision for a retroperitoneal approach for an open repair of AAA.

FIGURE 56.3 This drawing depicts a completed repair of the AAA using a tube graft.

that returns to a normal size proximal to the iliac bifurcation can have a tube graft sewn. One should use a bifurcated graft if the iliac arteries are aneurysmal. If more extensive iliac disease is present, other more complex options exist. The femoral arteries should be routinely avoided as distal landing targets to decrease the risk of wound and potential graft infection (Fig. 56.3).

Prior to removing all of the clamps, it is important to back bleed the iliac system and flush any residual or remaining debris out of the graft. After hemostasis is achieved, distal pulses should be assessed prior to beginning the closure. Typically, the aneurysm sac and then separately, the posterior peritoneum are closed over the graft in an effort to prevent intestinal contact with the aortic graft. The abdomen wall is then closed.

Many surgeons are more familiar with and thus prefer this approach to treat AAA. In addition, the transperitoneal method enables the surgeon the best exposure of the aneurysm, the renal arteries, both iliac, and both femoral arteries. This approach can be challenging in a patient who has undergone multiple prior abdominal surgeries and has a great deal of adhesions. In addition, juxta or suprarenal extension, the presence of ascites or inflammatory aneurysm can be challenging with the transabdominal approach.

Other surgeons prefer a retroperitoneal approach for repairing AAAs. The aorta is a retroperitoneal structure and avoiding the intraperitoneal contents is preferable in certain circumstances, especially in patients who have had prior intra-abdominal surgery. Typical situations where this approach is taken are a "hostile" abdomen secondary to multiple abdominal surgeries and adhesions, previous radiation therapy, abdominal wall stoma, a horseshoe kidney, or the need to extend the repair above the renal arteries. A left-sided retroperitoneal incision from lateral rectus margin up through the 11th or 12th intercostal space provide great exposure to the infrarenal juxta and suprarenal portions of the aorta (Fig. 56.4). A surgeon using this approach is limited in his exposure to the right renal artery, the right distal common iliac artery, and partially the right femoral artery. Also, any intra-abdominal pathology may be missed because the peritoneum is not entered. For a retroperitoneal incision, the patient is positioned in the right decubitus position and remains in that position with the assistance of a vacuum assisted bean bag device. The precise location of the incision depends on what procedure is planned. For an infrarenal or aorto-iliac exposure, the surgeon should make an incision medial but at the level on the umbilicus just lateral to the medial border of the rectus abdominus muscle. Based on the patient's size and body habitus, the incision should be extended in a curvilinear fashion superiorly and posteriorly to either the 12th rib or the interspace between the 11th and 12th ribs.

The peritoneum is mobilized until the left ureter and left gonadal vein are identified. The left ureter is then dissected and mobilized from the level of the renal pelvis down to the iliac artery bifurcation, looped with a vessel loop, and gently retracted medially to avoid an avulsion or traction injury. Care must also be taken not to devascularize the ureter, which can also lead to an ischemic injury. The gonadal vein is then dissected up to its insertion into the left renal vein and typically divided. Failure to ligate the gonadal vein can lead to avulsion injuries and further bleeding. Usually, both common iliac arteries can be dissected to allow for clamp placement. If the right common iliac artery is involved with aneurysmal dilatation, intraluminal control of the right iliac system can be accomplished with a balloon catheter. The use of self retaining retractors is also vital because it facilitates exposure and avoids unnecessary trauma to intra-abdominal organs, especially the spleen. The clamping sequence is the same as for a transperitoneal approach, the iliac arteries first, and then the proximal aortic clamp is applied.

Based on a patient's anatomy, either a tube graft or a bifurcated aortobi-iliac graft can be sewn into place. If an aortobifemoral bypass is required, we prefer to suture the common iliac arteries from within the aneurysm sac. We would complete the aortic anastomosis and then rotate the table to provide better access to both groins. A tunnel is made carefully directly on top of the iliac arteries and ureters from above and on top of the femoral arteries from below. It is critical to ensure that both femoral limbs are passed posterior to the patient's ureters to avoid ureteral injury or compression. The femoral anastomoses are usually performed in a standard end to side fashion. Once hemostasis has been achieved, the aneurysm sac is closed over the graft, if possible, and the abdominal lateral wall muscle and fascia are closed in two layers.

The two main complications specific to this approach are wound bulges or hernias and chronic incisional pain. LaCroix reported on a large series and found that only 5% had an incisional hernia, but 28% had a 2 cm or larger incision bulge [108]. Our group looked at more than 1,000 patients who underwent retroperitoneal approaches for AAA. Many described some level of incisional pain that ultimately resolved after 12–24 months, but fewer than 1% required nerve blocks to relieve the pain [109].

Postoperative Complications

AAA repair, regardless of the approach, does have its share of associated complications. Many patients undergoing EVAR are sent to a regular monitored floor and can be discharged the next day. Most patients undergoing an open AAA are followed immediately in an intensive care unit, with dedicated intensivists. Many patients will need some period of continued mechanical ventilation. Careful monitoring is also crucial to monitor fluid shifts, pain control and hemodynamic responses. Patients should have full laboratory values checked immediately postoperatively and any abnormalities, especially coagulopathies corrected immediately, along with ensuring adequate patient core body temperatures in the normal range. In addition, patients should have an ECG and a chest X-ray performed.

The perioperative complications from open AAA repairs can either be due to graft problems, such as bleeding, embolization, thrombosis, or kinking or due to organ system problems.

The most common organ complication is related to the heart and has been reported to as high as 15%, including arrhythmia, infarction, and congestive heart failure. In one series by Ali et al., which observed 43 consecutive patients who underwent elective open AAA repairs, found that 47% had troponin elevations postoperative, although only 26% met the criteria for a myocardial infarction [110]. Another study by Elkouri et al. reported on a large series of patients undergoing elective AAA repair and found cardiac complications in 22% [111]. Cardiac complications are certainly less in patients undergoing EVAR [68, 69, 71, 99].

Perioperative renal failure predicts a worse outcome. Preoperative renal dysfunction is the greatest predictor of perioperative or postoperative renal complications [112, 113]. Walsh et al. reported that in EVAR, perioperative renal dysfunction is attenuated. However, dialysis rates after EVAR are similar to those after open surgery. EVAR patients develop progressive deterioration in renal function, of unclear etiology, over time. It is most likely, multifactorial, including embolization, continued contrast media, and along with graft misplacement. They also felt that although the exact effect of a transrenal endograft fixation on long-term renal function is unknown, it may be associated with a significantly increased risk of renal infarction [114]. In open repairs, care must be taken to ensure adequate kidney perfusion to reduce this complication. Intraoperative measures, such as careful clamp placement to avoid renal embolization and flushing the proximal anastomosis, will aid in this. If flow to a kidney is halted for more than 30 min, topical packing of the kidney with ice along with flushing iced heparinized saline in the renal artery can help preserve renal function.

Pulmonary complications such as pneumonias or chronic ventilator dependence have also been reported. Elkouri also reported 16% of their patients had pulmonary complications [111]. A large series by Hertzer et al. at the Cleveland Clinic only reported 4.2% of their patients developing pulmonary complications, with the majority having pneumonia, although 1% developed adult respiratory distress syndrome [63]. Early extubation and aggressive pulmonary toilet and early ambulation can aid in preventing pulmonary complications. These complications are less for EVAR since most patients are extubated in the operating room and many of these cases are performed under spinal, epidural, or local anesthesia.

Perioperative procedure related complications include iatrogenic injuries, hemorrhage, renal and lower extremity embolization, and colonic ischemia. Hemorrhage usually results from technical problems with the proximal anastomosis or a missed arterial or venous injury. Venous bleeding is usually due to an iliac or renal vein injury during the initial exposure or clamp injury. In fact, some advocate that there is no need for circumferential dissection of the iliac vessels because the arteries can be adherent to the veins.

Colonic ischemia after AAA repair is rare, but it can be deadly and a high index of suspicion is required. A post op AAA patient with an unexplained fever, leukocytosis, and/or left lower quadrant pain, as well as, one with bloody rectal discharge should be urgently evaluated for colonic ischemia with a flexible sigmoidoscopy or colonoscopy. A study by Brandt et al. in 1997 reported that flexible sigmoidoscopy reliably predicts full thickness colonic ischemia for AAA repair. Patients with nonconfluent ischemia limited to the mucosa can be safely followed by serial endoscopic examinations [115]. Boley et al. have described three forms of ischemic colitis. In the mild version, which affects about 50% of the patients who underwent AAA repair, the ischemia is limited to the colonic mucosa and submucosa. Patients may have symptoms of abdominal pain, ileus, distention, or bloody diarrhea, but the disease process is self limited and resolves with adequate resuscitation. A worse case involves ischemia of the muscularis and may lead to stricture formation. The most catastrophic and concerning form of colonic ischemia affects less than 20% of the patients. Transmural ischemia and colonic infarction is present with free or contained colonic perforation being present. This necessitates a return to the operating room for a washout of the contamination, along with a Hartmann's procedure and a colostomy. Another issue here is graft infection [116, 117]. The overall incidence of clinically relevant ischemia has been reported to be 1–3% after elective AAA repairs, and much higher after ruptured AAA repairs [118–123]. Another study of 105 patients undergoing flexible sigmoidoscopy found colonic ischemia in 11.4% [124]. The classic presentation of bloody diarrhea in the early postoperative period only occurs in about 30% of cases [119].

AAA repair can alter sigmoid blood flow because ligation of the IMA or internal iliac artery, embolization of debris from the AAA, prolonged hypotension, or a retractor injury can affect the collateral branches to the colon. In patients undergoing open AAA repair, 50% have a patent IMA, which could be reimplanted or bypassed [125]. Most surgeons evaluate collateral colonic circulation by assessing the back bleeding of the IMA. Brisk back bleeding, along with a normal looking colon typically would indicate to a surgeon that it is safe to ligate the IMA. Several studies have shown that IMA reimplantation did not influence postoperative colonic ischemia [122, 123, 126, 127] but certainly was safe and may

be advantageous in selected patients. Preoperative imaging by CT angiography can be useful in assessing the potential need to reimplant the IMA, especially if evidence of chronic mesenteric arterial obstruction.

As for EVAR and colonic or visceral ischemia, many series report zero incidence of colonic ischemia [128–130]. Geraghty et al. reported on a large series of patients treated with bifurcated endovascular grafts. Of those, 19% underwent perioperative hypogastric artery embolization. They found that four patients (1.7%) had signs or symptoms of ischemic colitis, and three required a colectomy. All three patients who underwent a colectomy were found to have ischemia secondary to atheroemboli and all had bilateral patent hypogastric arteries. They therefore concluded that while elective embolization of one or both hypogastric arteries may contribute to pelvic ischemia and ischemic colitis, atheromatous debris rather than proximal hypogastric artery occlusion is the primary cause of ischemic colitis [131]. Another series by Mehta et al. found the incidence of ischemic colitis from endovascular repair to be less than their incidence from an open repair (2%) and also suggested that embolization was the most common cause of ischemic colitis [132].

Ureteral injury is rare, although if it occurs, it should be repaired at the time of discovery, over a double J stent using interrupted absorbable sutures. The spleen is another organ is often injured, usually because of retraction. The treatment for a fractured spleen, especially in the face of an ongoing coagulopathy is a splenectomy. Inadvertent enterotomies made during the initial opening should be repaired and the AAA portion should be aborted. One last complication that can occur, as with any wound closure, is the inadvertent capture of a piece of small or large intestine in the closure, lead to a fistula, an obstruction, or bowel ischemia.

Another complication, although usually more delayed, is sexual dysfunction as a result of injury to the autonomic nerves during the iliac dissection. It most frequently presents as retrograde ejaculation, although erectile dysfunction does occur too. Most men undergoing elective AAA repair have some component of this preoperatively. In the ADAM trial, 40% of men had impotence before AAA repair [133]. Careful dissection in the region of the distal left side of the aorta, especially near the IMA and the left common iliac artery has been shown to reduce this complication substantially, which has been reported as high as 25% [134, 135]. Another important component to preserve sexual function is the preservation of at least one internal iliac artery with antegrade blood flow.

One complication unique to EVAR is an endoleak. This refers to the persistent filling of the aneurysm sac despite the presence of a stent graft. It is the most common complication following EVAR and has been reported as high as 12–44% [136–140], but with newer grafts, the incidence is reported between 15 and 22% [98, 141–143] at 1 month. Endoleaks are divided into five types: Type I is perfusion of the sac from

CONTROVERSIAL CASE STUDY

A Complex AAA in an Elderly Patient Not Suitable for Open Repair

An 82-year-old African-American male with a past medical history of CAD, s/p CABG×4 6 years ago and PTCA and stenting 8 months ago, COPD on home oxygen at night, and poorly controlled hypertension presents to a vascular surgeon with a palpable and pulsatile abdominal mass. The patient denies abdominal or back pain and is otherwise asymptomatic. He states that he takes a long list of medications including aspirin, plavix, coreg, lasix, lipitor, and vasotec. His physical exam other than the palpable abdominal mass is unremarkable. A CT scan is obtained that shows an 8 cm infrarenal AAA that begins less than 1 cm below the renal arteries. His iliac arteries are very tortuous and heavily calcified. This patient is clearly not a suitable candidate for open AAA surgery and his anatomy is really unsuitable for standard EVAR techniques. Unfortunately, more and more patients present like this. What can be done for this and other patients like this? Some surgeons would attempt an open repair and hope that the patient can pull through it, although the patient would be at significant risk for postoperative cardiac or pulmonary complications. Others would try EVAR and potentially sacrifice one of the patient's kidneys and risk placing the patient on dialysis. Another option would be to refer the patient to one of the two or three centers in the country that can perform EVAR with the use of fenestrations (holes) or branches in the graft to allow for the preservation of the renal or visceral arteries. One final option is not to recommend any therapy. A discussion with the patient and his family would then need to occur describing the fact that the patient is at high risk for rupture but no one can predict when this may occur and some of his other comorbidities may lead to his death before his AAA. There is no correct option.

a proximal or distal endpoint due to inadequate fixation; type II is retrograde perfusion of the sac via collateral flow; type III is antegrade perfusion of the sac from a leak between components; type IV is antegrade perfusion from holes within the graft material; type V is serum transudation into the sac through the graft material. Type I and III are the most worrisome and require treatment rather urgently. Type II leaks are the most controversial. The majority will thrombose spontaneously over time. Many remain patent, but intervention is typically only indicated in the leak is associated with AAA enlargement [144].

Another unique complication of EVAR is graft migration after implantation. There is significant variability depending on the commercially available graft and over time with newer products, the incidence has been decreasing [98, 141, 143, 145].

One other complication related to EVAR is access-related injuries such as arterial dissection, rupture, thrombosis, pseudoaneurysm formation, and lymphocele. Each graft company has a unique set of complication rates from their IDE trials [98, 141, 143, 145].

One other dreaded complication with a very high postoperative morbidity and mortality is spinal cord ischemia and paralysis. This is much more common after thoracoabdominal or suprarenal AAA repairs, rather than infrarenal AAA repairs, because the accessory spinal artery normally takes off the aorta in the chest or proximal abdominal aorta, although it has been reported. These reports have stressed the value of preserving pelvic collaterals and internal iliac arteries if at all possible. Occlusion or division of these vessels combined with periods of severe hypotension can lead to spinal cord ischemia and paralysis [146]. Paralysis has also been reported after EVAR, although far less common with an estimated incidence of 0.21% [147, 148].

It has been estimated that 30–40% of patients with abdominal aortic aneurysms (AAA) are not candidates for endovascular repair using the current commercially available devices. The primary limitation has been unfavorable anatomy most often associated with the proximal aortic neck. Aortic necks with large diameter (>32 mm), severe angulation (>60°), a reverse taper or cone-shape, a short seal zone (<10 mm), or an absent infrarenal neck are not candidates for the currently available devices and open repair is the best option for those patients [149–154]. The mortality associated with conventional treatment of open pararenal and suprarenal aneurysms ranges from 2.5 to 8% [63, 111, 155–157] and for thoracoabdominal aneurysms is from 5 to 34% [158–162]. In addition, open surgery is associated with significant morbidity rates from 20 to 40% [157]. Notable complications include paraplegia, mesenteric ischemia, renal failure, cardiopulmonary complications, and wound complications [158–162]. This is even more relevant for elderly patients. While some may tolerate major open aortic surgery many will not, mainly because of poor cardiac or pulmonary function. Therefore, some other strategies are necessary to treat these patients effectively.

While not widely available nor approved in America for everyone's use, complex endovascular repairs involving the visceral segment do occur. These can be divided into two broad categories. A fenestrated endovascular repair is when a device is used to treat an aneurysm with an inadequate neck, yet the visceral vessels arise from a segment of normal aorta and the added length is required to provide an adequate proximal seal and secure attachment. Fenestrations are actual holes in the graft and vary in size depending on the need of a particular patient. Although fenestrated stent graft repairs do not typically require branches to ensure a tight seal, most visceral branches are stented open using balloon expandable stents to ensure proper alignment of the graft and the particular visceral branch vessel. Scallops are openings cut at the proximal end of a stent graft to allow for further extension of the graft cephalad, surrounding and encroaching onto a visceral vessel without actually it [152]. Branched endovascular repairs are currently performed using one of two methods. The main device can have cuffs that act as directional branches and serve as attachment sites for each visceral artery branch involved in the repair (cuffed-branched stent graft). On the other hand, the device may have multiple branches that arise from the aortic graft proximal to the target branch and are completed with a bridging covered stent extending into the target vessel [152, 163]. Aside from two major centers in the USA, these types of operations are performed either off label or the patients are not offered treatment because of their age and other comorbidities. FDA approved trials are just beginning at a few centers in the country to treat these complex AAA in patients not suited for open repair.

Open infrarenal AAA repairs have been performed for over many years with significant improvements in clinical outcomes. This repair has proven to be extremely safe and durable, especially in centers that perform a high volume of these cases each year. Even with the increasing popularity, success, and durability of endovascular repairs, some patients will not have the correct anatomy for a stent graft and thus require an open operation, although as technology and devices continue to improve, more and more patients are becoming candidates for EVAR. The knowledge and skill to perform both open AAA and EVAR is vital for today's vascular surgeon. Moreover, the knowledge about preoperative patient selection and optimization along with some of the pitfalls that can occur intraoperatively will further cut down a patient's perioperative morbidity and mortality regardless of the method employed. In addition, a keen eye to postoperative warning signs can potentially stave off major complications and improve long-term survival.

References

1. Johnston KW et al (1991) Suggested standards for reporting on arterial aneurysms. Subcommittee on Reporting Standards for Arterial Aneurysms, Ad Hoc Committee on Reporting Standards, Society for Vascular Surgery and North American Chapter, International Society for Cardiovascular Surgery. J Vasc Surg 13(3):452–458
2. Thompson RW (1996) Basic science of abdominal aortic aneurysms: emerging therapeutic strategies for an unresolved clinical problem. Curr Opin Cardiol 11(5):504–518
3. Thompson RW et al (1995) Production and localization of 92-kilodalton gelatinase in abdominal aortic aneurysms. An elastolytic metalloproteinase expressed by aneurysm-infiltrating macrophages. J Clin Invest 96(1):318–326
4. Thompson RW, Parks WC (1996) Role of matrix metalloproteinases in abdominal aortic aneurysms. Ann NY Acad Sci 800:157–174
5. Curci JA et al (1998) Expression and localization of macrophage elastase (matrix metalloproteinase-12) in abdominal aortic aneurysms. J Clin Invest 102(11):1900–1910
6. Osler W (1905) Aneurysm of the abdominal aorta. Lancet 2:1089
7. Osler W (1915) Remarks on arterio-venous aneurysm. Lancet 1:949
8. Leonardo R (1943) History of surgery. Froben Press, New York
9. Matas R (1940) Aneurysm of the abdominal aorta at its bifurcation into the common iliac arteries: a pictorial supplement illustrating the history of Corinne D., previously reported as the first recorded instance of cure of an aneurysm of the abdominal aorta by ligation. Ann Surg 112(5):909–922
10. Pearse HE (1940) Experimental studies on the gradual occlusion of large arteries. Ann Surg 112(5):923–937
11. Harrison PW, Chandy J (1943) A subclavian aneurysm cured by cellophane fibrosis. Ann Surg 118(3):478–481
12. Abbott OA (1949) Clinical experiences with the application of polythene cellophane upon the aneurysms of the thoracic vessels. J Thorac Surg 18(4):435–461
13. Power D (1921) The palliative treatment of aneurysms by wiring with Colt's apparatus. Br J Surg 9:27
14. Dente CJ, Feliciano DV (2005) Alexis Carrel (1873–1944): Nobel Laureate, 1912. Arch Surg 140(6):609–610
15. Edwards W (1979) Alexis Carrel 1873–1944. Contemp Surg 14:65–79
16. Carrel A (1902) La technique operatoire des anastomoses vasculaires et la transplation de viscere. Lyon Méd 98:859
17. Carrel A (1967) Suture of blood vessels and transplantation of organs. Nobel Lecture, 1912, in Nobel lectures in physiology-medicine. Elsevier, New York
18. Dubost C, Allary M, Oeconomos N (1952) Resection of an aneurysm of the abdominal aorta: reestablishment of the continuity by a preserved human arterial graft, with result after five months. AMA Arch Surg 64(3):405–408
19. DeBakey ME, Cooley DA (1953) Surgical treatment of aneurysm of abdominal aorta by resection and restoration of continuity with homograft. Surg Gynecol Pbstet 97:257–266
20. Voorhees AB Jr, Jaretzki A III, Blakemore AH (1952) The use of tubes constructed from vinyon "N" cloth in bridging arterial defects. Ann Surg 135(3):332–336
21. Friedman S (1989) A history of vascular surgery. Futura, Mt Kisco, NY
22. Levin SM (1987) Reminiscences and ruminations: vascular surgery then and now. Am J Surg 154(2):158–162
23. Blakemore AH, Voorhees AB Jr (1954) The use of tubes constructed from vinyon N cloth in bridging arterial defects; experimental and clinical. Ann Surg 140(3):324–334

24. De Bakey ME et al (1958) Clinical application of a new flexible knitted dacron arterial substitute. AMA Arch Surg 77(5):713–724

25. Creech O Jr (1966) Endo-aneurysmorrhaphy and treatment of aortic aneurysm. Ann Surg 164(6):935–946

26. Melton LJ III et al (1984) Changing incidence of abdominal aortic aneurysms: a population-based study. Am J Epidemiol 120(3):379–386

27. McFarlane MJ (1991) The epidemiologic necropsy for abdominal aortic aneurysm. JAMA 265(16):2085–2088

28. Bengtsson H, Bergqvist D, Sternby NH (1992) Increasing prevalence of abdominal aortic aneurysms. A necropsy study. Eur J Surg 158(1):19–23

29. Katz DJ, Stanley JC, Zelenock GB (1994) Operative mortality rates for intact and ruptured abdominal aortic aneurysms in Michigan: an eleven-year statewide experience. J Vasc Surg 19(5):804–815, discussion 816–817

30. LaMorte WW, Scott TE, Menzoian JO (1995) Racial differences in the incidence of femoral bypass and abdominal aortic aneurysmectomy in Massachusetts: relationship to cardiovascular risk factors. J Vasc Surg 21(3):422–431

31. Blanchard JF (1999) Epidemiology of abdominal aortic aneurysms. Epidemiol Rev 21(2):207–221

32. Wilmink AB et al (2001) The incidence of small abdominal aortic aneurysms and the change in normal infrarenal aortic diameter: implications for screening. Eur J Vasc Endovasc Surg 21(2):165–170

33. Lederle FA et al (2000) Yield of repeated screening for abdominal aortic aneurysm after a 4-year interval. aneurysm detection and management veterans affairs cooperative study investigators. Arch Intern Med 160(8):1117–1121

34. Verloes A et al (1995) Aneurysms of the abdominal aorta: familial and genetic aspects in three hundred thirteen pedigrees. J Vasc Surg 21(4):646–655

35. Johansen K, Koepsell T (1986) Familial tendency for abdominal aortic aneurysms. JAMA 256(14):1934–1936

36. Darling RC III et al (1989) Are familial abdominal aortic aneurysms different? J Vasc Surg 10(1):39–43

37. Cronenwett JL et al (1985) Actuarial analysis of variables associated with rupture of small abdominal aortic aneurysms. Surgery 98(3):472–483

38. Darling RC et al (1977) Autopsy study of unoperated abdominal aortic aneurysms. The case for early resection. Circulation 56(3 Suppl):II161–II164

39. Hammond EC, Garfinkel L (1969) Coronary heart disease, stroke, and aortic aneurysm. Arch Environ Health 19(2):167–182

40. Reed D et al (1992) Are aortic aneurysms caused by atherosclerosis? Circulation 85(1):205–211

41. Breckwoldt WL, Mackey WC, O'Donnell TF Jr (1991) The economic implications of high-risk abdominal aortic aneurysm. J Vasc Surg 13(6):798–803, discussion 803–804

42. Pasch AR et al (1984) Abdominal aortic aneurysm: the case for elective resection. Circulation 70(3 Pt 2):I1–I4

43. Cota AM et al (2005) Elective versus ruptured abdominal aortic aneurysm repair: a 1-year cost-effectiveness analysis. Ann Vasc Surg 19(6):858–861

44. Mehard WB, Heiken JP, Sicard GA (1994) High-attenuating crescent in abdominal aortic aneurysm wall at CT: a sign of acute or impending rupture. Radiology 192(2):359–362

45. Pennell RC et al (1985) Inflammatory abdominal aortic aneurysms: a thirty-year review. J Vasc Surg 2(6):859–869

46. Schermerhorn M et al (2008) Ultrasound screening for abdominal aortic aneurysm in medicare beneficiaries. Ann Vasc Surg 22(1):16–24

47. Derubertis BG et al (2007) Abdominal aortic aneurysm in women: prevalence, risk factors, and implications for screening. J Vasc Surg 46(4):630–635

48. Bengtsson H et al (1991) A population based screening of abdominal aortic aneurysms (AAA). Eur J Vasc Surg 5(1):53–57

49. Lindholt JS et al (1997) Mass or high-risk screening for abdominal aortic aneurysm. Br J Surg 84(1):40–42

50. Morris GE, Hubbard CS, Quick CR (1994) An abdominal aortic aneurysm screening programme for all males over the age of 50 years. Eur J Vasc Surg 8(2):156–160

51. Scott RA, Ashton HA, Kay DN (1991) Abdominal aortic aneurysm in 4,237 screened patients: prevalence, development and management over 6 years. Br J Surg 78(9):1122–1125

52. Scott RA, Bridgewater SG, Ashton HA (2002) Randomized clinical trial of screening for abdominal aortic aneurysm in women. Br J Surg 89(3):283–285

53. Vardulaki KA et al (2002) Late results concerning feasibility and compliance from a randomized trial of ultrasonographic screening for abdominal aortic aneurysm. Br J Surg 89(7):861–864

54. Lindholt JS et al (2002) Hospital costs and benefits of screening for abdominal aortic aneurysms. Results from a randomised population screening trial. Eur J Vasc Endovasc Surg 23(1):55–60

55. Heather BP et al (2000) Population screening reduces mortality rate from aortic aneurysm in men. Br J Surg 87(6):750–753

56. Ashton HA et al (2002) The Multicentre Aneurysm Screening Study (MASS) into the effect of abdominal aortic aneurysm screening on mortality in men: a randomised controlled trial. Lancet 360(9345):1531–1539

57. Kim LG et al (2007) A sustained mortality benefit from screening for abdominal aortic aneurysm. Ann Intern Med 146(10):699–706

58. Lederle FA et al (2002) Immediate repair compared with surveillance of small abdominal aortic aneurysms. N Engl J Med 346(19):1437–1444

59. Powell JT et al (2007) Final 12-year follow-up of surgery versus surveillance in the UK small aneurysm trial. Br J Surg 94(6):702–708

60. Heller JA et al (2000) Two decades of abdominal aortic aneurysm repair: have we made any progress? J Vasc Surg 32(6):1091–1100

61. Hua HT et al (2005) Early outcomes of endovascular versus open abdominal aortic aneurysm repair in the National Surgical Quality Improvement Program-Private Sector (NSQIP-PS). J Vasc Surg 41(3):382–389

62. Huber TS et al (2001) Experience in the United States with intact abdominal aortic aneurysm repair. J Vasc Surg 33(2):304–310, discussion 310–311

63. Hertzer NR et al (2002) Open infrarenal abdominal aortic aneurysm repair: the Cleveland Clinic experience from 1989 to 1998. J Vasc Surg 35(6):1145–1154

64. Lee WA et al (2004) Perioperative outcomes after open and endovascular repair of intact abdominal aortic aneurysms in the United States during 2001. J Vasc Surg 39(3):491–496

65. Akkersdijk GJ, Prinssen M, Blankensteijn JD (2004) The impact of endovascular treatment on in-hospital mortality following nonruptured AAA repair over a decade: a population based study of 16,446 patients. Eur J Vasc Endovasc Surg 28(1):41–46

66. Anderson PL et al (2004) A statewide experience with endovascular abdominal aortic aneurysm repair: rapid diffusion with excellent early results. J Vasc Surg 39(1):10–19

67. Bush RL et al (2007) Performance of endovascular aortic aneurysm repair in high-risk patients: results from the Veterans Affairs National Surgical Quality Improvement Program. J Vasc Surg 45(2):227–233, discussion 233–235

68. Blankensteijn JD et al (2005) Two-year outcomes after conventional or endovascular repair of abdominal aortic aneurysms. N Engl J Med 352(23):2398–2405

69. Greenhalgh RM et al (2004) Comparison of endovascular aneurysm repair with open repair in patients with abdominal aortic aneurysm (EVAR trial 1), 30-day operative mortality results: randomised controlled trial. Lancet 364(9437):843–848

70. Sicard GA et al (2006) Endovascular abdominal aortic aneurysm repair: long-term outcome measures in patients at high-risk for open surgery. J Vasc Surg 44(2):229–236

71. Lifeline Registry of EVAR Publications Committee (2005) Lifeline registry of endovascular aneurysm repair: long-term primary outcome measures. J Vasc Surg 42(1):1–10

72. Hirose Y, Hamada S, Takamiya M (1995) Predicting the growth of aortic aneurysms: a comparison of linear vs. exponential models. Angiology 46(5):413–419

73. Englund R et al (1998) Expansion rates of small abdominal aortic aneurysms. Aust N Z J Surg 68(1):21–24

74. Bengtsson H et al (1989) Ultrasound screening of the abdominal aorta in patients with intermittent claudication. Eur J Vasc Surg 3(6):497–502

75. Fillinger MF et al (2002) In vivo analysis of mechanical wall stress and abdominal aortic aneurysm rupture risk. J Vasc Surg 36(3):589–597

76. Fillinger MF et al (2003) Prediction of rupture risk in abdominal aortic aneurysm during observation: wall stress versus diameter. J Vasc Surg 37(4):724–732

77. Steyerberg EW et al (1995) Perioperative mortality of elective abdominal aortic aneurysm surgery. A clinical prediction rule based on literature and individual patient data. Arch Intern Med 155(18):1998–2004

78. Hallin A, Bergqvist D, Holmberg L (2001) Literature review of surgical management of abdominal aortic aneurysm. Eur J Vasc Endovasc Surg 22(3):197–204

79. Dardik A et al (1999) Results of elective abdominal aortic aneurysm repair in the 1990s: a population-based analysis of 2,335 cases. J Vasc Surg 30(6):985–995

80. Dimick JB et al (2003) Surgeon specialty and provider volumes are related to outcome of intact abdominal aortic aneurysm repair in the United States. J Vasc Surg 38(4):739–744

81. Larsson E et al (2008) A population-based case–control study of the familial risk of abdominal aortic aneurysm. J Vasc Surg 49(1):47–50

82. Scott RA et al (1998) Abdominal aortic aneurysm rupture rates: a 7-year follow-up of the entire abdominal aortic aneurysm population detected by screening. J Vasc Surg 28(1):124–128

83. Wanhainen A et al (2005) Risk factors associated with abdominal aortic aneurysm: a population-based study with historical and current data. J Vasc Surg 41(3):390–396

84. Hertzer NR, Mascha EJ (2005) A personal experience with factors influencing survival after elective open repair of infrarenal aortic aneurysms. J Vasc Surg 42(5):898–905

85. Crawford ES et al (1981) Infrarenal abdominal aortic aneurysm: factors influencing survival after operation performed over a 25-year period. Ann Surg 193(6):699–709

86. Sicard GA et al (2001) Endoluminal graft repair for abdominal aortic aneurysms in high-risk patients and octogenarians: is it better than open repair? Ann Surg 234(4):427–435, discussion 435–437

87. Johnston KW (1994) Nonruptured abdominal aortic aneurysm: six-year follow-up results from the multicenter prospective Canadian aneurysm study. Canadian Society for Vascular Surgery Aneurysm Study Group. J Vasc Surg 20(2):163–170

88. Roger VL et al (1989) Influence of coronary artery disease on morbidity and mortality after abdominal aortic aneurysmectomy: a population-based study, 1971–1987. J Am Coll Cardiol 14(5): 1245–1252

89. Fleisher LA et al (2007) ACC/AHA 2007 guidelines on perioperative cardiovascular evaluation and care for noncardiac surgery: a report of the American College of Cardiology/American Heart Association Task Force on Practice Guidelines (Writing Committee to Revise the 2002 Guidelines on Perioperative Cardiovascular Evaluation for Noncardiac Surgery): developed in collaboration with the American Society of Echocardiography, American Society of Nuclear Cardiology, Heart Rhythm Society, Society of Cardiovascular Anesthesiologists, Society for Cardiovascular Angiography and Interventions, Society for Vascular Medicine and Biology, and Society for Vascular Surgery. Circulation 116(17):e418–e499

90. Van Damme H et al (1997) Cardiac risk assessment before vascular surgery: a prospective study comparing clinical evaluation, dobutamine stress echocardiography, and dobutamine Tc-99m sestamibi tomoscintigraphy. Cardiovasc Surg 5(1):54–64

91. Poldermans D et al (2006) Should major vascular surgery be delayed because of preoperative cardiac testing in intermediate-risk patients receiving beta-blocker therapy with tight heart rate control? J Am Coll Cardiol 48(5):964–969

92. McFalls EO et al (2004) Coronary-artery revascularization before elective major vascular surgery. N Engl J Med 351(27):2795–2804

93. Kertai MD et al (2004) A combination of statins and beta-blockers is independently associated with a reduction in the incidence of perioperative mortality and nonfatal myocardial infarction in patients undergoing abdominal aortic aneurysm surgery. Eur J Vasc Endovasc Surg 28(4):343–352

94. Desiron Q et al (1995) Isolated atherosclerotic aneurysms of the iliac arteries. Ann Vasc Surg 9(Suppl):S62–S66

95. Conrad MF et al (2007) Long-term durability of open abdominal aortic aneurysm repair. J Vasc Surg 46(4):669–675

96. Barnes M et al (2008) A model to predict outcomes for endovascular aneurysm repair using preoperative variables. Eur J Vasc Endovasc Surg 35(5):571–579

97. Parodi JC, Palmaz JC, Barone HD (1991) Transfemoral intraluminal graft implantation for abdominal aortic aneurysms. Ann Vasc Surg 5(6):491–499

98. Zarins CK et al (1999) AneuRx stent graft versus open surgical repair of abdominal aortic aneurysms: multicenter prospective clinical trial. J Vasc Surg 29(2):292–305, discussion 306–308

99. EVAR trial participants (2005) Endovascular aneurysm repair and outcome in patients unfit for open repair of abdominal aortic aneurysm (EVAR trial 2): randomised controlled trial. Lancet 365(9478):2187–2192

100. Brewster DC et al (1998) Initial experience with endovascular aneurysm repair: comparison of early results with outcome of conventional open repair. J Vasc Surg 27(6):992–1003, discussion 1004–1005

101. Sanchez LA et al (1995) Placement of endovascular stented grafts via remote access sites: a new approach to the treatment of failed aortoiliofemoral reconstructions. Ann Vasc Surg 9(1):1–8

102. Krupski WC et al (1998) Contemporary management of isolated iliac aneurysms. J Vasc Surg 28(1):1–11, discussion 11–13

103. Clinical Update, Vol. 4, The AneuRx AAA Stent Graft System. 2007

104. Fairman RM et al (2008) Pivotal results of the Medtronic Vascular Talent Thoracic Stent Graft System: the VALOR trial. J Vasc Surg 48(3):546–554

105. Greenberg RK et al (2008) Zenith abdominal aortic aneurysm endovascular graft. J Vasc Surg 48(1):1–9

106. Peterson BG et al (2007) Five-year report of a multicenter controlled clinical trial of open versus endovascular treatment of abdominal aortic aneurysms. J Vasc Surg 45(5):885–890

107. Wang GJ, Carpenter JP (2008) The Powerlink system for endovascular abdominal aortic aneurysm repair: six-year results. J Vasc Surg 48(3):535–545

108. LaCroix H (1997) The optimal surgical approach for elective reconstruction of the infra- and juxtarenal abdominal aorta: a randomized prospective study. Acta Biomed Lovaniensia 157:1–131

109. Sicard GA et al (1995) Transabdominal versus retroperitoneal incision for abdominal aortic surgery: report of a prospective randomized trial. J Vasc Surg 21(2):174–181, discussion 181–183

110. Ali ZA et al (2007) Perioperative myocardial injury after elective open abdominal aortic aneurysm repair predicts outcome. Eur J Vasc Endovasc Surg 35(4):413–419

111. Elkouri S et al (2004) Perioperative complications and early outcome after endovascular and open surgical repair of abdominal aortic aneurysms. J Vasc Surg 39(3):497–505

112. Miller DC, Myers BD (1987) Pathophysiology and prevention of acute renal failure associated with thoracoabdominal or abdominal aortic surgery. J Vasc Surg 5(3):518–523

113. West CA et al (2006) Factors affecting outcomes of open surgical repair of pararenal aortic aneurysms: a 10-year experience. J Vasc Surg 43(5):921–927, discussion 927–928

114. Walsh SR, Tang TY, Boyle JR (2008) Renal consequences of endovascular abdominal aortic aneurysm repair. J Endovasc Ther 15(1):73–82

115. Brandt CP, Piotrowski JJ, Alexander JJ (1997) Flexible sigmoidoscopy. A reliable determinant of colonic ischemia following ruptured abdominal aortic aneurysm. Surg Endosc 11(2):113–115

116. Boley SJ, Brandt LJ, Veith FJ (1978) Ischemic disorders of the intestines. Curr Probl Surg 15(4):1–85

117. Boley SJ (1990) 1989 David H. Sun lecture. Colonic ischemia – 25 years later. Am J Gastroenterol 85(8):931–934

118. Brewster DC et al (1991) Intestinal ischemia complicating abdominal aortic surgery. Surgery 109(4):447–454

119. Bjorck M, Bergqvist D, Troeng T (1996) Incidence and clinical presentation of bowel ischaemia after aortoiliac surgery – 2,930 operations from a population-based registry in Sweden. Eur J Vasc Endovasc Surg 12(2):139–144

120. Longo WE et al (1996) Ischemic colitis complicating abdominal aortic aneurysm surgery in the U.S. veteran. J Surg Res 60(2):351–354

121. Levison JA et al (1999) Perioperative predictors of colonic ischemia after ruptured abdominal aortic aneurysm. J Vasc Surg 29(1):40–45, discussion 45–47

122. Pittaluga P et al (1998) Revascularization of internal iliac arteries during aortoiliac surgery: a multicenter study. Ann Vasc Surg 12(6):537–543

123. Van Damme H, Creemers E, Limet R (2000) Ischaemic colitis following aortoiliac surgery. Acta Chir Belg 100(1):21–27

124. Bast TJ et al (1990) Ischaemic disease of the colon and rectum after surgery for abdominal aortic aneurysm: a prospective study of the incidence and risk factors. Eur J Vasc Surg 4(3):253–257

125. Batt M, Ricco JB, Staccini P (2001) Do internal iliac arteries contribute to vascularization of the descending colon during abdominal aortic aneurysm surgery? An intraoperative hemodynamic study. Ann Vasc Surg 15(2):171–174

126. Kuttila K et al (1994) Tonometric assessment of sigmoid perfusion during aortobifemoral reconstruction for arteriosclerosis. Eur J Surg 160(9):491–495

127. Schiedler MG, Cutler BS, Fiddian-Green RG (1987) Sigmoid intramural pH for prediction of ischemic colitis during aortic surgery. A comparison with risk factors and inferior mesenteric artery stump pressures. Arch Surg 122(8):881–886

128. Mehta M et al (2004) Effects of bilateral hypogastric artery interruption during endovascular and open aortoiliac aneurysm repair. J Vasc Surg 40(4):698–702

129. Rhee RY et al (2002) Can the internal iliac artery be safely covered during endovascular repair of abdominal aortic and iliac artery aneurysms? Ann Vasc Surg 16(1):29–36

130. Wyers MC et al (2002) Internal iliac occlusion without coil embolization during endovascular abdominal aortic aneurysm repair. J Vasc Surg 36(6):1138–1145

131. Geraghty PJ et al (2004) Overt ischemic colitis after endovascular repair of aortoiliac aneurysms. J Vasc Surg 40(3):413–418

132. Mehta M et al (2001) Unilateral and bilateral hypogastric artery interruption during aortoiliac aneurysm repair in 154 patients: a relatively innocuous procedure. J Vasc Surg 33(2 Suppl):S27–S32

133. Lederle FA et al (2003) Quality of life, impotence, and activity level in a randomized trial of immediate repair versus surveillance of small abdominal aortic aneurysm. J Vasc Surg 38(4):745–752

134. Flanigan DP et al (1982) Elimination of iatrogenic impotence and improvement of sexual function after aortoiliac revascularization. Arch Surg 117(5):544–550

135. Weinstein MH, Machleder HI (1975) Sexual function after aortoiliac surgery. Ann Surg 181(6):787–790

136. Blum U et al (1997) Endoluminal stent-grafts for infrarenal abdominal aortic aneurysms. N Engl J Med 336(1):13–20

137. Buth J et al (2002) Outcome of endovascular abdominal aortic aneurysm repair in patients with conditions considered unfit for an open procedure: a report on the EUROSTAR experience. J Vasc Surg 35(2):211–221

138. Mialhe C, Amicabile C, Becquemin JP (1997) Endovascular treatment of infrarenal abdominal aneurysms by the Stentor system: preliminary results of 79 cases. Stentor Retrospective Study Group. J Vasc Surg 26(2):199–209

139. Moore WS, Rutherford RB (1996) Transfemoral endovascular repair of abdominal aortic aneurysm: results of the North American EVT phase 1 trial. EVT Investigators. J Vasc Surg 23(4):543–553

140. Stelter W, Umscheid T, Ziegler P (1997) Three-year experience with modular stent-graft devices for endovascular AAA treatment. J Endovasc Surg 4(4):362–369

141. Matsumura JS et al (2003) A multicenter controlled clinical trial of open versus endovascular treatment of abdominal aortic aneurysm. J Vasc Surg 37(2):262–271

142. Abraham CZ et al (2002) Abdominal aortic aneurysm repair with the Zenith stent graft: short to midterm results. J Vasc Surg 36(2):217–224, discussion 224–225

143. Carpenter JP (2002) Multicenter trial of the PowerLink bifurcated system for endovascular aortic aneurysm repair. J Vasc Surg 36(6):1129–1137

144. van Marrewijk CJ et al (2004) Is a type II endoleak after EVAR a harbinger of risk? Causes and outcome of open conversion and aneurysm rupture during follow-up. Eur J Vasc Endovasc Surg 27(2):128–137

145. Greenberg R (2003) The Zenith AAA endovascular graft for abdominal aortic aneurysms: clinical update. Semin Vasc Surg 16(2):151–157

146. Rosenthal D (1999) Spinal cord ischemia after abdominal aortic operation: is it preventable? J Vasc Surg 30(3):391–397

147. Berg P et al (2001) Spinal cord ischaemia after stent-graft treatment for infra-renal abdominal aortic aneurysms. Analysis of the Eurostar database. Eur J Vasc Endovasc Surg 22(4):342–347

148. Maldonado TS et al (2004) Ischemic complications after endovascular abdominal aortic aneurysm repair. J Vasc Surg 40(4):703–709, discussion 709–710

149. Boult M et al (2006) Predictors of success following endovascular aneurysm repair: mid-term results. Eur J Vasc Endovasc Surg 31(2):123–129

150. Dillavou ED et al (2003) Does hostile neck anatomy preclude successful endovascular aortic aneurysm repair? J Vasc Surg 38(4):657–663

151. Green RM (2002) Patient selection for endovascular abdominal aortic aneurysm repair. J Am Coll Surg 194(1 Suppl):S67–S73

152. Ricotta JJ II, Oderich GS (2008) Fenestrated and branched stent grafts. Perspect Vasc Surg Endovasc Ther 20(2):174–187, discussion 188–189

153. Sampaio SM et al (2004) Proximal type I endoleak after endovascular abdominal aortic aneurysm repair: predictive factors. Ann Vasc Surg 18(6):621–628

154. Schumacher H et al (1997) Morphometry and classification in abdominal aortic aneurysms: patient selection for endovascular and open surgery. J Endovasc Surg 4(1):39–44

155. Brewster DC et al (2003) Guidelines for the treatment of abdominal aortic aneurysms. Report of a subcommittee of the Joint Council of the American Association for Vascular Surgery and Society for Vascular Surgery. J Vasc Surg 37(5): 1106–1117

156. Sarac TP et al (2002) Contemporary results of juxtarenal aneurysm repair. J Vasc Surg 36(6):1104–1111

157. Greenberg RK et al (2006) Beyond the aortic bifurcation: branched endovascular grafts for thoracoabdominal and aortoiliac aneurysms. J Vasc Surg 43(5):879–886, discussion 886–887

158. Cambria RP et al (2002) Thoracoabdominal aneurysm repair: results with 337 operations performed over a 15-year interval. Ann Surg 236(4):471–479, discussion 479

159. Coselli JS (1994) Thoracoabdominal aortic aneurysms: experience with 372 patients. J Card Surg 9(6):638–647

160. Cowan JA Jr et al (2003) Surgical treatment of intact thoracoabdominal aortic aneurysms in the United States: hospital and surgeon volume-related outcomes. J Vasc Surg 37(6): 1169–1174

161. Cox GS et al (1992) Thoracoabdominal aneurysm repair: a representative experience. J Vasc Surg 15(5):780–787, discussion 787–788

162. Hines GL, Busutil S (1994) Thoraco-abdominal aneurysm resection. Determinants of survival in a community hospital. J Cardiovasc Surg (Torino) 35(6 Suppl 1):243–246

163. Chuter TA (2007) Fenestrated and branched stent-grafts for thoracoabdominal, pararenal and juxtarenal aortic aneurysm repair. Semin Vasc Surg 20(2):90–96

Section VIII
Gastrointestinal System

Chapter 57
Invited Commentary

Courtney M. Townsend Jr.

A 92-year-old widow, who lived alone, underwent a laparoscopic right hemicolectomy for a stage IIA cecal cancer found on workup after falling while climbing stairs at her home. Past history is important because of lack of systemic disease, no prescription medications, and only one visit to a doctor (for dog bite at an age of 86) in the past 57 years. She had no nasogastric tube and was disoriented periodically for the first two postoperative days with complete clearing without treatment and transferred to a rehabilitation floor on the seventh day for 2 weeks of reconditioning. She returned home where she resumed her activity, but with caregivers living with her. She had one postoperative visit with her doctor, then no further follow-up. At an age of 98, after 2 days of failure to eat and two episodes of vomiting, she was found to have a circumferential lesion in the mid-sigmoid colon that prevented retrograde passage of barium administered by enema. She had an emergency Hartmann's resection for a stage IIIB sigmoid colon cancer. Both the surgeon and anesthesiologist remarked that they had never taken part in an operation on a 98-year-old patient. The patient had no nasogastric tube, was disoriented periodically for the first three postoperative days, which cleared without treatment,

and she was discharged to a rehabilitation floor for 3 weeks. The patient required no narcotics after either operation. She then returned to her home where she resumed her activity and died 1 month short of her 101st birthday.

Abdominal surgery in elderly patients has made great strides in the past 30 years. More and more elderly patients have no or minimal comorbid conditions so that they are much more robust. Changes in operative and postoperative management as illustrated in this case have decreased complications and shortened the length of stay. Minimally invasive procedures, lack of use of drugs in expected postoperative disorientation, reduced use of narcotics, absent use of nasogastric tubes, and early ambulation have all improved outcomes in these patients. The absence of significant systemic disease must be recognized by surgeons and anesthesiologists as evidence that these patients can undergo required operations safely. Operations or other indicated treatments should not be withheld just because of a patient's advanced age. They should be treated as the conditions require. The chapters in this section reflect the significant advances in operative treatment of increasingly elderly patients.

C.M. Townsend Jr. (✉)
Department of Surgery, University of Texas Medical Branch, 301 University Blvd, Galveston, TX 77555-0527, USA
e-mail: ctownsen@utmb.edu

R.A. Rosenthal et al. (eds.), *Principles and Practice of Geriatric Surgery*,
DOI 10.1007/978-1-4419-6999-6_57, © Springer Science+Business Media, LLC 2011

Chapter 58
Age-Related Changes in the Gastrointestinal Tract

Nefertiti A. Brown, Joshua L. Levine, and Michael E. Zenilman

The multitude of changes that take place in the gastrointestinal tract throughout the life of a human have various clinical and surgical repercussions. Although our knowledge of age-related changes is growing, their consequences are still the subject of much debate and controversy. One problem when assessing the effects of aging on humans is the extreme physiologic variability seen among elderly individuals. As individuals age, differences among them increase, such as those relating to the genetic distinctions, exposure to toxins, and environmental, psychological, and physical factors. Additionally, it becomes increasingly difficult and to isolate control groups of healthy subjects because the elderly commonly have multiple medical problems. Many of these illnesses, such as diabetes, tend to confound study outcomes by adversely affecting the organs studied. Another obstacle to study age-related changes involves the vast reserve capacity with which to the human body is endowed. Some areas of the gastrointestinal tract and liver are capable of handling many times the quantitative functional capacity required during normal life and compensate well for normal physiological loss with aging, which makes it difficult to detect age-related changes in function even though they may be apparent on a microscopic level.

Esophagus

In the upper third of the human esophagus, the longitudinal and the circular muscles are striated. The second third is composed of both striated and smooth muscle fibers, and the lower third is entirely smooth muscle. Normal esophageal motor function is characterized by a peristaltic wave, which begins at the upper esophageal sphincter (UES) and propagates through the striated and smooth muscle layers to terminate in closure of the lower esophageal sphincter (LES). This peristaltic wave is initiated by swallowing, which is controlled centrally or by a bolus within the upper esophageal lumen (primary and secondary peristalsis, respectively). Activation of intrinsic peripheral control, which can function independently of the central control mechanism, helps propel the peristaltic wave forward (Fig. 58.1). The functions of the LES, which are controlled both locally and centrally, depend on various factors, including myogenic specialization, excitatory and inhibitory neural elements, and circulating hormones.

Difficulties with swallowing become more prevalent with increasing age. Problems with swallowing are multifactorial, ranging from physiologic parameters including oral, pharyngeal, and esophageal to neurologic conditions such as stroke, head injury, and other neurodegenerative diseases [1, 2]. Many comorbid conditions are involved with abnormal deglutition, which in itself carries increased complications of aspiration, pneumonia, dehydration, and malnutrition [3]. Ekberg and Feinberg found 84% of 56 healthy elderly subjects (mean age 83) to have swallowing abnormalities compared to that considered in normal young persons [4]. Evaluation of videofluoroscopy and radiographs with the subjects erect and recumbent found problems at each phase of swallowing. Altogether, 63% of the swallowing problems were due to oral abnormalities (difficulty ingesting, controlling, and delivering the bolus relative to swallowing initiation), 25% were due to pharyngeal dysfunction (bolus retention and lingual propulsion or pharyngeal constrictor paresis), 39% were due to pharyngoesophageal abnormalities (mostly cricopharyngeal muscle dysfunction), and 36% were due to intrinsic esophageal abnormalities (mostly motor in nature). Nilsson et al. compared 17 swallowing variables between young (average age 37) and nondysphagic elderly (average age 81.2) patients and found that oral transit time, pharyngeal delay time, and pharyngeal transit time in dentate elderly persons were prolonged significantly as they required more swallows to clear the oral cavity. Multiple swallows also predisposed them to increased inspiration resulting in increased coughing [5]. This lack of coordination may explain the increased incidence of aspiration that occurs with aging.

N.A. Brown (✉)
Department of Surgery, SUNY Downstate Medical Center,
450 Clarkson Avenue, Box 40, Brooklyn, NY 11203, USA
e-mail: nefertitibrownMD@aol.com

R.A. Rosenthal et al. (eds.), *Principles and Practice of Geriatric Surgery*,
DOI 10.1007/978-1-4419-6999-6_58, © Springer Science+Business Media, LLC 2011

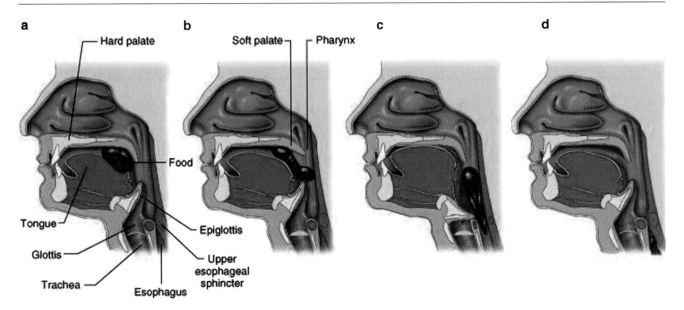

Figure 58.1 Movement of food through the pharynx and upper esophagus during swallowing. (**a**) The tongue pushes the food bolus to the back of the mouth. (**b**) The soft palate elevates to prevent food from entering the nasopharynx. (**c**) The epiglottis covers the glottis to prevent food from entering the airway and the upper esophageal sphincter relaxes. (**d**) Food descends into the esophagus (reprinted with permission from Barett et al. [96]).

Various UES abnormalities have been shown to be related to advance age. Mean resting UES pressure has been shown to be a decrease in elderly subjects, and UES relaxation is delayed [6]. Combined with the fact that the sensitivity of the cough reflex appears to be significantly reduced in elderly subjects [7] may increase the risk of aspiration pneumonia. Both increased age and aspiration are risk factors for nosocomial pneumonia, which is three times more prevalent in older age groups than in the general population [8]. Older subjects also tend to have markedly elevated pharyngeal contraction pressures, with a reduction in the duration of the upper esophageal contraction [9]. These findings help to explain dysphagia in some patients.

Presbyesophagus, or degenerating motor function in the esophagus, has long been associated with advanced age. Whether old age in and of itself is the cause, however, remains controversial. Early studies by Zboralske et al. [10] and Soergel et al. [11] found that a reduced rate of peristalsis following swallowing in the elderly is accompanied by an increase in nonpropulsive contractions. This results in discoordination of muscular activity in the esophagus. Other age-related changes found were a defect in the initiation of LES relaxation and a primary peristalsis shown by cineradiography, intraluminal manometry, and balloon kymography in nonagenarians. The studies found esophageal motor function to be disorganized and inefficient, with various abnormalities, including reduced or absent peristalsis, frequent and prominent tertiary contractions, delayed esophageal emptying, and dilation of the esophagus [11]. Radiographic evaluations on nonagenarians have also shown a higher incidence of intrathoracic LES (which normally straddles the diaphragmatic hiatus) [10].

These studies have been criticized for having included patients with diabetes and senile dementia, diseases that can contribute to esophageal dysmotility. However, a later study that controlled for these diseases but used younger subjects (70–87 years old) found decreased amplitude of esophageal peristalsis in the elderly but no increase in abnormal motility [12]. Adamek et al. confirm that age is of little significance in esophageal dysmotility. This study also showed, however, a tendency among the older subjects toward an increase in the following parameters: distal pressure amplitudes, quotient of distal and proximal pressure amplitudes, distal duration, and percentage of simultaneous waves. The percentage of propulsive waves and proximal pressure amplitude and duration tended to decrease in the subjects [13]. It should also be pointed out that the "older" subjects' median age in this study was just 62.4 years.

The contribution of aging to presbyesophagus remains to be fully elucidated. Some evidence suggests that dysphagia and aperistalsis can be attributed to aging alone in a distinct, small group of patients. Meshkinpour et al. performed esophageal manometry in 562 patients and found that in 29 aperistaltic patients no secondary explanation was detected. Of these patients, 26 were 65 years or older and only three were 40 years and younger. They concluded that aging remains a possible explanation [14].

Another study used only healthy volunteers to evaluate secondary esophageal peristalsis, which is believed to play an important role in the volume clearance of the esophagus of ingested material left behind after a swallow. This investigation found that in healthy elderly volunteers secondary peristalsis is either absent or its stimulation is inconsistent and significantly less frequent compared to that and younger volunteers. The frequency of stimulation of LES relaxation in response to intraesophageal air distention in the elderly was also significantly lower and that of the young. These elderly subjects demonstrated normal primary peristalsis, indicating an intact central, preganglionic, ganglionic, and postganglionic control mechanism. These findings suggest an intrinsic defect in the afferent neural pathway, reduced concentration (or absence) of tension-sensitive receptors within the esophageal wall, or both [15].

Degenerative esophageal neurologic changes in the elderly have also been suggested by the study of other esophageal functions. Graded intraesophageal balloon distension was used to evaluate the visceral pain threshold in patients older than 65 years compared to those in the young age group. Investigators found that upon inflation of the balloon 10 cm above the LES the mean pain threshold balloon volumes in the young subjects was 17.0 ± 0.8 ml of air, and for the elderly subjects it was 27.0 ± 1.4 ml ($P < 0.01$). In the elderly group, five patients felt no pain even at maximum inflatable volume of the balloon (30 ml). These data suggest an age-related decrease in visceral pain threshold [16].

Some studies have suggested neurologic loss as a possible mechanism to explain the facts in both motility and sensory thresholds. Histologic data have linked a decrease in the number of cells in Auerbach's plexus as part of the aging process in healthy elderly individuals [17]. Filho et al. showed that patients over 70 years had a decrease in the number of neurons along the esophagus compared to subjects aged 20–40 years. This decrease in number was accompanied by the increase in the size of the neurons, suggesting that compensatory growth may be an attempt to maintain neuronal density [18]. Recent studies indicate that neuronal losses occur in the myenteric as well as submucosal plexuses and are linked to the selective preservation of nitrergic over cholinergic neurons. The reasons for this specificity are unclear [19]. Despite evidence of these age-related changes, it has been difficult to show a significant correlation between these changes and clinical dysfunction. As more studies are done with a growing population of elderly subjects, this potential mechanism will be further elucidated.

Stomach

Many of the various functions of the stomach have been studied in the aging population. A brief overview of the normal stomach physiology follows.

The epithelial lining of the stomach lumen is characterized by thick folds called rugae, which contained microscopic gastric pits. The mucosal surface of the stomach and the linings of the gastric pits are composed of mucin-secreting columnar cells. The gastric glands are contained within the gastric pits and are responsible for secreting hydrochloric acid (HCl), pepsinogen, gastrin, intrinsic factor, mucus, and various gastrointestinal hormones. The capacity of the stomach to produce HCl is directly proportional to the parietal cell mass in the glands of the body and the fundus. The parietal cells secrete HCl by a process involving oxidative phosphorylation, the final step of which is accomplished by a sodium–potassium "proton pump" located in the apical membrane. Regulation of gastric acid secretion is controlled by histamine, gastrin, and postganglionic vagal fibers via muscarinic cholinergic receptors [20].

The motor activity of the stomach is essential to digestion in both the fasting and fed states. Between meals, contractile patterns clear the stomach of undigested material, and then the stomach relaxes and expands to receive a food bolus. The meal is ground and delivered to the small intestine for further digestion. This delivery is accomplished by a complex series of muscular contractions in the proximal and distal stomach [20]. These distinct physiologic regions of the stomach must coordinate contractile function to deliver the stomach contents to the duodenum. Gastric emptying has been found to depend on the type of food it contains: liquid, solid, or fat [20].

The cumulative effect of stress and exposure to various ingested substances over one's lifetime, such as ethanol, aspirin, and toxins, made me as the stomach mucosa and atrophic gastritis, gastric atrophy, achlorhydria, and intrinsic factor deficiency. These changes are difficult to distinguish from those resulting from age alone.

Acid Production

It is generally agreed that gastroduodenal secretory function changes with increased age, but the extent and the direction of the change remains controversial. Historically, it has been accepted that acid secretion declines as a consequence of normal aging. This observation, however, was based on studies that often included subjects with medical problems rather than healthy volunteers. The studies also predated understanding of the role of the bacterium *Helicobacter pylori* in acid production. *H. pylori*, found in more than 75% of individuals over the age of 60 [21], may cause transient hypochlorhydria in acutely infected patients (Fig. 58.2). Although long-term studies have not been conclusive, epidemiologic data suggest that long-standing *H. pylori infection* may result in reduced acid secretion secondary to atrophic changes in the gastric mucosa [22].

A large ($n = 437$) computer-selected family sample of the Finnish population aged 15 years or over was extensively studied in 1982 with pentagastrin stimulation and mucosal

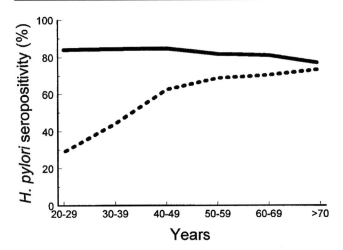

Figure 58.2 Age distribution of *Helicobacter pylori* seropositivity in gastric cancer cases (*bold line*) and normal controls (*dotted line*). In the control group, the prevalence of *H. pylori* increased significantly with advancing age. In patients with gastric cancer, *H. pylori* seropositivity is >70% in patients regardless of age, reflecting that *H. pylori* infection is a risk for development if gastric cancer (from Huang et al. [97] reprinted with permission from Elsevier).

biopsies. Gastric acid output, expressed as millimoles per hour (mmol/h), mmol/kg/h of total body weight (TBW), mmol/h/kg of lean body mass (LBM), and mmol/h/kg of fat-free body weight (FFB), correlated with the changes in the body mucosa but not with those of the antrum. This investigation also found that gastric acid secretion declines with age but did not attribute this change to aging alone. Reduced acid production did, however, correlate with atrophic gastritis (Table 58.1). Male patients with normal mucosa had no significant change in acid output, and female patients with normal mucosa actually demonstrated an increase in acid production when expressed in FFB (Table 58.2) [23].

More recently, Haruma et al. in 2000 studied the relationship between gastric acid secretion, age, and *H. pylori* infection in 280 patients with various grades of fundic atrophic gastritis (FAG) and found that basal and maximal acid output decreased with increasing age in *H. pylori*-positive patients while it had no effect on aging *H. pylori*-negative patients. The authors believe that these results correlate with the increased prevalence of FAG with age, with the progression of FAG directly proportional to the rate of gastric acid secretion [24]. This finding confirms that of prior studies that compared gastric acid secretion and *H. pylori* infection in young and old patients, concluding that gastric acid secretion does not decline as the result of healthy aging [22, 25]. Only gastritis had a negative effect on acid secretion, and *H. pylori* is commonly the causative agent [24, 26].

Studies finding a correlation between atrophic gastritis and reduced gastric acid secretion during old age are supported by the knowledge of the pathophysiology of pernicious anemia. Pernicious anemia is a disease of the elderly, the average

patient presenting near age 60. With this condition atrophy of the gastric mucosa results in decreased intrinsic factor secretion (also a product of the parietal cells), leading to reduced cobalamin uptake.

Gastric Emptying

Despite the abundance of data on gastric motility, the effect of aging on gastric emptying remains controversial. The importance of this finding extends beyond the obvious morbidity it causes in affected patients. For example, the rate of gastric emptying can influence the rate and extent of absorption of orally administered drugs, thereby influencing the rate and duration of their pharmacologic effect.

Various radioisotope methods have been employed in early studies to evaluate gastric emptying in the elderly (Table 58.3) [27, 28]. Horowitz et al. used a double isotope technique on healthy young ($n=22$; age 21–62, mean age 34) and elderly ($n=13$; age 70–84, mean age 77) subjects to evaluate gastric emptying of both liquids and solids. The data showed a statistically significant delay in both among the elderly subjects [29]. A similar study found that gastric emptying of solid foods did not change with age, but a delay in liquid phase emptying was observed [30]. In another study, Moore et al. also demonstrated a delay in gastric emptying of liquids in the elderly [28]. Evans et al. used a modified sequential scintiscanning after administration of the nonabsorbable chelated radiopharmaceutical technetium 99m-diethylenetriaminepentaacetic acid (^{99m}Tc-DTPA) to show that the rate of emptying was significantly longer in elderly subjects. The investigators concluded that it could explain a delay in absorption of drugs with aging. This study, however, did not control for the presence of concomitant chronic diseases such as parkinsonism, hypothyroidism, transient ischemic attacks, and strokes [27].

Clarkston et al. [31] used two isotopes to evaluate the gastric emptying of solid and liquid foods. The patients were healthy young ($n=19$, age 23–50) and old ($n=14$, age 70–84) volunteers who were evaluated sitting at a 45° angle. Gastric emptying of both solids and liquids was found to be delayed in the elderly patients. This investigation also found that the elderly had reduced hunger and desire to eat after a meal, which was thought to be in effect of delayed gastric emptying.

More recently Madsen and Graff [32] studied all segments of the GI tract, using the gamma camera technique, to observe the transit of radiolabeled liquid and solid meals. Compared to young, healthy subjects (aged 20–30, $n=16$), they found that advanced age ($n=16$, age 74–85) did not affect gastric emptying or the postprandial frequency of antral contractions or transit rate of the small intestine. They did find, however, that normal aging may decrease the colonic motility.

TABLE 58.1   Relation of acid output to age, sex, and morphology of the body mucosa acid output

Parameter	Men (ages ≤30 to≥70)				Women (ages ≤30 to≥70)				Units
	≤30	31–50	51–70	>70	≤30	31–50	51–70	>70	
Acid output per									
Total body weight	0.47±0.19	0.45±0.19	0.33±0.22	0.20±0.20	0.39±0.13	0.37±0.16	0.24±0.18	0.21±0.18	mmol/h/kg TBW
Fat-free body weight	0.60±0.23	0.59±0.25	0.46±0.31	0.29±0.29	0.54±0.18	0.58±0.24	0.40±0.28	0.34±0.29	mmol/h/kg FFBW
Lean body mass	0.62±0.23	0.62±0.27	0.46±0.31	0.28±0.28	0.52±0.17	0.55±0.23	0.37±0.27	0.32±0.28	mmol/h/kg LBW
Prevalence of atrophic gastritis (%)[a]	9	11	25	53	3	8	31	43	

Source: Adapted from Kekki et al. [23]

[a]Body gastritis

TABLE 58.2   Acid output in relation to morphologic state of the body mucosa

Mucosal status	Acid output (mmol/hr)		Acid output (mmol/hr/FFB)	
	Men	Women	Men	Women
Normal	36.5±13.2[a]	24.2±13.3[b]	0.63±0.20[c]	0.60±0.20[d]
Superficial gastritis	31.5±15.1[e]	21.1±17.9[f]	0.57±0.26[g]	0.51±0.22[h]
Slight atrophic gastritis	15.2±13.8[i]	10.33±18.4[j]	0.31±0.26[k]	0.25±0.28[l]
Moderate and severe atrophic gastritis	2.2±4.4[m]	1.38±4.0[n]	0.04±0.10[o]	0.03±0.09[p]

Source: Adapted from Kekki et al. [23]

a vs. b, $P<0.001$; c vs. d, NS; e vs. f, $P<0.001$; g vs. h, NS; i vs. j, NS; k vs. l, NS; m vs. n, NS; o vs. q, NS; a vs. e, $P<0.05$; c vs. g, NS; e vs. i, $P<0.001$; g vs. k, $P<0.001$; b vs. f, NS; d vs. h, $P<0.01$; f vs. j, $P<0.001$; h vs. l, $P<0.001$; j vs. n, $P<0.001$; l vs. q, $P<0.001$

TABLE 58.3   Gastric emptying studies using radiolabeled foods

Study	Year	Method	Mean age		Elimination time (min)		
			Elderly	Young	Elderly (solids)	Young (solids)	Elderly (liquids)
Evans et al. [27]	1981	^{99m}Tc-DTPA	77 ($n=11$)	26 ($n=7$)	–	–	123±23[a]
Moore et al. [28]	1982	Dual isotope	76.4 ($n=10$)	31 ($n=10$)	105±17[a]	104±10[a]	94±13[a]
Horowitz et al. [29]	1984	Dual isotope	77 ($n=13$)	34 ($n=22$)	103±8[a]	78±4[a]	25±3[a]
Kao et al. [30]	1993	^{99m}Tc-phylate	67 ($n=39$)	34 ($n=7$)	89±17.8[a]	88±18.2[a]	46.2±11[a]
Clarkston et al. [31]	1997	Dual isotope	76 ($n=14$)	30 ($n=19$)	182±26[a]	127±13[a]	47±4[a]
Madsen and Graff [32]	2004	^{111}In-DTPA/^{99m}Tc	81 ($n=16$)	24 ($n=16$)	183.5±9.2	150.5±7.5	150.66±7.5

[a]Half life of elimination of radiolabeled foods from the stomach

Gastric emptying is regulated in part by stomach myoelectric activity, which occurs at the membrane level of the gastric smooth muscle. The electrical membrane potentials of each region of the stomach differ as measured by electrogastrography (EGG). EGG abnormalities occur in various pathologic states of the stomach. For example, gastric dysrhythmias have been reported in patients with gastroparesis, idiopathic for diabetic peptic ulcer disease [20], functional dyspepsia (associated with tachygastria) [33], gastroesophageal reflux disease (associated with gastric dysrhythmias) [34], and chronic intestinal pseudoobstruction (associated with various gastric dysrhythmias). Despite these findings, abnormal EGG tracings alone do not necessarily correlate with symptoms.

The basal electrical rhythm (BER), or the slow wave, is a cyclic change in the membrane potential, which varies in different regions of the stomach (Fig. 58.3). The membrane potential is generated by the membrane sodium–potassium pump. The BER is associated with minimal contractile activity and does not result in detectable gastric peristalsis. The BER in the stomach, which originates in a pacemaker located in the mid-corpus along the greater curve, is propagated through gap junctions between adjacent smooth muscle cells. Vagotomy in humans has been shown to have no effect on the amplitude, rhythm, frequency, direction, or velocity of propagation of the electrical potentials, implying that the initiation of the current is a myogenic phenomenon [35]. This finding, along with an equally ineffectual denervation of nonvagal extrinsic stomach fibers, has also been confirmed in dogs [36].

In the distal stomach and duodenum, a cyclic contractile pattern called the interdigestive migrating motor complex (MMC) exists and is characterized by four phases. The contractions are associated with a myoelectric spike of attention superimposed on the basal electrical rhythm. The spikes are associated with rapid calcium influx into the cells. Phase I is characterized by a period of quiescence,

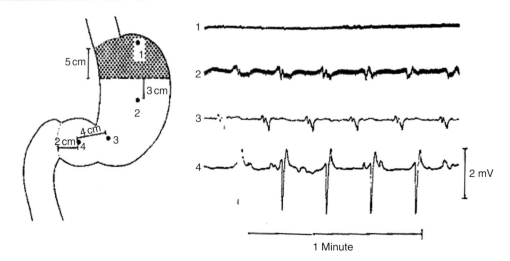

Figure 58.3 Myoelectric activity from the human stomach. Electrodes 1–4 were placed in the fundus, corpus, and proximal antrum and at the antral-pyloric juncture, respectively. The fundus is myoelectrically quiet. The BER is seen in tracings 2 and 3 and is associated with cyclic membrane depolarization. No contractions are associated with the BER. Rapid depolarizations of the proximal drive the myoelectric activity of the distal stomach. The pace-maker rests on the greater curvature of the stomach at the fundocorpal border. Spike potentials are seen in tracing 4 in the region of the antrum and pylorus. They are associated with contractions and therefore, emptying of the stomach (from Hinder and Kelly [35], with permission).

phase II is irregular motor activity, phase III is regular contraction that sweep the gastrointestinal tract in a peristaltic manner, and phase IV represents a brief period of irregular activity [20].

Abnormalities in gastric myoelectric activity have been associated with various gastric maladies, although patients with EGG disturbances alone do not necessarily have symptoms. There is evidence that the normal postprandial EGG frequency is less pronounced in elderly men [37].

Some studies have shown delayed gastric emptying in the elderly, but it has been difficult to show that it is associated with any clinical deficit. Other studies have found that there is no difference in gastric emptying between young and elderly subjects. Studies that evaluated only neuromuscular changes similarly were inconclusive about clinical relevance. If aging alone results in any gastric motility impairment, it is likely not clinically relevant.

Gastric Cancer

Because the peak incidence of gastric cancer is among patients older than 50 years, it is considered a disease primarily of the middle-aged and the elderly. Gastric cancer is also of interest to those studying the elderly because although its incidence in young patients has remained consistent, that in elderly patients as increased. Also, despite similarities in young and elderly patients in terms of tumor biology [characterized, e.g., by the magnitude of overexpression of the tumor suppressor gene p53 and the increased levels of other cellular markers, such as proliferating cell nuclear antigen (PCNA)], the survival rate after curative resection has been shown to be decreased in the elderly. Earlier studies suggested that elderly patients with gastric cancer have poorer survival than younger patients despite a similar rate of tumor extension [38], but more recent studies have shown that elderly patients do not have a worse prognosis than younger patients. Kim et al. [39] retrospectively reviewed the records of 331 patients [young groups (<36 years, $n=137$) and old groups (>70 years, $n=194$)] with gastric carcinoma who had undergone curative and noncurative resection from 1986 to 2000 (Fig. 58.4). The elderly and young patients had similar distributions with respect to depth of invasion, nodal involvement, hepatic metastasis, peritoneal dissemination, tumor stage at the initial diagnosis, and type of surgery. Based on these records, they found that at 5 years, the survival rates of elderly and young patients did not differ (noncurative: 52.8 vs. 46.5%, $P=0.5290$; curative: 67.0 vs. 60.0%, $P=0.3100$). Additional studies, such as those by Pisanu et al. compared elderly (age >75) and young subjects who had undergone curative gastrectomy and found that elderly patients have no worse prognosis than younger patients (the 5-year survival rate was 56.2% in the older group vs. 62.1% in the younger group). However, unlike younger patients, elderly patients often have more comorbidities and as such have a higher surgical risk, which, along with tumor stage and future quality of life, impacts operative planning [40]. As prognosis is dictated by tumor stage, others have postulated that the tumor is physiologically different than in younger patients as aged cells tend to undergo more methylation, apoptosis, and telomeric dysfunction.

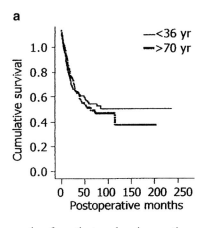
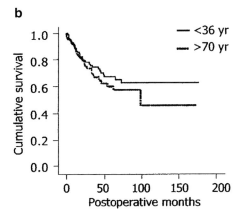

Figure 58.4 Survival curves time for patients undergoing curative resection for gastric cancer (**a**) noncurative resection or (**b**) curative resection in a Korean study. The patients were stratified to young (<36 years, $n = 137$,

thin line) and old groups (>70 years, $n - 194$, *heavy line*). The 5-year survival rates of young and elderly patients did not differ statistically regardless of surgery type. (From Kim et al. [39], with permission).

It is for this reason that gastric cancers in the elderly tend to be poorly differentiated [41].

Loss of gastric acidity is related to an increased risk of developing gastric cancer. It is manifested in the elderly by achlorhydria, atrophic gastritis, or pernicious anemia. It can also be the result of previous gastric resection for ulcer disease. The loss of gastric acidity may permit bacterial growth of the pathogen *H. pylori*, adding another independent risk factor for gastric cancer [42]. The risk of gastric cancer has been shown to be increased fourfold in *H. pylori*-positive persons. Although this may not reflect a causative relation, infection by *H. pylori* creates an environment of chronic gastritis and intestinal metaplasia to promote neoplastic change [43].

Mucosa-associated lymphoid tissue (MALT), which progresses to MALT lymphomas, has also been linked to *H. pylori* infection. Eradication of the *H. pylori* infection by oral antibiotic therapy has been shown to result in complete remission of the disease in some patients, especially those with early stage (stage I–II) MALT lymphomas [44].

Small Intestine

Over the course of an individual's life, enormous quantities of nutrients are processed through the small intestine. This makes the small intestine a likely place for potential changes with advancing age secondary to prolonged functioning and exposure to multitudes of potential carcinogens over time. Additionally, the small intestine is an organ of epithelial regeneration, turning over its cellular population often. This unique characteristic may be involved in the physiologic changes that occur with aging.

Motility

Advanced age is associated with a decrease in body weight, reduced caloric intake, and frequent gastrointestinal complaints. In fact, as many as 15% of adults have functional bowel complaints [45]. The effect of advanced age on the motility of the small intestine, however, is still unknown [46]. One way to evaluate small bowel motility is by studying the MMC, the ordered array of myoelectric activity and muscular contractions that travel down the small intestine in an aboral direction during fasting. The four phases of the MMC can be monitored by electrical activity, muscular contractions, intraluminal pressure, and intestinal transit times.

Husebye and Engedal [46] prospectively studied 15 healthy elderly subjects (age 81–91) and 19 young healthy controls, with ambulatory intraluminal manometry performed at home. This study found all subjects to have recurrent MMCs during fasting, with similar periodicity in old and young adults ($P = 0.4$) (Fig. 58.5). Duration of postprandial motility, amplitude, and frequency of contractions during phase III and the postprandial state was also preserved in the elderly subjects. Interestingly, the propagation velocity was slower (6.5 ± 0.8 vs. 10.8 ± 1.2 cm/min), and intermittent propagated clustered contractions were more frequent in the older subjects (Fig. 58.6). However, these minor-to-moderate changes were also within the range of healthy younger adults and are unlikely to have clinical relevance. The investigators concluded that small intestinal motility, for the most part, is preserved in healthy elderly subjects. Intestinal disorders such as maldigestion, malabsorption, and bacterial overgrowth should not be attributed to age-related hypomotility [46].

As previously mentioned, Madsen and Graff [32] confirmed these findings using solid and liquids meals with

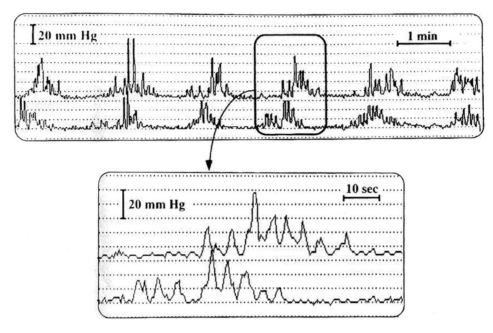

Figure 58.5 Propagated cluster contractions (PCCs) in the small intestine during the postprandial state in an old adult. A typical sequence of repeated PCCs at intervals of 1–2 min is shown. The *bottom tracings* in both *boxes* correspond to the duodenal sensor, and the top tracings show the recording from the proximal jejunum. These contractions are seen in increased frequency in the old person when compared with young controls (from Husebye and Engedal [46], with permission from Taylor and Francis).

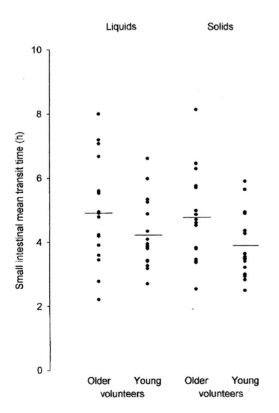

Figure 58.6 Small intestinal transit of liquid and solid marker in 16 older and 16 young volunteers. *Horizontal bars* indicate mean values (from Madsen and Graff [32], by permission of Oxford University Press).

radionucleotide tracers in healthy elderly subjects and compared it to that of younger subjects and found that advanced age did not affect small intestinal transit time (Fig. 58.6). This is also consistent with Argeny et al. who similarly evaluated transit times in ten young and nine elderly volunteers (using ^{99m}Tc-sulfur colloid-labeled eggs) and also found no difference between young and elderly subjects. The authors did note that there was a wide normal range of transit times in normal subjects and significant intrasubject biologic variability [47]. This is not uncommon in motility studies and is an important point highlighting the small bowels reserve capacity.

Morphology

There is little data concerning structural changes with increasing age on the human small bowel. In a study conducted in 1975, the jejunal mucosa for necropsies of 32 patients under the age of 60 (mean age 43) and 39 patients ages 67–90 (means age 80) were evaluated microscopically. Only minor differences were noted in the villous morphology between the young control group and older subjects. Specifically, broader, shorter villi were found to be more common in the elderly. This led the authors to postulate that

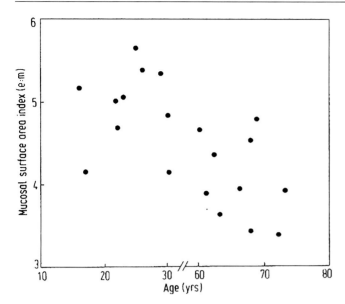

FIGURE 58.7 Relation of the intestinal mucosal surface area to the age of the patient. An indirect statistically significant correlation is noted (from Warren et al. [49], with permission from Elsevier).

this minor difference in total villous surface explains some absorption problems with age [48].

Warren et al. compared the small intestine histology of ten well-nourished elderly patients ages 60–73 to that of ten similar patients aged 16–30. A highly significant reduction in the mucosal surface area was found in the older age group (Fig. 58.7). The mean villous height was also slightly reduced and the breadth slightly increased, but these differences were not significant [49].

Corazza et al. evaluated the small bowel mucosa of 16 elderly patients and 22 younger controls (all with abdominal symptoms) to determine the surface area/volume ratio of jejunal mucosa using microscopic pointing techniques. This technique is performed by counting the number of times the standardized lines of a reticule intersects the jejunal mucosal surface under a set magnification. The surface area/volume ratio, which is an index of the extent of the mucosal surface area, was determined. No significant difference was found between the two groups for either parameter [50]. In a later study, Corazza et al. [51] showed through immunohistochemistry that this is likely linked to increased expression of a marker of enterocyte proliferation: proliferating nuclear cell antigen (PCNA) in both the crypts and villi of the human small bowel. The immunoreactivity and availability of PCNA results in a hyperproliferative state with rapid enterocyte migration. Ciccocioppo et al. [52] also suggests that in addition to the hyperproliferative state the maintenance of human intestinal morphology in the elderly is promoted by exaggerated apoptosis resulting in cellular immaturity. While these varying cascades allow the morphology of the small bowel to

remain intact with age, these authors surmise that it may be a contributing factor to the development of malabsorption in the elderly.

The integrity of small intestinal mucosa may age along with the host. The lactulose/mannitol test has been used to evaluate intestinal permeability in humans. The test is based on the comparison of the absorption of a monosaccharide (mannitol), which is absorbed transcellularly, to a disaccharide (lactulose), which is absorbed paracellularly. The urinary lactulose/mannitol ratio after oral administration is a reproducible measure of small intestine mucosal integrity. The ratio is increased when the mucosal integrity is disrupted. In a prospective cohort using healthy volunteers, Saltzman et al. found small intestinal permeability, or "leakiness," not significantly altered with age [53]. Riordan et al., using the same test, found that although intestinal permeability increases with small intestine bacterial overgrowth with colonic-type bacteria, this effect is independent of age [54]. Similarly, the thickness of the small bowel was found by deSouza et al. to be unchanged in the elderly. The latter investigation also found that the density of nerve cells in the myenteric plexus of the small bowel is decreased in the ages small intestine [55]. This implies that the intrinsic innervation of the human intestine is reduced during old age.

Absorption

Malnutrition in the elderly has been theoretically attributed to malabsorption at the level of the intestinal epithelium [56]. However, there is evidence that age alone does not adversely affect brush border enzymes. Wallis et al. collected 38 duodenal biopsy specimens from patients 55 to 91 years of age. Tissue was evaluated for the activity of the brush border enzymes maltase, sucrase, lactase, alkaline phosphatase, leucine aminopeptidase, and α-glucosidase. The study demonstrated no significant effect of age in the specific activities of these enzymes. It also found that glucose transport was not changed with extremes of age [58].

Using probe molecules that are absorbed by active and passive intestinal transport and are easily recovered in the urine, Beaumont et al. found no significant age-related decline in passive absorption of carbohydrate either in healthy nonhospitalized individuals or in elderly long-stay hospital residents [58]. In another study, Arora et al. investigated three aspects of intestinal absorption in the elderly and found no significant change. A series of 114 healthy adult volunteers (age 19–91) were started on a diet of 100 g of fat per day 1 day prior to testing. The subjects remained on the diet for the following 72 h as their stools were collected and tested for fecal fat. There was no change with advancing age. In another arm of the study, 25 g of D-xylose was given orally to 54 fasting volunteers (56–86 years; 20 men and 34 women). Serum and urinary xylose levels were measured. There was no significant difference in D-xylose serum levels between young and elderly volunteers. Although urinary excretion of D-xylose in the elderly was found to be significantly decreased ($P<0.02$), there was a concomitant decrease in the creatinine clearance with advancing age ($P<0.01$). This suggests a decrease in renal function rather than a problem with absorption as the reason for decreased D-xylose levels in the elderly. In the third part of the study, [^{14}C] glycocholate breath tests were performed in 60 healthy volunteers [30 were ≥30 years (15 men and 15 women) and 30 were ≥60 years (15 men and 15 women)]. This test is used to assess increased deconjugation of bile salts, which suggests bacterial overgrowth of the small intestine. There was no evidence of an age-associated increase in bile salt deconjugation by intestinal bacteria [59].

Malabsorption in the elderly has been shown to correlate with bacterial overgrowth. Vantrappen et al. [60] measured intraluminal pressures at the gastric antrum and at different levels of the upper small intestine to assess the interdigestive motor complex in 18 normal subjects (ages 18–71 years) with normal $^{14}CO_2$ acid breath test and 18 subjects with abnormal $^{14}CO_2$ acid breath test. Nine patients with various digestive diseases but negative $^{14}CO_2$ acid breath tests were studied as an additional control group. All but five patients had normal interdigestive motor complexes and the five patients in whom the motor complex was absent or greatly disordered had bacterial overgrowth as evidenced by $^{14}CO_2$ bile acid breath tests. These observations show that changes in interdigestive motor complexes occur in patients with bacterial overgrowth and as such it is a possible mechanism for malabsorption absence of structural abnormalities.

MacMahon et al. [61] evaluated 30 elderly patients between 68 and 90 years of age for small intestinal bacterial overgrowth (SIBO). Advancing age correlated significantly with rising counts of strict anaerobes in the small bowel. The investigators thought that malabsorption in these patients was not related to bacterial overgrowth because metabolic or nutritional abnormalities could be attributed to alternative causes. This refutes an earlier study done by McEvoy et al. who studied 490 patients over age 65 and found that 71% of the malnourished patients (those in whom poor diet alone was not a factor) had bacterial overgrowth [62].

Fat is a major source of caloric intake, and as such its absorption is an important area of investigation in the elderly. Fat absorption is a complex process involving four major phases: (1) Intraluminal processes (digestion and solubilization); (2) mucosal uptake; (3) intracellular reesterification and lipoprotein synthesis; and (4) export for the enterocyte into the lymph. Although disruption of any of these phases can lead to fat malabsorption, this too is rarely observed in elderly patients. In a study of 114 healthy, free-living subjects ages 19–91 years, Arora et al. found that on a diet of 100 g of fat per day, fecal fat in a 72-h collection did not increase with advancing age. Lipid digestion and absorption are well preserved in aging individuals [59].

Liver and Biliary Function

The liver is responsible for the synthesis of clotting factors and the metabolism of toxins, including anesthetics, analgesics, and sedatives, all of which are important in elderly surgical patients. The liver in adult men has been found to increase in size only marginally, from a median weight of 1,820 g at age 25 to a median weight of 1,840 g at age 55. It then decreases by 20% to a median weight of 1,480 g by age 75. The median weight of the female liver similarly changes from 1,430–1,460 g during the range of 20–60 years, to 1,180 g by 75 years (Fig. 58.8) [63]. At the microscopic level, the histology reveals a loss of mitochondria and smooth endoplasmic reticulum [64]. Blood flow to the liver is also reduced with aging. Sherloch et al. used the bromsulfalein technique to estimate hepatic blood flow in 29 men and found a decrease in flow with increasing age of about 1.5% per year. At age 65, hepatic blood flow would be expected to be reduced by about 40–45% compared with that of a 25-year- old [65]. There is some controversy as to whether a reduction in liver function with age is attributable to these physical changes or there is some intrinsic age-related cellular change [66].

In another branch of their study of 60 healthy, adult volunteers, Arora et al. performed [^{14}C] the aminopyrine breath test that measures the rate of demethylation by hepatic microsomes, thereby estimating the capacity of hepatic microsomal phase I monooxygenases. This study was unable to show a statistically significant difference between young and elderly subjects and concluded that hepatic functions are generally well preserved during the normal human aging process [59].

Many pharmacokinetic studies in human subjects have suggested that the clearance of drugs metabolized by oxidation–reduction is reduced in the elderly by 10–50% [65]. One way to evaluate liver function in aging is to study the liver's store of cytochrome P450 and its functional capacity. Sotaniemi et al. examined liver biopsy samples from 226 patients (102 women and 124 men) with equal histopathologic conditions. This was ensured by dividing the liver biopsies into three groups using standard histopathologic conditions: (1) apparently normal liver histologic diagnosis; (2) subjects with slight-to-moderate changes in the liver parenchyma (fatty liver, fatty liver with fibrosis, degree of fibrosis 1–3, and reactive changes such as granulomas or

FIGURE 58.8 Pattern of change in human liver weight with respect to age. At age 55–60, the mean weight begins to decline in both men and women (reprinted with permission from Boyd [63], Copyright © 1933 American Medical Association. All rights reserved).

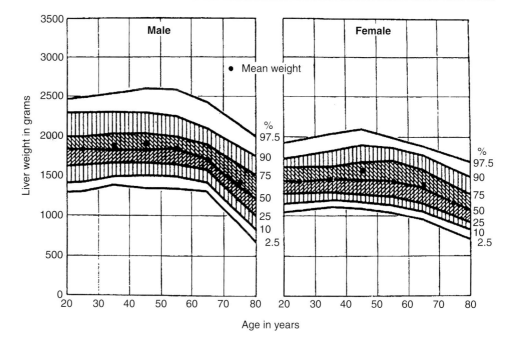

portal infiltrates); (3) subjects with severe changes (cirrhosis and hepatitis). They evaluated the cytochrome P450 contents in liver biopsy samples and the plasma antipyrine (phenzone) clearance rates, which tests for hepatic drug metabolizing capacity. The study found that cytochrome P450 content in subjects 20–29 years was 7.2 ± 2.6 mmol/g; it increased during the fourth decade to 7.6 ± 2.5 (+7.2%, $P=NS$) and declined after age 40 to 6.1 ± 2.2 (−16%, $P<0.01$), a level that remained relatively constant until age 69. It declined further to 4.8 ± 1.1 after age 70 (−32%, $P<0.001$). The antipyrine clearance rate in young subjects was 46.4 ± 18.5 ml/min, remained unaltered during the fourth decade, and declined after age 40 by a rate of 0.34 ml/min per year toward old age (−29%, $P<0.001$). The antipyrine half-life also changed during old age, increasing linearly from 9.6 ± 2.0 h in young subjects (20–29 years) to 12.1 ± 3.1 h in the elderly (>70 years) (+26%, $P<0.001$). There was also a decline in the apparent volume of distribution of the drug: 0.46 ± 0.12 l/kg in young subjects (20–29 years) and after a linear decline with aging 0.40 ± 0.07 l/kg in middle-aged subjects (60–69 years) and to 0.41 ± 0.09 l/kg in the elderly (70 years) (−11%). This reduction of liver drug metabolism with age, along with a decline in cytochrome P450 content in livers of the elderly, suggests primary hepatic aging. The authors concluded that caution is advisable when using drugs metabolized by the liver in the elderly and that elderly patients should be closely monitored for high blood levels caused by reduced drug metabolism, drug interactions, or both [67]. Aging of the liver may not be readily apparent in the healthy individual; and it is often unmasked only by stress, illness, or infection.

In addition to any changes due solely to aging, the liver is particularly susceptible to the toxic effects of environmental agents such as cigarettes and ethanol. Its decline in function is secondary to decreased size and blood flow can be attributed to nonhepatic factors, such as reduced cardiac output and age-related reduction of trophic factors from the pancreas via the portal system such as insulin and glucagon [65]. Here again it is difficult to determine how much functional decline can be attributed solely to age, as the liver has a large reserve capacity, but there is some evidence of physical change.

Increasing age is known to be associated with a high incidence of gallstones in both sexes. This was confirmed by a large ($n=1,000$) study in which multiple logistic regression was used to show that age was the most important variable associated with cholelithiasis [68]. Another study that supported this finding was the Multicenter Italian Study on Epidemiology of Cholelithiasis (MICOL). In this study, data from 29,584 individuals (15,910 men and 13,674 women) examined in 14 cohorts (with a participation rate above 50%) were collected. Increasing age was again found to be associated with an increased incidence of gallstone disease, by both univariate and multivariate analyses in men and women. Interestingly, gallstone disease was also associated with decreased serum cholesterol [69], which may be related to a high proportion of biliary cholesterol and the lithogenic index, which have been shown to be elevated in elderly women. Valdivieso et al. reported that 41.7% of elderly women had supersaturated bile compared to 8.3% of younger women [70].

Liver regeneration is known to occur after resection, and this effect has been studied in the elderly. The livers of aged rats have been found to have decreased regenerative capacity by PCNA [71] and [3H] thymidine incorporation [72]. This finding has been contradicted in human studies which found that there is no relation between advanced age and regenerative capacity.

Pancreas

Like the liver, the pancreas progressively atrophies with age. Histopathologic findings associated with it include increased ectasia of the pancreatic ducts as well as interlobular fibrosis, ductal hyperplasia, and narrowing of the pancreatic ducts [73]. Despite this, the pancreas, similar to other areas of the GI tract has enormous reserve capacity, making it difficult to attribute pancreatic changes solely to old age.

As acinar cells make up 80% of the pancreas, an effective way to assess pancreatic function is to test for exocrine output in response to infusion of secretin and cerulein. When this test was performed on 25 subjects over the age of 60, no statistically significant decrease in pancreatic output was observed compared with that in 30 young controls [74]. The same group subsequently confirmed their findings with an updated, elegant method of evaluating pancreatic function – the fluorescein dilaurate (pancreolauryl) test. For this test, subjects are given the synthetic, poorly water-soluble ester fluorescein dilaurate orally. In the duodenum, this compound is hydrolyzed by pancreatic arylesterases into lauric acid and free water-soluble fluorescein. The fluorescein is absorbed in the small intestine, conjugated in the liver, and excreted in the urine. Fluorescent activity in the urine output correlates with pancreatic function and digestive capacity. Sixty healthy elderly subjects (aged 66–88, mean age 78 years) were compared to 36 healthy younger subjects (aged 21–57, mean age 36 years). No significant differences in pancreatic function could be shown between the elderly under age 80 and those over age 80 [75].

Another way to evaluate pancreatic exocrine function is to determine serum levels of pancreatic enzymes. Carrere et al. compared immunoreactive tryspinogen and lipase in healthy elderly adults and younger adult controls. This investigation found that the pancreatic enzymes were similar in young and elderly adults, with no significant differences between the groups [76].

It has been established that humans become glucose intolerant with age. It is still somewhat controversial, though, whether this change is due to beta-cell failure, peripheral insulin resistance, or a combination of both. Discerning between each of these is difficult. Elahi et al. conducted a glucose clamp study, in which a hyperglycemic state is induced to differentiate the intrinsic functions of beta cells from peripheral insulin resistance. Two hundred and thirty hyperglycemic clamps were done on 85 young (age 24–39), 47 middle-aged (age 40–59), and 98 old (age 60–90) subjects [the latter group was further divided into old-normal and old-impaired, based on the results of the oral glucose tolerance tests (OGTT)]. Although OGTTs were worse in the elderly group, insulin responses during the clamp were not statistically different for this group as a whole. Additionally, insulin-dependent glucose uptake, a measure of tissue sensitivity to insulin, was decreased in the old-impaired group at each hyperglycemic plateau except the highest. This finding supports the view that glucose intolerance is due to insulin resistance [77].

Alteration in beta-cell function has also been shown in the elderly . Szoke et al. examined the effect of aging on insulin secretion (first phase and second phase) and insulin sensitivity in people with normal (NGT) and impaired glucose tolerance (IGT) tests. The study pool consisted of a total of 396 subjects (266 individuals with NGT and 130 individuals with IGT) aged 20–70 years. Changes in beta-cell function and insulin sensitivity were compared using the homeostasis model assessment HOMA indexes of beta-cell function, and insulin resistance calculated from fasting plasma insulin (in microunits per liter) and glucose (in millimoles per liter) concentrations. The authors found that beta-cell function was inversely correlated with age in the normal glucose tolerance group (NGT) ($P=0.003$) such that with each decade it decreased 11% (~1.1% per year). No significant correlation with age was found in the IGT group ($P=0.53$). First-phase insulin release was negatively correlated with age in both groups (all $P<0.05$) with the index for first- and second-phase insulin release decreased similarly at a rate of approximately 0.7% per year in people with NGT. In people with IGT, the disposition indexes for first- and second-phase insulin release decreased at greater rates (approximately 2.2 and 1.4% per year, $P=0.002$ and 0.009, respectively, vs. NGT), with the decrease in first phase being greater than that of second phase ($P=0.025$). Second-phase insulin release did not change with age in either group [78]. Therefore, it likely the combination of both decreased insulin secretion and insulin resistance that leads to glucose intolerance with advanced age.

Colon

Despite the abundance of data suggesting that colonic transit time is not decreased in the elderly, constipation, defined as fewer than three bowel movements per week [79], continues to be one of the most common chronic digestive complaints in this population [80]. About 9–34% of men and women over age 65 suffer from constipation compared to 4% of the younger population and 19% of the middle-aged population. The cause of constipation is typically ascribed to a low-fiber diet, sedentary lifestyle, and colonic motility disturbances [21] (Table 58.4). Of course, routine screening for colon cancer, including serial stool guiac tests, flexible endoscopy, or barium enema, is mandatory for the workup of new constipation.

There is a high rate of laxative use in the elderly (reported in 32% of nursing home patients). Constipation in the elderly may produce serious complications, such as acute mental confusion, urinary retention, urinary incontinence, fecal impaction, stercoral ulceration, and even bowel perforation. The primary symptom older people use to describe their constipation is the feeling of having to strain excessively to defecate. This may be due to outlet delay caused by pelvic dyssynergia, which is a paradoxical increase in anal canal pressure during attempts to defecate. This was found to be the predominant mechanism for constipation in ten of ten otherwise healthy patients over 65 in a study done by Cheskin et al. Colonic inertia, or total gut transit time over 67 h, was found in two of these patients, and rectosigmoid contractions in response to balloon distention was seen in only one subject [81].

The reasons for constipation in the elderly are multifactorial, resulting from decreased muscle tone and motor function of the colon causing decreased propulsive action. Madsen and Graff [32] studied gut motility and found that normal aging decreased colonic motility (age 74–85). Another possibility is a decrease in the neuron density in the myenteric plexus. Gomez et al. found that there was a 37% decrease in the number of neurons in the myenteric plexus in six colon specimens from elderly patients (average age 77.7 ± 7.6 years) with no previous digestive pathology [80]. Similarly, Koch et al. found a significant decrease in inhibitory junction potential in human colon with age, an association noted with other functional obstructions, as in Hirschsprung's disease [82]. This reduced propagation velocity likely explains the decreased rectal compliance often seen in elderly patients with constipation. A noncompliant rectum would be consistent with an infrequent urge to defecate, presence of stools in the rectum for a prolonged period of time, and finally, the straining often resulting in the passage of hard, pellet-like stools [83].

Constipation is also a side effect of many drugs commonly used in the elderly. In a study of 800 nursing homes, residents (age 65–105, mean 84.5 years) who were receiving psychoactive medication. Monane et al. evaluated the relation of these drugs to constipation based on reported frequency of laxative use. The investigators found that laxative use was significantly higher in residents taking highly anticholinergic antidepressants such as amitriptyline (odds ratio 3.12), diphenhydramine (odds ratio 2.18), or highly anticholinergic neuroleptics such as thioridazine (odds ratio 2.01); it was also high in the very old (age ≥85) (odds ratio 2.23). Among the factors that did not show a correlation with increased laxative use were gender, decreased functional status, impaired cognitive function, and the use of benzodiazepines or antiparkinsonian agents [84].

TABLE 58.4 Causes of constipation

Primary

Increased colonic mass movement of unknown etiology
Impaired relaxation of the pelvic floor
Congenital innervation disease (Hirschsprung's disease)
Rectocele
Prolapse

Secondary

Medications	Iron	
	Calcium	
	Opioids	
	Anti-cholingerics	
	Antipsychotics	
	Anticonvulsants	
	Tricyclic antidepressants	
	Calcium channel blockers	
Neurologic	CVA	Autonomic neuropathy
	Spinal cord lesions	Muscular dystrophies
	Parkinson's disease	Multiple sclerosis
Dietary and environmental	Low fiber diet	
	Irregular bowel habits	
	Immobility	
Mechanical	Colon cancer	
	Stricture	
	Intussusception	
	Extrinsic mass pressure	
	Volvulus	
	Sphincteric (fissure, hemorrhoids)	
Metabolic	Hypercalcemia	Hypocalcemia
	Hyperkalemia	Hypomagnesemia
	Uremia	
Endocrine	Diabetes	Hypothyroidism
	Hypoparathyroidism	Addison's disease
	Pheochromocytoma	
	Pregnancy	
Myopathies	Amyloidosis	
	Myotonic dystrophies	
Psychologic	Depression	
	Anxiety	

Source: Data from Cheskin [98]

Anorectum

Anorectal physiology plays a major role in the function of large bowel and in pelvic disorders [85]. The increase in fecal incontinence and constipation seen during old age is sometimes caused by mechanical changes in the rectum known as pelvic outlet obstruction [86]. Anal incontinence is seen predominantly in women, increases with advancing age, and is due to insufficient anal sphincter function. In a study of 61 healthy women with a mean age of 44 (age range 20–90), the anal pressure was recorded along with rectal compliance and sensation, through use of manometry, balloon distention, and a visual analog scale, respectively. Anal sphincter appearance and pelvic floor motion also were assessed by static and dynamic magnetic resonance imaging, respectively, in 38 of 61 females. Age-related changes were found along the length of the anal canal where the rectal compliance, anal resting and squeeze pressures, rectal compliance, rectal sensation, and perineal laxity were all reduced in older subjects [87].

In another study that explored the relationship between age and anorectal function, McHugh and Diamant [88] measured the resting anal canal pressures (RAP) and maximal squeeze pressures (MSP) of 143 incontinent patients and a control group of 157 healthy patients (aged 20–89). In healthy men and women age 40 and older, there was a decrease in RAP and MSP (women>men). For women, parity did not correlate with RAP or MSP. In the group with fecal incontinence (FI), 39% of females and 44% of males fell within the "normal" range for both the RAP and MSP. For all patients with FI, 41 and 17% had impairment of one or both parameters, respectively. As you can see, defining appropriate anorectal functioning is difficult, as a good deal of fecally incontinent men and women fell into the "normal" range.

Parity, however, may be associated with rectal prolapse that has a higher incidence in women and the elderly and is thought to be related to pelvic floor disease. In this condition, the rectum bulges into the perineum, tightening the puborectalis, and increasing anorectal angulation. The pudenal nerve is stretched as the rectum herniated through the weakened anal sphincter [89].

Anorectal physiology can also be evaluated in terms of recovery of function after an operative procedure. Young and elderly patients who have undergone an ileoanal reservoir procedure following a colectomy and ulcerative colitis or familial polyposis have been compared [90]. These patients were evaluated pre- and postoperatively with manometry for anorectal pressures and clinical outcomes by a questionnaire. No difference in preoperative anorectal pressures or in clinical outcome was found between the two groups. Also, despite the transient impairment of internal anal sphincter function seen in these patients, there is complete recovery after ileostomy closure.

Colorectal Cancer

The incidence of many types of neoplasia increases as humans age. The proliferative potential of the gastrointestinal tract, which turns over its entire epithelium every 24–72 h, makes it particularly susceptible to neoplasia [44].

The mean age of presentation is 71, and two-thirds of the 150,000 new cases of colon cancer each year occur in patients over age 65 [91].

Repeated and prolonged insults from environmental factors such as chemicals and radiation are external influences that affect genetic stability. Colon cancer is associated with genetic abnormalities such as mutations and, more commonly, deletions of tumor suppressor genes. Genomic entropy has been shown to increase with time, making genetic instability (and therefore the malfunction of genetic mechanisms such as DNA repair) more common in the elderly [92]. Even the pathology of aging itself may eventually give way to carcinogenesis.

Colorectal carcinomas appear to arise from adenomas, and the idea that carcinogenesis evolves in a multistage process is generally accepted [91]. It is described as a series of genetic alterations resulting in progressive derangement of the genetic factors that control normal growth. Vogelstein et al. looked at four genetic alterations in 172 colorectal tumor specimens representing various stages of neoplastic development: *ras* gene mutations and allelic deletions if chromosomes 5, 17, and 18. Specimens consisted of 40 predominantly early stage adenomas from seven patients with familial adenomatous polyposis (FAP), 40 adenomas (19 without associated foci of carcinoma and 21 with such foci) from 33 patients without FAP, and 92 carcinomas resected from 89 patients. The *ras* gene mutations were found to have occurred in a significantly higher proportion of adenomas >1 cm and in carcinomas (58 and 47%, respectively) than in adenomas <1 cm in size (9%). Sequences on chromosome 5 that are linked to the gene for FAP were present in adenomas from patients with polyposis but were lost in 29 and 35% of adenomas and carcinomas, respectively, from other patients. Carcinomas and advanced adenomas showed a higher rate of deletion of a specific region of chromosome 18 (73 and 47%, respectively) than in earlier-stage adenomas (11–13%). Chromosome 17p sequences were usually lost only in carcinomas (75%). The clinical progression of the tumors developed synchronously with these four genetic alterations. These findings are consistent with the model of tumorigenesis in which the development of cancer occurs in stepwise fashion, involving the mutational activation of an oncogene together with the loss of genes responsible for tumor suppression [93].

In addition to the higher incidence in the elderly, colon cancer also has been shown to have characteristically different locations of occurrence. In a review of 222 patients with colon cancer over age 60, Schub and Steinheber found that there was a higher incidence of right-sided lesions and a decreased incidence of rectosigmoid lesions as the population aged. For patients in their sixth decade, 8% of the tumors were located in the right colon, 9% in the transverse colon, 6% in the descending colon, and 77% in the rectosigmoid. During the seventh decade, 22% were located in the right colon, 11% in the transverse colon, and 58% in the rectosigmoid area. In the oldest group (older than 80 years) 29% were in the right colon, 14% in the transverse colon, 9% in the descending colon, and 49% in the rectosigmoid area. This trend was found to be statistically significant by chi-square analysis ($P < 0.05$). This "rightward" shift was also associated with a trend toward more favorable staging. The authors believed that it reflects an increase in the proportion of elderly patients with cancer and a predilection toward right-sided lesions with aging [94].

Similarly, Toyoda et al. did a retrospective study using patients from the Osaka Cancer Registry between 1974 and 2003 and found an increased incidence of proximal colon cancer in the elderly (from 22.5 to 34.6% among men and from 25.0 to 46.8% among women for age ≥80) over that time period. Among women, right colon cancer was more common in the elderly than in the young [95].

Conclusions

As technology and medical innovation continues to evolve, we will reap the benefits of longevity, and it is clear that our population reflects that the elderly promise to be one of its fastest growing segments. Despite these benefits, issues related to aging can often hinder one's quality of life and often times lack a definitive solution. The scientific explanation of these events eludes us, as for the most part there are no real differences in histology, motility, or mucosal structure. With continued study of aging as it relates to the gastrointestinal epithelial cell we can yield additional information on incidence of gastrointestinal malignancies. A better understanding of the factors related to aging will help us to improve the diagnosis and treatment of gastrointestinal ailments. The diagnosis and treatment of ailments in other organ systems are addressed in the chapters that follow.

References

1. Nicosia MA, Hind JA, Roecker EB, Carnes M, Doyle J, Dengel GA, Robbins J (2000) Age effects on the temporal evolution of isometric and swallowing pressure. J Gerontol A Biol Sci Med Sci 55(11):M634–M640
2. Ney DM, Weiss JM, Kind AJ, Robbins J (2009) Senescent swallowing: impact, strategies, and interventions. Nutr Clin Pract 24(3):395–413, Review
3. White GN, O'Rourke F, Ong BS et al (2008) Dysphagia: causes, assessment, treatment, and management. Geriatrics 63:15–20
4. Ekberg O, Feinberg MJ (1998) Altered swallowing function in elderly patients without dysphagia: radiologic findings in 56 cases. Am J Radiol 156:1181–1184
5. Nilsson H, Ekberg O, Olsson R, Hindfelt B (1996) Quantitative aspects of swallowing in an elderly nondysphagic population. Dysphagia 11(3):180–184
6. Fulp SR, Dalton CB, Castell JA, Castell DO (1990) Aging-related alterations in human upper esophageal sphincter function. Am J Gastroenterol 85:1569–1572
7. Newnham DM, Hamilton SJC (1997) Sensitivity of the cough reflex in young and elderly subjects. Age Ageing 26:185–188
8. Harkness GA, Bently DW, Roghmann KJ (1990) Risk factors for nosocomial pneumonia in the elderly. Am J Med 89:457–463
9. Wilson JA, Pryde A, Macintyre CCA, Maran AGD, Heasing RC (1990) The effects of age, sex, and smoking on normal pharyngesophageal motility. Am J Gastroenterol 85:686–691
10. Zboralske FF, Amberg JR, Sorgel KH (1964) Presbyesophagus cineradiographic manifestations. Radiology 82:463–467
11. Soergel KH, Zboralske FF, Amberg JR (1964) Presbyesophagus: esophageal motility in nonagenarians. J Clin Invest 43:1472–1479
12. Hollis JB, Castell DO (1974) Esophageal function in elderly men: a new look at "presbyesophagus". Ann Intern Med 80:371–374
13. Adamek JR, Wegener M, Weinbeck M, Gielen B (1994) Long term esophageal manometry in healthy subjects: evaluation of normal values and influence of age. Dig Dis Sci 39:2069–2073
14. Meshkinpour H, Haghhighat P, Dutton C (1994) Clinical spectrum of esophageal aperistalsis in the elderly. Am J Gastroenterol 89:1480–1483
15. Ren J, Shaker R, Kusano M et al (1995) Effect of aging on the secondary esophageal peristalsis: presbyesophagus revisited. Am J Physiol 268:G772–G779
16. Lasch HC, Castell DO, Castell JA (1997) Evidence for the diminished visceral pain with aging: studies using graded intraesophageal balloon distention. Am J Physiol 272:G1–G3
17. Ergun GA, Miskovitz P (1992) Aging and the esophagus: common pathologic conditions and their effect upon swallowing in the geriatric population. Dysphagia 7:58–63
18. Filho JM, Carvalho VC, deSouza RR (1995) Nerve cell loss in the myenteric plexus of the human esophagus in relation to age: a preliminary investigation. Gerontology 41:18–21
19. Phillips RJ, Powley TL (2007) Innervation of the gastrointestinal tract: patterns of aging. Auton Neurosci 136(1–2):1–19, Review
20. DelValle J, Lucey MR, Yamada T (1995) Gastric secretion. In: Yamada Y, Alpers DH, Powell DW, Owyang C, Silverstein FE (eds) Textbook on gastroenterology. Lippincott, Philadelphia, pp 295–326
21. Shamburek RD, Scott RB, Farrar JT (1990) Gastrointestinal and liver changes in the elderly. In: Katlic MR (ed) Geriatric surgery: comprehensive care of the elderly patient. Urban and schwarzenberg, Baltimore, pp 97–113
22. Katelaris PH, Seow F, Lin BPC, Napoli J, Ngu MC, Jones DB (1993) Effect of age, Helicobacter pylori infection, and gastritis with atrophy on serum gastrin and gastric secretion in healthy men. Gut 34:1032–1037
23. Kekki M, Samlott IM, Ihamaki T, Varis K, Siuala M (1982) Age and sex-related behaviour of gastric acid secretion at the population level. Scand J Gastroenterol 17:737–743
24. Haruma K, Kamada T, Kawaguchi H, Okamoto S, Yoshihara M, Sumii K, Inoue M, Kishimoto S, Kajiyama G, Miyoshi A (2000) Effect of age and Helicobacter pylori infection on gastric acid secretion. J Gastroenterol Hepatol 15(3):277–283
25. Goldschmiedt M, Barnett CC, Schwartz BE, Karnes WE, Redfern JS, Feldman M (1991) Effect of age on gastric acid secretion and serum gastrin concentrations in healthy men and women. Gastroenterology 101:990–997
26. Feldman M, Cryer B, Huet BA, Lee E (1996) Effects of aging and gastritis on gastric acid and pepsin secretion in humans: a prospective study. Gastroenterology 110:1043–1052
27. Evans MA, JE Triggs, GA Broe, Creasey H (1981) Gastric emptying rate in the elderly: implications for drug therapy. J Am Geriatr Soc 29:201–205
28. Moore JG, Tweedy C, Datz FL (1983) Effect of age on gastric emptying of liquid-solid meals in man. Dig Dis Sci 28:340–344

29. Horowitz M, Maddern GJ, Collins JP, Harding PE, Shearman DJ (1984) Changes in gastric emptying rates with age. Clin Sci 67:213–218

30. Kao CH, Lai TL, Chen GH, Yeh SH (1997) Influence of age on gastric emptying in health Chinese. Clin Nucl Med 19:401–404

31. Clarkston WK, Pantano MM, Horowitz M, Littlefield JM, Burton FR (1997) Evidence for the anorexia of aging: gastrointestinal transit and hunger in the healthy elderly vs. young adults. Am J Physiol 272:R243–R248

32. Madsen JL, Graff J (2004) Effects of ageing on gastrointestinal motor function. Age Ageing 33(2):154–159

33. Pfaffenbach B, Adamek RJ, Bartholomous C (1997) Gastric dsyrthmias and delayed gastric emptying in patients with functional dyspepsia. Dig Dis Sci 42:2094–2099

34. Cucchiara S, Salvia G, Borelli O et al (1997) Gastric electrical dysrhythmias and delayed gastric emptying in gastroesophageal reflux disease. Am J Gastroenterol 92:1103–1108

35. Hinder RA, Kelly KA (1977) Human gastric pacesetter potential: site of origin, spread, and response to gastric transection and proximal gastric vagotomy. Am J Surg 133:29–33

36. Spencer MP, Sarr MG, Hakim NS, Soper NJ (1989) Interdigestive gastric motility patterns: the role of vagal and nonvagal extrinsic innervation. Surgery 106:185193

37. Parkman HP, HArria AD, Fisher RS (1996) Influence of age, gender, and menstrual cycle on the normal electrogastrogram. Am J Gastroenterol 91:127–133

38. Kitamura K, Yamaguchi H, Taniguchi H et al (1996) Clinicopathologic characteristics of gastric cancer in the elderly. Br J Cancer 73:798–802

39. Kim DY, Joo JK, Ryu SY, Park YK, Kim YJ, Kim SK (2005) Clinicopathologic characteristics of gastric carcinoma in elderly patients: a comparison with young patients. World J Gastroenterol 11(1):22–26

40. Pisanu A, Montisci A, Piu S, Uccheddu A (2007) Curative surgery for gastric cancer in the elderly: treatment decisions, surgical morbidity, mortality, prognosis and quality of life. Tumori 93(5):478–484

41. Arai T, Takubo K (2007) Clinicopathological and molecular characteristics of gastric and colorectal carcinomas in the elderly. Pathol Int 57(6):303–314

42. Mayer RJ (2008) Gastrointestinal tract cancer. In: Fauci AS, Braunwald E, Kasper D et al (eds) Harrison's principles of internal medicine. McGraw Hill, New York, pp 570–579

43. Wu CY, Kuo KN, Wu MS, Chen YJ, Wang CB, Lin JT (2009) Early *Helicobacter pylori* eradication decreases risk of gastric cancer in patients with peptic ulcer disease. Gastroenterology 137(5):1641–1648

44. Andriani A, Miedico A, Tedeschi L et al (2009) Management and long-term follow-up of early stage *H. pylori*-associated gastric MALT-lymphoma in clinical practice: an Italian, multicentre study. Dig Liver Dis 41(7):467–473

45. Hasler W, Owyang C (2008) Approach to the patient with gastrointestinal disease. In: Fauci AS, Braunwald E, Kasper D et al (eds) Harrison's principles of internal medicine. McGraw Hill, New York, pp 1831–1835

46. Husebye E, Engedal K (1992) The patterns of motility are maintained in the human small intestine throughout the process of aging. Scand J Gastroenterol 27(5):397–404

47. Argeny EE, Soffer EE, Madsen MT, Berbaun KS, Walkner WO (1995) Scintigraphic evaluation of small bowel transit in healthy subjects: inter- and intrasubject variability. Am J Gasteroenterol 90:938–942

48. Webster SGP, Leeming JT (1975) The appearance of the small bowel mucosa in old age. Age Ageing 4:168–174

49. Warren PM, Pepperman MA, Montogomeryt RD (1978) Age changes in the small-intestinal mucosa. Lancet 2:849–850

50. Corazza GR, Frazzoni M, Gatto MRA, Gasbarrini G (1986) Ageing and small-bowel mucosa: a morphometric study. Gerontology 32:60–65

51. Corazza GR, Ginaldi L, Quaglione G, Ponzielli F, Vecchio L, Biagi F, Quaglino D (1998) Proliferating cell nuclear antigen expression is increased in small bowel epithelium in the elderly. Mech Ageing Dev 104:1–9

52. Ciccocioppo R, Di Sabatino A, Luinetti O, Rossi M, Cifone MG, Corazza GR (2002) Small bowel enterocyte apoptosis and proliferation are increased in the elderly. Gerontology 48:204–208

53. Saltzman JR, Kowdley KV, Russell RM (1995) Changes in small intestine permeability with ageing. J Am Geriatr Soc 43:160–164

54. Riordan SM, McIver CJ, Thomas DH, Duncombe VM, Bolin TD, Thomas MC (1997) Luminal bacterial and small intestinal permeability. Scand J Gastroenterol 32:556–563

55. DeSouza RR, Moratelli HB, Borges N, Liberti EA (1993) Age-induced nerve cell loss in the myenteric plexus of the small intestine in man. Gerontology 39:183–188

56. Holt PR (1985) The small intestine. Clin Gastroenterol 14:689–723

57. Wallis JL, Lipski PS, James OFW, Hirst BH (1993) Duodenal brush border mucosal glucose transport and enzyme activities in aging man and effect of bacterial contamination of the small intestine. Dig Dis Sci 38:403–409

58. Beaumont DM, Cobden I, Sheldon WL (1987) Passive and active carbohydrate absorption by the ageing gut. Age Ageing 16:294–300

59. Arora S, Kassarijan Z, Krasinski SD, Croffey B, Kaplan MM, Russell RM (1989) Effect of age on test of intestinal and hepatic function on healthy humans. Gastroenterology 96:1560–1565

60. Vantrappen G, Janssens J, Hellemans J, Ghoos Y (1977) The interdigestive motor complex of normal subjects and patients with bacterial overgrowth of the small intestine. J Clin Invest 59:1158–1166

61. MacMahon M, Lynch M, Mullins E et al (1994) Small intestinal bacterial overgrowth – an incidental finding. J Am Geriatric Soc 42:146–149

62. McEvoy S, Dutton J, James OFW (1983) Bacterial contamination of the small intestine is an important cause of occult malabsorption on the elderly. BMJ 287:789–793

63. Boyd E (1933) Normal variability in weight of the adult human liver and spleen. Arch Pathol 16:350–572

64. Schmuker DL (1998) Aging and the liver: an update. J Gerontol A Biol Sci Med Sci 53:B315–B320

65. Sherloch S, Bearn AG, Billing BH, Paterson JCS (1950) Splanchnic blood flow in man by the bromsulfalein method: the relation of peripheral plasma bromsulfalein level to the calculated flow. J Lab Clin Med 35:923–932

66. MacMahon MM, James OFW, Holt PR (1994) Liver disease in the elderly. J Clin Gastroenterol 18:330–334

67. Sotaniemi EA, Arranto AJ, Pelkonen O (1997) Age and cytochrome P450-linked drug metabolism in humans: an analysis of 226 subjects with equal histopathologic conditions. Clin Pharmacol Ther 61:331–339

68. De Pancorbo CM, Carballo F, Horcajo P et al (1997) Prevalence and associated factors for gallstone disease: results of a population survey in Spain. J Clin Epidemiol 50:1347–1355

69. Attili AF, Capocaccia R, Carulli N et al (1997) Factors associated with gallstone disease in the MICOL experience. Hepatology 26:809–818

70. Valdivieso V, Palma R, Wunkaus R, Antezana C, Severin C, Contreras A (1978) Effect of aging on biliary lipid composition and bile acid metabolism in normal Chilean woman. Gastroenterology 74:871–874

71. Tanno M, Ogihara M, Taguchi T (1996) Age-related changes in proliferating cell nuclear antigen levels. Mech Ageing Dev 92:53–66

72. Fry M, Silber J, Loeb LA, Martin GM (1984) Delayed and reduced cell replication and diminishing levels of DNA polymerase – α in regenerating liver of aging mice. J Cell Physiol 118:225–232

73. Anand BS, Vij JC, Mac MS et al (1989) Effect of aging on the pancreatic ducts: a study based on endoscopic retrograde pancreatography. Gastrointest Endosc 35:210–213

74. Gullo L, Priori P, Daniele C, Ventrucci M, Gasbarrini GL (1983) Exocrine pancreatic function in the elderly. Gerontology 29:407–411

75. Gullo L, Ventrucci M, Naldoni P, Pezzilli R (1986) Aging and exocrine pancreatic function. J Am Geriatr Soc 34:790–792

76. Carrere J, Serre G, Vincent C et al (1987) Human serum pancreatic lipase and trypsin I in aging: enzymatic and immunoenzymatic assays. J Gerontol 42:315–317

77. Elahi D, Muller DC, McAloon-Dyke M, Tobin JD, Andres R (1993) The effect of age in insulin response and glucose utilization during four hyperglycemic plateaus. Exp Gerontol 28:393–409

78. Szoke E, Shrayyef MZ, Messing S, Woerle HJ et al (2008) Effect of aging on glucose homeostasis: accelerated deterioration of beta-cell function in individuals with impaired glucose tolerance. Diabetes Care 31(3):539–543

79. Camilleri M, Murray JA (2008) Diarrhea and constipation. In: Fauci AS, Braunwald E, Kasper D et al (eds) harrison's principles of internal medicine. McGraw Hill, New York, pp 245–254

80. Gomez OA, deSouza RR, Liberti EA (1997) A preliminary investigation of the effects of aging on the nerve cell number in the myenteric ganglia of the human colon. Gastroenterology 43:210–217

81. Cheskin LJ, Kamal N, Crowell MD, Schuster MM, Whitehead WE (1995) Mechanisms of constipation in older persons and effect of fiber compared with placebo. J Am Geriatr Soc 43:666–669

82. Koch TR, Go VLW, Szurszewski JH (1986) Changes in some electrophysical properties of circular muscle from normal sigmoid colon of the aging patient [abstract]. Gastroenterology 90:1497

83. Orr WC, Chen WL (2002) Aging and neural control of the GI tract: IV. Clinical and physiological aspects of gastrointestinal motility and aging. Am J Physiol Gastrointest Liver Physiol 283(6):G1226–G1231

84. Monane M, Avorn J, Beers MH, Everitt DE (1993) Anticholinergic drug use and bowel function in nursing home patients. Arch Intern Med 153:633–638

85. Jameson JS, Chia YW, Kamm MA, Speakman CTM, Chye YH, Henrey MM (1994) Effect of age, sex, and parity on anorectal function. Br J Surg 81:1689–1692

86. Lovat LB (1996) Age related status changes in gut physiology and nutritional status. Gut 38:306–309

87. Fox JC, Fletcher JG, Zinsmeister AR, Seide B, Riederer SJ, Bharucha AE (2006) Effect of aging on anorectal and pelvic floor functions in females. Dis Colon Rectum 49(11):1726–1735

88. McHugh SM, Diamant NE (1987) Effect of age, gender, and parity on anal canal pressures. Contribution of impaired anal sphincter function to fecal incontinence. Dig Dis Sci 32(7):726–736

89. Read NW, Celik AF, Katsinelos P (1995) Constipation and incontinence in the elderly. J Clin Gastroenterol 20:61–70

90. Jorges JMN, Wexner SD, James K, Nogueras JJ, Jagelman GD (1994) Recovery of anal sphincter function after ileoanal reservoir procedure in patients over the age of fifty. Dis Colon Rectum 37:1002–1005

91. Horner MJ, Ries LAG, Krapcho M, Neyman N et al (1975–2006) SEER cancer statistics review. National Cancer Institute, Bethesda, MD

92. Riggs JE (1993) Aging, genomic entropy and carcinogenesis: implications derived from longitudinal age-specific colon cancer mortality rate dynamics. Mech Ageing Dev 72:165–181

93. Vogelstein B, Fearon E, Hamilton SR et al (1988) Genetic alterations during colorectal-tumor development. N Engl J Med 3119:525–532

94. Schub R, Steinheber FU (1986) Rightward shift of colon cancer: a feature of the aging gut. J Clin Gastroenterol 8:630–634

95. Toyoda Y, Nakayama T, Ito Y, Ioka A, Tsukuma H (2009) Trends in colorectal cancer incidence by subsite in Osaka, Japan. Jpn J Clin Oncology 39(3):189–191

96. Barett KE, Barman S, Boitano S, Brooks H (eds) (2009) Ganong's review of medical physiology, 23rd edn. New York, McGraw Hill Companies, INC

97. Huang JQ, Sridhar S, Chen Y, Hunt RH (1998) Meta-analysis of the relationship between *Helicobacter pylori* seropositivity and gastric cancer. Gastroentereology 114(6):1169–1179

98. Cheskin LJ (1999) Constipation and diarrhea. In: Barker LR, Burton JR, Zieve PD (eds) Principles of ambulatory medicine, 5th edn. Williams & Wilkins, Baltimore, pp 498–503

Chapter 59
Benign Esophageal Diseases in the Elderly

Prathima Kanumuri and Neal E. Seymour

Introduction

Noncancer conditions of the esophagus and esophagogastric region may have implications in elderly patients that differ from those encountered in younger age groups. Special consideration must be given to the unique presentations as well as to the physiologic impact of treatments and treatment complications in this vulnerable population. Minimally invasive approaches are now preferred for most esophageal diseases that require surgical treatment. Despite these and other improvements in therapy, benign esophageal disorders continue to present great challenges to practitioners treating the geriatric population.

Gastroesophageal Reflux Disease

The full spectrum of gastroesophageal reflux disease (GERD) symptoms and complications are observed in elderly patients and present specific management considerations. Although GERD does not itself present a significant risk for mortality in the elderly, it may impair quality of life and lead to considerable complication-related morbidity. Patient tolerance of severe symptoms is often poor, and complications such as chronic upper aerodigestive manifestations, esophagitis with ulceration, peptic stricture, and Barrett's esophagus may pose significant management challenges in the elderly.

Pathophysiology

The antireflux barrier at the gastroesophageal junction (GEJ) is an anatomically and physiologically complex zone, which consists of (1) the intrinsic lower esophageal sphincter (LES) pressure (10–30 mmHg), (2) intra-abdominal location of the LES (3–4 cm below the diaphragm), (3) extrinsic compression of LES by the crural diaphragmatic sphincter, (4) integrity of the phrenoesophageal ligament, and (5) maintenance of an acute angle of His. Disruption of the antireflux barrier and abnormal clearance of esophageal contents results in increased exposure of the esophageal lumen to gastric refluxate (acidic or alkaline) [1] (Table 59.1).

Asymptomatic elderly patients differ physiologically from their younger counterparts (Table 59.2) [2–10]. They may have decreased LES pressure, abnormal esophageal motility and clearance, and an increased pain threshold. Older patients may be more likely to take medications that decrease LES tone and potentiate reflux events. These include nitrates, calcium channel blockers, theophylline, benzodiazepines, anticholinergics, and tricyclic antidepressants. Translocation of the esophagogastric junction and LES into the mediastinum through the esophageal hiatus (type 1, sliding hiatal hernia) (Fig. 59.1) occurs more frequently with increasing age [11] and is thought to contribute to pathologic reflux by exposing the LES a decrement in extraluminal pressure in the chest as compared to the abdomen. This relatively lower extraluminal pressure permits LES tone to be more easily overcome by intragastric pressure, leading to reflux. Marco et al. have shown that the degree of reflux symptoms, LES dysfunction, and esophagitis increase with hiatal hernia size [12].

Clinical Presentation

A population-based study in Olmsted County, Minnesota defined the general incidence of GERD symptoms as 19.8% without significant differences with age [13]. Triadafilopoulos and Sharma similarly reported no clear age-related difference in clinical prevalence of GERD above and below age 65 [14]. However, GERD symptom severity may not correlate as well with the severity of pathology in elderly patients. Johnson and Fennerty reported that 34% of patients >70 years old had severe heartburn with a 37% incidence of endoscopically evident severe esophagitis. In contrast, 82% of patients <21 years old with severe heartburn had severe esophagitis only 12% of the time [15]. Furthermore, Collen et al. reported

P. Kanumuri (✉)
Department of Surgery, Baystate Medical Center,
759 Chestnut Street, Springfield, MA 01199, USA
e-mail: philip.rascoe@uphs.upenn.edu

R.A. Rosenthal et al. (eds.), *Principles and Practice of Geriatric Surgery*,
DOI 10.1007/978-1-4419-6999-6_59, © Springer Science+Business Media, LLC 2011

TABLE 59.1 Pathophysiologic factors contributing to GERD

Increased frequency and duration of transient LES relaxation

Hypotensive LES (0–4 mmHg) leading to free reflux

Disruption of phrenoesophageal ligament and diaphragmatic sphincter (Hiatal hernia)

Shortening of intra-abdominal LES

Decreased clearance of esophageal contents due to loss of primary and secondary esophageal peristalsis

Decrease in rate of salivation and salivary bicarbonate

Decreased gastric emptying and increased intra-gastric pressure

GERD gastroesophageal reflux disease, *LES* lower esophageal sphincter

TABLE 59.2 Physiological changes of the esophagus in the elderly

LED

  Decreased LES pressure [2]

  Decreased LES length [3]

  Increase in gastroesophageal reflux events during the postprandial period from pharyngeal stimulation [3]

Esophageal motility

  Aperistalsis without any specific etiology [4]

  Absent or decreased secondary peristalsis with esophageal distention [5]

  Increased tertiary contractions (multiple, simultaneous, nonperistaltic contractions) [6]

  Decreased amplitude and velocity of peristaltic waves [2, 7]

  Impaired esophageal clearance [8, 9]

Higher pain threshold with esophageal distension [10]

LES lower esophageal sphincter

TABLE 59.3 Symptoms and complications associated with GERD

Typical

Heartburn

Regurgitation

Atypical symptoms

Chest pain

Dysphagia

Dyspepsia

Anorexia, weight loss

Dental problems

Atypical symptoms: Respiratory

Globus sensation

Laryngitis

Hoarseness

Chronic cough

Asthma

Bronchitis

Aspiration pneumonia

Pulmonary fibrosis

Complications

Esophagitis

Gastrointestinal bleeding

Peptic strictures

Barrett's esophagitis

GERD gastroesophageal reflux disease

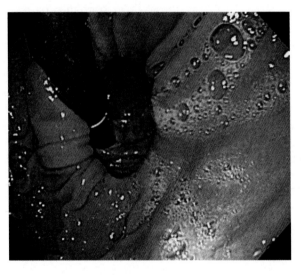

FIGURE 59.1 Retroflexed endoscopic view of type I sliding hiatal hernia. The endoscope is seen emerging from the true esophagogastric junction into the hernia above the muscular ring of the hiatus.

that for a given level of severe reflux symptoms, patients >60 years old had more severe esophagitis compared to younger patients [16]. Zhu et al. reported that 21% of patients >65 years with GERD present with endoscopically severe esophagitis, while only 3.4% of patients under 65 years have severe esophagitis [17]. Patients with GERD present with symptoms which can be described as typical or atypical or a combination of both (Table 59.3). Atypical symptoms may be more prevalent in the elderly [13, 18]. Alkaline reflux may also be more frequent and can be associated with respiratory

symptoms more often than with heartburn [19]. Pellegrini et al. found that individuals with alkaline reflux have less heartburn, regurgitation, and dysphagia but at least as much esophagitis and stricture risk as those with acid reflux, as well as a higher frequency of pulmonary symptoms [20].

Long-standing GERD can result in complications which may lead to significant morbidity. The incidence of erosive esophagitis (45.4%), esophageal ulcers (6%), and esophageal strictures (8.4%) all increase with age. Furthermore, patients with esophageal ulcers or strictures are generally older than patients with uncomplicated esophagitis [21]. In one report, esophagitis was the cause of upper gastrointestinal bleeding in 21% of patients >80 years [22].

Barrett's esophagus, or columnar metaplasia, is a marker of severe chronic esophageal mucosal injury and has been reported to occur in as many as 10–12% of patients with GERD [23, 24]. The prevalence of Barrett's esophagus increases with age and plateaus by the seventh decade [25]. It occurs more frequently in patients greater than 60 years of age (34 vs. 12%) [16]. Elderly patients with Barrett's esophagus experience less severe symptoms compared to younger patients, which may lead to delayed recognition of the condition [14]. The outcome of Barrett's esophagus which is of utmost concern is its progression to adenocarcinoma, but there are no compelling data that define this risk in the elderly. In a meta-analysis of 41 Barrett's esophagus surveillance studies, the reported cancer incidence was found to be between 6 and 9 per 1,000 person-years follow-up [26]. The presence of ulcers, strictures, and nodules was associated with increased cancer incidence. Patients who developed cancer had significantly longer Barrett's segments compared to patients who did not. However, these data did not stratify risk by age, and it is uncertain to what extent age may be an independent risk factor either dysplasia or cancer.

Treatment for Barrett's esophagus is close surveillance, and either medical or surgical control of reflux with the aim to avoid progression of disease. Standard therapy for high-grade dysplasia in Barrett's is esophagectomy. Mucosal ablative therapies (photodynamic therapy, argon plasma coagulation, and cryoablation) for high-grade dysplasia have seen expanded use and could offer benefits to elderly patients, if the morbidity and mortality risk associated with esophagectomy can be avoided. However, uncertain efficacy and potential to undertreat cancer present at the time of the therapy remain a matter of concern.

Diagnostic Studies

Tests to diagnose GERD, GERD complications, and responses to therapy are listed in Table 59.4. GERD symptoms are frequently under treatment with proton pump inhibitors (PPI) or histamine receptor antagonists (HRA) before any diagnostic tests are done. There should be a low threshold to proceed with endoscopy in elderly patients because of the recognized risk of more advanced disease in the face of less severe or atypical symptoms in comparison to younger patients. Endoscopy with biopsy is currently the only study that can effectively identify esophagitis, rule out Barrett's and cancer, as well as document healing of esophagitis

Table 59.4 Diagnostic studies for GERD

Test	Purpose of study
Cine esophagram	Evaluate anatomical causes for dysphagia; document presence of hiatal or paraesophageal hernia; rule out achalasia, scleroderma, strictures, diverticuli, webs and masses
Endoscopy	Evaluate endoscopy positive vs. negative reflux disease; documentation of healing esophagitis; rule out complications of GERD (esophagitis, stricture, and BE), peptic ulcer disease and cancer
Esophageal manometry	Evaluate LES function; rule out esophageal dysmotility before proceeding with antireflux surgery
pH monitoring	Document abnormal acid exposure in symptomatic endoscopy negative patients being evaluated for endoscopic or surgical antireflux therapy; evaluation of patients on PPI therapy with persistent typical symptoms; document adequacy of PPI therapy in patients with complications due to GERD
Esophageal impedance testing	Evaluation of endoscopy negative patients with persistent symptoms despite PPI therapy
Bile acid reflux monitoring	Evaluation of patients with persistent reflux symptoms with normalization of distal esophageal acid exposure confirmed by pH studies

GERD gastroesophageal reflux disease, *BE* Barrett's esophagus, *PPI* proton pump inhibitor

with therapy. Ciné esophagography can help characterize anatomic and functional features of the esophagus during the passage of ingested barium materials of varying consistencies. Some motility characteristics and disorders (Table 59.4) as well as esophagogastric junction anatomy can be defined with the study, and it can be particularly useful in evaluating dysphagia.

Complex or suspected reflux disease and persistent or atypical symptoms should be further evaluated using more objective tests, especially when antireflux surgery is being considered. 2007 American College of Gastroenterology practice guidelines recommend ambulatory pH monitoring to identify pathologic esophageal acid exposure in endoscopy negative patients being considered for endoscopic or surgical antireflux procedures and patients who are symptomatic on PPI therapy. Symptom correlation index can establish likelihood of causality in the relationship between symptom occurrence and episodes of esophageal acid exposure. Although pH monitoring can also be used to evaluate effectiveness of PPI therapy, a specific threshold value for adequate suppression of esophageal acid exposure has not been defined [27], and no age-specific guidelines for the use of this test are available.

Ambulatory pH monitoring can be performed using a nasopharyngeal catheter system or a wireless pH capsule ("Bravo" probe, Medtronic, Minneapolis, MN) that transmits information to an external receiver. Results from the two systems correlate well, but there may be advantages with wireless pH monitoring. The most important is that the modality is associated with less discomfort, less interference with daily activities, and better patient satisfaction compared to the traditional catheter system. Less interference with daily activities will provide more accurate information about reflux episodes [28]. Furthermore, pH monitoring can be performed for more than 24-h periods, and it may be more feasible to study patients on and off PPI therapy. Disadvantages include the need to place the capsule endoscopically, which adds cost and the potential problems of an invasive procedure. Some patients may have severe chest pain, and the capsule may either dislodge early or not dislodge at all, both of which are problematic situations. Wireless pH monitoring might offer advantages in elderly patients based on improved tolerance, but there are no data that specifically support this assumption.

Esophageal impedance monitoring detects changes in resistance to electrical current across adjacent electrodes with the movement of solids, liquids, and gases. It can detect both acid and alkaline reflux (even very weak patterns of reflux) and evaluate esophageal bolus transit when combined with motility studies. Specific monitoring of bile acid reflux is possible by using a probe that detects bile by spectrophotometry. AGA guidelines suggest that these tests may be useful in patients with reflux symptoms despite PPI therapy and normal pH monitoring studies [27]. They are not widely used at this time because the long-term clinical implications of non-acid reflux are not well studied. It is unclear at this time how recognition of this entity might change management in elderly patients.

Chest pain symptoms in the elderly deserve special mention. The most obvious concern lies in the physician's ability to distinguish cardiac from noncardiac chest pain (NCCP) and to institute the appropriate treatment. Although most patients with GERD-induced chest pain will give a history of antecedent reflux symptoms, the possibility of myocardial ischemia ought to be considered and basic investigations conducted so as not to miss this diagnosis. There is considerable overlap in symptoms that could be attributable to either GERD or pain of cardiac origin. DeMeester et al. performed 24-h pH probe studies in patients with typical angina pectoris symptoms and normal cardiac catheterizations and demonstrated reflux to be present in 46% [29]. A positive correlation between chest pain episodes and acid reflux during the pH probe study can be demonstrated in up to 50% of patients with NCCP [30].

Treatment

Irrespective of patient age, the goals in the treatment of GERD are to ameliorate symptoms, promote healing of esophagitis, maintain remission, and prevent long-term complications. These goals maybe achieved using various modalities.

Nonsurgical Treatment

Life style or behavioral modifications can alleviate symptoms in mild reflux disease when employed alone or with medical therapies. These might include the elevation of the head and chest during sleep, avoidance of supine position or sleep less than 3 h after meals, weight loss in overweight patients, smoking cessation, and avoidance of foods associated with reflux (e.g., high fat foods, chocolate, peppermint, coffee, and alcohol). As mentioned previously, selected medications may decrease LES tone. Caution with these as well as with medications that might predispose to pill esophagitis (potassium tablets, iron sulfate, and alendronate) should be exercised.

Histamine receptor antagonists (cimetidine, ranitidine, famotidine, and nizatidine) may be effective but are used less frequently than proton pump inhibitors (PPIs) as first-line therapy. PPIs (omeprazole, lansoprazole, rabeprazole, pantoprazole, and esomeprazole) inhibit the H^+/K^+ ATPase proton pump. They have become the mainstay of medical therapy for significant GERD and are now available over-the-counter (omeprazole). If symptoms are suggestive, empiric treatment is usually started before diagnostic tests are done, and prompt clinical improvement is generally taken as confirmatory of the GERD diagnosis. Historical exceptions to prompt use of PPIs rather than investigations include long-standing GERD and alarm symptoms such as anemia, weight loss, and dysphagia [31]. Since elderly patients may present with more advanced disease and less severe symptoms, an argument can be made for the use of endoscopy prior to starting prolonged acid suppression in order to clearly establish the presence of esophagitis.

Almost 50% of patients with GERD suffer frequent relapses and need some form of maintenance therapy. PPIs are currently regarded as the most effective medications available for acute as well as maintenance therapy for GERD [32], although H_2 receptor antagonists may also be effective if PPI treatment cannot be given. Since PPIs are long-acting medications, dosing is convenient for older patients. Added potential advantages include easy administration in older patients with swallowing problems (granules can be mixed in soft food or liquids) and the fact that dose adjustments are not necessary in hepatic and renal insufficiency [33]. Some studies have shown an increased risk for respiratory infections, Clostridium difficile colitis, and osteoporosis with PPI use [34].

Cisapride is a prokinetic agent which may be available for use in GERD outside the USA, having been removed from the US market in 2000 due to increased risk for cardiac arrhythmias. Metoclopramide can be problematic in elderly patients due to CNS side effects (sedation and tardive dyskinesia). Other promotility drugs such as Tegaserod (serotonin agonist) and Baclofen (GABA agonist) may have some efficacy in GERD but are not standard therapies.

Surgical Treatment

Indications for surgical treatment of GERD include (1) patient choice in order to discontinue medical therapy, (2) intolerance of medical therapy, (3) persistence of symptoms on medical therapy, and (4) complications of GERD including persistent esophagitis on medication, peptic strictures, and Barrett's esophagus (although the latter indication may be controversial). The goals of surgery are to repair any associated hiatal hernia, establish an intra-abdominal length of esophagus, and perform a fundoplication as a barrier to reflux. Nissen or 360° fundoplication (Fig. 59.2) is the most frequently performed

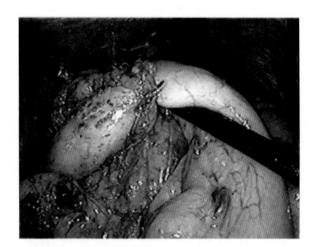

FIGURE 59.2 Laparoscopic Nissen fundoplication. The loose nature of this complete (360°) wrap of gastric fundus around the esophagogastric junction and distal esophagus is demonstrated by the insertion of an instrument below the left-sided fundic component of the wrap.

antireflux procedure. Toupet or 270° fundoplication has generally been reserved for GERD patients with ineffective esophageal motility, although its efficacy as compared to a loose Nissen fundoplication is controversial [35, 36]. There are numerous other types of antireflux procedure intended for use via transabdominal or transthoracic access methods, but a full discussion of surgical antireflux treatments is beyond the scope of this chapter. It can currently be stated that laparoscopic antireflux procedures represent the surgical standard of care for GERD, and advantages relative to open procedures are well established [37]. Investigations of surgical treatment of GERD in the elderly have generally shown that outcomes are favorable. Table 59.5 summarizes eight studies that compare surgical outcomes in "older" (>60 years) and "younger" patients (<60 years of age) [38–45]. These have established that postoperative symptom relief is not adversely affected by advancing age with mean follow-up of between 3 months and 5 years. There may be a perception that postoperative complication rates are higher and length of hospital stay are greater for patients >60 years of age, but this has not been consistently observed for antireflux surgery. Although patients >60 years had significantly higher American Society of Anesthesia (ASA) score in four studies and a higher rate of comorbidities in one study, this did not closely correlate with an increase in complication rate and length of stay. The likelihood of mortality with antireflux surgery is very close to zero in both populations.

Current data suggest that antireflux surgery can improve formally measured quality of life in elderly patients. Kamolz et al. reported the use of the gastrointestinal quality of life index (GIQLI) to assess postoperative outcomes in 72 patients greater than 65 years of age. Scores were significantly improved 3 months after surgery compared to preoperative values. This improvement persisted 1 and 3 years after surgery and was similar to scores in healthy individuals [46]. Fernando et al. [41] and Wang et al. [45] showed that SF 36 health survey and GIQLI assessments of global and disease-associated quality of life postsurgical outcomes were not significantly different in patients <60 years and >60 years of age. The overwhelming weight of evidence indicates that antireflux surgery is both effective and safe in the elderly, and that outcomes are comparable to those achieved in younger patients.

Intraoperative complications of antireflux surgery are uncommon. Esophageal perforation is rare and may result from dissection or bougie injuries. Common causes of intraoperative bleeding are adhesiolysis, or injury to the left lobe of liver or the spleen. Bleeding is generally controlled by local measures and rarely requires conversion to an open procedure. Splenic injuries and splenectomy, which were surprisingly common events with open fundoplication (2–5%), are rare occurrences in laparoscopic antireflux surgery. Pneumothorax is also rare and is thought to be due to extensive dissection into the mediastinum. Chest tube placement is rarely required due to the rapid uptake of CO_2. Conversion rates from laparoscopic to open procedures are less than 5%.

Coelho et al. evaluated complications of laparoscopic fundoplication in 77 patients >70 years of age and reported 7.8% gas bloat syndrome, 5.2% dysphagia, and 2.6% gastric ulceration incidences [47]. Although most dysphagia after fundoplication either resolves or responds well to modest dietary measures, severe dysphagia symptoms may on rare occasions require endoscopic dilatation or surgical revision of fundoplication. Technical considerations that minimize the likelihood of postoperative dysphagia include routine division of the gastrosplenic ligament and short-gastric vessels, and adequate fundic mobilization for a loose wrap. The incidence of anatomic failure of antireflux procedures ranges from 3 to 6%. These cases include fundoplication disruption or slipping, or axial herniation of the fundoplication into the mediastinum. Pledgeted suture repair of the hiatus and reinforcement of the defect with a mesh may decrease incidence of some types of anatomic failure [48].

Endoscopic Treatment

Endoscopic therapy for GERD has shown to significantly decrease PPI use, improve symptoms, and decrease but never normalize acid exposure in patients with mild forms of GERD. Proposed exclusion criteria include hiatal hernias greater than 2 cm, esophagitis greater than grade II, and disease refractory to PPI therapy [49]. Currently there are three FDA approved devices available for GERD endoluminal therapy: (1) EndoCinch (Bard, Davol, Inc., Cranston, RI),

TABLE 59.5 Laparoscopic antireflux surgery outcomes in elderly (>60 years) vs. adult (<60 years) patients

Year	Author	Age (years)	n	Symptom relief	Complications	LOS (days)	Mortality in elderly
1998	Trus et al. [38]	69 (65–79)	42	=	=	=	None
1999	Brunt et al. [39]	65 (65–82)	36	=	> (13.9% vs. 2.6%)	> (2.3 vs. 1.6)	None
2002	Khajanchee et al. [40]	71 ± 6 (SD)	30	=	=	=	NA
2003	Fernando et al. [41]	68 (60–80)	43	=	=	> (2.9 vs. 1.6)	None
2006	Cowgill et al. [42]	70 (70–90)	108	=	=	> (4.3 vs. 2.6)	One patient
2006	Brehant et al. [43]	70 (65–94)	369	=	> (7.6% vs.4.5%)	> (5.9 vs. 4.6)	None
2006	Tedesco et al. [44]	69 (65–88)	63	=	=	=	None
2008	Wang et al. [45]	73 (70–76)	33	=	> (9% vs. 0.5%)	=	None

SD standard deviation; n total number of elderly patients in the study, = Similar to adult patients; > Greater than adult patients; LOS length of stay; NA not available

PARAESOPHAGEAL HERNIA

Case Study: Part 1

Presentation: An 81-year-old man with mild dementia, hypertension, and atrial fibrillation cared for at home by his 74-year-old spouse was brought to the emergency department with a 12 h history of vomiting and chest pain. He was accompanied by his wife, who provided most of the health history information. He had significant short-term memory loss, but walked for exercise and enjoyed fishing and watching televised baseball games. The patient's knowledge of recent events was very incomplete, although he answered question appropriately and was oriented to time and place. His wife reported that he had had recent difficulties with tolerance of certain ingested foods and beverages. Over the past 2 months, he had increasingly frequent interruption of meals with agitation and "spitting up" small amounts of undigested food. He complained of substernal chest discomfort with some of these episodes but was unable to provide more specific information on this symptom. He had been able to take his oral medications until the present episode. At presentation, the patient was comfortable, but had not eaten and had only taken in minimal fluids over the previous 12 h. Three weeks prior to presentation, in investigation of his symptoms, he had a 12-lead EKG that showed his usual rate-controlled atrial fibrillation and a radionuclide cardiac perfusion scan was normal. He also had a chest X-ray that showed an air–fluid level suspected to be stomach occupying the lower half of the left lung field. His medications included warfarin, hydrocholorothiazide, and lisinopril. He had no abdominal surgery history, but had bilateral knee replacements 12 years previously. The remainder of his review of systems was negative, with the exception of knee and back pain for which he took acetaminophen.

Physical examination: The patient was a pleasant, Caucasian man of medium build. He had irregular heart rhythm with a rate of 75 bpm and BP 147/85. Breath sounds were present, but when he rocked front-to-back, a splashing sound was auscultated at the left lung base. His abdomen was soft and nontender. The remainder of his examination was unremarkable. Diagnostic studies: Serum electrolytes, BUN, and creatinine were normal. His automated WBC count was 7,200 with 68% leukocytes, and his hematocrit was 38%. INR is 1.9. His chest X-ray was available for review, and based on suspicion of the presence of a paraesophageal hernia, an immediate barium esophagram was obtained (Fig. 59.3), which identified a Type III paraesophageal hernia.

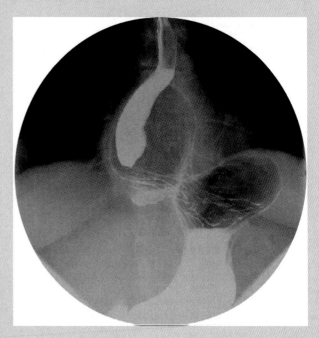

FIGURE 59.3 Barium esophagram of a type III (paraesophageal) hiatal hernia. In this case, there is clear demonstration of the relationship between the axially rotated gastric fundus and the adjacent esophagus, which tapers at the expected location of the diaphragmatic hiatus.

(2) Plicator (NDO surgical, Inc., Mansfield, MA), and (3) Stretta (Curon Medical, Inc., Fremont, CA). The principles by which these devices operate are (1) Plication of the submucosa at the GEJ (EndoCinch). (2) Full-thickness serosa-to-serosa plication at the GEJ (Plicator). (3) Radiofrequency thermal therapy delivered to LES (Stretta). Potential advantages in elderly patients include performance with conscious sedation, and relatively short-procedure duration. There may be applications in poor surgical candidates or as a bridge between medical and surgical therapy. However, based on current literature, there are no clear indications based on perceived or measured superiority relative to traditional surgical measures. Published studies have been small and more focused on safety and feasibility than on long-term durability and efficacy. With increasing experience, evolving techniques and hardware, as well as more thorough investigation, endoluminal therapies may become a viable option in the treatment of GERD, with specific applications in the elderly.

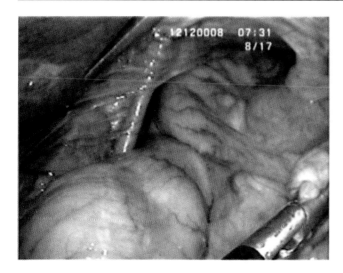

FIGURE 59.4 Laparoscopic view of a type III (paraesophageal) hiatal hernia, with the herniated body and fundus of the stomach above the right crural pillar.

Paraesophageal hernia is primarily a disease of the elderly and the average age of diagnosis is 60–70 years. The true incidence of hiatal hernias is difficult to determine because majority of patients remain asymptomatic and therefore undiagnosed. There are four types of hiatal hernias. (1) Type I (Sliding hiatal hernia): Esophagogastric junction migrates through the hiatus and is commonly associated with GERD. (2) Type II: Gastric fundus herniates through the hiatus with esophagogastric junction in an intra-abdominal position. This is a true paraesophageal hernia. (3) Type III (combination of Type I and II). In this hernia type, gastric fundus and esophagogastric junction herniate into the mediastinum (Fig. 59.4). (4) Type IV: Type III hernia with herniation of other viscera such as spleen or colon [50]. Type II, III, and IV hiatal hernias are called paraesophageal hernias, and Type III hernia is the most common among them (90%). Type I or sliding hiatal hernias are at least seven times more common than paraesophageal hernias [51].

Pathophysiology

Paraesophageal hernias occur more frequently with advancing age and are believed to result from progression of a sliding hiatal hernia. Prolonged repetitive stretching of the phrenoesophageal membrane due to movement of the esophagus during swallowing, as well as increased intra-abdominal pressure due to conditions such as morbid obesity, COPD, asthma and chronic constipation, may contribute to more complex patterns of gastric herniation into the chest [51].

Clinical Presentation

Symptoms associated with paraesophageal hernias are primarily related to partial or complete gastric obstruction. Patients present with nausea, bloating, early satiety, chest pain, and fullness relieved with vomiting and dysphagia. Fifteen to thirty percent of patients with paraesophageal hernias complain of GERD symptoms [52, 53]. Patients with larger hernias may suffer from chest pain and shortness of breath. Paraesophageal hernias may be associated with chronic blood loss and anemia due to gastric erosions from prolonged trauma [54]. Gastric volvulus is a possible complication of paraesophageal hernias, with rotation either along the long axis of the stomach (organoaxial) or along a perpendicular axis (mesenteroaxial). Patients with completed volvulus can present emergently with acute gastric obstruction and potentially with gastric strangulation. Symptoms associated with this presentation are epigastric pain, persistent retching and vomiting, bloody vomitus due to gastric ischemia and ulceration, and an acute abdomen and sepsis, if a gastric perforation has occurred. Previous studies have reported an acute presentation in 29% of patients with paraesophageal hernias [55, 56]. However, a recent study by Stylopoulos et al. looked at five studies and estimated the probability of developing acute symptoms to be 1.16% per year. The lifetime risk for developing acute symptoms is 18% for 65 years and decreases as patent's age increases [57]. Arguments for mandatory surgical treatment of paraesophageal hernia are generally based on the need to avoid this variably estimated risk, which may be favorably affected by advancing patient age.

Diagnostic Studies

Chest radiograph may demonstrate an air–fluid level in the left chest. Upper gastrointestinal contrast study with barium is the study of choice to diagnose paraesophageal hernias (Fig. 59.3). Computed tomography can also establish the diagnosis (Fig. 59.5). Upper endoscopy can aid in recognition of a paraesophageal component of a hiatal hernia and will provide other information such as the presence of esophagitis or ulcerations. Twenty-four hours pH monitoring and esophageal manometry can be considered in patients with GERD symptoms, but may not influence surgical planning.

Treatment

Surgical management of symptomatic and asymptomatic paraesophageal hernias has historically represented a mandatory standard of care. This is based largely on reports of a

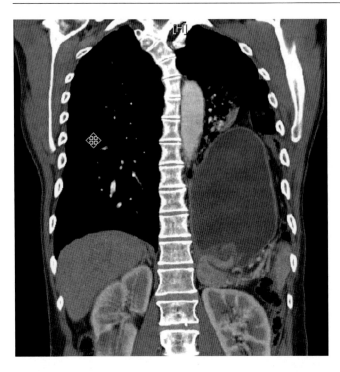

Figure 59.5 CT chest coronal section of a type III hiatal hernia (paraesophageal), with adjacent contrast-filled esophagus between the distended, herniated stomach, and the thoracic vertebrae. Such studies have become increasingly valuable in more precisely defining anatomic relationships in complex hernias of this type. This information can be used to better understand the condition, or as an aid in operative planning.

high (28–30%) incidence of acute symptoms necessitating emergency operations, which were associated with high rates of morbidity and mortality [55, 56]. Surgery continues to be the treatment of choice for symptomatic paraesophageal hernias. However, the treatment of asymptomatic and minimally symptomatic hernias has become more controversial. Allen et al. followed 23 patients managed nonoperatively for an average of 78 months and reported that only four developed progression of symptoms and that the two patients who underwent elective repair did well [52]. Stylopoulos et al. assessed outcomes of elective laparoscopic hernia repair vs. watchful observation in patients with asymptomatic and minimally symptomatic indications based on information from 20 published studies. Using a predictive model, it was determined that less than one in five 65-year-old patients and only one in ten 85-year-old patients will benefit from elective surgical treatment [57].

The goals of operative treatment of paraesophageal hernias are (1) reduction of the herniated stomach (or other viscera), (2) reduction and excision of the hernia sac, (3) hiatal hernia repair with or without prosthetic mesh, and (4) secure subdiaphragmatic positioning of the stomach. Although the use of fundoplication in paraesophageal hernia repair remains controversial, it is frequently used on the assumption that it may reduce recurrent hernia risk as well as reduce

postoperative GERD occurrence. As many as 60% of patients with type III hernias have diminished LES pressures and abnormal esophageal pH monitoring studies [59]. Willekes et al. reported that as many as 30% of patients had preoperative reflux symptoms and that some patients develop postoperative reflux despite the absence of preoperative reflux symptoms. He concluded that GEJ and LES physiology cannot be predicted once it has been surgically disturbed and all phrenoesophageal supporting attachments are divided [53]. Despite these observations, there are no compelling data to support either the use or omission of fundoplication in this clinical situation, and no specific data in elderly patients to guide this decision.

Minimally invasive surgery has become the preferred method of management for paraesophageal hernias, with the well-founded expectation of decreased postoperative pain, length of stay, and morbidity and mortality compared to open surgical methods [59–62]. A recent large series (203 patients) of laparoscopic repair for giant paraesophageal hernia (1/3 or more of stomach herniation into chest) suggests a pattern of disease skewed toward more elderly patients. The mean patient age was 67 years (34–91 years) and median follow-up was 18 months. The median length of hospital stay was 3 days, morbidity was 28%, and mortality was 0.5. Postoperative symptom relief was excellent to good in 92% of patients [61].

Bammer et al. and Grotentuis et al. evaluated outcomes of laparoscopic paraesophageal hernia repair in patients >80 years of age and >70 years of age, respectively. Results were comparable to studies with mixed age groups [63, 64]. Gangopadhyay et al. compared results of laparoscopic paraesophageal hernia repair in three age groups <65 years (Group 1), 65–74 years (Group 2), and >74 years (Group 3). Group 3 had significantly higher ASA scores and hospital length of stay but their postoperative complication rate, symptom relief, and recurrence rates were comparable to other groups [65]. In a retrospective review of 1,005 patients (>80 years of age) who underwent diaphragmatic hernia repair, 43% of procedures were emergent. Emergency operations were more common among older patients, and the concurrent finding of CHF and was associated with longer hospital length of stay and mortality (14 ± 1 days and 16%) compared to patients who underwent elective repair (7 ± 1 days and 2.5%) [66]. Laparoscopic paraesophageal hernia repair is a safe and effective option in the elderly and they should not be denied surgery based on age alone, because emergency surgery in this population is associated with significant mortality. In elderly and debilitated patients with multiple comorbidities, one should consider shorter, less invasive techniques such as anterior gastropexy or placement of percutaneous endoscopic gastrostomy after the reduction of paraesophageal hernias. Agwunobi et al. and Kercher et al. performed these techniques in small series of high-risk patients (13 and 11 patients) with minimal complications and low recurrence rates [67, 68].

CASE STUDY: PART 2

Treatment plan: The patient was admitted to the Surgical Service and maintenance intravenous fluids were started. Although there was discussion of placement of a nasogastric tube, this was not done as the patient was comfortable and there were deemed to be risks associated with any attempt to position this tube given potential obstructive pathology associated with the hernia. A Geriatric Medicine consult was obtained, and it was decided to observe the patient on a telemetry unit and not to give any of his home medications. If he became tachycardic, this would be treated with intravenous beta-blockers. The decision was made to hold anticoagulation and to give Vitamin K 10 mg and 2 U fresh frozen plasma in anticipation of surgical intervention. On the second hospital day, the patient underwent successful laparoscopic repair of a large paraesophageal hernia, with pledgeted repair of the esophageal hiatus, and Toupet fundoplication. Postoperative care: In the postanesthesia care unit (PACU), he developed rapid atrial fibrillation (130 bpm) with a blood pressure of 105/60. There was no evidence of acute bleeding, and operative blood loss was minimal. He was given two 2 mg doses of intravenous morphine sulfate and three 5 mg doses of intravenous Metoprolol over a 2-h period, and better rate control was achieved, with increase in BP to 135/80. Troponin, CPK, and CPK-MB levels were nonelevated, and a 12-lead EKG showed no change from a preoperative study. After discharge from PACU, he returned to the telemetry unit. On postoperative day #1,

he started a clear liquid diet along with his home medications, including Warfarin. He remained in atrial fibrillation at 70 bpm and telemetry was discontinued. On postoperative day #2, a soft diet was started, which the patient tolerated well. He ambulated well with assistance and was discharged home to follow-up with his surgeon and primary care physician in 1–2 weeks.

Salient Points

1. Although nasogastric tube placement is not absolutely contraindicated in paraesophageal hernia, risk of perforation in this setting should temper use, and placement may be best deferred until operative visualization of the reduced stomach can be achieved. There is no indication for postoperative use of a nasogastric tube after laparoscopic paraesophageal hernia repair.
2. Despite advanced age, repair a paraesophageal hernia ought to be with the expectation of a good postoperative result, although special precautions with comorbidities is required. In a highly symptomatic patient, prompt surgical treatment is suggested to avoid obstructive issues or more dire complications such as completed volvulus with strangulation.
3. A succussion splash, described in the examination findings, can be found in some patients with a large hiatal hernia, but does not identify hernia type, or necessarily suggest the need for intervention.

Esophageal Motility Disorders

Esophageal motility may undergo various physiological changes with aging. Among these are decreased secondary esophageal peristalsis, increased ineffective tertiary contractions, and diminished velocity and amplitude of peristaltic waves (Table 59.2). Esophageal dysmotility may be primary, such as in achalasia, diffuse esophageal spasm (DES) and nutcracker esophagus or secondary to conditions such as systemic sclerosis, polymyositis and diabetes mellitus [69].

Achalasia

Achalasia has two incidence peaks: The first between ages 20 and 40 and the second in more elderly patients. Sonnenberg et al. reported an average age of 78 years for patients with

achalasia based on hospital admission codes, with a steady increase in hospitalization rates between the ages of 65 and 94 years [70].

Pathophysiology

Achalasia is a primary functional disorder of the esophagus characterized by the absence of peristalsis and incomplete relaxation of the LES during swallowing. These characteristics contribute to a functional obstruction at the GEJ [71]. Although occasional familial clustering of achalasia cases has been reported, most are sporadic and of uncertain etiology [72]. The esophageal manifestations of Chaga's disease (Tripanisoma Cruzi), which is endemic in South America, can be considered a form of achalasia, but is accompanied by a host of other infection-related problems. It can be observed in elderly patients and presents particular management challenges largely due to the broader range of systems affected and overall poorer prognosis.

Viral infection has been proposed as a causative factor in achalasia [73, 74]. Reported histologic characteristics are based on resected and autopsy esophageal specimens, and most likely reflect advanced disease findings. Wallerian degenerative changes, loss of myenteric ganglion cells, microscopic degeneration of the vagus nerve, and hypertrophy of the muscularis propria of the distal esophagus have been described [75]. A loss of nitric oxide and vasoactive intestinal peptide (VIP)-containing postganglionic inhibitory neurons in the myenteric plexus may be responsible for impairment of LES relaxation due to unopposed cholinergic stimulation [76–78]. Goin et al. have suggested an autoimmune etiology based on the identification of circulating antimuscarinic antibodies in chagasic achalasia [79]. The presence of Lewey bodies in the myenteric plexus and loss of neurons in the dorsal motor nucleus of the vagus in both achalasia and Parkinson's disease suggests a possible link between the two diseases, which appear with high prevalence in the elderly.

Aperistalsis in achalasia is not clearly understood. Inhibitory innervation is believed to be critical to the phasic sequence of esophageal muscular contractions and it is possible that loss of inhibitory neurons abolishes peristatic motor function. Long-term aperistalsis and functional GEJ obstruction can eventually result in a massively dilated and tortuous esophagus devoid of any discernible motor function [71].

Clinical Presentation

The most common symptoms of achalasia are dysphagia to solid food, regurgitation of esophageal contents, weight loss, and various patterns of chest pain. Dysphagia is progressive in achalasia and may also interfere with ingestion of liquids. Other clinical complaints may include cervical level dysphagia and difficulty belching. It has been suggested that some symptoms are related to impaired upper esophageal sphincter relaxation [80, 81].

Dysphagia and impaired esophageal emptying in achalasia is due to both impaired LES relaxation and loss of esophageal peristalsis. There is stasis of varying amounts of undigested food proximal to the LES depending on the capacitance of the dilated esophagus and the rate and quantity of food intake. Patients develop techniques to facilitate esophageal emptying, including slow, purposeful swallowing, avoidance of firm foods, postural changes (twisting, stretching), and ingestion of warm liquids with meals. Approximately 40% of patients have chest pain in the xiphoid or substernal areas, which often prompts evaluation for cardiac problems. This pain may be increased by exercise and relieved by rest [82]. Achalasia patients also commonly describe "heartburn," which is most likely related to esophageal stasis [83]. Clouse et al. compared clinical presentations of achalasia in patients greater and lesser than 70 years of age. Although symptom patterns were similar in the two groups, fewer of the older patients complained of chest pain [84].

Patients with achalasia are at risk for developing chronic inflammation, ulceration, perforation, and fistulas as a result of chronic stasis and retention. It has been shown that there is a 33-fold increased risk of esophageal carcinoma in these patients, with a yearly incidence of 3.4/1,000. The patients at highest risk are elderly patients with a long-standing history of dysphagia and a markedly dilated esophagus [85].

Diagnosis

A plain chest radiograph may demonstrate a widened mediastinum and an air–fluid level in the posterior mediastinum due to esophageal dilation. A barium esophogram effectively demonstrates the gross esophageal changes, which can include dilation, tortuosity, retention of food and barium, and a symmetric smooth tapering of the esophagus resembling a bird's beak (Fig. 59.6). The most striking gross feature of achalasia is massive esophageal dilation known as sigmoid esophagus or megaesophagus seen in advanced cases (Fig. 59.7).

Upper endoscopy should be considered a mandatory study to exclude peptic stricture and malignancy. The latter condition may be associated with clinical changes similar to those of achalasia, particularly in patients over 60 years of age [86, 87]. A diagnosis of pseudoachalasia can be firmly established only by biopsy and histologic demonstration of carcinoma.

Of all currently available studies, esophageal manometry establishes the diagnosis of achalasia most effectively. Although the resting LES pressure is normal in 40% of patients, up to 80% have absent or incomplete LES relaxation with wet swallows. It must be emphasized that the presence of LES relaxation does not exclude achalasia. Postdeglutitive relaxations may appear complete but usually are of short duration [88, 89]. Loss of normal esophageal body peristalsis is manifested by simultaneous contractions following wet swallows. Contractile amplitudes are low (10–40 mmHg) with frequent prolonged and repetitive waves. Studies have shown increased basal LES pressure in older patients with achalasia compared to younger patients [90, 91]. Chuah et al. demonstrated a linear correlation between age and LES basal pressure in achalasia patients [91].

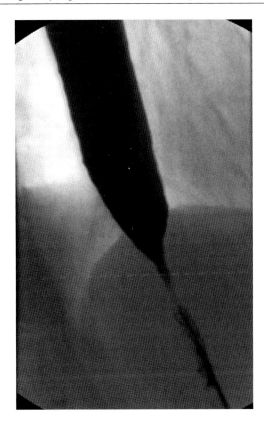

FIGURE 59.6 Bird's beak deformity of the distal esophagus in a patient with achalasia seen on a barium esophagram. This characteristic appearance in a patient with the clinical features of achalasia is strongly suggestive of this condition.

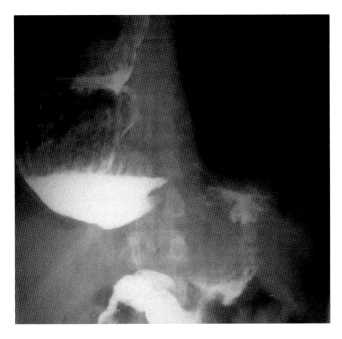

FIGURE 59.7 Barium esophagram of a megaesophagus in a patient with advanced achalasia. The barium column may be diluted by retain fluid and food in the enlarged and sometimes tortuous esophagus.

Vigorous achalasia is a variant of achalasia characterized by high amplitude (>60 mmHg) simultaneous esophageal contractions, which may be associated with intense chest pain. This form of achalasia may be less frequent in elderly patients.

Treatment

Treatment of achalasia is primarily palliative and is geared towards adequate symptom relief from functional LES obstruction [71]. Variety of nonsurgical and surgical options are available.

Nonsurgical Treatment

Calcium channel blockers and nitrates are the most commonly used pharmacological agents in the treatment of achalasia. Clinical improvement with both sublingual isosorbide dinitrite and nifedipine treatment has been reported; however, symptom relief is variable 53–87% and 0–75%, respectively [92, 93]. These agents must be taken sublingually immediately prior to meals to achieve the desired result. The major potential side effects that might limit this treatment are headache, hypotension, and tachyphylaxis. However, oral pharmacotherapy has not gained popularity because of its short-lived effects, poor symptom relief, and decreasing efficacy with time. They are definitely an option in patients awaiting definitive therapy and the elderly who have failed botulinum toxin therapy and are poor candidates for pneumatic dilatation and surgery.

Intrasphincteric injection of botulinum toxin type A has shown to effectively reduce LES pressure by inhibiting cholinergic receptors. Pasricha et al. reported a 70% symptomatic relief in patients treated with botulinum toxin with 40% requiring more than one injection [94]. Despite impressive early results, the long-term efficacy of this treatment has been questioned based on high 1 year relapse rates and less successful repeat injection. Older patients and patients with vigorous achalasia have a better response to botulinum therapy [95]. Elderly patients (>60 years) with significant medical problems tolerate this treatment modality well [96, 97]. Advantages of this procedure are: it is well tolerated with minimal complications and is a good option in elderly patients that cannot tolerate dilatation and surgery. On the other hand, relapse rates are high and frequent injections may be necessary which could lead to patient discomfort and increased costs.

Pneumatic balloon dilatation has wide acceptance and is a mainstay of treatment for achalasia. This technique employs a rapidly inflated balloon in the distal esophagus to dilate and disrupt the circular smooth muscle fibers of the LES.

The procedure is well tolerated with a short-hospital stay. The first dilatation results in symptom relief in 50–65% of patients [71]; however, 15–48% of patients require repeat procedures [98–100]. Patients older than 40 years had better 2-year results than patients younger than 40 (67 vs. 29%) [101]. The principal risk of pneumatic dilation is esophageal perforation, which in skilled hands is less than 2%. The risk of perforation is highest with the first dilatation.

Surgical Treatment

Surgical treatment of achalasia consists of longitudinal division of the LES muscle fibers also referred to as *myotomy* or *esophagomyotomy*. This procedure lowers LES pressure and esophageal intraluminal pressure, but most importantly eradicates the effects of incomplete LES relaxation. Good-to-excellent results have been reported in as high as 90% of patients with 1–36 years' follow-up of. Follow-up studies have demonstrated an improvement in esophageal emptying, increased LES diameter, and decreased esophageal diameter [102–105]. Although the point in a patient's care at which surgery should be offered is undefined, superior results with laparoscopic myotomy as initial therapy, as compared to pneumatic dilatation and botulinum toxin, have been suggested [106]. Furthermore, Smith et al. reported that complication rates after laparoscopic Heller myotomy were higher among patients who underwent previous endoscopic treatment with GI perforation being the most common complication (9.7 vs. 3.6%) [107].

Laparoscopic esophagomyotomy is currently the most frequently used surgical approach for achalasia, with decreased postoperative pain, length of hospitalization, and technical ease, compared to open and thoracoscopic methods. Current data indicate that laparoscopic myotomy is a safe and effective option in elderly patients. Kilic et al. reported that in 57 patients >70 years of age who underwent laparoscopic Heller myotomy, there were no perioperative deaths and that there was a 19.3% complication rate and median hospital stay of 3 days. At a mean follow-up of 23.5 months 96.5% reported improvement in symptoms [108]. Severe preoperative dysphagia, dilated esophagus, and absence of all motility are predictors of poor outcome, and LES pressure >35 mmHg is a predictor of good outcome after Laparoscopic Heller myotomy [109, 110]. The overall complication rate for esophagomyotomy is 10%, with GERD being the most common postoperative problem followed by dysphagia from insufficient myotomy [102]. Although partial fundoplication (Dor vs. Toupet) may substantially reduce postoperative reflux with esophagomyotomy, the potential for residual dysphagia has tempered its use.

Diffuse Esophageal Spasm

Diffuse esophageal spasm (DES) is a primary esophageal hypermotility disorder characterized by dysphagia and episodic substernal chest pain. It is a rare condition, the etiology of which is unknown. Although the mean age of occurrence is in the 5th decade, it can in the elderly patients up to the 8th decade of life. Because the symptom that most often brings DES patients to medical attention is angina-like chest pain, formal workup for a cardiac etiology is almost always undertaken. The principal manometric findings in DES are frequent simultaneous and repetitive contractions of abnormally high amplitude or long duration. The finding of 20% or more simultaneous contractions per 10 wet swallows is considered diagnostic of the disorder [111]. LES resting pressures and relaxation with swallows are usually normal. DES activity is intermittent and ambulatory 24-h manometry allows patients to go about their daily activities and receive whatever typical stimuli are necessary to precipitate an episode [112]. Many patients with DES have an underlying psychiatric history with diagnoses that include depression, psychosomatic complaints, and anxiety. These diagnoses have been reported in 80% of patients with manometric contraction abnormalities [113].

A barium esophagram can help in the characterization of DES. Occasionally, a "corkscrew" esophagus caused by segmental contractions of circular muscle is identified. The finding of an esophageal pulsion diverticulum in a patient with characteristic chest pain is virtually diagnostic of DES. Esophagoscopy should be performed in all patients to exclude the possibility of a tumor, fibrosis, or esophagitis, which might cause esophageal narrowing that may be associated with proximal tertiary esophageal contractions.

Treatment of this condition may be difficult. As with achalasia, some patients respond to sublingual nitrates or calcium channel blockers before meals [114, 115]. Esophageal dilation may alleviate symptoms of dysphagia for days to months and can be repeated for continued relief [116]. However, there is an increased risk of perforation with multiple dilations of a hypertrophic, spastic esophagus.

Surgical treatment is generally reserved for medical and endoscopic treatment failures. This consists of a long myotomy aimed at reducing simultaneous contractions and improving compliance, at the cost of peristaltic loss and reduced residual muscular contraction amplitude [117]. It can be accomplished thoracoscopically [118], with an 80% rate of diminished symptoms during the early postoperative period. Fundoplication may be performed to avoid reflux, but with the same concerns expressed for achalasia. With long durations of follow-up (5.0–10.7 years), surgically treated patients can remain free of chest pain and dysphagia [119].

Other Esophageal Disorders

Nutcracker esophagus is another primary esophageal hypermotility disorder that like DES presents as episodic dysphagia and chest pain. It tends to occur later than DES (5th and 6th decades of life) and can occur in elderly patients as well. It is diagnosed by manometry when average peristaltic pressures are above 180 mmHg and have a prolonged duration. Treatment is similar to DES.

Secondary esophageal dysmotility disorders occur in conjunction with systemic diseases such as diabetes, hypo- and hyperthyroidism, systemic sclerosis, polymyositis, and amyloidosis. These diseases are prevalent in the elderly and should be kept in mind while working up a patient for a suspected esophageal motility disorder [120].

Benign Tumors of the Esophagus

Benign tumors of the esophagus often go unreported and undiagnosed, their exact incidence is not known. In two large autopsy series, the reported incidences of these tumors were 0.45 and 0.59% [121, 122]. They can be intraluminal, intramural, or extramural. The most common benign tumors of the esophagus are leiomyomas, followed by fibrovascular polyps.

Leiomyomas

Leiomyomas are mesenchymal in origin and account for two-thirds of all benign esophageal tumors. The peak incidence for leiomyomas is between the ages of 30 and 59, but can occur in much older patients [123]. In a review of 838 cases, 56% were found in the lower third of the esophagus, 33% in the middle third, and 11% in the upper third [124]. Majority of leiomyomas are intramural and arise from the muscularis propria, but they can also rise from the muscularis mucosa. Esophageal leiomyomas grow slowly and 50% of cases are less than 5 cm in size [124] and in some instances maybe as large as 15 cm. They can be single or multiple, spherical well-circumscribed intramural, pedunculated intraluminal, or annular masses.

The most common symptoms are dysphagia (46.9%) and retrosternal or epigastric pain (46.7%). Other symptoms associated with leiomyomas are weight loss, nausea, vomiting, reflux, ulceration, and bleeding [123]. Symptoms do not necessarily correlate with size [123, 125].

Large leiomyomas may present as rounded or lobulated lateral mediastinal growths on chest radiography, this is usually an incidental finding in asymptomatic patients. Barium swallow is the first diagnostic test performed in patients with symptoms suspicious for benign esophageal tumors. Leiomyomas present as a well-circumscribed smooth filling defects with normal overlying mucosa on swallows. Endoscopy confirms the tumor location and further evaluates the mucosa overlying the mass. Mucosa is usually normal and moves freely over the mass in leiomyomas, one may observe luminal narrowing. However, mucosal irregularity, ulceration, and luminal stenosis with obstruction are suspicious for a malignant lesion. Endoscopic ultrasonography is useful in differentiating extrinsic vs. esophageal wall tumors and in delineating their layer of origin. Leiomyomas are well-demarcated, uniform, hypoechoic masses, which may arise from the muscularis mucosa or muscularis propria [126, 127]. Identification of leiomyomas that originate in the muscularis mucosa permits consideration of endoscopic removal, while those that originate from the muscularis propria require more invasive surgical enucleation [128]. Computed tomography provides information regarding size, location, and anatomic relationships that may aid in operative planning. Endoscopic biopsy or endoscopic ultrasound guided fine needle aspiration may provide a definitive tissue diagnosis. This should be reserved for lesions suspicious for malignancy as preoperative endoscopic biopsy is associated with an increased incidence of intraoperative mucosal tears [129].

Indications for surgical treatment are unremitting symptoms, increasing tumor size, mucosal ulceration to obtain histological diagnosis and facilitation of other procedures. Although controversial, asymptomatic patients should be managed nonoperatively with periodic radiological follow-up [130]. Symptomatic leiomyomas should be enucleated after performing a longitudinal esophageal myotomy, care should be taken to avoid mucosal injury. Myotomy should be reapproximated to avoid mucosal bulging and postoperative dysphagia. Tumors in the upper and middle third of the esophagus are approached from the right side of the chest, tumors in the lower third are approached from the left, and tumors at the GEJ can be resected through an upper midline abdominal incision. Tumors larger than 8 cm and those that are firmly adherent to the mucosa may necessitate esophageal resection [124, 131]. Resection can be achieved via open and minimally invasive techniques. Thoracoscopic approach has been gaining popularity because of its association with decreased hospital length of stay and postoperative pain in comparison to open procedures [129]. Overall patients tolerate resection well with minimal complications, good symptom relief, and no recurrences [130].

Fibrovascular Polyps

Fibrovascular esophageal polyps are intraluminal polyploid lesions that appear most commonly in the upper esophagus near the cricopharyngeus muscle. These lesions occur predominantly in men during the sixth and seventh decades, but are also encountered in much older patients. As a group they include fibromas, fibrolipomas, myomas, myxofibromas, pedunculated lipomas, and fibroepithelial polyps [132, 133]. Early lesions consist of nodular submucosal tissue that may over time elongate into a pedunculated polyp. The geometric forces of peristalsis eventually cause the tip of the polyp to reach the distal esophagus.

Fibrovascular polyps come to medical attention when large enough to cause intermittent dysphagia, substernal fullness, or regurgitation of recently ingested material. The presentation may be more acute if a pedunculated polyp obstructs the esophagogastric junction or becomes ulcerated and bleeds. Although rare, regurgitation of the tumor and asphyxiation secondary to acute glottic obstruction are an additional concern [134]. A barium esophogram demonstrates the smooth polyploid intraluminal filling defect. Upper endoscopy can also be used to visualize the polyp and permits the stalk to be traced to its level of attachment [135].

Fibrovascular polyps are resected to relieve symptoms and prevent aspiration and asphyxiation. The greatest polyp size that might be amenable to endoscopic excision is dictated by the polyp's architecture and location and by the endoscopist's skill. Surgical treatment is undertaken when endoscopic removal is unfeasible. The standard approach is through a cervical incision on the side of the neck opposite the stalk attachment. An esophagomyotomy is performed below the cricopharyngeal muscle, and the polyp is delivered into the wound and amputated at the stalk base. If the base is a significant distance below the cricopharyngeus, a right transthoracic approach can be used.

References

1. Kahrilas PJ (1997) Anatomy and physiology of the gastroesophageal junction. Gastroenterol Clin North Am 26(3):467–486
2. Grande L, Lacima G, Ros E et al (1999) Deterioration of esophageal motility with age: a manometric study of 79 healthy subjects. Am J Gastroenterol 94(7):1795–1801
3. Xie P, Ren J, Bardan E, Mittal RK, Sui Z, Shaker R (1997) Frequency of gastroesophageal reflux events induced by pharyngeal water stimulation in young and elderly subjects. Am J Physiol 272(2Pt 1): G233–G237
4. Meshkinpour H, Haghighat P, Dutton C (1994) Clinical spectrum of esophageal aperistalsis in the elderly. Am J Gastroenterol 89(9): 1480–1483
5. Ren J, Shaker R, Kusano M et al (1995) Effect of aging on the secondary esophageal peristalsis: presbyesophagus revisited. Am J Physiol 268(5 Pt 1):G772–G779
6. Grishaw EK, Ott DJ, Frederick MG, Gelfand DW, Chen MY (1996) Functional abnormalities of the esophagus: a prospective analysis of radiographic findings relative to age and symptoms. AJR Am J Roentgenol 167(3):719–723
7. Nishimura N, Hongo M, Yamada M et al (1996) Effect of aging on the esophageal motor funcions. J Smooth Muscle Res 32(2):43–50

8. Ferrioli E, Dantas RO, Oliveira RB, Braga FJ (1996) The influence of ageing on esophageal motility after ingestion of liquids with different viscosities. Eur J Gastroenterol Hepatol 8(8):793–798
9. Ferriolli E, Oliveira RB, Matsuda NM, Braga FJ, Dantas RO (1998) Aging, esophageal motility, and gastroesophageal reflux. J Am Geriatr Soc 46(12):1534–1537
10. Lasch H, Castell DO, Castell JA (1997) Evidence for diminished visceral pain with aging: studies using graded intraesophageal balloon distension. Am J Physiol 272(1 Pt 1):G1–G3
11. Stilson WL, Sanders I, Gardiner GA, Gorman HC, Lodge DF (1969) Hiatal hernia and gastroesophageal reflux. A clinicoradiological analysis of more than 1, 000 cases. Radiology 93(6): 1323–1327
12. Patti MG, Goldberg HI, Arcerito M, Bortolasi L, Tong J, Way LW (1996) Hiatla hernia size affects lower esophageal sphincter function, esophageal acid exposure, and the degree of mucosal injury. Am J Surg 171(1):182–186
13. Locke GR III, Talley NJ, Fett SL, Zinsmeister AR, Melton LJ (1997) Prevalence and clinical spectrum of gastroesophgeal reflux: a population-based study in Olmsted County Minnesota. Gastroenterology 112(5):1448–1456
14. Triadafilopoulos G, Sharma R (1997) Features of symptomatic gastroesophageal reflux disease in elderly patients. Am J Gastroenterol 92(11):2007–2011
15. Johnson DA, Fennerty MB (2004) Heartburn severity underestimates erosive esophagitis severity in elderly patients with gastroesophageal reflux disease. Gastroenterology 126(3):660–664
16. Collen MJ, Abdulian JD, Chen YK (1995) Gastroesophageal reflux disease in the elderly: more severe disease that requires aggressive therapy. Am J Gastroenterol 90(7):1053–1057
17. Zhu H, Pace F, Sanaletti O, Bianchi Porro G (1993) Features of symptomatic gastroesophageal reflux in the elderly patients. Scand J Gastroenterol 28(3):235–238
18. Pilotto A, Franceschi M, Leondro G et al (2006) Clinical features of reflux esophagitis in older people: a study of 840 consecutive patients. J Am Geriatr Soc 54(10):1537–1542
19. Mold JW, Reed LE, Davis AB, Allen ML, Decktor DL, Robinson M (1991) Prevalence of gastroesophageal reflux in elderly patients in a primary care setting. Am J Gastroenterol 86(8):965–970
20. Pellegrini CA, DeMeester TR, Wernly JA, Johnson LF, Skinner DB (1978) Alkaline gastroesophageal reflux. Am J Surg 135(2):177–184
21. El-Serag HB, Sonnenberg A (1997) Associations between different forms of gastroesophageal reflux disease. Gut 41(5): 594–599
22. Zimmerman J, Shohat V, Tsvang E, Arnon R, Safadi R, Wenrower D (1997) Esophagitis is a major cause of upper gastrointestinal hemorrhage in the elderly. Scand J Gastroenterol 32(9):906–909
23. Winters C Jr, Spurling TJ, Chobanian SJ et al (1987) Barrett's esophagus. A prevalent occult complication of gastroesophageal reflux disease. Gastroenterology 92(1):118–124
24. Mann NS, Tsai MF, Nair PK (1989) Barrett's esophagus in patients with symptomatic reflux esophagitis. Am J Gastroenterol 84(12): 1494–1496
25. Cameron AJ, Lomboy CT (1992) Barrett's esophagus: age, prevalence, and extent of columnar epithelium. Gastroenterology 103(4):1241–1245
26. Thomas T, Abrams KR, De Caestecker JS, Robinson RJ (2007) Meta analysis: Cancer risk in Barrett's oesophagus. Aliment Pharmacol Ther 26(11–12):1465–1477
27. Hirano I, Richter JE (2007) ACG practice guidelines: esophageal reflux testing. Am J Gastroenterol 102(3):668–685
28. Wong WM, Bautista J, Dekel R et al (2005) Feasibility and tolerability of transnasal/per-oral placement of the wireless pH capsule vs, traditional 24-h oesophageal pH monitoring – a randomized trial. Aliment Pharmacol Ther 21(2):155–163

29. DeMeester TR, O'Sullivan GC, Bermudez G, Midell AI, Cimochowski GE, O'Drobinak J (1982) Esophageal function in patients with angina-type chest pain and normal coronary angiograms. Ann Surg 196(4):488–498

30. Hewson EG, Sinclair JW, Dalton CB, Richter JE (1991) Twenty-four hour esophageal pH montoring: the most useful test for evaluating non-cardiac chest pain. Am J Med 90(5):576–583

31. Wilcox CM, Heudebert G, Klapow J, Shewchuk R, Casebeer L (2001) Survey of primary care physicians approach to gastroesophageal reflux disease in elderly patients. J Gastroenterol 56(8):M514–M517

32. De Vault KR, Castell DO (2005) Updated guidelines for the diagnosis and treatment of gastroesophageal reflux disease. Am J Gastroenterol 100:190–200

33. Pilotto A, Paris FF (2005) Recent advances in the treatment of GERD in the elderly: focus on proton pump inhibitors. Int J Clin Pract 59(10):1204–1209

34. Schuler A (2007) Risks versus benefits of long-term proton pump inhibitor therapy in the elderly. Geriatr Nurs 28(4):225–229

35. Richter JE (2007) Gastrooesophageal reflux disease. Best Prac Res Clin Gastroenterol 21(4):609–631

36. Karim SS, Panton ON, Finley RJ et al (1997) Comparison of total versus partial laparoscopic fundoplication in the management of gastroesophageal reflux disease. Am J Surg 173(5):375–378

37. Richards KF, Fisher KS, Flores JH, Christensen BJ (1996) Laparoscopic Nissen fundoplication: cost, morbidity, and outcome compared to open surgery. Surg Laparosc Endosc 6:140–143

38. Trus TL, Laycock WS, Wo JM et al (1998) Laparoscopic antireflux surgery in the elderly. Am J Gastroenterol 93:351–353

39. Brunt LM, Quasebarth MA, Dunnegan DL, Soper NJ (1999) Is Laparoscopic antireflux surgery for gastroesohageal reflux disease in the elderly safe and effective? Surg Endosc 13:838–842

40. Khajanchee YS, Urbach DR, Butler N, Hansen PD, SWanstrom LL (2002) Laparoscopic antireflux surgery in the elderly: surgicaloutcome and effect on quality of life. Surg Endosc 16:25–30

41. Fernando HC, Schauer PR, Buenaventura PO et al (2003) Outcomes of minimally invasive antireflux operations in the elderly: a comparative review. JSLS 7:311–315

42. Cowgill SM, Arnaoutakis D, Villadolid D et al (2006) Results after laparoscopic fundoplication: does age matter? Am Surg 72(9):778–784

43. Brehant O, Pessaux P, Arnaud JP et al (2006) Long-term outcome of laparoscopic antireflux surgery in the elderly. J Gastroenterol Surg 10(3):439–444

44. Tedesco P, Lobo E, Fisichella PM, Way LW, Patti MG (2006) Laparoscopic fundoplication in elderly patients with gastroesophageal reflux disease. Arch Surg 141:289–292

45. Wang W, Huang MT, Wei PL, Lee WJ (2008) Laparoscopic antireflux surgery for the elderly: a surgical and quality-of-life study. Surg Today 38:305–310

46. Kamolz T, Bammer T, Granderath FA, Pasiut M, Pointner R (2001) Quality of life and surgical outcome after laparoscopic antireflux surgery in the elderly gastroesophageal reflux disease patient. Scand J Gastroenterol 36(2):116–120

47. Coelho JCU, Campos ACL, Costa MAR, Soares RV, Faucz RA (2003) Complications of laparoscopic fundoplication in the elderly. Surg Laparosc Endosc Percutan Tech 13(1):6–10

48. Grandernath FA, Kamolz T, Schweiger UM et al (2002) Long-term results of laparoscopic antireflux surgery. Surg Endosc 16(5):753–757

49. Rothstein RI, Ducowicz AC (2005) Endoscopic therapy for gastroesophageal reflux disease. Surg Clin N Am 85:949–965

50. Lal DR, Pellegrini CA, Oelschlager BK (2005) Laparoscopic repair of paraesophageal hernia. Surg Clin N Am 85:105–118

51. Hashemi M, Sillin LF, Peters JH (1999) Current concepts in the management of paraesophageal hiatal hernia. J Clin Gastroenterol 29(1):8–13

52. Allen MS, Trastek VF, Deschamps C et al (1993) Intra-thoracic stomach. Presentation and results of operation. J Thorac Cardiovasc Surg 105(2):253–258

53. Willekes CL, Edoga JK, Frezza EE (1997) Laparoscopic repair of the paraesophageal hernia. Ann Surg 225:31–38

54. Cameron AJ, Higgins JA (1986) Linear gastric erosion: a lesion associated with large diaphragmatic hernia and chronic blood loss anemia. Gastroenterology 91:338–342

55. Skinner DB, Belsey RHR (1967) Surgical management of esophageal reflux and hiatus hernia. J Thorac Cardiovasc Surg 53(1):33–54

56. Hill LD (1973) Incarcerated paraesophageal hernia. A surgical emergency. Am J Surg 126(2):33–54

57. Stylopoulos DB, Gazelle GS, Rattner DW (2002) Paraesophageal hernias: operation or observation? Ann Surg 236(4):492–500

58. Walther B, DeMeester TR, Lafontaine E et al (1984) Effect of paraesophageal hernia on sphincter function and its implication on surgical therapy. Am J Surg 147:111–116

59. Wiechmann RJ, Ferguson MK, Naunheim KS et al (2002) Laparoscopic management of giant paraesophageal herniation. Ann Thorac Surg 71(4):1080–1087

60. Mattar SG, Bowers SP, Galloway KD, Hunter JG, Smith CD (2002) Long-term outcome of laparoscopic repair of paraesophageal hernia. Surg Endosc 16:745–749

61. Pierre AF, Luketich JD, Fernando HC et al (2002) Results of laparoscopic repair of giant paraesophageal hernias: 200 consecutive patients. Ann Thorac Surg 74(6):1909–1915

62. Diaz S, Brunt LM, Klingensmith ME et al (2003) Laparoscopic paraesophageal hernia repair, a challenging operation: medium-term outcome of 116 paients. J Gastrointest Surg 7(1):59–66

63. Bammer T, Hinder RA, Klaus A, Libbey JS, Napoliello DA, Rodriquez JA (2002) Safety and long-term outcome of laparoscopic antireflux surgery in patients in their eighties and older. Surg Endosc 16:40–42

64. Grotentuis BA, Wijnhoven BPL, Bessel JR, Watson DI (2008) Laparoscopic antireflux surgery in the elderly. Surg Endosc 22:1807–1812

65. Gangopadhyay N, Perrone JM, Soper NJ et al (2006) Outcomes of laparoscopic paraesophageal hernia repair in elderly and high-risk patients. Surgery 140:491–419

66. Poulose BK, Gosen C, Marks JM et al (2008) Inpatient mortality analysis of paraesophageal hernia repair in octogenarians. J Gastrointest Surg 12:1888–1892

67. Agwunobi AO, Bancewicz J, Attwood SE (1998) Simple laparoscopic gastropexy as the initial treatment of paraesophageal hiatal hernia. Br J Surg 85:604–606

68. Kercher KW, Matthews BD, Ponsky JL et al (2001) Minimally invasive management of paraesophageal herniation in the high-risk surgical patient. Am J Surg 182:510–514

69. Johnston RD (2005) Upper gastrointestinal disease in the elderly patient. Rev Clin Gerontol 15:175–185

70. Sonnenberg A, Massey BT, McCarty DJ, Jacobsen JT (1993) Epidemiology of hospitalization for achalasia in the United States. Dig Dis Sci 38:233–244

71. Bruley des Varannes S, Scarpignato C (2001) Current trends in the management of achalasia. Digest Liver Dis 33:266–277

72. Bosher L, Shaw A (1981) Achalasia in siblings: clinical and genetic aspects. Am J Dis Child 84:1329–1330

73. Robertson C, Martin B, Atkinson M (1993) Varicella zoster virus DNA in the oesophageal myenteric plexus in achalasia. Gut 34:299–302

74. Jones D, Mayberry F, Rhodes J, Munro J (1983) Preliminary report of an association between measles virus and achalasia. J Clin Pathol 36:655–657

75. Goldblum JR, Whyte RI, Orringer MB, Appelman HD (1994) Achalasia: a morphologic study of 42 resected specimens. Am J Surg Pathol 18:327–337

76. Aggestrup S, Uddman R, Sundler F et al (1983) Lack of vasoactive intestinal peptide nerves in esophageal achalasia. Gastroenterology 84:924–927

77. Mearin F, Mourelle M, Guarner F et al (1993) Patients with achalasia lack nitrous oxide synthase in the gastro-esophageal junction. Eur J Clin Invest 23:724–728

78. Holloway RH, Dodds WJ, Helm JF et al (1986) Integrity of cholinergic stimulation to the lower esophageal sphincter in achalasia. Gastroenterology 90:924–929

79. Goin JC, Sterin-Borda L, Bilder CR et al (1999) Functional implications of circulating muscarinic cholinergic receptor autoantibodies in chagasic patients with achalasia. Gastroenterology 117:798–805

80. Massey BT, Hogan WJ, Dodds WJ, Dantas RO (1992) Alteration of the upper esophageal sphincter belch reflex in patients with achalasia. Gastroenterology 103:1574–1579

81. Dudnick RS, Castell JA, Castell DO (1992) Abnormal upper esophageal sphincter function in achalasia. Am J Gastroenterol 87:1712–1715

82. Howard PJ, Maher L, Pryde A et al (1992) Five year prospective study of the incidence, clinical features, and diagnosis of achalasia in Edinburgh. Gut 33:1011–1015

83. Smart HL, Foster PN, Evans DF et al (1987) Twenty-four hour oesophageal acidity in achalasia before and after pneumatic dilatation. Gut 28:883–887

84. Clouse RE, Abramson BK, Todorczuk JR (1991) Achalasia in the elderly: effects of aging on clinical presentation and outcome. Dig Dis Sci 36:225–228

85. Meijssen MAC, Tilanus HW, van Blankenstein M et al (1992) Achalasia complicated by oesophageal squamous cell carcinoma: a prospective study in 195 patients. Gut 33:155–158

86. Kahrilas PJ, Kishk SM, Helm JF et al (1987) Comparison of pseudoachalasia and achalasia. Am J Med 82:439–446

87. Rozman RW Jr, Achkar E (1990) Features distinguishing secondary achalasia from primary achalasia. Am J Gastroenterol 85:1327–1330

88. Cohen S, Lipshutz W (1971) Lower esophageal sphincter dysfunction in achalasia. Gastroenterology 61:814–820

89. Katz PO, Richter JE, Cowan R, Castell DO (1986) Apparent complete lower esophageal sphincter relaxation in achalasia. Gastroenterology 90:978–983

90. Hashemi N, Banwait KS, Dimarino AJ, Cohen S (2005) Manometric evaluation of achalasia in the elderly. Aliment Pharmacol Ther 21:431–434

91. Chuah S, Changchien C, Wu K et al (2007) Esophageal motility differences among aged patients with achalasia: A Taiwan report. J Gastroenterol Hepatol 22:1737–1740

92. Gelfond M, Rozen P, Gilat T (1982) Isosorbide dinitrite and nifedipine treatment of achalasia: a clinical, manometric and radionuclide evaluation. Gastroenterology 83:963–969

93. Vaezi MF, Richter JE (1998) Current therapies for achalasia: comparison and efficacy. J Clin Gastroenterol 27:21–35

94. Pasricha PJ, Ravich WJ, Hendrix TR et al (1995) Intrasphincteric botulinum toxin for the treatment of achalasia. N Engl J Med 322:774–778

95. Pasricha PJ, Rai R, Ravich J et al (1996) Botulinum toxin for achalasia: long-term outcome and predictors of response. Gastroenterology 110:1410–1415

96. Gordan JM, Eaker EY (1997) Prospective study of esophageal botulinum toxin injection in high-risk achalasia patients. Am J Gastroenterol 92:1812–1817

97. Dughera L, Battaglia E, Maggio D et al (2005) Boulinum toxin treatment of esophageal achalasia in the old and oldest old. Drugs Aging 22:779–783

98. Barkin JS, Guelrud M, Reiner DK et al (1990) Forceful balloon dilation: an outpatient procedure for achalasia. Gastrointest Endosc 36:123–126

99. Kadakia SC, Wong RKH (1993) Graded pneumatic dilation using Rigiflex achalasia dilators in patients with primary esophageal achalasia. Am J Gastroenterol 88:34–38

100. Wehrmann T, Jacobi V, Jung M et al (1995) Pneumatic dilation in achalasia with a low compliance balloon: results of a 5 year prospective evaluation. Gastrointest Endosc 42:31–36

101. Eckhardt VF, Aignherr C, Bernhard G (1992) Predictors of outcome in patients with achalasia treated with pneumatic dilatation. Gastroenterology 103:1732–1738

102. Ellis FH Jr (1993) Oesophagomyotomy for achalasia: a 22 year experience. Br J Surg 80:882–885

103. Malthaner RA, Todd TR, Miller L, Pearson FG (1994) Long term results in surgically managed esophageal achalasia. Ann Thorac Surg 58:1343–1347

104. Csendes A, Braghetto I, Mascaro J, Henriquez A (1988) Late subjective and objective evaluation of the results of esophagomyotomy in 100 patients with achalasia of the esophagus. Surgery 104:469–475

105. Little AG, Soriano A, Ferguson MK et al (1988) Surgical treatment of achalasia: results with esophagomyotomy and Belsey repair. Ann Thorac Surg 45:489–494

106. Spiess AE, Kahrilas PJ (1998) Treating achalasia: from whalebone to laparoscope. J Am Med Assoc 280:638–642

107. Smith CD, Stival A, Howell DL, Swafford V (2006) Endoscopic therapy for achalasia before heller myotomy results in worse outcomes than heller myotomy alone. Ann Surg 243:579–584

108. Kilic A, Schuchert MJ, Pennathur A et al (2008) Minimally invasive myotomy for achalalsia in the elderly. Surg Endosc 22:862–865

109. Khajanchee YS, Kanneganti S, Leatherwood AE, Hansen PD, Swanstrom LL (2005) Laparoscopic heller myotomy with toupet fundoplication: outcome predictors in 121 consecutive patients. Arch Surg 140:827–833

110. Torquati A, Richards WO, Holzman MD, Sharp KW (2006) Laparoscopic myotomy for achalasia: predictors of successful outcomes after 200 cases. Ann Surg 243:587–591

111. Dent J, Holloway RH (1996) Esophageal motility and reflux testing. Gastroenterol Clin N Am 25:50–73

112. Barham CP, Gotley DC, Fowler A et al (1997) Diffuse oesophageal spasm: diagnosis by ambulatory 24 hour manometry. Gut 41:151–155

113. Clouse RE, Lustman PJ (1983) Psychiatric illness and contraction abnormalities of the esophagus. N Engl J Med 309:1337–1342

114. Kikendall JW, Mellow MH (1980) Effect of sublingual nitroglycerin and long acting nitrate preparations on esophageal motility. Gastroenterology 79:703–706

115. Drenth JP, Bos LP, Engels LG (1990) Efficacy of diltiazem in the treatment of diffuse esophageal spasm. Aliment Pharmacol Ther 4:411–416

116. Irving D, Owen WJ, Linsell J et al (1992) Management of diffuse esophageal spasm with balloon dilatation. Gastrointest Radiol 17:189

117. Eypasch EP, DeMeester TR, Klingman RR et al (1992) Physiologic assessment and surgical management of diffuse esophageal spasm. J Thorac Cardiovasc Surg 104:859–869

118. Patti MG, Pellegrini CA, Arcerito M et al (1995) Comparison of medical and minimally invasive surgical therapy for primary esophageal motility disorders. Arch Surg 130:609–616

119. Henderson RD, Ryder D, Marryatt G (1987) Extended esophageal myotomy and short total fundoplication hernia repair in diffuse esophageal spasm: five year review in 34 patients. Ann Thorac Surg 43:25–31

120. Lock G (2001) Physiology and pathology of the oesophagus in the elderly patient. Best Prac Res Clin Gastroenterol 15: 919–941

121. Plachta A (1962) Benign tumors of the esophagus. Review of literature and report of 99 cases. Am J Gastroenterol 38:639–652

122. Moersch HJ, Harrington SW (1944) Benign tumor of the esophagus. Ann Otol Rhinol Laryngol 53:800–817

123. Hatch GF III, Wertheimer-Hatch L, Hatch KF et al (2000) Tumors of the esophagus. World J Surg 24:401–411

124. Seremetis MG, Lyons WS, DeGuzman VC et al (1976) Leiomyomata of the esophagus: an analysis of 838 cases. Cancer 38:2166

125. Fountain SW (1986) Leiomyoma of the esophagus. Thorac Cardiovasc Surg 34:194–195

126. Tio TL, Tygat GNJ (1990) denHartog Jager FCA. Endoscopic ultrasonography for the evaluation of gastrointestinal smooth muscle tumors in the upper gastrointestinal tract: an experience with 42 cases. Gastrointest Endosc 36:342

127. Rosch T, Lorenz R, Dancygier H et al (1992) Endosonographic diagnosis of submucosal upper gastrointestinal tract tumor. Scand J Gastroenterol 27:1–8

128. Takada N, Higashino M, Osugi H, Tokuhara T, Kinoshita H (1999) Utility of endoscopic ultrasonography in assessing the indications for endoscopic surgery of submucosal esophageal tumors. Surg Endosc 13:228–230

129. Bonavina L, Segalin A, Rosati R, Pavanello M, Peracchia A (1995) Surgical Therapy of esophageal Leiomyoma. J Am Coll Surg 181:257–262

130. Lee LS, Singhal S, Brinster CJ et al (2004) Current Management of Esophageal Leiomyoma. J Am Coll Surg 198:136–146

131. Rendeina EA, Venuta F, Pescarmona ED et al (1990) Leiomyoma of the esophagus. Scand J Thorac Cardiovasc Surg 24:79

132. Avezzano EA, Fleischer DE, Merida MA et al (1990) Giant fibrovascular polyps of the esophagus. Am J Gastroenterol 85:299

133. Patel J, Kieffer RN, Martin M et al (1984) Giant fibrovascular polyp of the esophagus. Gastroenterology 87:953

134. Cochet B, Hohl P, Sans M et al (1980) Asphyxia caused by laryngeal impaction of an esophageal polyp. Arch Otolaryngol Head Neck Surg 106:176

135. Vrabec DP, Colley AT (1983) Giant intraluminal polyps of the esophagus. Ann Otol Rhinol Laryngol 92:344

Chapter 60
Esophageal Cancer in the Elderly

Philip A. Rascoe, John C. Kucharczuk, and Larry R. Kaiser

Neoplasms of the esophagus and gastroesophageal junction are aggressive tumors that often present at an advanced stage and that historically have been associated with poor survival despite therapy. Survcillance, Epidemiology and End Results (SEER) data from the National Cancer Institute estimate that 16,470 Americans are diagnosed with and 14,280 die of esophageal cancer annually. Moreover, the incidence of esophageal cancer is increasing, with an annual percentage change of +0.5% between 1975 and 2005. SEER data also demonstrate that esophageal cancer is primarily a disease of the elderly. From 2001 to 2005, the median age at diagnosis for cancer of the esophagus was 69 years, with 61.5% of those diagnosed being age 65 or older (Fig. 60.1) [1]. According to US Census Bureau projections, we can expect our population to be older by midcentury. In 2000, 12% of the population was 65 or older. In 2030, when all of the baby boomers will be 65 or older, this age group will represent 20% of the US population. This age group is projected to increase to 88.5 million in 2050, more than doubling the number in 2008 (38.7 million) [2]. It is apparent that surgeons should expect to see an ever-increasing number of patients with esophageal cancer. With earlier identification due to surveillance of premalignant disease and improved treatment strategies, some improvement in survival has been made over the past two decades (Fig. 60.2). However, most patients still present at an advanced stage. Surgeons will continue to play a significant role in the management of these patients, performing potentially curative extirpation in those with early stage disease, and palliative procedures in those with advanced malignancy.

CASE STUDY

A 79-year-old Caucasian gentleman was referred by his gastroenterologist for a surgical opinion. He had suffered with severe gastroesophageal reflux for many years, despite therapy with antacids, H2-blockers, and proton-pump inhibitors. One year ago, while taking 20 mg of omeprazole daily, he underwent upper endoscopy which revealed Barrett's esophagus and low-grade dysplasia. His daily dose of omeprazole was escalated to 40 mg. Upper endoscopy was recently repeated revealing progression of disease, with biopsy-proven multifocal high-grade dysplasia. Examination in the office revealed a slightly obese, but otherwise healthy-appearing individual. His past medical history was significant only for hypertension and hypercholesterolemia, both of which were well-controlled with medication. Detailed discussion focused on the premalignant nature of his disease, and his significant risk (40–50%) of harboring esophageal adenocarcinoma. He was loath to undergo less-proven options such as endoscopic PDT or mucosal resection. He accepted advisement that he have an esophagectomy after careful discussion of the risks, including morbidity as high as 40% and mortality of at least 5%. Preoperative serology, hemogram, CXR, and CT of the chest, abdomen, and pelvis were unremarkable. He was referred to a cardiologist for preoperative clearance and a noninvasive stress test revealed no evidence of reversible cardiac ischemia. He underwent transhiatal esophagectomy (THE), esophagogastric anastomosis, and feeding jejunostomy. His postoperative course was complicated by atrial fibrillation requiring management with amiodarone but was otherwise uneventful. Barium esophagram on postoperative day 7 revealed no evidence

(continued)

P.A. Rascoe (✉)
Department of Thoracic Surgery, University of Pennsylvania,
3400 Spruce St., 6 Silverstein, Philadelphia, PA 19104, USA
e-mail: philip.rascoe@gmail.com

R.A. Rosenthal et al. (eds.), *Principles and Practice of Geriatric Surgery*,
DOI 10.1007/978-1-4419-6999-6_60, © Springer Science+Business Media, LLC 2011

Histologic Classification, Location, and Incidence

Malignant neoplasms of the esophagus include epithelial tumors (such as adenocarcinoma, squamous cell carcinoma, and small-cell carcinoma), sarcomas, lymphomas, and metastatic lesions from distant primary sites (Table 60.1). Adenocarcinoma and squamous cell carcinoma are the most frequent malignant lesions, and adenocarcinoma has emerged in recent years as the more common lesion (Fig. 60.3). In fact, the incidence of esophageal adenocarcinoma has increased in the last 25 years greater than the incidence of any other major malignancy in the USA (Fig. 60.4) [3]. Most thoracic surgeons will complete an entire career without seeing the less common types of esophageal malignancies. In this chapter, the focus is diagnosis and management of esophageal squamous cell carcinoma and adenocarcinoma.

The distribution of esophageal cancers along the esophagus is different and somewhat characteristic. Squamous cell cancer occurs most commonly in the middle third of the

esophagus. Postlethwaite [4], in a collective review of more than 28,000 patients with squamous tumors, reported these tumors to be in the upper, middle, and lower esophagus in 15, 50, and 35% of patients, respectively. Adenocarcinoma, on the other hand, tends to involve the lower esophagus. Ming [5], reviewing a series of 4,783 patients with adenocarcinoma, showed the tumor to be in the lower third in 67%. Small-cell cancers occur with equal frequency in the middle and lower thirds, with the upper third involved in fewer than 5% of cases [6]. Esophageal melanoma and choriocarcinoma, though rare, seem to be most prevalent in the lower third. No specific pattern of distribution has been noted for esophageal sarcomas, lymphomas, or metastases.

There have been several consequences of the increasing prevalence of adenocarcinoma. Patients with adenocarcinoma are more likely to be treated surgically than patients with squamous cell carcinoma. Therefore the predominance of adenocarcinoma in many US surgical series results from two factors: an overall increase in the prevalence of adenocarcinoma since 1978 and an increase in the likelihood of resection

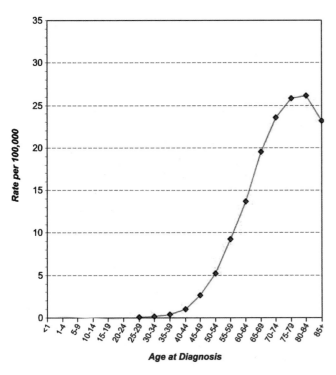

Figure 60.1 Age-specific incidence of esophageal cancer (2000–2005) [1].

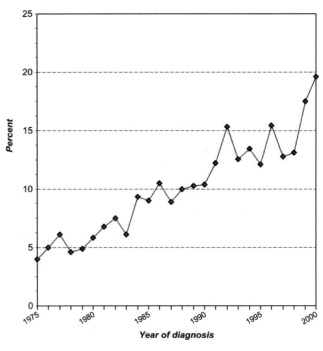

Figure 60.2 5-year survival rates of esophageal cancer by year of diagnosis (1975–2000) [1].

TABLE 60.1   Classification of esophageal tumors

Epithelial
   Squamous cell
   Adenocarcinoma
   Small cell

Non-Epithelial
   Melanoma
   Choriocarcinoma
   Metastatic tumors
   Lymphoma
   Sarcoma

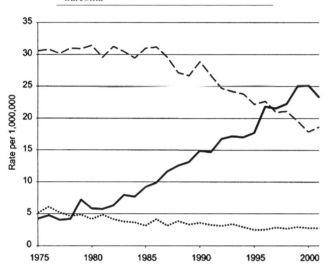

FIGURE 60.3   Histology and esophageal cancer incidence (1975–2001). Data from the National Cancer Institute's Surveillance, Epidemiology, and End Results program with age-adjustment using the 2000 US standard population. *Solid black line* = adenocarcinoma; *dashed line* = squamous cell carcinoma; *dotted line* = not otherwise specified (from [3], reprinted with permission of Oxford University Press).

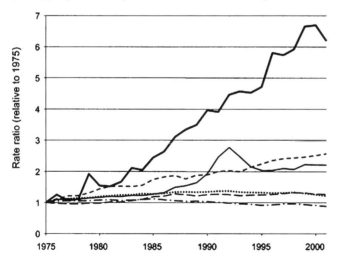

FIGURE 60.4   Relative change in incidence of esophageal adenocarcinoma and other malignancies (1975–2001). Data from the National Cancer Institute's Surveillance, Epidemiology, and End Results program with age-adjustment using the 2000 US standard population. Baseline was the average incidence between 1973 and 1975. *Solid black line* = esophageal adenocarcinoma; *short dashed line* = melanoma; *line* = prostate cancer; *dashed line* = breast cancer; *dotted line* = lung cancer; *dashes and dotted line* = colorectal cancer (from [3], reprinted with permission of Oxford University Press).

for patients with these tumors. As adenocarcinoma invariably involves the lower third of the esophagus and esophagogastric junction, both the tumor and the regional lymph nodes are accessible through an abdominal approach and are suitable for resection using the THE technique. With the option of avoiding thoracotomy (using the THE approach), many elderly patients who otherwise may not have been a candidate for surgical therapy may now be offered esophagectomy.

Pathogenesis

The exact etiology of esophageal cancer is unknown. The data support the hypothesis that the more common epithelial tumors arise as a result of chronic irritation of the esophagus from a wide range of behavioral, nutritional, and environmental sources, and that the likelihood of developing cancer may be increased in immunocompromised patients. Tobacco, alcohol, and obesity are all risk factors associated with the development of esophageal cancer [7]. Table 60.2 shows the additional risk factors associated with esophageal cancer and their contributions to the development of either squamous cell carcinoma or adenocarcinoma.

The relationship between smoking and the development of squamous cell cancers is well documented for both men and women [8–12]. Choi and Kahyo [9] have shown a

TABLE 60.2   Risk factors for the development of esophageal cancer with their relevant contribution to both squamous cell and adenocarcinoma of the esophagus

Risk factor	Squamous cell carcinoma	Adenocarcinoma
Tobacco use	+ + +	+ +
Alcohol use	+ + +	–
Barrett's esophagus	–	+ + + +
Weekly reflux symptoms	–	+ + +
Obesity	–	+ +
Poverty	+ +	–
Achalasia	+ + +	–
Caustic injury to the esophagus	+ + + +	–
Nonepidermolytic palmoplantar keratoderma (tylosis)	+ + + +	–
Plummer–Vinson syndrome	+ + + +	–
History of head and neck cancer	+ + + +	–
History of breast cancer treated with radiotherapy	+ + +	+ + +
Frequent consumption of extremely hot beverages	+	–
Prior use of beta-blockers, anticholinergic agents, or aminophyllines	–	±

+, increase in the risk by a factor of less than two; + +, increase by a factor of two to four; + + +, increase by a factor of more than four to eight; + + + +, increase by a factor of more than eight; ±, conflicting results have been reported; –, no proven risk

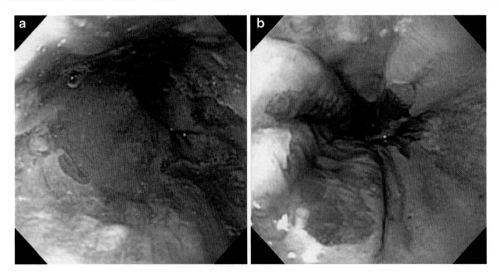

Figure 60.5 (a) The typical endoscopic appearance of Barrett's metaplasia at the GE junction. Note the "salmon-colored" areas of erosion extending proximally from the GE junction. Also, note the intervening areas of normal-appearing mucosa (image courtesy of Micheal L. Kochman, M.D., Professor of Medicine, University of Pennsylvania).

(**b**) Vital staining with methylene blue. Vital stains are used to highlight the mucosal changes at the time of endoscopy (image courtesy of Micheal L. Kochman, M.D., Professor of Medicine, Univeristy of Pennsylvania).

dose-dependent relation between the amount of smoking and the risk of developing cancer, and they have shown that this risk decreases with smoking cessation. Smokeless tobacco products have also been shown to increase the risk of cancer of the oropharynx, larynx, and esophagus [13]. Numerous studies have documented the relationship between alcohol consumption and squamous cell cancer [9–12, 14, 15]. As with smoking, the risk appears to be dose dependent. These risk factors, alcohol consumption and smoking, are additive. Other factors implicated in the development of squamous cell cancer are diet, including meal composition, consistency, temperature, and rate of consumption, achalasia, lye ingestion, radiation therapy, Plummer–Vinson syndrome, and prior head and neck squamous cell cancer. Although many have postulated a genetic predisposition to esophageal cancer, tylosis is the only recognized familial syndrome that predisposes to the development of esophageal cancer. This is an autosomal dominant disorder, which has been mapped to chromosome 17q25 [16]. Patients have hyperkeratosis of the palms of their hands and the soles of their feet. The risk of developing squamous cell carcinoma of the esophagus by age 70 is 95% in this cohort of patients [17].

Obesity and Barrett's or columnar-lined esophagus are associated with an increased risk of developing adenocarcinoma of the esophagus. Chronic gastroesophageal reflux disease (GERD) is considered the predominant contributor to the development of Barrett's metaplasia. The frequency, severity, and duration of reflux symptoms are correlated with an increased risk of developing esophageal adenocarcinoma [18]. Patients with recurring symptoms of reflux have an eightfold increase in the risk of esophageal adenocarcinoma. Barrett's esophagus develops in about 5% of patients

with GERD. Endoscopically, it is recognized by inflamed salmon-colored mucosa extending proximally from the GE junction. Often there are intervening areas of normal-appearing mucosa, or so-called skip areas. Figure 60.5a shows the typical endoscopic appearance; Fig. 60.5b shows the same patient with methylene blue vital stain, which can be used to highlight the mucosal changes. Microscopic evaluation reveals replacement of the normal stratified squamous epithelium of the esophagus with columnar epithelium more typical of other parts of the gastrointestinal tract. Thus, these changes are often referred to as "intestinalization" of the mucosa. With progression to dysplasia, the nuclei become "crowded" and the normal glandular architecture is lost. Histologically, patients with high-grade dysplasia carry a significant risk for esophageal carcinoma and should be considered candidates for resection. Approximately 10–30% of patients with high-grade dysplasia will develop invasive adenocarcinoma within 5 years of the initial diagnosis; moreover, in patients undergoing esophagectomy for presumed high-grade dysplasia, invasive carcinoma is identified in 30–40% of the pathologic specimens [19]. Barrett's esophagus increases the risk of esophageal adenocarcinoma 30- to 40-fold when compared with the general population [20]. The annual rate of neoplastic transformation to adenocarcinoma in patients with Barrett's is 0.5% [21]. A great deal of progress has been made in understanding columnar-lined esophagus since the entity was first described by Barrett in 1950 [22]. However, many questions remain including why Barrett's esophagus and adenocarcinoma affect primarily Caucasian men, why only some patients progress to dysplasia and adenocarcinoma, and how long this process takes.

Diagnosis

Unfortunately, early esophageal carcinoma is largely asymptomatic. As a distensible muscular tube, a significant portion of the esophageal lumen must be obstructed to impede passage of a food bolus and produce symptoms. Dysphagia is the primary manifestation of esophageal cancer in 80% of patients and up to 20% have odynophagia. Vague symptoms of retrosternal discomfort and transient dysphagia are often overlooked by the patient and the physician. On retrospective evaluation, many patients have significantly altered their eating habits by avoiding foods such as meats and breads while increasing their intake of semisolid foods and liquids. About one-half of patients have significant weight loss. Weight loss of more than 10% of body mass is an independent predictor of poor prognosis [23].

Pulmonary symptoms may be caused by aspiration of regurgitated food or by direct invasion of the airway by esophageal tumor, resulting in an esophagorespiratory fistula. Direct invasion through the membranous airway can occur with locally advanced lesions, usually involving the trachea or left mainstem bronchus as it passes anterior to the esophagus. Patients with cancers involving the upper thoracic esophagus must undergo preoperative bronchoscopy to rule out airway involvement as this precludes resection. Although flexible bronchoscopy may demonstrate gross airway invasion, rigid bronchoscopy is much more sensitive in determining adherence to the membranous trachea. Loss of the normal "ripple" effect as the rigid scope slides over the membranous trachea and left main bronchus suggests the tumor is fixed to the airway and is not resectable.

New hoarseness due to vocal cord paralysis is indicative of left recurrent nerve involvement and suggests unresectability. Virchow's node, a palpable left supraclavicular lymph node, may be apparent in some patients. Fine-needle aspiration with positive cytology confirms the pathologic involvement of Virchow's node, which is considered distant metastatic

disease and precludes resection. Symptoms of metastatic disease vary depending on the site. The most common sites and associated symptoms include celiac lymph nodes or liver with epigastric or right upper quadrant pain, pulmonary or pleural space metastases with shortness of breath and chest pain, and bone metastases with localized, severe pain.

The evaluation of a patient with suspected esophageal cancer involves securing the diagnosis, clinically staging the patient, and determining the medical operability of patients with stage-appropriate lesions for resection. Barium swallow and esophagoscopy remain the most important diagnostic tools for assessing the patient with esophageal symptoms. Barium swallow is usually the first study obtained. It provides both anatomic and functional information. A localized, concentric, "apple-core" narrowing of the esophagus is highly suggestive of carcinoma. Some benign diseases, such as a peptic stricture and achalasia, may mimic cancer. Therefore, flexible esophagogastroduodenoscopy (EGD) and biopsy are required to confirm the diagnosis, precisely locate the lesion, and rule out concurrent gastric disease that would preclude using the stomach as a conduit. Endoscopic information that should be noted and recorded includes the proximal and distal extent of the tumor and the presence and location of concurrent esophageal or gastric pathology (e.g., Barrett's mucosa). In patients considered for surgical resection, endoscopic ultrasonography (EUS) is the single most valuable test in determining tumor size and depth of penetration (T stage). EUS successfully predicts the T stage in greater than 80% of cases confirmed at surgery, and generally performs better for advanced (T4) than local (T1) disease. Regional lymph nodes are also visualized during EUS and can be sampled by FNA to determine the cytologic presence or absence of metastatic nodal disease (N stage). The sensitivity of EUS alone to predict N stage is 85% and improves to greater than 95% with FNA [24]. Figure 60.6 is an example of EUS for esophageal cancer.

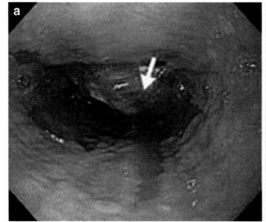
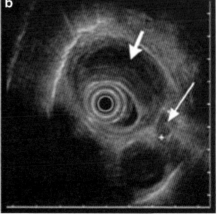

Figure 60.6 Endoscopic image (**a**) and endoscopic ultrasound (**b**) showing a transmural adenocarcinoma of the esophagus associated with Barrett's esophagus (*short arrows*), with lymph-node metastasis (*long arrow*) (image courtesy of John R. Saltzman, M.D., Assistant Professor of Medicine, Harvard Medical School; from [7]).

A computed tomographic (CT) scan of the chest, abdomen, and pelvis with intravenous contrast is valuable for assessing lung and liver metastasis. However, it is not accurate for determining T stage or assessing regional lymph node involvement.

Positron emission tomography (PET) with 18F-flourode-oxyglucose (FDG) is a physiologic test unique in its ability to detect increased metabolic activity within tissues. It is increasingly used to detect distant metastasis (M stage) in patients with esophageal cancer. It has been reported that PET will detect otherwise radiographically occult metastatic disease in up to 15% of patients who were thought to have only localized disease by conventional studies, thus making them more appropriately managed by nonsurgical interventions [25]. We now routinely obtain a PET scan as part of the preoperative staging evaluation in patients under consideration for esophagectomy. Increasingly, PET is being used to restage patients and evaluate response after neoadjuvant chemoradiation. Several studies have shown promising results in demonstrating that decreased FDG avidity after neoadjuvant therapy predicts pathologic response and increased survival [26, 27].

The use of combined thoracoscopy and laparoscopy for preoperative staging has been advocated by some centers. Periesophageal mediastinal lymph nodes and celiac lymph nodes can be sampled with a high degree of accuracy using these techniques [28]. This practice has largely been replaced by the combination of EUS–FNA and PET. We currently do not use these techniques as part of our standard evaluation.

Unfortunately, no serum tumor markers have been consistently found in patients with esophageal cancers. Standard serum cancer markers including CEA, CA 19-9, and CA 125 have no value in the preoperative evaluation of patients with esophageal cancer.

Staging

Esophageal cancers are staged according to the American Joint Committee on Cancer (AJCC) TNM staging system [29]. The staging system for esophageal cancer has recently undergone revision. Pathologic stage according to the updated system is dependent upon the number of nodes containing metastasis, tumor grade, tumor location, and histologic cell type. The current (seventh edition) AJCC TNM definitions are shown in Table 60.3. The stage groupings according to histology are displayed in Table 60.4. It is clear that the outcome in esophageal cancer is strongly associated with the stage of disease. Thus, accurate clinical staging is of paramount importance in formulating an appropriate

TABLE 60.3 American Joint Committee on Cancer (AJCC) staging of esophageal cancer: TNM definitions

Stage	Description
Primary tumor (T)	
TX	Primary tumor cannot be assessed
T0	No evidence of primary tumor
Tis	High-grade dysplasia[a]
T1	Tumor invades lamina propria, muscularis mucosa, or submucosa
T1a	Tumor invades lamina propria or muscularis mucosa
T1b	Tumor invades submucosa
T2	Tumor invades muscularis propria
T3	Tumor invades adventitia
T4	Tumor invades adjacent structures
T4a	Resectable tumor invading pleura, pericardium, or diaphragm
T4b	Unresectable tumor invading other adjacent structures, such as aorta, vertebral body, trachea, etc.
Regional lymph nodes (N)	
NX	Regional lymph nodes cannot be assessed
N0	No regional lymph node metastasis
N1	Metastasis in 1–2 regional lymph nodes
N2	Metastasis in 3–6 regional lymph nodes
N3	Metastasis in seven or more regional lymph nodes
Distant metastasis (M)	
M0	No distant metastasis
M1	Distant metastasis

Source: Used with permission of the AJCC, Chicago, Illinois. The original source for this material is the AJCC Cancer Staging Manual, Seventh Edition (2010) published by Springer Science and Business Media, LLC, http://www.springerlink.com
[a]High-grade dysplasia includes all noninvasive neoplastic epithelia that was formerly called carcinoma in situ, a diagnosis that is no longer used for columnar mucosa anywhere in the gastrointestinal tract

treatment plan and providing the patient with information regarding prognosis. In stage-appropriate candidates, plans are made to optimize the patient from a medical standpoint and proceed to resection. The role of preoperative therapy followed by operation remains ill defined and hotly debated.

Analysis of Comorbidities and Medical Clearance

Esophagectomy for carcinoma is a major surgical endeavor and causes significant physiologic stress to the patient. As such, it is associated with considerable morbidity and mortality. As the majority of patients presenting for resection are

TABLE 60.4 AJCC staging of esophageal cancer: anatomic stage/prognostic groups

Squamous cell carcinoma[a]

Stage	T	N	M	Grade	Tumor location[b]
0	Tis (HGD)	N0	M0	1, X	Any
IA	T1	N0	M0	1, X	Any
IB	T1	N0	M0	2–3	Any
	T2-3	N0	M0	1, X	Lower, X
IIA	T2-3	N0	M0	1, X	Upper, middle
	T2-3	N0	M0	2–3	Lower, X
IIB	T2-3	N0	M0	2–3	Upper, middle
	T1-2	N1	M0	Any	Any
IIIA	T1-2	N2	M0	Any	Any
	T3	N1	M0	Any	Any
	T4a	N0	M0	Any	Any
IIIB	T3	N2	M0	Any	Any
IIIC	T4a	N1-2	M0	Any	Any
	T4b	Any	M0	Any	Any
	Any	N3	M0	Any	Any
IV	Any	Any	M1	Any	Any

Adenocarcinoma

Stage	T	N	M	Grade
0	Tis (HGD)	N0	M0	1, X
IA	T1	N0	M0	1–2, X
IB	T1	N0	M0	3
	T2	N0	M0	1–2, X
IIA	T2	N0	M0	3
IIB	T3	N0	M0	Any
	T1-2	N1	M0	Any
IIIA	T1-2	N2	M0	Any
	T3	N1	M0	Any
	T4a	N0	M0	Any
IIIB	T3	N2	M0	Any
IIIC	T4a	N1-2	M0	Any
	T4b	Any	M0	Any
	Any	N3	M0	Any
IV	Any	Any	M1	Any

Source: Used with permission of the AJCC, Chicago, Illinois. The original source for this material is the AJCC Cancer Staging Manual, Seventh Edition (2010) published by Springer Science and Business Media, LLC, http://www.springerlink.com
[a] Or mixed histology including a squamous component or NOs
[b] Location of the primary cancer site is defined by the position of the upper (proximal) edge of the tumor in the esophagus

over the age of 65, they commonly have comorbidities such as hypertension, diabetes mellitus, cardiac disease, and pulmonary dysfunction. Moreover, all elderly patients have measurable diminution in cardiovascular, pulmonary, and renal physiology [30]. Careful patient selection and medical optimization of existing comorbidities is of paramount importance in maintaining acceptable surgical outcomes, especially in the elderly. All patients have basic laboratory tests (serum chemistries, CBC, and PT/PTT), EKG, CXR, and pulmonary function studies preoperatively. Younger patients with cardiac risk factors and all elderly patients are referred to a cardiologist for operative clearance. Most

undergo provocative screening to identify reversible ischemic heart disease. Unless contraindicated, perioperative beta-blockade is implemented.

Therapy

The goal of any therapy designed to manage patients with esophageal cancer is to relieve symptoms and treat the underlying cancer. The purpose of this chapter is not to present an exhaustive review of all treatment modalities but to cover those which are applicable in the elderly patient. It is important for elderly patients and their families to be aware of their treatment options so the choice of therapy fits the patient's desires, lifestyle, and personal and family support systems.

Surgery

Surgery has emerged as the best single-modality therapy for patients with esophageal cancer in terms of durable control of dysphagia and survival. Multiple factors influence the surgical approach to an esophageal malignancy. These include the nature and location of the neoplasm, the overall health of the patient, and the expertise of the surgeon. Several surgical approaches have been described. These include the transhiatal approach [31], the transabdominal transthoracic approach (Ivor Lewis) [32], the three-stage or "three-hole" approach (McKeown) [33], the thoracoabdominal approach, and the minimally invasive approach. These operations all include subtotal esophageal resection and resection of the esophagogastric junction, gastric cardia, and regional lymph nodes (Fig. 60.7). The incisions used for these techniques are demonstrated in Fig. 60.8. Each approach has its own set of risks and benefits as well as outspoken opponents and proponents. Selection of the appropriate approach requires experienced surgical judgment. Despite the rhetoric, several studies have shown equivalent outcome among the multiple approaches. It appears that the experience of the surgeon [34] and the number of cases performed at a particular institution are the leading factors determining outcome [35]. Clearly, failures in technique that occur during the performance of an esophagectomy are associated with increased length of hospital stay and increased in-hospital mortality and are predictive of a poorer overall long-term survival [36].

Options for reconstruction include gastric tube, colonic interposition, and small intestinal free graft. Because of its ample blood supply, ease of mobilization, and sufficient length to reach the neck, the gastric tube is the usual conduit of choice for reconstruction. The use of colon is more complex and has increased morbidity when compared to gastric pull-up [37]. We reserve the use of colon or jejunum for patients with an unusable stomach due to previous surgery, tumor extension, or other technical considerations.

The esophageal anastomosis requires meticulous attention. Many esophageal operations are plagued by high anastomotic leak rates and a significant number of postoperative strictures. At present, the modified stapled anastomosis [38] as described by Orringer appears to have the lowest leak rate, about 3% as compared with sutured techniques, which are as high as 15%. Many thoracic surgeons have adopted this anastomotic technique.

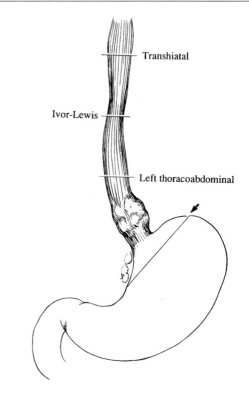

Figure 60.7 Standard esophagectomy for cancer involves subtotal esophagogastric resection along with removal of the regional lymph nodes. Different incisional approaches result in variations in the amount of resected esophagus and the level of the esophageal anastomosis (reprinted from [67], with permission from Elsevier).

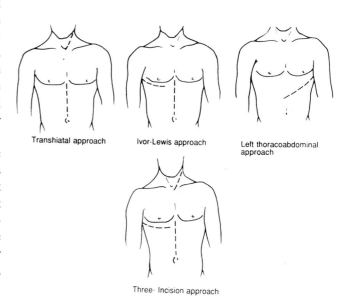

Figure 60.8 Incisions used for the more common esophagectomy techniques (from [68], with permission).

The transhiatal approach. The THE was reintroduced by Orringer and Sloan [31] in 1978 and continues to be refined [38–40]. THE does not require a thoracotomy. As such, THE may be cautiously offered to some elderly and high-risk patients who otherwise would not be candidates for surgery. Indications for THE include benign or malignant esophageal pathology usually involving the distal half of the intrathoracic esophagus in which there are options for long-segment esophageal replacement. The procedure is performed through an upper midline laparotomy and left cervical incision. A gastric conduit based on the right gastroepiploic artery is used to establish gastrointestinal continuity. If the stomach is unusable, a colonic interposition can be performed. Advantages of the THE approach are that (1) it avoids thoracotomy, which results in less short-term incisional pain, reduced narcotic requirement, and greater mobility and independence; (2) it uses a cervical esophageal anastomosis, which minimizes the adverse consequences of anastomotic leakage; and (3) gastric pull-up with cervical esophagogastric anastomosis results in reliable and durable quality of swallowing. Disadvantages are that (1) it requires long-segment esophageal replacement; (2) it is associated with a risk of ipsilateral recurrent laryngeal nerve injury; (3) there is a chance of intrathoracic injury from the "blunt" transhiatal dissection; and (4) complete intrathoracic lymphadenectomy is difficult to achieve.

The Ivor Lewis approach. Partial esophagogastrectomy using midline abdominal and right thoracotomy incisions, also known as the Ivor Lewis [32] technique, is designed to optimize exposure of the intrathoracic esophagus, which passes through the upper two-thirds of the chest along the right posterior mediastinum. The involved portion of esophagus is freed from the mediastinum and resected along with the esophagogastric junction, proximal cardia, and regional lymph nodes. The resected esophageal segment is replaced most commonly by stomach, which is mobilized and passed into the chest along the esophageal bed and anastomosed to the proximal esophagus near the level of the azygous vein. The advantage of Ivor Lewis esophagectomy (ILE) is the excellent exposure of the mid- to upper intrathoracic esophagus and lymph nodes. The disadvantages are (1) postthoracotomy pain; (2) the potential for intrathoracic esophageal anastomotic leak; and (3) a moderate amount of thoracic esophagus is retained with this approach and may be at risk of recurrent disease, specifically in the setting of severe Barrett's esophagus.

Three-field esophagectomy. This approach is carried out through separate laparotomy, right thoracotomy, and cervical incisions [33]. Proponents of this approach fall into two categories. The first group utilizes this approach to resect large intrathoracic lesions of the mid-esophagus. Exposure, especially at the level of the carina and left mainstem bronchus, is superior as compared with the transhiatal approach. Because visualization is improved, the injury rate to nearby structures, especially the airway and azygous vein, is lower. This approach has the benefits of both ILE and THE, as direct visualization of the mid-esophagus is obtained

while allowing for cervical esophagogastric anastomosis. The second group utilizes this approach to perform a complete two- or three-field lymph node dissection, suggesting that this approach provides a more complete resection and thus improves long-term survival. This approach has been shown to have acceptable morbidity and mortality as compared with other approaches; however, the often-cited report was from a single US center [41]. On the other hand, a large randomized Dutch trial comparing transhiatal resection with extended transthoracic resection showed that the transhiatal approach was associated with a lower morbidity and no statistically different overall, disease-free, and quality-adjusted survival [42]. Patients who underwent thoracotomy had an increased incidence of chyle leak and pulmonary complications, as well as longer ventilator-dependence, ICU stay, and hospital stay. A meta-analysis by the same group demonstrated no difference in survival at 3 and 5 years [43]. The statistically significant differences in morbidity and mortality from the meta-analysis are demonstrated in Table 60.5. In a recent retrospective review of 2,303 esophageal cancer patients treated with R0 resection without adjuvant or neoadjuvant therapy, the number of nodes removed was an independent predictor of survival. The authors concluded that to maximize this survival benefit, a minimum of 23 nodes should be removed at esophagectomy [44]. The true value of extensive lymphadenectomy in esophageal cancer remains undefined.

The thoracoabdominal approach. The left thoracoabdominal approach is probably the least utilized of all approaches to the esophagus. It is performed by making an oblique incision from the midpoint between the xiphoid and umbilicus across the costal arch to the tip of the scapula. The abdomen is opened, the costal arch is divided, and the chest is entered through the seventh intercostal space. The diaphragm is opened in a circumferential manner along the chest wall to avoid any damage to the phrenic nerve branches. At least a 2-cm rim of diaphragm is preserved on the chest wall to aid in reconstruction of the diaphragm at the completion of the

Table 60.5 Transthoracic esophagectomy vs. transhiatal esophagectomy for carcinoma – a meta-analysis (7,527 patients)

	Transthoracic	Transhiatal
In-hospital mortality	9.2%	5.7%
Blood loss (mL)	1,001	728
Pulmonary complications	18.7%	12.7%
Chylothorax	2.4%	1.4%
Intensive care unit stay (days)	11.2	9.1
Hospital stay (days)	21.0	17.8
Anastomotic leak	7.2%	13.6%
Vocal cord paralysis	3.5%	9.5%
3-year survival	26.7%	25.0% (ns)
5-year survival	23.0%	21.7% (ns)

Source: From [43], reprinted with permission from Elsevier

procedure. This approach offers superior exposure to the left upper quadrant, including the hiatus, and is our approach of choice in patients with previous extensive hiatal or proximal gastric surgery. For patients with distal tumors and inadequate conduit for total esophageal replacement, the anastomosis can be placed in the left chest below the inferior pulmonary vein or up to the level of the aortic arch. For those with adequate conduit, a separate left cervical incision can be made and the cervical esophagastric anastomosis can be placed in the neck. A consecutive case series of 64 thoracoabdominal esophagectomies reported no anastomotic leaks and a 2% mortality rate [45].

Minimally invasive esophagectomy. A number of minimally invasive techniques to esophagectomy have been described. These include laparoscopic, hand-assisted, thoracoscopic, and robotic-assisted esophagectomy. The hope of these procedures is that minimizing the incision size will decrease the morbidity of the operation while at the same time providing adequate resection. The largest study included 217 patients from the University of Pittsburgh who underwent esophagectomy via thoracoscopy, laparoscopy, and a left neck incision [46]. The investigators observed equivalent results as compared to open techniques and suggest development of a multicenter trial to define the role of minimally invasive esophagectomy. At present, the advantage of this approach remains to be determined.

Esophagectomy in the Elderly

As previously stated, elderly patients presenting for esophagectomy often have pre-existing cardiopulmonary comorbidities. However, whether postsurgical outcome in the elderly is worse than for younger patients remains controversial.

In a retrospective review by Ruol et al., of 1,400 patients presenting with esophageal cancer over the course of 13 years, there was no difference in morbidity (~49%), 30-day mortality (1.9%), or 5-year survival (~34%) in postesophagectomy patients 70 or older when compared to the group younger than 70 [47]. As discussed in this paper, a significantly higher percentage of patients in the younger age group underwent esophagectomy, indicating that these results were obtained in a highly selected group of elderly patients. This underscores the importance of preoperative risk assessment, but also demonstrates that long-term survival of elderly esophageal cancer patients who tolerate esophagectomy is independent of age alone.

A retrospective review of the experience at Roswell Park Cancer Institute revealed similar results. The percentage of patients older than 70 who were deemed surgical candidates was statistically lower than younger patients. Overall morbidity, mortality, and survival were equivalent in the two surgical groups, with only atrial fibrillation and myocardial infarction being increased in the elderly [48].

In contrast to the previous two studies, experience at Memorial Sloan-Kettering Cancer Center revealed that older patients had longer length of hospital stay and worse postoperative mortality. In particular, their octogenarian cohort had a perioperative mortality of almost 20%, as well as an overall shorter disease-free survival [49].

In analyzing surgical outcome in 1,777 esophagectomy patients from the Veterans Affairs (VA) Medical Centers, the largest cohort to date, Bailey et al. documented a 10% mortality and 50% morbidity rate. Multivariate analysis revealed increasing age to be one of eight preoperative and intraoperative variables predictive of 30-day mortality [50].

In a retrospective cohort study analyzing outcomes from two large national databases, Finlayson and colleagues demonstrated higher mortality, lower 5-year survival, and greater probability of transfer to extended-care facilities among octogenarians undergoing esophagectomy for cancer when compared to patients aged 65–69 [51]. They identified similar results for patients undergoing pancreatectomy and lung resection for malignancy.

Finally, Ra and colleagues similarly analyzed the SEER-Medicare national database and found that age greater than 80, increasing Charlson comorbidity index, and operation at a low esophagectomy volume hospital were statistically significant predictors of postoperative mortality after esophagectomy for cancer [52].

The above-mentioned studies demonstrate well the ongoing controversy regarding postsurgical outcome in elderly esophageal cancer patients. Series of highly selected elderly patients at tertiary referral centers appear to demonstrate equivalent outcome when compared to younger patients. However, when national series are obtained from retrospective analyses of the VA and SEER-Medicare databases, increasing age appears to be an independent predictor of morbidity and mortality. It seems likely that the best possible surgical outcomes are obtained in elderly patients who are meticulously screened, medically optimized with regards to existing comorbidities, and undergo surgery in a high-volume tertiary referral center.

Neoadjuvant Therapy

The role of preoperative therapy followed by operation for Stage II and III disease remains ill-defined and hotly debated. The current information on neoadjuvant treatment can be divided into studies evaluating preoperative radiation, preoperative chemotherapy, and combined preoperative chemoradiation therapy. In operable patients with resectable tumors, the results of any preoperative therapy followed by resection must be compared with the results of primary resection alone. Importantly, this analysis must take into account the toxicities associated with multimodality therapy and the impact on the intended resection and quality of life.

A number of randomized trials have failed to show any benefit from preoperative radiation therapy alone. Proponents of preoperative radiotherapy argue that the trials are too small to demonstrate the advantages of this approach. A meta-analysis of available randomized trials comprising 1,147 patients, however, found no improvement in survival with preoperative radiotherapy alone in patients with resectable esophageal cancer [53]. At this time, there is no indication for preoperative radiation therapy alone followed by resection.

The utility of preoperative chemotherapy alone is much more poorly defined. A large multicenter randomized trial in the USA (Intergroup Trial) of 440 patients failed to show any improvement in survival after three cycles of combined cisplatin and fluorouracil followed by surgery and two postoperative cycles when compared to surgery alone [54]. This is in contrast to a large randomized European study (Medical Research Council), which suggested that neoadjuvant chemotherapy resulted in nearly a 10% improvement in survival at 2 years [55]. Unfortunately, the preoperative staging techniques and duration of treatments were quite different, making the two studies difficult to compare. More recently, another European neoadjuvant chemotherapy trial (MAGIC trial) demonstrated improved survival with perioperative chemotherapy vs. surgery alone (36 vs. 23% at 5 years) [56]. Of note, 75% of the MAGIC trial participants had gastric cancer, while only 25% had either distal esophageal or GE junction adenocarcinoma. Also, only 41.6% of patients randomized to perioperative chemotherapy were able to complete all six prescribed cycles of therapy. In the most recent Cochrane Review of the topic, 11 randomized controlled trials with 2,051 patients suggested that preoperative chemotherapy plus surgery may offer a survival advantage compared to surgery alone for resectable esophageal cancer [57]. There was no demonstrable difference in the rate of resection, tumor recurrence, or postoperative morbidity. There was some chemotherapy-related morbidity. Presumably based on the relative success of the MRC and MAGIC trials, chemotherapy alone is utilized quite commonly as neoadjuvant therapy in Europe, while combined chemotherapy and radiation is utilized more commonly in the USA.

Several small randomized trials have evaluated combined preoperative chemoradiation followed by surgical resection. The most widely cited trial to justify the use of combined treatment followed by surgery was published by Walsh et al. in 1996 [58]. This study projected a 3-year survival of 32% in the neoadjuvant treatment group as compared to 6% in the surgery alone group for patients with adenocarcinoma. Critics were quick to point out the lack of appropriate staging, the poor survival in the surgical group as compared with other surgical series, and the small study size. A more recent study found equivalent median and 3-year survival in patients

with squamous cell carcinoma of the esophagus randomized to either preoperative chemoradiation followed by surgery or surgery alone [60]. An increased complication rate was noted in the patients undergoing preoperative chemoradiation therapy. A recent meta-analysis of ten randomized controlled trials of neoadjuvant chemoradiotherapy vs. surgery alone demonstrated an absolute survival advantage of 13% at 2 years favoring neoadjuvant therapy [60]. Despite a paucity of conclusive data, there seems to be an evolving consensus at most centers that patients with T3 and/or N1 disease should receive neoadjuvant chemoradiation. This issue remains unresolved, and operation remains the standard treatment for localized esophageal cancer outside of a clinical trial. At this time we consider neoadjuvant chemoradiotherapy to be investigational. Unfortunately, a large intergroup trial designed to answer this question was closed because of poor accrual.

Very little data exists regarding neoadjuvant chemoradiation in the elderly. Elderly patients are often not offered neoadjuvant therapy due to concerns of susceptibility to treatment-related toxicities. Moreover, octogenarians are often excluded from neoadjuvant trials. The M.D. Anderson Cancer Center group has reported their experience with combined modality therapy in elderly patients. They compared three groups of patients: (1) patients 70 years or older who received neoadjuvant chemoradiation; (2) patients younger than 70 who received neoadjuvant chemoradiation; and (3) patients 70 years or older who received surgery alone. Elderly patients receiving preoperative chemoradiation were more likely to require perioperative blood transfusions and had a higher incidence of postoperative atrial arrhythmias. Otherwise, postoperative outcome as well as median, 1-year, and 3-year survival were similar in the three groups [61].

Palliation

The goal of esophageal resection, whether as primary treatment or as part of a multimodality plan, is cure, though this goal remains elusive. Palliative esophagectomy is associated with mortality rates in excess of 20% and morbidity rates as high as 50% and should therefore be avoided [62]. Very effective palliation can be obtained with chemotherapy, radiation therapy, and endoscopic interventions such as stenting. The intent of palliation is to maintain comfort, restore swallowing function, and support nutrition. Establishment of alternative enteral access is helpful in maintaining nutritional status and hydration. When possible, this is provided by a percutaneous gastrostomy (PEG) tube placed under endoscopic guidance. For patients with bulky obstructing lesions who cannot undergo PEG, an open or laparoscopic gastrostomy or jejunostomy tube is required.

Radiation

Palliative radiotherapy relieves dysphagia in up to 75% of patients. The dose is 4,000–5,000 cGy delivered over 4 weeks. This allows patients with advanced disease and severe dysphagia to handle secretions and to swallow liquids as well as dietary supplements. Unfortunately, relief is not immediate and maximal improvement occurs at about 4 weeks following completion of treatment. In patients with a life expectancy greater than 3 months, combined chemotherapy with radiation is utilized. Short-term side effects from radiation therapy include skin irritation and erythema. Esophagitis with painful swallowing also occurs with some frequency. Additional complications include stricture formation, radiation pneumonitis, and fistulization to the airway.

Chemotherapy

Esophageal cancers are usually responsive to chemotherapeutic drugs, providing some palliation. Agents currently in use include fluorouracil and taxanes either alone or in combination with platin-based agents. Palliative chemotherapy requires time to effectively reduce symptoms of dysphagia and must be balanced with the associated risks of systemic treatment in usually debilitated, malnourished patients. Chemotherapy has been used in combination with radiation therapy with the goal of increasing response rates, lengthening the disease-free interval, and improving survival. The Radiation Therapy Oncology Group (RTOG) compared four cycles of cisplatinum+5-fluorouracil (5-FU)+50 Gy of radiation to radiotherapy alone with 64 Gy [63]. The trial was stopped early because the interim results demonstrated a significant survival advantage in the chemotherapy group, with median survival of 12.5 and 8.9 months and 2-year survival of 50 and 38% for the chemoradiation and radiotherapy groups, respectively. Therefore patients with locally advanced disease who are not considered surgical candidates as a result of unresectable tumors or medical risks should be considered for chemoradiation therapy rather than irradiation alone.

Endoscopic Palliation

Endoscopic techniques to restore luminal patency are palliative procedures that may be used in patients who are not candidates for primary surgical therapy, in an adjuvant setting for patients receiving combination therapy, or in the setting of locally recurrent cancer following surgery.

Endoscopic techniques include dilatation, thermal ablation with laser or coagulation probes, intubation with self-expanding stents, and photodynamic therapy (PDT). The variables that must be considered when selecting the specific method are cost, tumor location and length, whether the tumor is circumferential, and the presence or absence of an esophagorespiratory fistula.

Stenting

Palliative endoscopic intubation of inoperable malignant esophageal strictures was first described in the 1970s [64]. Currently, self-expanding coated and uncoated nitinol stents are utilized for palliation. These stents can be inserted either radiologically or endoscopically on an outpatient basis. Following insertion, the lumen can be balloon-dilated to an acceptable diameter to provide palliation. Cook and Dehn [65] cited four major benefits of covered expandable stent use: (1) shorter hospital stay compared with rigid tube insertion; (2) single hospital stay; (3) lack of readmission for recurrent obstruction from tumor ingrowth or food impaction; and (4) no procedure-related morbidity or mortality.

Neodymium: Yttrium–Aluminum–Garnet Laser Fulguration

Endoscopic neodymium:yttrium–aluminum–garnet (Nd:YAG) laser fulguration can be used to provide temporary relief of esophageal obstruction in patients with unresectable obstructing tumors. A flexible quartz fiber is passed through the working channel of the esophagoscope to deliver the laser energy at the fiber tip. Multiple sessions are usually required to achieve debulking and functional success. Laser fulguration is often combined with endoluminal stenting and radiation therapy. It can also be useful in patients who have undergone uncovered stenting procedures with ingrowth of tumor through the stent. To be a candidate for this therapy, the endoscope must be able to traverse the tumor. Contraindications for laser therapy include completely obstructing cancers and esophagorespiratory fistulae.

Photodynamic Therapy

Intraluminal PDT is a nonthermal ablative technique that can be used to palliate patients. This technique requires the systemic administration of a hematoporphyrin, which is concentrated within the malignant cells. Approximately 48 h after administration of the photosensitizer, patients undergo endoscopy and an argon-pump dye-laser is used to deliver endoluminal light at a wavelength of 630 nm. This results in the generation of oxygen radicals, which quickly lead to tumor necrosis. The depth of penetration is relatively limited and this decreases the risk of full-thickness necrosis with perforation. Unfortunately, the photosensitizing agents are retained by the reticuloendothelial system in skin; thus, patients are sensitive to infrared wavelength light, including sunlight, radiant heat, fluorescent light, and strong incandescent light. Depending on the photosensitizing agent used, this sensitivity can persist up to 3 months, a challenging problem in patients with short life expectancies.

A recent series of 215 patients treated with palliative endoluminal PDT revealed a procedure-related mortality rate of 1.8%, effective palliation for patients with obstructing cancers in 85% of the treatment courses, and median survival of 4.8 months [66]. A number of patients in this series also required stenting, suggesting that PDT has a role in multimodality palliation of obstructing esophageal cancers.

Summary

- 16,470 Americans are diagnosed with and 14,280 die of esophageal cancer annually.
- Esophageal cancer is primarily a disease of the elderly. The median age at diagnosis for cancer of the esophagus is 69 years, with 61.5% of those diagnosed being age 65 or older.
- The incidence of esophageal adenocarcinoma has increased in the last 25 years greater than the incidence of any other major malignancy in the USA.
- Careful patient selection and medical optimization of existing comorbidities is of paramount importance in maintaining acceptable surgical outcomes, especially in the elderly.
- Despite a paucity of conclusive data, there seems to be an evolving consensus at most centers that patients with T3 and/or N1 disease should receive neoadjuvant chemoradiation.
- Whether postsurgical outcome in the elderly is worse than for younger patients remains controversial. It seems likely that the best possible surgical outcomes are obtained in elderly patients who are meticulously screened, medically optimized with regards to existing comorbidities, and undergo surgery in a high-volume tertiary referral center.
- Palliative esophagectomy is associated with mortality rates in excess of 20% and morbidity rates as high as 50% and should therefore be avoided. Very effective palliation can be obtained with chemotherapy, radiation therapy, and endoscopic interventions such as stenting.

References

1. Surveillance, Epidemiology and End Results (2008) http://seer.cancer.gov/statfacts/html/esoph.html. Accessed 2 Nov 2008
2. U.S. Census Bureau (2008) http://www.census.gov/Press-Release/www/releases/archives/population/012496.html. Accessed 2 Nov 2008
3. Pohl H, Welch G (2005) The role of overdiagnosis and reclassification in the marked increase of esophageal adenocarcinoma incidence. J Natl Cancer Inst 97:142–146
4. Postlethwaite RW (1986) Squamous cell carcinoma of the esophagus. In: Postlethwaite RW (ed) Surgery of the esophagus, 2nd edn. Appleton & Lange, Norwalk, CT, pp 369–442
5. Ming S (1992) Adenocarcinoma and other epithelial tumors of the esophagus. In: Ming S, Goldman H (eds) Pathology of the gastrointestinal tract. Saunders, Philadelphia, pp 459–477
6. Ibrahim NB, Briggs JC, Corbishley CM (1984) Extrapulmonary oat cell carcinoma. Cancer 54:1645–1661
7. Enzinger C, Mayer J (2003) Esophageal cancer. N Engl J Med 349:2241–2252
8. Newcomb PA, Carbone PP (1992) The health consequences of smoking. Med Clin North Am 76:305–331
9. Choi SY, Kahyo H (1991) Effect of cigarette smoking and alcohol consumption in the etiology of cancers of the digestive tract. Int J Cancer 49:381–386
10. Francheschi S, Talamini R, Barra S et al (1990) Smoking and drinking in relation to cancers of the oral cavity, pharynx, and esophagus in northern Italy. Cancer Res 50:6502–6507
11. DeStefani E, Munoz N, Esteve J et al (1990) Mate drinking, alcohol, tobacco, diet, and esophageal cancer in Uruguay. Cancer Res 50:426–431
12. Gray JR, Coldman AJ, MacDonald WC (1992) Cigarette and alcohol use in patients with adenocarcinoma of the gastric cardia or lower esophagus. Cancer 69:2227–2231
13. Christen AG, McDonald JL Jr, Olsen BL, Christen JA (1989) Smokeless tobacco addiction: a threat to the oral and systemic health of the child and adolescent. Pediatrician 16:170–177
14. Adami HO, McLaughlin JK, Hsing AW et al (1992) Alcoholism and cancer risk: a population-based cohort study. Cancer Causes Control 3:419–425
15. Kato I, Nomura AM, Stemmermenn GN, Chyon PH (1992) Prospective study of the association of alcohol with cancer of the upper aerodigestive tract and other sites. Cancer Causes Control 3:145–151
16. Risk JM, Mills HS, Garde J et al (1999) The tylosis esophageal cancer (TOC) locus: more than just a familial cancer gene. Dis Esophagus 12:173–176
17. Ellis A, Field JK, Field EA et al (1994) Tylosis associated with carcinoma of the oesophagus and oral leukoplakia in a large Liverpool family – a review of six generations. Eur J Cancer B Oral Oncol 30:102–112
18. Lagergren J, Bergström R, Lindgren A et al (1999) Symptomatic gastroesophageal reflux as a risk factor for esophageal adenocarcinoma. N Engl J Med 340:825–831
19. Spechler SJ (2005) Dysplasia in Barrett's esophagus: limitations of current management strategies. Am J Gastroenterol 100(4):927–935
20. Solaymani-Dodaran M, Logan RF, West J et al (2004) Risk of oesophageal cancer in Barrett's oesophagus and gastro-oesophageal reflux. Gut 53:1070–1074
21. Shaheen N, Ransohoff DF (2002) Gastroesophageal reflux, Barrett esophagus, and esophageal cancer: scientific review. JAMA 287:1972–1981
22. Barrett NR (1950) Chronic peptic ulcer of the oesophagus and "oesophagitis". Br J Surg 38:175–182

23. Fein R, Kelsen DP, Geller N et al (1985) Adenocarcinoma of the esophagus and gastroesophageal junction: prognostic factors and results of therapy. Cancer 56:2512–2518

24. Puli SR, Reddy JB, Bechtold ML et al (2008) Staging accuracy of esophageal cancer by endoscopic ultrasound: a meta-analysis and systematic review. World J Gastroenterol 14(10):1479–1490

25. Flamen P, Lerut A, Van Cutsem E et al (2000) Utility of positron emission tomography for the staging of patients with potentially operable esophageal carcinoma. J Clin Oncol 18:3202–3210

26. Swisher SG, Maish M, Erasmus JJ et al (2004) Utility of PET, CT, and EUS to identify pathologic responders in esophageal cancer. Ann Thorac Surg 78:1152–1160

27. Cerfolio RJ, Bryant AS, Buddhiwardhan O et al (2005) The accuracy of endoscopic ultrasonography with fine-needle aspiration, integrated positron emission tomography with computed tomography, and computed tomography in restaging patients with esophageal cancer after neoadjuvant chemoradiotherapy. J Thorac Cardiovasc Surg 129:1232–1241

28. Krasna MJ, Flowers JL, Attar S et al (1996) Combined thoracoscopic/laparoscopic staging of esophageal cancer. J Thorac Cardiovasc Surg 111:800–806, discussion 806–807

29. (2010) Esophagus. In: Edge SE, Byrd DR, Compton CC, Fritz AG, Greene FL, Trotti A (eds) AJCC cancer staging manual, 7th edn. Springer, New York, NY

30. Loran DB, Zwischenberger JB (2004) Thoracic surgery in the elderly. J Am Coll Surg 199(5):773–784

31. Orringer MB, Sloan H (1978) Esophagectomy without thoracotomy. J Thorac Cardiovasc Surg 76:643–654

32. Lewis I (1946) The surgical treatment of carcinoma of the esophagus with special reference to a new operation for growths of the middle third. Br J Surg 34:18

33. McKeown KC (1976) Total three-stage esophagectomy for cancer of the esophagus. Br J Surg 51:259–262

34. Bolten JS, Teng S (2002) Transthoracic or transhiatal esophagectomy for cancer of the esophagus – does it matter. Surg Oncol Clin N Am 11:365–375

35. Dimick JB, Pronovost PJ, Cowan JA et al (2003) Surgical volume and quality of care for esophageal resection: do high-volume hospitals have fewer complications? Ann Thorac Surg 75:337–341

36. Rizk NP, Bach PB, Schrag D et al (2004) The impact of complications on outcomes after resection for esophageal and gastroesophageal junction carcinoma. J Am Coll Surg 198:42–50

37. Davis PA, Law S, Wong J (2003) Colonic interposition after esophagectomy for cancer. Arch Surg 138:303–308

38. Orringer MB, Marshall B, Iannettoni MD (2000) Eliminating the cervical esophagogastric anastomotic leak with a side-to-side stapled anastomosis. J Thorac Cardiovasc Surg 119:277–288

39. Marshall OMB, Iannettoni MD B (1999) Transhiatal esophagectomy: clinical experience and refinements. Ann Surg 230:392–400, discussion 400–403

40. Orringer MB, Marshall B, Chang AC et al (2007) Two thousand transhiatal esophagectomies: changing trends, lessons learned. Ann Surg 246:363–374

41. Altorki N, Kent M, Ferrara C, Port J (2002) Three-field lymph node dissection for squamous cell and adenocarcinoma of the esophagus. Ann Surg 236:177–183

42. Hulscher JB, van Sandick JW, de Boer AG et al (2002) Extended transthoracic resection compared with limited transhiatal resection for adenocarcinoma of the esophagus. N Engl J Med 374:1662–1669

43. Hulscher JB, Tijssen JG, Obertop H, van Lanschot JJ (2001) Transthoracic versus transhiatal resection for carcinoma of the esophagus: a meta-analysis. Ann Thorac Surg 72:306–313

44. Peyre CG, Hagen JA, DeMeester SR et al (2008) The number of lymph nodes removed predicts survival in esophageal cancer: an international study on the impact of extent of surgical resection. Ann Surg 248:549–556

45. Heitmiller RF (1992) Results of standard left thoracoabdominal esophagogastrectomy. Semin Thorac Cardiovasc Surg 4:314–319

46. Luketich JD, Alvelo-Rivera M, Buenaventura PO et al (2003) Minimally invasive esophagectomy: outcomes in 222 patients. Ann Surg 238:486–494

47. Ruol A, Portale G, Zaninotto G et al (2007) Results of esophagectomy for esophageal cancer in elderly patients: age has little influence on outcome and survival. J Thorac Cardiovasc Surg 133:1186–1192

48. Sabel MS, Smith JL, Nava HR et al (2002) Esophageal resection for carcinoma in patients older than 70 years. Ann Surg Oncol 9(2):210–214

49. Moskovitz AH, Rizk NP, Venkatraman E et al (2006) Mortality increases for octogenarians undergoing esophagogastrectomy for esophageal cancer. Ann Thorac Surg 82:2031–2036

50. Bailey SH, Bull DA, Harpole DH et al (2003) Outcomes after esophagectomy: a ten-year prospective cohort. Ann Thorac Surg 75:217–222

51. Finlayson E, Fan Z, Birkmeyer JD (2007) Outcomes in octogenarians undergoing high-risk cancer operation: a national study. J Am Coll Surg 205:729–734

52. Ra J, Paulson EC, Kucharczuk J et al (2008) Postoperative mortality after esophagectomy for cancer: development of a preoperative risk prediction model. Ann Surg Oncol 15(6):1577–1584

53. Arnott SJ, Duncan W, Gignoux M, Girling DJ, Hansen HS, Launois B, Nygaard K, Parmar MKB, Rousell A, Spiliopoulos G, Stewart LA, Tierney JF, Wang M, Rhugang Z (Oeosphageal Cancer Collaborative Group) (2005) Preoperative radiotherapy for esophageal carcinoma. Cochrane Database Syst Rev (4). Art. No: CD001799. doi: 10.1002/14651858.CD001799.pub2

54. Kelsen DP, Ginsberg R, Pajak TF et al (1998) Chemotherapy followed by surgery compared with surgery alone for localized esophageal cancer. N Engl J Med 339:1979–1984

55. Medical Research Council Oesophageal Cancer Working Group (2002) Surgical resection with or without postoperative chemotherapy in oesophageal cancer: a randomised controlled trial. Lancet 359:1727–1733

56. Cunningham D, Allum WH, Stenning SP et al (2006) Perioperative chemotherapy versus surgery alone for resectable gastroesophageal cancer. N Engl J Med 355(1):11–20

57. Malthaner RA, Collin S, Fenlon D (2006) Preoperative chemotherapy for resectable thoracic esophageal cancer. Cochrane Database Syst Rev (3) Art. No: CD001556. doi: 10.1002/14651858.CD001556.pub2

58. Walsh T, Noonan N, Hollywood D et al (1996) A comparison of multimodal therapy and surgery for esophageal adenocarcinoma. N Engl J Med 335:462–467

59. Bosset J-F, Gignoux M, Triboulet J-P et al (1997) Chemoradiotherapy followed by surgery compared with surgery alone in squamous-cell cancer of the esophagus. N Engl J Med 337:161–167

60. Gebski V, Burmeister B, Smithers BM et al (2007) Survival benefits from neoadjuvant chemoradiotherapy or chemotherapy in oesophageal carcinoma: a meta-analysis. Lancet Oncol 8:33–34

61. Rice DC, Correa AM, Vaporciyan AA et al (2005) Preoperative chemoradiotherapy prior to esophagectomy in elderly patients is not associated with increased morbidity. Ann Thorac Surg 79:391–397

62. Orringer MB (1984) Substernal gastric bypass of the excluded esophagus – results of an ill-advised operation. Surgery 96:467–470

63. Herskovic A, Martz K, Al-Sarraf M et al (1992) Combined chemotherapy and radiotherapy compared with radiotherapy alone in patients with cancer of the esophagus. N Engl J Med 326:1593–1598

64. Atkinson M, Ferguson R (1997) Fibreoptic endoscopic palliative intubation of inoperable oesophagogastric neoplasms. Br Med J 1:266–267

65. Cook TA, Dehn CB (1996) Use of covered expandable metal stents in the treatment of oesophageal carcinoma and tracheo-oesophageal fistula. Br J Surg 83:1417–1418

66. Litle VR, Luketich JD, Christie NA et al (2003) Photodynamic therapy as palliation for esophageal cancer: experience in 215 patients. Ann Thorac Surg 76:1687

67. Heitmiller RF (1994) Cancer of the esophagus. In: Bayless TM (ed) Current therapy in gastroenterology and liver disease, 4th edn. Mosby, St. Louis, pp 81–85

68. Reichle R, Nixon M, Heitmiller RF, Fishman E (1993) Post surgical evaluation of the esophagus: normal radiographic appearance and complications. Invest Radiol 28:247–257

Chapter 61
Benign Diseases of Stomach and Duodenum

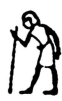

Daniel Borja-Cacho and Selwyn M. Vickers

Normal Anatomy and Physiology of the Stomach

The stomach comprises five anatomical regions: the cardia, fundus, body or corpus, antrum, and pylorus. The cardia is contiguous to the lower esophageal sphincter and is the transition between the esophagus and the stomach. The cardia is used to create a reference horizontal plane that delimits the second and third regions of the stomach, the fundus, and corpus, respectively. The fundus is located above this horizontal plane. The body is delimited proximally by the horizontal plane at the level of the cardia and distally by the incisura angularis. The incisura angularis is located at the abrupt right angle created by the lesser curvature in the distal portion of the stomach; it marks the transition between the body and the antrum. The pylorus delimits the transition between the stomach and duodenum; it controls gastric emptying [1].

Microscopically, the stomach has four different layers. The external layer or serosa is an extension of the visceral peritoneum that covers the entire stomach. Underneath the serosa is the second layer known as muscularis propia which is formed by three different layers of muscle: an inner oblique layer, a middle circular layer and an outer longitudinal layer. The middle muscular layer forms the pylorus at the end of the stomach. The muscularis propia contains many ganglion cells that create a neuronal plexus known as myenteric or Auerbach's plexus. The third layer or submucosa is a firm matrix of collagen and elastin that contains plasma cells, lymphocytes, lymphatics, and blood vessels. Numerous ganglion cells are also located in this layer; they form the submucosal or Meissner's plexus. The gastric lumen is lined internally by the last layer or gastric mucosa which is formed by a columnar epithelium that covers a layer of connective tissue (lamina propia) and a thin muscular layer known as

muscularis mucosa. The columnar epithelium invaginates and contains different gastric pits. Each gastric pit opens to four or five different gastric glands [2].

Each region has a different function and histology, the whole surface of the stomach is lined with glands, but the epithelial cells that create these glands are different in each region. Gastric glands can be classified as oxyntic or antral based on the main type of cell present in them. Oxyntic glands are present in the proximal stomach (fundus and body) while antral glands are found in the distal stomach (antrum). Oxyntic glands produce pepsin and gastric acid. The major function of antral glands is to produce gastrin [3].

Mucous cells are the most common type of gastric cell and are present in the surface of the stomach. The mucous and bicarbonate secreted by them create a neutral mucous film that prevents back diffusion of hydrogen ions (H^+) from the gastric lumen to the cells. This film is very viscous owing to a high content of long chain oligosaccharides. Mucous cells also produce a hydrophobic film of phospholipids that blocks back diffusion of hydrogen ions [4].

The main component of oxyntic glands are parietal cells. These cells contain multiple mitochondria that generate the energy required for acid secretion. The apical membrane of parietal cells contains the H^+/K^+-ATPase pump, responsible of gastric acid secretion. Parietal cells are mainly present in the proximal stomach (fundus and the body) [1].

Chief cells are located at the base of the oxyntic glands in the fundus and the body. They store pepsinogen inside intracytoplasmic granules that get secreted shortly after eating. This effect is mediated by acetylcholine. Pepsinogen is converted to pepsin in the gastric lumen; it breaks the ingested proteins into small peptides. Pepsin has an optimal activity at a pH 2.5, but if the intraluminal pH raises above 5, pepsin gets deactivated [5].

The body of the stomach also contains enterochromaffin like cells (ECL) that express histidine decarboxylase. ECL cells secrete histamine in response to acetylcholine release during the cephalic or vagal phase of gastric secretion. Histamine is also secreted in response to gastric distention. This effect is mediated by gastrin. Histamine induces the release of gastric acid by parietal cells [2].

S.M. Vickers (✉)
Department of Surgery, University of Minnesota, 420 Delaware St.
SE, MMC 195, Minneapolis, MN 55455, USA
e-mail: vickers@umn.edu

R.A. Rosenthal et al. (eds.), *Principles and Practice of Geriatric Surgery*,
DOI 10.1007/978-1-4419-6999-6_61, © Springer Science+Business Media, LLC 2011

G cells are the major component of antral glands. They secrete gastrin in response to gastric distention, vagal stimulation, or on increase of the intraluminal concentration of peptides and amino acids. Gastrin increases the secretion of gastric acid and pepsinogen. It also induces cell growth and differentiation of parietal cells.

D cells release somatostatin into the bloodstream when the concentration of gastric acid increases. The primary location of these cells is the antrum, but the body of the stomach also has D cells. Somatostatin inhibits the secretion of gastric acid, histamine, and gastrin [5].

Immature or undifferentiated cells are intercalated between other cells in the isthmus of gastric glands. They migrate and differentiate into other type of cells.

Effect of Age on Gastric Physiology

Gastric diseases are influenced by age. The surgeon caring for elderly patients has to understand that not only co-morbidities influence the clinical scenario; aging affects the normal physiology, histology, and pathology of the stomach.

The major changes in gastric physiology and histology associated with normal aging are:

1. *Gastric motility.* Aging is associated with normal gastric emptying of liquids but slower gastric emptying with solid foods. The accommodation reflex is slower in elderly patients. In healthy subjects the presence of nutrients in the small intestine decreases antral contractions, increases the pyloric tone, and induces relaxation of the gastric fundus. These responses are mediated by different hormones but cholecystokinin (CCK) is most responsible for this response. The plasma concentrations of CCK are persistently elevated in older patients before and after meals. As a consequence, they experience decreased appetite and slower gastric emptying [6]. The decrease in gastric motility can influence drug absorption. This is one of the reasons why older patients have more side effects as compared to younger patients [7].

2. *Bicarbonate secretion.* Aging decreases both the basal and induced secretion of bicarbonate in the human stomach which decreases acid neutralization in elderly patients [6].

3. *Mucous.* The quality of the mucus in the stomach decreases with age; this effect is independent of *Helicobacter pylori* infection and any medication. In vivo studies with rats have shown that the population of mucous cells decreases in older animals. In humans, the total number of mucous secreting cells only decreases after *H. pylori* infection [7].

4. *Prostaglandins (PG) synthesis.* The main types of PGs identified in the gastric mucosa are PGE2 and PGI2 and lesser amounts of PGF2 and PGD2 [4]. Mucous cells release PGE2 and PGI2 on epithelial injury. Both molecules increase the mucosal blood flow and induce the release of mucous and bicarbonate secretion. The mucous and bicarbonate create a preepithelial barrier that keeps the pH neutral [5]. Gastric biopsies from elderly patients showed a decrease in PGE2 and PGF2 α levels [8]. Studies in rats have shown that the constitutive expression of COX (COX-1), the enzyme that catalyzes the conversion of arachidonic acid to PGs decreases in older animals. This finding has yet to be confirmed in humans [9].

5. *Pepsin.* Studies evaluating the secretory function of the stomach have indicated that pepsin secretion decreases in elderly subjects [9].

6. *Mucosal blood flow.* There is no evidence that mucosal blood flow changes in older healthy patients [9].

7. *Gastric acid secretion.* Studies prior to 1983 demonstrated that gastric acid secretion decreases in elderly patients. However these studies were completed before *H. pylori* was identified. The prevalence of *H. pylori* infection increases with age (up to 80% in patients older than 80 years). Chronic infection with *H. pylori* induces atrophic gastritis, therefore the hypochlorhydria previously described in older patients is a consequence of *H. pylori* infection, not a consequence of aging. Current evidence suggests that gastric acid secretion is not influenced by aging [10].

CASE STUDY

A 77-year-old white female arrives to the emergency department complaining of 3 days with multiple episodes of melena and seven episodes of hematemesis during the last day. She denies any other symptom. Her family affirms that she has longstanding diabetes mellitus complicated with renal insufficiency and coronary artery disease that required treatment with two stents 3 years ago. She also had total right knee replacement 6 months ago. Her current medications are insulin, lisinopril, ibuprofen, and clopidogrel.

She appears initially stable, with normal vital signs, no acute distress but while being examined she has an episode of massive hematemesis. The heart rate increases to 120 bpm, blood pressure decreases to 70/50, respiratory rate 20, the saturation decreases to 85%.

1. What is the initial management required by this patient?

At an upper endoscopy a 2-cm ulcer is seen in the duodenum. Bleeding is successfully controlled and remains hemodynamically stable; however, 10 h later

(continued)

CASE STUDY (continued)

she develops a new episode of hematemesis with hypotension and tachycardia.

2. What treatment should be offered to this patient now?

  (a) Repeat upper endoscopy
  (b) Emergent laparotomy

The bleeding continues and the patient is taken to the OR.

3. Where is the most common location of duodenal ulcers that require surgery?

The patient recovers successfully after surgery; however, she is concerned about continuing treatment with clopidogrel and ibuprofen.

4. What is the medical treatment required by this patient?

Peptic Ulcer Disease

Epidemiology

The number of admissions, surgeries, and mortalities related to peptic ulcer disease (PUD) has generally decreased; however, the proportion of patients older than 65 years admitted for duodenal or gastric ulcer complications is increasing [11]. The first clinical manifestation of PUD is an acute abdomen in up to 50% of elderly patients [12]. Acute upper gastrointestinal (GI) bleeding related to PUD is more frequent in elderly patients [13, 14].

Physiopathology

In the early 1900s, Schwarz dictated: "no acid, no ulcer"; however, the advances in gastric physiology during the past 40 years now establish that PUD results from multiple factors that either injure the mucosal barrier in the stomach and duodenum or increase the production of gastric acid. In the healthy gastric mucosa the mucous and bicarbonate form a hydrophobic preepithelial barrier that prevents backflow of H⁺ and maintains a neutral pH even if the intraluminal concentration of gastric acid is increased [5]. Mucosal injury occurs regularly but secondary components of the mucosal defense repair it. Elderly cells in the gastric mucosa are replaced continuously; the epithelium is renewed every 2–4 days. The normal response after epithelium damage is migration of healthy cells from the gastric pits to denude areas of the basement membrane, increase in the release of mucous by damaged cells, and the release of plasma by the mucosal vessels. When mucous and plasma mix, they create a mucoid cap that protects the denuded area. Although the basement membrane is highly sensitive to gastric acid, the mucoid cap prevents further damage because it has a neutral pH. This response is dependent on mucosal blood flow. Sensory afferent nerve endings in the mucosa release calcitonin gene-related peptide (CGRP) if the gastric mucosa gets exposed to gastric acid. CGRP vasodilates mucosal vessels. The increase in blood flow is mediated by nitric oxide. The enhanced blood flow buffers, dilutes, and removes gastric acid. PGs are crucial for this defense because they induce the release of mucous, bicarbonate, and phospholipids from the mucous cells. PGE2 and PGI2 also increase blood flow to the gastric mucosa [4]. True ulcers occur if the insult continues and extends into the muscularis propia.

Classification of Gastric Ulcers

Gastric ulcers are classified according to location and possible physiopathology in four types: Type I are gastric ulcers located in the lesser curvature; Type II are gastric ulcers associated with a history of previous or active duodenal ulcer; Type III are prepyloric ulcers; Type IV are ulcers located near the GE junction. While Type II and III are associated with increased acid production, Type I and IV are associated either with malignancy or decreased mucosal defense [15].

Etiology

The main factors that predispose to PUD are as follows:

Helicobacter pylori

This microaerophilic gram-negative spiral bacterium colonizes the preepithelial mucous layer of the stomach. It is one of the most common human chronic infections worldwide; humans are the only known reservoir for *H. pylori*. The transmission is either fecal–oral or oral–oral. Prevalence is influenced by socioeconomic status, ethnicity, and age. Around 30–40% of the US population is infected with *H. pylori* (50% African Americans, 60% Mexican Americans, 26% in Caucasians) [16, 17]. Approximately 50% of the world's population is infected; the frequency is higher in developing countries with poor sanitation and household hygiene, and with low family income and educational level. The infection is acquired during childhood in developing countries. In high-income countries, the rate of seroconversion is approximately 0.5–1% per annum. In the USA, the prevalence increases with age: less than 10% before 30 years, 50% around 50 years, and up to 80% in patients older than 80 years [7, 11, 18]. *H. pylori* always produces inflammation (gastritis) but only 15% of the patients develop PUD [16]. *H. pylori* secretes urease, which produces ammonium, that favors gastric colonization with *H. pylori* and damages epithelial cells. *H. pylori* also produces proteases and phospholipases that affect the efficacy of the mucous-bicarbonate layer. *H. pylori* has a rich catalase activity that blocks the neutrophil response [19]. These bacteria also release toxins that generate a chronic inflammatory response which results in type B atrophic gastritis.

Why *H. pylori* induces duodenal inflammation is not fully understood. Some studies suggest that gastric metaplasia in the first portion of the duodenum facilitates *H. pylori* colonization and further inflammation. Other studies posit that antral *H. pylori* infection increases gastric acid secretion because the ammonia produced by *H. pylori* increases the pH to which G cells are exposed and because the population of the D cells decreases with *H. pylori* infection. Duodenal *H. pylori* infection decreases bicarbonate secretion in the duodenal cells [16, 19].

Nonsteroidal Anti-inflammatory Drugs (NSAIDs)

At least 40% of the patients older than 65 years use NSAIDs. Between 1 and 8% of these patients will require a hospitalization to treat a NSAID-related complication. Duodenal and gastric ulcers develop in 5–8% and 15–20% of patients taking NSAIDs, respectively. Proton pump inhibitors (PPI) or misoprostol decrease the risk of PUD but only 10–20% of the patients receive prophylaxis [13]. The risk of NSAIDs' toxicity increases with age; the risk of serious GI complications after 1 year of NSAIDs ingestion is 0.32% in patients older than 65 as compared to 0.039% in younger patients [20]. NSAIDs significantly decrease the production of mucous, bicarbonate, and phospholipids in the stomach and duodenum because these drugs inhibit the activity of COX-1 and COX-2. The final result is a preepithelial barrier that cannot prevent H^+ backflow.

NSAIDs also delay mucosal healing because they decrease PG synthesis, therefore the mucoid cap cannot be formed, and the increase in mucosal flow and mucosal regeneration cannot occur. COX-1 inhibition also releases endothelin-1, a potent vasoconstrictor, and for that reason blood flow to the mucosa decreases in patients with mucosal injury induced by NSAIDs [20]. NSAIDs also increase the expression of leukocyte adhesion molecules and neutrophil

adherence. Neutrophils cause further damage because they release proteases and reactive oxygen metabolites [4].

The toxic effects of NSAIDs are mainly systemic but these drugs also induce topical cytotoxic injury in the gastric mucosa because they increase cellular permeability with diffusion of the drugs to mucosal cells [4].

NSAIDs ingestion and *H. pylori* infection are independent risk factors for PUD, but if both factors coexist the risk of PUD is synergistically increased [21]. This is particularly likely in elderly patients because both risk factors are more prevalent in older populations [11].

Zollinger–Ellison Syndrome

This syndrome is associated with neuroendocrine tumors that secrete excessive amounts of gastrin into the bloodstream. Gastric acid greatly increases in these patients. Zollinger–Ellison syndrome (ZE syndrome) accounts for 0.1–1% of all peptic ulcers. The diagnosis requires an elevated gastrin (>500 pg/ml) in the presence of an acid gastric pH (pH < 5). In patients with nondiagnostic gastric elevations (>150 but less than 500 pg/ml) a rise of more than 120 pg/ml after the intravenous administration of secretin (0.2 µg/kg) is diagnostic. The tumor can be localized with CT, MRI, endoscopic ultrasound, selective arterial secretin stimulation test, and somatostatin receptor scintigraphy but surgical exploration of the gastrinoma triangle with intraoperative ultrasound is the best method to localize the tumor. This entity is more common in young patients (mean age 41) but it should be considered in patients with atypical PUD localization (ulcers in the second, third, or fourth portion of the duodenum, jejunum), severe gastroesophageal reflux, diarrhea, PUD refractory to treatment and recurrent disease in patients without *H. pylori* infection or NSAID ingestion [22, 23].

Smoking

Smoking decreases wound-healing, increases the risk of *H. pylori* infection and is an independent risk factor that predicts failure to antibiotic treatment [24].

Clinical Manifestations of Noncomplicated Peptic Ulcer Disease

The cardinal symptom is epigastric pain without any irradiation. This pain is frequently described as "burning," "gnawing," or "hunger pain." It is usually exacerbated with fasting and relieved with the ingestion of food or anti-acids. The presence of other symptom than pain such as weight loss, anorexia, melena, hematemesis, constant pain or pain irradiated to the back suggests complicated PUD. Differential diagnosis includes dyspepsia, upper GI malignancies, cholelithiasis, pancreatitis, and GERD.

Elderly patients always require an extensive workup because the risk of malignancy increases with age. The conservative approach recommended for young patients without complications is not recommended for elderly patients. The gold standard test to diagnose PUD is an upper endoscopy. Duodenal ulcers typically occur in the first portion of the duodenum; they are usually not associated with malignancy (risk less than 1%). The presence of multiple ulcers or ulcers located beyond the second portion of the duodenum suggests ZE syndrome. Gastric adenocarcinoma exists in up to 5% of the patients with gastric ulcers with gross benign appearance, therefore all gastric ulcers should be biopsied [15].

Medical Treatment for Noncomplicated Peptic Ulcer Disease

The mainstay of treatment is to inhibit gastric acid secretion. This can be achieved with proton pump inhibitors (PPIs) or with Histamine-2 receptor antagonists (H2RA). PPIs are irreversible inhibitors of the H^+/K^+-ATPase. They should be given before meals. The recommended therapy for duodenal ulcers is 4–6 weeks, the healing rate is between 80 and 100%, for gastric ulcers the recommended therapy is 8 weeks, and the healing rate is 70 and 85%. In case the ulcer is associated to hypergastrinemia or NSAIDs ingestion, the treatment should be continued. H2RA are reversible inhibitors of the H2 receptor in the membrane of parietal cells. The healing rate is 70–80% in duodenal ulcers and 55–65% in gastric ulcers. The duration of treatment is the same than PPIs [5]. An alternative in the treatment of PUD is sucralfate, this agent improves mucosal healing because it creates a protective barrier in the ulcer, stimulates bicarbonate, mucous, and growth factor release. Misoprostol is a PG analogue that improves ulcer healing; however, it is frequently associated to GI side effects such as diarrhea.

The presence of *H. pylori* infection is associated with a high recurrence rate; in duodenal ulcers the recurrence rate is 95% without *H. pylori* eradication compared to 12% for those patients who receive eradication treatment. The recurrence rate for gastric ulcers without *H. pylori* eradication is 74% vs. 13% after eradication [19]. The two most common techniques to diagnose *H. pylori* infection are urea breath test or detection in the biopsy; other tools are rapid urease testing, culture, polymerase chain reaction, antibody testing, and the fecal antigen test. Eradication treatment is always indicated in patients with PUD complicated or uncomplicated. The current regimens

TABLE 61.1 FDA approved regimens for *Helicobacter pylori* eradication*

Regimen	Duration (days)
1. Omeprazole 20 mg b.i.d. + Clarithromycin 500 mg b.i.d. + Amoxicillin 1 g b.i.d.	10
2. Lansoprazole 30 mg b.i.d. + Clarithromycin 500 mg b.i.d. + Amoxicillin 1 g b.i.d.	10
3. Esomeprazole 40 mg q.d + Clarithromycin 500 mg b.i.d. + Amoxicillin 1 g b.i.d.	10
4. Rabeprazole 20 mg b.i.d. + Clarithromycin 500 mg b.i.d. + Amoxicillin 1 g b.i.d.	7
5. Bismuth 525 mg q.i.d. + Metronidazole 250 mg q.i.d. + Tetracycline 500 mg q.i.d. + Histamine-2 Receptor Antagonists**	14

*The success rate is around 80%
**In this regimen the total duration of Histamine-2 receptor antagonists therapy is 4 weeks

approved by the FDA for the eradication of *H. pylori* are in Table 61.1. The success rate is approximately 80% [16, 17].

Patients with gastric or duodenal ulcers associated with NSAIDs require replacement of the NSAIDs with narcotics or acetaminophen plus the administration of a PPI. Prophylaxis with misoprostol or PPIs is indicated in elderly patients that cannot stop NSAIDs. The incidence of ulceration decreases from 20 to 4.5% [4].

Clinical Manifestations of Complicated Peptic Ulcer Disease

The first clinical manifestation is a complication in 50–60% of elderly patients[20]. Elderly patients frequently have comorbidities that affect the mental status or pain perception (uncompensated diabetes, stroke, dementia) or they are receiving drugs that create or mask PUD (i.e., NSAIDs, narcotics, steroids). The diagnosis is frequently challenging because the normal systemic inflammatory response (fever, leukocytosis) is often absent in elderly patients or is affected by drugs (steroids, beta blockers) [12, 14]

PPI, H2RA, and antibiotic therapy for *H. pylori* have decreased the number of elective surgical procedures required for PUD, but the incidence of complications such as perforation or bleeding has not changed significantly over time.

Perforation

The incidence of perforation in PUD has remained stable or slightly increased in elderly patients, especially women [25]. Between 2 and 10% of the patients with duodenal ulcers present as a perforated ulcer.

Elderly patients frequently present to the emergency room without any history of PUD. The diagnosis is suggested by acute epigastric pain that rapidly becomes generalized. The patient is often diaphoretic and tachycardic; low grade fever can also occur. The presence of generalized tenderness, positive rebound, and abolished peristalsis is usually evident, but the physical examination in very old or immunocompromised patients can be nonspecific. The diagnosis is confirmed with chest radiography because 70 and 80% of the patients have free subdiaphragmatic air. If the physical examination is nonconclusive or in the absence of free air the most useful test is a CT scan of the abdomen and pelvis; this study excludes other diagnosis and is highly sensitive to detect free intra-abdominal air.

Despite conservative treatment with antibiotics and IV fluids has been described in hemodynamically stable patients with contained perforations, elderly patients usually require surgical treatment. After the initial evaluation, an aggressive IV fluid resuscitation is crucial. Elderly patients frequently have cardiovascular co-morbidities that require measurement of central venous pressure (CVP) and urine output. Broad spectrum antibiotics should be started on diagnosis. The initial assessment and medical therapy should not delay surgery. The most frequent surgical procedure for perforated ulcers is primary closure plus reinforcement with an omental patch. The treatment for perforated ulcers is summarized in Fig. 61.1.

Primary Closure Reinforced with Omental Patch

The patient is placed in supine position; under general anesthesia an endotracheal and nasogastric tube, and a Foley catheter are placed. Our preferred approach is a midline supraumbilical incision because it provides easy access to the stomach and duodenum; in case a different pathology is found the incision can be easily extended. After an exploratory laparotomy has ruled out other diagnoses, the gastrocolic ligament is divided to enter the lesser sac. This maneuver allows a complete visualization of the anterior and posterior surfaces of the stomach. If the perforation is in the stomach, the margins of the perforation are debrided (Fig. 61.2). Ulcer biopsies must be sent for definitive diagnosis because gastric cancer can simulate perforated PUD. The defect is closed with a full-thickness single layer of interrupted 3-0 silk stitches (Fig. 61.3). The primary closure is reinforced with omentum (Omental patch) (Fig. 61.4). The tails of the sutures are used to hold the omental pedicle, avoiding ischemia while the sutures are tied (Fig. 61.5). It is important to avoid vascular injury to the omentum during dissection of the gastrocolic ligament. The abdominal cavity is copiously irrigated. The fascia is closed with a running suture. The subcutaneous tissue is also irrigated. The skin is usually not closed due to high risk of infection.

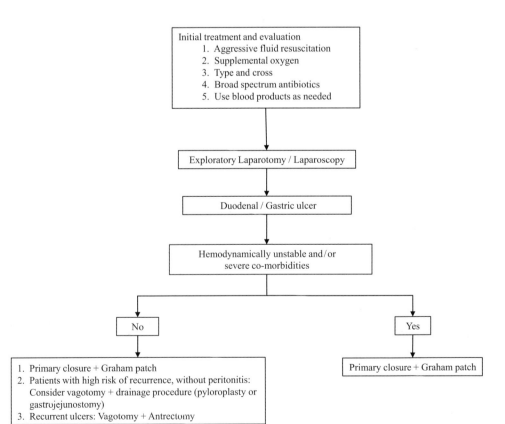

FIGURE 61.1 Algorithm for the management of perforated peptic ulcers in elderly patients.

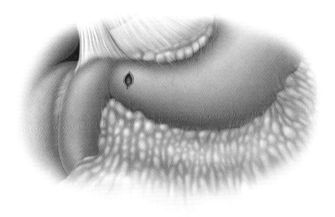

FIGURE 61.2   Debridement of the ulcer margins.

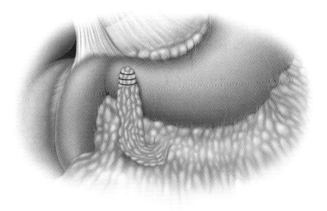

FIGURE 61.5   Final view of the primary repair of a perforated ulcer with an omental patch.

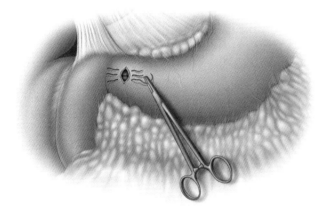

FIGURE 61.3   Primary closure of a perforated ulcer.

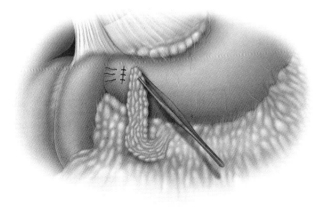

FIGURE 61.4   Reinforcement of the primary closure using an omental patch.

For duodenal ulcers, after a complete exploratory laparotomy is done, the duodenum is mobilized anteriorally and medially (Kocher maneuver). This maneuver avoids excessive tension on the primary closure. Both the anterior and posterior surfaces are carefully inspected. Routine biopsies are not required because the risk of malignancy in duodenal ulcers is very low; however, adequate debridement of the margins is required. The duodenal defect is closed following the same principles for a gastric ulcer: interrupted full-thickness sutures reinforced with an omental patch. Duodenal ulcers are associated with more inflammation and defects larger than gastric ulcers, so if the primary closure is not possible, a true omental patch (Graham patch) is used. In this repair the ulcer margins are not approximated, the orifice is only plugged with omentum sutured to the duodenal defect, avoiding ischemia in the omentum. The abdominal cavity is closed following the same principles described for gastric ulcers. Patients are usually extubated unless they have persistent hemodynamic instability and/or if the patient has any oxygenation problem. The nasogastric tube is kept to prevent gastric or duodenal distention and it is pulled out once the bowel function is normal. The integrity of the repair is evaluated with an upper GI study done with hydrosoluble contrast.

Additional procedures that decrease gastric acid secretion are not recommended because elderly patients frequently present with shock and severe co-morbidities that require a rapid intervention to control the damage. Often, these patients have a delay in diagnosis and generalized peritonitis is found during the laparotomy, therefore further dissection of the hiatus increases the risk of other complications such as mediastinitis. It is important to consider also that PPIs and *H. pylori* eradication treatment decrease the risk of recurrence.

The morbidity and mortality associated with perforated PUD are between 25–89% and 4–30%, respectively. Risk factors associated with increased morbidity and mortality are age, delay in diagnosis, high ASA score (III and IV), and shock during surgery. Age is crucial because patients older than 65 years have a mortality rate of 37.7% as compared with 1.4% in younger patients. A delay in diagnosis (>24 h) increases the mortality rate in elderly patients. The most common causes of mortality are myocardial infarct, arrhythmias, septic shock, and pneumonia. Resection procedures (i.e., antrectomy) are also associated with more mortality than primary closure in these patients [26].

Bleeding

Bleeding is the most common complication of PUD, which in turn is the most common source of upper GI bleeding. It is seen in 15–20% of the patients [27, 28]. The frequency of acute upper GI bleeding has decreased in general but the proportion of patients older than 60 years that bleed is increasing; recent studies have published that 65 and 25% of the patients are older than 65 and 80 years old, respectively [13, 14]. This trend is a result of increased life expectancy: older patients have more co-morbidities that predispose them to PUD (i.e., chronic renal failure, myeloproliferative disorders, portal hypertension) or that require anticoagulation. Elderly patients ingest more NSAIDs either as analgesics or as a preventive measure for other disorders.

The most important risk factor to develop GI bleeding is NSAIDs ingestion. These drugs decrease the mucosal defense to gastric acid and inhibit platelet aggregation by decreasing thromboxane A2 production. The risk is dose dependent, but bleeding occurs also with low aspirin doses (75–325 mg/day) [29]. The risk of bleeding is considerably lower with COX-2 inhibitors as compared with nonselective NSAIDS, but COX-2 inhibitors can induce bleeding when they are combined with anticoagulants, aspirin, or any other NSAIDs [27]. The risk of bleeding significantly increases in patients taking anticoagulants, serotonin reuptake inhibitors, or drugs that prevent platelet aggregation [20]. *H. pylori* infection marginally increases the risk of bleeding; however, concomitant NSAIDs use and *H. pylori* infection significantly increase the risk of bleeding [21].

The main symptom is melena and/or hematochezia. The main focus during the initial evaluation is to assess the hemodynamic status. The presence of tachycardia, systolic blood pressure <100 mmHg, postural hypotension or altered mental status suggests a significant blood loss so an aggressive fluid resuscitation should start immediately. The initial goals of resuscitation are to establish a secure airway if needed, to ensure proper breathing, and to administer IV fluids. Fluid resuscitation is challenging in elderly patients with preexistent cardiac or renal failure; the placement of a central line

and Foley catheter is particularly useful but should not delay further treatment. It is mandatory to obtain a complete blood count, glucose, blood urea nitrogen, creatinine, electrolytes, INR, type and cross-match in all patients. The use of blood products needs to be individualized for each patient; any history of coronary artery disease lowers the threshold for packed red blood cells. Plasma should be given to any patient with a coagulopathy associated with drugs or co-morbidities. Once the patient is hemodynamically stable, he or she should be thoroughly examined. In the absence of any other disease the physical examination of the abdomen is usually unremarkable.

Upper GI endoscopy is the gold standard for diagnosis and initial therapy because it indicates the source of the bleeding, rules out other diagnoses, and because bleeding can be stopped using hemoclips, sclerosing agents, epinephrine, thrombin or fibrin glue, or thermal contact with bipolar electrocoagulation, heater probe or argon plasma. Except for epinephrine, all these techniques can be used either to stop active bleeding or to prevent it in visible vessels. Epinephrine injection can partially control the bleeding before implementation of other techniques. Endoscopic therapy has a low complication rate (0.5%) [30]. The two most common complications are perforation or induced bleeding.

Most duodenal ulcers that bleed are in the posterior wall of the first portion of the duodenum; the bleeding almost always arises from the gastroduodenal artery (GDA) [11]. The most common vessels that bleed in the stomach branch off the inferior branch of the left gastric artery in the lesser curvature [15].

Approximately 20% of the patients will rebleed after endoscopy. For these patients, a second endoscopy is indicated because the success rate is high without significant morbidity; however, if bleeding persists, surgery is necessary. The frequency of surgery depends on the endoscopist's experience; the failure rate in high volume centers is less than 3%; however, most centers report a failure rate between 5 and 10–20% [14, 15, 19].

Another indication for surgery is a persistent blood requirement, if more than 4 units are given during 24 h. Because elderly patients develop coagulopathy associated to active bleeding faster than younger patients and active bleeding aggravates preexistent co-morbidities (myocardial infarct, renal failure, and stroke) faster than in younger patients, surgery needs to be considered in elderly patients before 4 units of blood are required.

Ulcer size is not considered a surgical indication but ulcers bigger than 2 cm are associated with greater risk of rebleeding. If an ulcer >2 cm presents with persistent hypotension, surgical treatment should be considered [14].

Adequate platelet aggregation and hemostasis require an intragastric pH>6. Diffcrent studies have shown that high doses of PPI decrease the re-bleeding rate by 54% and the need for surgery by 41%. The recommended regimens are

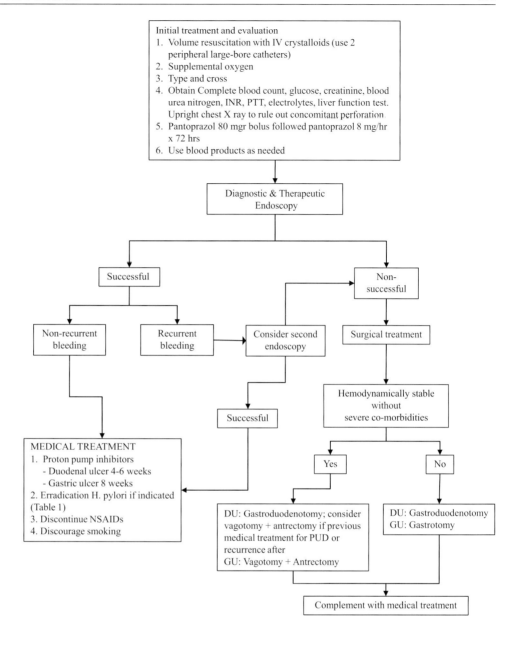

FIGURE 61.6 Algorithm for the management of acute peptic ulcer bleeding in elderly patients.

pantoprazol 80 mg IV bolus followed by 8 mg/h for 3 days; pantoprazol 80 mg bolus followed by pantoprazol 40 mg every 12 h [31]. Figure 61.6 summarizes the diagnosis and treatment of bleeding ulcers.

Surgical Treatment of Bleeding Duodenal Ulcers

The anesthesia, positioning, and incision are the same as per-forated ulcers. A full Kocher maneuver follows an explor-atory laparotomy. Profuse bleeding in the first portion of the duodenum can be partially stopped by compressing the duo-denal bulb. The pylorus is identified by the palpation of the concentric ring between the stomach and the duodenum, or by visual identification of the pyloric vein that crosses anterior to the pylorus (Mayo's vein). Two 3-0 silk sutures are placed in the superior and inferior borders of the anterior surface of the pylorus. A 3-cm longitudinal gastrotomy per-pendicular to the pylorus is followed by 3-cm extension toward the duodenum. The most common bleeding vessel is the GDA, which is located in the posterior duodenal wall (Fig. 61.7). Three stitches are placed to stop bleeding: two initial figure 8 stitches in the superior and inferior margin of the ulcer followed by a third figure 8 or U-stitch that controls the pancreatic branch of the GDA (Fig. 61.8). Each suture must be placed carefully to avoid injury to the common bile duct. Once vascular control is achieved, the duodenum and stomach are carefully inspected to rule out any other source of bleeding. The aperture is closed transversely. The internal layer is a full-thickness continuous closure with an absorbable

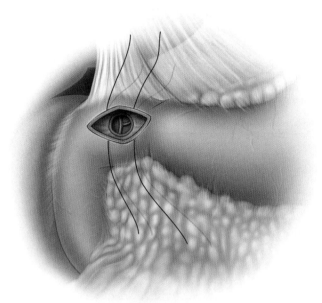

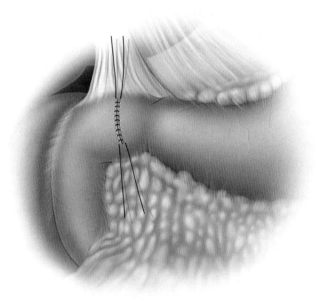

Figure 61.7 Bleeding ulcer in the posterior wall of the first portion of the duodenum.

Figure 61.9 Primary closure of the duodenotomy.

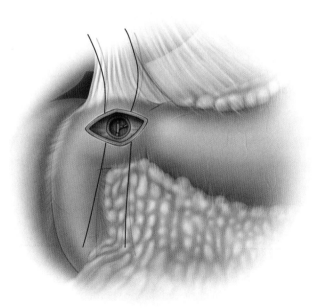

Figure 61.8 Haemostasis of the GDA using 3-0 silk stitches.

3-0 suture reinforced by a second layer of interrupted seromuscular stitches using 3-0 silk (Lembert type) (Fig. 61.9). The closure can be reinforced with omentum, similar to a Graham patch.

Additional procedures that decrease acid secretion are controversial. The recurrence rate was high before predisposing risk factors to develop PUD were fully understood. Not all patients require anti-acid procedures; the surgeon has

to consider additional interventions based on other factors. The most important factor is the patient's hemodynamic condition. In case of patients with severe co-morbidities or refractory shock the only aim of surgery is to stop the bleeding. Additional factors to be considered are NSAIDs use, *H. pylori* infection, and previous surgical or medical treatment for PUD. Two randomized trials have shown that eradicating *H. pylori* decreases bleeding recurrence after 1 year of follow-up [32, 33]. In patients without history of PUD or *H. pylori* infection, we recommend only to control the bleeding. In stable patients with previous medical or surgical PUD treatment or who require NSAIDs, a truncal vagotomy with or without antrectomy should be considered. These procedures will be described in the treatment of bleeding gastric ulcers. The postoperative management is the same as described for the perforated ulcers.

Surgical Treatment of Bleeding Gastric Ulcers

Most gastric ulcers that bleed are type I. The anesthesia, patient's position, and incision are similar to duodenal bleeding ulcers. Treatment depends on the hemodynamic status of the patient. For those with shock, a conservative approach that only aims to control bleeding is recommended. Through an anterior gastrotomy, the ulcer is biopsied and oversown with figure 8 stitches. The gastrotomy is closed in two layers using the same technique described for closing bleeding duodenal ulcers.

Stable patients are treated with truncal vagotomy plus an antrectomy. The gastrocolic ligament is divided to enter the lesser sac; this dissection begins in the middle point between the pylorus and the cardia and continued distally to the pylorus where the right gastroepiploic vessels are transected. Adhesions between the posterior gastric wall and the pancreas are divided. The gastrohepatic ligament is divided in order to control the inferior branch of the left gastric artery. The proximal and distal margins of this dissection are the incisura angularis and the beginning of the first portion of the duodenum, respectively. The stomach is divided proximally with a gastrointestinal anastomosis (GIA) stapler. The first portion of the duodenum is divided immediately after the pylorus with a transverse anastomosis (TA) stapler. The integrity can be restored with a Billroth I, Billroth II, or a Roux en Y gastrojejunostomy.

The first option to reconstruct is a gastroduodenostomy, or Billroth I, which requires a complete Kocher maneuver to avoid tension in the anastomosis. The duodenum is mobilized close to the gastric remnant. The anastomosis is done in two layers. The internal layer is a continuous full-thickness layer using a 3-0 absorbable suture reinforced by a second layer of interrupted seromuscular sutures with 3-0 silk (Lembert type). This anastomosis is considered the most physiological reconstruction as the normal transit of the stomach goes to the duodenum; however, alkaline gastritis can occur. Previous scarring can limit the Kocher maneuver and the anastomosis cannot be done without tension.

The second reconstruction is a Billroth II procedure or gastrojejunostomy, which is preferred in cases with excessive scarring that, prevents duodenal mobilization. This side-to-side anastomosis is created between the posterior gastric wall and the anti-mesenteric border of a jejunal limb (10–20 cm distal to Treitz ligament). The jejunum is brought close to the stomach, anterior or posterior to the transverse colon (antecolic or retrocolic, respectively). There is no functional difference in benign diseases. The anastomosis is done with a stapler or manually using the Hofmeister technique. The anastomosis is stapled through a small gastrotomy and enterostomy. The stapler is introduced through these defects, and the anastomosis is created. Both orifices are closed manually with a continuous full-thickness layer reinforced by an interrupted seromuscular layer. The mesenteric defect in the mesocolon is closed with interrupted 3-0 silk stitches in order to avoid internal hernias. The two most common options to restore are Billroth I or II, but both anastomoses predispose patients to alkaline gastritis or reflux; therefore, some surgeons recommend a reconstruction using a Roux en Y gastrojejunostomy for benign conditions.

A truncal vagotomy follows the anastomosis. This step requires mobilization of 4–5 cm of the intra-abdominal esophagus. The initial step is liver mobilization; the falciform ligament is followed posteriorly until the left triangular ligament can be identified and sectioned. Right traction of segments II and III of the liver allows direct visualization of the cardia. The proximal

gastrohepatic ligament is divided, and dissection is continued proximally until the phreno-esophageal membrane is identified and sectioned; this allows the right wall of the esophagus to be visualized. The division continues proximally 4–5 cm; the peritoneum is then transected transversally and continued through the left border of the esophagus which has to be mobilized also 4–5 cm. This dissection is done carefully to avoid any splenic injury or bleeding from the short gastric vessels. The placement of a Penrose drain around the esophagus facilitates exposure. The left vagus nerve is easily identified if the esophagus is retracted posteriorly and inferiorly. At least 2 cm of nerve are clipped and divided. The right vagus, in the posterior wall, is located if the esophagus is retracted inferiorly and to the left. At least 2 cm are divided. Both nerves are sent to pathology to confirm the vagotomy. Once the dissection is completed the abdomen is closed using a standard technique. Postoperative management is similar to duodenal bleeding ulcers.

Outcome

This complication has a mortality rate that ranges between 10 and 35% in patients older than 60 years as compared with 10% in younger patients. Bleeding is the most common complication that causes death in PUD. Risk factors that predict high mortality are increased age, severe co-morbidities associated, re-bleeding, or patients that present with hypotension, shock, or in-hospital bleeding [11, 13, 15].

Gastric Outlet Obstruction

Gastric outlet obstruction (GOO) is the final result of chronic edema, scarring, and fibrosis of the distal stomach or duodenum. The area proximal to the stenosis is chronically dilated; gastric dilation induces gastrin release, which is further aggravating because it increases gastric acid production. The incidence of GOO has declined with the advances in the medical therapy for PUD. GOO accounts for less than 5–8% of all PUD complications. The typical symptoms are early satiety, nausea, vomit of undigested food, heartburn, and weight loss.

The most common GOO etiology is malignancy (60–80%), therefore multiple biopsies from the stenosis need to be taken [34]. Only 5–8% of patients with GOO have PUD [28]. Other diagnoses to consider are external duodenal or gastric compression (i.e. pancreatic pseudocysts, tumors), GOO caused by a large gallstone (Bouveret syndrome), bezoars, and gastroparesis. The initial evaluation relies on an upper endoscopy with multiple biopsies plus a hydrosoluble-contrast upper GI series ; however, if external compression is suspected, a CT scan is required.

The initial treatment is conservative and uses an NG tube to decompress the stomach, IV infusion of PPIs, and corrects any electrolyte or acid–base disorder. Prokinetics are contraindicated. If *H. pylori* infection is proven, antibiotic therapy is indicated because some studies report that symptoms improve after *H. pylori* eradication [34]. Nutritional status is crucial; a liquid diet should be attempted unless the patient cannot tolerate ingestion. Severe GOO requires total parenteral nutrition. Medical treatment improves GOO obstruction in 50% of the patients [35]. Endoscopic therapy with endoscopic balloons increases the success rate up to 70% [36, 37]. Serial dilations can be attempted in patients with recurrent stenosis, but the failure rate is proportional to the number of dilations attempted. The most common complication is perforation. Although our experience with endoscopic stenting for malignancies is increasing, current data on benign disease is limited [38].

Elderly patients benefit from conservative therapy because they have multiple co-morbidities; however, in refractory cases a truncal vagotomy plus antrectomy may be necessary. Chronic gastric obstruction dilates the stomach with subsequent accumulation of food and secretions; this condition predisposes patients to aspiration pneumonia, and wound infection due to bacterial overgrowth, so decompressing stomach with an NG tube is indicated before surgery. The technique for truncal vagotomy plus antrectomy is the same as described previously. Prolonged gastric dilation increases the risk of delayed gastric emptying which can be aggravated by narcotics or co-morbidities such as Parkinson disease or diabetes. These patients benefit from an intraoperative gastrostomy to decompress the stomach or a feeding jejunostomy to avoid the risk of TPN.

Duodenal dissection can be difficult in patients with chronic scarring; in these patients we recommend a truncal vagotomy plus a Hofmeister type gastrojejunostomy. The risk of fistula rate from the duodenal stump is also increased in these patients, so duodenal decompression through a lateral duodenostomy in the second portion of the duodenum decreases the risk in elderly patients.

Gastric Polyps

Gastric polyps are nodules of tissue, either sessile or pedunculated, that protrude into the gastric lumen [39]. Gastric polyps are seen in 0.5–2% of all endoscopies; most of them are asymptomatic but occasionally gastric polyps can grow, erode, and bleed. Large polyps can produce GOO [40–42]. Several types of gastric polyps can be found but the three most common in elderly patients are hyperplastic polyps, fundic gland polyps, and adenomatous polyps. Uncommon type of polyps include inflammatory fibroid polyps, xanthomas, Peutz-Jegher type hamartomatous polyps, juvenile polyps, gastric polyps associated with Cowden disease, and finally gastric polyps associated with Cronkhite–Canada Syndrome [43].

Hyperplastic Polyps

Hyperplastic polyps are the most common variety found during endoscopies [41–43]. The incidence increases with age (mean age of diagnosis is 64–75 years) and they are more prevalent in women. Hyperplastic polyps are usually asymptomatic but are associated with other gastric diseases such as *H. pylori* infection, autoimmune gastritis, ZE syndrome, antral vascular ectasia, gastric amyloidosis, or cytomegalovirus gastritis [43]. Gastrin plasma levels are higher than controls [39]. The most common location is the antrum followed by the fundus and body. The mean size is 1 cm, although larger hyperplastic polyps have been reported. The diagnosis is usually incidental and, while an upper endoscopy is being done for another reason. These polyps are usually sessile. The typical histological findings show elongated, dilated, tortuous foveolae lined by mucin-containing epithelium and edema of the lamina propia [42]. The natural history is variable. *H pylori* eradication is associated with regression [40]. Most hyperplastic polyps are benign and asymptomatic, though a routine biopsy is recommended because the final histology reports dysplasia or carcinoma in 1.5–4% of the patients. This risk of malignancy is higher in polyps larger than 2 cm [42, 43].

Fundic Gland Polyps

These polyps are the second most common type of benign gastric polyps. They can be found sporadically or associated with familiar adenomatous polyposis at any age. The most common location is in the fundus. Gastrin values are usually normal and are not strongly associated to *H. pylori* infection [39, 41]. Histology reveals cystic dilated glands lined by parietal and chief cells [42]. These polyps can regress spontaneously; routine follow-up is not required because they are not premalignant [39].

Adenomatous Polyps

The incidence of these polyps increases with age. They are associated with atrophic gastritis and are more prevalent in countries with high incidence of gastric cancer [42]. The median age of diagnosis is 67 years [40]. The most common location is the antrum, and gastrin levels do not differ from controls. The risk of malignancy is higher in adenomatous polyps than any other gastric polyp, especially if the size is greater than 2 cm (40–50% risk of malignancy) [41]. *H. pylori* eradication does not cause regression. Routine excision is recommended because they may be malignant [40].

Dieulafoy Lesion/Malformation

Dieulafoy lesion is an abnormal submucosal artery associated with a minute mucosal defect frequently associated with bleeding. It causes between 1 and 5.8% of acute nonvariceal upper GI bleeding. The most common location is the stomach followed by the first portion of the duodenum but they can occur throughout GI tract or in the bronchial tree. The most common location in the stomach is the fundus and body [44]. The histology reveals a submucosal artery that does not undergo the usual ramification within the wall of the stomach or failure to diminish to the minute size of the mucosal capillary vasculature without any inflammation or defect in the mucosa [45]. It is more common in men. The mean age of diagnosis is 63 years, so they are frequently associated with co-morbidities. Most patients develop melena and hematemesis associated with hemodynamic stability. The treatment follows the same principles described previously for bleeding peptic ulcers; the initial goal is hemodynamic stabilization followed by an upper endoscopy. The same endoscopic techniques described for PUD are used to stop bleeding. The success rate is >90% [46]. In patients who do not respond to endoscopic therapy, local wedge resection of the lesion is indicated.

Gastroparesis

Gastroparesis indicates impaired transit of intraluminal content from the stomach to the duodenum without a mechanical obstruction [47]. It affects 4% of the population.

Etiology

The most common causes of gastroparesis are diabetes, idiopathic, and surgery; however, the most common etiologies in the elderly patient are as follows:

1. *Diabetes.* Gastroparesis is present in 30% of the patients with type 2 diabetes [48]. Different theories explain this effect. Since gastroparesis is seen in patients with other manifestations of autonomic neuropathy, it is believed that autonomic neuropathy contributes to the development of gastroparesis. Diabetes decreases the number of interstitial Cajal cells, induces smooth muscle fibrosis and decreases the neurons present in Auerbach's plexus. Hyperglycemia decreases gastric emptying [48]. Diabetes is the most common cause of gastroparesis in elderly patients because diabetes is one of the most common co-morbidities seen in this population.
2. *Upper GI surgery.* Any surgery that involves the distal esophagus, stomach, or duodenum can be complicated by delayed gastric emptying. Unfortunately upper GI malignancies that require surgery are more common in older patients. This complication is also seen in benign diseases; gastroparesis may occur after any surgery for PUD or anti-reflux procedures.
3. *Neurological diseases.* Parkinson disease and cerebrovascular accidents are associated with gastroparesis. Parkinson disease is present in 7% of patients with gastroparesis [48].
4. *Drugs.* Elderly patients often require drugs that delay gastric emptying such as calcium channel antagonists, L-dopa, opiates, tricyclic antidepressants, and aluminum antacids [47].
5. *Other co-morbidities.* Renal insufficiency, hypothyroidism, previous abdominal irradiation, cirrhosis, chronic pancreatitis, and paraneoplastic syndromes can produce gastroparesis.

Clinical Manifestation

The most common symptoms are nausea, vomiting, bloating, early satiety, epigastric pain, and belching. Although in severe gastroparesis the previous symptoms present with liquid meals, they are more frequent with solid meals. The physical examination usually shows abdominal distention, mild pain, and tympanic percussion in epigastrium, but in severe cases dehydration is evidenced by tachycardia, orthostatic hypotension, poor skin turgor, and dry mucous membranes. Succussion splash is also present in severe cases.

Gastroparesis should be suspected in any patient with predisposing conditions associated with the symptoms previously described. An extensive workup can rule out cancer, dyspepsia, GOO secondary to PUD, pancreatitis, GERD, cyclic vomiting syndrome, chronic pancreatitis, superior mesenteric, and rumination syndrome. An upper GI radiographic study with contrast plus an upper endoscopy are frequently required to rule out any anatomical obstruction. Retained food in the stomach (with proper fasting) without anatomical obstruction increases the probability of gastroparesis. The gold standard for diagnosis is gastric emptying scintigraphy. In this test the patient receives a solid meal (typically scrambled eggs) mixed with ^{99}Technitium sulfur colloid. Gastric emptying is measured after 2, 3, and 4 h. The diagnosis is confirmed if more than 60 or 10% of the meal is retained after 2 and 4 h, respectively [49]. Other useful diagnostic tools are ^{13}C-labeled octanoate breath test, abdominal ultrasound evaluating gastric emptying of liquid meals, magnetic resonance imaging, single-photon emission CT, radiopaque markers, swallowed capsule telemetry, antroduodenal manometry, and electrogastrography. These techniques are available in specialized centers [50].

Treatment

The initial goal of therapy is to correct any preexisting dehydration or electrolyte disorders. The medical treatment has different components: dietary recommendations, control of predisposing conditions, and drug therapy.

In elderly patients, predisposing conditions are irreversible or difficult to treat. However, good metabolic control and replacement of any drug that delays gastric emptying is required. Meals rich in fiber or fat should be avoided because they delay gastric emptying; carbonated beverages should also be avoided. Frequent small meals are better tolerated than larger meals [48]. Prokinetic drugs improve gastric emptying. In the USA only two prokinetic agents, erythromycin and metoclopramide, are FDA approved for gastroparesis. Different studies have shown that erythromycin is the most potent agent because it activates motilin receptors and increases both antral peristalsis and gastric emptying. Metoclopramide is a benzamide that increases the contraction in the esophagus, fundus, and antrum; it also elevates the lower esophageal sphincter pressure and improves antral–pylorus–duodenal coordination. It is also helpful to control vomit [51]. Nausea and vomit are present in 92 and 84% of the patients, respectively, therefore antiemetics are also indicated. The most useful agents are phenothiazines (prochlorperazine and tiethyperazine). Serotonin 5-HT3 receptor antagonists may be helpful because they do not affect gastric emptying. Muscarinic M1 receptors antagonists and H2RA are not recommended because they inhibit gastric emptying [48]. Tricyclic antidepressants have anticholinergic activity, therefore they decrease gastric emptying; however, low doses can improve nausea and vomit. There are no prospective studies evaluating this effect [50].

The role of surgery in gastroparesis is limited to patients with severe gastroparesis that require multiple hospitalizations plus enteral or parenteral nutrition and those patients who fail medical treatment. Surgery relies on the placement of gastric stimulation devices that alter the gastric myoenteric neural network and interrupt gastric arrhythmias [52]. Through laparoscopy or open approach, two electrodes are placed 1 cm apart in the muscularis propia along the greater curvature 10 cm proximal to the pylorus. The electrodes are connected to a neurostimulator located in a subcutaneous pocket in the left flank [52]. This device has only been implanted in patients with severe gastroparesis. A recent study showed that gastric electrical stimulation produces a good outcome in 70% of the patients, most of whom are able to tolerate oral diets after surgery and have a significant increase in the body mass index [52].

For patients with refractory symptoms placement of a palliative gastrostomy or feeding jejunostomy should be considered.

Complications After Gastric Surgery

It is not uncommon for elderly patients to develop complications after gastric surgery. Each region has a particular response to food ingestion, which are mediated by the vagus nerve. The proximal stomach (fundus) is the main reservoir for liquids; and shortly after liquid ingestion there is a decrease in the tone in the fundus which allows liquid storage. Antral motility is increased by the ingestion of solid meals, it triturates large particles; only 1–2 mm particle pass through the duodenum. The pylorus controls the transit of food particles to the duodenum and limits alkaline reflux. Any surgery that involves the intra-abdominal esophagus, stomach, and duodenum can affect the motor functions of the stomach. The most common postgastrectomy syndromes are as follows:

Dumping Syndrome

It can present after any vagotomy, drainage procedure, or gastric resection. Between 25 and 50% of the patients have some manifestations related to dumping syndrome. In approximately 5–10% of the patients these symptoms are significant and in 1–5% of the patients produce disability. After vagal denervation, the stomach loses the relaxation and accommodation reflexes; therefore, it cannot function as a reservoir. In case a drainage procedure is added, gastric emptying cannot be controlled because the size of the particles is no longer regulated. In healthy persons, the presence of food in the duodenum exerts a negative feedback in gastric emptying, this loop is lost after drainage procedures such as a Billroth II. Dumping syndrome can be divided into early and late dumping syndrome.

Early dumping syndrome presents 10–30 min after food ingestion, the rapid emptying of hyperosmolar meals into the duodenum or jejunum induces water diffusion from the intravascular space to the intraluminal space and the release of serotonin, pancreatic polypeptide, enteroglucagon, peptide YY, glucagon like peptide, vasoactive inhibitory peptide, neurotensin, and epinephrine. These substances induce diaphoresis, weakness, dizziness, flushing, palpitations, fullness, crampy abdominal pain, nausea, vomit, and diarrhea.

Late dumping is seen after 2–4 h after the ingestion of food. The rapid increase of carbohydrate concentration in the intestinal lumen induces a rapid absorption of carbohydrates with hyperinsulinism which creates reactive hypoglycemia. The clinical difference is that patients present only with vasomotor symptoms and no GI symptoms [53].

The diagnosis is suspected in patients with a previous gastric surgery, it can be confirmed with a glucose oral challenge test, with a hydrogen breath test after glucose ingestion or with gastric emptying scintigraphy. Late dumping syndrome is diagnosed measuring the concentration of glucose 60–180 min after the ingestion of food [54].

The mainstay of treatment are diet modifications, liquids should be ingested 30 min after the ingestion of solids, simple carbohydrates should be avoided, supplemental fiber is recommended, because it decreases gastric emptying. In case symptoms are persistent, octreotide or acarbose can help to control the symptoms. At least 1 year of medical treatment is recommended before surgery is considered. The best surgical therapy is to convert the previous procedure to a Roux en Y gastrojejunostomy, because this procedure decreases gastric emptying [54].

Postvagotomy Diarrhea

It is seen after vagotomy. The physiopathology is unclear, some theories that can explain this complication are denervation of the small intestine, gallbladder, and common bile duct; another theory is rapid gastric emptying associated with rapid intestinal transit that leads to malabsorption. The diagnosis should be suspected in every patient with the antecedent of gastrectomy and a negative workup that rules out other causes of diarrhea. The initial treatment is dietary modification (avoid lactose, decrease liquid ingestion before meals), use of anti-diarrheal agents (loperamide). For refractory untreatable diarrhea the anti-peristaltic interposition of a jejunal limb after 100 cm of the gastrojejunostomy is a possible treatment [55].

Gastroparesis or Delayed Gastric Emptying

Gastric surgery is responsible approximately of 10% of all gastroparesis cases [47]. This complication was described previously.

Afferent Loop Syndrome

It is the result of an obstructed afferent limb secondary to stomal edema, anastomosis, kinking, scarring, stricture, adhesions, internal hernias, or cancer. It can occur acutely 1 or 2 weeks after surgery or chronically. It occurs in 0.3% of the patients that had a Billroth II. The manifestations are abdominal pain most of the time in the right upper quadrant, nausea, nonbilious vomit; however, if the limb is partially obstructed the abdominal pain is relieved after vomit. In severe cases the chronic obstruction can result in jaundice or pancreatitis. The diagnosis is confirmed with an endoscopy that demonstrates the obstruction. The initial treatment can

be endoscopic using balloon dilation, but if it persists the gastrojejunostomy should be converted to a Roux en Y gastrojejunostomy. A second option is a Braun entero-enterostomy between the afferent and the efferent limb [56].

Efferent Syndrome

It results when the efferent limb of a gastrojejunostomy is obstructed. It can also be acute or chronic and it is manifested as abdominal pain, epigastric distention, and bilious vomit. The diagnosis can be done with an upper GI endoscopy or an upper GI transit study that show the obstruction. Possible etiologies are limb kinking, retroanastomotic herniation of the efferent limb or adhesions. The treatment is surgical, either converting a Billroth II procedure into a Roux en Y gastrojejunostomy or revising the initial anastomosis [55].

Duodenal Stump Leak

It presents in patients that have undergone an antrectomy. It is the dehiscence of the initial duodenal closure, and it is common when there is previous inflammation and scarring in this area but can also be a consequence of an incomplete duodenal mobilization or distal obstruction. It can be avoided with a Kocher maneuver to ensure that the closure is tension free; however, if the area has important fibrosis or acute inflammation, a lateral duodenostomy in the second portion of the duodenum help to create a controlled duodenal fistula.

Alkaline Gastritis

After a Billroth II, Billroth I, or pyloroplasty, 5–15% of the patients develop gastritis associated with bilious reflux. Patients complain of epigastric pain, nausea, and bilious vomit. The diagnosis is done with an endoscopy that shows gastric inflammation in the presence of bile. For patients with severe symptoms the previous anastomosis can be converted to a Roux en Y gastrojejunostomy.

Summary

- The major risks factors to develop PUD in elderly patients are *H. pylori* infection and NSAIDs ingestion.
- 50–60% of elderly patients will have an acute complication (bleeding or perforation) as the first clinical manifestation of PUD.

- *H. pylori* eradication decreases the risk of recurrence of PUD complications.
- The outcome associated with PUD complications in elderly patients is worse than young patients.
- Hyperplastic polyps are the most common type of polyps found in the stomach of elderly patients.
- Adenomatous gastric polyps have increased risk of malignancy.
- Diabetes is the most common etiology of gastroparesis in elderly patients.

References

1. Soybel DI (2005) Anatomy and physiology of the stomach. Surg Clin North Am 85:875–894
2. Russo MA, Redel CA (2006) Anatomy, histology, embryology, and developmental anomalies of the stomach and duodenum. In: Feldman M, Friedman LS, Brandt LJ (eds) Sleisenger & Fordtran's gastrointestinal and liver disease, 8th edn. Saunders Elsevier, Philadelphia, PA, pp 981–998
3. Mulholland MW (2006) Gastric anatomy and physiology. In: Mullholand MW, Lillemoe KD, Doherty GM, Maier RV, Upchurch JR (eds) Greenfield's surgery, 4th edn. Lippincott Williams & Wilkins, Philadelphia, pp 722–735
4. Wallace JL (2008) Prostaglandins, NSAIDs, and gastric mucosal protection: why doesn't the stomach digest itself? Physiol Rev 88:1547–1565
5. Eswaran S, Roy MA (2005) Medical management of acid-peptic disorders of the stomach. Surg Clin North Am 85:895–906
6. Kuo P, Rayner CK, Horowitz M (2007) Gastric emptying, diabetes, and aging. Clin Geriatr Med 23:785–808
7. Newton JL (2005) Effect of age-related changes in gastric physiology on tolerability of medications for older people. Drugs Aging 22:655–661
8. Morley JE (2007) The aging gut: physiology. Clin Geriatr Med 23:757–767
9. Newton JL (2004) Changes in upper gastrointestinal physiology with age. Mech Ageing Dev 125:867–870
10. Salles N (2007) Basic mechanisms of the aging gastrointestinal tract. Dig Dis 25:112–117
11. van Leerdam ME (2008) Epidemiology of acute upper gastrointestinal bleeding. Best Pract Res Clin Gastroenterol 22:209–224
12. Martinez JP, Mattu A (2006) Abdominal pain in the elderly. Emerg Med Clin North Am 24:371–388
13. Theocharis GJ, Arvaniti V, Assimakopoulos SF et al (2008) Acute upper gastrointestinal bleeding in octogenarians: clinical outcome and factors related to mortality. World J Gastroenterol 14:4047–4453
14. Gralnek IM, Barkun AN, Bardou M (2008) Management of acute bleeding from a peptic ulcer. N Engl J Med 359:928–937
15. Martin RF (2005) Surgical management of ulcer disease. Surg Clin North Am 85:907–929
16. Vilaichone RK, Mahachai V, Graham DY (2006) *Helicobacter pylori* diagnosis and management. Gastroenterol Clin North Am 35:229–247
17. Chey WD, Wong BC (2007) American College of Gastroenterology guideline on the management of *Helicobacter pylori* infection. Am J Gastroenterol 102:1808–1825
18. Lehours P, Yilmaz O (2007) Epidemiology of *Helicobacter pylori* infection. Helicobacter 12(Suppl 1):1–3
19. Behrman SW (2005) Management of complicated peptic ulcer disease. Arch Surg 140:201–208
20. Go MF (2006) Drug injury in the upper gastrointestinal tract: nonsteroidal anti-inflammatory drugs. Gastrointest Endosc Clin N Am 16:83–97
21. Huang JQ, Sridhar S, Hunt RH (2002) Role of *Helicobacter pylori* infection and non-steroidal anti-inflammatory drugs in peptic-ulcer disease: a meta-analysis. Lancet 359:14–22
22. Fendrich V, Langer P, Waldmann J et al (2007) Management of sporadic and multiple endocrine neoplasia type 1 gastrinomas. Br J Surg 94:1331–1341
23. Ellison EC (2008) Zollinger-Ellison syndrome: a personal perspective. Am Surg 74:563–571
24. Egan BJ, Katicic M, O'Connor HJ et al (2007) Treatment of *Helicobacter pylori*. Helicobacter 12(Suppl 1):31–37
25. Robson AJ, Richards JM, Ohly N et al (2008) The effect of surgical subspecialization on outcomes in peptic ulcer disease complicated by perforation and bleeding. World J Surg 32:1456–1461
26. Kocer B, Surmeli S, Solak C et al (2007) Factors affecting mortality and morbidity in patients with peptic ulcer perforation. J Gastroenterol Hepatol 22:565–570
27. Esrailian E, Gralnek IM (2005) Nonvariceal upper gastrointestinal bleeding: epidemiology and diagnosis. Gastroenterol Clin North Am 34:589–605
28. Ramakrishnan K, Salinas RC (2007) Peptic ulcer disease. Am Fam Physician 76:1005–1012
29. Yuan Y, Padol IT, Hunt RH (2006) Peptic ulcer disease today. Nat Clin Pract Gastroenterol Hepatol 3:80–89
30. Laine L, McQuaid KR (2009) Endoscopic therapy for bleeding ulcers: an evidence-based approach based on meta-analyses of randomized controlled trials. Clin Gastroenterol Hepatol 7:33–47
31. Boparai V, Rajagopalan J, Triadafilopoulos G (2008) Guide to the use of proton pump inhibitors in adult patients. Drugs 68:925–947
32. Jaspersen D, Koerner T, Schorr W et al (1995) *Helicobacter pylori* eradication reduces the rate of rebleeding in ulcer hemorrhage. Gastrointest Endosc 41:5–7
33. Rokkas T, Karameris A, Mavrogeorgis A et al (1995) Eradication of *Helicobacter pylori* reduces the possibility of rebleeding in peptic ulcer disease. Gastrointest Endosc 41:1–4
34. Brandimarte G, Tursi A, di Cesare L, Gasbarrini G (1999) Antimicrobial treatment for peptic stenosis: a prospective study. Eur J Gastroenterol Hepatol 11:731–734
35. Yusuf TE, Brugge WR (2006) Endoscopic therapy of benign pyloric stenosis and gastric outlet obstruction. Curr Opin Gastroenterol 22:570–573
36. Kozarek RA, Botoman VA, Patterson DJ (1990) Long-term follow-up in patients who have undergone balloon dilation for gastric outlet obstruction. Gastrointest Endosc 36:558–561
37. Solt J, Bajor J, Szabo M, Horvath OP (2003) Long-term results of balloon catheter dilation for benign gastric outlet stenosis. Endoscopy 35:490–495
38. McLoughlin MT, Byrne MF (2008) Endoscopic stenting: where are we now and where can we go? World J Gastroenterol 14:3798–3803
39. Borch K, Skarsgard J, Franzen L et al (2003) Benign gastric polyps: morphological and functional origin. Dig Dis Sci 48:1292–1297
40. Ljubicic N, Kujundzic M, Roic G et al (2002) Benign epithelial gastric polyps–frequency, location, and age and sex distribution. Coll Antropol 26:55–60
41. Morais DJ, Yamanaka A, Zeitune JM, Andreollo NA (2007) Gastric polyps: a retrospective analysis of 26,000 digestive endoscopies. Arq Gastroenterol 44:14–17
42. Park do Y, Lauwers GY (2008) Gastric polyps: classification and management. Arch Pathol Lab Med 132:633–640

43. Jain R, Chetty R (2009) Gastric hyperplastic polyps: a review. Dig Dis Sci 54(9):1839–1846
44. Linhares MM, Filho BH, Schraibman V et al (2006) Dieulafoy lesion: endoscopic and surgical management. Surg Laparosc Endosc Percutan Tech 16:1–3
45. Pathan NF, El-Fanek H (2006) A 70-year-old man with episodes of upper gastrointestinal bleeding. Dieulafoy lesion/malformation. Arch Pathol Lab Med 130:e27–e29
46. Sone Y, Kumada T, Toyoda H et al (2005) Endoscopic management and follow up of Dieulafoy lesion in the upper gastrointestinal tract. Endoscopy 37:449–453
47. Lacy BE, Weiser K (2005) Gastric motility, gastroparesis, and gastric stimulation. Surg Clin North Am 85:967–987
48. Hasler WL (2007) Gastroparesis: symptoms, evaluation, and treatment. Gastroenterol Clin North Am 36:619–647
49. Guo JP, Maurer AH, Fisher RS, Parkman HP (2001) Extending gastric emptying scintigraphy from two to four hours detects more patients with gastroparesis. Dig Dis Sci 46:24–29
50. Waseem S, Moshiree B, Draganov PV (2009) Gastroparesis: current diagnostic challenges and management considerations. World J Gastroenterol 15:25–37
51. Park MI, Camilleri M (2006) Gastroparesis: clinical update. Am J Gastroenterol 101:1129–1139
52. Mason RJ, Lipham J, Eckerling G et al (2005) Gastric electrical stimulation: an alternative surgical therapy for patients with gastroparesis. Arch Surg 140:841–846
53. Pedrazzani C, Marrelli D, Rampone B et al (2007) Postoperative complications and functional results after subtotal gastrectomy with Billroth II reconstruction for primary gastric cancer. Dig Dis Sci 52:1757–1763
54. Ukleja A (2005) Dumping syndrome: pathophysiology and treatment. Nutr Clin Pract 20:517–525
55. Eagon JC, Miedema BW, Kelly KA (1992) Postgastrectomy syndromes. Surg Clin North Am 72:445–465
56. Wise SW (2000) Case 24: afferent loop syndrome. Radiology 216:142–145

Chapter 62
Gastric Cancer in the Elderly

Daniel Albo, Daniel A. Anaya, and David H. Berger

In recent decades, improved socioeconomic conditions, medical progress, and preventive medicine have lengthened life expectancy in our society and consequently increased the elderly population. Despite an overall drop in the incidence of gastric cancer in the Western world, increased life expectancy has resulted in a growing proportion of elderly patients with gastric cancer. Today, more than 30% of patients with gastric cancer are older than 70 years. Although some characteristics of this disease are similar in younger and older patients, management of gastric cancer in the elderly exhibits some significant differences and presents unique challenges compared to management in younger patients. In this chapter, we will explore some of the unique epidemiological and pathological features of this disease in the elderly. Furthermore, we will try to elucidate the ideal surgical treatment strategies and the role of multimodality management in this challenging group of patients.

Gastric Cancer in the Elderly: Epidemiological and Pathological Considerations

Worldwide, gastric cancer is the second most common cause of cancer-related death with over 700,000 deaths annually. In the USA, over 21,500 new cases of gastric cancer were estimated to occur in 2008 [2]. Advancing age is a risk factor for the development of gastric cancer. The incidence of gastric cancer increases linearly with advancing age. In the USA the age-adjusted risk of developing gastric cancer for an individual between the ages of 40 and 49 is 3.6 per 100,000. The incidence increases to 20.9 per 100,000 for

people between the ages of 60 and 69 and to over 50 cases per 100,000 population above the age of 80 (Fig. 62.1). Similarly, the mortality rate for gastric cancer increases with age and is similar to the incidence rate (Fig. 62.2) [1]. This is likely due to the fact that most patients with gastric cancer in the USA present at an advanced stage. The majority of patients with gastric adenocarcinoma will present with either regional (30%) or distant (35%) disease [2].

The overall incidence of gastric cancer has been decreasing over the past 30 years. This decrease in the incident rate is age related. There has been a greater than 40% decline in the incidence of gastric cancer in Americans aged 65 and older compared to only a 7% decrease in the incidence of gastric cancer in patients younger than 65 (Fig. 62.3) [3]. The age-related decline in gastric cancer incidence may be due to an increase in the incidence of proximal gastric cancer compared to distal gastric cancer [4]. Proximal gastric cancer appears to occur more frequently in younger individuals. The mean age of patients diagnosed with proximal gastric cancer is 67.7 years compared to a mean age of 71.5 years for patients with distal gastric cancer. Additionally, more than 60% of patients with distal gastric cancer are aged 70 years or while only 49.5% of patients with proximal gastric cancer are in this age group [5].

The characteristic pathological features of gastric carcinoma in elderly people are somewhat different than in younger patients [6, 7]. Gastric cancer in the elderly tends to involve the lower third of the stomach and shows a higher incidence of histopathologically well-differentiated adenocarcinoma. Multiple and metastatic cancers are more common in aged people. In a comprehensive analysis of 994 surgical patients aged 65 years or older, Arai et al. studied the pathologic characteristics of gastric cancer in the elderly [8]. Pathological findings in the very old group (older than 85 years; $n = 126$) were compared with those in younger groups (65–74 years [young-old group]; $n = 356$) and (75–84 years [middle-old group]; $n = 512$). While the male-to-female ratio significantly decreased with advancing age, the relative odds of gastric cancer in men was higher than that in women across all age groups. In the very old

D. Albo (✉)
Department of Surgery, Baylor College of Medicine,
Michael E. DeBakey Veterans Affairs Medical Center,
OCL 112A, 2002 Holcombe Blvd, Houston, TX 77030, USA
e-mail: albo@bcm.tmc.edu

R.A. Rosenthal et al. (eds.), *Principles and Practice of Geriatric Surgery*,
DOI 10.1007/978-1-4419-6999-6_62, © Springer Science+Business Media, LLC 2011

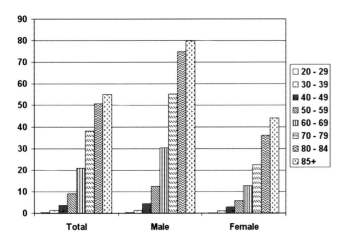

Figure 62.1 Age-adjusted incidence of stomach cancer per 100,000 population, United States Cancer Statistics 2001–2005 [1].

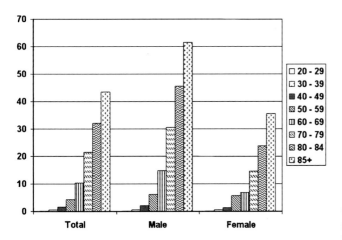

Figure 62.2 Age-adjusted mortality from stomach cancer per 100,000 population, United States Cancer Statistics 2001–2005 [1].

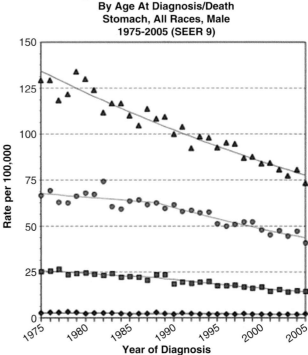

Cancer sites include invasive cases only unless otherwise noted.
Incidence source: SEER 9 areas (San Francisco, Connecticut, Detroit, Hawaii, Iowa, New Mexico, Seattle, Utah, and Atlanta).
Rates are per 100,000 and are age-adjusted to the 2000 US Std Population (19 age groups-Census P25-1130). Regression lines are calculated using the Joinpoint Regression Program Version 3.3, April 2008, National Cancer Institute.

Figure 62.3 Gastric cancer age-adjusted SEER incidence rates by age at diagnosis/death. Stomach, all races, male, 1975–2005 (SEER 9). Cancer sites include invasive causes only unless otherwise noted. Incidence source SEER 9 areas (San Francisco, Connecticut, Detroit, Hawaii, New Mexico, Seattle, Utah, and Atlanta). Rates are per 100,000 and age-adjusted to the 2000 US Std population (19 age groups – Census P25-1130). Regression lines are calculated using the Joinpoint Regression Line Program Version 3.3, April 2008, National cancer Institute.

group, cancer of the lower third of the stomach tended to increase with advancing age, and accounted for 43.7% of cases. In the overall population, differentiated-type adenocarcinoma accounted for 89.6% in the early cancers and 50.3% in the advanced cancers. The proportion of cases involving differentiated-type carcinoma significantly increased with advancing age in early cancer and female advanced cancer cases, whereas no significant change was found in male advanced-cancer patients. In the very old group, lymph node metastasis was found in 5.4% of early cancers and 72.7% in advanced cancers. The incidence of multiple cancers significantly increased with advancing age ($P<0.05$; 10.7% in the younger-old group, 12.7% in the middle-old group, and 19.0% in the very old group).

Chronic infection with *Helicobacter pylori* is a risk factor for distal but not proximal gastric cancer. Proximal gastric cancer has been associated with alcohol use, gastroesophageal reflux disease, and obesity [9]. Epidemiological

and clinical studies indicate that *H. pylori* infection is associated with a greater risk of distal gastric cancer. The International Agency for Research on Cancer and The World Health Organization have characterized *H. pylori* as a group I carcinogen. It has been postulated that *H. pylori* infection contributes to gastric cancer, through a sequence of events: infection → acute gastritis → chronic superficial gastritis → atrophic gastritis → atrophy → intestinal metaplasia → dysplasia → adenocarcinoma [10]. The seroprevalance of *H. pylori* increases with age. Whereas only 16.7% of individuals aged 20–29 have clinical evidence of *H. pylori* infection, greater than 56% of individuals above age 70 are infected. The association of *H. pylori* infection with age likely explains the increased incidence of distal gastric cancer seen in the elderly population. Furthermore, the declining incidence of gastric cancer in the elderly is likely a result of the declining prevalence of *H. pylori* infection in the USA.

Surgical Therapy for Gastric Cancer in the Elderly (Table 62.1)

Age Alone is not a Contraindication for Gastrectomy

A German study from Gretschel et al. investigated the value of individual risk-adapted therapy in geriatric patients [11]. They performed a consecutive analysis of 363 patients undergoing potentially curative surgery for gastric cancer. All patients underwent extensive preoperative workup to assess surgical risk. Comorbidities, tumor characteristics, type of resection, postoperative morbidity and mortality, recurrence rate, overall survival, and disease-free survival were evaluated in three age groups: <60 years, 60–75 years,

and >75 years. Not surprisingly, investigators found that there was an increased rate of comorbidities in the higher age groups (51% vs. 76% vs. 83%; $P<0.05$). Cardiovascular and pulmonary diseases were the most common comorbid conditions. With advancing age there was a decrease in the rate of both total gastrectomy (74, 54, 46%; $P<0.05$) and D2 lymphadenectomy (78, 53, 31%; $P<0.05$). The 30-day mortality in the three age groups was 0, 1, and 8%, respectively ($P<0.05$). There was only a slight difference in tumor recurrence rate (35, 37, and 27%; $P=0.437$), with no significant difference in 5-year cancer-related survival (61, 53, 61%; $P=0.199$). The authors concluded that patient selection and risk-adapted surgery in elderly patients results in acceptable therapeutic results comparable to younger patients. Additionally, these authors stated that limited surgery in elderly gastric cancer patients with high comorbidities does not necessarily compromise oncological outcome.

Looking to define the risk factors that predict 30-day morbidity and mortality after gastrectomy for cancer in Veterans Affairs (VA) Medical Centers, Grossman et al. reported data gathered prospectively by the VA National Surgical Quality Improvement Program on 708 patients

TABLE 62.1 Tailored surgical therapy for the elderly with gastric cancer

Study origin	N	Perioperative morbidity (elderly vs. young)	Perioperative mortality (elderly vs. young)	DFS (elderly vs. young)	OS (elderly vs. young)	Notes	References
Germany	363	Higher	Higher	Minimal decrease	Same	Limited surgery does not compromise oncological outcomes in the elderly with comorbidities	[10]
USA	708	Higher	Same	–	–	VA study evaluated risks factors for perioperative morbidity and mortality	[11]
China	2,613	–	–	Same	Higher	Limitations: age cutoff at 60; no analysis of comorbidities	[12]
Japan	289	Higher	Higher	–	Lower	Lower rate of curative surgery observed in the elderly	[13]
China	433	Higher	Higher	Same	Same	Limited resection recommended in the very old	[14]
Korea	719	Higher	Same				[15]
Japan	93	All patients >80 years old	–	D2 > D1	D2 > D1	D1 vs. D2 Resections compared. Recommended D2 in patients with good functional status	[16]
Italy	110	All patients >80 years old	–			Higher comorbidities resulted in higher mortality; radical resection recommended only for fit patients	[17]
United Kingdom	180	Higher	Same	–	–	By tailoring the extent of resection and balancing risk and radicality, gastric cancer surgery can be performed with low mortality in the elderly	[19]

VA veterans administration, *DFS* disease free survival, *OS* overall survival

undergoing gastrectomy for cancer in 123 participating VA medical centers from 1991 to 1998 [12]. Independent variables analyzed by the authors included 68 preoperative patient characteristics and 12 intraoperative variables; the dependent variables were 21 defined adverse outcomes and death. Predictive models for 30-day morbidity and mortality were constructed by using stepwise logistic regression analysis. Overall, the 30-day morbidity rate was 33.3% (236 of 708). The overall 30-day mortality rate was 7.6% (54 of 708). Significant positive predictors of morbidity (P<0.05) included current pneumonia, American Society of Anesthesiologists class IV (threat to life), partially dependent functional status, dyspnea on minimal exertion, preoperative transfusion, extended operative time, and increasing age. Significant positive predictors of mortality (P<0.05) included do not resuscitate status, prior stroke, intraoperative transfusion, preoperative weight loss, preoperative transfusion, and elevated preoperative alkaline phosphatase level. Although they found an increase in overall morbidity, age alone was not an independent risk factor for increased perioperative mortality after gastrectomy in elderly patients.

In one of the largest series published on outcomes after resection for gastric cancer, Chinese investigators analyzed the factors influencing the prognosis of patients with gastric cancer after surgical treatment [13]. In this retrospective study, 2,613 consecutive patients with gastric cancer were studied. Of these patients, 2,301 received operations, and of these, 1,975 underwent surgical resection of the tumors (891 received palliative resection and 1,084 received curative resection). Of the patients with surgical resection of the tumors, the overall 1-, 3-, and 5-year survival rates were 82.7, 46.3 and 31.1%, respectively, with the 5-year survival rate being 51.2% in patients with curative resection, and 7.8% for those with palliative resection. The 5-year survival rate was 32.5% for patients with total gastrectomy, and 28.3% for those with total gastrectomy plus resection of the adjacent organs. The factors that independently correlated with poor survival in this study included advanced stage, upper third location, palliative resection, poor differentiation, Bormann classification type IV, tumor metastasis (N3), tumor invasion into the serosa and/or contiguous structures, proximal subtotal gastrectomy for upper third carcinoma, and D1 lymphadenectomy after curative treatment. Age alone was not found to be an adverse independent prognostic factor of outcome. Moreover, 5-year survival was higher in patients over the age of 60 compared to younger patients (36.2% vs. 29.2%, respectively; P = 0.05). The limitations of this study include a relative young age of cutoff to define the elderly population (60 years and older), the lack of analysis on comorbidities in the different age groups, and the lack of information on tumor characteristics specific to the different age groups. Nonetheless, the authors concluded that primary gastric cancer should be resected with a radical operation as long as the local conditions permitted in order to prolong patient survival and improve their quality of life regardless of age at the time of presentation.

A study from Japan analyzed outcomes after gastrectomy for gastric cancer on 50 patients ≥80 years of age compared to 239 patients ≤60 years of age [14]. The incidence of advanced gastric cancer in the older vs. younger groups was 59.6% vs. 27.9%, respectively (P<0.01). The tumor size was significantly larger in the older group. The tumor location in the older group predominantly involved the upper third of the stomach, while in the younger group, the middle third of the stomach was primarily involved. Histologically, the incidence of differentiated tumor types was 65.1% vs. 50.5% (P<0.05), and undifferentiated types, 34.9% vs. 49.5% (P<0.05), in the older and younger groups, respectively. Retrospective comparisons conducted between the older and younger groups revealed the following curative resectability rates: 52.0% vs. 74.5% (P<0.01); hospital mortality rate: 2% vs. 0%; overall 5-year survival rate: 46.1% vs. 71.1% (P<0.01); and a 5-year survival rate in patients who underwent curative resection of 65.0% vs. 88.8% in the older vs. younger age groups, respectively. These results suggest that the survival of elderly patients with gastric cancer is worse than that of younger patients because of a lower curative resection rate of advanced cancers. However, the survival rate in elderly patients is similar to that in younger patients if a curative resection is performed.

The Case for Tailoring the Extent of Resection According to Patient Factors

Contrary to the above reports, a study from China found an increase in operative mortality after gastrectomy in the elderly [15]. In this study, 433 patients aged >65 years who underwent gastric resection for gastric adenocarcinoma were analyzed. Two groups were considered: patients aged 65–74 years and those >74 years. Most of the patients (78.1%) had advanced disease, and nearly half (41.3%) had associated chronic conditions. Resections with curative intention were performed in 83.6% of patients. The overall operative morbidity and mortality rates were 21.7 and 5.1%, respectively. Although operative procedures were similar in both groups, patients aged >74 years had a higher mortality rate than those aged 65–74 years (10.1% vs. 3.5%; P = 0.034). Age and extent of gastric resection were two independent factors negatively affecting mortality. The cumulative survival rates for patients who underwent curative resection were 86.2, 72.4, 67.2, 62.9, and 60.0% at 1, 2, 3, 4, and 5 years, respectively. Nearly all patients (96%) after surgery had normal work and daily activities. Some patients appeared to lack energy (16%) or experienced a period of anxiety or depression. There was no statistical difference in survival and quality of life assessed by the Spitzer index after curative resection between the two groups. The authors concluded that resection with curative intention can be performed for the elderly with acceptable morbidity and mortality rates, possible long-term survival, and good quality of life, but a limited operation should be considered in the very elderly patients.

Another study from Korea on 719 consecutive patients who underwent operations for gastric cancer also found an increased risk of perioperative morbidity, but no increase in mortality after surgical resection for gastric cancer in elderly patients [16]. Overall morbidity and mortality rates were 17.4 and 0.6%, respectively, and the rates of surgical and nonsurgical complications were 14.7 and 3.3%. Morbidity rates were higher in patients aged over 50 years (odds ratio 1.04, 95% confidence interval 1.02–1.06), when the gastric tumor was resected with another organ (36% for combined resection vs. 15.4% for gastrectomy only; odds ratio 3.25, 95% confidence interval 1.76–6.03) and when gastrojejunostomy was used for reconstruction after subtotal gastrectomy (17.0% for Billroth II vs. 9.5% for Billroth I; odds ratio 2.00 (95% confidence interval 1.05–3.79). The authors concluded that age, combined resection, and Billroth II reconstruction after radical subtotal gastrectomy were independently associated with the development of complications after gastric cancer surgery.

A study on 93 patients who underwent gastrectomy for gastric cancer evaluated the benefit of R2 vs. R1 gastrectomy for gastric cancer in Japanese patients over 80 years of age [17]. The clinical and pathological characteristics of the patients in the two groups were comparable at the time of surgery, except that the group who underwent R1 gastrectomy was older. R2 gastrectomy involved a significantly longer operation time ($P<0.01$) and greater intraoperative blood loss ($P<0.05$) when compared to R1 gastrectomy, but no patient undergoing this extensive surgery died. The difference in the morbidity rate between the two groups was not statistically significant. The 5-year survival rate was 55.8% in the R1 group and 65.4% in the R2 group. When gastric cancer invaded the serosa and/or secondary nodes, a substantial increase in survival time was gained with R2 gastrectomy when compared to an R1 operation. These findings suggested that an R2 gastrectomy is feasible, even for patients over 80 years, but seems to be indicated mainly when the carcinoma had invaded the serosa and/or secondary nodes and the patients are at good risk for major surgery.

A group of Italian surgeons recently reported on their 18-year experience with 110 patients aged 80 years and over affected with gastric cancer [18]. Postoperative morbidity and mortality rates and risk factors affecting their incidence were examined by univariate and multivariate analysis. Operability and resectability rates were 70.9 and 47.3%, respectively. Of the resective procedures, 78.8% were subtotal gastrectomies. In 9.6% of cases, combined resections

were performed. Twenty-five patients (32.1%) experienced postoperative complications; overall mortality rate was 12.8%. In resective procedures, morbidity and mortality were 26.9 and 3.8%, respectively. Statistical analysis identified the number of preexisting medical illnesses as an independent predictor of morbidity and mortality. The crude 5 year survival rate of curatively resected cases was 43%. Although multiple medical illnesses led to higher operative mortality, neither the presence of postoperative complications nor the number of preexisting medical illnesses significantly influenced the 5-year survival rate of curatively resected patients. The authors concluded that with careful patient selection, gastric surgery provides good immediate and long-term results even in very old patients. However, the authors also concluded that subtotal gastrectomy with limited lymphadenectomy should be the preferred procedure; total gastrectomy, combined resections and extended lymphadenectomy should be performed only when necessary, in patients with fewer than two illnesses. Surgery should be avoided in elderly patients with highly advanced disease, if multiple medical illnesses are present.

Another Japanese study evaluated the relationship between operative procedures for treatment of patients with gastric carcinoma and complications with special reference to the age of patients [19]. In this study, the patients were divided into four age groups: 50–59; 60–69; 70–79; and over 80 years. In elderly patients, proximal gastrectomies were not performed, resection of the neighboring organs was seldom performed and lymph node dissection was usually limited to the primary and secondary nodes. There was no significant difference in the rate of postoperative complications between groups. Although only limited surgery was performed for patients of 80 years and over, there was no significant difference in age-corrected cumulative survival rate between groups. This study concluded that limited resection may allow safe surgical treatment for patients of 80 years and over with gastric carcinoma, without a negative effect on prognosis.

In a study from the UK of 180 consecutive patients undergoing resection for gastric adenocarcinoma with curative intent the balance between risk and radicality of resection was evaluated [20]. The extent of lymphadenectomy was based upon preoperative and intraoperative staging and balanced against the patient's age and fitness. In this study, 83 patients underwent subtotal or distal partial gastrectomy and 97 patients underwent total or proximal partial gastrectomy. Operative procedures were as follows: D1 lymphadenectomy ($n=62$); modified (spleen and pancreas preserving) D2 lymphadenectomy ($n=73$); D2 lymphadenectomy ($n=42$); and extended resection ($n=3$). The TNM classification for these patients was: stage 1 ($n=45$); stage 2 ($n=37$); stage 3 ($n=61$); and stage 4 ($n=37$). Of the patients, 48 developed postoperative complications including 17 patients with a major surgical complication. The in-hospital mortality was

1.7%. Predicted mortality was 21.4 and 7.8%, respectively. Disease-specific 5-year survival according to stage was 85.4, 64.2, 33.3, and 6.9%. The authors concluded that by tailoring the extent of resection and balancing risk and radicality, gastric cancer surgery can be performed with low mortality in Western patients.

Adjuvant and Neoadjuvant Therapies in Gastric Cancer

Despite improvements in diagnosis and surgical management of patients with gastric cancer, cure rates are still extremely low and long-term survival has remained stagnant over the last few decades [21]. Studies using worldwide [22] and national US cancer registries [2] have revealed current 5-year overall survival (OS) rates of 20–24%, a modest increase as compared to 17% seen in the early 1970s [2]. Similarly, outside Asian countries, and with no formal standardized screening programs, most patients with gastric cancer are diagnosed with advanced stages with less than a quarter (24%) presenting with early gastric cancer at time of diagnosis [2]. Additionally, even in the setting of curative resection, at least 50% of patients develop early (within 2 years) recurrence, generally evenly distributed between distant and locoregional sites [23]. Considering these outcomes, it is not surprising that additional therapies have been and continue to be evaluated as a means to achieve better long-term outcomes. During the last decade two pivotal studies [24, 25] helped define a milestone in the approach to patients with gastric cancer and have contributed to shifting the standard of care from surgery alone to multimodality therapy.

History and Current Standards in the General Population

More than 30 randomized clinical trials have been performed evaluating the role of different chemotherapy agents in the adjuvant setting with inconclusive results regarding its benefit and impact on OS. Most are old studies evaluating outdated regimens including single or combination therapies of mytomicin C, cytarabine, methyl-lomustine, 5-fluorouracil, doxorubicin, and epirubicin among other agents. Although some of these trials were able to show improved OS, [26–29] others revealed contradictory results [30–32]. In an attempt to clarify this, multiple meta-analysis have been performed [33–36] and although most have shown a benefit of adjuvant chemotherapy, albeit small, the heterogeneity of the studies included in all, as well as the selective benefit

of chemotherapy in some (Asian patients only [36] and nodal-positive disease [34]) precluded any definitive recommendation for the standard use of chemotherapy.

Given the high rate of locoregional recurrence after curative resection, radiation therapy in different settings, has also been explored. A randomized trial by the British Stomach Cancer Group evaluated the role of external beam radiation therapy (EBRT) after resection in patients with stage II and III gastric cancer [37]. Five-year OS was lower for those in the radiation therapy arm as compared to patients having surgery alone or surgery followed by chemotherapy. The effect of intraoperative radiation therapy (IORT) in the treatment of gastric cancer has also been evaluated with studies revealing no effect on OS either [38]. Another strategy has been the use of chemotherapy with radiation therapy in the postoperative setting. A series of studies have been conducted in the past trying to address this strategy for gastric cancer [39–41]. Although two of these trials showed a difference in survival benefiting the treatment arm [40, 41], multiple methodological flaws limited the validity of their results. More recently, a well-designed randomized controlled trial, the Gastrointestinal Cancer Intergroup Trial (INT-0116) [24], assessed the role of postoperative chemoradiation (5-FU/leucovorin and 45Gy of EBRT) in 556 patients with stage IB-IVM0 gastric and gastroesophageal adenocarcinoma after complete (R0) resection. Although the study is criticized due to the high proportion of patients unable to tolerate treatment (~30%) as well as to issues regarding adequacy of radiation technique and surgical resection (>50% of patients had <D-1 lymphadenectomy), results were encouraging revealing a 9% absolute benefit in the 3-year OS of patients in the treatment group as compared to those having surgery alone (3-year OS 50% vs. 41%, respectively, $P = 0.005$). This study was the first one showing a clear benefit in OS for patients with gastric cancer and marked the transition from resection alone to multimodality therapy as the standard of care for the management of patients with gastric cancer.

Neoadjuvant approaches have also been evaluated in an attempt to improve survival in patients with resectable gastric cancer as well as an alternative approach for patients presenting with initially unresectable tumors. Proponents of this approach argue that with neoadjuvant therapy, foci of micrometastatic disease can be targeted earlier, tumor response can be assessed, down-sizing can be achieved possibly leading to higher rates of resectability as well as to higher R0 resections and that it allows to select out the patients who will progress while on therapy due to the aggressive behavior of their tumors. An additional benefit is that neoadjuvant therapy tends to be better tolerated, a potentially relevant feature when considering multimodality therapy in elderly or debilitated patients. More recently, investigators from MD Anderson Cancer Center have shown the prognostic value of response to preoperative chemotherapy as well [43]. The use of preoperative chemotherapy has been well studied in multiple phase I and phase II trials and its feasibility and safety have been well delineated [43–47]. Although a recent phase III study led by the Dutch Gastric Cancer Group evaluating the effect of preoperative chemotherapy in resectable gastric cancer failed to demonstrate any long-term benefit in survival with this strategy [48], a more recent and well-designed study utilizing perioperative chemotherapy has become the gold standard in managing gastric cancer in many places worldwide [26]. The MAGIC trial (Medical Research Council Gastric Infusional Chemotherapy Trial) randomized 503 patients with ≥stage II nonmetastatic gastric and gastroesophageal cancer to surgery alone vs. perioperative chemotherapy [epirubicin/cisplatin/5-FU (ECF) pre- and postoperatively] and surgery. Despite only 42% of patients in the treatment arm completing both pre- and postoperative therapy, intention-to-treat analysis revealed a significant benefit in 5-year OS (36% vs. 23% for the surgery alone group, $P=0.009$). Similarly, patients in the perioperative chemotherapy group were found to have smaller size tumors, more early stage tumors, and had a higher rate of curative resection, arguing in favor of some of the added benefits of response to preoperative chemotherapy. Postoperative complications were similar for both groups. Although this regimen was not tolerated by all patients and only 42% completed therapy, it is hard to argue against the benefit of this strategy and this should currently be considered the standard of care in eligible patients.

More recently, a randomized controlled trial from Japan evaluated the role of adjuvant chemotherapy for 1 year with the oral fluoropyrimidine S-1 as compared to surgery alone in patients with stages II (excluding T1 tumors), IIIA and IIIB gastric cancer undergoing D-2 resections [49]. They randomized a total of 529 patients and found a survival benefit in the treatment arm with 3-year OS of 80.1% vs. 70.1% in the surgery alone group ($P=0.003$) and a relatively low incidence of major toxicities. Although this trial confirms the benefit of multimodality therapy for gastric cancer it is limited by the extent of the operation (100% of patients had D-2 resections), since this type of operation is the exception rather than the rule in western countries, as evidenced by the findings from the INT-0116 trial [25].

Current studies are focusing on the role of preoperative chemoradiation [50, 51], combinations of the MAGIC and INT-0116 trials regimens (CALBG 80101 trial) evaluated in the postoperative setting, and addition of targeted therapies (bevacizumab) to MAGIC-type chemotherapy (MAGIC-B trial) [52]. Additionally, current effective regimens (i.e., ECF) are being evaluated with newer agents such as capecitabine and oxaliplatin, which have shown similar or better response rates with the added benefit of more favorable toxicity profiles [53]. Future strategies will very likely be characterized by the use of multimodality therapy both in the preoperative and postoperative settings with the emergence of biologic agents as a promising addition to these recent positive findings.

Data on Adjuvant and Neoadjuvant Therapies in the Elderly

When approaching elderly patients with the diagnosis of gastric adenocarcinoma, specific considerations must be included in the decision-making strategy for both the surgical approach and the use of adjuvant/neoadjuvant therapies. At least 60% of patients diagnosed with gastric adenocarcinoma are over the age of 65 and multiple studies have confirmed increasing age as an important predictor of worse long-term outcomes (Fig. 62.2). The specific reason driving this prognostic difference is not clear; however, a series of studies have shown that in the elderly, substandard surgical and systemic therapy is often the rule in patients with colorectal carcinoma [54] as well as in those diagnosed with other gastrointestinal malignancies, including gastric cancer [55, 56]. Specifically, a population level study originated from the analysis of two large cancer registries in France revealed that in patients over the age of 80 years, regardless of the specific gastrointestinal cancer site, chemotherapy was administered in an extremely low number of patients (1.6–5.1%) [55]. These findings have also been confirmed in other larger US registry studies evaluating the use of adjuvant chemotherapy for stage III colorectal cancer, in which increasing age has been identified as independently associated with lower use of this proven effective strategy [57].

In parallel to patient selection in randomized trials from other sites [58], elderly patients are underrepresented in adjuvant and neoadjuvant trials for the management of gastric cancer, complicating the strength of potential inferences made regarding the benefit and/or toxicity of these regimens in this subset of patients. For example, in the INT-0116 trial the median age of patients was 60 and 59 years in the treatment and control arms, respectively, and no additional analysis regarding effectiveness or toxicities was done based on age [25]. The MAGIC trial [26] and the Japanese trial evaluating the role of S-1 [49] had a median age of 62 and 63 years, respectively, and although in the latter there was a set limit of age over 80 for eligibility and in both, patients were well selected to minimize the number of comorbidities (a rare situation in the elderly), both of these trials did have at least 20% of their population over the age of 70 years. Although this proportion does not reflect the typical age distribution of this disease and despite no specific subset analysis being done to evaluate age as a predictor of response or toxicity, the inclusion of such proportion of elderly patients, albeit small, allows to consider that regimens may be tolerated as well and that their clinical effect on survival may in fact be applicable to older patients too.

To better establish this observation, at least five recent phase II trials have been performed evaluating the tolerability of different regimens for advanced gastric cancer (locally advanced and metastatic) in the elderly and to define the response rates in these patients [58–63]. In 2003, Graziano et al. reported adequate safety with the use of cisplatin/leucovorin/fluorouracil in the elderly population.

More recently [58], with the emergence of the newer platinum class agent oxaliplatin, investigators have evaluated different oxaliplatin-based regimens in the elderly population. The advantage of this newer agent includes better response rates as well as a more favorable toxicity profile with dose-limiting toxicity due to peripheral neuropathy rather than other more complicated and potentially lethal toxicities (i.e., hematologic). These reports have recently shown an overall tumor control rate of approximately 70–80% with overall responses of 32–45%, complete response rates in the range of 2–8%, and grade III toxicities of 7–15% with no reported chemotherapy-induced deaths [59, 61]. The effectiveness of these regimens compares well to those used in the general population and based on these preliminary studies, they appear safe when used for managing elderly patients. The caveats to some of these reports includes the strict selection criteria of patients characterized by good performance status (ECOG 0-1) and the low number of comorbidities, a feature often unrealistic when managing older populations. Additionally, the clinical effectiveness (i.e., impact on survival) of these regimens still needs to be tested specifically for resectable nonmetastatic disease, ideally in the setting of multi-institutional randomized controlled trials with a higher proportion of patients over the age of 65 years.

In summary, multimodality therapy for the management of nonmetastatic gastric cancer has become the standard of care with postoperative chemoradiation and perioperative chemotherapy being the most commonly used approaches. Adjuvant chemotherapy with S-1 for a more prolonged period of time in patients having had a D-2 curative resection is also a proven effective strategy. None of these studies have addressed the effectiveness and/or toxicity profiles of these regimens in the elderly specifically; however, a reasonable proportion of older patients were included and appeared to benefit similarly to younger patients from the two multimodality approaches. Further, perioperative chemotherapy (MAGIC-type regimen), although not tolerated

well by all patients, has the advantage of being started prior to surgery, which can theoretically be better tolerated than after a large operation with all the potential side effects that this could have on older patients as described earlier. Newer regimens with more effective agents and better toxicity profiles have proven to be a safe approach in the elderly specifically. As additional phase III trials evaluating these newer regimens are completed with consistent information regarding their benefit on survival, more solid data will become available to shift the management of older patients from current regimens to those newly tested. Finally, with the improvements in diagnosis, staging, and perioperative care as well as with the worldwide effects of the demographic transition and the so-called increase in the "graying" population, future trials evaluating multimodality approaches in combination with biologic agents need to include a higher proportion of elderly patients that more realistically represent the demographic characteristics of patients with gastric cancer.

Practical Application

Based on these data, we have developed a selective approach to the surgical management of gastric cancer in the elderly. In order to decide the extent of surgical resection (total vs. subtotal gastrectomy) and the extent of lymphadenectomy (D1 vs. D2 lymphadenectomy; Table 62.2 compares the extent of lymphadenectomy in these two techniques) we do not necessarily consider the patient's chronological age, but his/her biological age. Factors considered in this decision making process include the number and type of comorbidities, functional status, and nutritional status. For the latter, we consider the extent of weight loss and the patient's albumin level. The following two cases illustrate this selective approach to the surgical management of gastric cancer in the elderly in our practice (Table 62.3).

TABLE 62.2 "D" nomenclature: extent of lymphadenectomy during gastrectomy for gastric cancer

Description	Regions included in resection
D1	Removal of all nodal tissue within 3 cm of the primary tumor
D2	D1 plus clearance of hepatic, splenic, and left gastric lymph nodes
D3[a]	D2 plus omentectomy, splenectomy, distal pancreatectomy, and clearance of celiac and porta hepatis lymph nodes

[a] D3 resections are not currently recommended

CASE STUDY 1

The patient is an 80-year-old male who was status post-antrectomy and truncal vagotomy with a Billroth II reconstruction for peptic ulcer disease over 20 years ago. Over the last 3 months, he developed progressive dysphagia, lost approximately 10 pounds, and reported vague epigastric discomfort. His past medical history included hypertension (well controlled) and gastro esophageal reflux disease. He did not smoke or drink alcohol. He lived independently and was very active. He underwent an esophagogastroduodenoscopy, which revealed a mass in the gastric remnant involving the body and fundus of the stomach. A biopsy of this mass revealed a well-differentiated adenocarcinoma. His serum albumin level was 3.6 mg/dl. A CT scan of the chest, abdomen, and pelvis revealed a thickening of the stomach remnant with no evidence of regional adenopathy, visceral metastases or carcinomatosis (Fig. 62.4). An endoscopic ultrasound revealed this mass was a eusT3, N0, M0.

Although this patient's chronological age was advanced, he was in excellent functional state, had no severe comorbidities and a good nutritional status. His gastric cancer was potentially curable with multimodality therapy. Therefore, we took an aggressive approach with him, with modern perioperative chemotherapy and radical surgery. He underwent Magic-type perioperative chemotherapy and had a completion gastrectomy with a D2 lymphadenectomy and a Roux-en-Y esophagojejunostomy reconstruction. His final pathology report showed a well-differentiated adenocarcinoma with negative margins and 0/24 lymph nodes positive. The final pathological staging was a T3N0M0. Twenty-six months later he is alive and disease-free and in good functional state.

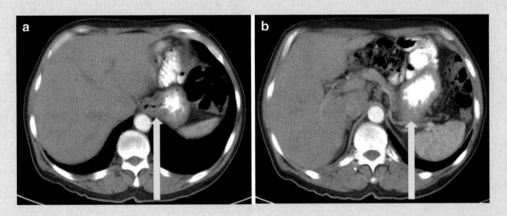

FIGURE 62.4 CT of the abdomen of an 80-year-old patient with gastric adenocarcinoma. The *arrows* show thickening of the stomach at the level of the fundus and gastro esophageal junction (**a**) and the body of the stomach (**b**).

TABLE 62.3 Case presentations: tailoring the radicality of surgery and adjuvant therapy to the patient's functional state

	Case 1	Case 2
Age	80	82
Symptoms	Dysphagia; mild weight loss	Bleeding requiring multiple transfusions; significant weight loss
Comorbidities	HTN, GERD	HTN, COPD, CAD, DM, AAA
	No smoking or alcohol intake	Significant smoking and alcohol consumption
Functional state	Excellent	Poor
Nutritional state	Excellent	Poor
Albumin level	3.6 mg/dl	2.3 mg/dl
Type of gastrectomy	Total gastrectomy	Distal gastrectomy
Extent of lymphadenectomy	D2	D1
Adjuvant therapy	Magic-type, perioperative	Postoperative therapy not tolerated
Surgical pathology report	T3N0M0; 0/24 lymph nodes	T3N1M0; 1/10 lymph nodes
Current status	Disease-free 26 months after surgery; excellent functional state	Disease-free 14 months after surgery; baseline fair functional state

HTN hypertension, *GERD* gastro esophageal reflux diseased, *COPD* chronic obstructive pulmonary disease, *CAD* coronary artery disease, *DM* diabetes mellitus, *AAA* abdominal aortic aneurysm

CASE STUDY 2

The patient is an 82-year-old male with repeated episodes of upper gastrointestinal bleed requiring several hospitalizations and multiple blood transfusions. He had extensive comorbidities, including severe chronic obstructive pulmonary disease, coronary artery disease, diabetes, hypertension, and an abdominal aortic aneurysm (4.5 cm, stable, nonsymptomatic). He was an active heavy smoker with a history of significant alcohol consumption (quit 5 years prior). He reported a recent weight loss of 15 pounds. He lived in an assisted-living home and his functional state was only fair. His most recent hemoglobin was 8.2 mg/dl after transfusion of two units of blood. His albumin level was 2.3 mg/dl. An esophago-gastroduodenoscopy reveled an ulcer in the antrum of the stomach with raised borders and stigmata of a recent bleed. Biopsies revealed a moderately differentiated adenocarcinoma. A CT scan showed thickening of the antrum and no evidence of visceral metastases or carcinomatosis (Fig. 62.5).

This patient had multiple, severe comorbidities, and a poor functional and nutritional status. The ongoing bleeding was of concern, though, and we decided on a less radical approach with him. We did not consider him a candidate for neoadjuvant therapy. We performed a distal gastrectomy with a limited D1 lymphadenectomy and a Billroth II gastrojejunostomy anastomosis. His final pathology report showed a moderately differentiated gastric adenocarcinoma with negative margins of resection and 1/10 lymph nodes positive for metastatic disease. The final pathological staging was T3N1M0. Although an attempt to administer postoperative chemoradiation was made by our hematology/oncology colleagues, the patient did not tolerate it well and it had to be stopped. Fourteen months after surgery he has not had any more episodes of gastrointestinal bleed and is back to his baseline functional state. He remains cancer-free.

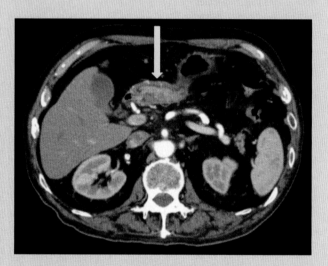

Figure 62.5 CT of the abdomen of an 82-year-old patient with gastric adenocarcinoma. The *arrow* shows thickening of the stomach at the level of the antrum.

Conclusion

Gastric cancer remains one of the most common and aggressive malignancies worldwide. Since the incidence of gastric cancer increases linearly with age, and since the average lifespan of the population is increasing steadily, gastric cancer is a significant problem in the elderly. Gastric cancer presents unique challenges in this age group: a distinctive pathological profile, higher incidence of advanced disease, and higher incidence of significant comorbidities that make radical surgical options riskier. Although age alone is not a contraindication for aggressive surgical and adjuvant therapy, the preponderance of the evidence suggests a tailored approach to this disease in the elderly, with radical surgery and aggressive adjuvant and/or neoadjuvant therapy reserved for patients with good performance status, and less radical surgery and adjuvant therapy for debilitated patients with multiple concomitant comorbidities.

References

1. US Cancer Statistics Working Group (2009) United States Cancer Statistics: 1999–2005 Incidence and Mortality Web-based Report. US Department of Health and Human Services, Centers for Disease Control and Prevention and National Cancer Institute, Atlanta. Available at: http://www.cdc.gov/uscs
2. Jemal A, Siegel R, Ward E et al (2008) Cancer statistics, 2008. CA Cancer J Clin 58(2):71–96
3. Ries LAG, Melbert D, Krapcho M, Stinchcomb DG, Howlader N, Horner MJ, Mariotto A, Miller BA, Feuer EJ, Altekruse SF, Lewis DR, Clegg L, Eisner MP, Reichman M, Edwards BK (2007) SEER Cancer Statistics Review, 1975–2005. National Cancer Institute, Bethesda, MD
4. Brown LM, Devesa SS (2002) Epidemiologic trends in esophageal and gastric cancer in the United States. Surg Oncol Clin N Am 11(2):235–256
5. Wilkinson NW, Howe J, Gay G, Patel-Parekh L, Scott-Conner C, Donohue J (2008) Differences in the pattern of presentation and treatment of proximal and distal gastric cancer: results of the 2001 gastric patient care evaluation. Ann Surg Oncol 15(6):1644–1650

6. Inoshita N, Yanagisawa A, Arai T, Kitagawa T, Hirokawa K, Kato Y (1998) Pathological characteristics of gastric carcinomas in the very old. Jpn J Cancer Res 89(10):1087–1092

7. Kitamura K, Yamaguchi T, Taniguchi H et al (1996) Clinico-pathological characteristics of gastric cancer in the elderly. Br J Cancer 73(6):798–802

8. Arai T, Esaki Y, Inoshita N et al (2004) Pathologic characteristics of gastric cancer in the elderly: a retrospective study of 994 surgical patients. Gastric Cancer 7(3):154–159

9. Lambert R, Hainaut P (2007) The multidisciplinary management of gastrointestinal cancer. Epidemiology of oesophagogastric cancer. Best Pract Res Clin Gastroenterol 21(6):921–945

10. Wang C, Yuan Y, Hunt RH (2007) The association between *Helicobacter pylori* infection and early gastric cancer: a meta-analysis. Am J Gastroenterol 102(8):1789–1798

11. Gretschel S, Estevez-Schwarz L, Hunerbein M, Schneider U, Schlag PM (2006) Gastric cancer surgery in elderly patients. World J Surg 30(8):1468–1474

12. Grossmann EM, Longo WE, Virgo KS et al (2002) Morbidity and mortality of gastrectomy for cancer in Department of Veterans Affairs Medical Centers. Surgery 131(5):484–490

13. Zhang XF, Huang CM, Lu HS et al (2004) Surgical treatment and prognosis of gastric cancer in 2,613 patients. World J Gastroenterol 10(23):3405–3408

14. Hanazaki K, Wakabayashi M, Sodeyama H et al (1998) Surgery for gastric cancer in patients older than 80 years of age. Hepatogastroenterology 45(19):268–275

15. Wu CW, Lo SS, Shen KH, Hsieh MC, Lui WY, P'Eng FK (2000) Surgical mortality, survival, and quality of life after resection for gastric cancer in the elderly. World J Surg 24(4):465–472

16. Park DJ, Lee HJ, Kim HH, Yang HK, Lee KU, Choe KJ (2005) Predictors of operative morbidity and mortality in gastric cancer surgery. Br J Surg 92(9):1099–1102

17. Korenaga D, Baba H, Kakeji Y et al (1991) Comparison of R1 and R2 gastrectomy for gastric cancer in patients over 80 years of age. J Surg Oncol 48(2):136–141

18. Roviello F, Marrelli D, De Stefano A, Messano A, Pinto E, Carli A (1998) Complications after surgery for gastric cancer in patients aged 80 years and over. Jpn J Clin Oncol 28(2):116–122

19. Tsujitani S, Katano K, Oka A, Ikeguchi M, Maeta M, Kaibara N (1996) Limited operation for gastric cancer in the elderly. Br J Surg 83(6):836–839

20. Lamb P, Sivashanmugam T, White M, Irving M, Wayman J, Raimes S (2008) Gastric cancer surgery – a balance of risk and radicality. Ann R Coll Surg Engl 90(3):235–242

21. Crane SJ, Locke GR III, Harmsen WS, Zinsmeister AR, Romero Y, Talley NJ (2008) Survival trends in patients with gastric and esophageal adenocarcinomas: a population-based study. Mayo Clin Proc 83(10):1087–1094

22. Kamangar F, Dores GM, Anderson WF (2006) Patterns of cancer incidence, mortality, and prevalence across five continents: defining priorities to reduce cancer disparities in different geographic regions of the world. J Clin Oncol 24(14):2137–2150

23. D'Angelica M, Gonen M, Brennan MF, Turnbull AD, Bains M, Karpeh MS (2004) Patterns of initial recurrence in completely resected gastric adenocarcinoma. Ann Surg 240(5):808–816

24. Macdonald JS, Smalley SR, Benedetti J et al (2001) Chemoradiotherapy after surgery compared with surgery alone for adenocarcinoma of the stomach or gastroesophageal junction. N Engl J Med 345(10):725–730

25. Cunningham D, Allum WH, Stenning SP et al (2006) Perioperative chemotherapy versus surgery alone for resectable gastroesophageal cancer. N Engl J Med 355(1):11–20

26. Imanaga H, Nakazato H (1977) Results of surgery for gastric cancer and effect of adjuvant mitomycin C on cancer recurrence. World J Surg 2(1):213–221

27. Grau JJ, Estape J, Alcobendas F, Pera C, Daniels M, Teres J (1993) Positive results of adjuvant mitomycin-C in resected gastric cancer: a randomised trial on 134 patients. Eur J Cancer 29A(3):340–342

28. The Gastrointestinal Tumor Study Group (1982) Controlled trial of adjuvant chemotherapy following curative resection for gastric cancer. The Gastrointestinal Tumor Study Group. Cancer 49(6):1116–1122

29. Neri B, de Leonardis V, Romano S et al (1996) Adjuvant chemotherapy after gastric resection in node-positive cancer patients: a multicentre randomised study. Br J Cancer 73(4):549–552

30. Macdonald JS, Fleming TR, Peterson RF et al (1995) Adjuvant chemotherapy with 5-FU, adriamycin, and mitomycin-C (FAM) versus surgery alone for patients with locally advanced gastric adenocarcinoma: a Southwest Oncology Group study. Ann Surg Oncol 2(6):488–494

31. Engstrom PF, Lavin PT, Douglass HO Jr, Brunner KW (1985) Postoperative adjuvant 5-fluorouracil plus methyl-CCNU therapy for gastric cancer patients. Eastern Cooperative Oncology Group study (EST 3275). Cancer 55(9):1868–1873

32. Higgins GA Jr, Amadeo JH, McElhinney J, McCaughan JJ, Keehn RJ (1984) Efficacy of prolonged intermittent therapy with combined 5-fluorouracil and methyl-CCNU following resection for carcinoma of the large bowel. A Veterans Administration Surgical Oncology Group report. Cancer 53(1):1–8

33. Hermans J, Bonenkamp JJ, Boon MC et al (1993) Adjuvant therapy after curative resection for gastric cancer: meta-analysis of randomized trials. J Clin Oncol 11(8):1441–1447

34. Earle CC, Maroun JA (1999) Adjuvant chemotherapy after curative resection for gastric cancer in non-Asian patients: revisiting a meta-analysis of randomised trials. Eur J Cancer 35(7):1059–1064

35. Mari E, Floriani I, Tinazzi A et al (2000) Efficacy of adjuvant chemotherapy after curative resection for gastric cancer: a meta-analysis of published randomised trials. A study of the GISCAD (Gruppo Italiano per lo Studio dei Carcinomi dell'Apparato Digerente). Ann Oncol 11(7):837–843

36. Janunger KG, Hafstrom L, Nygren P, Glimelius B (2001) A systematic overview of chemotherapy effects in gastric cancer. Acta Oncol 40(2–3):309–326

37. Hallissey MT, Dunn JA, Ward LC, Allum WH (1994) The second British Stomach Cancer Group trial of adjuvant radiotherapy or chemotherapy in resectable gastric cancer: five-year follow-up. Lancet 343(8909):1309–1312

38. Martinez-Monge R, Calvo FA, Azinovic I et al (1997) Patterns of failure and long-term results in high-risk resected gastric cancer treated with postoperative radiotherapy with or without intraoperative electron boost. J Surg Oncol 66(1):24–29

39. Dent DM, Werner ID, Novis B, Cheverton P, Brice P (1979) Prospective randomized trial of combined oncological therapy for gastric carcinoma. Cancer 44(2):385–391

40. Moertel CG, Childs DS, O'Fallon JR, Holbrook MA, Schutt AJ, Reitemeier RJ (1984) Combined 5-fluorouracil and radiation therapy as a surgical adjuvant for poor prognosis gastric carcinoma. J Clin Oncol 2(11):1249–1254

41. Bleiberg H, Goffin JC, Dalesio O et al (1989) Adjuvant radiotherapy and chemotherapy in resectable gastric cancer. A randomized trial of the gastro-intestinal tract cancer cooperative group of the EORTC. Eur J Surg Oncol 15(6):535–543

42. Lowy AM, Mansfield PF, Leach SD, Pazdur R, Dumas P, Ajani JA (1999) Response to neoadjuvant chemotherapy best predicts survival after curative resection of gastric cancer. Ann Surg 229(3):303–308

43. Ajani JA, Mansfield PF, Lynch PM et al (1999) Enhanced staging and all chemotherapy preoperatively in patients with potentially resectable gastric carcinoma. J Clin Oncol 17(8):2403–2411

44. Melcher AA, Mort D, Maughan TS (1996) Epirubicin, cisplatin and continuous infusion 5-fluorouracil (ECF) as neoadjuvant chemotherapy in gastro-oesophageal cancer. Br J Cancer 74(10): 1651–1654

45. Fink U, Schuhmacher C, Stein HJ et al (1995) Preoperative chemotherapy for stage III-IV gastric carcinoma: feasibility, response and outcome after complete resection. Br J Surg 82(9):1248–1252

46. Barone C, Cassano A, Pozzo C et al (2004) Long-term follow-up of a pilot phase II study with neoadjuvant epidoxorubicin, etoposide and cisplatin in gastric cancer. Oncology 67(1):48–53

47. Hartgrink HH, van de Velde CJ, Putter H et al (2004) Neo-adjuvant chemotherapy for operable gastric cancer: long term results of the Dutch randomised FAMTX trial. Eur J Surg Oncol 30(6):643–649

48. Sakuramoto S, Sasako M, Yamaguchi T et al (2007) Adjuvant chemotherapy for gastric cancer with S-1, an oral fluoropyrimidine. N Engl J Med 357(18):1810–1820

49. Lowy AM, Feig BW, Janjan N et al (2001) A pilot study of preoperative chemoradiotherapy for resectable gastric cancer. Ann Surg Oncol 8(6):519–524

50. Ajani JA, Mansfield PF, Janjan N et al (2004) Multi-institutional trial of preoperative chemoradiotherapy in patients with potentially resectable gastric carcinoma. J Clin Oncol 22(14):2774–2780

51. Lim L, Michael M, Mann GB, Leong T (2005) Adjuvant therapy in gastric cancer. J Clin Oncol 23(25):6220–6232

52. Sumpter K, Harper-Wynne C, Cunningham D et al (2005) Report of two protocol planned interim analyses in a randomised multicentre phase III study comparing capecitabine with fluorouracil and oxaliplatin with cisplatin in patients with advanced oesophagogastric cancer receiving ECF. Br J Cancer 92(11):1976–1983

53. Chang GJ, Skibber JM, Feig BW, Rodriguez-Bigas M (2007) Are we undertreating rectal cancer in the elderly? An epidemiologic study. Ann Surg 246(2):215–221

54. Bouvier AM, Launoy G, Lepage C, Faivre J (2005) Trends in the management and survival of digestive tract cancers among patients aged over 80 years. Aliment Pharmacol Ther 22(3):233–241

55. Msika S, Tazi MA, Benhamiche AM, Couillault C, Harb M, Faivre J (1997) Population-based study of diagnosis, treatment and prognosis of gastric cancer. Br J Surg 84(10):1474–1478

56. Jessup JM, Stewart A, Greene FL, Minsky BD (2005) Adjuvant chemotherapy for stage III colon cancer: implications of race/ethnicity, age, and differentiation. JAMA 294(21): 2703–2711

57. Hutchins LF, Unger JM, Crowley JJ, Coltman CA Jr, Albain KS (1999) Underrepresentation of patients 65 years of age or older in cancer-treatment trials. N Engl J Med 341(27):2061–2067

58. Graziano F, Santini D, Testa E et al (2003) A phase II study of weekly cisplatin, 6S-stereoisomer leucovorin and fluorouracil as first-line chemotherapy for elderly patients with advanced gastric cancer. Br J Cancer 89(8):1428–1432

59. Santini D, Graziano F, Catalano V et al (2006) Weekly oxaliplatin, 5-fluorouracil and folinic acid (OXALF) as first-line chemotherapy for elderly patients with advanced gastric cancer: results of a phase II trial. BMC Cancer 6:125

60. Nardi M, Azzarello D, Maisano R et al (2007) FOLFOX-4 regimen as fist-line chemotherapy in elderly patients with advanced gastric cancer: a safety study. J Chemother 19(1):85–89

61. Liu ZF, Guo QS, Zhang XQ et al (2008) Biweekly oxaliplatin in combination with continuous infusional 5-fluorouracil and leucovorin (modified FOLFOX-4 regimen) as first-line chemotherapy for elderly patients with advanced gastric cancer. Am J Clin Oncol 31(3):259–263

62. Zhao JG, Qiu F, Xiong JP et al (2009) A phase II study of modified FOLFOX as first-line chemotherapy in elderly patients with advanced gastric cancer. Anticancer Drugs 20(4):281–286

Chapter 63
Small Bowel Obstruction in the Elderly

Kelley A. Sookraj and Wilbur B. Bowne

Introduction

Small bowel obstruction (SBO) is a common surgical entity that can occur at any patient age. Although the general principles of diagnosis and treatment of SBO has remained consistent across all age groups, recent shifts in both incidence and etiology among patients of more advanced years now requires focused treatment considerations [1]. Historically, the classical dilemmas associated with management of SBO has remained steadfast for the elderly and include (1) differentiating strangulated from nonstrangulated SBO; (2) delineating ileus from SBO; and (3) determining optimal duration of nonoperative management for partial SBO. Indeed, a better understanding and approach to these clinical scenarios is especially pertinent for the elderly due to their increased risk for perioperative morbidity and mortality [2].

To date, no current data suggest much change in the primary etiologic causes of SBO which remains adhesions, neoplasms, and hernias [2, 3]. Likewise, standard operative management still includes an "open" exploratory approach along with adhesiolysis, herniorraphy, enteric by-pass, and/or bowel resection. Similarly, laparoscopic surgery, yet still a promising alternative, remains controversial. Importantly, advances in clinical imaging (e.g., multidetector computed tomography or MDCT) and biotechnology now provide more effective modalities for accurate detection along with preventative measures for reducing recurrence of SBO following major abdominal surgery; ultimately leading to better patient management and outcome.

This chapter will focus on fundamentals for approaching the assessment and timely management of SBO in the geriatric population. Operative vs. nonoperative management in the elderly will be addressed. This review will also highlight the important pathophysiology of adhesion formation and resultant SBO as well as current data supporting selected minimally invasive approaches for the treatment of this disease. Moreover, operative intervention coupled with recent developments in preventative measures, e.g., biological barriers, will be discussed. Throughout, an algorithmic, evidence-based approach for the evaluation and appropriate therapeutic management will be emphasized.

Epidemiology

Geriatric persons are now the largest growing segment of our population, with the number of persons 65 years of age and older more than doubling by the middle of this century, to approximately 80 million [4]. What remains problematic is accurately determining the actual incidence of SBO among this cohort. Previously, patient statistics were typically derived from population-based samples, primarily through national hospital-based discharge registries predicated upon imprecise coding schema for SBO; now seemingly more standardized in the updated International Classification of Diseases (ICD-10 CM) [5]. Therefore, current data likely reflect an underestimation of this escalating clinical problem.

Nevertheless, recent trends in aging have shown that patients 65 years of age and older make up 38% of all hospital discharges accounting for nearly 43% of in-patient care days [4]. These rising figures remain in accord with overall age-adjusted national rates of hospitalization for intestinal obstruction occurring in 44.8 per 10,000 [4]. Similarly, census data based upon National Health Statistics for 2008 report an increasing rise in intestinal obstruction with advancing age (see Fig. 63.1) [6]. These upward trends remain in accord with previously published data derived from state hospital-based discharge registries correlating age-specific increases of SBO with gender, whereby females (age > 75 years) had a greater predilection (Fig. 63.2) [7], in part, attributed to a larger number of operative procedures performed on woman, both abdominal and gynecologic.

K.A. Sookraj (✉)
Department of Surgery, SUNY Downstate Medical Center,
107-45 87th St. Ozone Park Queens, Brooklyn, NY 11417, USA
e-mail: kelley.sookraj@downstate.edu

R.A. Rosenthal et al. (eds.), *Principles and Practice of Geriatric Surgery*,
DOI 10.1007/978-1-4419-6999-6_63, © Springer Science+Business Media, LLC 2011

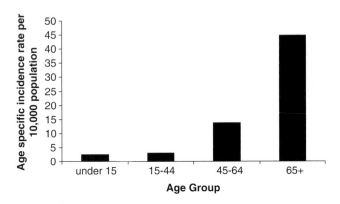

Figure 63.1 Age-specific incidence of small bowel obstruction showing an increase in persons aged 65 and older. National Center for Health Statistics Report, No. 5 pp. 1–20, 2008.

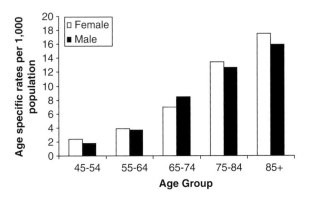

Figure 63.2 Data derived from state-based discharge registries show that as age increases, so does the incidence of obstruction, with women having an increased predilection with age. National Center for Health Statistics, 2004.

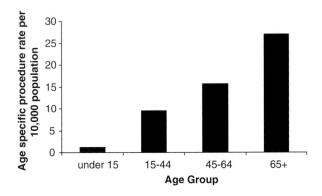

Figure 63.3 Rate of age-specific reported procedures (lysis of adhesions) performed following a diagnosis of small bowel obstruction. National Health Statistics Report, No. 5 pp. 1–20, 2008.

Moreover, as small bowel obstruction increases with age, so also does the rate of reported operative procedures (lysis of adhesions, only) performed on elderly patients (Fig. 63.3) [6]. However, more concerning is recent data on the actual incidence of intestinal obstruction (without mention of

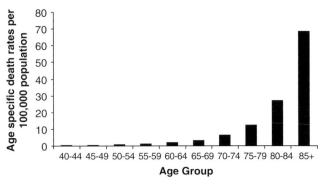

Figure 63.4 Occurrence of US age-specific death rates in the elderly with small bowel obstruction. National Center for Health Statistics, 2004.

hernia) derived from the National Center for Health Statistics; demonstrating US age-specific death rates from SBO being more likely to occur in the elderly; especially among individuals over age 70 (Fig. 63.4) [7].

Etiology-Specific Considerations in the Elderly

To predict the etiology of SBO and direct its treatment, it is first useful to classify SBO using several defining characteristics. Upon initial presentation, the degree of luminal obstruction should be described as either partial or complete. Equally important is *where* along the axis of the small bowel does the obstruction occur (e.g., proximal, mid, or distal). Underscoring the importance of these descriptors is the clinical scenario of the worrisome "closed" loop obstruction where two areas of complete obstruction prevent axial flow of intestinal contents from the involved bowel loop in either the aborad or orad direction. Similarly, structures causing obstruction can also be classified by their anatomic location as they relate to the perpendicular axis of the bowel. These structures may be either extrinsic and/or intrinsic to the bowel wall [8–10], both capable of comprising the entire lumen – as seen in obturation obstruction. Table 63.1 depicts some of the more common etiologies for SBO, keeping in mind that increasing age is a risk factor for most [11].

By definition, mechanical bowel obstruction is an abnormal decrease in the caliber of the involved bowel such that the passage of liquid or solid intestinal contents is impeded. In the majority of cases, SBO starts out as a simple mechanical obstruction with adequate blood supply to the intestinal wall such that the bowel remains viable. However, SBO can progress to strangulation where local bowel ischemia occurs either by direct compression of the affected segment by the obstructing lesion or by extreme dilation and increased

TABLE 63.1   Etiology of small bowel obstruction in the elderly

Extrinsic lesions

Postoperative adhesions

Hernias
  Inguinal, femoral, obturator, umbilical, internal

Malignancy
  Intra-abdominal, extra-abdominal

Volvulus

Intrinsic lesions

Inflammatory bowel disease
  Crohn's disease

Primary small bowel tumors

Radiation enteritis/strictures

Bowel wall abscess

Bowel wall hematoma

Intraluminal obstruction

Gallstones

Fecal Impaction

Bezoars

Foreign body
  Stents

Common Etiologies of Small Bowel Obstruction in the Elderly

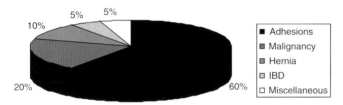

FIGURE 63.5 Percentage of most common causes of small bowel obstruction in the elderly.

pressure in the bowel just proximal to the obstruction, leading to mesenteric occlusion and diminished vascular perfusion.

By comparison, the etiology and pathophysiology of large bowel obstruction (LBO) is considerably different from those of SBO; due to the mostly retroperitoneal nature of the large bowel, it's relatively short mesentery, along with the competency of the ileocecal valve. Indeed, both types of obstruction occur frequently in the elderly, but nearly 80% of intestinal obstruction involves the small bowel; the predominant cause of obstruction in the elderly being due to adhesions from prior abdominal surgery [12]. Thus emphasis of this chapter will focus on the pathophysiology, management, and measures to prevent intra-abdominal adhesions. Figure 63.5 illustrates the incidence of the three most common causes of SBO in the elderly – postoperative adhesions, neoplasms, and hernias – again all have increasing prevalence in the elderly population [10].

Adhesions

More than 90% of abdominal adhesions develop after surgery [13, 14]. The formation of adhesive bands following surgical manipulation is a dynamic process that can occur within several days after surgically traumatized tissues appose one another. Under *normal* circumstances, following nonsurgical traumatic injury, an inflammatory response ensues with recruitment and release of pro-inflammatory cells and cytokines (e.g., interleukin-1) along with activation of the coagulation cascade resulting in the deposition of a fibrinous matrix between apposing tissue surfaces. This fibrin matrix consists primarily of polymorphonuclear cells (PMNs), macrophages, eosinophils, red blood cells, platelets, and tissue debris encased within fibrinous strands. In most cases, such an *early* fibrin matrix is temporary and undergoes fibrinolysis following activation of tissue plasminogen; whereafter degradation occurs within 72 h leading to tissue remodeling and repair as mesothelial and mesenchymal cells proliferate to restore peritoneal defects. This process occurs 4–5 days after tissue injury preventing permanent attachment of adjacent tissue surfaces. In contrast, following surgically induced trauma, these involved tissues become ischemic from reduced blood flow resulting in suppression of fibrinolytic activity. With an absence of fibrin degradation (days 5 through 7), the fibrinous matrix now matures into an adhesive band from continued deposition of collagen and organization by fibroblasts. Over time, these adhesive bands represent a well-organized composition of connective tissues containing arterioles, venules, capillaries, and nerve fibers.

Remarkably, postoperative adhesions account for approximately 60% of all cases of intestinal obstruction in the elderly since many patients by the age of 65 have already undergone some form of abdominal surgery [15]. Whereby, the remaining causes of adhesions are typically secondary to inflammatory processes: such as pelvic inflammatory disease, diverticulitis, tuberculosis, and peritonitis.

The onset of adhesion-associated SBO may occur from several days up to 65 years from the initial operation. However, most SBOs develop earlier on during this interval period with reported median times to occurrence between 1.5 and 5.0 years [16–18] Interestingly, the incidence of SBO after abdominal surgery appears to decrease over time; however, the cumulative risk remains substantial over the increasing lifetime of the patient. Nieuwenhuijzen et al. reported on a series of 234 patients who underwent colectomy and found that 11% of patients developed SBO within the first postoperative year and 30% within the first 10 years [19]. Similarly, a series from Norway demonstrated a 9% cumulative incidence of SBO after colorectal resection over 5 years [20].

Associated procedure-related formation of adhesions typically results after colorectal procedures, appendectomies, as well as multiple prior abdominal surgeries (including adhesiolysis for SBO) each accounting for 20–25% occurrence of adhesive SBO. Gynecologic procedures comprise the remaining 10–15% [18, 21, 22]. These procedures have been found to lead to the formation of single and multiple matted adhesive bands. Interestingly, vascular procedures have also been found to contribute substantially to the occurrence of adhesive SBO [23–25]. Therefore, not surprisingly, more than half of all adhesions causing SBO typically involves the ileum and occur within the pelvis. Moreover, in a recent Mayo Clinic series report, 48% of adhesion-associated SBO resulted from only single bands, whereas nearly 40% were multiple, among these 10% were categorized as dense [16]. In part, these findings clearly support adopting a less traumatic surgical approach (e.g., laparoscopy) in the treatment of certain diseases.

Neoplasms represent the second most common cause of SBO and are responsible for nearly 20% of intestinal obstruction in the elderly. Malignant obstruction occurs by the following mechanism (s): (1) via direct tumor extension causing extrinsic compression of bowel, (2) bulky lymphatic metastases which impinge on adjacent bowel, (3) and, more commonly, peritoneal implants (e.g., carcinomatosis); typically ovarian in origin, leading to a large burden of peritoneal disease and SBO [10]. Tumors intrinsic to the bowel wall, such as carcinoids or lymphomas, do occur and can cause obstruction, although this is extremely uncommon.

The third most common etiology found in the geriatric population is derived from hernias, which accounts for the remaining 10% of cases of SBO. Clinically, hernias are more often associated with bowel strangulation than adhesive bands [8]: these include ventral, umbilical, incisional, inguinal, and internal hernias. In addition, there are certain hernias that occur more frequently in the elderly, also requiring special consideration if a diagnosis of hernia-associated small bowel obstruction is suspected; these include femoral and obturator hernias. There is a well-known preponderance of femoral hernias among female patients, therefore a high incidence of suspicion is warranted and femoral hernias should never be overlooked. By comparison, obturator hernias, however less common, should also be considered in the aging population with chronic disease, also more prevalent in the elderly and often associated with bowel strangulation [10].

Other miscellaneous causes of small bowel obstruction (10%) in older patients include inflammatory disease processes; such as Crohn's disease, diverticulitis, and radiation-induced colitis. Moreover, gallstone ileus which is rare in the general population, is more common in the elderly and can lead to SBO. Volvulus, bezoars (particularly in edentulous patients with prior gastrectomy), foreign bodies, fecal impaction, intestinal wall hematomas from blunt traumas (i.e., traumatic falls), and intestinal wall abscesses are also potential causes of small bowel obstruction in the elderly. Clinicians must be aware of these possibilities when differentiating an underlying cause for small bowel obstruction.

Moreover, as minimally invasive techniques become a larger part of our diagnostic and treatment armamentarium, application of these techniques is likewise expanding in the elderly due to the potential advantages for reduced morbidity. However, with these changes, new etiologic subclasses of iatrogenic causes of SBO are now being reported with increasing frequency. For example, endoscopically placed foreign objects, such as percutaneous endoscopic gastrostomy tubes [26–28] and endoscopic retrograde cholangiopancreatography (ERCP) stents [29–31], can become dislodged and lead to obturation obstruction. Similarly, SBO after laparoscopic procedures is well established [32]. Hernias can occur in trocar sites as well as through peritoneal defects created during laparoscopic procedures [33, 34]. Although postoperative adhesions are less likely, they also can occur. Because of the different etiologies of obstruction after laparoscopy, the general approach to SBO after laparoscopy may differ from that after laparotomy. One recent report examining a series of patients with early postoperative SBO after laparoscopy found that all patients eventually required surgical intervention [35].

Pathophysiology of SBO and Evaluation

Mechanical small bowel obstruction, (e.g., adhesion, neoplasia, and hernia) is accompanied by proximal intestinal distension which is a result of the accumulation of normal gastrointestinal secretions and gas above the obstructed segment. Initially, hyperperistalsis of the bowel is stimulated from intestinal distension leading to frequent loose bowel movements distal to the point of obstruction. Typically, this occurs in the early onset both in partial and complete obstruction. Paradoxically, presentation of frequent bowel movements in the elderly has been found to contribute to high rates of misdiagnosis, delayed treatment, and resultant increased morbidity and mortality [36–38].

As the distension becomes more severe, intraluminal hydrostatic pressures increase leading to the compression of the intestinal mucosal villus lymphatics. This results in the hindrance of lymphatic flow and development of bowel wall lymphedema. Consequently, the venules of the capillaries become congested from the increased hydrostatic pressure at the level of the capillary bed. Resultant fluids accumulate intraluminally as luminal pressures exceed 20 cm H_2O thereby inhibiting absorption and stimulating secretions of salt and water into the lumen, proximal to the obstruction. Moreover, other causes of accumulation of intraluminal fluid may include (1) release of endocrine and paracrine substances, (2) changes in mesenteric circulation, (3) luminal release of bacterial toxins and (4) excess release of prostaglandins. These may all contribute to promoting small bowel epithelial secretion, therefore, inhibiting absorption [36–38]. As a result, loss of intravascular fluid into the bowel manifests clinically as dehydration and hypovolemia. Consequently, prolonged dehydration can result in oliguria, azotemia, hemoconcentration, and eventually hypotension and hypovolemic shock. Furthermore, congested loops of bowel may twist upon themselves and accompanying mesentery resulting in vascular occlusion. In turn, bowel ischemia and necrosis develop and if untreated perforation, peritonitis, and sepsis may occur.

In general, the pathophysiologic changes that occur in small bowel obstruction are similar between the nongeriatric and geriatric patient population. However, and very importantly, as a result of inherent comorbidities found in the elderly, any delay in diagnosis may negatively impact on patient outcome with mortality exceeding 20% [11].

Clinical Features of SBO in the Elderly

Symptoms of SBO are primarily determined by the anatomic level and degree of obstruction. These include nausea and emesis, abdominal distension, abdominal pain, and obstipation (lack of passage of stool or flatus). Proximal SBO is characterized by frequent vomiting of bilious material and dehydration early in the course of disease with relatively little abdominal distension. With distal SBO, swallowed air and gastrointestinal secretions leads first to small bowel and abdominal distension. Only later do patients develop vomiting, usually after bacterial overgrowth has resulted in a feculent character to the enteric content. Partial obstruction is accompanied by continued, though potentially diminished, passage of flatus or stool. Early complete obstruction may also be accompanied by seemingly normal bowel movements, but eventually obstipation occurs.

Strangulation is notoriously difficult to detect reliably. Classic signs include fever, tachycardia, hypotension, and severe pain or focal tenderness which are especially unreliable in the elderly, whereby the inflammatory response may be muted. Similarly, an elevated white blood cell (WBC) count may be absent in the elderly patient. From a previous Mayo Clinic series [16], strangulation was present in 13% of patients operated for SBO and was most commonly seen with the etiologies of hernia and small bowel volvulus. Only 52% of patients with strangulation had an elevated WBC count, and the mean WBC count for patients with strangulation was just 2,000 cells/mm [3] higher than that observed for patients with simple obstruction.

Diagnostic Considerations for the Elderly

Symptoms of SBO are common presenting complaints of elderly patients. The differential diagnosis for abdominal pain, nausea, and vomiting includes gastroenteritis, food poisoning, pancreatitis, biliary colic, porphyria, diabetic ketoacidosis, intestinal ischemia, constipation, paralytic ileus, and intestinal pseudo-obstruction. Compounding this problem in the elderly are age-related concurrent comorbidities that have been shown in a recent large retrospective study to be attributed to misdiagnosis, delay in surgical evaluation, and increased mortality [39]. Among these diagnoses, SBO is fairly common. In a review of ER visits to a regional trauma center by patients over 65 years of age, 12% of patients presenting with nontraumatic abdominal pain were ultimately found to have SBO [40]. Patients should be asked about any history of abdominal surgery or SBO; and during the physical examination, evidence of abdominal wall hernias should be vigilantly elicited. Laboratory values that can aid in the diagnosis and management of these patients include a complete blood count (CBC), basic metabolic profile, and serum amylase. As the classic signs of strangulation are often absent in the elderly, a leukocytosis, elevated hematocrit, and blood urea nitrogen (BUN) levels are often seen as a consequence of dehydration. Serum bicarbonate may be elevated because of loss of chloride-rich emesis and as part of a contraction alkalosis. These findings indicate a significant fluid deficit, which should be aggressively corrected upon initial presentation.

Diagnostic imaging is an important part of the evaluation of every patient with suspected SBO. Supine and upright abdomen and upright PA chest films are typically all that is required to confirm the diagnosis of complete SBO and to plan its treatment. Dilation of small bowel, paucity of colon and rectal gas, and air-fluid levels suggest complete SBO. Forty eight percent of patients with proven SBO will have abdominal plain films that are consistent with SBO [16]. This, of course, means that almost half of patients with SBO have equivocal or even normal plain films, with residual colonic or rectal gas.

When these films are not diagnostic of complete SBO, the decision has traditionally been to rely on the clinical examination and serial plain films. In our experience, as well as other CT scans has been useful in equivocal cases as an early diagnostic test [41] and alters management in up to 20% of patients [42]. Some centers have reported high accuracy of CT in identifying strangulation obstruction. A prospective evaluation of CT in 60 patients with high-grade SBO (with 48% strangulation rate) showed that CT had 100% sensitivity and 61% specificity for detecting bowel ischemia [43]. The CT findings consistent with strangulation included bowel thickening and a high attenuation bowel wall on nonenhanced CT and abnormal bowel wall enhancement and mesenteric fluid on enhanced CT. A similar series of 100 patients from a different institution found a sensitivity of 83% and a specificity of 93% [44]. In contradistinction to these studies, several studies have compared CT with plain radiography and have found only modest differences in the overall accuracy of these tests when evaluating the grade of obstruction [45, 46]. CT also is helpful in patients with closed loop obstructions and patients who swallow little air and thus have a gasless proximal bowel, as these problems are difficult to detect on plain films. At our institution, contrast-enhanced CT scans are not routinely used in the decision-making process except when the clinical history, physical examination, and plain films are not conclusive for a SBO diagnosis.

In our experience, CT scans are more likely to demonstrate the cause of SBO, particularly when the obstruction is not secondary to adhesions. Current generation multidetector computed tomography or MDCT now permit high-quality reformatted images to be obtained in multiple planes which facilitate identification of the transition point and other findings in SBO: presence of a high degree of SBO and abnormal vascular course around the transition zone. Ultimately, MDCT may result in a paradigm shift toward earlier cross-sectional imaging in the elderly by its inherent ability to better predict the necessity for emergent surgery (i.e., ischemia) in the elderly when SBO is caused by adhesions [47, 48].

Less often used diagnostic imaging modalities in the acute setting include ultrasonography [49–52] and MRI [53]. In the more subacute and chronic setting in patients with an intermittent or partial SBO, enteroclysis (small bowel enema) and small bowel follow-through may be useful [54, 55]. The passage of water-soluble oral contrast into the cecum within 4 h after CT or small bowel follow-through, remains highly predictive of nonsurgical resolution of SBO [56, 57]. Interestingly, there have also been two randomized controlled trials examining whether water-soluble contrast speeds the resolution of partial SBO. Assalia et al. found a therapeutic benefit in terms of a shorter hospital stay in those patients receiving oral contrast with SBO from a variety of etiologies [58], whereas Feigin et al. reported no therapeutic benefit in patients with postoperative SBO [59].

A special case of the diagnostic dilemma between SBO and paralytic ileus may occur during the early postoperative period. At 1–6 weeks after abdominal surgery, inflammatory adhesion can be thick and highly vascular. For these reasons, the morbidity of reoperation can be considerable. Because these early adhesions are also in a fluid state of constant remodeling, there is also a good chance of resolution of even high-grade partial obstructions without surgical intervention. It therefore becomes even more critical to define the degree of obstruction in these patients to avoid the higher morbidity of reoperation. In such circumstances, MDCT scanning may prove more beneficial for accurately distinguishing these equivocal cases [47, 48]. In very selected cases, when persistent partial SBO is a problem, endoscopic placement of a long intestinal tube may prove to be therapeutic and allow for a high-quality small bowel contrast study that more clearly characterizes the site of partial obstruction.

Initial Treatment

Surgery, like aviation, in itself is not inherently dangerous. But to an even larger degree than the air, it is terribly unforgiving of any carelessness, incapacity or neglect.

Peter K. Kottmeier, M.D., Chief of Pediatric Surgery, SUNY-HSCB (1965–1999)

Inscribed on the entrance of the Peter K. Kottmeier Library, SUNY-HSCB

The traditional adage of "never let the sun set or rise on a small bowel obstruction" [16], in part, underscores the severity of this diagnosis, particularly in the elderly. Recently, however, this has been largely modified by a multifactorial assessment and approach that first considers the physiologic abnormality that has occurred since the onset of the SBO (i.e., hemodynamic status), type of SBO (partial, complete, strangulated), and patient comorbidities/performance status (cardiac, pulmonary, renal, malignancy).

Even the patient who clearly has a complete bowel obstruction benefits from initial nonsurgical measures including proximal decompression, aggressive fluid resuscitation, and correction of electrolyte abnormalities. A Foley catheter is critical in the elderly to assess organ perfusion and fluid status. Generally, a nasogastric tube is adequate to decompress the gastrointestinal (GI) tract, but in some patients in whom a prolonged course of nonoperative management is contemplated, as for early postoperative SBO or the patient with multiple previous laparotomies or known severe adhesions, a long nasointestinal tube may be considered.

Patients with complete SBO or with obvious signs of strangulation should be expeditiously resuscitated and then brought to the operating room. This strategy particularly applies to patients in whom the etiology is thought unlikely due to adhesions or neoplasm. In this case, *not letting the sun rise or set*, certainly applies. However, most patients admitted for an SBO do not fall into this category. Two-thirds to three-fourths of patients with partial (primarily adhesive) SBO can be treated conservatively, with resolution of their acute episode [60–63]. In patients with a partial SBO, the duration of medical therapy continues to be a hotly debated issue. Recent series examining this question have consistently shown that partial SBOs that ultimately resolve generally do so within 24–72 h. Delays beyond 48 h have been associated with increased morbidity in some series [63], whereas others have shown no increased morbidity with even longer delays [64].

The potential arguments against maintaining a nonoperative approach are that the diagnosis of strangulation is inaccurate [65] and the duration of medical treatment may be proportional to the incidence of strangulation or need for bowel resection and the subsequent higher incidence of complications. These concerns are particularly relevant in elderly patients. Adhesive SBO requiring surgery in elderly patients ultimately requires bowel resection in up to 50% of

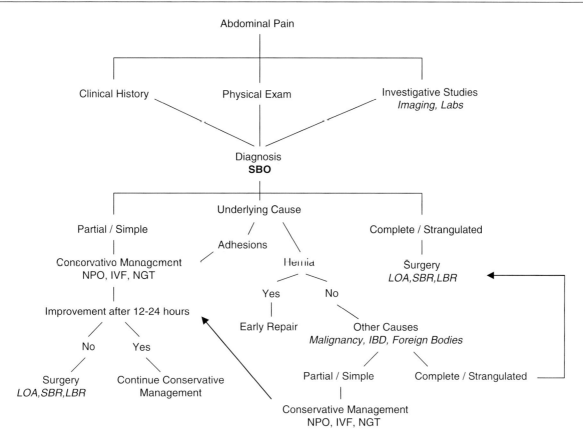

FIGURE 63.6 Algorithm for management of small bowel obstruction in the elderly. *SBO* small bowel obstruction, *IVF* intravenous fluid, *NGT* nasogastric, *LOA* lysis of adhesions, *SBR* small bowel resection, *LBR* large bowel resection, *NPO* nil per os (nothing by mouth), *IVF* intravenous fluids, *IBD* inflammatory bowel disease.

cases [66], whereas only 8% of patients of all ages required bowel resection in the Mayo Clinic series [16]. In that series, among patients in whom strangulation was found, delays of more than 4 h from presentation to surgery were associated with higher morbidity rates. Much emphasized is the importance of the underlying etiology when determining the mortality risk of delayed surgical intervention [16]. Data from the Mayo Clinic series showed that in the case of obstruction due to hernia, the time from presentation to operation was directly related to the mortality rate, but this relation with mortality did not exist for SBO caused by adhesions or malignancy.

We favor a selective approach in the elderly patient with SBO. The immediate strategy should be determined by consideration of (1) the evidence for current bowel ischemia and (2) the presumed etiology of the SBO and degree of obstruction. Patients with two or more signs of strangulation, radiographic signs of complete SBO, or both are operated on as soon as possible after adequate resuscitation is carried out. Nasogastric decompression and serial examinations are then planned for those in whom an adhesive SBO is likely. For those in whom the diagnosis of SBO is unclear or the etiology is in question, CT is performed. The longer-term strategy in patients initially treated nonoperatively should include both the above factors as well as (3) the likelihood of intraopera-

tive and postoperative complications. These factors should be weighed against the likelihood of success using continued nonsurgical management. Figure 63.6 shows our diagnostic and treatment algorithm for patients with SBO.

Surgical Treatment: General Principles

Preoperative antibiotic coverage to cover enteric organisms should be administered, as a number of cases involve bowel resection or inadvertent enterotomy. Although elderly patients are more likely to have underlying cardiovascular disease, increasing the risk of a perioperative cardiac event, invasive monitoring devices are rarely required. Hypotension upon induction of anesthesia should be avoided by attention to adequate preoperative fluid resuscitation often requiring 3–4 L of intravenous isotonic crystalloid.

Laparotomy should be performed through a midline approach with at least part of the initial incision over virgin skin, if possible. Entry through the fascia is done with extreme care, avoiding the use of cautery, as transmitted heat can injure underlying bowel. Adhesions are usually stronger than the junctions between the small bowel muscle layers and the muscularis propria and submucosa, and this seems particularly true in the elderly patient. Sharp dissection with scissors or knife should therefore be performed to avoid seromuscular injuries. We generally lyse adhesions from the anterior abdominal wall first and then proceed to run the small bowel lysing adhesions as we progress from the terminal ileum to the ligament of Treitz.

While running the bowel, the etiology of the SBO and local bowel viability are assessed. The commonly available parameters include bowel color, peristalsis, and mesenteric pulsations. Although clearly viable and clearly nonviable extremes are easy to identify, many gradations of color are difficult to judge, and assessment of ultimate viability is prone to error. Adjuncts to these methods continue to include Doppler flow probe assessment of mesenteric and antimesenteric blood flow [67, 68], intravenous fluorescein perfusion [67, 69], and electromyography (EMG). Although these methods have their advocates, none has consistently been shown to have higher accuracy than "clinical judgment" using visual and manual inspection. Our general strategy is to resect questionable bowel if possible. If resection would result in less than 4–5 ft of clearly viable intestine, questionable segments with the highest likelihood of viability should be left in situ with a planned "second-look" reoperation within 24–48 h.

To allow abdominal wall closure, frequently the bowel must be decompressed. This can be achieved with a long nasointestinal tube, but we favor gentle retrograde milking of the intestine toward the duodenum with fluid evacuation via a nasogastric tube. To minimize excessive distension and the risk of serosal tears, this process is first started in the midjejunum. The proximal jejunal segment is then evacuated of luminal content. The process is then repeated starting progressively more distally on the bowel. Prior to closing the abdomen, the bowel loops should be laid back in the abdomen in gentle folds. Some have advocated the use of long intestinal tubes to act as stents, particularly in the patient with recurrent SBO or pervasive adhesions [70]. Another option gaining popularity is the application of hyaluronidase-containing films to inhibit adhesion formation [71]. Clinical trial data (see section "Biological Barriers") demonstrate safety and potential efficacy for reducing adhesions and adhesion-associated SBO.

Laparoscopic Treatment of SBO

Laparoscopic surgery has theoretic advantages over open surgery including decreased postoperative pain, reduced wound complications, decreased respiratory complications, and shorter hospital stay. These advantages are particularly attractive in elderly patients and have likely led to a decreased threshold for elderly patients seeking surgical management by a minimally invasive approach. Thus far the laparoscopic approach to SBO has not been widely accepted, although recent reports of SBO management using a laparoscopic approach have been documented [72–76]. The challenge for laparoscopy for treating SBO rests not in the diagnostic efficiency which is between 60 and 100%, but the therapeutic efficacy which is generally low (40–88%). Not surprisingly, the conversion rate to laparotomy has been reported to be as high as 52%.

Several factors make laparoscopic treatment of SBO difficult and have prevented many surgeons from adopting this approach to SBO. Exposure can be problematic because of diffuse adhesions to the anterior abdominal wall and because distended bowel may have already increased the intra-abdominal pressure and decreased the volume of pneumoperitoneum that can be achieved. Therefore, it is generally best to use an open insertion technique and to select an initial insertion site remote from previous scars. Bowel distension should be minimized by preoperative nasogastric decompression, and in selected cases using a long intestinal tube prior to attempting laparoscopic treatment. Perhaps the most common reason for reluctance to use laparoscopy for SBO is a concern that treatment may ultimately require an extensive adhesiolysis or resection that is problematic to achieve laparoscopically. Therefore, proper patient selection is paramount before choosing a minimally invasive approach. A recent Medline, Embase, Cochrane review from 1980 to 2007 identified predictive factors for a successful laparoscopic adhesiolysis which includes: ≤2 previous laparotomies, adhesions associated with appendectomy, single adhesive band, early <24 h laparoscopic management from onset of symptoms, no peritonitis, and surgical expertise [73].

The laparoscopic approach is particularly attractive for adhesive SBOs where there is a single adhesive band. Conventional laparotomy is recommended for malignant SBOs and hernia-related SBOs, where there is a high rate of strangulation. The general principles of the laparoscopic approach are similar to those of the open approach. Adhesions are dissected sharply, and after adhesiolysis the bowel is inspected from the ileocecal valve to the ligament of Treitz.

Although one-half to two-thirds of patients may be treatable laparoscopically, one must anticipate a high conversion rate to open laparotomy; moreover, the mastery of laparoscopic skills is essential. A study by Bailey et al. compared SBOs treated in two surgical units, one with a special interest in laparoscopy [77]. The laparoscopy unit attempted laparoscopic treatment in 80% of SBOs, and among those cases, they completed treatment laparoscopically in 56%. The laparoscopically treated patients left the hospital 5 days earlier than the open procedure patients, but they also had a higher rate of unplanned reoperation (14% vs. 5%).

In 2010, the safety and efficacy of diagnostic laparoscopy for SBO appears well established from retrospective studies, whereas laparoscopic adhesiolysis requires careful patient selection with an operative plan that includes converting to an open approach if extensive adhesions or nonadhesive causes are encountered. Ultimately, prospective randomized trials assessing all clinically relevant outcomes are needed.

Outcomes of Treatment of SBO

Most studies of the outcomes of treatment of SBO have centered on traditional surgical outcomes, such as perioperative mortality, survival, and postoperative complications. Increased age is a risk factor for mortality from SBO (Fig. 63.4). Perioperative mortality is also related to the etiology of the SBO. For example, SBO with a malignant etiology has an in-hospital mortality of 21% and a median survival of 6 months compared to a 4–5% mortality risk for hernia and adhesive etiologies. Similarly, a large prospective experience by Miner et al. from Memorial Sloan Kettering [78] showed that the potential benefits of palliative surgery are minimized by the inherent morbidity (29%) and mortality (11%) of these procedures. Of note, delay from symptom onset to presentation is not generally related to mortality risk except in the case of hernias, where there is also a higher risk of strangulation; overall in-hospital morbidity is 30% but is increased in patients with strangulation to 60%.

As adhesions represent the most common cause of SBO in the elderly, identifying pertinent risk factors for adverse outcome following surgery for adhesion-associated SBO may provide the clinician with important information for stratifying the risk-to-benefit ratio for clinical decision making especially in the more concerning elderly population. A recent VA National Surgical Quality Improvement Program developed a morbidity and mortality risk index assessment based on a cumulative score that predicts the probability of an adverse outcome [79]. Not surprisingly, the odds of mortality in a patient 70–79 years of age are increased by a factor of 1.855 compared to a patient younger than 50 years. Similarly, better outcomes are associated with adhesiolysis only, compared to bowel resection.

Attempts were also made to ascertain the longevity of treatment of SBO. Specifically, for patients treated nonsurgically, the likelihood and timing of recurrence, and how this compares to patients treated surgically? These questions were largely addressed from a state-wide longitudinal population-based outcome analysis derived from 32,583 hospitalized patients (mean age 63 years) admitted with a diagnosis of SBO (index admission). From this study, Foster et al.

[63], showed that in California, from data derived from patients hospitalized in 1997, SBO was primarily managed nonoperatively in 76% of these patients. Of the patients that underwent operative management (24%), there was a longer length of stay, lower mortality rate, fewer SBO readmissions, and longer time to readmission. In general, patients who did not have operations were usually older and with more comorbidities. However, regardless of the treatment, 81% of patients had no subsequent SBO requiring readmission over the 5-year study follow-up period. Similarly, Landercasper et al. [80] retrospectively reviewed 309 consecutive patients with SBO and followed them for recurrence [55]. The SBOs recurred in 34% by 4 years and in 42% by 10 years. Those who were operated on had a lower recurrence rate (29%) than those who were treated nonoperatively (53%). Among those who had surgery, recurrences differed by etiology: malignant (56%), adhesive (28%), and hernia (0%). In this study, the number of prior obstructive episodes was not a risk factor for recurrence. However, Fevang et al. [81] retrospectively studied 500 patients with adhesive-associated SBO (ASBO) for up to 40 years for recurrence [56]. They found that the cumulative recurrence rate for patients operated once for ASBO was 18% after 10 years and 29% at 30 years. The likelihood of a recurrent ASBO was highest within 5 years after the previous one, but a considerable risk was still present 10–20 years after an ASBO episode.

In addition to recurrence risk, treatment choice affects the cost of care and utilization of health-care resources. The costs of caring for patients with SBO are considerable. From a Swedish study, 60% of all bowel obstructions were due to adhesions; 65% of them required more than a 1-day hospital stay, and 45% of these required surgery. Calculating direct costs and extrapolating these data, $13 million are spent on adhesive SBO in Sweden (a country of 8.5 million population) annually [82]. In many cases, treatment choice is determined solely by the initial clinical presentation. Either the decision to undergo surgery occurs early or an initial short duration of medical management results in rapid clinical improvement and resolution of the SBO. However, in patients with high-grade partial obstruction likely due to adhesions, an early decision to treat surgically is likely to have a favorable clinical outcome but may result in a longer hospital stay and higher cost of care compared to a nonsurgical approach. As one might expect, retrospective analysis of patients treated medically and surgically show that surgically treated patients have clinical outcomes similar to those treated medically but with longer lengths of stay [17]. The additional costs of care in patients ultimately treated surgically may be as much as eight times higher than nonsurgically treated patients. This differential makes tests with improved diagnostic accuracy such as CT or MDCT more cost-effective for questionable partial SBO [83].

Biological Barriers

Barriers are biosynthetic membranes or gels that have been shown to be effective in decreasing surgically induced adhesions. One of the first prototypes that was successful in reducing postoperative adhesions in humans was Interceed® which was composed of modified oxidized regenerated cellulose. This particular barrier was found to be applicable following gynecologic procedures; however, its use in general surgical procedures is unknown. Another type of biological barrier is expanded polytetrafluoroethylene (PTFE). This was shown to prevent pelvic adhesions. However, PTFE was not cost-effective or bioabsorbable and required a large piece of material and suturing to keep it in place for adhesion prevention.

To date, the most efficacious barrier is a hyaluronan and carboxymethylcellulose bioresorbable membrane called Seprafilm®. The mechanism of action of adhesion prevention is believed to occur by one of the components known as sodium hyaluronate. It is believed to improve peritoneal healing by increasing the proliferation of mesothelial cells and facilitating their detachment and migration thereby leading to the restoration of the mesothelial lining within the peritoneal cavity. It is also thought to increase the fibrinolytic response of mesothelial cells which may aid in adhesion prevention.

Seprafilm® is typically prepared as a membranous sheet that is applied over potential sites of ahesion formation, (e.g., traumatized tissue), prior to closure following an abdominal surgical procedure. Placement of the membrane requires that the peritoneal cavity, as well as the instruments and gloves used to handle the barrier be as dry as possible. Approximately 1–2 cm of the membrane should be exposed from its holder prior to application. When entering the abdominal cavity the membrane can be curved or slightly folded to facilitate placement over the desired area. To ensure adequate adherence to the tissue a dry instrument or gloved hand can be used to gently press down on the membrane. Seprafilm® should be sufficiently placed over the margins of the incision or surgically traumatized tissue and overlapped to achieve sufficient coverage. Importantly, a bowel anastomosis should not be wrapped with Seprafilm® as this practice has been associated with adverse events. Seprafilm® slowly resorbs within 7 days of placement and is fully excreted by 28 days.

Seprafilm® was evaluated in a number of prospectively, randomized, controlled, multicenter studies and consistently demonstrated overall safety [84–89] (Table 63.2). The larger clinical trials did show a significant reduction in the formation of adhesions and adhesion-associated SBO [84–89] (Table 63.3). These barriers potentially provide an excellent form of adjunctive therapy for preventing postoperative adhesions which is the number one cause of SBO, not only in the elderly but also in the general population.

TABLE 63.2 Seprafilm® safety and efficacy for small bowel obstruction

References	Number of patients	Patient/disease cohort	Occurrence of ASBO (Seprafilm vs. no Seprafilm)		Reoperation of ASBO (Seprafilm vs. no Seprafilm)		Complications (Seprafilm vs. no Seprafilm)	
Becker et al. [84]	183	Ulcerative colitis/FAP	42	85	NR	NR	82	86
Diamond et al. [85]	127	Uterine fibroids	27	54	NR	NR	NR	NR
Beck et al. [86]	1,791	IBD	NR	NR	NR	NR	249	223
Fazio et al. [87]	1,791	IBD	15	29	8	4	249	223
Kusunoki et al. [88]	62	Rectal cancer	2	5	1	3	NR	NR
Hayashi et al. [89]	150	Gastric cancer	4	7	0	1	23	22

ASBO adhesive small bowel obstruction, *IBD* inflammatory bowel disease, *NR* not recorded

TABLE 63.3 Seprafilm® reported clinical trial statistical outcomes

References	Occurrence of ASBO (Seprafilm vs. no Seprafilm p-value)	Complications (Seprafilm vs. no Seprafilm p-value)
Becker et al. [84]	$p < 0.00000000001$	$p > 0.05$
Diamond et al. [85]	$p < 0.0001$	NR
Beck et al. [86]	NR	$P < 0.05^{a}$
Fazio et al. [87]	$p < 0.05$	NR
Kusunoki et al. [88]	$p = 0.220$	NR
Hayashi et al. [89]	$p = 0.534$	$p = 0.722$

ASBO adhesive small bowel obstruction, *NR* not recorded
[a] Overall complication

Summary

Small bowel obstruction is a common pathological process that can occur in any patient population. Its effects, however, are devastating in the elderly and warrants prompt appropriate management. Utilization of a thorough clinical history, physical examination, and investigative studies provide the necessary information to determine a diagnosis and direct the next step in treatment. Immediate aggressive resuscitation is required with monitoring of hemodynamic parameters especially in older patients because of their limited physiologic reserve and comorbidities.

Based on the type of SBO, a trial of conservative management may be initiated or definitive surgery may be performed. Either, the standard open laparotomy or minimally invasive surgical technique may be used dependent on surgeon experience, patient stability or underlying cause. Recent developments of biosynthetic products have made a positive impact in the management of SBO that help in the prevention of surgically induced adhesions in the elderly.

References

1. Yen EL, McNamara RM (2007) Abdominal pain. Clin Geriatr Med 23:255–270
2. Duties EH, Katz PR, Malone ML (2007) Gastroenterological disorders. Practice of geriatrics, 4th edn. pp 578–580
3. Sanson TG, O'Keefe KP (1996) Evaluation of abdominal pain in the elderly. Emerg Med Clin North Am 14:615–627
4. Martinez JP, Mattu A (2006) Pain in the elderly. Emerg Med Clin North Am 24:371–388
5. International Classification of Diseases, Tenth Revision, Clinical Modification (ICD-10-CM), CDC, National Center for Health Statistics, 2009
6. National Center for Health Statistics (2008) National hospital ambulatory medical care survey. Hyattsville: NCHS, Report, No. 5, pp 1–20. ftp://ftp.cdc.gov/pub/HealthStatistics/NCHS/Datasets/NHAMCS/ed2008.exe
7. National Center for Health Statistics (2004) National hospital ambulatory medical care survey. NCHS, Hyattsville. ftp://ftp.cdc.gov/pub/HealthStatistics/NCHS/Datasets/NHAMCS/ed2004.exe
8. Neugut AI, Marvin MR, Rella VA, Chabot JA (1997) An overview of adenocarcinoma of the small intestine. Oncology (Huntingt) 11:529–536
9. Gutstein DE, Rosenberg SJ (1997) Nontraumatic intramural hematoma of the duodenum complicating warfarin therapy. Mt Sinai J Med 64:339–341
10. Miller G, Boman J, Shirer L et al (2000) Etiology of small bowel obstruction. Am J Surg 180:33–36
11. Eagon CJ (2001) Small bowel obstruction in the elderly. Principles and Practice of Geriatric Surgery, 569–579
12. Hendrickson M, Naparst TR (2003) Abdominal surgical emergencies in the elderly. Emerg Med Clin North Am 21:937–969
13. Attard JP, Maclean AR (2007) Adhesive small bowel obstruction: epidemiology, biology and prevention. Can J Surg 50:291–300
14. Miller G, Boman J, Shrier I et al (2000) Natural history of patients with adhesive small bowel obstruction. Br J Surg 87:1240–1247
15. Tjandra JJ, Gordon CJA, Kaye AH et al (2006) Small bowel obstruction. Textbook of surgery, 3rd edn. pp 159–177
16. Mucha P (1987) Small intestinal obstruction. Surg Clin North Am 67:597–620
17. Wilson MS, Hawkswell J, McCloy RF (1998) Natural history of adhesional small bowel obstruction: counting the cost. Br J Surg 85:1294–1298
18. Matter I, Khalemsky L, Abrahamson J, Nash E, Sabo E, Eldar S (1997) Does the index operation influence the course and outcome of adhesive intestinal obstruction? Eur J Surg 163:767–772
19. Nieuwenhuijzen M, Reijnen MM, Kuijpers JH, van Goor H (1998) Small bowel obstruction after total or subtotal colectomy: a 10-year retrospective review. Br J Surg 85:1242–1245
20. Edna TH, Bjerkeset T (1998) Small bowel obstruction in patients previously operated on for colorectal cancer. Eur J Surg 164:587–592
21. Cox MR, Gunn IF, Eastman MC, Hunt RF, Heinz AW (1993) The operative aetiology and types of adhesions causing small bowel obstruction. Aust NZ J Surg 63:848–852
22. Meagher AP, Moller C, Hoffmann DC (1993) Non-operative treatment of small bowel obstruction following appendectomy or operation on the ovary or tube. Br J Surg 80:1310–1311
23. Franko E, Cohen JR (1991) General surgical problems requiring operation in postoperative vascular surgery patients. Am J Surg 162:247–250
24. Siporin K, Hiatt JR, Treiman RL (1993) Small bowel obstruction after abdominal aortic surgery. Am Surg 59:846–849
25. Rijken AM, Butzelaar RM (1996) Compression of the descending duodenum after reconstruction of infrarenal aortic aneurysm. J Vasc Surg 24(1):178–179
26. Khan S, Gatt M, Petty D, Stojkovic S (2008) Intestinal obstruction after PEG tube replacement: implications to daily clinical practice. Surg Laparosc Endosc Percutan Tech 18(1):80–81
27. Schrag SP, Sharma R, Jaik NP, Seamon MJ, Lukaszczyk JJ, Martin ND, Hoey BA, Stawicki SP (2007) Complications related to percutaneous endoscopic gastrostomy (PEG) tubes. A comprehensive clinical review. J Gastrointestin Liver Dis 16(4):407–418
28. Lambertz MM, Earnshaw PM, Short J, Cumming JG (1995) Small bowel obstruction caused by a retained percutaneous endoscopic gastrostomy gastric flange. Br J Surg 82:951
29. Barton RJ (2006) Migrated double pigtail biliary stent causes small bowel obstruction. J Gastroenterol Hepatol 21(4):783–784
30. Ikeda T, Nagata S, Ohgaki K (2004) Intestinal obstruction because of a migrated metallic biliary stent. Gastrointest Endosc 60(6):988–989
31. Simpson D, Cunningham C, Paterson-Brown S (1998) Small bowel obstruction caused by a dislodged biliary stent. J R Coll Surg Edinb 43:203
32. Spier LN, Lazzaro RS, Procaccino A, Geiss A (1993) Entrapment of small bowel after laparoscopic herniorrhaphy. Surg Endosc 7:535–536
33. Boughy JC, Nottingham JM, Walls AC (2003) Richter's hernia in the laparoscopic era: four case reports and review of the literature. Surg Laparosc Endosc Percutan Tech 13:55–58
34. McKay R (2008) Preperitoneal herniation and bowel obstruction post laparoscopic inguinal hernia repair: case report and review of the literature. Hernia 12:535–537
35. Velasco JM, Vallina VL, Bonomo SR, Hieken TJ (1998) Postlaparoscopic small bowel obstruction: rethinking its management. Surg Endosc 12:1043–1045
36. DiMizio R, Scaglione M (2007) Computed tomography: pathophysiology of imaging, mechanisms of small bowel obstruction. Small bowel obstruction, 1st edn.
37. Evers MB (2004) Small intestine. Sabiston textbook of surgery. 17th edn. pp 1323–1380
38. Campbell KA (2008) Small bowel obstruction. Cameron current surgical therapy. 9th edn. pp, 117–120

39. Laurell H, Hansson LE, Gunnarsson U (2006) Acute abdominal pain among elderly patients. Gerontology 52(6):339–344

40. Bugliosi TF, Meloy TD, Vukov LF (1990) Acute abdominal pain in the elderly. Ann Emerg Med 19:1383–1386

41. Donckier V, Closset J, Van Gansbeke D et al (1998) Contribution of computed tomography to decision making in the management of adhesive small bowel obstruction. Br J Surg 85:1071–1074

42. Taourel PG, Fabre JM, Pradel JA, Seneterre EJ, Megibow AJ, Bruel JM (1995) Value of CT in the diagnosis and management of patients with suspected acute small-bowel obstruction. Am J Roentgenol 165:1187–1192

43. Frager D, Baer JW, Medwid SW, Rothpearl A, Bossart P (1996) Detection of intestinal ischemia in patients with acute small-bowel obstruction due to adhesions or hernia: efficacy of CT. Am J Roentgenol 166:67–71

44. Balthazar EJ, Liebeskind ME, Macari M (1997) Intestinal ischemia in patients in whom small bowel obstruction is suspected: evaluation of accuracy, limitations, and clinical implications of CT in diagnosis. Radiology 205:519–522

45. Maglinte DD, Reyes BL, Harmon BH et al (1996) Reliability and role of plain film radiography and CT in the diagnosis of small-bowel obstruction. Am J Roentgenol 167:1451–1455

46. Fukuya T, Hawes DR, Lu CC, Chang PJ, Barloon TJ (1992) CT diagnosis of small-bowel obstruction: efficacy in 60 patients. Am J Roentgenol 158:765–769, discussion 771–772

47. Hwang JY, Lee JK, Lee JE, Baek SY (2009) Value of multidetector CT in decision making regarding surgery in patients with small-bowel obstruction due to adhesion. Eur Radiol 19:2425–2431

48. Desser TS, Gross M (2008) Multidetector row computed tomography of small bowel obstruction. Semin Ultrasound CT MR 29:308–21

49. Ko YT, Lim JH, Lee DH, Lee HW, Lim JW (1993) Small bowel obstruction: sonographic evaluation. Radiology 188:649–653

50. Ogata M, Imai S, Hosotani R, Aoyama H, Hayashi M, Ishikawa T (1994) Abdominal ultrasonography for the diagnosis of strangulation in small bowel obstruction. Br J Surg 81:421–424

51. Czechowski J (1996) Conventional radiography and ultrasonography in the diagnosis of small bowel obstruction and strangulation. Acta Radiol 37:186–189

52. Schmutz GR, Benko A, Fournier L, Peron JM, Morel E, Chiche L (1997) Small bowel obstruction: role and contribution of sonography. Eur Radiol 7:1054–1058

53. Regan F, Beall DP, Bohlman ME, Khazan R, Sufi A, Schaefer DC (1998) Fast MR imaging and the detection of small-bowel obstruction. Am J Roentgenol 170:1465–1469

54. Makanjuola D (1998) Computed tomography compared with small bowel enema in clinically equivocal intestinal obstruction. Clin Radiol 53:203–208

55. Maglinte DD, Nolan DJ, Herlinger H (1991) Preoperative diagnosis by enteroclysis of unsuspected closed loop obstruction in medically managed patients. J Clin Gastroenterol 13:308–312

56. Joyce WP, Delaney PV, Gorey TF, Fitzpatrick JM (1992) The value of water-soluble contrast radiology in the management of acute small bowel obstruction. Ann R Coll Surg Engl 74:422–425

57. Chung CC, Meng WC, Yu SC, Leung KL, Lau WY, Li AK (1996) A prospective study on the use of water-soluble contrast follow-through radiology in the management of small bowel obstruction. Aust NZ J Surg 66:598–601

58. Assalia A, Schein M, Kopelman D, Hirshberg A, Hashmonai M (1994) Therapeutic effect of oral Gastrografin in adhesive, partial small-bowel obstruction: a prospective randomized trial. Surgery 115:433–437

59. Feigin E, Seror D, Szold A et al (1996) Water-soluble contrast material has no therapeutic effect on postoperative small-bowel obstruction: results of a prospective, randomized clinical trial. Am J Surg 171:227–229

60. Brolin R (1984) Partial small bowel obstruction. Surgery 95:145–149

61. Peetz DJ, Gamelli RL, Pilcher DB (1982) Intestinal intubation in acute, mechanical small-bowel obstruction. Arch Surg 117:334–336

62. Nova FM, McGory ML, Zingmond DS, Ko CY (2006) Small bowel obstruction: a population-based appraisal. J Am Coll Surg 203:170–176

63. Sosa J, Gardner B (1993) Management of patients diagnosed as acute intestinal obstruction secondary to adhesions. Am Surg 59:125–128

64. Cox MR, Gunn IF, Eastman MC, Hunt RF, Heinz AW (1993) The safety and duration of non-operative treatment for adhesive small bowel obstruction. Aust NZ J Surg 63:367–3

65. Sarr MG, Bulkley GB, Zuidema GD (1983) Preoperative recognition of intestinal strangulation obstruction: prospective evaluation of diagnostic capability. Am J Surg 145:176–182

66. Zadeh BJ, Davis JM, Canizaro PC (1985) Small bowel obstruction in the elderly. Am Surg 51:470

67. Mann A, Fazio VW, Lucas FV (1982) A comparative study of the use of fluorescein and the Doppler device in the determination of intestinal viability. Surg Gynecol Obstet 154:53–55

68. Cooperman M, Pace WG, Martin EW Jr et al (1978) Determination of viability of ischemic intestine by Doppler ultrasound. Surgery 83:705–710

69. Bulkley GB, Zuidema GD, Hamilton SR (1981) Intraoperative determination of small intestinal viability following ischemic injury. Ann Surg 193:628–637

70. Rodriguez-Ruesga R, Meagher AP, Wolff BG (1995) Twelve-year experience with the long intestinal tube. World J Surg 19:627–630, discussion 630–631

71. DeCherney AH, diZerega GS (1997) Clinical problem of intraperitoneal postsurgical adhesion formation following general surgery and the use of adhesion prevention barriers. Surg Clin North Am 77:671–688

72. Cirocchi R, Abraha I, Farinella E, Montedori A, Sciannameo F (2010) Laparoscopic versus open surgery in small bowel obstruction. Cochrane Database Syst Rev 2: CD007511

73. Farinella E, Cirocchi R, La Mura F, Morelli U, Cattorini L, Delmonaco P, Migliaccio C, De Sol AA, Cozzaglio L, Sciannameo F (2009) Feasibility of laparoscopy for small bowel obstruction. World J Emerg Surg 4:3

74. Zerey M, Sechrist CW, Kercher KW, Sing RF, Matthews BD, Heniford BT (2007) Laparoscopic management of adhesive small bowel obstruction. Am Surg 73:773–778

75. Kirshtein B, Roy-Shapira A, Lantsberg L, Avinoach E, Mizrahi S (2005) Laparoscopic management of acute small bowel obstruction. Surg Endosc 19(4):464–467

76. Franklin ME Jr, Gonzalez JJ, Miter DB, Glass JL, Paulson D (2004) Laparoscopic diagnosis and treatment of intestinal obstruction. Surg Endosc 18(1):26–30

77. Bailey IS, Rhodes M, O'Rourke N, Nathanson L, Fielding G (1998) Laparoscopic management of acute small bowel obstruction. Br J Surg 85:84–87

78. Miner TJ, Brennan MF, Jaques DP (2004) A prospective, symptom related, outcome analysis of 1022 palliative procedures for advanced cancer. Ann Surg 240:719–727

79. Margenthaler JA, Longo WE, Virgo KS, Johnson FE, Grossman EM, Schiffner TL, Henderson WG, Khuri SF (2006) Risk factors for adverse outcomes following surgery for small bowel obstruction. Ann Surg 243:456–464

80. Landercasper J, Cogbill TH, Merry WH et al (1993) Long-term outcome after hospitalization for small-bowel obstruction. Arch Surg 128:765–770

81. Fevang B, Fevang J, Lie S, Soreide O, Svanes K, Viste A (2004) Long-term prognosis after operation for adhesive small bowel obstruction. Ann Surg 240:193–201

82. Ivarsson ML, Holmdahl L, Franzen G, Risberg B (1997) Cost of bowel obstruction resulting from adhesions. Eur J Surg 163: 679–684

83. Ogata M, Mateer JR, Condon RE (1996) Prospective evaluation of abdominal sonography for the diagnosis of bowel obstruction. Ann Surg 223:237–241

84. Becker JM, Dayton MT, Fazio VW, Beck DE, Stryker SJ, Wexner SD, Wolff BG, Roberts PL, Smith LE, Sweeney SA, Moore M (1996) Prevention of postoperative abdominal adhesions by a sodium hyaluronate-based bioresorbable membrane: a prospective, randomized, double-blind multicenter study. J Am Coll Surg 183: 297–306

85. Diamond MP (1996) Reduction of adhesions after uterine myomectomy by seprafilm membrane (HAL-F): a blinded, prospective, randomized, multicenter study. Fertil Steril 66:904–910

86. Beck DE, Cohen Z, Fleshman JW, Kaufman HS, Goor HV, Wolff BG (2003) A prospective, randomized, multicenter, controlled study of the safety of seprafilm adhesion barrier in abdominopelvic surgery of the intestine. Dis Colon Rectum 46:1310–1319

87. Fazio VW, Cohen Z, Fleshman JW et al (2005) Reduction in Adhesive small-bowel obstruction by seprafilm adhesion barrier after intestinal resection. Dis Colon Rectum 49:1–11

88. Kusunoki M, Ikeuchi H, Yanagi H et al (2005) Bioresorbable hyaluronate-carboxymethycellulose membrane (seprafilm) in surgery for rectal carcinoma: a prospective randomized clinical trial. Surg Today 35:940–945

89. Hayashi S, Takayama T, Masuda H, Kochi M, Ishii Y, Matsuda M, Yamagata M, Fujii M (2008) A bioresorbable membrane to reduce postoperative small bowel obstruction in patients with gastric cancer. A randomized clinical trial. Ann Surg 247:766–770

Chapter 64
Lower Gastrointestinal Bleeding in the Elderly

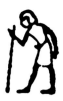

Sylvia S. Kim and Michael E. Zenilman

Introduction

Lower gastrointestinal bleeding is a commonly encountered surgical problem that increasingly affects the elderly. This is not surprising given that the two most commonly cited causes of lower gastrointestinal bleeding, diverticula and arterio-venous malformations (AVMs) have an increasing incidence with increased age. One large population-based study found that the incidence of acute lower gastrointestinal hemorrhage increased over 200-fold from the third to ninth decades of life [1] with an incidence of 500 episodes per 100,000 people per year in the elderly population. Increased age has also been demonstrated to be an independent predictor of both increased length of stay as well as cost of hospitalization in resource utilization studies [2].

The goals of therapy for an elderly patient presenting with a lower gastrointestinal bleed are the same as those for a younger patient: resuscitation and stabilization, localization of the bleeding source, and definitive therapy. However, elderly patients do merit special consideration. Comorbidities are common and can translate into adverse outcomes in elderly surgical patients [3]. Polypharmacy often includes antiplatelet agents such as aspirin or other anticoagulants such as warfarin which may impact the severity of gastrointestinal hemorrhage. Impairments in nutrition, cognition, and functional status may also be present to various degrees and should be considered in the assessment of any geriatric patient.

Etiology

Gastrointestinal changes associated with aging include prolonged intestinal motility, mucosal atrophy, and sequelae of atherosclerosis and decreased splanchnic blood flow.

Diverticular disease and vascular ectasias, both acquired lesions related to aging, account for the majority of cases of lower gastrointestinal bleeding in elderly patients. Other conditions causing intestinal bleeding to which the elderly are predisposed include ischemic colitis and neoplasms.

Diverticula

In most large case series, diverticular bleeding is the leading etiology of lower gastrointestinal bleeding (see Table 64.1) [1, 4–15]. Colonic diverticula are false or pulsion diverticula comprised of mucosa and serosa outpouching in areas where the colonic wall is inherently weaker – at the entrance points of the vasa rectae (see Fig. 64.1). These vessels penetrate through the muscular wall of the colon to supply the colonic muscosa. It is rupture of these vasa rectae that account for diverticular bleeding (see Fig. 64.2). Displacement of the vessel by the enlarging diverticulum and subsequent vessel rupture causes hemorrhage into the diverticulum [16]. Colonic diverticula are quite common in Western societies, affecting at least one half of the elderly population. It accounts for 17–67% of all lower gastrointestinal bleeding (see Table 64.1) and an estimated one third of cases of lower gastrointestinal bleeding in the elderly [8, 11, 17]. The estimated lifetime risk of bleeding caused by diverticular disease ranges between 4–48% [18]. The largest literature review to date, examining over 6,000 cases, placed the estimated risk of significant lower gastrointestinal bleeding from diverticulosis to be 17% [19]. The relative risk for diverticular bleeding is increased for regular users of NSAIDS and acetaminophen [20].

While diverticula are most commonly found on the left colon, they can occur throughout the colon, and there is a greater propensity for bleeding to occur on the right side of the colon [21]. Typically, diverticular bleeding is painless and abrupt in onset. It resolves spontaneously in an estimated 80% of patients [22]. Severity of bleeding can be minimal or massive and life-threatening. Approximately, one third will require blood transfusion and/or invasive evaluation while 5% ultimately require surgical intervention [18].

M.E. Zenilman (✉)
Department of Surgery Johns Hopkins Medicine, Baltimore, MD
and
SUNY Downstate School of Public Health, Brooklyn NY
e-mail: mzenilm1@jhmi.edu

R.A. Rosenthal et al. (eds.), *Principles and Practice of Geriatric Surgery*,
DOI 10.1007/978-1-4419-6999-6_64, © Springer Science+Business Media, LLC 2011

TABLE 64.1 Etiology of lower gastrointestinal bleeding

Author	Mean age Years	Etiology % Diverticular	AVM	Cancer/polyp	Colitis/ulcer	Anorectal	Other	Unknown
Al Qahtani (2002)	70	38	10	2	8	3	3	35
Chaudry (1998)	75	22	12	13	34	18	0.01	0
Czymek (2008)	">65"	66	7	2	5	19	0	0
Green (2005)	70	67	6	3	10	0	0	14
Jensen (1988)	65	17	30	11	9	0	27	6
Kaplan (2001)	73	23	7	20	14	0	11	24
Kok (1998)	63	29	2	9	26	8	5	21
Leitman (1989)	63	33	30	11	13	2	11	0
Longstreth (1997)	67	42	3	9	15	4	14	12
Richter (1995)	70	47	12	11	6	3	7	14
Rios (2005)	80	42	16	7	2	9	5	19
Strate (2003)	66	30	3	13	25	12	9	9
Schmulewitz (2003)	67	35	3	10	14	12	6	23

Source: Data from refs: [1, 4–15]

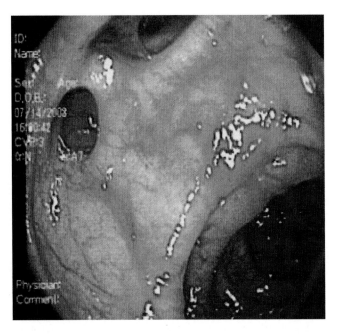

FIGURE 64.1 Endoscopic view of colonic diverticula. Bowel lumen is visible on the right with wide-mouthed diverticula seen on the left.

Arteriovenous Malformations

Arteriovenous malformations (AVMs), also known as vascular ectasias or angiodysplasias, are degenerative lesions that can occur anywhere in the gastrointestinal tract. They are postulated to be caused by chronic, intermittent, low grade obstruction of submucosal veins leading to dilation and tortuosity of submucosal veins, then venules, capillaries, and finally arteries. Ultimately, as precapillary sphincters lose their competency, small arteriovenous communications form (see Fig. 64.3) [22]. Within the colon, they are more commonly found within the right colon, particularly in the cecum

[23, 24]. It is postulated that the increased wall tension found in the cecum as determined by Laplace's Law explains the greater incidence of cecal AVM [25]. An estimated 15% of all massive lower gastrointestinal hemorrhage is attributed to AVM [26] with case series reporting rates from 2 to 30% (see Table 64.1). More commonly, the bleeding is subacute and stops spontaneously, but with a high rate of recurrence – at least 25% in most series [27].

Colitis

Inflammatory bowel disease has a bimodal peak incidence with a second peak incidence in the seventh decade. Both Crohn's disease and ulcerative colitis can manifest as bloody diarrhea. The incidence of massive lower intestinal bleeding attributed to inflammatory bowel disease varies, ranging from 2 to 34% (see Table 64.1).

Ischemic colitis is a condition characterized by impaired perfusion of the colon, typically at the "watershed" areas of the vascular supply such as at the splenic flexure where the distribution of the superior mesenteric artery and inferior mesenteric artery overlap. It is typically a multifactorial process and predominantly a diagnosis of the elderly. Patients often present with bloody diarrhea and abdominal pain. The diagnosis is often made based on clinical presentation. CT scan may be suggestive of colitis. The definitive diagnosis is often made at the time of endoscopy, where mucosal ischemia is evident. Treatment is often supportive with bowel rest, fluid resuscitation and intravenous antibiotics. Patients who present with pneumoperitoneum or peritonitis are manifesting signs of bowel infarction and necrosis and warrant urgent laparotomy. While bloody diarrhea is a hallmark of ischemic colitis, it is an unlikely source of massive blood loss.

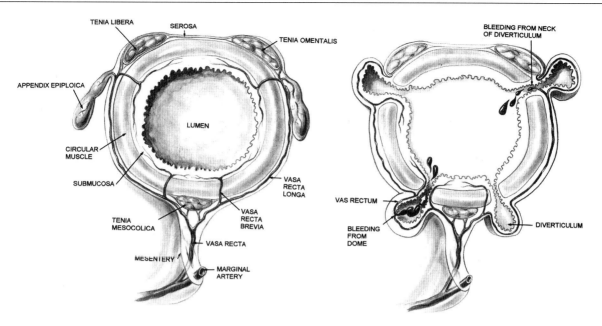

Figure 64.2 Acquired colonic diverticula. Increased intraluminal pressure causes herniation of mucosa and muscularis mucosa through inherently weak sites of the bowel wall where vasa recta pierce the muscularis propria between the teniae coli. Hemorrhage occurs when the vessel ruptures either into the dome or neck of a diverticula.

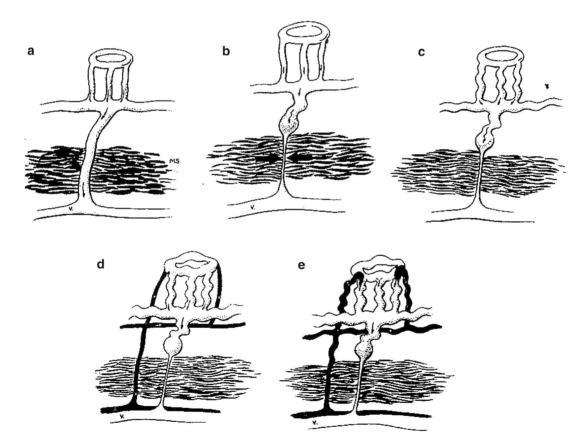

Figure 64.3 Proposed concept of the development of vascular ectasias. (**a**) Normal state of vein perforating muscular layers. (**b**) With muscular contraction or increased intraluminal pressure, the vein is partially obstructed. (**c**) After repeated episodes over many years the submucosal vein becomes dilated and tortuous. (**d**) Later the veins and venules draining into the abnormal submucosal vein become similarly involved. (**e**) Ultimately, the capillary ring becomes dilated, the precapillary sphincter becomes incompetent, and a small arteriovenous communication is present through the ectasia. (From Boley et al. [23] with permission).

Neoplasia

Neoplasms typically present with more insidious blood loss and anemia, and do not ordinarily cause major hemorrhage. However, the passage of blood per rectum in an elderly patient, especially in the setting of anemia, needs to be evaluated completely in order to exclude malignancy, even in the presence of more benign anorectal pathology such as internal hemorrhoids. Classically, right-sided colon cancers present with insidious weakness and anemia, left-sided colon cancers present with obstruction, and rectal cancers present with more bright red blood per rectum and sometimes a palpable mass on rectal exam. While massive hemorrhage is uncommon, it can account for up to 2–20% of lower gastrointestinal bleeding (see Table 64.1). It is an important diagnosis to exclude since surgical intervention is often a mainstay of treatment either for curative intent or even in advanced, palliative settings.

Initial Assessment

The fundamental principles guiding the management of acute lower gastrointestinal bleeding remain the same for nonelderly and elderly patients: initial resuscitation, localization of bleeding site, and definitive therapeutic intervention (see Fig. 64.4).

After initial assessment of hemodynamic stability, resuscitation efforts should begin with intravenous fluid resuscitation via large bore peripheral access. A foley catheter is useful in recording strict intake and outtake levels including the urine output – a commonly used indicator of adequate volume resuscitation. Additional monitoring with a central venous pressure (CVP) monitor may be of particular use in the elderly patient. Cardiac function in the elderly is characterized by a number of significant alterations. Both the chronotropic and inotropic response of aged myocardium to adrenergic stimuli are blunted [28]. As a result, both the maximal heart rate and increase in ejection fraction in response to stress are depressed [29]. In addition, due to preexisting comorbidities, the elderly patient may also be taking beta blockers which could impair their tachycardic response to hypovolemia. Older persons are thus more dependent upon preload to maintain cardiac output in the face of increased demand, making them especially sensitive to the dangers of hypovolemia [30]. Adequate fluid resuscitation is therefore of paramount importance in the elderly patient who presents with gastrointestinal bleeding.

An adequate history and physical exam may help in identifying the etiology of the gastrointestinal bleed. In an elderly patient with impaired cognition or memory lapses, communication with the patient's primary physician or geriatrician and family members may provide additional crucial information. An important aspect of the history-taking is the discovery of use of any anticoagulant or antiplatelet medications. Warfarin toxicity precipitating intestinal bleeding may be amenable to treatment with reversal through transfusion of clotting factors. While NSAID use is more typically associated with upper gastrointestinal bleeding, it can contribute to lower gastrointestinal bleeding as well and has been associated in some series, with an increased need for blood transfusion [31]. History of past episodes of gastrointestinal bleeding from either an upper or lower source should also be elicited. Symptoms such as abdominal pain may be more indicative of an inflammatory process such as ischemic colitis or inflammatory bowel disease. Associated tenderness on physical exam, especially when coupled with leukocytosis on laboratory studies, may warrant further study with imaging modalities such as a CT scan, which are not necessarily considered a standard diagnostic tool in patients presenting with presumed lower gastrointestinal bleeding.

Excluding the possible diagnosis of an upper gastrointestinal bleed is then the next priority in the management algorithm. Brisk blood loss from an upper gastrointestinal source can manifest as apparent bright red blood loss via the rectum in part due to the cathartic effect of the blood itself. Up to 15% of cases of presumed lower gastrointestinal bleeding are actually found to be due to upper gastrointestinal sources [32]. Discriminating between an upper and lower source of bleeding can be accomplished typically either with a nasogastric lavage or upper endoscopy. Bilious, nonbloody nasogastric aspirate typically ensures a lower intestinal source. Nonbilious aspirates are equivocal and should be further evaluated with upper endoscopy.

Rigid proctosigmoidoscopic or anoscopic evaluation is also recommended to rule out potential anorectal sources. If an anorectal source such as hemorrhoids or anal fissure is found, then management is the same as for the general population. Stable patients with minimal symptoms may respond to conservative management with hydration, fiber bulking agents and stool softeners, since these processes are typically associated with constipation and straining. Actively bleeding hemorrhoids, especially in the face of anticoagulation, may require immediate therapy with either banding ligation or formal hemorrhoidectomy.

Diagnosis and Treatment

Attempts to isolate colonic etiologies of gastrointestinal bleeding typically begin with either a colonoscopic evaluation or tagged red cell nuclear medicine study. Most patients who present with lower gastrointestinal bleeding have stopped actively bleeding by the time they present to the hospital for further evaluation.

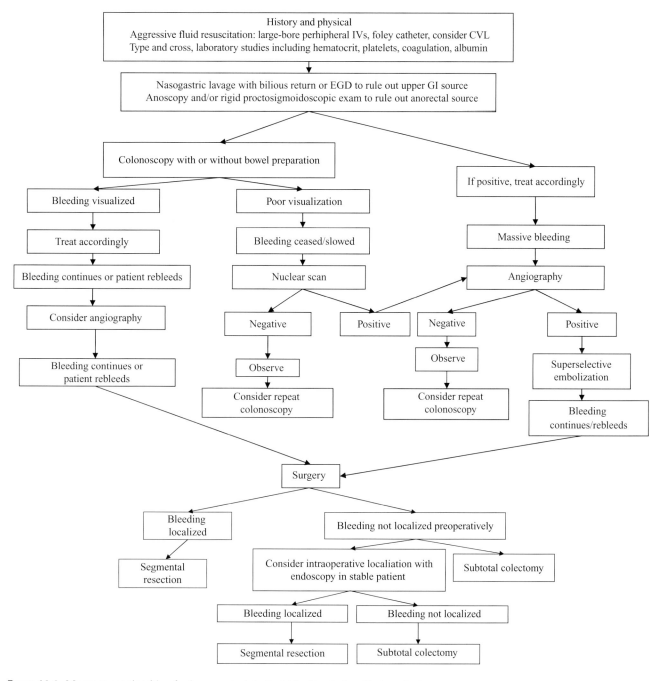

Figure 64.4 Management algorithm for lower gastrointestinal bleeding in the elderly patient.

Colonoscopy

Colonoscopy is a vital diagnostic and potentially therapeutic tool in the management of patients with lower gastrointestinal bleeding. It is the study of choice for patients in whom bleeding has slowed or ceased, and its role in the initial evaluation of actively bleeding patients is increasingly advocated as well. The diagnostic yield varies from 45 to 97% (see Table 64.2) [4, 5, 7, 8, 12, 14, 15, 17, 33–44]. Positive localization of bleeding by endoscopy typically depends on visualization of either active bleeding or stigmata of recent blood loss such as adherent clot, oozing, or presence of a visible vessel.

A number of studies have demonstrated that colonoscopy can be safely and successfully performed in the elderly, with morbidity rates similar to that of the general population [45–47].

Table 64.2 Colonoscopy for the diagnosis of lower gastrointestinal bleeding

Study	Number of patients	Number of positive studies (%)
Al Qahtani	152	45
Angtuaco	39	74
Caos	35	69
Chaudry	85	97
Dell'Abate	80	86
Goenka	166	85
Green	50	96
Gupta	32	84
Jensen (1988)	80	74
Jensen (2000)	121	96
Lin	55	67
Machicado	100	74
Ohyama	345	89
Richter	78	90
Rossini	409	76
Schmulewitz	415	89
Strate	144	89
Tada	206	89
Vellacott	21	95
Wang	205	95

Source: Data from refs: [4, 5, 7, 8, 12, 14, 15, 17, 33–44]

Tolerance of sedation in this patient population should be given extra consideration since the elderly are more sensitive to and require less sedative compared to younger patients with similar body mass index [48]. The American Society for Gastrointestinal Endoscopy [49] guideline for endoscopic practice in the elderly recommends lower initial doses of sedatives and more gradual titration with intensified monitoring when dealing with elderly patients [50]. Careful monitoring with pulse oximetry and aspiration precautions and suctioning should be implemented.

Use of a colonic purge, usually in the form of GoLYTELY (Braintree Laboratories, Inc., Braintree, MA), has been a topic of some debate. The use of bowel preparation is fairly common and appears to be well tolerated when given as either a rapid purge (GoLYTELY given via nasogastric tube over 1 h) [8] or more slowly (GoLYTELY administered as 4 ounces every 5 min until clear) [17]. While studies have shown the safety of colon purge, even in the setting of acute bleeding [17], others argue that any prep may be unnecessary due to the cathartic effect of the blood itself. Proponents of early colonoscopy in an unprepped colon have reported accurate identification of bleeding sources in 76–97% of cases [5, 41].

The therapeutic potential of colonoscopy makes it especially appealing in the management of lower gastrointestinal bleeding, especially in elderly patients whose performance status may place them at a higher operative risk. Colonic AVMs or angiodysplasias are particularly amenable to endoscopic treatment. After a bleeding AVM is identified at colonoscopy, an attempt is made to stop the bleeding with

coagulation by heater probe, bipolar coagulation, or Nd:YAG (Neodymium:Yttrium aluminum garnet) laser therapy. Injection of vasoconstrictors such as epinephrine, may also be used. Success rates of 68–87% have been reported [36, 51, 52]. Endoscopic therapy has become first-line therapy for hemorrhage from angiodysplasia, especially in the elderly [53]. Rates of rebleeding vary and range from 13 to 53% [18, 52, 54]. Rebleeding is often amenable to repeat endoscopic treatment although surgery may be necessary in some patients. Surgical considerations will be discussed later in this chapter. Complications have been reported after endoscopic coagulation and include risk of perforation in approximately 2% of patients [55].

Endoscopic coagulation of hemorrhage from diverticulosis had not been considered feasible in the past; however, some small series have reported successful endoscopic coagulation of bleeding diverticula [37, 56]. It is now reasonable to consider colonoscopy as a plausible approach to this common cause of lower gastrointestinal hemorrhage.

Patients in whom endoscopic evaluation is not feasible may benefit from further study with a nuclear medicine bleeding scan or mesenteric angiography.

Radionuclide Scintigraphy

A nuclear medicine bleeding scan utilizes technetium-99m (99mTc)-labelled sulfur colloid or red blood cells as the imaging tracer for radionuclide scanning. Sulfur colloid marker can be prepared immediately and is rapidly cleared from the circulation; however, rapid uptake in the spleen, liver, and bone marrow can impair localization of bleeding sites. The use of tagged red cells requires some prep time, but the longer half-life of the tracer allows for repeated imaging study that may detect recurrent bleeding.

Both modalities are quite sensitive for the detection of active lower GI bleeding at rates as slow as 0.1 ml/min (see Fig. 64.5) [57]. While the sensitivity of radionuclide imaging for detecting bleeding is widely accepted, the accuracy rates at localizing bleeding are quite variable (see Table 64.3) [58–65]. There are studies that report radionuclide scanning accurately localized active bleeding in over 90% of patients who subsequently underwent surgical resection [66]. These results are not uniform, however, and other studies have shown that when used as a single localizing modality, 42% of patients had an incorrect resection when surgery was based on radionuclide scanning alone [61]. Recognizing this variable accuracy rate, most surgeons will prefer to perform a confirmatory study before proceeding with a segmental resection based on radionuclide scintigraphy alone. In fact, some advocate that the role of radionuclide scanning is to function as a screening test to

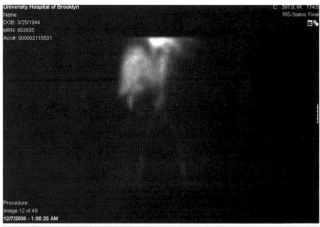

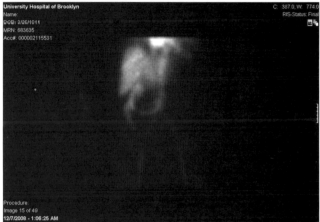

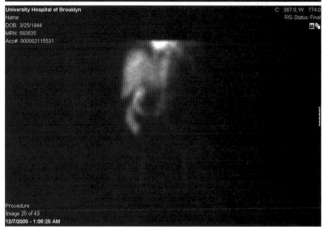

FIGURE 64.5   99mTC-labelled RBC scan images demonstrating tracer uptake at the hepatic flexure suggestive of active bleeding.

TABLE 64.3   Radionuclide imaging for the detection of bleeding

Study	Numberstudies	% Positive	% Correct
Bentley	162	60	52
Bunker	100	41	93
Gutierrez	105	40	88
Hunter	203	26	41
Kester	62	60	82
Levy	287	70	47
McKusick	80	64	83
Suzman	224	51	78

Source: Data from refs: [58–65]

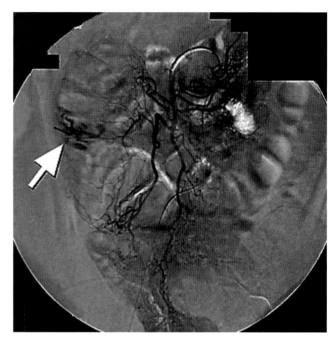

FIGURE 64.6   Mesenteric angiogram showing contrast extravasation at the hepatic flexure suggestive of active bleeding.

demonstrate any increase in rate of positive angiograms when radionuclide scanning was used to screen patients [58, 68].

Mesenteric Angiography

Selective mesenteric angiography utilizes a percutaneous femoral artery catheter to inject radiocontrast dye to allow angiographic visualization of the celiac, superior mesenteric, and inferior mesenteric arterial systems. Active gastrointestinal bleeding is visualized as contrast extravasation into the bowel lumen (see Fig. 64.6). It is less sensitive than radionuclide scintigraphy, with an active bleeding rate of at least 1.0 ml/min required for detection [69]. Bleeding detection rates with angiography vary from 27 to 86% (see Table 64.4) [11, 66, 68, 70–74].

select patients for angiography. The noninvasive, sensitive radionuclide study can select out patients with active bleeding who may benefit from the more invasive, but potentially therapeutic angiogram. This is an area of some debate. The argument in favor of utilizing screening radionuclide scanning is that it increases the yield of positive angiograms following a positive radionuclide scan. One study demonstrated an increase from 22 to 53% in angiography yield when screening radionuclide scans were used [67]. Other studies, however, failed to

TABLE 64.4 Angiography for the diagnosis of lower GI bleeding

Study	Number of studies	% Bleeding sites localized
Cohn	75	35
Colacchio	98	41
Leitman	68	40
Nath	14	86
Ng	49	45
Pennoyer	131	34
Rantis	30	27
Uden	28	57

Source: Data from refs: [11, 66, 68, 70–74]

Positive studies may guide segmental resection in patients who require surgery. Angiography has the additional benefit of being a potentially therapeutic as well as diagnostic intervention. When active bleeding has been identified and the bleeding site localized, transcatheter vasopressin or embolization may be utilized to try to stop the bleeding. Vasopressin acts as a vasoconstrictor and is typically infused at a rate of 0.2–0.4 units/min. If bleeding is controlled, infusion continues for an additional 12–24 h before repeat study and catheter removal. Small series report success rates approaching 90% in controlling hemorrhage utilizing this method [75, 76]. Reported rebleeding rates are not insignificant, ranging from 18 to 57% [77–79]. Infusion of vasopressin should be approached with extreme caution, especially in the elderly population. Systemic absorption of the vasoconstrictor can potentially precipitate myocardial ischemia or peripheral ischemia. Severe coronary artery disease or peripheral vascular disease is considered a contraindication to its use. Other potential complications of vasopressin infusion include hypertension, arrhythmias, hyponatremia, mesenteric thrombosis, and bowel infarction [18].

Another angiographic modality for controlling bleeding is embolization. Historically, early use of transcatheter therapy for colonic bleeding was discouraged due to high rates of colonic infarcts. With the advent of superselective embolization therapy and subsequently lower complication rates, this technique is now widely used. When active bleeding is identified, the catheter is advanced as far distally as possible utilizing even smaller microcatheters. Superselective embolization of individual vessels may then be possible using a variety of agents (microcoils, polyvinyl alcohol particles, and gelfoam). This approach has been used with success for lower gastrointestinal bleeding from a variety of sources including the most common etiologies, namely diverticulosis, angiodysplasia, ulcers, and malignancy [78] and may be an appropriate treatment option for elderly patients with significant comorbidities and moderate to high operative risk. Reported success rates for superselective embolization of active colonic hemorrhage range from 50 to 90%, with rebleeding rates of 10–35% [76, 77, 80–83]. Approximately 20% of patients may have complications from the procedure, including abdominal pain, intestinal ischemia or rarely, intestinal infarction. Late complications of intestinal stricture secondary to ischemia have also been reported.

Angiography may also function as a guide or bridge to surgery. In cases where bleeding has been localized but not controlled, surgery in the form of a segmental resection is indicated. Even temporary control via embolization may be beneficial. If for instance, a large AVM unamenable to complete embolization due to multiple feeding arteries is encountered, angioembolization may provide initial temporary cessation of bleeding, allowing for stabilization of the patient and optimization for definitive surgical treatment. A segmental colon resection can then be offered to the stabilized patient. In this manner, an emergency surgery situation with its inherent high morbidity and mortality is converted into a more elective and thereby safer surgical situation. Surgical intervention will be addressed in the following section.

Surgery

Indications for surgery in patients with lower gastrointestinal bleeding typically include: hemodynamic instability, persistently active bleeding, recurrent bleeding, and significant transfusion requirements typically stated as more than six units of packed red blood cells in a 24-h period [49]. With these guidelines in mind, one should also consider that because of the diminished physiologic reserve found in elderly patients and the significantly increased morbidity and mortality associated with surgery in an emergency setting, early surgical intervention is sometimes preferable. While elective surgery may be well tolerated in an elderly patient, the same procedure done in an emergency setting is accompanied by significant morbidity and mortality.

In patients meeting surgical criteria in whom bleeding is localized, a segmental resection should be done. The decision to proceed with an anastomosis versus creation of an ostomy is multifactorial and should be tailored to the individual patient. In an emergency setting and in the face of hemodynamic instability, most surgeons would not risk creation of an anastomosis and would opt for creation of a colostomy or ileostomy. Patients in whom bleeding has not been localized require a subtotal colectomy. Blind segmental colectomy in such instances is associated with rebleeding rates up to 75% and subsequent mortality rates approaching 50% [84].

The presence of associated comorbidities and need for urgent surgery are cited as independent factors associated with increased morbidity and mortality in patients with severe, acute lower gastrointestinal bleeding, regardless of age [85]. One large study of octogenarians undergoing major intestinal surgery demonstrated that ASA (American Society of Anesthesiologists) score and emergency status were the best predictors of surgical outcome in the elderly. Those who underwent emergency surgery had a statistically significant increased mortality rate, 32% vs. 1.7% [86]. While emergency surgery for lower gastrointestinal bleeding has consistently been associated with an increased mortality, the impact may be even more pronounced in the elderly population undergoing emergency colectomy for bleeding. One retrospective study of emergency colectomy for LGIB found an increase in mortality from 21% for patients less than 70 years to 37% for patients aged 70 years and older [87]. Postoperative complications have also been found to portend a worse prognosis and high mortality rate as evidenced by the Veterans Administration National Surgical Quality Improvement Project (VA-NSQIP). In their database of elderly patients who underwent surgery, patients with more than 48 h of ventilatory assistance, acute renal failure, and systemic sepsis had mortality rates of 39%, 52%, and 45% respectively [88]. Other studies have found similar postoperative mortality rates of about 50% in patients who required postoperative ICU care [89].

Patients who undergo surgery may not be able to return home when they are ready for discharge from the hospital. Elderly patients undergoing abdominal surgery may require nursing home or rehabilitation facility placement at least 50% of the time [89]. Again, whether the surgery is done in an emergency setting is an important factor. In elderly patients who undergo emergency surgery, discharge to skilled nursing facilities instead of home is even higher; in one series 90% compared to over 70% of patients were able to go home after surgery done in an elective setting [86].

Small Intestinal Bleeding

Bleeding from the small bowel can be a diagnostic and therapeutic challenge. Small bowel sources are classified as lower gastrointestinal bleeding since by definition they occur distal to the Ligament of Treitz. However, some advocate considering them as a separate entity given the intrinsic difficulties inherent to adequate small bowel evaluation [90]. Small bowel bleeding accounts for 2–15% of lower gastrointestinal bleeding [8] and is usually secondary to AVMs [90, 91]. Other potential small bowel sources include tumors, lymphoma, ulcers, and Crohn's disease. The length of small bowel, distance from a natural orifice, and redundancy make it difficult to evaluate thoroughly in its entirety. Most commonly used tools to evaluate the small bowel are push enteroscopy, contrast radiography, and capsule endoscopy. Capsule endoscopy is becoming the preferred modality for evaluating the small bowel for sources of bleeding. The diagnostic yield has been demonstrated to be superior to both push endoscopy (55–70% vs. 25–30%) [92, 93] and small bowel contrast radiography (31% vs. 5%) [94].

CASE STUDY

An 81-year-old female presented with bright red blood per rectum and light-headedness. Her past history was significant for hypertension and diabetes. She lived at home with her daughter but functioned quite independently, requiring no assistance with her Activities of Daily Living. On arrival in the Emergency Room, the patient was found to be hypotensive, but with a normal heart rate. On physical examination, the patient was lethargic, but arousable and able to answer questions appropriately. She appeared to be well-nourished. Her lung and heart sounds were clear. Her abdomen was soft and nontender, and the digital rectal examination was unremarkable. Immediate fluid resuscitation was started with large bore peripheral access, and a foley catheter was inserted. Her laboratory studies showed a 10-point decrease in her hematocrit compared to baseline values from routine studies one year prior. Coagulation panel was normal. Blood transfusion was initiated with improvement in her blood pressure and urine output. Nasogastric lavage demonstrated bilious, nonbloody return, and rigid proctosigmoidoscopic evaluation showed normal-appearing internal hemorrhoids without fresh blood in the anal canal. The patient was admitted to the intensive care unit for close monitoring, continued resuscitation, and further workup. A central line was placed for central venous pressure monitoring and continued fluid resuscitation. Colonoscopy without bowel preparation was done later the same day and demonstrated pandiverticular disease and old blood, but no evidence of active bleeding. The patient remained stable with no further passage of blood per rectum. The following day the patient had passage of a large amount of blood per rectum and transient hypotension. Immediate resuscitation with IV fluid and additional blood transfusion resulted in stabilization of the patient. Urgent angiogram was obtained and demonstrated bleeding from diverticula in the area of the sigmoid colon. Superselective embolization was performed with cessation of bleeding.

(continued)

CASE STUDY (continued)

The patient was transferred back to the ICU for further stabilization, monitoring, and optimization for surgery. She had no further episodes of bleeding and developed no abdominal symptoms. She was started on a diet which she tolerated. Patient and family were counselled that given the risk of rebleeding, surgery was recommended. The benefit of elective surgical intervention compared to the increased morbidity and mortality associated with a possible emergency scenario was emphasized to them as well. She was medically optimized and several days later underwent a mechanical bowel prep followed by an elective sigmoid resection with primary anastomosis. She tolerated the surgery well. Her subsequent postoperative course was unremarkable. She worked with the in-house physical therapists and was eventually discharged to home.

CASE STUDY: DISCUSSION

This case demonstrates several key features in the evaluation of an elderly patient who presents with lower gastrointestinal bleeding. First, while the patient is clearly volume-depleted due to her acute blood loss, she does not manifest tachycardia. This may be due to both diminished chronotropic response seen in the elderly as well as her prescribed beta blocker. Restoration of adequate preload is of paramount importance, and in this patient, was guided by both urine output and central venous monitoring. Nasogastric lavage or upper endoscopy is used to rule out an upper gastrointestinal source which can account for up to 15% of presumed lower gastrointestinal hemorrhages [32]. Early colonoscopy is being used increasingly and is well-tolerated in the elderly population. While the diagnostic yield for colonoscopy ranges from 45 to 97% [4, 5, 7, 8, 12, 14, 15, 17, 33–44], in our patient, it failed to localize the bleeding. Subsequent angiography when our patient had recurrent bleeding was able to localize and control the bleeding. Superselective embolization is being used increasingly in cases of colonic hemorrhage, and remains an attractive treatment modality especially for patients who are at high risk for surgical intervention. In patients who are surgical candidates, embolization can also be utilized as a bridge to surgery, allowing time for adequate resuscitation and optimization, as was the case here. In light of the risk of recurrent bleeding from her diverticula, surgery was advised. It has been shown that some elderly patients can tolerate even major abdominal surgery well when done in an elective setting [86]. Emergency surgery, however, is not well tolerated, as evidenced by significant morbidity and mortality. Postoperative mortality rates for emergency colon resection in elderly patients are typically over 30% [86, 87]. Therefore, an elective segmental resection after medical optimization was offered to this patient. Avoiding the potential increased morbidity of an emergency surgery likely contributed to the ultimate disposition home for this patient. Being discharged to home would have been unlikely in the aftermath of an emergency colectomy. Most patients (up to 90%) who do survive such a scenario are ultimately discharged to a nursing home or rehabilitation facility [86]. This transition from independent living to institutional care can be distressing for some elderly patients.

References

1. Longstreth GF (1997) Epidemiology and outcome of patients hospitalized with acute lower gastrointestinal hemorrhage: a population-based study. Am J Gastroeneterol 92:419–424
2. Comay D, Marshall JK (2002) Resource utilization for acute lower gastrointestinal hemorrhage: the Ontario GI bleed study. Can J Gastroeneterol 16(10):677–82
3. Extermann M (2000) Measurement and impact of comorbidity in older cancer patients. Crit Rev Oncol Hematol 35(3):181–200
4. Al Qahtani AR, Satin R, Stern J et al (2002) Investigative modalities for massive lower gastrointestinal bleeding. World J Surg 26(5):620–625
5. Chaudhry V, Hyser MJ, Gracias VH et al (1998) Colonoscopy: the initial test for acute lower gastrointestinal bleeding. Am Surg 64(8):723–728
6. Czmek R, Kempf A, Roblick UJ et al (2008) Surgical treatment concepts for acute lower gastrointestinal bleeding. J Gastrointest Surg 12(12):2212–2220
7. Green BT, Rockey DC, Portwood G (2005) Urgent colonoscopy for evaluation and management of acute lower gastrointestinal hemorrhage: a randomized controlled trial. Am J Gastroenterol 100(11):2395–2402
8. Jensen DM, Machicado GA (1988) Diagnosis and treatment of severe hematochezia. The role of urgent colonoscopy after purge. Gastroenterology 95(6):1569–1574
9. Kaplan RC, Heckbert SR, Koepsell TD et al (2001) Risk factors for hospitalized gastrointestinal bleeding among older persons. Cardiovascular Health Study Investigators. J Am Geriatr Soc 49(2):126–133
10. Kok KY, Kum CK, Goh PM (1998) Colonoscopic evaluation of severe hematochezia in an Oriental population. Endoscopy 30(8):675–680

11. Leitman IM, Paull DE, Shires GT III (1989) Evaluation and management of massive lower gastrointestinal hemorrhage. Ann Surg 209(2):175–180

12. Richter JM, Christensen MR, Kaplan LM et al (1995) Effectiveness of current technology in the diagnosis and management of lower gastrointestinal hemorrhage. Gastrointest Endosc 41(2):93–98

13. Rios A, Montoya MJ, Rodriguez JM et al (2005) Acute lower gastrointestinal hemorrhages in geriatric patients. Dig Dis Sci 50(5):898–904

14. Schmulewitz N, Fisher DA, Rockey DC (2003) Early colonoscopy for acute lower GI bleeding predicts shorter hospital stay: a retrospective study of experience in a single center. Gastrointest Endosc 58(6):841–846

15. Strate LL, Sungal S (2003) Timing of colonoscopy: impact on length of hospital stay in patients with acute lower intestinal bleeding. Am J Gastroenterol 98(2):317–322

16. Meyers MA, Baer JW, Alonso DR et al (1976) Pathogenesis of bleeding colonic divertiulosis. Gastroenterology 71:577–583

17. Caos A, Benner KG, Manier J et al (1986) Colonoscopy after Golytely preparation in acute rectal bleeding. J Clin Gastroenterol 8(1):46–49

18. Vernava AM, Moore BA, Longo WE et al (1997) Lower gastrointestinal bleeding. Dis Colon Rectum 40:846–858

19. Rushford AJ (1956) The significance of bleeding as a symptom in diverticulitis. J R Soc Med 49:577–579

20. Aldoori WH, Giovannucci EL, Rimm EB et al (1998) Use of acetaminophen and non-steroidal anti-inflammatory drugs: a prospective study and the risk of symptomatic diverticular disease in men. Arch Fam Med 7:255–260

21. Stollman NH, Raskin JB (1999) Diverticular disease of the colon. J Clin Gastroenterol 29:241–252

22. Bokhari M, Vernava AM, Ure T et al (1996) Diverticular hemorrhage in the eldery – is it well tolerated? Dis Colon Rectum 39:191–195

23. Boley SJ, Sammartano R, Adams A et al (1977) On the nature and etiology of vascular ectasias of the colon. Degenerative lesions of aging. Gastroenterology 72:650–660

24. Sorbi D, Conio M, Gostout CJ (1999) Vascular disorders of the small bowel. Gastrointest Endosc Clin N Am 9(1):71–92

25. Boley SJ, Brandt LJ, Frank MS (1981) Severe lower intestinal bleeding: diagnosis and treatment. Clin Gastroenterol 10(1):65–91

26. Reinus JF, Brandt LJ (1994) Vascular ectasias and diverticulosis. Common causes of lower intestinal bleeding. Gastroenterol Clin North Am 23(1):1–20

27. Breen E, Murray JJ (1997) Pathophysiology and natural history of lower gastrointestinal bleeding. Semin Colon Rectal Surg 8:128–138

28. Lernfelt B, Wikstrand J, Svanborg A et al (1991) Aging and left ventricular function in elderly healthy people. Am J Cardiol 68:547–549

29. Fleg JL, O'Connor F, Gerstenblit G et al (1995) Impact of age on the cardiovascular response to dynamic upright exercise in healthy men and women. J Appl Physiol 78:890–900

30. Rodeheffer RJ, Gerstenblith G, Becker LC et al (1984) Exercise cardiac output is maintained with advancing age in healthy human subjects: cardiac dilatation and increased stroke volume compensate for a diminished heart rate. Circulation 69:203–213

31. Yong D, Grieve P, Keating J (2003) Do nonsteroidal anti-inflammatory durgs affect the outcome of patients admitted to hospital with lower gastrointestinal bleeding? N Z Med J 116(1178):517

32. Reinus J, Brandt L (1991) Lower intestinal bleeding in the elderly. Clin Geriatr Med 7:301–319

33. Angtuaco TL, Reddy SK, Drapkin S et al (2001) The utility of urgent colonoscopy in the evaluation of acute lower gastrointestinal tract bleeding: a 2-year experience from a single center. Am J Gastroenerol 96(6):1782–1785

34. Dell'Abate P, Del Rio P, Soliani P et al (2002) Value and limits of emergency colonoscopy in cases of severe lower gastrointestinal haemorrhage. Chir Ital 54(2):123–126

35. Goenka MK, Kochhar R, Mehta SK (1993) Spectrum of lower gastrointestinal hemorrhage: an endoscopic study of 166 patients. Indian J Gastroenterol 12(4):129–131

36. Gupta N, Longo WE, Vernava AM III (1995) Angiodysplasia of the lower gastrointestinal tract: an entity readily diagnosed by colonoscopy and primarily managed nonoperatively. Dis Colon Rectum 38(9):979–982

37. Jensen DM, Machicado GA, Jutabha R et al (2000) Urgent colonoscopy for the diagnosis and treatment of severe diverticular hemorrhage. N Engl J Med 342(2):78–82

38. Lin CC, Lee YC, Lee H et al (2005) Bedside colonoscopy for critically ill patients with acute lower intestinal bleeding. Intensive Care Med 31(5):743–746

39. Machicado GA, Jensen DM (1997) Acute and chronic management of lower gastrointestinal bleeding: cost-effective approaches. Gastroenterologist 5(3):189–201

40. Ohyama T, Sakura Y, Ito M et al (2000) Analysis of urgent colonoscopy for lower gastrointestinal tract bleeding. Digestion 61(3):189–192

41. Rossini FP, Ferrari A, Spandre M et al (1989) Emergency colonoscopy. World J Surg 13(2):190–192

42. Tada M, Shimizu S, Kawai K (1991) Emergency colonoscopy for the diagnosis of lower intestinal bleeding. Gastroenterol Jpn 26(Suppl 3):121–124

43. Vellacott KD (1986) Early endoscopy for acute lower gastrointestinal haemorrhage. Ann R Coll Surg Engl 68(5):243–244

44. Wang CY, Won CW, Shieh MJ (1991) Aggressive colonoscopic approaches to lower intestinal bleeding. Gastroenterol Jpn 26(Suppl 3):125–128

45. Zerey M, Paton BL, Khan PD et al (2007) Colonoscopy in the very elderly: a review of 157 cases. Surg Endosc 21(10):1806–1809

46. Karajeh MA, Sanders DS, Hurlstone DP (2006) Colonoscopy in elderly people is a safe procedure with a high diagnostic yield: a prospective comparative study of 2000 patients. Endoscopy 38(3):226–230

47. Clarke GA, Jacobsen BC, Hammett RJ et al (2001) The indications, utilization and safety of gastrointestinal endoscopy in an extremely elderly patient cohort. Endoscopy 33(7):580–584

48. Yano H, Iishi H, Tatsuta M et al (1998) Oxygen desaturation during sedation for colonoscopy in elderly patients. Hepatogastroenterology 45(24):2138–2141

49. Davila RE, Rajan E, Adler DG et al (2005) ASGE Guideline: the role of endoscopy in the patient with lower-GI bleeding. Gastrointest Endosc 62(5):656–660

50. Qureshi WA, Zuckerman MJ, Adler DG et al (2006) ASGE guideline: modifications in endoscopic practice for the elderly. Gastrointest Endosc 63(4):566–569

51. Trudel JL, Fazio VW, Sivak MV (1988) Colonoscopic diagnosis and treatment of arteriovenous malformations in chronic lower gastrointestinal bleeding. Clinical accuracy and efficacy. Dis Colon Rectum 31(2):107–110

52. Santos JC, Aprilli F, Guimaraes AS (1988) Angiodysplasia of the colon: endoscopic diagnosis and treatment. Br J Surg 75(3):256–258

53. Sharma R, Gorbien MJ (1995) Angiodysplasia and lower gastrointestinal tract bleeding in elderly patients. Arch Intern Med 155(8):807–812

54. Richter JM, Hedberg SE, Athanasoulis CA et al (1984) Angiodysplasia. Clinical presentation and colonoscopic diagnosis. Dig Dis Sci 29(6):481–485

55. Naveau S, Aubert A, Poynard T et al (1990) Long-term results of treatment of vascular malformations of the gastrointestinal tract by neodymium YAG laser photocoagulation. Dig Dis Sci 35(7):821–826

56. Bloomfeld RS, Rockey DC, Shetzline MA (2001) Endoscopic therapy of acute diverticular hemorrhage. Am J Gastroenterol 96:2367–2372
57. Alavi A, Dann RW, Baum S et al (1977) Scintigraphic detection of acute gastrointestinal bleeding. Radiology 124:753–756
58. Bentley DE, Richardson JD (1991) The role of tagged red blood cell imaging in the localization of gastrointestinal bleeding. Arch Surg 126(7):821–824
59. Bunker SR, Lull RJ, Tanasescu DE et al (1984) Scintigraphy of gastrointestinal hemorrhage: superiority of 99Tc red blood cells over 99mTc sulfur colloid. Am J Roentgenol 143(3):543–548
60. Gutierrez C, Mariano M, Vander Laan T et al (1998) The use of technetium-labeled erythrocyte scintigraphy in the evaluation and treatment of lower gastrointestinal hemorrhage. Am Surg 64(10):989–992
61. Hunter JM, Pezim ME (1990) Limited value of technetium 99m-labeled red cell scintigraphy in localization of lower gastrointestinal bleding. Am J Surg 159(5):504–506
62. Kester RR, Welch JP, Sziklas JP (1984) The 99m-labeled RBC scan. A diagnostic method for lower gastrointestinal bleeding. Dis Colon Rectum 27(1):47–52
63. Levy R, Barto W, Gani J (2003) Retrospective study of the utility of nuclear scintigraphic-labeled red cell scanning for lower gastrointestinal bleeding. ANZ J Surg 73(4):205–209
64. McKusick KA, Froelich J, Callahan RJ et al (1981) 99mTc red blood cells for detection of gastrointestinal bleeding: experience with 80 patients. Am J Roentgenol 137(6):1113–1118
65. Suzman MS, Talmor M, Jennis R et al (1996) Accurate localization and surgical management of active lower gastrointestinal hemorrhage with technetium-labeled erythrocyte scintigraphy. Ann Surg 224(1):29–36
66. Ng DA, Opelka FG, Beck DE et al (1997) Predictive value of technetium Tc99m-labeled red blood cell scintigraphy for positive angiogram in massive lower gastrointestinal hemorrhage. Dis Colon Rectum 40:471–477
67. Gunderman R, Leef JA, Lipton MJ et al (1998) Diagnostic imaging and the outcome of acute lower gastrointestinal bleeding. Acad Radiol 5(Suppl 2):S303–S305
68. Pennoyer WP, Vignati PV, Cohen JL (1997) Mesenteric angiography for lower gastrointestinal hemorrhage: are there predictors for a positive study? Dis Colon Rectum 40:1014–1018
69. Steer ML, Silen W (1983) Diagnostic procedures in gastrointestinal hemorrhage. N Engl J Med 309:646–650
70. Cohn SM, Moller BA, Zieg PM et al (1998) Angiography for preoperative evaluation in patients with lower gastrointestinal bleeding: are the benefits worth the risks? Arch Surg 133(1):50–55
71. Colacchio TA, Forde KA, Patsos TJ et al (1982) Impact of modern diagnostic methods on the management of active rectal bleeding: ten year experience. Am J Surg 143(5):607–610
72. Nath RL, Sequeira JC, Weitzman AF et al (1981) Lower gastrointestinal bleeding: diagnostic approach and management conclusions. Am J Surg 141(4):478–481
73. Rantis PC Jr, Harford FJ, Wagner Rh et al (1995) Technetium-labelled red blood cell scintigraphy: is it useful in acute lower gastrointestinal bleeding? Int J Colorectal Dis 10(4):210–215
74. Uden P, Jiborn H, Jonsson K (1986) Influence of selective mesenteric arteriography on the outcome of emergency surgery for massive, lower gastrointestinal hemorrhage. A 15-year experience. Dis Colon Rectum 29(9):561–566
75. Kickuth R, Rattunde H, Gschossmann J et al (2008) Acute lower gastrointestinal hemorrhage: minimally invasive management with microcatheter embolization. J Vasc Interv Radiol 19(9):1289–1296
76. Silver A, Bendick P, Wasvary H (2005) Safety and efficacy of superselective angioembolization in control of lower gastrointestinal hemorrhage. Am J Surg 189:361–363
77. Koh D, Luchtefeld M, Kim D et al (2008) Efficacy of transarterial embolization as definitive treatment in lower gastrointestinal bleeding. Colorectal Dis 11:53–59
78. Tan K, Wong D, Sim R (2008) Superselective embolization for lower gastrointestinal hemorrhage: an institutional review over 7 years. World J Surg 32:2707–2715
79. Karanicolas P, Colquhoun P, Dahike E et al (2008) Mesenteric angiography for the localization and treatment of acute lower gastrointestinal bleeding. Can J Surg 51(6):437–441
80. Guy GE, Shetty PC, Sharma RP et al (1992) Acute lower gastrointestinal hemorrhage: treatment by superselective embolization with polyvinyl alcohol particles. Am J Roentgenol 159(3):521–526
81. Peck DJ, McLoughlin RF, Hughson MN et al (1998) Percutaneous embolotherapy of lower gastrointestinal hemorrhage. J Vasc Interv Radiol 9(5):747–751
82. Patel TH, Cordts PR, Abcarian P et al (2001) Will transcather embolotherapy replace surgery in the treatment of gastrointestinal bleeding? Curr Surg 58(3):323–327
83. Gady JS, Reynolds H, Blum A (2003) Selective arterial embolization for control of lower gastrointestinal bleeding: recommendations for a clinical mananagement pathway. Curr Surg 60(3):344–347
84. Eaton AC (1981) Emergency surgery for acute colonic haemorrhage – a retrospective study. Br J Surg 68(2):109–112
85. Rios A, Montoya M, Rodriguez J et al (2007) Severe acute lower gastrointestinal bleeding: risk factors for morbidity and mortality. Langenbecks Arch Surg 392:165–171
86. Louis DJ, Hsu A, Brand MI et al (2009) Morbidity and mortality in octogenarians and older undergoing major intestinal surgery. Dis Colon Rectum 52:59–63
87. Bender JS, Wiencek RG, Bouwman DL (1991) Morbidity and mortality following total abdominal colectomy for massive lower gastrointestinal bleeding. Am Surg 57(8):536–540
88. Hamel MB, Henderson WG, Khuri SF et al (2005) Surgical outcomes for patients aged 80 and older: morbidity and mortality from noncardiac surgery. J Am Geriatr Soc 53(3):424–429
89. Ganai S, Lee F, Merrill A et al (2007) Adverse outcomes of geriatric patients undergoing abdominal surgery who are at high risk for delirium. Arch Surg 142(11):1072–1078
90. Prakash C, Zuckerman GR (2003) Acute small bowel bleeding: a distinct entity with significantly different economic implications compared with GI bleeding from other locations. Gastrointest Endosc 58:330–335
91. Zuckerman GR, Prakash C, Askin MP et al (2000) Technical review: the evaluation and management of occult and obscure GI bleeding. Gastroenterology 118:201–221
92. Adler DG, Knipschield M, Gostout C (2004) A prospective comparison of capsule endoscopy and push enteroscopy in patients with GI bleeding of obscure origin. Gastrointest Endosc 59(4):492–498
93. Ell C, Remke S, May A et al (2002) The first prospective controlled trial comparing wireless capsule endoscopy with push enteroscopy in chronic gastrointestinal bleeding. Endoscopy 34(9):685–689
94. Costamagna G, Shah SK, Riccioni ME et al (2002) A prospective trial comparing small bowel radiographs and video capsule endoscopy for suspected small bowel disease. Gastroenterology 123(4):999–1005

Chapter 65
Ischemic Disorders of the Large and Small Bowel

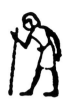

Jack R. Oak and Gregorio A. Sicard

CASE STUDY

The patient is a 76-year-old male with a history of coronary artery disease who presents with an 18 month history of vague abdominal pain. The patient reports of pain after meals and approximately a 70 lbs weight loss over this time. The patient has been seen by the local gastroenterologist and has undergone both upper and lower endoscopy, which were both normal. The patient presented back to the emergency room with more complaints of abdominal pain and bloating. As part of his emergency room workup, the patient had a CT scan of the abdomen and pelvis. This revealed a tight stenosis in the superior mesenteric artery (SMA) as well as a large 6 cm abdominal aortic aneurysm (Figs. 65.1 and 65.2). Vascular surgery was consulted. It was decided that, since the patient was a poor open surgical candidate and that the patient had suitable aortic anatomy for an aortic endograft, a staged endoluminal procedure to address both the SMA stenosis and the large abdominal aortic aneurysm was recommended.

The patient first underwent a percutaneous mesenteric angiography with successful stent placement in the SMA (Fig. 65.3). The following day after an uneventful recovery, the patient underwent successful endoluminal repair of his abdominal aortic aneurysm.

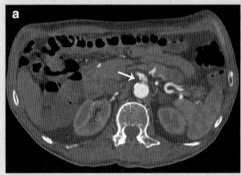 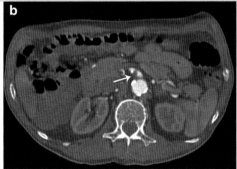

Figure 65.1 (a, b) Axial images from CT scan at the level of the superior mesenteric artery. *Arrow* pointing at the stenotic lesion at the origin of the SMA.

(continued)

J.R. Oak (✉)
Department of Vascular Surgery, Barnes-Jewish Hospital,
University of Washington School of Medicine,
St. Louis, MO, USA
e-mail: jroak@stanfordalumni.org

R.A. Rosenthal et al. (eds.), *Principles and Practice of Geriatric Surgery*,
DOI 10.1007/978-1-4419-6999-6_65, © Springer Science+Business Media, LLC 2011

CASE STUDY (continued)

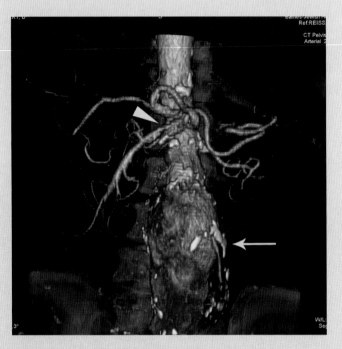

FIGURE 65.2 3D reconstruction from the CT scan demonstrating both the SMA lesion (*arrowhead*) and the large infrarenal abdominal aortic aneurysm (*arrow*).

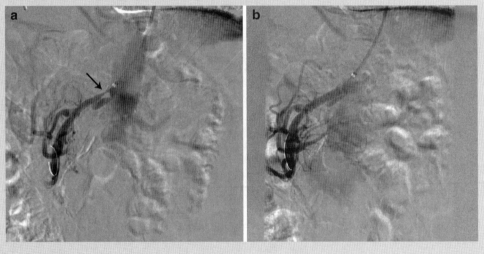

FIGURE 65.3 (**a**) Transbrachial mesenteric angiogram demonstrating the tight stenosis at the origin of the SMA. Note that an 0.018″ wire was able to traverse across the lesion. (**b**) Angiogram after successful deployment of a balloon expandable stent across the lesion.

Anatomy

Intestinal ischemia is usually a disease that affects the elderly. It is useful to categorize it as acute or chronic because of the different presentations of patients and the urgency of treatment. It can also be further subdivided by etiology; causes include arterial insufficiency secondary to thrombosis or embolus, venous thrombosis, and nonocclusive mesenteric ischemia (NOMI).

To understand the etiology of mesenteric ischemia, it is helpful to review the basic vascular anatomy of the gastrointestinal (GI) tract. The gut is supplied basically by three arteries: celiac axis (CA), SMA, and inferior mesenteric artery (IMA). The celiac axis branches almost immediately into the common hepatic, left gastric, and splenic arteries. The celiac axis communicates with the SMA recirculation via the gastroduodenal artery and the pancreaticoduodenal arcades. The SMA originates from the aorta usually approximately 1 cm below the celiac axis. This occurs at the level of the L1 vertebra. The SMA supplies the midgut, and its major branches are the inferior pancreaticoduodenal branches, middle colic artery, right colic artery, ileal branches, and ileocolic artery. The middle colic artery comes off the proximal SMA and supplies the transverse colon. It also communicates directly with branches of the IMA. The ileocolic artery is the terminal branch of the SMA and supplies the terminal ileum, cecum, and ascending colon. The IMA is the most distal and smallest of the mesenteric arteries and is also a ventral branch of the aorta. It arises approximately 6–7 cm below the SMA, which corresponds to the level of the L3 vertebra. It supplies the hindgut, which includes the distal transverse colon, descending colon, sigmoid colon, and rectum. The left colic artery communicates with the SMA via the marginal artery.

To understand the pathophysiology of mesenteric ischemia, it is important to understand the anatomic collateral pathways. For collateral circulation between the CA and the SMA, the principle pathways are the gastroduodenal and pancreaticoduodenal arteries. Unusual anatomic variations can also provide collateral flow, such as a replaced right hepatic artery or a pancreatic or middle colic artery originating from the CA. In addition, there is an infrequent but well-recognized collateral pathway known as the arc of Buhler, which represents a direct collateral pathway between the CA and the SMA. This is thought to be due to persistence of an embryonic ventral segmental artery.

There are three major anastomotic pathways between the SMA and the IMA, the most significant of which is the marginal artery of Drummond. This artery runs within the mesentery of the colon and gives rise to the vasa recta. It receives branches from the ileocolic, right colic, middle colic, and the left colic arteries. It usually runs close to the mesenteric border of the colon. Normally, this artery is not particularly large; but with occlusion of the SMA, it can enlarge significantly. The arc of Riolan also lies within the mesentery, but is much closer to its base. This collateral connects the middle and left colic arteries (Fig. 65.4). The final potential collateral pathway between the SMA and IMA is the meandering or wandering mesenteric artery. Occasionally, this is markedly hypertrophied arc of Riolan, and other times, there is a distinct anastomotic pathway between the SMA and IMA. The IMA can be collateralized not only by the SMA, but also by the lumbar branches of the aorta, as well as from the hypogastric artery and its branches.

The venous drainage of the gut is principally via the splenic vein for the foregut, the superior mesenteric vein (SMV) for the midgut, and the inferior mesenteric vein (IMV) for the hindgut. These vessels all drain into the portal vein and hence through the liver.

Mesenteric blood vessels are highly reactive; and, accordingly, mesenteric blood flow can fluctuate between 10 and 35% of cardiac output [1]. They react to a large variety of endogenous cytokines and exogenous medications. The teleological reason given for the vasoreactivity is the widely varying metabolic needs of the gut based on the fasting and fed states. Absolute blood flow through the CA and the SMA ranges from 300 to 1,200 ml/min [2]. At rest (fasting state), the mesenteric flow is low due to high resistance with low diastolic flow with flow reversal, which is typical of high resistance beds. In the fed state, there is both systolic and continuous diastolic flow.

Although the nutritional state of the individual is often the principle determinant of blood flow, there is also extensive extrinsic and intrinsic control of splanchnic blood flow. Sympathetic tone to the gut is supplied by preganglionic cholinergic fibers of the greater splanchnic nerves [3]. These synapse in the paired celiac ganglia next to the CA. Postganglionic adrenergic fiber stimulation of the celiac axis ganglia results in vasoconstriction of the mesenteric arteries and arterioles [4, 5]. The rennin–angiotensin axis and vasopressin can both cause profound vasoconstriction. These substances are released in settings of hypovolemia [6]. The net effect of their secretion is to preserve cerebral and renal circulation at the expense of the mesenteric circulation.

Arterial Mesenteric Ischemia

Acute Mesenteric Ischemia

The most dramatic and feared form of mesenteric ischemia is *acute* mesenteric ischemia. Despite broad advances in diagnostic capabilities, surgical techniques, and perioperative management, the mortality associated with acute mesenteric ischemia is high, ranging from 60 to 90% in most series [7, 8]. The risk factors for acute mesenteric ischemia are essentially those associated with advanced age, including cardiac arrhythmias, low cardiac output states secondary to congestive heart failure, severe valvular cardiac disease or recent myocardial infarction, generalized atherosclerosis, and intra-abdominal malignancy.

Acute arterial insufficiency to the small bowel results from occlusion of the SMA. Approximately 50% of acute SMA occlusions are due to emboli [9]. Most of the emboli are cardiac in origin. They originate from left atrial or ven-

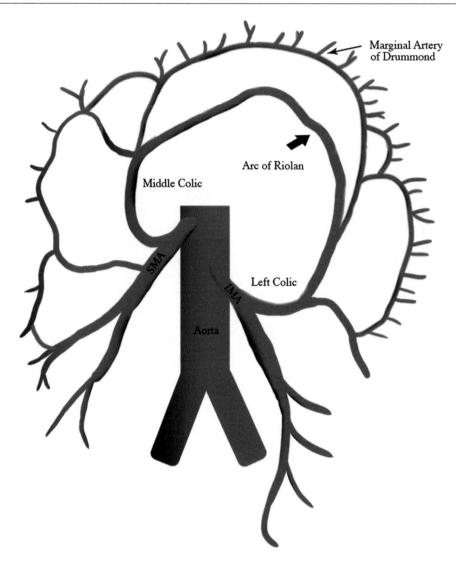

Figure 65.4 Collateral pathways between the SMA and IMA. The more constant marginal artery of Drummond connects the SMA and IMA via distal branches, giving of the vasa recta branches to the bowel. The more variable arc of Riolan connects the SMA to the IMA more proximally, usually through the middle colic artery to the left colic artery.

tricular mural thrombi or from cardiac valvular lesions. They often occur in the setting of cardiac arrhythmias, particularly atrial fibrillation, or immediately following acute myocardial infarction. Although the emboli can lodge at the origin of the SMA, approximately 85% lodge more distally, usually 3–10 cm beyond the origin of the SMA where it begins to taper. The typical point of occlusion is just distal to the middle colic artery (Fig. 65.5). It is important to realize that in approximately 20% of cases, patients with SMA emboli also have emboli to other vascular beds [10]. Often intestinal ischemia caused by the embolus is exacerbated or compounded by reflexive mesenteric vasoconstriction. This compounds the ischemic insult to the bowel. Other more unusual causes include dissections of the SMA occurring in isolation or as part of extensive aortic dissection [11].

Acute mesenteric ischemia can occur up to 25% of the time in the setting of acute in situ thrombosis superimposed on preexisting atherosclerotic lesions. Although the SMA is most commonly affected, the celiac axis may be involved. Often even though these patients present acutely, on questioning they give a history consistent with chronic mesenteric ischemia (CMI), which will be discussed later in this chapter. Anatomically, these lesions occur at the origin of the SMA and not distally, as with embolic disease.

Acute mesenteric ischemia can also be nonocclusive (NOMI).. The cause of NOMI is usually a low-flow state in the setting of preexisting atherosclerotic lesions, often coupled with the administration of vasoconstricting medications or digitalis. Such causes of low-flow states are most often seen in the setting of cardiac failure or sepsis. The diagnosis of

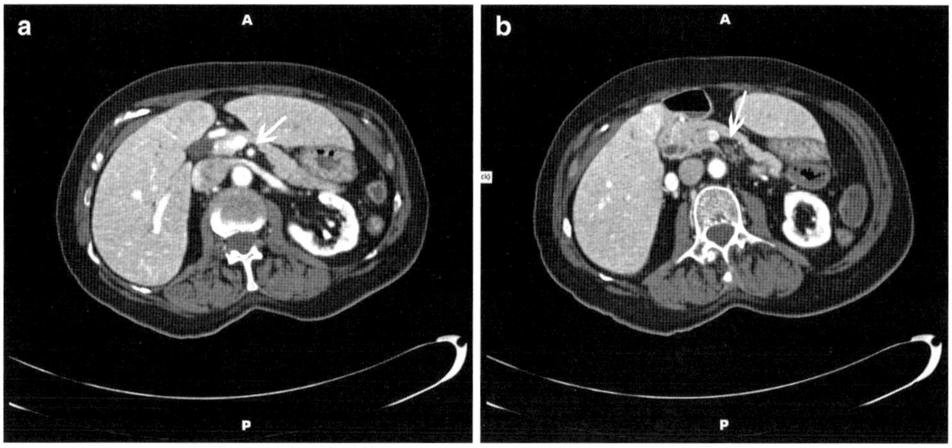

Figure 65.5 CT angiogram view of a patient who presented with a history of acute abdominal pain in the setting of atrial fibrillation. Patient had to be off anticoagulation due to upcoming knee surgery. (**a**) *White arrow* pointing to SMA at the level right above middle colic artery as it courses behind the neck of pancreas. (**b**) *White arrow* showing acute occlusion in the SMA at the level of the uncinate process.

NOMI is based on a high index of clinical suspicion followed by arteriography. It requires an even higher index of suspicion than other causes of acute mesenteric ischemia because the presentation is sometimes more insidious. Mortality in the setting of NOMI is high, approaching 70%, and reflects not only the morbidity associated with mesenteric ischemia, but also probably more likely the underlying medical conditions that precipitated the episode of mesenteric ischemia [12].

The overall incidence of NOMI is decreasing despite the aging population. The likely reasons are the widespread use of systemic vasodilators in coronary care units and the improved treatment for cardiogenic shock [13]. The best chance for avoiding poor clinical outcome with NOMI resides in making the correct diagnosis and treating the underlying precipitating cause of the NOMI. It has been postulated that low flow results in peripheral hypoxemia and a paradoxical splanchnic vasospasm, which precipitates intestinal ischemia. Laboratory studies have confirmed that mesenteric vasoconstriction, intestinal hypoxia, and ischemia/reperfusion injury may play a role in the pathogenesis of NOMI. In low-flow states, the neurohormonal mediators of mesenteric vasoconstriction appear to be vasopressin and angiotensin [14]. The use of digoxin is common in patients with NOMI, and in in vitro and in vivo studies it has been shown to enhance mesenteric arterial vasoconstriction [15]. Once set in motion, mesenteric vasospasm can become persistent, even after correcting the underlying precipitating event. The persistence of prolonged vasoconstriction is responsible for the development of intestinal ischemia and subsequent infarction in NOMI [16].

Chronic Mesenteric Ischemia

Chronic mesenteric ischemia (CMI) is a relatively rare diagnosis, and there is a paucity of surgical literature involving its treatment. This being said, it appears that the number of elective operations for CMI is increasing; and given the general aging population, it is expected to continue to increase [17]. CMI is most common during late middle age. Most patients are smokers; and in contradistinction to vascular disease in other beds, most of the patients (60%) are female. In addition, there is a high incidence of other factors for vascular disease, including a high incidence of hypertension, coronary artery disease, and cerebrovascular disease [18]. It is interesting to note that, although clinically significant CMI is uncommon, asymptomatic atherosclerosis of the mesenteric circulation is common, with autopsy series showing significant stenoses in approximately 50% of celiac axes, in 30% of the superior mesenteric arteries, and in 30% of inferior mesenteric arteries [19]. The prevalence of mesenteric atherosclerotic disease increases with age, with two-thirds of patients over 80 years of age having significant stenoses.

Councilman's report was the first to recognize the syndrome of CMI with its pathognomonic symptom of postprandial pain [20]. He described three patients who presented with epigastric and midabdominal pain following eating. Typically, this pain occurs 1–2 h after a meal. The degree of pain correlates well with the quantity and the fat content of the ingested meal. Although the pain is typically described as a dull, cramping pain, there is some variability in presentation, with symptoms ranging from vague pain to severe sharp pains that can penetrate to the back. In advance cases, patients may have persistent or continuous pain, and sometimes it progresses to acute mesenteric ischemia (in situ thrombosis of mesenteric vessels in the setting of advanced occlusive disease) [21]. Because of the postprandial pain, the patients often experience what has been termed "food fear." Food fear results in the patient being unwilling to eat, which in turn results in the most common physical finding of CMI: weight loss. The weight loss has been described as malignant cachexia without malignancy. Frequently, these patients have been evaluated for a GI malignancy prior to making the correct diagnosis of mesenteric ischemia [22]. It is worthwhile to note, however, that a few patients present without weight loss. Presenting symptoms other than abdominal pain and weight loss that are also GI in nature, include nausea, vomiting, diarrhea, and constipation. It is thought that the symptoms may relate to the distribution of the vascular occlusive disease, with foregut ischemia (celiac distribution) leading to nausea and vomiting, midgut ischemia (SMA) leading to the common postprandial abdominal pain and subsequent weight loss, and hindgut ischemia (inferior mesenteric ischemia) leading to constipation [23].

On physical exam, the most obvious and common finding in patients with CMI is evidence of weight loss. Signs of peripheral vascular disease may also be noted as well as the presence of an abdominal bruit. Unfortunately, the diagnosis of CMI is often delayed. Given the nonspecific symptoms with which patients present, they are often evaluated for other more common diseases, such as cholecystitis, liver disease, peptic ulcer disease, and occult malignancy. These patients have undergone extensive evaluations prior to being referred to a vascular surgeon for evaluation. Due to the prolonged nature of their illnesses, nonspecific laboratory findings may include evidence of malnutrition, such as anemia, hypoalbumenemia, hypocholesterolemia, and evidence of impaired immune function. Patients have frequently undergone both plain and contrast radiologic studies of their abdomen and GI tract, but these tests are of little value. They have also often undergone both upper and lower endoscopy, which may occasionally document evidence of ischemia.

Diagnosis

Regardless the etiology of mesenteric ischemia, the key to improved patient outcome is diagnosis in a timely fashion. Unfortunately, the signs and symptoms of mesenteric arterial disease may be protean in nature, and by the time a definite diagnosis is reached, the patient may have already sustained bowel necrosis. Acute mesenteric occlusion must be considered in any patient who presents with acute onset of abdominal pain and a history of cardiac disease or recent arterial catheterization.

In regards to CMI, the most common scenario is an elderly female with a history of tobacco abuse, abdominal pain, and weight loss. Careful questioning will usually elucidate a history of postprandial pain in the periumbilical or epigastric location. This "intestinal angina" is thought to result from inability of the stenotic or occluded visceral vessels to meet the hyperemic demands of active digestion. Patients come to associate pain with eating, and this may induce a pattern of food avoidance that results in profound malnutrition.

In NOMI, the diagnosis should be entertained when elderly patients present with the risk factors previously mentioned, including acute myocardial infarction with cardiogenic shock, congestive heart failure, arrhythmias, hypovolemic shock from sepsis, or hemorrhage or in the setting of burns and pancreatitis. In addition, the use of splanchnic vasoconstrictors including digitalis and alpha agonists are commonly seen in patients who develop NOMI. Although patients with SMA occlusion usually present with pain out of proportion to their physical findings, a significant portion of patients with NOMI (20–25%) may not have severe abdominal pain [24]. When present, the pain is often less severe or more variable in intensity, character, and location than it is in classic occlusive arterial mesenteric ischemia. Even in patients without pain, if there is unexplained abdominal distension, GI bleeding, fever, diarrhea, nausea, or vomiting, the diagnosis of NOMI should be entertained in these high-risk patients. As with other forms of mesenteric ischemia, once a patient develops abdominal tenderness or localized peritonitis, it indicates that the mesenteric ischemia has progressed to bowel infarction.

Leukocytosis and elevated serum lactate levels are nonspecific findings that may help to confirm the diagnosis of acute mesenteric ischemia. Typically, the history and physical exam reveals pain that is severe, unrelenting, and usually not well localized – usually "pain out of proportion to exam." Progression to localized peritonitis is a late finding that suggests the presence of transmural infarction or perforation. Indeed, time is of the essence, and in those settings where detailed radiographic imaging is not readily available, a history and physical exam strongly suggestive of acute mesenteric ischemia mandates exploratory laparotomy for revascularization and assessment of bowel viability.

Imaging Modalities

Radiographic imaging plays an increasingly significant role in the diagnosis of mesenteric ischemia. Plain radiographs are commonly used to exclude other causes of the acute abdomen, such as bowel obstruction or a perforated viscus. As an early diagnostic aid in acute mesenteric ischemia, plain radiographs lack sensitivity, being reported as normal in up to 25% of cases involving acute mesenteric ischemia [25]. Unfortunately, definitive plain radiographic findings of acute mesenteric ischemia are those associated with progressive loss of tissue integrity, such as pneumatosis and portal venous air and with a much poorer prognosis at this stage.

Duplex Ultrasound

Duplex ultrasound of the mesenteric vessels is noninvasive and does not require administration of nephrotoxic contrast agents. Its utilization has primarily been in the diagnosis of CMI. As with all duplex examination, this modality is operator-dependent. An optimal patient setting, such as a thin patient with minimal bowel gas, is required to achieve quality results. Duplex ultrasonography accurately identifies high-grade stenoses of the celiac artery and SMA. In nonselected patient groups, adequate visualization may be 60%, but in more selected studies of patients thought to have CMI, the reported technical adequacy approaches 100% [26, 27].

Studies from Dartmouth and the Oregon Health Sciences University attempted to established duplex criteria for the diagnosis of splanchnic artery stenosis and occlusion [28]. Based on repeat studies, they have determined the peak systolic velocity (PSV) and end-diastolic velocity (EDV) that correlates with a significant degree of stenosis. For the SMA, a PSV of >275 cm/s correlated with a >70% angiographic stenosis with sensitivity of 92% and specificity of 96% [29]. An EDV of >45 cm/s correlated with a >50% angiographic stenosis with sensitivity of 90% and specificity of 91% [27]. For the celiac artery, a PSV of >200 cm/s suggests a stenosis of >70% with sensitivity of 90% and specificity of 91%. Retrograde hepatic artery flow is 100% predictive of a severe celiac artery stenosis or occlusion. Celiac EDV >55 cm/s indicates a stenosis of >50% with sensitivity of 93% and specificity of 100%.

CT Angiography

Catheter angiography has long been the gold standard in delineating mesenteric arterial anatomy. However, as the availability of multidetector helical CT scans has spread, the ability to rapidly acquire high-quality CT angiographic images has made this modality the study of choice when evaluating a patient with possible mesenteric ischemia [30]. A significant amount of information can be obtained about the central arterial and venous circulation with CT angiography. Accurate timing of contrast injection and fine slices (0.5–1.5 mm) through the upper abdomen usually provides excellent visualization of the celiac artery and SMA distributions (Fig. 65.6). Other causes of abdominal pathology can also be assessed with CT. Nonspecific findings for bowel ischemia or infarction may include mesenteric stranding, bowel wall edema, or even air within the bowel wall or mesenteric vessels. The exact timing of intravenous contrast administration is tailored to the specific clinical question. Usually, a noncontrasted study is performed first to establish a baseline of the appearance of the bowel wall. The traditional use of "positive" oral contrast agents detracts from

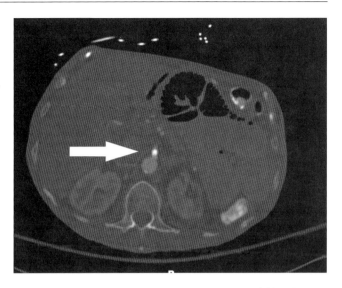

Figure 65.6 CT angiogram demonstrating heavily calicific plaque at the origin of the SMA.

image quality, and most visceral computed tomography angiography (CTA) protocols recommend the use of a "negative" oral contrast agent, such as water, given before the scan. The negative contrast agent prevents image artifact from pooled areas of high opacification within the intestinal tract and actually enhances the ability to see bowel wall enhancement (or lack thereof) in the late arterial phase of the contrast bolus. Three-dimensional reconstructions may be generated from the raw CT data set, yielding a spatially oriented image that allows for the clinician to evaluate the diseased segments from different perspectives (Fig. 65.7). Some protocols may offer the use biphasic scanning, a technique borrowed from standard pancreatic and liver studies. A delayed set of images are acquired approximately 1 min after the administration of IV contrast to obtain portal venous phase imaging.

Magnetic Resonance Angiography

Magnetic resonance angiography (MRA) provides excellent evaluation of the splanchnic vessels (Fig. 65.8). MRI/MRA is noninvasive and avoids the risk of allergic reaction with iodinated contrast agents. There are several caveats to the use of MRI/MRA, such as avoidance of patients with ferrous-containing implants and concern for gadolinium-induced nephrogenic systemic fibrosis (NSF) in patients with impaired renal function.

Anatomic imaging of the visceral vessels relies on contrast-enhanced MRI techniques; noncontrast three-dimensional phase-contrast MRA identifies only 66% of angiographic stenoses and creates some false-positive results [31]. The most common error of visceral MRA is overestimation of the stenosis. This weakness may result from the

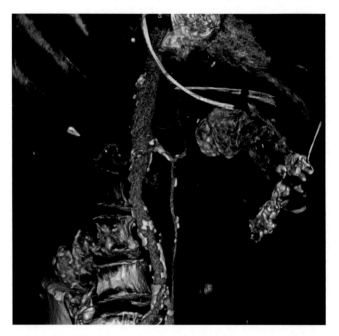

Figure 65.7 3D reconstruction from CT angiogram of the mesenteric vessels. Lateral projection. Notice common trunk for both SMA and celiac axis. Also note heavy calicification at the common trunk.

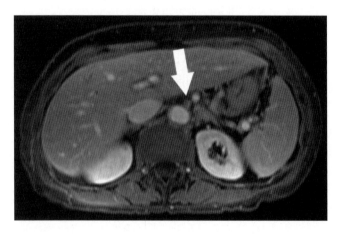

Figure 65.8 MR angiogram demonstrating nonfilling of the SMA secondary to calcific plaque at the origin. *White arrow* demonstrating non-opacified SMA.

relatively poor spatial resolution of MRA. Even on the best systems, resolution is limited to 1 mm³. Gadolinium-enhanced MRA currently does not provide sufficient resolution to show distal emboli; nonocclusive, low-flow states; small vessel occlusion; or vasculitis [32]. Meaney and associates evaluated 14 patients with CMI; three-dimensional contrast-enhanced MRA had a sensitivity of 100% and a specificity of 87% in the overall detection of 50% or greater visceral artery stenosis [33]. The lack of specificity was due to false-positive diagnosis of IMA stenoses. Looking only at the subset of celiac artery and SMA data, the sensitivity and specificity were 100% for the detection of 50% or greater stenosis. In a

similar, more recent study by Carlos et al., two blinded observers reviewed gadolinium-enhanced MRA studies and compared them with conventional angiography in 26 patients suspected to have CMI. The overall accuracies for the detection of 50% or greater stenosis or occlusion in the celiac artery, SMA, or IMA were 95 and 97%.

Secondary signs of mesenteric ischemia, such as fat or bowel wall thickening, which are routinely delineated by CT, are more difficult to assess with MRI. In general, the anatomic evaluation of the mesenteric arteries is limited to the proximal celiac artery and SMA only, and the evaluation of SMA branches or IMA is limited by the spatial resolution of MRI techniques. MRA is not routinely the first imaging study to obtain in the setting of AMI because of time delay. The utility of MRA in CMI depends on the quality of the instrumentation, the sophistication of the software, and the skill of the interpreting radiologist, especially when other modalities are available.

Catheter-Based Arteriography

Finally, catheter-based arteriography is a time-tested modality offers superbly detailed images of the visceral arterial tree, and venous patency may also be assessed on delayed images. Due to the time urgency in the treatment of AMI, as well as the burgeoning availability of CTA, the use of catheter angiography prior to laparotomy is now distinctly uncommon. In the setting of CMI, diagnostic angiography may be combined with therapeutic intervention in selected candidates (Fig. 65.9). To document stenoses of the origins of the SMA and celiac axes, lateral views are best. Usually, involvement of at least two mesenteric vessels is required to diagnose symptomatic CMI. It is unusual for a patient to be symptomatic from occlusion of only one vessel. Additional evidence of chronic ischemia is evidenced by hypertrophy of collateral pathways, including the marginal artery of Drummond and the arc of Riolan (Fig. 65.10). Relative drawbacks of this technique include the need for arterial instrumentation and administration of nephrotoxic contrast agents.

Treatment

Once the diagnosis of mesenteric ischemia is made, prompt surgical intervention is necessary. However, the approach for acute mesenteric thrombosis from an embolus is entirely different from that of thrombosis.

Unfortunately in the acute setting, the patient has usually presented with advanced stages of ischemia and thus emergent exploration is warranted. The abdomen is explored through a generous midline incision, typically extending from xiphoid to pubic symphysis. The main goal of the

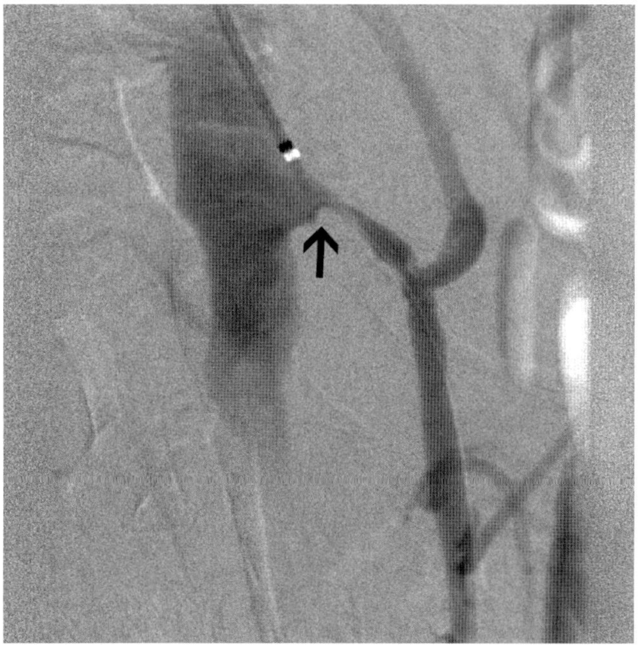

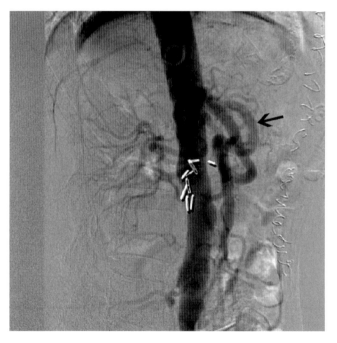

Figure 65.9 Lateral projection of SMA during catheter arteriography. Note wire crossing lesion in preparation for deployment of a stent.

Figure 65.10 *Lateral view* of SMA angiogram. Note large collateral between celiac axis and SMA as demonstrated by *black arrow.*

but potentially viable bowel and infarcted bowel. Obvious signs of bowel necrosis include bowel wall that is an ashen, dull gray color, lacking the normal glistening sheen, and bowel that does not exhibit peristalsis. Other adjunctive measures include trying to obtain Doppler signals along the antimesenteric side of the bowel wall, intravenous administration of fluorescein, and using a Wood's lamp to see the extent of bowel perfusion. Unfortunately, some patients have such obvious, extensive bowel infarction that after resection they would be left with insufficient bowel to sustain life. In such cases, it is appropriate to close without attempting to restore blood flow or resect the infarcted bowel.

Bowel that appears severely ischemic may be viable after revascularization. Thus, in all but the case of obvious bowel necrosis, the surgeon should proceed with revascularization before resecting any intestine. The questionable bowel should be kept moist in well covered with warmed saline solution during the remainder of the case. At any time after revascularization that there is any questionable appearing bowel, it is always safe to plan for a "second-look" laparotomy after 24–48 h to see if more bowels can be either saved or sacrificed during this second exploration.

Exposure of the SMA for embolectomy is achieved by retraction of the transverse colon cephalad and the small bowel and its mesentery inferiorly. One can trace the middle colic artery down to its junction to the SMA as a means to identify the SMA. An incision is made in the small bowel mesentery near the root of the mesentery, directly over the area where the superior mesenteric vessels lie. A segment of the proximal SMA and its branches (jejunal branches and the middle colic artery) are controlled. The artery is opened transversely if direct repair after embolectomy is planned, or longitudinally if the vessel is diseased and may need to be closed with a potentially saphenous vein patch. Proximal embolectomy is performed with a 3 or 4 French (F) embolectomy balloon catheter. With extraction of the embolus, pulsatile inflow should be expected. Distal embolectomy is performed with a smaller catheter, typically 2 or 3 French embolectomy catheter. Difficulty in passing a catheter down multiple branches of small size adds to the complexity of performing the distal embolectomy (Fig. 65.11). An alternative or adjunct to balloon embolectomy of the distal mesenteric vessels is for the surgeon to place a hand on either side of the mesentery and "milk" thrombotic material out of the vessels. When all thrombus is removed, the arteriotomy is closed primarily or with vein patch, and flow is reestablished.

In regards to CMI, it is indicated to offer revascularization whenever a patient is symptomatic. The ultimate goal is to restore a normal mesenteric circulation, thereby allowing normalization of the nutritional status and alleviation of abdominal pain. Three basic techniques are available for revascularization: bypass grafting, transaortic endarterectomy, and more recently, angioplasty with possible stenting.

explorations is to (1) determine and confirm the cause of the extent of the mesenteric disease and (2) assess the viability of the bowel. The extent and pattern of bowel ischemia can offer valuable clues concerning the cause of bowel ischemia, thereby aiding in planning for revascularization.

The bowel assessment for viability is made by visual inspection, with an attempt to differentiate between ischemic

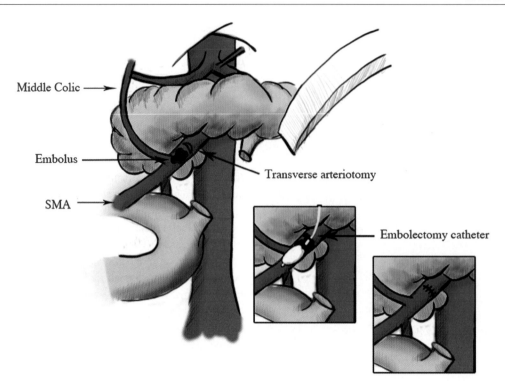

Middle Colic

Embolus

SMA

Transverse arteriotomy

Embolectomy catheter

Figure 65.11 Embolectomy for acute mesenteric ischemia. Embolus typically lodged at the takeoff of middle colic from SMA. A small transverse arteriotomy is made with an 11-blade. Passing a 2 or 3 French embolectomy catheter distally to remove lodged embolus and a 3 or 4 French catheter proximally will usually restore pulsatile inflow. The arteriotomy is then closed with nonabsorbable monofilament suture.

The choice of therapy must be individualized not only to the patient's anatomic lesions, but also to the patient's comorbidities. The ideal procedure for CMI remains a subject of debate [34]. Preoperative evaluation of patients for mesenteric revascularization is not different from preparing for any other major vascular reconstruction. As indicated by the patient's general medical condition, he or she should be evaluated for coronary artery disease, cerebrovascular disease, or renal vascular disease.

It is also important to realize that these patients are often nutritionally debilitated and as a result are both volume-contracted and anemic. These conditions should be approached in an urgent, aggressive manner prior to surgery. Because of the high incidence of multisystem disease, invasive intraoperative monitoring with radial artery and pulmonary artery catheters is recommended. As part of this goal, it is hoped that the progression of mesenteric ischemia to visceral infarction is avoided as well. In unusual circumstances, prophylactic mesenteric revascularization is undertaken in patients undergoing major aortic reconstruction who have had incidentally identified significant mesenteric artery stenoses [35]. The rationale for doing this is that the patient may be at increased risk for perioperative visceral infarction due to unexpected hypovolemia, hypotension, or disruption of the collateral circulation by the periaortic dissection. In the absence of performing aortic procedures, prophylactic mesenteric revascularization is not usually

recommended. As previously noted, mesenteric artery occlusive disease is widely present in autopsy series, but most of it was asymptomatic.

Mesenteric Bypass

Several techniques are available for performing mesenteric bypasses. Because mesenteric ischemia usually results from multiple-vessel disease, multiple-vessel reconstruction is usually recommended. Bypasses are generally categorized into two broad techniques: antegrade and retrograde. Antegrade bypass grafts generally originate from the supraceliac aorta, which is an excellent site for originating a bypass graft because it is usually spared significant atherosclerotic or aneurysmal disease. Autologous material or synthetic grafts can be used without any documented difference in efficacy. Polytetrafluoroethylene (PTFE) and Dacron grafts have been used. If there is any question about contamination at the time of surgery (e.g., if bowel resection is necessary), an autologous conduit, usually the saphenous vein, should be used.

The supraceliac aorta is usually exposed transabdominally, which can be done through either a midline incision or bilateral subcostal incisions. After thorough exploration of the abdomen, the supraceliac aorta is exposed by first mobilizing the lateral segment of the left lobe of the liver, which is retracted inferiorly and to the right. The gastrohepatic omentum is divided and the lesser sac entered. Care is taken not to injure the esophagus, which is easily identified by palpating the nasogastric tube within its lumen. The right crus of the diaphragm is divided with electrocautery. In this fashion, approximately 7–110 cm of distal thoracic and proximal abdominal supraceliac aorta can be isolated. The celiac axis and SMA are skeletonized. The rationale for doing multivessel revascularization is to maximize symptomatic relief and prevent symptomatic recurrence and visceral infarction, which may result from single-graft failure [36]. Supraceliac aortic control is obtained with a partially occluding clamp if possible. This step helps limit the large increase of afterload on the heart that can result from supraceliac cross-clamping, as well as renal and visceral ischemia. If a synthetic graft is used, a bifurcated graft of appropriate size is chosen. The proximal anastomosis is sewn in an end-to-side fashion to the aorta. One limb is then sewn in end-to-end to the celiac axis. In a similar fashion, an end-to-end anastomosis is performed to the SMA. Sometimes it is necessary to completely cross-clamp the supraceliac aorta, but the proximal anastomosis can usually be completed in 20 min or less, and this amount of visceral and renal ischemia time is well tolerated. A straight graft to the SMA is placed with reimplantation of the celiac axis onto that graft. In addition, as mentioned, the SMA anastomosis can usually be performed to the proximal SMA anterior to the pancreas. If necessary, due to extensive disease within the proximal SMA, the graft can be tunneled behind the pancreas with construction of the distal anastomosis to the SMA distal to the point where the SMA has passed through the uncinate process of the pancreas.

An alternative technique uses an autologous conduit. This is done in the setting of the contaminated or clean-contaminated case secondary to the need for bowel resection. One effective and simple technique is to perform an inline bypass using saphenous vein to the SMA, with the hood of the vein graft forming a patch angioplasty at the origin of the celiac axis. In this fashion, both the celiac axis and the SMA are revascularized. Once revascularization is completed, blood flow is restored to the viscera. This is done in coordination with the anesthesia team to avoid declamping hypotension. Following this step, the bowel is carefully inspected to ensure that adequate flow has been restored.

Occasionally, the supraceliac aorta is not suitable as the origin for the antegrade bypass because of aneurysmal or atherosclerotic disease or secondary to previous surgery at the diaphragmatic hiatus. Also, some patients cannot tolerate supraceliac cross-clamping. In this situation, retrograde bypass from either the infrarenal aorta or the iliac vessels can be performed. The infrarenal aorta is also often used as the inflow source if mesenteric revascularization is being performed at the time of concomitant infrarenal aortic reconstruction. The synthetic aortic prosthesis provides an excellent inflow vessel. Standard transperitoneal exposure of the iliac vessels or of the infrarenal aorta is performed. It is necessary to mobilize the ligament of Treitz fully, and then the proximal SMA is isolated below the inferior border of the pancreas at the base of the small bowel mesentery. Once again, the choice of conduit can be saphenous vein or prosthetic graft. The proximal anastomosis is performed to either the distal infrarenal aorta or the proximal common iliac artery in an end-to-side fashion. The conduit is left with a long, gentle curve around the base of the mesocolon, which not only facilitates the anastomosis to the SMA, but also helps avoid kinking, which tends to occur with short grafts, particularly saphenous vein grafts [37]. The anastomosis to the SMA can be performed in an end-to-end or end-to-side fashion. In the event that the celiac axis is to be revascularized at the same time, a bifurcated graft can be used, or a "piggyback" graft can be sewn onto the SMA graft. The celiac axis is exposed as previously described. Once again the graft is tunneled to a retropancreatic tunnel and can be anastomosed to the celiac axis or the common hepatic artery.

These operations, as might be expected, are associated with significant perioperative mortality, which averages approximately 6% for patients undergoing revascularization for CMI [38]. These patients, despite their significant comorbidities, have an approximately 75–80% 3-year survival following surgery. Graft thrombosis with visceral infarction is a significant cause of both early and late mortality [39]. The rate of symptomatic graft failure has been documented to be 15% at an average follow-up of 38 months. Another more recent series by McMillan et al. has shown that an objective primary patency rate of 89% at 72 months was obtained in a single series. In that series, there was no difference between primary patency rates in patients undergoing retrograde or antegrade bypass. There were also no differences noted for the type of conduit used. Overall, given the extensive comorbidities of these patients and their underlying atherosclerotic disease, visceral revascularization is a durable procedure, and the morbidity and mortality of the procedure are acceptable.

Transaortic Mesenteric Endarterectomy

For occlusive disease limited to the origins of the visceral vessels, transaortic mesenteric endarterectomy is a well-described technique for mesenteric revascularization. The advantages of endarterectomy are that (1) it eliminates the occlusive lesion; (2) it is an anatomic revascularization and is therefore not subject to turbulent flow or problems with graft compression or alignment; and (3) it provides an autogenous method for multiple-vessel reconstruction [40]. The patients are prepped for surgery in a similar manner with all the precautions mentioned earlier. The visceral abdominal aorta can be exposed through a thoracoabdominal incision or a midline or extended left subcostal incision using medial visceral rotation. The advantage of medial visceral rotation is that it avoids entering the thoracic cavity. Exposure of the upper abdominal aorta is accomplished via left-sided medial visceral rotation. First, the splenic flexure of the colon is mobilized by dividing its peritoneal attachments, and then the descending colon is mobilized along its lateral peritoneal reflection. In a similar fashion, the spleen is mobilized by dividing its lateral peritoneal attachments, and it is rotated medially. The dissection plane is established in the retroperitoneum and lies between Gerota's fascia and the peritoneal envelope and posterior to the tail of the pancreas. Once the spleen and pancreas are mobilized medially, the left renal vein is identified and is dissected free from the renal hilum to the vena cava. Division of the adrenal and lumbar branches of the renal vein allows the vein to be retracted inferiorly, thereby providing optimal exposure of the perirenal aorta. The left crus of the diaphragm is divided along the left anterior lateral aorta. Once it is divided, the distal thoracic aorta is exposed, which is the site of proximal aortic control. The side of distal control depends on the extent of the planned endarterectomy. Usually, infrarenal aortic control is necessary because of the proximity of the SMA to the renal arteries. The origins of all the visceral vessels are circumferentially dissected free. When circumferentially dissecting the vessels, care is taken to palpate the vessels to make sure the dissection proceeds beyond the margins of the disease. If the disease goes well beyond the ostium, aortic endarterectomy is not possible.

Once vascular isolation is obtained, an aortotomy is performed. The extent of the aortotomy depends on whether endarterectomy of the renal vessels is planned. A standard endarterectomy is performed around the base of each vessel. Usually with ostial disease, gentle eversion endarterectomy suffices and good endpoints are obtained. Once the endarterectomy is completed, the aortotomy is closed. On occasion, it is not possible to complete the SMA endarterectomy through the transaortic incision. In this case, an arteriotomy can be made on the SMA, and a good endpoint can be obtained. If the more distal SMA is diseased, and it is thought that endarterectomy cannot suffice, a longitudinal arteriotomy can be performed and then closed with a patch angioplasty using saphenous vein.

This operation has proved to be durable. Its drawback is that the patient must be able to tolerate an extensive abdominal dissection as well as a supraceliac aorta cross-clamp. In addition, there is the anatomic constraint that the occlusive disease must be limited to the ostium.

Percutaneous Options

The final option for mesenteric revascularization is percutaneous transluminal mesenteric angioplasty. The application of angioplasty techniques to mesenteric ischemia is in its infancy. Currently, there are no standard guidelines for the application of angioplasty, and the literature suggest that it is being reserved for patients considered to be "extremely poor surgical candidates," which historically have included the elderly [41]. However, most of the reports, coming from small, single-center experiences, do seem to implicate that the percutaneous approach may offer advantages in the short term, such as shorter hospital stay and less perioperative complications than the open surgical approach [42]. The benefits from the percutaneous approach, however, come at the cost of lower primary patency rates and higher reintervention rates [43]. For such reasons, percutaneous options may be ideal for the high-risk elderly patient – where long-term durability is not the main concern; but rather achieving symptomatic relief to help improve the nutritional status of the patient at minimal morbidity to the patient [44]. The improving technology for angioplasty, including better catheters, guidewires, low-profile balloons, and stent technology, have made angioplasty more applicable to increasingly complex lesions. Ideal lesions for angioplasty are short-segment ones that are not being caused by extrinsic constriction. It goes without saying that any patient who presents with acute mesenteric ischemia and evidence of intestinal infarction requires immediate laparotomy, not angioplasty. The technique for angioplasty of a mesenteric vessel is similar to that of any other lesion. Unlike most other peripheral vascular interventions that are accessed via a femoral approach, a left brachial approach may be easier given the acute angle of the SMA takeoff from the aorta. The lesion must be able to be crossed with a guidewire. Following placement of the guidewire, a balloon must be passed over the wire across the lesion. In addition, if necessary, a stent may be placed.

Moreover, using a percutaneous approach can be a useful adjunct when treating patients with NOMI. Once the diagnosis of NOMI is made, intra-arterial papaverine infusion into the SMA is possible. The usual dose is in the range of 30–60 mg/h. The patient's response to vasodilator therapy is monitored by clinical and angiographic criteria. Of importance is that there is a resolution of abdominal pain. Arteriography should be repeated to document that the vasospasm has been broken. Once the vasospasm is broken, papaverine treatment should continue for another 24 h. It is important to carefully monitor the patients receiving intra-arterial vasodilator therapy, as marked hypotension can result. These patients obviously must be cared for in the intensive care unit.

Mesenteric Venous Thrombosis

Mesenteric venous thrombosis is the least common form of mesenteric ischemia. It currently accounts for only 5–15% of all cases of mesenteric ischemia [45]. As with arterial ischemia, mesenteric venous thrombosis can be divided into acute and chronic presentations. Acute mesenteric venous thrombosis is a process in which the patient presents with <4 weeks of symptoms. Patients who present with more than 4 weeks of symptoms without evidence of bowel infarction, or those who have a diagnosis of mesenteric venous thrombosis made incidentally and it is clinically insignificant, are classified as having chronic mesenteric venous thrombosis [46].

The etiology of mesenteric venous thrombosis is classified into one of two categories: primary or secondary. Primary mesenteric venous thrombosis is a spontaneous, idiopathic event with thrombosis of the mesenteric veins that is not associated with any other disease process or a hypercoagulable state [47]. The frequency of this diagnosis has decreased with the improved ability to diagnose hypercoagulable states. The conditions associated with secondary mesenteric venous thrombosis are hypercoagulability, malignancy, cirrhosis, splenomegaly, intra-abdominal infection, trauma, and pancreatitis. The hypercoagulable states are usually related to hematologic disorders and include protein C and S deficiency, antithrombin III deficiency, dysfibrinogenemia, abnormal plasminogen, polycythemia vera, thrombocytosis, sickle cell disease, and factor V Leiden mutation.

Although patients with acute mesenteric venous thrombosis can present with a picture similar to that of acute arterial thrombosis, their presentation is usually not as dramatic and the symptoms not as severe. Therefore, there is often a delay in diagnosis. This delay is a major contributory factor to the relatively high mortality reported in the literature secondary to mesenteric venous thrombosis [48]. Patients usually present with a several-day to several-week history of diffuse, nonspecific, and often intermittent abdominal pain. Typically, these symptoms are gradually progressive. Aside from abdominal pain, other symptoms occur much less frequently. Physical findings are often vague, with abdominal distension being the most common, but it is seen in only approximately 50% of patients. Peritonitis is present only in advanced cases that have progressed to bowel infarction. Studies have indicated that along with bowel infarction requiring resection, advanced age, underlying malignancy, and prolong duration of symptoms (more than 5 days) are usually predictive of a poor outcome [49].

As with NOMI, laboratory tests are usually not helpful for diagnosing acute mesenteric venous ischemia. Leukocytosis is seen in some patients, as are elevated amylase and LDH levels; but once again, this is in the setting of mesenteric infarction.

Diagnosis

Mesenteric venous thrombosis is diagnosed by radiographic means. Plain abdominal films are usually nonspecific and help

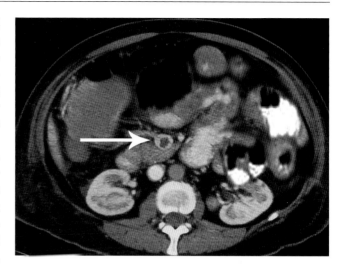

FIGURE 65.12 CT angiogram, delayed venous phase. *White arrow* is pointing to thrombus within the superior mesenteric vein.

little with the diagnosis. The most common finding is a nonspecific ileus. Computed tomography (CT) scanning has proved to be the most sensitive diagnostic test for mesenteric venous thrombosis. CT scanning accurately identified thrombus within the SMV and the portal vein [50] (Fig. 65.12). Magnetic resonance imaging has also proved to be sensitive [51]. Duplex scanning of the mesenteric veins can be performed as well, but has a slightly lower sensitivity than CT scanning.

Unlike with other forms of mesenteric ischemia, mesenteric arteriography has proved not to be diagnostically sensitive. Evidence of venous thrombosis can only be seen on the venous phase of a selective SMA injection. As with other forms of mesenteric ischemia, any patient who presents with evidence of peritonitis or other signs of bowel infarction should undergo emergent exploratory laparotomy. If mesenteric venous thrombosis is diagnosed prior to surgery, anticoagulation with intravenous heparin should be started immediately. If it is diagnosed at the time of laparotomy, heparin should be initiated immediately.

Treatment

The guidelines for bowel resection are the same as with any other form of mesenteric ischemia. Frankly necrotic segments are removed. If there are questionable areas, a second-look laparotomy is performed. In general, venous thrombectomy is not recommended, as it is almost uniformly unsuccessful; although it may be indicated in a few selective circumstances, such as when it can be clearly documented that there is thrombus within the SMV within 1–3 days of the initial symptoms [52]. More recently, thrombolytic therapy has been used, but its efficacy is unclear, and its use remains controversial [53]. In patients who do not present with peritonitis or who have evidence of bowel necrosis, optimal management consists of anticoagulation and observation. Anticoagulation with intravenous heparin acutely is followed by chronic anticoagulation with warfarin. Chronic anticoagulation is associated with improved survival compared with the survival of those who did not undergo anticoagulation [25]. The underlying cause of the mesenteric venous thrombosis does not appear to affect survival. It is recommended that this regimen continue for the life of the patient [54].

Chronic mesenteric venous thrombosis is different from acute mesenteric venous thrombosis. Patients usually present with vague abdominal pain or slight distension. The most frequent presentation is asymptomatic, with the thrombosis being an incidental finding on diagnostic imaging for another complaint. No specific therapy is generally indicated.

Ischemic Colitis

The final category of mesenteric ischemia in the elderly to be considered here is ischemic colitis. As with other causes of mesenteric ischemia, ischemic colitis can be caused by occlusive or nonocclusive lesions. The colon is normally supplied on the right side by the SMA and on the left by the IMA and branches of the hypogastric arteries. The collateral pathways that exist among the SMA, the IMA, and the hypogastric arteries were described earlier in this chapter. Ischemic colitis results when there is obviously decreased flow in one of these vascular beds. Patients susceptible to this problem are those who have absent or poorly developed collateral pathways. It is important to know that previous colonic surgery can interfere with these pathways. The splenic flexure of the colon is in a watershed area between the IMA and SMA. It is more susceptible than the rest of the colon to ischemic injury. In 5% of the population, the marginal artery of Drummond is absent or diminutive, and it is also poorly developed in the right colon of nearly 50% of the population. This helps explain the relatively frequent occurrence of right-sided ischemic colitis [55]. Ischemic colitis results when the colon is rendered ischemic for any of the reasons presented previously.

Ischemic colitis tends to produce local and systemic symptoms. In particular, there is a release of inflammatory cytokines and other mediators of inflammation, which is thought to be secondary to endotoxemia and portal bacteremia. These situations result from the increased mucosal permeability caused by ischemia [56]. Also, if there is reperfusion of the ischemic areas, there can be release of oxygen-free radicals and other toxins, resulting in further systemic symptoms. Moreover, recent studies suggest that neutrophils activated during the ischemia/reperfusion process play an important role [57]. It is therefore not surprising that patients with ischemic colitis can be extremely ill and that their mortality is often secondary to multisystem organ failure.

Diagnosis

The typical patient who presents with ischemic colitis is an elderly man with comorbid conditions, including cardiac disease, peripheral vascular disease, diabetes mellitus, or renal insufficiency. The presentation of ischemic colitis can be insidious, with patients complaining of abdominal pain, distension, and diarrhea. Progression to lower GI hemorrhage occurs at an advanced stage of ischemic injury. It usually results from sloughing of the mucosa.

Three degrees of severity of ischemic colitis have been described [58]. The mildest form involves only the colonic mucosa and submucosa. It is estimated that more than half of all patients with ischemic colitis have experienced this degree of the disease. These patients typically have abdominal pain and bloody diarrhea, but the symptoms typically resolve with conservative measures and surgery is not required [59]. The most severe form of ischemic colitis, which only affects 10–20% of patients, involves full thickness necrosis of the colon, requiring immediate surgical resection. The intermediate of ischemic colitis involves the mucosa, submucosa, and the muscularis layer of the colon. It can lead to chronic stricture due to scarring when the lesion heals or to persistent symptoms. Often, in patients with the two milder forms of ischemic colitis, the initial presenting symptoms are vague and nonspecific. Once again, as with other forms of mesenteric ischemia, a high index of suspicion should be maintained in patients who present with GI symptoms.

As with other forms of mesenteric ischemia, blood tests, although providing collaborative evidence of colonic ischemia, are nonspecific. As with midgut ischemia, the presence of metabolic acidosis and elevated CPK and LDH levels are indicative of advanced colonic ischemia. The most definitive way to diagnose ischemic colitis is by endoscopic evaluation. Acutely, pale mucosa with areas of petechial hemorrhage is seen with mild ischemia; more severe degrees of ischemia are indicated by a dark (blue to black) mucosa, which may be accompanied by mucosal sloughing and ulceration [60]. Because the findings at the time of endoscopy can be confused with other forms of colitis, biopsy and histological examination may prove to be useful. With ischemic colitis, there is destruction of the crypts, sloughing of the epithelium, edema, thrombosis of the capillaries, and a relative lack of inflammatory cells. Later findings include stricture and fibrosis; biopsy reveals extensive transmural fibrosis with mucosal atrophy [61].

Unlike other forms of mesenteric ischemia due to arterial lesions, angiography is usually not helpful in this setting. This is because often the lesion leading to ischemic colitis is more peripheral and therefore more difficult to detect [62]. CT scans are often obtained due to the unclear diagnosis in the patient presenting with abdominal pain; they are often normal in these patients, particularly those who present early in the course of their illness [63]. A late finding highly suggestive of ischemic colitis is pneumotosis [65]. The most frequent positive finding is circumferential thickening of the colonic wall, which is secondary to edema or hemorrhage, but it is nonspecific [65]. The use of other imaging studies remains to be experimental, and so far they have proved to be insensitive [66, 67] as with other forms of ischemia; findings on plain films are not often seen, are usually nonspecific, and when seen, usually are due to advanced ischemia. Contrast studies are infrequently used to evaluate patients with acute abdominal pain; if obtained, thumb printing due to submucosal edema and hemorrhage is the classic finding of ischemic colitis.

Treatment

The management of patients with ischemic colitis is individualized and depends on the patient's presentation. Most patients who present with ischemic colitis do not have an acute abdomen, and therefore emergent surgery is usually not necessary. These patients are managed with intravenous fluids, administration of broad-spectrum antibiotics, and stopping oral intake. The precipitating events for ischemic colitis, which are often low-flow states, should be corrected. Within 1 week, most patients with mild form of ischemic colitis respond well to treatment [68]. In the patient who presents with ischemic colitis with no clear cause, visceral angiography can be considered; but once again it has a relatively low yield.

Any patient who presents with an acute abdomen requires emergent surgery. Those who fail to respond to conservative measures and who have persistent bleeding or low-grade sepsis require surgical intervention. Surgical treatment involves resecting the ischemic segments of colon. It is recommended that patients have a colostomy or an ileostomy, with a subsequent procedure to restore intestinal continuity [69]. Patients with ischemic colitis have a relatively high mortality, but it is usually due to the underlying condition that precipitated the ischemic colitis. In this sense, it is similar to NOMI. Obviously, patients who require surgery have an even higher mortality rate [70]. Elective aortic reconstruction for aneurysm disease is associated with a 1–2% incidence of ischemic colitis [71]. In the emergent setting of a ruptured abdominal aortic aneurysm, the incidence of ischemic colitis has been reported to be as high as 60% [72]. This association with ischemic colitis and aortic reconstruction has often been centered around the IMA. Replanting the IMA in aortic

surgery to prevent ischemic colitis has been discussed, and few randomized trials have been done to compare the incidence of ischemic colitis in patients with and without IMA revascularization. One recent prospective study, however, found that there was no significant reduction in postoperative ischemic colitis in patients with IMA revascularization, however, found that age and intraoperative blood loss correlated with an increased risk of developing ischemic colitis [73]. Ischemic colitis following aortic surgery is associated with a high mortality rate, which has been reported to be in excess of 50% [74]. In the subgroup of patients who require emergent colectomy, mortality is nearly 90%. As with other forms of mesenteric ischemia, the key to a successful clinical outcome is a timely diagnosis, which requires a high index of clinical suspicion. Therefore, in any patient who has undergone aortic reconstruction and develops bloody or heme-positive diarrhea, has an unexplained high fluid resuscitation requirement, presents with fever and leukocytosis of unknown origin, or has an unexplained acidosis, the diagnosis of colitis should be suspected and evaluation including endoscopy should be undertaken.

References

1. McMillan WD, McCarthy WJ, Bresteker MR et al (1995) Mesenteric artery bypass: objective patency determination. J Vasc Surg 21:720–741
2. Schwartz LB, Puret CM, Craig DM, et al (in press) Input impedance of revascularized skeletal muscle, renal, and mesenteric vascular beds. Vasc Surg
3. Ahlborg G, Weitzberg E, Lundberg JM (1995) Circulating endothelin-1 reduces splanchnic and renal blood low and splanchnic glucose productions in humans. J Appl Physiol 79:141–145
4. VanHoutte PM (1978) Heterogeneity in vascular smooth muscle cells. In: Caley G, Altura BM (eds) Microcirculation. University Park Press, Baltimore, pp 181–308
5. Reilly PM, Buckley GB (1993) Vasoactive mediators and splanchnic perfusion. Crit Care Med 21:S55–S68
6. Granger DN, Richardson PDI, Kvietys PR, Mortillaro NA (1980) Intestinal blood flow. Gastroenterology 78:837–863
7. Heys SD, Brittenden J, Crofts TJ (1993) Acute mesenteric ischemia: the continuing difficulty and early diagnosis. Postgrad Med J 69:48–51
8. Kaleya RN, Boley SJ (1992) Acute mesenteric ischemia: an aggressive diagnostic and therapeutic approach: 1993 Roussel lecture. Can J Surg 5:613–623
9. Stoney RJ, Cunningham CG (1993) Acute mesenteric ischemia. Surgery 114:489–490
10. Kaleya RN, Sammartano RJ, Boley SJ (1992) Aggressive approach to acute mesenteric ischemia. Surg Clin North Am 72:157–182
11. Cambria RP, Brewster DC, Gertler J et al (1988) Vascular complications associated with spontaneous aortic dissection. J Vasc Surg 7:199–209
12. Deehan DJ, Heys SD, Brittenden J, Eremin O (1995) Mesenteric ischaemia: prognostic factors and influence of delay upon outcome. J R Coll Surg Edinb 40:112–115

13. Bassiouny HS (1997) Nonocclusive mesenteric ischemia. Surg Clin North Am 77:319–326
14. McNeil JR, Stark RD, Greenway CV (1970) Intestinal vasoconstriction after hemorrhage: roles of vasopressin and angiotensin. Am J Physiol 219:1342–1347
15. Mikkelsen E, Andersson DK, Pedersen OL (1979) Effects of digoxin on isolated human mesenteric vessels. Acta Pharmacol Toxicol (Copenh) 5:249–256
16. Gewertz BL, Zarins CK (1991) Postoperative vasospasm after antegrade mesenteric revascularization: a report of three cases. J Vasc Surg 14:382–385
17. Hallet JW, James ME, Ahlquist DA et al (1990) Recent trends in the diagnosis and management of chronic intestinal ischemia. Ann Vasc Surg 4:126–132
18. Calderon M, Reul GJ, Gregoric ID et al (1992) Long term results of the surgical management of symptomatic chronic intestinal ischemia. J Cardiovasc Surg 33:723–728
19. Derrick JR, Pollard HS, Moore RM (1959) The pattern of atherosclerotic narrowing of the celiac and superior mesenteric arteries. Ann Surg 149:684–689
20. Councilman WT (1894) Three cases of occlusion in the superior mesenteric artery. Boston Med Surg J 130:410–411
21. Lye CR (1988) Chronic mesenteric ischemia. Can J Surg 31:159–161
22. Gluecklich B, Deterling RA, Matsumoto GH et al (1979) Chronic mesenteric ischemia masquerading as cancer. Surg Gynecol Obstet 148:49–56
23. Watt JK (1968) Arterial diseases of the gut. Br Med J 3:231–233
24. Howard TJ, Plaskon LA, Wiebke EA, Wilcox MG (1996) Nonocclusive mesenteric ischemia remains a diagnostic dilemma. Am J Surg 171:405–408
25. Smerud MJ, Johnson CD, Stephens DH (1990) Diagnosis of bowel infarction: a comparison of plain films and CT scans in 23 cases. Am J Roentgenol 154:99
26. Sabba C, Ferraioli G, Sarin SK et al (1990) Feasibility spectrum for Doppler flowmetry of splanchnic vessels: in normal and cirrhotic populations. J Ultrasound Med 9:705
27. Zwolak RM, Fillinger MF, Walsh DB et al (1998) Mesenteric and celiac duplex scanning: a validation study. J Vasc Surg 27:1078
28. Bowersox JC, Zwolak RM, Walsh DB et al (1991) Duplex ultrasonography in the diagnosis of celiac and mesenteric artery occlusive disease. J Vasc Surg 14:780
29. Moneta GL, Lee RW, Yeager RA et al (1993) Mesenteric duplex scanning: a blinded prospective study. J Vasc Surg 17:79
30. Fleischmann D (2003) Multiple detector-row CT angiography of the renal and mesenteric vessels. Eur J Radiol 45(Suppl):79–87
31. Wasser MN, Geelkerken RH, Kouwenhoven M et al (1996) Systolically gated 3D phase contrast MRA of mesenteric arteries in suspected mesenteric ischemia. J Comput Assist Tomogr 20:262
32. Carlos RC, Stanley JC, Stafford-Johnson D, Prince MR (2001) Interobserver variability in the evaluation of chronic mesenteric ischemia with gadolinium-enhanced MR angiography. Acad Radiol 8:879
33. Meaney JF, Prince MR, Nostrant TT, Stanley JC (1997) Gadolinium-enhanced MR angiography of visceral arteries in patients with suspected chronic mesenteric ischemia. J Magn Reson Imaging 7:171
34. Stanley CJ, Ozaki KC, Zelenock GB (1997) Bypass grafting for chronic mesenteric ischemia. Surg Clin North Am 7:381–395
35. Reiner L, Himinez FA, Rodriquez FL (1963) Atherosclerosis in the mesenteric circulation: observations and correlations with aortic and coronary atherosclerosis. Am Heart J 66:200–209
36. McMillan WD, McCarthy WJ, Bresticker MR et al (1995) Mesenteric artery bypass: objective patency determination. J Vasc Surg 21:729–740, discussion 740–741
37. Taylor LM Jr, Moneta GL (1991) Intestinal ischemia. Ann Vasc Surg 5:403–406
38. Johnston KW, Lindsay TF, Walker PM, Kalman PG (1995) Mesenteric arterial bypass grafts: early and late results on suggested surgical approach for chronic and acute mesenteric ischemia. Surgery 118:1–7
39. Cunningham CG, Reilly LM, Stoney R (1992) Chronic visceral ischemia. Surg Clin North Am 72:231–244
40. Hansen KJ, Deitch S (1997) Transaortic mesenteric endarterectomy. Surg Clin North Am 77:397–407
41. Allen R, Maratin G, Rees C et al (1996) Mesenteric angioplasty in the treatment of chronic intestinal ischemia. J Vasc Surg 24:415–423
42. Kougias P, El Sayed HF, Zhou W, Lin PH (2007) Management of chronic mesenteric ischemia. The role of endovascular therapy. J Endovasc Ther 14:395–405
43. Brown DJ, Schermerhorn ML, Cronenwett JL et al (2005) Mesenteric stenting for chronic mesenteric ischemia. J Vasc Surg 42(2):268–274
44. Zerbib P, Lebuffe G, Chambon JP et al (2008) Endovascular versus open revascularization for chronic mesenteric ischemia: a comparative study. Langenbecks Arch Surg 393(6):865–870
45. Rhee RY, Gloviczki P, Mendonca CT et al (1994) Mesenteric venous thrombosis: still a lethal disease in the 1990s. J Vasc Surg 20:688
46. Rhee RY, Gloviczki P (1997) Mesenteric venous thrombosis. Surg Clin North Am 77:327
47. Kitchens CS (1992) Evolution of our understanding of the pathophysiology of primary mesenteric venous thrombosis. Am J Surg 163:346
48. Grieshop RJ, Dalsing MC, Ckrit DF et al (1991) Acute mesenteric venous thrombosis: revisited in time of diagnostic clarity. Am J Surg 57:53
49. Hedayati N, Riha GM, Lin PH et al (2008) Prognostic factors and treatment outcome in mesenteric vein thrombosis. Vasc Endovasc Surg 42(3):217–224
50. Rhmouni A, Mathieu D, Golli M et al (1992) Value of CT and sonography in the conservative management of acute splenoportal and superior mesenteric venous thrombosis. Gastroint Radiol 17:135
51. Gehl HB, Bohndorf K, Flose KC et al (1990) Two-dimensional MR angiography in the evaluation of abdominal vein with gradient refocused sequences. J Comput Assist Tomogr 14:619
52. Inhara T (1971) Acute superior mesenteric venous thrombosis: treatment by thrombectomy. Ann Surg 74:956
53. Bilbao JI, Rodriquez-Cabello J, Longo J et al (1989) Portal thrombosis: percutaneous transhepatic treatment with urokinase: a case report. Gastrointest Radiol 14:326
54. Boley SJ, Kaleya RN, Brandt LJ (1992) Mesenteric venous thrombosis. Surg Clin North Am 72:183
55. Sonneland J, Anson LJ, Beaton LE (1958) Surgical anatomy of the arterial supply of the colon from the superior mesenteric artery based upon a study of 60 specimens. Surg Gynecol Obstet 106:385–397
56. Turnage RH, Guice KS, Oldham KT (1994) Endotoxemia and remote organ injury following intestinal reperfusion. J Surg Res 56:571–578
57. Sisley AC, Desai T, Harig JM, Gewertz BL (1994) Neutrophil depletion attenuates human intestinal reperfusion injury. J Surg Res 57:192–196
58. Bradbury AW, Brittenden J, McBride K, Ruckley CV (1995) Mesenteric ischemia in multi-disciplinary approach. Br J Surg 82:1446–1459
59. Booley SJ, Brandt LF, Veith SJ (1978) Ischemic disorders of the intestines. Curr Probl Surg 15:1–85
60. Longo WE, Ballantyne GH, Gusberg BJ (1992) Ischemic colitis: patterns and prognosis. Dis Colon Rectum 35:726–730
61. Price AB (1990) Ischemic colitis. Curr Top Pathol 81:229–246
62. Robert JH, Mentha G, Rohner A (1993) Ischaemic colits: two distinct patterns of severity. Gut 34:4–6

63. Alpern MB, Glazer PM, Francis IR (1988) Ischemic or infracted bowel: CT findings. Radiology 66:149–152
64. Philpotts LE, Heiken JP, Westcott MA, Gore RM (1994) Colitis: use of CT findings and differential diagnosis. Radiology 190:445–449
65. Jacobs JE, Birnbaum BA (1995) CT of inflammatory disease of the colon. Semin Ultrasound CT MR 16:91–101
66. Teefey SA, Roarke NC, Brink JA et al (1996) Bowel wall thickening: differentiation of inflammation from ischemia with color Doppler and duplex, ultrasound. Radiology 198:547–551
67. Wilkerson DK, Mezrich R, Drake C et al (1990) MR imaging of acute occlusive intestinal ischemia. J Vasc Surg 11:567–571
68. Scholz FJ (1993) Ischemic bowel disease. Radiol Clin North Am 31:1197–1218
69. Toursarkissian B, Thompson RW (1997) Ischemic colitis. Surg Clin North Am 77:461–470
70. Guttormson N, Brubrick MP (1989) Mortality from ischemic colitis. Dis Colon Rectum 342:469–472
71. Ernst CB, Hagihara PF, Dougherty ME et al (1976) Ischemic colitis incidence following abdominal aortic reconstruction: a prospective study. Surgery 80:417–421
72. Hagihara PF, Enrst CB, Griffen WO Jr (1979) Incidence of ischemic colitis following abdominal aortic reconstruction. Surg Gynecol Obstet 149:571–573
73. Senekowitsch C, Assadian A, Assadian O et al (2006) Replanting the inferior mesentery artery during infrarenal aortic aneurysm repair: influence on postoperative colon ischemia. J Vasc Surg 43:689–694
74. Longo WE, Lee TC, Barnett MG et al (1996) Ischemic colitis complicating abdominal aortic aneurysm surgery in the U.S. veteran. J Surg Res 60:351–354

Chapter 66
Surgery for Inflammatory Bowel Disease in the Elderly

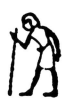

Stefan D. Holubar and Bruce G. Wolff

Early in the twenty-first century, inflammatory bowel diseases (IBD) remain idiopathic chronic conditions and are often considered afflictions of the young. However, significant and growing proportions of those either presenting with or requiring surgery for Crohn's disease (CD) or chronic ulcerative colitis (CUC) are elderly. Currently, it is estimated that >1.1 million persons in the United States suffer from IBD [1], of which an estimated 13–16% are over the age of 60 years. In addition, an estimated 65% of all CD patients and 25% of all CUC patients require surgery within 10 years of diagnosis [2]. Thus, as the proportion of the American population over age 60 increases, surgeons and other health-care providers who care for IBD patients can expect to see a relative increase in elderly patients with IBD who require surgical intervention [3].

Understanding the differences in disease presentation, indications for surgery, and physiologic differences in the elderly as compared to the young patients with IBD is an important consideration to deliver the highest quality care possible in timely manner, thus optimizing the risk of morbidity in this at-risk population [4]. In addition, minimally invasive operative approaches, which are increasingly being applied to patients with IBD, must be tailored to the needs of the elderly patient. In this chapter, we review the epidemiology of IBD (including the natural history and presentation), differential diagnosis, indications for surgery, and operative principles (including minimally invasive [laparoscopic] techniques), which are relevant to elderly patients with IBD. A summary of the highlights of this chapter is provided in Table 66.1.

Epidemiology

Several factors influence the interpretation of data regarding the incidence of inflammatory bowel disease (IBD) in the elderly: the source of the data (population-based studies versus clinical series), the geographic setting (incidence rates vary between countries [5]), the definition of elderly, the historic age of the series, and the disease definition [3]. More accurate data on the incidence of IBD in the elderly are derived from population-based studies because clinical series are typically retrospective descriptions of patients from a single institution, often a tertiary center where complicated cases may be overrepresented. Late-onset cases are variably defined in patients ranging from >40 years to those >65 years of age.

Crohn's Disease Incidence

Crohn's disease (CD) has been called a disease of the twentieth century, having first been described by Crohn and his colleagues in 1932 at Mount Sinai Hospital, New York [6]. The incidence of the disease ranges from 3.1 to 14.6 per 100,000 person-years [7] and usually accounts for one-third to one-half of cases of IBD. Multiple studies have indicated that the incidence of CD in Western society is increasing, and North America is considered a high-incidence area [7]. Interestingly, although CD is known to be more prevalent in persons of North-European and Ashkenazi-Jewish genetic origin [8], a recent population-based study from Korea demonstrated the incidence of CD has increased from 0.05 in 1986 to 1.34 in 2005 [9]: the incidence of CD in non-Western populations is now approaching those seen in Western countries, although Asians with IBD may require surgery less often [10].

The proportion of elderly patients with CD varies in population-based studies from 5.9 to 30.7% [3] with a mean of 16.0% [11], the age of late-onset being variably defined as 50–60 years of age. A recent population-based series from Stockholm, Sweden noted an increase in the proportion of elderly patients (≥60 years) from 3.4 to 12.0% between 1955 and 1989 [12]. Similarly, in a study from Olmsted County, Minnesota, the incidence increased from 3.0 from 1940 to 1949 to 10.8 from 1990 to 2000 [1]. Considering this rise in incidence, combined with an increased overall life expectancy, we anticipate a significant increase in the prevalence of CD in the elderly in the coming decades.

S.D. Holubar (✉)
Division of Colon and Rectal Surgery, Dartmouth Medical School, Dartmouth-Hitchcock Medical Center, Lebanon, NH, USA
e-mail: stefan.holubar@hitchcock.org

R.A. Rosenthal et al. (eds.), *Principles and Practice of Geriatric Surgery*,
DOI 10.1007/978-1-4419-6999-6_66, © Springer Science+Business Media, LLC 2011

TABLE 66.1 Summary table

- It is estimated that >1.1 million North Americans suffer from inflammatory bowel disease of which approximately 15% are over the age of 60 years
- Population-based studies suggest that the incidence of inflammatory bowel disease is increasing, including in the elderly
- The diagnosis of inflammatory bowel disease that presents in the elderly may be confused with other age-related colonic pathologies such as diverticular disease and ischemic colitis, but elderly patients with IBD may be less likely than younger patients to require surgery
- The surgical approach to elderly patients with Crohn's disease who require surgery parallels the surgical approach to young patients
- The surgical approach to elderly patients with ulcerative colitis who require surgery is significantly different than in young patients, with age-related cancers, age-related comorbidities, age-related fecal incontinence, altered lifestyle and decreased life-span, and anticipated need for pelvic radiation, all more likely to contribute to a nonrestorative approach to proctocolectomy with permanent ileostomy
- A significant proportion of elderly patients with permanent stoma will experience a stoma-related complication
- Advanced age alone should not be an absolute contraindication to ileal pouch-anal anastomosis
- Advanced age alone should not be an absolute contraindication to laparoscopic colectomy
- Elderly patients who require surgery for IBD are at increased risk of postoperative complications relative to young patients

Ulcerative Colitis Incidence

Ulcerative colitis was recognized as early as 1859 by Samuel Wilks who first described ulcerative colitis in a young woman [8, 13]. Since then, CUC has been shown to have an incidence rate in North America ranging from 3.0 to 14.3, almost identical to that seen for CD [14]. Also similar to CD, the incidence of UC shows interesting geographic differences. There has been a stable incidence throughout Europe, and greater incidence of both UC and CD in northern Europe was confirmed by the European Collaborative Study on IBD (EC-IBD) [15]. Also paralleling CD, the findings of increased incidence of CUC in Asia have also been observed. The incidence of CUC in the Songpa-Kangdong district of Seoul, Korea ranged from 0.34 in 1986 to 3.08 in 2005, lower than that observed in the West, but nonetheless on the rise [9]. Similar results have been seen in Hong Kong, China [16]. However, incidence data for UC may be influenced by inclusion or exclusion of patients with ulcerative proctitis, as available data suggest this entity is more common in elderly individuals [17].

Population-based studies suggest that the proportion of patients with late-onset UC (defined variably as >50 to >70 years) ranges from 8.1 to 43.9% with a mean of 12.0%. The EC-IBD study also found that the age-specific incidence of UC decreases with age in women, but not in men, confirming reports by others [17, 18].

Unimodal vs. Bimodal Age Distribution

Although in the past many epidemiologic studies demonstrated a bimodal distribution in the age at diagnosis for both UC [19, 20] and CD [20], more recent studies have not and this postulate is currently considered controversial [1, 7, 21]. As this issue is particularly pertinent to elderly patients with IBD, in the following sections we review the evidence for and against bimodality.

In older studies, the first age peak (mode) typically occurred during the third decade, whereas the second varied between the age of 50 and 80 years. The reason for the observed bimodality was not known, although several theories have been proposed. One is that the two peaks represent two types of disease, or a differential effect of age on the underlying disease. The variation in the anatomic distribution of CD depending on the patient's age is an example of the latter: CD of the terminal ileum tends to present in young patients [22], producing a unimodal age distribution for small bowel CD, with a peak during the third and fourth decades [23]. Conversely, older patients tend to have purely colonic disease, and the second peak has been found to be comprised predominantly of elderly women with Crohn's colitis, often left-sided [24, 25].

Another earlier theory that misdiagnosis was responsible for the second peak has gained less credence with time. As Crohn's colitis and UC came to be recognized as distinct clinical and pathologic entities during the middle part of the twentieth century, some authors ascribed the second peak to misclassification of such other conditions as ischemic and infectious colitis [26]. That may possibly have been so at one time, as was well shown in a retrospective review by Brandt et al. [27], where of 81 patients >50 years with a diagnosis of colitis, only 14% were thought to have UC and 5% to have CD after further consideration; ischemic colitis was the diagnosis assigned to three-fourths of the series. However, even exclusion of ischemic colitis did not abolish the second peak in UC; the incidence of UC in the elderly appears to have continued to increase, not decrease, in the face of improved diagnostic ability.

In 1996, Shivananda et al. reported for the EC-IBD project. In that study, which included 2,201 patients from across Europe from 1991 to 1993, no bimodality for either CD or CUC was observed [21]. Similarly in 2007, Loftus et al. updated the Olmsted County, MN experience with IBD from 1940 to 2000 [1]. Regarding bimodality, this pattern was *only* observed in men with CUC, and this subgroup (i.e., men with CUC) presented later in life than women with CUC. Changes in smoking patterns over the decades may play a role in the etiology of these age and gender observations [28]. Further study will be needed to refute or corroborate the suggestion that both CD and CUC actually have a unimodal, and not bimodal, age distribution.

Presentation and Natural History

Presentation

Overall, the presentation of CD and UC in the elderly does not vary significantly from that in the young population. A review of the clinical features in patients more than 50 years of age with CD found abdominal pain (82%), diarrhea (70%), weight loss (56%), and rectal bleeding (26%) to be the most common presenting features [29]. Toxic dilatation at presentation was rare. However, the initial diagnosis of IBD in the elderly is more often incorrect (64% of patients older than 65 years versus 96% of younger patients [30]) or delayed (despite clinical characteristics similar to those in younger patients) because of confusion caused by a higher incidence of diverticular disease and cardiovascular disease [31]. This delay in final diagnosis may in part result in the higher observed complication rate, which is seen in elderly as compared with younger IBD patients (36% vs. 16%, respectively), and a higher mortality rate [30].

Natural History

There are conflicting reports on the natural history vis-à-vis surgical intervention for CD and UC in the elderly. Gupta et al. [32], in a series of patients with both CD and UC, found that few patients required operation. This concurred with the findings of Fabricius et al. [33], who found that in elderly patients with CD, the course of the disease was largely dependent on the site of the lesion. Most of those with distal ileal disease required laparotomy for obstruction, peritonitis, or to rule out carcinoma, but thereafter, the prognosis was good. In contrast, patients with colonic disease rarely required operation and were managed medically. This contrasted with findings from others [34, 35] where 40–91% of those with colitis required surgery.

The natural history in UC is also the subject of controversy. Jones and Hoare [36] found that elderly patients were admitted more often with their first attack and were more likely to receive intravenous steroids than younger patients, but none required emergent surgery, and mortality on follow-up was no greater than that expected in the general population of the same age. The prognosis was found to be the same as in younger patients. This differs from Brandt et al. [37], who noted that in a group of 11 patients with UC, two developed toxic dilatation, three underwent operation, and three died during the first admission, leading to the conclusion that the prognosis was worse in the elderly as compared with younger patients. This conclusion has been supported by a study that utilized the Nationwide Inpatient Sample which

found that IBD patients >65 had higher mortality (odds ratio 3.9, 95% confidence interval [2.5–6.1]) even after adjusting for comorbidities [4]. Thus, current evidence supports that the elderly with IBD may have an equivalent, and likely worse, prognosis as compared with younger patients.

Differential Diagnosis

The majority of elderly patients with IBD will present with classic symptoms such as weight loss, abdominal pain, or bleeding and may prompt a workup for, and confusion with, more common pathology such as diverticular disease, ischemic colitis, or colorectal carcinoma as mentioned in the section "Natural History." However, due to effects of aging on physiology, elderly patients may present with atypical signs and symptoms. IBD should be considered during the evaluation of elderly patients with digestive complaints, particularly chronic diarrhea with or without bleeding. Symptoms in the elderly may not suggest IBD for reasons that include blunted response to pain, poor communication because of altered comprehension or hearing, fear of the medical system, and focus on cancer as the most likely cause of symptoms [11]. A delay in diagnosis is common in old patients with IBD and may result in inappropriate treatment and a higher rate of complications [4, 30].

The differential diagnosis of IBD in the elderly includes ischemic colitis, diverticular disease, infectious colitis such as *Clostridium difficile* colitis (antibiotic-associated colitis) or cytomegalovirus (CMV) colitis, and of course, colorectal and other cancers. Less common entities that should be considered are collagenous colitis, lymphocytic colitis, radiation enterocolitis, lymphoma, carcinoid, vasculitis, and drug-induced colitis [11]. Diagnostic evaluation is generally unaffected by age, although elderly patients may be more likely to have underlying renal insufficiency precluding intravenous contrast, especially in the face of dehydration. Nonetheless, prompt diagnostic evaluation may be particularly important in elderly patients who may present with atypical symptoms. Two particularly common sources of diagnostic confusion are ischemic colitis and diverticulitis.

Ischemic Colitis

A history of cardiovascular disease may suggest a diagnosis of ischemic colitis. Occasionally, there is difficulty distinguishing ischemia from IBD. Brandt et al., in a study of 81 patients, found that half were originally diagnosed with CD, UC, or nonspecific colitis, but on retrospective review, ischemic colitis was diagnosed in 75% of the series [37]. The authors raised the question as to whether such incorrect diagnoses might explain why colitis is reported to behave differently in the elderly. It is known that ischemic changes may mimic UC or CD. Computed tomography (CT) scanning of the abdomen and pelvis may not be able to differentiate the etiology of colitis. The addition of CT angiography (CTA) to the diagnostic armamentarium may assist clinicians in ruling out macrovascular ischemic colitis by allowing visualization of the patency of the mesenteric arteries and veins without formal angiography, at a lower dye load than traditional angiography. If ischemic colitis is strongly considered, clinicians should consider nonintravenous CT initially, or followed by, or proceeding directly to CTA if ischemic colitis is strongly suspected.

Diverticulitis

In addition to often being confused with ischemic colitis, IBD in the elderly presenting as segmental colitis may also be confused with segmental colitis associated with diverticular disease (SCAD) [38, 39]. Distinguishing segmental CD with diverticula from pure diverticulitis may be difficult, as each may have abdominal pain, diarrhea, fistula, and abdominal mass; blood in the stool, especially if in small amounts and frequent, should suggest CD. Peppercorn et al. described eight patients with segmental chronic active colitis associated with sigmoid diverticula [40]. These patients were all over 60 years of age, and none had features of CD. Endoscopy reveals a characteristic appearance with patchy areas of hemorrhage in the sigmoid colon; biopsy demonstrates focal chronic active colitis without granulomata. It is important to consider this differential diagnosis, as major complications may be increased following surgery for suspected diverticulitis in elderly patients with unrecognized CD [41].

Surgical Therapy

Many aspects of the surgical therapy of Crohn's disease and ulcerative colitis are similar. This is particularly true with regard to indications (especially emergent ones), preoperative evaluation, and preoperative preparation. There are many excellent book chapters and atlases that deal with operative details [8, 42] but few describe adjustments that must be considered when operating on the elderly patient. This section highlights factors that may influence decision making in the older patient. A summary of recent studies of Crohn's disease in the elderly is presented in Table 66.2.

Crohn's Disease: Indications for Elective Surgery

Despite advances in the medical therapy of Crohn's disease, most patients undergo surgical intervention at some point during their lifetime. The National Cooperative Crohn's Disease Study reported operative rates of 78% at 20 years

TABLE 66.2 Summary of recent studies of Crohn's disease in the elderly

Author	Institution	Year	Study design	Age (years)	Elderly (N)	Major findings/comments
Heresbach et al. [107][a]	Hospital Pontchillou, France	2004	Population-based, comparative	≥60	63	Elderly with similar overall incidence, more colonic involvement, more likely to also have diverticular disease and granulomas, and had more easy-to-manage flares
Triantafillidis et al. [108]	Saint Panteleimon, Greece	2000	Case-control	>60	19	Terminal ileal involvement most common. Elderly more likely to present with acute abdomen, had higher complication rate, and lower rate of surgery for perianal disease. No difference in postoperative recurrence patterns
Norris et al. [109]	University of Sydney, Australia	1999	Subgroup comparisons	>55	33	Bimodal age distribution. Elderly with more colonic involvement, fewer ileocecal resections, and higher rate of cardiopulmonary complications
Wagtmans et al. [110]	Leiden University, The Netherlands	1998	Case-control	>40	98	Elderly were less likely to present with abdominal pain, shorter time from symptoms to diagnosis, more likely to be misdiagnosed, had a shorter interval from diagnosis to first operation, and recurred faster but less frequently. In summary, CD in elderly with a more rapid onset and time course

[a]High quality/recommended

and 90% at 30 years from diagnosis [43]. The form of this intervention is determined by the operative indication, extent of disease, and site within the gastrointestinal tract.

For CD, but not ulcerative colitis, the risk of surgery for non-neoplastic IBD decreases with increasing age at diagnosis, irrespective of disease distribution and history of cigarette smoking [44].

Fistulas and Abscesses

Fistulas and abscesses, hallmark manifestations of Crohn's disease, are the most common indications for surgical intervention. The presence of fistulizing disease, with or without accompanying abscess, was the reason for operation in 35% of 482 patients in an early series reported by Farmer et al. [45] More recent series, including multicenter studies, have confirmed the prominence of this complication as an indication for operation. The risk of developing fistulas is to some extent related to the site of the underlying Crohn's disease. Fistulas appear to arise more commonly from the ileocolic distribution; 44% occurs in patients with ileocolitis, compared with 32% in patients with more proximal small bowel distribution, and 23% in those with colonic disease alone.

Fistulas may develop between diseased bowel and any structure or surface adjacent to the inflammatory process. They may be internal or external. Internal fistulas may, for example, be classified as enteroenteric, enterocolic, enterovesical, or enterovaginal. External fistulas are enterocutaneous, perianal, and perirectal. Accompanying abscesses may be within the peritoneal cavity (enteroparietal), interloop, intramesenteric, retroperitoneal, or perianal.

Symptomatic fistulas generally require operative intervention. Corticosteroids rarely result in fistula closure. Fistulas have been demonstrated to heal in 30–40% of patients given 6-mercaptopurine [46] but only in the absence of obstruction. Similarly, the Food and Drug Administration (FDA)-approved antitumor necrosis factor-α antibody (anti-TNF-α) antibody infliximab has been shown to be efficacious in healing fistulas in up to 55% of patients [47]. Percutaneous drainage under antibiotic coverage is the first-line therapy for abscesses, followed by resection of the affected bowel. Long-standing fistula and chronic pelvic abscess cavities can harbor scirrhous type adenocarcinoma.

Obstruction

Obstruction is the second most common indication for operation; in one report, it occurred in 34% of patients undergoing surgical therapy of Crohn's disease [45]. It is seen in 55% of patients requiring operation for small bowel disease, 35% where there is ileocolic disease, and 12% in patients with Crohn's colitis. Early obstructive symptoms may improve with steroid therapy, but longer-standing symptoms generally indicate a fibrotic stricture that does not respond to medical therapy. These long-standing strictures, especially colonic but also in the small bowel, are worrisome for harboring adenocarcinoma.

Carcinoma

There is an established association between Crohn's disease and carcinoma of the colon and the small bowel. The magnitude of this association is, however, controversial. Carcinoma complicating the inflammatory state can be difficult to recognize on preoperative radiologic studies and even macroscopically at operation. For this reason, it is advised that all sites of stricturing undergoing stricturoplasty, rather than resection, should be biopsied to exclude underlying malignancy. Resection of malignancy that occurs in a background of Crohn's disease unfortunately has poor results, particularly in the small intestine [48].

Refractory to Medical Therapy

In the absence of indications mandating prompt surgical therapy, patients with symptomatic Crohn's disease undergo medical therapy. The severity and extent of disease determine the role of sulfasalazine, 5-aminosalicylic acid (5-ASA) compounds, antibiotics, steroids, immunosuppressive drugs, and biologic agents such as anti-TNF-α antibodies. Operative intervention is indicated if the response to medical therapy is incomplete, side effects develop, or planned withdrawal of steroids, for example, is not possible once a response has been induced.

Indications for Emergency Surgery

Toxic Colitis

A diagnosis of toxic colitis mandates emergent treatment. One of the most useful definitions includes a subjective and an objective component [42]. Toxic colitis is defined as an acute "flare" of Crohn's disease accompanied by two of the following: fever (>38.6°C), hypoalbuminemia (<3.0 g/dl), leukocytosis ($>10.5 \times 10^9$ cells/l), tachycardia (>100 beats/min). Megacolon is additionally diagnosed by colonic dilatation of more than 5 cm. A low threshold of suspicion is important in the elderly, where age alone can mask classic abdominal symptoms and signs, even in the absence of steroids or immunosuppressive agents, which may also conceal symptoms.

Therapy should be instituted as soon as the diagnosis is suspected. Emergent operative intervention is necessary in the presence of perforation, peritonitis, sepsis, and massive hemorrhage. In the absence of these findings, medical therapy is initiated with intravenous rehydration, high-dose parenteral corticosteroids or other immunosuppressive drugs, bowel rest, and broad-spectrum antibiotics. A vital component of treatment is frequent serial abdominal examinations and abdominal radiographs. Deterioration during therapy is a further indication for operation, as is failure to improve after 5–7 days of conservative treatment, or 24–48 h in the case of megacolon. Surgical management should be pursued aggressively in the elderly, who have little physiologic reserve and are less well able to survive the consequences of colonic perforation.

Perforation

Free perforation is unusual but may occur in the setting of acute disease or chronic disease. With acute toxic colitis, perforation occurs in the presence of a dilated, friable colon with transmural inflammation. Perforation in patients with chronic disease occurs in the presence of an acute exacerbation of small bowel disease often in association with obstruction. Perforation occurs in fewer than 2% of patients with small bowel CD [49]. More commonly, the fistulizing nature of CD results in adhesions to adjacent loops of bowel that contain the process and prevent free perforation; an abscess so formed may itself perforate and result in purulent peritonitis or fecal peritonitis if there is a free connection to the bowel lumen.

Hemorrhage

Hemorrhage, a relatively unusual complication of CD, should be treated in a fashion similar to that for significant gastrointestinal bleeding due to other causes. The patient's condition should be stabilized while investigations proceed to determine the site of bleeding. Emergent operative intervention is indicated for persistent hemodynamic instability after transfusion with 4–6 units of blood, recurrent bleeding, or an additional indication for resection of the diseased bowel. The elderly, particularly those with coexisting cardiopulmonary disease, have little physiologic reserve, and early operative intervention should be considered in those who have demonstrated unstable vital signs.

Preoperative Preparation

Completion of Workup

Initial studies are guided by the patient's symptoms. Once the primary site of Crohn's disease has been identified, the remainder of the gastrointestinal tract should be evaluated to identify the presence of coexistent sites of disease, which may determine the nature and extent of the operative approach. For example, the individual with obstructive-type symptoms may undergo a CT, CT-enterography, or small bowel series indicating ileocecal disease; the operative approach is different depending on whether the disease is localized or there is also coexistent extensive colitis demonstrated on colonoscopy. The Montreal classification of CD is especially useful is classifying the extent of disease (Table 66.3). Such information is important when discussing the nature of the operative approach, the extent of resection, and the likely postoperative course.

Preoperative Discussion

Knowing the extent and severity of disease assists in preoperative discussions with the patient and family. Procedure-specific risks should be discussed and tailored to the patient and to the procedure contemplated. Such risks may include bleeding with the attendant risks of blood transfusion, wound infection, anastomotic leak and possible abscess,

TABLE 66.3 Montreal (Revised Vienna) classification of Crohn disease

Category	Abbreviation	Description
Age (of diagnosis)	A1	<16 Years old
	A2	17–40 Years old
	A3	≥40 Years old
Location (pre-surgical)	L1	Terminal ileum
	L2	Colon
	L3	Ileocolonic
	L4[a]	Upper gastrointestinal tract
Behavior	B1[b]	Non-stricturing, non-penetrating
	B2[b]	Stricturing
	B3[b]	Penetrating

Source: Reproduced with permission, Can J Gastroenterol 2005;19 (Suppl A):5A–36A

[a]May be added to L1, L2, or L3 for synchronous disease (e.g., L2+L4= colon+upper)

[b]May add "p" as a perianal disease modifier (e.g., B3p=penetrating+ perianal)

enterocutaneous fistula, or peritonitis, and the likelihood of the need for a temporary or permanent stoma. Comorbidities, more prevalent in the elderly, need to be thoroughly assessed, and increase the risk of operation and anesthesia and should be discussed with the patient.

Bowel Preparation

Recent level I evidence suggests that mechanical bowel preparations (MBP) can be safely omitted during elective colorectal resections and anastomoses as MBP may be associated with increased anastomotic leakage rates [50]. This has been postulated to be related to the presence of liquid (as opposed to solid) stool, or nutritional/metabolic/toxic alteration of the enterocolonic mucosa.

Currently, MBP is widely practiced and remains the standard of care. For elective MBP or for constipated patients, most commonly recommended is a clear liquid diet for 24 h preoperatively with 2–4 L of polyethylene glycol with oral rehydration the evening before surgery. Nil per os (NPO) after midnight is still routine despite evidence that clear liquids up to 4 h preoperatively increases gastric emptying and reduces the risk of aspiration, and important consideration in elderly patients who may be at increased risk of delayed gastric emptying.

The MBP regimen must be modified in the patient with obstructive symptoms and may include a longer period of clear liquids in addition to low volume cathartics such as milk of magnesia (30 cc), magnesium citrate, or phospho-soda. However, surgeons must be aware that phospho-soda, although generally well tolerated by most patients, is contraindicated in those with known renal impairment (such as the elderly), electrolyte abnormalities, cardiovascular disease, bowel obstruction or otherwise altered GI motility or permeability, and in the elderly in whom it has been associated with acute phosphate nephropathy [51]. Tap water or phospho-soda enemas may be more helpful, particularly in the presence of obstructive symptoms. Despite the now routine use of bowel preparation in the outpatient setting, selected elderly patients, particularly those with cardiac disease such as aortic stenosis, may require hospitalization to prevent dehydration and avoid dramatic fluid shifts.

Intravenous antibiotic preparation does not differ from routine bowel surgery and typically consists of a second- or third-generation cephalosporin (e.g., Cefoxitin), or a quinolone (e.g., Ciprofloxacin) with metronidazole and in the case of penicillin, quinolone, or metronidazole allergy, vancomycin is used. Antibiotics must be administered within ½ h prior to skin incision and redosed intraoperatively after 4–6 h, and in the absence of an indication for ongoing antibiotic treatment discontinued within 24 h postoperatively.

Steroid Preparation

Recent level I data suggests that with the exception of patients with primary diseases of the hypothalamic–pituitary–adrenal axis, stress-dose steroids may be safely omitted as long as the patient continues to receive their usual daily dose [52]. However, current standard of care is for perioperative stress doses of corticosteroids to be administered if the patient has been treated with steroids within the preceding 6 months, a common occurrence in IBD patients. Our current preference is to administer methylprednisone 40 mg IV on call to the operating room, 30 mg every 12 h for the next 24 h, and then 20 mg daily; an alternative regimen is 50 mg of hydrocortisone on call to the OR, then 50 mg every 12 h in the first 24 h, 25 mg every 12 h the 2nd day, 12.5 mg every 12 h (or equivalent of the patients' usual dose) on the 3rd day, and the equivalent of the patients' usual dose the 4th day. Continuation of the taper depends on the preoperative dose and duration of steroid therapy but generally occurs slowly over a period of 6 weeks.

Electrolyte and Nutritional Deficits

Appropriate preoperative testing may reveal abnormalities. Electrolyte derangements, anemia, dehydration, and coagulation deficits should be corrected in both elective and emergent settings. Correction of nutritional deficits, as evidenced by weight loss, hypoalbuminemia, and negative nitrogen balance, is controversial. The use of total parenteral nutrition (TPN) has been shown in some series to improve nutritional parameters but does not significantly reduce postoperative complications [53].

One randomized study of severely nutritionally depleted patients undergoing GI surgery, a category which often applies to IBD patients, demonstrated a reduction in postoperative complications when such patients received 10 days of enteral nutrition preoperatively [54]. In addition, one series [55] did show that the extent of small bowel resection was less in patients receiving preoperative TPN, but this finding is possibly of clinical value only in patients who would otherwise be at risk of short bowel syndrome.

Enterostomal Therapy

Preoperative preparation of the patient for a stoma is invaluable, regardless of whether an ileostomy or colostomy is being considered and whether it is to be temporary or permanent. Preparation consists of marking the abdomen preoperatively and patient education. Such marking guides the correct site of the stoma within the rectus muscle, away from bony prominences and skin creases and scars.

Preoperative education and counseling, preferably from an enterostomal therapist, is valued by patients.

Operative Principles

Resection, Stricturoplasty, Diversion, or Bypass

Resection, with the goal of preserving as much absorptive bowel length as possible, is generally the approach of choice in patients whose symptoms are sufficient to merit operative intervention. In elderly patients, the colon is the most common site of disease, and with rare exceptions, symptomatic disease is resected. The surgery may take the form of segmental resection with primary anastomosis with or without diverting ostomy for limited colonic disease, or a subtotal colectomy with or without anastomosis, or proctocolectomy and Brooke ileostomy. Controversially, some centers construct ileal pouch-anal anastomosis (IPAA) in the setting of known CD; at our institution, CD is considered an absolute contraindication to IPAA, especially in the elderly. With small bowel disease, the ileocecal region is often affected most severely and merits resection.

Stricturoplasty is generally employed in the small bowel to avoid resection. It is usually not necessary at a first operation but can be employed at subsequent procedures to widen the lumen of the bowel at short strictures, and multiple to many stricturoplasties may be performed concurrently. Although active Crohn's disease is left in situ by this method, it does not appear to increase the rate of subsequent reoperation and has proven invaluable for preserving small bowel length in patients who would otherwise be at risk of short bowel syndrome. Stricturoplasty is less commonly used at anastomotic strictures but can be useful in this situation. It is advisable to obtain frozen section biopsy of the stricture being left in situ, as although quite rare (less than 0.1%), small bowel cancer has been observed in strictures [56].

In rare cases, when a resection or stricturoplasty of the diseased segment cannot be safely performed, diversion of the fecal stream or enteroenteric (internal) bypass may be the only remaining options and used as temporizing measures to improve the patients' condition [42]. Specifically, in the case of phlegmonous involvement of vital (vascular) structures (e.g., the iliac artery and vein), several options exist including exclusion with proximal external diversion and distal mucus fistula construction (to avoid creating a closed loop), or internal bypass, which allows the fecal stream proximal to the diseased segment to be diverted to a healthy segment while allowing the area distal to drain normally. As the patients' condition allows these, temporizing may allow sufficient healing to occur to allow more definitive surgical options.

Extent of Resection: Macroscopic vs. Microscopic Margins

The extent of resection is essentially based on the surgeon's judgment at operation and the ability to recognize macroscopically diseased bowel. Typical small bowel disease is manifested by bowel wall thickening and induration; serositis and prominent vessels running on the surface of the serosa; "creeping fat" or encroachment of mesenteric fat over the bowel wall; and thickening along the mesenteric edge of the bowel (Figs. 66.1 and 66.2). Correlating with these changes in the bowel are a characteristic thickening of

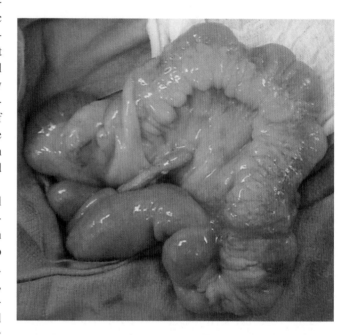

FIGURE 66.1 Crohn's disease, gross specimen, terminal ileitis. Note the creeping fat, serosal hyperemia, mesenteric lymphadenopathy, and ileo-ileal fistulization.

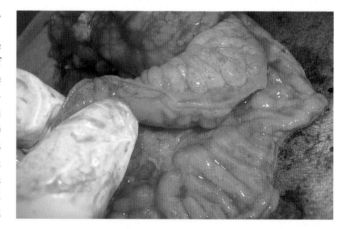

FIGURE 66.2 Crohn's disease, sectioned gross specimen, terminal ileitis. Note the transmural inflammation, strictured lumen, and linear (cat-scratch) ulceration which are typically pathognomonic for Crohn's disease, as compared to ulcerative colitis.

the mesentery, with enlarged lymph nodes that may occur diffusely throughout the small bowel mesentery but are usually more prominent at sites of active disease. Establishing the extent of disease in the colon may be more problematic by inspection of the external appearance alone, and intraoperative colonoscopy may prove invaluable in such cases.

Adequate margins are obtained by resecting back to macroscopically normal bowel. Once a subject of controversy, radical margins of resection now are thought to sacrifice more functioning small bowel than is of benefit for reducing recurrence. Several retrospective series have demonstrated no relation between the presence of microscopic disease at resection margins and the rate of recurrence [57, 58]. Hamilton et al. [59] compared patients undergoing frozen section evaluation of margins with a group whose margins were judged macroscopically free of disease; at 10 years, the clinical recurrence rates were not significantly different (60 and 66%, respectively), nor were the reoperative rates (36 and 32%, respectively). More recently, a randomized prospective trial comparing macroscopically free margins of 2 cm versus 12 cm has revealed no difference in clinical or operative recurrence rates at 5 years [60]. The advent of postoperative medical prophylaxis with mesalamine, azathioprine, and other medications has made microscopic disease-free resection margins moot [61].

Type of Anastomosis: Hand sewn vs. Stapled

Standard surgical principles apply to the creation of any anastomosis, ensuring good blood supply, lack of tension, and correct orientation. Use of suturing or stapling techniques depends on the surgeon's preference. Recent level I data demonstrated that the anastomotic technique had no impact on postoperative outcomes [62], while a meta-analysis found side-to-side (linear stapled) anastomoses to be superior. This finding is especially relevant for surgeons who do not perform a high volume of hand-sewn anastomoses or who do not see a high volume of CD patients. As anastomotic staples are not intended to be hemostatic (least they induce tissue necrosis), it is important to check the suture line for excessive oozing.

Operative Approach: Minimally Invasive (Laparoscopic) Surgery

Laparoscopic (LAP) or minimally invasive surgery (MIS) techniques are being increasingly used for Crohn's disease, a disease that was once thought not to be compatible with the laparoscopic approach. Initial concerns centered on the inherent inflammatory nature of the disease, with its attendant thickened bowel and mesentery and frequent association with fistulas and abscesses, which can make even open surgery

challenging. As experience with the technique has grown to include hand-assisted laparoscopic surgery (HALS), the feasibility and benefits of this approach in selected patients are becoming even more apparent. To date, several randomized trials and a meta-analysis have demonstrated the benefits of a MIS resection for ileocecal and small bowel disease [63]. Although these procedures take longer to perform, patients had shorter lengths of stay and lower morbidity. The presence of fistulas and abscesses do not necessarily preclude a successful laparoscopic approach, this being possible in up to 75% of such patients. A similar success rate was demonstrated in patients who had undergone prior abdominal operations. The procedure results in statistically significant and clinically relevant benefits, with patients exhibiting less pain, more rapid resolution of ileus, and earlier discharge [64]. Similar benefits have been demonstrated after MIS colectomy for Crohn's colitis [66] and also in elderly patients. A case-control series from the Mayo Clinic [64] of laparoscopic resection versus matched open resection found in the former group that postoperative ileus resolved more rapidly, patients had fewer postoperative complications, and they were discharged sooner. In addition, a significantly larger percentage of patients in the laparoscopy group were discharged to their own homes and remained independent after operation, an important consideration in the elderly.

It is now understood that age alone is not a contraindication to laparoscopic colon and rectal surgery [66], and several studies have examined the benefits of laparoscopic colorectal surgery in the elderly. Law et al. reported on the outcomes in a series of 65 patients over the age of 70 compared with 89 patients who had undergone open surgery [67]. They found benefits typical of a laparoscopic approach including earlier return of GI function and earlier discharge, but also found that LAP elderly patients had fewer cardiopulmonary complications. Similarly, Frasson et al. reported the results of a subgroup comparison from a randomized study of laparoscopic colorectal surgery of which 201 were >70 years of age [68]. They also found that the benefits of laparoscopic surgery are more pronounced in elderly patients; specifically, elderly patients who underwent LAP had lower morbidity and short lengths of stay. Although care must be taken to assess the impact of pneumoperitoneum on the cardiopulmonary comorbidities frequently seen in the elderly, clearly age alone is not a contraindication to LAP, and at our institution, is the preferred approach.

Management by Anatomic Site

Gastric and Duodenal Disease

Primary gastric disease is an unusual manifestation of CD [69]. Endoscopy may reveal gastric dilatation and superficial ulceration. The findings may be suggestive of peptic ulcer disease or may be difficult to distinguish from carcinoma. Biopsy may reveal characteristic granulomas. Patients may undergo gastrectomy if carcinoma cannot be excluded.

The duodenum may be the site of primary or secondary manifestations of CD. Primary CD is unusual; the early nonspecific symptoms are suggestive of peptic ulcer disease and may respond to antacids and systemic treatments for CD such as corticosteroids, immunomodulators, and biologic agents. In terms of definitive surgical management in the era of proton pump inhibitors, laparoscopic gastrojejunostomy with or without vagotomy has become an attractive alternative to open gastrojejunostomy and in experienced hands is the procedure of choice [70] for the palliation of CD-related gastric outlet obstruction. The omission of vagotomy (in lieu of PPI treatment in the face of complications) or performing a highly selective vagotomy prevents the marginal ulceration associated with bypass alone and avoids the postvagotomy diarrhea associated with truncal vagotomy. Duodenal stricturoplasty is technically challenging and rarely performed, even in tertiary referral centers.

More commonly, the duodenum may be secondarily affected as a bystander adjacent to fistulizing disease in the ileum or colon, especially from a previous ileocolic anastomosis. This complication may be reduced by performing an ileoascending anastomosis, preserving as much of the right colon as possible at the time of ileocecal resection. The omentum should be used whenever possible to separate the anastomosis from the duodenum. Bystander duodenum may be closed primarily in a transverse manner.

Jejunoileal Disease

Manifestations of CD in the small bowel may be localized or diffuse. Most commonly, localized disease occurs distally and is generally amenable to resection, particularly at first operation. This also holds true for several segments of disease concentrated in one area, where a single resection and anastomosis is preferred rather than several anastomoses. Although sparing of the terminal ileum is relatively unusual with distal ileal disease, the ileocecal valve should be preserved if there is a distal disease-free area of more than 5 cm allowing an anastomosis to avoid ischemia to the anastomosis.

Surgical judgment faces stronger challenges in the event of diffuse small bowel disease. Occasionally, areas of small bowel dilatation serve as guides to points of significant stricturing, but often with diffuse disease, it is difficult to distinguish small bowel that is thickened secondary to CD from bowel that is thickened from chronic obstruction proximal to a stricture, In such instances, it is helpful to make an enterotomy distally and perform direct enteroscopy to evaluate the proximal bowel. An alternative is to insert a Baker tube (a long tube bearing an inflatable balloon near its tip) proximally as far as the ligament of Treitz. The balloon is then inflated to a diameter of 1.5–2.0 cm and withdrawn slowly. The balloon is held up at points of stricturing that can be marked with seromuscular sutures, and stricturoplasties are performed at these sites.

Ileocecal Disease

Ileocecal disease is the commonest indication for operative intervention in all patients but is less common in older than in young patients. Frequently, the right colon is affected only to the level of the ileocecal valve, and it is possible to perform an ileoascending anastomosis, preserving most of the right colon.

Colonic Disease

The surgical approach to colonic disease is determined primarily by three factors: extent of disease (localized or diffuse), presence of rectal sparing, and function of the anal sphincter in preserving continence.

Localized Colitis

Among patients with disease limited to the colon, only 10% [71] exhibit limited or segmental disease of the colon. Unlike the situation with the small intestine, segmental resection of the colon was in the past considered controversial because of the impression that recurrence rates were high and that an ileostomy would ultimately be required [42]. A series from the Mayo Clinic [72] of 49 patients undergoing limited colonic resection for segmental disease showed that only 14% of patients over a mean follow-up period of 14 years ultimately required stoma construction. Those who ultimately required a stoma enjoyed a mean stoma-free interval of 23 months. Thus, a stoma was avoided in most of the patients. Even those in whom a stoma was eventually necessary benefited from an extended period of stoma avoidance. Social and body image arguably may be of more importance to young patients for avoiding a stoma. The elderly also benefit from this approach, particularly those in whom a previous small bowel resection has been performed and who potentially might be debilitated by profuse small bowel effluent through an ileorectal anastomosis or an ileostomy. The use of segmental colonic resection may increase with more widespread prescription of immunosuppressive drugs, such as azathioprine or 6-mercaptopurine for diffuse colitis; areas of most severe ulceration appear in some instances to heal with focal stricturing.

Diffuse Colitis

In the elective setting, the choice of procedure for treating pancolitis is determined in part by the presence or absence of rectal disease. In the patient with proctocolitis, the preferred option is proctocolectomy and Brooke ileostomy. Although some have suggested use of a low Hartmann closure of the rectum to allow perianal disease to regress, 40% of the patients (10/25) required a later perineal proctectomy, and three of these patients still exhibited wound problems [73]. The use of ileostomy alone improves general well-being in about two-thirds of patients but does not consistently avoid later proctocolectomy, and fewer than 10% ever experience restoration of intestinal continuity. Diversion alone may be a consideration in an elderly patient who refuses or who would not tolerate proctocolectomy.

The elderly patient with pancolitis but rectal sparing deserves careful evaluation. Measurement of anal canal pressures is not predictive of postoperative function, although Keighley et al. [74] found assessment of rectal compliance (by identifying those whose maximum tolerated rectal volume was >150 ml) to be helpful. The individual who remains continent despite loose stool during attacks of colitis has undergone the most rigorous physiologic test of continence and would be a candidate for total abdominal colectomy (subtotal colectomy) with ileosigmoid or ileorectal anastomosis. Those occasionally incontinent of loose stool probably have less than perfect control, but this situation may be preferable to having a stoma; it merits discussion with the patient. The individual who is frankly incontinent would be best served by a proctocolectomy or a subtotal colectomy, ileostomy, and retained rectal stump. Although some authors have suggested use of an ileal pouch to improve compliance if resection is necessary to the level of the mid-rectum [42], this procedure is highly controversial, as known Crohn's disease is widely considered an absolute contraindication to use of a pouch, given the 45% risk of pouch failure secondary to complications [75].

In the emergent setting, the guiding principle is to remove the site of disease as expeditiously as possible, avoid further complications, and perform a later staged procedure if necessary. In the setting of diffuse colonic involvement and megacolon, perforation, or hemorrhage, a subtotal colectomy with ileostomy is performed, and the rectum is either left long as a mucus fistula or short as an extraperitoneal stump. If hemorrhage is arising from the rectum in the face of diffuse disease, however, proctocolectomy cannot be avoided. Perforation resulting from localized disease in the colon is addressed with resection, proximal stoma, and mucus fistula or exclusion of the distal bowel. Perforation of localized rectal disease is approached by proximal colostomy and drainage of the pelvis, with proctectomy 3–6 months later.

Perianal Disease

Crohn's disease manifestations in the perianal region include skin tags, fissures, ulcers, abscesses, fistulas, and anorectal stricture. These findings frequently occur after intestinal symptoms have resulted in a diagnosis of CD, but when perianal findings precede other symptoms, the diagnosis can present difficulties. Examination includes digital assessment, anoscopy, and rigid or flexible sigmoidoscopy. Discomfort may necessitate examination under anesthesia for full evaluation. Biopsy infrequently yields evidence of a granuloma, but other features are suggestive of CD: edematous, violaceous skin tags; fissures at sites other than the midline; indolent abscesses; complex fistulas; and stricturing without evidence of malignancy or prior anorectal surgery. A new diagnosis of CD should prompt evaluation of the entire gastrointestinal tract, although it is unclear whether disease activity more proximally affects perianal disease [76].

Therapy must be individualized, bearing in mind treatment principles of relief of symptoms and avoidance of additional complications. Careful consideration should be given to appropriate medical and surgical approaches. Perianal skin tags and hemorrhoids are best approached conservatively, with control of diarrhea, sitz baths, and analgesia; surgical therapy of either is associated with a high rate of poor outcomes [77]. Symptomatic fissures should be evaluated to rule out underlying sepsis and then approached initially with medical therapy. In selected cases and when conservative therapy has failed, lateral internal sphincterotomy may be beneficial. Careful consideration must be given to issues of continence, however, particularly in the elderly. Abscesses should be treated with incision and drainage, making the incision into the abscess cavity as close to the anus as possible to keep any subsequent fistula as short as possible.

Management of perianal fistulas is often challenging. As with other situations, therapy is aimed at relieving symptoms; hence, in the absence of associated sepsis, an asymptomatic fistula may require no specific therapy. Simple low fistulas without accompanying proctitis may be managed successfully with fistulotomy [78], particularly when combined with therapy such as metronidazole or sulfasalazine [79]. When it is thought that sphincterotomy may result in fecal continence because the fistula is high or complex or because the elderly patient has borderline continence, other approaches are necessary. Noncutting setons achieve drainage without compromise of continence; despite the presence of a foreign body, most patients tolerate setons far better than undrained fistulas, particularly if the seton is of a soft material such as Silastic vessel loops [42]. If the rectal mucosa does not exhibit active disease, the patient may be a candidate for a rectal mucosal advancement flap. An overall success rate of 60% has been reported for this approach to low fistulas [80], but the success rate falls to approximately one-third in high, complex fistulas [81]. An alternative approach is the use of fibrin glue, which has a lower success rate than with non-Crohn's fistulas after a single application, but repeated applications may result in success and there is no risk of compromising the sphincter. Although anti-TNF-Ab therapy (infliximab) is showing promise in therapy of perianal CD that would otherwise be considered an indication for proctectomy; data in the elderly are still limited or absent. Creation of a diverting ileostomy is occasionally a useful means for controlling severe perianal disease, but only one-third of patients ever achieve successful reversal [42].

Ulcerative Colitis: Indications for Elective Surgery

Failure of Medical Therapy

An algorithmic approach to the surgical management of CUC is presented in Fig. 66.3. Medical therapy may be considered to have failed when maximal therapy has not controlled symptoms or when symptoms are abolished only at the expense of side effects from the medications themselves. The inability to wean steroids completely or to an acceptable level is also an indication for operation. Inability or unwillingness to comply with a medical regimen may prompt surgical intervention.

Presence or Risk of Carcinoma

An increased risk of colorectal cancer has been documented in those with extensive long-standing ulcerative colitis [82, 83]. The magnitude of this risk is controversial, with population-based studies suggesting that the risk is lower than previously thought and most dependent on the extent and duration of colitis. It is best defined in patients whose disease onset occurred during childhood or the teenage years, those with extensive disease, and those whose duration of disease is more than 10 years; in these patients, the risk of developing cancer is reported to be 2% per year [84]. The risk in patients with later age of onset is not well defined. Monitoring by screening colonoscopy for dysplasia has limitations, including patient compliance and the finding that carcinoma may not have evidence of preceding dysplasia [85]. At the time of colectomy for dysplasia, more than 50% already have invasive cancer [86]. In the absence of an absolute indication (i.e., stricture, evidence of dysplasia or a dysplasia-associated mass, existing cancer [87]), the role of surgery is less clear, despite results of a decision analysis that suggest prophylactic colectomy improves survival more than surveillance [88]. In the elderly, later onset of disease and shorter duration of remaining life compared with younger patients probably results in surgery being used more for specific indications than for prophylaxis.

Indications for Emergency Surgery

Fulminant Colitis

The definition of fulminant colitis is identical to that described for CD, although the Truelove and Witts' criteria may be useful in stratifying disease severity in CUC (Table 66.4) [89]. It is important to remember, particularly in the patient presenting with a fulminant first attack, that the differentiation

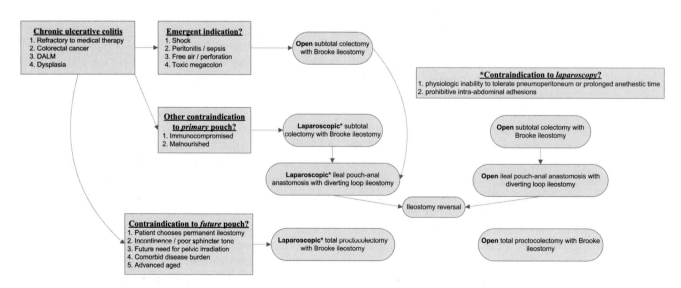

Figure 66.3 Surgery for elderly patients with chronic ulcerative colitis treatment algorithm.

TABLE 66.4 Modified Truelove and Witts' criteria of ulcerative colitis disease severity [89, 111]

Variable	Mild disease	Moderate disease	Severe disease	Fulminant disease
No. stools (per 24 h)	<4	4–6	>6	>10
Blood in stool	Intermittent	Occasional	Frequent	Continuous
Temperature (°C)	Normal	>37.5	>37.5	>37.5
Pulse (beats/min)	Normal	>90	>90	>90
Hemoglobin	Normal	Anemia	<75% of normal	Transfusion requirement
ESR (mm/h)	<30	–	>30	>30
Colonic features on X-ray	–	–	Wall edema, thumbprinting	Dilatation
Clinical signs	–	–	Abdominal tenderness	Abdominal distention and tenderness

ESR erythrocyte sedimentation rate
Source: Mahadevan et al. [89]. Reprinted with permission of John Wiley & Sons, Inc.

between CD and UC may not be possible. The surgical approach is the same, whichever the underlying diagnosis. Although this diagnosis previously has been associated with a high mortality rate, mortality is now less than 3% [90] due in part to aggressive surgical intervention and probably to changes in medical management.

Toxic Megacolon, Perforation, Hemorrhage, Obstruction

In emergent settings, UC is often indistinguishable from CD. The principles of therapy outlined for CD, including the appropriate extent of resection in emergent settings, apply equally to either diagnosis.

Preoperative Preparation

Many of the principles of preoperative preparation discussed for patients with CD apply equally to those with UC. They include correction of electrolyte abnormalities and severe anemia, bowel preparation, use of antibiotics, and stress doses of steroids. Possibly, the most important aspect differentiating the patient with UC from the one with CD is consideration given to reconstructive surgery in the form of the ileal pouch-anal anastomosis (IPAA), which should be avoided in the acute setting.

Operative Procedure

Essentially, the choice of procedure (Table 66.5, Fig. 66.3) depends on the presentation of the patient (e.g., disease severity) and how much of the rectum is to be removed (all, part, or none), and if the anal sphincter is competent.

If the patient is incontinent of stool due to an incompetent sphincter (and not to poor compliance in a diseased rectum), the decision is simple: proctocolectomy and Brooke ileostomy. In the individual without compromise of the sphincter, consideration may be given to proctocolectomy and ileostomy, subtotal colectomy, (Fig. 66.4) and ileorectal anastomosis, or proctocolectomy, and IPAA (or ileal pouch-distal rectal anastomosis).

Multiple studies have examined the role of restorative proctocolectomy in the elderly [91–102]. These have been summarized in Table 66.6. Advanced age has generally been considered a contraindication to IPAA because of the high risk of fecal incontinence in the elderly. The clinical results in carefully selected patients over the age of 50, however, are equivalent to those of younger patients. Anal sphincter strength does decline after the age of 70 [103], and few, if any, patients beyond this age are candidates for this operation.

Operative Approach: Minimally Invasive (Laparoscopic) Surgery

Similar to as seen in CD, MIS techniques are being increasingly used in CUC. Several recent studies from Mayo Clinic have demonstrated the applicability of MIS techniques to CUC, including subtotal colectomy, IPAA, TPC with BI [104–106]. In a case series of 50 patients with severe-to-fulminant CUC who underwent MIS subtotal colectomy with Brooke ileostomy, the majority (95%) who subsequently underwent IPAA were performed laparoscopically with a median length of stay of 4 days for each procedure. Similarly in a case-matched study comparing open and LAP IPAA, the benefits typical of a LAP approach were demonstrated. Finally, in a case series of 43 patients who underwent MIS TPC-BI, and in whom the median age was 66 years, this procedure was demonstrated to be safe and feasible. Our preferred port placement for both LAP and HALS approaches to colectomy for CUC is shown in Fig. 66.5.

TABLE 66.5 Choice of operation for ulcerative colitis in elderly patients

Typical no. of stages	Procedure	Contraindications	Comments
3-, 2-, or 1-stage[a] IPAA	TPC with IPAA and DLI; 3-stage if follows STC with BI, rarely, if ever 1-stage without DLI	Incompetent sphincter Advanced age (relative) Need for pelvic irradiation	Risks related to multiple operations and general anesthestics Complete excision of disease Risk of pouchitis Risk of cancer in retained mucosa
2-Stage (modified) IPAA	STC with BI followed by IPAA *without* DLI	None	Easier/faster operation to perform Complete excision of disease Risk of pouchitis; increased risk of leak? Risk of cancer in retained mucosa
1-Stage[a]	TPC with BI	None	Easier/faster operation to perform Complete excision of disease Risk of stoma-related complications
2-, or 1-stage	TPC with IRA (straight IRA or ileal pouch-rectal anastomosis); infrequently 2-stage with DLI	Incompetent sphincter Advanced age (relative) Need for pelvic irradiation Noncompliant for follow-up	Easier/faster operation to perform Risk of pouchitis Increased risk of cancer in retained rectal mucosa
2-, or 1-stage	TPC with K-pouch; 2-stage if follows STC with BI	Most patients	Frequent reoperation Rarely recommended, even in young patients
2-, or 1-stage	STC with IRA; infrequently 2-stage with DLI	Incompetent sphincter Active rectal disease Noncompliant for follow-up	Incomplete excision of disease At risk for proctitis or development of rectal cancer
2-, or 1-stage	STC with BI	None	Easier/faster operation to perform Incomplete excision of disease At risk for proctitis or development of rectal cancer
2-, or 1-stage	Segmental colectomy with primary anastomosis	Most patients	Rarely if ever recommended due to incomplete excision of disease, even in young patients
Temporizing procedure	Turnbull procedure (ileostomy with blowhole colostomy)	Almost all patients	Generally of historic interest only for the treatment of toxic megacolon in unstable patients; however, success with this procedure has recently been reported in 2 pregnant women with toxic megacolon [112]

TPC total proctocolectomy, *BI* Brooke ileostomy, *DLI* diverting loop ileostomy, *IPAA* ileal pouch-anal anastomosis, *IRA* ileorectal anastomosis, *STC* subtotal colectomy, *K-pouch* continent ileostomy (Kock pouch)
[a]Most commonly preferred surgical approaches in elderly patients

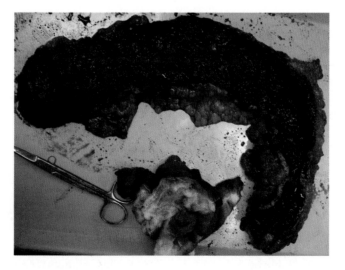

FIGURE 66.4 Chronic ulcerative colitis, subtotal colectomy, gross specimen. Note the complete carpeting of the colonic mucosa with pseudopolyps and foreshortening of the right, transverse, and left colon from an elderly woman with long-standing CUC.

TABLE 66.6 Summary of recent studies of ileal pouch-anal anastomosis in the elderly

Author	Institution	Year	Study design	Age (years)	Elderly (N)	Major findings/comments
Ho et al. [102][a]	Cleveland Clinic, Florida	2006	Subgroup comparisons	>70	17	No difference in length of stay, complications (40%), or pouch failure between >70 and <70 years old cohorts
Chapman et al. [101]	Mayo Clinic, Rochester	2005	Subgroup comparisons	>55	65	No difference in complications. Incontinence more common, but did not affect QoL
Longo et al. [99][a]	St. Louis University	2003	Population-based (Veterans) subgroup comparisons	>50	158	Of 46 patients >70 years, no IPAA's were performed. 22% overall surgical morbidity; 4% mortality (all non-IPAA patients)
Delaney et al. [100][a]	Cleveland Clinic, Ohio	2003	Subgroup comparisons	56–65 >65	154 42	Increased incontinence, night-time seepage in older groups; QoL decreased but not statistically
Farouk et al. [97][a]	Mayo Clinic, Rochester	2000	Subgroup comparisons	>45	204 (1 year) 33 (12 years)	At 1 and 12 years, incontinence affected older group more often. Incontinence increased with time in older, but not younger, patients. Pouch excision due to incontinence not statistically different between group (<45, $n=11$ vs. >45, $n=3$)
Church [98]	Cleveland Clinic, Ohio	2000	Case report, 10-year follow-up	85	1	Bowel function, QoL remained relatively stable; age is not necessarily a contraindication to IPAA
Takao et al. [96]	Cleveland Clinic, Florida	1998	Subgroup comparisons	>60	17	Postoperative minor and transient functional impairment is not an age-related phenomenon
Tan et al. [95]	Queen Elizabeth Hospital	1997	Subgroup comparisons	>50	28	Included 4 non-CUC patients. Higher incidence of IPAA stenosis in the elderly. Age did not impact functional outcomes
Bauer et al. [94]	Mount Sinai	1997	Subgroup comparisons	>50	66	Elderly group with longer duration of disease, more dysplasia. Age did not impact functional outcomes
Reismann et al. [93]	Cleveland Clinic, Florida	1996	Subgroup comparisons	>60	14	Older patients experience more nocturnal movements (2 vs. 1.1, $p<0.05$) than younger patients. Morbidity and manometry did not differ
Jorge et al. [92]	Cleveland Clinic, Florida	1994	Subgroup comparisons	Mean 56	22	Transient, statistically significant decrease in internal anal sphincter function in older group, but recovered completely
Lewis et al. [91][a]	General Infirmary, Leeds	1993	Matched case-control	>50	18	Anorectal manometry not statistically different between age groups before/after surgery. Age alone is not a contraindication to restorative surgery if anal sphincter is completely intact

[a]High quality/recommended

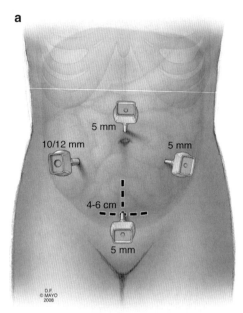 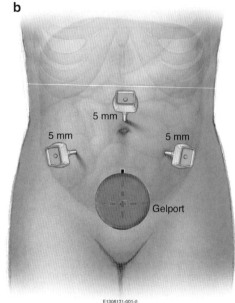

Figure 66.5 Laparoscopic port placement for total proctocolectomy. (**a**) Laparoscopic-assisted surgery; IPAA, TPC-BI, STC-EI. (**b**) Hand-assisted surgery; IPAA, TPC-BI, STC-EI. *Dashed lines* represent potential specimen extraction sites (copyrighted and used with permission of Mayo Foundation for Medical Education and Research, used with permission, all rights reserved).

CASE STUDY: REFRACTORY ULCERATIVE COLITIS IN AN OCTOGENARIAN

An 83-year-old male with a 2-month history of CUC presented to the surgical service with refractory colitis despite 5-aminosalicylate dose escalation and 30 mg of prednisone daily. The patient complained of 8–14 bloody bowel movements per day. The patient's body mass index was 25 kg/m². The patient had multiple comorbidities including steroid-induced diabetes mellitus, chronic renal insufficiency, hyperlipidemia, iron-deficiency anemia, and a history of a type 5 peptic ulcer disease. Preoperatively, the patient's Charlson score was 8 points, and American Society of Anesthesiology (ASA) score was 3. The patient has a history of a radical prostatectomy with postoperative external beam irradiation. Endoscopy revealed moderately active pancolitis with no evidence of dysplasia. Given the patient's, age, comorbidities, and history of pelvic surgery and irradiation, we recommended a total proctocolectomy with end ileostomy.

The patient underwent an uneventful laparoscopic total proctocolectomy, intersphincteric dissection, and Brooke ileostomy. Given the history of pelvic surgery and irradiation, the pelvic dissection was tedious; overall operative time was 444 min, estimated blood loss was 450 ml, and he was transfused one unit of pack cells. There were no intraoperative complications, and the procedure was completed laparoscopically. Gross pathology revealed severely active pancolitis with a tubular adenoma with low-grade dysplasia in the descending colon.

Postoperatively, the patient's stoma began functioning on day 3, and he tolerated a regular diet. The patient was discharged home on postoperative day 4 but 2 days later returned to the hospital with left lower extremity swelling and was found to have an ileofemoral deep vein thrombosis, treated with anticoagulation. He suffered no other complications within 30 days. Subsequently, the patient had developed a partial small bowel obstruction related to a parastomal hernia, which was initially managed with a hernia belt. The hernia was enlarged, and the patient underwent an uneventful mesh repair and remains asymptomatic.

This case demonstrates that:

1. Age alone is not a contraindication to laparoscopic colectomy (nor is it an absolute contraindication to IPAA).
2. Prior treatment of age-related cancers may affect surgical decision making and recommendations for restorative proctocolectomy.

(continued)

CASE STUDY (continued)

3. The timing of surgical intervention for elderly patients with moderate-to-severe CUC must take into account the patients physiologic reserve and ability to tolerate ongoing bloody diarrhea. In the face of worsening anemia, renal insufficiency, a lower threshold for operation may be appropriate for elderly patients with active CUC.

4. The risks and benefits of surgical therapy for elderly patients with CUC must be weighted against the risks and benefits of escalated medical therapy with agents such as corticosteroids and infliximab. These agents in particular may be associated with increased postoperative infectious complications and less well tolerated in elderly, as compared with younger patients.

5. Elderly patients with long-standing IBD colitis are likely to be at increased risk of inflammatory-associated cancer.

6. A 1-stage procedure with permanent ileostomy may obviate the need for subsequent planned operations, but this advantage must be weighted against the long-term risk of stoma-related complications and need for reoperation.

References

1. Loftus CG, Loftus EV Jr, Harmsen WS et al (2007) Update on the incidence and prevalence of Crohn's disease and ulcerative colitis in Olmsted County, Minnesota, 1940–2000. Inflamm Bowel Dis 13(3):254–261

2. Jess T, Riis L, Vind I et al (2007) Changes in clinical characteristics, course, and prognosis of inflammatory bowel disease during the last 5 decades: a population-based study from Copenhagen, Denmark. Inflamm Bowel Dis 13(4):481–489

3. Robertson DJ, Grimm IS (2001) Inflammatory bowel disease in the elderly. Gastroenterol Clin North Am 30(2):409–426

4. Ananthakrishnan AN, McGinley EL, Binion DG (2008) Inflammatory bowel disease in the elderly is associated with worse outcomes: a national study of hospitalizations. Inflamm Bowel Dis 15(2):182–189

5. Jess T (2008) Prognosis of inflammatory bowel disease across time and countries. An epidemiological study of population-based patient cohorts. Dan Med Bull 55(2):103–120

6. Crohn BB, Ginzburg L (1932) Regional ileitis: a pathologic and clinical entity. JAMA 99:1323–1329

7. Loftus EV Jr, Schoenfeld P, Sandborn WJ (2002) The epidemiology and natural history of Crohn's disease in population-based patient cohorts from North America: a systematic review. Aliment Pharmacol Ther 16(1):51–60

8. Corman ML (2005) Colon and rectal surgery, 5th edn. Lippincott Williams & Wilkins, Philadelphia

9. Yang SK, Yun S, Kim JH et al (2008) Epidemiology of inflammatory bowel disease in the Songpa-Kangdong district, Seoul, Korea, 1986–2005: a KASID study. Inflamm Bowel Dis 14(4):542–549

10. Thia KT, Loftus EV Jr, Sandborn WJ, Yang SK (2008) An update on the epidemiology of inflammatory bowel disease in Asia. Am J Gastroenterol 103(12):3167–3182

11. Fleischer DE, Grimm IS, Friedman LS (1994) Inflammatory bowel disease in older patients. Med Clin North Am 78(6):1303–1319

12. Lapidus A, Bernell O, Hellers G et al (1997) Incidence of Crohn's disease in Stockholm County 1955–1989. Gut 41(4):480–486

13. Wilks S (1859) The morbid appearance of the intestines of Miss Bankes. Med Times Gaz 2:264

14. Loftus EV Jr, Silverstein MD, Sandborn WJ et al (2000) Ulcerative colitis in Olmsted County, Minnesota, 1940–1993: incidence, prevalence, and survival. Gut 46(3):336–343

15. Stockbrugger RW, Russel MG, van Blankenstein M, Shivananda S (2000) EC-IBD: a European effort in inflammatory bowel disease. Eur J Intern Med 11(4):187–190

16. Lok KH, Hung HG, Ng CH et al (2008) Epidemiology and clinical characteristics of ulcerative colitis in Chinese population: experience from a single center in Hong Kong. J Gastroenterol Hepatol 23(3):406–410

17. Softley A, Myren J, Clamp SE et al (1988) Inflammatory bowel disease in the elderly patient. Scand J Gastroenterol Suppl 144:27–30

18. Langholz E, Munkholm P, Nielsen OH et al (1991) Incidence and prevalence of ulcerative colitis in Copenhagen county from 1962 to 1987. Scand J Gastroenterol 26(12):1247–1256

19. Evans JG, Acheson ED (1965) An epidemiological study of ulcerative colitis and regional enteritis in the Oxford area. Gut 6(4):311–324

20. Garland CF, Lilienfeld AM, Mendeloff AI et al (1981) Incidence rates of ulcerative colitis and Crohn's disease in fifteen areas of the United States. Gastroenterology 81(6):1115–1124

21. Shivananda S, Lennard-Jones J, Logan R et al (1996) Incidence of inflammatory bowel disease across Europe: is there a difference between north and south? Results of the European Collaborative Study on Inflammatory Bowel Disease (EC-IBD). Gut 39(5):690–697

22. Kyle J (1971) Prognosis after ileal resection for Crohn's disease. Br J Surg 58(10):735–737

23. Lee FI, Costello FT (1985) Crohn's disease in Blackpool – incidence and prevalence 1968–80. Gut 26(3):274–278

24. Lockhart-Mummery HE (1972) Crohn's disease of the large bowel. Br J Surg 59(10):823–826

25. Lee FI, Giaffer M (1987) Crohn's disease of late onset in Blackpool. Postgrad Med J 63(740):471–473

26. Shapiro PA, Peppercorn MA, Antoniolo DA et al (1981) Crohn's disease in the elderly. Am J Gastroenterol 76(2):132–137

27. Brandt L, Boley S, Goldberg L et al (1981) Colitis in the elderly. A reappraisal. Am J Gastroenterol 76(3):239–245

28. Loftus EV Jr (2007) Inflammatory bowel diseases. In: Talley NJ, Locke GR III, Saito YA (eds) GI epidemiology. Blackwell, Malden

29. Eisen GM, Schutz SM, Washington MK et al (1993) Atypical presentation of inflammatory bowel disease in the elderly. Am J Gastroenterol 88(12):2098–2101

30. Stalnikowicz R, Eliakim R, Diab R, Rachmilewitz D (1989) Crohn's disease in the elderly. J Clin Gastroenterol 11(4):411–415

31. Harper PC, McAuliffe TL, Beeken WL (1986) Crohn's disease in the elderly. A statistical comparison with younger patients matched for sex and duration of disease. Arch Intern Med 146(4):753–755

32. Gupta S, Saverymuttu SH, Keshavarzian A, Hodgson HJ (1985) Is the pattern of inflammatory bowel disease different in the elderly? Age Ageing 14(6):366–370

33. Fabricius PJ, Gyde SN, Shouler P et al (1985) Crohn's disease in the elderly. Gut 26(5):461–465

34. Elliott PR, Ritchie JK, Lennard-Jones JE (1985) Prognosis of colonic Crohn's disease. Br Med J (Clin Res Ed) 291(6489):178

35. Serpell JW, Johnson CD (1991) Complicated Crohn's disease in the over 70 age group. Aust N Z J Surg 61(6):427–431

36. Jones HW, Hoare AM (1988) Does ulcerative colitis behave differently in the elderly? Age Ageing 17(6):410–414

37. Brandt LJ, Boley SJ, Mitsudo S (1982) Clinical characteristics and natural history of colitis in the elderly. Am J Gastroenterol 77(6): 382–386

38. Van Rosendaal GM, Andersen MA (1996) Segmental colitis complicating diverticular disease. Can J Gastroenterol 10(6):361–364

39. Hadithi M, Cazemier M, Meijer GA et al (2008) Retrospective analysis of old-age colitis in the Dutch inflammatory bowel disease population. World J Gastroenterol 14(20):3183–3187

40. Peppercorn MA (1992) Drug-responsive chronic segmental colitis associated with diverticula: a clinical syndrome in the elderly. Am J Gastroenterol 87(5):609–612

41. Tchirkow G, Lavery IC, Fazio VW (1983) Crohn's disease in the elderly. Dis Colon Rectum 26(3):177–181

42. Strong SA (2007) Surgery for Crohn's disease. The ASCRS textbook of colon and rectal surgery. Springer, New York, pp 584–600

43. Mekhjian HS, Switz DM, Watts HD et al (1979) National Cooperative Crohn's Disease Study: factors determining recurrence of Crohn's disease after surgery. Gastroenterology 77(4 Pt 2):907–913

44. Tremaine WJ, Timmons LJ, Loftus EV Jr et al (2007) Age at onset of inflammatory bowel disease and the risk of surgery for non-neoplastic bowel disease. Aliment Pharmacol Ther 25(12): 1435–1441

45. Farmer RG, Hawk WA, Turnbull RB Jr (1976) Indications for surgery in Crohn's disease: analysis of 500 cases. Gastroenterology 71(2):245–250

46. O'Brien JJ, Bayless TM, Bayless JA (1991) Use of azathioprine or 6-mercaptopurine in the treatment of Crohn's disease. Gastroenterology 101(1):39–46

47. Present DH, Rutgeerts P, Targan S et al (1999) Infliximab for the treatment of fistulas in patients with Crohn's disease. N Engl J Med 340(18):1398–1405

48. Michelassi F, Testa G, Pomidor WJ et al (1993) Adenocarcinoma complicating Crohn's disease. Dis Colon Rectum 36(7):654–661

49. Abascal J, Diaz-Rojas F, Jorge J et al (1982) Free perforation of the small bowel in Crohn's disease. World J Surg 6(2):216–220

50. Slim K, Vicaut E, Panis Y, Chipponi J (2004) Meta-analysis of randomized clinical trials of colorectal surgery with or without mechanical bowel preparation. Br J Surg 91(9):1125–1130

51. Markowitz GS, Stokes MB, Radhakrishnan J, D'Agati VD (2005) Acute phosphate nephropathy following oral sodium phosphate bowel purgative: an underrecognized cause of chronic renal failure. J Am Soc Nephrol 16(11):3389–3396

52. Marik PE, Varon J (2008) Requirement of perioperative stress doses of corticosteroids: a systematic review of the literature. Arch Surg 143(12):1222–1226

53. Heyland DK, Montalvo M, MacDonald S et al (2001) Total parenteral nutrition in the surgical patient: a meta-analysis. Can J Surg 44(2):102–111

54. Bozzetti F, Gavazzi C, Miceli R et al (2000) Perioperative total parenteral nutrition in malnourished, gastrointestinal cancer patients: a randomized, clinical trial. JPEN J Parenter Enteral Nutr 24(1):7–14

55. Lashner BA, Evans AA, Hanauer SB (1989) Preoperative total parenteral nutrition for bowel resection in Crohn's disease. Dig Dis Sci 34(5):741–746

56. Yamamoto T, Fazio VW, Tekkis PP (2007) Safety and efficacy of strictureplasty for Crohn's disease: a systematic review and meta-analysis. Dis Colon Rectum 50(11):1968–1986

57. Papaioannau N, Piris J, Lee ECG (1979) The relationship between histological inflammation in the cut ends after resection of Crohn's disease and recurrence. Gut 20:A916

58. Kotanagi H, Kramer K, Fazio VW, Petras RE (1991) Do microscopic abnormalities at resection margins correlate with increased anastomotic recurrence in Crohn's disease? Retrospective analysis of 100 cases. Dis Colon Rectum 34(10):909–916

59. Hamilton SR, Reese J, Pennington L et al (1985) The role of resection margin frozen section in the surgical management of Crohn's disease. Surg Gynecol Obstet 160(1):57–62

60. Fazio VW, Marchetti F, Church M et al (1996) Effect of resection margins on the recurrence of Crohn's disease in the small bowel. A randomized controlled trial. Ann Surg 224(4):563–571, discussion 571–573

61. McLeod RS, Wolff BG, Steinhart AH et al (1995) Prophylactic mesalamine treatment decreases postoperative recurrence of Crohn's disease. Gastroenterology 109(2):404–413

62. McLeod RS, Wolff BG, Ross S et al (2009) Recurrence of Crohn's disease after ileocolic resection is not affected by anastomotic type: results of a multicenter, randomized, controlled trial. Dis Colon Rectum 52(5):919–927

63. Tan JJ, Tjandra JJ (2007) Laparoscopic surgery for Crohn's disease: a meta-analysis. Dis Colon Rectum 50(5):576–585

64. Young-Fadok TM, HallLong K, McConnell EJ et al (2001) Advantages of laparoscopic resection for ileocolic Crohn's disease. Improved outcomes and reduced costs. Surg Endosc 15(5):450–454

65. Holubar SD, Privitera A, Dozois EJ, et al (2010) Minimally invasive colectomy for Crohn colitis: a single institution experience. Inflamm Bowel Dis 6(11):1940–1946

66. Schwandner O, Schiedeck TH, Bruch HP (1999) Advanced age – indication or contraindication for laparoscopic colorectal surgery? Dis Colon Rectum 42(3):356–362

67. Law WL, Chu KW, Tung PH (2002) Laparoscopic colorectal resection: a safe option for elderly patients. J Am Coll Surg 195(6):768–773

68. Frasson M, Braga M, Vignali A et al (2008) Benefits of laparoscopic colorectal resection are more pronounced in elderly patients. Dis Colon Rectum 51(3):296–300

69. Poggioli G, Stocchi L, Laureti S et al (1997) Duodenal involvement of Crohn's disease: three different clinicopathologic patterns. Dis Colon Rectum 40(2):179–183

70. Shapiro M, Greenstein AJ, Byrn J et al (2008) Surgical management and outcomes of patients with duodenal Crohn's disease. J Am Coll Surg 207(1):36–42

71. Goligher JC (1985) The long-term results of excisional surgery for primary and recurrent Crohn's disease of the large intestine. Dis Colon Rectum 28(1):51–55

72. Prabhakar LP, Laramee C, Nelson H, Dozois RR (1997) Avoiding a stoma: role for segmental or abdominal colectomy in Crohn's colitis. Dis Colon Rectum 40(1):71–78

73. Sher ME, Bauer JJ, Gorphine S, Gelernt I (1992) Low Hartmann's procedure for severe anorectal Crohn's disease. Dis Colon Rectum 35(10):975–980

74. Keighley MR, Buchmann P, Lee JR (1982) Assessment of anorectal function in selection of patients for ileorectal anastomosis in Crohn's colitis. Gut 23(2):102–107

75. Sagar PM, Dozois RR, Wolff BG (1996) Long-term results of ileal pouch-anal anastomosis in patients with Crohn's disease. Dis Colon Rectum 39(8):893–898

76. Wolff BG (1986) Crohn's disease: the role of surgical treatment. Mayo Clin Proc 61(4):292–295

77. Jeffery PJ, Parks AG, Ritchie JK (1977) Treatment of haemorrhoids in patients with inflammatory bowel disease. Lancet 1(8021):1084–1085

78. Fry RD, Shemesh EI, Kodner IJ, Timmcke A (1989) Techniques and results in the management of anal and perianal Crohn's disease. Surg Gynecol Obstet 168(1):42–48

79. Williamson PR, Hellinger MD, Larach SW, Ferrara A (1995) Twenty-year review of the surgical management of perianal Crohn's disease. Dis Colon Rectum 38(4):389–392

80. Makowiec F, Jehle EC, Becker HD, Starlinger M (1995) Clinical course after transanal advancement flap repair of perianal fistula in patients with Crohn's disease. Br J Surg 82(5):603–606

81. Crim RW, Fazio VW, Lavery IC (1990) Rectal advancement flap repair in Crohn's patients – factors predictive of failure. Dis Colon Rectum 33:P3

82. Ekbom A, Helmick C, Zack M, Adami HO (1990) Ulcerative colitis and colorectal cancer. A population-based study. N Engl J Med 323(18):1228–1233

83. Jess T, Loftus EV Jr, Velayos FS et al (2006) Risk of intestinal cancer in inflammatory bowel disease: a population-based study from Olmsted county, Minnesota. Gastroenterology 130(4):1039–1046

84. Devroede G (1980) Colorectal cancer: prevention, epidemiology, and screening. Lippincott-Raven, Philadelphia

85. Reiser JR, Waye JD, Janowitz HD, Harpaz N (1994) Adenocarcinoma in strictures of ulcerative colitis without antecedent dysplasia by colonoscopy. Am J Gastroenterol 89(1):119–122

86. Blackstone MO, Riddell RH, Rogers BH, Levin B (1981) Dysplasia-associated lesion or mass (DALM) detected by colonoscopy in long-standing ulcerative colitis: an indication for colectomy. Gastroenterology 80(2):366–374

87. Lennard-Jones JE (1995) Colitic cancer: supervision, surveillance, or surgery? Gastroenterology 109(4):1388–1391

88. Provenzale D, Kowdley KV, Arora S, Wong JB (1995) Prophylactic colectomy or surveillance for chronic ulcerative colitis? A decision analysis. Gastroenterology 109(4):1188–1196

89. Mahadevan U, Loftus EV Jr, Tremaine WJ et al (2002) Azathioprine or 6-mercaptopurine before colectomy for ulcerative colitis is not associated with increased postoperative complications. Inflamm Bowel Dis 8(5):311–316

90. Hawley PR (1988) Emergency surgery for ulcerative colitis. World J Surg 12(2):169–173

91. Lewis WG, Sagar PM, Holdsworth PJ et al (1993) Restorative proctocolectomy with end to end pouch-anal anastomosis in patients over the age of fifty. Gut 34(7):948–952

92. Jorge JM, Wexner SD, James K et al (1994) Recovery of anal sphincter function after the ileoanal reservoir procedure in patients over the age of fifty. Dis Colon Rectum 37(10):1002–1005

93. Reissman P, Teoh TA, Weiss EG et al (1996) Functional outcome of the double stapled ileoanal reservoir in patients more than 60 years of age. Am Surg 62(3):178–183

94. Bauer JJ, Gorfine SR, Gelernt IM et al (1997) Restorative proctocolectomy in patients older than fifty years. Dis Colon Rectum 40(5):562–565

95. Tan HT, Connolly AB, Morton D, Keighley MR (1997) Results of restorative proctocolectomy in the elderly. Int J Colorectal Dis 12(6):319–322

96. Takao Y, Gilliland R, Nogueras JJ et al (1998) Is age relevant to functional outcome after restorative proctocolectomy for ulcerative colitis?: prospective assessment of 122 cases. Ann Surg 227(2):187–194

97. Farouk R, Pemberton JH, Wolff BG et al (2000) Functional outcomes after ileal pouch-anal anastomosis for chronic ulcerative colitis. Ann Surg 231(6):919–926

98. Church JM (2000) Functional outcome and quality of life in an elderly patient with an ileal pouch-anal anastomosis: a 10-year follow up. Aust N Z J Surg 70(12):906–907

99. Longo WE, Virgo KS, Bahadursingh AN, Johnson FE (2003) Patterns of disease and surgical treatment among United States veterans more than 50 years of age with ulcerative colitis. Am J Surg 186(5):514–518

100. Delaney CP, Fazio VW, Remzi FH et al (2003) Prospective, age-related analysis of surgical results, functional outcome, and quality of life after ileal pouch-anal anastomosis. Ann Surg 238(2):221–228

101. Chapman JR, Larson DW, Wolff BG et al (2005) Ileal pouch-anal anastomosis: does age at the time of surgery affect outcome? Arch Surg 140(6):534–539, discussion 539–540

102. Ho KS, Chang CC, Baig MK et al (2006) Ileal pouch anal anastomosis for ulcerative colitis is feasible for septuagenarians. Colorectal Dis 8(3):235–238

103. McHugh SM, Diamant NE (1987) Effect of age, gender, and parity on anal canal pressures. Contribution of impaired anal sphincter function to fecal incontinence. Dig Dis Sci 32(7):726–736

104. Holubar S, Larson D, Dozois E et al (2009) Minimally invasive subtotal colectomy and ileal pouch-anal anastomosis for fulminant ulcerative colitis: feasibility and short-term outcomes. Dis Colon Rectum 52(2):187–192

105. Larson DW, Dozois EJ, Piotrowicz K et al (2005) Laparoscopic-assisted vs. open ileal pouch-anal anastomosis: functional outcome in a case-matched series. Dis Colon Rectum 48(10):1845–1850

106. Holubar S, Privitera A, Cima R et al (2009) Minimally invasive total proctocolectomy with Brooke ileostomy for ulcerative colitis. Inflamm Bowel Dis 15(9):1337–1342

107. Heresbach D, Alexandre JL, Bretagne JF et al (2004) Crohn's disease in the over-60 age group: a population based study. Eur J Gastroenterol Hepatol 16(7):657–664

108. Triantafillidis JK, Emmanouilidis A, Nicolakis D et al (2000) Crohn's disease in the elderly: clinical features and long-term outcome of 19 Greek patients. Dig Liver Dis 32(6):498–503

109. Norris B, Solomon MJ, Eyers AA et al (1999) Abdominal surgery in the older Crohn's population. Aust N Z J Surg 69(3):199–204

110. Wagtmans MJ, Verspaget HW, Lamers CB, van Hogezand RA (1998) Crohn's disease in the elderly: a comparison with young adults. J Clin Gastroenterol 27(2):129–133

111. Truelove SC, Witts LJ (1955) Cortisone in ulcerative colitis; final report on a therapeutic trial. Br Med J 2(4947):1041–1048

112. Ooi BS, Remzi FH, Fazio VW (2003) Turnbull-Blowhole colostomy for toxic ulcerative colitis in pregnancy: report of two cases. Dis Colon Rectum 46(1):111–115

Chapter 67
Diverticulitis and Appendicitis in the Elderly

Scott C. Thornton

CASE STUDY

MS is a 90-year-old woman with no significant comorbidities who lives on her own at home. She was hospitalized five times over 4 months with an initial diagnosis of unrelenting ischemic colitis of the descending colon. This was diagnosed by multiple CT scans and with endoscopic confirmation. Despite antibiotics and enteral supplementation, she had slow and progressive weight loss and increasing inability to eat. Indication for operation was failure to progress with medical therapy and inability to eat. Her albumin, prealbumin, and initial weight were 2.0, 9, and 92 pounds, respectively. She underwent a left colectomy with primary anastomosis and protective loop ileostomy. Operative finding, confirmed by pathologic examination, was retroperitoneal perforated diverticulitis with contained abscess (Hinchey class II). Her postoperative course was complicated by ileostomy dysfunction, resulting in watery diarrhea, which caused dehydration and electrolyte imbalance. She developed a lower extremity deep venous thrombosis and was started on warfarin after a vena cava filter was placed. After a single 5-mg dose of warfarin, her INR rose to ten, and she had a spontaneous intra-abdominal bleed requiring transfusion. Aging does not alter the pharmacokinetics of warfarin but may increase sensitivity to its anticoagulant effects. She was unable to eat due to newly diagnosed, severe esophagitis. This was treated medically, and a PEG was placed for enteral nutrition. She was ultimately discharged to an extended care facility 1 month after surgery. She maintained mental acuity throughout her illness and is anxiously awaiting the reversal of her ostomy.

Elderly patients are often difficult to be correctly diagnosed due to nonroutine presentations. Once treated, they more frequently have complications with medical therapies aimed at cure. The following case presentation illustrates many of these problems found when treating older patients.

This chapter deals with diverticular disease and appendicitis in the elderly. Diverticular disease increases in incidence with age and also appears to present with diffuse peritonitis more frequently in old than in young patients. Acute appendicitis in the elderly accounts for 5–10% of all appendicitis, and old patients tend to present more frequently with advanced disease than do young groups. There is good evidence that the elderly present more frequently in an atypical fashion with both of these diseases compared with their younger counterparts. Abdominal pain may be absent or not greatly perceived in older patients. Physiologic responses to stress and infection are also blunted in the elderly. Older patients are burdened with more comorbid conditions and less mental and physical reserves compared with their younger counterparts. Furthermore, it is well known that emergency operations in the elderly are associated with significantly higher mortality and morbidity rates than similar operations on younger patients. Thus, old patients present atypically, often with more advanced disease and have higher complication and death rates than the young. This chapter attempts to explain these findings.

S.C. Thornton (✉)
Department of General Surgery, Bridgeport Hospital, Yale University, Bridgeport, CT, USA
e-mail: scottthorntonmd@yahoo.com

R.A. Rosenthal et al. (eds.), *Principles and Practice of Geriatric Surgery*,
DOI 10.1007/978-1-4419-6999-6_67, © Springer Science+Business Media, LLC 2011

Diverticular Disease

Etiology

Diverticular disease is the fifth most costly digestive disease in the USA [1]. The cause of diverticulosis is unknown. Colonic diverticula are mucosal (and submucosal) herniations through the muscle wall of the colon. The sigmoid colon is affected in 96% of patients, with this area being the only site of diverticulosis in two-thirds of patients [2]. Acute diverticulitis can occur anywhere in the colon and has been reported in the rectum [3, 4]. Diverticula occur at the points of weakness where the blood supply to the mucosa penetrates the bowel wall. Most commonly, they occur between the mesenteric and antimesenteric taenia coli. Less commonly, they occur between the two antimesenteric taenia. Strong epidemiologic evidence suggests that a low-fiber diet has a substantial etiologic role in the development of diverticulosis [5, 6], and low-fiber intake has long been implicated as a cause of diverticulosis [5, 7]. In the USA, the incidence of diverticular disease has increased with decreasing fiber intake [8]. Vegetarians have been found to have a lower incidence of diverticular disease than nonvegetarians [9]. Other studies have confirmed these findings [10–14].

The current speculation is that a diet low in fiber decreases stool bulk. This in turn causes narrowing of the colonic lumen, prolongs intestinal transit time, and increases intraluminal pressures. Painter et al. [15] combined manometry and cineradiography and found that the increased intraluminal pressure may be due to simultaneous contractions of circular muscular bands causing occlusion of short segments of bowel. Contraction rings are thus formed in the sigmoid colon, which produces "segmentation" of these short segments of bowel. Contraction of the muscle wall of these sections can result in intraluminal pressures of 90 mmHg or more. This pulsion pressure may lead to mucosal herniation along the weak points of the bowel wall, resulting in diverticula. Others have found that the contractile response to eating is exaggerated in people with diverticulosis [16]. Although consistent with the speculation that elevated pressures are particularly significant in combination with or potentiated by low-fiber stools, experimentation with colomyotomy showed that decreased muscular activity did not affect intraluminal pressures [17]. Stool bulk may be related to intraluminal pressure only in that stool bulk increases the radius of the colon, thereby decreasing wall tension. Painter et al. suggested that a low-fiber diet causes a narrower colonic lumen, which allows the colon to segment more efficiently, increasing the segmental intraluminal pressures [15]. Low-fiber diets in rats has been shown to result in diverticulosis in 45% of subjects compared with only 9% in a group fed the highest fiber diet [18]. Further, a large, longitudinal study of males in the USA revealed a relatively straight line correlation between fiber intake and diverticular symptoms [19]. Exercise may also have a protective effect on the development of symptoms from diverticular disease [20].

Colonic dysmotility may contribute to diverticular disease. Abnormally slow wave patterns have been found in patients with symptomatic diverticular disease [21]. Furthermore, patients with symptomatic diverticular disease return to normal motility patterns with ingestion of bran, whereas those with asymptomatic diverticulosis have no change in motility with bran intake [22]. Others have disputed these findings [23]. Colonic transit times can be decreased by adding bran to the diet [24–26], and water-retaining fiber can decrease intraluminal pressure [27]. These findings lead to dietary modifications in attempts to alleviate diverticular symptoms.

One report [28] implicated localized ischemia as a causative factor for antimesenteric free perforation of the colon from diverticulitis. In patients with multiple bilateral pseudo-diverticula arranged in a double row about the antimesenteric taenia, the vascular supply to the middle area of the antimesenteric wall is compromised. Careful histologic studies showed that free perforation associated with diverticulitis has the same histologic characteristics as ischemic bowel perforations. It is well known that microvascular changes predisposing to microvascular ischemia occur in the elderly. The more aggressive disease and higher perforation rates found in the elderly [29–32] may be related to this ischemic process. Perhaps this is the reason why the elderly have higher free perforation rates when compared with younger patients.

Investigators have also touched on whether an intrinsic change in bowel wall composition is necessary for the development of diverticula. Young people with collagen vascular diseases such as Marfan's syndrome [33] have been reported with diverticular disease. Several authors have also documented an association of diverticular disease with degenerative disorders such as varicose veins [34], hiatal hernias [35], and arthritis [36]. The most important element with regard to strength of the colon wall is collagen [37]. Collagen fibrils in the left colon become more numerous but smaller in width with age, and this difference is greater with diverticular disease [38]. Similarly, elastin fibrils increase in number but decrease in quality with age [39]. Pace [39] found that colon wall thickness increases with age and is thickest in the distal colon. These factors combined to result in decreased tensile strength and decreased expandability of the aging colon wall [40]. Electron microscopic examination reveals that there is a two-time increase in elastin deposition and normal muscle cells in the muscle layer of diverticular diseased colon. The elastin is in a shortened form, which may account for the thickened, foreshortened bowel typically found at surgery [41].

The distal sigmoid is the narrowest portion of the colon, and the distal sigmoid narrows with age [42]. The law of Laplace states that wall tension is directly proportional to the pressure times the diameter. Thus, as contractile pressures (as measured by wall tension) remain the same and the diameter is decreased, there is an increase in pressure delivered to the bowel wall. A simple example of Laplace's law is blowing up a balloon. It is most difficult when there is no air in the balloon and becomes easier as the diameter increases. Similarly, increased pressures are required in the narrower distal sigmoid to propel stool. As the lumen narrows with age, higher pressures are required. This increased stress further damages the colon, causing decreased elasticity and more loss of tensile strength [40]. Comparison studies show that populations with a low incidence of diverticular disease have stronger, more elastic distal colons than industrialized populations [42], presumably due to years of more bulky stools keeping the lumen diameter large. Furthermore, with increasing wall tension pressures, there must be a concomitant decrease in microvascular perfusion [43], possibly adding further weight to the vascular theory of free perforation of diverticulitis [15]. The resulting increased intraluminal pressure causes long-term changes in the bowel wall, including decreased tensile strength, decreased diameter, and vascular changes which predispose to diverticular disease and the more frequent perforation seen in the elderly.

Epidemiology

Diverticulosis is an entity particular to the dietary patterns of Western society. There are linear increases in size, number, incidence, and symptoms of diverticula with age [6, 44]. Diverticulae are commonly 5–10 mm in size and can occasionally be >2 cm. Giant diverticula have been described. Diverticulosis occurs in 2–5% of patients under age 40 and up to one-third of people over age 45. Two-thirds of people over age 85 have radiographic or pathologic evidence of diverticulosis [45]. Deckman and Cheskin [46] cited a prevalence in the USA as high as 33% with similar figures in European countries. In comparison, the prevalence in populations with higher per capita fiber intake is much lower. Diverticulosis is uncommon in developing parts of Africa and Asia and may be as low as 1% in Korea [35], with low incidences found in other similar populations [47–52].

Independent of age, prevalence is thought to be similar in men and women. However, in a large single institutional series by Rodkey and Welch [53], when sex and age were examined jointly, women over 70 years of age predominated over men by more than 3:1. The reverse was found in patients under 50 years of age, with more than twice as many men affected as women. This ratio was also substantiated by Ouriel and Schwartz [54], who found a predominance of men in the under-40 age group.

Nonsteroidal anti-inflammatory drugs (NSAIDs) have also been linked to diverticular disease [55], and others have implicated NSAIDs as a potential cause of acute diverticulitis [56–58]. Steroids have been linked to diverticulitis as well. Steroids also mask symptoms of infection which may cause delays in diagnosis, resulting in poor prognosis [59–61].

Pathogenesis

Diverticulitis is the inflammatory process that originates within colonic pseudodiverticula. The particular mechanisms of both the local and systemic infections have not been well characterized. It has been hypothesized that diverticulitis constitutes the same end point of localized luminal obstruction found with other intraabdominal visceral inflammatory processes such as appendicitis and cholecystitis [62–64]. Obstruction of the neck of the diverticula, presumably with inspissated stool, creates a closed microenvironment characterized by fluid sequestration, stasis, and bacterial overgrowth. Deitch [65] showed that even in the absence of perforation, obstruction alone is sufficient for bacterial translocation across the intestinal barrier. As the diameter of the diverticulum expands to accommodate the increased intraluminal pressure, venous and then arterial pressures are overcome. This results in congestion, ischemic necrosis, and perforation. Others cannot find supporting pathologic evidence and suggest that perforation is likely the result of increased intraluminal pressure [46]. Activation of local and systemic inflammatory mediators, in combination with microscopic or macroscopic perforation and soiling of the peritoneum, leads to the clinical manifestations of the disease. The role of localized ischemia was discussed earlier [28].

Atypical, painful or chronic diverticular disease is a difficult-to-describe entity. It is described as chronic, intermittent left lower abdominal pain, not usually associated with typical findings of acute inflammation. Motility patterns may be abnormal in this subset of patients [67]. Pain is usually chronic, intermittent, and not associated with acute symptoms. Narrow stools and other changes in bowel habits may result. Attacks may come and go. Symptoms may be confused with irritable bowel syndrome. The diagnosis is difficult, with barium enema showing only diverticulosis and possibly spasm of the sigmoid colon. CAT scan does not reveal acute inflammation, and it does not respond to antibiotics or dietary modification. Endoscopic findings are generally nonspecific, although a tortuous colon may be found. Endoscopy may show edema or associated patchy colitis.

Treatment is aimed at relieving symptoms. Bulk agents (psyllium seed) and a high-fiber diet are usually helpful. Differentiating between irritable bowel syndrome and painful diverticular disease is difficult as symptoms of bloating, distention, and intermittent nonspecific abdominal pain are common. Fortunately, IBS and painful diverticular disease are treated similarly with high-fiber diet and symptom control with moderate success. Uncommonly, sigmoid resection is required to produce relief. Appropriate patient selection is paramount in identifying who may respond to operative intervention and those who will not. When well chosen, sigmoid resection will relieve pain in 79–80% of patients [67].

Symptoms

The spectrum of disease produced by diverticula ranges from completely symptom-free to vascular collapse secondary to systemic sepsis from peritonitis. About 10–25% of patients with diverticulosis progress to diverticulitis [68, 69]. Most of these patients never come to surgical attention [68, 69]. A small number, estimated at fewer than 25% of those with diverticulitis, require inpatient management of their disease [70]. Complicated cases involving sepsis, obstruction, fistula formation, or peritonitis constitute approximately 40% of all those admitted. Older patients present more often with complicated disease. The elderly present with diffuse peritonitis up to twice as frequently as younger patients [29, 31].

Typically, patients with diverticulitis seek medical care owing to mild or moderate peritoneal irritation often accompanied by a change in bowel habits. Crampy left lower quadrant pain is also common. Approximately two-thirds of patients complain of constipation or diarrhea [71]. Other associated symptoms may include a palpable mass, abdominal distension, dysuria, excessive flatus, nausea, and vomiting. About 30–40% of patients have occult blood in their stool [3]. Fever and pain are the most consistent indicators of acute disease, occurring 45% of the time. Septic shock with diffuse peritonitis may be the presenting picture. With the presence of a redundant sigmoid colon, suprapubic or right lower quadrant pain may manifest. Occasionally, the diagnosis of appendicitis is the indication for surgical exploration when a redundant sigmoid colon with diverticulitis is found to be the culprit.

Considerable diagnostic overlap exists between diverticulitis and other acute abdominal processes. The spectrum of differential diagnoses ranges from relatively common urinary tract infections in the elderly to inflammatory bowel disease, colon cancer, closed loop obstruction, and ischemic bowel. These diagnoses and causes of abdominal pain must always be kept in mind during the initial evaluation.

Symptoms of diverticular fistulas may lead to an accurate preoperative diagnosis. Pneumaturia and fecaluria are diagnostic of an enteric-vesical fistula and in the appropriate patients are highly suggestive of a diverticular origin. Similarly, flatus or stool via the vagina leads to common bowel sources. Thigh abscesses, especially those with foul-smelling anaerobic pus, may originate from a diverticular abscess with tracking along the psoas muscle onto the skin.

Many investigators have found atypical presentations of diverticular disease in the elderly [29, 72–76]. Wroblewski and Mikulowski [74] noted the absence of typical manifestation of peritonitis in the elderly to be associated with a poor outcome. They also found an absence of abdominal pain in half of their patients with peritonitis. Intraabdominal abscesses are the most common cause of fever of unknown origin in the elderly [77]. Others noted that elderly patients with intraabdominal infections have hypothermic temperatures more frequently than young patients. Similarly, old patients have less nausea, vomiting, diarrhea, and fever compared to the young [72]. Acute abdominal pain is more likely to require surgery in the elderly [78, 79]. France et al. [73] examined 12 old patients who died of diverticulitis: 75% did not have symptoms typical of their disease, 3 of the 12 did not have abdominal symptoms, and another's symptoms did not warrant further investigation. Generalized peritonitis occurs in up to one-half of old patients [29, 30]. Old patients require operations more frequently, have free perforation more commonly, and have higher mortality rates than young patients [29–32, 80]. Watters et al. [29] attempted to explain this difference. They found that the mean time from the onset of symptoms to hospitalization for old and young patients with generalized diverticular peritonitis was the same. Thus, old patients have peritonitis and free perforation more frequently than the young do, and it is not due to a delay in seeking medical care. This finding suggests that the severity of disease in the elderly is determined early in its course and is independent of the passage of time. Another possible explanation is that symptoms begin later in the course of the disease in the elderly. The former explanation further supports the theory that ischemia is the cause of the more frequent diffuse peritonitis found in the elderly.

Diagnosis

Diverticulitis is usually diagnosed based completely on clinical grounds. This presents a unique problem in the elderly because, as previously shown, they often present atypically, and abdominal pain is minimal or absent. A history of known diverticula seen by barium enema or endoscopy often aids the clinician. However, it is unnecessary to have previous knowledge of diverticula in a particular patient, as more elderly patients have diverticula than do not [46]. Useful serologic and hematologic tests include a complete blood count, serum electrolytes, urinalysis, and in the case of suspected ischemic bowel, arterial blood gas measurement for acid–base disturbances. White blood cell (WBC) can be normal in almost one-half of older patients [32]. Physical examination usually reveals peritoneal irritation to some extent. Mild left lower quadrant tenderness to generalized peritonitis may be found. Rectal examination may reveal a pelvic abscess.

Several diagnostic modalities are helpful for establishing the diagnosis of diverticular disease and assessing the extent of inflammation. In preceding decades, contrast enema was the test of choice for diagnosis. Previous practice parameters of the American Society of Colon and Rectal Surgeons [81] cite a sensitivity of 94%, an accuracy of 77%, and a false-negative rate of 2–15% with water-soluble enemas. Contrast enemas in the setting of diverticular disease have been shown to be less reliable in identifying neoplastic growth compared with colonoscopy [82]. Radiographic findings include intramural or extramural sinus tracts, filling of the abscess cavity, or inferred extramural compression or spasm of the bowel lumen.

Ultrasonography may also provide useful information in the setting of suspected diverticular disease. Investigators have found it to be 84–98% sensitive [83–85]. Ultrasonography can detect abnormal segments of bowel, those with mural thickening, peridiverticular inflammation and abscess, and linear echogenic foci suggestive of fistulous tracts. Unfortunately, this technique is both operator-dependent and limited by the body habitus of the patient. Zielke et al. [86] found that surgical residents were able to accurately diagnose diverticulitis in 84% of patients, with a 16% false-negative rate.

Computed tomography (CT) has emerged as the imaging modality of choice for evaluating suspected diverticulitis [87–91]. Though in some studies it is comparable to contrast enema, other investigators have found a clear advantage regarding its diagnostic sensitivity and specificity [92]. Hulnick et al. [91] found that CT not only stages the extent of the inflammatory process more accurately, but it also better differentiates the varying gradations of pericolic inflammation. Furthermore, CT has the distinct advantage over a contrast enema because of its ability to identify both the intraluminal and extraluminal components of diverticular disease. It is also the diagnostic modality of choice for identifying colovesical and colovaginal fistulas. Findings suggestive of diverticulitis include inflammation of the pericolic fat, thickening of the sigmoid mesocolon, pericolic phlegmon, visualization of colonic diverticula themselves, and thickening of the colonic wall (see Fig. 67.1). CT is helpful for demonstrating the manifestations of intraabdominal abscess, particularly abscesses amenable to percutaneous drainage [87–91]. Despite these modalities, the diagnosis of diverticulitis can be obscure in the elderly [74].

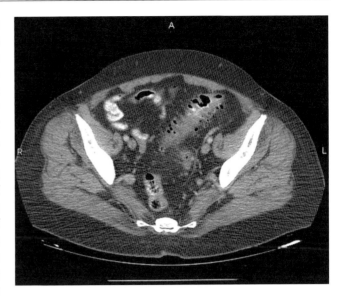

Figure 67.1   Acute diverticulitis of the sigmoid colon with paracolonic fat stranding.

Endoscopic evaluation is reserved until after the acute phase has resolved; it is used mainly to rule out carcinoma. CT colography is a new modality that noninvasively evaluates the contour of the colon lumen. It is especially helpful in cases where, due to stricture or obstruction, a colonoscope cannot traverse the diseased bowel. Colography can ensure that the proximal bowel does not harbor unsuspected neoplastic lesions.

Treatment

Prevention of Symptoms

High-fiber diet has been shown to decrease the formation of diverticulae in rats [19]. Examination of population-based per capita fiber intake reveals less diverticular disease with high average fiber intake [47, 50, 51]. High fiber intake in American males decreases the risk of diverticular symptoms. There is no evidence that increasing fiber intake can cause diverticulae to regress. It follows that high-fiber diet should be suggested to decrease the chance of diverticular symptoms [93]. There is no evidence to support the concept of avoiding food particles that can obstruct the neck of diverticulae. Accordingly, avoidance of seeds, nuts, popcorn, etc., has not been shown to cause acute disease. Most physicians suggest a high-fiber diet with bulk-producing supplements (psyllium seed) for patients with asymptomatic diverticulosis [94]. Fiber has been shown to decrease intraluminal pressures and colonic transit time [27, 95–97]. It also decreases symptoms attributed to diverticular disease [94, 95, 97–100]. Antispasmodic medications have not been shown to help.

Uncomplicated Diverticulitis

Most acute diverticulitis are treated by primary physicians on an outpatient basis. Those with only mild tenderness, no clinical peritoneal signs, and the ability to achieve satisfactory pain control and tolerate adequate fluids orally may be treated empirically on an outpatient basis [6]. Treatment consists of oral antibiotics covering anaerobic and gram-negative bacteria for at least 7 days and liquid diet until resolution of symptoms. Significant systemic signs of infection including high fever and leukocytosis suggest the need for hospital treatment. Resolution is common. There is no place for outpatient management in the setting of significant concurrent medical disease, immune compromise, or in those with altered mental status, or patients without appropriate supervision.

Immune-compromised patients have a more aggressive disease path, are more likely to present with perforation, and have higher morbidity and mortality rates [60, 101]. Perkins et al. [101] found a 100% failure rate with conservative treatment of immune-compromised patients. Early surgical management is appropriate in this patient population. Due to the aggressive nature of diverticulitis, some have suggested elective sigmoid resection in patients with a single prior attack when they are candidates for organ transplantation with its attendant long-term immune suppression [102]. Patients on continuous peritoneal dialysis represent a special dilemma. CT scanning is usually nondiagnostic, and delay in treatment results in poor outcomes. After treatment, very few will be able to remain on peritoneal dialysis [103].

Patients who fail in outpatient therapy or who present with significant systemic symptoms should be admitted to the hospital. Hospital treatment consists of complete bowel rest and parenteral broad-spectrum antibiotics to cover anaerobic and gram-negative bacteria. Triple-antibiotic or single-agent therapy are both effective. Nasogastric suction is required only with persistent vomiting or evidence of bowel obstruction. Laboratory evaluation includes a complete blood count and urinalysis. CT should be done to confirm the diagnosis, quantify the extent of inflammation, and identify possible complicated diverticular disease. Conservative treatment of acute uncomplicated diverticulitis leads to resolution of symptoms in 70–100% of cases [2, 3, 46, 47, 53, 87, 104]. Oral intake is resumed with disappearance of symptoms. Following hospital discharge, oral antibiotics should be continued for 7–10 days. With complete resolution of the inflammation, patients should have endoscopic or radiographic evaluation of their colon to rule out carcinoma, and they should be started on long-term fiber supplementation. Psyllium seed or hydrophilic colloids have been shown to reduce recurrence by up to 70% [100]. Old studies suggest that one-fourth of patients who recover from their first attack will have further attacks requiring hospitalization [2, 105]. A recent study with a median 5-year follow-up revealed that <2% of patients reported more than mild symptoms [106].

The goal of elective sigmoid resection is to reduce the potential for re-presentation with complicated disease requiring emergency colon surgery with its attendant increased complication and mortality rates. Hartmann's resection with temporary ostomy formation is often a result of these emergent operations. Ostomies formed during emergency operations are not reversed in a significant minority of patients [107]. Over the last decade, there has been a major shift in decision making regarding elective resection and diverticulitis. The natural history of disease is not well known. Practice parameters from the American College of Gastroenterology, American Society of Colon and Rectal Surgeons, and the Eurogean Association of Endoscopic Surgeons have all supported elective resection after 1–2 attacks, especially in younger patients [108–110].

A recent population-based study of first-event-hospitalized diverticulitis patients [111] showed that only 5% of older patients who did not require emergency surgery at first presentation ultimately required emergent colectomy/colostomy formation. Some have estimated the risk of colostomy after one attack of mild diverticulitis at one in 2,000 patient years of follow up [112]. A multicenter Kaiser Permanente study [113] followed 3,165 patients admitted with diverticulitis for a mean of 8.9 years. They found a 13.3% recurrence rate in patients treated nonoperatively, one quarter had re-recurrences. Old age was associated with a lower recurrence rate (12.2%). They also noted an increased risk of further attacks with each additional recurrence. They believe that no patients had colostomies in this group.

These findings have led to a change in the traditional suggestion that patients undergo elective sigmoid resection after 1–3 documented attacks. The frequency and severity of attacks, crescendo attacks, and the medical comorbidities should be considered when deciding to suggest elective sigmoid resection. The number of attacks should not be a major factor in decisions regarding timing of surgery. Most patients with perforating diverticular disease present with such at their first attack [111–116].

As seen above, very few patients require colostomies after initial successful nonoperative management. Further, the severity of disease, as measured by CAT scan during the first attack, may be a predictor of aggressive disease and the future need for operative intervention [117]. The number of attacks required to suggest elective resection is in dispute at this time. Salem [114] used a Markov model to evaluate the lifetime risk of death and colostomy as well as care cost and quality of life and elective resection for diverticulitis. They conclude that performing colectomy after a fourth attack in 50-year-old patients would result in 0.5% fewer deaths, 0.7% fewer colostomies, and save over $1,000.00 per patient.

Using 35-year-old patients in the model resulted in 0.1% fewer deaths, 2% fewer colostomies, and over $5,400.00 saved per patient. Clearly, delaying elective resection appears beneficial to patients and the cost of health care.

Elective resection for diverticulitis results in acceptable results. Thorn et al. [118] followed 75 consecutive elective sigmoid resections for diverticulitis. They found 13% major perioperative complications. Eight percent had recurrent diverticulitis during the follow-up period. Two-thirds of patients classified their results as good or excellent. IBS type symptoms in the preoperative period predicted less successful outcomes. Further along this line, a 21-year retrospective postresection study [119] showed that patients without histologic evidence for acute or chronic inflammation were seven times more likely to have persistent postoperative pain and twice as likely to have recurrent "diverticulitis" as those with histologic evidence of inflammation. Elective resection after one attack in patients requiring long-term immunosuppression is appropriate to prevent future sepsis. Elective resection may be required if cancer cannot be ruled out [62].

Surgical Technique

Elective sigmoid resection after resolution of the acute inflammation should include adequate mobilization of the proximal bowel to provide a tension-free anastomosis. The proximal bowel need not be devoid of diverticulosis, but the bowel must be soft, supple, and free of diverticular thickening. Resection should include all thickened, diseased bowel. Splenic flexure mobilization is occasionally required to achieve these goals. Distal resection must include removal of the entire sigmoid to the rectum to significantly reduce recurrent attacks [120]. No diverticula should be left distal to the anastomosis. The site of distal transection should be at the point where the taenia coli are lost, signifying the beginning of the intraperitoneal rectum.

Laparoscopic techniques have evolved significantly in recent years. Laparoscopy has been used in all types of diverticular resections and to drain abscesses not amenable to percutaneous CAT approaches. Laparoscopic colectomy in the elderly is safe and effective as well [121]. Laparoscopy is safe with complicated diverticulitis as well [122]. Laparoscopic surgery is successful in treating fistula disease as well, with laparoscopic colovesicle and colovaginal fistula operations becoming more common [123, 124]. Many studies have showed that laparoscopic approach to this disease is safe and effective and may confer benefits to patients compared with traditional open surgery. Decreased complications, faster recovery of bowel function, and oral intake have been seen in older patients [125, 126]. Pulmonary function is better preserved, and a host of stress measurements show

that less stress is imparted to laparoscopically treated patients compared with open techniques [127]. These benefits have been shown to be enhanced in older patients compared with younger ones [128]. Older patients also enjoy fewer cardiopulmonary complications with laparoscopy [129]. Laparoscopy has allowed more elderly patients to be discharged home rather than to rehab facilities compared with open surgery [125, 130]. Finally, Senagore [131] showed a lower direct cost in elderly patients undergoing laparoscopic resection compared with those having open surgery.

As experience and instrumentation improves, laparoscopy will most likely become the standard approach for most elective diverticular surgery and many urgent and emergent procedures as well. The most recent Practice Parameters published by the American Society of Colon and Rectal Surgeons conclude: When a colectomy for diverticular disease is performed, a laparoscopic approach is appropriate in selected patients [132].

Up to one-third of all patients admitted to the hospital require urgent or emergent surgery [2, 44, 45, 56, 105]. Up to one-half of elderly patients present with generalized peritonitis requiring operative intervention [29]. Similarly, more older patients with diverticulitis require urgent or emergent operations compared with younger patients [30]. Most patients requiring urgent or emergent surgery are undergoing their initial episode of diverticulitis [3, 113]. Hinchey et al. [133] described a grading system for acute diverticulitis. Stage I is confined pericolic abscess. Stage II is distant abscess. Stage III is generalized peritonitis caused by rupture of a pericolic or pelvic abscess, "noncommunicating" with bowel lumen because of obliteration of diverticular neck by inflammation. Stage IV is fecal peritonitis caused by free perforation of a diverticulum ("communication"). Emergent surgical treatment aims to relieve sepsis, remove the diseased bowel, minimize mortality and morbidity, and avoid stomas with their concomitant second operation to restore bowel continuity. Options include resection with primary anastomosis, resection with proximal colostomy and closure of the distal end (Hartmann's procedure), and diversion with drainage alone. The latter plays only a small role today, with only the most ill and unstable patients unable to tolerate removal of the infectious foci. Diversion alone leaves a column of undrained stool above the perforation that can further contribute to the septic process [134, 135].

Resection with primary anastomosis for acute disease is often possible with gentle preoperative bowel preparation and localized sepsis [134]. Mobilization of the colon should begin in an unaffected area to facilitate entrance into normal planes of dissection. The retroperitoneal structures (ureters and gonadal vessels) can be swept dorsally, elevating the sigmoid colon. Ureteral catheters can be helpful for acute inflammation and occasionally for elective resections [136]. Hartmann's resection with diverting colostomy has been traditionally reserved for patients with unprepared bowel. Hartmann's procedure carries significant complication and mortality rates [137].

More recently, primary resection and anastomosis in well-selected acute disease has been successful [138]. Selection includes minimal local sepsis and well-nourished patients. On-table lavage is an option in patients with proximal solid stool and minimal contamination. Adequate diverticular resection requires removal of the distal sigmoid from the rectum when restoring bowel continuity after Hartmann's procedure. Removing the sigmoid from the rectum decreases recurrences of diverticular disease [120]. Furthermore, using the distal sigmoid instead of rectum for the anastomosis was found to be a risk factor in the development of postoperative colocutaneous fistulas [139].

Complicated Diverticular Disease

Complicating factors associated with diverticular disease include abscess formation, free perforation, fistula formation, obstruction, and bleeding. The presentation of complicated diverticular disease occurs in up to 32% of hospitalized patients [87] and in more than 50% of the elderly [29]. Bleeding diverticular disease is discussed in Chap. 45. The vast majority of perforating diverticulitis occurs during the first attack [140, 141], and the incidence of nonperforating complicated diverticulitis is decreasing compared with past studies [117]. In contrast, the incidence of perforating diverticulitis may be increasing [141]. Complicated diverticulitis is associated with significant morbidity and mortality, and the need for operative intervention should be continually reassessed. Treatment of complicated diverticular disease requires accurate diagnosis and staging. The goal of treatment of complicated diverticular disease is to minimize morbidity and mortality, avoid ostomy formation and the number of subsequent operations. To achieve these goals, nonoperative techniques can convert complicated disease to medically manageable disease, thereby allowing elective resection with primary anastomosis.

Hartmann's procedure is associated with high morbidity and mortality rates [136, 142, 143]. Retained colostomy rates after Hartmann's operation range from 5 to 58% [136, 144]. A large review of Hartmann's procedure [107], where diverticulitis was the indication for almost 60% of operations, found a 14% mortality rate and that more than 40% of colostomies were not reversed. In a related study [145], a higher than expected mortality rate was found in older patients undergoing colostomy reversal. And, in these older patients, only 30% of colostomies created were reversed! Surgeons operating emergently on the elderly need to ensure proper placement and construction of these temporary ostomies, as many of

them are permanent to the patient. Furthermore, colostomy closure is associated with significant complication and death rates, especially in the elderly [144]. Eisenstat et al. [146] recorded a lower mortality rate for complicated diverticular disease treated with elective resection than that treated with staged surgical procedures. Avoiding a stoma with its concomitant second operation is a major goal of operative treatment for complicated diverticular disease. Accurate preoperative diagnosis is helpful, as up to 25% of patients explored for abscess or fistula have a perforated cancer [147].

Abscess formation is the most common complication of acute diverticulitis, occurring in 32–68% of complicated diverticular cases [88–90, 148]. A wide spectrum of presentations may result: small occult abscesses; scrotal, buttock, or thigh abscess; and sepsis due to a large abscess. Diagnosis is best made with CT [8, 149]. Treatment is aimed at relief of the sepsis and the diverticulitis. Small pericolic abscesses or phlegmon may be managed conservatively with bowel rest and broad-spectrum intravenous antibiotics. Elective, single-stage sigmoid resection with primary anastomosis can be done with resolution of symptoms. If symptoms worsen or are not alleviated, repeat CT scan with percutaneous drainage of the abscess should be considered (see Figs. 67.2 and 67.3). Exploration is reserved for patients whose abscesses are not amenable to percutaneous drainage or who fail in conservative management. Primary anastomosis is possible if the proximal and distal bowel is healthy and the perforation is contained, and if a gentle preoperative mechanical preparation has been done [144]. The patient's underlying medical diseases and acute physiologic status must obviously be considered.

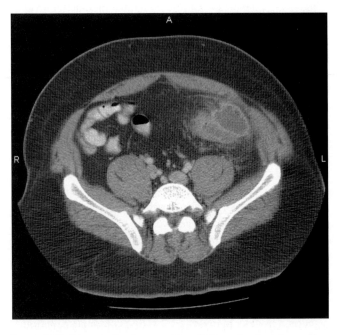

Figure 67.2 Diverticular abscess with well-formed, enhancing wall.

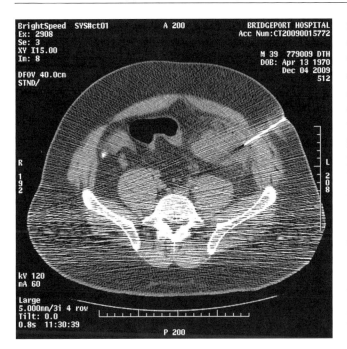

Figure 67.3 Percutaneous drainage of the abscess.

Large abscesses, including more distant pelvic abscesses, and smaller ones that do not respond to conservative treatment should be referred quickly for possible percutaneous drainage under CT guidance [150]. Percutaneous drainage of diverticular abscesses is associated with a success rate of 62–100% [88, 89, 150–154]. Following placement of a drainage catheter and aspiration of the pus, repeat radiologic evaluation should be undertaken to assess not only resolution of the abscess cavity but also to identify potential fistulous communications to the small or large bowel. In the setting of appropriate drainage, treatment should progress as for uncomplicated diverticulitis. The catheter may be removed when the drainage stops or when complete collapse of the abscess cavity has been shown by sinography. At discharge, the catheter may also be left in place and removed during subsequent elective sigmoid resection [88]. The presence of a persistent colocutaneous fistula does not preclude elective resection with primary anastomosis [136]. Such a course of treatment allows complicated disease to be transformed nonoperatively to disease that responds to medical treatment, thereby avoiding emergent surgery with stoma formation. Subsequent elective sigmoid resection with primary anastomosis after resolution of inflammation (in about 6 weeks) becomes the only operative intervention required [154]. This has become the standard treatment for diverticulitis complicated by abscess formation.

Stabile et al. [88] followed three patients who refused surgery after catheter drainage for large abscesses. One required resection after a repeat diverticulitis attack 7 months later. The second required permanent catheter drainage for

recurrent and persistent abscesses. The third died in hospital of sepsis. Ambrosetti et al. [32] followed one patient without operation after percutaneous drainage who required elective resection 11 months later owing to stenosis. The authors suggested that occasional small mesocolic abscesses can be managed without operation, but they stated that pelvic and abdominal abscesses behave aggressively and require surgical treatment. Kaiser [155] found that 41% of patients who managed with percutaneous abscess drainage without surgery developed severe sepsis. Conversely, Broderick-Villa [113] found no increase in recurrence rates after abscesses were percutaneously drained and treated without elective operation compared with uncomplicated diverticulitis followed nonoperatively. Others suggest a conservative approach after drainage is appropriate as well [156]. As with elective resection after uncomplicated diverticulitis, there may be a change of surgical decision making. At this time, all patients, with the possible exception of those with small mesocolic abscesses, which are treated with percutaneous drainage, should have elective sigmoid resection after resolution of inflammation to prevent future complications [132].

Pelvic abscesses can be drained transrectally and transvaginally in women as well. These techniques are being replaced by CT-guided drainage but should remain in the surgeon's arsenal. If large abscesses cannot be drained adequately or if sepsis does not resolve, operative exploration is required. Gentle preoperative mechanical bowel preparation can be performed in well-selected patients, and with normal proximal and distal bowel, resection and primary anastomosis can be performed safely [144]. The use of Hartmann's procedure is reserved for most other patients. One should remember that restoring bowel continuity after Hartmann's procedure has high morbidity and mortality rates, and a large percentage of "temporary" stomas become permanent [134, 143–145].

A few important technical aspects of resection must be emphasized. When possible, care should be taken in the face of peritonitis to avoid opening noninfected tissue planes such as the presacral space and the splenic flexure area. These areas are known to invite abscess formation and are best left intact and free from contamination by the infectious process. Ureteral catheters may be employed, as the inflammatory process may obliterate the normal tissue planes and allow the ureters to be drawn into the inflammatory process [157]. The reader is referred to standard surgical textbooks for other technical aspects of sigmoid resection.

Perforating diverticular disease is the most virulent form of this disease. The vast majority of patients with perforating diverticulitis have no previous history of diverticulitis [112–114]. It is important to consider these patients separately from other complicated diverticulitis patients. Perforating diverticulitis has higher operative mortality (12–21% vs. 0–2.6%)

compared with nonperforating complicated diverticulitis [53, 116]. Free perforation of diverticulitis generally presents as acute sepsis or an acute abdominal crisis and some degree of shock. It occurs in approximately 10% of complicated cases [88]. More importantly, up to 50% of elderly patients present with diffuse peritonitis [29, 30]. Rapid hydration with correction of electrolyte abnormalities is necessary. Broad-spectrum antibiotics are administered preoperatively. Immunocompromised patients may not exhibit classic abdominal findings. Physical examination and CT scans generally yield the diagnosis. A large number of old patients with peritonitis lack abdominal pain as a finding [74], so a high index of suspicion is required when treating them. Emergent exploration with aspiration of pus, cleansing of fecal material, resection of the diseased bowel, and proximal end colostomy with oversewing of the distal stump (Hartmann's operation) are performed [158–160]. Only rarely are patients so sick that diversion and drainage without resection is appropriate [159, 161]. In fact, one study [134] found higher mortality among patients treated with diversion only compared to those who underwent resection, despite more steroid use and fecal peritonitis in the resection group. The mortality rate associated with fecal peritonitis is as high as 35% [134, 159, 161].

Fistula formation occurs in approximately 2% of diverticulitis cases but accounts for up to 22% of patients requiring surgery [144, 159, 162, 163]. Multiple fistulas are uncommon [163]. Fistulas develop when inflammation or abscesses develop in close proximity to adjacent organs. The inflammatory process invades the adjacent normal organs and causes decompression, which spontaneously converts the acute complicated infectious process to controlled, drained, simple diverticulitis. It is diagnosed often on clinical grounds, and diagnostic tests are used to rule out cancer and other diagnoses. Expensive, complex testing is often unnecessary. In general, single-stage resection with primary anastomosis can be performed in a fashion similar to that used for complicated diverticulitis treated with percutaneous abscess drainage.

The bladder is affected most commonly [164, 165]. Symptoms include pneumaturia and fecaluria. Sepsis can also occur. Diagnosis is made most commonly by the patient's history. CT scan is most accurate for diagnosis, showing air in the uninstrumented bladder and inflammation of the sigmoid colon and dome of the bladder [159]. Contrast enema or endoscopic evaluation is required to rule out colon cancer. Cystoscopy may be performed to rule out a neoplastic process originating in the bladder. In some patients, the fistula cannot be demonstrated. Elective sigmoid resection with primary anastomosis is curative [164]. The fistula is pinched off the bladder. A small bladder defect is best treated by Foley catheter drainage for 7–10 days. Large defects should be closed in two layers with absorbable suture and drained by Foley catheter for a similar length of time. Bladder resection should be reserved for malignant disease [165].

Colovaginal fistulas occur most commonly in women who have had a hysterectomy. Diagnosis is simply made by the history, including flatus or stool per vagina. It is confirmed by transvaginal and transanal endoscopy. Air may be heard exiting from the vagina during sigmoidoscopy. Contrast enema or endoscopic evaluation of the colon is required to rule out neoplastic and inflammatory bowel disorders. Patients generally are not septic at the time of presentation and may undergo elective sigmoid resection with primary anastomosis. The vagina can be left open for drainage or may be closed with absorbable sutures and omentum interposed between the vagina and the anastomosis. Other organs, including the uterus, may be involved with the fistulous process. Hysterectomy may be required if the uterus is involved with the infectious process or if a neoplastic process is suspected [166]. Spontaneous colocutaneous fistulization is uncommon and can be treated with resection and primary anastomosis if sepsis is controlled.

Obstruction complicating diverticulitis occurs uncommonly [167]. Repeated episodes of edema, spasm, and inflammation cause a chronically strictured bowel lumen to become narrowed. Acute inflammation can then complete the luminal obstruction. Gentle water-soluble enema or endoscopy by a skilled endoscopist with minimal air insufflation can confirm the diagnosis and exclude a neoplasm. With proper diagnosis and treatment, the inflammation usually resolves, and the obstruction abates. This allows it to be treated as uncomplicated diverticulitis with preoperative bowel preparation followed by elective resection and primary anastomosis after complete resolution of inflammation. Emergency operation for obstruction due to diverticulitis generally requires removing the diseased bowel with creation of an end colostomy. The unprepared and dilated proximal bowel often precludes safe primary anastomosis. On-table lavage has been used more frequently in selected cases to allow primary anastomosis [168].

Right-Sided Diverticulitis

Right-sided diverticulitis has a different etiology, pathophysiology and affects a different patient population group compared with left-sided disease. Right-sided diverticula are true diverticula, with all layers of the bowel wall involved with the outpouching. They most commonly affect Far-Eastern populations. Presentation mimics appendicitis with right-sided pain and infectious systems. Preoperative diagnosis is uncommon. X-ray findings often suggest neoplastic diseases. Nonoperative treatment is usually effective if accurate diagnosis is made before surgery. Not infrequently, the diagnosis is in doubt at time of operation, and right colon resection is performed with a presumed diagnosis of tumor. Resection, diverticulectomy, and inversion of the diverticulum have been reported.

In conclusion, diverticulitis is common in the elderly. Symptoms may be avoided with a high-fiber diet and fiber (psyllium) supplement intake. Older patients frequently present atypically and are difficult to be accurately diagnosed. Diverticulitis appears to be a more virulent disease at initial presentation in the elderly. More than one-half of patients require emergent operation with many having ostomy formation. Ostomies are commonly permanent in these old patients. CAT drainage of abscesses allow for safer, elective resection. Most patients who avoid surgery at initial presentation can be managed without subsequent operation. Laparoscopic approaches allow for decreased morbidity, mortality, shorter hospital stays, and early discharge to home, and these advantages are more pronounced in the elderly.

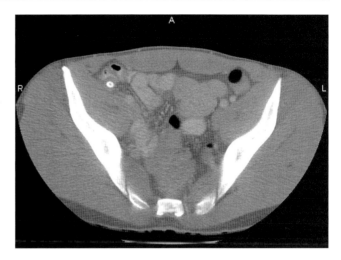

FIGURE 67.4   Fecalith within an acutely inflamed appendix.

Appendicitis

Many investigators have tried to assign an immune function to the appendix, as it does secrete immunoglobins, but the appendix is an organ whose function is unknown. Certainly, normal life results after its removal. Inflammation and neoplastic transformation are by far the most common afflictions that affect the human appendix. Infectious diseases (typhoid and tuberculosis), regional enteritis, and congenital defects of the appendix are beyond the scope of this chapter. Similarly, neoplasms of the appendix are not addressed. Appendectomy is one of the most common operations performed, with more than 500,000 appendices removed annually in the USA; 5–10% of acute appendicitis occurs in the elderly. Old patients delay presentation, present atypically, and suffer delay in diagnosis and treatment more often than young patients. Perforation is found more frequently in the elderly. Higher mortality rates and prolonged hospital stays result. The following section attempts to explain these findings.

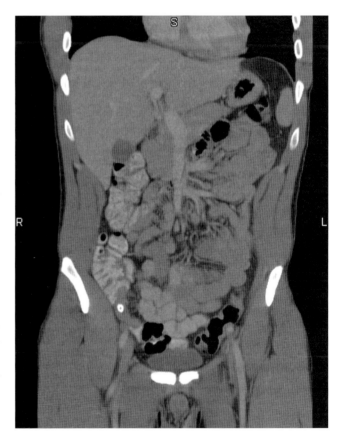

FIGURE 67.5   Same patient, coronal view.

Etiology

Obstruction of the lumen of the appendix is the predominant cause of appendicitis, and fecaliths are a common cause of obstruction (Figs. 67.4 and 67.5). After the lumen has been obstructed, a closed microenvironment is produced, which allows fluid sequestration, stasis, distension, and bacterial overgrowth. Mucosal secretion and bacterial multiplication increase the distension and intraluminal pressure. As the diameter of the lumen expands to accommodate the increased pressure, venous and then arterial pressures are overcome. Ischemia, necrosis, bacterial translocation, and appendiceal perforation result. Interestingly, humans are one of the few animals able to secrete fluid into the lumen of the appendix at pressures high enough to produce necrosis and perforation [169].

Perforation occurs owing to vascular compromise, causing necrosis, usually on an antimesenteric border. There are thought to be many differences in the elderly appendix that predispose it to obstruction and perforation. The appendiceal lumen is small or obliterated, and the blood supply is decreased, predisposing to necrosis; the mucosa is thinned, and there is fatty infiltration of the wall [170]. These changes may lead to increased rupture rates with decreased pressures, thus altering the natural history of appendicitis in the elderly. NSAIDs have been implicated in appendicitis as well. Campbell and DeBeaux [171] found that 37% of patients over the age of 50, with the diagnosis of acute appendicitis, were on NSAIDs compared with only 11% of a similar age group admitted with other emergencies.

Epidemiology

Appendicitis is the most common acute surgical condition of the abdomen. Six to eight percent of the population will suffer from acute appendicitis in their lifetime [172–174]. Life-table analysis estimates that 12% of males and 23% of females have their appendixes surgically removed [173]. Acute appendicitis occurs at all ages but is most frequent during the teenage years [173, 175]. This age peak is thought to result from the peak in lymph tissue in the appendix during these years. The extra lymph tissue presumably narrows the lumen, predisposing it to obstruction and the resulting appendicitis. Males are more commonly affected at young age, but during later adult life, the male/female ratio equals out [176]. There is a decrease in the incidence of acute appendicitis in the young over recent decades, and the reason is unknown [170, 173, 175–177]. Five to ten percent of all acute appendicitis occurs in the elderly [172, 175, 177, 178], and in fact, the incidence of acute appendicitis in the elderly is increasing [170, 176, 177]. It may be due to longer life spans, as Thorbjarnarson and Loehr [170] found that old patients accounted for only 1% of appendicitis between 1932 and 1937, whereas this percentage increased to 6–8% after 1957. Altogether, 1 of 35 women and 1 of 50 men over age 50 years develop acute appendicitis [174]. Furthermore, appendicitis accounted for 2.5–5.0% of all acute abdominal disease in patients over 60–70 years of age [74, 178].

Acute appendicitis is the third most common cause of abdominal pain in the elderly after gallbladder disease and small bowel obstruction [179, 180]. It is the leading source of intraabdominal abscess, which in turn is the most common cause of fever of unknown origin in the elderly [77]. About 33–50% of the mortality due to acute appendicitis occurs in the elderly [172, 173, 181]. Whereas mortality from appendicitis in general has been decreasing, the percentage of deaths among the elderly is on the rise [170], often due to delays in diagnosis and treatment. Also, lowered immune responses to foreign antigens and decreased production of lymphocytes with advancing age limits the older patients' ability to wall off peritoneal inflammation and fight overall infectious events [182, 183]. It has been postulated that changes occur in the appendix as we age, including atrophy of the intraluminal lymphoid tissue and thinning of the appendiceal wall, which render the appendix more susceptible to inflammation. Atherosclerosis diminishes the blood supply, narrowing the lumen. Small changes in intraluminal pressure can produce rapid ischemia, gangrene, and perforation at rates much quicker in older persons than the young [184].

Symptoms and Diagnosis

Abdominal pain, fever, and leukocytosis are the hallmarks of acute appendicitis. Distension of the obstructed appendix stimulates visceral afferent nerve fibers, producing vague, dull, midabdominal pain. Pain classically begins in the periumbilical area and migrates to the right lower quadrant within hours [169, 185]. This pain is peritoneal in origin and as such is constant and increases with time. Anorexia is common. Vomiting occurs up to 75% of the time. Protracted vomiting and diarrhea should lead the clinician away from the diagnosis. There are many variations in presentation.

Physical examination reveals the site of peritoneal inflammation. Usually, tenderness is found at McBurney's point. Rovsing's sign (pain referred to the right lower quadrant with palpation of the left side) indicates localized peritoneal irritation. The appendix may be found anywhere in the abdomen and thus can cause pain during psoas muscle stretch, obturator muscle stretch, rectal examination, or palpation of any abdominal site [185]. Continued irritation results in rebound and referred peritoneal irritation. Frank peritonitis can ultimately result with perforation. Elevated core temperature is usually not more than 39°C. The WBC count is generally between 10,000 and 18,000/mm^3 with a left shift [169]. Higher or lower counts and extreme left shifts are indications of diffuse peritonitis. Acute-phase reactants are being examined in an attempt to increase the accuracy of the preoperative diagnosis. Urinalysis should be done but may be abnormal if the appendix is adjacent to the bladder or ureter.

The presentation and difficulty with diagnosis of acute appendicitis in the elderly deserves special consideration. Most importantly, older patients more frequently delay seeking medical attention for a variety of reasons: difficulty leaving home, fear of hospitalization, decreased ability to appreciate or express symptoms. An elderly patient with a perforated appendicitis who was incorrectly treated for alcohol withdrawal for 5 days prior to being accurately diagnosed has been reported [186]. Burns et al. [187] found that 20% of older patients with acute appendicitis had WBC counts <10,000/mm^3 and neutrophil counts <75%. Lau et al. [188] found only 43% of old patients with simple appendicitis to have elevated WBC counts. Thorbjarnarson and Loehr [170] recorded an average duration of symptoms prior to admission in patients over age 60 to be 2.5 days. Horattas et al. [189] found that one-third of patients over 60 years of age waited more than 48 h from onset of symptoms before presenting to the hospital. Fewer than two-thirds had "typical" right lower quadrant pain, and one-half had a temperature <37.6°C. Similarly, Smithy et al. [190] found that only 55% of patients over age 80 had right lower quadrant pain, and 18% did not have abdominal pain. They also noted that only 1 of 13 patients had "typical" periumbilical pain localizing in the right lower quadrant. They hypothesized that because of the smaller lumen diameter of the elderly appendix, which requires less pressure to produce rupture, the old patient does not necessarily experience the prodromal phase of appendicitis with the generalized abdominal pain, anorexia, nausea, and vomiting thought to be caused by visceral distension. Nausea, vomiting, fever, and anorexia were found to be uncommon in old patients by others as well [72, 186]. Burns et al. [187] compared the presentations of young and old patients. They found that twice as many young patients presented "classically," and old patients were more than two times more likely to delay presentation for more than 72 h after onset of symptoms. Furthermore, in their study, old patients were three times likely to have operation delayed more than 24 h after admission than were the young. Horattas et al. [189] found that 13% of patients had their operations delayed more than 48 h after admission, further illustrating the difficulty of correctly diagnosing this age group. Samiy [191] described a blunted or absent pain response in the elderly and, perhaps more importantly, found that doctors often minimize the importance of the old patient's pain, attributing it to old age or concomitant diseases [192–194]. Clinicians must be more cognizant of the abdominal complaints in old patients if prompt diagnosis and treatment with resultant decreased morbidity and mortality are to be expected.

The confident diagnosis of acute appendicitis is difficult, and the experienced clinician is wrong 5–25% of the time [175, 195]. Many books and articles have been written describing techniques for diagnosing acute appendicitis [175, 196–198]. The combination of appropriate history, physical examination, and elevated WBC count is thought to be most important for diagnosing appendicitis correctly [199]. Unfortunately, these factors are not often present together [198]. Ultrasonography and focused CT have been used extensively for presurgical evaluation of patients [196, 197, 200]. Despite numerous advances in radiographic techniques, the rate of unnecessary explorations remains at 5–20% [196, 197, 201].

C-reactive protein (CRP) has been studied as a tool to aid in the accurate diagnosis of appendicitis [202]. There is a decline in the production of inflammatory mediators and in the immune system with aging [182, 183, 203]. CRP is preserved with age [202]. CRP has been found to be consistently elevated only in patients with perforation, perhaps since it first appears in the serum about 8 h after the initial insult and takes 24–48 h to reach peak blood levels [202]. Thus, elevated serum levels are often found only with prolonged symptoms, which correspond to high perforation rates. Obviously, if symptoms progress rapidly, there is no time for serum CRP levels to rise. CRP is not specific for appendicitis: It also increases with any inflammation, surgical trauma, and acute myocardial infarcts [202].

CT scanning has made accurate diagnosis easier. More liberal use of CT scanning can lead to the diagnosis of appendicitis in older patients where this diagnosis was not entertained [204]. Despite this, outcomes including perforation rates and duration of hospitalization may not be affected.

Exploratory laparotomy or laparoscopy remains the diagnostic test of choice in appropriately chosen patients. Despite the advances in preoperative modalities, an accurate diagnosis of acute appendicitis is made in only 30–77% of the elderly on admission and in only 70% preoperatively [186, 189, 190, 195, 205]. Between 14 and 33% of older patients have operations more than 24 h after admission [187–190, 205].

Treatment and Outcomes

Nonoperative care of acute appendicitis is appropriate only if emergent surgical expertise is unavailable. Recurrence within 18 months is seen in at least 35% of patients treated only with antibiotics [206]. Early, aggressive treatment is imperative to minimize mortality in the elderly. In fact, Burns et al. [187] suggested "based on the lack of significant complications in those patients with a false positive diagnosis and the 65% perforation rate in older patients, we feel an even earlier and more aggressive surgical approach is warranted." Operative treatment for acute appendicitis remains resection of the offending organ. Hydration and correction of electrolyte imbalances prior to urgent operation is prudent. Untoward delay before exploration may allow progression of the disease and ultimately free rupture of the organ with resultant peritonitis. Preoperative broad-spectrum antibiotics are administered intravenously and are continued postoperatively if necrosis or perforation is discovered. All pus should be evacuated, localized abscess cavities irrigated thoroughly, and appropriate closed-suction drains employed if abscess cavities are encountered [187]. The skin should be left open in complicated cases. When a normal appendix is discovered, the abdomen should be systematically examined to search for the origin of the symptoms; resection of the normal appendix is usually appropriate. Nonoperative management of abdominal abscesses is well known. CT-guided drainage of abscesses allows resolution of the acute septic process followed by elective, internal operative treatment, thereby avoiding emergency surgery with its attendant morbidity (Figs. 67.6 and 67.7) [88, 89, 151, 207]. Acute appendicitis with a contained abscess

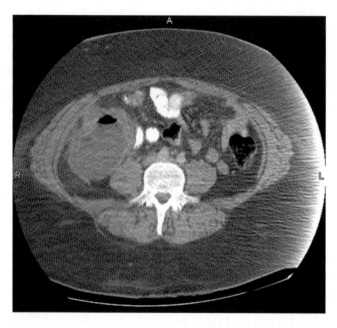

FIGURE 67.6 Acute appendiceal abscess with enhancing wall and air within the abscess.

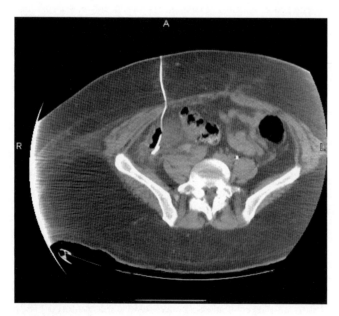

FIGURE 67.7 Percutaneously placed drain within this abscess.

responds well to drainage [208], and most patients with appendicitis respond to antibiotics [207, 209]. Interval appendectomy 6–12 weeks later, after resolution of the infectious process, is suggested because of the high recurrence rates. Some question the need for interval resection [207–209]. Recurrence rates in adult age groups approach 35% [207]. With the well-known delay in presentation, difficulty with accurate and timely diagnosis, and the increased morbidity and mortality seen in the elderly, interval appendectomy is suggested in all but the frailest. Neoplasm must be ruled out in those managed conservatively. Furthermore, elective interval appendectomy lends itself well to the laparoscopic approach, as stressed by Greig and Nixon [209].

Ileocecal resection and primary anastomosis are reserved for the markedly inflamed cecum. Rarely, resection cannot be performed safely because of the inflammatory reaction. In these cases, irrigation and drainage are performed, and interval appendectomy is scheduled for 6–12 weeks later. The reader is referred to general surgical textbooks for the detailed operative technique.

More than 75% of young patients are found to have simple appendicitis at operation [29, 186, 206]. This is in contrast to 48–63% of patients over 50 years of age having a ruptured appendicitis [205, 210] and 49–92% of patients over 70 years age having perforation, an abscess, or both [29, 176, 179, 190, 192, 193, 209]. Luckmann [175] found an age-related increase in complex appendicular disease in a California population-based study. About 1.8–32.0% of the older patients succumb to their disease, mostly owing to sepsis [170, 173, 175, 178, 188, 190, 195, 205]. In a countrywide population-based study, the mortality was 4.6% for patients over 65 years of age and only 0.2% for those <65 [173].

It is debated whether appendicitis in the elderly progresses more quickly than that in younger patients, which may account for the higher perforation rates found in old patients. Children with symptoms for more than 48 h have perforation rates up to 98% [211]. Franz et al. [205] studied a Veterans Administration hospital population and found that those with simple appendicitis had symptoms lasting a mean of 22 h, perforated appendicitis patients a mean of 50 h, and those with abscesses an average 66 h prior to presentation. They concluded that the delay in seeking care accounts for the increased perforation and abscess rates in old patients. Watters et al. [29] agreed that prehospital delay accounted for the increased rate of perforation found in the elderly compared with the young. Paajanen et al. [212] agreed that duration of symptoms within an age group corresponds well with perforation rates for that group, thus dispelling the concept that in old patients appendicitis progresses more rapidly than in young patients. Others have found an increased rate of perforation in pregnant women, with symptoms lasting longer than 24 h [213], and in children, with symptoms more than 48 h prior to operation [211]. Similarly, Temple et al.

[214] examined 95 consecutive patients and found an average of 31 h from onset of pain to operation for simple appendicitis, whereas patients with perforation had symptoms for 63 h before operation. Interestingly, those with perforation spent less time in the hospital before operation. In contrast, Smithy et al. [190] observed a 92% perforation rate in patients more than 80 years of age, with an average time from admission to operation of 15 h, bespeaking the difficulty of making the diagnosis in the elderly. Thus, the rate of evolution of appendicitis is not different in the elderly. Old patients more frequently delay seeking treatment, increasing the rate of perforation.

Lau et al. [188] found a 38% perforation rate in old patients operated on within 24 h of the onset of symptoms, suggesting aggressive disease. Wolff and Hindman [215] agreed finding a perforation rate of 41% in old patients with onset of symptoms within 24 h of operation. However, Burns et al. [187] found that one-third of young and old patients operated on within 24 h had perforation. Von Tittle et al. [216] also found that roughly one-third of old patients with perforation had symptoms for <24 h. Thus, an equal number of their young and old patients progressed rapidly to advanced disease. They concluded that physicians are responsible for almost two-thirds of older patients' delays in diagnosis and treatment of appendicitis, with the patients themselves being responsible for the rest. Obviously, duration of symptoms correlates with perforation rates in all age groups. Luckmann [175] found that only 53% of patients over 80 years of age in California had their operation on the day of admission, compared to more than 80% of young patients. More impressively, in patients with abscesses, more than 85% of young patients had operations within 1 day of admission, compared to only 57% of those older than 80 years. This further attests to the difficulty accurately diagnosing and treating acute appendicitis in the elderly. One study revealed that 17% of elderly patients were treated without accurate diagnosis prior to being admitted with acute appendicitis [187]. Incorrect diagnosis rates in the elderly are as high as 25% [217].

Most studies show that the progression of appendicular disease in the elderly is similar to that in younger groups. However, old patients frequently present with longer duration of symptoms and are more commonly misdiagnosed, resulting in delayed operation. This prolonged time from onset of symptoms to operation accounts for the increased perforation rates found in the elderly. Their concomitant medical problems most likely account for the high mortality rates reported. Incidental appendectomy should not be performed in patients over 60 years of age and probably not in those over 35 years of age [173].

In-hospital observation has been shown to decrease negative operative rates safely without increasing the perforation rate [217, 218]. This suggests that the out-of-hospital delay is most important for determining the aggressiveness of disease. Lau et al. [188] found a statistically significant increase in perforation rates in elderly patients when surgeons delayed operation for more than 25 h. Klein et al. [195] also found increased perforation and abscess rates in old patients with increasing delays of operation. Because of the difficulty diagnosing old patients, attempting to decrease perforation rates through hospital observation in the elderly is unwise.

Many authors have examined laparoscopic vs. open appendectomy [198, 219–223]. One prospective randomized study found that patients used fewer analgesics and returned to full activity sooner compared to those exposed to conventional operative techniques [222]. Some have found fewer wound infections with laparoscopic techniques [224–226]. This good record is usually achieved with increased hospital cost. Others have found an increase in abdominal abscesses in laparoscopically treated patients [227]. A recent large comparative study and a prospective randomized study both has found advantages for laparoscopic approach to appendicitis, without increased abdominal abscesses [228, 229]. One obvious advantage of laparoscopic appendectomy is the ability to view the entire abdomen and pelvis in cases where the diagnosis is in question.

Konstantinos [230] examined more than 1,000 consecutive laparoscopic operations for suspected appendicitis. They had a conversion rate of <1 and 1.1% wound infection rate with no intraabdominal abscesses or deaths, despite a 14% ruptured or gangrenous appendix rate and 4% having intraabdominal abscesses. They also found significantly shorter hospital stays and quicker return of bowel function. Paranjape [231] examined three different time periods and how laparoscopy changed outcomes in the elderly. They found an increased use of CT scanning, fewer patients presenting with classic symptoms, increased correct admission diagnoses, fewer perforations, and fewer complications in the most recently treated group. They also found shorter hospital stays with laparoscopy. Their operative time was similar for both open and laparoscopic approaches.

Laparoscopic appendicitis in elderly North Carolina residents has been studied as well [232]. The patients who underwent conventional and laparoscopic operations were comparable with regard to age, gender, and comorbidities. Fifty-five percent presented with perforated appendicitis. There was a steady increase in laparoscopic use over time, rising from 11.9% in 1997 to 26.9% in 2003. Advantages found in the laparoscopic group includes: shorter length of stay (4.6 vs. 7.3 days), higher rate of discharge to home (91.4 vs. 78.9%), fewer complications (16.3 vs. 20.8%), and a lower mortality (0.4 vs. 2.1%). As important is overall hospital cost, which shows a trend for lower total cost for the laparoscopic group, $17,031 vs. $19,587.

In conclusion, 10% of all appendicitis occurs in the elderly. Older patients present atypically and often delay seeking medical treatment. Diagnosis is difficult owing to blunted symptoms and response to inflammation. Perforation occurs more frequently and possibly faster than in younger patients. High index of suspicion and liberal use of CT scanning can facilitate correct diagnosis. Laparoscopic technique decreases complications, shortens hospital stay, increases home discharge, and is not associated with increased hospital cost.

References

1. Sandler RS, Everhart JE, Donowitz M et al (2002) The burden of selected digestive diseases in the United States. Gastroenterology 122:1500–1511
2. Parks TG (1969) Natural history of diverticular disease of the colon: a review of 521 cases. Br Med J 4:639–642
3. Chiu TT, Bailey HR, Hernandez AJ Jr (1983) Diverticulitis of the midrectum. Dis Colon Rectum 26:59–60
4. Hackford AW, Veidenheimer MC (1985) Diverticular disease of the colon: current concepts and management. Surg Clin North Am 65:347–363
5. Painter NS, Burkitt DP (1971) Diverticular disease of the colon: a deficiency disease of Western civilization. Br Med J 2:450–454
6. Painter NS, Burkitt DP (1975) Diverticular disease of the colon, a 20th century problem. Clin Gastroenterol 4:3–21
7. Burkitt DP (1969) Related disease-related cause? Lancet 2:1229–1231
8. Trowell H (1976) Definition of dietary fiber and hypotheses that it is a protective factor in certain diseases. Am J Clin Nutr 29:417–427
9. Gear JSS, Fursdon P, Nolan DJ et al (1979) Symptomless diverticular disease and intake of dietary fiber. Lancet 1:511–514
10. Segal I, Solomon A, Hunt JA (1977) Emergence of diverticular disease in the urban South African Black. Gastroenterology 72:215–219
11. Aktan H, Ozden A, Kesim E et al (1984) Colonic function in rural and urban populations of Turkey. Dis Colon Rectum 27:538–541
12. Dabestani A, Aliabadi P, Shah-Rookh FD et al (1982) Prevalence of colonic diverticular disease in southern Iran. Dis Colon Rectum 24:385–387
13. Manousos O, Day NE, Tzonou A et al (1985) Diet and other factors in the aetiology of diverticulosis: an epidemiological study in Greece. Gut 26:544–549
14. Brodribb AJM, Humphreys DM (1976) Diverticular disease: three studies. Part I. Relation to other disorders and fibre intake. BMJ 1:424–425
15. Painter NS, Truelove SC, Ardran GM et al (1965) Segmentation and the localization of intraluminal pressures in the human colon, with special reference to the pathogenesis of colonic diverticula. Gastroenterology 29:169–177
16. Trotman IF, Misiewicz JJ (1988) Sigmoid motility in diverticular disease and the irritable bowel syndrome. Gut 29:218–222
17. Attisha RP, Smith A (1696) Pressure activity of the colon and rectum in diverticular disease before and after sigmoid myotomy. Br J Surg 56:891–894
18. Fisher N, Berry CS, Fearn T et al (1985) Cereal dietary fibre consumption and diverticular disease: a lifespan study in rats. Am J Clin Nutr 43:788–804
19. Aldoori WH, Giovannucci EL, Rockett HRH et al (1998) A prospective study of dietary fiber types and symptomatic diverticular disease in men. J Nutr 128:714–719
20. Aldoori WH, Giovannucci EL, Rimm EB et al (1995) Prospective study of physical activity and the risk of symptomatic diverticular disease in men. Gut 36:276–282
21. Snape WJ Jr, Carlson GM, Cohen S (1976) Colonic myoelectric activity in the irritable bowel syndrome. Gastroenterology 70:326–332
22. Findlay JM, Smith AN, Mitchell WD et al (1974) Effects of unprocessed bran on colon function in normal subjects and in diverticular disease. Lancet 1:146–149
23. Painter NS (1967) Diverticulosis of the colon: fact and speculation. Am J Dig Dis 12:222–227
24. Almy TP, Howel DA (1980) Medical progress: diverticular disease of the colon. N Engl J Med 302:324–330
25. Muller-Lissner SA (1988) Effect of wheat bran on weight of stool and gastrointestinal transit time: a meta analysis. Br Med J 296:615–617
26. Kirwan WO, Smith AN (1977) Colonic propulsion in diverticular disease, idiopathic constipation, and the irritable colon syndrome. Scand J Gastroenterol 12:331–335
27. Smith AN, Drummond E, Eastwood MA (1981) The effect of coarse and fine Canadian red spring wheat and French soft wheat bran on colonic motility in patients with diverticular disease. Am J Clin Nutr 34:2460–2463
28. Tagiacozzo S, Tocchi A (1997) Antimesenteric perforation of the colon during diverticular disease. Dis Colon Rectum 40:1358–1361
29. Watters JM, Blakslee JM, March RJ et al (1996) The influence of age on the severity of peritonitis. Can J Surg 39:142–146
30. Freischlag J, Bennion RS, Thompson JE Jr (1986) Complications of diverticular disease of the colon in young people. Dis Colon Rectum 29:639–643
31. Ambrosetti P, Robert JH, Witzig JA et al (1994) Acute left colonic diverticulitis in young patients. J Am Coll Surg 179:156–160
32. Ambrosetti P, Robert JH, Witzig JA et al (1994) Acute left colonic diverticulitis: a prospective analysis of 226 consecutive cases. Surgery 115:546–550
33. Mielke JE, Becker KL, Gross JB (1965) Diverticulitis of the colon in a young man with Marfan's syndrome. Gastroenterology 48:379–382
34. Latto C (1975) Diverticular disease and varicose veins. Am Heart J 90:274–275
35. Kim EH (1964) Hiatus hernia and diverticulum of the colon: their low incidence in Korea. N Engl J Med 271:764–768
36. Klein S, Mayer L, Present DH et al (1988) Extraintestinal manifestations in patients with diverticulitis. Ann Intern Med 108:700–702
37. Fung YC (1981) Biomechanics: mechanical properties of living tissues. Springer, New York
38. Thomson HJ, Busuttil A, Eastwood MA et al (1987) Submucosa collagen changes in the normal colon and in diverticular disease. Int J Colorectal Dis 2:208–213
39. Pace JL. Cited by Watters DAK, Smith AN. (1990) Strength of the colon wall in diverticular disease. Br J Surg 77:257–259
40. Iwasaki T (1970) Tensile properties of the large intestine. In: Yamada H (ed) Strength of biological materials. Williams & Wilkins, Baltimore
41. Whiteway J, Morson BC (1985) Elastosis in diverticular disease of the sigmoid colon. Gut 26:258–266
42. Watters DAK, Smith AN, Eastwood MA et al (1985) Mechanical properties of the colon: comparison of the features of the African and European colon in vitro. Gut 26:394–397
43. Watters DAK, Smith AN (1990) Strength of the colon wall in the diverticular disease. Br J Surg 77:257–259
44. Sugihar K, Muto T, Morioka Y et al (1984) Diverticular disease of the colon: a review of 615 cases. Dis Colon Rectum 27:531–537
45. Welch CE, Allen AW, Donaldson GA (1953) An appraisal of resection of the colon for diverticulitis of the sigmoid. Ann Surg 138:332–343
46. Deckman RC, Cheskin LJ (1993) Diverticular disease in the elderly. J Am Geriatr Soc 40:986–993

47. Vajrabukka T, Saksornchai K, Jimakorn P (1980) Diverticular disease of the colon in a far-eastern community. Dis Colon Rectum 23:151–154
48. Fatayer WT, Alkhalaf MM, Shalan KA et al (1983) Diverticular disease of the colon in Jordan. Dis Colon Rectum 26:247–249
49. Calder JF (1979) Diverticular disease of the colon in Africans. Br Med J 1:1465–1466
50. Coode PE, Chan KW, Chan YT (1985) Polyps and diverticula of the large intestine: a necropsy survey in Hong Kong. Gut 26:1045–1048
51. Chia JG, Chintana WC, Ngoi SS et al (1991) Trends of diverticular disease of the large bowel in a newly developed country. Dis Colon Rectum 34:498–501
52. Lee YS (1986) Diverticular disease of the large bowel in Singapore: an autopsy survey. Dis Colon Rectum 29:330–335
53. Rodkey GV, Welch CE (1984) Changing patterns in the surgical treatment of diverticular disease. Ann Surg 200:466–478
54. Ouriel K, Schwartz SI (1983) Diverticular disease in the young patient. Surg Gynecol Obstet 156:1–5
55. Rampton DS (1987) Non-steroidal anti-inflammatory drugs, and the lower gastrointestinal tract. Scand J Gastroenterol 22:1–4
56. Coutrot S, Roland D, Barbier J et al (1978) Acute perforation of colonic diverticula associated with short-term indomethacin. Lancet 2:1055–1057
57. Corder A (1987) Steroids, non-steroidal anti-inflammatory drugs, and serious septic complications of diverticular disease. Br Med J 295:1238
58. Campbell K, Steele RJC (1991) Non-steroidal anti-inflammatory drugs and complicated diverticular disease: a case-control study. Br J Surg 78:190–191
59. Warshaw AL, Welch JP, Ottinger LW (1976) Acute perforation of colonic diverticula associated with chronic corticosteroid therapy. Am J Surg 131:442–446
60. Remine SG, McIlrath DC (1984) Bowel perforation in steroid-treated patients. Ann Surg 192:581–586
61. Arsura EL (1990) Corticosteroid-associated perforation of colonic diverticula. Arch Intern Med 150:1337–1338
62. Schoetz DJ Jr (1993) Uncomplicated diverticulitis. Surg Clin North Am 73:965–974
63. Chappuis CW, Cohn I Jr (1988) Acute colonic diverticulitis. Surg Clin North Am 68:301–313
64. Rege RV, Nahrwold DL (1989) Diverticular disease. Curr Probl Surg 26:133–189
65. Deitch EA (1990) Strength of the colon wall in diverticular disease. Br J Surg 77:257–259
66. Cortesini C, Pantalone D (1991) Usefulness of colonic motility study in identifying patients at risk for complicated diverticular disease. Dis Colon Rectum 34:339–342
67. Horgan AF, McConnell EJ, Wolff BG et al (2001) Atypical diverticular disease. Dis Colon Rectum 44:1315–1318
68. Cheskin LJ, Bohlman M, Schuster MM (1990) Diverticular disease in the elderly. Gastroenterol Clin North Am 19:391–403
69. Parks TG (1975) Natural history of diverticular disease of the colon. Clin Gastroenterol 4:53–69
70. Sarin S, Boulos PB (1994) Long-term outcome of patients presenting with acute complications of diverticular disease. Ann R Coll Surg Engl 76:117–120
71. Zollinger RW (1968) The prognosis in diverticulitis of the colon. Arch Surg 97:418–422
72. Cooper GS, Shlaes DM, Salata RA (1994) Intraabdominal infection: differences in presentation and outcome between younger patients and the elderly. Clin Infect Dis 19:146–148
73. France MJ, Vuletic JC, Koelmeyer TD (1992) Does advancing age modify the presentation of disease. Am J Forensic Med Pathol 13:120–123
74. Wroblewski M, Mikulowski P (1991) Peritonitis in geriatric inpatients. Age Ageing 20:90–94
75. Fenyo G (1982) Acute abdominal disease in the elderly: experience from two series in Stockholm. Am J Surg 143:751–754
76. Telfer S, Fenyo G, Holt PR, DeDombal FT (1988) Acute abdominal pain in patients over 50 years of age. Scand J Gastroenterol Suppl 23:47–50
77. Esposito AL, Gleckman RA (1978) Fever of unknown origin in the elderly. J Am Geriatr Soc 26:498–505
78. Brewer BJ, Golden GT, Hitch DC et al (1976) Abdominal pain: an analysis of 1000 consecutive cases in a university hospital emergency room. Am J Surg 131:219–223
79. Eisenberg RL, Montgomery CK, Margulis AR (1979) Colitis in the elderly: ischemic colitis mimicking ulcerative and granulomatous colitis. Am J Roentgenol 133:1113–1118
80. Kahn AL, Heys SD, Ah-See AK et al (1995) Surgical management of the septic complications of diverticular disease. Ann R Coll Surg Engl 77:16–20
81. Roberts P, Abel M, Rosen L et al (1995) Practice parameters for sigmoid diverticulitis – supporting documentation. Dis Colon Rectum 38:126–132
82. Boulos PB, Karamanolis DG, Salmon PR et al (1984) Is colonoscopy necessary in diverticular disease. Lancet 1:95–96
83. Schwerk WB, Schwarz S, Rothmund M (1992) Sonography in acute colonic diverticulitis: a prospective study. Dis Colon Rectum 35:1077–1084
84. Verbanck J, Lambrecht S, Rutgeerts L et al (1989) Can sonography diagnose acute colonic diverticulitis in patients with acute intestinal inflammation? A prospective study. J Clin Ultrasound 17:661–666
85. Taylor KJ, Wasson JF, de Graaff C et al (1978) Accuracy of grey scale ultrasound diagnosis of abdominal and pelvic abscesses in 220 patients. Lancet 1:3–4
86. Zielke A, Hasse C, Bandorski T et al (1997) Diagnostic ultrasound of acute colonic diverticulitis by surgical residents. Surg Endosc 12:1194–1197
87. Hachigian MP, Honickman S, Eisenstat TE et al (1992) Computed tomography in the initial management of acute left-sided diverticulitis. Dis Colon Rectum 35:1123–1129
88. Stabile BE, Puccio E, vanConnenberg E, Neff CC (1990) Preoperative percutaneous drainage of diverticular abscesses. Am J Surg 159:99–104
89. Ambrosetti P, Robert J, Witzig JA et al (1992) Incidence, outcome, and proposed management of isolated abscesses complicating acute left-sided colonic diverticulitis. Dis Colon Rectum 35:1072–1076
90. Ambrosetti P, Robert J, Witzig JA et al (1992) Prognostic factors from computed tomography in acute left colonic diverticulitis. Br J Surg 79:117–119
91. Hulnick DH, Megibow AG, Balthazar EJ et al (1984) Computed tomography in the evaluation of diverticulitis. Radiology 152:491–495
92. Stefansson T, Nyman R, Nilsson S et al (1997) Diverticulitis of the sigmoid colon: a comparison of CT, colonic enema, and laparoscopy. Acta Radiol 38:313–319
93. Mendeloff AI (1986) Thoughts on the epidemiology of diverticular disease. Clin Gastroenterol 15:855–877
94. Brodribb AJM, Humphries DM (1976) Diverticular disease. Part II. Treatment with bran. Br Med J 1:425–428
95. Hodgson J (1972) Effect of methylcellulose on rectal and colonic pressures in the treatment of diverticular disease. Br Med J 3:729–731
96. Taylor I, Duthie HL (1976) Bran tablets and diverticular disease. Br Med J 1:988–990
97. Andersson H, Bosaeus I, Falkheden T et al (1979) Transit time in constipated geriatric patients during treatment with a bulk laxative and bran: a comparison. Scand J Gastroenterol 14:821–826
98. Srivastava GS, Smith AN, Painter NS (1976) Sterulica bulk-forming agent with smooth-muscle relaxant versus bran in diverticular disease. Br Med J 1:315–318

99. Hyland JMP, Taylor I (1980) Does a high fibre diet prevent the complications of diverticular disease? Br J Surg 76:77–79

100. Brodribb AJM (1977) Treatment of symptomatic diverticular disease with a high-fibre diet. Lancet 1:664–666

101. Perkins JD, Shield CF III, Chang FC et al (1984) Acute diverticulitis: comparison of treatment in immunocompromised and nonimmunocompromised patients. Am J Surg 148:745–748

102. Tyau ES, Prystowsky JB, Joehl RJ et al (1991) Acute diverticulitis: a complicated problem in the immunocompromised patient. Arch Surg 126:855–859

103. Carmeci C, Muldowney W, Mazbar SA, Bloom R (2001) Emergency laparotomy in patients on continuous ambulatory peritoneal dialysis. Am Surg 67:615–618

104. Parks TG, Connell AM (1970) The outcome in 455 patients admitted for treatment of diverticular disease of the colon. Br J Surg 57:775–778

105. Kirson SM (1988) Diverticulitis: management patterns in a community hospital. South Med J 81:972–977

106. Salem TA, Molloy RG, O'Dwyer PJ (2007) Prospective, five-year follow-up study of patients with symptomatic uncomplicated diverticular disease. Dis Colon Rectum 50:1460–1464

107. Desai DC, Brennan EJ Jr, Reilly JF, Smink RD Jr (1998) The utility of the Hartmann procedure. Am J Surg 176:86

108. Stollman NH, Raskin JB (1999) Diagnosis and management of diverticular disease of the colon in adults. Ad hoc practice parameters of the American College of Gastroenterology. Am J Gastroenterol 94:3110–3121

109. Wong WD, Wexner SD, Lowry A et al, The Standards Task Force, The American Society of Colon and Rectal Surgeons (2000) Practice parameters for sigmoid diverticulitis-supporting documentation. Dis Colon Rectum 43:290–297

110. Kohler L, Sauerland S, Neugebauer E (1999) Diagnosis and treatment of diverticular disease: results of a consensus development conference. The Scientific Committee of the European Association for Endoscopic Surgery. Surg Endosc 13:430–436

111. Anaya DA, Flum DR (2005) Risk of emergency colectomy and colostomy in patients with diverticular disease. Arch Surg 140:681–685

112. Janes S, Meagher A, Frizelle FA (2005) Elective surgery after acute diverticulitis. Br J Surg 92:133–144

113. Broderick-Villa G, Burchette MA, Collins C et al (2005) Hospitalization for acute diverticulitis does not mandate routine elective colectomy. Arch Surg 140:576–583

114. Salem L, Veenstra DL, Sullivan SD et al (2004) The timing of elective colectomy in diverticulitis: a decision analysis. J Am Coll Surg 199:904–912

115. Guzzo J, Hyman N (2004) Diverticulitis in young patients: is an aggressive approach really justified? Dis Colon Rectum 47:1187–1191

116. Chapman J, Davies M, Wolff B et al (2005) Complicated diverticulitis: is it time to rethink the rules? Ann Surg 242:576–581

117. Ambrosetti P, Grossholz M, Becker C et al (1997) Computed tomography in acute left colonic diverticulitis. Br J Surg 84:532–534

118. Thorn M, Graf W, Stefansson T, Pahlman L (2002) Clinical and functional results after elective colonic resection in 75 consecutive patients with diverticular disease. Am J Surg 183:7–11

119. Moreaux J, Vons C (1990) Elective resection for diverticular disease of the sigmoid. Br J Surg 77:1036–1038

120. Benn PL, Wolff BG, Ilstrup DM (1986) Level of anastomosis and recurrent colonic diverticulitis. Am J Surg 151:269–271

121. Tuech JJ, Pessaux P, Rouge C et al (2000) Laparoscopic vs. open colectomy for sigmoid diverticulitis: a prospective comparative study in the elderly. Surg Endosc 14:1031–1033

122. Scheidbach H, Schndieder C, Rose J et al (2004) Laparoscopic approach to treatment of sigmoid diverticulitis: changes in the spectrum of indications and results of a prospective, multicenter study on 1545 patients. Dis Colon Rectum 47:1883–1888

123. Bartus CM, Lipof T, Shahbaz Sarwar CM et al (2005) Colovesical fistula: not a contraindication to elective laparoscopic colectomy. Dis Colon Rectum 28:233–236

124. Laurent SR, Detroz B, Detry O et al (2005) Laparoscopic sigmoidectomy for fistulized diverticulitis. Dis Colon Rectum 48:148–152

125. Stocchi L, Nelson H, Young-Fadok TM et al (2000) Safety and advantages of laparoscopic vs. open colectomy in the elderly: matched-control study. Dis Colon Rectum 43:326–332

126. Delgado S, Lacy AM, Garcia Valdecasas JC et al (2000) Could age be an indication for laparoscopic colectomy in colorectal cancer? Surg Endosc 14:22–26

127. Braga M, Vignali A, Zuliani W et al (2002) Metabolic and functional results after laparoscopic colorectal surgery. A randomized controlled trial. Dis Colon Rectum 45:1070–1077

128. Frasson M, Braga M, Vignali A et al (2008) Benefits of laparoscopic colorectal resection are more pronounced in elderly patients. Dis Colon Rectum 51:296–300

129. Law WL, Chu KW, Ming Tung PH (2002) Laparoscopic colorectal resection: a safe option for elderly patients. J Am Coll Surg 195:768–773

130. Vignali A, DiPalo S, Tamburini A et al (2005) Laparoscopic vs. open colectomies in octogenarians: a case-matched control study. Dis Colon Rectum 48:2070–2075

131. Senagore AJ, Madbouly KM, Fazio VW et al (2003) Advantages of laparoscopic colectomy in older patients. Arch Surg 138:252–256

132. Rafferty J, Shellito P, Hyman NH, Buie WD (2006) Practice parameters for sigmoid diverticulitis. Dis Colon Rectum 49:939–944

133. Hichey EJ, Schaal PH, Richards MB (1978) Treatment of perforated diverticular disease of the colon. Adv Surg 12:85–109

134. Nagorney DM, Adson MA, Pemberton JH (1985) Sigmoid diverticulitis with perforation and generalized peritonitis. Dis Colon Rectum 28:71–75

135. Krukowski ZH, Matheson NA (1984) Emergency surgery for diverticular disease complicated by generalized and faecal peritonitis: a review. Br J Surg 71:921–927

136. Fazio VW, Church JM, Jagelman DG et al (1987) Colocutaneous fistulas complicating diverticulitis. Dis Colon Rectum 30:89–94

137. Chandra V, Nelson H, Larson DR, Harrington JR (2004) Impact of primary resection on the outcome of patients with perforated diverticulitis. Arch Surg 139:1121–1124

138. Lee EC, Murray JJ, Coller JA et al (1997) Intraoperative colonic lavage in nonelective surgery for diverticular disease. Dis Colon Rectum 40:669–674

139. Finlay IG, Carter DC (1987) A comparison of emergency resection and staged management in perforated diverticular disease. Dis Colon Rectum 30:929–933

140. Salem TA, Molloy RG, O'Dwyaer PJ (2006) Prospective study on the management of patients with complicated diverticular disease. Colorectal Dis 8:173–176

141. Hart AR, Kennedy HJ, Stebbings WS et al (2000) How frequently do large bowel diverticula perforate? An incidence and cross-sectional study. Eur J Gastroenterol Hepatol 12:661–665

142. Labow JM, Salvati EP, Rubin RJ (1978) The Hartmann procedure in the treatment of diverticular disease. Dis Colon Rectum 16:392–394

143. Belmonte C, Klas JV, Perez JJ et al (1996) The Hartmann procedure: first choice or last resort in diverticular disease? Arch Surg 131:612–615

144. Berry AL, Turner WH, Mortensen NJM, Kettlewell MGW (1989) Emergency surgery for complicated diverticular disease: a five-year experience. Dis Colon Rectum 32:849–855

145. Salem L, Anaya DA, Robert KE, Flum DR (2005) Hartmann's colectomy and reversal in diverticulitis: a population-level assessment. Dis Colon Rectum 48:988095

146. Eisenstat TE, Rubin RJ, Salvati EP (1983) Surgical management of diverticulitis: the role of the Hartmann procedure. Dis Colon Rectum 26:429–432

147. Colcock BP (1958) Surgical management of complicated diverticulitis. N Engl J Med 259:570–573

148. Alexander J, Karl RC, Skinner DB (1983) Results of changing trends in the surgical management of complications of diverticular disease. Surgery 94:683–690

149. Labs JD, Sarr MG, Ek F et al (1988) Complications of acute diverticulitis of the colon: improved early diagnosis with computerized tomography. Am J Surg 155:331–336

150. Schechter S, Eisenstat TE, Oliver GC et al (1994) Computerized tomographic scan-guided drainage of intra-abdominal abscesses. Dis Colon Rectum 37:984–988

151. Hemming A, Davis NL, Robins RE (1991) Surgical versus percutaneous drainage of intraabdominal abscesses. Am J Surg 161:593–595

152. Mueller PR, Siani S, Wittenberg J et al (1987) Sigmoid diverticular abscesses: percutaneous drainage as an adjunct to surgical resection in twenty-four cases. Radiology 164:321–325

153. Neff CC, van Sonnengerb E, Casola G et al (1987) Diverticular abscesses: percutaneous drainage. Radiology 163:15–18

154. Saini S, Mueller PR, Wittenberg J et al (1986) Percutaneous drainage of diverticular abscess. Arch Surg 121:475–478

155. Kaiser AM, Kaing JK, Lake JP et al (2005) The management of complicated diverticulitis and the role of computed tomography. Am J Gastroenterol 100:910–917

156. Franklin ME, Dorman JP, Jacobs M, Plasencia G (1997) Is laparoscopic surgery applicable to complicated diverticular disease? Surg Endosc 11:1021–1025

157. Leff EI, Groff FW, Rubin RJ et al (1982) Use of ureteral catheters in colonic and rectal surgery. Dis Colon Rectum 25:457–460

158. Rothenberger DA, Wiltz O (1993) Surgery for complicated diverticulitis. Surg Clin North Am 73:975–992

159. Smirniotis V, Tsoutsos D, Totopoulos A et al (1992) Perforated diverticulitis: a surgical dilemma. Int Surg 77:44–47

160. Kronborg O (1993) Treatment of perforated sigmoid diverticulitis: a prospective randomized trial. Br J Surg 80:505–507

161. Hackford AW, Schoetz DJ Jr, Coller JA et al (1985) Surgical management of complicated diverticulitis: the Lahey Clinic experience, 1967 to 1982. Dis Colon Rectum 65:347–363

162. Woods RJ, Lavery IC, Fazio VW et al (1988) Internal fistulas in diverticular disease. Dis Colon Rectum 31:591–596

163. Elliot TB, Yego S, Irvin TT (1997) Five-year audit of the acute complications of diverticular disease. Br J Surg 84:535–539

164. Pontari MA, McMillen MA, Garvey RH et al (1992) Diagnosis and treatment of entero-vesical fistulae. Am J Surg 58:258–263

165. Kirsh GM, Hampel N, Shuck JM, Resnick MI (1991) Diagnosis and management of vesicoenteric fistulas. Surg Gynecol Obstet 173:91–97

166. Chaikof EL, Cambria RP, Warshaw AL (1985) Colouterine fistula secondary to diverticulitis. Dis Colon Rectum 28:358–360

167. Greenlee HB, Pienkos FJ, Vanderbilt PC et al (1974) Proceedings: acute large bowel obstruction: comparison of county, Veterans' Administration and community hospital publications. Arch Surg 108:470–476

168. Dudley HA, Radcliffe AG, McGeehan D (1980) Intra-operative irrigation of the colon to permit primary anastomosis. Br J Surg 67:80–81

169. Schwartz SI (1989) Appendix. In: Schwartz SI (ed) Principles of surgery, 5th edn. McGraw-Hill, New York

170. Thorbjarnarson B, Loehr WJ (1967) Acute appendicitis in patients over the age of sixty. Surg Gynecol Obstet 125:1277–1280

171. Campbell KL, DeBeaux AC (1992) Non-steroidal anti-inflammatory drugs and appendicitis in patients over 50 years. Br J Surg 79:967–968

172. Norman DC, Yoshikawa TT (1983) Intraabdominal infections in the elderly. J Am Geriatr Soc 31:677–684

173. Addis DG, Shaffer N, Fowler BS, Tauxe RV (1990) The epidemiology of appendicitis and appendectomy in the United States. Am J Epidemiol 132:910–925

174. Peltokallio P, Jauhiainen K (1970) Acute appendicitis in the aged patient. Arch Surg 100:140–143

175. Luckmann R (1989) Incidence and case fatality rates for acute appendicitis in California. J Epidemiol 129:905–918

176. Nockerts SR, Detmer DE, Fryback DG (1980) Incidental appendectomy in the elderly? No. Surgery 88:301–306

177. Peltokallio P, Tykka H (1981) Evolution of the age distribution and mortality of acute appendicitis. Arch Surg 116:153–156

178. Owens WB, Hamit HF (1978) Appendicitis in the elderly. Ann Surg 187:392–396

179. Bott DE (1960) Geriatric surgical emergency. BMJ 1:832–836

180. Williams JS, Hale HW Jr (1965) Acute appendicitis in the elderly. Ann Surg 162:208–212

181. Hall A, Wright TM (1976) Acute appendicitis in the geriatric patient. Am Surg 42:147–150

182. Weksler ME (1994) Immune senescence. Ann Neurol 35:S35–S37

183. Roberts-Thomson IC, Whittingham S, Young-Chaiyud U, MacKay IR (1974) Ageing, immune response and mortality. Lancet 2:368

184. Podnos YD, Jimenez JC, Wilson SE (2002) Intra-abdominal sepsis in elderly persons. Clin Infect Dis 35:62–68

185. Silen W (ed) (1996) Cope's early diagnosis of the acute abdomen, 19th edn. Oxford University Press, New York

186. Agafonoff S, Hawke I, Khadra M et al (1987) The influence of age and gender on normal appendicectomy rates. Aust NZ J Surg 57:843–846

187. Burns RP, Cochran JL, Russell WL, Bard RM (1985) Appendicitis in mature patients. Ann Surg 201:695–702

188. Lau WY, Fan ST, Yiu TF et al (1985) Acute appendicitis in the elderly. Surg Gynecol Obstet 161:157–160

189. Horattas MC, Guyton DP, Wu D (1990) A reappraisal of appendicitis in the elderly. Am J Surg 160:291–293

190. Smithy WB, Wexner SD, Dailey TH (1986) The diagnosis and treatment of acute appendicitis in the aged. Dis Colon Rectum 29:170–173

191. Samiy AH (1983) Clinical manifestations of disease in the elderly. Med Clin North Am 76:333–344

192. Harkins SW, Chapman CR (1976) Detection and decision factors in pain perception in young and elderly men. Pain 2:253–264

193. Hodgkinson HM (1980) Common symptoms of disease in the elderly, 2nd edn. Blackwell, Oxford

194. Hunt TE (1976) Management of chronic non-rheumatic pain in the elderly. J Am Geriatr Soc 24:402–406

195. Klein SR, Layden L, Wright JF, White RA (1988) Appendicitis in the elderly. A diagnostic challenge. Postgrad Med 83:247–254

196. Birnbaum BA, Balthazar EJ (1994) CT of appendicitis and diverticulitis. Radiol Clin North Am 32:885–898

197. Yacoe ME, Jeffrey RB Jr (1994) Sonography of appendicitis and diverticulitis. Radiol Clin North Am 32:899–912

198. Hale DA, Molloy M, Pearl RH et al (1997) Appendectomy: a contemporary appraisal. Ann Surg 225:252–261

199. Eskelinen M, Ikonen J, Lipponen P (1995) The value of history-taking, physical examination, and computer assistance in the diagnosis of acute appendicitis in patients over 50 years old. Scand J Gastroenterol 30:349–355

200. Lane MJ, Katz DS, Ross BA et al (1997) Unenhanced helical CT for suspected acute appendicitis. Am J Roentgenol 168:405–409

201. Andersson RE, Hugander A, Thulin AJG (1992) Diagnostic accuracy and perforation rate in appendicitis: association with

age and sex of the patient and with appendicectomy rate. Eur J Surg 158:37–41

202. Paajanen H, Maniskka A, Laato M et al (1997) Are serum inflammatory markers age dependent in acute appendicitis? J Am Coll Surg 184:303–308

203. Sansoni P, Cossarizza A, Brianti V et al (1993) Lymphocyte subsets and natural killer cell activity in healthy old people and centenarians. Blood 82:2767–2773

204. Hui TT, Major KM, Avital I et al (2002) Outcome of elderly patients with appendicitis. Arch Surg 127:995–1000

205. Franz MG, Norman J, Fabri PJ (1995) Increased morbidity of appendicitis with advancing age. Am Surg 61:40–44

206. Erkisson S, Granstrom L (1995) Randomized controlled trial of appendicectomy versus antibiotic therapy for acute appendicitis. Br J Surg 82:166–169

207. Hurme T, Nylamo E (1995) Conservative versus operative treatment of appendicular abscess. Ann Chir Gynaecol 84:33–36

208. Ein SH, Shandling B (1996) Is interval appendectomy necessary after rupture of an appendiceal mass? J Pediatr Surg 31:849–850

209. Greig JD, Nixon SJ (1995) Correspondence: randomized controlled trial of appendicectomy versus antibiotic therapy for acute appendicitis. Br J Surg 82:1000

210. Ricci MA, Trevisani MF, Beck WC (1991) Acute appendicitis: a 5 year review. Am Surg 57:301–305

211. Rappaport WD, Peterson M, Stanton C (1989) Factors responsible for the high perforation rate seen in early childhood appendicitis. Am Surg 55:602–605

212. Paajanen H, Kettunen J, Kostianinen S (1994) Emergency appendectomies in patients over 80 years. Am Surg 60:951–953

213. Tamir LL, Bongard FS, Klein SR (1990) Acute appendicitis in the pregnant patient. Am J Surg 160:571–576

214. Temple CL, Huchcroft SA, Temple WJ (1995) The natural history of appendicitis in adults. Ann Surg 221:278–281

215. Wolff WI, Hindman R (1952) Acute appendicitis in the aged. Surg Gynecol Obstet 94:239–247

216. Von Tittle SN, McCabe CJ, Ottinger LW (1996) Delayed appendectomy for appendicitis: causes and consequences. Am J Emerg Med 14:620–622

217. Thomson HJ, Jones PF (1985) Active observation in acute appendicitis. J R Coll Surg Edinb 30:290–293

218. White JJ, Santillana M, Haller JA (1975) Intensive in-hospital observation: a safe way to decrease unnecessary appendectomy. Am Surg 41:793–798

219. Vallina VL, Velasco JM, McCulloch CS (1993) Laparoscopic versus conventional appendectomy. Ann Surg 218:685–692

220. Attwood SE, Hill AD, Murphy PG et al (1992) A prospective randomized trial of laparoscopic versus open appendectomy. Surgery 112:497–501

221. Frazee RC, Roberts JW, Symmonds RE et al (1994) A prospective randomized trial comparing open versus laparoscopic appendectomy. Ann Surg 219:725–731

222. Minne L, Varner D, Burnell A et al (1997) Laparoscopic vs open appendectomy. Arch Surg 132:708–712

223. Hansen JB, Smithers BM, Schache D et al (1996) Laparoscopic vs. open appendectomy: prospective randomized trial. World J Surg 20:17–21

224. McAnena OJ, Austin O, O'Connell PR et al (1992) Laparoscopic versus open appendectomy: a prospective evaluation. Br J Surg 79:818–819

225. Tate JJT, Dawson JW, Chung SCS et al (1993) Laparoscopic versus open appendectomy: prospective randomized trial. Lancet 342:633–637

226. Ortega AE, Hunter JG, Peters JH et al (1995) A prospective randomized comparison of laparoscopic appendectomy with open appendectomy. Am J Surg 169:208–213

227. Slim K, Pezet D, Chipponi J (1998) Laparoscopic or open appendectomy? Dis Colon Rectum 41:398–403

228. Olmi S, Magnone S, Bertolini A, Croce E (2005) Laparoscopic vs. open appendectomy in acute appendicitis. A randomized prospective study. Surg Endosc 19:1193–1195

229. Yau KK, Siu WT, Tang CN et al (2007) Laparoscopic versus open appendectomy for complicated appendicitis. J Am Coll Surg 205:60–65

230. Konstantinos K, Konstantinidis M, Anastasakou KA et al (2006) A decade of laparoscopic appendectomy: presentation of 1026 patients with suspected appendicitis treated in a single surgical department. J Laparoendos Adv Surg Tech A 18:248–258

231. Paranjape C, Dalia S, Pan J, Horattas M (2007) Appendicitis in the elderly: a change in the laparoscopic era. Surg Endosc 21:777–781

232. Harrell AG, Lincourt AE, Novitsky YW et al (2006) Advantages of laparoscopic appendectomy in the elderly. Am Surg 72:474–480

Chapter 68
Benign Colorectal Disease

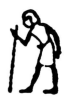

Elisa H. Birnbaum

The incidence of benign medical and surgical diseases of the colon and rectum increases with age. Although constipation, fecal incontinence, and several other associated benign conditions increase in frequency with aging, a paucity of information exists regarding the normal aging effect on gastrointestinal pathophysiology. Studies documenting anatomic, physiologic, and pathologic changes that occur in the aging colon have not been definitive, and many studies have reported conflicting results. Mucosal atrophy, atrophy of circular muscles, thickening of longitudinal muscles (taeniae coli), increased elastin deposition, and atherosclerosis are several of the changes seen in the aging bowel [1]. These changes may factor into the development of several disease states (i.e., diverticular disease and angiodysplasia). Medications affect gastrointestinal function and many have constipation as a side effect. Preexisting diseases (cardiac, pulmonary, renal, neurologic, psychiatric) may affect colonic motility directly or secondarily. In addition, these comorbidities affect medical and surgical therapy, making geriatric operative risks higher. Early diagnosis and treatment is crucial even for seemingly benign diseases or symptoms. In this chapter, we address benign colorectal diseases frequently encountered in the elderly patient and which may increase as the population ages. Diseases common to both young and old persons, such as hemorrhoids and fissures, are not discussed.

Constipation and Pelvic Floor Abnormality

Constipation is a frequent complaint in the USA and has been estimated to affect more than four million people. Complaints of constipation increase with age and are more common in women, blacks, and persons of lower socioeconomic status [2, 3]. The overall prevalence of reported constipation in

the elderly Western population is approximately 20–25%, but differs according to the source of the sample [3–5]. The incidence of constipation is approximately 12% in the ambulatory geriatric population vs. 41% in acute-care facilities and more than 80% in geriatric nursing homes and extended-care facilities. Elderly women are more likely to report symptoms of constipation than elderly men [5]. Further studies indicate large variation in bowel habits and frequent use of laxatives in as many as 30–50% of the elderly population [6–8]. Subjective complaints of constipation and laxative use increase with age, but true epidemiologic data suggest that clinical constipation does not [9]. Although complaints of constipation increase in those over age 65, about 80–90% of subjects over age 60 report at least one bowel movement per day [6, 7]. Although there may be normal physiologic aging of the colon and rectum, asymptomatic geriatric patients do not seem to differ significantly from their younger cohorts.

It is important to define constipation, as patients and their physicians frequently have different definitions [10]. Several investigators have attempted to define "normal" bowel function in the elderly [6, 8]. The normal number of bowel movements within the elderly population ranges from three per week to two or three per day and does not differ from that found among the young population [11]. It is generally accepted that patients with a reduced frequency in the number of bowel movements (fewer than three per week) are considered constipated [12]. A consensus definition of constipation was developed by a group of experts at an international congress of gastroenterology and is known as the Rome II criteria (Table 68.1) [13].

Decreased motility or prolonged transit diffusely throughout the colon can be caused by several factors. Dietary factors (fluid and fiber) have frequently been implicated. Inadequate fluid intake may decrease the fecal bulk causing decreased intraluminal pressures in the colon, which in turn may decrease the number of propagating motor complexes generated [9]. Fiber plays a questionable role in the development and treatment of constipation. A meta-analysis showed that bran did not affect the stool output or transit time in constipated patients [14]. Many medications taken by the elderly

E.H. Birnbaum (✉)
Department of Surgery, Barnes Jewish Hospital,
Washington University School of Medicine,
St. Louis, MO, USA
e-mail: Birnbaume@wustl.edu

R.A. Rosenthal et al. (eds.), *Principles and Practice of Geriatric Surgery*,
DOI 10.1007/978-1-4419-6999-6_68, © Springer Science+Business Media, LLC 2011

TABLE 68.1 Rome II criteria for defining chronic functional constipation in adults

Two or more of the following for at least 12 weeks in the preceding 12 months:

Straining in more than 25% of defecations

Lumpy or hard stools in more than 25% of defecations

Sensation of incomplete evacuation in more than 25% of defecations

Sensation of anorectal obstruction or blockade in more than 25% of defecations

Manual maneuvers (e.g., digital evacuation, support of the pelvic floor) to facilitate more than 25% of defecations

Fewer than three defecations per week

Source: Reprinted from [13], with permission from MacMillan Publishers, Ltd

are known to cause constipation [15]. Anticholinergics, tricyclic antidepressants, β-blockers, and calcium channel blockers are commonly implicated. Over-the-counter medications, such as aluminum and calcium antacids and laxatives, may also contribute to patients' symptoms. Chronic medical diseases such as hypothyroidism, diabetes, scleroderma, multiple sclerosis, and Parkinson's disease can result in decreased colonic motility. Psychiatric conditions (depression and dementia) have been associated with constipation, which may be behaviorally related [2]. Inability to ambulate to the bathroom because of arthritis, for example, or ignoring the call to defecate because of dementia may contribute to symptoms of fecal impaction, constipation, and the development of a megarectum [2, 7]. Constipation is probably not a normal consequence of aging but is associated with and possibly caused by the immobility, chronic illnesses, and increased neuropsychiatric problems of the elderly population.

Generally, patients with constipation can be separated into three groups. The first are those with normal transit or functional constipation. These patients complain of hard, dry stools that are difficult to evacuate and should be treated with life style manipulation: increased fiber, increased fluid, and exercise. The second group is patients with slow transit or colonic inertia. These patients have minimal to no motility of their colon and rarely have spontaneous bowel movements. Many of these patients report going for days and occasionally weeks without bowel function. Patients with colonic inertia commonly report a long history of laxative use and abuse. Chronic laxative use, particularly with the anthracene laxatives, can cause degeneration of the myoneural chains and may impede motility irreversibly over time [16]. The third group are the patients with anorectal dysfunction or pelvic floor abnormalities. The pelvic floor abnormality can be identified with colonic transit marker studies, scintidefecography and dynamic MRI. These patients have normal transit to the sigmoid colon but are unable to evacuate their rectums easily despite having soft stool. Within this group are patients with rectal intussusception, pelvic organ prolapse, rectocele and obstructed defecation (nonrelaxing puborectalis or anismus).

Rectal intussusception results from a loss of fixation of the rectum from the sacrum. The rectum folds in onto itself and acts as a valve that prevents normal emptying. Symptoms vary from mild constipation with rectal pressure to severe constipation with rectal pain and a "plugging" sensation. Incomplete evacuation and discharge of mucus and blood per rectum are frequent complaints. Other associated disease entities are colitis cystica profunda, solitary rectal ulcer syndrome, and mucosal prolapse. Rectal intussusception may be identified as a component of pelvic organ prolapse. The etiology of outlet obstruction is unclear, although dysfunction and discoordination of the pelvic floor muscles is the most common explanation. In patients with chronic fecal impaction, the rectal capacity increases over time and rectal sensation becomes blunted. These patients cannot feel the urge to defecate until a fecal bolus is too large to pass. These patients often report the need to use digital maneuvers, suppositories, or enemas to evacuate to their satisfaction.

Patients with complaints of severe constipation should be completely evaluated. Initially, a history and physical examination are performed. A detailed medication list, including all over-the-counter medications, is imperative. A diet and defecation diary is helpful to attempt to define the extent of the problem. The American Gastroenterological Association consensus guideline recommends that most patients with severe constipation have a complete blood count, serum glucose, calcium and creatinine, and thyroid-stimulating hormone levels checked [17].

A digital rectal examination should be done to exclude low rectal carcinomas, anal strictures, and other anorectal abnormalities. Contrast studies or colonoscopy should be performed to rule out obstructing colonic lesions, particularly if the symptoms of constipation are recent or associated with bleeding, mucus, or altered stool caliber. On proctosigmoidoscopic examination, the typical patient with significant intussusception is found to have an erythematous anterior rectal wall approximately 5–8 cm from the mucocutaneous junction. Patients with solitary rectal ulcer syndrome frequently have more severe symptoms of straining, passage of bloody mucus per rectum, and incomplete evacuation. On examination, the solitary rectal ulcer appears as a heaped-up lesion in the anterior midline 5–8 cm from the mucocutaneous junction. This lesion can often be palpated and may be mistaken for a rectal carcinoma. Biopsy of the lesion reveals cystic proliferation of fibroblasts and muscle hypertrophy in the lamina propria, epithelial hyperplasia, colitis cystica profunda, or excess mucosal collagen [18].

Several tests are available for assessment of constipation and can aid in creating a strategy for management although it is not uncommon that patient's complaints and concerns do not correlate well with colonic and anorectal physiologic tests. Colonic transit time is a simple radiographic test which helps assess the bowel motility and can identify patients with colonic inertia or outlet obstruction. Patients are placed on a high-fiber diet and taken off all laxatives and enemas for several days prior to testing. A capsule with 24 radiopaque markers is given to the patient to take orally on day 0. A plain radiograph is obtained on the third and fifth days. The markers are counted and their location should be noted. The presence of more than 10% of the markers on the fifth day is considered to be an abnormal study. It is important to ensure that the patient took the capsule, did not take laxatives, and did not have abnormal bowel function (i.e., diarrhea) during the study period, as these possibilities may give a false normal examination. Patients with colonic inertia have markers scattered diffusely throughout the colon that remain through the fifth day. In patients with rectal intussusception or outlet obstruction, the markers move through the colon and are held up in the rectosigmoid region. Total colonic transit times in healthy asymptomatic elderly subjects show no change with aging but are prolonged in healthy elderly subjects who report symptoms of constipation [19, 20].

Physical examination is limited in the complete evaluation of the pelvic floor and can miss a significant number of rectoceles, enteroceles, sigmoidoceles, and cystoceles [21]. Scintidefecography may identify patients with severe rectal intussusception or rectal prolapse and can identify patients with significant rectoceles and enteroceles if vaginal contrast is used. This test is done by placing a thickened barium paste in the rectosigmoid to simulate a bowel movement. The patient is then placed on a commode and asked to evacuate the paste while radiographs are obtained. In a normal test the rectosigmoid remains stable along the presacral space, and the puborectalis is seen to relax as the patient passes the contrast bolus. With an abnormal test, the rectosigmoid falls away from its attachments to the presacral space, and the

proximal rectum is seen to infold (intussuscept) (Fig. 68.1). Internal intussusception of the rectum can block the rectal outlet, resulting in incomplete evacuation of the rectal contrast. With severe straining, the intussusception may worsen, and occasionally the entire rectum is seen prolapsing through the anorectal ring.

One of the shortcomings of defecography is the utilization of ionizing radiation. MRI is noninvasive, does not use ionizing radiation, has a larger field of view, has improved soft tissue contrast, and has multiplanar capability. Dynamic MR imaging has been used to assess the complex pelvic anatomy and changes in these structures during attempts at evacuation. Older methods had long acquisition times (6–12 s) which did not allow for real-time evaluation. Newer techniques have near real-time continuous imaging and can be performed in less than 2 min [22, 23]. Dynamic radiologic examinations of the endopelvis may reveal multicompartmental dysfunction [24]. Segregation of the pelvic floor into posterior, middle and anterior compartments, however, is artificial because these structures are closely interrelated [25]. Pelvic organ prolapse can be detected and characterized using dynamic MR imaging but cine defecography is more sensitive in detecting parietal alterations [26].

Anal manometry has limited value in the workup of constipation in the elderly. In select cases, anal manometry, rectal anal inhibitory reflex, minimal sensory rectal volume, and balloon expulsion may identify patients with megarectum and patients with nonrelaxing puborectalis muscle. These tests require specialized manometric instruments and can be done utilizing a capillary perfusion system or microballoon system.

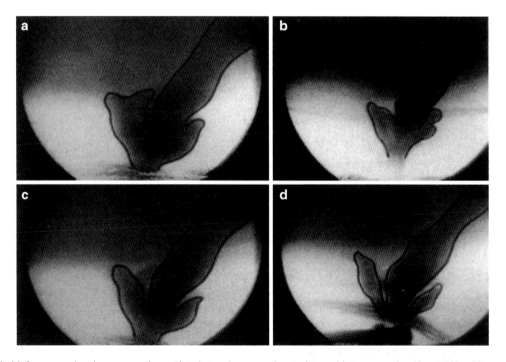

FIGURE 68.1 Scintidefecogram showing progressive outlet obstruction secondary to internal intussusception (from [72], with permission from the McGraw-Hill Companies).

The systems measure the pressures within the anal canal and test the function of the anal sphincter mechanism. Anal sensation is tested by inserting a rectal balloon just above the anal sphincter and insufflating increasing amounts of air until the patient notes sensation. Patients with megarectums require large amounts of distension before any sensation is noted. The rectoanal inhibitory reflex is absent in the setting of Hirschsprung's disease and is also absent in patients with megarectum who require large volumes to induce the inhibitory reflex. A rectal examination performed on an "unprepped" patient with megarectum may reveal a rectum full of stool. The inability to expel the rectal balloon is tested by asking the patient to evacuate a rectal balloon filled with 60 cc of air in the privacy of the bathroom. If patients have an outlet obstruction and the puborectalis muscle does not relax properly they have difficulty doing this simple task. The inability to relax the puborectalis muscle and evacuate the contrast on scintidefecography helps confirm the diagnosis.

Treatment of constipation in the younger population is generally medical, and treatment of the elderly constipated patient is no different. A trial of dietary fiber and increased fluid intake should be initially instituted once a malignancy has been ruled out (Fig. 68.2). The daily recommended fiber intake is 20–35 g daily, even in the elderly [27]. By adding approximately 5 g of fiber per week until the goal is met the excessive gas and bloating that occurs with high-fiber diets can be minimized [28]. A bowel evacuation routine is often helpful for those patients with outlet obstruction. The patient is instructed to take bulk-forming agents daily and to use a glycerine suppository or tap water enema at the same time daily. To maximize the effect of the gastrocolic reflex patients are encouraged to perform this evacuation routine upon wakening in the morning and approximately 15–20 min after drinking a warm beverage. Biofeedback has had some success in the treatment of pelvic floor outlet obstruction but requires a motivated patient [29, 30]. Surgical intervention is rarely necessary for older patients with constipation. A total colectomy with ileorectal anastomosis has been successful in the treatment of severe colonic inertia if there is no element of outlet obstruction. This operation should be reserved for the younger, medically stable patient. Other patients with colonic inertia are probably best treated by accepting the need for continuous laxative use.

Treatment of patients with intussusception is primarily medical. Surgery should be limited to patients who are incapacitated because of the pressure or who have a persistent solitary rectal ulcer after intensive medical therapy. Surgery involves low anterior resection or retrorectal sacral fixation of the mobile rectum. Many patients have persistent postoperative symptoms of constipation and difficulty emptying. Patients with symptoms of nonrelaxing puborectalis or colonic inertia must have these symptoms addressed and treated preoperatively to have a successful surgical result [31]. Patients with pelvic organ prolapse, enterocele, cystocele combined with intussusception may benefit from a combined procedure. Women with severe symptomatic rec-

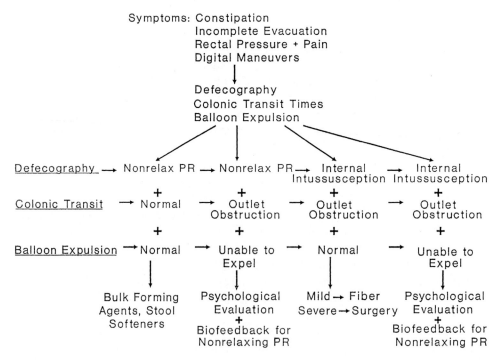

FIGURE 68.2 Management plan for the treatment of severe constipation. PR, puborectalis muscle (from [73], with permission of The McGraw-Hill Companies).

tal intussusception and pelvic organ prolapse may benefit from a multidiscipline approach including urology and gynecology. The decision for surgical intervention for pelvic organ prolapse should not be determined by age alone [32].

Rectal Prolapse

The most severe rectal abnormality of the pelvic floor is rectal prolapse. Rectal prolapse can be partial (mucosal) or full (complete extrusion of the rectum through the anal canal). Circumferential rings are typical of a full rectal prolapse, whereas radial folds are more typical of mucosal prolapse or prolapsing hemorrhoids. Rectal prolapse is associated with chronic constipation and straining and is more frequent in elderly women and institutionalized patients who often have neurologic or psychiatric comorbidities [33]. In addition, since the prevalence of this abnormality increases with age, many patients have other significant medical problems [33, 34].

Rectal pressure, mucous discharge, rectal bleeding, and fecal incontinence are frequent symptoms of rectal prolapse. Once the prolapse begins to occur the patients complain more of fecal incontinence and rectal bleeding than they do of constipation [35]. Often the patient does not mention that the rectum extrudes through the anal canal, and it is not uncommon for the symptoms to be attributed to prolapsing hemorrhoids. Direct questioning may result in the history that the patient's rectum protrudes with bowel movements (especially with straining) and occasionally when assuming an upright position. Manual replacement by the patient or their caretakers is common. A lax anal sphincter and prolapsing rectum are usually found on physical examination. Incarceration or strangulation of the prolapsed rectum is a rare presentation but can occur if there is normal tone to the anal sphincter or the prolapsed rectum has become extremely edematous. An erythematous edematous circumferential region (the "leading edge") may be seen approximately 5–8 cm from the dentate line on proctosigmoidoscopic examination. Asking patients to strain to evacuate their rectum may allow visualization of the prolapse by the examiner. If the prolapse cannot be demonstrated in the office setting, defecography, or dynamic MRI may be done to demonstrate the redundant prolapsing rectosigmoid. A complete evaluation with contrast studies or colonoscopy is necessary to rule out a tumor as a lead point of the rectal prolapse. Occasionally a solitary rectal ulcer is seen at the leading edge of the prolapsing rectum and may be confused with a rectal tumor. Biopsy of the ulcer should give a more definitive diagnosis. The anal sphincter may be assessed using anal manometry and electromyography although the results typically show extremely low rest and squeeze efforts. Unilateral or bilateral neurogenic injury may result from chronic stretching of the pudendal nerve. Stretch injury may also be a direct result of repeated trauma to the anal sphincter by the prolapsing rectum. Preoperative motility studies with colonic transit times should be done in patients with complaints of severe constipation to identify a group of patients with colonic inertia and prolapse who may require more extensive resection [36].

The surgical approach to rectal prolapse is transabdominal or perineal; more than 100 operations have been cited as forms of treatment for rectal prolapse. Surgical therapy must be tailored to the individual patient. Abdominal suture rectopexy with or without sigmoid resection can be done in patients who are good surgical risks [36, 37]. Low anterior resection may improve the bowel habits of patients who complain of preoperative constipation in whom a markedly redundant distal colon is found [36, 38] (Fig. 68.3a). Complete encirclement of the rectum with a band of mesh (Ripstein procedure) can be modified to leave the anterior bowel wall free [39, 40] (Fig. 68.3b), which minimizes the stenosis by the foreign material and may decrease postoperative fecal impaction at the level of the mesh. Resection should not be done in the presence of foreign material. Modifications using the laparoscope to perform rectopexy have been described [41].

The functional and recurrence rates are similar if the rectopexy is done laparoscopically or open, the benefit is in the shorter hospital stay [42, 43]. Recurrence rates after abdominal procedures are generally less than those after perineal procedures but morbidity can be higher. Abdominal procedures are generally reserved for patients who can tolerate general anesthesia. Recurrence rates do increase over time with both the perineal approach and abdominal approach [44, 45].

Perineal procedures (anal encirclement or proctosigmoidectomy) can be done under regional anesthesia, minimizing the anesthetic risk in the high-risk patient. Thiersch wire or other synthetic material may be used to encircle the anal canal to prevent rectal prolapse (Fig. 68.3c). The synthetic material acts as an obstruction to defecation and prevents the rectum from prolapsing through the anal canal. The anal encirclement procedures do not treat the underlying condition, and the symptoms of rectal intussusception persist in most patients. It is not uncommon for patients to require laxatives and enemas for fecal evacuation after anal encirclement, as the synthetic material acts as an obstruction to defecation. Because septic and mechanical complications are high, anal encirclement as a primary treatment for rectal prolapse is generally reserved for moribund patients with limited life expectancy.

Perineal proctosigmoidectomy, first described in 1889 by Mikulicz [46], has been modified and popularized by others [33, 47] (Fig. 68.4). It can easily be performed under regional anesthesia in either prone jackknife or lithotomy position. The redundant rectum and portion of sigmoid colon can be

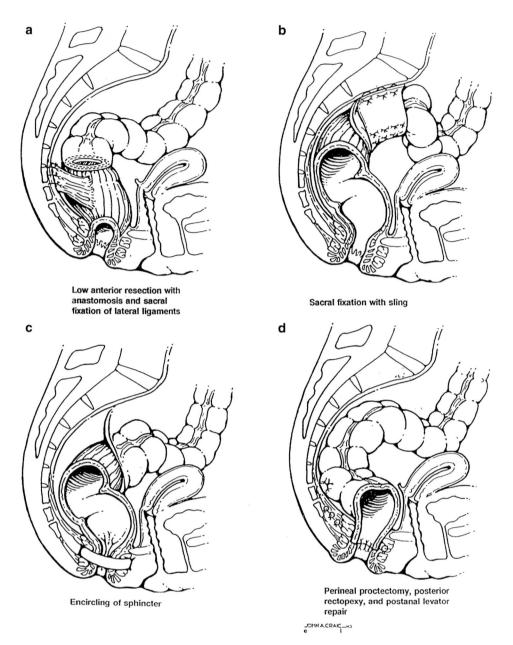

a

Low anterior resection with
anastomosis and sacral
fixation of lateral ligaments

b

Sacral fixation with sling

c

Encircling of sphincter

d

Perineal proctectomy, posterior
rectopexy, and postanal levator
repair

JOHN A.CRAIG—MD

FIGURE 68.3 Surgical options for the treatment of rectal prolapse (from [73], with permission of The McGraw-Hill Companies).

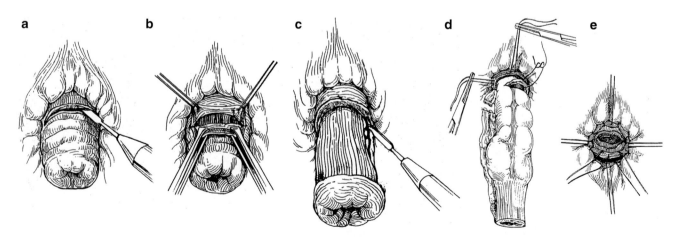

a   **b**   **c**   **d**   **e**

FIGURE 68.4 Perineal proctosigmoidectomy (reprinted with permission from The ASCRS textbook of colon and rectal surgery, publisher Springer 2007, Chap. 47 Rectal prolapse, pp. 665–677).

easily removed via the anal incision. Addition of a posterior levator repair described by Prasad et al. re-creates the anatomic anorectal angle and may help patients gain fecal control postoperatively [47]. Minimal pain and little physiologic alteration are associated with this procedure, and most patients can be discharged from the hospital within 3–4 days. The recurrence rate of a perineal proctosigmoidectomy is related to the length of follow-up and ranges from 0 to 22% [33, 34, 47]. The morbidity is 3–12%, and mortality is less than 5% [33, 34, 47].

Another perineal approach, the Delorme procedure, has been recommended for the treatment of rectal prolapse since the morbidity and mortality is relatively low [48]. This procedure is not a full thickness rectal resection but rather the redundant rectal mucosa is stripped circumferentially. The remaining, redundant outer rectal wall is then plicated with a series of circumferential sutures which then allows the mucosal edges to be reapproximated. It has not been used as widely for the treatment of full rectal prolapse because of concerns for recurrence [49]. A recent study found that the Delorme procedure could be done with minimal morbidity, a short hospital stay and a recurrence rate of 14.5%. The mean time to recurrence was 31 months. They found that the recurrence rate was relatively low in patients under 50 (8%) and felt that this procedure could be offered to younger patients as well [35].

Stercoral Ulceration

Ischemic pressure necrosis by a large fecal mass causing fecal peritonitis is a rare cause of free perforation of the colon. Mortality can be as high as 35% in patients presenting with perforation [50]. Although considered a disease of the elderly, the average age of patients presenting with stercoral ulceration is in the fifties. Associated medical diseases occur in about one-third of patients, and almost all patients complain of chronic constipation requiring laxatives. The sigmoid and rectosigmoid are the most common sites of perforation, which almost always occurs along the antimesenteric border [50]. The symptoms of abdominal pain and peritonitis start acutely and the clinical picture is usually one of sepsis. If there is a free perforation, an upright chest radiograph will show free air under the diaphragm. A CT scan, if done before free perforation, may show focal colonic wall thickening and mild pericolonic fat stranding indicating a localized process. Small air bubbles in the vicinity of a large fecal bolus indicate wall compromise and perforation [51]. The actual diagnosis is rarely made preoperatively. At exploration, the bowel wall adjacent to the perforation is usually thin and rarely inflamed, in contrast to the colonic findings of diverticulitis. Irrigation of the abdominal cavity and distal

rectal stump help to decrease the fecal load. Several surgical procedures are recommended for treatment in the literature. Resection with end colostomy, with a mucous fistula or Hartmann's procedure has the lowest operative mortality rate (23%). A proximal colostomy with closure of the perforation is rarely done and carries a mortality of approximately 44%. Proximal loop colostomies and exteriorization of the perforation have the highest mortality rate (71%) [52]. Since this is an uncommon diagnosis and there are limited reports in the literature, morbidity and mortality rates may only reflect the small numbers of very ill patients with this diagnosis.

Volvulus

Colonic volvulus occurs when an air-filled segment of colon twists about its elongated mesentery. In the USA, colonic volvulus is a rare cause of intestinal obstruction and accounts for approximately 3% of colonic obstructions [53]. In parts of Iran and Russia, colonic volvulus is one of the predominant causes of intestinal obstruction. The high incidence of sigmoid volvulus in other parts of the world has been attributed to the high-fiber diets of those regions. Chagas' disease, which causes megacolon, may play a role in the development of sigmoid volvulus, particularly in countries where the disease is common [54]. In North America, the incidence increases over the age of 50. The disease is associated with chronic constipation, laxative use, psychiatric illness, and institutionalization [53]. A dilated, redundant colon with a narrow mesocolon is a prerequisite for a volvulus to occur, and therefore the intra-abdominal portions of colon are at risk. Colonic volvulus most commonly occurs in the sigmoid colon; cecal volvulus and volvulus of the transverse colon occur less frequently (<10%) and are generally seen in young patients.

Patients with sigmoid volvulus usually present with abdominal distension, obstipation, and pain. Peritoneal irritation on physical examination, fever, or an elevated white blood cell count indicates ischemic or gangrenous bowel. Plain abdominal radiographs may show an inverted, U-shaped, air-filled bowel loop ("bent inner tube"), with a dense line running toward the point of torsion. This radiologic finding is highly suggestive of a sigmoid volvulus. If peritonitis is not present, sigmoidoscopy should be performed to the point of obstruction. The volvulus can often be reduced by inserting a soft rectal tube past the point of obstruction. A release of gas and liquid stool follows successful detorsion. The rectal tube should be left in place for several days to assist with further decompression. The success rate with this technique is good, and reduction of the volvulus can be expected with approximately 75% of attempts. The colonoscope may be used to attempt reduction, but its use should be limited to patients in whom a rigid proctoscope has been unsuccessful in reaching

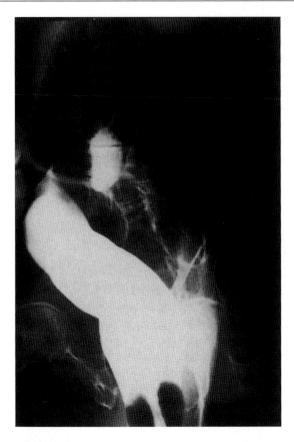

Figure 68.5 Hypaque enema showing sigmoid volvulus. Note the "bird's beak" deformity (*arrow*) (from [73], with permission of The McGraw-Hill Companies).

the point of torsion. Contrast enemas may be necessary when plain radiographs are not diagnostic for volvulus but suggest a colonic obstruction. The column of contrast tapers at the point of torsion ("bird's beak" deformity) (Fig. 68.5). Occasionally, reduction occurs with contrast enemas, but detorsion occurs in fewer than 10% of attempts [55]. Evidence of mucosal ischemia, bloody discharge, or unsuccessful detorsion indicates strangulation and possibly gangrene. If the patient has signs of peritoneal irritation or if gangrene is suspected, contrast studies and tube decompression should not be attempted and the patient should undergo emergency exploration.

Nonoperative reduction is successful in approximately 90% of patients but does not constitute adequate treatment in good risk patients [56]. Recurrence rates following nonoperative reduction range from 20 to 60% but can be as high as 90% [56, 57]. Once the volvulus is reduced, medically stable patients should undergo mechanical bowel preparation and elective resection. The choice of operation depends on the adequacy of the bowel preparation and the viability of the colon. A sigmoid resection with primary anastomosis can be done after bowel preparation and if the colon shows no signs of ischemia. The presence of ischemic or gangrenous bowel is an indication for resection and colostomy.

Mortality is related to the presence of gangrenous bowel and to delay in decompressing the ischemic bowel. The operative mortality following elective resection of a primary volvulus is approximately 6 vs. 21% for recurrent volvulus [56]. Some investigators have found high mortality rates associated with elective resection and recommend elective resection only in good risk, young patients [58]. Patients who require emergency operation for sigmoid volvulus have a mortality rate of more than 30% [56].

Cecal and transverse colonic volvuluses are less common than sigmoid volvulus. Anomalous fixation of the cecum may be an important reason why cecal volvulus occurs in a young age group [59]. Other predisposing factors, such as prior abdominal surgery, pregnancy, and distal obstruction, have been implicated as causes of cecal volvulus. Ninety percent of patients with cecal volvulus have a full axial volvulus twisting the associated mesentery and blood vessels [53]. In the remaining patients, the cecum folds in an anterior cephalad direction (cecal bascule). Although a bascule is not a true volvulus around the mesentery, gangrene can result from tension on the bowel wall. Patients with cecal volvulus clinically appear to have a small bowel obstruction. Abdominal pain, nausea, vomiting, and obstipation are common symptoms. Many patients give a history of chronic intermittent symptoms of partial bowel obstruction [53]. Plain abdominal radiographs show the cecum as an air-filled, kidney-shaped structure pointing to the left upper quadrant. Multiple air-fluid levels are suggestive of a distal small bowel obstruction. Contrast enemas may show the "bird's beak" tapered edge of the contrast pointing toward the site of torsion (Fig. 68.6). Contrast studies are useful in difficult cases but should not be performed routinely if the diagnosis of cecal volvulus is clear. Contrast studies and colonoscopy have rarely been successful in reducing a cecal or transverse volvulus.

Once a cecal volvulus is diagnosed operative intervention should be undertaken. Operative detorsion alone has high recurrence and mortality rates and should not be performed as the sole procedure. Cecopexy, cecostomy, and resection have variable rates of recurrence and morbidity. The highest rates of postoperative complications, mortality, and recurrence are seen with cecostomy [60]. Cecostomy or appendicostomy allows decompression of the distended bowel and fixation of the cecum. Although the recurrence rate is similar to that for cecopexy, the intra-abdominal and wound complications are more than 25% [60]. Cecopexy is done by anchoring the right colon to the parietal peritoneum by direct suture or by making a peritoneal flap. This technique eliminates the cecal hypermobility but is technically challenging to perform if the cecum is dilated and thin-walled. The recurrence rate after cecopexy is variable, with some series reporting recurrence as high as 28% [61]. Patients who are medically stable should undergo a right hemicolectomy with primary

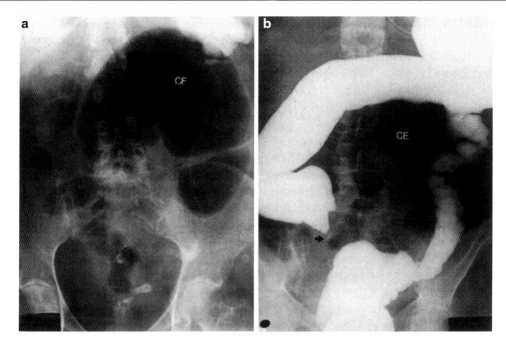

FIGURE 68.6 (**a**) Cecal volvulus, plain radiograph, *CE* cecum. (**b**) Barium enema. *Arrow* indicates the point of obstruction, *CE* cecum.

anastomosis if there is no evidence of gangrenous bowel. Resection, ileostomy, and mucous fistula are indicated if there is evidence of ischemia or gangrene. Mortality is increased in the presence of gangrenous bowel and is higher with cecal volvulus than with sigmoid volvulus (33 vs. 7%). This increased mortality rate with cecal volvulus is due to the increased presence of gangrenous bowel seen with cecal volvulus (21% vs. 7%) [53].

Fecal Incontinence

Fecal incontinence is a disabling problem in the elderly and in institutionalized patients [62]. A community-based prevalence study estimated that fecal incontinence affects 2.2% of the general population although the incidence and prevalence is probably underestimated [63]. More than 60% of patients who complain of fecal incontinence are women [63]. In community-based women older than 60 it is estimated that the prevalence varies from 12 to 33% depending on the definition used [64].

Incontinence may be neurogenic, mechanical, mixed, or secondary to other medical conditions. Anal sphincter injuries are the leading cause of mechanical incontinence and are most commonly the result of a midline episiotomy. Fecal incontinence may not occur immediately after the injury but rather the presentation may be delayed for years. The majority of women with late onset fecal incontinence have an anatomic sphincter defect [65]. Neurogenic incontinence may be due to central or peripheral denervation of the puborectalis muscle or external anal sphincter. Rectal prolapse or descending perineum syndrome may denervate the sphincter by a stretch injury to the pudendal nerve. Injury to the sphincter mechanism, traumatic or surgical, may lead to fecal incontinence immediately after the injury or during the ensuing years. Decreased anorectal sensation caused by radiotherapy or diabetes mellitus may lead to incontinence as well. Certain physiologic factors have been shown to occur with aging: decreased rectal tone and weakening of the anal sphincter mechanism [66, 68]. The anal sphincter may decrease in strength secondary to loss of muscle mass or neuropathy. These differences are more pronounced in elderly women. It may be due to weakening of connective tissues, possibly from decreased estrogen secretion. Physical limitations and poor general health are other predisposing factors that contribute to fecal incontinence [62, 63]. A common cause of fecal incontinence in the elderly, however, is fecal impaction with overflow incontinence [63]. Systemic diseases such as scleroderma, polymyositis, multiple sclerosis, and diabetes melitis can be associated with fecal incontinence. Colorectal carcinoma, colonic ischemia, and inflammatory bowel disease may cause symptoms of fecal urgency, and incontinence may be a result of the patient's inability to respond quickly.

On initial evaluation, constipation with overflow incontinence must be ruled out by history and digital rectal examination. A complete colonic evaluation with colonoscopy or contrast enema should be done especially if the symptoms of fecal incontinence have a short history. The anal physiology laboratory can objectively evaluate the anal sphincter mechanism to determine the cause of fecal incontinence and direct treatment. Anal manometry, electromyography, and transrectal ultrasonography can help differentiate neurogenic from mechanical injury to the anal sphincter. Anal manometry assesses the rest and squeeze pressures generated by the anal sphincter. The sphincter length can be determined, and some systems can identify the specific quadrant involved in a sphincter defect. The minimal sensory rectal volume is useful for identifying patients with megarectum who do not sense the presence of a large bolus of fecal material in their rectum. Electromyography is used to evaluate the pudendal nerve terminal motor latency. The pudendal nerve innervates the external anal sphincter and the puborectalis muscle. Both muscles are involved in maintaining fecal continence; and denervation of these muscles, represented by prolonged pudendal nerve terminal motor latency, may cause neurogenic incontinence. Transrectal endoluminal ultrasonography has replaced needle electromyography as the preferred method for evaluating the anal sphincter for defects. Using this modality, the puborectalis muscle and the external and internal anal sphincters can be thoroughly evaluated for defects.

CASE STUDY

Rectal Prolapse

An 86-year-old woman with a several year history of hemorrhoidal complaints presents with increased rectal bleeding, mucous discharge, and fecal incontinence. She has a long history of constipation and currently takes MiraLax and Milk of Magnesia. She complains of prolapsing rectal tissue which occurs daily with defecation. The problem has been ongoing for several years and the rectum is becoming harder to reduce. She uses a pessary for a cystocele and has urinary incontinence. Her past medical history is significant for an irregular heartbeat and coronary artery disease. Her past surgical history is significant for a total abdominal hysterectomy and bilateral salpingo-oophorectomy done years prior. She is gravida 3, para 3. Her current medications include Verapamil, Synthroid, and Digoxin.

On physical exam, she is an alert, elderly woman. Abdominal exam is benign. There is a well-healed Pfannenstiel incision. On digital rectal examination, she has lax anal tone, diminished squeeze efforts, and a normal proctosigmoidoscopic examination. There is hard stool in her rectal vault and full rectal prolapse upon straining on the toilet.

Workup

Anal physiology (including anal manometry, EMG, and transrectal ultrasound) is not needed for evaluation of fecal incontinence in this patient. The full rectal prolapse dilates the anal canal stretching the anal sphincters. The rectal tone is often diminished in patients with longstanding prolapse and is a cause of fecal incontinence.

Defecography is not needed in this patient since the full rectal prolapse is visible on examination. If the rectal prolapse is not reproduced by having the patient strain on the toilet, then defecography or dynamic MRI would be indicated to assess for full rectal prolapse. These tests can also evaluate for enteroceles and vaginal prolapse.

Colonic transit time may be indicated in this patient if she had significant symptoms of constipation. If her complaints were that she had no bowel movements without the use of laxatives or if she had bowel movements every 5–7 days, a colonic transit time would be indicated to assess for colonic inertia.

Medical evaluation is done to determine whether the patient can withstand general anesthesia. If the patient is too frail or general anesthesia is medically contraindicated, then spinal anesthesia and a perineal approach is the preferred approach.

If the patient is extremely frail and medical conditions preclude anesthesia, it is possible to place a Thiersch wire under local anesthesia. However, the performance of a Thiersch wire causes obstruction at the outlet and the patients will need to have continued evacuations. This procedure is not recommended for patients whose life expectancy exceeds 6 months.

If the patient is in poor health and cannot undergo general anesthesia, then a perineal proctectomy would be the operation of choice.

If the patient is in good health with no constipation but elderly and frail, a perineal proctectomy would be a good choice.

If the patient has significant constipation and is in good health, then a resection rectopexy would be the operation of choice.

If the patient is in good health with no complaints of constipation but a urogyn procedure is necessary, then a sutured rectopexy can be done in conjunction with a sacral colpopexy or other urogynecologic treatment.

Initial treatment may be as simple as dietary alteration (avoidance of milk products and food with high fat content) and a bowel evacuation regimen (bulk-forming agents and glycerine suppositories) [68]. Biofeedback has had some success in patients but requires the understanding and cooperation of the patient [69]. Combined pharmacologic and physical therapy may be more beneficial when combined in appropriate patients [70]. Anterior sphincter reconstructions with direct muscle repair has had success in the elderly population [71]. Older women undergoing pelvic floor surgery can expect similar results and outcomes as younger patients [32]. A diverting colostomy is rarely necessary for control of the fecal stream in the elderly population. If the rectum is severely damaged by radiation injury, a diverting colostomy is probably the best treatment option for severely incontinent patients.

References

1. Whiteway J, Morson B (1985) Pathology of the aging: diverticular disease. Clin Gastroenterol 14:829–846
2. Everhart JE, Go VL, Johannes RS et al (1989) A longitudinal survey of self-reported bowel habits in the United States. Dig Dis Sci 34:1153–1162
3. Stewart WF, Liberman JN, Sandler RS et al (1999) Epidemiology of constipation (EPOC) study in the United States: relation of clinical subtypes to sociodemographic features. Am J Gastroenterol 94:3530–3540
4. Read NW, Celik AF, Katsinelos P (1995) Constipation and incontinence in the elderly. J Clin Gastroenterol 20:61–70
5. Stewart RB, Moore MT, Marks RG, Hale WE (1992) Correlates of constipation in an ambulatory elderly population. Am J Gastroenterol 87:859–864
6. Connell AM, Hilton C, Irvine G et al (1965) Variation of bowel habit in two population samples. Br Med J 2:1095–1099
7. Milne JS, Williamson J (1972) Bowel habit in older people. Gerontol Clin 14:56–60
8. Donald IP, Smith RG, Cruikshank JG et al (1985) A study of constipation in the elderly living at home. Gerontology 31:112–118
9. Harari D, Gurwitz JH, Minaker KL (1993) Constipation in the elderly. J Am Geriatr Soc 41:1130–1140
10. Moore-Gillon V (1984) Constipation: what does the patient mean? J R Soc Med 77:108–110
11. Merkel IS, Locher J, Burgio K et al (1993) Physiologic and psychologic characteristics of an elderly population with chronic constipation. Am J Gastroenterol 88:1854–1859
12. Johanson JF, Sonnenberg A, Koch TR (1989) Clinical epidemiology of chronic constipation. J Clin Gastroenterol 11:525–536
13. Thompson WG, Longstreth GF, Drossman DA et al (1999) Functional bowel disorders and functional abdominal pain. Gut 45(suppl 2):1143–1147
14. Muller-Lissner SA (1988) Effect of wheat bran on weight of stool and gastrointestinal transit time: a meta-analysis. Br Med J 296:615–617
15. Campbell AJ, Busby WJ, Horwath CC (1993) Factors associated with constipation in a community based sample of people aged 70 years and over. J Epidemiol Community Health 47:23–26
16. Smith B (1968) Effect of irritant purgatives on the myenteric plexus in man and the mouse. Gut 9:139–143
17. Locke GR III, Pemberton JH, Phillips SF (2000) American Gastroenterological Association Medical Position Statement: guidelines on constipation. Gastroenterology 119:1791–1796
18. Tjandra JJ, Fazio VW, Church JM et al (1992) Clinical conundrum of solitary rectal ulcer. Dis Colon Rectum 35:227–234
19. Metcalf A, Phillips S, Zinsmeister A et al (1987) Simplified assessment of segmental colonic transit. Gastroenterology 92: 40–47
20. Melkersson M, Andersson H, Bosaeus I, Falkheden T (1983) Intestinal transit time in constipated and nonconstipated geriatric patients. Scand J Gastroenterol 18:593–597
21. Kelvin FM, Hale DX, Maglinte DD et al (1999) Female pelvic organ prolapse: diagnostic contribution of dynamic cystoproctography and comparison with physical examination. AJR Am J Roentgenol 173:31–37
22. Lienemann A, Anthuber C, Baron A et al (1997) Dynamic MR colpocystorectography assessing pelvic floor descent. Eur Radiol 7:1309–1317
23. Hecht EM, Lee VS, Tanpitukpongse TP et al (2008) MRI of pelvic floor dysfunction: dynamic true fast imaging with steady state precision versus HASTE. AJR Am J Roentgenol 191:352–358
24. Maglinte DD, Kelvin FM, Fitzgerald K et al (1999) Association of compartment defects in pelvic floor dysfunction. AJR Am J Roentgenol 172:439–444
25. Stoker J, Halligan S, Bartram CI (2001) Pelvic floor imaging. Radiology 218:621–641
26. Modot L, Movellas S, Senni M et al (2007) Pelvic prolapse: static and dynamic MRI. Abdom Imaging 32:775–783
27. Thomas DR, Forrester L, Gloth MF et al (2003) Clinical consensus: the constipation crisis in long-term care. Ann Longterm Care 11(suppl):3–14
28. Shariati A, Maceda JS, Hale DS (2008) High-fiber diet for treatment of constipation in women with pelvic floor disorders. Obstet Gynecol 111:908–913
29. Fleshman J, Dreznik Z, Meyer K et al (1992) Outpatient protocol for biofeedback therapy of pelvic floor outlet obstruction. Dis Colon Rectum 35:1–7
30. Harrington KL, Haskvitz EM (2006) Managing a patient's constipation with physical therapy. Phys Ther 86:1511–1519
31. Kuijpers HC, Schreve RH, ten Cate Hoedemakers H (1986) Diagnosis of functional disorders of defecation causing the solitary rectal ulcer syndrome. Dis Colon Rectum 29:126–129
32. Gerten KA, Markland AD, Lloyd LK et al (2008) Prolapse and incontinence surgery in older women. J Urol 179:2111–2118
33. Altemeier WA, Culbertson WR, Schowengerdt C, Hunt J (1971) Nineteen years' experience with the one-stage perineal repair of rectal prolapse. Ann Surg 173:993–1006
34. Williams JG, Rothenberger DA, Madoff RD, Goldberg SM (1992) Treatment of rectal prolapse in the elderly by perineal rectosigmoidectomy. Dis Colon Rectum 35:830–834
35. Lieberth M, Kondyllis LA, Reilly JC et al (2009) The Delorme repair for full thickness rectal prolapse: a retrospective review. Am J Surg 197:418–423
36. Watts JD, Rothenberger DA, Bulls JG et al (1985) The management of procidentia: 30 years' experience. Dis Colon Rectum 28: 96–102
37. Kuijpers HC (1992) Treatment of complete rectal prolapse: to narrow, to wrap, to suspend, to fix, to encircle, to plicate or to resect? World J Surg 16:826–830
38. McKee RF, Lauder JC, Poon FW et al (1992) A prospective randomized study of abdominal rectopexy with and without sigmoidectomy in rectal prolapse. Surg Gynecol Obstet 174: 145–148
39. Ripstein CB (1952) Treatment of massive rectal prolapse. Am J Surg 83:68–71

40. Kuijpers JHC, DeMorree H (1988) Toward a selection of the most appropriate procedure in the treatment of complete rectal prolapse. Dis Colon Rectum 31:355–357

41. Berman IR (1992) Sutureless laparoscopic rectopexy for procidentia: technique and implications. Dis Colon Rectum 35:689–693

42. Kariv Y, Delaney CP, Casillas S et al (2006) Long term outcome after laparoscopic and open surgery for rectal prolapse: a case control study. Surg Endosc 20:35–42

43. Carpelan-Holmstrom M, Kruuna O, Scheinin T (2006) Laparoscopic rectal prolapse surgery combined with short hospital stay is safe in elderly and debilitated patients. Surg Endosc 20:1353–1359

44. Madiba TE, Baig MK, Wexner SD (2005) Surgical management of rectal prolapse. Arch Surg 140:63–73

45. Raftopoulous Y, Senagore AJ, DiGiuroetal G (2005) Recurrence rates after abdominal surgery for complete rectal prolapse: a multicenter pooled analysis of 643 individual patient data. Dis Colon Rectum 48:1200–1206

46. Mikulicz J (1889) Zur operativen behandlung des prolapsus recti et coli invaginati. Arch Klin Chir 38:74–97

47. Prasad ML, Pearl RK, Abcarian H et al (1986) Perineal proctectomy, posterior rectopexy, and postanal levator repair for the treatment of rectal prolapse. Dis Colon Rectum 29:547–552

48. Delorme E (1985) On the treatment of total rectal prolapse of the rectum by excision of the rectal mucous membranes or recto-colic. Dis Colon Rectum 28:544–553

49. Watkins BP, Landercasper J, Belzer GE et al (2003) Long-term follow-up of the modified Delorme procedure for rectal prolapse. Arch Surg 138:498–503

50. Serpell JW, Nicholls RJ (1990) Stercoral perforation of the colon. Br J Surg 77:1325–1329

51. Heffernan C, Pachter HL, Megbow AJ et al (2005) Stercoral colitis leading to patal peritonitis: CT findings. AJR Am J Roentgenol 184:1189–1193

52. Guyton DP, Evans D, Schreiber H (1985) Stercoral perforation of the colon: concepts of operative management. Am Surg 51:520–522

53. Ballantyne GH, Brandner MD, Beart RW, Ilstrup DM (1985) Volvulus of the colon; incidence and mortality. Ann Surg 202:83–92

54. Habr Gama A, Haddad J, Simonsen O, Warde P et al (1976) Volvulus of the sigmoid colon in Brazil: a report of 230 cases. Dis Colon Rectum 19:314–320

55. Ballantyne GH (1982) Review of sigmoid volvulus: history and results of treatments. Dis Colon Rectum 25:494–501

56. Bak MP, Boley SJ (1986) Sigmoid volvulus in elderly patients. Am J Surg 151:71–75

57. Hines JR, Geurkink RE, Bass RT (1967) Recurrence and mortality rates in sigmoid volvulus. Surg Gynecol Obstet 124:567–570

58. Arnold GJ, Nance FC (1973) Volvulus of the sigmoid colon. Ann Surg 177:527–533

59. Wolfer JA, Beaton LE, Anson BJ (1942) Volvulus of the cecum: anatomical factors in its etiology; report of a case. Surg Gynecol Obstet 74:882–894

60. Rabinovici R, Simansky DA, Kaplan O et al (1990) Cecal volvulus. Dis Colon Rectum 55:765–769

61. Todd GJ, Forde KA (1979) Volvulus of the cecum: choice of operation. Am J Surg 138:632–634

62. Barrett JA, Brocklehurst JC, Kiff ES et al (1989) Anal function in geriatric patients with faecal incontinence. Gut 30:1244–1251

63. Nelson R, Norton N, Cautley E, Furner S (1995) Community-based prevalence of anal incontinence. JAMA 274:559–561

64. Norton C, Whitehead WE, Bliss DZ et al (2005) Conservative and pharmacologic management of fecal incontinence in adults. In: Abrams P, Cardozo L, Khoury S, Wein A (eds) Incontinence, 3rd international consultation on incontinence. Health Publications, Paris, pp 1521–1564

65. Oberwalder M, Dinnewitzer A, Baig MK et al (2004) The association between late-onset fecal incontinence and obstetric anal sphincter defects. Arch Surg 139:429–432

66. McHugh SM, Diamant NE (1987) Effect of age, gender, and parity on anal canal pressures; contribution of impaired anal sphincter function to fecal incontinence. Dig Dis Sci 32:726–736

67. Bannister JJ, Abouzekry I, Read NW (1987) Effect of aging on anorectal function. Gut 28:353–357

68. Roach M, Christie JA (2008) Fecal incontinence in the elderly. Geriatrics 63:13–22

69. Whitehead WE, Burgio KL, Engel BT (1985) Biofeedback treatment of fecal incontinence in geriatric patients. J Am Geriatr Soc 33:320–324

70. Markland AD, Richter HE, Burgio KL et al (2008) Outcomes of combination treatment of fecal incontinence in women. Am J Obstet Gynecol 199:699.el–699.e7

71. Simmang C, Birnbaum EH, Kodner IJ et al (1994) Anal sphincter reconstruction in the elderly: does advancing age affect outcome? Dis Colon Rectum 37:1065–1069

72. Nyhus LM (ed) (1992) Surgery annual, vol 24. McGraw-Hill, New York

73. Schwartz SI (ed) (1998) Principles of surgery, 6th edn. McGraw-Hill, New York

Chapter 69
Neoplastic Diseases of the Colon and Rectum

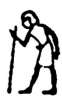

Aundrea L. Oliver, Stanley W. Ashley, and Elizabeth Breen

Colorectal cancer, like many neoplasms, is primarily a disease of aging. The incidence of both colorectal carcinoma and its precursor lesions increases progressively with age. Although there is no evidence that the biologic aggressiveness of colorectal cancer increases with age, delays in diagnosis contribute to the presence of relatively advanced disease at presentation, and therefore a poorer prognosis, in the elderly [1]. These delays in diagnosis may also result in the development of complications of colorectal cancer, requiring emergent surgery, with its higher morbidity and mortality rates. Although recently reported series document excellent results for some elderly patients undergoing elective operations for colorectal cancer, many elderly patients are more likely to have comorbid conditions and fare poorly with treatment. Elderly patients, thus, represent a heterogeneous group of patients with issues of comorbidity, vulnerability, and life expectancy that can pose unique challenges in the treatment of their colorectal cancer [1–3].

In this chapter, the epidemiology, pathology, diagnosis, and therapy of colorectal neoplasms are reviewed, with an emphasis on elderly patients. A common scenario involving an elderly patient with colorectal cancer would be as follows.

Clinical Vignette

An 82-year-old man with a history of CAD complicated by congestive heart failure with an ejection fraction of 35% and who has smoked 1 pack of cigarettes a day for 60 years presents to his physician with 6 months of increasing rectal bleeding. Colonoscopy reveals only a 3×2 cm posterior tumor 8 cm proximal to his dentate line. Biopsies reveal a moderately differentiated adenocarcinoma. Endoanal magnetic resonance imaging (MRI) scan stages the lesion as T2N0. Abdominal and chest CT scans do not reveal any evidence of metastatic spread to the liver, lungs, or bones.

How would this patient be best treated? Decisions, as detailed in the following chapter, relate to the goals of treatment-curative intent versus palliative and the potential methods used to try and achieve these goals. The invasiveness of potential treatments and their likelihood of producing a lasting effect together with the patients' comorbidities and resulting ability to tolerate treatment along with their life expectancy all need to be carefully considered before a treatment plan is made.

Epidemiology

Colorectal cancer remains the third most frequently diagnosed cancer and the second leading cause of cancer-related mortality in the USA, where it accounts for about 8–9% of cancer-related deaths. Altogether, 148,810 new cases and 49,960 deaths due to colorectal cancer were estimated to have been diagnosed in the USA in 2008 [4]. Its incidence progressively increases in populations with advancing age, consistent with the hypothesis that colorectal cancer arises as the result of multiple genetic mutations accumulated in patients over time. The median age at which patients in the USA diagnosed with colorectal cancer is 71 years. The overall incidence of colorectal cancer in the USA is approximately 50 per 100,000. In individuals under the age of 65, the incidence is 18 per 100,000 compared with 273 per 100,000 for those over 65 years. The 5-year survival rate for men and women over 75 is 59.7% compared with 66% for individuals under 65. The cumulative lifetime risk of developing colorectal cancer is approximately 5%, with the lifetime risk of dying from colorectal cancer remaining less than 0.1% [5].

E. Breen (✉)
Department of Surgery, Brigham and Women's Hospital, Harvard Medical School, Boston, MA, USA

Adenomatous polyps of the colon and rectum, which have the potential to undergo transformation into cancers, are found in approximately 40% of people by the age of 60 years, and their prevalence increases with advancing age. The prevalence of large (>1 cm in diameter) polyps, which have the greatest probability of harboring cancer, also appears to be related to age. In one series, such large polyps were found in 4.6% of patients of age more than 54 years and in 15.6% of patients of age more than 75 years [3]. This may be related to the fact that for adenomas >1 cm in diameter the risk of progression to cancer is 1% per year [6].

Not only are the elderly at greater risk of developing colorectal cancer, but they are also likely to have more advanced disease at the time of diagnosis. In one report, patients over 75 years of age were twice as likely to present with advanced, untreatable colorectal cancer as those under 65 years of age [7]. The relative contributions of physician bias, limited access to health care, poor social support, and impaired cognition to this observation are not clear. Comorbid conditions play a significant role in survival for elderly patients with colorectal cancer. A recent review article outlined the fact that for individuals over 67 years with stage III disease at the time of diagnosis, the life expectancy could range from approximately 8.5–7 to 4.5 years with zero, one to two, and three or more comorbidities, respectively. Interestingly, patients still fared better with adjuvant therapy versus none regardless of the degree of comorbidity [8].

Risk Factors

Epidemiologic studies have suggested that an increase in the consumption of dietary fiber, fruits, and cruciferous vegetables as well as a reduction in the consumption of fat is associated with a decrease in mortality from colorectal cancer. However, the efficacy of modifications in diet in preventing colorectal cancer has not yet been demonstrated in prospective trials. Similarly there have been several studies investigating the chemopreventative effects of NSAIDs, aspirin, calcium, and folate. Unfortunately there is little compelling data to support such claims as independent preventative measures for colorectal cancer, Again, the efficacy of modifying these risk factors in colorectal cancer prevention remains to be shown [9, 10].

In addition to older age, factors clearly associated with an increased incidence of colorectal cancer include a history of colorectal cancer, either in oneself or in one's relatives. Patients with colorectal cancer are more likely to develop a subsequent (metachronous) lesion than is the general population to develop primary cancer. Patients who have a first-degree relative with colorectal cancer, but not one of the specific genetic syndromes discussed below, have approximately twice the probability of developing colorectal cancer as those without

such a family history. This probability is higher if more than one first-degree relative is affected or if the age at diagnosis of the relative's cancer is less than 55 years. A similar increase in risk is found for patients with a first-degree relative found to have an adenomatous polyp prior to the age of 60 [6].

In the USA, approximately 25% of cases of colorectal cancer occur in individuals with a family history of the disease or an underlying condition specifically associated with the development of colorectal cancer. Patients who have first-degree relatives with colorectal cancer, but not any of the defined genetic syndromes, account for most of these cases (15–20%). Hereditary nonpolyposis colon cancer (HNPCC) accounts for 4–7% of cases, and familial adenomatous polyposis (FAP) accounts for 1%. An additional 1% of cases are accounted for by a combination of patients with inflammatory bowel disease, Peutz–Jeghers syndrome, and familial juvenile polyposis. Keeping in mind that the majority of patients who develop colorectal cancer will not have an identifiable risk factor, screening remains an important part of minimizing the incidence of this disease [11]. The main relevance of potential inherited risk and familial syndromes for elderly patients is to mainly to inform younger family members of their diagnosis should changes in screening recommendations be appropriate for those younger family members.

Pathology

Polyps

Polyps are mucosal masses in the colon and rectum. There are several histologically distinct types of polyps of varying clinical significance, including adenomatous polyps (which are premalignant and represent 50–66% of all colorectal polyps), hyperplastic polyps (which have no malignant potential and represent 10–30% of all polyps), mucosal tags (which are of no clinical significance and represent 10–30% of polyps), and a variety of more unusual other histologic types, such as lipomas and hamartomas. Polyps in which the bulk of the lesion projects into the bowel lumen and is tethered to the mucosal surface through a narrow stalk of submucosa surrounded by mucosa are characterized as pedunculated. Polyps that are flat and have a broad base are characterized as sessile.

Adenomatous polyps can be found throughout the colon and rectum, with approximately 30% occurring proximal to the splenic flexure. With advancing age, a larger percentage of adenomatous polyps are found in the proximal colon. Histologically, adenomatous polyps are subclassified as tubular, tubulovillous, and villous. Tubular and tubulovillous adenomas tend to be pedunculated, whereas villous adenomas tend to be sessile. The potential for malignant transformation is least for tubular adenomas and highest for villous adenomas.

The size of an adenomatous polyp is directly related to the probability that it is harboring high-grade dysplasia, which is likely to be the direct precursor of preinvasive carcinoma, and that the patient will develop other adenomatous polyps and colorectal cancer. In one report, 11% of adenomatous polyps <5 mm in diameter, 4.6% of those 5–9 mm in diameter, and 20.6% of those ≥1 cm exhibited high-grade dysplasia [12]. Fewer than 1% of adenomatous, polyps <1 cm in diameter harbor invasive carcinoma, whereas more than 10% of larger adenomatous polyps do so.

Colorectal Cancer

Approximately 95% of all colorectal cancers are adenocarcinomas. Macroscopically, the lesions can have a polypoid, infiltrative, or ulcerated appearance. Histologically, they are characterized as being well differentiated, moderately differentiated, or poorly differentiated. Lesions that have an infiltrative or ulcerated appearance and are less well differentiated are associated with poorer prognosis. Cancers associated with increased production of mucin are typically characterized by the presence of signet ring cells. The prognostic implication of these signet ring cells is not well-defined.

Extension of colorectal cancers occurs through three routes: (1) via the bloodstream to distant sites, particularly the liver; (2) via the lymphatics to regional lymph nodes and ultimately the systemic circulation; and (3) by direct extension into adjacent organs, such as the posterior vaginal wall, uterus, prostate, bladder, small intestine, stomach, and retroperitoneal structures.

The anatomic distribution of cancers is as follows: ascending colon 18%, transverse colon 9%, descending colon 5%, sigmoid colon 25%, and rectum 43%. Cancers are currently found with greater frequency in the proximal colon than they were earlier during the twentieth century. It is unknown whether the advent of colonoscopy (and its ability to detect more proximally located cancers) or a change in the biologic behavior of colorectal cancer explains this shift.

Pathogenesis

Most colorectal cancers presumably arise via transformation of preexisting adenomatous polyps. Several lines of circumstantial evidence support this assertion: (1) cancers and adenomatous polyps occur with the same anatomic distribution; (2) cancers rarely arise in the absence of adenomatous polyps; (3) the average age of onset of adenomatous polyps precedes that of cancer by several years; (4) patients found to have large polyps are at increased risk for subsequently developing cancer, with most of these cancers arising at sites where these polyps are left in place; (5) patients with FAP are at markedly increased risk of developing cancer; and (6) the

detection and removal of adenomatous polyps reduces the incidence of colorectal cancer.

The strongest evidence for the clinical relevance of the concept that most cancers arise from precursor adenomatous polyps is derived from the National Polyp Study. A group of 1,418 patients was followed for an average of 5.9 years after the removal of all identifiable colonic polyps. Only five subsequent malignant polyps (all being Dukes' stage A lesions) were found, and no deaths from colorectal cancer occurred during 8,401 person-years of follow-up [13]. The incidence of malignant transformation of adenomatous polyps has been estimated to be 2.5 polyps per 1,000 per year. The mean time required for an individual polyp to undergo such transformation has been estimated to be 10 years [14].

The transformation of an adenomatous polyp to invasive cancer (and that of normal mucosa to adenomatous polyp) is associated with an accumulation of acquired genetic mutations. This model of tumorigenesis, proposed by Fearon and Vogelstein, is shown in Fig. 69.1. Genetic changes include mutational activation of dominantly acting cellular oncogenes and mutational inactivation of recessive tumor-suppressor genes. Protooncogenes are present in normal cells; their protein products tend to be positive regulators of cell growth. When these genes undergo mutation, they can become oncogenes, whose protein products are produced in excessive quantities or act in an unregulated manner, thereby promoting tumor formation. The protein products of tumor-suppressor genes, on the other hand, tend to suppress cell growth, and their loss may promote tumor development.

Mutations characteristic of colorectal cancer have begun to be identified. Approximately 50% of colorectal cancers and adenomatous polyps >1 cm in diameter have been found to harbor mutations in the *ras* oncogene [15–17], whereas fewer than 10% of adenomas <1 cm in diameter are associated

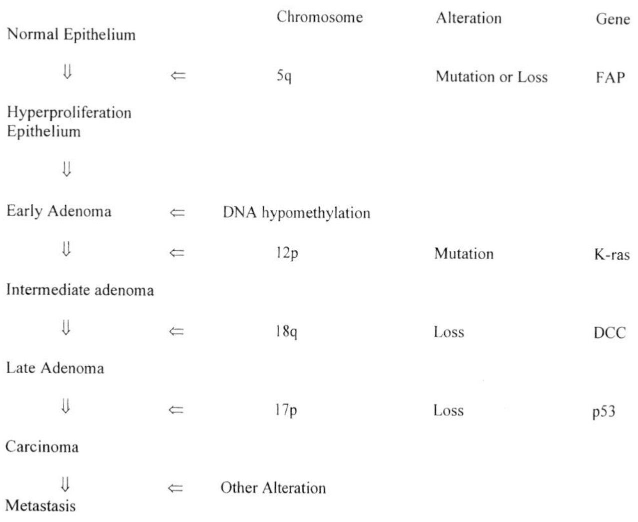

		Chromosome	Alteration	Gene
Normal Epithelium				
⇓	⇐	5q	Mutation or Loss	FAP
Hyperproliferation Epithelium				
⇓				
Early Adenoma	⇐	DNA hypomethylation		
⇓	⇐	12p	Mutation	K-ras
Intermediate adenoma				
⇓	⇐	18q	Loss	DCC
Late Adenoma				
⇓	⇐	17p	Loss	p53
Carcinoma				
⇓	⇐	Other Alteration		
Metastasis				

FIGURE 69.1 Genetic model for colorectal tumorigenesis as proposed by Fearon and Vogelstein (from Vogelstein et al. [15]. © Massachusetts Medical Society, with permission).

with such mutations. The highly conserved *ras* protooncogenes (N-*ras*, H-*ras*, and K-*ras*) encode for the production of signal transduction G-proteins (guanosine triphosphate-binding proteins). Mutations in the *ras* gene result in the production of an abnormal G-protein that is associated with unregulated cell growth. In vitro and animal studies have suggested that mutations in the *ras* gene may also inhibit programmed cell death (apoptosis).

The development of colorectal cancer is also associated with the deletion of chromosomal fragments. This phenomenon is also known as *allelic loss* or *loss of heterozygosity*. This process primarily affects chromosomes 17 and 18 and to a lesser degree chromosome 5. The DNA lost in such deletions may contain tumor-suppressor genes. One such gene whose loss is associated with FAP has been localized to chromosome 5q and is known as the adenomatous polyposis coli (*APC*) gene. The *APC* gene is thought to be a tumor-suppressor gene, although the function of its protein product is not yet known. Therefore, allelic loss of *APC* may promote neoplastic transformation. Allelic loss of chromosome 5q is present in approximately 20–50% of sporadic colorectal carcinomas and 30% of sporadic adenomatous polyps.

The loss of chromosome 17p, which contains the *p53* tumor-suppressor gene, is seen in 75% of sporadic colorectal cancers but rarely in adenomas of any size. Therefore, loss of chromosome 17p may be particularly associated with the progression of an adenoma to cancer. The allelic loss of chromosome 17p is also seen in a wide range of cancers, including those of the brain, breast, lung, and bladder. Evidence has indicated that reconstitution of wild-type *p53* expression in human and murine cell lines inhibits growth through induction of cell cycle arrest, apoptosis, or both.

Approximately 70% of colorectal cancers and 50% of large adenomatous polyps are associated with allelic deletions of chromosome 18q. *DCC* (deleted in colorectal carcinoma) is a candidate tumor-suppressor gene that has been mapped to chromosome 18q. The protein product of the *DCC* gene has significant homology to the neural cell adhesion molecule (N-CAM). It has been speculated that deletion of the *DCC* gene may modify cell–cell or cell–basement membrane interactions (or both), which are important for regulating cell growth and differentiation.

Several germ-line mutations (*MLH1*, *MSH2*, *PMS1*, *PMS2*) on chromosomes 2, 3, and 7 have been identified in patients with HNPCC. These genes are human homologues of the bacterial mutHLS complex, which is involved in genetic proof-reading (the repair of mismatched basepairs in DNA). Loss of this function is thought to allow basepair mismatches to accumulate, resulting in a replication-error phenotype, which is seen in a high percentage of patients with HNPCC and approximately 15% of those with sporadic colorectal cancer.

It is likely that specific mutations, for sporadic and familial forms of colorectal cancer, will be identified at an increasingly rapid pace in the years to come. Tailoring therapies to specific mutations is becoming a reality in the treatment of colorectal cancer [18]. Furthermore, as the functions of the protein products of these abnormal genes are characterized, genetic interventions may become a reality.

Staging

A variety of pathologic staging systems have been used. Dukes, a pathologist, in 1932 proposed a staging system for rectal cancer based on the depth of invasion of the bowel wall by the primary tumor. The TNM, however, recommended by the American Joint Committee on Cancer is the most widely used system. With the TNM system, staging is based on the depth of invasion of the primary tumor (T), status of regional lymph nodes (N), and the presence of distant metastasis (M). The advantage of the TNM staging system is its applicability to both presurgical clinical-diagnostic staging and postsurgical resection-pathologic staging [19].

Screening

The terms screening, diagnosis, and surveillance have distinct clinical definitions. *Screening* identifies those patients who are at risk for having colorectal cancer or adenomatous polyps from among the population who are without signs or symptoms of the disease. *Diagnosis* classifies patients who, because of a positive screening test or symptoms, are suspected of having colorectal cancer or adenomatous polyps into those with and without the disease. *Surveillance* monitors patients with previously diagnosed colorectal disease (polyps, colorectal cancer, or inflammatory bowel disease, for example) for the development of adenomatous polyps or colorectal cancer.

Screening for a disease is justified when the following four criteria are met: (1) the disease is common and associated with serious morbidity and/or mortality; (2) screening tests are accurate for detecting early stage disease; (3) treatment after detection by screening improves prognosis relative to the treatment after diagnosis in the absence of screening; and (4) potential benefits outweigh the potential harms and costs of screening. Several screening modalities for colorectal cancer fulfill all of these criteria [14].

Screening for colorectal cancer has clearly been demonstrated to have efficacy in reducing cancer-related mortality. There has been controversy, however, related to which screening and surveillance methods are optimal, how frequently the tests should be done, who should undergo testing, and the cost-effectiveness of the various strategies. In addition, only a small number of the elderly population undergo screening of any kind for colorectal cancer. The Behavioral Risk Factor Surveillance System (BRFSS), a telephone-based survey designed to monitor utilization of preventative services, has indicated that from 1991 to 2004 consistently less than 60% of individuals over 50 years of age have utilized colorectal screening modalities according to recommended guidelines. The 2004 BRFSS data indicated that only 57% of older individuals had either an FOBT within the prior year or sigmoidoscopy/colonoscopy within the last 10 years. The same study indicated that socioeconomic factors and consistent health care (insurance and services) were key predictors of compliance with screening recommendations [20]. Education (for both patients and physicians) and investigation related to screening would likely have a major impact on the overall management of colorectal cancer. In this section, the terminology related to screening is defined, tests and strategies used for screening are discussed, and recommendations are outlined.

Fecal Occult Blood Testing

The rationale for using FOBT to screen for colorectal cancer is based on the observation that colonic neoplasms have a greater tendency to bleed than does normal mucosa. This propensity increases with polyp size and cancer stage, although the bleeding is usually intermittent and unevenly distributed in the stool.

The most widely used test to detect fecal occult blood is the guaiac-based assay for peroxidase activity. Hemoglobin, which has pseudoperoxidase activity, in blood yields a positive test result. This test has considerable limitations. The test is not specific for cancer, as nonneoplastic processes such as gum disease, gastritis, peptic ulcer disease, and hemorrhoids can also cause gastrointestinal hemorrhage. The test is also not specific for blood, as other substances with peroxidase or pseudoperoxidase activity such as red meat, bacteria, and some fruits and vegetables can cause false-positive reactions. False-negative tests may result if the cancer did not bleed when the sampled stool was being formed or if the quantity of bleeding is below the limits of test detection. The antioxidant activity of vitamin C can interfere with the test reaction, causing a false-negative result. Iron supplements do not interfere with the reaction; but by making the stool dark they interfere with the interpretation of test results. The patient should therefore observe a diet restricted from these confounding substances for 2 days prior to stool sampling.

The sensitivity of FOBT is increased with the number of samples per stool and the number of stools sampled. Therefore, it is recommended that patients provide several specimens from several consecutive stools and that each stool be sampled at two sites. A single specimen obtained by digital rectal examination has questionable value and should not be considered adequate when screening for colorectal cancer. Typically, several days elapse between stool collection and testing it for blood. The sensitivity of a guaiac-based test is increased if the test slide is rehydrated with a few drops of water before performing the test. The best available evidence that FOBT is effective in preventing death caused by colorectal cancer is from a study with rehydrated tests on two samples from each of three consecutive stools in patients who followed a restricted diet prior to testing [21].

In a program of repeated screening (rather than a single test), the nonhydrated form of FOBT has a reported sensitivity for detecting cancer that ranges from 72 to 78%, a specificity of 98%, and a positive predictive value of 10–17%. Rehydrating the slides increases the sensitivity to 88–92% but decreases the specificity to 90–92%, and the positive predictive value to 2–6% [14, 22].

The FOBT for detecting colon cancer has been reported to be of lower specificity for patients over 60 years of age than for younger patients. This observation may be related to a higher prevalence of other etiologies for gastrointestinal hemorrhage with increasing age. On the other hand, there is no evidence that the value of FOBT is diminished in the very elderly. In fact, the positive predictive value of FOBT has been reported to increase with age from 1.6% for those under 60 years of age to 3.6% for those over 70 years of age [23].

Fecal Immunochemical Testing

Fecal immunochemical testing (FIT) was originally developed in the 1970s. It is a screening technique based on immunochemical detection of human globin in stool. This test sheds some of the false negative and false positives caused by the peroxidase-based stool testing influenced by dietary factors or medications. In addition it has a higher sensitivity for colonic blood due to the fact that upper gastrointestinal bleeding is subject to degradation by digestive enzymes and would not be detected in the stool sample by this technique. A large study comparing a high-sensitivity guaiac-based study with FIT found no clear superiority in performance. The one-time sensitivity FIT was evaluated in another study of over 20,000 patients scheduled for colonoscopy. This particular study found 5.6% of patients to be FIT positive with a sensitivity of 27.1% for advanced neoplasia and 65.8% for cancer. Another study evaluating the sensitivity of FIT in both asymptomatic and symptomatic patients scheduled for colonoscopy, the sensitivity and specificity was raised to 94.1 and 87.5% respectively when the sample number was increased to 3 and a hemoglobin threshold set to 75 ng/ml. Overall the specificity appears to be higher with FIT in comparison to high-sensitivity FOBT; however, the FOBT has higher sensitivity for adenomas. The advantage to the FIT includes the lack of dietary restriction prior to testing, and with some assays, greater ease of sampling procedures in comparison to the FOBT [22].

sDNA

The most recent development in the stool assay arena is the stool DNA test. It is based on the principle that cancers and adenomas harbor known DNA alterations in the transformation of adenoma to carcinoma in colorectal cancer. This DNA is continuously shed in the stool, and remains stable in the feces for reliable detection. This tool relys on a multiple marker array targeting mutations in K-*ras*, APC, and p53, as well as markers of microsatellite instability and DNA integrity to assess for possible adenomatous or carcinomatous changes. Of note this test requires at least 30 g of stool for assay. Sensitivity has ranged from 52 to 91% and specificity from 93 to 97%. The majority of effect on sensitivity relates to DNA degradation after obtaining the specimen, usually during transport. When compared with low-sensitivity FOBT in the setting of colonoscopy, sDNA was found to have superior sensitivity for detecting cancer and high-grade dysplasia (40% vs. 14% for FOBT). However, since this is a relatively new modality and there are no programmatic studies to evaluate screening technique or frequency, no definitive recommendations can be offered at this time. It may prove a modality that could benefit from combination with high-sensitivity FOBT or FIT [22].

Sigmoidoscopy

Although supporting data from randomized trials are lacking, several case–control studies support the efficacy of screening sigmoidoscopy for reducing mortality due to colorectal cancer. As a screening method, sigmoidoscopy has three advantages over FOBT: (1) the bowel is directly visualized; (2) lesions can be biopsied during the procedure; and (3) it has high sensitivity and specificity for detecting polyps in the bowel examined. Its primary limitation is that only the rectum and distal colon are examined.

Patients usually do not require sedation or full bowel preparation for screening sigmoidoscopy. Although lesions are biopsied, full polypectomies are not routinely done, as cautery used for polypectomies can result in complications in colons subjected to less than full bowel preparation. Prophylactic antibiotics are given to patients at risk for developing endocarditis.

The performance of the flexible 60 cm sigmoidoscope is superior to that of the 25 cm rigid scope. With the flexible scope, a larger area of colon can be examined, the optics are better, and there is more comfort for both patient and examiner. Within the area of reach, nearly all cancers and all polyps >1 cm in diameter and 70–85% of smaller polyps are detected by flexible sigmoidoscopy. False-positive findings are rare, although many polyps identified prove to be nonadenomatous. The 60 cm scope, which reaches up to or beyond the proximal sigmoid colon in 80% of examinations, should be able to detect 40–60% of adenomatous polyps and cancers based on the known anatomic distribution of these lesions. The rigid scope would be able to detect only 20–30% of these lesions.

What constitutes a positive finding on screening sigmoidoscopy requiring full colonoscopy is somewhat controversial. Cancer or an adenomatous polyp >1 cm in diameter should be followed by colonoscopy. Polyps shown to be hyperplastic and normal mucosa do not require follow-up. It is not yet clear whether a small adenoma (<1 cm in diameter), especially if it is tubular and without high-grade dysplasia, needs follow-up. When an adenomatous polyp is found in the rectosigmoid, there is an approximately 33% probability that more proximally located adenomatous polyps are present. However, if the rectosigmoid adenoma is <1 cm in diameter, it is unlikely that adenomas >1 cm or with high-grade dysplasia will be found more proximally.

Barium Enema

Barium enema examination allows the entire colon and all but the most distal rectum to be evaluated, although there are no specific data that its use as a screening test is associated with a reduction in mortality from colorectal cancer. This test can be performed in two ways: as a single-contrast study using barium alone or as a double-contrast study, in which air is instilled into the colon after most of the barium is removed. With the single-contrast study lesions appear as filling defects, whereas with the double-contrast study lesions are outlined by the retained barium against a background of air. The double-contrast study has considerably more sensitivity and specificity than the single-contrast study and has generally replaced it, except in patients who are not able to tolerate the more complicated and uncomfortable study. The sensitivity of double-contrast barium enema has been reported as 50–80% for polyps <1 cm in diameter, 70–90% for polyps >1 cm in diameter, and 55–85% for TNM stage 1 and 2 cancers. False-negative results are related to inadequate visualization of segments of bowel, especially the sigmoid colon, and to errors in interpretation. False positives are the result of stool in the bowel and of nonneoplastic mucosal irregularities. When a finding on double-contrast barium enema is interpreted as cancer, the false-positive rate is less than 1%; the rate ranges from 5 to 10% when the interpretation is a large polyp and 50% when it is a small polyp. Another limitation of the test is that 5–10% of studies are technically unsatisfactory, requiring another attempt at barium enema or colonoscopy.

Colonoscopy

Colonoscopy is the only screening technique that offers the potential to both detect and remove premalignant lesions throughout the colon and rectum. With respect to technical difficulty and the risk to the patient, it is more formidable than either sigmoidoscopy or barium enema. Colonoscopy is poorly tolerated without intravenous sedation. Because there is potential for the development of cardiorespiratory complications, elderly patients, particularly those with significant comorbidities, should undergo cardiorespiratory monitoring. As is the case for sigmoidoscopy, patients at risk for developing bacterial endocarditis should undergo appropriate antibiotic prophylaxis.

Sensitivity rates for colonoscopy are difficult to discern, as colonoscopy itself is often used as the gold standard for the presence or absence of lesions. However, studies in which colonoscopy is done prior to surgical resection for polyps and cancers suggest that colonoscopy misses 3% of such lesions. In comparison to barium enema, colonoscopy has more sensitivity for detecting small polyps, but its ability to detect polyps >1 cm is equivalent. It is unclear which procedure causes less discomfort and is therefore associated with greater patient acceptability. Models of diagnostic strategies for patients with a positive screening FOBT have shown that barium enema and colonoscopy are associated with comparable cost-effectiveness [14].

A limitation of colonoscopy is that in only 80–95% of procedures the entire colon is visualized. The probability of reaching the proximal colon depends primarily on the skill of the examiner and the adequacy of the bowel preparation. If the entire colon cannot be visualized, another examination is required: another attempt at colonoscopy or a barium enema.

Computed Tomographic Colonoscopy

Computed tomographic colonoscopy (CTC) or virtual colonoscopy was introduced in the mid-1990s as a minimally invasive technique to visualize the colon for possible neoplasm. This technique generates both high-resolution 2D and 3D reconstructions of the large bowel allowing for both polyp detection and limited investigation of adjacent structures (Fig. 69.2). A recent meta-analysis of both screening and high-risk cohorts of a sensitivity and specificity of large versus small (>10 mm vs. 6–9 mm) polyps was 85–93% and 97% vs. 70–86% and 86–93%, respectively. The sensitivity of invasive CRC was 96% when compared with standard colonoscopy. The advantages of this technique are the lack

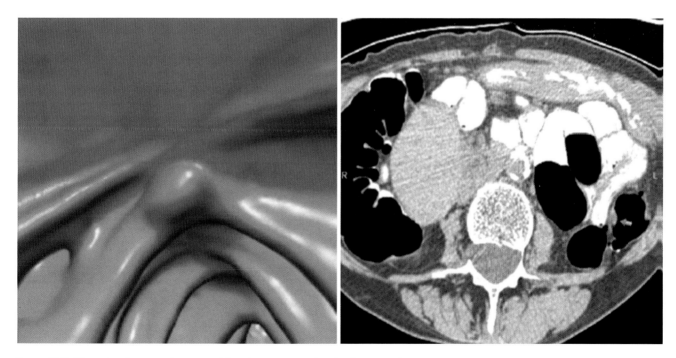

Figure 69.2 Example of computed tomographic colonoscopy or virtual colonoscopy image.

of sedation required and the speed of the test as well as the ability to immediately refer for colonoscopy for positive tests without requiring an additional bowel preparation. The disadvantages are the requirement of a second intervention for polypectomy/biopsy as well as the lack of reimbursement in some states. Furthermore, the radiation dose delivered with multiple studies for screening has not yet been evaluated in terms of independent risk. The perforation rate is as much as 22 times less than with standard colonoscopy (1 in 22,000 vs. 1 in 1–2000) [22]. Although this may be a promising modality, there is not enough data at this time to recommend it as a screening tool when compared with standard colonoscopy.

Digital Rectal Examination

A common practice is to screen for colorectal cancer by performing digital rectal examination, followed by a test for fecal occult blood if stool is present in the rectum. Based on the anatomic distribution of cancers, only 5–10% of lesions would be within reach of the examining finger. In addition, stool obtained from the digital rectal examination represents inadequate sampling and is associated with high false-negative rates. Digital rectal examination, by itself, is not an effective method of screening for colorectal cancer.

Screening Recommendations

Screening for colorectal cancer and adenomatous polyps should be offered to all men and women without special risk factors beginning at age 50. A positive screening test should be followed by a diagnostic evaluation. Five screening options have been proposed in guidelines defined by a multidisciplinary panel [14, 22, 24]. These guidelines have been endorsed by a wide range of organizations, including the American Cancer Society, the American Gastroenterological Association, and the American Society of Colon and Rectal Surgeons; and they represent the current standard of care (Table 69.1).

1. *Yearly fecal occult blood screening.* Those with a positive test should undergo diagnostic evaluation with colonoscopy or double-contrast barium enema (with flexible sigmoidoscopy).
2. *Flexible sigmoidoscopy every 5 years.* If polyps >1 cm in diameter are found, colonoscopy should be done. Polyps <1 cm in diameter should be biopsied, and if adenomatous polyps or cancers are found, colonoscopy should be done. It is not clear whether patients with small tubular adenomas (<1 cm in diameter) should undergo colonoscopy.
3. *Combined fecal occult blood testing and flexible sigmoidoscopy.* The combination of these two methods theoretically compensates for some of the deficiencies of each. However, there are no good data proving that combining the two methods offers any advantage over either alone.
4. *Double-contrast barium enema every 5–10 years.* No data exist to support that this method reduces mortality due to colorectal cancer.
5. *Colonoscopy every 10 years.* No data exist to support that this method reduces mortality due to colorectal cancer.

When to Stop Screening

The recommendations for screening in elderly patients, however, may differ from those of younger patients. Given the more limited life expectancy and the potential for more comorbidities making elderly patients more vulnerable to the risks of screening procedures, the benefits may not outweigh the risks. A recent set of guidelines published by the US Preventative Services Task Force states that for individuals over age 75, the benefit of screening is questionable and for those over age 85 it is not recommended [25].

TABLE 69.1 Screening guidelines for colorectal cancer

Symptoms	Family history	Age to begin (years)	Evaluation
None	None	50	DRE; stool guaiac; colonoscopy: if negative repeat in 3–5 years, otherwise repeat in 1 year to ensure no new lesions
None	One or more FDR	40	As above
None	FAP	10	DRE; colonoscopy: repeat annually if polyps found or at 3 years if no polyps
None	HNPCC	Late teens	As for FAP
Present	None	25	DRE; stool guaiac; colonoscopy: if negative repeat in 3–5 years, otherwise repeat in 1 year to ensure no new lesions

DRE digital rectal examination, *FDR* first-degree relative, *FAP* familial adenomatous polyposis, *HNPCC* hereditary nonpolyposis colorectal carcinoma
Source: Byers et al. [24]. This material is reproduced with permission of Wiley-Liss, Inc., a subsidiary of John Wiley & Sons, Inc.

Clinical Presentation

Symptoms of colorectal cancer are nonspecific and include abdominal pain, change in bowel movement patterns, and rectal bleeding (Table 69.2). In elderly patients, particularly, the presentation may be varied and insidious, with vague symptoms such as apathy and weight loss sometimes being the only clue to the existence of cancer. Unfortunately, the incidence of benign colonic diseases associated with such nonspecific symptoms is increased in the elderly, and there is a tendency to procrastinate when proceeding with an appropriate diagnostic evaluation in this patient population.

There is some correlation between the location of the cancer and its resulting symptoms. Lesions in the right colon are frequently associated with such symptoms as a dull, aching pain in the right lower quadrant and fatigue and dizziness, which are related to the iron-deficiency anemia of chronic blood loss. Colonic obstruction is rare with cancers of the right colon. Transverse colon cancer frequently manifests as signs of obstruction or pain in the mid-epigastrium. Lesions of the left colon are often associated with an alteration in bowel habits and a decrease in stool caliber, with these changes being related to the narrower lumen and the presence of more solid stool in the left colon. Overt bleeding and colonic obstruction occur more frequently with rectosigmoid cancers than they do with more proximal lesions. Low rectal cancer can be associated with the presence of tenesmus, urgency, and pain.

Signs of colorectal cancer include the presence of an abdominal or rectal mass or tenderness, anemia, and weight loss. Approximately 15% of colorectal cancers are first diagnosed in patients presenting with evidence of complete colonic obstruction. A smaller percentage of cancers present as colonic perforation, with most perforations occurring at the site of the tumor.

TABLE 69.2 Signs and symptoms of colorectal cancer

Right colon
Chronic anemia
Occult gastrointestinal bleeding
Fungating lesion
Left colon
Obstructing symptoms
Grossly bloody stool
Change in bowel habits
Circumferential lesion
Rectum
Tenesmus, perineal pain
Gross bleeding
Change in bowel habits
Palpable tumor

On occasion, signs and symptoms of metastatic disease are the first indication of the presence of colorectal cancer. Metastasis to the liver may manifest as jaundice and pruritus. Metastatic pulmonary disease may be seen on a chest radiograph in an otherwise asymptomatic patient. Signs of metastatic disease include the presence of ascites, hepatomegaly, and lymphadenopathy (in the supraclavicular and periumbilical areas, for example).

Treatment of Polyps

In general, sigmoidoscopy allows biopsy of polyps but not their complete removal. Full bowel preparation and colonoscopy are required for polypectomy. The current literature on the need for colonoscopy for small distal tubular adenomas found at sigmoidoscopy is controversial. Markowitz and Winawer [26], in a review of the management of colorectal polyps, proposed the following guidelines. If a small polyp (<1 cm in diameter) biopsied on sigmoidoscopy is an adenoma, colonoscopic polypectomy with examination of the entire colon should be performed to look for synchronous neoplastic lesions. Read et al. [27], in a prospective study of asymptomatic average-risk individuals, reported that 31% of patients with benign adenomas on flexible sigmoidoscopy were found to have a synchronous neoplasm, and 8% with adenomas >1 cm in diameter had invasive cancers. If the polyp is >1 cm on sigmoidoscopy, however, rather than biopsy the lesion, colonoscopic polypectomy with examination of the proximal colon for synchronous lesions should be performed. Finding a nonneoplastic polyp at sigmoidoscopy requires no further evaluation. Radiographic detection of a polyp warrants full colonoscopy to resect the polyp and to examine the entire colon for the presence of synchronous lesions.

Polyps seen on colonoscopy should be excised endoscopically, unless their configuration or size renders them too difficult to be removed endoscopically for technical reasons. For sessile polyps with invasive carcinoma, the incidence of lymph node metastasis is 15%, and the incidence of residual tumor after attempted endoscopic removal is 6%. A local recurrence rate of 21% can be anticipated if formal bowel resection is not done. For pedunculated lesions, polypectomy has the potential to be both diagnostic and therapeutic; although if invasive carcinoma is present in the polyp, further therapy is indicated. Invasive carcinoma in a pedunculated polyp implies invasion of the cancer through the muscularis mucosa. The incidence of lymph node metastases in this circumstance ranges from 8 to 16%. Tumor features predictive of nodal metastasis are the presence of positive or close margins of resection, invasion of the neck or stalk of the polyp, poor differentiation status, and the presence of vascular and lymphatic invasion.

Rectal polyps can be challenging. Unless invasion is proven, transanal sphincter-sparing excision is the procedure of choice.

Treatment of Colorectal Cancer

Colorectal Surgery in the Elderly

Most reported series of operations for colorectal cancer document a higher postoperative mortality rate in the elderly. This age-related increase in postoperative mortality rate is likely to be related to two factors: (1) the higher prevalence of coexisting illnesses in elderly patients; and (2) the higher incidence of emergency operations in elderly patients, as they are more likely to present with complications of colorectal cancer, such as intestinal obstruction and perforation. In one study, the subgroup of patients who were 70 years of age or older, who were without concomitant pulmonary, renal, hemopoietic, or cardiac disease had a postoperative mortality rate of 4% following colon surgery; those younger than age 70 had a postoperative mortality rate of 3.2% [28]. In another review of 357 patients over the age of 50 undergoing colon resection, the postoperative mortality rate was directly correlated with the number of preexisting illnesses; age was not an independent risk factor for postoperative mortality. The postoperative mortality rate for all studies was 4.8%. For patients with no or one concomitant disease, the postoperative mortality rate for patients younger than age 70 was 0%, and it was 1.5% for those older than age 70 [29]. In this study, for all age groups mortality for elective colon surgery was 3.4%, but it was 18% for emergency surgery. In another report of 101 colon resections in patients 70 years of age or older, the postoperative mortality rate was 5%, but no deaths occurred following elective procedures [30].

It appears, as demonstrated in contemporary series, that elective colon resection can be performed safely in the elderly and that age is an independent risk factor for postoperative mortality following surgery for colorectal cancer. Existing data also suggest that early detection of colorectal cancer, allowing elective rather than emergent surgery, with careful preoperative assessment and optimization of organ system function, should be the goal in elderly patients.

When cancer stage is taken into account, the long-term survival rates following curative resection for colorectal cancer are comparable in elderly and younger patients. In one reported series, 3-year survival following surgery for colorectal cancer in patients older than 80 years was equivalent to that for patients under age 80, although increased age was associated with longer hospitalization and higher hospital costs [31]. Although there are few data regarding quality of life issues following surgery for colorectal cancer in the elderly, in one report of patients older than 80 years, 82% of those who were admitted to the hospital from home for colon surgery were able to resume their normal level of activity postoperatively [1–3, 32]. When surgical treatment of colorectal cancer can potentially be most influenced by a patient's age, therefore, is when the patients comorbidities makes them unable to withstand aggressive surgical management and/or their life expectancy is not expected to be long enough that they will develop significant symptoms from their tumor. Trade-offs and compromises in surgical treatment options are discussed further below within each specific treatment.

Preoperative Evaluation

Prior to surgery, elderly patients should undergo careful evaluation to diagnose and treat preexisting medical illnesses and to detect the presence of synchronous lesions and metastatic disease. The operative approach to be taken depends on the results of the preoperative evaluation.

Once a cancer in the colon or rectum has been diagnosed, the incidence of synchronous cancer is 5%, and the incidence of a synchronous adenomatous polyp is 28%. Preoperative colonoscopy or barium enema to detect such lesions is the standard of care. In general, colonoscopy is preferable. Barium enema or virtual colonoscopy can be performed if the cancer is nearly obstructing and prevents proximal passage of a colonoscope.

The hematocrit should be checked because of the possibility of anemia, which might require correction prior to surgery. Liver function tests should be checked, as they may indicate the presence of metastatic disease in the liver. Tumor markers such as carcinoembryonic antigen (CEA), CA 19-9, and CA-50 have been used for patients with colon cancer. Of these, CEA has had the most clinical application. Its preoperative concentration correlates well with tumor stage, as well as postoperative survival and recurrence rates. Elevated CEA concentrations are not specific for colorectal cancer, however. The CEA concentration in normal individuals ranges from 0 to 2.5 ng/ml. Benign elevations in CEA concentration are usually less than 10 ng/ml and are reversible. Known benign conditions associated with elevations in CEA concentration include biliary obstruction, hepatocellular dysfunction, cigarette smoking, bronchitis, gastric ulcer, gastritis, inflammatory bowel disease, diverticulitis, adenomatous polyps, renal disease, and benign prostatic hyperplasia. CEA concentration can also be elevated with noncolorectal cancers.

A preoperative chest radiograph is obtained to detect the presence of lung metastases and cardiopulmonary disease.

For colon cancers, a preoperative computed tomography (CT) scan is not necessary as information that would change the operative plan is rarely found, although in some practice settings it is obtained routinely. It would be indicated in patients with abnormal liver function tests or who have a palpable mass on physical examination, potentially indicating that the patient had a burden of metastatic disease or technically unresectable disease that would signal a nonoperative approach to their diagnosis.

Rectal cancers should undergo a somewhat different preoperative evaluation from cancers of the colon to clarify curative versus palliative intent, to determine whether preoperative neoadjuvant therapies might be indicated, or if a more conservative surgical approach can be used. A careful digital rectal examination should be done to evaluate tumor size, fixation, and ulceration and to evaluate possible extension of the cancer to pararectal lymph nodes or adjacent organs. A woman should have a complete pelvic examination to determine if the tumor has invaded the vagina or has spread to the ovaries. Rigid sigmoidoscopy is done to assess size, ulceration, and distance of the distal edge of the tumor to the anal verge. Flexible instruments are unreliable for assessing distance. CT scanning is indicated in patients with rectal cancer to evaluate pelvic extension and to look for distant metastases. Transrectal ultrasound or endoanal MRI examinations are the best attempts to accurately determine the depth of cancer invasion (T stage) and nodal involvement (N stage) helping to determine which patients are candidates for preoperative chemoradiation to allow for more sphincter-sparing operations and reduce local recurrence of their disease [33].

Preoperative Bowel Preparation

In the past, it had been standard to perform a mechanical bowel preparation prior to surgical intervention under the premise that it would reduce the risk of anastomotic leak and fecal soilage resulting in abscess or surgical site infection rates by reducing bacterial load. This has not been borne out in statistical analyses [34]. Moreover, there have been case reports, including an FDA alert in May 2006, regarding sodium phosphate products in particular. The case reports have described renal failure, in particular, acute phosphate nephropathy after oral sodium phosphate, even in patients with normal creatinine clearance. A recent consensus statement was published by the combined task force of ASCRS, ASGE, and SAGES outlining the evidence for various bowel preparations and their efficacy specifically for colonoscopy where preparation is necessary for adequate screening. In an addendum, they outlined particular groups at risk with sodium phosphate preparations. In particular, the elderly independent of renal function were considered at increased risk of acute renal failure with the oral preparation [35].

Statistically significant changes in serum Na, K, and PO_4 were seen; however, all within the range of normal. In addition, a statistically significant correlation between rise in serum phosphate and age was found in patients with normal creatinine clearance [36]. Due to this increasing volume of evidence, the author's institution has phased out phosphosoda preparations in general and has moved away from aggressive preoperative mechanical bowel preparation for colorectal surgery.

Surgical Technique

Colon Cancer

Surgery with curative intent is possible in approximately 85% of patients diagnosed with colorectal cancer. The goal of curative resection is en bloc excision of the primary tumor along with its regional lymphatic system. Prophylactic extensive central or retroperitoneal lymph node dissections are associated with increased operative morbidity but no survival advantage. Tumor-free margins proximal and distal to the lesion along the length of the intestine are most often easily achievable for colon cancer, as pathology studies have shown that longitudinal spread of the disease rarely exceeds 4 cm. Local extension into organs contiguous with the large intestine is found in approximately 10% of cases. Excision with tumor-free margins is still the goal in such cases, as 67% 5-year survival has been reported for patients undergoing curative resection of such lesions.

Traditional resections for colon cancer are based on the pattern of lymphatic drainage. As the lymphatics course together with the major vascular supply of the colon, resection of lymphatic channels draining a particular colonic segment necessitates devascularization of that segment. This approach sometimes requires resection of segments of colon beyond what longitudinal margins alone would require.

Cancers of the cecum and ascending colon are treated with a right hemicolectomy. The ileocolic artery, right colic artery, and right branch of the middle colic artery are ligated. This requires resection of the distal 5–8 cm of the ileum, cecum, ascending colon, and proximal transverse colon.

For cancers of the transverse colon, transverse colectomy with ligation of the middle colic artery and anastomosis between the ascending colon and the descending colon can be done, although there may be tension at the anastomosis, even after full mobilization of the colon. Cancers of the proximal and mid-transverse colon can be resected with an extended right hemicolectomy, with ligation of the ileocolic artery, right colic artery, and middle colic artery. The terminal ileum, cecum, ascending colon, hepatic flexure, transverse colon, and splenic flexure are resected; and an anastomosis between the ileum and the descending colon is performed.

Cancers of the splenic flexure and descending colon are treated by left hemicolectomy. The left colic artery is ligated, the splenic flexure and the descending colon are resected, and an anastomosis is created between the transverse colon and sigmoid colon.

A sigmoid colectomy is performed for sigmoid cancers. The inferior mesenteric artery is ligated distal to the origin of the left colic artery, and an anastomosis is created between the descending colon and the rectum.

Rectal Cancer

Surgical options for curable rectal cancer are summarized in Table 69.3. The surgical approach to rectal cancer is different from that for colon cancer, largely because of anatomic factors. Wide excision of the cancer and surrounding structures, possible in colon cancer, is difficult for rectal cancer, as the rectum resides within the confines of the pelvis. The proximity of the anal sphincter mechanism, organs of the urogenital tract, and enervation of the urogenital system pose significant challenges.

The desired distal margin in rectal cancer excisions has been the focus of much interest. A 5 cm margin of normal tissue distal to the grossly visible lesion was once the standard of care. This concept was based on observations by Dukes, who failed to detect submucosal or lymphatic spread more than 4.5 cm distal to the tumor. Unfortunately, tumor differentiation status was not considered in his study. More recent pathology studies have shown that for well-differentiated and moderately well-differentiated rectal cancers, a 2 cm distal margin is adequate. In recent years, the importance of margins lateral to the rectum has received greater attention. Clearance of these margins can be difficult to achieve, a factor that may account for the high local recurrence rates observed for rectal cancer.

Cancers of the upper rectum are treated by anterior resection, during which the proximal rectum is resected through an abdominal incision, and intestinal continuity is reestablished by colorectal anastomosis. Resection of the rectosigmoid colon performed proximal to the pelvic peritoneal reflection is known as a high anterior resection, whereas an operation in which it is necessary to open the pelvic peritoneum is known as a low anterior resection. Typically, the sigmoid colon is resected in continuity with the rectum, as the inferior mesenteric artery has been divided. The more generous collateral circulation to the descending colon provides a safer anastomosis.

Cancers of the lower rectum (<4 cm from the anorectal junction) have traditionally been treated by abdomino-perineal resection (APR). Patients should understand that a permanent colostomy, which is integral to APR, does not signify a hopelessly advanced cancer. Other surgical options for low rectal cancers include a low anterior resection with coloanal anastomosis or local excision of the tumor, usually via a transanal approach. The option for these procedures is based on the preoperative stage. Elderly patients, however, in whom a curative goal is being superseded by a limited life expectancy might undergo a local procedure (see below) even if it is of palliative rather than curative intent as local procedures are much better tolerated by patients.

Cancers of the middle third of the rectum require the most surgical judgment to determine whether a sphincter-sparing procedure can be done. Clearly, with the advent of stapling devices and an understanding that a distal margin of 2 cm is adequate, sphincter-sparing operations are more prevalent. Although the distance from the distal edge of the tumor to the anal verge is clinically the most often used criterion for determining whether a patient is a candidate for low anterior resection, other factors also play a role. These factors include body habitus, tumor size, mobility, histologic grade, the presence of metastatic disease, the preoperative continence status, the patient's willingness to accept a stoma and his or her ability to care for a stoma, and the general medical condition of the patient. Elderly patients may have compromised sphincter function and might experience poor bowel control following a low coloanal anastomosis. Careful consideration of this possibility is needed when deciding whether to recommend such an anastomosis over a permanent stoma. Furthermore, in those patients in whom a permanent stoma is determined to provide the best bowel control, the bowel distal to the tumor can be stapled off and left in place as a short rectal stump to avoid the lengthy perineal dissection and morbid perineal wound found in a traditional APR.

TABLE 69.3 Treatment options for curable rectal cancer

Mid and upper rectum (6–15 cm)
Anterior resection, stapled, or hand-sutured

Lower rectum (0–5 cm)
Coloanal anastomosis, with or without a pouch
Transanal excision
Transsphincteric and parasacral approaches
Diathermy
Abdominal perineal resection
Primary radiation therapy

All sites
Adjuvant radiation therapy

Source: DeCosse J, Tsioulias G, Jacobson J (1994) Colorectal cancer: detection, treatment, and rehabilitation. CA Cancer J Clin 44:27–42. This material is reproduced with permission of Wiley-Liss, Inc., a subsidiary of John Wiley & Sons, Inc.

Total Mesorectal Excision

Given the probable contribution of inadequate lateral clearance of rectal cancers to high local recurrence rates, modifications of the traditional surgical techniques have been proposed. The technique of total mesorectal excision (TME) has been advocated initially by Heald [37]. With TME, the envelope of lymphovascular fatty tissue surrounding the rectum and mesorectum are completely excised under direct vision. The avascular plane between the mesorectum and the surrounding tissues is developed using sharp dissection. The excised specimen includes the whole posterior, distal, and lateral mesorectum; the inferior hypogastric plexuses are preserved. Anteriorly, Denonvilliers' fascia is included as part of the excised specimen.

Using TME, local recurrence rates of 4–8% have been reported [37, 38]. These rates are significantly lower than those for historical controls, for whom recurrence rates range from 20 to 45%. However, TME has been associated with a high anastomotic leak rate ($\geq$17%), leading some to advocate routine proximal colonic diversion following the procedure. Although many have proposed TME as the standard of care, its overall role in the management of patients with rectal cancer is not yet clear, particularly given the improvements in neoadjuvant therapies [39].

Local Therapies

Although radical surgery is the treatment of choice for most patients, local treatment is a satisfactory alternative under defined conditions. Local resection should be considered with curative intent for early stage rectal cancers that are too distal to allow a restorative resection and as a palliative measure in patients with metastatic disease or comorbid medical conditions who may not be able to tolerate the stress of general anesthesia and a major abdominal operation.

Local techniques include excision, ablation, and irradiation. Local excision can be performed through transanal, transsacral, or transsphincteric approaches, with the transanal approach being used most frequently [40]. Transanal endoscopic microsurgery (TEMS) has allowed local excision to be performed in slightly more proximal lesions. In patients who are particularly poor surgical candidates, transanal electrocoagulation, possibly in multiple stages, offers effective palliation [41].

For curative resections, the success of local excision depends on stringent selection criteria, as described by Ogunbiyi and Fleshman [42] (Table 69.4). Transrectal ultrasonography or endoanal magnetic resonance imaging should be performed to stage the lesions preoperatively. Candidate lesions should be small (<3 cm in diameter), mobile, confined to the rectal wall (T1 or T2), without evidence of regional or distant metastasis (N0 and M0), exophytic, and well or moderately well differentiated, without lymphovascular or perineural invasion. Graham et al. reported a 5-year cancer-specific survival of 89% in their series of local excisions for rectal cancer using such selection criteria [43] The local recurrence in this series was 19%.

Special Cases

Synchronous Lesions

Total abdominal colectomy with an ileal to rectal anastomosis may be performed when synchronous lesions or multiple adenomatous polyps are present. This operation is also recommended for patients with HNPCC. Although this operation can be associated with initial postoperative diarrhea, intestinal adaptation allows good long-term function. Total proctocolectomy with mucosal proctectomy and ileoanal anastomosis is done for younger patients with FAP; there is less experience with this operation in the elderly.

Colonic Obstruction

Complete obstruction of the colon or rectum by an obstructing carcinoma is a surgical emergency. Obstructing cancer of the right or transverse colon can be treated by resection and anastomosis without proximal diversion, but treatment of left-sided obstruction is more controversial. The preferred approaches are resection without anastomosis, resection and anastomosis with a proximal diverting ileostomy, or subtotal colectomy with ileorectal anastomosis. In the presence of an extensively dilated proximal colon and unstable patient, a temporary proximal decompressing stoma may be appropriate. The preliminary experience with colonic stenting in patients with advanced tumors presenting with obstruction has been reported to be promising [39]. Such stents, although not long-term solutions, can be used for palliation or for recanalization to allow bowel preparation and safer elective surgery.

Perforated Colon Carcinoma

The surgical approach is resection of the perforated segment of the bowel, together with involved adjacent structures. An anastomosis in a contaminated field should be protected by a proximal diverting stoma. Although the prognosis is poor, a curative operation should be attempted.

TABLE 69.4 Criteria for local management of rectal cancer

Diameter <3 cm

Mobile tumor

Exophytic

Confined to rectal wall (maximum T2) on transrectal ultrasonography

No evidence of extrarenal spread or distant metastases on computed tomography

Well-differentiated or moderately differentiated histology

No lymphovascular or perineural invasion

Laparoscopy for Colorectal Cancer

Laparoscopic surgery has integrated into most realms of surgery; however, its progress into oncologic procedures has been slower and more heavily scrutinized than in other arenas. To answer the question of the efficacy of laparoscopic approach to colorectal cancer surgery, a large multicenter trial was established to prospectively evaluate outcomes. The Clinical Outcomes of Surgical Therapy (COST) study group designed a multicenter, randomized, prospective trial to specifically answer the question of the appropriateness of laparoscopy in colorectal surgery. Their most recent update from 2007 includes follow-up data where they found no statistical difference in 5-year overall or disease-free survival overall, or site-specific recurrence between laparoscopic and open colorectal surgery. Of note this study was restricted to cancer of the right/left or sigmoid colon, and excluded those with locally (T4) or systemically (stage IV) advanced disease. This data provides needed level 1 evidence that laparoscopic colon surgery is equivalent to the standard technique with no higher incidence of tumor seeding than with an open procedure [44]. A recent Canadian study reviewed their center experience with laparoscopic resection for colon cancer between the elderly (>74 years) and their younger counterparts (50–74 years). In their experience, age was not an independence factor predicting poorer outcome after laparoscopy. Furthermore, they found no difference in conversion rate in comparison to the younger cohort. However, they found as others that the elderly were likely to present with more advanced stage of cancer, more comorbidities which would affect their outcome as it would for a younger patient. They concluded that laparoscopy should be considered in the elderly. They were not able to show decreased length of stay with laparoscopy versus open in the elderly but they did find no significant difference based on age alone [45].

Adjuvant Therapies

Adjuvant therapies are designed to eradicate micrometastases present at the time of surgery, with the goal of reducing local recurrence rates and prolonging survival. Several chemotherapy regimens based on 5-fluorouracil (5-FU) have been shown to prolong survival in selected groups of patients following curative resection for colon cancer. For example, the American National Cancer Institute Intergroup Study reported a 41% reduction in tumor recurrence and a 33% reduction in cancer-related mortality during a 3-year observation period in node-positive patients treated with levamisole and 5-FU [46]. Recent advances with more complex regimens adding chemotherapeutic agents in combination potentially along with monoclonal antibodies targeting specific tumor antigens has led to improvements in survival for stage III patients [47].

Ongoing trials are designed to identify chemotherapeutic agents with more antitumor efficacy and to define which patients would benefit from such treatments. Although standard treatment for colon cancer includes adjuvant chemotherapy for patients with stage III disease but not for patients with stage II tumors (who have no lymph node metastases), 20% of patients with stage II tumors die of recurrent disease. The challenge is to identify the subset of patients with stage II disease who would benefit from adjuvant chemotherapy. In a recent report, 192 lymph nodes from 26 consecutive patients with stage II colorectal cancer were examined using a CEA-specific nested reverse-transcriptase polymerase chain reaction (RT-PCR) to detect the presence of micrometastases not otherwise identified by routine histologic methods. Micrometastases were detected by PCR in one or more lymph nodes from 14 of 26 patients (54%). The 5-year survival rate was 36% in this group, but it was 75% in the group without micrometastases. The groups were similar with respect to age, sex, tumor location, tumor differentiation, and tumor size [48].

The proper use of adjuvant chemotherapy in elderly patients raises several issues. Patients are often seen as having more limited life expectancies and thus less potential advantages of adjuvant therapy and more vulnerable to toxicity. Studies have documented that elderly patients are receiving chemotherapy less often that their younger counterparts [49]. Toxicities, aside from myelosuppression and fatigue, however, have not been demonstrated to be more severe in elderly patients (same reference as prior). In addition, many studies do show a benefit from chemotherapy in the small groups of elderly patients that have been studied that age alone has not been recommended to be a criterion on which adjuvant chemotherapy is limited. It is rather the patients' life expectancy and comorbidities that are most helpful to assess when making this determination.

Adjuvant radiation therapy is rarely used following curative resection of colon cancers, as local recurrence rates are low and adjacent structures (e.g., small intestine) are sensitive to radiation-induced toxicity. For rectal cancer, however, the reported local recurrence rates are usually 30–35% for stage II disease and 40–60% for stage III disease. The use of adjuvant radiation therapy has clearly been shown to be associated with a reduction in local recurrence rates [50–52]. Postoperative adjuvant radiation therapy and chemotherapy for transmural and node-positive rectal cancer is the current standard of care. However, the optimal timing of adjuvant therapy for rectal cancer remains controversial.

The advantage of postoperative radiotherapy is that it allows patient selection based on surgical and histopathologic findings. Preoperative radiation therapy protocols may include patients who do not need such adjuvant treatments, given the limitations of currently available imaging studies. However, preoperative radiation therapy has the potential to downstage tumors and allows sphincter-sparing surgery in patients who otherwise might have required abdominoperineal resection.

At least ten modern randomized trials of preoperative radiation therapy for resectable rectal cancer have been reported. In five reports, the authors found a significant reduction in the rate of local recurrence. In some studies, a significant improvement in survival, as determined in subgroup analyses, was reported. In only one trial, a significant survival advantage for the whole group of treated patients was reported [53]. In this trial, done in Sweden, 1,168 patients received either a short course (five fractions over 1 week) of radiation therapy preoperatively combined with surgery or surgery alone. Irradiation was not associated with an increase in postoperative mortality. The local recurrence rate was 11% in the group who underwent irradiation and 27% in the group who were subjected to surgery alone. The difference in local recurrence rate was statistically significant for lesions of all stages. The overall 5-year survival rate was 58% in the group who received radiation and 48% in the surgery-alone group ($p = 0.004$).

The Swedish trial has been criticized, as more than 100 surgeons at 70 hospitals participated, with each surgeon, on average, performing fewer than four operations per year [53]. The local recurrence rate for stage I cancers in the trial (4% after irradiation and 12% after surgery alone) was higher than is typically reported, and radiation delivered all in 5 days rather than 4–6 weeks is not the protocol used most often in the USA. This study also did not address the role of preoperative irradiation in combination with preoperative chemotherapy. Additional studies are required to define the optimal adjuvant therapy regimens for rectal cancer.

Postoperative Surveillance

There are two goals of postoperative surveillance: (1) to increase the detection of recurrent carcinoma at a potentially curable stage and (2) to detect metachronous lesions. Recurrent disease following resection for colorectal cancer, even at distant sites, is potentially treatable. Hepatic resection for metastatic lesions is safe and appears to prolong survival in selected patients. In a report of 128 patients over the age of 70 undergoing major hepatic resections for colorectal metastasis, those over 80 years of age had perioperative outcomes and 5-year survival rates equivalent to those of younger patients. Hepatic resection for colorectal metastases with clear margins of resection is associated with a 5-year survival of 25–48% and mean survival of 20–40 months. The lung is the second most common site of metastases from colorectal cancers. In selected patients, complete resection of pulmonary metastases is associated with a 5-year survival of 20–44%.

The best surveillance strategies remain to be determined. Postoperative surveillance following surgery for colorectal cancer is highly variable in clinical practice. In one report,

the number of office visits during the first 5 years ranged from 6 to 18, CEA measurements ranged from 0 to 44, liver ultrasound examinations ranged from 0 to 10, and sigmoidoscopy ranged from 0 to 13 [54].

Traditional surveillance protocols have included periodic history and physical examination, FOBT, complete blood count, liver function tests, tumor marker sampling, colonoscopy, and chest radiography. Surveillance tests are generally performed more frequently during the initial postoperative period, as 80–90% of all recurrences become evident during the first 2–3 years after surgery. One standard textbook of surgery has recommended that the history, physical examination, FOBT, and blood studies be obtained every 3 months during the first 3 years and every 6 months for an additional 2 years. Tumor markers are measured every 8 weeks by some investigators and monthly by others for 3 years and then every 3 months for another 2 years. Traditionally, colonoscopy has been done 6–12 months after resection, at yearly intervals for an additional 2 years, and at less frequent intervals thereafter.

In another recent report, the efficacy of a surveillance strategy using the history, physical examination, liver function tests, CEA assay, and colonoscopy 5 years postoperatively is as good as a more intensive strategy using yearly colonoscopy, CT, and chest radiography [55]. Survival rates were equivalent, regardless of the surveillance strategy used.

In guidelines recently published by a multidisciplinary panel, patients in whom large (>1 cm in diameter) or multiple adenomatous polyps have been removed should have an examination of the entire colon 3 years after the initial examination. If the first follow-up is normal or if only a single, small, tubular adenoma is found, the next examination can be at 5 years.

Patients with a colorectal cancer who has been resected with curative intent (but who did not undergo complete adequate colonoscopic examination preoperatively) should have a complete examination of the colon within 1 year after resection. If this or a complete preoperative examination is normal, subsequent examination should be offered after 3 years and then, if normal, every 5 years [56]. As with original cancers, subsequent cancers are preceded by adenomatous polyps that occur with increased frequency. There is no evidence to suggest that these polyps progress to cancer at a different rate from those in average-risk people.

References

1. Janssen-Heijnen MLG, Huub AAMM, Houterman S et al (2007) Comorbidity in older surgical cancer patients: influence on patient care and outcome. Eur J Cancer 43:2179–2193
2. Pasetto LM, Monfardini S (2007) Colorectal cancer screening in elderly patients: when should be more useful? Cancer Treat Rev 33:528–532

3. Clark AJ, Stockton D, Elder A et al (2004) Assessment of outcomes after colorectal cancer resection in the elderly as a rationale for screening and early detection. Br J Surg 91:1345–1351

4. Jemal A, Siegel R, Ward E et al (2008) Cancer statistics 2008. CA Cancer J Clin 58:71–96

5. Ries LAG, Melbert D, Krapcho M et al SEER Cancer Statistics Review, 1975–2005. National Cancer Institute, Bethesda, MD. http://seer.cancer.gov/csr/1975_2005/, based on November 2007 SEER data submission, posted to the SEER web site, 2008

6. Levine JS, Ahnen DJ (2006) Adenomatous polyps of the colon. N Engl J Med 355(24):2551–2557

7. Kingston RD, Jeacock J, Walsh S et al (1995) The outcome of surgery for colorectal cancer in the elderly: a 12-year review from the Trafford databases. Eur J Surg Oncol 21:514–516

8. Raferty L, Sanoff HK, Goldberg R (2008) Colon cancer in older adults. Semin Oncol 35(6):561–568

9. Coyle YM (2009) Lifestyle, genes, and cancer. Methods Mol Biol 472:25–56

10. Dube C, Rostom A, Lewin G et al (2007) The use of aspirin for primary prevention of colorectal cancer: a systematic review prepared for the U.S. Preventive Services Task Force. Ann Intern Med 146(5):365–375

11. Vasen HF, Mechlin JP, Khan PM et al (1991) The International Collaborative Group on Hereditary Non Polyposis Colorectal Cancer (ICG-HNPCC). Dis Colon Rectum 34:424–425

12. O'Brien MJ, Winawer SJ, Zauber AG et al (1990) The National Polyp Study: patient and polyp characteristics associated with high-grade dysplasia in colorectal adenomas. Gastroenterology 98:371–379

13. Winawer SJ, Zauber AG, Ho MN et al (1993) Prevention of colorectal cancer by colonoscopic polypectomy. N Engl J Med 329:1977–1981

14. Winawer SJ, Fletcher RH, Miller L et al (1997) Colorectal cancer screening: clinical guidelines and rationale. Gastroenterology 112:594–642

15. Vogelstein B, Fearon ER, Hamilton SR et al (1988) Genetic alterations during colorectal-tumor development. N Engl J Med 319:525–532

16. Bos JL, Fearon ER, Hamilton SR et al (1987) Prevalence of ras gene mutations in human colorectal cancers. Nature 327:293–297

17. Forrester K, Almoguera X, Han K et al (1987) Detection of high incidence of K-ras oncogenes during human colon tumorigenesis. Nature 327:298–303

18. Karapetis CS, Khambata-Ford S, Jonker DJ et al (2008) K-ras mutations and benefit from cetuximab in advanced colorectal cancer. N Engl J Med 359:1757–1766

19. AJCC Cancer Staging Manual, 7th edn. In Edge SB, Byrd DR, Compton CC et al (eds). Springer, New York, 2010

20. Beydoun HA, Beydoun MA (2008) Predictors of colorectal cancer screening behaviors among average-risk older adults in the United States. Cancer Causes Control 19:339–359

21. Mandel JS, Bond JH, Church TR et al (1993) Reducing mortality from colorectal cancer by screening for fecal occult blood: Minnesota Colon Cancer Control Study. N Engl J Med 328:1365–1371

22. Levine B, Lieberman DA, McFarland B et al (2008) Screening and surveillance for the early detection of colorectal cancer and adenomatous polyps, 2008: a joint guideline from the American Cancer Society, the US Multi-Society Task Force on Colorectal Cancer, and the American College of Radiology. CA Cancer J Clin 58:130–160

23. Mandel JS, Bond JH, Bradley M et al (1989) Sensitivity, specificity, and positive predictivity of the hemoccult test in screening for colorectal cancers: the Minnesota Colon Cancer Control Study. Gastroenterology 17:597–600

24. Byers T, Levin B, Rothenberger D et al (1997) American Cancer Society guidelines for screening and surveillance for early detection of colorectal polyps and cancer: update 1997, American Cancer Society Detection and Treatment Advisory Group on Colorectal Cancer. CA Cancer J Clin 47:154–160

25. Whitlock EP, Lin JS, Liles E, Beil TL, Fu R (2008) Screening for colorectal cancer: a targeted, updated systematic review for the US Preventative services Task Force. Ann Intern Med 149:638–658

26. Markowitz AJ, Winawer SJ (1997) Management of colorectal polyps. CA Cancer J Clin 47:93–113

27. Read TE, Read JD, Butterfly LF (1997) Importance of adenomas 5 mm or less in diameter that are detected by sigmoidoscopy. N Engl J Med 336:8–12

28. Greenberg AG, Salk RP, Pridhom D (1985) Influence of age on mortality of colon surgery. Am J Surg 150:65–70

29. Boyd JB, Bradford B Jr, Watne AL (1980) Operative risk factors of colon resection in the elderly. Ann Surg 192:743–746

30. Cohen H, Willis I, Wallack M (1986) Surgical experience of colon resection in the extreme elderly. Ann Surg 52:214–217

31. Hobler KE (1986) Colon surgery for cancer in the very elderly: cost and 3 year survival. Ann Surg 203:129–131

32. Morel P, Egeli RA, Wachtl S et al (1989) Results of operative treatment of gastrointestinal tract tumors in patients over 80 years of age. Arch Surg 124:662–664

33. Tatli S, Mortele KJ, Breen E et al (2006) Local staging of rectal cancer using combined pelvic phased-array and endorectal coil MRI. J Magn Reson Imaging 23:534–540

34. Guenaga KK, Matos D, Wille-Jørgensen P. Mechanical bowel preparation for elective colorectal surgery. Cochrane Database Syst Rev (1):CD001544. DOI: 10.1002/14651858.CD001544.pub3

35. Wexner SD, American Society of Colon and Rectal Surgeons (ASCRS); American Society for Gastrointestinal Endoscopy (ASGE); Society of American Gastrointestinal and Endoscopic Surgeons (SAGES) et al (2006) A consensus document on bowel preparation before colonoscopy: prepared by a task force from the American Society of Colon and Rectal Surgeons (ASCRS), the American Society for Gastrointestinal Endoscopy (ASGE), and the Society of American Gastrointestinal and Endoscopic Surgeons (SAGES). Surg Endosc 20:1147–1161

36. Gumurdulu Y, Serin E, Ozer B et al (2004) Age as a predictor of hyperphosphatemia after oral phosphosoda administration for colon preparation. J Gastroenterol Hepatol 19(1):68–72

37. Heald RJ (1986) Recurrence and survival after total mesorectal excision for rectal cancer. Lancet 1:1479–1482

38. MacFarlane JK, Ryall RD, Heald RJ (1993) Mesorectal excision for rectal cancer. Lancet 341:457–460

39. Stamos MJ (1998) Colon and rectal surgery. J Am Coll Surg 186:134–140

40. Bailey HR, Huval WV, Max E et al (1992) Local excision of carcinoma of the rectum for cure. Surgery 111:555–561

41. Madden JL, Kandalaft SI (1983) Electrocoagulation as a primary curative method in the treatment of carcinoma of the rectum. Surg Gynecol Obstet 157:164–179

42. Ogunbiyi OA, Fleshman JW (1997) Colorectal cancer and laparoscopic colorectal surgery in the elderly patient. Probl Gen Surg 13: 154–162

43. Graham RA, Garnsey L, Jessup JM (1990) Local excision of rectal carcinoma. Am J Surg 160:306–312

44. Fleshman J, Sargent DJ, Green E et al (2007) Laparoscopic colectomy for cancer is not inferior to open surgery based on 5-year data from the COST Study Group trial. Ann Surg 246(4):655–664

45. Devon KM, Vergara-Fernandez O, Victor JC, McLeod RS (2009) Colorectal cancer surgery in elderly patients: presentation, treatment, and outcomes. Dis Colon Rectum 52:1272–1277

46. Moertel CG, Fleming TR, MacDonald JS et al (1990) Levamisole and fluorouracil for adjuvant therapy of resected colon carcinoma. N Engl J Med 322:352–358

47. Wolpin BM, Mayer RJ (2008) Systemic treatment of colorectal cancer. Gastroenterology 134:1296–1310

48. Liefers GJ, Cleton-Jansen AM, van de Velde CJ et al (1998) Micrometastases and survival in stage II colorectal cancer. N Engl J Med 339:223–228

49. Schrag D, Cramer LD, Bach PB et al (2001) Age and adjuvant chemotherapy use after surgery for stage III colon cancer. J Natl Cancer Inst 93:850–857

50. Kodner IJ, Shemesh EI, Fry RD et al (1989) Preoperative irradiation for rectal cancer: improved local control and long-term survival. Ann Surg 209:194–199

51. Mendenhall WM, Bland KI, Copeland EM et al (1992) Does preoperative radiation enhance the probability of local control and survival in high risk distal rectal cancer? Ann Surg 215:696–706

52. Roe JP, Kodner IJ, Walz BJ et al (1982) Preoperative radiation therapy for rectal carcinoma. Dis Colon Rectum 25:471–473

53. Swedish Rectal Cancer Trial (1997) Improved survival with preoperative radiotherapy in resectable rectal cancer. N Engl J Med 336:980–988

54. Lavery IC, Fazio VW, Lopez-Kostner R et al (1997) Correspondence. N Engl J Med 337:346

55. Graham RA, Wang S, Catalano PJ et al (1998) Postsurgical surveillance of colon cancer; preliminary cost analysis of physician examination, carcinoembryonic antigen testing, chest x-ray, and colonoscopy. Ann Surg 228:59–63

56. Schoemaker D, Black R, Giles L (1998) Yearly colonoscopy, liver CT, and chest radiography do not influence 5-year survival of colorectal cancer patients. Gastroenterology 114:7–14

Chapter 70
Abdominal Wall Hernia in the Elderly

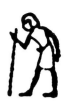

Catherine Straub and Leigh Neumayer

CASE STUDY: PART 1

The following case study, woven throughout the chapter, highlights the nuances and difficulties that inguinal hernias present in the elderly.

A 70-year-old male presented to the General Surgery clinic at the VA Hospital with complaints of a new bulge in his right groin. He first noticed the bulge 2 months ago after moving heavy boxes into a new home. Though initially painful it has not bothered him in weeks. He has not had any symptoms of obstruction. His past medical history is significant for well-controlled hypertension and a 30-pack-year smoking history. He is not enthusiastic about surgery and wants to know if he truly needs it.

Abdominal wall hernia repair is the most common surgical procedure in the USA. More than 1,000,000 herniorrhaphies are performed annually. Of these 750,000 are inguinal, 166,000 are umbilical, 97,000 are incisional, and 25,000 are femoral [1]. The incidence of groin hernias, in men over age 65 is approximately 13 per 1,000 population [2]. The incidence in women is 12–25% that of men. In a British study of more than 30,000 inguinal hernia repairs, 27% were in an elderly population; 85.5% of repairs on patients aged 65 or older were elective, and the remaining 14.5% were classified as emergency procedures [3]. Since the majority of all hernias are inguinal or femoral, the focus of this chapter will be on the preoperative evaluation, repair options and complications of groin hernias. Incisional, umbilical, and other hernias will be discussed separately at the end of the chapter.

C. Straub (✉)
Department of General Surgery, University of Utah,
Salt Lake City, UT, USA
e-mail: catherine.straub@hsc.utah.edu

Inguinal Hernias

The inguinal and femoral canals are anatomically one of the most confusing areas of the human body (Fig. 70.1). The inguinal canal is bordered anteriorly by the external oblique fascia and posteriorly, also called the floor of the canal, by the transversalis fascia. The superior border is the transverses abdominus and the inferior border is the inguinal ligament, which is itself the inferior edge of the external oblique muscle. The spermatic cord in males or round ligament in females, courses through the inguinal canal from deep to superficial inguinal rings. The spermatic cord itself is composed of cremasteric muscle, pampiniform plexus, testicular artery, genital branch of the genitofemoral nerve, ductus deferens, cremasteric artery, lymphatics, and processus vaginalis.

An important concept in groin anatomy is the myopectineal orifice (Fig. 70.2). Through this anatomic opening, structures traverse from the pelvis to the leg. The spermatic cord and the femoral vessels pass through this orifice anterior and deep to the inguinal ligament, respectively. The myopectineal orifice can further be divided into three triangles – the medial, lateral, and femoral [4]. The medial and lateral triangles are separated from the femoral triangle by the inguinal ligament. The majority of groin hernias in older individuals occur through a weakening in the floor of the medial triangle. The majority of recurrences occur through the lateral triangle when it is not dealt with appropriately during the primary operation [5]. Accordingly, femoral hernias occur through the femoral triangle, more specifically through the empty space of the femoral canal medial to the femoral vessels.

Inguinal hernias are divided into two types: direct and indirect. Indirect hernias pass through the deep inguinal ring, lie anterior and medial to the vas deferens within the spermatic cord, and descend through the inguinal canal to the scrotum. These are more commonly congenital and arise from a patent processus vaginalis. Direct hernias pass directly through the floor of the inguinal canal and point anteriorly. This area in the floor of the canal is referred to as Hesselbach's triangle and is bordered by the lateral border of the rectus abdominis muscle, the inferior epigastric vessels and the

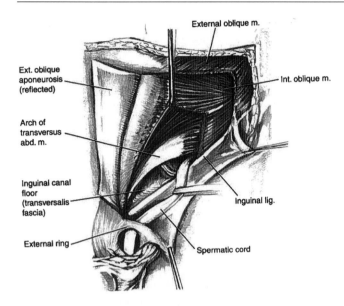

Figure 70.1 Anatomy of the inguinal region (reprinted from Mulvihill; Surgery: Basic Science and Clinical Evidence; 2001, with kind permission of Springer Science + Business Media).

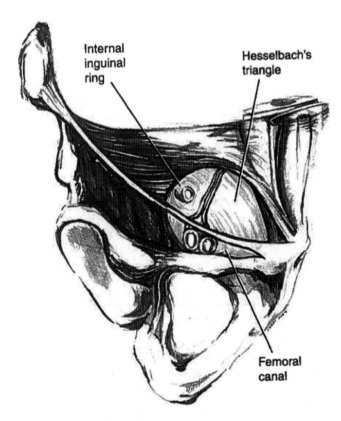

Figure 70.2 Myopectineal orifice (reprinted from Mulvihill; Surgery: Basic Science and Clinical Evidence; 2001, with kind permission of Springer Science + Business Media).

inguinal ligament. These are acquired hernias that are due to a weakness of the inguinal floor. A pantaloon hernia has both a direct and indirect component. Femoral hernias are a variation of direct hernias in which the inguinal ligament prevents

the sac from protruding through the inguinal floor. Instead, the sac passes through the femoral canal [6].

Inguinal hernias in elderly persons present very specific challenges. For example, they are frequently long-standing. Many have been present for 10–20 years, although some may have occurred as long as 50–60 years prior to presentation for repair [7–9]. As a result of the chronic nature of these hernias, the surrounding normal anatomic architecture is disrupted and there is loss of appropriate tissue planes to facilitate repair. Furthermore, with age comes the anticipated loss of muscle mass and tissue strength, making an anatomic repair more difficult. By the age of 80 up to 40% of muscle mass may be lost, with a proportional increase in body fat [10]. Increased co-morbidities in this age group can make elective repair challenging, but operative morbidity and mortality is still remarkably low. Prolonged neglect, however, can result in a high incidence of preoperative complications, such as bowel obstruction, incarceration, and strangulation. These conditions frequently necessitate emergency treatment. In a Swedish study, patients undergoing emergent operation for inguinal hernias were on average 12 years older than those undergoing elective repair (70 vs. 58 years old) [11]. However, new data suggest that watchful waiting is a viable option in this population [12]. There are also new and emerging techniques for hernia repair, including laparoscopic and the use of biologics, that may be of particular interest to this demographic. These issues will be discussed in more detail later in the chapter.

Etiology and Distribution

The etiology of abdominal wall hernias differs somewhat in the elderly population. Indirect inguinal hernias, which are often congenital, comprise 90% of the hernias in young men, account for only 50–60% of hernias in older men. The incidence of direct hernias increase to 35% in men over age 65 [8]. Furthermore, the incidence of sliding hernias also increases from 0.5% during the third decade of life to as much as 13% during the sixth to eighth decades [13]. In youth indirect hernias are repaired by a simple herniotomy, the Marcy repair; however, indirect hernias in the adult population treated this way have a significant rate of recurrence indicating additional factors are present. Studies have shown that the presence of a persistent processus vaginalis does not change with age – roughly 20% [14]. Autopsy studies have shown that despite this high number, a very low proportion of patients suffered from a hernia in their life [15]. In addition, increased intra-abdominal pressure from such activities as coughing and straining put tremendous forces on the abdominal wall where there are natural weaknesses such as the internal inguinal ring and the transversalis fascia. Given the high proportion of patent processus vaginalises and the physiologic necessity of increased intra-abdominal pressure, more patients suffer from inguinal hernias. Abrahamson describes a mechanism that may explain why this is not so. The "shutter mechanism" explains that when intra-abdominal pressure increases the muscles of the abdominal wall contact and the fibers of the aponeuroses within the inguinal region shorten. This essentially tightens around physiologic weaknesses such as the inguinal ring and the myopectineal orifice [16].

Acquired hernias are more common with increasing age and are often associated with other physiologic changes or disease processes. In most cases the pathophysiologic mechanism of an acquired hernia is a structural inadequacy of the inguinal floor, which manifests as a direct inguinal hernia. A recent study compared the structure of the rectus sheath in patients undergoing inguinal hernia repair and those undergoing appendectomy. There was a significant difference in the alignment and quality of collagen and elastic fibers. In those with inguinal hernias there was increased disorganization of collagen fibrils, thinning of elastic fibrils, and generalized replacement with ground matter [17]. A similar study showed that these changes were present in the transversalis fascia of both the herniated side as well as the nonherniated side [18].

The inguinal floor may therefore be weakened by any factors that interfere with normal collagen and elastin production. These include congenital connective tissue disorders such as Marfan and Ehler–Danlos Syndromes, as well as metabolic defects in collagen formation. Cigarette smoking also plays a significant role in hernia formation. The same proteases and elastases found in the lungs of smokers that lead to emphysema are also found in their serum and can bring about the destruction of elastin and collagen in other tissues. Systemic illnesses with an enhanced leukocyte response can also lead to the release of proteases and antioxidants having a similar effect [16, 18, 19].

Other factors associated with groin hernia formation involve conditions that lead to chronically increased intra-abdominal pressure, such as long-standing constipation and straining, bladder outlet obstruction, chronic cough, obesity, and kyphoscoliosis. In the elderly patient it is not uncommon for several of these factors to be present simultaneously. Occasionally, this confluence of factors contributes to the development of a giant hernia or one with a large scrotal component. These hernias can become extremely large and may contain a significant portion of the abdominal viscera. When forced reduction of the viscera into the contracted abdominal cavity is attempted, severe respiratory compromise due to increased intra-abdominal pressure and decreased diaphragmatic excursion may occur.

Approximately 15–30% of all herniorrhaphies in the elderly are performed on an emergent basis as a result of incarceration. Overall, 50–60% are indirect and 17–25% are femoral. When separated by gender, 73% of incarcerated hernias in men are indirect and 15% are femoral, whereas femoral hernias account for 50% of incarcerations in women [7, 20, 21]. Although rare, once strangulation has occurred, the hernia changes from a simple mechanical problem to a complex life-threatening systemic illness, and the repair changes from correction of a simple mechanical defect to reversal of a major abdominal catastrophe.

Diagnosis

In most cases, the diagnosis of inguinal hernia in the elderly is clear. More than 70% of patients with groin hernias complain of a groin or scrotal mass and pain in the inguinal region. The pain may wax and wane if the hernia is reducible. In many cases the patient has been aware of, or diagnosed with, a hernia for many years. Symptomatic control is often achieved at the expense of physical activity. Trusses have been historically used to palliate the symptoms of a hernia; however, recent studies have shown that they are infrequently worn, uncomfortable, improperly fitted, and under the best circumstances only provide appropriate relief in 31% of patients [22].

The presence of a femoral hernia, however, is more difficult to recognize. Typically, poorly localized pain is present in the groin area without an obvious, visible bulge. Unfortunately, because of the subtle findings, femoral hernias are frequently not diagnosed until they incarcerate. In 1 review of 83 femoral hernias over 40% were repaired emergently for incarceration [23].

Historic factors that contribute to the development of inguinal hernias should always be elicited. Respiratory symptoms with chronic cough, chronic constipation, and symptoms of bladder outlet obstruction are most prevalent in an older population.

Examination for the presence of groin hernias should be part of the standard physical exam. Patients should be examined in the erect position, as a reducible hernia is sometimes more difficult to appreciate in the supine position. The only visible abnormality may be groin asymmetry. Indirect inguinal hernias appear as a small mass in the region of the deep ring, midway between the pubic tubercle and the anterior superior iliac spine. Direct hernias appear more medially, although this distinction is not always clear. Invaginating the skin of the scrotum and introducing the examining finger along the spermatic cord structures into the external inguinal ring is usually necessary for accurate diagnosis. Prolonged standing or increasing intra-abdominal pressure by coughing or with Valsalva maneuver causes the sac and its contents to descend toward the examining finger, where it is felt as a mass or a transmitted impulse. A small hernia defect or a sac that is difficult to reduce presents the greatest risk for future incarceration. In women, inguinal hernias may be difficult to diagnose until they become quite large.

It is important when examining the groin to include an examination of the upper thigh below the inguinal ligament as well. Most femoral hernias can be felt as a soft mass medial to the femoral vessels. Frequently, hernias in this location are mistaken for inguinal lymph nodes or lipomas. Increased intra-abdominal pressure may transmit an impulse through the sac, but this too can be mistaken for normal transmission of the increased pressure in the femoral vein.

A rectal exam to assess prostate size, the presence of a rectal mass, and fecal occult blood, is an essential part of every physical exam for hernia, particularly in elderly patients. Although there is no association between inguinal hernia and colonic abnormalities, the high risk of colon neoplasm in these patients, in general, justifies a screening procedure, such as flexible sigmoidoscopy, for all patients over age 50 (see Elective Surgical Repair).

The differential diagnosis of a groin mass is extensive and includes hernias as well as lipomas, lymphadeonpathy, abscess, varicocele, hydrocele, testicular mass, testicular torsion, epididymitis, and femoral artery aneurysm [24]. For this reason a imaging modality for the diagnosis of groin hernias has been sought for years. Herniography consists of injecting a small amount of contrast material directly into the peritoneal cavity and taking a radiograph during a valsalva maneuver. This is an accurate but invasive and painful technique with a complication rate reported at 5.8% [25]. Ultrasound has been shown to have an accuracy of 92% for all groin hernias and a 75% accuracy for those without a palpable bulge (Fig. 70.3) [26]. Therefore, it may be a useful adjunct in qualified hands. Computed tomography and MRI scans may also be beneficial in the evaluation of the difficult groin, but history and physical examination remain the mainstays of groin hernia diagnosis (Fig. 70.4).

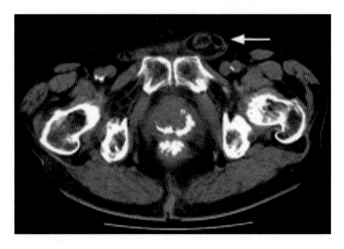

Figure 70.4 CT image of inguinal hernia (reprinted with permission from [91]. Copyright © Radiological Society of North America).

The diagnosis of an incarcerated hernia is usually not difficult to establish. Most often patients present with a previously recognized hernia that has recently become increasingly painful and "stuck out." In the case of a femoral hernia, a painful mass in the groin may be the first indication. Obstructive symptoms such as nausea, vomiting, and obstipation may not be present early in the course but develop if the incarceration goes untreated. Strangulation, or ischemia to the incarcerated portion, is indicated by increasing pain and signs of systemic sepsis. On physical examination, a tender, nonreducible mass is present in the groin. Erythema and edema of the overlying skin are suggestive of strangulation of bowel in a hernia sac, as is severe tenderness to palpation.

CASE STUDY: PART 2

The 70-year-old veteran is not too concerned about his hernia and knows many of his friends who have been ignoring theirs for years. He has never had surgery and does not want to start now. He is hoping you are going to tell him not to worry about it.

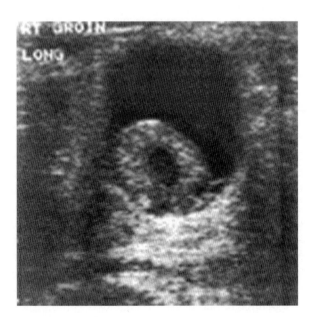

Figure 70.3 Ultrasound of inguinal hernia (reprinted from [90], with kind permission of Springer Science + Business Media).

Watchful Waiting

Surgical repair has been the gold standard for even asymptomatic hernias for decades. However, awareness of complications from hernia repairs including recurrence and chronic groin pain are now better defined and so also should carry weight when determining the benefits of operative intervention. It is also apparent that the risk of incarceration and strangulation from these minimally symptomatic hernias may have been previously overstated. For these reasons the concept of watchful waiting has recently been considered as a viable option. Fitzgibbons et al. performed a trial of over 700 patients where patients were randomized to either open mesh repair or watchful waiting. Thirty-three percent of patients in each group were over 65 years of age. After 3 years of follow-up, pain and health outcomes were similar is each group. Eighty-five patients crossed over to the repair arm mostly because their hernias became more symptomatic. The rate of hernia accident was only 1.8 per 1,000. There were no deaths associated with hernia accidents [12]. This study seems to support a trial of watchful waiting in all asymptomatic or minimally symptomatic patients. A cost analysis performed as part of the Fitzgibbons study showed that a 2-year watchful waiting was a cost-effective option for such patients [27].

An additional study by O'Dwyer sought to answer a similar question looking at the geriatric population. One hundred and sixty patients over the age of 55 were randomized to watchful waiting or operation. There were 23 patients who crossed over to the repair arm, which is over 20% of those randomized to watchful waiting. This article argues that given longer follow-up there would be more cross-over to surgery and that elderly patients' health would only deteriorate over that time, making the risks associated with a hernia accident more severe [28]. In this study, like that of Fitzgibbons, the incidence of hernia accident (strangulation) was rare. There were two patients who crossed over from watchful waiting to repair and experienced significant postoperative complications not related directly to the hernia repair (myocardial infarction and stroke) but presumably to the decrease in the patient's overall health. Clearly as a patient ages, his or her general risks for undergoing any type of procedure increases.

CASE STUDY: PART 3

Upon further questioning the veteran has enough discomfort from his hernia that it limits his daily activities around the house. He lives over an hour from the nearest VA hospital and after hearing the potential complications of not repairing his hernia he has elected to proceed with repair.

Elective Surgical Repair

Prior to elective repair, conditions that may cause increased intra-abdominal pressure should be investigated and corrected if possible. Increased intra-abdominal pressure puts stress on the repair, interferes with normal wound healing, and may

predispose to recurrence. Constipation, symptoms of prostatic hypertrophy, chronic cough, and obesity are common conditions associated with increased tension on the abdominal wall. Managing the first three conditions with medications sufficiently to proceed with operation can often be accomplished in several weeks. Obesity cannot, however, and should not be controlled rapidly. Therefore, significant weight loss should not be used as an absolute prerequisite for repair.

Although there was a previously made association between inguinal hernias and colon cancer, those theories have been proven incorrect by multiple studies [29]. Current recommendations are to follow colon cancer screening guidelines. However, the majority of the elderly population does not currently follow these guidelines and their presentation with a hernia may be one of the best ways to enter them into the system. In a recent study, polyps were found in 62% of patients over the age of 60 undergoing screening colonoscopy, 86% of which were asymptomatic. Colon cancer was detected in 2.4% of patients [30]. The high incidence of colonic abnormalities in the elderly justifies screening. For patients with primary-care providers, this screening can be accomplished at any time. For those who enter the health-care system primarily to have the hernia repaired, screening should be part of the preoperative assessment. Elective repair should not be extensively delayed, however, to perform a screening procedure.

Anesthesia

The first step in elective hernia repair is the choice of anesthesia. Avoiding anesthetic techniques that place unnecessary stress on cardiac, pulmonary, and renal reserves may minimize the surgical morbidity and mortality. This is more important in elderly patients who often present with multiple co-morbidities. Both general and spinal anesthetic techniques are associated with perioperative complications. Guillen and Aldrete reported that in men over age 70 undergoing elective inguinal hernia repair the incidences of hypotension with spinal and inhaled anesthetic were 43 and 36%, respectively [31]. In a randomized trial of local vs. general and regional anesthesia, those patients receiving local anesthesia had less postoperative pain, fewer micturation complications, and shorter hospital stays. These results have been backed up by multiple other studies [32–34]. These data support the concept that local field block is the ideal anesthesia method for elective hernia repair in the geriatric age group. There are, however, a few limitations to this method. Patients with dementia or those who for other reasons are unable to understand commands and lie still on the operative table, as well as those who are unusually anxious, are considered poor candidates for local blocks. The excessive use of sedation necessary to control these patients frequently worsens the confusion and results in respiratory complications, which defeats the whole purpose of using local anesthetic. Further problems are encountered in obese patients for whom adequate local anesthesia may not be achievable because of limitations in dose and absorption.

With a detailed understanding of the neuroanatomy of the inguinal region, painless inguinal herniorrhaphy may be accomplished in the elderly patient. The innervation of the inguinal region is complex (Fig. 70.5). A clear understanding of the intercostal nerve supply is paramount. Following the pattern of dermatome distribution, the tenth thoracic nerve innervates the umbilicus, the first lumbar nerve innervates the inguinal area, and the twelfth thoracic nerve innervates the area in between. The iliohypogastric and ilioinguinal nerves lie deep to the external oblique fascia and lateral to the anterior superior iliac spine. The iliohypogastric originates at the first lumbar nerve and lies under the external oblique aponeurosis after penetrating the internal oblique muscle. This nerves supplies sensory fibers to the suprapubic region. The ilioinguinal nerve follows the same course as the iliohypogastric nerve but lies closer to the crest of the ileum and inguinal ligament. The ilioinguinal nerve penetrates the internal oblique muscle approximately 1.0 cm from the

antero superior iliac spine and supplies sensory innervation to the base of the penis and part of the scrotum (and comparable areas in the female body). The penile skin and a small area of the scrotum are supplied by sensory fibers from the sacral plexus. When repairing a femoral hernia, more attention must be paid to the ilioinguinal nerve and the femoral branch of the genitofemoral nerve, which supply the upper thigh. The genitofemoral nerve originates from the first and second lumbar nerves to supply sensory fibers to the scrotum and upper thigh and motor fibers to the cremasteric muscle via the genital branch. The genital branch reaches the inguinal canal at the internal abdominal ring. When performing herniorrhaphy under local anesthesia, pain is also felt when traction is applied to the sac or the spermatic cord or when a finger is inserted into the peritoneal cavity. Knowledge of this anatomy is also paramount during the operation to avoid injury to these nerves and thusly postoperative inguinodynia (see below).

A simple five-step method has been advocated for the use of local anesthetic during inguinal herniorrhaphy. Appropriate use of this method requires minimal IV sedation with Midazolam and does not necessarily require monitoring or the use of anesthesia staff. A 50:50 mixture of 1% Lidocaine and 0.5% Bupivicaine is used. (1) Approximately, 5 mL of solution is injected subdermally along the entire length of the proposed incision. (2) A skin wheal is then raised using an additional 3 mL along the same path. (3) A total of 10 mL is then injected subcutaneously 2 cm apart. (4) After making the skin incision and beginning to expose the external oblique fascia, 10 mL of solution is injected directly underneath the fascia. This bathes the entire inguinal canal and should anesthetize all three major nerves in this area. (5) Additional injections of a few milliliters of solution may also be injected into the pubic tubercle and the hernia sac and additional solution may be used to bathe the incision prior to closure of the external oblique as well as the skin (Fig. 70.6a, b) [35].

In this era of cost analysis and health-care economics, inguinal herniorrhaphy is becoming predominantly an outpatient procedure. Even though outpatient general anesthesia is possible, local block facilitates earlier ambulation and is associated with fewer immediate postoperative complications.

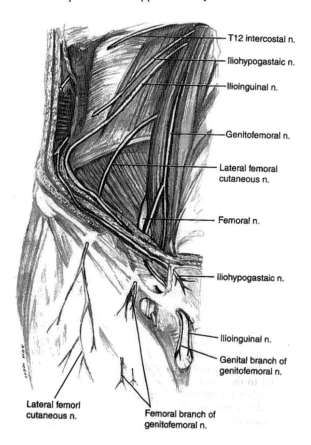

T12 intercostal n.

Iliohypogastric n.

Ilioinguinal n.

Genitofemoral n.

Lateral femoral cutaneous n.

Femoral n.

Iliohypogastric n.

Ilioinguinal n.

Genital branch of genitofemoral n.

Lateral femorl cutaneous n.

Femoral branch of genitofemoral n.

Figure 70.5 Nerve supply to the groin (from Mulvihill, Surgery: Basic Science and Clinical Evidence; 2001, reprinted with kind permission of Springer Science + Business Media).

Tissue Repairs

Inguinal hernia repair has previously been dominated by an anterior, open approach that was first proposed by Bassini, who introduced the concept of repair of the inguinal floor in 1887. This basic tenet of hernia repair has undergone many modifications, with various combinations of suturing the transversalis fascia, conjoined tendon, internal oblique, or transversus abdodinis to the inguinal or Cooper's ligament.

a

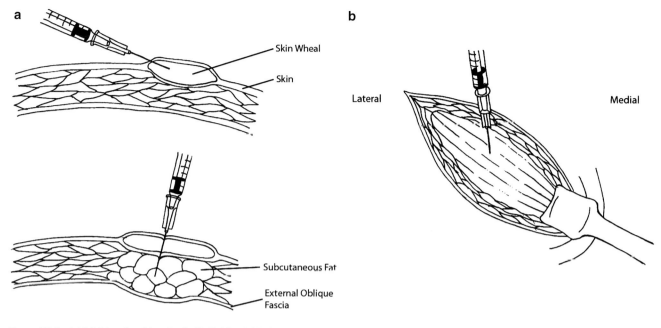

Skin Wheal

Skin

Subcutaneous Fat

External Oblique Fascia

b

Lateral

Medial

FIGURE 70.6 (a) Making the skin wheal. (b) Subfascial infiltration.

The choice of herniorrhaphy technique must take into account the risk of recurrence and patient tolerance of the procedure. The actual rate of recurrence is difficult to establish. There are, however, no randomized, prospective studies comparing the various techniques with comparable lengths of follow-up in the world's literature. The best reported recurrence rates by conventional tissue repairs range between 1 and 20%. Prospective data on hernia repair in the elderly are even more difficult to interpret. There is no good evidence that the choice of technique significantly affects outcome. There is, however, a general move away from tissue repairs toward "tension-free" repairs using synthetic patches.

CASE STUDY: PART 4

Many of the veteran's friends have undergone hernia repairs and he has heard about the use of synthetic materials in the repairs. He is concerned about the use of a foreign material and wants the best and most up-to-date method for repairing his hernia.

Synthetic Repairs

In 1909, McGavin was the first to use a prosthetic material, a filigree of silver wire, to repair an inguinal hernia [36]. Throckmorton introduced tantalum gauze for use when there was insufficient tissue for adequate primary tissue repair.

This material, however, did not prove to be durable. During the 1950s and 1960s, Usher et al. used polypropylene mesh to bolster primary tissue repairs of direct and indirect hernias [37–39].

The premise behind using synthetic materials is to provide a tension-free repair with fewer recurrences and a quicker to return to normal activity. It was not until 1986, with the published work of Lichtenstein and Shulman, that synthetic mesh became accepted for primary hernia repair without approximation of the underlying hernia margins (Fig. 70.7) [40]. With this technique, one single layer piece of mesh is secured over the inguinal floor with a slit to go around the internal ring. Data regarding recurrences with a particular hernia repair technique can be difficult to interpret because so much of it comes from specialized hernias center. However in a recent study comparing the Shouldice (a tissue repair) and the Lichtenstein repair in a general surgery practice, recurrence rates for the mesh repair were 0.7% compared to 4.7% for the tissue repair [41]. A meta-analysis comparing over 11,000 patients from various institutions demonstrated an overall recurrence rate of 2.0% for Lichtenstein mesh repair compared with 4.9% for various tissue repairs and persistent groin pain in 5.1 and 10.1% of patients, respectively [42].

Since the institution of the Lichtenstein method was first described, a multitude of other methods have attempted to supplant it. The plug-and-patch system was first described in 1993 and utilizes a polypropylene mesh plug to obliterate the defect in the internal ring or the inguinal floor. An additional patch is often used to provide additional support to the inguinal floor (Fig. 70.8) [43]. Recurrences remain as low as

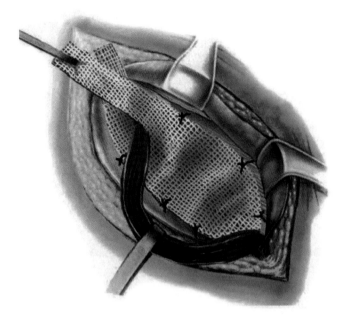

FIGURE 70.7 Lichtenstein repair (from Fitzgibbons RJ, Jr., Abdominal Wall Hernias, Fig. 8. Available at: http://knol.google.com/k/bob/abdominal-wall-hernias/Ilo7ZexB/MyZquQ#What_is_an_abdominal_wall_hernia(3F). Reprinted with kind permission of Springer Science + Business Media).

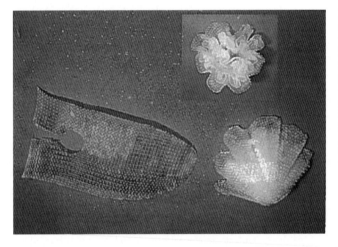

FIGURE 70.8 Plug and patch repair (from Mulvihill; Surgery: Basic Science and Clinical Evidence; 2001, Chap. 43; reprinted with kind permission of Springer Science + Business Media).

the Lichtenstein method but complications of plug migration and shrinkage were reported [44]. This remains a simple and viable method for hernia repair. The Kugel Patch consists of two layers of mesh placed preperitoneally through an anterior approach, thus placing the mesh where it would be placed during a laparoscopic approach. A small muscle splitting incision is used to gain access to the pre-peritoneal space [43]. Though initial results were very promising showing a recurrence rate of 0.45, these results have never been reproduced and there is a very steep learning curve with recur-

rence rates as high as 18.2% in the initial learning period and rates as high as 27.8% for recurrent hernias [45, 46].

The Prolene Hernia System (PHS) is another method of prosthetic repair. It consists of two pieces of mesh that serve to overlay and underlay the inguinal floor attached by a mesh connector that is placed either through the internal ring or a defect in the transversalis fascia. The benefits of the PHS are that it touts to repair indirect, direct, and femoral hernias all at once by covering the entire myopectineal orifice preperitoneally [43]. Theoretically, this should reduce hernia recurrence through the lateral triangle of the orifice. As of now, studies demonstrating long-term recurrences with the PHS have not been performed but preliminary results show similar operating times and short-term recurrence rates as both the Lichtenstein and plug-and-patch methods. Some studies have demonstrated less pain with the PHS (Fig. 70.9) [47, 48].

Currently there are no studies comparing any of the above techniques specifically in the elderly population. In fact, the majority of studies exclude elderly patients or those with elevated ASA status. It would stand to reason though that any repair amenable to local anesthesia with a relatively short operating time would suit the elderly population well. Currently all of the above techniques qualify.

CASE STUDY: PART 5

On further examination, our veteran has a small asymptomatic hernia on the opposite side. He wants to get them both repaired at once but is worried about the increase in pain and inactivity if he has incisions in both of his groins.

Laparoscopic Repairs

Shortly after the success of laparoscopic cholecystectomy became apparent, surgeons began to apply minimal access techniques to a wide variety of other surgical procedures. This approach has become generally accepted for some procedures, whereas for others there is still considerable disagreement. Hernia repair is one of the latter group. Although some skilled laparoscopists prefer the approach for all inguinal hernias, many others believe the benefits do not outweigh the risks, particularly in the elderly.

The advantages of laparoscopic inguinal herniorrhaphy include less postoperative pain, reduced recovery time and earlier return to full activity, easier repair of recurrent hernia through unoperated tissues, the ability to treat bilateral inguinal hernias simultaneously through a single set of incisions, and improved cosmesis [49–52].

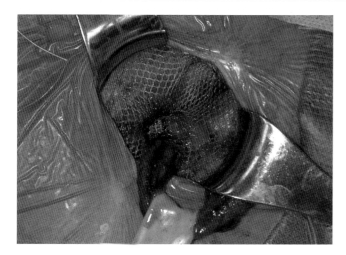

Figure 70.9 Placement of the Prolene Hernia System.

The laparoscopic approach to the inguinal hernia may be performed by either a transabdominal preperitoneal (TAPP) approach or a totally extraperitoneal (TEP) approach. In a TAPP repair the abdomen is entered in the typical laparoscopic fashion and once anatomy is appropriately identified a peritoneal flap is made. The hernia sac is then reduced and dissected free. A piece of mesh is then rolled out over the entire myopectineal orifice and in most instances is tacked in place being careful to avoid the bladder and the epigastric vessels. The peritoneal flap is then replaced and tacked in place as well (Fig. 70.10). In the TEP repair the preperitoneal space is entered. This is most often done with a balloon dissector placed through the umbilical port (Fig. 70.11).

Once the preperitoneal space is insufflated the anatomy of the groin is identified and the hernia sac dissected in a similar fashion as the TAPP repair. Mesh is placed and may be tacked in place. Any defects in the peritoneum are repaired. Previous lower abdominal incisions and radiation are a relative contradiction to the TEP repair, due to the difficulty of dissecting the peritoneum free from the abdominal wall [53].

The difficulty when operating from either of these approaches is the ability to obtain adequate exposure of the inguinal anatomy. Most recurrences are due to incomplete dissection of the region or inadequate placement of mesh to cover the defect. The TAPP repair provides the largest operating space and the most unobstructed view of the inguinal region and is probably the procedure of choice when learning to perform laparoscopic herniorrhaphy and master the elements of the preperitoneal space. There is no doubt that the more proficient a surgeon is in either of these techniques the fewer complications they will encounter. A recent study examining the experience of the surgeon demonstrated that surgeon age (>45 years old) and laparoscopic inexperience were risk factors for recurrence; however, the only risk factor for recurrence in open mesh repairs was a PGY level <3 [54].

A meta-analysis performed in 2003 examined 41 facilities with a total of over 7,000 patients comparing open to laparoscopic herniorraphy. Operating time was longer for the laparoscopic groups. The rate of injury, both visceral and vascular, was higher in the laparoscopic groups but was consistent (<0.3%) for both groups. Return to work, postoperative pain and postoperative numbness were both significantly decreased in the laparoscopic group [55].

Figure 70.10 View of inguinal anatomy (printed with permission from Charles H. Booras, M.D., All about Inguinal Hernias: Symptoms and Causes 5/16/98 http://jaxmed.com/articles/surgery/inguinalhernia.htm).

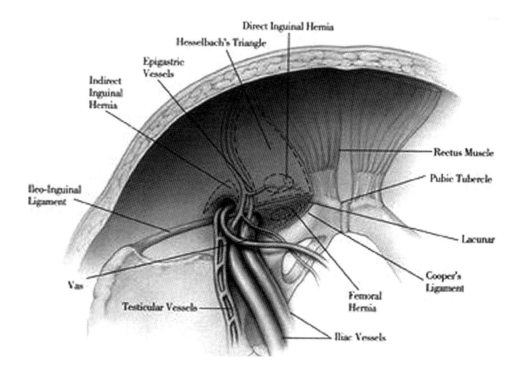

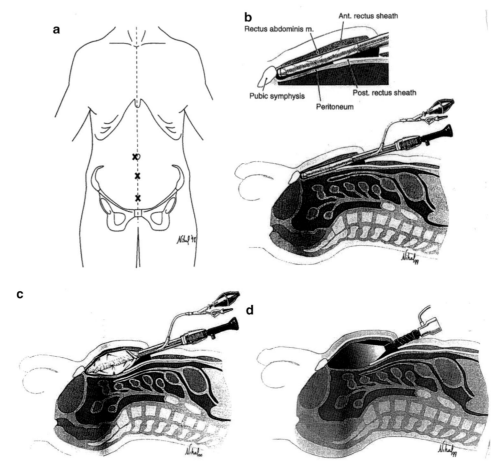

FIGURE 70.11 Use of balloon dissector during TEP repair (from Mulvihill; Surgery: Basic Science and Clinical Evidence; 2001, Chap. 43; Fig. 43.18, reprinted with kind permission of Springer Science + Business Media).

There are some significant disadvantages to the laparoscopic approach. Laparoscopic herniorrhaphy requires general anesthesia, is frequently performed by a transperitoneal route, is technically more difficult to understand and learn than mesh repairs, and in most hands, takes considerably longer. In comparisons of anesthetic techniques for open hernia repair, general anesthesia in the elderly is associated with far higher complication rates than local anesthesia. Therefore, the need for general anesthesia alone could obviate most of the benefits of the laparoscopic approach in some elderly patients. In addition, the transperitoneal route exposes the patient to the risk of inadvertent bowel injury, which in any age group could be devastating. Although the increased time to return to full activity may be an important consideration in a young person, the length of recovery may not be as important in old patients so long as mobility is not significantly compromised. Postoperative pain after the tension-free open approach is rarely severe enough to curtail activity.

There are a paucity of studies specifically involving the elderly population and laparoscopic hernia repair. One study evaluated 110 patients over 65 years old with an ASA of either 2 or 3. Operative time was longer than that for open repairs;

however, return to work was similar. Fifteen percent of patients experienced complications, the overwhelming majority of which were urinary retention. There was an alarmingly high recurrence rate of 9.7%. Hospital length of stay correlated with ASA status, but recurrences, complications, and return to activities did not [56]. Though the overall conclusion of this paper was that laparoscopic hernia repair in the elderly was safe, there was no assertion that it was in fact superior to open

CASE STUDY: PART 6

The veteran decided to postpone his surgery but was then lost to follow-up. He returned to the Emergency Room 2 years later stating that his hernia is now "stuck out" he is having significant pain from it. He cannot remember the last time he had a bowel movement. On exam, his hernia is incarcerated, and due to some crythema over his groin there is concern for strangulation. He is taken urgently to the operating room.

repair in this population. A review of laparoscopic surgery in geriatric patients reached the same conclusions [57]. It is clear that until further investigation is performed, laparoscopic hernia repair in the elderly should be reserved for the most experienced surgeons and the most appropriate patients, those with lower ASA status and recurrent or bilateral hernias.

Emergency Repair

The consequences of emergency surgery in the elderly population cannot be understated. There is a threefold increase in morbidity and mortality after emergent operation, regardless of the type of procedure [58]. Accordingly, there is also an increase in the need for intensive care and extended hospital stay in these patients, as well as rehabilitative services.

A representative study reports incidence of incarcerated inguinal hernia as 16.8% in patients over age 65, compared to only 4.4% in younger patients [59]. Unfortunately, acute incarceration and the sequela, strangulation, are also less well tolerated in the elderly. Strangulation occurs when the blood supply to the incarcerated organ becomes occluded at the neck of the hernia sac. Initially there is venous compression with subsequent edema, venous occlusion, and eventually arterial occlusion. Strangulation occurs in 1.3–3.0% of all groin hernias, most often in the elderly and children [60]. Indirect inguinal and femoral hernias are the most likely hernias to strangulate. The probability that an indirect inguinal hernia will strangulate is reported as 2.8% within 3 months of diagnosis and 4.5% after 2 years, compared to 22% at 3 months and 45% at 21 months for femoral hernias [61].

Kuleh et al. examined risk factors for strangulation and bowel resection in elderly patients with acutely incarcerated hernias. In examining 189 patients over 65 years old, it was found that femoral hernias were more frequently strangulated and required bowel resection at presentation. Although males were more likely to present with incarcerted hernias, females were likely to have strangulated hernias, possibly due to the increase in femoral hernias in this population. Late admission was also a significant risk factor for strangulation, bowel resection, and hospital stay. Morbidity increased from 15 to 33% when admission was delayed 48 h after symptoms began, and mortality increased from 2 to 9%. ASA status >3 was only a risk factor for prolonged hospital stay and morbidity but not mortality [11].

The approach to an incarcerated hernia in the elderly depends on the nature of the incarceration. Chronic incarcerations pose less of a threat of strangulation and can be treated on an elective basis. Acute incarcerations, on the other hand, require immediate surgical treatment. Forceful attempts at nonoperative reduction may result in an en masse reduction of a compromised loop of intestine within the hernia sac. This ischemic bowel may not produce significant abdominal findings in the older patient until full-thickness necrosis and perforation occur. Any patient with skin changes or systemic symptoms – tachycardia, hypotension, fever, leukocytosis, or lactic acidosis – should raise suspicion for progression to strangulation.

The type of repair for incarcerated hernias depends to some extent on the viability of the contents of the hernia sac. A general or regional anesthetic is usually necessary. In the presence of inflammation, local anesthetic agents are usually not effective. In addition, the muscle relaxation provided by regional or general anesthesia may facilitate reduction of the incarcerated organ. If the incarceration is of short duration and there is no erythema or induration of the overlying skin suggesting strangulation, the choice of approach is less critical. Open anterior repair, which allows careful inspection of the sac contents outside the peritoneal cavity, is usually preferred. Frequently, a recently incarcerated hernia is reduced spontaneously or with minimal force when anesthesia is induced. In this setting, identifying the incarcerated loop of bowel through the hernia defect may be difficult but is usually not impossible. Skilled laparoscopists may prefer to inspect the bowel and repair the hernia laparoscopically through a transperitoneal approach. A recent study examining TAPP repair of 28 strangulated inguinal hernias demonstrated a conversion to open rate of 10.7%, for either extensive adhesions or bowel distention. Morbidity was only 4% and there were no deaths or recurrences [62]. The same precautions mentioned previously for laparoscopic herniorrhaphy should be considered here.

If the incarceration is of longer duration or there are signs of local inflammation suggestive of strangulation, an open procedure is safest and most expeditious. Many surgeons prefer a direct anterior approach to the hernia. If ischemic bowel is found in the hernia sac, resection can generally be accomplished through the hernia defect. The not infrequent need to use synthetic materials to repair the hernia defect in the presence of dead bowel creates a difficult clinical dilemma. Every attempt is then made to repair the defect with tissue rather than synthetic material, accepting the higher risk of recurrence in exchange for a lower chance for infection. Others advise that if there is high suspicion for compromised bowel preoperatively, a small lower midline laparotomy or laparoscopy should be performed for more careful inspection of the bowel and a more controlled resection. After the abdomen is closed, an open anterior repair of the hernia with mesh can be accomplished through a reprepared field.

A new innovation in hernia repair is the use of acellular dermal matrix. Most often made of cadaveric or porcine skin, these biologics are composed entirely of basement membrane and collagen bundles. They are highly resistant to infection and have been used for the repair of ventral hernias for years. They are uniquely helpful when there is compromised bowel and the potential for contamination. A small retrospective study examined 12 patients with strangulated hernias and contaminated operative fields where bio-prosthesis (specifically Alloderm™) was used. Two patients developed superficial wound infections that were treated conservatively and in a short follow-up there were no recurrences [63]. This may represent a viable option in elderly patients with compromised bowel to avoid further infectious complications.

CASE STUDY: PART 7

The veteran underwent a mesh repair of his incarcerated hernia and did not require bowel resection. He followed up in clinic for a few months but once again became lost to follow-up. He called the general surgery clinic 3 years later to say he thought his hernia was back. The resident on call reminds him of the signs and symptoms of incarceration and makes an appointment for him the following week.

Recurrence

When performing hernia repairs, the primary focus of success is determined by the incidence of recurrence. There is a wide variation in the time frame over which recurrences are reported. There is, however, general agreement that follow-up should be at regular intervals and recurrence determined by direct examination rather than by patient report. Hernias recur for one or more reasons: tension on the tissues created by the repair, inherent abnormalities in collagen that predispose to the development of new hernias, an unrecognized second hernia component at the time of the initial repair (usually a small indirect component), and technical error.

Hernia recurrences can be classified as early or late. Most early recurrences are due to undue tension on the repair. For instance, when a hernia is due to a defect of the musculofascial abdominal wall, covering the defect with endogenous tissues results in suturing together tissues that are not normally juxtaposed. This then subjects these structures to undue tension [64]. Suture lines under tension exhibit an inadequate fibroblastic response for healing, which results in a weak scar and a subsequent recurrence of the hernia. Furthermore, these suture lines are subject to the same degenerative process that resulted in the initial herniation. The increasing use of tension-free repairs has significantly reduced this type of recurrence.

Late recurrences are usually due to missed components or new hernias at the site of a previous repair or in a new location. This type of recurrence is more appropriately termed

reherniation. Following a mesh repair, reherniation occurs because the mesh was not sutured in place or it was not of sufficient size to cover beyond the inguinal floor. Progression of tissue degeneration is of great concern and can be compensated for by placing a large sheet of mesh underneath the external oblique aponeurosis well beyond Hesselbach's triangle. This dissection is extensive but can be necessary, particularly in some patients with severe tissue loss. This is of particular importance when performing a preperitoneal or laparoscopic repair. Appropriate and extensive dissection of the entire myopectineal orifice is necessary to facilitate choosing the right size mesh and performing appropriate fixation. The most common causes of failure are mesh size being too small or inappropriate fixation either infero-medially or infero-laterally [65, 66]. Another study found that the vast majority of recurrences after laparoscopic herniorrhaphy were medial. For this reason a large piece of mesh should be chosen, sufficient enough to cross the midline with multiple tacks in the pubic tubercle and Cooper's Ligament (Fig. 70.12). Bilateral hernias should be managed with a single piece of mesh, large enough to cover both groins, the so-called bikini repair [67].

Risk factors for recurrence of hernias are similar to those for the formation of primary hernias. It would stand to reason that the elderly would be more susceptible to recurrence because of an increased risk of those factors already known to cause hernias: Obesity, chronic cough, constipation, bladder outlet obstruction, and general degradation of tissue. Age >50 has been shown to be an independent risk factor as well. Those undergoing repair for a recurrent hernia are at greater

---

CASE STUDY: PART 8

The veteran was an appropriate candidate for a laparoscopic repair and during his TAPP repair was noted to have a small indirect hernia on the opposite side. Both the recurrence and the incidental hernia were repaired laparoscopically with mesh.

CASE STUDY: PART 9

Two weeks after the above-mentioned laparoscopic repair, the patient is still complaining of significant pain. Rather than incisional, his pain shoots down his medial thigh. On physical exam there is no evidence of occurrence or infection, but there is significant numbness in the skin over his thigh.

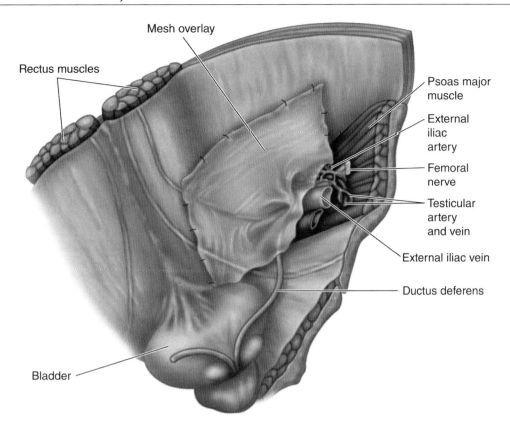

FIGURE 70.12 Appropriate placement of mesh in a laparoscopic hernia repair (from Online Laparoscopic Technical Manual, Laparoscopic Inguinal-Femoral Hernia Repair, Step 5, Deploying and Anchoring the Mesh; http://www.laparoscopy.net/inguinal/ingher11.htm).

risk for recurrence than those undergoing a primary repair, as are those with two or more relative who also suffered from a recurrence [68].

Inguinodynia

As recurrence rates continue to decrease with advances in inguinal hernia repair techniques, a greater emphasis is being placed on other complications of the surgery. The most common is inguinodynia or inguinal pain. Although not proven, the potential causes include partial transection or entrapment of a nerve, which eventually leads to neuroma formation and chronic pain. In an open repair the most common nerves involved are the ilioinguinal, iliohypogastric and genital branch of the genitofemoral nerve. All three of these nerves supply sensation to the genitals and medial upper thigh. Refer to the previous section on anesthesia for a more in-depth discussion of this anatomy. The nerves most commonly injured during laparoscopic herniorrhaphy are the lateral femoral cutaneous nerve (supplying the upper lateral thigh), and the femoral branch of the genitofemoral nerve (supplying the skin over the femoral triangle). These nerves lie near each other in a space nicknamed the "triangle of pain" (Fig. 70.13).

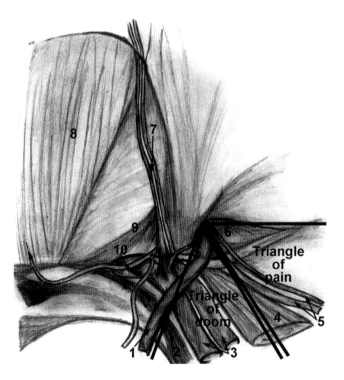

FIGURE 70.13 Triangles of doom and pain – representing where injuries to vessels and nerves occur, respectively, during a laparoscopic inguinal hernia repair (from [92] © Moore and Hasenboehler; licensee BioMed Central Ltd. Available from: http://www.pssjournal.com/content/1/1/3).

A study from the Swedish Hernia register examined 3,000 patients undergoing unilateral primary hernia repair. All techniques (tissue, mesh, laparoscopic) were examined. Overall 30% of patients were still experiencing pain over a year after surgery and 6% were having significant enough pain to impair their activities of daily life. Risk factors for inguinodynia included age, with those >59 years old having significantly less pain than those younger (21 vs. 33%). Patients having pain prior to their operation were more likely to continue to experience pain afterwards. Operative technique was also important. Anterior approaches, either tissue repair or mesh repair, had the highest incidence (~30%), whereas preperitoneal repair, either open or laparoscopic, had a significantly lower incidence (~20%) [69].

During an open repair careful dissection and identification of all the nerves is the best way to avoid injury. If injury is already suspected, complete transection of the nerve is preferable. During laparoscopic repair careful dissection is also important, as well as judicious tack placement avoiding the "triangle of pain." Some have advocated not securing the mesh, which effectively alleviates this problem [23]. Recent studies have advocated prophylactic ilioinguinal neurectomy during open hernia repair. A double-blind randomized study showed a significant reduction in groin pain in the neurectomy group (8 vs. 28%) without any difference in postoperative numbness [70].

Patients suffering from injury to these nerves typically have pain in the immediate postoperative period, which intensifies over the next few weeks. In most cases it will regress over 2 months. Initial management consists of injections of local anesthetic and corticosteroids, as well as analgesics and anti-convulsants. In refractory cases the surgical treatment of choice is a triple neurectomy of the ilioinguinal, iliohypogastric, and genitofemoral nerves. This has shown 85% complete resolution and 15% partial resolution of pain in some case series [71].

CASE STUDY: PART 10

Initial conservative management with anti-inflammatory medications fail to alleviate the veterans pain. He is seen again 1 month later and lidocaine injection is prescribed. At 6 month follow-up his pain has been largely relieved and his quality of life has returned to normal.

Other Hernias

Although groin hernias are by far the most common, there are several other types of hernias that are also of concern in the elderly: some because of the frequency and technical challenge they present, and others because they are relatively uncommon and are not discovered until they incarcerate.

Incisional Hernias

Incisional hernias in the elderly are common and can often be challenging to repair. The incidence of hernias in patients with a midline surgical incision is 2–11% [72]. The etiology of these hernias is often multifactorial. Wound infection, suture failure, malnutrition, increased age, obesity, excessive straining, smoking, ascites or peritoneal dialysis, chemotherapy, steroids, and tension on the wound closure are factors that have been implicated. The symptoms of incisional hernia often begin with a noticeable bulge in a previously healed incision. Incarceration is the presenting symptom in 17% of patients leading to a perioperative mortality rate three times higher than that for elective repair [73].

Technically, these hernias may be challenging for several reasons. First, it is possible for most of the abdominal contents to become a fixed part of the hernia, which may result in a decrease in the intra-abdominal compartment volume. This in turn complicates complete reduction of the contents at the time of repair. This is known as a loss of domain. Second, the defects are usually multiple, reflecting failure of wound healing throughout the length of the incision. Identifying all the defects in the "Swiss cheese"-type abdominal wall and freeing all of the underlying adhesions may be tedious and time-consuming. Finally, extreme care must be exercised not to enter the bowel lumen during dissection because most incisional hernias are large and require synthetic materials for repair without tension. Biologic materials mentioned previously are now used to repair these hernia defects, especially in the presence of the contaminated operative field. They may also be used to overlay primary repairs to provide additional stability to weakened tissues, not uncommon to the elderly.

Laparoscopic techniques are being used with increased frequency to repair these large defects. Unlike laparoscopic inguinal hernia repair, there is a clear benefit to utilizing this technique in elderly patients, as long as preexisting comorbidities does not preclude the use of laparoscopic techniques. A recent meta-analysis shows that operative times are similar between open and laparoscopic groups while complications and hospital length of stay were significantly decreased in the laparoscopic group [74].

Umbilical Hernias

The umbilical hernia was first noted in 1 AD by the Hindu physician Charaka, who mistakenly believed it to be an abdominal tumor. The treatment of umbilical hernia has run the gamut from external compression devices to amputation. Umbilical hernias occur in 10–30% of live births but defects <2 cm are likely to close spontaneously. When repairs become necessary they are performed primarily. In adults, umbilical hernias occur through an umbilical canal that is bordered by the umbilical fascia, the linea alba, and the two rectus sheaths [75]. Because of the tight limitations of this canal, this type of hernia is apt to incarcerate and strangulate. For years the "vest over pants" method of repair as first described by Mayo was the standard of care. As with inguinal hernias, mesh repairs have begun to supplant primary repairs. There are a variety of meshes available, from simple sheets, to plugs and a combination of the two. Studies have shown that while complication rates between primary and mesh repairs are similar, recurrence rates are vastly lower in mesh repairs, 1% compared to 11% for primary repairs [76].

Umbilical hernias are common in cirrhotic patients and in those with ascites of other etiologies because of the increased intra-abdominal pressure against a thinned umbilical ring and fascia. An incidence as high as 24% has been reported in this patient population [77]. Umbilical hernia is also an important consideration in patients on peritoneal dialysis. Dialysis must be interrupted and ascites controlled prior to repair to decrease the incidence of recurrence. There are significant difficulties in closing this type of hernia, in order to prevent complications such as ascitic leak, wound infection and recurrence. Therefore every effort should be made to avoid strangulation and protect the thin skin over the defect. When necessary, these hernias may be repaired under local or regional anesthesia. Primary repair is optimal, but occasionally a prosthetic or biologic material is needed for tension-free closure.

Richter's Hernia

A partial enterocele is a form of hernia that bears the name Richter's hernia after August Gottlieb Richter, who first described it in 1785. This hernia is unique because only one side of the bowel wall becomes entrapped in the hernia defect (Fig 70.14). The classic signs and symptoms of small bowel obstruction that usually accompany incarceration are absent. The first indication of the incarceration may not become apparent until strangulation and necrosis occur. There is some concern that the incidence of Richter's hernia may be

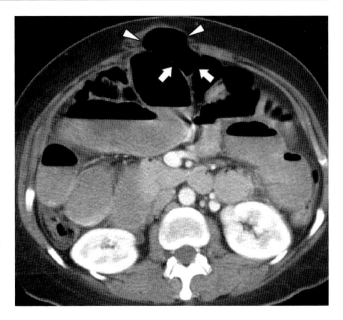

Figure 70.14 Richter's hernia (from [93], reprinted with permission of the American Journal of Roentgenology).

increasing as laparoscopic surgery becomes more prevalent. Small port-site hernias are the perfect size to involve only a small portion of the bowel [78].

Kadirov and associates reviewed 350 incarcerated hernias at their institution between 1977 and 1994 [79]. Of the 350 patients, 14 had Richter's-type hernias (4%). These 14 cases were compared to 14 non-Richter's incarcerated hernias matched for location of the hernia and the age and sex of the patient. The average patient's age was 69 years. In the Richter's group, there was a significantly longer delay to diagnosis and treatment (15.8 vs. 4.4 h). As a result of this delay, 50% of the Richter's hernias required bowel resection compared to only 7.1% of the non-Richter's incarcerations. Mortality reflected the degree of established sepsis by the time of operation, with 21.4% of Richter's patients dying; none of the non-Richter's patients succumbed. Imaging modalities add little to the diagnosis of a Richter's hernia. Only astute clinical examination and a high level of suspicion identify these hernias before devastating necrosis and perforation have occurred, especially devastating in the elderly population.

Obturator Hernias

Arnaud de Ronsil first described the obturator hernia in 1724 at the Royal Academy of Science in Paris. This hernia is rare, accounting for 0.05% of all hernias and 0.2% of bowel obstructions [80]. It is usually found in frail, elderly debilitated women, but may also be associated with profound weight loss in other groups. Obturator hernias may be bilateral or associated with hernias through the femoral canal. The obturator foramen, through which the hernia occurs, is the largest foramen in the body. The obturator membrane, however, occludes most of the foramen. The obturator canal consists of a 1–2 cm long and 1 cm wide opening in the superolateral part of the foramen. Usually, this canal is obliterated with fat, which prevents herniation of abdominal contents. In the frail and malnourished, this fat disappears and the potential space is unmasked.

A preoperative diagnosis is difficult because the complaints are not specific and the physical manifestations are minimal. A history of symptoms suggestive of intermittent or partial intestinal obstruction may be elicited. The Howship–Romberg sign – pain radiating down the medial aspect of the leg to the knee due to compression of the obturator nerve – is pathognomonic and is present in up to 50% of cases [23]. However, this sign is often overlooked in the elderly or attributed to other causes. The optimal way to look for an obturator hernia is with the patient supine and the thigh flexed, abducted, and externally rotated. The hernia mass is often concealed underneath the adductor muscles in the thigh. Occasionally, it is possible to feel a small mass on vaginal or rectal examination. The four indicators of obturator hernia – intestinal obstruction, Howship–Romberg sign, prior similar symptoms, a palpable mass on vaginal or rectal examination – are rarely seen together.

Ijiri and colleagues reviewed 17 obturator hernias [81]. There were 16 women and 1 man with an average age of 79.9 years (range 69–89 years) and an average body weight of 35 kg (range 25–43 kg). The average duration from onset of symptoms to surgery was 6 days (range 1–13 days). The diagnostic modalities ranged from computed tomography (CT) scans to exploratory laparotomy. The diagnosis of an obturator hernia was made in eight of eight cases when CT scan of the pelvis was performed (Fig. 70.15). An additional study showed that the use of CT decreased the time from symptoms to surgery by 3 days. In addition, bowel resection was performed half as often, and perioperative mortality decreased from 30 to 5%. This highlights not only the utility of CT scans in the diagnosis of obturator hernias but also the benefit of early diagnosis [82]. Others have supported the use of Ultrasonography, especially in the diagnosis of strangulation [83]. Even so diagnosis is only made prior to laparotomy in 10% of cases, and surgery should not be delayed while attempting to make the diagnosis.

Primary repair of an obturator hernia is impossible because the surrounding tissues are immobile. Some studies have reported using sac ligation alone or flaps of bladder, periosteum, uterine ligament, or rib cartilage to close the defect [84–86]. These repairs are unsuitable for large or bilateral hernias and may lead to postoperative pain and bladder dysfunction. A synthetic material is usually necessary. A plug system has been described as tension free

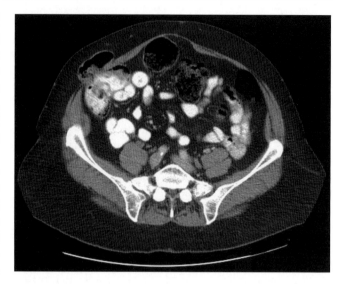

Figure 70.15 CT scan of obturator hernia (reprinted with permission from [91], Copyright © Radiological Society of North America. Available at: http://radiographics.rsnajnls.org/cgi/content-nw/full/21/2/341/F8).

and easy to perform; however, there is the potential for chronic obturator neuralgia [87]. If the diagnosis has been established preoperatively, the most suitable approach is an open preperitoneal repair, as described by Stoppa et al. [88]. With this repair, a large piece of mesh is placed extraperitoneally to cover both sides of the pelvic floor. If the viability of the incarcerated bowel is questioned once the hernia is reduced, the peritoneum may be opened. In the usual case where the diagnosis is not known preoperatively, an initial transabdominal approach with a preperitoneal mesh repair is optimal. The use of laparoscopic methods has also been described, but there is no current data supporting benefits of this approach.

Spigelian Hernias

The Spigelian hernia, another unusual abdominal wall hernia, is named for Adriaan van den Spiegel, who was the first to describe the semilunar line. The semilunar line is the demarcation from muscle to aponeurosis in the transversus abdominis muscle. Protrusion of a peritoneal sac, organ, or preperitoneal fat from its normal location through this aponeurosis, is termed a spigelian hernia. These hernias are usually superior to the inferior epigastric vessels. Once they enter Hesselbach's triangle, they are termed low Spigelian hernias. These hernias are often located within different aspects of the abdominal wall and may also be termed interparietal, interstitial, intermuscular, intramuscular, or intramural. Most Spigelian hernias occur in individuals 40 70 years of age.

The etiology of these hernias is most often related to the inherent weakness in the transversus abdominis aponeurosis. Increased intra-abdominal pressure further increases the incidence. Erect posture puts most of the pressure on the lower abdomen, which could be another cause of hernias in this region. In their earliest form, these hernias are small protrusions of fat or omentum with a peritoneal covering. They may progress to include more fat or even bowel. The symptoms are usually localized abdominal pain, although signs of obstruction or a palpable mass on the abdominal wall may occur.

The diagnosis is difficult in patients with defects too small to produce overt manifestations on the abdominal wall. It is best to examine patients by having them alternately tense and relax the abdominal wall.

Imaging studies are usually necessary to elucidate the source of the localized symptoms. Ultrasonography is a good method for determining a hernia orifice and locating hernia contents. CT scan may also be used to examine the abdominal wall, but the sections must be close together to enable localization of the hernia orifice. Helical CT scans may increase the diagnostic yield. The CT scans may also provide information about the hernia sac and the nature of the abdominal contents in the sac (Fig. 70.16).

When the hernia itself is palpable and open approach may be performed. There is often enough laxity in the surrounding tissues to allow for primary closure, although mesh can be used [23]. As with all hernia repairs there have been recent advances in the use of laparoscopic techniques for the repair of these hernias as well. A recent prospective randomized trial comparing open vs. extraperitoneal laparoscopic repair showed significant improvement in complications and hospital stay in the laparoscopic group [89].

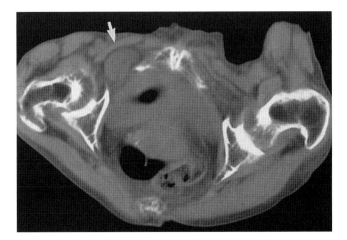

Figure 70.16 Preoperative CT showing Spigelian hernia (from [94]. Available at: http://www.rcsed.ac.uk/Journal/vol45_3/4530046.htm).

> **CASE STUDY: PART 11**
>
> Despite his complicated course, the veteran has ultimately returned to his normal level of activity. In follow-up he has had no further recurrences and he has had resolution of his inguinodynia.

Conclusions

Abdominal wall hernias in the elderly, whether common or unusual, are ultimately surgically correctable disorders. Recent studies have shown that watchful waiting is safe for asymptomatic or minimally symptomatic inguinal hernias. Other hernias wherein the fascial defect is large can also be managed nonoperatively if not symptomatic. Pain is frequently what leads the patient to operative repair.

Elective repair of inguinal hernias, in particular, is safe even in patients with significant co-morbidity. With local anesthesia and tension-free repairs, nearly all patients can ambulate immediately; and they can obtain excellent pain control with minimal oral pain medication. Complications are uncommon, and mortality is nearly zero in many large series. For elderly patients with significant co-morbidities, a complete preoperative evaluation of their fitness for surgery is in order.

Patients with chronically incarcerated hernias are not at significant risk for strangulation while those with an acute incarceration do have some risk of progressing to strangulation. Therefore, acutely incarcerated hernias present more of an urgent to emergent situation and surgical consultation early in the patient's course is of upmost importance.

Once strangulation has occurred, a hernia is no longer just a defect in the abdominal wall, and repair is not just patching the hole. The systemic consequences of bowel obstruction and ischemic tissue stress the limited reserves that define the physiologic state of the older patient. Once the inflammatory state is initiated, the cascade of events demands a response that the elderly are frequently unable to mount. Fluid and electrolyte imbalance, dehydration, and systemic sepsis become the major problems, and the mechanical issue of fixing the hernia defect fades in comparison. Morbidity and mortality rates soar.

For those hernias that are rare or the presentation more obscure, an increased level of awareness is necessary to avoid the consequences of incarceration. Although we may have to accept the higher complication rates that accompany the unusual hernia, we should never allow the common hernia to progress from a simple mechanical problem to a deadly systemic illness.

References

1. Rutkow IM (2003) Demographic and socioeconomic aspects of hernia repair in the United States in 2003. Surg Clin North Am 83:1045

2. Deysine M, Grimson R, Soroff HS (1987) Herniorrhaphy in the elderly: benefits of a clinic for the treatment of external abdominal wall hernias. Am J Surg 153:387–391

3. Primatesta P, Goldacre MJ (1996) Inguinal hernia repair: incidence of elective and emergency surgery, readmission and mortality. Int J Epidemiol 25:835–839

4. Fagan SP (2004) Abdominal wall anatomy: the key to a successful inguinal hernia repair. Am J Surg 188:3S–8S

5. Gilbert AI (1994) Pitfalls and complications of inguinal hernia repair. In: Arregui ME, Nagan R (eds) Inguinal hernia, advances or controversies? Radcliffe Medical, New York, pp 205–212

6. Zollinger RM Jr, Zollinger RM (1993) Atlas of surgical operations. McGraw Hill, New York, p 425

7. Nehme AE (1983) Groin hernias in the elderly patients: management and prognosis. Am J Surg 146:257–260

8. Ponka JL, Bush BE (1974) Experience with the repair of groin hernia in 200 patients aged 70 or older. J Am Geriatr Soc 22:18–24

9. Williams JS, Hale HW (1966) The advisability of inguinal herniorrhaphy in the elderly. Surg Gynecol Obstet 122:100–104

10. Argenta LC (2004) Basic science for surgeons. Saunders, Philadelphia

11. Kulah B (2001) Emergency hernia repairs in elderly patients. Am J Surg 182:455–459

12. Fitzgibbons R (2006) Watchful waiting vs repair of inguinal hernia in minimally symptomatic men: a randomized clinical trial. JAMA 295:285–292

13. Ryan EA (1982) An analysis of 313 consecutive cases of indirect sliding inguinal hernias. Surg Gynecol Obstet 154:704–706

14. van Wessem KJP (2003) The etiology on indirect inguinal hernias: congenital and/or acquired. Hernia 7:76–79

15. Hughson W (1925) The persistent or preformed sac in relation to oblique inguinal hernia. Surg Gynecol Obstet 41:610

16. Abrahamson J (1998) Etiology and pathophysiology of primary and recurrent groin hernia formation. Surg Clin North Am 78:953–972

17. Szczeny W (2006) Etiology of inguinal hernia: ultrastructure of rectus sheath revisted. Hernia 10:266–271

18. Pans A, Pierard GE (1998) Immunohistochemical study of the rectus sheath and transversalis fascia in adult groin hernias. Hernia 2(Suppl 1):13

19. Read RC (1998) The metabolic role in the attenuation of transversalis fascia found in patients with groin herniation. Hernia 2(Suppl 1):17

20. Green WW (1969) Bowel obstruction in the aged patient: a review of 300 cases. Am J Surg 118:541–545

21. Fenyo G (1974) Diagnostic problems of acute abdominal disease in the aged. Acta Chir Scand 140:396–405

22. Law NW (1992) Does a truss benefit a patient with inguinal hernia. Br Med J 304:6834

23. Alimoglu O (2005) Femoral hernia: a review of 83 cases. Hernia 10:70–73

24. Scott D (2001) Hernia and abdominal wall defects. In: Norton J (ed) Surgery: basic science and clinical evaluation. Springer, New York

25. Ekberg O (1983) Complications after herniography in adults. AJR Am J Roentgenol 140:491–495

26. Lilly MC (2002) Ultrasound of the inguinal floor for evaluation of hernias. Surg Endosc 16:659–662

27. Stroupe K (2006) Tension-free repair versus watchful waiting for men with asymptomatic or minimally symptomatic inguinal hernias: a cost-effective analysis. J Am Coll Surg 203:458–468

28. O'Dwyer P (2006) Observation or operation for patients with an asymptomatic inguinal hernia: a randomized clinical trial. Ann Surg 244:167–173

29. Avidan B (2004) Colorectal cancer screening in patients with an inguinal hernia: is it necessary? Gastrointest Endosc 59:369–373

30. Wan J (2002) Colonoscopic screening and follow-up for colorectal cancer in the elderly. World J Gastroenterol 8:267–269

31. Guillen J, Aldrete JA (1970) Anesthetic factors influencing morbidity and mortality of elderly patients undergoing inguinal herniorrhaphy. Am J Surg 120:760–763

32. Nordin D (2003) Local, regional, or general anesthesia in groin hernia repair: multicentre randomized trial. Lancet 362:853–858

33. van Reen RN (2008) Spinal or local anesthesia in lichtenstein hernia repair: a randomized controlled trial. Ann Surg 247:428–433

34. Ozgün H, Kurt MN, Kurt I, Cevikel MH (2002) Comparison of local, spinal and general anesthesia for inguinal herniorrhaphy. Eur J Surg 168:455–459

35. Amid PK (1994) Local anesthesia for inguinal hernia repair step-by-step procedure. Ann Surg 222:735–737

36. McGavin L (1909) The double filigree operation for the radical cure of inguinal hernia. Br Med J 2:357–363

37. Usher FC, Cogan JE, Lowry TI (1960) A new technique for the repair of inguinal and incisional hernias. Arch Surg 81:187–194

38. Usher FC, Hill JR, Ochsner JL (1959) Hernia repair with Marlex mesh: a comparison of techniques. Surgery 46:718–724

39. Usher FC (1970) The repair of incisional and inguinal hernias. Surg Gynecol Obstet 131:525–530

40. Lichtenstein IL, Shulman AG (1986) Ambulatory (outpatient) hernia surgery including a new concept: introducing tension-free repair. Int Surg 71:1–4

41. Nordin P (2002) Randomized trial of Lichtenstein versus Shouldice hernia repair in general surgery practice. Br J Surg 89:45–49

42. EU Hernia Trialists Collaberation (2002) Repair of groin hernias with synthetic mesh: meta analysis if randomized control trials. Ann Surg 235:322–332

43. Awad S (2004) Current approaches to hernia repair. Hernia 188:9S–16S

44. Dieter RA (1999) Mesh plug migration into scrotum: a new complication of hernia repair. Int Surg 84:57–59

45. Kugel RD (2003) The Kugel repair for groin hernias. Surg Clin North Am 83:1119–1139

46. Shroder DM (2004) Inguinal hernia recurrence following Kugel patch repair. Am Surg 70:132–136

47. Vironen J (2005) Randomized clinical trial of Lichtenstein patch or Prolene Hernia System for inguinal hernia repair. Br J Surg 93:33–39

48. Huang CS (2004) Prolene Hernia System compared with mesh plug technique: a prospective study of short- to mid-term outcomes in primary groin hernia repair. Hernia 9:167–171

49. Fitzgibbons RJ Jr, Salerno GM, Filipi CJ et al (1994) Laparoscopic intraperitoneal onlay mesh technique for the repair of an indirect inguinal hernia. Ann Surg 219:144–156

50. McKernan JB, Laws HL (1993) Laparoscopic repair of inguinal hernias using a totally extraperitoneal prosthetic approach. Surg Endosc 7:26–28

51. Ger R, Mishrick A, Hurwitz J et al (1993) Management of groin hernias by laparoscopy. World J Surg 17:46–50

52. Felix EL, Michas C (1993) Double-buttress laparoscopic herniorraphy. J Laparoendosc Surg 3:1–8

53. Feldman L (2005) Laparoscopic hernia repair. ACS Surgery: Principles and Practices 20:1–20

54. Neumayer LA (2005) Proficiency of surgeons in inguinal hernia repair: effect of experience and age. Ann Surg 242:344–348

55. McCormack K (2003) Laparoscopic techniques versus open techniques for inguinal hernia repair. Cochrane Database Syst Rev 1:CD 001785

56. Velasco JM (1998) Laparoscopic herniorraphy in the geriatric population. Am Surg 64:633–637

57. Efrom DT (2001) Laparoscopic surgery in older adults. J Am Geriatr Soc 49:658–663

58. Rosenthal RA (1998) Physiologic considerations in the elderly patient. In: Miller TA (ed) Modern surgical care, 2nd edn. Quality Medical, St. Louis, pp 1362–1384

59. Lewis DC, Moran CG, Vellacot KD (1989) Inguinal hernia repair in the elderly. J R Coll Surg Edinb 34:101–103

60. Wantz GE (1997) A 65 year old man with an inguinal hernia. JAMA 277:663–668

61. Gallegos NC, Dawson J, Jarvis M, Hobstey M (1991) Risk of strangulation in groin hernias. Br J Surg 78:1171–1173

62. Rebuffat C (2006) Laparoscopic repair of strangulated hernias. Surg Endosc 20:131–134

63. Albo D (2006) Decellularized human cadaveric dermis provides a safe alternative for primary inguinal hernia repair in contaminated surgical fields. Am J Surg 192:e12–e17

64. Wexler MJ (1997) Symposium on the management of inguinal hernias: overview; the repair of the inguinal hernia: 110 years after Bassini. Can J Surg 40:186–191

65. Felix E (1998) Causes of recurrence after laparoscopic hernioplasty. Surg Endosc 12:226–231

66. Lowham AS (1997) Mechanisms of hernia recurrence after preperitoneal mesh repair, traditional and laparoscopic. Ann Surg 225:422–431

67. Deans GT (2005) Recurrent inguinal hernia after laparoscopic repair: possible cause and prevention. Br J Surg 82:539–541

68. Junge K (2006) Risk factors related to recurrence in inguinal hernia repair: a retrospective analysis. Hernia 10:309–315

69. Franneby U (2006) Risk factors for long-term pain after hernia surgery. Ann Surg 244:212–219

70. Lik-Man M (2006) Prophylactic ilioinguinal neurectomy in open inguinal hernia repair: a double-blind randomized controlled trial. Ann Surg 244:27–33

71. Amid P (2007) New understanding of the causes an surgical treatment of postherniorrhaphy inguinodynia and orchalgia. J Am Coll Surg 205:381–385

72. Santora TA (1993) Incisional hernia. Surg Clin North Am 73:557–570

73. Heydorn WH (1990) A five year US Army experience with 36, 250 abdominal hernia repairs. Am Surg 56:596–600

74. Goodney PP (2002) Short-term outcomes of laparoscopic and open ventral hernia repair. Arch Surg 137:1161–1165

75. Blumberg NA (1980) Infantile umbilical hernia. Surg Gynecol Obstet 150:187

76. Arroyo A (2002) Randomized clinical trial comparing suture and mesh repair of umbilical hernia in adults. Br J Surg 88:1321–1323

77. Chapman CB, Snell AM, Rowntree L (1931) Decompensated portal cirrhosis: report of one hundred and twelve cases. N Engl J Med 97:237

78. Boughley J (2003) Richter's hernia in the laparoscopic era: four case reports and review of the literature. Surg Laparosc Endosc Percutan Tech 13:1

79. Kadirov S, Sayfan J, Friedman S, Orda R (1996) Richter's hernia: a surgical pitfall. J Am Coll Surg 182:60–62

80. Ziegler DW (1995) Obturator hernia needs a laparotomy, not a diagnosis. Am J Surg 170:67–68

81. Ijiri R, Kanamura H, Yokoyama H, Shirakawa M, Hashimoto H, Yoshino G (1996) Obturator hernia: the usefulness of computed tomography in diagnosis. Surgery 119:137–140

82. Kammori M (2004) Forty-three cases of obturator hernia. Am J Surg 187:549–552

83. Yokoyama T (1997) Preoperative diagnosis of strangulated obturator hernia using ultrasonography. Am J Surg 174:76–78

84. Short AR (1923) The treatment of strangulated obturator hernia. Br Med J 1:718

85. Franklin RH (1938) Obturator hernia. Lancet 1:721–722

86. Fakim A, Walker MA, Byrne DJ, Forrester JC (1991) Recurrent strangulated obturator hernia. Ann Chir Gynaecol 80:317–320

87. Bergstein JM (1996) Obturator hernia: current diagnosis and treatment. Surgery 119:133–136

88. Stoppa RE, Rives JL, Warlaumont CR et al (1984) The use of Dacron in the repair of hernias of the groin. Surg Clin North Am 64:269–285

89. Moreno-Egea A (2002) Open vs laparoscopic repair of spigelian hernias: a prospective randomized trial. Arch Surg 137:1266–1268

90. Middlebrook MR (1992) Sonographic findings in Richter's hernia. Gastrointest Radiol 17:229–230

91. Furukawa A, Yamasaki M, Furuichi K et al (2001) Helical CT in the diagnosis of small bowel obstruction. Radiographics 21:341–355

92. Moore JB, Hasenboehler EA (2007) Orchiectomy as a result of ischemic orchitis after laparoscopic inguinal hernia repair: case report of a rare complication. Patient Saf Surg 1:3

93. Aguirre DA, Casola G et al (2004) Abdominal wall hernias: MDCT findings. AJR Am J Roentgenol 183:681–690

94. Rehman JM, Seo'm CS, O'Dwyer PJ (2000) A case of a Spigelian hernia at an unusually high anatomical location. J R Coll Surg Edinb 46:196–197

Section IX
Hepatobiliary System

Chapter 71
Invited Commentary

Seymour I. Schwartz

Almost a decade has past since the original publication of this reference work. As the population continues to enjoy increasing longevity, the need to consider the unique elements in the surgical care of those advanced in years becomes more evident. As was the case in my previous commentary, the two major issues are the substitution of physiologic status for chronologic age as a criterion for undertaking the more extensive elective resections of the liver and pancreas, and the broader application of minimally invasive procedures.

Laparoscopic cholecystectomy remains the gold standard. This has led to surgical training issues; namely, providing residents with experience in performing open cholecystectomy. In reference to cholecystectomy, a new approach has been introduced. NOTES, Natural Orifice TransEndoscopic Surgery. Successful removal of the Gall bladder transendoscopically through the gastric wall remains a curiosity and has not gained broad enthusiasm. It is doubtful that it will. Endoscopic palliation of jaundice secondary to malignant obstruction of the extrahepatic bile ducts has become increasingly successful.

Symptomatic nonparasitic cysts of the liver are preferentially unroofed by laparoscopy. Similarly, smaller nonanatomic hepatic resections and segmentectomies are readily performed by minimally invasive techniques. With the introduction of improved techniques of hemostasis during transection of the hepatic parenchyma, laparoscopic resection with hand-assist has been extended to hemihepatectomy. In regard to resection for primary and, in some instances, secondary hepatic malignancies, the argument continues as to whether major resection or orthotopic transplantation is preferable. Another visible change related to hepatic pathology is the disappearance of surgical portal-systemic procedures, which have been replaced by trancscutaneous intrahepatic portal systemic shunts (TIPS). But one recent assessment indicates that the operation is preferable.

An increasing number of pancreaticoduodenectomies are being performed disregarding the nodal status and the involvement of the adjacent major veins suggesting that better palliation is achieved. This remains to be affirmed by irrefutable evidence. Distal pancreatic resection is readily performed laparoscopically and several series of laparoscopic pancreaticoduodenectomy have been reported.

Splenectomy, in the face of a normal sized or minimally enlarged spleen should be performed laparoscopically. In the case of splenectomy for hematologic disease and particularly Idiopathic Thrombocytopenic Purpura deliberate inspection of the peritoneal cavity to identify accessory spleens is mandated. The massively enlarged spleens associated with myeloproliferative disorders are more safely removed by open operation and these patients should be protected by the preoperative administration of anti-platelet-aggregating drugs.

S.I. Schwartz (✉)
Department of Surgery, University of Rochester,
Strong Memorial Hospital, Rochester, NY, USA
e-mail: Seymour_Schwartz@URMC.Rochester.edu

R.A. Rosenthal et al. (eds.), *Principles and Practice of Geriatric Surgery*,
DOI 10.1007/978-1-4419-6999-6_71, © Springer Science+Business Media, LLC 2011

Chapter 72
Hepatobiliary and Pancreatic Function: Physiologic Changes

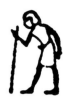

Vadim Sherman and F. Charles Brunicardi

Morphologic and physiologic changes in hepatolbiliary and pancreatic function observed in elderly persons

Parameter	Change with age	Functional impact
Liver		
Organ size (absolute and relative)	↓	No significant change?
Hepatocyte number	↓	↓ Metabolic function
Cell volume, ploidy, organelle constituents	↑	↓ Metabolic function
Hepatic blood flow	↓	↓ Metabolic function
Liver function tests	No change	No significant change?
Biliary system		
Bile duct size	↑	None
Gallbladder contractility	↓	↑ Gallstone incidence
Gallbladder absorptive capacity	No change	None
Cholecystokinin plasma levels	↑	No significant change?
Gallbladder cholecystokinin sensitivity	↓	No significant change?
Bile cholesterol saturation	↑	↑ Gallstone incidence
Pancreas		
Organ size	↓	None
Ductal size	↑	None
Acinar glands	↓	None
Exocrine function	?	None
β-Cell function	↓	↑ Incidence of glucose intolerance
Glucagon levels	↑?	↑ Incidence of glucose intolerance
Pancreatic polypeptide levels	↑	Unknown

↑, increased; ↓, decreased; ?, not proven or consistent

The normal variation in physiologic parameters of the hepatobiliary system and pancreas should be taken into account when managing an elderly patient. Appreciation of these alterations allows the surgeon to distinguish between expected physiologic variation and intercurrent pathophysiology in the clinical setting. A review of normal versus expected aging hepatobiliary and pancreatic physiology, as well as a review of select pathophysiology, will be presented in these organ systems.

V. Sherman (✉)
Department of Surgery, Baylor College of Medicine,
1709 Dreyden Suite 1500, Houston, TX 77030, USA
e-mail: vsherman@bcm.tmc.edu

Liver and Biliary System

Liver Anatomy

The liver is the largest solid organ in the body and is situated in the right upper quadrant of the abdomen. Protected by the thoracic cage, its borders extend from the level of the nipples to slightly below the costal margin. The horizontal axis spans the right hemidiaphragm and a portion of the left hemidiaphragm. The Couinaud nomenclature is currently accepted as the main classification system of liver anatomy, rather than historic classifications based on external topography (Fig. 72.1). The gross anatomical landmarks include the ligamentum teres (round ligament of the liver) which appears to divide the liver into a small left and larger right lobe. However, the anatomic classification divides the left and

Figure 72.1 Anatomic division
of the liver into right and left
lobes by the interlobar line of
Cantlie extending from the
gallbladder fossa to the inferior
vena cava. (From Feldman M
et al (eds) (2006) Sleisenger &
Fordtran's Gastrointestinal and
liver disease, 8th edn. Saunders,
Philadelphia. Reprinted with
permission from Elsevier).

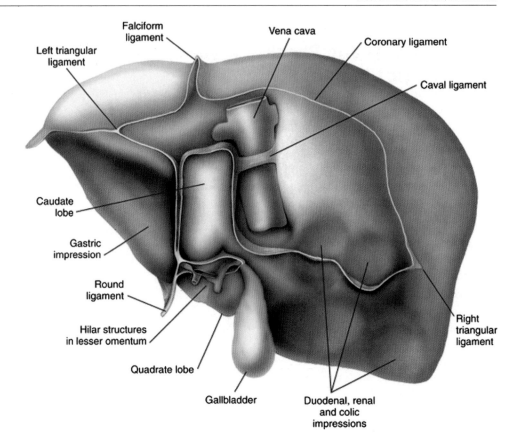

right lobe of the liver based on Cantlie's line, which represents the plane of the middle hepatic vein and the primary bifurcation of the portal vein. Cantlie's line can also be visualized as the plane extending from the gallbladder fossa to the inferior vena cava. The liver benefits from dual vascularization from the portal and systemic vasculature. The portal vein, hepatic artery, and biliary ductal system generally run in parallel, each bifurcating just before entry into the hilum and sending major branches to each hepatic lobe. Couinaud's functional anatomical classification divides the liver into eight segments according to the anatomic relation of portal vein and hepatic vein branches (Fig. 72.2) [1]. The right lobe is divided into an anterior and posterior segment by the right hepatic vein and the left lobe is divided into a medial and lateral segment by the left hepatic vein. The lobes are divided into their eight subsegments based on the transverse plane through the bifurcation of the portal vein.

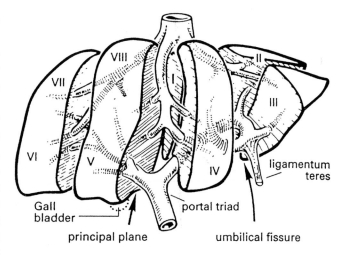

Figure 72.2 Hepatic segmental anatomy as defined by Couinaud, based on the anatomic relation of the portal vein and hepatic vein branches (reprinted with permission from Blumgart LH (ed) Surgery of the liver and biliary tract. Edinburgh: Churchill Livingstone, © Elsevier, 1994).

Hepatic Physiology

The liver is vital to a number of processes aimed at maintaining health and homeostasis. The functions of the liver include detoxification, protein synthesis, bile acid synthesis, storage of substances, and metabolism of proteins, carbohydrates, and lipids. Whether toxins originate internally or result from external sources, the liver is integral in filtering the toxins from the blood. Toxins are cleared through a series of enzymatic reactions that render the toxins water- or fat-soluble, thereby allowing for their secretion in urine or bile. The liver's production of bile further adds to the process of detoxification by providing a vehicle of export for various offending agents.

In addition to toxins, bile also transports bilirubin, cholesterol, bile salts, and phospholipids to the intestinal tract for excretion. Moreover, bile acids aid in the digestion of fats, thereby facilitating their absorption. Approximately 500–1,000 ml of bile is secreted per day. The amount of hepatocyte bile acid synthesis is the determining factor of the amount of secretion; however, additional secretion is aided by vagal stimulation, gastrin, secretin, and cholecystokinin (CCK) [1]. Once bile acids are excreted into the intestines, they undergo transformation into secondary bile acids. In the jejunum and ileum, these bile acids are then absorbed into the portal venous system and ultimately 90% are extracted by hepatocytes. This extremely efficient extraction of bile acids prevents their loss into the systemic circulation. The hepatocytes reconjugate the extracted product into the formation of new bile, thereby completing the circuit. This is referred to as the enterohepatic circulation of bile acids. The rate of new bile acid formation is therefore dependent on the rate of intestinal reabsorption and hepatocyte extraction. At the level of hepatocytes, bile is formed by the oxidation of cholesterol. The cholesterol secretion rate of the liver is dependent on the activity of two hepatocyte enzymes: 3-hydroxy-3-methylglutaryl coenzyme A (HMG-CoA) reductase, which catalyzes the rate-limiting step in the synthesis of cholesterol, and cholesterol 7-α-hydroxylase, which converts hepatic cholesterol to bile salts. Dietary intake and availability of lipoprotein carriers also affect cholesterol metabolism. Although insoluble in water, cholesterol remains soluble in bile if the relative concentrations of bile salts and phospholipids are maintained within certain limits. As first presented by Admirand and Small in 1968, the solubility characteristics of cholesterol are depicted by plotting the percentages of bile constituents on triangular coordinates [2] (Fig. 72.3). The area under the curve represents relative percentages of bile constituents that are required to maintain cholesterol in solution. If the relative percentages fall outside this area, supersaturation and crystallization of cholesterol can occur, which of course, can be a prelude to gallstone formation.

Carbohydrate metabolism is centered in the liver where it manages the surplus or deficit of metabolic fuels by engaging in storage or distribution of glucose. Both the liver and muscle are capable of glucose storage; however, only the liver is involved in the conversion of glycogen to glucose for systemic use. Other catabolic functions of the liver include gluconeogenesis and ketogenesis. Anabolic functions of the liver include glycogenesis and synthesis of plasma proteins, such as albumin, transferrin, haptoglobin, and numerous coagulation factors.

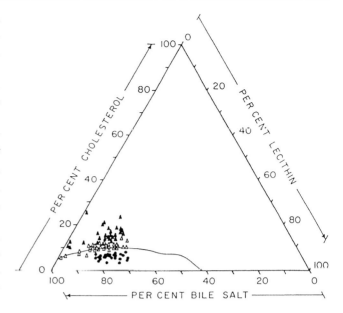

FIGURE 72.3 Triangular coordinates of the primary bile constituents for prediction of cholesterol solubility or crystallization. Any single point within the triangle represents a solution of bile with unique relative proportions of cholesterol, phospholipid (lecithin), and bile salt. Solutions represented by points under the curve are likely to maintain cholesterol in solution, whereas points above the curve are likely to represent solutions with cholesterol supersaturation and propensity to crystallization (reprinted with permission from Admirand and Small [2]).

Hepatic Function in the Elderly

Grossly, the change in liver size in elderly subjects is referred to as "brown atrophy." This brown discoloration is caused by accumulation of pigmented lipofuscin granules in hepatocytes and Kupffer cells. These granules are thought to be the depository of residues, predominantly exogenous dietary contaminants, that the liver cannot metabolize. Few studies have examined the structural and functional changes associated with normal liver aging. The pertinent morphologic and physiologic changes are summarized in the physiology table at the beginning of this chapter. On average, liver weight is decreased 6.5% in males and 14.3% in females [3]. The absolute number of hepatic lobules remains constant, but they undergo a decrease in the size of each lobule. Consequently, the number of hepatocytes decreases, yet each hepatocyte assumes an increased volume. Postmortem liver tissue analysis in subjects over 60 years old demonstrates decreased microsomal enzyme activity and a decreased hepatic concentration of smooth endoplasmic reticulum [4]. Furthermore, the number of mitochondria per hepatocyte decreases with age [5]. Although these are not significant changes on their own, when coupled with a decreased hepatic blood flow, this may account for a reduced capacity for metabolism of certain drugs and toxins. Hepatic blood flow, measured with dye clearance tests, shows a corresponding decrease with age at an estimated 0.3–1.5% decline per year. Reduced blood flow is attributed to the diminution of hepatic parenchymal mass with aging. As a result of this decline, individuals aged 65 years have 40–45% less total hepatic blood flow than they had at age 25 [6].

Examination of human and rat hepatocytes has provided insight into mechanisms of impaired drug metabolism by the aging liver. Hepatocytes isolated from young and old rats and humans demonstrated no difference in rates of oxidative phase I drug metabolism and phase II conjugation reactions [7]. In contrast, in vivo rates of oxidative phase I drug metabolism was impaired in older rats, yet glucuronidation was preserved [8]. A possible explanation for these observations is that older animals experience a degree of hypoxia. The decreased oxygen delivery may be a result of the creation of a diffusion barrier secondary to pseudocapillarization of hepatic sinusoids. The sinusoids of older rats has been found to have thicker endothelium and increased deposition of type IV collagen. Therefore, the pseudocapillarization and subsequent relative hypoxia in older rats may have implications for elderly humans. That is, this finding may impact drug therapy in the elderly, specifically those drugs whose clearance involves undergoing oxidative metabolism [9].

Despite the morphologic changes the liver undergoes with normal aging, the great functional reserve of this organ allows little or no clinical impairment. Several studies have documented that standard liver function tests (LFTs) do not vary significantly with increasing age alone [3, 10, 11]. Therefore, presence of abnormal liver chemistries in the elderly should not be considered normal and investigation of possible hepatobiliary disease should be undertaken. Regardless, standard LFTs – including serum bilirubin, aminotransferases, and alkaline phosphatase – do not reflect the true dynamic function of the liver. Evaluation of dynamic hepatic function requires measuring clearance of anionic dyes, such as sodium sulfobromophthalein (Bromsulphthalein or BSP) and ^{131}I-rose bengal, or various drugs that require hepatic microsomal enzyme activity. Prior studies investigating hepatic clearance or retention in the elderly have been controversial and conflicting, requiring control for multiple comorbid diseases, medications, and decreased hepatic blood flow [10, 12, 13]. To date, the most definitive study is that of Kampmann and associates, which demonstrated no significant variation in retention of anionic dyes in 43 carefully-selected patients aged 50–88 years when compared with younger persons [11]. Patients who were obese, alcoholic, receiving potentially hepatotoxic medicines, or showing evidence of renal, hepatic, or bone disorders were excluded from this study. Additionally, liver biopsies were performed in all patients to rule out hepatic pathology that could secondarily elevate dye retention rates, such as fatty degeneration, cirrhosis, or chronic hepatitis.

Although the liver is prone to the aging process, the changes it undergoes are less significant than those seen in other organ systems. Studies in old rats have demonstrated that although hepatic regeneration following hepatectomy is slower, these livers will eventually achieve their original volume [14]. In humans, clinical data has also demonstrated the longevity of aging livers through results garnered from liver transplants. Five patients whose transplanted livers were from donor patients over 80 years old experienced similar clinical outcomes to the group ($n=35$) that received livers from patients under 80 years old [15]. In terms of function, synthesis of most hepatic proteins remains intact with some impaired catabolism. Also, the activities of certain hepatic enzymes necessary for cholesterol metabolism are thought to be affected by the aging process. These age-related changes in hepatic enzyme activity may well be contributing factors in the pathogenesis of gallstone formation in the elderly.

Biliary Anatomy

After being secreted by the hepatocyte, bile drains along canaliculi that form into progressively larger intrahepatic ducts. These continue to coalesce within each lobe to form the right and left lobar ducts, which then exit the hilum and join to form the common hepatic duct (CHD). The CHD, in its course to the intestine, becomes the common bile duct (CBD) once it joins with the cystic duct from the gallbladder. The gallbladder is a pear-shaped, blind-ended, organ lying on the inferior surface of the liver that receives and drains bile through the cystic duct. The CBD then courses toward the second portion of the duodenum, where it empties into the ampulla of Vater within the duodenal wall. Shortly before entering the duodenum, the CBD also joins with the pancreatic duct, although variations to this anatomy are common. The sphincter of Oddi is a complex muscular structure surrounding the distal portions of the CBD, main pancreatic duct, and ampulla of Vater that is separate from the duodenal musculature. This sphincter coordinates appropriate release of biliary and pancreatic secretions during a meal while preventing harmful reflux of duodenal contents into the CBD.

Biliary Physiology

The purpose of the gallbladder is to store and concentrate bile during the fasting state. Following ingestion of a meal, the secretion of gastrointestinal hormones such as secretin, gastrin, and CCK results in the release of bile from the gallbladder into the intestinal tract. Although the gallbladder generally holds only 40–50 ml of bile, its remarkable absorptive capacity allows it to accommodate the 500–1,000 ml of bile produced by the liver each day [1]. The electrolyte and water content of bile secreted from the liver is modified during passage through the extrahepatic biliary system by the biliary ductal epithelium. In comparison, the mucosa of the gallbladder results in significantly more efficient absorption of sodium and water than cholesterol and calcium. The active transport of sodium leads to passive absorption of water, yet each is more significant than the gallbladder's capacity to reabsorb calcium. As the concentration of calcium increases in bile, it also affects the solubility of cholesterol. In turn, the increased concentrations of cholesterol and calcium may result in precipitation and creation of gallstones.

Between meals, the gallbladder passively fills with bile that is continuously produced and pumped into the extrahepatic biliary system. With the sphincter of Oddi contracted, the pressure within the common bile duct increases above that of the gallbladder lumen, thereby facilitating passive movement of bile into the cystic duct. Periodically, a small amount of bile (10–30%) is released from the gallbladder. This process of partial emptying and filling seems to be coordinated with late phase II and phase III activity of the gastrointestinal migrating myoelectric complex (MMC), which is associated with increases in plasma concentrations of the hormone motilin [16]. The turnover of gallbladder bile during fasting may serve as a mechanism to prevent or expel cholesterol crystals prior to macroscopic stone formation.

Following a meal of fatty acids or amino acids, vagal stimulation and CCK result in contraction of the gallbladder and the release of approximately 50–70% of the stored bile. The presence of intraluminal gastric acid, fatty acids, and certain amino acids triggers the release of CCK from epithelial cells in the proximal intestine, primarily in the duodenum. In addition to the release of bile from the gallbladder, CCK also impacts the contraction and relaxation of the sphincter of Oddi. This coordinated reflex allows the flow of bile and pancreatic juice into the duodenum to aid in the digestive process. At physiologic levels, CCK seems to influence vagal cholinergic innervation of the gallbladder by means of CCK-A receptors on postganglionic neurons [17]. This neurohumoral interaction may provide control of basal gallbladder smooth muscle tone and coordination of postprandial gallbladder contraction.

Biliary Function in the Elderly

The gallbladder undergoes minor changes with aging. There is little effect on size, contractility, or absorptive capacity. The effect of a decreased responsiveness to CCK may not have clinical significance. Khalil et al. demonstrated that gallbladder sensitivity to CCK decreases with age, but

fasting and fat-stimulated plasma levels of CCK are significantly higher in older individuals. These physiologic alterations appear to offset each other functionally, as the rate of gallbladder emptying in the elderly is similar to that of younger individuals [18]. The age-related increase in serum concentration of pancreatic polypeptide may also depress gallbladder emptying; however, the data to date is conflicting and further studies are needed to clarify the role of this hormone in hepatobiliary function in the elderly [19].

The most significant age-related change involving the hepatobiliary system involves the common bile duct. Namely, the duct increases in size, in a similar fashion to the pancreatic duct. One study by Nagase and associates used intravenous cholangiography to measure the CBD size in 84 healthy Japanese persons and documented a mean diameter of 9.2 mm at age 70 compared to 6.8 mm at age 20 [20]. Other studies have confirmed the upper normal size of the CBD as 10 mm in patients over 75 years old and 14 mm postcholecystectomy [21]. The distal portion of the CBD and the sphincter of Oddi become progressively narrower with age, possibly predisposing to stone impaction. Biliary obstruction in older adults is usually due to malignancy rather than to choledocholithiasis. The most common malignancy is adenocarcinoma of the pancreas but may be caused by other malignancies such as ampullary, gallbladder, bile duct, duodenal, and metastatic cancers. Benign strictures can result from cholangitis or common duct injuries. Primary sclerosing cholangitis is rare in those older than 65 years of age.

Gallstone Pathogenesis

Gallstone disease is a significant health-care problem in the United States, with an overall prevalence of 10–12%, translating to 25–30 million people. Risk factors for gallstone development include female sex, obesity, ethnicity, and age [22]. Epidemiological studies have shown that cholesterol gallstones occur infrequently in adolescence and the presence increases linearly with age (Table 72.1) [23–27]. The incidence of gallstones increases approximately 1–3% per year [28]. Recent studies have indicated that the incidence of gallstones in females approaches 50% by age 70 [29]. In fact, the most common abdominal operation performed in the geriatric population is cholecystectomy, with the total number of cases performed annually for nonfederal inpatients 65 years of age and over approximating 161,000 [30]. Furthermore, the risk of complications from gallstone disease is increased in elderly patients, with an increased incidence of CBD obstruction, perforation, and gangrene [31].

As discussed earlier, gallstone formation is dependent on relative concentrations of cholesterol, calcium, and other

Table 72.1 Prevalence of gallstones at autopsy in women in various countries

Age (Years)	Prevalence of gallstones (%)			
	UK [14]	USA [15]	Sweden [16]	Chile [17]
10–19	–	0	–	7.2
20–29	6.8	4.2	14.3	25.1
30–39	–	8.6	16.7	26.4
40–49	9.7	12.1	15.0	46.5
50–59	28.0	23.3	27.6	55.6
60–69	31.5	27.5	40.0	65.3
70–79	33.6	30.6	52.7	63.7
80–89	42.6	34.9	51.9	77.1
90+	42.7	44.4	58.4	–

Sources: Data from Bateson [23], Lieber [24], Lindström [25], and Marinovic et al. [26]

The table illustrates the geographic variation of gallstone disease and increasing prevalence with advancing age

Table 72.2 Factors contributing to cholesterol gallstone formation

Cholesterol supersaturation
  Cholesterol hypersecretion
  Diminished bile acid pool
  Ileal disease or resection
Nucleation
  Mucin glycoproteins
  Pronucleating substances: phospholipase C, fibronectin
  Nucleation-inhibiting substances: apolipoprotein A1
  Calcium concentration
Gallbladder dysmotility
  Altered cholecystokinin (CCK) plasma levels or receptors
  Neurohumoral influences: CCK somatostatin, estrogen
  Vagolysis, mechanical or functional

biliary solutes. Gallstones are classified according to their cholesterol content as either cholesterol stones or pigment stones. Pigment stones are further classified as black or brown. In the United States, gallstones are most commonly composed of cholesterol (70–80%) with pigment stones accounting for the remaining 20–30% [1].

Cholesterol Gallstone Pathogenesis

Three independent but mutually inclusive processes appear to be necessary for gallstone formation are as follows: (1) cholesterol supersaturation, (2) nucleation (also known as crystallization), and (3) stone growth. As previously mentioned, cholesterol is a highly hydrophobic molecule requiring appropriate relative concentrations of bile salts and phospholipids to remain soluble in bile. These biliary solutes are arranged in cholesterol–phospholipid vesicles and mixed micelles when in solution. Excess biliary cholesterol can result from hypersecretion of cholesterol with a normal bile acid pool or with normal cholesterol secretion in conjunction with a diminished bile acid pool. Therefore, cholesterol supersaturation can be produced by decreased activity of cholesterol 7-α-hydroxylase (decreasing the conversion of hepatic cholesterol to bile acids), overactivity of HMG-CoA reductase (the rate-controlling enzyme in the synthesis of cholesterol), or terminal ileal disease or resection (interrupting the enterohepatic conservation of bile acids).

In addition to cholesterol supersaturation, the second necessary requirement for gallstone formation is the process of crystallization. Cholesterol supersaturation alone is a common finding in normal patients free of biliary pathology [32, 33]. Nucleation, or the precipitation of supersaturated bile cholesterol into solid cholesterol monohydrate crystals, usually occurs due to a combination of depressed biliary kinetics and procrystalizing protein action on the bile. Nucleation

time, the rate at which cholesterol crystals form, is decreased from approximately 15 days in control patients free of biliary disease to 3 days in patients with gallstones [34]. Mucin glycoproteins secreted under prostaglandin control and immunoglobulins secreted by the gallbladder mucosa are thought to serve as pronucleating agents, perhaps using the mucous gel coating on the mucosa as a nucleation matrix. Other substances that have demonstrated pronucleating effects in vitro include phospholipase C, fibronectin, and a low-density lipoprotein, whereas apolipoprotein A-I has been shown to inhibit nucleation [23]. Concentration of bile within the gallbladder causes the formation of large, cholesterol-rich multilamellar vesicles that can precipitate cholesterol crystals. Also, concentration of calcium salts within the gallbladder leading to saturation may serve as a nidus for nucleation.

Lastly, the gallstone attains clinical significance when its size grows to the point at which it causes an obstruction of the biliary system. Macroscopic stone formation from cholesterol crystals results from progressive enlargement of individual crystals with deposition of insoluble material onto its outer surface or by fusion of crystals into a larger conglomerate. However, patients may present with typical biliary disease symptoms, yet routine radiological assessment may not visualize a definite stone formation. This biliary "sludge," also known as biliary microlithiasis, is a precipitation of cholesterol crystals and calcium bilirubinate granules in bile with a high mucin content, not infrequently observed in states of prolonged bowel rest or with use of total parenteral nutrition (TPN). Nevertheless, the pathogenesis of cholesterol gallstones is clearly multifactorial (Table 72.2).

The effects of aging on hepatic and biliary cholesterol metabolism are difficult to elucidate; however, it has become increasingly clear that gallbladder mucosal function and contractility play key roles in this process. Gallbladder hypomotility with infrequent or incomplete emptying of the gallbladder contents may predispose to bile stasis and crystal formation. As previously discussed, gallbladder kinetics are decreased in the elderly population, thereby increasing the risk of development of cholelithiasis. It is also important to consider other mechanisms that predispose to cholelithiasis, that may be present within a comorbid illness in the elderly patient. For instance, the elderly patient may require TPN, which further delays gallbladder emptying. Another notable condition that may predispose a patient to gallstone formation is rapid weight loss, which may be due to poor dietary intake or chronic illness [35, 36].

Although gallstones are associated with abnormal gallbladder contractility, it is not known whether altered motility is the primary problem or a secondary consequence. The presence of cholesterol-supersaturated bile alone has been shown to impair gallbladder emptying before cholesterol crystals or gallstones are evident [34]. Mechanisms proposed to explain the apparent effect of cholesterol-rich bile or gallstones on gallbladder motility, include a possible myotoxic or neurotoxic effect of cholesterol or bile salts, the development of hypertrophic myopathy with chronic inflammation or inflammatory mediator release, and disordered regulation of hormonal influences, such as CCK, motilin, or somatostatin [34, 37].

As part of a series of studies evaluating the characteristics and regulation of gallbladder motility in patients with and without gallstones, Thompson et al. reported that most gallbladders containing gallstones contract like normal controls when evaluated by ultrasonography after a lipid meal [38]. These "contractors" exhibited a diminished release of endogenous CCK measured with plasma bioassay, but an increased sensitivity to the hormone was apparent relative to controls. A few patients with gallstones displayed depressed gallbladder contractility but with CCK output equivalent to that of the controls. Gallbladder muscle strips obtained from these "noncontractors" were subsequently shown to have significantly reduced in vitro responsiveness to CCK [39] and a decrease in the number of CCK receptors [40]. The cause-and-effect relation between gallstones, gallbladder dysmotility, and neurohumoral influences is an area of active investigation.

Pigment Gallstone Pathogenesis

Although pigment stones comprise approximately 20% of the total in the Western population, the rate is much higher in the Asian population. Pigment stones are formed by the precipitation of bilirubin in bile. Like cholesterol, bilirubin is insoluble in water. The liver conjugates bilirubin, making it soluble, and secretes it into bile. A small percentage (3%) remains unconjugated. However, in healthy patients, this amount of insoluble bilirubin does not lead to formation of pigment stones. Hyperparathyroidism may predispose a patient to pigment stones by increasing the level of ionized calcium. Pigment stones may also occur secondary to an increase in unbound bilirubinate. This is due to chronic hemolysis (cirrhosis or sickle cell disease) or increased synthesis of unconjugated bilirubin as a result of increased activity of β-glucuronidase (which converts conjugated bilirubin to

unconjugated) [41]. When an increase in insoluble bilirubin comes into contact with insoluble calcium, a black pigment stone of solid consistency forms. Brown pigment stones are more common in Asian populations and are associated with chronic biliary tract infections or bile stasis. They are almost always associated with colonization of bile by *Escherichia coli*, *Bacteroides*, or *Clostridium* [42]. The stones are much more fragile than cholesterol or black pigment stones, crumbling readily when manipulated. Brown pigment stones are usually found in the bile ducts where β-glucuronidase produced by bacteria hydrolyzes conjugated bilirubin to the free form, a hydrophobic solute that readily combines with calcium to produce a nidus for gallstone formation.

Lithogenic Factors in the Elderly

A multitude of factors is responsible for the increased incidence of gallstones in the elderly. Einarsson and associates demonstrated age-associated changes of biliary cholesterol saturation and bile acid kinetics in a group of nonobese, normolipidemic subjects known to be gallstone-free [43]. Specifically, this investigation was able to show a direct correlation between advancing age and increasing cholesterol saturation of bile, presumably due to an increased rate of hepatic cholesterol secretion (Fig. 72.4). Additionally, bile acid synthesis and pool sizes were noted to decrease with advancing age (Fig. 72.5). Each of these changes contributes to the enhanced lithogenicity of bile in the elderly.

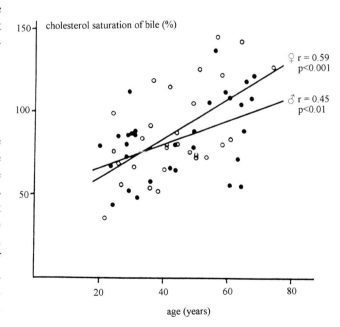

Figure 72.4 Relation between age and cholesterol saturation of bile. *Open symbols* denote women, and *closed circles* denote men (reprinted with permission from Einarsson et al. [43]. © Massachusetts Medical Society. All rights reserved).

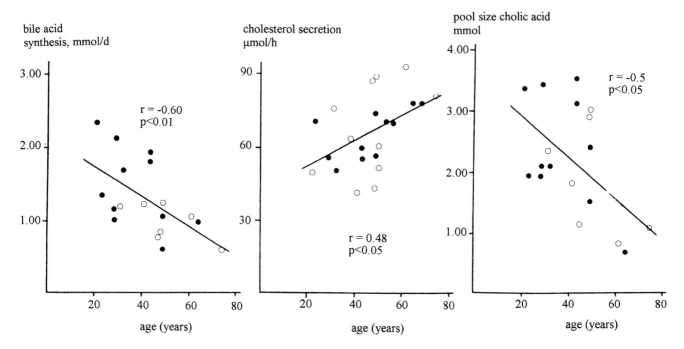

FIGURE 72.5 Relation between age and hepatic cholesterol secretion, total bile acid synthesis, and size of the cholic acid pool. *Open circles* denote women, and *closed circles* denote men (reprinted with permis- sion from Einarsson et al [43]. © Massachusetts Medical Society. All rights reserved).

The relation of these physiologic changes with possible age-related changes in hepatocyte enzyme activity for HMG-CoA reductase and 7-α-reductase has been investigated, with studies available that both support [44] and refute [45] this position.

To explore whether aging increases cholesterol supersaturation of bile and gallstone prevalence, Wang studied age-related changes in hepatic and biliary lipid metabolism in gallstone-susceptible and resistant mice of varying ages [29]. The rats were fed a lithogenic diet for 8 weeks and then evaluated for gallstone prevalence, gallbladder size, biliary lipid secretion, and HMG-CoA reductase activity. These outcomes were all increased in the gallstone-susceptible mice. Furthermore, increasing age-augmented biliary secretion and intestinal absorption of cholesterol, reduced hepatic synthesis and biliary secretion of bile salts, and decreased biliary contractility, all of which increased susceptibility to cholesterol gallstones in susceptible mice. The research concluded that aging was an independent risk factor for cholesterol gallstone formation.

As previously mentioned, gallbladder stasis may play an active role in formation of gallstones. Factors that may lead to gallbladder dysmotility in older patients include increasing saturation of bile with cholesterol and altered sensitivity of the gallbladder smooth muscle to CCK. Reviews of CCK receptor stimulants, motilin agonists, and procholinergic agents provide encouragement for emerging pharmacotherapy as treatment options for gallbladder hypomotility [34, 46].

Pancreas

Pancreatic Development and Anatomy

The pancreas is a retroperitoneal organ in the upper abdomen. It lies posterior to the stomach, with its head nestled at the C loop of the duodenum and tail extending toward the hilum of the spleen. Pancreatic tissue is of endodermal origin and develops in tandem with the hepatobiliary system. During the 4th week of gestation, two buds develop from the duodenum, a hepatic diverticulum and a dorsal bud. The anterior bud develops into the liver and biliary system while the dorsal bud eventually forms the body and tail of the pancreas. During the 32nd week of gestation, the hepatic diverticulum gives rise to the ventral bud, which ultimately forms the uncinate process. It then rotates 180° clockwise around the duodenum and fuses with the dorsal pancreatic bud to form the mature pancreas (Fig. 72.6). The main pancreatic duct of Wirsung, formed by fusion of the ventral duct and the distal portion of the dorsal pancreatic duct, drains most of the pancreas into the duodenum at the ampulla of Vater. The diameter of the main pancreatic duct is 2.0–3.5 mm in healthy young adults [47]. The common bile duct joins with the main pancreatic duct at the ampulla of Vater and empties through the greater duodenal papilla. The proximal ductal system of the dorsal bud persists as the accessory pancreatic duct of Santorini, draining the superior portion of the

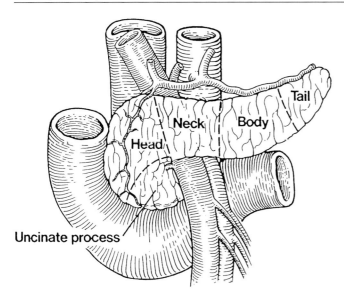

Figure 72.6 Anatomy of the mature pancreas, relative to surrounding structures (reprinted with permission from Trede M, Carter DC, (eds). Surgery of the pancreas. Edinburgh: Churchill Livingstone, © Elsevier, 1993).

pancreatic head via the lesser papilla into the duodenum proximal to the greater papilla.

Pancreatic Physiology

The pancreas has dual functions, both exocrine and endocrine. The exocrine activity is geared toward facilitating digestion, neutralizing gastric acid, and regulating intraintestinal pH. Pancreatic endocrine activity is vital for glucose homeostasis. Because of the great functional reserve of this organ, 90% of pancreatic function can be lost before signs of insufficiency become clinically evident [48].

Exocrine Function

The exocrine pancreas accounts for approximately 85% of the total mass and produces 500 ml of secretions per day. The acinar cells of the pancreas secrete enzymes responsible for digestion, and centroacinar cells and the ductal system direct the exocrine secretions to the duodenum, modifying the electrolyte concentration and water content of the pancreatic fluid as it passes. The acinar cells are innervated by the sympathetic and parasympathetic nervous systems. The parasympathetic system increases secretions, whereas the sympathetic system inhibits them [49]. The enzymes produced by the acinar cells include amylase (isoamylase type P), lipase, trypsinogen, chymotrypsinogen, procarboxypeptidases A and B, deoxyribonuclease, ribonuclease, proelastase, and trypsin inhibitor.

Pancreatic juices are secreted based on a three-phase response to a meal, including a cephalic phase, a gastric phase, and an intestinal phase. The cephalic phase accounts for 10–15% of meal-stimulated pancreatic secretion and occurs in response to the sight, smell, or taste of food. This is thought to be mediated by direct stimulation and increased gastric acid secretion in the stomach, which indirectly stimulates pancreatic secretion due to duodenal acidification and secretin release. The gastric phase also accounts for 10–15% of meal-stimulated pancreatic secretion and is due to gastric distention brought on by the ingested meal. This can lead to release of gastrin and vagal stimulation, both thought to have a weak direct effect on the pancreas. More importantly, the gastrin and vagal stimulation increases gastric acid content, leading to duodenal acidification, which triggers the release of secretin. This, in turn, leads to pancreatic secretions aimed at raising the pH. Pancreatic secretions are alkaline and have a pH that varies from 7.6 to 9.0, depending on the rate of bicarbonate secretion from the ductal epithelium. This alkaline pH is necessary to maintain the inactive proteolytic enzymes and transport them to the appropriate acidic milieu of the duodenum where they undergo activation. Secretin is the major stimulant for pancreatic electrolyte and water secretion, with CCK, gastrin, and peripherally released acetylcholine acting as weaker stimulants. Lastly, the intestinal phase is secondary to food and gastric contents entering the proximal intestine, which again increases secretin release. Dietary fats and proteins in the duodenum also stimulate the release of CCK, which then stimulates acinar secretion. The intestinal phase is the most important determinant of pancreatic secretion.

In addition to the water and electrolyte secretions, the exocrine pancreas secretes digestive enzymes. The major proteolytic enzyme is trypsin, initially secreted within the pancreas in an inactive form but activated within the duodenum by increasing acidity and enterokinase, a hormone produced by duodenal mucosa. Only amylase is secreted directly from the acinus in an active form. The other enzymes are initially secreted as inactive proenzymes, requiring trypsin and the acidic environment of the duodenum for activation. Inappropriate early activation of enzymatic action can result in autodigestion of the pancreatic substance, as may be seen in acute pancreatitis. The protein, fat, and carbohydrate constituents of diet alter the absolute amount and ratio of enzymes secreted. Regulation of enzyme secretion is primarily through the hormones CCK and acetylcholine. Secretin, vasoactive intestinal peptide (VIP), and pancreatic islet hormones weakly stimulate acinar secretion [47].

Endocrine Function

The main physiologic function of the endocrine pancreas is the regulation of energy through the hormonal regulation of carbohydrate metabolism. This is achieved via the islets of Langerhans, clusters of specialized endocrine cells which are scattered throughout the exocrine tissue. Most islets contain approximately 3,000 to 4,000 cells, consisting of four major cell types: alpha cells which secrete glucagon, beta cells which secrete insulin, delta cells which secrete somatostatin, and PP or F cells which secrete pancreatic polypeptide.

The predominant and most studied pancreatic hormone is insulin. Insulin, a 51-amino-acid polypeptide, is synthesized as a preprohormone in the beta cells of Langerhans islets. The proinsulin is synthesized in the endoplasmic reticulum, then travels to the Golgi complex where the C peptide is cleaved from it to create the insulin molecule. Upon stimulation, insulin is transported into secretory granules and released into the bloodstream by extrusion of the 6-kd polypeptide through the cell membrane. Insulin secretion occurs in response to elevated blood glucose levels and is suppressed by hypoglycemia. Insulin secretion is greater in response to orally administered glucose than intravenous glucose, even when serum glucose levels are equal. Insulin secretion occurs in two phases, the first being the release of stored insulin. The first phase is short (approximately 5 min) and is in response to a glucose challenge, whereas the second phase is longer and related to the sustained release of newly produced insulin. Maximal secretion of insulin occurs at serum glucose concentrations of 400–500 mg/dl. Type I diabetes results from a combination of genetic, environmental, and autoimmune factors which lead to selective destruction of β-cells. The endocrine tissue of the pancreas has excellent reserve, thereby requiring destruction of at least 80% of the tissue before clinical manifestations are evident [50].

Insulin binds to specific membrane-associated glycoprotein receptors that effect an increase in membrane-bound glucose transporters (GLUT-1 to GLUT-5), thereby facilitating glucose transport from the blood into cells. Skeletal muscle accounts for the majority of insulin-mediated glucose uptake and impaired insulin action at the level of the muscle is the cause of insulin resistance in type II diabetes [51]. In the liver, insulin facilitates glycogen deposition while inhibiting gluconeogenesis and glycogenolysis, resulting in a net increase in glucose uptake. Insulin also promotes lipogenesis and protein synthesis. As part of the insulin resistance syndrome, malfunction of insulin at the level of the liver can lead to abnormal lipid accumulation in hepatocytes, leading to non-alcoholic steatohepatitis (NASH) [52].

Glucagon is also synthesized as a 29-amino-acid propeptide and its purpose is to counteract the effects of insulin and increase the concentration of blood glucose. Similar to insulin, glucose is the primary regulator of glucagon secretion, although with glucagon, it causes an inhibitory effect. Furthermore, insulin and somatostatin also serve as negative regulators of glucagon secretion. Secretion is stimulated by hypoglycemia, acetylcholine, and generalized stressed states such as that occur with infection, trauma, or inflammation.

Glucagon promotes an elevation of blood glucose levels, with mobilization of intracellular fuels by hepatic glycogenolysis, gluconeogenesis, ketogenesis, and lipolysis. It is the provision of metabolic fuels during times of stress that resulted in glucagon being grouped with epinephrine, cortisol, and growth hormone as stress hormones.

Somatostatin is a 14-amino-acid polypeptide that has a wide anatomic distribution in neurons, pancreas, intestines, and other organs. It was originally isolated in 1973 as a hypothalamic extract that inhibited the release of growth hormone. Endocrine release of somatostatin occurs during a meal, in response to intraluminal fat; however, its exact role in the pancreas remains unclear, but it has been shown to inhibit the release of almost all peptide hormones and to inhibit gastric, pancreatic, and biliary secretion. Some researchers have suggested that somatostatin may regulate adjacent islet cell functions, but this has not been proven in vivo. The potent inhibitory effects of somatostatin and octreotide, a long-acting synthetic analogue, have been used to treat a variety of endocrine and exocrine disorders.

Pancreatic polypeptide (PP) is a 36-amino-acid polypeptide secreted in response to protein and less so to glucose from F cells. Although they are distributed throughout the pancreas, the predominance of these cells is concentrated in the pancreatic head and uncinate process. One of its most important roles may be as a mediator of the hepatic response to insulin. It has been demonstrated that abnormal glucose homeostasis associated with PP deficiency in patients with chronic pancreatitis is due to impaired suppression of hepatic glucose production by insulin [53]. This relative hepatic resistance to insulin is a consequence of diminished insulin receptor concentration, rather than altered receptor affinity, and can be ameliorated by administration of PP [54]. This mechanism of glucose metabolism has been further clarified by studies suggesting that hepatic insulin resistance in chronic pancreatitis is due to impaired transcription of the insulin receptor gene. Additionally, PP increases hepatic insulin-binding sites perhaps by upregulating insulin receptor gene expression [55]. PP is known to inhibit pancreatic exocrine secretion, choleresis, and motilin release [56]. PP release is augmented by cholinergic stimulation, with the normal postprandial rise in PP levels being ablated by vagotomy, antrectomy, or both [47].

PP is part of the polypeptide-fold family of peptide hormones, along with the central nervous system peptide, neuropeptide Y, and peptide tyrosine-tyrosine (PYY). Each of these is believed to play an important role in the regulation of appetite. PP was the first of these hormones to be isolated, from an impure insulin extraction. PP functions as a component of the "ileal brake" since it acts in various ways to slow the transit of food through the gut. It delays gastric emptying, attenuates pancreatic exocrine secretion and inhibits gallbladder contraction [57]. The role of PP in obesity is undergoing increasing investigation. Preliminary data suggest that PP reduced postprandial secretion is associated with obesity, whereas elevated postprandial levels of PP are found in patients with anorexia nervosa [58].

Pancreatic Anatomy in the Elderly

The pancreas undergoes an aging process resulting in minimal amounts of atrophy, fatty infiltration and fibrosis. One of the main age-related changes occurs with ductal anatomy, specifically an increase in the caliber of the main pancreatic duct and ectasia of branched ducts. One review by Kreel and Sandin [59] of in situ retrograde pancreatography at necropsy in 120 subjects older than 30 years revealed the main pancreatic duct width to increase with age at a rate of 8% per decade. A study using ultrasonography demonstrated an increasing pancreatic duct diameter with age. Regardless, the pancreatic duct was not found to be more than 3 mm, which if detected, should be considered a pathologic finding and not solely age-related [60]. The pancreatic duct widens proportionally along its entire length such that a uniform taper in caliber is maintained. This ductal anatomy can be distinguished from ductal dilatation associated with obstruction as seen with chronic pancreatitis and periampullary cancer. In some elderly patients, ductal ectasia becomes cystic as a variant of the aging pancreas. Acinar atrophy, an increased amount of intralobular fibrosis and fatty infiltration, and calcified pancreatic ductal calculi [61] seem to be common findings in the pancreas over the age of 70. Because of the increasing frequency of intercurrent disease states and degrees of malnutrition in the elderly, the proportion of these morphologic changes that are due to age alone vs. pathology has yet to be determined. In summary, the morphologic changes of the aging pancreas can be considerable, requiring clinicians to take caution when interpreting ERCP and computed tomography (CT) findings in the elderly (see physiology table at the beginning of this chapter).

Aging of the Exocrine Pancreas

Regarding the body of literature addressing physiologic changes in pancreatic function, conflicting data has emerged owing largely to a lack of consensus on defining pancreatic exocrine insufficiency. For instance, Laugier determined that patients over 65 years of age demonstrated a decrease in the volume and bicarbonate output of pancreatic secretion and the concentrations of pancreatic protein and lipase in response to stimulation from secretin and CCK stimulation [62]. In contrast, Gullo and associates failed to show any decrease in bicarbonate, trypsone, or lipase in response to continuous stimulation in elderly patients when compared to younger controls [63]. Regardless of the contrasting results, the

clinical significance of age-related changes in exocrine function is limited to a decrease of 10–30%. Therefore, the presence of steatorrhea in the elderly patient must be considered outside of expected aging and in the greater scope of other pathologies such as intraductal papillary mucinous neoplasms or pancreatic carcinoma [64].

Aging of the Endocrine Pancreas

Insulin Resistance in the Elderly

It has long been recognized that persons over 60 years of age more commonly exhibit dysfunction of glucose regulatory mechanisms in response to a glucose challenge [65]. Minimal morphologic alteration occurs in the aging endocrine pancreas, but a number of functional tests suggest progressive impairment of glucose tolerance in the elderly [66–68]. Clinical studies show an age-related increase in fasting blood glucose levels of about 1–2 mg/dl per decade, which may be less marked in lean, physically active individuals [66, 69]. The prevalence of diabetes over the past decade has increased enormously, largely due to a concomitant rise in the prevalence of obesity. As the aging population continues to grow and their life expectancy increases, so too does the rate of diabetes. Currently, about 20% of patients over 65 years suffer from diabetes [70].

Type II diabetes results from a multifactorial, progressive disease state and decompensation. Patients begin with impaired glucose tolerance as a result of the β-cell's attempts to maintain glucose homeostasis under chronic hyperglycemia and elevated free fatty acids. Once the β-cell can no longer compensate for peripheral hormone resistance, frank diabetes ensues. The interaction of many factors associated with aging contributes to the development of diabetes. Proposed mechanisms include altered insulin metabolism (depressed secretion, increased clearance, or diminished prohormone activation), increased resistance of peripheral tissues to insulin (receptor aberration, altered postreceptor pathways, or altered glucose transporter), loss of hepatic sensitivity to insulin, causing reduced glycogenesis, increased glucagon levels, and an age-associated increase in adipose tissue [72]. Studies which have specifically examined age-related effects on β-cell function have demonstrated variable results. This may be due to the small magnitude of the age effect, different techniques of measurement, and the presence of confounding factors such as obesity.

Current theories involving aging and insulin secretion highlight the interplay between a decreased β-cell secretory function and failure of peripheral glucose uptake mechanisms. The number and affinity of insulin receptors are similar across the spectrum of age groups [72]. Therefore, in absence of other risk factors, insulin resistance in the elderly is also due to impairments at the postreceptor level and β-cell dysfunction. A number of age-related effects on β-cells are known, such as decreased sensitivity to incretins and impaired compensation to insulin resistance, thereby predisposing older people to develop impaired glucose tolerance and diabetes [73]. Future studies aimed at delineating β-cell function may shed additional light on the subject.

Glucagon

Little is known about glucagon metabolism and actions in the elderly. Berger and associates reported that fasting plasma glucagon levels are significantly higher after age 30 when compared to those of a younger cohort [69]. However, after age 30, plasma glucagon levels did not significantly increase with advancing age. These findings are compared with those from the more recent work of Simonson and DeFronzo [74], who showed no correlation between advancing age and glucagon levels in 111 subjects aged 21–75 years. Additionally, this study demonstrated no difference in glucagon concentrations or clearance in young and old subjects receiving glucagon infusion, but hepatic sensitivity to the hormone appeared to be enhanced in the older age groups. Although the mechanism for this effect is not known, heightened hepatic sensitivity to glucagon in the elderly may be one of several factors contributing to progressive glucose intolerance of aging. Although some follow-up studies have confirmed no age-related changes in glucagon concentrations, other studies have shown reduced and elevated glucagon levels in the elderly [75].

Pancreatic Polypeptide

It has been previously noted that plasma levels of immunoreactive PP increase linearly with patient age [69]. The functional consequence of the age-related rise in PP levels is unknown. Studies using an isolated perfused human pancreas model reaffirmed this phenomenon and suggested that elevated PP levels in the elderly are due to enhancement of basal PP secretion, not reduced PP clearance [56].

References

1. Klein AS, Lillemoe KD, Yeo CJ, Pitt HA (1996) Liver, biliary tract, and pancreas. In: O'Leary JP (ed) The physiologic basis of surgery, 2nd edn. Williams & Wilkins, Baltimore, pp 441–478
2. Admirand WH, Small DM (1968) The physicochemical basis of cholesterol gallstone formation in man. J Clin Invest 47: 1043–1052
3. Popper H (1986) Aging and the liver. Prog Liver Dis 8:659–683
4. Schmucker DL (1990) Hepatocyte fine structure during maturation and senescence. J Electron Microsc Tech 14(2):106–125, Review
5. Tauchi H, Sato T (1968) Age changes in size and number of mitochondria of human hepatic cells. J Gerontol 23(4):454–461
6. Mooney H, Roberts R, Cooksley WGE et al (1985) Alterations in the liver with aging. Clin Gastroenterol 14:757–771
7. Williams D (1996) Age-related changes in O-deethylase and aldrin epoxidase activity in mouse skin and liver microsomes. Age Ageing 25(5):377–380
8. Le Couteur DG, McLean AJ (1998) The aging liver. Drug clearance and an oxygen diffusion barrier hypothesis. Clin Pharmacokinet 34(5):359–373
9. Junaidi O, Di Bisceglie AM (2007) Aging liver and hepatitis. Clin Geriatr Med 23(4):889–903
10. Thompson EN, Williams R (1965) Effect of age on liver function with particular reference to Bromsulphalein excretion. Gut 6:266–269
11. Kampmann JP, Sinding J, Møller-Jørgensen I (1975) Effect of age on liver function. Geriatrics 30:91–95
12. Rafsky HA, Newman B (1943) Liver function tests in the aged (the serum cholesterol partition, Bromsulphalein, cephalinflocculation and oral and intravenous hippuric acid tests). Am J Dig Dis 10:66–69
13. Koff RS, Garvey AJ, Burney SW et al (1973) Absence of an age effect on sulfobromophthalein retention in healthy men. Gastroenterology 65:300–302
14. Sawada N, Ishikawa T (1988) Reduction of potential for replicative but not unscheduled DNA synthesis in hepatocytes isolated from aged as compared to young rats. Cancer Res 48(6):1618–1622
15. Zapletal Ch, Faust D, Wullstein C, Woeste G et al (2005) Does the liver ever age? Results of liver transplantation with donors above 80 years of age. Transplant Proc 37(2):1182–1185
16. Qvist N (1995) Motor activity of the gallbladder and gastrointestinal tract as determinants of enterohepatic circulation: a scintigraphic and manometric study. Dan Med Bull 42:426–440
17. Gadacz TR (1993) Biliary anatomy and physiology. In: Greenfield LJ (ed) Surgery: scientific principles and practice. Lippincott, Philadelphia, pp 925–936
18. Khalil T, Walker JP, Wiener I et al (1985) Effect of aging on gallbladder contraction and release of cholecystokinin-33 in humans. Surgery 98:423–429
19. Rajan M, Wali JP, Sharma MP et al (2000) Ultrasonographic assessment of gall bladder kinetics in the elderly. Indian J Gastroenterol 19(4):158–160
20. Nagase M, Hikasa Y, Soloway RD et al (1980) Surgical significance of dilatation of the common bile duct: with special reference to choledocholithiasis. Jpn J Surg 10:296–301
21. Kaim A, Steinke K, Frank M, Enriquez R et al (1998) Diameter of the common bile duct in the elderly patient: measurement by ultrasound. Eur Radiol 8(8):1413–1415
22. Valdivieso V, Palma R, Wünkhaus R et al (1978) Effect of aging on biliary lipid composition and bile acid metabolism in normal Chilean women. Gastroenterology 74:871–874
23. Bateson MC (1984) Gallbladder disease and cholecystectomy rate are independently variable. Lancet 2:621–624
24. Lieber MM (1952) The incidence of gallstones and their correlation with other diseases. Ann Surg 135:394–405
25. Lindström CG (1977) Frequency of gallstone disease in a well-defined Swedish population. Scand J Gastroenterol 12:341–346
26. Marinovic I, Guerra C, Larach G (1972) Incidencia de litiasis biliar en material de autopsias y analisis de composicion de los calculos. Rev Med Chil 100:1320–1327
27. Heaton KW (1973) The epidemiology of gallstones and suggested aetiology. Clin Gastroenterol 2:67–83
28. Attili AF, Capocaccia R, Carulli N et al (1997) Factors associated with gallstone disease in the MICOL experience. Multicenter Italian Study on Epidemiology of Cholelithiasis. Hepatology 26(4):809–818
29. Wang DC (2002) Aging per se is an independent risk factor for cholesterol gallstone formation in gallstone susceptible mice. J Lipid Res 43(11):1950–1959

30. National Center for Health Statistics (1994) National Hospital Discharge Survey: Annual Summary. Series 13: Data from the National Health Care Survey, No. 128. DHHS Publ No. (PHS) 97–1789. National Center for Health Statistics, Hyattsville, MD, May 1997
31. Reiss R, Deutsch AA (1985) Emergency abdominal procedures in patients above 70. J Gerontol 40:154–158
32. Tang WH (1996) Serum and bile lipid levels in patients with and without gallstones. J Gastroenterol 31:823–827
33. Holan KR, Holzbach RT, Hermann RE et al (1979) Nucleation time: a key factor in the pathogenesis of cholesterol gallstone disease. Gastroenterology 77:611–617
34. Portincasa P, Stolk MFJ, van Erpecum KJ et al (1995) Cholesterol gallstone formation in man and potential treatments of the gallbladder motility defect. Scand J Gastroenterol 30(Suppl 212):63–78
35. Festi D, Colecchia A, Orsini M et al (1998) Gallbladder motility and gallstone formation in obese patients following very low calorie diets. Use it (fat) to lose it (well). Int J Obes Relat Metab Disord 22(6):592–600
36. Shiffman ML, Shamburek RD, Schwartz CC et al (1993) Gallbladder mucin, arachidonic acid, and bile lipids in patients who develop gallstones during weight reduction. Gastroenterology 105(4):1200–1208
37. Schneider H, Sänger P, Hanisch E (1997) In vitro effects of cholecystokinin fragments on human gallbladders: evidence for an altered CCK-receptor structure in a subgroup of patients with gallstones. J Hepatol 26:1063–1068
38. Thompson JC, Fried GM, Ogden WS et al (1982) Correlation between release of cholecystokinin and contraction of the gallbladder in patients with gallstones. Ann Surg 195:670–676
39. Zhu XG, Greely GH, Newman J et al (1985) Correlation of in vitro measurements of contractility of the gallbladder with in vivo ultrasonographic findings in patients with gallstones. Surg Gynecol Obstet 161:470–472
40. Upp JR, Nealon WH, Singh P et al (1987) Correlation of cholecystokinin receptors with gallbladder contractility in patients with gallstones. Ann Surg 205:641–648
41. Carey MC (1993) Pathogenesis of gallstones. Am J Surg 165(4):410–419, Review
42. Lambou-Gianoukos S, Heller SJ (2008) Lithogenesis and bile metabolism. Surg Clin North Am 88(6):1175–1194
43. Einarsson K, Nilsell K, Leijd B, Angelin B (1985) Influence of age on secretion of cholesterol and synthesis of bile acids by the liver. N Engl J Med 313:277–282
44. Bowen JC, Brenner HI, Ferrante WA, Maule WF (1992) Gallstone disease: pathophysiology, epidemiology, natural history, and treatment options. Med Clin North Am 76:1143–1157
45. Ahlberg J, Angelin B, Einarsson K (1981) Hepatic 3-hydroxy-3-methylglutaryl coenzyme A reductase activity and biliary lipid composition in man: relation to cholesterol gallstone disease and effects of cholic acid and chenodeoxycholic acid treatment. J Lipid Res 22:410 422
46. Patankar R, Ozmen MM, Bailey IS, Johnson CD (1995) Gallbladder motility, gallstones, and the surgeon. Dig Dis Sci 40:2323–2335
47. Anderson DK, Brunicardi FC (1993) Pancreatic anatomy and physiology. In: Greenfield LJ (ed) Surgery: scientific principles and practice. Lippincott, Philadelphia, pp 775–791
48. DiMagno EP, Vay LWG, Summerskill WHJ (1973) Relations between pancreatic enzyme outputs and malabsorption in severe pancreatic insufficiency. N Engl J Med 288:813–815
49. Havel PJ, Taborsky GJ Jr (1989) The contribution of the autonomic nervous system to changes of glucagon and insulin secretion during hypoglycemic stress. Endocr Rev 10(3):332–350, Review
50. Diabetes Control and Complications Trial/Epidemiology of Diabetes Intervention and Complication (DCCT/EDIC) Study Research Group (2005) Intensive diabetes treatment and cardiovascular disease in patients with type 1 diabetes. N Engl J Med 353:2634
51. Lara-Castro C (2008) Intracellular lipid accumulation in liver and muscle and the insulin resistance syndrome. Endocrinol Metab Clin North Am 37(4):841–856
52. Viljanen AP (2009) Effect of weight loss on liver free fatty acid uptake and hepatic insulin resistance. J Clin Endocrinol Metab 94(1):50–55
53. Brunicardi FC, Chaiken RL, Ryan AS et al (1996) Pancreatic polypeptide administration improves abnormal glucose metabolism in patients with chronic pancreatitis. J Clin Endocrinol Metab 81:3566–3572
54. Seymour NE, Volpert AR, Lee EL et al (1995) Alterations in hepatocyte insulin binding in chronic pancreatitis: effects of pancreatic polypeptide. Am J Surg 169:105–110
55. Spector SA, Frattini JC, Zdankiewicz PD et al (1997) Insulin receptor gene expression in chronic pancreatitis: the effect of pancreatic polypeptide. In: Surgical forum. Proceedings for the 52nd annual sessions of the Owen H. Wangensteen surgical forum; 1997 Oct 12–17; Chicago. Allen, Lawrence, pp 168–171
56. Brunicardi FC, Druck P, Sun YS et al (1988) Regulation of pancreatic polypeptide secretion in the isolated perfused human pancreas. Am J Surg 155:63–69
57. Kojima S, Ueno N, Asakawa A et al (2007) A role for pancreatic polypeptide in feeding and body weight regulation. Peptides 28:459–463
58. Jayasena CN (2008) Role of gut hormones in obesity. Endocrinol Metab Clin North Am 37(3):769–787
59. Kreel L, Sandin B (1973) Changes in pancreatic morphology associated with aging. Gut 14:962–970
60. Glaser J, Stienecker K (2000) Pancreas and aging: a study using ultrasonography. Gerontology 46(2):93–96
61. Nagai H, Ohtsubo K (1984) Pancreatic lithiasis in the aged. Gastroenterology 86:331–338
62. Laugier R, Sarles H (1985) The pancreas. Clin Gastroenterol 14:749–756
63. Gullo L, Ventrucci M, Naldoni P, Pezzilli R (1986) Aging and exocrine pancreatic function. J Am Geriatr Soc 34:790–792
64. Walsh RM (2006) Innovations in treating the elderly who have biliary and pancreatic disease. Clin Geriatr Med 22(3):545–558
65. Spence JC (1921) Some observations on sugar tolerance, with special reference to variations found at different ages. Q J Med 14:314–326
66. Davidson MB (1979) The effect of aging on carbohydrate metabolism: a review of the English literature and a practical approach to the diagnosis of diabetes mellitus in the elderly. Metabolism 28:688–705
67. Bennett PH (1984) Diabetes in the elderly: diagnosis and epidemiology. Geriatrics 39:37–41
68. Taylor R, Agius L (1988) The biochemistry of diabetes. Biochem J 250:625–640
69. Berger D, Crowther RC, Floyd JC Jr et al (1978) Effect of age on fasting plasma levels of pancreatic hormones in man. J Clin Endocrinol Metab 47:1183–1189
70. Mazza AD (2008) Insulin resistance syndrome and glucose dysregulation in the elderly. Clin Geriatr Med 24(3):437–454
71. Timiras PS (1994) The endocrine pancreas and carbohydrate metabolism. In: Timiras PS (ed) Physiological basis of aging and geriatrics, 2nd edn. CRC Press, Boca Raton, FL, pp 191–197
72. Goldfine ID (1987) The insulin receptor: molecular biology and transmembrane signaling. Endocr Rev 8:235–255
73. Chang AM, Halter JB (2003) Aging and insulin secretion. Am J Physiol Endocrinol Metab 284(1):E7–E12, Review
74. Simonson DC, DeFronzo RA (1983) Glucagon physiology and aging: evidence for enhanced hepatic sensitivity. Diabetologia 25:1–7
75. Pagano G, Marena S, Scaglione L, Bodoni P et al (1996) Insulin resistance shows selective metabolic and hormonal targets in the elderly. Eur J Clin Invest 26(8):650–656

Chapter 73
Benign Disease of the Gallbladder and Pancreas

Jennifer A. Wargo and Kim U. Kahng

Benign diseases of the gallbladder and pancreas represent significant causes of morbidity and mortality worldwide, particularly in elderly patients. Additionally, asymptomatic benign lesions of the gallbladder and pancreas are diagnosed more frequently with the increased use of imaging, and require thoughtful consideration for appropriate and timely treatment or follow-up. A critical understanding of these diseases is mandatory for proper patient care in the geriatric population.

Benign Disease of the Gallbladder

Disease of the biliary tract is common among adults in the USA: 10–15% of the adult population has gallstones, accounting for approximately 20 million people, and one million new cases are discovered annually. Gallstone disease is the most common and most costly digestive disease causing hospitalization, with an estimated annual cost exceeding $5 billion [1]. Among the elderly, biliary disease is the most common indication for abdominal surgery [2]. This is undoubtedly related to the progressive increase in the prevalence of cholelithiasis with advancing age (Fig. 73.1), which in some reports exceeds 50% in those older than age 70 [3]. In addition to being common, gallbladder disease in the elderly is more severe than in the young, as indicated by the higher proportion of elderly patients requiring cholecystectomy for acute rather than chronic cholecystitis [4]. Biliary tract disease in the elderly is further complicated by the greater incidence of choledocholithiasis. Common duct stones are found at the time of cholecystectomy in up to 30% of those in their 60s and in up to 50% of those in their 70s [5].

Manifestations of biliary disease in the elderly differ significantly from those in the young, which may contribute to the higher morbidity and mortality in older patients [6]. The atypical presentation in elderly patients and the frequency of coincidental gastrointestinal complaints often lead to delays in diagnosis [7]. These delays contribute to the higher incidence of the known complications of cholelithiasis and the increased mortality of gallstone disease in the aged population [8]. Recognizing the frequency and understanding the clinical presentation of biliary disease in the elderly is thus imperative for the proper care and treatment of these patients.

Cholelithiasis

Incidence and Epidemiology

The prevalence of cholelithiasis varies widely among populations of the world. The considerable variation in the incidence of cholelithiasis among ethnic groups is perhaps best illustrated by the markedly increased rate of gallstone disease in Pima Indians. The prevalence of cholelithiasis in female Pima Indians exceeds 60% for those over 35 years of age [9]. To a lesser degree, an increased propensity for gallstone formation is also seen in the Scandinavian countries, Chile, and among Native Americans [10]. The prevalence of gallstones in blacks, however, is roughly one-half that of whites [5] and is as low as 3% in some African tribes [11].

Regardless of geographic site or ethnicity, the two primary factors associated with the development of gallstones are gender and age. Female gender unquestionably contributes to an increased incidence of cholelithiasis, as women are twice as likely as men to develop gallstones [10]. Differences in the hormonal milieu have been

J.A. Wargo (✉)
Division of Surgical Oncology, Harvard Medical School,
Massachusetts General Hospital Cancer Center,
55 Fruit Street, YAW 7B, Boston, MA 02114, USA
e-mail: jwargo@partners.org

R.A. Rosenthal et al. (eds.), *Principles and Practice of Geriatric Surgery*,
DOI 10.1007/978-1-4419-6999-6_73, © Springer Science+Business Media, LLC 2011

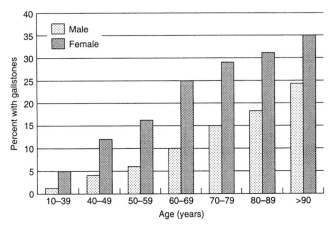

Figure 73.1 Incidence of gallbladder disease by age.

implicated by studies showing that estrogen and progesterone increase the lithogenicity of bile and alter gallbladder motility [11]. Exogenous estrogen induces hypersecretion of cholesterol into bile in both men [12] and women [13] and affects the motility of the sphincter of Oddi in animal models [14].

Advancing age is clearly associated with an increased prevalence of cholelithiasis. This is true regardless of gender [4] or ethnicity. The effect of age may be magnified in the institutionalized elderly as indicated by a report that cholelithiasis was present in 60% of institutionalized women aged 80–89 years and 80% of those older than 90 years [15].

Classification

Most gallstones in Western countries, including the USA, are composed of a mixture of both cholesterol and pigment. Pure cholesterol stones account for only 10% and pure pigment stones for about 15% of gallstones in the USA [16]. Most mixed stones contain cholesterol as their principal constituent, with alternating layers of mucin glycoproteins [10].

Pigment stones are composed mainly of bilirubin, usually in the form of calcium bilirubinate. These stones may be further categorized as either black or brown, with black stones seen more commonly in the presence of hemolytic disease or hepatic cirrhosis. Brown pigment stones are typically seen in Asian patients and are associated with biliary infection [16]. At the time of cholecystectomy, the percentage of stones that are pigmented increases with advancing age [17]. Whether the type of stone is related to the subsequent development of symptoms is debatable, but the differentiation between cholesterol and pigment stones is important when nonoperative management is considered, as black pigment stones are resistant to dissolution therapy [18].

Pathogenesis

Cholesterol Stones

The pathogenesis of cholesterol stones involves a series of defects that ultimately lead to the formation of stones. These pathogenic factors include cholesterol hypersecretion with subsequent supersaturation of bile, gallbladder hypomotility leading to bile stasis, cholesterol crystallization in bile serving as a nidus for stone formation, hypersecretion of gallbladder mucus [19], and increased concentration of biliary calcium [20].

Hypersecretion of cholesterol is considered the primary requisite factor for the development of cholesterol gallstones in the Western world [21]. Advancing age is associated with increased biliary secretion of cholesterol and decreased hepatic bile salt synthesis [22]. These changes in cholesterol secretion and bile salt synthesis may contribute to the increased prevalence of cholelithiasis in the elderly population.

In addition to factors related to bile composition, decreased gallbladder motility plays a significant role in gallstone formation. The risk of gallstone formation is significantly increased by conditions that impair normal gallbladder emptying, such as pregnancy [23], treatment with total parenteral nutrition (TPN) [24], octreotide therapy for acromegaly [25], diabetes mellitus [26], sickle cell anemia [27], and in patients who have suffered spinal cord injury [28] or who have undergone truncal vagotomy [29].

Normally, there is a continuous flow of bile in and out of the gallbladder. The greatest flow of gallbladder bile is stimulated by food consumption [30], which causes gallbladder contraction in a triphasic pattern of emptying, refilling, then emptying again [4]. Gallbladder emptying and refilling also occurs during fasting. Nearly 10% of gallbladder volume is ejected during fasting in association with migrating motor complexes (MMCs) in the duodenum [31]. This facilitates exchange of bile between the common duct and the gallbladder and may prevent stratification of bile within the gallbladder itself [14]. Gallbladder motility is influenced by several neurohumoral mechanisms. The entry of food into the duodenum stimulates the release of cholecystokinin (CCK) by intestinal endocrine cells. CCK has several effects, including increasing the flow of hepatic bile into the biliary tree and contracting the gallbladder with concomitant relaxation of the sphincter of Oddi [14]. Nearly three-fourths of the gallbladder volume is ejected in response to CCK [32], with approximately 15% released prior to the onset of gastric emptying. The effect of CCK is modulated by several other peptide hormones as well. Secretin has no intrinsic effect on gallbladder motility, but it significantly potentiates the effects of CCK [33]. Somatostatin inhibits CCK-mediated gallbladder contraction and is thought to act as a physiologic "brake" [32]. Other inhibitors of CCK-mediated gallbladder contraction include vasoactive intestinal polypetide (VIP) [34], pancreatic polypeptide [35], and peptide YY [36].

In addition to neurohumoral control mechanisms, gallbladder motility may be influenced by the degree of cholesterol saturation of bile. Animal and human studies suggest that cholesterol hypersaturation of bile attenuates gallbladder motility. In animal models, 1 week of cholesterol feeding reduces the gallbladder ejection fraction from 76 to 26% [37]. Gallbladder contraction is considerably diminished in patients with cholesterolosis, or "strawberry gallbladder" [38]. The ability to contract both spontaneously and in response to stimulation with CCK, acetylcholine, and potassium chloride is markedly reduced in gallbladders from patients with cholesterol cholelithiasis [38].

Bile stasis may also lead to the formation of biliary sludge, a viscous aggregate composed of mucin glycoproteins, calcium bilirubinate, and cholesterol crystals [14]. The presence of sludge in the gallbladder can be detected by ultrasonography, and its formation is typically related to the presence of lithogenic bile and gallbladder hypomotility [39]. Biliary sludge has been found in 50% of patients receiving TPN for a period of 6 weeks and in nearly 100% of those receiving TPN for more than 6 weeks [40]. This is thought to be related to the lack of oral intake during therapy with TPN, as enteral feeding may reverse the process of biliary sludge deposition [40]. The formation of both cholesterol and pigment stones is virtually always anteceded by the presence of biliary sludge [6].

Investigation into the effects of aging on gallbladder motility have been confined primarily to changes in neurohumoral control mechanisms, particularly age-related changes in CCK sensitivity. In animal studies, aging is associated with a decrease in the gallbladder contractile response to CCK, which appears to be related to a decrease in the number of CCK receptors [41]. The increased incidence of gallstone formation seen in old animals can be prevented by the administration of exogenous CCK [42]. Human studies have also demonstrated markedly reduced gallbladder sensitivity to CCK with aging, but there appears to be a compensatory elevation in the level of serum CCK [43]. In addition to changes in CCK activity, aging is associated with increased levels of pancreatic polypeptide [44], which may contribute to bile stasis because of decreased gallbladder contractility and increased sphincter of Oddi pressures.

Pigmented Stones

Despite their relatively low incidence in the USA, pigment stones are the most common type of gallstone worldwide [45]. The etiology and pathogenesis differ between black

and brown pigment stones. Black pigment stones form in the presence of increased secretion of bilirubin conjugates, which typically occurs with chronic hemolysis and to some degree with hepatic cirrhosis. Normally, unconjugated bilirubin produced by the action of β-glucuronidase constitutes less than 1% of the total bile pigments [46]. In patients with hemolytic disease, the percent of unconjugated bilirubin may increase more than tenfold [47], thus exceeding its solubility in bile. The unconjugated bilirubin precipitates with calcium ions, leading to the formation of insoluble calcium salts [48]. Most pigment stones are composed primarily of calcium bilirubinate and generally form in sterile bile [49].

Brown pigment stones form in the presence of chronic anaerobic infection of bile [50]. This particular type of pigment stone is endemic to Asia, probably owing to the high incidence of biliary infection in this area of the world [51]. The finding of significantly increased bacterial β-glucuronidase activity in the bile of patients with brown pigment stones is supporting evidence that biliary infection is an important etiologic factor [52]. The pathogenesis of brown pigment stones also involves biliary stasis, which predisposes to biliary infection. The incidence of brown pigment stones in the common bile duct in the presence of preexisting cholelithiasis increases with age, probably owing to decreased biliary motility with subsequent stasis and infection of bile [53].

Natural History

Asymptomatic Cholelithiasis

Few studies have addressed the natural history of gallstone disease, particularly in the aged population. Understanding the natural history of cholelithiasis has become increasingly important with the widespread use of abdominal ultrasonography and computed tomography, as the incidental finding of gallstones occurs with significant frequency [54]. This is particularly pertinent in elderly patients in whom the prevalence of cholelithiasis is known to be much higher than in the general population.

Several studies have attempted to describe the natural history of asymptomatic gallstone disease, mainly focusing on the rate of symptom development and complications. Gallstone disease is considered symptomatic with the development of biliary pain or any of its associated complications such as acute cholecystitis, biliary obstruction, or biliary pancreatitis [55].

An early report from the 1940s cited the development of symptoms in nearly 50% of patients with known gallstones when followed for 10–20 years. The complication rate in this study was roughly 19% over 15 years, accounting for an annual complication rate of approximately 1.4% [56]. In contrast, Gracie and Ransohoff reported much lower rates for the development of symptoms and associated complications [57]. The probability of symptom development in the presence of cholelithiasis in this study was estimated to be only 15% at 10 years and 18% at 15 and 20 years; the complication rate was approximately 20% in those who became symptomatic. Based on these findings, Gracie and Ransohoff introduced the concept of the "innocent gallstone." The population in their study, however, consisted of exclusively white, predominantly male subjects with a mean age of 54 years who had documented gallstone disease on oral cholecystography [57]. Attili et al. [58] questioned the results of Gracie and Ransohoff and reviewed the natural history of both asymptomatic and symptomatic gallstones in a much more representative population. The probability of symptom development in asymptomatic individuals in their study was nearly 12% at 2 years, 16.5% at 4 years, and close to 26% at 10 years. The complication rate in this study was approximately 3% after 10 years. The authors concluded that the natural history of gallstone disease is less benign than suggested by the studies of Gracie and Ransohoff. A conservative annual rate of symptom development of approximately 2% with about 1.5% requiring cholecystectomy was reported by McSherry et al. in their study of 691 patients with gallstone disease enrolled in a large health maintenance organization [59]. Based on all of these studies it can be estimated that serious symptoms and complications of gallstone disease are likely to occur at an annual rate of about 2% in those with cholelithiasis, with roughly two-thirds of patients remaining asymptomatic over a period of 20 years [60]. In light of this information, prophylactic cholecystectomy for asymptomatic cholelithiasis in the general population is not recommended [61].

The natural history of asymptomatic gallstones in the elderly is much less well defined. Studies that have included a significant number of older individuals have shown that elderly patients are more likely to present with complications of gallstone disease. In a study of 750 patients with gallstone disease, Wenckhert and Robertson demonstrated that nearly half of these patients developed severe complications within 11 years after the diagnosis of cholelithiasis [62]. Additionally, the complications of biliary disease are much less likely to be preceded by the typical symptoms ordinarily exhibited by younger individuals with biliary tract disease. In one study, nearly 80% of those who died from complications of gallbladder disease were previously classified as "asymptomatic" [63].

Gallstones may be discovered when patients undergo laparotomy for other reasons. Incidental cholecystectomy is generally not recommended in elderly patients undergoing abdominal surgery. Though early small studies in the 1970s suggested that it could be done safely [64], other studies demonstrated a slightly higher rate of wound infection and increased length of hospital stay [65].

Symptomatic Cholelithiasis

The natural history of symptomatic gallstones is understandably different from that of asymptomatic gallstones. Studies on the natural history of symptomatic cholelithiasis are somewhat sparse, as treatment is customarily recommended for patients within this population. Some studies are available, however. Annual rates of severe symptom development and cholecystectomy in patients with mildly symptomatic cholelithiasis were 44.0 and 3.2%, respectively, in the National Cooperative Gallstone Study [66]. Annual rates for cholecystectomy in patients with severe symptoms are typically 6–8% [67]. The rate of complications is not significantly different between patients with symptomatic and asymptomatic gallstone disease, suggesting that the presence or absence of symptoms is not a reliable prognostic indicator for the development of complications in cholelithiasis.

The typical initial presentation of symptomatic gallstone disease is that of biliary colic or chronic cholecystitis. Elderly patients are less likely to present with the "typical" symptoms of gallstone disease experienced by younger individuals [2]. Furthermore, elderly patients may present with complications of gallstone disease without any precursor symptoms of chronic cholecystitis. Morrow et al. [68] reported minimal or absent prior symptoms in nearly 40% of elderly patients presenting with grave complications, such as gangrenous cholecystitis, gallbladder empyema, or gallbladder perforation. Because of atypical symptomatology and the predilection for presenting with complicated gallstone disease, clinicians must have a high index of suspicion for biliary tract disease when caring for elderly patients.

Chronic Cholecystitis

The pain associated with chronic cholecystits, often referred to as biliary colic, is produced by a stone obstructing the cystic duct. The term "colic" is deceiving, as the pain is abrupt in onset and constant in nature, unlike true "colicky" pain that is characterized by a waxing and waning course. The pain is typically located in the right upper quadrant or epigastrium. Although radiation of pain is classically to the right shoulder or the inferior angle of the scapula, the pain may also radiate to other areas of the thorax or abdomen. The pain usually occurs at night, often around midnight, and lasts several hours. The frequency of recurrent pain varies among individuals, with intervals between attacks of pain ranging from days to weeks to occasionally months [69].

Patients may also present with nonspecific symptoms, such as bloating, gassiness, indigestion, nausea, and fatty food intolerance [70, 71]. Elderly patients are more likely to present with dyspepsia and vague epigastric discomfort [73]. The nonspecific nature of biliary symptoms commonly seen in aged patients, along with the multiplicity of coexisting gastrointestinal problems, clearly contribute to delays in diagnosis and treatment.

Physical examination of the symptomatic patient may yield right upper quadrant tenderness but is likely to be normal when the patient is not experiencing symptoms. Laboratory values are usually normal with chronic cholecystitis.

Based primarily on the history, a diagnosis of chronic cholecystitis is confirmed by establishing the presence of gallstones. The use of ultrasonography to detect cholelithiasis is clearly established. Gallstones are best visualized when the gallbladder is examined in both axial and sagittal planes after 8 h of fasting [73]. Gallstones typically appear as echogenic foci that demonstrate acoustic shadowing and gravitational dependence. Ultrasonogrphy may detect stones as small as 1–2 mm in size, which when multiple, are often characterized as "gravel." Gallbladder sludge, in contrast to gravel, appears as an echogenic layer that does not cast an acoustic shadow and is less gravitationally dependent. The sensitivity and specificity of ultrasonography for cholelithiasis when chronic cholecystitis is suspected are 0.95 and 0.97, respectively [74].

In addition to detecting the presence of gallstones, ultrasonography provides structural information about the gallbladder itself and the biliary ductal system. The ability to detect significant biliary ductal dilatation is particularly useful in the elderly because of the high incidence of common bile duct stones. Furthermore, information is provided about the liver, kidneys, and pancreas. For all these reasons, ultrasonography is the diagnostic study of choice for gallstone disease.

Several other radiologic studies can yield information about the biliary tree but have little role in the diagnosis of chronic cholecystitis. Plain roentgenography alone has limited usefulness in the diagnosis of cholelithiasis, as most of the stones are radiolucent. Fewer than 20% of gallstones can be visualized on plain radiographs of the abdomen [75]. Abdominal CT is far less sensitive than ultrasonography for detecting gallstones [76], as most stones are of the same attenuation as bile and therefore not well visualized. Cholescintigraphy has limited usefulness in the routine diagnosis of chronic cholecystitis, as it cannot provide anatomic information or identify gallstones. In atypical cases of classic biliary symptomatology with no ultrasonographic abnormalities, the functional information provided by cholescintigraphy becomes important. In such cases, analyzing gallbladder motility in response to a prokinetic agent may be the only means of establishing gallbladder pathology. It must be emphasized, however, that these atypical cases are rare.

When considering treatment for patients with symptomatic cholelithiasis, the natural history of the disease, the general life expectancy and medical condition of the individual, and the risks and benefits of the various treatment modalities are all factors that must be noted [77]. Expectant management of symptomatic gallstone disease is generally not advisable, as severe symptom development in patients with mildly symptomatic cholelithiasis is reported to be as high as 44% per year [66]. Particularly in the elderly, the risk of developing complicated biliary disease requiring emergent treatment with attendant high mortality, weighs strongly in favor of definitive treatment of symptomatic gallstones in an elective setting.

The definitive treatment for gallstone disease is cholecystectomy, which is performed in patients with chronic cholecystitis to relieve symptoms and prevent potentially life-threatening complications. Prior to the introduction of laparoscopic cholecystectomy, open cholecystectomy had been the gold standard for treating cholelithiasis for more than a century [16]. A comprehensive review by Roslyn et al. [78] of 42,474 open cholecystectomies performed at all nonveterans administration (VA) acute care hospitals in California and Maryland for a 12-month period, indicated that open cholecystectomy was a safe, effective treatment for gallstone disease. The study, which included patients undergoing emergent and elective cholecystectomy, reported an overall mortality rate of 0.17%. This is significantly lower than the mortality rate of 1.77% reported by Glenn more than 15 years prior [79]. In this more contemporary study, however, advanced age (more than 65 years) was associated with significantly higher mortality (0.5 vs. 0.03%) and complication (25.7% vs. 10.1%) rates than for the less than 65-year-old group. Significant increases in length of stay and in-hospital charges were also noted in aged patients [78].

Several factors contribute to the increased mortality and complication rates following open cholecystectomy in aged patients. A primary factor is the larger proportion of elderly patients compared to younger patients requiring emergency rather than elective cholecystectomy. Pigott and Williams [80] studied a group of 347 patients over 65 years of age who underwent open cholecystectomy for symptomatic gallstone disease. More than half of the patients in this study presented with an acute complication of gallstone disease, and they often required emergent surgical procedures. There may be multiple reasons for the greater tendency of the elderly to present with complicated gallstone disease. The early diagnosis of symptomatic gallstone disease at an uncomplicated stage (i.e., simple chronic cholecystitis) may not be made as readily, as elderly patients are more likely to present with atypical symptoms such as dyspepsia and vague epigastric discomfort. Elderly patients often present without antecedent symptoms of chronic cholecystitis. Finally, the increased incidence of choledocholithiasis adds to the complexity of biliary disease in the elderly.

Laparoscopic cholecystectomy has changed the surgical management of symptomatic cholelithiasis dramatically since its advent during the late 1980s [81]. First performed in France by Dr. Phillipe Mouret in 1987 [82], and in the USA by McKernan and Saye in 1988 and Olsen and Reddick in 1989 [83], laparoscopic cholecystectomy is now established as the procedure of choice for symptomatic gallstone disease. The laparoscopic approach offers many advantages when compared to open cholecystectomy, including reduced postoperative pain, shorter hospital stay and recovery, improved cosmetic results, and lower cost. The reduction of postoperative pain is a major benefit, resulting in decreased analgesic requirement and improved pulmonary function following surgery [84].

Mortality rates for laparoscopic cholecystectomy are reportedly lower than those of open cholecystectomy in reviews of both European [85] and US experiences [86], averaging about 0.1%. One of the largest reported series is that of the Southern Surgeons Club, which included more than 1,500 patients who underwent laparoscopic cholecystectomy for symptomatic cholelithiasis [87]. This study reported a 4.7% conversion rate to open cholecystectomy and a complication rate of 5.1%. The most significant complication of laparoscopic cholecystectomy is major bile duct injury, which is reported to occur in 5–10 per 1,000 cases [88]. Bile duct injury tends to occur early in a surgeon's experience with laparoscopy [89]. An updated study by the Southern Surgeons Club reported that 90% of bile duct injuries occurred during the first 30 cases performed by individual surgeons, clearly supporting the existence of a learning curve for laparoscopic cholecystectomy [90]. The overall complication rate for laparoscopic cholecystectomy is noted to be significantly lower than that of open cholecystectomy [91].

Conversion to open cholecystectomy is generally required in approximately 5% of patients undergoing laparoscopic cholecystectomy [92], most commonly because adhesions and chronic inflammation preclude the laparoscopic approach. Advanced age, male gender, obesity, acute cholecystitis, and the presence of a thickened gallbladder wall on ultrasonography are factors associated with a significantly increased rate of conversion from laparoscopic to open cholecystectomy [93]. A study based on the Connecticut Laparoscopic Cholecystectomy Registry, reported a correlation between conversion rates and age among elderly patients. Conversion was necessary in roughly 8% of those aged 70–74 years, 12% of those aged 75–80 years, and more than 12% of those over 80 years of age [94]. Although conversion to an open procedure is not a complication of laparoscopic

surgery and should never have a negative connotation, an appreciation for the likelihood of conversion is important when considering the risk of laparoscopic surgery in an elderly patient.

Laparoscopic cholecystectomy has significant implications in the treatment of elderly patients with gallstone disease. Several studies have reported favorable results in elderly individuals undergoing the laparoscopic procedure compared to those with the open approach [95–98]. A study of 233 patients by Massie et al. [95], demonstrated a sevenfold reduction in postoperative morbidity following laparoscopic cholecystectomy compared to open cholecystectomy in elderly patients and younger patients with clinically significant associated illnesses. A more extensive study of 1,677 patients at McGill University reported similar results [96]. As expected, elderly patients in this study were much more likely to present with evidence of complicated gallstone disease and were nearly twice as likely to require conversion to open cholecystectomy. The mortality rate of 0.6% for elderly patients was roughly five times higher than that for patients under 65 years of age [96] but was markedly lower than rates reported for open cholecystectomy in the same age group [5]. Complication rates were also significantly lower after laparoscopic cholecystectomy in the elderly compared to the historical complication rate following open cholecystectomy [96]. In particular, laparoscopic cholecystectomy in the older patients results in less postoperative impairment of pulmonary function compared to open cholecystectomy [99].

There are few absolute contraindications to laparoscopic cholecystectomy. These include an uncorrected coagulopathy and the inability to tolerate general anesthesia [16]. Conditions that may increase a patient's risks for postoperative complications of laparoscopic cholecystectomy include cardiopulmonary disease, immunosuppression, and cirrhosis with portal hypertension [100]. These factors are particularly pertinent during the preoperative risk assessment of elderly patients, as their presence is associated with an increased frequency of complications [98].

For those patients who are unwilling or unable to tolerate cholecystectomy, the nonoperative methods for treating chronic cholecystitis are primarily oral and contact dissolution as well as extracorporeal shock wave lithotripsy. These methods are limited by their variable efficacy, requiring careful patient selection. Furthermore, even when they successfully achieve clearance of gallstones, the rate of recurrent cholelithiasis approaches 50% over 5 years [16]. It must be noted that although these methods may find application in the treatment of uncomplicated symptomatic cholelithiasis, they should not be used to treat complicated gallstone disease [101].

Oral dissolution therapy involves the use of litholytic bile acids. These substances act primarily by inhibiting the enzyme HMG-CoA reductase, thus decreasing the biosynthesis of cholesterol and the saturation of cholesterol in bile [101]. Chenodeoxycholic acid (CDCA) was the first of these agents to be used in the dissolution of gallstones [102]. CDCA had an unfavorable side effect profile and poor efficacy and in 1988 was replaced by ursodeoxycholic acid (UDCA) [103]. Patients eligible for UDCA therapy include those with a history of biliary colic, radiolucent stones less than 1.5–2.0 cm in diameter, and a functional gallbladder. By these selection criteria, only 10–20% of those undergoing cholecystectomy would be eligible for UDCA therapy [5]. The dose is 8–10 mg/kg/day [102], and the expense of therapy is approximately $2,000 per year [5]. Although better than the results with CDCA, treatment with UDCA has limited efficacy, with complete dissolution occurring in 10% and partial dissolution in 20% after 2 years of therapy [104].

Contact dissolution therapy was first described in the late 1800s and is of historical interest only since it is not used today [105]. In this technique, a catheter is placed transhepatically into the gallbladder, and organic solvents are infused to dissolve gallstones. Its use was reevaluated in 1972 when Admirand and Way reported use of contact dissolution therapy to eradicate retained common duct stones [106]. The most commonly used solvent is methyl *tert*-butyl ether (MTBE). The efficacy of contact dissolution with MTBE is reported to be quite high, with complete dissolution of stones in more than 90% of patients [107]. Disadvantages of this technique, however, include a relatively high recurrence rate [108] and cost.

Extracorporeal shock wave lithotripsy (ESWL) for the treatment of gallstones was introduced in 1985 [109]. It is used to fragment gallstones into particles small enough to be expelled by a functional gallbladder and often requires the use of general or epidural anesthesia. Patients eligible for ESWL include those with a history of biliary colic who have one to three radiolucent stones with a combined diameter not exceeding 3 cm and a functional gallbladder [5]. Again, this topic is mostly of historical interest, as it is rarely used in the era of laparoscopic cholecystectomy.

In summary, laparoscopic cholecystectomy has found wide application for treatment of chronic cholecystitis, regardless of age, and has supplanted open cholecystectomy as the new gold standard. The overall improvement in mortality rates and the clear demonstration of the benefits of laparoscopic compared to open cholecystectomy specifically in the elderly, makes it the preferred procedure for definitive treatment of chronic cholecystitis even in the elderly. The crux is diagnosing symptomatic gallstone disease at an early stage to allow elective rather than emergency cholecystectomy. Although it must be acknowledged that age increases the risk for cholecystectomy, it is crucial to understand how this risk is magnified when emergency surgery is required.

Acute Cholecystitis

Acute cholecystitis is by far the most common complication of gallstone disease. It typically results from cystic duct obstruction due to impaction of a stone in the cystic duct itself or in Hartmann's pouch, with resultant bile stasis and distension of the gallbladder. The consequent mucosal release of lysolecithin, prostaglandins, and phospholipase A result in local inflammation. Bile becomes secondarily infected, resulting in positive bile cultures in nearly three-fourths of patients with acute cholecystitis [16]. The organisms most commonly isolated include *Escherichia coli*, *Klebsiella*, and *Enterococcus* species [3].

The classic presentation of acute cholecystitis includes fever and localized right upper quadrant abdominal pain [4]. Initially the pain may resemble that of biliary colic, but it differs in its longer duration and greater propensity to localize to the right upper quadrant. Patients often have associated nausea and vomiting. Physical examination typically yields right upper quadrant tenderness and a positive Murphy's sign. Laboratory values usually reveal a mild to moderate polymorphonuclear leukocytosis and may demonstrate a mild rise in transaminases, bilirubin, and alkaline phosphatase [3], but liver function studies are not universally elevated in those patients experiencing acute cholecystitis.

Acute cholecystitis in the elderly can be a diagnostic challenge, as the presentation is commonly atypical [110] and may vary widely. Abdominal pain remains a common presenting symptom but is often not accompanied by nausea, vomiting, fever, or leukocytosis [6]. Symptoms, however, may be minimal and the presentation may be nonspecific mental and physical disability alone. At the opposite end of the spectrum, nearly 12% of elderly patients with acute cholecystitis present in septic shock [111]. The physical examination may also be misleading. Morrow et al. reported that nearly 40% of elderly patients presenting with acute cholecystitis were afebrile, and more than half did not have peritoneal signs on examination. The absence of these findings did not correlate with milder disease, as 40% of the patients studied had severe complications including gallbladder empyema, gangrenous cholecystitis, and gallbladder perforation [68]. Given the variability and atypical features of presentation, the initial diagnostic accuracy of acute abdominal pain in patients over age 80 is only 29%, which is significantly lower than in younger patients [112].

When acute cholecystitis is suspected, the diagnosis may be established by the ultrasonographic findings of gallbladder distension and wall thickening with intramural sonolucency, pericholecystic fluid, cholelithiasis or gallbladder sludge (or both), and a sonographic Murphy's sign. Ultrasonography may also provide valuable information about the status of the pancreas and biliary tree [4]. It is important to recognize, however, that the presence of gallbladder wall thickening or fluid around the gallbladder may not be specific for acute cholecystitis. A review by Shea et al. [74] reported the sensitivity and specificity of ultrasonography for acute cholecystitis as 94 and 78%, respectively.

Cholescintigraphy is also useful in the diagnosis of acute cholecystitis. Visualization of the gallbladder typically occurs within half an hour of the administration of tracer. If the gallbladder fails to visualize after 45 min, an intravenous dose of morphine may facilitate visualization by promoting sphincter of Oddi contraction, thereby diverting flow of tracer into the gallbladder [113], assuming that the cystic duct is patent. Nonvisualization of the gallbladder indicates obstruction of the cystic duct, a finding that is highly suggestive of acute cholecystitis. The sensitivity and specificity of cholescintigraphy for acute cholecystitis are 93 and 91%, respectively [74].

As mentioned previously, laparoscopic cholecystectomy is now considered the new gold standard treatment for elective management of cholecystitis, both chronic and acute. The results of laparoscopic cholecystectomy in elderly patients with acute cholecystitis have been encouraging. Lo et al. [114] reported morbidity and mortality rates of 26.7 and 0%, respectively, in their study of elderly patients undergoing laparascopic cholecystectomy for acute cholecystitis. The conversion rate to open cholecystectomy was comparable to that for the general population. Common bile duct stones were present in four of ten elderly patients evaluated by endoscopic retrograde cholangiopancreatography (ERCP). Elderly patients, however, had a longer hospital stay than those under age 65, owing to greater delays in resumption of regular diet and return to ambulatory status [114].

Although cholecystectomy is the treatment of choice for acute cholecystitis, patients for whom the risk of immediate definitive surgery is considered too high may benefit from several forms of limited intervention. These methods are frequently used as temporizing procedures in critically ill patients who later can tolerate cholecystectomy [115]. Traditionally, decompression of the gallbladder by placing a tube that drained externally (cholecystostomy) was the operative alternative to cholecystectomy. The surgical approach to cholecystostomy has even been reported to be effective as a curative procedure in patients unable to tolerate a more extensive operation [116]. Percutaneous cholecystostomy may be performed under ultrasound guidance at a patient's bedside [117]. Van Steenbergen et al. assessed the outcomes of elderly patients treated with cholecystostomy for complicated acute cholecystitis and demonstrated rapid improvement in all patients after percutaneous decompression of the gallbladder. Half of the patients studied underwent elective cholecystectomy 1–12 weeks after cholecystostomy [118]. Mortality rates for cholecystostomy are typically about 10% and relate largely to the severity of illness in

patients requiring this procedure [119]. Morbidity is also acceptably low for this procedure. Once acute cholecystitis has resolved, the role of elective laparoscopic cholecystectomy remains a topic of debate. While it seems self-evident that cholecystectomy would be definitive treatment, it is difficult to recommend routine cholecystectomy in this high-risk group, even under elective circumstances, particularly when no impact on overall survival can be demonstrated [120]. The decision regarding interval cholecystectomy must be made on an individual basis, weighing the likelihood of recurrent acute cholecystitis (feasibility of percutanous extraction of stones, size of residual stones), the presence of coincident common bile duct stones, and the degree of risk related to comorbidities. For those who are not surgical candidates, cholecystostomy tubes may be removed 4 weeks after resolution in elderly or debilitated patients [119].

Gallbladder Perforation and Gallstone Ileus

Elderly patients are more likely than the young to suffer complications of acute cholecystitis, such as gangrenous cholecystitis, gallbladder perforation, and emphysematous cholecystitis [4]. Rates of gallbladder perforation in acute cholecystitis are reportedly as high as 8% in some series [121], with associated mortality rates approaching 40% for acute rupture [122]. Perforation of the gallbladder may be categorized using the Niemeier classification as acute (type I) with associated bile peritonitis, subacute (type II) with abscess formation in the area of the gallbladder, or chronic (type III) with perforation and fistula formation between the gallbladder and either the skin, bile duct, or digestive tract [123]. Perforation typically occurs at the site of the gallbladder fundus, the area of least blood supply [124]. A study by Roslyn and Busuttil demonstrated that this condition occurs more commonly in elderly patients, probably relating to gallbladder wall ischemia associated with atherosclerotic splanchnic vessels and limitations in cardiac output [125]. The mechanisms implicated in the development of gallbladder perforation involve obstruction of the cystic duct leading to gallbladder distension with subsequent vascular impairment resulting in ischemia, necrosis, and perforation of the wall [126]. It has also been noted that acute perforation is more common in young patients, whereas elderly patients are more likely to develop chronic perforation with fistula formation [127]. Complications of chronic perforation arise when gallstones traverse the fistulous tract and cause obstruction in areas of the gastrointestinal tract. Gallstone ileus accounts for nearly one-fourth of all cases of intestinal obstruction in aged patients [128].

The clinical presentation of acute gallbladder perforation is similar to that of acute cholecystitis. Patients frequently present with abdominal pain, nausea, and fever. Laboratory findings typically include polymorphonuclear leukocytosis and elevations in transaminases as well as in alkaline phosphatase, γ-glutamyl transpeptidase, and bilirubin. The diagnosis of gallbladder perforation can be aided by several diagnostic modalities, including plain abdominal films, ultrasonography, computed tomography (CT), cholangiography, and radionuclide scanning. Radiographic findings may include calculi within the right upper quadrant (representing spilled gallstones) or soft tissue masses within the area (suggesting the presence of a pericholecystic abscess) [129]. Typical findings in gallstone ileus include evidence of a small bowel obstruction, air in the biliary tree, and a radiopaque density in the right lower quadrant [4]. Ultrasonographic findings of pericholecystic fluid collections with free peritoneal fluid, disappearance of the gallbladder wall, and findings consistent with emphysematous cholecystitis are highly suggestive of gallbladder perforation [130]. CT scanning has been shown to be superior to ultrasonography for diagnosing gallbladder perforation, using criteria of pericholecystic fluid collection, streaky omentum, and a gallbladder wall defect on CT [131].

The treatment of gallbladder perforation relates mainly to the acuteness of the problem and the presence of associated disease. Acute perforation is often not diagnosed preoperatively in patients undergoing cholecystectomy for acute cholecystitis. One should have a high index of suspicion for acute perforation in any patient with a history of immune suppression or vascular disease who presents with abdominal tenderness localized to the right upper quadrant [125]. Initial management in patients with suspected acute perforation consists of intravenous hydration, and antibiotic coverage followed by cholecystectomy. Chronic perforation tends to occur in older individuals with a history of long-standing cholelithiasis and is often only recognized when patients present with small bowel obstruction related to the gallstone. Patients with this condition are treated by removal of the offending stone at laparotomy to relieve the obstruction. Cholecystectomy with fistula repair at the time of laparotomy is generally not recommended for elderly patients with significant comorbidities in the absence of acute biliary tract disease.

Emphysematous Cholecystitis

Another complication of acute cholecystitis that occurs with greater frequency in the elderly population is emphysematous cholecystitis [132], which is a peculiar variant of acute cholecystitis caused by gas-forming bacteria [133]. It is characterized by the appearance of gas in the gallbladder lumen or wall on abdominal radiographs [134] and has an overall mortality rate approaching 15% [12]. It occurs more frequently in diabetic patients and is less likely to be associated

with stones than is the usual form of acute cholecystitis [133]. It is believed to be caused by bacterial invasion of the gallbladder wall, most frequently by bacteria of the *Clostridium* species with *E. coli* often found as a copathogen. This form of acute cholecystitis often progresses to gallbladder gangrene and perforation.

Patients with emphysematous cholecystitis present with signs and symptoms consistent with acute cholecystitis and few added features [134]. In fact, patients are less likely to be febrile and often do not exhibit severe localized abdominal tenderness. Laboratory findings may reveal leukocytosis of less than 16,000/mm [3]. The most distinguishing characteristic in these patients is the presence of air within the gallbladder lumen or wall [132]. Three stages of emphysematous cholecystitis have been described radiographically and relate to the progression of disease, including findings of gas in the gallbladder lumen, the gallbladder wall, and finally the pericholecystic space. The latter two stages are pathognomonic for emphysematous cholecystitis. Ultrasonography has limited application in the diagnosis of emphysematous cholecystitis, as air within the tissues may lead to nonvisualization of the gallbladder [135]. CT scan findings include visualization of gas within the gallbladder or gallbladder wall (Fig. 73.2) [132].

Treatment of emphysematous cholecystitis is surgery after the patient has been adequately stabilized. Delays in surgical treatment of this condition can be devastating. Appropriate antibiotic coverage both pre- and postoperatively is imperative and should include coverage for anaerobes and gram-negative pathogens as well as for *Clostridium* organisms. Although there is some controversy regarding timing of laparotomy, all agree that rapid clinical deterioration with a palpable mass in the right upper quadrant sanctions immediate cholecystectomy. Reports suggest that a laparoscopic approach is feasible in these patients [136].

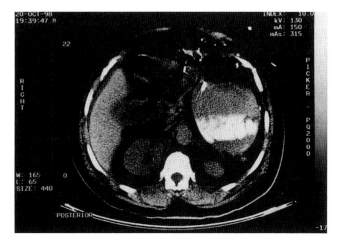

FIGURE 73.2 Computed tomography scan showing air within the gallbladder wall consistent with emphysematous cholecystitis.

Choledocholithiasis

Common duct stones are classified as primary or secondary depending on their site of origin. Primary duct stones, or stones that form within the common bile duct, are rare and account for a small fraction of cases of choledocholithiasis. This subtype of common duct stone is typically associated with infection [5]. Most cases of choledocholithiasis are due to the presence of secondary stones that arise in the gallbladder and later migrate into the common bile duct. The composition of these stones is similar to that of stones found primarily in the gallbladder, consisting of cholesterol and varying degrees of calcium bilirubinate [16].

The incidence of choledocholithiasis increases considerably with age. Common duct stones are reported to occur in 10% of the general population undergoing cholecystectomy and in up to 50% of patients in their 70s requiring surgery for symptomatic cholelithiasis [5]. Additionally, elderly patients with common bile duct stones are more likely to have positive bile cultures [137]. The reasons for this discrepancy are yet to be elucidated. Untreated common duct stones may lead to complications of cholangitis, pancreatitis, and obstructive jaundice [134].

The clinical presentation of patients with choledocholithiasis varies depending on the degree of ductal obstruction and the severity of associated complications. The range of symptoms is broad, as patients may be completely asymptomatic or may present with symptoms typical of life-threatening conditions such as ascending cholangitis. Choledocholithiasis should certainly be suspected in any patient who presents with cholelithiasis and associated jaundice. This presentation is common in patients with common duct stones; however, 10–20% of patients present with symptoms of cholangitis or pancreatitis [138]. Patients who present with cholangitis may exhibit the classic triad of fever, right upper quadrant abdominal pain, and jaundice; but it is important to recognize that more than half of the patients who present with cholangitis do not exhibit all three of these findings [16]. Laboratory values commonly reveal significant elevations in alkaline phosphatase, bilirubin, and γ-glutamyl transpeptidase [139], with elevations in the leukocyte count, amylase, and lipase in patients presenting with complications of choledocholithiasis [5]. Abnormal liver function tests, however, are absent in some individuals with documented common duct stones.

Several studies have attempted to identify predictors of choledocholithiasis. Factors that may lead one to suspect the presence of common duct stones include common bile duct dilation on ultrasonography, age exceeding 60 years, serum bilirubin higher than 2.5 mg/dl [140], and the presence of acute or chronic cholecystitis [141]. The sensitivity of ultrasonography in the evaluation of choledocholithiasis is fairly low, however, with highest estimates around 60% [142]. CT may reveal biliary ductal dilatation but is typically used to evaluate malignant rather than benign common duct

obstruction. ERCP and percutaneous transhepatic cholangiography (PTC) provide the most accurate means of diagnosing choledocholithiasis [5]. Intraoperative cholangiography is useful for this diagnosis in patients undergoing cholecystectomy [143]. MR cholangiography may be helpful in evaluating for choledocholithiasis (Fig. 73.3).

When considering treatment for patients with choledocholithiasis, one must consider the specific conditions under which they occur as well as the advantages and disadvantages of the various forms of treatment. Various endoscopic, radiologic, and surgical methods are available for the treatment of common duct stones. The presence of choledocholithiasis has a major impact on patient outcome in those undergoing cholecystectomy for symptomatic gallstone disease and therefore must be carefully assessed preoperatively [144].

Most agree that patients who are suspected of harboring common duct stones prior to elective or emergent cholecystectomy should have ERCP. Patients who are found to have stones at this time may then undergo endoscopic sphincterotomy (ES) with possible stone extraction [145]. ES has been shown to be the treatment of choice for patients with acute cholangitis [146] or acute pancreatitis [147] before cholecystectomy is performed. Successful stone clearance is possible in more than 90% of patients undergoing ES [148]. Mortality and complication rates for ES are reported to be 0.3 and 4.0%, respectively, for patients under 65 years of age. These rates increase to 0.4 and 6.5% in patients age 65 years or older [149]. Complication rates are noted to be higher when ES is performed in the absence of common duct dilation [150].

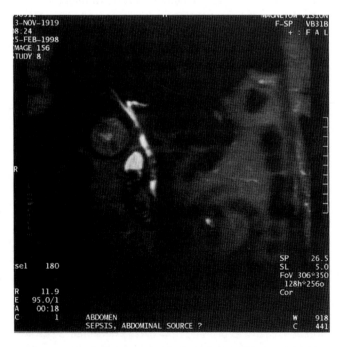

Figure 73.3 Magnetic resonance image demonstrating acute cholecystitis and common bile duct stones.

Choledochotomy at the time of open cholecystectomy was the treatment of choice for choledocholithiasis before the advent of laparoscopic cholecystectomy, endoscopic sphincterotomy, and other nonsurgical methods [151]. When open cholecystectomy is performed, common bile duct exploration (CBDE) is effective in clearing the duct of stones in 98% of cases. Unfortunately, this procedure is associated with a significant increase in operative morbidity and mortality, particularly in elderly patients. Because of this additional risk, intraoperative cholangiography is used to avoid unnecessary CBDE. In the critically ill patient, management of choledocholithiasis during open cholecystectomy may be restricted to placement of a T-tube. Subsequent clearance of common bile duct stones can be achieved by ES or radiologic manipulation via the T-tube tract, which is successful in more than 70% of patients [152].

The presence of associated choledocholithiasis complicates laparoscopic treatment of symptomatic gallstone disease. Ideally, patients with common duct stones are identified preoperatively and undergo ES with stone removal. Roughly 2–3% of patients with choledocholithiasis, however, do not have any associated laboratory or ultrasonographic evidence of common duct pathology [153]. The routine use of intraoperative cholangiography (IOC) may identify these patients and prevent the occurrence of retained common duct stones [154]. In the past, patients in whom common duct stones have been identified have traditionally undergone either conversion to open cholecystectomy with CBDE or completion of the cholecystectomy laparoscopically followed by ES in 1–2 weeks. More recently, laparoscopic CBDE has become part of the armamentarium against choledocholithiasis. Although still not widely used, this method has been shown to be effective in clearing more than 90% of common bile duct stones [155]. Choledocholithiasis discovered after cholecystectomy is best treated by ES.

There are several nonsurgical treatment modalities for treating choledocholithiasis in elderly and debilitated patients who also have cholelithiasis, but who are poor surgical candidates. ES has become the treatment of choice for common bile duct stones in this situation [156]. Adjunctive therapies to ES in the case of unretrievable common duct stones include the use of both intra- and extracorporeal lithotripsy [157] and temporary biliary stenting [158]. Permanent biliary stenting is associated with a high incidence of late complications and should be reserved for elderly patients with a short life expectancy [158]. The decision to forego cholecystectomy following ES for choledocholithiasis should be made not on the basis of chronologic age alone, but rather on an assessment of surgical risk [159].

Endoscopic sphincterotomy can be challenging in elderly patients. In their study of 182 patients, Deenitchin et al. [160] reported that elderly patients had a higher frequency of periampullary diverticula and were much more likely to require lithotripsy, nasobiliary drainage, and biliary stenting than younger patients. Elderly patients typically had larger and more abundant stones.

Acalculous Cholecystitis

Symptoms of gallstone disease may arise in the absence of documented cholelithiasis. Patients with chronic acalculous cholecystitis typically describe pain identical to that noted by patients with calculous biliary disease and often tell of extrabiliary symptoms of nausea, vomiting, and fatty food intolerance [161]. Although ultrasonography reveals no abnormalities, cholecystokinin-stimulated cholescintigraphy (CSC) characteristically reveals pain after CCK injection associated with a low gallbladder ejection fraction (<35%), nonvisualization of the gallbladder, or an absence of gallbladder emptying [162]. The treatment of chronic acalculous cholecystitis is identical to that for chronic cholecystitis secondary to cholelithiasis, which is either laparoscopic or open cholecystectomy [163]. Histologic examination of gallbladders following cholecystectomy for chronic acalculous cholecystitis often reveals evidence of chronic inflammation, cholesterolosis, and microscopic cholesterol crystallization. Predictors of symptom relief following cholecystectomy include a convincing history of true biliary colic in conjunction with cholescintigraphic evidence of gallbladder dysfunction.

Acute acalculous cholecystitis is a grave complication of critical illness and trauma [164] that has also been associated with extensive surgical procedures [165], total parenteral nutrition [166], and the acquired immunodeficiency syndrome (AIDS) [167]. This form of cholecystitis is also associated with high rates of gangrene and perforation [168]. Mortality rates for acute acalculous cholecystitis are high, reaching 50% in some reports.

Factors thought to be implicated in the pathogenesis of acute acalculous cholecystitis involve bile stasis, hyper-alimentation, gallbladder ischemia, and systemic infection [168]. Bile stasis in critically ill individuals may be related to prolonged narcotic use or mechanical ventilation, resulting in increased biliary concentration of lysophosphatydil choline, which may in turn lead to inflammatory changes in the gallbladder wall [169]. Total parenteral nutrition has also been implicated in the pathogenesis of acalculous cholecystitis, with gallbladder sludge occurring in 100% of patients after 6 weeks of hyper-alimentation.

The clinical presentation of acute acalculous cholecystitis is similar to that of acute cholecystitis due to calculous gallbladder disease. It has been suggested that this diagnosis be entertained in any critically ill septic patient with no apparent source of their sepsis [167]. Ultrasonography, cholescintigraphy, and CT are useful for supporting a diagnosis of acute acalculous cholecystitis (AAC). Ultrasonographic findings supportive of a diagnosis of AAC include gallbladder wall thickness exceeding 3.5 mm, the presence of sludge within the gallbladder, pericholecystic fluid, or the presence of gas within the gallbladder wall. These criteria also apply to the diagnosis of AAC by CT scan.

Acute acalculous cholecystitis is often treated with percutaneous cholecystostomy, as most patients with this condition are too ill to tolerate general anesthesia. In fact, there are some who suggest that percutaneous cholecystostomy may obviate the need for cholecystectomy in patients with acalculous cholecystitis [170].

Benign Disease of the Pancreas

With increased use of imaging, including computed tomography, pancreatic neoplasms are diagnosed more frequently and are often identified in elderly individuals. The natural history of pancreatic neoplasms is widely variable, with a relatively favorable prognosis for some and a dismal outlook for others. The appropriate management of these neoplasms requires a comprehensive knowledge of benign, premalignant, and malignant lesions. The most frequently identified of these lesions are cystic neoplasms, thus will be the focus of the discussion in this chapter. The management of acute pancreatitis and malignant disease of the pancreas in geriatric patients is beyond the scope of this review.

Previously accounting for less than 5% of recognized pancreatic neoplasms, cystic neoplasms of the pancreas are now diagnosed more frequently, certainly because of the increased use of abdominal imaging [171]. The cystic neoplasms include serous cystadenomas (SCA), mucinous cystic neoplasms (MCN), and intraductal papillary mucinous neoplasms (IPMN), with these three families (benign and malignant varieties) comprising more than 95% of pancreatic cystic neoplasms (Table 73.1). Many are diagnosed incidentally on abdominal imaging, although some patients present with abdominal pain and/or pancreatitis [172]. It is critical to differentiate inflammatory pseudocyst from cystic neoplasms of the pancreas, as pseudocysts still account for the majority of cystic lesions of the pancreas [173] and the treatments are completely different.

Serous Cystadenoma

Serous cystadenomas account for 32–39% of all cystic pancreatic neoplasms [174]. They occur more frequently in women, with a peak incidence between 50 and 80 years of age [175], and may also be associated with the von Hippel–Lindau syndrome [176]. A significant proportion of these neoplasms are diagnosed incidentally by ultrasound or CT scan done for other reasons. Symptoms occur in 50–80% of patients, most often abdominal pain [177, 178]. When large and located in the head of the gland, they may produce obstructive jaundice. The location of SCA is fairly evenly distributed throughout the pancreas, with a slightly higher predominance in the body and tail. Serous cystadenomas, once termed microcystic adenomas, may appear either spongiform (honeycomb), multicystic, or unilocular on CT or MRI. The presence of a central scar (sunburst calcification) is highly suggestive for this neoplasm, though it is found in only 20% of cases (Fig. 73.4) [179, 180]. Histologically, serous cystadenomas are characterized by simple, glycogen-rich cuboidal epithelium and have a very low potential for malignancy, with only a few cases reported in the literature [181]. ERCP or MRCP may be useful for distinguishing serous cystadenomas from other cystic lesions in that the serous tumors almost never communicate with the duct system whereas communication is common in pancreatic pseudocysts, IPMNs, and perhaps MCNs. When imaging is equivocal, cyst aspiration may be performed with cytologic analysis of the fluid for a variety of biochemical and tumor markers [182]. Growth rates are variable, though tumors that are <4 cm at presentation have been shown to grow at a rate of 0.12 cm/year whereas tumors 4 cm or larger at presentation grow at a much faster rate (2 cm/year) [183]. Recommendations based on this natural history data include resection for patients with serous cystadenomas 4 cm or larger who have a reasonable life expectancy [183]. Observation of serous cystadenomas with serial imaging is feasible if there are no symptoms or complicating circumstances [180], but some authors recommend resection in all patients with acceptable operative risk [184].

TABLE 73.1 Epidemiologic and biologic characteristics of pancreatic cystic neoplasms [173]

Type	Sex predilection	Peak decade of life	% of cystic neoplasms	Malignant potential/natural history
Serous cystadenoma	Female	7th	32–39	Resection curative, cystadenocarcinoma very rare
Mucinous cystic neoplasm	Female	5th	10–45	Resection curative if adenoma or borderline, diminished prognosis if invasive cancer present
Intraductal papillary mucinous neoplasm	Equal distribution	6–7th	21–33	Excellent prognosis if adenoma or borderline, diminished prognosis if invasive cancer present

Source: Data from Brugge et al. [173]

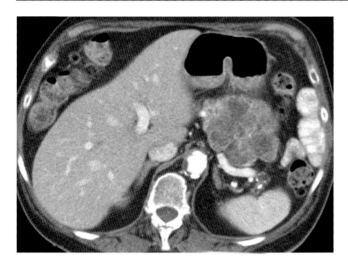

Figure 73.4 CT scan of serous cystadenoma (adapted with permission from Wargo and Warshaw [207]).

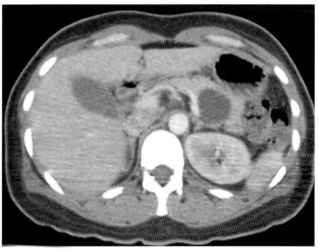

Figure 73.5 CT scan of a mucinous cystic neoplasm.

In the elderly population, these lesions can be followed with serial imaging if the diagnosis is certain and if they are under 4 cm. If lesions are over 4 cm, a careful assessment of risk of resection must be weighed against patient comorbidities. Lesions in the tail are commonly treated with distal pancreatectomy with or without splenectomy, while lesions in the head of the gland are treated with conventional pancreaticoduodenectomy. Lesions in the neck or body may be treated with middle-segment pancreatectomy [185]. Enucleation has been described for small cystic lesions but has been associated with excessive numbers of pancreatic fistulas [186]. Enucleation with the use of intraoperative ultrasound and closure of the pancreatic defect may be safer in some situations [187].

Mucinous Cystic Neoplasm

Mucinous cystic neoplasms account for 10–45% of all cystic pancreatic neoplasms [183]. Three stages are described by the World Health Organization: benign (adenomatous), low-grade malignant (borderline), and malignant (carcinoma in situ and invasive cancer) [188]. They are much more common in women than men, 90–100% in all series, and are generally found in the pancreatic body and tail in individuals between the ages of 50 and 70 years of age [185, 188]. Patients with MCN often present with symptoms of abdominal pain [188]. The lesions may be unilocular or multilocular [189]. Peripheral calcification on CT scan is specific for this lesion (Fig. 73.5), and when present, is suggestive for the presence of malignancy [190]. Because MCN infrequently communicate with the duct system, ERCP or MRCP may be helpful in distinguishing these from IPMNs. Cyst aspiration, most often guided by EUS, is used to demonstrate the presence of mucin, malignant cells, or elevated tumor markers such as CA 72-4

[191], CA 19-9 [192], or CEA. The most reliable and accessible indicators of MCN are a positive stain for mucin and a CEA level >192 ng/ml [191]. Histologically, they are characterized by a dense ovarian-like stroma, which differentiates them from IPMNs. As a group, MCN have a relatively high malignant potential. A recent study identified several risk factors for malignancy in mucinous cystic neoplasms, including advanced age, presence of symptoms, and the presence of large cysts and mural nodules on CT scan [193]. Five-year survival rates for patients undergoing resection for mucinous cystic neoplasms are excellent (100%) if histology reveals adenoma to minimally invasive carcinoma but are much lower (37%) if invasive cancer is present [193]. These lesions are less commonly found in the elderly population; however, do warrant resection if the operative risk is acceptable.

Intraductal Papillary Mucinous Neoplasm

Intraductal papillary mucinous neoplasms are mucus-producing tumors of the epithelial lining of the pancreatic duct and at present account for 21–33% of pancreatic cystic neoplasms [173]. It may be difficult to distinguish between branch-duct IPMNs and mucinous cystic neoplasms. IPMN occur at least as often in males and are usually diagnosed in patients between 60 and 70 years of age [194]. Most patients are symptomatic; at least 25% of patients report epigastric discomfort or backache [195] and almost as many have experienced at least one episode of pancreatitis [196]. The pathogenesis of acute pancreatitis is thought to be due to blockage of the pancreatic duct with viscid mucus.

IPMNs occur most frequently in the head of the pancreas and are classified into three types based on location in the duct system: main duct, side-branch, and mixed types [196]. CT or MRI may demonstrate evidence of a cystic pancreatic mass with or without dilation of the main pancreatic duct, and MRCP can assess the degree of ductal dilation, the presence of mural nodules, and any communication between the cystic lesion and the pancreatic duct (Fig. 73.6) [197]. Mucin extruding from a dilated pancreatic duct orifice, seen at endoscopy, is pathognomonic for IPMN, probably of the main-duct type. Injection of contrast into the pancreatic duct may show ductal dilation, filling defects (mucin or papillary growths), and cystic dilation of side branches off the main pancreatic duct [171]. Side-branch IPMN may not be visualized by pancreatography, making the distinction from MCN uncertain. In some cases, endoscopic pancreatoscopy has been used to visualize the duct directly and to assess for mural nodules [198]. Interestingly, IPMNs are often associated with other malignancies at extra-pancreatic sites [199].

The malignant potential of these lesions is significant. Over 40% of patients in recent series who underwent resection for main-duct IPMN had evidence of invasive carcinoma [200], and as many more had borderline tumors or carcinoma in situ. A number of studies suggest that main-duct IPMNs are more likely than branch-duct IPMNs to harbor malignancy [201].

Several factors have been identified which may be helpful in predicting malignancy in IPMNs. Involvement of the main pancreatic duct (in main-duct or mixed-type) is an independent predictor of malignancy [202]. A large combined study from the University of Verona and the Massachusetts General Hospital identified cancer in 60% of patients with main-duct IPMNs [200]. Factors associated with a higher risk of malignancy in patients with main-duct IPMNs in this study included older age, the presence of jaundice or new onset/worsening of diabetes [200]. Risk factors associated with malignancy in main-duct, branch-duct, and mixed-type variants were identified in other studies and include the presence of mural nodules, jaundice, the presence of symptoms at presentation, and main pancreatic duct diameter >7 mm [202]. In branch-duct variants, the presence of mural nodules and tumor diameter >30 mm were predictive of invasive carcinoma [202]. The presence of mucus at the time of endoscopy was associated with benign disease in one study, though this remains controversial [203].

The surgical management of IPMN is evolving as we gain more experience. An essential question is whether or not the neoplasms represent a localized process within an otherwise normal pancreas or if they arise within a field defect with the potential to give rise later to more neoplastic tissue in seemingly unaffected portions of the duct [204]. If IPMNs are part of a larger field defect involving the entire pancreas, it would be rational to consider total pancreatectomy to eradicate all disease. However, the significant morbidity associated with total pancreatectomy, including the management challenges of complete endocrine and exocrine insufficiency, must give pause. To date, most surgeons, including ourselves, subscribe to a policy of image-guided resection of the affected anatomic segment with intraoperative frozen sections to ensure noninvolvement of the resection margins [200, 202, 205]. It is generally accepted that most main-duct lesions should be resected in patients who are appropriate surgical candidates [200].

IPMNs have a natural history that is very different than that of pancreatic adenocarcinoma. In the combined series with the Massachusetts General Hospital and the University of Verona, the overall survival for those undergoing resection for IPMNs with adenoma, borderline tumors, or carcinoma in situ was excellent: 100% at 5 years. Sixty percent of those with IPMNs and invasive cancer were alive at 5 years, and 50% at 10 years. Not surprisingly, those patients with invasive cancer and positive nodes (41%) had decreased survival compared to those with negative nodes, though in contrast to pancreatic adenocarcinoma, their survival was reasonable (45% at 5 years). Recurrences in the remnant pancreas occurred in only 7% [200]. These data were corroborated by the Hopkins group, though the percentage of patients presenting with invasive cancer and positive lymph nodes was slightly higher [205].

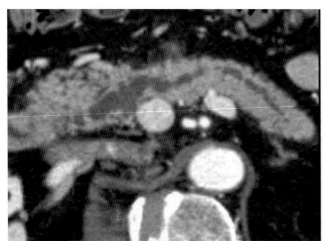

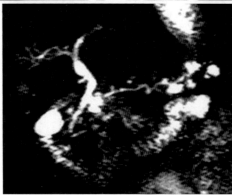

Figure 73.6 MRI/MRCP of intraductal papillary mucinous neoplasm (IPMN) (adapted with permission from Wargo and Warshaw [207]).

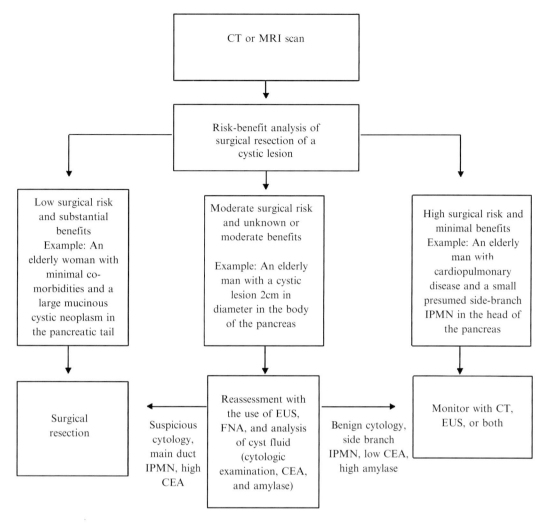

FIGURE 73.7 Algorithm for management of pancreatic cystic neoplasms (adapted with permission from Wargo and Warshaw [207]).

Management recommendations for branch-duct IPMNs are not quite as clearcut. In virtually all series, branch-duct IPMNs were less likely to harbor malignancy. In the recent series published from Johns Hopkins, 70% of branch-duct IPMNs were noninvasive compared to 50% of main-duct IPMNs [205]. Based on this, some have proposed a somewhat more selective approach for patients with branch-duct IPMNs. In general, branch-type IPMNs should be excised when they extend to the main duct, cause symptoms (such as acute pancreatitis), are large (>3 cm), when mural nodules are present, and when the main pancreatic duct diameter exceeds 7 mm [206]. If patients are asymptomatic and do have any of the above findings, they may be observed with close surveillance with CT scan every 6 months to 1 year. Others recommend a more aggressive posture, performing anatomic oncologic resections for any branch-duct IPMN in a suitable operative candidate [204]. Management strategies are likely to become clearer with more prospective data from specialized centers. An algorithm for management of cystic pancreatic lesions is shown in Fig. 73.7.

Conclusions

Benign disease of the gallbladder and pancreas remain major causes of morbidity and mortality worldwide, particularly in the elderly population. Their varied presentation in these patients clearly contributes to the complexity in treating these disorders. Advances in the diagnosis and therapy of biliary and pancreatic disease are likely to contribute to improvements in the care of elderly patients, but it is only with an astute understanding of the pathophysiology and treatment of these disorders that one can best manage these conditions in the elderly patient.

CASE STUDY

Eighty-four-year old female is admitted to the hospital with a 24 h history of confusion. PMH is significant for coronary artery disease, chronic renal insufficiency, and obstructive sleep apnea. Initially she is afebrile and has no abdominal findings. Labs are unremarkable. Forty-eight hours into her hospital course, she develops a fever, RUQ pain, and WBC 18,000. PE now reveals a tender RUQ mass. U/S reveals a distended gallbladder, cholelithiasis,

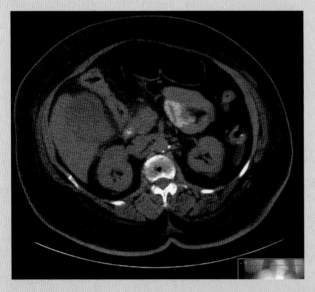

FIGURE 73.8 Computed tomography scan without intravenous contrast showing a distended gallbladder and surrounding inflammation.

and wall thickening. CT (done without contrast) shows a distended gallbladder with inflammatory changes in the mesocolon of the hepatic flexure (Fig. 73.8). There is no evidence of biliary ductal dilatation.

A diagnosis of acute cholecystitis is made. Because of concern about her cardiac function and renal insufficiency, CT-guided percutaneous cholecystostomy is performed. In addition, intravenous antibiotics are administered. She shows initial improvement in her fever, elevated WBC, and RUQ pain; however, within 24 h, her fever and WBC begin to rise. She is taken to the OR for an open cholecystectomy. The cholecystostomy tube is in good position; however, the gallbladder is gangrenous with frank areas of necrosis. A cholecystectomy is performed, and the subhepatic space is drained.

After an initial 48 h in the SICU, the patient is transferred to the floor. She is discharged 5 days later.

Key Points

- The clinical presentation of acute cholecystitis in the elderly may be atypical and/or subtle. In this case, the patient presented with mental status changes rather than the usual RUQ pain and fever.
- Imaging studies may be limited particularly in situations where contrast cannot be administered.
- After placement of a cholecystostomy tube, the patient's clinical course must be closely monitored. Lack of clinical resolution must lead to considering the possibility of gangrenous and/or perforated cholecystitis.

References

1. National Institutes of Health (1993) Consensus statement on gallstones and laparoscopic cholecystectomy. Am J Surg 165:390–393
2. Sanson TG, O'Keefe KP (1996) Evaluation of abdominal pain in the elderly. Emerg Med Clin North Am 14:615–627
3. Harness JK, Strodel WE, Talsma SE (1986) Symptomatic biliary tract disease in the elderly patient. Am J Surg 52:442–446
4. Kahng KU, Roslyn JJ (1994) Surgical issues for the elderly patient with hepatobiliary disease. Surg Clin North Am 74:345–373
5. Krasman ML, Gracie WA, Strasius SR (1991) Biliary tract disease in the aged. Clin Geriatr Med 7:347–370
6. Rosenthal RA, Andersen DK (1993) Surgery in the elderly: observations on the pathophysiology and treatment of cholelithiasis. Exp Gerontol 28:459–472
7. Cooper GS, Shlaes DM, Salata RA (1994) Intraabdominal infection: differences in presentation and outcome between younger patients and the elderly. Clin Infect Dis 19:146–148
8. Ingber S, Jacobson IM (1990) Biliary and pancreatic disease in the elderly. Gastroenterol Clin North Am 19:433–457

9. Sampliner RE, Bennett PH et al (1970) Gallbladder disease in Pima Indians: demonstrations of high prevalence and early onset by cholecystography. N Engl J Med 283:1358–1364
10. Johnston DE, Kaplan MM (1993) Pathogenesis and treatment of gallstones. N Engl J Med 328:412–421
11. Bowen JC, Brenner HI, Ferrante WA et al (1992) Gallstone disease: pathophysiology, epidemiology, natural history, and treatment options. Med Clin North Am 76:1143–1157
12. Henriksson P, Einarsson K, Eriksson A et al (1989) Estrogen-induced gallstone formation in males: relation to changes in serum and biliary lipids during hormonal treatment of prostate carcinoma. J Clin Invest 84:811–816
13. Everson GT, McKinley C, Kern F Jr (1991) Mechanisms of gallstone formation in women: effects of exogenous estrogen (Premarin) and dietary cholesterol on hepatic lipid metabolism. J Clin Invest 87:237–246
14. Tierney S, Pitt HA, Lillemoe KD (1993) Physiology and pathophysiology of gallbladder motility. Surg Clin North Am 73:1267–1290
15. Ratner J, Lisbona A, Rosenbloom M et al (1991) The prevalence of gallstone disease in very old institutionalized persons. JAMA 265:902–903

16. Giurgiu DI, Roslyn JJ (1996) Treatment of gallstones in the 1990s. Prim Care Clin North Am 23:497–513
17. Trotman BW, Sotoway RD (1975) Pigment vs. cholesterol cholelithiasis: clinical epidemiological aspects. Dig Dis 20:735–740
18. Pazzi P, Morsiani E, Sighinolfi D et al (1989) Pigment vs. cholesterol cholelithiasis: clinical and epidemiological aspects. Ital J Gastroenterol 21:310
19. Apstein MD, Carey MC (1996) Pathogenesis of cholesterol gallstones: a parsimonious hypothesis. Eur J Clin Invest 26:343–352
20. Portincasa P, Stolk MF, Van Erpecum KJ et al (1995) Cholesterol gallstone formation in man and potential treatments of the gallbladder motility defect. Scand J Gastroenterol 30:63S–78S
21. Nilsell K, Angelin B, Liljeqvist L et al (1985) Biliary lipid output and bile acid kinetics in cholesterol gallstone disease: evidence for an increased hepatic secretion of cholesterol in Swedish patients. Gastroenterology 89:287–293
22. Einarsson K, Nilsell K, Leijd B et al (1985) Influence of age on secretion of cholesterol and synthesis of bile acids by the liver. N Engl J Med 313:277–282
23. Friedman GD, Kannel WB, Dawber TR (1996) The epidemiology of gallbladder disease: observations in the Framingham study. J Chronic Dis 19:273–292
24. Roslyn JJ, Pitt HA, Mann LL, Ament ME, DenBesten L (1993) Gallbladder disease in patients on long-term parenteral nutrition. Gastroenterology 84:148–154
25. Ho KY, Weissberger AJ, Marbach P, Lazarus L (1990) Therapeutic efficacy of the somatostatin analog SMS 201-995 (octreotide) in acromegaly. Ann Intern Med 112:173–181
26. Shaw SJ, Hajnal F, Lebovitz Y et al (1993) Gallbladder dysfunction in diabetes mellitus. Dig Dis Sci 38:490–496
27. Everson GT, Nemeth A, Kourourian S et al (1989) Gallbladder function is altered in sickle cell hemoglobinopathy. Gastroenterology 96:1307–1316
28. Nino Murchia M, Burton D et al (1990) Gallbladder contractility in patients with spinal cord injuries: a sonographic investigation. AJR Am J Roentgenol 154:521–524
29. Masclee AA, Jansen JB, Dreissen WM et al (1990) Effect of truncal vagotomy on cholecystokinin release, gallbladder contraction, and gallbladder sensitivity to cholecystokinin in humans. Gastroenterology 98:1338–1344
30. Patankar R, Ozmen MM, Bailey IS et al (1995) Gallbladder motility, gallstones, and the surgeon. Dig Dis Sci 40:2323–2335
31. Howard PJ, Murphy GM, Dowling RH (1991) Gallbladder emptying patterns in response to a normal meal in healthy subjects and patients with gallstones: ultrasound study. Gut 32:1406–1411
32. Fisher RS, Rock E, Levin G et al (1987) Effects of somatostatin on gallbladder emptying. Gastroenterology 92:885–890
33. Cameron AJ, Phillips SF, Summerskill WH (1968) Effect of cholecystokinin, gastrin, secretin, and glucagon on human gallbladder in vitro. Proc Soc Exp Biol Med 131:149
34. Kalfin R, Milenov K (1991) The effect of vasoactive intestinal polypeptide (VIP) on the canine gallbladder motility. Comp Biochem Physiol 100:513–517
35. Conter R, Roslyn JJ, Muller EL et al (1985) Effect of pancreatic polypeptide on gallbladder filling. J Surg Res 38:461–467
36. Conter R, Roslyn JJ, Taylor IL (1987) Effects of peptide YY on gallbladder motility. Am J Physiol 252:G736–G741
37. Pellegrini C, Ryan T, Broderick W, Way LW (1986) Gallbladder filling and emptying during cholesterol gallstone formation in the prairie dog. Gastroenterology 90:143–149
38. Behar J, Lee KY, Thompson WR et al (1989) Gallbladder contraction in patients with pigment and cholesterol stones. Gastroenterology 97:1479–1484
39. Maringhini A, Ciambra M, Baccelliere P et al (1993) Biliary sludge and gallstones in pregnancy: incidence, risk factors, and natural history. Ann Intern Med 119:116–120
40. Messing B, Bories C, Kunstlinger F et al (1983) Does total parenteral nutrition induce gallbladder sludge formation and lithiasis? Gastroenterology 84:1012–1019
41. Poston GJ, Singh P, Maclellan D et al (1988) Age related contractility and gallbladder cholecystokinin receptor population in the guinea pig. Mech Ageing Dev 46:225–236
42. Poston GJ, Draviam EJ, Yao CZ et al (1990) Effect of age and sensitivity to cholecystokinin on gallstone formation in the guinea pig. Gastroenterology 98:939–999
43. Khalil T, Walker PJ, Wiener I et al (1985) Effects of aging on gallbladder contraction and release of cholecystokinin-33 in humans. Surgery 98:423–429
44. Berger D, Crowther RC, Floyd JC Jr et al (1978) Effect of age on fasting plasma levels of pancreatic hormones in man. Am J Surg 47:1183–1189
45. Moser AJ, Abedin MZ, Roslyn JJ (1993) The pathogenesis of gallstone formation. Adv Surg 26:357–386
46. Cahalane MJ, Neubrand MW, Carey MC (1988) Physical-chemical pathogenesis of pigment stones. Semin Liver Dis 8:317–328
47. Trotman BW, Bernstein SE, Bove KE et al (1980) Studies on the pathogenesis of pigment gallstones in hemolytic anemia. J Clin Invest 65:1301–1308
48. Ostrow JD (1984) The etiology of pigment gallstones. Hepatology 4:215S–222S
49. Carey MC (1993) Pathogenesis of gallstones. Am J Surg 165:410–419
50. Cetta F (1991) The role of bacteria in pigment gallstone formation. Am Surg 213:315–326
51. Nagase M, Hikaro Y, Soloway RD et al (1980) Gallstones in western Japan: features affecting the prevalence of intrahepatic gallstones. Gastroenterology 78:684–690
52. Ho KJ (1996) Biliary electrolytes and enzymes in patients with and without gallstones. Dig Dis Sci 41:2409–2416
53. Apstein MD, Carey MC (1993) Biliary tract stones and associated diseases. In: Stein JH (ed) Internal medicine, 4th edn. Mosby Yearbook, St. Louis
54. Cucchiaro G, Rossitch JC, Bowie J et al (1990) Clinical significance of ultrasonographically detected coincidental gallstones. Dig Dis Sci 35:417–421
55. Gibney EJ (1990) Asymptomatic gallstones. Br J Surg 77:368–372
56. Comfort MW, Gray HK, Wilson JM (1948) The silent gallstone: a ten to twenty year follow-up study of 112 cases. Ann Surg 128:931–937
57. Gracie WA, Ransohoff DF (1982) The natural history of silent gallstones: the innocent gallstone is not a myth. N Engl J Med 307:798–800
58. Attili AF, DeSantis A, Capri R, Repice AM, Maselli S (1995) GREPCO group. The natural history of gallstones: the GREPCO experience. Hepatology 21:656–660
59. McSherry CK, Ferstenberg H, Calhoun WF et al (1985) The natural history of diagnosed gallstone disease in symptomatic and asymptomatic patients. Ann Surg 202:59–63
60. Friedman GD (1993) Natural history of asymptomatic and symptomatic gallstones. Am J Surg 165:399–404
61. Fendrick AM, Gleeson SP, Cabana MD, Schwartz JS (1993) Asymptomatic gallstones revisited: is there a role for laparoscopic cholecystectomy? Arch Fam Med 2:959–968
62. Wenckhert A, Robertson B (1966) The natural course of gallstone disease. Gastroenterology 50:376–381
63. Cucchiaro G, Walters CR, Rossitch JC et al (1989) Deaths from gallstones: incidence and associated clinical factors. Ann Surg 209:149–151
64. Schreiber H, Macon WL, Pories WJ (1978) Incidental cholecystectomy during major abdominal surgery in the elderly. Am J Surg 135:196

65. Green JD, Birkhead G, Herbert J et al (1990) Increased morbidity in surgical patients undergoing secondary (incidental) cholecystectomy. Ann Surg 211:50–54

66. Thistle JL, Cleary PA, Lachin JM et al (1984) The natural history of cholelithiasis: the National Cooperative Gallstone Study. Ann Intern Med 101:171–175

67. Friedman GD, Raviola CA, Fireman B (1989) Prognosis of gallstones with mild or no symptoms: 25 years of follow-up in a health maintenance organization. J Clin Epidemiol 42:127–136

68. Morrow DJ, Thompson J, Wilson SE (1978) Acute cholecystitis in the elderly: a surgical emergency. Arch Surg 113:1149–1152

69. Moscati RM (1996) Cholelithiasis, cholecystitis, and pancreatitis. Emerg Med Clin North Am 14:719–736

70. Zollinger RM (1933) Observations following distension of the gallbladder and common duct in man. Proc Soc Exp Biol Med 30:1260–1261

71. Fenster LF, Lonborg R, Thirlby RC et al (1995) What symptoms does cholecystectomy cure? Insights from an outcomes measurement project and review of the literature. Am J Surg 169:535–538

72. Gilliland TM, Traverso W (1990) Cholecystectomy provides longterm symptom relief in patients with acalculous cholecystitis. Am J Surg 159:489–492

73. Zeman RK, Garra BS (1991) Gallbladder imaging: the state of the art. Gastroenterol Clin North Am 20:127–156

74. Shea JA, Berlin JA, Escarce JJ et al (1994) Revised estimates of diagnostic test sensitivity and specificity in suspected biliary tract disease. Arch Intern Med 154:2573–2581

75. Ros E, Valderrama R, Bru C et al (1994) Symptomatic versus silent gallstones: radiographic features and eligibility for nonsurgical treatment. Dig Dis Sci 39:1697–1703

76. Baron RL, Rohrmann CA, Lee SP et al (1988) CT evaluation of gallstones in vitro: correlation with chemical analysis. Am J Radiol 151:1123–1128

77. Tierney S, Pitt HA, Lillemoe KD (1993) Physiology and pathophysiology of gallbladder motility. Surg Clin North Am 73:1267–1290

78. Roslyn JJ, Binns GS, Hughes EFX et al (1993) Open cholecystectomy: a contemporary analysis of 42,474 patients. Ann Surg 218:129–137

79. Glenn F (1980) The incidence and causes of death following surgery for nonmalignant biliary tract disease. Ann Surg 191:271–275

80. Pigott JP, Williams GB (1988) Choleystectomy in the elderly. Am J Surg 155:408–410

81. Gadacz TR, Talamini MA, Lillemoe KD et al (1990) Laparoscopic cholecystectomy. Surg Clin North Am 70:1249–1262

82. Dubois F, Icard P, Barthelot G et al (1990) Coelioscopic cholecystectomy: preliminary report of 36 cases. Ann Surg 211:60–62

83. Reddick EJ, Olsen DO (1989) Laparoscopic laser cholecystectomy: a comparison with mini-lap cholecystectomy. Surg Endosc 3:131–133

84. McMahon AJ, Russell IT, Ramsay G et al (1994) Laparoscopic and minilaparotomy cholecystectomy: a randomized trial comparing postoperative pain and pulmonary function. Surgery 115:533–539

85. Perissat J (1993) Laparoscopic cholecystectomy: the European experience. Am J Surg 165:444–449

86. Gadacz TR (1993) U.S. experience with laparoscopic cholecystectomy. Am J Surg 165:450–454

87. Southern Surgeons Club (1991) A prospective analysis of 1518 laparoscopic cholecystectomies. N Engl J Med 324:1073–1078

88. Deziel DJ, Milikan KW, Economou SG et al (1996) Complications of laparoscopic cholecystectomy: a national survey of 4292 hospitals and an analysis of 77,604 cases. Am J Surg 165:9–14

89. Nenner RP, Imperato PJ, Alcorn CM (1992) Serious complications of laparoscopic cholecystectomy in New York State. NY State J Med 92:179–181

90. Southern Surgeons Club, Moore MJ, Bennett CL (1995) The learning curve for laparoscopic cholecystectomy. Am J Surg 170:55–59

91. Williams LF, Chapman WC, Bonau RA et al (1993) Comparison of laparoscopic cholecystectomy with open cholecystectomy in a single center. Am J Surg 165:459–465

92. Lee VS, Chari RS, Cucchiaro G et al (1993) Complications of laparoscopic cholecystectomy. Am J Surg 165:527–532

93. Fried GM, Barkum JS, Sigman HH et al (1994) Factors determining conversion to laparotomy in patients undergoing laparoscopic cholecystectomy. Am J Surg 167:35–41

94. Orlando R, Russell JC, Mattie A (1993) Connecticut laparoscopic cholecystectomy registry. Laparoscopic cholecystectomy: a statewide experience. Arch Surg 128:494–499

95. Massie MT, Massie LB, Marrangoni AG et al (1993) Advantages of laparoscopic cholecystectomy in the elderly and in patients with high ASA classifications. J Laparoendosc Surg 3:467–476

96. Fried GM, Clas D, Meakins JL (1994) Minimally invasive surgery in the elderly patient. Surg Clin North Am 74:375–387

97. Askew AR (1995) Surgery for gallstones in the elderly. Aust N Z J Surg 65:312–315

98. Ido K, Suzuki T, Kimura K et al (1995) Laparoscopic cholecystectomy in the elderly: analysis of pre-operative risk factors and postoperative complications. J Gastroenterol Hepatol 10:517–522

99. Milheiro A, Sousa FC, Oliveira L et al (1996) Pulmonary function after laparoscopic cholecystectomy in the elderly. Br J Surg 83:1059–1061

100. Soper NJ (1993) Effect of nonbiliary problems on laparoscopic cholecystectomy. Am J Surg 165:522–526

101. Salen G, Tint GS, Shefer S (1991) Treatment of cholesterol gallstones with litholytic bile acids. Gastroenterol Clin North Am 20:171–181

102. Danzinger RG, Hofmann AF, Schoenfield LJ et al (1972) Dissolution of cholesterol gallstones by chenodeoxycholic acid. N Engl J Med 286:1–8

103. Bachrach WH, Hofmann AF (1982) Ursodeoxycholic acid in the treatment of cholesterol lithiasis. Dig Dis Sci 27:333–356

104. Salen G (1991) Clinical perspective on the treatment of gallstones with ursodeoxycholic acid. J Clin Gastroenterol 10:S12–S17

105. Walker JW (1891) The removal of gallstones by ether solution. Lancet 1:874–875

106. Admirand WH, Way LW (1972) Medical treatment of retained gallstones. Trans Assoc Am Physicians 85:382–387

107. Thistle JL, May GR, Bender CE et al (1989) Dissolution of cholesterol gallbladder stones by methyl tert-butyl ether administered by percutaneous transhepatic catheter. N Engl J Med 320:633–635

108. Pauletzki J, Holl J, Sackman M et al (1995) Gallstone recurrence after direct contact dissolution with methyltert-butyl ether. Dig Dis Sci 40:1775–1781

109. Albert MB, Fromm H, Borstelmann R et al (1990) Successful outpatient treatment of gallstones with piezoelectric lithotripsy. Ann Intern Med 113:164–166

110. Norman DC, Yoshikawa TT (1983) Intraabdominal infections in the elderly. J Am Geriatr Soc 31:677–684

111. Hafif A, Gutman M, Kaplan O et al (1991) The management of acute cholecystitis in elderly patients. Am Surg 57:648–652

112. De Dombal FT (1994) Acute abdominal pain in the elderly. J Clin Gastroenterol 19:331–335

113. Kim EE, Pjura G, Lowry P et al (1986) Morphine augmented cholescintigraphy in the diagnosis of acute cholecystitis. Am J Radiol 147:1177–1179

114. Lo CM, Lai ECS, Fan ST et al (1996) Laparoscopic cholecystectomy for acute cholecystitis in the elderly. World J Surg 20:983–987

115. Cohen SA, Siegel JH (1995) Biliary tract emergencies: endoscopic and medical management. Crit Care Clin 11:273–294

116. Kaufman M, Weissberg D, Schwartz I et al (1990) Cholecystostomy as a definitive operation. Surg Gynecol Obstet 170:533–537

117. Goodacre B, van Sonnenberg E, D'Agostino H et al (1991) Interventional radiology in gallstone disease. Gastroenterol Clin North Am 20:209–227

118. Van Steenbergen W, Rigauts H, Ponette E et al (1993) Percutaneous cholecystostomy for acute complicated calculous cholecystitis in elderly patients. J Am Geriatr Soc 41:157–162

119. Browning PD, McGahan JP, Gerscovich EO (1993) Percutaneous cholecystostomy for suspected acute cholecystitis in the hospitalized patient. J Vasc Inter Radiol 4:531–538

120. Ha JPY, Tsui KK, Tang CN et al (2008) Cholecystectomy or not after percutaneous cholecystostomy for acute calculous cholecystitis in high-risk patients. Hepatogastroenterology 55:1497–1502

121. Strohl EL, Diffenbaugh WG, Baker JH et al (1962) Collective reviews: gangrene and perforation of the gallbladder. Int Abstr Surg 114:1–7

122. Felice PR, Trowbridge PE, Ferrara JJ (1984) Evolving changes in the pathogenesis and treatment of the perforated gallbladder: a combined hospital study. Am J Surg 149:466–473

123. Niemeier OW (1934) Acute free perforation of the gallbladder. Ann Surg 99:922–924

124. Abu-Dalu J, Urca I (1971) Acute cholecystitis with perforation into the peritoneal cavity. Arch Surg 102:108–111

125. Roslyn JJ, Busuttil RW (1979) Perforation of the gallbladder: a frequently mismanaged condition. Am J Surg 137:307–312

126. Madrazo BL, Francis I, Hricak H et al (1982) Sonographic findings in perforation of the gallbladder. AJR Am J Roentgenol 139:491–496

127. Roslyn JJ, Thompson JE Jr, Darvin H et al (1987) Risk factors for gallbladder perforation. Am J Gastroenterol 82:636–640

128. Cooperman AM, Dickson ER, ReMine WH (1968) Changing concepts in the surgical treatment of gallstone ileus. Ann Surg 167:377–383

129. Siskind BN, Hawkins HB, Cinti DC et al (1987) Gallbladder perforation: an imaging analysis. J Clin Gastroenterol 9:670–678

130. Soiva M, Pamilo M, Paivansalo M et al (1988) Ultrasonography in acute gallbladder perforation. Acta Radiol 29:41–44

131. Kim PN, Lee KS, Kim IY et al (1994) Gallbladder perforation: comparison of US findings with CT. Abdom Imaging 19:239–242

132. Andreu J, Perez C, Caceres J et al (1987) Computed tomography as the method of choice in the diagnosis of emphysematous cholecystitis. Gastrointest Radiol 12:315–318

133. Mentzer RM, Golden GT, Chandler JG et al (1975) A comparative appraisal of emphysematous cholecystitis. Am J Surg 129:10–15

134. Yeatman TJ (1986) Emphysematous cholecystitis: an insidious variant of acute cholecystitis. Am J Emerg Med 4:163–166

135. Parulekar SG (1982) Sonographic findings in acute emphsematous cholecystitis. Radiology 145:117–119

136. Banwell PE, Hill ADK, Menzies-Gow N et al (1994) Laparoscopic cholecystectomy: safe and feasible in emphysematous cholecystitis. Surg Laparosc Endosc 4:189–191

137. Csendes A, Burdiles P, Maluenda F et al (1996) Simultaneous bacteriologic assessment of bile from gallbladder and common bile duct in control subjects and patients with gallstones and common duct stones. Arch Surg 131:389–394

138. Bernhoft RA, Pelligrini CA, Moston RW et al (1984) Composition and morphologic and clinical features of common duct stones. Am J Surg 148:77–79

139. Anciaux ML, Pelletier G, Attali P et al (1986) Prospective study of clinical and biochemical features of symptomatic choledocholithiasis. Dig Dis Sci 31:449–451

140. Hauer-Jensen M, Karesen R, Nygaard K et al (1993) Prospective randomized study of routine intraoperative cholangiography during open cholecystectomy: long-term follow-up and predictors of choledocholithiasis. Surgery 113:318–323

141. Hunguier M, Bornet P, Charpak Y et al (1991) Selective contraindication based on multivariate analysis for operative cholangiography in biliary lithiasis. Surg Gynecol Obstet 172:470–474

142. Cronan JJ (1986) US diagnosis of choledocholithiasis: a reappraisal. Radiology 161:133–134

143. Phillips EH (1993) Routine versus selective intraoperative cholangiography. Am J Surg 165:505–507

144. Perissat J, Huibregtse K, Keane FBV et al (1994) Management of bile duct stones in the era of laparoscopic cholecystectomy. Br J Surg 81:799–810

145. Boulay J, Schellenberg R, Brady PG (1992) Role of ERCP and therapeutic biliary endoscopy in association with laparoscopic cholecystectomy. Am J Gastroenterol 87:837–842

146. Lai ECS, Mok FPT, Tan ESY et al (1992) Endoscopic biliary drainage for severe acute cholangitis. N Engl J Med 326:1582–1586

147. Fan ST, Lai ECS, Mok FPT et al (1993) Early treatment of acute biliary pancreatitis by endoscopic papillotomy. N Engl J Med 328:228–232

148. Lezoche E, Paganini AM, Carlei F et al (1996) Laparoscopic treatment of gallbladder and common bile duct stones: a prospective study. World J Surg 20:535–542

149. Vaira D, D'Anna L, Ainley C et al (1989) Endoscopic sphincterotomy in 1000 consecutive patients. Lancet 2:431–434

150. Sherman S, Ruffolo TA, Hawes RH et al (1991) Complications of endoscopic sphincterotomy: a prospective series with emphasis on the increased risk associated with sphincter of Oddi dysfunction and nondilated bile ducts. Gastroenterology 101:1068–1075

151. Pitt HA (1993) Role of open choledochotomy in the treatment of choledocholithiasis. Am J Surg 165:483–486

152. Moston RW, Wetter LA (1990) Operative choledochoscopy: common bile duct exploration is incomplete without it. Br J Surg 77:975–979

153. Phillips EH (1993) Routine versus selective intraoperative cholangiography. Am J Surg 165:505–507

154. Levine SB, Lerner SJ, Leifer ED et al (1983) Intraoperative cholangiography: a review of indications and analysis of age-sex groups. Ann Surg 198:692–697

155. Petelin JB (1993) Laparoscopic approach to common duct pathology. Am J Surg 165:487–491

156. May GR, Shaffer EH (1991) Should elective endoscopic sphincterotomy replace cholecystectomy for the treatment of high-risk patients with gallstone pancreatitis? J Clin Gastroenterol 13:125–128

157. Adamek HE, Maier M, Jakobs R et al (1996) Management of retained bile duct stones: a prospective open trial comparing extracorporeal and intracorporeal lithotripsy. Gastrointest Endosc 44:40–47

158. Costi R, DiMauro D, Mazzeo A et al (2007) Routine laparoscopic cholecystectomy after endoscopic sphincterotomy for choledocholithiasis in octogenarians: is it worth the risk? Surg Endosc 21:41–47

159. Hammarstrom LE, Holmin T, Stridbeck H et al (1995) Long-term follow-up of prospective randomized study of endoscopic versus surgical treatment of bile duct calculi in patients with gallbladder in situ. Br J Surg 82:1516–1521

160. Deenitchin GP, Konomi H, Kimura H et al (1995) Reappraisal of safety of endoscopic sphincterotomy for common bile duct stones in the elderly. Am J Surg 170:51–54

161. Jones DB, Soper NJ, Brewer JD et al (1996) Chronic acalculous cholecystitis: laparoscopic treatment. Surg Laparosc Endosc 6:114–122

162. Barron LG, Rubio PA (1995) Importance of accurate preoperative diagnosis and role of advanced laparoscopic cholecystectomy in relieving chronic acalculous cholecystitis. J Laparoendosc Surg 5:357–361

163. Gilliland TM, Traverso LW (1990) Cholecystectomy provides long-term symptom relief in patients with acalculous gallbladders. Am J Surg 159:489–492

164. Raunest J, Imhof M, Rauen U et al (1992) Acute choecystitis: a complication in severely injured intensive care patients. J Trauma 32:433–440

165. Savoca P, Longo W, Zucker K et al (1990) The increasing prevalence of acalculous cholecystitis in outpatients: results of a 7-year study. Ann Surg 211:433–437

166. Peterson SR, Sheldon GF (1984) Acute acalculous cholecystitis: a complication of hyperalimentation. Arch Surg 119:1389–1392

167. Barie PS, Fischer E (1995) Acute acalculous cholecystitis. J Am Coll Surg 180:232–244

168. Orlando R, Gleason E, Drezner AD (1983) Acute acalculous cholecystitis in the critically ill patient. Am J Surg 145:472–476

169. Niderheiser DH (1986) Acute acalculous cholecystitis induced by lysophosphatidyl choline. Am J Pathol 124:559–563

170. Melin MM, Sarr MG, Bender CE et al (1995) Percutaneous cholecystostomy: a valuable technique in high-risk patients with presumed acute cholecystitis. Br J Surg 82:1274–1277

171. Megibow AJ, Lombardo FP, Guarise A, Carbognin G, Scholes J, Macari NM, Balthazar EJ, Rocacci C (2001) Cystic masses: cross-sectional imaging observations and serial follow-up. Abdom Imaging 26:640–647

172. Talamini MA, Pitt HA, Hruban RH, Boitnott JK, Coleman J, Cameron JL (1992) Spectrum of cystic tumors of the pancreas. Am J Surg 163:117–124

173. Brugge WR, Lauwers GY, Sahani D, Fernandez-del Castillo C, Warshaw AL (2004) Cystic neoplasms of the pancreas. N Engl J Med 351:1218–1226

174. Fernandez-del Castillo C, Targarona J, Thayer SP, Rattner DW, Brugge WR, Warshaw AL (2003) Incidental pancreatic cysts: clinicopathologic characteristics and comparison with symptomatic patients. Arch Surg 138:427–434

175. Yang EY, Joehl RJ, Talamonti MS (1994) Cystic neoplasms of the pancreas. J Am Coll Surg 179:747–757

176. Mohr VH, Vortmeyer AO, Zhuang Z et al (2000) Histopathology and molecular genetics of multiple cysts and microcystic (serous) cystadenomas of the pancreas in von Hippel-Lindau patients. Am J Pathol 157:1615–1621

177. Sarr MG, Kendrick ML, Nagorney DM et al (2001) Cystic neoplasms of the pancreas: benign to malignant epithelial neoplasms. Surg Clin North Am 81:497–509

178. Warshaw AL, Compton CC, Lewandrowski K, Cardenosa G, Mueller PR (1990) Cystic tumors of the pancreas: new clinical, radiologic, and pathologic observations in 67 patients. Ann Surg 212:432–445

179. Fernandez-del Castillo C, Warshaw AL (2000) Current management of cystic neoplasms of the pancreas. Adv Surg 34:237–248

180. Santos LD, Chow C, Henderson CJ et al (2002) Serous oligocystic adenoma of the pancreas, a clinicopathological and immunohistochemical study of three cases with ultrastructural findings. Pathology 34:148–156

181. Pyke CM, van Heerden JA, Colby TV, Sarr MG, Weaver AL (1992) The spectrum of serous cystadenoma of the pancreas: clinical, pathologic, and surgical aspects. Ann Surg 215:132–139

182. Centeno BA, Warshaw AL, Mayo-Smith W, Southern JF, Lewandrowski K (1997) Cytologic diagnosis of pancreatic cystic lesions: a prospective study of 28 percutaneous aspirates. Acta Cytol 41:972–980

183. Tseng JF, Warshaw AL, Sahani DV, Lauwers GY, Rattner DW, Fernandez-del Castillo C (2005) Pancreatic serous cystadenoma: tumor growth rates and recommendations for treatment. Ann Surg 242(3):413–419

184. Horvath KD, Chabot JA (1999) An aggressive resectional approach to cystic neoplasms of the pancreas. Am J Surg 178:269–274

185. Warshaw AL, Rattner DW, Fernandez-del Castillo C, Z'graggen K (1998) Middle segment pancreatectomy: a novel technique for conserving pancreatic tissue. Arch Surg 133:327–331

186. Talamini MA, Moesinger R, Yeo CJ, Poulose B, Hruban RH, Cameron JL, Pitt HA (1998) Cystadenomas of the pancreas: is enucleation an adequate operation? Ann Surg 227:896–903

187. Kiely JM, Nakeeb A, Komorowski RA, Wilson SD, Pitt HA (2003) Cystic pancreatic neoplasms: enucleate or resect? J Gastrointest Surg 7:890–897

188. Kloppel G, Solcia E, Longnecker DS, Capella C, Sobin LH (1998) Histologic typing of tumors of the exocrine pancreas: World Health Organization international histological classification of tumours, 2nd edn. Springer-Verlag, New York

189. Buetow PC, Rao P, Thompson LD (1998) Mucinous cystic neoplasms of the pancreas: radiologic-pathologic correlation. Radiographics 18:433–449

190. Curry CA, Eng J, Horton KM et al (2000) CT of primary cystic pancreatic neoplasms: can CT be used for patient triage and treatment? AJR Am J Roentgenol 175:99–103

191. Brugge WR, Lewandrowski K, Lee-Lewandrowski E et al (2004) Diagnosis of pancreatic cystic neoplasms: a report of the cooperative pancreatic cyst study. Gastroenterology 126:1330–1336

192. Frossard JL, Amouyal P, Amouyal G et al (2003) Performance of endoscopically-guided fine needle aspiration and biopsy in the diagnosis of pancreatic cystic lesions. Am J Gastroenterol 98:1516–1524

193. Suzuki Y, Atomi Y, Sugiyama M, Isaji S, Inui K, Kimua W, Sunamura M, Fuurukawa T, Yanagisawa A, Ariyama J, Takada T, Watanabe H, Suda K (2004) Cystic neoplasms of the pancreas: a Japanese multiinstitutional study of intraductal papillary mucinous tumors and mucinous cystic tumor. Pancreas 28(3):241–246

194. Sheehan MK, Beck K, Pickleman J, Aranha GV (2003) Spectrum of cystic neoplasms of the pancreas and their surgical management. Arch Surg 138:657–662

195. Yamaguchi K, Ogawa Y, Chijiwa K et al (1996) Mucin-hypersecreting tumors of the pancreas: assessing the grade of malignancy preoperatively. Am J Surg 171:427–431

196. Tanaka M (2004) Intraductal papillary mucinous neoplasm of the pancreas: diagnosis and treatment. Pancreas 28(3):282–288

197. Koito K, Namieno T, Ichimura T et al (1998) Mucin-producing pancreatic tumors: comparison of MR cholangiopancreatography with endoscopic retrograde cholangiopancreatography. Radiology 208:231–237

198. Hara T, Yamaguchi T, Ishihara T et al (2002) Diagnosis and patient management of intraductal papillary mucinous tumor of the pancreas by using peroral pancreatoscopy and intraductal ultrasonography. Gastroenterology 122:34–43

199. Sugiyama M, Atomi Y, Kuroda A (1997) Two types of mucin-producing cystic tumors of the pancreas: diagnosis and treatment. Surgery 122:617–625

200. Salvia R, Fernandez-del Castillo C, Bassi C, Thayer SP, Falconi M, Mantovani W, Pederzoli P, Warshaw AL (2004) Main-duct intraductal papillary mucinous neoplasms of the pancreas: clinical predictors of malignancy and long-term survival following resection. Ann Surg 239(5):678–687

201. Kobari M, Egawa S, Shibuya K et al (1999) Intraductal papillary mucinous tumors of the pancreas comprise 2 clinical subtypes: differences in clinical characteristics and surgical management. Arch Surg 134:1131–1136

202. Sugiyama M, Izumisato Y, Abe N, Masaki T, Mori T, Atomi Y (2003) Predictive factors for malignancy in intraductal papillary mucinous tumours of the pancreas. Br J Surg 90:1244–1249

203. Kitagawa Y, Unger TA, Taylor S, Kozarek RA, Traverso LW (2003) Mucus is a predictor of better prognosis and survival in patients with intraductal papillary mucinous tumor of the pancreas. J Gastrointest Surg 7(1):12–19

204. Sarr MG, Murr M, Smyrk TC, Yeo CJ, Fernandez-del-Castillo C, Hawes RH, Freeny PC (2003) Primary cystic neoplasms of the pancreas: neoplastic disorders of emerging importance – current state-of-the-art and unanswered questions. J Gastrointest Surg 7(3):417–428

205. Sohn TA, Yeo CJ, Cameron JL, Hruban RH, Fukushima N, Campbell KA, Lillimoe KD (2004) Intraductal papillary mucinous neoplasms of the pancreas: an updated experience. Ann Surg 239(6):788–799

206. Maguchi H, Osania M, Yanagawa N et al (1998) Therapeutic strategy for mucin-producing tumor of the pancreas. Geka 60:1152–1157

207. Wargo JA, Warshaw AL (2005) Surgical approach to pancreatic exocrine neoplasms. Minerva Chir 60(6):445–468

Chapter 74
Malignant Diseases of the Gallbladder and Bile Ducts

Steven A. Ahrendt and Thomas H. Magnuson

Gallbladder and bile duct cancers are relatively uncommon malignancies and tend to occur primarily in elderly patients. Although the overall prognosis of these malignancies remains poor, recent advances in hepatobiliary surgery, perioperative care, and adjuvant therapy have helped to improve overall survival and quality of life. A multidisciplinary approach in the management of these patients, including surgery, medical oncology, radiation oncology, and invasive radiology, is critical to achieving favorable results.

Gallbladder Cancer

Cancer of the gallbladder is an aggressive malignancy that occurs predominantly in elderly patients. It is strongly associated with gallstones but is also linked with other geographic and genetic factors. With the exception of early-stage cases detected incidentally at the time of cholecystectomy for gallstone disease, the prognosis is poor. Most patients present with unresectable tumors, and most can be managed nonoperatively. Recently, an aggressive surgical approach for patients with gallbladder cancer has produced encouraging results at several centers with acceptable morbidity and mortality in the predominantly elderly patient population.

Incidence

Gallbladder cancer is the fifth most common gastrointestinal malignancy following cancer of the colon, pancreas, stomach, and esophagus [1, 2]. Cancer of the gallbladder is two to three times more common in women than in men, in part due to the higher incidence of gallstones in women [1–3]. With the increase in age of the American population, the incidence of gallbladder cancer has gradually increased, with approximately 5,000 new cases diagnosed annually [4]. The overall incidence of gallbladder cancer in the USA is 2.5 cases per 100,000 residents [1], with the incidence varying considerably with both ethnic background and geographic location [5, 6]. In the USA, gallbladder cancer is more common in American Indians than in the non-Indian populations [6]. The annual incidence of gallbladder cancer in American Indian women with gallstones approaches 75 cases per 100,000 [6]. Similarly, in Chile, where more than 50% of women over age 50 have gallstones, adenocarcinoma of the gallbladder is the leading cause of cancer deaths among women [7, 8].

Cancer of the gallbladder is a disease of the elderly. More than 75% of patients with this malignancy are over age 65 [3]. The peak incidence of gallbladder cancer occurs within the 75- to 79-year age group. The median age for patients with gallbladder cancer (73 years) is more than the median age for patients with pancreatic (67 years) or extrahepatic bile duct (69 years) cancer.

Etiology

Several factors have been associated with an increased risk of developing gallbladder cancer. Mayo was the first who recognized an association between gallstones and gallbladder cancer [9]. More recently, an anomalous pancreatobiliary duct junction (APBDJ) and other biliary disorders, such as choledochal cysts and primary sclerosing cholangitis, have been associated with gallbladder cancer.

A strong association has long been noted between gallbladder cancer and cholelithiasis, which is present in 75–90% of cases [3]. The incidence of gallstones increases with age, and by age 75 about 35% of women and 20% of men in the USA have developed gallstones [4]. The incidence of

S.A. Ahrendt (✉)
Department of Surgery, University of Pittsburgh,
UPMC Cancer Center, 9100 Babcock Blvd, Pittsburgh,
PA 15090, USA
e-mail: ahresa@ph.upmc.edu

R.A. Rosenthal et al. (eds.), *Principles and Practice of Geriatric Surgery*,
DOI 10.1007/978-1-4419-6999-6_74, © Springer Science+Business Media, LLC 2011

gallbladder cancer is approximately seven times more common in the presence of cholelithiasis and chronic cholecystitis than in people without gallstones [6]. Approximately 1% of all patients with elective cholecystectomies performed for chronic cholecystitis and cholelithiasis harbor an occult gallbladder cancer [1, 10]. In the elderly patient population, this percentage is certainly higher [11].

The risk of developing gallbladder cancer is higher in patients with symptomatic gallstones than in those with asymptomatic gallstones [4]. In a review, Ransohoff and Gracie estimated the risk of developing gallbladder cancer in patients with symptomatic or asymptomatic gallstones [4]. The risk of developing gallbladder cancer (0.08% per year) was fourfold higher in patients with symptomatic gallstones over age 50 years than in those who were asymptomatic. Similar results have been observed in a multicenter study evaluating 196 patients with gallbladder cancer [12]. Twenty-eight percent of patients developing gallbladder cancer had undergone a medical evaluation for gallbladder disease in the past. A history of symptoms suggestive of gallbladder disease occurred significantly less frequently in control subjects without cancer.

Pathology and Staging

Ninety percent of cancers of the gallbladder are classified as adenocarcinoma [3]. Six percent of gallbladder cancers demonstrate papillary features on histologic examination. These tumors are commonly diagnosed while localized to the gallbladder and are also associated with an improved overall survival [3]. At diagnosis, 25% of cancers are localized to the gallbladder wall, 35% have associated metastases to regional lymph nodes or extension into adjacent organs, and 40% have already metastasized to distant sites [3].

Lymphatic drainage from the gallbladder occurs in a reproducible, predictable fashion and correlates with the pattern of lymph node metastases seen with gallbladder cancer [13, 14]. Lymph flow from the gallbladder initially drains to the cystic duct node and then descends along the common bile duct to the pericholedochal lymph nodes. The flow then proceeds to nodes posterior to the head of the pancreas and then to the interaortocaval lymph nodes. Secondary routes of lymphatic drainage include the retroportal and right celiac lymph nodes [14].

Hepatic involvement with gallbladder cancer can occur by direct invasion through the gallbladder bed, angiolymphatic portal tract invasion, or distant hematogenous spread [15]. Spread via the angiolymphatic portal tracts is the predominant mode of hepatic metastases; it may extend more

Table 74.1 TNM staging for gallbladder cancer [16]

TX	Primary tumor cannot be assessed
T0	No evidence of primary tumor
Tis	Carcinoma in situ
T1	Tumor invades lamina propria (T1a) or muscular (T1b) layer
T2	Tumor invades perimuscular connective tissue, no extension beyond serosa or into liver
T3	Tumor perforates the serosa (visceral peritoneum) and/or directly invades the liver and/or one other adjacent organ or structure, such as the stomach, duodenum, colon, pancreas, omentum, or extrahepatic bile ducts
T4	Tumor invades main portal vein or hepatic artery or invades two or more extrahepatic organs or structures
NX	Regional lymph nodes cannot be assessed
N0	No regional lymph node metastasis
N1	Metastases to nodes along the cystic duct, common bile duct, hepatic artery, and/or portal vein
N2	Metastases to periaortic, pericaval, superior mesenteric artery, and/or celiac artery lymph nodes
M0	No distant metastases
M1	Distant metastases

Stage grouping

0	Tis	N0	M0
I	T1	N0	M0
II	T2	N0	M0
IIIa	T3	N0	M0
IIIb	T1–3	N1	M0
IVa	T4	N0–1	M0
IVb	Any T	N2	M0
	Any T	Any N	M1

Source: Used with permission of the American Joint Committee on Cancer (AJCC), Chicago, IL. The original source for this material is the *AJCC Cancer Staging Manual*, 7th edition (2010) published by Springer Science and Business Media, LLC, http://www.springerlink.com

than 1 cm from the main tumor mass and correlates well with the depth of direct invasion of the liver. Distant spread beyond the region of the gallbladder is associated with hematogenous metastases elsewhere.

The current TNM classification of the American Joint Committee on Cancer is shown in Table 74.1 [16]. Stage I tumors are confined to the lamina propria, the gallbladder mucosa, submucosa, or muscularis. Stage II tumors extend into the perimuscular connective tissue without penetrating the gallbladder serosa or liver. Stage III tumors penetrate the serosa and can invade the liver or another adjacent organs or structures, such as the stomach, duodenum, colon, pancreas, omentum, or extrahepatic bile ducts. Stage IV tumors have extensive liver invasion, metastatic spread to second-order lymph nodes, or distant metastases.

Diagnosis

Clinical Presentation

Gallbladder cancer most often presents with right upper quadrant abdominal pain often mimicking other, more common biliary and nonbiliary disorders [1]. Weight loss, jaundice, and an abdominal mass are less common presenting symptoms. Piehler and Crichlow described five presenting clinical syndromes occurring in a review of more than 1,000 patients with gallbladder cancer [2]. Altogether, 16% of patients presented with symptoms of acute cholecystitis with a short duration of pain associated with vomiting, fever, and tenderness; 43% presented with symptoms of chronic cholecystitis often with a recent change in the quality or frequency of the painful episodes; 34% had signs and symptoms of malignant biliary obstruction with jaundice, weight loss, and right upper quadrant pain. An additional 29% of patients had symptoms of nonbiliary malignancies with anorexia and weight loss in the absence of jaundice, and a small percentage of patients had signs of gastrointestinal bleeding or obstruction.

The preoperative diagnosis of gallbladder cancer is difficult, particularly in the elderly population. In one series, only 8% of 53 patients with carcinoma of the gallbladder were diagnosed correctly preoperatively [17]. The most common misdiagnoses included chronic cholecystitis (28%), pancreatic cancer (13%), acute cholecystitis (9%), choledocholithiasis (8%), and gallbladder hydrops (8%).

Radiologic Evaluation

Ultrasonography is often the first diagnostic modality used for evaluating patients with right upper quadrant abdominal pain. Ultrasonographic features of advanced gallbladder cancer include a heterogeneous mass replacing the gallbladder lumen (40–65% of cases) or thickening of the gallbladder wall (20–30% of cases) [18]. Most patients have coexistent gallstones, gallbladder wall thickening, or both, suggesting benign biliary disease. Ultrasonography can determine the level of obstruction in patients with biliary ductal involvement. Overall, the sensitivity of ultrasonography for detecting gallbladder cancer ranges from 70 to 100% [18, 19].

Computed tomography (CT) has also improved the detection rate for gallbladder cancer with a sensitivity in the range of 55–100% (Fig. 74.1) [18]. CT scanning can demonstrate extension into the liver parenchyma but can overestimate hepatic involvement because of large perfusion defects. CT is less accurate for determining peritoneal seeding or lymph node involvement.

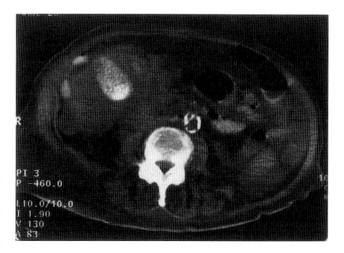

FIGURE 74.1 Computed tomography (CT) scan demonstrates large gallbladder cancer with extension into the duodenum. Gallstones (calcifications) are present within the mass.

Magnetic resonance imaging (MRI) is also sensitive for detecting gallbladder cancer, but its exact role in preoperative staging remains unclear (Fig. 74.2) [9, 18]. Hepatic artery and portal vein encasement may also be identified by MRI. Dilatation of the biliary tract that may occur with direct extension of gallbladder cancer into the biliary tree can be detected by standard MRI. In the elderly jaundiced patient with gallbladder cancer, the extent of biliary tract involvement should be further defined with cholangiography [9]. Percutaneous transhepatic cholangiography, endoscopic retrograde pancreatography, or magnetic resonance cholangiography are all helpful for the preoperative staging. A typical finding in the jaundiced patient with gallbladder cancer is a long stricture of the common hepatic duct [9].

Resection

The primary treatment of patients with localized gallbladder cancer is resection of the primary tumor along with areas of regional lymphatic involvement. After preoperative staging, patients with clinical stage I–IVa tumors warrant exploration if they are otherwise suitable operative candidates. Most of these patients are elderly, but the patient's general medical condition is more important than age when determining operative risk. Preexisting cirrhosis may dramatically increase the risk of surgery particularly if liver resection is contemplated [9].

Simple Cholecystectomy

The appropriate operative procedure for the patient with localized gallbladder cancer is determined by the pathologic

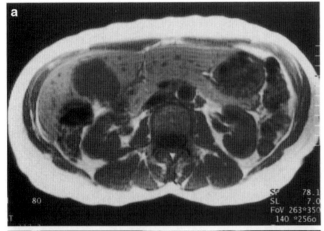

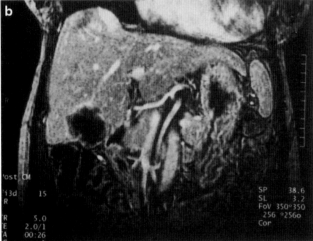

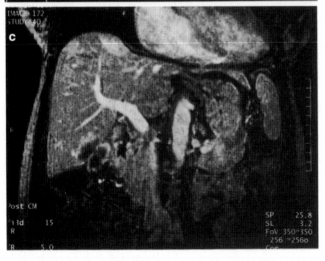

FIGURE 74.2 (a) Magnetic resonance imaging (MRI) scan demonstrating a mass arising within the gallbladder with extension into the hepatic parenchyma. (b) MR angiogram from the same patient demonstrating the relation between the hepatic artery and the mass. (c) MR angiogram from the same patient showing the relation between the main and right portal vein and the mass.

stage. Patients with tumors confined to the gallbladder mucosa or submucosa (stage Ia) have a negligible incidence of lymph node metastases and an overall 5-year survival approaching 100% [20–22]. These early-stage tumors are usually identified postoperatively by the pathologist and following open cholecystectomy, have had an excellent prognosis. More recently, with widespread use of the laparoscopic approach, recurrent cancer at port sites and peritoneal carcinomatosis have been reported following cholecystectomy even for patients with in situ disease [10]. The correct management of patients undergoing laparoscopic cholecystectomy with or without bile spillage for an incidental gallbladder cancer remains unclear.

Extended Cholecystectomy

Cancer of the gallbladder with invasion into or beyond the gallbladder muscularis is associated with an increasing incidence of regional lymph node metastases and should be managed with an extended lymphadenectomy as part of the operative procedure [22–26]. In addition, local extension into the hepatic parenchyma, colon, or duodenum requires en bloc resection of these structures to achieve an adequate resection margin.

The extent of the lymphadenectomy is based on the operative findings and knowledge of the patterns of lymphatic spread in patients with gallbladder cancer [13, 14]. This dissection should include the cystic duct, pericholedochal, portal, right celiac, and posterior pancreatoduodenal lymph nodes. In patients without grossly involved lymph nodes, the common bile duct, hepatic artery, and portal vein are skeletonized from the porta hepatis to the pancreas and celiac axis, respectively [24]. Following an extensive Kocher maneuver, the posterior pancreatoduodenal lymph nodes are included with the specimen. In the presence of any grossly enlarged pericholedochal lymph nodes, consideration should be given to resecting the common bile duct to avoid leaving a positive margin [24]. Biliary enteric continuity is restored with a Roux-en-Y hepaticojejunostomy. Several authors have advocated a pancreatoduodenectomy in the setting of pancreatoduodenal lymph node metastases, but this approach increases the operative mortality substantially in the elderly and should be considered in only the good risk patient with no evidence of metastasis to the liver, celiac, or interaortocaval lymph nodes [24, 25, 27].

Extension of more advanced staged lesions into the hepatic parenchyma is common, and extended cholecystectomy should incorporate at least a 2-cm margin beyond the palpable or sonographic extent of the tumor to include any angiolymphatic extension from the main tumor mass [15]. For smaller tumors, this can be incorporated into a wedge resection of the liver.

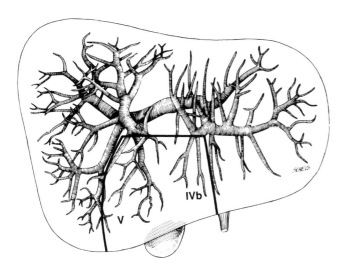

Figure 74.3 Extent of bisegmentectomy (segments IVb and V) in patients with T4 gallbladder cancer (from Gall et al. [28] with permission).

Extended Resections

For stage IV tumors invading more than 2 cm into the liver, an anatomic liver resection may be required to achieve a histologically negative margin. Cancers originating in the gallbladder fundus can usually be adequately treated with resection of segments IVb and V (Fig. 74.3) [28]. Tumor extension into the right hepatic artery or portal vein may be resectable only with a right hepatic lobectomy or trisegmentectomy [24, 29, 30].

Locally advanced lesions can also extend into adjacent structures. In the absence of distant lymph node, peritoneal, or hepatic metastases, these lesions may still be resectable for cure. Extension into the right colon should be managed with segmental colectomy, whereas duodenal invasion may require a pancreatoduodenectomy.

Palliative Therapy

Adequate palliation of the symptoms of advanced gallbladder cancer is eventually required in most elderly patients with this disease [9, 31]. Pain, jaundice, and gastric outlet obstruction are the common symptoms requiring palliation and can be managed nonoperatively or operatively. Survival in patients with unresectable gallbladder cancer is just 2–6 months, and therefore operative exploration should be avoided in patients with unresectable disease [1, 17, 22]. Narcotics should be given when necessary. Percutaneous celiac ganglion block may be helpful in reducing the need for narcotics. Chemical splanchnicectomy can be performed

in patients whose lesions are found to be unresectable at the time of operative exploration [9].

The presence of jaundice is a poor prognostic sign in patients with gallbladder cancer and usually signifies involvement of at least the common hepatic duct or hepatic duct bifurcation (or both). More than 70% of gallbladder cancers that present with jaundice and are explored with an intent to resect are unresectable for cure [29, 32]. Nonoperative biliary decompression to relieve jaundice and pruritus can be achieved percutaneously or endoscopically by placing metallic or nonmetallic stents [9]. In patients with hilar or intrahepatic ductal involvement, the percutaneous route is preferred. Relief of gastric outlet obstruction is difficult to achieve nonoperatively and usually requires gastrojejunostomy.

Survival

Extended cholecystectomy is reasonably well tolerated in the elderly patient population with gallbladder cancer. Operative mortality in several series was 0–1% [24, 29]. Common postoperative complications include wound or intraabdominal infection, hemorrhage, or delayed gastric emptying. Mortality increases with the magnitude of the operative procedure. Extended cholecystectomy, combined with a major hepatectomy or pancreatoduodenectomy, has a mortality rate of 10–15% and adds the risks of biliary or pancreatic anastomotic leaks to the procedure [25].

Survival in elderly patients with gallbladder cancer is strongly influenced by the pathologic stage at presentation. Patients with gallbladder cancer limited to the gallbladder mucosa and submucosa (stage Ia) have a uniformly excellent prognosis [20–22]; 35 patients with incidentally discovered stage Ia gallbladder cancer reported by Shirai et al. had an overall 5-year survival of 100% [20]. Invasion into the muscular wall of the gallbladder increases the risk of recurrent cancer after curative resection. The reported 5-year survival for patients with stage Ib gallbladder cancer varies widely, ranging from 20 to 100% (Table 74.2) [20–22]. In a survey of 172 major hospitals in Japan, the 5-year survival for patients with stage Ib tumors was 72%, with many patients undergoing simple cholecystectomy, suggesting that this procedure is an inadequate therapy once muscular invasion is present.

Invasion into the muscularis or the subserosa increases the risk of regional lymph node metastases to 15 and 50%, respectively. Tsukada et al. reported a 5-year overall survival of 80% for patients with stage II disease with extended cholecystectomy [24]. Similar results have been reported with an aggressive surgical approach at Memorial Sloan–Kettering [29]. In patients with tumors confined to the gallbladder wall

TABLE 74.2 Actuarial survival with stage I gallbladder cancer

Study	Year	Number	T stage	5-year survival (%)	Cholecystectomy (%)	Extended cholecystectomy (%)
Cubertafond et al. [22]	1994	23	T1a	93	100	0
		20	T1b	20	100	0
Donohue et al. [21]	1990	6	T1	100	83	17
Gall et al. [28]	1991	7	T1a	80	100	0
Ogura et al. [25]	1991	201	T1a	83	71	29
		165	T1b	72	54	46
Ouchi et al. [26]	1994	5	T1a	80	100	0
		5	T1b	40	100	0
Shirai et al. [20]	1991	35	T1a	100	100	0
		4	T1b	100	100	0

FIGURE 74.4 Actuarial survival for patients with gallbladder cancer by pathologic stage (see Table 74.1). Survival of patients with stage I and stage II tumors was significantly better than that of patients with stage III tumors. In addition, stage III patients survived significantly longer than patients with stage IV disease (from Tsukada et al. [24] with permission).

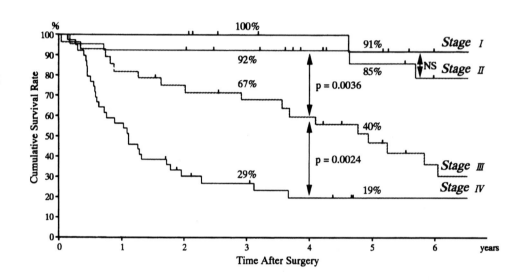

or with local extension into the liver or other adjacent organs (stages III and IV), long-term survival with extended cholecystectomy is possible [24, 29]. Several groups have reported 5-year overall survival for patients with stage III and stage IV gallbladder cancer of 40–63% and 19–25%, respectively (Fig. 74.4) [24, 29].

Tsukada et al. identified curative, margin-negative resection as the most significant factor in predicting prognosis [24]. Their 5-year survival of 52% in patients undergoing resection with microscopically negative margins was significantly higher than the 5-year survival (5%) in patients with a microscopically positive margin (Fig. 74.5). In the Memorial Sloan–Kettering series, the presence of lymph node metastases was a significant predictor of treatment failure [29]. Eighty-one percent of patients without lymph node metastases were alive 5 years after radical resection, whereas all of the patients with lymph node metastases died within 18 months. In the Japanese series, 11 of the 35 five-year survivors had lymph node metastases [24]. Age was not predictive of survival following surgery for gallbladder cancer [29].

Adjuvant Therapy

The results of chemotherapy in patients with gallbladder cancer have been poor owing to the limited responsiveness to these agents. Partial response rates to oral 5-fluorouracil (5-FU) alone or in combination with methyl-CCNU or streptozotocin range from 5 to 13% with a median survival of 10–21 weeks in patients receiving treatment [33]. The combination of intravenous 5-FU, high-dose levofolinic acid, and oral hydroxyurea has achieved a partial response rate of 30% with a median survival of 8 months in patients with unresectable gallbladder cancer [34]. Toxicity was limited, and the regimen was well tolerated in this group of patients (median age 60).

Both external beam and intraoperative radiation therapy have been used for management of patients with gallbladder cancer. In the postoperative adjuvant setting, no randomized data have demonstrated improved survival with external beam radiation alone [9]. In a retrospective review of 38 patients with gallbladder cancer managed with postoperative

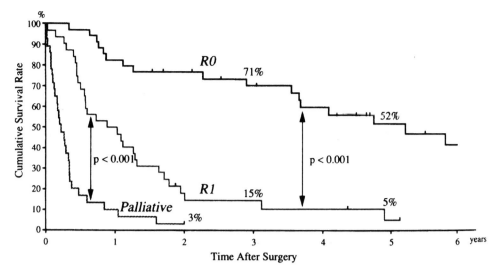

Figure 74.5 Actuarial survival for patients with stage III and stage IV gallbladder cancer by resection margin status. Results are shown for patients managed with curative (negative margins) resection (R0), noncurative (microscopically positive margin) resections (R1), and palliative (grossly positive margin) resections (R2). Patients managed with R0 resection survived significantly longer than patients undergoing R1 resection. In addition, patients with extensive tumor resected with palliative intent survived a significantly shorter time than patients with microscopic positive margins (from Tsukada et al. [24] with permission).

adjuvant therapy, overall survival was improved in patients receiving more than 4,000 cGy compared with patients receiving less than 4,000 cGy [35]. However, the response to the radiation therapy in this series was difficult to differentiate from the effect of resection alone. Overall survival was not influenced by patients' age in this series. The use of intraoperative radiation therapy (IORT) in one Japanese series has been reported to provide a slight survival benefit in patients with locally advanced gallbladder cancer [36]. In a collective review of unresectable gallbladder cancers, patients undergoing IORT had a longer survival (11.0 vs. 6.3 months) than patients with standard external beam radiotherapy [37].

Cholangiocarcinoma

Cholangiocarcinomas may occur anywhere along the intrahepatic or extrahepatic biliary tree. The hepatic duct bifurcation is the most frequently involved site, and approximately 60–80% of cholangiocarcinomas encountered at tertiary referral centers are found in the perihilar region [9, 38–41]. Cholangiocarcinoma is an uncommon tumor and occurs in conditions in which bile is stagnant, infected, or both. These clinical situations include primary sclerosing cholangitis, choledochal cysts, and hepatolithiasis. Cholangiocarcinoma usually presents with painless jaundice, so this diagnosis should be considered in every case of obstructive jaundice. Perihilar cholangiocarcinomas involve the region of the hepatic duct bifurcation and frequently also involve major portal vascular structures, making resection difficult. When possible, surgical resection offers a chance for long-term disease-free survival. Many patients, however, are candidates only for palliative bypass or operative or nonoperative intubation aimed at providing biliary drainage and preventing cholangitis and hepatic failure.

Incidence

Approximately 15,000 new cases of liver and biliary tract cancer are diagnosed annually in the USA, and they account for more than 12,000 deaths per year. About 15–25% of these cancers are bile duct tumors or cholangiocarcinomas. The incidence of cholangiocarcinoma increases with age, and these tumors occur with similar frequency in men and women. Approximately two-thirds of patients diagnosed with cholangiocarcinoma are of age 50–70 years [42, 43]. Overall, the incidence of cholangiocarcinoma in the USA is approximately 1 per 100,000 people per year [9, 44].

Etiology and Associated Diseases

A number of diseases and environmental agents have been linked to cholangiocarcinoma including primary sclerosing cholangitis, choledochal cysts, and hepatolithiasis. Factors common to a number of these etiologic factors include stones, biliary stasis, and infection [9]. Bile duct cancers in patients with primary sclerosing cholangitis are most often extrahepatic, commonly occur near the hepatic duct bifurcation, and are difficult to differentiate from the multiple, benign strictures associated with this disease [45]. The mean age at presentation in patients with cholangiocarcinoma and primary sclerosing cholangitis is the fifth decade of life, and these tumors occur only rarely in the elderly population. Similarly, choledochal cysts are usually diagnosed during childhood or early adult life. However, choledochal cysts are occasionally diagnosed in the elderly, and the risk of cholangiocarcinoma increases steadily with patients' age [46]. Hepatolithiasis occurs in the elderly population and is a known risk factor for cholangiocarcinoma. Cholangiocarcinoma develops in 5–10% of patients with hepatolithiasis [9, 47–49]. Cholangiocarcinoma has been reported to develop a mean 8 years following treatment for hepatolithiasis and may occur despite complete stone clearance from the intrahepatic biliary tree [49].

Staging and Classification

Cholangiocarcinoma is best classified into three broad groups (1) intrahepatic, (2) perihilar, and (3) distal. This classification correlates with the anatomic distribution and implies the preferred treatment for each site. Intrahepatic tumors are treated like liver lesions, with hepatectomy when possible. Distal tumors are managed in a fashion similar to that for other periampullary malignancies, with pancreatoduodenectomy. The perihilar tumors make up the largest group and are managed with local resection of the bile duct with or without hepatic resection.

Cancers of the hepatic duct bifurcation were further classified by Bismuth et al. according to their anatomic location [50]. With this system, type I tumors are confined to the common hepatic duct; type II tumors involve the right and left hepatic ducts; type IIIa and IIIb tumors extend into the right or left secondary intrahepatic ducts, respectively; and type IV tumors involve the secondary intrahepatic ducts on both sides.

Cholangiocarcinoma is also staged according to the tumor, node, metastasis (TNM) classification of the American Joint Commission on Cancer (Tables 74.3 and 74.4) [16]. Using this system, stage I tumors are limited to the bile duct mucosa or muscular layer; stage II tumors invade periductal tissues; stage III tumors have regional lymph node metastases; and stage IV tumors invade adjacent structures (IVa) or have distant metastases (IVb).

TABLE 74.3 TNM staging for tumors of the perihilar bile ducts

TX	Primary tumor cannot be assessed
T0	No evidence of primary tumor
Tis	Carcinoma in situ
T1	Tumor confined to the bile duct, with extension up to the muscle layer or fibrous tissue
T2	(a) Tumor invades beyond the wall of the bile duct to surrounding adipose tissue; (b) tumor invades adjacent hepatic parenchymal
T3	Tumor invades unilateral branches of the portal vein or hepatic artery
T4	Tumor invades main portal vein or its branches bilaterally; or the common hepatic artery; or the second-order biliary laterals bilaterally; or unilateral second-order biliary radicals with contralateral portal vein or hepatic artery involvement
NX	Regional lymph nodes cannot be assessed
N0	No regional lymph node metastasis
N1	Regional lymph node metastasis (including nodes along the cystic duct, hepatic artery, and portal vein)
N2	Metastasis to periaortic, pericaval, superior mesenteric artery, and/or celiac artery lymph nodes
M0	No distant metastasis
M1	Distant metastasis

Stage grouping

0	Tis	N0	M0
I	T1	N0	M0
II	T2a–b	N0	M0
IIIa	T3	N0	M0
IIIb	T1–3	N1	M0
IVa	T4	N0–1	M0
IVb	Any T	N2	M0
	Any T	Any N	M1

Source: Used with permission of the American Joint Committee on Cancer (AJCC®), Chicago, IL. The original source for this material is the *AJCC Cancer Staging Manual*, 7th edition (2010) published by Springer Science and Business Media, LLC, http://www.springerlink.com

Diagnosis

Clinical Presentation

More than 90% of patients with perihilar or distal tumors present with jaundice. Patients with intrahepatic cholangiocarcinoma rarely present with jaundice until late in the course of the disease. Less common presenting clinical features include pruritus, fever, mild abdominal pain, fatigue, anorexia, and weight loss [9]. Cholangitis is not a frequent presentation but most commonly develops after biliary manipulation by endoscopic or percutaneous techniques.

TABLE 74.4 TNM staging for tumors of the distal bile ducts

TX	Primary tumor cannot be assessed
T0	No evidence of primary tumor
Tis	Carcinoma in situ
T1	Tumor confined to the bile duct histologically
T2	Tumor invades beyond the wall of the bile duct
T3	Tumor invades the gallbladder, pancreas, duodenum, or other adjacent organs without involvement of the celiac axis, or the superior mesenteric artery
T4	Tumor involved the celiac axis, or the superior mesenteric artery
NX	Regional lymph nodes cannot be assessed
N0	No regional lymph node metastasis
N1	Regional lymph node metastasis
M0	No distant metastasis
M1	Distant metastasis

Stage grouping

0	Tis	N0	M0
IA	T1	N0	M0
IB	T2	N0	M0
IIA	T3	N0	M0
IIB	T1	N1	M0
III	T1	N1	M0
	T2	N1	M0
	T3	N1	M0
IV	Any T	Any N	M1

Source: Used with permission of the American Joint Committee on Cancer (AJCC®), Chicago, IL. The original source for this material is the *AJCC Cancer Staging Handbook*, 7th edition (2010), pp. 211–213, published by Springer Science and Business Media, LLC, http://www.springerlink.com

Laboratory Data

At the time of presentation, most patients with perihilar or distal cholangiocarcinoma have a total serum bilirubin level higher than 10 mg/dl [9]. Marked elevations are also observed in serum alkaline phosphatase and γ-glutamyl transferase levels. Patients with long-standing biliary obstruction may also have a low serum albumin or prolonged prothrombin time. The serum tumor markers carcinoembryonic antigen (CEA) and α-fetoprotein (AFP) are typically normal. Serum CA 19-9 and CA 50 may be elevated in patients with cholangiocarcinoma and may be useful for screening patients in high-risk groups for developing cholangiocarcinoma [51].

Radiologic Evaluation

The goals of radiologic evaluation in patients with cholangiocarcinoma include delineation of the overall extent of the tumor, including involvement of the bile ducts, liver, portal vessels, and distant metastases. An ordered sequence of tests can usually achieve these goals. The initial radiographic studies consist of either abdominal ultrasonography or CT scanning. Intrahepatic cholangiocarcinomas are easily visualized on CT scans. A hilar cholangiocarcinoma gives a picture of a dilated intrahepatic biliary tree, a normal or collapsed gallbladder and extrahepatic biliary tree, and a normal pancreas. Distal tumors lead to dilation of the gallbladder and intra- and extrahepatic biliary tree.

Perihilar tumors are often difficult to visualize on ultrasonography and standard CT scans [52]. Duplex ultrasonography has been reported to visualize the primary tumor in more than 85% of patients, whereas bolus contrast-enhanced CT scans were able to define the primary tumor in only 59% of patients [53, 54]. Duplex sonography has also been able to determine accurately the extent of bile duct involvement in 87% of patients and the presence or absence of portal vein involvement in 86% [55]. A study comparing enhanced CT scans and MRI in 15 patients with perihilar cholangiocarcinoma managed at Johns Hopkins suggested that MRI is more sensitive than CT scans for detecting these small tumors [56]. However, newer spiral CT techniques are better at detecting the parenchymal extent of the tumor.

After documentation of bile duct dilation, biliary anatomy traditionally has been defined cholangiographically through the percutaneous transhepatic or endoscopic retrograde routes. The most proximal extent of the tumor is the most important feature when determining resectability in patients with perihilar tumors. Percutaneous transhepatic cholangiography is favored in these patients because it defines the proximal extent of tumor involvement most reliably [9]. This approach also allows preoperative placement of percutaneous transhepatic catheters. Recently, magnetic resonance cholangiopancreatography (MRCP) has been documented to have a diagnostic accuracy comparable to those of percutaneous and endoscopic cholangiography. In a series of 14 patients with cholangiocarcinoma, diagnostic quality MRCP images were better at visualizing intrahepatic biliary anatomy than endoscopic retrograde cholangiopancreatography (ERCP) [57]. MRCP also has the advantage of obtaining two-dimensional images to define an obstructing lesion. The sensitivity, specificity, and overall accuracy of MRCP at determining the level of biliary obstruction and the presence of a benign or malignant lesion are similar to those for ERCP.

The advantages of transhepatic catheter placement include (1) assistance in the technical aspects of hilar dissection by allowing palpation of the catheter within the biliary tree at the time of exploration and (2) facilitation of intraoperative Silastic transhepatic stent placement. Currently available randomized studies do not support the practice of placing preoperative transhepatic catheters in an effort to reduce operative mortality [58–60]. However, if a liver resection is contemplated, preoperative drainage may be justified.

Biopsy/Cytology

Efforts to establish a tissue diagnosis including percutaneous fine-needle aspiration (FNA) biopsy, brush and scrape biopsy, and cytologic examination of bile have been used [61–64]. Prolonged efforts to obtain a preoperative tissue diagnosis are not indicated unless the patient is not an operative candidate. Bile obtained from a percutaneous catheter demonstrates malignant cells in approximately 30% of cases [62]. This yield may be improved to approximately 40% by brush cytologic techniques through transhepatic stents or at the time of endoscopic procedures and to 67% by percutaneous FNA. Even with these efforts, up to one-third of patients with cholangiocarcinoma have negative biopsy and cytologic results.

Assessment of Resectability

A careful evaluation of the overall general medical condition of the elderly patient and an accurate staging evaluation are necessary prior to selecting the appropriate management for the patient with cholangiocarcinoma. The preoperative assessment should include the usual evaluation of cardiac risk factors, respiratory status, and renal function, as well as overall performance status. Patients with obstructive jaundice often have decreased hepatic protein synthesis and altered hemostatic mechanisms, and they are at increased risk for infectious complications.

Several studies have defined preoperative risk factors associated with an increase in morbidity and mortality in patients undergoing treatment for malignant biliary obstruction [39, 60, 65, 66]. In 1981, Pitt and colleagues identified eight risk factors predictive of mortality, including serum albumin less than 3.0 g/dl [65]. Little also defined a mortality index predictive of procedure-related mortality in a prospective analysis of patients with obstructive jaundice [60]. The mortality index was derived from the preoperative serum creatinine and albumin levels and the severity of the cholangitis. Several large series of patients undergoing resection for perihilar cholangiocarcinoma have also identified low preoperative serum albumin concentration and perioperative sepsis as factors contributing to operative mortality [65, 66]. Control of sepsis and intensive nutritional support should be undertaken preoperatively in the malnourished elderly patient with cholangiocarcinoma.

The preoperative evaluation also includes careful staging to determine the extent of the cholangiocarcinoma [38, 53–55,

67–69]. In the past, the combination of an abdominal CT scan, cholangiography, and visceral angiography was useful for determining the extent of disease. CT or MRI scan findings signifying unresectable disease include peripheral hepatic metastases or extrahepatic disease. Findings on traditional or MRI cholangiography suggestive of unresectable disease in patients with perihilar cholangiocarcinoma include proximal extension of tumor into second-order bile ducts in both hepatic lobes. The angiographic or MRI findings of tumor encasement or occlusion of the proper hepatic artery, main portal vein, or both right and left portal venous branches or hepatic arterial branches are also considered contraindications to resection by most.

The combination of angiography and cholangiography provides better data than cholangiography alone for staging the elderly patient with perihilar cholangiocarcinoma [70]. More recently, MRI has provided all the data previously obtained by these two studies and CT scanning [71, 72]. For patients with distal cholangiocarcinoma, a good-quality spiral CT scan can provide sufficient information to predict resectability.

Palliative Therapy

Palliative therapy in elderly patients with perihilar and distal cholangiocarcinoma is directed at relieving obstructive jaundice and pruritus, preventing recurrent cholangitis, and avoiding hepatic failure secondary to unrelieved biliary obstruction. In addition, palliative therapy in patients with distal cholangiocarcinoma is aimed at preventing or relieving gastric outlet obstruction. Palliation can be achieved nonoperatively with percutaneous or endoscopic techniques or by using an operative approach.

Nonoperative Palliation

Patients with unequivocal evidence of unresectable cholangiocarcinoma at initial evaluation are palliated nonoperatively. Tumor extension into the secondary biliary radicals of both right and left hepatic lobes, the main portal vein, or the main hepatic artery or the presence of distant metastases excludes patients from curative resection. In addition, elderly patients in poor general medical condition may also not be operative candidates. Nonoperative palliation can be achieved endoscopically and percutaneously. A significant proportion of the functioning hepatic parenchyma should be decompressed, and this philosophy may require two or three percutaneously or endoscopically placed catheters in patients with hilar cholangiocarcinoma [70, 74, 74].

Percutaneous biliary drainage has several advantages over endoscopic management in patients with perihilar cholangiocarcinoma. Stent placement is more reliably achieved percutaneously than via endoscopic means [75]. In addition, occluded percutaneous stents are easily changed over a guidewire on an outpatient basis, whereas replacement of an endoprosthesis requires an additional invasive procedure. In contrast, endoscopic palliation is the preferred approach in patients with distal cholangiocarcinoma. Placement of an endoprosthesis in experienced centers has been technically successful in approximately 95% of patients with advanced periampullary cancer, with relief of jaundice and pruritus in 80%. More recently, percutaneous or endoscopically placed metallic stents have been used to palliate patients with malignant biliary obstruction [76–78]. Metallic stents remain patent longer than plastic stents and require fewer subsequent manipulations in patients with distal malignant biliary obstruction [79]. Self-expanding metallic stents have also been effective in patients with unresectable perihilar tumors, with median stent patency rates of up to 1 year [77].

Operative Palliation

In good-risk patients without preoperative evidence of unresectable cholangiocarcinoma, operative exploration is undertaken in an attempt to resect the primary tumor. At Johns Hopkins, approximately 45% of patients with perihilar cholangiocarcinoma were found at exploration to have intraperitoneal or liver metastases (15%) or extensive tumor involvement of the porta hepatis (30%), precluding resection [38, 42, 70, 80–82]. Ten percent of patients with distal cholangiocarcinoma have unresectable lesions at operative exploration. Patients with peritoneal carcinomatosis undergo minimal operative intervention. Cholecystectomy is performed to prevent the subsequent development of acute cholecystitis from cystic duct obstruction related to the percutaneous catheter [83]. Postoperatively, the preoperatively placed transhepatic catheters are replaced with larger, softer transhepatic stents [84].

In patients with locally advanced unresectable perihilar tumors, several operative approaches are available for palliation, including Roux-en-Y choledochojejunostomy with intraoperative placement of Silastic biliary catheters or a segment III cholangiojejunostomy. The operative procedure for placing transhepatic Silastic catheters begins with obtaining a tissue diagnosis of cholangiocarcinoma. A tissue diagnosis is required prior to initiating postoperative irradiation or chemotherapy.

The gallbladder is then mobilized, and the distal common bile duct is divided and oversewn. Next, the Ring catheters are exchanged for larger Silastic biliary catheters. A hepaticojejunostomy is then performed to a Roux-en-Y limb of jejunum (Fig. 74.6). The advantages of this approach over nonoperative palliation include (1) removal of the gallbladder [83], (2) placement of larger, softer Silastic stents with a lower risk of hemobilia and improved patient comfort, and (3) positioning the stent into a defunctionalized Roux-en-Y jejunal limb to reduce the incidence of subsequent cholangitis.

In patients with locally unresectable or metastatic distal cholangiocarcinoma, operative palliation is directed at relieving both biliary and gastric outlet obstruction. Symptomatic gastroduodenal obstruction occurs prior to death in approximately 30% of patients with periampullary malignancies. Gastrojejunostomy at the time of initial presentation prevents this complication without increasing the operative morbidity or mortality. Biliary-enteric continuity is restored most often with a hepaticojejunostomy or a choledochojejunostomy.

Surgical Resection

Curative treatment of patients with cholangiocarcinoma is possible only with complete resection. For patients with anatomically resectable intrahepatic cholangiocarcinoma and without advanced cirrhosis, partial hepatectomy is the procedure of choice. After careful exploration of the peritoneal surfaces and regional lymph nodes for metastatic disease, the liver is mobilized and examined with intraoperative ultrasonography. Approximately 40% of resectable intrahepatic cholangiocarcinomas are multiple or involve both hepatic lobes. Hepatic resection is planned to remove completely all tumor with an adequate margin. Most commonly it involves a formal lobectomy or trisegmentectomy.

Elderly patients with tumors involving the hepatic hilum or proximal common hepatic duct (Bismuth types I or II) that have no vascular invasion are candidates for local tumor excision [38]. Preoperatively, bilateral transhepatic Ring catheters are placed to aid in the intraoperative identification of the right and left hepatic ducts [38, 81, 82, 84]. After excluding the presence of metastatic disease, the common bile duct (CBD) is dissected free and encircled just proximal to the suprapancreatic portion. The CBD is then divided, and the distal end is oversewn. It is then reflected cephalad, skeletonizing the portal vein and proper hepatic artery. Once the entire common hepatic duct has been elevated off the portal vasculature, the left and right hepatic ducts can be identified by palpating the diverging Ring catheters. The left and right hepatic ducts are then divided above the extent of palpable tumor. Frozen section examination is used to determine the adequacy of the surgical margin. The percutaneous transhepatic catheters are then exchanged for 16F Silastic catheters. A 60-cm retrocolic Roux-en-Y limb is then constructed, and bilateral hepaticojejunostomies are performed over the Silastic stents.

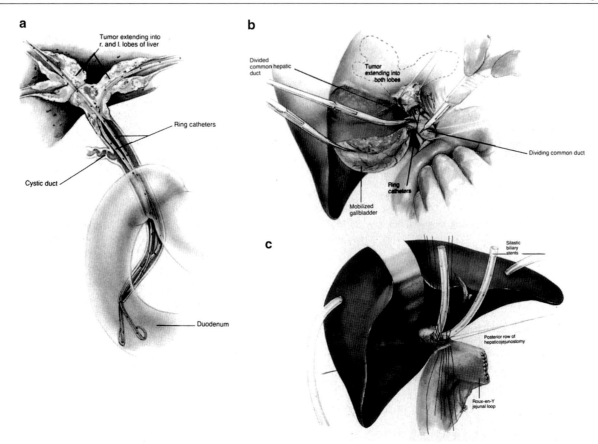

FIGURE 74.6 (**a**) Palliative intubation of Bismuth type IV unresectable perihilar cholangiocarcinoma with preoperatively placed transhepatic stents changed over guidewires. (**b**) Common bile duct is divided distal to the tumor and a cholecystectomy is performed. (**c**) Roux-en-Y choledochojejunostomy is constructed over Silastic transhepatic stents distal to the tumor (from Cameron [100] with permission).

Proximal extension of a hilar cholangiocarcinoma into either the intrahepatic segments of the right or left hepatic duct renders these tumors incurable by local tumor resection. Complete resection in these patients is achievable only with combined resection of the extrahepatic biliary tree and major liver resection. Improvements in operative morbidity and mortality and in long-term survival when negative surgical margins are achieved support the use of this approach when complete tumor resection is possible [38, 41, 50, 52, 85–99].

The need for hepatic resection can usually be predicted on the basis of preoperative angiography, cholangiography, or MRI. When unilateral neoplastic involvement of the right or left portal vein or hepatic ducts is visualized radiographically, the initial hilar dissection is performed as described previously with division of the uninvolved hepatic duct. A frozen section should be examined to confirm a negative hepatic duct margin on the uninvolved side. Next, the extrahepatic segments of the hepatic vein, portal vein, and hepatic artery to the involved lobe are divided or occluded with vascular clamps. The hepatic parenchyma is then divided using the ultrasonic dissector or cautery. Extension of the tumor into the caudate lobe frequently necessitates caudate lobec-

tomy to achieve negative tumor margins. Biliary enteric continuity is restored to a Roux-en-Y limb of jejunum (see Fig. 74.7).

Elderly patients with resectable distal cholangiocarcinoma are managed similarly to patients with other periampullary malignancies with pancreatoduodenectomy. More than 85% of these patients are suitable for the pylorus-preserving modification, and gastrointestinal continuity is restored with an end-to-end pancreatojejunostomy, an end-to-side hepaticojejunostomy, and an end-to-side duodenojejunostomy. The hepaticojejunostomy is usually stented with a T-tube to decompress the system in the event of a biliary or pancreatic leak.

Survival

Procedure-related morbidity and mortality, quality of survival, and long-term survival are highly dependent on the stage of disease at presentation and on whether the patient is treated by a palliative procedure or complete tumor resection.

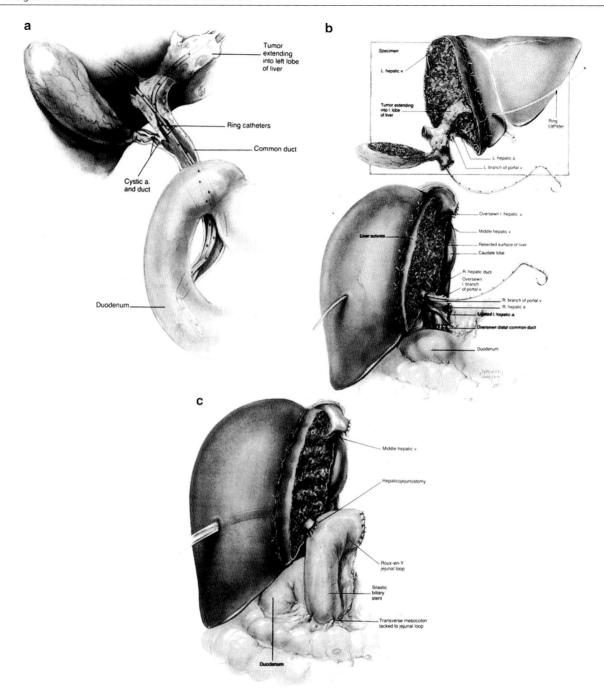

Figure 74.7 (**a**). Left hepatic and hilar resection of Bismuth type IIIb cholangiocarcinoma with preoperatively placed transhepatic stents. (**b**). Resected left hepatic lobe and hilum with perihilar cholangiocarcinoma (*top*) and right hepatic lobe with divided right hepatic duct prior to reconstruction (*bottom*). (**c**) Silastic transhepatic stent is placed through a right Roux-en-Y cholangiojejunostomy after left hepatic lobectomy (from Cameron [100] with permission).

Palliative Therapy

Between 1973 and 1989, a group of 65 patients with unresectable hilar cholangiocarcinoma underwent nonoperative percutaneous stenting or operative palliation at The Johns Hopkins Hospital [38, 70]. Altogether, 21 patients were managed with percutaneous biliary stents; 44 patients underwent laparotomy, with placement of large-bore Silastic transhepatic stents in 33. The procedure-related morbidity was similar for patients undergoing nonoperative palliation and those undergoing laparotomy. Hospital mortality was 14% in the nonoperatively palliated group and 7% in those managed operatively.

Mean survival was 8 months for the patients managed with operative palliation and 5 months for those managed with percutaneous stenting ($p < 0.05$).

Quality of survival measured by the number of readmissions per month of survival, hospital days per month of survival, and episodes of cholangitis was better in the patients undergoing operative palliation. In addition, patients managed nonoperatively required more frequent stent changes than patients managed operatively. On the other hand, eight patients (15%) managed operatively required late operations. These procedures were most frequently required for small bowel or duodenal obstruction. None of the patients managed nonoperatively required laparotomy during the follow-up period.

Several additional studies have examined the results of palliative therapy for hilar cholangiocarcinoma [74, 97, 99, 101]. In a French report, the operative mortality and long-term survival were similar for patients managed with operatively placed biliary stents and those managed with palliative biliary-enteric anastomosis [97]. Guthrie et al. demonstrated more effective palliation with a segment III cholangiojejunostomy than with endoscopic or percutaneous stenting [101]. The operatively managed patients had a lower incidence of cholangitis and jaundice than the patients managed with nonoperative stenting. Lai et al. demonstrated lower procedure-related mortality among patients managed operatively than among those palliated with endoscopic stenting [74]. Overall survival and quality of survival assessed by frequency of cholangitis attacks, episodes of jaundice, and days in the hospital were similar for the two groups. Patients managed with endoscopic stents had a higher incidence of catheter-related problems than patients managed with cholangioenteric bypass. In contrast, Washburn et al. demonstrated better survival in patients palliated nonoperatively than in surgically palliated patients [99]. All of these retrospective analyses are limited, however, by biases in selecting patients for each treatment group.

Several randomized, prospective trials have compared operative vs. nonoperative palliation in patients with periampullary cancer [102]. In general, these trials demonstrated lower procedure-related morbidity and mortality rates for the nonoperatively managed patients. However, the procedure-related mortality in the operatively managed patients ranged from 15 to 24%. In addition, a higher rate of recurrent jaundice or gastric outlet obstruction occurred in the nonoperatively managed patients. Survival was similar among the two treatment groups in each study (mean survival 12–22 weeks).

Between 1987 and 1991, a series of 118 patients with unresectable periampullary tumors were explored at The Johns Hopkins Hospital [102]. Seventy percent of the patients were over age 60. The most common operative procedure was choledochojejunostomy and hepaticojejunostomy, which were performed in 67% of patients. Perioperative mortality was 2.5%, and gastric outlet obstruction or recurrent jaundice developed prior to death in only 4.0 and 2.5% of patients, respectively.

Surgical Resection

A series of 34 patients with intrahepatic cholangiocarcinoma managed with surgical resection was recently reported by Casavilla et al. [103]; 53% of these patients were over age 60. Multiple tumors were present in 44% of the patients, and 41% had involvement of both hepatic lobes. Histologically negative surgical margins were obtained in 71% of patients. Operative mortality was 6%. Overall patient survival was 60% at 1 year, 37% at 3 years, and 31% at 5 years after resection. Significant predictors of postoperative treatment failure were positive surgical margins, multiple tumors, and metastatic disease in regional lymph nodes. Age was not predictive of operative or long-term mortality.

A group of 109 patients with perihilar cholangiocarcinoma was managed with resection at The Johns Hopkins Hospital between 1973 and 1995 [39]. Following resection, 36 patients had obvious gross tumor remaining, and 81 patients had a positive microscopic surgical margin. Of the 109 patients, 94 underwent local hilar excision, and 15 were managed with hepatic lobectomy with resection of the extrahepatic biliary tree. Four operative deaths (3.6%) occurred among these 109 patients, including one death (6.6%) among the 15 managed with hepatic lobectomy. Actuarial survival among the 109 patients undergoing resection was 68% at 1 year, 30% at 3 years, and 11% after 5 years of follow-up. Survival was significantly prolonged in patients without residual microscopic tumor at the surgical margin. In the 28 patients with a negative margin, the actuarial survival was 68% at 1 year, 56% at 3 years, and 19% after 5 years. Patients' age did not influence operative morbidity or mortality or the long-term survival. Fifty-three percent of these patients also received a combination of external beam radiotherapy, a boost of internal irradiation utilizing iridium 192, or both.

In recent years, the trend around the world has been to perform more hepatic resections for perihilar cholangiocarcinoma. More than 580 patients with perihilar cholangiocarcinoma have been reported in the literature since 1989 (Table 74.5) [39, 50, 66, 88, 90, 92, 94–99, 104]. For 233 patients undergoing local hilar resection, the operative mortality rate was 6%; and for 352 patients managed with combined hilar and hepatic resection, the operative mortality was 8%. The mean age of these 585 patients undergoing aggressive surgical resection for perihilar cholangiocarcinoma was 60 years, with half of them in their seventh, eighth, or ninth

TABLE 74.5   Operative mortality of hilar vs. hepatic resection for perihilar cholangiocarcinoma (1989 to present)

| Study | Year | Age (years) | | Hilar resection | | Hepatic resection[a] | |
		Mean	Range	Number	Operative mortality (%)	Number	Operative mortality (%)
Baer et al. [92] (Berne, Switzerland)	1993	62	34–85	12	0	9	11
Bismuth et al. [50] (Paris, France)	1992	50	22–82	10	0	13	0
Fortner et al. [88] (Memorial Sloan–Kettering)	1989	60	33–81	7	0	7	0
Hadjis et al. [90] (London, England)	1990	55	33–74	11	0	16	12
Kawasaki et al. [94] (Matsumoto, Japan)	1994	58	39–72	–	–	9	0
Klempnauer et al. [104] (Hanover, Germany)	1997	57	25–79	31	6	77	8
Nagino et al. [95] (Nagoya, Japan)	1995	55	44–64	–	–	4	0
Nakeeb et al. [39] (Johns Hopkins)	1996	62	23–84	94	3	15	7
Nimura et al. [96] (Nagoya, Japan)	1991	60	33–76	–	–	45	2
Reding et al. [97] (French Surgical Association)	1991	64		47	17	50	14
Su et al. [66] (Taipei, Taiwan)	1996	62	32–74	21	5	28	14
Sugiura et al. [98] (Tokyo, Japan)	1994	60	33–78	–	–	61	7
Washburn et al. [99] (Boston)	1995	60	25–86	–	–	18	11
Total		60	22–86	233	6	352	8

[a]Does not include patients also undergoing portal vein or hepatic artery resection and reconstruction

decade of life. The mean survival rate in the locally resected patients ranged from 19 to 36 months. Similarly, the mean survival of patients undergoing combined hilar and hepatic resection ranged from 16 to 32 months.

Several factors may be important when determining long-term prognosis following curative resection for hilar cholangiocarcinoma. Achieving negative histologic margins is important for determining overall long-term survival [41, 87, 92, 99]. Bengmark et al. initially reported several 10-year survivors following hepatic resection with negative histologic margins for hilar cholangiocarcinoma [87]. In two large series of patients managed with attempted curative resection for perihilar cholangiocarcinoma, both Klempnauer et al. and Sugiura et al. reported a 33% overall 5-year survival for patients with negative histologic margins, whereas no patient with microscopic cancer at the surgical margins survived 5 years (Fig. 74.8) [98, 99, 102–104]. Among patients with negative histologic margins, the addition of a caudate lobectomy significantly prolonged the 5-year survival (46 vs. 12%). In addition, the presence of regional lymph node metastases adversely affected survival. In several large series, multivariate analysis found that patients' age did not influence overall survival.

Seventy-three patients with distal cholangiocarcinoma undergoing pancreatoduodenectomy have been reported from The Johns Hopkins Hospital [39]. The 1-, 3-, and 5-year survival rates were 70, 31, and 28%, respectively. Factors associated with prolonged survival of these patients include tumor differentiation and lymph node status. Negative nodes increased the median survival from 17 to 27 months, whereas poorly differentiated tumors had a lower median survival (10 vs. 22 months).

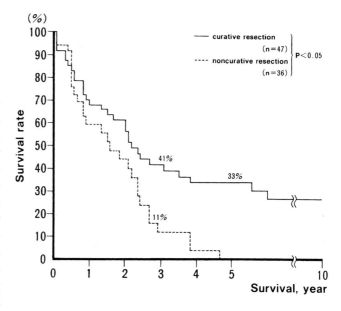

FIGURE 74.8   Actuarial Kaplan–Meier survival of patients with perihilar cholangiocarcinoma undergoing curative or noncurative resection (microscopic tumor at surgical margin). Survival was improved ($p < 0.05$) in the curatively resected patients (from Sugiura et al. [98] with permission).

Adjuvant Therapy

Radiation therapy has been evaluated in patients with perihilar cholangiocarcinoma using a variety of methods including external beam radiotherapy, intraoperative radiotherapy, internal radiotherapy, radioimmunotherapy, and charged particle radiation. External beam radiotherapy has been the most commonly used modality and is typically administered to a total dose of 45–60 Gy [38, 105–107]. Internal radiotherapy is normally delivered through percutaneous or endoscopically placed biliary stents using iridium 192 as the radiation source [38, 108, 109]. Multiple retrospective analyses have suggested that radiation therapy may provide some benefit in patients with perihilar cholangiocarcinoma administered via one of these techniques.

In a prospective analysis from The Johns Hopkins Hospital, 23 patients underwent irradiation and 27 did not [110]. The radiation dose ranged from 45 to 63 Gy and consisted of external beam plus iridium 192 seeds. None of the patients underwent adjuvant chemotherapy. Patients undergoing curative resection survived significantly longer than patients undergoing operative palliation. Among those with resection, irradiation had no effect on the mean (24 vs. 24 months), median, or actuarial survival. Similarly, among palliated patients irradiation had no effect on the mean (10 vs. 13 months), median, or actuarial survival. Multivariate analysis identified resection as the only positive predictive factor for prolonged survival.

The use of chemotherapy (along with 5-FU, mitomycin C, or cisplatin) has not been shown to improve survival in patients with resected or unresected cholangiocarcinoma. Response rates using multidrug chemotherapeutic regimens also remain low. Given the potential radiosensitization effect of 5-FU, the combination of irradiation and chemotherapy may be more effective than either agent alone. Preliminary data in relatively small numbers of patients have been reported, but no randomized data are available [35, 111–114].

Conclusions

Despite overall advances in the ability to diagnose and treat elderly patients with malignant tumors of the gallbladder and biliary tract, the prognosis for patients with these malignancies remains poor. Improvements in diagnostic CT scanning, duplex ultrasonography, and MRI will improve our ability to diagnose noninvasively and stage gallbladder cancer or cholangiocarcinoma in the elderly patient. Complete surgical resection remains the only curative treatment for malignancy of the biliary tract. Aggressive surgical approaches are likely to continue, and the challenge remains in being able to perform these procedures safely in jaundiced and sometimes septic elderly patients. Unfortunately, for most patients with malignant tumors of the biliary tract, curative resection is not possible, and optimal palliation remains the goal of therapy. Finally, advances in adjuvant chemotherapy and radiotherapy are required to improve the overall prognosis of patients with gallbladder cancer or cholangiocarcinoma.

References

1. Jones RS (1990) Carcinoma of the gallbladder. Surg Clin North Am 70:1419–1428
2. Piehler JM, Crichlow RW (1978) Primary carcinoma of the gallbladder. Surg Gynecol Obstet 147:929–939
3. Carriaga MT, Henson DE (1995) Liver, gallbladder, extrahepatic bile ducts, and pancreas. Cancer 75:171–190
4. Ransohoff DF, Gracie WA (1993) Treatment of gallstones. Ann Intern Med 119:606–619
5. Strom BL, Soloway RD, Rios-Dalenz JL et al (1995) Risk factors for gallbladder cancer: an international collaborative case-control study. Cancer 76:1747–1756
6. Lowenfels AB, Lindstrom CG, Conway MJ et al (1985) Gallstones and risk of gallbladder cancer. J Natl Cancer Inst 75:77–80
7. De Aretxabala X, Roa I, Burgos L et al (1992) Gallbladder cancer in Chile: a report on 43 potentially resectable tumors. Cancer 69:60–65
8. Nervi F, Duarte I, Gomez G et al (1988) Frequency of gallbladder cancer in Chile: a high-risk area. Int J Cancer 41:657–660
9. Pitt HA, Dooley WC, Yeo CJ et al (1995) Malignancies of the biliary tree. Curr Probl Surg 32:1–90
10. Wibbenmeyer LA, Wade TP, Chen RC et al (1995) Laparoscopic cholecystectomy can disseminate in situ carcinoma of the gallbladder. J Am Coll Surg 181:504–510
11. Liu KJM, Richter HM, Cho MJ et al (1997) Carcinoma involving the gallbladder in elderly patients presenting with acute cholecystitis. Surgery 122:748–756
12. Zatonski WA, Lowenfels AB, Boyle P et al (1997) Epidemiologic aspects of gallbladder cancer: a case-control study of the SEARCH program of the international agency for research on cancer. J Natl Cancer Inst 89:1132–1138
13. Fahim RB, McDonald JR, Richards JC et al (1962) Carcinoma of the gallbladder: a study of its modes of spread. Ann Surg 156:114–123
14. Shirai Y, Yoshida K, Tsukada K et al (1992) Identification of the regional lymphatic system of the gallbladder by vital staining. Br J Surg 79:659–662
15. Shirai Y, Tsukada K, Ohtani T et al (1995) Hepatic metastases from carcinoma of the gallbladder. Cancer 75:2063–2068
16. Edge SE, Byrd DR, Carducci MA, Compton CA (eds) (2010) AJCC cancer staging manual, 7th edn. Springer, New York
17. White K, Kraybill WG, Lopez MJ (1988) Primary carcinoma of the gallbladder: TNM staging and prognosis. J Surg Oncol 39:251–255
18. Soyer P, Gouhiri M, Boudiaf M et al (1997) Carcinoma of the gallbladder: imaging features with surgical correlation. AJR Am J Roentgenol 169:781–785
19. Mizuguchi M, Kudo S, Fukahori T et al (1997) Endoscopic ultrasonography for demonstrating loss of multiple-layer pattern of the thickened gallbladder wall in the preoperative diagnosis of gallbladder cancer. Eur Radiol 7:1323–1327
20. Shirai Y, Yoshida K, Tsukada K et al (1992) Inapparent carcinoma of the gallbladder: an appraisal of a radical second operation after simple cholecystectomy. Ann Surg 215:326–331
21. Donohue JH, Nagorney DM, Grant CS et al (1990) Carcinoma of the gallbladder: does radical resection improve outcome? Arch Surg 125:237–241
22. Cubertafond P, Gainant A, Cucchiaro G (1994) Surgical treatment of 724 carcinomas of the gallbladder: results of the French Surgical Association survey. Ann Surg 219:275–280
23. Tsukada K, Kurosaki I, Uchida K et al (1997) Lymph node spread from carcinoma of the gallbladder. Cancer 80:661–667
24. Tsukada K, Hatakeyama K, Kurosaki I et al (1996) Outcome of radical surgery for carcinoma of the gallbladder according to the TNM stage. Surgery 120:816–822

25. Ogura Y, Mizumoto R, Isaji S et al (1991) Radical operations for carcinoma of the gallbladder: present status in Japan. World J Surg 15:337–343
26. Ouchi K, Suzuki M, Tominaga T et al (1994) Survival after surgery for cancer of the gallbladder. Br J Surg 81:1655–1657
27. Nakamura S, Nishiyama R, Yokoi Y et al (1994) Hepatopancreatoduodenectomy for advanced gallbladder carcinoma. Arch Surg 129:625–629
28. Gall FP, Kockerling F, Scheele J et al (1991) Radical operations for carcinoma of the gallbladder: present status in Germany. World J Surg 15:328–336
29. Bartlett DL, Fong Y, Fortner JG et al (1996) Long-term results after resection for gallbladder cancer: implications for staging and management. Ann Surg 224:639–646
30. Bloechle C, Izbicki JR, Passlick B et al (1995) Is radical surgery in locally advanced gallbladder carcinoma justified? Am J Gastroenterol 90:2195–2200
31. Jones RS (1991) Palliative operative procedures for carcinoma of the gallbladder. World J Surg 15:348–351
32. Miyazaki M, Itoh H, Ambiru S et al (1996) Radical surgery for advanced gallbladder carcinoma. Br J Surg 83:478–481
33. Falkson G, MacIntyre JM, Moertel CG (1984) Eastern Cooperative Oncology Group experience with chemotherapy for inoperable gallbladder and bile duct cancer. Cancer 54:965–969
34. Gebbia V, Majello E, Testa A et al (1996) Treatment of advanced adenocarcinomas of the exocrine pancreas and the gallbladder with 5-fluorouracil, high dose levofolinic acid and oral hydroxyurea on a weekly schedule. Cancer 78:1300–1307
35. Kraybill WG, Lee H, Picus J et al (1994) Multidisciplinary treatment of biliary tract cancers. J Surg Oncol 55:239–245
36. Todoroki T, Iwasaki Y, Orii K et al (1991) Resection combined with intraoperative radiation therapy (IORT) for stage IV (TNM) gallbladder carcinoma. World J Surg 15:357–366
37. Todoroki T (1997) Radiation therapy for primary gallbladder cancer. Hepatogastroenterology 44:1229–1239
38. Cameron JL, Pitt HA, Zinner MJ et al (1990) Management of proximal cholangiocarcinoma by surgical resection and radiotherapy. Am J Surg 159:91–98
39. Nakeeb A, Pitt HA, Sohn TA et al (1996) Cholangiocarcinoma: a spectrum of intrahepatic, perihilar, and distal tumors. Ann Surg 224:463–475
40. Tompkins RK, Saunders K, Roslyn JJ et al (1990) Changing patterns in diagnosis and management of bile duct cancer. Ann Surg 211:614–621
41. Nagorney DM, Donohue JH, Farnell MB et al (1993) Outcomes after curative resections of cholangiocarcinoma. Arch Surg 128:871–877
42. Broe PJ, Cameron JL (1981) The management of proximal biliary tract tumors. Adv Surg 15:47–62
43. Sons HU, Borchard F (1987) Carcinoma of the extrahepatic bile ducts: a postmortem study of 65 cases and review of the literature. J Surg Oncol 34:6–12
44. Miller BA, Ries LAG, Hankey BF et al (1993) SEER cancer statistics review: 1973–1990 (NIH Publ No. 93-2789). National Cancer Institute, Bethesda
45. Ahrendt SA, Pitt HA, Kalloo AN et al (1998) Primary sclerosing cholangitis: resect, dilate, or transplant? Ann Surg 227:412–423
46. Lipsett PA, Pitt HA et al (1994) Choledochal cyst disease: a changing pattern of presentation. Ann Surg 220:644–652
47. Sheen-Chen SM, Chou FF, Eng HL (1991) Intrahepatic cholangiocarcinoma in hepatolithiasis: a frequently overlooked disease. J Surg Oncol 47:131–135
48. Fan ST, Lai EC, Wong J (1993) Hepatic resection for hepatolithiasis. Arch Surg 128:1070–1074
49. Chijiiwa K, Ichimiya H, Kuroki S et al (1993) Late development of cholangiocarcinoma after the treatment of hepatolithiasis:

50. Bismuth H, Nakache R, Diamond T (1992) Management strategies in resection for hilar cholangiocarcinoma. Ann Surg 215:31–38
51. Ramage JK, Donaghy A, Farrant JM (1995) Serum tumor markers for the diagnosis of cholangiocarcinoma in primary sclerosing cholangitis. Gastroenterology 108:865–869
52. Langer JC, Langer B, Taylor BR et al (1985) Carcinoma of the extrahepatic bile ducts: results of an aggressive surgical approach. Surgery 98:752–759
53. Looser CH, Stain SC, Baer HU et al (1992) Staging of hilar cholangiocarcinoma by ultrasound and duplex sonography: a comparison with angiography and preoperative findings. Br J Radiol 65:871–877
54. Yamashita Y, Takahashi M, Kanazawa S et al (1992) Parenchymal changes of the liver in cholangiocarcinoma: CT evaluation. Gastrointest Radiol 17:161–166
55. Hann LE, Graetrex KV, Bach AM et al (1997) Cholangiocarcinoma at the hepatic hilus: sonographic findings. AJR Am J Roentgenol 168:985–989
56. Saeki M, Pitt HA, Tempany CM (1992) Magnetic resonance imaging of hilar cholangiocarcinoma (abstract). In: Proceedings of the international hepatobiliary pancreatic association, 100A
57. Lomanto D, Pavone P, Laghi A et al (1997) Magnetic resonance-cholangiopancreatography in the diagnosis of biliopancreatic disease. Am J Surg 174:33–38
58. Pitt HA, Gomes AS, Lois JF et al (1985) Does preoperative percutaneous biliary drainage reduce operative risk or increase hospital cost? Ann Surg 201:545–553
59. Nakeeb A, Pitt HA (1995) The role of preoperative biliary decompression in obstructive jaundice. Hepatogastroenterology 42:332–339
60. Little JM (1987) A prospective evaluation of computerized estimates of risk in the management of obstructive jaundice. Surgery 102:473–476
61. Cope C, Marinelli DL, Weinstein JK (1988) Transcatheter biopsy of lesions obstructing the bile ducts. Radiology 169:555–560
62. Desa LA, Akosa AB, Lazzara S et al (1991) Cytodiagnosis in the management of extrahepatic biliary stricture. Gut 32:1188–1191
63. Ferrucci JT, Chuttani R (1995) Magnetic resonance cholangiopancreatography (MRCP): comparison to invasive cholangiopancreatography. Hepatology 22:107A
64. Foutch PG, Kerr DM, Horlan JR et al (1990) Endoscopic retrograde wire-guided brush cytology for diagnosis of patients with malignant obstruction of the bile duct. Am J Gastroenterol 85:791–795
65. Pitt HA, Cameron JL, Postier RG et al (1981) Factors influencing mortality in biliary tract surgery. Am J Surg 141:66–72
66. Su CH, Tsay SH, Wu CC et al (1996) Factors influencing postoperative morbidity, mortality, and survival after resection for hilar cholangiocarcinoma. Ann Surg 223:384–394
67. Lynn RB, Wilson JAP, Cho KJ (1988) Cholangiocarcinoma: role of percutaneous transhepatic cholangiography in determination of resectability. Dig Dis Sci 33:587–592
68. Dooley WC, Pitt HA, Venbrux AD et al (1992) Is angiography useful in patients with perihilar cholangiocarcinoma (abstract). In: Proceedings of the international hepatobiliary pancreatic association, 32A
69. Dooley WC, Cameron JL, Pitt HA et al (1990) Is preoperative angiography useful in patients with periampullary tumors? Ann Surg 211:649–655
70. Nordback IH, Pitt HA, Coleman JA et al (1994) Unresectable hilar cholangiocarcinoma: percutaneous versus operative palliation. Surgery 115:597–603

71. Soto JA, Carish MA, Yucel EK et al (1996) Magnetic resonance cholangiography: comparison with endoscopic retrograde cholangiopancreatography. Gastroenterology 110:589–597

72. Lee MG, Lee HJ, Kim MH et al (1997) Extrahepatic biliary diseases: 2D MR cholangiography compared with endoscopic retrograde cholangiopancreatography. Radiology 202:663–669

73. Hausegger KA, Kleinert R, Lammer J et al (1992) Malignant biliary obstruction: histologic findings after treatment with self-expandable stents. Radiology 185:461–464

74. Lai EC, Chu KM, Lo CY et al (1992) Choice of palliation for malignant hilar obstruction. Am J Surg 163:208–212

75. Lamere JS, Stoker J, Dees J et al (1987) Non-surgical palliative treatment of patients with malignant biliary obstruction: the place of endoscopic and percutaneous drainage. Clin Radiol 38:603–608

76. Schima W, Prokesch R, Osterreicher C et al (1997) Biliary wall-stent endoprosthesis in malignant hilar obstruction: long-term results with regard to the type of obstruction. Clin Radiol 52:213–219

77. Peters RA, Williams SG, Lombard M et al (1997) The management of high-grade hilar structures by endoscopic insertion of self-expanding metal endoprosthesis. Endoscopy 29:10–16

78. O'Brien S, Hatfield AR, Craig PI et al (1995) A three year follow up of self-expanding metal stents in the endoscopic palliation of long-term survivors with malignant biliary obstruction. Gut 36:618–621

79. Becker CD, Glattie A, Mailbach R et al (1993) Percutaneous palliation of malignant obstructive jaundice with wall stent endoprosthesis: follow-up and reintervention in patients with hilar and non-hilar obstruction. J Vasc Interv Radiol 4:597–604

80. Pitt HA (1993) Proximal bile duct: resection and palliation. In: Daly JM, Cady B (eds) Atlas of surgical oncology. Mosby-Year Book, St. Louis, pp 417–437

81. Yeo CJ, Pitt HA, Cameron JL (1990) Cholangiocarcinoma. Surg Clin North Am 70:1429–1447

82. Ahrendt SA, Pitt HA (1993) Cholangiocarcinoma. In: Niederhuber JE (ed) Current therapy in oncology. Mosby-Year Book, St. Louis, pp 410–414

83. Lillemoe KD, Pitt HA, Kaufmann SL et al (1989) Acute cholecystitis occurring as a complication of percutaneous transhepatic drainage. Surg Gynecol Obstet 168:348–352

84. Crist DW, Kadir S, Cameron JL (1987) Proximal biliary tract reconstruction: the value of preoperatively placed percutaneous biliary catheters. Surg Gynecol Obstet 165:421–426

85. Stain SC, Baer HU, Dennison AR et al (1992) Current management of hilar cholangiocarcinoma. Surg Gynecol Obstet 175:579–588

86. Ouchi K, Matsuno S, Sato T (1989) Long-term survival in carcinoma of the biliary tract. Arch Surg 124:248–252

87. Bengmark S, Ekberg H, Evander A et al (1988) Major liver resection for hilar cholangiocarcinoma. Ann Surg 207:120–128

88. Fortner JG, Vitelli CE, Maclean BJ (1989) Proximal extrahepatic bile duct tumors: analysis of a series of 52 consecutive patients treated over a period of 13 years. Arch Surg 124:1275–1282

89. Lai ECS, Tompkins RK, Roslyn JJ et al (1987) Proximal bile duct cancer: quality of survival. Ann Surg 205:111–118

90. Hadjis NS, Blenkhard JI, Alexander N et al (1990) Outcome of radical surgery in hilar cholangiocarcinoma. Surgery 107:597–604

91. Boerma EJ (1990) Research into the results of resection of hilar bile duct cancer. Surgery 108:572–580

92. Baer HU, Stain SC, Dennison AR et al (1993) Improvements in survival by aggressive resections of hilar cholangiocarcinoma. Ann Surg 217:20–27

93. Vauthey JN, Baer HU, Guastella T et al (1993) Comparison of outcome between extended and nonextended liver resections for neoplasms. Surgery 114:968–975

94. Kawasaki S, Makuuchi M, Miyagawa S et al (1994) Radical operation after portal embolization for tumor of hilar bile duct. J Am Coll Surg 178:480–486

95. Nagino M, Nimura Y, Kamiya J et al (1995) Right or left trisegmental portal vein embolization before hepatic trisegmentectomy for hilar bile duct carcinoma. Surgery 117:677–681

96. Nimura Y, Hayakawa N, Kamiya J et al (1991) Combined portal vein and liver resection for carcinoma of the biliary tract. Br J Surg 78:727–731

97. Reding R, Buard JL, Lebeau G et al (1991) Surgical management of 552 carcinomas of the extrahepatic bile ducts: results of the French Surgical Association survey. Ann Surg 213:236–241

98. Sugiura Y, Nakamura S, Iida S et al (1994) Extensive resection of the bile ducts combined with liver resection for cancer of the main hepatic duct junction: a cooperative study of the Keio Bile Duct Cancer Study Group. Surgery 115:445–451

99. Washburn WK, Lewis DW, Jenkins RL (1995) Aggressive surgical resection for cholangiocarcinoma. Arch Surg 130:270–276

100. Cameron JC (1990) Atlas of surgery, vol 1. B.C. Decker, Philadelphia

101. Guthrie CM, Haddock G, de Beaux AC et al (1993) Changing trends in the management of extrahepatic cholangiocarcinoma. Br J Surg 80:1434–1439

102. Lillemoe KD, Sauter PK, Pitt HA et al (1993) Current status of surgical palliation of periampullary carcinoma. Surg Gynecol Obstet 176:1–10

103. Casavilla FA, Marsh JW, Iwatsuki S et al (1997) Hepatic resection and transplantation for peripheral cholangiocarcinoma. J Am Coll Surg 195:429–436

104. Klempnauer J, Ridder GJ, von Wasielewski R et al (1997) Resectional surgery of hilar cholangiocarcinoma: a multivariate analysis of prognostic factors. J Clin Oncol 15:947–954

105. Hayes JK Jr, Sapozink MD, Miller FJ (1988) Definitive radiation therapy in bile duct carcinoma. Int J Radiat Oncol Biol Phys 15:735–740

106. Verbeek PC, van Leeuwen DJ, van der Heyde MN et al (1991) Does additive radiotherapy after hilar resection improve survival of cholangiocarcinoma: an analysis in sixty-four patients. Ann Chir 45:350–354

107. Shiina T, Mikuriya S, Uno T et al (1992) Radiotherapy of cholangiocarcinoma: the roles for primary and adjuvant therapies. Cancer Chemother Pharmacol 31(Suppl):S115–S118

108. Ede RJ, Williams SJ, Hatfield ARW et al (1989) Endoscopic management of inoperable cholangiocarcinoma using iridium-192. Br J Surg 76:867–871

109. Koyama K, Tanaka J, Sato S et al (1989) New strategy for treatment of carcinoma of the hilar bile duct. Surg Gynecol Obstet 168:523–529

110. Pitt HA, Nakeeb A, Abrams RA et al (1995) Perihilar cholangiocarcinoma: postoperative radiotherapy does not improve survival. Ann Surg 221:788–798

111. Minsky BD, Kemeny N, Armstrong JG et al (1991) Extrahepatic biliary system cancer: an update of a combined modality approach. Am J Clin Oncol 14:433–439

112. Koyama K, Tanaka J, Sato Y et al (1993) Experience in twenty patients with carcinoma of hilar bile duct treated by resection, targeting chemotherapy and intercavitary irradiation. Surg Gynecol Obstet 176:239–245

113. Robertson JM, Lawrence TD, Dworzanin LM et al (1993) Treatment of primary hepatobiliary cancer with conformal radiation therapy and regional chemotherapy. J Clin Oncol 11:1286–1292

114. Whittington R, Neuberg D, Teste WJ et al (1995) Protracted intravenous fluorouracil infusion with radiation therapy in the management of localized pancreaticobiliary carcinoma: a phase I Eastern Cooperative Oncology Group trial. J Clin Oncol 13:227–234

Chapter 75
Benign and Malignant Neoplasms of the Exocrine Pancreas

Kathryn M. Dalbec and Keith D. Lillimoe

Introduction

Pancreatic neoplasms represent a major health-care problem for the aging population. The elderly are at risk for the entire spectrum of benign and malignant pancreatic tumors. Pancreatic adenocarcinoma is the most frequent and clinically significant of these tumors. It is the fourth leading cause of cancer death in the United States, and its incidence is associated with advancing age. The diagnosis and treatment of pancreatic cancer often represents a significant clinical challenge in the elderly, as there is a significant bias against aggressive surgical treatment in this population. In recent years, however, advances in diagnostic techniques, improved outcomes with regionalization of care, and a deeper understanding of prognostic factors have improved our ability to treat this challenging disease. In addition to pancreatic adenocarcinoma, the recognition and diagnosis of benign and premalignant pancreatic tumors has become more common in the elderly. These tumors require a thorough understanding of their clinical behavior as one weighs these risks with the risk of surgery in the elderly population. Fortunately, many of these tumors are amenable to less invasive therapeutic procedures with lessened perioperative morbidity and mortality.

Epidemiology

According to the National Cancer Institute, the incidence of pancreatic cancer is approximately 37,000 new cases per year, with 34,000 deaths per year from the disease [1]. Pancreatic adenocarcinoma is also one of the most lethal cancers, with a 5-year survival rate for 1996–2004 of only 5%, due to the fact that more than half of patients have distant metastases at diagnosis, and only 7% of cases are diagnosed at a stage where the cancer is confined to the pancreas. The incidence of pancreatic cancer among persons aged 55–59 is 18 per 100,000, while the incidence among 75–79 year-olds is 72 per 100,000. Above age 85, the incidence rises to 91 per 100,000 (Fig. 75.1).

Cystic neoplasms represent less than 10% of pancreatic tumors and include a spectrum of benign and malignant lesions. The last two decades have seen a striking increase in the diagnosis of cystic neoplasms, with many detected due to the widespread use of abdominal imaging studies. Intraductal papillary mucinous neoplasms (IPMNs) comprise a significant portion of all cystic neoplasms. The peak incidence of IPMN is in the sixth and seventh decade of life, and IPMNs are more likely to be malignant in patients older than 60 years [2].

Risk Factors

Environmental and genetic factors have been implicated as risk factors for pancreatic cancer. As noted above, advanced age is a significant risk factor for both pancreatic cancer and IPMNs. Male gender and African American race are also associated with higher rates of pancreatic cancer. Among many potential environmental risk factors, cigarette smoking has been confirmed as a major contributor, with a twofold greater risk of developing pancreatic cancer among smokers compared with nonsmokers. Recently, a pooled analysis of cohort studies has found a modestly increased risk of pancreatic cancer associated with the consumption of 30 or more grams of alcohol per day [3]. Chemical and radiation exposure is also associated with increased pancreatic cancer risk. Several preexisting medical conditions are associated with increased risk of pancreatic cancer: chronic pancreatitis, primary sclerosing cholangitis, obesity, and prior gastric surgery. Diabetes mellitus has been shown in some studies to confer an increased risk of pancreatic cancer, but it is also possible that diabetes is an early symptom of the cancer, rather than a risk factor. Thus, new-onset diabetes in an

K.M. Dalbec (✉)
Department of Surgery, Indiana University Hospital,
545 Barnhill Drive, EH 203, Indianapolis, IN 46202, USA
e-mail: kdalbec@iupui.edu

R.A. Rosenthal et al. (eds.), *Principles and Practice of Geriatric Surgery*,
DOI 10.1007/978-1-4419-6999-6_75, © Springer Science+Business Media, LLC 2011

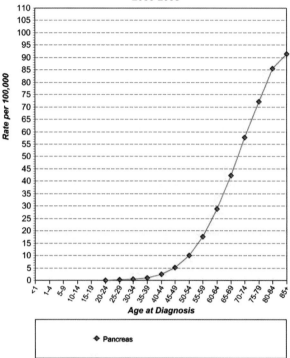

**Age-Specific (Crude) SEER Incidence Rates
By Cancer Site
All Ages, All Races, Both Sexes
2000–2005**

◆ Pancreas

Cancer sites include invasive cases only unless otherwise noted.
Incidence source: SEER 17 areas (San Francisco, Connecticut, Detroit, Hawaii, Iowa, New Mexico, Seattle, Utah, Atlanta, San Jose-Monterey, Los Angeles, Alaska Native Registry, Rural Georgia, California excluding SF/SJM/LA, Kentucky, Louisiana and New Jersey).
Rates are per 100,000.
Datapoints were not shown for rates that were based on less than 16 cases.

Figure 75.1 Increased pancreatic cancer incidence by age. (SEER Cancer Stat Fact Sheets [1]).

otherwise asymptomatic elderly patient could be an early clue to the presence of pancreatic malignancy.

Genetic factors often play a role in the development of pancreatic cancer. There are multiple inherited familial cancer syndromes that increase the risk of pancreatic cancer, including Peutz–Jeghers, hereditary pancreatitis, hereditary nonpolyposis colon cancer (HNPCC), ataxia-telangiectasia, familial atypical mole and multiple melanoma (FAMMM) syndrome, familial breast cancer 2, and familial adenomatous polyposis. There is also a significantly increased risk of developing pancreatic cancer in patients with a family history of the disease without association with a specific syndrome. Patients who have two first-degree relatives with pancreatic cancer have a 6-fold increase in risk, while patients with three affected first-degree relatives have a 32-fold higher risk of developing pancreatic cancer [4]. It is also important to note that age becomes a significant factor in these kindreds, as the age of cancer diagnosis in subsequent generations actually becomes progressively younger.

While the genetic significance in these cancer syndromes is apparent, recent advances in molecular genetics have led to the identification of frequent genetic mutations even among sporadic pancreatic cancers. These include inactivated tumor-suppressor genes such as p53, p16, and DPC4, each of which are found in >50% of sporadic pancreatic cancers. Mutations in K-ras, an oncogene involved in signal transduction, are found in over 90% of pancreatic cancer, which may prove diagnostically important in the future.

Perhaps the most increasingly identified risk factor for pancreatic cancer is the presence of a precancerous lesion, such as IPMNs or other mucinous cystic neoplasms. The increasingly frequent identification of these tumors, primarily in asymptomatic patients, has led to the development of management algorithms for the management of precancerous lesions and surveillance for disease progression. The optimal techniques and interval for follow-up may vary based on patient-specific characteristics including age. Nevertheless, for IPMNs, both the incidence of malignancy and invasiveness increases with age.

Pathology

Solid Tumors

Solid tumors of the exocrine pancreas are classified according to their cell of origin; which may include the pancreatic ductal epithelium or the acinar cell. Solid tumors can be either malignant or premalignant or benign. Ductal adenocarcinoma is the most common neoplasm of the exocrine pancreas, accounting for more than 75% of all malignant pancreatic tumors. Ductal adenocarcinoma arises most commonly in the pancreatic head (65%) but may also be present in the body or tail (15%) or diffusely involve the whole pancreas (20%). Tumors of the head tend to be smaller at diagnosis, as they are more likely to cause obstructive jaundice earlier in their development. Adenocarcinomas arise from pancreatic ductal tissue, often obstructing ductal branches and causing a desmoplastic reaction with associated fibrosis and chronic pancreatitis. They often infiltrate into vascular, lymphatic, and perineural spaces, leading to early local and metastatic spread. Common sites of local invasion are duodenum, stomach, transverse mesocolon, colon, spleen, and adrenal glands. Pancreatic cancer typically metastasizes to regional lymph nodes and then liver, peritoneum, lungs, and adrenal glands. Pathologic examination of resected specimens often reveals the presence of precursor lesions (see below) in close proximity to the cancer. The recognition of these lesions has broadened our understanding of the development of adenocarcinoma.

Pancreatic adenocarcinoma is staged based on the tumor characteristics, node involvement, and metastatic disease (TNM) classification system, as outlined by the American Joint Commission on Cancer (AJCC) [5]. This system has considerable prognostic significance, with

Stages I and II representing resectable, and therefore potentially curable, disease.

In addition to ductal adenocarcinoma, a very small percentage of solid exocrine tumors is comprised of adenosquamous carcinoma, acinar cell carcinoma, giant cell carcinoma, and pancreatoblastoma. Pancreatoblastoma should rarely be considered in the differential in an elderly patient, however, as it is found almost exclusively in children less than 15 years of age.

Cystic Tumors

Cystic tumors make up less than 10% of all exocrine pancreas neoplasms, although they are being diagnosed with increasing frequency in recent decades. Cystic tumors of the pancreas include serous cystic neoplasms, mucin-producing cystic neoplasms (MCN and IPMN), solid pseudopapillary or Hamoudi tumors, and lymphoepithelial cysts [6].

Serous cystic neoplasms, or serous cystadenomas, are the most common cystic neoplasm of the pancreas, comprising 30–60% of cystic tumors (Fig. 75.2). They are more common in women and elderly and are often located in the body and tail of the pancreas. Serous cystadenomas have both microcystic and oligocystic variants, both of which are benign. Serous cystadenocarcinoma is a rare malignant variant that is difficult to distinguish histologically from its benign relative.

Unlike serous neoplasms, which are almost always benign, mucin-producing cystic tumors of the pancreas are considered either premalignant or frankly malignant. There are two distinct types of mucin-producing pancreatic tumors, mucinous cystic neoplasms (MCNs, or mucinous cystadenomas) and intraductal papillary mucinous neoplasms (IPMNs). Both types are characterized by abnormal growth of mucin-producing epithelial cells, but IPMNs involve the main pancreatic duct or ductal branches, while MCNs do not. MCNs occur almost exclusively in women and are most common between age 40 and 50. They are typically found in the body or tail and contain a distinctive subepithelial ovarian-type stroma (Fig. 75.3). The degree of dysplasia of MCNs can vary from benign to malignant,

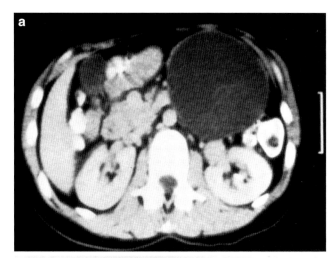

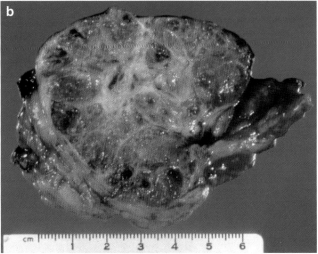

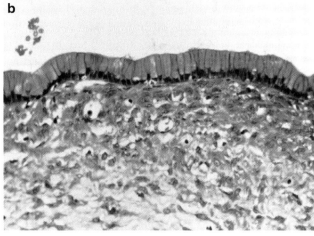

Figure 75.2 Serous cystadenoma seen in (**a**) cross-sectional imaging and (**b**) histologic section.

Figure 75.3 Mucinous cystic neoplasm seen in (**a**) cross-sectional imaging and (**b**) histologic section showing typical histologic feature of "ovarian stroma".

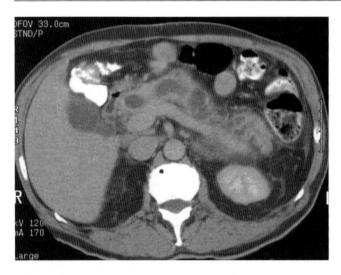

Figure 75.4 Multidetector CT (MDCT) scan with IV contrast showing main-duct type IPMN.

Table 75.1 Comparison between MCN and IPMN [6, 7]

	MCN	IPMN
Age (years)	40–50	60–80
Gender	F>M	M>F
Location	Body/tail	Head
Pancreatic duct involvement	No	Yes
Mucin found at ampulla	No	Yes
Ovarian-like stroma	Yes	No

Table 75.2 Likelihood of malignancy in main duct IPMN [2]

	Benign	Malignant	Total	P (benign vs. malignant)
n	57	83	140	–
Gender (M/F)	31/26	40/43	71/69	NS
Median age	60.9	67.3	64.8	0.042
Smoking history (%)	35 (61%)	43 (52%)	78 (56%)	NS
Abdominal pain (%)	43 (76%)	47 (57%)	90 (65%)	0.038
Jaundice (%)	2 (3.5%)	21 (26%)	23 (16.5%)	0.001
Weight loss (%)	23 (40%)	39 (47%)	62 (44%)	NS

Source: Data from Salvia et al. [2]

with up to one-third containing an invasive component. In contrast to MCNs, IPMNs are found more commonly in males, do not contain ovarian stroma, and are more common in the pancreatic head, neck, and uncinate process (Fig. 75.4 and Table 75.1). IPMNs represent about 25% of cystic neoplasms and are classified into 3 types: main duct, branch duct, and mixed type. Histologically, IPMNs can range from benign to intermediate to malignant, with about 35% of resected IPMNs showing a component of invasive carcinoma. Features associated with increased likelihood of malignancy are increased patient age, main duct involvement, jaundice, and diabetes [7] (Table 75.2). Much less common than MCN or IPMN, the solid pseudopapillary tumor, also known as Hamoudi tumor, or solid cystic neoplasm, is found predominantly in young women. This tumor is always considered to be malignant but with very low metastatic potential.

Precancerous Lesions

The recent increase in identification and understanding of premalignant lesions of the pancreas has elucidated the processes associated with the progression from benign to

malignant disease. Multiple precursors to adenocarcinoma exist, including pancreatic intraepithelial neoplasia (PanIN), and the cystic precursors IPMN and MCN. PanIN is divided into three grades of increasing dysplasia. PanIN-1 is characterized as a proliferative lesion without nuclear atypia; PanIN-2 is associated with a moderate degree of architectural and cytonuclear abnormalities; PanIN-3 has severe nuclear abnormalities with abnormal mitoses, but without invasion through the basement membrane. PanIN-3 is also referred to as carcinoma in situ and is almost always found in close proximity to an invasive cancer [8]. The prevalence of PanIN lesions increases with age, with one-third of patients greater than 60 years of age, without any known pancreatic disease, having a PanIN-1 lesion. It is proposed that advanced age, in addition to other factors, must be present for a PanIN-1 lesion to progress to PanIN-3 and then to invasive cancer [8]. These factors include genetic events such as telomere shortening, K-ras and p16 mutations, and clonal expansion [9].

IPMNs are macroscopic precursor lesions, which can also progress from benign to malignant histologically. About half the resulting invasive neoplasms are actually colloid (mucinous) carcinomas, with the remainder being the typical tubular adenocarcinoma. The progression to malignant IPMN is directly related to age, with multiple clinical studies demonstrating an increased percentage of malignant lesions in patients of increasing age [2, 10].

Clinical Presentation

History and Physical

Tumors of the exocrine pancreas in their early stage are often asymptomatic or present with the insidious onset of nonspecific symptoms. Tumors in the head of the pancreas typically lead to obstructive jaundice (80%), which is often the only specific symptom pointing to the diagnosis. In an elderly patient, the development of jaundice, with dark urine, light stools, and pruritis, should lead to prompt diagnostic workup with a high index of suspicion for malignancy. Abdominal/back pain (72–87%) and weight loss (90–100%) are also common presenting symptoms, although these often signify locally advanced disease. New-onset diabetes or the presentation with "acute pancreatitis"-like symptoms may also be the presenting clinical features of pancreatic cancer. Nonspecific gastrointestinal symptoms may also exist, such as nausea, decreased appetite, constipation, or diarrhea.

One interesting trend in the presentation of pancreatic neoplasms has been that of the pancreatic 'incidentaloma.' Increased use of computed tomography scanning in the United States has led to increased identification of asymptomatic pancreatic lesions [11]. This has been especially true in the early detection of cystic lesions. The ability of CT scans to distinguish benign vs. malignant cystic disease or risk-stratify patients with very small solid lesions remains unknown, but there is likely some benefit in the early identification of these often asymptomatic lesions [12].

Physical examination of the jaundiced patient may show only a palpable gallbladder. Signs suggestive of advanced cancer, such as cachexia, ascites, abdominal mass, migrating thrombophlebitis, palpable supraclavicular lymphadenopathy (Virchow's node), periumbilical lymphadenopathy (Sister Mary Joseph's Node), and pelvic drop metastases (Blumer's shelf) are obvious evidence of advanced disease with a poor prognosis. Among elderly patients, the presenting signs and symptoms of pancreatic cancer are not significantly more different than in younger patients [13, 14].

Laboratory Studies

Unfortunately, there is no screening test or definitive laboratory diagnostic test for pancreatic cancer. In patients with cancer in the body or tail of the pancreas, laboratory values are typically normal. In patients presenting with jaundice, laboratory studies will reveal an increase in total bilirubin and alkaline phosphatase, with occasional mildly elevated transaminases. Biliary obstruction can also lead to malabsorption of fat-soluble nutrients, which can lead to malnutrition and subsequent decreases in albumin, iron, hemoglobin, and vitamin-K-dependent clotting factors.

The most widely used tumor marker to aid in the diagnosis of pancreatic cancer is CA 19-9, a Lewis blood-group-related mucin glycoprotein. CA 19-9 is present at low levels (<38 U/ml) in most healthy patients, but if elevated, its level often correlates with the presence and even aggressiveness of pancreatic cancer. CA 19-9, however, may be falsely elevated in patients with obstructive jaundice, cirrhosis, pancreatitis, and other malignancies. CA 19-9 has an overall sensitivity of 83% and specificity of 82%, but by raising the cutoff value to 200 U/ml and combining it with other testing modalities, the accuracy increases to 95–100% [15].

Management of Malignant Neoplasms

Diagnosis and Staging

When clinical symptoms or laboratory abnormalities are suspicious for a malignant pancreatic neoplasm, the first step toward diagnosis is noninvasive imaging. Computed tomography (CT) scan or magnetic resonance imaging (MRI) with or without cholangiopancreatography (MRCP) are noninvasive imaging studies that may aid in the diagnosis of pancreatic cancer. Transabdominal ultrasound can confirm obstructive jaundice by demonstrating a dilated biliary tree but lacks the sensitivity of CT and MRI in actually defining a pancreatic mass. Most clinicians regard CT scan with multiphase intravenous (IV) contrast enhancement as the initial imaging modality of choice. In recent years, the development of multidetector CT (MDCT) scanners has reduced acquisition time and drastically enhanced image resolution, resulting in submillimeter slices [16] (Fig. 75.5). In addition, when dual phases of IV contrast are used, both arterial and venous structures can be well visualized to determine

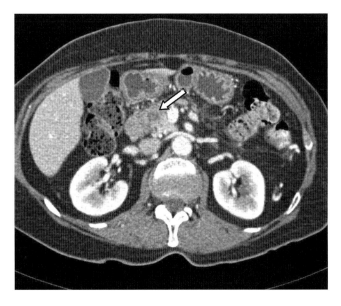

FIGURE 75.5 Multidetector CT (MDCT) scan with IV contrast revealing a 1cm tumor in the head of the pancreas (*arrow*).

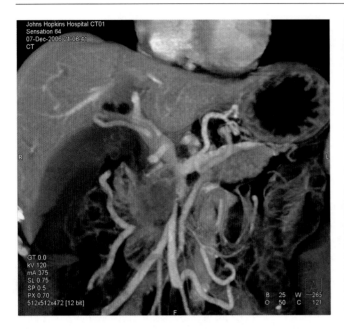

Figure 75.6 Dual-phase contrast MDCT allows clear delineation of peripancreatic vessels, showing a detailed angiographic reconstruction. Note the tumor encroachment of the superior mesenteric vein.

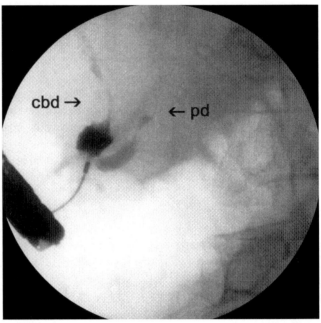

Figure 75.7 ERCP of patient with adenocarcinoma of the pancreatic head. Note the involvement of both the common bile duct (cbd) and pancreatic duct (pd).

local involvement by the tumor that defines resectability (Fig. 75.6). The inclusion of a "pancreatic phase" of IV contrast often leads to improved pancreas-to-lesion distinction. As well as visualizing the lesion and any associated blood vessels, MDCT is able to detect extrapancreatic disease, including liver, lung, and peritoneal metastases, to again provide preoperative staging with respect to resectability [17]. In spite of these advantages, many clinicians are hesitant to expose elderly patients to the potential toxicity of IV contrast. Recently, Itoh et al. have examined the effect of patient age on contrast enhancement during CT scans of the pancreatobiliary region. Results indicate that the ideal dose of IV contrast in the elderly may be about 10% less, or 0.07 mL/kg instead of 0.08 mL/kg. This dose, which takes into account changes in cardiac output and blood volume in the elderly, optimizes tumor enhancement and lessens the risk of nephrotoxicity [18].

Most studies have found no advantage of MRI over MDCT, with the exception of possible improved visualization of small liver metastases and peritoneal implants [17]. MRCP has the added benefit of 3D visualization of both the bile and pancreatic ducts, often revealing the "double duct" pattern of obstruction and can eliminate the need for invasive cholangiography. Another potential modality for the diagnosis and staging of pancreatic cancer is the positron emission tomography (PET) scan. Although PET scanning shows increased uptake of the glucose tracer by both the primary tumor and metastases in other cancers, it has not been shown to reliably provide useful diagnostic information in patients with pancreatic cancer [19].

When noninvasive studies reveal a malignant pancreatic lesion , or when noninvasive studies are inconclusive, invasive studies may be indicated to confirm the diagnosis of pancreatic adenocarcinoma. Endoscopic retrograde cholangiopancreatography (ERCP) provides an endoscopic view of the ampulla and visualizes the biliary and pancreatic ductal systems (Fig. 75.7). ERCP can also be used to obtain cytologic brushings of suspicious areas in the pancreatic ductal system. While cytology results approach 99% specificity, the sensitivity is <50% due to a high false-negative rate [20, 21]. ERCP has been shown to be safe and well tolerated in elderly patients [22]. Rodriguez-Gonzalez et al. studied 159 ERCPs performed on patients 90 years of age or older. Complication rate (2.5%) and procedure-related mortality (0.7%) were low, and therapeutic interventions were able to be performed in 96% of indicated cases [23]. Although ERCP can be a safe and valuable tool in many patients, its use as a diagnostic tool has diminished with the use of MRCP. Therefore, ERCP is now currently used predominantly for endoscopic stent placement, for both palliative and preoperative biliary decompression.

Endoscopic ultrasound (EUS) has recently become a valuable tool in both the diagnosis and staging of pancreatic cancer. EUS sensitivity and specificity in detecting pancreatic cancer are 85–100 and 80–100%, respectively (Fig. 75.8). Multiple studies have demonstrated greater diagnostic accuracy of EUS compared to MDCT, particularly in the detection of small tumors less than 2 cm in size [24–27]. EUS can also be used to obtain a cytologic diagnosis via fine needle aspiration (FNA). This technique is typically more accurate

Figure 75.8 Endoscopic Ultrasound. (**a**) The tumor (*black arrow*) is clearly visualized, as well as its relationship to the superior mesenteric artery (sma) and vein (smv). (**b**) Fine-needle aspiration of the tumor for cytologic examination.

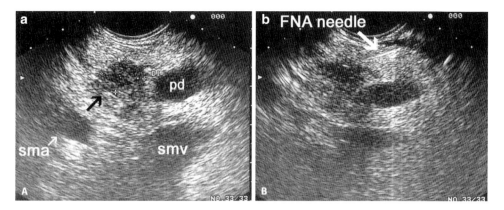

than ERCP brushings, with a sensitivity ranging from 75 to 90%, with a specificity approaching 100% [16, 17]. Complications of EUS are uncommon, even in the elderly.

A preoperative histologic or cytologic diagnosis of pancreatic cancer is not necessary in patients with a clearly defined presentation – obstructive jaundice and a pancreatic mass on CT — in a patient who is considered to be a candidate for surgical resection, regardless of age. When a tissue diagnosis is indicated, EUS-guided FNA has become the preferred method of choice. Yet, even in the elderly patient, a high level of clinical suspicion should override a negative cytologic diagnosis. EUS offers the advantage of the close proximity to the tumor, and for cancers of the pancreatic head, the needle traverses the duodenum, which will be resected. Conversely, percutaneous fine needle aspiration has fallen out of favor both due to the fact that the distance of the pancreatic tumor from the skin surface leads to a higher incidence of false-negative aspirations, as well as the risk of seeding of the tumor along the needle tract, leading to intraperitoneal spread of the tumor.

Surgical resectability of a pancreatic cancer requires that the tumor both shows no evidence of metastatic disease (liver, peritoneal cavity) or local invasion of key adjacent structures. For most surgeons, direct extension of tumor into adjacent organs, encasement of the celiac or superior mesenteric arteries, significant encasement or occlusion of the portal – superior mesenteric vein (SMV) complex, involvement of distant lymph nodes, or obvious metastatic disease will preclude resection of a cancer of the head of the pancreas [28–30]. For cancers of the pancreatic body and tail, extension into the celiac axis or SMA, the SMV/portal vein, or into adjacent organs or metastatic disease renders the tumor unresectable, whereas isolated splenic vein or splenic artery involvement does not preclude resection. MDCT is the most useful imaging modality in detecting obvious vessel invasion and/or metastatic disease, leading to excellent accuracy in predicting unresectability (90–100%), but its specificity in predicting resectabilty is relatively low, about 30–50% [16]. Some studies indicate that EUS may be more

accurate in determining local invasion precluding resection of pancreatic cancer, owing to its increased ability to detect tumor invasion into adjacent vessels [17, 24, 27].

Unfortunately, neither MDCT nor EUS is able to detect small peritoneal or liver metastases, which are common with pancreatic cancer. This problem has led to the use of diagnostic laparoscopy at some centers for staging purposes. The role of routine laparoscopy has been controversial as the sensitivity of CT scanning has increased. Several reports have shown that routine laparoscopy for pancreatic head cancer would spare very few patients from a laparotomy (5–15%) [31, 32]. The value of laparoscopy is increased in evaluating cancers of the body and tail, however, as these patients are found to have occult metastatic disease at operation 50% of the time [33]. Diagnostic laparoscopy in the management of pancreatic cancer must be used on an individualized basis, taking into account the age and comorbidities of the patient, as well as the likelihood of finding occult metastatic disease. It would seem appropriate, however, if suspicion exists in an elderly patient that laparoscopy, to spare the patient an unnecessary laparotomy, might be in order. It has been suggested that markedly elevated CA 19-9 levels may correlate with advanced cancer stage [15, 34]. Finally, the need for surgical palliation of biliary and duodenal obstruction must also be taken into account, as patients who require palliative bypass will not benefit from laparoscopy. On the other hand, as the endoscopic and laparoscopic technical ability has advanced, many palliative procedures can be performed using these techniques, avoiding the need for open surgical procedures.

Preparation for Operation

If the decision is to proceed with an operation for pancreatic cancer in an elderly patient, proper preoperative preparation is required. Thorough assessment of cardiopulmonary status, renal and hepatic function, the state of hydration, nutrition, anemia, and coagulation abnormalities is necessary. All efforts should be made to optimize the patient's overall health prior to proceeding with operation for resection or palliation. Nutritional status can have a major impact on surgical outcome after major abdominal surgery. The method of perioperative nutritional supplementation is controversial, as many methods are currently available. Meta-analyses regarding the use of preoperative total parenteral nutrition (TPN) for at least 7 days show varying results. Some studies have shown a reduction in serious postoperative complications, whereas several other studies show no benefit of preoperative TPN [35]. A recent Evidence Based Medicine Review notes that perioperative TPN is associated with a higher mortality and complication rate after pancreaticoduodenectomy, and recommends cyclic enteral nutrition for the optimal outcome in patients undergoing pancreatic resection [36].

Another major controversy in the preoperative management patients with pancreatic cancer presenting with obstructive jaundice is the role of preoperative biliary decompression. Biliary decompression can be performed by percutaneous transhepatic drainage or by placement of an endoscopic stent at the time of ERCP. In recent years, endoscopic stent placement has become the preferred method, as it is usually accomplished with less pain and complications and is better tolerated by patients. The benefit of routine preoperative biliary drainage is questionable, however, with multiple series suggesting that the use of preoperative stenting increases the incidence of perioperative complications, especially wound infection [32, 37]. Therefore, preoperative biliary drainage is indicated only in selected patients, including the elderly, with advanced malnutrition, sepsis, or correctable medical conditions. Preoperative biliary drainage may be useful in allowing time for improvement of the patient's overall health status, particularly in an elderly patient. Furthermore, if surgery is to be delayed to facilitate referral of the patient to a high-volume center, endoscopic biliary stenting is advantageous. Finally, if preoperative neoadjuvant therapy is considered, biliary drainage is necessary before such therapy can be initiated.

Resection of Lesions of the Pancreatic Head

Pancreaticoduodenectomy (Whipple procedure) is the appropriate procedure for resectable cancers of the head of the pancreas, regardless of the age of the patient (Fig. 75.9) [38]. While many clinicians have regarded advanced age as a relative contraindication for major surgery, recent evidence suggests that age alone should not preclude surgery for pancreatic cancer. Prior to 1980, when the morbidity and mortality for pancreatic resection were substantially higher in all age groups, several studies found that elderly populations fared worse than their younger counterparts. Herter et al. observed that operative deaths rose from 7.7% in patients in the 41- to 50-year age group to 25% in patients 61–70 years of age [39].

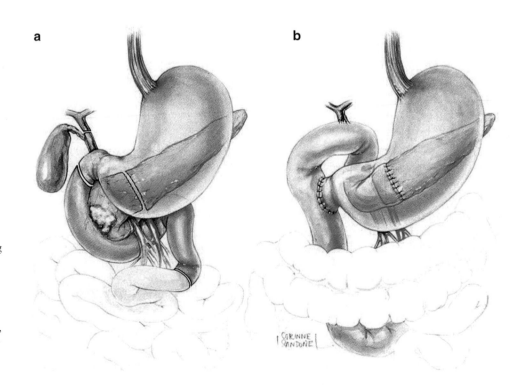

FIGURE 75.9 Pylorus preserving pancreaticoduodenectomy (**a**) Depicts the extent of resection for a pylorus-preserving pancreaticoduodenectomy for cancer of the head of the pancreas. (**b**) depicts reconstruction with an end-to-end pancreaticojejunostomy, end-to-side hepaticojejunostomy, and a retrocolic duodenojejunostomy. (Reprinted with permission from Cameron [38]).

Lerut and colleagues also noted a significant increase in mortality, 41% versus 5% ($p<0.001$), and morbidity, 58.8% versus 16.3% ($p<0.01$), in patients undergoing pancreaticoduodenectomy over the age of 65 when compared to that in younger patients [40]. Finally, Obertop et al. reported 33% mortality following pancreaticoduodenectomy in patients over age 70 compared to 4% in younger patients [41].

Over the past two decades, however, numerous studies have challenged the view that pancreaticoduodenectomy may be contraindicated in elderly patients. One of the first series to show equivalent outcomes in elderly patients was a report from The Johns Hopkins Hospital, which reported 145 consecutive pancreaticoduodenectomies performed without mortality. Subgroup analysis, which separated patients by age (≥70, $n=37$; <70, $n=108$), revealed no significant difference in the incidence of postoperative complications. No specific complication was significantly more frequent in the older group, and for many serious complications, patient over the age of 70 had a lower incidence. Operating time, blood loss, and length of stay were also statistically equivalent between the two groups, and no deaths occurred in either group [42].

Since 1990, numerous single-center series have been published, reporting the perioperative outcome of pancreatic resection in elderly (Table 75.3) [14, 43–58]. Most of these studies found equivalent or acceptable morbidity and mortality rates in elderly patients compared with younger cohorts, suggesting that age alone should not be seen as a contraindication to surgery.

In one such study, Delcore et al. reported a series of 42 patients between age 70 and 80 who underwent pancreaticoduodenectomy. The incidence of major complications was 14%, with 2 operative deaths (5%) [59]. Hannoun and colleagues reported perioperative morbidity and mortality in 223 patients undergoing pancreaticoduodenectomy, with 44 patients who were of age 70 and over. Perioperative morbidity was similar in the two groups (35%), while mortality was actually decreased in the older patients (4.5% vs. 10%) [46]. In a large series from Memorial Sloan–Kettering Cancer Center, Fong et al. analyzed the results of 138 elderly patients (≥70 who underwent major pancreatic resection compared to 350 patients under age 70 [47]. Length of stay (20 days vs. 20 days), frequency of complications (39% vs. 45%), and perioperative mortality (4% vs. 6%)

TABLE 75.3 Summary of publications comparing perioperative outcome between elderly and young patients undergoing pancreatic resection

Author (Year)	Comparison groups	Complication rate (%), older vs. young (p)	Perioperative mortality rate (%), older vs. young (p)
Hannoun et al. (1993) [46]	≥70 ($n=44$) vs. <70 ($n=179$)	36 vs. 34 (NS)	4.5 vs. 10 (NS)
Fong et al. (1995) [47]	≥70 ($n=138$) vs. <70 ($n=350$)	45 vs. 39 (NS)	6 vs. 4 (NS)
Vickers et al. (1996) [48]	≥70 ($n=21$) vs. <70 $n=49$)	43 vs. 53 (NS)	8 vs. 0 (NS)
Sohn et al. (1998) [49]	≥80 ($n=46$) vs. <80 ($n=681$)	57 vs. 41 (0.05)	4.3 vs. 1.6 (NS)
DiCarlo et al. (1998) [50]	≥70 ($n=33$) vs. <70 ($n=85$)	39 vs. 33 (NS)	6 vs. 4 (NS)
Bottger et al. (1999) [51]	>70 ($n=57$) vs. ≤70 ($n=243$)	56 vs. 40 (NS)	5.3 vs. 2.9 (NS)
Al-Sharaf et al. (1999) [52]	≥70 ($n=27$) vs. <70 ($n=47$)	45 vs. 46 (NS)	7 vs. 4 (NS)
Bathe et al. (2000) [53]	≥75 ($n=16$) vs. 65–74 ($n=54$)	69 vs. 52 (NS)	25 vs. 3.7 (NS)
Bathe et al. (2001) [45]	>74 ($n=19$) vs. 65–74 ($n=47$) vs. <65 ($n=38$)	57 vs. 38 (NS)[a]	21 vs. 2 (NS)[a]
Hodul et al. (2001) [44]	≥70 ($n=48$) vs. <70 ($n=74$)	40 vs. 35 (NS)	0 vs. 1.4 (NS)
Richter et al. (2002) [14]	≥70 ($n=93$) vs. <70 ($n=426$)	24 vs. 22 (NS)	3 vs. 3 (NS)
Lightner et al. (2004) [43]	≥75 ($n=30$) vs. <75 ($n=188$) (at UCSF)	70 vs. 56 (NS)	3 vs. 3 (NS)
	≥75 ($n=515$) vs. <75 ($n=2,598$) (in CA)	Data unavailable	10 vs. 7 (<0.05)
Brozzetti et al. (2006) [54]	≥70 ($n=57$) vs. <70 ($n=109$)	49 vs. 46 (NS)	10.6 vs. 3.7 (NS)
Makary et al. (2006) [55]	≥90 ($n=10$) vs. 80-89 ($n=197$) vs. <80 ($n=2,491$)	53 vs. 42 (<0.05)[b]	4.1 vs. 1.7 (<0.05)[b]
Scurtu et al. (2006) [56]	≥75 ($n=32$) vs. 70-75 ($n=38$)	50 vs. 37 (NS)	6.2 vs. 0 (NS)
Casadei et al. (2006) [57]	≥70 ($n=35$) vs. <70 ($n=53$)	40 vs. 26 (NS)	8.6 vs. 3.8 (NS)
Riall et al. (2008) [58]	≥80 ($n=214$) vs. 70–79 ($n=855$) vs. 60–69 ($n=887$) vs. <60 ($n=1,780$)	Data unavailable	11.4 vs. 7.4 vs. 5.8 vs. 2.4 (<0.0001)[c]

UCSF Patients from University of California San Fransisco, *CA* Patients from a California statewide database

[a] Age >74 vs. 65–74. Complications and mortality of age group <65 years old (55% and 3%, respectively) were not significantly different from the other two age groups

[b] Age 80–89 vs. <80. After controlling for comorbidities, complication rate and mortality rate were not statistically significant between age groups

[c] ≥80 vs. 70–79 vs. 60–69 vs. <60. The mean values of all four groups were compared using analysis of variance (ANOVA)

were no different in the younger vs. older groups. In fact, there were no deaths among the 24 patients aged over 80 years who underwent pancreatic resection. Analysis of the complications in this study identified that a history of cardiopulmonary disease, abnormal preoperative ECG or chest radiograph, and operative blood loss of >2,000 ml were most powerful predictors of a complication [47].

Ultimately, experienced groups of pancreatic surgeons have extended the operative indications for resection to patients over 80 years of age. A series of 46 patients aged 80 and over, undergoing pancreaticoduodenectomy over a 10-year period at Johns Hopkins, were compared to 681 patients under 80 who underwent the procedure during the same time period [49]. The two groups were similar with respect to gender, race, intraoperative blood loss, transfusions, and type of resection performed. The older patients had a shorter mean operative time (6.3 ± 1.3 vs. 7.1 ± 4.0 hours, $p < 0.05$) but a longer postoperative length of stay (median 15.0 vs. 13.0 days, $p < 0.05$) than their younger counterparts. A higher incidence of overall complications was seen in the older patients (57% vs. 41%, $p = 0.05$), with a statistically significant increase in delayed gastric emptying among the elderly (33% vs. 18% $p = 0.03$). Perioperative mortality was slightly higher among the elderly patients (4.3% vs. 1.6%), but this was not statistically significant. Another study several years later by the same group examined the outcomes of pancreaticoduodenectomy in the very elderly, which included patients aged 90 and older [55]. Three groups that underwent pancreaticoduodenectomy between 1970 and 2005 were compared: under age 80 ($n = 2,491$), age 80–89 ($n = 197$), and age ≥ 90 ($n = 10$). While the patients aged 80–89 did have a higher mortality rate (4.1% vs. 1.7%, $p < 0.05$) and complication rate (52.8% vs. 41.6%, $p < 0.05$) than their younger counterparts, these differences were not significant after adjusting for preoperative comorbidities. Multivariate analysis found that coronary artery disease and COPD were independent risk factors for mortality after pancreaticoduodenectomy, but age alone was not.

In addition to these numerous studies that looked specifically at patient age, several large series examined all patients after major pancreatic resection to elucidate overall prognostic indicators for outcome. One such study came from the Massachusetts General Hospital, in which 733 consecutive pancreatic resections performed from 1990 to 2000 were reviewed. The authors found that mean age of patients increased significantly over that time period, from 57 to 65 years of age. Multivariate analysis of this series of patients did not identify age as a significant prognostic indicator of poor outcome [60]. A series published from our institution reviewed 516 pancreaticoduodenectomies performed over a period of 20 years. Multivariate analysis of multiple demographic and preoperative variables revealed several prognostic factors of poor outcome, none of which were age-related. These include preoperative serum total bilirubin level, blood loss, operation type, diagnosis, and lymph node status [61]. Another large series from Memorial Sloan–Kettering studied 555 pancreatic resections for pancreatic adenocarcinoma performed over a period of 17 years. Cox multivariate analysis did not find age to be an independent risk factor ($p = 0.695$) [62]. House and colleagues examined preoperative factors among 356 patients who underwent pancreaticoduodenectomy for pancreatic adenocarcinoma between 2000 and 2005. Multivariate analysis again revealed that age was not an independent predictor of complications, but body mass index (BMI) and visceral fat thickness were predictors of pancreatic fistulas, infectious complications, and increased overall complication rate [63].

A number of factors have accounted for the overall improvement in surgical outcomes following pancreatic resection including improvements in surgical technique, anesthesia, and management of complications. However, the "regionalization" of pancreatic surgery to "high-volume" centers is believed to be a major factor by many. The first data supporting this theory came from a study of patients who underwent pancreatic surgery in all nonfederal hospitals in Maryland that revealed that decreased procedural volume was associated with a significantly increased in-hospital mortality rate [64]. Similar results have been reported by numerous other investigators [65–69]. Perhaps the most convincing data, however, has come from Birkmeyer and colleagues, who drew national medical attention by publicizing major disparities between high- and low-volume centers with regard to outcome after major surgeries including pancreatectomy [70].

The effect of "regionalization" to high-volume centers has also been analyzed with respect to older patients. Several groups have published population-based studies to study the effects of both age and hospital volume on postpancreatectomy outcome. Using a statewide database, Lightner and colleagues studied four groups of patients who underwent pancreatic resection for neoplasia: patients from any California hospital younger than 75 years of age ($n = 2,491$), patients from any California hospital aged 75 and older ($n = 515$), patients from UCSF <75 ($n = 188$), and patients from UCSF ≥ 75 years of age ($n = 30$). Results revealed a striking difference in outcome between older patients who were treated at UCSF, a high-volume referral center, compared with those from a statewide database. While mortality was no different between younger and older patients at UCSF (3%), elderly patients had higher mortality rates statewide compared to their younger counterparts (10% vs. 7%, $p = 0.006$). Length of stay was statistically equivalent for young and old patients at UCSF (16 vs. 15 days), whereas elderly patients statewide had a longer length of stay (21.4 vs. 19.8 days, $p<0.05$). Even at UCSF, complications were more frequent in the elderly (70% vs. 56%), and they were more likely to be discharged to a skilled nursing facility (17% vs. 1%, $p<0.05$) [43].

More recently, Riall et al., using a population-based cohort in Texas, have stratified patients undergoing pancreatic resection in Texas from 1999 to 2005 ($n=3,736$) by age into 4 groups: <60, 60–69, 70–79, and ≥80 years of age. Hospitals with low volume (≤10 pancreatic resections/year) and high volume (>10 pancreatic resections/year) were also compared. Mortality increased with increasing age in both types of hospitals, but low-volume hospitals had a more significant increase (Table 75.4). Unfortunately, this study also found that elderly patients were less likely to be resected at high-volume hospitals (62.3% of <60 year-olds vs. 53.7% of ≥80 year-olds, $p=0.01$). Bivariate and multivariate analysis were performed, which revealed older age as an independent predictor for increased mortality, longer length of stay, and increased discharge to nursing facility [58]. These population-based studies suggest that elderly patients who undergo pancreatic resection would be best served in a high-volume referral hospital and that surgeons must carefully weigh all patient factors before making the decision to operate.

Resection of Lesions of the Body and Tail

The opportunity to resect cancers of the body and tail of the pancreas is typically more limited than that of the pancreatic head, due to high frequency of advanced disease at diagnosis. If an elderly patient appears to have resectable disease based on available imaging, many surgeons favor diagnostic laparoscopy to look for occult metastatic disease before proceeding with resection. In the absence of metastatic disease, distal pancreatectomy with splenectomy is the operation of choice. Although less well studied than outcomes after

pancreatic head resection in the elderly, available data indicate that elderly patients tolerate distal pancreatectomy well. In a study of the risk factors predicting outcome after distal pancreatectomy, multivariate analysis found that age was not an independent predictor of outcome [71].

Palliation

Unfortunately, many cancers of the pancreas are unresectable at the time of diagnosis. Thus, optimal palliation of symptoms to maximize the quality of life is of primary importance. The three primary symptoms warranting palliation are obstructive jaundice, gastric outlet obstruction, and pain. Palliation in patients with unresectable pancreatic carcinoma has evolved over the last few decades with the increased use of endoscopic biliary stenting. Early prospective randomized trials showed that nonoperative biliary stent placement for palliation of obstructive jaundice had both lower complication and mortality rates. Many surgeons pointed out, however, that the mortality rate in the surgical arms (15–24%) was much higher than typical mortality rates for surgical biliary bypass. None the less, nonoperative palliation of periampulary carcinoma, especially in older patients, has become routine. Advocates for surgical bypass, however, remark that most surgical series report mortality rates of less than 5% and a much lower incidence of late jaundice when compared to endoscopic palliation [72]. Furthermore, when Nuzzo and colleagues compared the outcomes of elderly people (over age 70) undergoing surgical vs. endoscopic palliation, surgical palliation resulted in better long-term outcomes with similar morbidity [73]. Mean survival after surgery was significantly higher than that after stent placement (13.2 months vs. 7.29, $p<0.001$), and total readmissions were fewer after surgery than stenting (1 vs. 25, $p=0.001$) (Table 75.5).

Although the role of nonoperative palliation in patients found to be unresectable during preoperative evaluation has been well defined, most surgical groups favor performing surgical biliary bypass, should the tumor be determined to be unresectable at the time of laparotomy. This is best

Table 75.4 Mortality by age after pancreatic resection at high-volume and low-volume hospitals in Texas

Age	<60	60–69	70–79	≥80	Overall
Mortality: low-volume (%)	3.0	9.5	11.4	14.7	7.3[a]
Mortality: high-volume (%)	2.0	3.5	4.5	8.7[b]	3.2
Mortality: overall (%)	2.4	5.8	7.4	11.4[c]	

Source: Data from Riall et al. [58]
[a] $p<0.0001$ overall mortality at low-volume vs. high-volume institution
[b] $p<0.0001$ the difference in mortality between low- and high-volume institutions was accentuated with each increasing age group
[c] $p<0.0001$ All age groups compared to each other using ANOVA

Table 75.5 Palliative biliary bypass vs. biliary stenting in patients >70 years of age with unresectable pancreatic cancer [73]

	Surgery ($n=24$)	Stent ($n=35$)	p Value
Mortality (%)	1	3	NS
Morbidity (%)	6	10	NS
Patients readmitted	1	15	0.006
Number of readmissions	1	25	0.001
Mean survival (months)	13.2±8.06	7.29±2.25	<0.001

Source: Data from Nuzzo et al. [73]

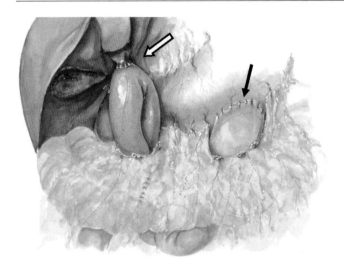

Figure 75.10 Roux-en-Y hepaticojejunostomy (*white arrow*) is performed for biliary decompression, and a retrocolic gastrojejunostomy (*black arrow*) relives gastric outlet obstruction. (Reprinted with permission from Cameron [38]).

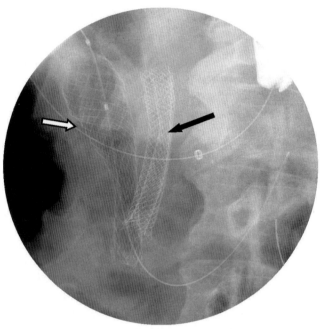

Figure 75.11 Enteric palliation using an endoscopically placed duodenal stent (*white arrow*) and relief of biliary obstruction with biliary stent (*black arrow*).

accomplished by an anastomosis of the bile duct to the small intestine as a hepaticojejunostomy. If patients have duodenal obstruction, a retrocolic gastrojejunostomy should be performed (Fig. 75.10) [38].

The role of prophylactic gastrojejunostomy for palliation in patients found to have unresectable pancreatic carcinoma at laparotomy has been considered controversial. The question, however, appears to have been answered by two prospective randomized trials. One such study was performed at Johns Hopkins which evaluated 87 patients with unresectable periampullary cancer who were randomized at the time of laparotomy to either prophylactic retrocolic gastrojejunostomy or no gastrojejunostomy. None of the patients who underwent gastrojejunostomy developed late gastric outlet obstruction, whereas the patients without gastrojejunostomy had a 19% rate of late gastric outlet obstruction requiring intervention ($p < 0.01$). Length of stay, morbidity, mortality, and long-term survival were comparable between the two groups [75]. In a second prospective, randomized multicenter trial, patients with unresectable cancer at the time of laparotomy underwent either a biliary bypass alone (single bypass) with hepaticojejunostomy or a double bypass with both a hepaticojejunostomy and a retrocolic gastrojejunostomy [75]. The group who underwent double bypass had significantly decreased incidence of late gastric outlet obstruction without any increase in complication rate, providing evidence that prophylactic double bypass should be routinely performed in these patients.

Traditionally, patients who present with unresectable cancer and duodenal obstruction required an open gastrojejunostomy to provide palliation. Recent developments including both laparocopic gastrojejunostomy and endoscopic metallic stent placement offer less invasive alternatives. A number of series have shown excellent results with laparoscopic gastrojejunostomies [76, 77]. In addition, the role of endoscopic stenting for duodenal obstruction has quickly expanded over the last decade (Fig. 75.11). Several retrospective studies have compared outcome after duodenal stent placement vs. gastrojejunostomy (GJJ). In one study, 42 patients who underwent GJJ were compared to 53 patients who underwent stent placement [78]. There were no differences between the groups as far as minor complications, early major complications, and long-term survival, although the surgical group had fewer late complications (22% vs. 60%), and the stented group had a shorter length of hospital stay (6 days vs. 18 days, $p < 0.001$). This study suggests that gastrojejunostomy is associated with better long-term outcomes, while endoscopic stent placement is associated with better short-term outcomes, with no difference in long-term survival. For many patients, primarily with advanced unresectable disease or elderly patients with poor performance status, duodenal stent placement has become the procedure of choice.

The management of pain in patients with advanced pancreatic adenocarcinoma is one of the most important aspects of their care, and multiple complementary treatment strategies are available. Most patients can be successfully managed with a combination of short- and long-acting oral opiates, often combined with topical sustained-release opiates. However, appropriate dosing of opioids in the elderly must be considered. In a recent review of the pharmalogical management of cancer pain in the elderly, the authors note frequent undertreatment of elderly patients with cancer-related pain [79]. Unrelieved cancer pain in the elderly can lead to disturbances in mood, sleep, appetite, and cognition. Many health-care providers have misconceptions about pain perception in the elderly, tolerance and addiction, and increased potency of medications. In general, opioid use in the elderly should start at low doses and be titrated according to the patient's response and adverse effects. Choice of medication should take into account duration of action, ease of administration, and overall health of the patient. Long-acting morphine preparations are commonly used for cancer pain, but its use in the elderly with renal impairment must be weighed carefully, as renal failure may lead to the buildup of a toxic, antagonistic metabolite. Meperidine is ill-advised in the elderly due to its short duration of action, poor oral availability, and neurotoxic metabolites. Oxycodone is appealing for use in the elderly, as its pharmacokinetics is usually independent of age, renal function, and albumin concentration. Transdermal fentanyl is an analgesic that has also been shown to be well tolerated in the elderly population.

When pancreatic cancer pain is intractable in spite of appropriate opioid analgesics, several invasive techniques are available for pain control. These techniques target either the celiac plexus or the splanchnic nerves. Two methods are available for absolute alcohol neurolysis of the celiac plexus: standard needle placement through the midback (with CT or fluoroscopic guidance) or endoscopic ultrasound (EUS)-guided needle placement. Both methods have been shown to significantly reduce pain for sustained periods of time, with the EUS-guided approach having fewer complications [80–82]. When a pancreatic cancer is determined to be unresectable at laparotomy, intraoperative chemical splanchnicectomy with direct injection into the area of the celiac axis (Fig. 75.12)

[38] should be performed. Lillemoe and colleagues performed a prospective, randomized, double-blind, placebo-controlled trial comparing chemical splanchnicectomy with 50% alcohol to a sham saline injection [83]. The patients who received alcohol injections had significantly improved pain scores compared to those who received saline at 2-, 4-, and 6-month follow-up assessments, as well as at the final assessment ($p<0.05$). This procedure can also be performed during laparoscopic staging for pancreatic cancer. Neurolytic celiac plexus block also improved multiple quality-of-life measures in those patients. In the elderly population, EUS-guided neurolytic celiac plexus block likely delivers the least invasive, most effective option for intractable pancreatic cancer pain.

Post-Op Care and Complications

Adequate fluid and electrolyte maintenance, glucose regulation, pulmonary toilet, nutritional evaluation and support, and provision of appropriate perioperative antibiotic prophylaxis are routine. Unfortunately, complications are common in all age groups after pancreaticoduodenectomy, with typical rates of 30–40%. The difference in complication rates between elderly and younger patients has been addressed by multiple retrospective comparisons [13, 14, 43–58]. Although numerous studies have found no difference in complication rates between these two groups, others have reported higher rates of delayed gastric emptying [49, 56], bleeding complications [50], cardiac morbidity [43, 55], or pancreaticojejunostomy leaks [14] in older patients. Several studies report that elderly patients with comorbidities have increased complication rates compared to younger patients with the same comorbidities [54, 55]. Similarly, unpublished data from Indiana University demonstrates that elderly patients with few comorbidities and in better overall health (albumin>3 g/dl, hemoglobin>10 g/ml) had equivalent outcomes as younger patients, while elderly patients with more comorbidities and poor overall health had significantly worse outcomes than younger patients [84]. This suggests that careful preoperative patient selection and increased postoperative diligence are warranted in elderly patients who undergo major pancreatic resection.

Chemotherapy/Radiation Therapy

Many surgeons believe that the future improvement in outcome of pancreatic cancer will come through advances in adjuvant and neoadjuvant chemoradiation therapy. Traditionally, in the United States, standard adjuvant therapy following pancreatic resection has consisted of external

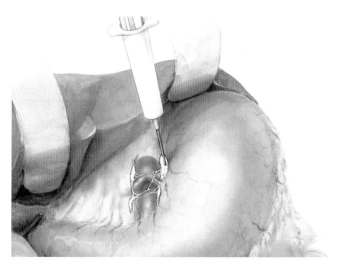

Figure 75.12 Chemical Splanchnicectomy. After identification of the celiac axis in the lesser sac, 50% ethanol is injected into the celiac plexus for pain control. (Reprinted with permission from Cameron [38]).

beam radiotherapy with concomitant 5-fluorouracil (5-FU) chemotherapy. In recent years, gemcitabine has been substituted for 5-FU. These recommendations have been based on a somewhat outdated prospective randomized trial conducted in the 1980s (GITSG trial) [85]. More recently, a large prospective, randomized multi-institutional trial in Europe (ESPAC) has confirmed the benefit of postoperative adjuvant chemotherapy with 5-FU following pancreatic resection [86]. However, this study showed that the addition of radiation showed no benefit and perhaps led to a worsening of outcomes when combined with chemotherapy alone. While neither study specifically addressed age as a factor in determining outcome in patients who were included in these trials, traditionally, a major factor determining the ultimate success of any chemotherapy regimen is the functional status of the patient and their ability to complete the treatment regimen. Elderly patients following pancreatic resection might tend to have a slower overall recovery of functional status limiting either their inclusion in or full completion of adjuvant therapy regimens. Similarly, recent results have suggested that neoadjuvant therapy with preoperative chemotherapy and radiation therapy can be applied safely to patients prior to pancreaticoduodenectomy for cancer of the pancreas [87, 88]. These studies have shown no increase in perioperative complications and comparable long-term survival. Again, the selection criteria for these studies have not defined age as being a prohibitive factor in inclusion in the trials.

In patients with unresectable pancreatic cancer, systemic chemotherapy, usually with gemcitabine is typically applied alone in patients with metastatic disease or in combination with radiation for locally advanced tumors. Traditionally, concerns have been raised that chemotherapeutic side effects may be prohibitive, particularly with concurrent radiation therapy, in elderly patients. Morizane and colleagues reviewed outcome data from pancreatic cancer patients <70 (n=39) and ≥70 (n=19) who underwent 5-FU therapy with concurrent radiotherapy [89]. In spite of lower pretreatment albumin levels and more weight loss in the elderly group, there were no significant differences in toxicity or discontinuation of treatment between groups. In fact, the median survival time was longer in the elderly patients (11.3 months vs. 9.5 months, p=0.04). Another study evaluated the tolerance of gemcitabine regimens in patients aged over 70 years with advanced pancreatic cancer [90]. The elderly patients (n=42) had a higher incidence of neutropenia and peripheral neuropathy than their younger counterparts, resulting in more frequent dose reductions (62% vs. 40%, p=0.03) in the elderly. Overall tolerance was equivalent between the groups, however, and efficacy was similar. In a study investigating the economics of the often-expensive chemoradiation therapy in elderly patients with pancreatic cancer, combination treatment with radiation and chemotherapy was determined to be a cost-effective alternative to no treatment [91]. These results indicate that standard chemoradiation modalities should be strongly considered in elderly patients who have a suitable performance status.

Long-Term Outcomes

Despite improvements in surgical management and perioperative mortality, long-term survival remains poor following resection for pancreatic adenocarcinoma in patients of all ages. Even the best 5-year actuarial survival rates after pancreaticoduodenectomy only approach 20%. Several large series that have applied multivariate statistical analysis have shown that age is not an independent prognostic factor for survival [61, 62, 92, 93]. In contrast, one large study of a statewide database of 2,230 patients diagnosed with pancreatic cancer found that advanced age at diagnosis was an independent risk factor for decreased survival (hazard ratio 1.23, CI 1.18–1.29), although this may be a result of elderly patients not undergoing surgical resection [94]. Most analyses find tumor characteristics and stage to be the most influential prognostic factors for survival, such as tumor size, nodal status, margin status, and tumor differentiation.

Numerous single-institution studies have examined long-term outcome after pancreatic resection in the elderly compared to younger patients (Table 75.6). The majority of series found similar 5-year survival rates in elderly patients as those in younger patients [14, 49, 50, 52, 53, 56, 57, 95]. In contrast, a review performed at the Memorial Sloan–Kettering Cancer Center, the 5-year survival rate for patients ≥70 who underwent pancreatic resection (n=138) was significantly lower than the 5-year survival of patients under age 70 (n=350) (21% vs. 29%, p=0.03) [45, 47, 55]. As with short-term outcomes, hospital volume is an important determining factor in long-term outcome after pancreatic resection. High-volume, single-institution series report postresection 5-year survival rates as high as 29%, while population-based studies report rates of 15–16% [47, 95]. A study by Birkmeyer and colleagues investigated the relationship between hospital volume and 5-year survival after major cancer surgery. This study showed that for pancreatic cancer resection, there was a difference in long-term survival between low- and high-volume hospitals (10.8% vs. 15.9%) [96]. These data, like those regarding perioperative outcome, suggest that elderly patients are best served at high-volume institutions.

Failure to Operate on Early Stage Cancer

Unfortunately, most patients with pancreatic cancer (52%) are found to have distant disease at the time of diagnosis.

TABLE 75.6 Survival among older versus younger patients after pancreatic resection for pancreatic adenocarcinoma

Author (year)	Comparison groups	Median survival (months), old vs. young (p value)	5-Year overall survival (%), old vs. young (p value)
Hannoun et al. (1993) [46]	≥70 (n=21) vs. <70 (n=71)	16 vs. 16 (NS)	17 vs. 19 (NS)
Fong et al. (1995) [47]	≥70 (n=138) vs. <70 (n=350)[a]	18 vs. 24 (0.03)	21 vs. 29 (NS)
Vickers et al. (1996) [48]	≥70 (n=15) vs. <70 (n=17)	–	47 vs. 26 (NS)[b] (4 years)
Sohn et al. (1998) [49]	≥80 (n=25) vs. <80 (n=282)	18 vs. 17 (NS)	46 vs. 36 (NS)[b] (2 years)
DiCarlo et al. (1998) [50]	≥70 (n=29) vs. <70 (n=69)	14 vs. 16 (NS)	0 vs. 9[b]
Al-Sharaf et al. (1999) [52]	≥70 (n=14) vs. <70 (n=27)	9.7 vs. 8.3 (NS)	0 vs. 11[b]
Bathe et al. (2001) [45]	>74 (n=19) vs. 65-74 (n=47)	11 vs. 25 (0.022)	–
	>74 (n=19) vs. <65 (n=38)	11 vs. 12 (NS)	
Richter et al. (2002) [14]	≥70 (n=42) vs. <70 (n=205)	23 vs. 14 (NS)	39 vs. 25 (NS) in R0 resections
Makary et al. (2006) [55]	80-89 (n=102) vs. <80 (n=1,022)	11 vs.18	12 vs. 19 (0.002)
Scurtu et al. (2006) [56]	≥75 (n=20) vs. 70-75 (n=27)	–	7 vs. 17 (NS) (3 years)
Casadei et al. (2006) [57]	≥70 (n=26) vs. <70 (n=38)	20 vs. 15 (NS)	0 vs. 13 (NS)

[a] Includes patients with other periampullary malignancies, islet cell malignancy, and other cancers metastatic to the pancreas
[b] Actuarial survival

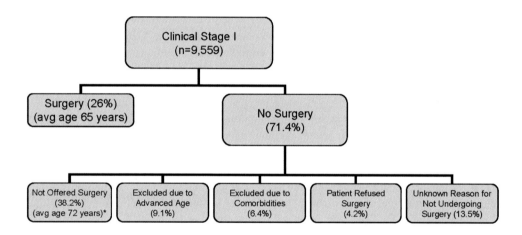

FIGURE 75.13 Failure to operate on stage I pancreatic cancer. Note the role of age in the chances that a patient will be offered surgery. *p<0.0001 compared to age of patients who underwent surgery (Data from Bilimoria et al. [97]).

The dismal prognosis for these patients has led to an overall pessimism for the aggressive treatment of this disease. Of the 38,000 pancreatic cancer patients in the SEER National Cancer Registry database, 7% have localized disease, and 26% present with regional disease. When these 33% patients with locoregional disease have been studied, only about half of them underwent any form of surgical or radiation treatment [97, 98]. Even among Stage I patients, who are potentially curable with resection, Bilimoria et al. found that 71% did not undergo surgery. Analysis of these patients showed that 6.4% were excluded due to comorbidities, 4.2% refused, 9.1% were excluded due to age alone, and 38.2% were not offered surgery for undetermined reasons [97]. In addition to the 9.1% who were excluded due to age, the average age of patients who were not offered surgery was significantly higher, 71.7 vs. 62.1 (p<0.0001). This study suggests that age has a major influence in the management options that are offered to patients, including referral to a surgeon (Fig. 75.13). Gawron et al. found similar differences, with a much higher percentage of older patients treated nonoperatively [99]. This age-related referral bias did not appear to be related to increased comorbidities in the elderly, since the group of patients who were offered surgery had significantly more comorbid conditions than those who were not offered surgery (p<0.0001) [97]. Furthermore, the pattern of not offering surgery to elderly patients did not change over the time period of the study (1995–2004) despite significant decreases in surgical morbidity/mortality during that time and multiple reports of successful pancreatic resection in elderly patients. This unfortunate trend is true for cancer-directed surgery in other diseases as well, with underutilization in elderly populations [100].

Management of Benign and Premalignant Neoplasms

Diagnosis

The diagnosis and management of benign pancreatic neoplasms has become an increasingly frequent problem over the last decade. This is in part due to the increased detection of asymptomatic lesions due to the widespread application of cross-sectional imaging studies. The challenge is determining which lesions are malignant, benign but premalignant, or benign with no malignant potential. The majority of the asymptomatic lesions is cystic and includes mucinous cystic neoplasm (MCN), intraductal papillary mucinous neoplasm (IPMN), and serous cystadenoma (SCA). Cross-sectional imaging (with or without pancreatography), endoscopic ultrasound, and cyst fluid analysis are the principal methods for evaluating cystic lesions of the pancreas.

Multidetector CT scan is generally the first technique used, whether it reveals an incidental, asymptomatic lesion, or has been obtained in the workup of abdominal symptoms. CT can often help discern between several types of cysts, based on specific characteristics. For example, the presence of multiple small-diameter microcysts, stellate scar, and sunburst calcifications is characteristic of SCAs and distinguishes these lesions from mucinous cystic tumors (Fig. 75.2). In addition to aiding in classification of cysts, several findings on cross-sectional imaging can predict the likelihood of malignancy of a cystic pancreatic lesion: peripheral calcification, dilated pancreatic duct, and presence of a solid component [101]. A noninvasive alternative to CT is MRCP, as this technique can determine if the lesion communicates with the pancreatic ductal system. IPMNs typically communicate with the pancreatic ductal system, whereas MCNs do not. MRCP or ERCP, as an invasive procedure, can classify IPMN into main duct type, branch duct type, or mixed type IPMN, which has important implications with respect to management [6, 102]. Endoscopic ultrasound with fine-needle aspiration (EUS-FNA) has also become an important method used to differentiate between cyst types. The viscosity of aspirated fluid is the first clue to diagnosis, as mucinous neoplasms have a higher fluid viscosity than serous ones. Fluid analysis revealing a high mucin content and high carcinoembryonic antigen (CEA) is diagnostic of a mucinous neoplasm, with an accuracy of 79% [11]. This differentiation between mucinous and nonmucinous is essential, as serous tumors are very rarely malignant and in most cases can be managed without surgery.

Estimating the Malignant Potential

When a pancreatic cystic lesion has been classified as mucinous, whether it be MCN or IPMN, the clinician must then determine the likelihood of malignancy. Certain clinical and morphologic features of mucinous cystic lesions are associated with a higher likelihood of malignancy. When cross-sectional imaging of MCN or IPMN reveals a tumor size >3 cm, calcification, or presence of a solid component, there is an increased chance of malignancy [6, 102]. In patients with IPMN, a main-duct subtype, side branch tumors with a dilated main pancreatic duct, elevated serum CEA or CA19-9, presence of jaundice, and new-onset diabetes have all been shown to be predictors of malignancy [2, 7, 101]. In addition, cyst fluid analysis revealing markedly elevated levels of CEA or PGE_2 is associated with malignancy [103, 104]. Cytology of the cyst aspirate may also be used, which has a specificity of 83%, but the high false-negative rate creates a low sensitivity (34.5%) [105]. Finally, advanced age is also associated with increased likelihood of malignancy, as most series find the average age of patients with malignant lesions to be 5–6 years older than patients with benign tumors [106].

Indications for Resection

In elderly patients, the decision to proceed with surgical resection must take into account the patients symptoms, the likelihood of malignancy, the patient's general medical condition, and the expected morbidity and even mortality of the procedure. In patients with serous cystadenoma, the likelihood of malignancy is less than 1%, so surgery should only be offered to symptomatic patients in relatively good heath or for tumors demonstrating significant growth. In the case of mucinous cystic neoplasms (MCNs), resection is indicated in symptomatic patients and in cases with a high suspicion of malignancy. Because it is impossible to determine malignancy preoperatively with absolute certainty, many surgeons advocate surgical resection for all patients with MCN who are suitable operative candidates [6]. For patients with branch duct IPMN, malignancy is extremely rare in asymptomatic patients with lesions less than 3 cm. Therefore, only those patients who are symptomatic or have large (>3 cm) lesions should undergo resection. In contrast, main-duct IPMN has a malignancy rate of 60–92%, leading to most authors recommending resection for all patients [2, 7, 107].

Resection

When the decision is made to resect a benign or premalignant tumor of the pancreas, most resections are performed using traditional pancreaticoduodenectomy or distal pancreatectomy. However, in recent years, multiple new minimally invasive and/or pancreas-sparing techniques have become popular options for surgical management. These include laparoscopic distal pancreatectomy with or without splenic preservation, central pancreatectomy, and enucleation of the lesion. For lesions of the body and tail of the gland, laparoscopic distal pancreatectomy, with or without the spleen-preserving procedure, has gained favor with many surgeons [108, 109]. The laparoscopic technique has become widely applied for benign tumors or small tumors of undetermined malignant status. In patients considered to have a high probability of malignancy, splenectomy should be considered. For benign small lesions in the midpancreas, a central pancreatectomy may be an appropriate choice, as it preserves as much pancreatic tissue as possible to ensure maintenance of endocrine and exocrine function. An even less invasive option for benign neoplasms is enucleation, in which the lesion is essentially 'cored' out from the pancreatic parenchyma. This procedure is most appropriate for lesions that are not in communication with the main pancreatic duct [110].

Outcomes

Theoretically, the long-term survival after resection of a benign or premalignant pancreatic tumor should be comparable to age-matched controls. However, patients with IPMNs are at risk for recurrent disease in the remnant gland after partial pancreatectomy. The extent of surgical resection of IPMNs should be determined by the extent of disease (especially the presence of multifocal lesions) and intraoperative frozen section of resection margins. After resection, patients with even benign or noninvasive IPMNs require careful follow-up for recurrent disease, which has been reported in approximately 10% of patients [2]. Survival for patients with resected invasive IPMNs is substantially better than for pancreatic ductal carcinoma and in some series approaches 50% at 5 years [10]. The role of postoperative adjuvant therapy for invasive IPMN has not been specifically determined but in general has been applied similarly to ductal carcinoma.

Conclusions

Tumors of the exocrine pancreas are a significant issue in the elderly. In general, older patients should be treated aggressively with similar indications for surgery and similar procedures as in younger patients. The morbidity and mortality of major pancreatic resection have decreased among all age groups over the last three decades, making safer surgery an option. Great care should be taken, however, in assessing an older patient's preoperative risk factors, potential for increased life expectancy, and hospital volume before proceeding with major surgical resection. In patients with malignant tumors, primary-care physicians and surgeons alike must recognize that surgical resection offers the only chance for cure and must not be withheld based on age alone.

CASE STUDY

Mr. Smith is an 80-year-old man who presented with painless jaundice, dark urine, clay-colored stools, and pruritus. His workup at an outside hospital consisted of a CT scan, which showed a potentially resectable 2.5 cm mass in the head of the pancreas, and an ERCP, which demonstrated pancreatic and biliary ductal obstruction. A biliary endostent was placed. Finally, an endoscopic ultrasound was performed, which showed a pancreatic mass with no evidence of visceral vessel invasion. Fine-needle aspirate performed at the time of EUS was positive for pancreatic cancer. The patient was referred for surgical evaluation.

The patient's past medical history is significant for a 40-year smoking history, although he stopped smoking 20 years ago. He has long-standing atrial fibrillation and has been on anticoagulation with warfarin. The patient has an internal cardiac defibrillator in place. He has type II diabetes managed with oral medications. He has a history of prostate cancer treated with radiation therapy, which has resulted with neuropathic bladder, which requires self-catheterization. He also has a history of a left hip replacement.

After determining that the patient was indeed a potential candidate for surgical management, follow-up with his cardiologist was obtained where echocardiogram revealed an ejection fraction of 20–25%, likely due to a

(continued)

CASE STUDY (continued)

nonischemic cardiomyopathy. His medications included avandia, corgard, glucosamine, iron, lasix, metformin, and norvasc. On review of systems, he denied chest pain, but exercise tolerance was limited with shortness of breath at one block or one flight of stairs. He had no history of cerebral vascular accident or stroke. He had lost a total of 10 pounds since the presentation. He denied nausea, vomiting, or blood in his stool.

The patient was evaluated preoperatively by cardiology as well as in our preoperative assessment and testing center and was brought to the operating room for a planned pancreaticoduodenectomy. His warfarin was stopped five days before surgery and on the morning of admission, he had a normal INR. General anesthesia was induced following placement of an epidural catheter for intraoperative anesthesia and perioperative pain control. After general anesthesia was obtained, the patient underwent a diagnostic laparoscopy, which showed no evidence of metastatic disease. A classic pancreaticoduodenectomy was then performed with an estimated blood loss of 400 ml and no intraoperative complications. After the reconstruction, a feeding jejunostomy was placed. At completion of the surgical procedure, the patient was extubated and transferred to the ICU. He was maintained in the ICU overnight and then transferred to a progressive care unit in the morning following surgery. On postoperative day two, tube feeds were initiated, and on postoperative day three, the patient was started on a clear liquid diet. The patient was maintained with perioperative prophylaxis with lovenox, and on postoperative day four, with no evidence of bleeding in the drains, the patient

was started on therapeutic heparin for the remainder of his hospitalization. On postoperative day five, he developed an episode of atrial fibrillation with rapid ventricular response, and cardiology follow-up was obtained. His heart rate was eventually controlled with digoxin and beta blockers which were not associated with hemodynamic instability. Perioperatively, he had some confusion, thought to be due to intervenous narcotic PCA, but this cleared, and his pain was eventually well controlled with tylenol. He was able to tolerate a diet although oral intake was only marginal, and he was, therefore, maintained on cycled tube feeds throughout the remainder of his hospitalization. The patient was discharged to a rehab center on postoperative day 10 with drains removed and on therapeutic lovenox until his anticoagulation was adequate on oral warfarin.

The patient was seen in follow-up on 1 month after discharge. He has recently been returned to his home where he lives independently with family nearby. He tolerates a diet although we are still using the feeding jejunostomy for daily boluses of tube feeds but felt that his oral intake was adequate. He had no new cardiac events and was therapeutically anticoagulated with warfarin. His feeding tube jejunostomy was removed. His incision was well healed.

Final pathology revealed a 2.7×2.2×1.6 cm ductal carcinoma of the pancreas. All margins were negative. One of 13 pancreatic lymph nodes showed direct invasion by the cancer, but all other lymph nodes were negative. (A.J.C.C. State pT3, N1, M0). After consultation with the patient and his family, it was felt that his recovery was adequate for referral to medical oncology for consideration of postoperative adjuvant chemotherapy.

References

1. Ries LM, D; Krapcho, M; Stinchcomb, DG; Howlader, N; Homer, MJ; Mariotto, A; Miller, BA; Fuer, EJ; Altekruse, SF; Lewis, DR; Clegg, L; Eisner, MP; Reichman, M; Edwards, BK (eds) (2007) SEER Cancer Stat Fact Sheets – Cancer of the Pancreas. http://www.seer.cancer.gov/statfacts/html/pancreas. Accessed 29 November 2008.
2. Salvia R, Fernandez-del Castillo C, Bassi C et al (2004) Main-duct intraductal papillary mucinous neoplasms of the pancreas: clinical predictors of malignancy and long-term survival following resection. Ann Surg 239(5):678–685
3. Genkinger JM, Spiegelman D, Anderson KE, Bergkvist L, Bernstein L, van den Brandt PA (2009) Alcohol intake and pancreatic cancer risk: a pooled analysis of fourteen cohort studies. Cancer Epidemiol Biomarkers Prev 18(3):765–776

4. Klein AP, Brune KA, Petersen GM et al (2004) Prospective risk of pancreatic cancer in familial pancreatic cancer kindreds. Cancer Res 64(7):2634–2638
5. Katz MH, Hwang R, Fleming JB et al (2008) Tumor-node-metastasis staging of pancreatic adenocarcinoma. CA Cancer J Clin 58(2): 111–125
6. Katz MH, Mortenson MM, Wang H et al (2008) Diagnosis and management of cystic neoplasms of the pancreas: an evidence-based approach. J Am Coll Surg 207(1):106–120
7. Tanaka M, Tanaka M (2004) Intraductal papillary mucinous neoplasm of the pancreas: diagnosis and treatment. Pancreas 28(3):282–288
8. Hruban RH, Takaori K, Klimstra DS et al (2004) An illustrated consensus on the classification of pancreatic intraepithelial neoplasia and intraductal papillary mucinous neoplasms. Am J Surg Pathol 28(8):977–987
9. Takaori K, Hruban RH, Maitra A, Tanigawa N (2004) Pancreatic intraepithelial neoplasia. Pancreas 28(3):257–262

10. Sohn TA, Yeo CJ, Cameron JL et al (2004) Intraductal papillary mucinous neoplasms of the pancreas: an updated experience. Ann Surg 239(6):788–797, discussion 797–789

11. Brugge WR, Lewandrowski K, Lee-Lewandrowski E et al (2004) Diagnosis of pancreatic cystic neoplasms: a report of the cooperative pancreatic cyst study. Gastroenterology 126(5):1330–1336

12. Winter JM, Cameron JL, Lillemoe KD et al (2006) Periampullary and pancreatic incidentaloma: A single institution's experience with an increasingly common diagnosis. Ann Surg 243(5): 673–683

13. Spencer MP, Sarr MG, Nagorney DM (1990) Radical pancreatectomy for pancreatic cancer in the elderly. Is it safe and justified? Ann Surg 212(2):140–143

14. Richter A, Niedergethmann M, Lorenz D et al (2002) Resection for cancers of the pancreatic head in patients aged 70 years or over. Eur J Surg 168(6):339–344

15. Kau SY, Shyr YM, Su CH, Wu CW, Lui WY (1999) Diagnostic and prognostic values of CA 19-9 and CEA in periampullary cancers. J Am Coll Surg 188(4):415–420

16. Nichols MT, Russ PD, Chen YK, Nichols MT, Russ PD, Chen YK (2006) Pancreatic imaging: current and emerging technologies. Pancreas 33(3):211–220

17. Sahani DV, Shah ZK, Catalano OA et al (2008) Radiology of pancreatic adenocarcinoma: current status of imaging. J Gastroenterol Hepatol 23(1):23–33

18. Itoh S, Ikeda M, Satake H et al (2006) The effect of patient age on contrast enhancement during CT of the pancreatobiliary region. AJR Am J Roentgenol 187(2):505–510

19. Friess H, Erkan M, Kleef J, Haberkorn U, Buchler MW (2008) Role of positron emission tomography in diagnosis of pancreatic cancer and cancer recurrence. In: Beger HG, Warshaw A, Buchler M, Kozarek R, Lerch M, Neoptolemos J, Shiratori K, Whitcomb D (eds) The pancreas: an integrated textbook of basic science, medicine, and surgery. Blackwell, Oxford, pp 648–655

20. Fogel EL, deBellis M, McHenry L et al (2006) Effectiveness of a new long cytology brush in the evaluation of malignant biliary obstruction: a prospective study. Gastrointest Endosc 63(1): 71–77

21. Brugge WR (2006) Advances in the endoscopic management of patients with pancreatic and biliary malignancies. South Med J 99(12):1358–1366

22. Fritz E, Kirchgatterer A, Hubner D et al (2006) ERCP is safe and effective in patients 80 years of age and older compared with younger patients. Gastrointest Endosc 64(6):899–905

23. Rodriguez-Gonzalez FJ, Naranjo-Rodriguez A, Mata-Tapia I et al (2003) ERCP in patients 90 years of age and older. Gastrointest Endosc 58(2):220–225

24. DeWitt J, Devereaux B, Chriswell M et al (2004) Comparison of endoscopic ultrasonography and multidetector computed tomography for detecting and staging pancreatic cancer. Ann Intern Med 141(10):753–763

25. Rafique A, Freeman S, Carroll N (2007) A clinical algorithm for the assessment of pancreatic lesions: utilization of 16- and 64-section multidetector CT and endoscopic ultrasound. Clin Radiol 62(12):1142–1153

26. Agarwal B, Krishna NB, Labundy JL et al (2008) EUS and/or EUS-guided FNA in patients with CT and/or magnetic resonance imaging findings of enlarged pancreatic head or dilated pancreatic duct with or without a dilated common bile duct. Gastrointest Endos 68(2):237–242, quiz 334

27. Tamm EP, Loyer EM, Faria SC et al (2007) Retrospective analysis of dual-phase MDCT and follow-up EUS/EUS-FNA in the diagnosis of pancreatic cancer. Abdom Imaging 32(5):660–667

28. Lall CG, Howard TJ, Skandarajah A et al (2007) New concepts in staging and treatment of locally advanced pancreatic head cancer. AJR Am J Roentgenol 189(5):1044–1050

29. Dewitt J, Devereaux BM, Lehman GA et al (2006) Comparison of endoscopic ultrasound and computed tomography for the preoperative evaluation of pancreatic cancer: a systematic review. Clin Gastroenterol Hepatol 4(6):717–725, quiz 664

30. Clarke DL, Thomson SR, Madiba TE et al (2003) Preoperative imaging of pancreatic cancer: a management-oriented approach. J Am Coll Surg 196(1):119–129

31. Barreiro CJ, Lillemoe KD, Koniaris LG et al (2002) Diagnostic laparoscopy for periampullary and pancreatic cancer: what is the true benefit? J Gastrointest Surg 6(1):75–81

32. Pisters PW, Lee JE, Vauthey JN, Charnsangavej C, Evans DB (2001) Laparoscopy in the staging of pancreatic cancer. Br J Surg 88(3):325–337

33. Stefanidis D, Grove KD, Schwesinger WH, Thomas CR Jr (2006) The current role of staging laparoscopy for adenocarcinoma of the pancreas: a review. Ann Oncol 17(2):189–199

34. Kilic M, Gocmen E, Tez M et al (2006) Value of preoperative serum CA 19-9 levels in predicting resectability for pancreatic cancer. Can J Surg 49(4):241–244

35. Howard L, Ashley C, Howard L, Ashley C (2003) Nutrition in the perioperative patient. Annu Rev Nutr 23:263–282

36. Goonetilleke KS, Siriwardena AK, Goonetilleke KS, Siriwardena AK (2006) Systematic review of peri-operative nutritional supplementation in patients undergoing pancreaticoduodenectomy. JOP 7(1):5–13

37. Sewnath ME, Karsten TM, Prins MH et al (2002) A meta-analysis on the efficacy of preoperative biliary drainage for tumors causing obstructive jaundice. Ann Surg 236(1):17–27

38. Cameron JL (1990) Atlas of surgery, vol 1. BC Decker, Philadelphia

39. Herter FP, Cooperman AM, Ahlborn TN, Antinori C (1982) Surgical experience with pancreatic and periampullary cancer. Ann Surg 195:274–281

40. Lerut JP, Gianello PR, Otte JB, Kestens PJ (1984) Pancreaticoduodenal resection: surgical experience and evluation of risk factors in 103 patients. Ann Surg 199:432–437

41. Obertop H, Bruining HA, Schattenkerk ME et al (1982) Operative approach to cancer of the head of the pancreas and the periampullary region. Br J Surg 69:573–576

42. Cameron JL, Pitt HA, Yeo CJ (1993) One hundred and forty-five consecutive pancreaticoduodenectomies without mortality. Ann Surg 217:430–438

43. Lightner AM, Glasgow RE, Jordan TH et al (2004) Pancreatic resection in the elderly. J Am Coll Surg 198(5):697–706

44. Hodul P, Tansey J, Golts E, Oh D, Pickleman J, Aranha GV (2001) Age is not a contraindication to pancreaticoduodenectomy. American Surgeon 67(3):270–275, discussion 275–276

45. Bathe OF, Caldera H, Hamilton KL et al (2001) Diminished benefit from resection of cancer of the head of the pancreas in patients of advanced age. J Surg Oncol 77(2):115–122

46. Hannoun L, Christophe M, Ribeiro J et al (1993) A report of forty-four instances of pancreaticoduodenal resection in patients more than seventy years of age. Surg Gynecol Obstet 177(6):556–560

47. Fong Y, Blumgart LH, Fortner JG, Brennan MF (1995) Pancreatic or liver resection for malignancy is safe and effective for the elderly. Ann Surg 222(4):426–434, discussion 434–427

48. Vickers SM, Kerby JD, Smoot TM et al (1996) Economics of pancreatoduodenectomy in the elderly. Surgery 120(4):620–625, discussion 625–626

49. Sohn TA, Yeo CJ, Cameron JL et al (1998) Should pancreaticoduodenectomy be performed in octogenarians? J Gastrointest Surg 2(3):207–216

50. DiCarlo V, Balzano G, Zerbi A, Villa E (1998) Pancreatic cancer resection in elderly patients. Br J Surg 85(5):607–610

51. Bottger TC, Engelmann R, Junginger T (1999) Is age a risk factor for major pancreatic surgery? Hepatogastroenterology 46:2589

52. Al-Sharaf K, Andren-Sandberg A, Ihse I (1999) Subtotal pancreatectomy for cancer can be safe in the elderly. Eur J Surg 165(3): 230–235

53. Bathe OF, Levi D, Caldera H et al (2000) Radical resection of periampullary tumors in the elderly: evaluation of long-term results. World J Surg 24(3):353–358

54. Brozzetti S, Mazzoni G, Miccini M et al (2006) Surgical treatment of pancreatic head carcinoma in elderly patients. Arch Surg 141(2):137–142

55. Makary MA, Winter JM, Cameron JL et al (2006) Pancreaticoduodenectomy in the very elderly. J Gastrointest Surg 10(3):347–356

56. Scurtu R, Bachellier P, Oussoultzoglou E et al (2006) Outcome after pancreaticoduodenectomy for cancer in elderly patients. J Gastrointest Surg 10(6):813–822

57. Casadei R, Zanini N, Morselli-Labate AM et al (2006) Prognostic factors in periampullary and pancreatic tumor resection in elderly patients. World J Surg 30(11):1992–2001

58. Riall TS, Reddy DM, Nealon WH et al (2008) The effect of age on short-term outcomes after pancreatic resection: a population-based study. Ann Surg 248(3):459–467

59. Delcore R, Thomas JH, Hermreck AS (1991) Pancreaticoduodenectomy for malignant pancreatic and periampullary neoplasms in elderly patients. Am J Surg 162:532–536

60. Balcom JHT, Rattner DW, Warshaw AL, Chang Y, Fernandez-del Castillo C (2001) Ten-year experience with 733 pancreatic resections: changing indications, older patients, and decreasing length of hospitalization. Arch Surg 136(4):391–398

61. Schmidt CM, Powell ES, Yiannoutsos CT et al (2004) Pancreaticoduodenectomy: a 20-year experience in 516 patients. Arch Surg 139(7):718–725, discussion 725–717

62. Brennan MF, Kattan MW, Klimstra D et al (2004) Prognostic nomogram for patients undergoing resection for adenocarcinoma of the pancreas. Ann Surg 240(2):293–298

63. House MG, Fong Y, Arnaoutakis DJ et al (2008) Preoperative predictors for complications after pancreaticoduodenectomy: impact of BMI and body fat distribution. J Gastrointest Surg 12(2):270–278

64. Sosa JA, Bowman HM, Gordon TA et al (1998) Importance of hospital volume in the overall management of pancreatic cancer. Ann Surg 228(3):429–438

65. Bilimoria KY, Talamonti MS, Sener SF, Bilimoria MM, Stewart AK, Winchester DP, Ko CY, Bentrem DJ (2008) Effect of hospital volume on margin status after pancreaticoduodenectomy for cancer. J Am Coll Surg 207(4):510–519

66. Goodney PP, Stukel TA, Lucas FL et al (2003) Hospital volume, length of stay, and readmission rates in high-risk surgery. Ann Surg 238(2):161–167

67. Balzano G, Zerbi A, Capretti G, Rocchetti S, Capitanio V, Di Carlo V (2007) Effect of hospital volume on outcome of pancreaticoduodenectomy in Italy. Br J Surg 95(3):357–362

68. Allareddy V, Allareddy V, Konety BR (2007) Specificity of procedure volume and in-hospital mortality association. Ann Surg 246(1):135–139

69. van Heek NT, Kuhlmann KFD, Scholten RJ, deCastro SMM, Busch ORC, van Gulik TM, Obertop H, Gouma DJ (2005) Hospital volume and mortality after pancreatic resection: A systematic review and an evaluation of intervention in the Netherlands. Ann Surg 242(6):781–790

70. Birkmeyer JD, Siewers AE, Finlayson EV et al (2002) Hospital volume and surgical mortality in the United States. N Engl J Med 346(15):1128–1137

71. Sledzianowski JF, Duffas JP, Muscari F, Suc B, Fourtanier F (2005) Risk factors for mortality and intra-abdominal morbidity after distal pancreatectomy. Surgery 137(2):180–185

72. Lillemoe KD, Sauter PK, Pitt HA, Yeo CJ, Cameron JL (1993) Current status of surgical palliation of periampullary carcinoma. Surg Gynecol Obstet 176(1):1–10

73. Nuzzo G, Clemente G, Greco F, Ionta R, Cadeddu F (2004) Is the chronologic age a contra-indication for surgical palliation of unresectable periampullary neoplasms? J Surg Oncol 88(4):206–209

74. Lillemoe KD, Cameron JL, Hardacre JM et al (1999) Is prophylactic gastrojejunostomy indicated for unresectable periampullary cancer? A prospective randomized trial. Ann Surg 230(3): 322–328, discussion 328–330

75. Van Heek NT, deCastro SMM, van Eijck CH, van Geenen RCI, Hesselink EJ, Breslau PJ, Tran TCK, Kazemier G, Visser MRM, Busch ORC, Obertop H, Gouma DJ (2003) The need for a prophylactic gastrojejunostomy for unresectable periampullary cancer: A prospective randomized multicenter trial with special focus on assessment of quality of life. Ann Surg 238(6):894–905

76. Navarra G, Musolino C, Venneri A, De Marco ML, Bartolotta M (2006) Palliative antecolic isoperistaltic gastrojejunostomy: a randomized controlled trial comparing open and laparoscopic approaches. Surg Endosc 20(12):1831–1834

77. Kazanjian KK, Reber HA, Hines OJ (2004) Laparoscopic gastrojejunostomy for gastric outlet obstruction in pancreatic cancer. Am Surg 70(10):910–913

78. Jeurnink SM, Steyerberg EW, Hof G et al (2007) Gastrojejunostomy versus stent placement in patients with malignant gastric outlet obstruction: a comparison in 95 patients. J Surg Oncol 96(5):389–396

79. Mercadante S, Arcuri E, Mercadante S, Arcuri E (2007) Pharmacological management of cancer pain in the elderly. Drugs Aging 24(9):761–776

80. Wong GY, Schroeder DR, Carns PE et al (2004) Effect of neurolytic celiac plexus block on pain relief, quality of life, and survival in patients with unresectable pancreatic cancer: a randomized controlled trial. JAMA 291(9):1092–1099

81. Levy MJ, Wiersema MJ, Levy MJ, Wiersema MJ (2003) EUS-guided celiac plexus neurolysis and celiac plexus block. Gastrointest Endosc 57(7):923–930

82. Yan BM, Myers RP, Yan BM, Myers RP (2007) Neurolytic celiac plexus block for pain control in unresectable pancreatic cancer. Am J Gastroenterol 102(2):430–438

83. Lillemoe KD, Cameron JL, Kaufman HS, Yeo CJ, Pitt HA, Sauter PK (1993) Chemical splanchnicectomy in patients with unresectable pancreatic cancer. A prospective randomized trial. Ann Surg 217(5):447–455, discussion 456–447

84. Turrini O, Lillemoe KD, Schmidt CM. Preoperative score predicting survival of elderly patients undergoing pancreaticoduodenectomy for pancreatic adenocarcinoma. (manuscript in preparation). Vol 2009.

85. Kalser M, Ellenberg SS (1985) Pancreatic cancer: Adjuvant combined radiation and chemotherapy following curative resection. Arch Surg 120(8):899–903

86. Neoptolemos JP, Dunn JA, Stocken DD, Almond J, Link K, Beger H (2001) Adjuvant chemoradiotherapy and chemotherapy in resectable pancreatic cancer. A randomised controlled trial. Lancet 358:1576–1585

87. Palmer D, Stocken DD, Hewitt H, Markham CE, Hassan AB, Johnson PJ, Buckels JA, Bramhall SR (2007) A randomized phase 2 trial of neoadjuvant chemotherapy in resectable pancreatic cancer: gemcitabine alone versus gemcitabine combined with cisplatin. Ann Surg Oncol 14(7):2088–2096

88. Heinrich S, Pestalozzi BC, Schafer M, Weber A, Bauerfeind P, Knuth A, Clavien PA (2008) Prospective phase II trial of neoadjuvant chemotherapy with gemcitabine and cisplatin for resectable adenocarcinoma of the pancreatic head. J Clin Oncol 26(15):2526–2531

89. Morizane C, Okusaka T, Ito Y et al (2005) Chemoradiotherapy for locally advanced pancreatic carcinoma in elderly patients. Oncology 68(4–6):432–437

90. Marechal R, Demols A, Gay F et al (2008) Tolerance and efficacy of gemcitabine and gemcitabine-based regimens in elderly patients with advanced pancreatic cancer. Pancreas 36(3):e16–e21

91. Krzyzanowska MK, Earle CC, Kuntz KM et al (2007) Using economic analysis to evaluate the potential of multimodality therapy for elderly patients with locally advanced pancreatic cancer. Int J Radiat Oncol Biol Phys 67(1):211–218

92. Millikan KW, Deziel DJ, Silverstein JC et al (1999) Prognostic factors associated with resectable adenocarcinoma of the head of the pancreas. Am Surg 65(7):618–623, discussion 623–614

93. Lim JE, Chien MW, Earle CC, Lim JE, Chien MW, Earle CC (2003) Prognostic factors following curative resection for pancreatic adenocarcinoma: a population-based, linked database analysis of 396 patients. Ann Surg 237(1):74–85

94. Eloubeidi M, Desmond R, Wilcox C, Wilson RJ et al (2006) Prognostic factors for survival in pancreatic cancer: a population study. Am J Surg 192(3):322–329

95. Finlayson E, Fan Z, Birkmeyer JD, Finlayson E, Fan Z, Birkmeyer JD (2007) Outcomes in octogenarians undergoing high-risk cancer operation: a national study. J Am Coll Surg 205(6):729–734

96. Birkmeyer JD, Sun Y, Wong SL et al (2007) Hospital volume and late survival after cancer surgery. Ann Surg 245(5):777–783

97. Bilimoria KY, Bentrem DJ, Ko CY et al (2007) National failure to operate on early stage pancreatic cancer. Ann Surg 246(2):173–180

98. Baxter NN, Whitson BA, Tuttle TM, Baxter NN, Whitson BA, Tuttle TM (2007) Trends in the treatment and outcome of pancreatic cancer in the United States. Ann Surg Oncol 14(4):1320–1326

99. Gawron AJ, Gapstur SM, Fought AJ et al (2008) Sociodemographic and tumor characteristics associated with pancreatic cancer surgery in the United States. J Surg Oncol 97(7):578–582

100. O'Connell JB, Maggard MA, Ko CY, O'Connell JB, Maggard MA, Ko CY (2004) Cancer-directed surgery for localized disease: decreased use in the elderly. Ann Surg Oncol 11(11):962–969

101. Goh BK, Tan YM, Thng CH et al (2008) How useful are clinical, biochemical, and cross-sectional imaging features in predicting potentially malignant or malignant cystic lesions of the pancreas? Results from a single institution experience with 220 surgically treated patients. J Am Coll Surg 206(1):17–27

102. Khalid A, Brugge W, Khalid A, Brugge W (2007) ACG practice guidelines for the diagnosis and management of neoplastic pancreatic cysts. Am J Gastroenterol 102(10):2339–2349

103. Shami VM, Sundaram V, Stelow EB et al (2007) The level of carcinoembryonic antigen and the presence of mucin as predictors of cystic pancreatic mucinous neoplasia. Pancreas 34(4):466–469

104. Schmidt CM, Yip-Schneider MT, Ralstin MC et al (2008) PGE(2) in pancreatic cyst fluid helps differentiate IPMN from MCN and predict IPMN dysplasia. J Gastrointest Surg 12(2):243–249

105. Brugge WR (2004) Evaluation of pancreatic cystic lesions with EUS. Gastrointest Endosc 59(6):698–707

106. Traverso WL, Kozarek RA (2008) Diagnosis and natural history of intraductal papillary mucinous neoplasms. In: Beger HG, Warshaw A, Buchler M, Kozarek R, Lerch M, Neoptolemos J, Shiratori K, Whitcomb D (eds) The pancreas: an integrated textbook of basic science, medicine, and surgery. Blackwell, Oxford

107. Goh BK, Tan YM, Cheow PC et al (2006) Cystic lesions of the pancreas: an appraisal of an aggressive resectional policy adopted at a single institution during 15 years. Am J Surg 192(2):148–154

108. Rodriguez JR, Madanat MG, Healy BC et al (2007) Distal pancreatectomy with splenic preservation revisited. Surgery 141(5):619–625

109. Kooby DA, Gillespie T, Bentram D, Nakeeb A, Schmidt CM, Merchant NB, Parikh AA, Martin RCG, Scoggins CR, Ahmad S, Kim HJ, Park J, Johnston F, Strouch MJ, Menze A, Rymer J, McClaine R, Strasberg SM, Talamonti MS, Staley SA, McMasters KM, Lowy AM, Byrd-Sellers J, Wood WC, Hawkins WG (2008) Left-sided pancreatectomy: A multicenter conmparison of laparoscopic and open approaches. Ann Surg 248(3):438–446

110. Madura JA, Yum MN, Lehman GA et al (2004) Mucin secreting cystic lesions of the pancreas: treatment by enucleation. Am Surg 70(2):106–112

Chapter 76
Benign and Malignant Tumors of the Liver

Anita Kit Wan Chiu and Yuman Fong

A decade ago, one eighth of the population of the United States was over the age of 65, and this small portion suffered one half of all cancers diagnosed [1]. It is projected by the U.S. Census Bureau that by the year 2030, more than 20% of the U.S. population will be over the age of 65. This demographic change alone will increase the number of cancers in America by approximately 30% [2, 3], making no other single factor as important as age for cancer incidence.

Advanced age has also long been associated with higher risk during surgical therapy. Brooks in 1937 reported operative results of 287 patients over the age of 70 years who underwent surgical procedures that today would be considered minor [4, 5]. The mortality rate was remarkably high (19%), with approximately one third of the patients who had undergone abdominal operations having in-hospital deaths. Brooks foretold that with a rapid increase of the elderly population, surgeons would increasingly be confronted with surgical problems among the elderly and should strive to improve their results by becoming more accustomed to the physiologic changes associated with aging. It has been approximately seven decades since his paper, and with improvements in anesthetic and surgical technique, there has been substantial improvement in surgical outcomes of elderly patients after routine surgical procedures [5]. High-risk procedures such as cardiac operations and liver resections are now being routinely performed on the elderly population with good outcomes [6]. Advances in surgical technology have also increased the potential for curative cancer surgeries in older patients [7]. However, although elderly patients do favorably when carefully selected, they generally are wrought with more preoperative comorbidities, which can cause an increase in morbidity and mortality. Turrentine in 2006, in an institutional review of ACS NSQIP data, acknowledges that increasing age itself remains an important risk factor for postoperative morbidity and mortality [8]. In 2007, Finlayson

commented on population-based outcomes after high-risk cancer operations in the elderly to be worse than previously reported in the literature with a point that patients in this population need to be carefully selected [9].

Surgical extirpation is the only curative therapy for malignant disease of the liver. Although thermal destruction techniques such as radiofrequency ablation are utilized, resection is still the gold standard for potential cure. In approximately 50,000 cases of hepatic colorectal metastasis encountered annually in the United States, and the more than one million cases of primary hepatocellular carcinoma seen worldwide, surgical excision has been shown to result in long-term survival for more than one third of patients [10]. Because the number of elderly persons in the United States is growing and the incidence of many liver tumors increases with age, increasing numbers of patients are presenting for consideration for resection of primary or secondary liver cancers. This chapter summarizes the current data on morbidity and mortality after liver operations in the elderly and the pathophysiology that may underlie the increased risk of complications in this age group. The current approaches for the most common tumors seen in the elderly are then summarized.

Perioperative Outcome After Liver Resection in the Elderly

The past four decades have seen a dramatic decline in mortality rates after liver resection [11–14]. Major liver resections are routinely performed at major centers with perioperative mortality rates less than 5%. In the past, elderly patients were thought to be at particularly high risk for perioperative complications (Table 76.1). Studies published during the late 1980s still reported mortality rates of 11–41% [15–17]. Extensive resections consisting of trisegmentectomy were associated with operative mortality of more than 30% [17]. The higher operative mortality and morbidity rates in elderly patients can be explained partly by associated conditions in elderly patients such as diabetes mellitus, cardiopulmonary

Y. Fong (✉)
Department of Surgery, Memorial Sloan Kettering Cancer Center,
New York, NY, USA

R.A. Rosenthal et al. (eds.), *Principles and Practice of Geriatric Surgery*,
DOI 10.1007/978-1-4419-6999-6_76, © Springer Science+Business Media, LLC 2011

TABLE 76.1 Clinical studies of liver resection in the elderly

Study	Year	No.	Years of study	Age[a]	Cancer type	No. with cirrhosis	Operative mortality (%)	5-Year survival (%)	LOS (days)	Cause of death
Ezaki et al. [15]	1987	37	6	≥66	HCC	25/37 (68%)	5	18	NS	Liver failure, infection
Yanaga et al. [16]	1988	27	13	≥65	HCC	17/27 (63%)	41	NS	NS	Liver failure (3), sepsis (8)
Fortner and Lincer [17]	1989	90	18	≥65	Mixed	NS	11.1	NS	15 ± 9[b]	Liver failure (6), MI, infection (2), hemorrhage (1)
Mentha et al. [23]	1992	52	23	≥65	Mixed	4/52 (8%)	6	NS	21[c]	Liver failure (2), MI
Nagasue et al. [20]	1993	32	10	≥70	HCC	31/32 (97%)	19	18	NS	Hemorrhage (2), pneumonia, abscess
Takenaka et al. [21]	1994	39	14	≥70	HCC	31/39 (79%)	5	76	NS	Liver failure (2)
Karl et al. [24]	1994	16	6	≥70	Mixed	NS	0	NS	NS	None
Fong et al. [5]	1995	128	10	≥70	CR mets	7/128	4	35	13[c]	Liver failure (3), sepsis (2)
Fong et al. [25]	1998	133	3	≥65	Mixed	8/133 (6%)	4	NS	11[c]	Liver failure (3), infection
Zacharias et al. [86]	2004	61	10	>70	CRLM (1st, recurrent)	NS	0	22	NS	None
Nagano et al. [87]	2005	62	12	>70	CRLM	NS	0	34.1	NS	None
Brand et al. [88]	2000	126	24	>70	CRLM	NS	2.4	NS	16.6	NS
Menon et al. [6]	2006	127	11	>70	Mixed	NS	7.9	NS	15.2	NS
Figueras et al. [89]	2007	160	16	>70	CRLM	NS	8	36	NS	Liver failure, sepsis, hemorrhage, MI
Mann et al. [27]	2008	49	49	>70	CRLM	0	0	31	11	None
Riffat et al. [90]	2006	15	15	>80	Mixed	NS	0.1	NS	12	Cerebrovascular accident

HCC hepatocellular carcinoma; CR mets colorectal metastasis; LOS length of hospital stay; MI myocardial infarction; NS not stated

[a]Criterion for being elderly (age in years)

[b]Mean

[c]Median

disease, and renal disease [18]. Other studies have implicated high American Society of Anesthesiologist grades, intraoperative transfusions, tumor size, and gender to be predictors of overall survival [6, 19]. A more important factor for such high complication and mortality rates in these series is the high incidence of the concomitant hepatic disorders of hepatitis and cirrhosis [5, 15, 20–22]. Several studies suggest that if these factors were excluded, there would be no difference in morbidity and mortality between old and young patients [20]. In more recent studies, in predominantly noncirrhotic elderly patients, the perioperative mortality mirrored that expected in a younger population [5, 6, 20, 21, 23–26].

We have reported two large series where resections in the elderly were performed with an operative mortality less than 4% and a complication rate less than 35% [5, 25]. The major cause of mortality continues to be postoperative hepatic insufficiency; therefore, elderly patients with cirrhosis should be scrutinized closely before an operation is performed. Chronologic age alone should not be considered a contraindication to liver resection. In fact, many studies suggest that an aggressive surgical policy in the elderly is associated with low perioperative morbidity and mortality, as well as good long-term outcomes [27]. However, because associated medical conditions are more frequently encountered in patients with advanced age, we routinely refer patients of age 65 and over for cardiopulmonary evaluation prior to liver resection. Contrary to recommendations of others [17, 24], we do not believe that trisegmentectomies carry prohibitive risk in the elderly, and routinely offer such extensive resections to medically fit patients of advanced age. Postoperative medical monitoring is based on objective evaluation of medical fitness and not on age alone. In a series of 128 patients undergoing liver resection for metastatic colorectal cancer, only 7% required intensive-care unit (ICU) admission at any time during the

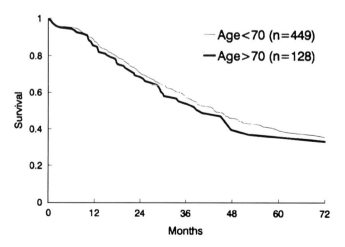

FIGURE 76.1 Survival after liver resection for colorectal metastases for patients age 70 years or older ($n=128$) compared with that of patients younger than age 70 ($n=449$; $p=$ NS) (from Fong et al. [5] with permission from Lippincott Wilkins & Williams).

hospitalization, and the median hospital stay was only 13 days [5]. Liver resection in the elderly can, therefore, be performed with low mortality and morbidity and with expenditure of health-care resources similar to that for resections performed in a younger age group. In fact, the long-term survival of elderly patients undergoing liver resection for malignancy mirrors that of younger patients (Fig. 76.1).

Pathophysiologic Basis of Liver Complications in the Elderly

The liver undergoes physiologic changes during aging, such as a decrease in size and blood flow [1, 2, 28]. There is an observed increase in mean cellular and mitochondrial volume and a decrease in cell number. There is also a decrease in mitochondrial DNA [29]. Under normal conditions, these changes do not seem to be clinically significant, as hepatocyte functions such as detoxification, demethylation, conjugation, and hepatic extraction remain normal. However, during periods that require increased hepatocyte function, the liver of an older patient may not be able to respond by increasing synthetic or metabolic function, and hence, hepatic insufficiency may result [1, 3, 30]. One clinically important scenario requiring increased hepatocyte function is the immediate postresection period, when a reduced hepatocyte mass must perform the physiologic tasks of the preoperative liver until such time as regeneration may restore the liver to preoperative capacities. The reduced hepatocyte protein synthesis in the elderly may be a factor contributing to postoperative hepatic insufficiency [31, 32]. This may help explain the higher incidence of liver failure, particularly in cirrhotic elderly patients after liver resection [16, 20]. Elderly patients with cirrhosis should therefore be considered discriminantly for surgical resection.

Postoperative liver insufficiency may also be explained by a reduced "regenerative" capacity in the aged. The basis for major liver resection is the potential for the liver to undergo compensatory hypertrophy and hyperplasia, or "regeneration," as it is more often termed. Resection of up to 80% of the hepatic mass is followed by liver regeneration, such that within a 3-week period, a liver of approximately the same size as the preresection liver can be expected, with normalization of liver functions usually within 6 weeks. This regeneration, however, may be altered by the processes of aging. Numerous animal studies have demonstrated retarded liver regeneration in aged animals, as measured by mitotic index, tritiated thymidine uptake, and restoration of liver mass [33, 34]. Such alterations in liver regeneration and function in aged animals are particularly dependent on the nutritional status of the animal [32], making nutritional support particularly important in this age group. One possible mechanism of such retardation of regeneration is a reduction of thymidine kinase expression in aged animals [34]. In addition, levels of DNA polymerase-α, a key enzyme for DNA synthesis, are diminished in aged animals [35]. These and other enzymes are necessary for maintenance of DNA synthesis in animals. There is also decreased fidelity of DNA synthesis by DNA polymerase-α [36], which may very well be related to the alterations in histone function that have long been recognized [37, 38]. Whether such cellular changes are seen in human regenerating livers is not known, as studies evaluating cellular alterations during liver regeneration in the elderly patient are sparse. For the noncirrhotic patient, the alterations in liver regeneration seen in animals cannot be clinically relevant in humans, as most reports suggest that there is little difference in the hepatic regeneration rate measured by size when the old patient is compared to young individuals. In patients with cirrhosis, it is this parenchymal abnormality that has the greatest influence over the regenerative capacity.

Treatment of Liver Tumors

In the following section, we discuss the most commonly encountered liver tumors in the elderly patient, beginning with benign tumors. The latter usually do not require therapy but are discussed because patients of advancing age are more likely to be subjected to the wide variety of imaging modalities now available. Benign liver tumors are often discovered incidentally and lead to emotional distress and diagnostic confusion. Our discussion then concentrates on the two malignant tumors most commonly encountered: metastatic colorectal cancer and hepatocellular carcinoma.

Benign Liver Tumors

Most benign liver tumors are asymptomatic and are discovered incidentally at the time of laparotomy or detected on an imaging examination done for other indications. When a patient presents with an incidentally discovered liver mass, a workup should begin as always with a thorough history and physical examination. A history of previous cancers is elicited, as are any symptoms suggestive of gastrointestinal malignancy. Patients should be questioned for a history of hepatitis, alcohol abuse, and familial history of liver disease. Most patients are asymptomatic. It is a highly unusual situation when a patient presents with definable symptoms from a benign tumor, which are usually related to encroachment on adjacent structures or the stretching of Glisson's capsule by a large tumor. On physical examination, signs of portal hypertension such as caput medusae and ascites are sought, and a stool guaiac test is done for occult blood. Serum transaminase levels are sometimes elevated as a consequence of tissue

necrosis in hepatic cell adenomas. Alkaline phosphatase levels may be elevated because of impingement of tumor on the biliary tree. Most liver function tests, however, are normal in patients with benign tumors. Hepatitis screen – hepatitis B surface antigen (HBsAg) and hepatitis C antibody – is assayed along with α-fetoprotein (AFP) and carcinoembryonic antigen (CEA). The most common imaging test employed is computed tomography (CT) scanning because it is the most commonly available and most uniform in quality. Ultrasonography is performed if cystic lesions are suspected, but for most other lesions, it is not specific enough for a confident diagnosis [39]. Magnetic resonance imaging (MRI) is currently the most accurate noninvasive diagnostic tool used for differentiating various benign lesions including adenomas, fibronodular hyperplasia (FNH), and hemangiomas, and with the recent addition of MR cholangiography, MR techniques have proven to be even more powerful for evaluating liver tumors [40]. Occasionally, angiography is still called on to diagnose a hemangioma, adenoma, or FNH more confidently.

Bile Duct Adenomas

Bile duct adenomas are sometimes referred to as bile duct hamartomas and are presumed to be developmental defects. They are usually small lesions that rarely exceed 1 cm in diameter. Often discovered at the time of laparotomy and confused with metastatic cancers, they are grayish white and firm to palpation. Microscopically, they are composed of fibrous stroma surrounding bile ducts. It is estimated that approximately one third of the population has these lesions [41]. Bile duct hamartomas are universally asymptomatic and require no therapy.

Hepatocellular Adenomas

Hepatocellular adenomas are soft and fleshy with a yellowish-tan color. They are sometimes quite vascular and can grow to an enormous size. These rare tumors have been associated with the use of oral contraceptives. Liver enzyme abnormalities are nonspecific, and tumor markers are usually negative. On CT scan, the adenoma is typically a low-density solid mass. Even with imaging by MR and angiogram, and occasionally even after biopsy, these lesions are still not distinguishable from a well-differentiated hepatocellular cancer.

Management of the asymptomatic patient presents an interesting and slightly controversial conundrum. There are growing concerns about leaving adenomas in situ, with recent reports suggesting that adenomas are premalignant lesions [42]. Adenomas may also rupture, and the resultant hemorrhage is associated with high mortality [42]. In young individuals, we almost always resect adenomas for fear of rupture and malignant transformation. Oral contraceptives should also be discontinued. In the elderly individual, enthusiasm for resection must be moderated by the medical risks of surgery. Certainly, if the tumor was symptomatic, the decision would be easier. Asymptomatic tumors in a patient with significant associated medical illnesses may warrant observation.

Hemangiomas

Hemangioma is the most common benign tumor of the liver. Cavernous hemangiomas in most autopsy series have a reported incidence of approximately 7% [43]. The age range associated with hemangiomas is usually 55 years or above in most clinical series, although it is probably due to the higher chance for abdominal imaging in patients with advanced age.

Hemangiomas usually present as a solitary lesion but are multiple in about 10% of cases. They usually measure less than 2 cm in diameter but occasionally grow to enormous size and in some cases even replace an entire lobe of the liver. Most of the lesions remain asymptomatic, and hemangiomas <4 cm in diameter rarely become clinically relevant. Sixty percent of patients with large tumors present with abdominal pain or discomfort, digestive problems, and the sensation of an abdominal mass or distension [44]. Rarely, platelet trapping in the large tumors results in thrombocytopenia, which may manifest as ecchymoses and purpura.

Liver function is almost always normal, and tumor markers are consistently negative. On CT scans, hemangiomas present as low-density areas within the liver parenchyma which upon intravenous injection of contrast show early peripheral opacification followed by variable degrees of enhancement of the central portion. Even though ultrasonography and CT scanning are usually the first imaging tests used in the investigation of hemangiomas, MRI scans have been shown to improve specificity. A combination of T1-weighted, T2-weighted, and gadolinium-enhancedf dynamic scans provide the diagnosis of hemangioma with an accuracy of more than 95% (Fig. 76.2) [40]. MRI has

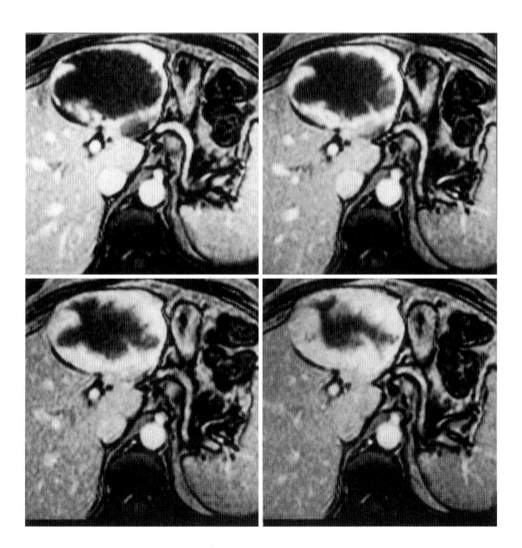

FIGURE 76.2 Gadolinium-enhanced magnetic resonance imaging (MRI) scans of a hemangioma. The peripheral nodular enhancement pattern seen is diagnostic of a hemangioma.

replaced the tagged red blood cell (RBC) scan as the modality of choice for evaluating patients with suspected hemangiomas. MRI can provide information for diagnosis of other liver lesions and provide anatomic details not possible on tagged-RBC scans. Percutaneous needle biopsy should be avoided, as it is associated with severe, sometimes fatal, hemorrhage.

In the elderly, asymptomatic hemangiomas require no treatment. Indications for treatment include pain, discomfort, early satiety, rapid increase in size, thrombocytopenia, or evidence of bleeding intraperitoneally or intraparenchymally [45, 46]. There are a few documented reports of significant reduction in tumor size with the use of external beam radiation, but those results are inconsistent [47, 48]. Hepatic artery embolization has also been attempted but has only occasionally been successful [49]. Symptomatic lesions should be resected. Because hemangiomas are usually surrounded by compressed hepatic parenchyma, lesions are often amenable to enucleation, though deep lesions are usually best treated with a formal resection along anatomic planes.

Malignant Liver Tumors

Hepatic cancers may be subdivided into primary and metastatic cancers. Primary hepatic cancers arise within the liver and include hepatocellular carcinoma (HCC) and cholangiocarcinoma. Metastatic cancers are derived from a variety of primary sites, with metastatic colorectal cancer being predominant and few other types being appropriate for surgical therapy. The challenges of treating elderly patients with HCC or metastatic colorectal cancer are discussed.

Hepatocellular Carcinoma

Hepatocellular carcinoma is the most common solid organ tumor worldwide and comprises approximately 90% of all primary liver cancers in the elderly population. Most of these tumors are associated with chronic liver disease, such as viral hepatitis or alcoholic cirrhosis. HCCs may be unifocal or multifocal. Most patients are relatively asymptomatic until the tumor reaches an advanced stage when it causes symptoms, usually right upper quadrant pain. It is then found as a highly vascular, large tumor that is susceptible to rupture and intraperitoneal hemorrhage. The most common physical finding is hepatomegaly with tenderness. Bile duct obstruction and invasion with tumor embolus may cause jaundice.

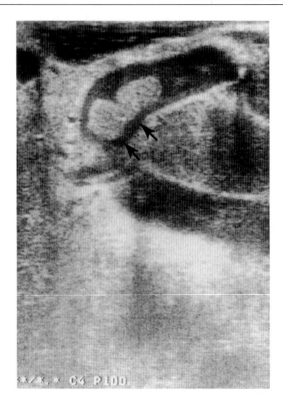

FIGURE 76.3 Portal vein invasion and intraportal extension by hepatocellular carcinoma (HCC) as demonstrated by intraoperative ultrasonography (*arrows*). HCC has a great propensity for intraluminal growth and extension along major blood vessels and bile ducts.

At an advanced stage, these tumors cause a host of other symptoms, including abdominal distension, weight loss, fatigue, anorexia, and fever. Occasionally, hepatic decompensation, ascites, Budd–Chiari syndrome, variceal bleeding, severe jaundice, or encephalopathy is the presentation of HCC in a previously well-compensated cirrhotic patient [50]. Not infrequently, the cause of such decompensation is portal vein invasion and thrombo-occlusion by the tumor (Fig. 76.3).

Diagnosis

The triad diagnostic of HCC consists of hepatic mass by imaging, positive serologic markers for hepatitis B or C, and a strongly positive AFP level [50]. At presentation, patients should be evaluated for a history of chronic liver disease or a familial history of liver disease. Questions and the examination should be directed at uncovering signs and symptoms of hepatic insufficiency. Blood tests should include liver function tests, renal functions, hepatitis screen, AFP, and CEA. An AFP > 500 ng/dl is diagnostic of HCC.

The goals of diagnostic imaging are to distinguish primary liver cancer, metastatic cancers, and benign liver tumors, to assess the extent of spread of the tumor, and to define local resectability. The patient is usually evaluated by CT scan before referral. CT scanning is a widely available test that allows examination of hepatic and tumor anatomy, as well as the presence of cirrhosis or fatty infiltration in uninvolved segments of the liver [51]. Of note, a noncontrast CT is essential for evaluating HCC in addition to the contrast-enhanced scans. This is because an HCC often is isodense to the liver parenchyma on contrast-enhanced images and requires noncontrast scans for imaging.

If the portal veins and hepatic veins are well visualized, a CT scan alone may be sufficient for evaluating the liver tumor. Most often, though, an ultrasound examination or MRI should be performed because of the propensity for HCCs to invade and grow along major vasculature, even when they are small tumors. We prefer abdominal ultrasonography for this evaluation because of the lower cost and the accuracy of this test in experienced hands, acknowledging that the results are highly dependent on the skill of the ultrasonographer. In general practice, MRI is of more uniform quality and should be the test performed. MRI with magnetic resonance angiography (MRA) and magnetic resonance cholangiopancreatography (MRCP) [52] allows not only characterization of various tumors, assessment of the tumor extent, and proximity to vascular structures but also proximity to biliary structures. Hepatic angiography is now rarely used because of the quality of current noninvasive imaging studies; it is reserved largely for patients requiring embolization as treatment of the HCC.

Surgical Treatment

Surgical resection is the only potentially curative treatment for patients with HCC. However, because small HCCs are usually asymptomatic, most patients do not present until the disease is far advanced, and only 30% of patients with suspected HCC are candidates for surgical exploration. In the elderly, surgical therapy is further restricted because liver transplantation is not an available option. In the general population, liver transplantation is considered for those patients with small tumors but with liver reserve considered too risky for partial hepatectomy. However, most transplant centers do not give liver transplants to patients aged 65 or more, and therefore, total hepatectomy and liver transplantation are not an option for this age group.

Technical aspects of partial hepatectomy are largely as for patients of a younger age group, and the reader is referred to textbooks of liver surgery for a general discussion [53]. The differences are modifications to suit not only elderly patients but also cirrhotic patients who usually comprise the population undergoing HCC resection. Bilateral subcostal incisions are usually employed with a xiphoid extension although we advocate a midline incision with a right transverse extension. This high incision and the likelihood of a right pleural effusion after liver resection are the main reasons elderly patients should be evaluated carefully for pulmonary status. Respiratory compromise and pneumonia are frequent complications in patients undergoing liver resection, compounded in the elderly patient by the normal loss of pulmonary reserve with advancing age. At exploration, the entire liver should be mobilized from its ligamentous attachments to evaluate resectability. Exposure is constantly maintained with a retractor fixed to the table, enabling excellent exposure and decreasing the chances of needing to enter the chest. Intraoperative ultrasonography is performed to determine the relation of the tumor to the major vascular structures and to identify additional sites of disease in the liver not appreciated by conventional preoperative imaging [54]. Inflow and outflow vasculature to the section of liver to be removed is usually controlled. We avoid total vascular exclusion (TVE), in general, but are even more adamant about it in the elderly. The hemodynamic changes often associated with TVE are particularly poorly tolerated in elderly patients who may have cardiopulmonary disease. The porta hepatis is controlled to allow application of the Pringle maneuver. A Pringle maneuver is performed to decrease bleeding when dividing the liver parenchyma [55]. We prefer use of the Pringle maneuver intermittently, releasing the Pringle every 5 min to allow reperfusion of the liver.

Operative mortality in cirrhotic patients of any age undergoing liver resection in a major center continues to be in the 10% range [56]. In elderly cirrhotic patients, the mortality rate has been reported to be as high as 19–41% [16, 20] and as low as 5% [15, 21]. Most of the complications following liver resections are usually cardiopulmonary (angina, arrhythmia, myocardial infarction, transient ischemic attacks, pneumothorax, pulmonary embolism) [2]. Patient selection is key to a favorable outcome. Although many sophisticated tests have been proposed for preoperative evaluation of liver function, none has been demonstrated to be better than Child's criteria. We routinely consider Child's A patients for surgical resection. Patients with Child's B liver functional status are considered for resection only if the lesion is peripheral and requires resection of little functional liver. Elderly Child's C patients are offered only supportive care, as transplantation is generally not an option in the elderly, and even ablative therapies are associated with prohibitive risk in patients with such little liver functional reserve [57].

Unfortunately, only 30% of patients explored have resectable lesions. Among patients who undergo resection, long-term survival is achieved in up to 76% (Table 76.1), though most series of HCC resections report long-term survival in one third of patients.

Nonsurgical Treatment

Many ablative therapies have been developed for the treatment of nonresectable HCC. Transarterial embolization or chemoembolization has had the most extensive record. It involves use of a foam, gelatin particles, thrombin-soaked foam, plastic particles, or metallic coils injected into the hepatic artery to selectively occlude blood flow to the tumor (Fig. 76.4) [58]. Others have also attempted to increase antitumor efficacy by soaking the various particles in a

chemotherapeutic drug [59], though such chemoembolizations have not been demonstrated objectively to have improved efficacy over plain particle embolization. Embolization is associated with low morbidity and mortality and with 2- to 3-year survival rates of up to 30% [60]. This compares favorably with resection results; enthusiasm to supplant potentially curative resection in otherwise healthy patients of advanced age should be tempered. Prospective randomized trials to compare these modalities with surgical resection are ongoing.

Ablative therapies have recently increased in popularity among surgeons as treatment for HCC. The most used forms at present for HCC are alcohol injection and radiofrequency ablation (RFA) [61]. Alcohol injection involves chemical killing of tumor by percutaneous or operative injection. This method is very safe but suffers from the fact that multiple treatments are necessary for effective ablation.

Percutaneous ethanol injection ablates tumor by using CT- or ultrasound-guided direct injection of ethanol into the tumor. This technique is limited by the size and number of tumors that can be treated. Few investigators treat tumors >4 cm and more than four in number. For small tumors, however, such ablation can be highly effective [62]. The morbidity associated with such treatment includes pain, fever, and infection of the dead tumor. Mortality rates are low. Approximately 40% of these lesions are not detectable on CT scan at 6–12 months. Although this treatment is effective, there is a significant recurrence rate associated with the technique. Recent efforts have combined this technique with transarterial embolization, a combination that appears to be complementary in action. These ablative techniques should be considered for patients who are medically unfit or anatomically unsuitable for partial hepatectomy. Irradiation and systemic chemotherapy are of limited value for treating HCCs [63].

RFA kills tumors by generation of heat to ablate the malignancy. Reports with thousands of patients have shown this to be a safe and effective therapy. This technique has great potential for managing high-risk elderly patients with concomitant medical problems or cirrhosis (or both) who might not tolerate a resection. Several preliminary reports suggest that RFA may be as effective as liver resection for small tumors, though it has not been formally compared to other therapies. When a patient clearly has an unresectable tumor, we prefer nonsurgical ablative approaches that do not require anesthesia, abdominal incisions, and the associated risks. When patients are explored for resection, we usually have the RFA instrument prepared in case more tumor than is resectable is encountered, since in such cases, the risks of general anesthesia and laparotomy have already been incurred [64].

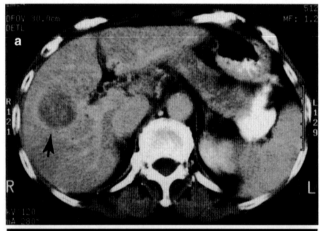

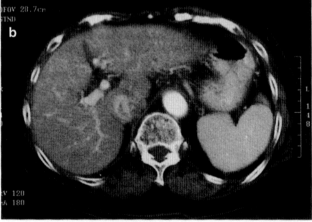

Figure 76.4 Embolization as ablative treatment for hepatocellular carcinoma. A large solitary right lobe HCC in a 91-year-old woman is seen on CT before (**a**) and 3 months after (**b**) embolization.

Metastatic Colorectal Cancer

There are an estimated 150,000 new cases of colorectal cancer diagnosed annually [10]. Of these patients, 25% are over the age of 70, and 6% are over 80 years old. It is believed that 40–45% experience recurrence within 5 years. About 75–80% of these patients have the liver as one of the involved sites of recurrence and 15–20% have the liver as the first or only site of recurrence [65]. Advances in liver surgery and an increasing proportion of elderly patients have encouraged hepatic resection in this ever-growing segment of the population. Early studies on hepatic resection in the elderly reported significant mortality rates, with cirrhosis and concomitant medical problems being the most commonly identified associated factors [17]. Later studies in predominantly noncirrhotic patients, however, reported mortality rates in the elderly population similar to those reported in younger patients [5]. There is little doubt now whether liver resection is a potentially curative option for treating metastatic colorectal cancer of the liver and such resections can be performed safely in the elderly and with good long-term results.

Natural History

Several studies have analyzed in a retrospective fashion patients who were not treated for metastatic colon cancer to the liver [66]. In most of these series, even when patients had liver metastases that were solitary and clearly resectable by radiologic criteria, fewer than 40% of untreated patients were alive at 3 years, and nearly all of the patients were dead at 5 years. Chemotherapy, whether based on 5-fluorouracil [67, 68] or irinotecan (CPT-11) [69, 70], improves survival but is not curative. The demonstration that resection can provide 10-year disease-free survivors for this disease [71] has led to acceptance of surgical resection as the treatment of choice for liver metastases.

Preoperative Evaluation

Preoperative evaluation of the elderly patient with colorectal metastases to the liver should address several concerns. As with any major operation, a comprehensive initial examination is paramount. Particular attention should be directed to the cardiopulmonary status of the patient, as nearly 50% of all postoperative deaths that occur in the elderly are related to cardiovascular or pulmonary disease. There have been several predictive risk indices and functional assessments reported that can identify with fairly accurate certainty the elderly patients at increased risk for cardiopulmonary complications [72]. As stated above, the elderly patient undergoing liver resection is at particularly high risk for pulmonary complications because of decreased pulmonary reserve with aging, a high abdominal incision and increased discomfort with the respiratory effort, and postoperative pleural effusion. In series that have examined liver resection for metastatic colorectal cancer, the risk of pneumonia is 2–8% [73, 74].

Generally, patients undergoing evaluation for resection of hepatic colorectal metastases do not have associated cirrhosis. In the noncirrhotic patient, there is enormous liver reserve, and resections of up to 80% of liver parenchyma can be performed with confidence of full recovery. In patients with associated liver parenchymal disease such as from alcohol abuse or viral hepatitis, thorough evaluation with a physical examination, liver function tests, coagulation studies, and nutritional assessment for degree of baseline hepatic insufficiency may identify patients intolerant of a liver resection. No test of greater sophistication than these have proved to be clinically useful for distinguishing patients at high risk for liver failure. Tests such as bromosulfophthalein retention, indocyanine green retention, and hepatic wedge pressure [76] have advocates but are not accepted universally.

Selection of patients is also based on clinical details of the colorectal cancer. Risk factors for recurrence after liver resection include regional lymph node involvement by the primary tumor [65, 76, 77], symptomatic liver tumors [65, 66], synchronous presentation of liver metastases with the primary tumor [12, 76, 78], large numbers of tumors [12, 76], the presence of satellite nodules [12, 78], high preoperative CEA level [78], and the extent of liver involvement of more than 50% [77, 79]. Whereas none of these criteria alone is a complete contraindication for resection, increasing numbers of these criteria, particularly in a patient with medical problems, should lead one to be circumspect when recommending resection. The two criteria considered by most liver surgeons to be absolute contraindications to resection are the presence of extrahepatic disease and the presence of the technical inability to clear all of liver tumor. The preoperative evaluation must therefore include adequately imaging areas with the highest likelihood of disease spread and adequate imaging for the distribution of tumors within the liver. The radiologic techniques available are the same used for evaluating primary liver cancer. Before surgery, the extent of disease workup should include chest radiography, abdominal and pelvic CT scans, and colonoscopy. CT portography is also highly recommended as the most sensitive test for imaging metastatic tumors within the liver. MRI or sonography is used occasionally if proximity to the vena cava or hepatic veins is a major concern. Routine use of angiography has declined with the increasing use of MRI technology.

Surgical Treatment

The technical concerns are as for resection of HCCs, except liver failure is less of a concern in this predominantly non-cirrhotic population, and up to 80% of the liver can be resected with confidence for recovery. Following entry of the abdomen with bilateral subcostal incisions with xiphoid extension, a complete abdominal exploration is performed. If extrahepatic disease is identified, resection is not justified by the data. Intraoperative ultrasonography is performed to identify lesions missed on preoperative scans and to confirm the relations of known lesions to vascular structures. Resection is then performed using standard inflow and outflow vascular control and low central venous pressure as previously described [80]. In a series of 128 consecutive resections in patients aged over 70 with metastatic colorectal cancer, the operative mortality was 4% [5]. This was no different from a cohort of patients less than 70 years of age operated on during the same time period. Of particular note, long-term survival was also no different between the two groups (Fig. 76.5). In fact, among six series of patients analyzing long-term outcome after liver resection for metastatic colorectal cancer [13, 71, 73, 77, 78, 81], only one demonstrated a more adverse outcome for elderly patients [13]. Thus, resection of metastatic colorectal cancer in the elderly is safe and can result in long-term survival.

For metastatic colorectal cancer, large resections can be undertaken with safety and potential eradication of the tumor.

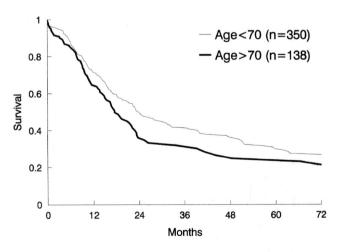

Figure 76.5 Survival of patients of age 70 or more undergoing liver resection for metastatic colorectal cancer compared to those less than 70 years of age (from Fong et al. [5] with permission from Lippincott Wilkins & Williams).

Thus, unlike the situation with HCCs, where enthusiasm for resection is tempered by the risks of such resections, ablative techniques do not have established roles in metastatic colorectal cancer. Cryoablation has been performed with safety but has not been shown to have an advantage. We reserve cryoablation for the rare patient with widely scattered disease isolated to the liver that is not resectable or for the patient with an unresectable recurrence. In otherwise fit patients regardless of age, we routinely resect up to ten tumors even if they are bilateral. Medically fit patients who can have complete extirpation of disease are offered potentially curative resections.

Minimally invasive liver therapies have advanced greatly in the last decade with the improvements in the field of laparoscopic surgery. Initially, laparoscopic liver resections were described for small, benign peripheral lesions, but as the field has evolved, experienced teams are performing anatomic resections for cancer [82]. Buell's group at the University of Louisville conducted a retrospective review at their liver center with data supporting that laparoscopic hepatic resection is a viable alternative to open resection with superior results compared to radiofrequency ablation for the treatment of cancer [83]. However, as exposure is limited compared with an open surgical approach, certain groups advocate careful selection of patients based on various factors, such as tumor location [84, 85]. Our record is that we find approximately 5–10% of patients to be candidates for laparoscopic resection.

Conclusions

The aging process generally does not lead to clinically evident compromised liver function under normal conditions, and age alone is not a contraindication for most surgical procedures. For liver resections, clinicians have long feared that the physiologic decrease in liver function with age and a decrease in regenerative capacity would compromise recovery. In clinical practice, these fears have not been substantiated except in the cirrhotic patient. Liver resection remains the only potentially curative therapy for liver tumors of any type. In our advancing technological age, minimally invasive liver therapies are becoming safer and more widespread as an alternative at some centers. In the noncirrhotic patient, associated medical conditions, measured physiologic function, and clinical case history should be the criteria for patient selection for surgery, not simply chronologic age. A much more cautious approach is recommended in the cirrhotic patient, and ablative therapies are often chosen for physically resectable liver tumors.

CASE STUDY

The patient is an 80-year-old male with a past medical history significant for atrial fibrillation on anticoagulation and digoxin, scarlet fever, coronary artery disease, diabetes mellitus, hypertension, arthritis, and DVT who was referred by his primary-care physician for evaluation and management of a right-sided liver mass. The patient had undergone a routine physical exam entailing basic laboratory tests and X-rays, which were suggestive of a liver mass. A CT scan at that time revealed a large 10-cm mass in the right aspect of his liver. A biopsy was performed prior to referral that was read as a well-differentiated hepatocellular carcinoma versus adenoma. His past surgical history included tonsillectomy, appendectomy, hydrocele repair, knee replacement, and laparoscopic cholecystectomy. At the initial consultation, a right hepatic lobectomy was offered to the patient as the lesion occupied the right posterior sector all the way up to the right hepatic vein and the right anterior sectoral vessels were on the tumor. The options of resection, embolization, radiofrequency ablation, chemotherapy, and biologic therapies were all discussed. The risks of liver surgery including liver failure, bleeding, and death were discussed as well. The patient was then referred to cardiology for clearance because of atrial fibrillation and coronary artery disease. At the time, the patient was clinically alive with disease, Karnofsky's score 100.

He was evaluated by cardiology 2 days after initial consultation. A recent ECHO and a prior Persantine stress test were reviewed. He was deemed an intermediate-to-high-risk patient given his advanced age, well-controlled arrhythmia, and insulin-dependent diabetes for the upcoming liver resection, approximated to take 2 h. No further cardiac testing was thought to decrease his risk. No anticoagulation bridging was recommended. The proposed plan was to monitor postoperative telemetry, to start low-molecular-weight heparin with warfarin as soon as possible postoperatively, and to continue digoxin for rate control up until the morning of surgery. Perioperative beta blockade was recommended. He was

received again in the clinic 5 days after cardiac evaluation and clearance for consenting and preadmission testing and anesthesia evaluation. He was deemed ASA III.

The patient was taken to the operating room for a right hepatic lobectomy 1 week after initial consultation with no complications and an estimated blood loss of 300 cc. In the immediate postoperative period, he was also assessed by respiratory therapy for ventilator management as well as hospital chaplaincy services. He was extubated without difficulty in the PACU. Postoperatively, the patient did well. He was followed by the cardiology service. He was advanced to clears on POD#1. FFP was administered for an elevated INR of 1.47. Pain was controlled with a fentanyl PCA pump. He was noted by hospital staff to be confused at times but easily oriented. He was maintained on fall precautions. On POD#2, the patient was evaluated by physical therapy services. That evening, he was confused and pulled out his triple lumen catheter and arterial line. He was placed on 1:1 precautions for his own safety. He was cleared from telemetry by cardiology. Additional FFP was administered for an elevated INR of 1.7. POD#3 was uneventful. PT recommended that he be discharged to a subacute rehabilitation facility or with home PT and concurrent 24-h care. He was advanced to a regular diet on POD#4 with return of bowel function. PCA was discontinued, and he was converted to oral pain medications. Reassessment by PT recommended home PT with home-care services. The Foley catheter was discontinued on POD#6. The patient was evaluated by the hospital dietitian for a low-nutrition risk assessment, and recommendations were made for a discharge diet. On POD#8, he was discharged with VNS for RN and PT services. His daughter was present and was also given discharge medications and instructions.

The patient returned for a postoperative visit in the clinic 4 days following discharge. He was tired but otherwise oriented and doing better. He was sent for routine blood work. He was clinically with no evidence of disease, with a Karnofsky's score of 70.

Final pathology was consistent with hepatocellular carcinoma confined to the liver.

References

1. Killen DA (1988) Cardiac surgery in the elderly. In: Adkins RB Jr, Scott HW Jr (eds) Surgical care for the elderly. Williams and Wilkins, Baltimore, pp 203–220
2. Koruda MJ, Sheldon GF (1992) Surgery in the aged. Curr Surg 293–331
3. Greenfield LJ (1975) Surgery of the aged. W.B. Saunders, Philadelphia
4. Brooks B (1937) Surgery in patients of advanced age. Ann Surg 105:481–501
5. Fong Y, Blumgart LH, Fortner JG, Brennan MF (1995) Pancreatic or liver resection for malignancy is safe and effective for the elderly. Ann Surg 222(4):426–434
6. Menon KV, Al-Mukhtar A, Aldouri A, Prasad RK, Lodge PA, Toogood GJ (2006) Outcomes after major hepatectomy in elderly patients. J Am Coll Surg 203(5):677–683
7. Kemeny MM (2004) Surgery in older patients. Semin Oncol 31(2): 175–184

8. Turrentine FE, Wang H, Simpson VB, Jones RS (2006) Surgical risk factors, morbidity, and mortality in elderly patients. J Am Coll Surg 203(6):865–877

9. Finlayson E, Fan Z, Birkmeyer JD (2007) Outcomes in octogenarians undergoing high-risk cancer operation: a national study. J Am Coll Surg 205(6):729–734

10. Parker SL, Tong T, Bolden S, Wingo PA (1996) Cancer statistics, 1996. CA Cancer J Clin 46(1):5–27

11. Fortner JG, Silva JS, Cox EB, Golbey RB, Gallowitz H, Maclean BJ (1984) Multivariate-analysis of a personal series of 247 patients with liver metastases from colorectal-cancer. 2. Treatment by intrahepatic chemotherapy. Ann Surg 199(3):317–324

12. Rosen CB, Nagorney DM, Taswell HF, Helgeson SL, Ilstrup DM, Van Heerden JA et al (1992) Perioperative blood transfusion and determinants of survival after liver resection for metastatic colorectal carcinoma. Ann Surg 216:492–505

13. Gayowski TJ, Iwatsuki S, Madariaga JR, Selby R, Todo S, Irish W et al (1994) Experience in hepatic resection for metastatic colorectal cancer: analysis of clinical and pathologic risk factors. Surgery 116:703–711

14. de Liguori CN, van Leeuwen BL, Ghaneh P, Wu A, Audisio RA, Poston GJ (2008) Liver resection for colorectal liver metastases in older patients. Crit Rev Oncol Hematol 67(3):273–278

15. Ezaki T, Yukaya H, Ogawa Y (1987) Evaluation of hepatic resection for hepatocellular carcinoma in the elderly. Br J Surg 74:471–473

16. Yanaga K, Kanematsu T, Takenaka K, Matsumata T, Yoshida Y, Sugimachi K (1988) Hepatic resection for hepatocellular carcinoma in elderly patients. Am J Surg 155:238–241

17. Fortner JG, Lincer RM (1990) Hepatic resection in the elderly. Ann Surg 211:141–145

18. Fong Y, Blumgart LH, Cohen A, Fortner J, Brennan MF (1994) Repeat hepatic resections for metastatic colorectal cancer. Ann Surg 220(5):657–662

19. Virani S, Michaelson JS, Hutter MM, Lancaster RT, Warshaw AL, Henderson WG et al (2007) Morbidity and mortality after liver resection: results of the patient safety in surgery study. J Am Coll Surg 204(6):1284–1292

20. Nagasue N, Chang YC, Takemoto Y, Taniura H, Kohno H, Nakamura T (1993) Liver resection in the aged (seventy years or older) with hepatocellular carcinoma. Surgery 113:148–154

21. Takenaka K, Shimada M, Higashi H, Adachi E, Nishizaki T, Yanaga K et al (1994) Liver resection for hepatocellular carcinoma in the elderly. Arch Surg 131:71–76

22. Schwartz SI (1981) Biliary tract surgery and cirrhosis: a critical combination. Surgery 90:577–583

23. Mentha G, Huber O, Robert J, Klopfenstein C, Egeli R, Rohner A (1992) Elective hepatic resection in the elderly. Br J Surg 79:557–559

24. Karl RC, Smith SK, Fabri PJ (1995) Validity of major cancer operations in elderly patients. Ann Surg Oncol 2:107–113

25. Fong Y, Brennan MF, Cohen AM, Heffernan N, Freiman A, Blumgart LH (1997) Liver resection in the elderly. Br J Surg 84(10):1386–1390

26. Aldrighetti L, Arru M, Catena M, Finazzi R, Ferla G (2006) Liver resections in over-75-year-old patients: surgical hazard or current practice? J Surg Oncol 93(3):186–193

27. Mann CD, Neal CP, Pattenden CJ, Metcalfe MS, Garcea G, Dennison AR et al (2008) Major resection of hepatic colorectal liver metastases in elderly patients – an aggressive approach is justified. Eur J Surg Oncol 34(4):428–432

28. Wynne HA, Cope LH, Mutch E, Rawlins MD, Woodhouse KW, James OFW (1989) The effect of age upon liver volume and apparent blood flow in healthy man. Hepatology 9:297–301

29. Asano K, Nakamura M, Asano A, Sato T, Tauchi H (1992) Quantitation of changes in mitochondrial DNA during aging and regeneration of rat liver using non-radioactive DNA probes. Mech Ageing Dev 62:85–98

30. Mooney H, Roberts R, Cooksley WGE, Halliday JW, Powell LW (1985) Alterations in the liver with ageing. Clin Gastroenterol 14:757–771

31. Yamamoto K, Takenaka K, Matsumata T, Shimada M, Itsaka H, Shirabe K et al (1997) Right hepatic lobectomy in elderly patients with hepatocellular carcinoma. Hepatogastroenterology 44:514–518

32. Carrillo MC, Carnovale CE, Favre C, Monti JA, Scapini C (1996) Hepatic protein synthesis and serum aminoacid levels during liver regeneration in young and old malnourished rats. Mech Ageing Dev 91:55–64

33. Schapiro H, Hotta SS, Outten WE, Klein AW (1982) The effect of aging on rat liver regeneration. Experientia 38:1075–1076

34. Beyer HS, Sherman R, Zieve L (1991) Aging is associated with reduced liver regeneration and diminished thymidine kinase mRNA content and enzyme activity in the rat. J Lab Clin Med 117:101–108

35. Fry M, Silber J, Loeb LA, Martin GM (1984) Delayed and reduced cell replication and diminishing levels of DNA polymerase-alpha in regenerating liver of aging mice. J Cell Physiol 118:225–232

36. Taguchi T, Ohashi M (1996) Age-associated changes in the template-reading fidelity of DNA polymerase alpha from regenerating rat liver. Mech Ageing Dev 92:143–157

37. Piantanelli L, Ermini M, Ricciotti R (1974) Histone phosphorylation after partial hepatectomy in young and old rats. Experientia 30(2):210–211

38. Oh YH, Conard RA (1972) Effect of aging on histone acetylation of the normal and regenerating rat liver. Life Sci 11(2):1207–1214

39. Ferrucci JT (1991) Liver tumor imaging. Cancer 67:1189–1195

40. Larson RE, Semelka RC (1995) Magnetic resonance imaging of the liver. Top Magn Reson Imaging 7(2):71–81

41. Nichols FC, Van Heerden JA, Weiland LA (1989) Benign liver tumors. Surg Clin North Am 69:290–313

42. Leese T, Farges O, Bismuth H (1988) Liver cell adenomas: a 12 year surgical experience from a specialist hepatobiliary unit. Ann Surg 208:558–564

43. Schwartz SI, Husser WC (1987) Cavernous hemangioma of the liver. Ann Surg 205:456

44. Kuo PC, Lewis WD, Jenkins RL (1994) Treatment of giant hemangiomas of the liver by enucleation. J Am Coll Surg 178:49

45. Trastek VF, Van Heerden JA, Sheedy PFI, Adson MA (1983) Cavernous hemangiomas of the liver: resect or observe? Am J Surg 145:49

46. Yamagata M, Kanematsu T, Matsumata T, Utsunomiya T, Ikeda Y, Sugimachi K (1991) Management of hemangioma of the liver: comparison between surgery and observation. Br J Surg 78:1223

47. Gaspar L, Mascarenhas F, de Costa MS, Dias JS, Afonso JG, Silvestre ME (1993) Radiation therapy in the unresectable cavernous hemangioma of the liver. Radiother Oncol 29:45–50

48. Biswal BM, Sandhu M, Lal P, Bal CS (1995) Role of radiotherapy in cavernous hemangioma of liver. Indian J Gastroenterol 14:95–98

49. Yamamoto T, Kawarda Y, Yano T, Noguichi T, Mizumoto R (1991) Spontaneous rupture of hemangioma of the liver: treatment with transcatheter hepatic arterial embolization. Am J Gastroenterol 86:1645–1649

50. RJSr McKenna, Murphy GP (1994) Cancer surgery. J.B. Lipincott, Philadelphia

51. Farmer DG, Rosove MH, Shaked A, Busuttil RW (1994) Treatment of hepatocellular carcinoma. Ann Surg 219:236–247

52. Takayasu K, Moriyama N, Muramatsu Y, Makuuchi M, Hasegawa H, Okazaki N et al (1990) The diagnosis of small carcinomas: efficacy

of various imaging procedures in 100 patients. Am J Radiol 155:49–54

53. Blumgart LH (1988) Liver resection-liver and biliary tumours. In: Blumgart LH (ed) Surgery of the liver and biliary tract, 1st edn. Churchill Livingstone, New York, pp 1251–1280

54. Parker GA, Lawrence W Jr, Horsley JS III, Neifeld JP, Cook D, Walsh J et al (1989) Intraoperative ultrasound of the liver affects operative decision making. Ann Surg 209:569–577

55. Iwatsuki S, Starzl TE (1988) Personal experience with 411 hepatic resections. Ann Surg 4:421–434

56. Fong Y, Blumgart LH (1996) Surgical therapy of liver cancer. In: Zakim D, Boyer TD (eds) Hepatology, 3rd edn. W.B.Saunders, Philadelphia, pp 1548–1564

57. Iwatsuki S, Gordon RD, BWJr S, Starzl TE (1985) Role of liver transplantation in cancer therapy. Ann Surg 202:401–407

58. Bismuth H, Morino M, Sherlock D, Castaing D, Miglietta C, Cauquil P et al (1992) Primary treatment of hepatocellular carcinoma by arterial chemoembolization. Am J Surg 163:387–394

59. Raoul JL, Heresbach D, Bretagne JF, Bentue Ferrer D, Duvauferrier R, Bourguet P et al (1992) Chemoembolization of hepatocellular carcinomas. Cancer 70:585–589

60. Brown K, Nevins AB, Getradjman G, Brody LA, Kurtz RC, Fong Y et al (1998) Particle embolization of hepatocellular carcinoma. J Vasc Interv Radiol 9(5):822–828

61. Livraghi T, Solbiati L, Meloni MF, Gazelle GS, Halpern EF, Goldberg SN (2003) Treatment of focal liver tumors with percutaneous radio-frequency ablation: complications encountered in a multicenter study. Radiology 226(2):441–451

62. Livraghi T, Bolondi L, Lazzaroni S, Marin G, Morabito A, Rapaccini GL et al (1992) Percutaneous ethanol injection in the treatment of hepatocellular carcinoma in cirrhosis. A study on 207 patients. Cancer 69:925–929

63. Sitzman JV, Abrams R (1993) Improved survival for hepatocellular cancer with combination surgery and multimodal treatment. Ann Surg 217:149–154

64. Liang HH, Chen MS, Peng ZW, Zhang YJ, Zhang YQ, Li JQ et al (2008) Percutaneous radiofrequency ablation versus repeat hepatectomy for recurrent hepatocellular carcinoma: a retrospective study. Ann Surg Oncol 15(12):3484–3493

65. Hughes KS, Simon R, Songhorabodi S, Adson MA, Ilstrup DM, Fortner JG et al (1986) Resection of the liver for colorectal carcinoma metastases: a multi-institutional study of patterns of recurrence. Surgery 100:278–284

66. Wood CB, Gillis CR, Blumgart LH (1976) A retrospective study of the natural history of patients with liver metastases from colorectal cancer. Clin Oncol 2:285–288

67. Doroshow JH, Multhauf P, Leong L, Margolin K, Litchfield T, Akman S et al (1990) Prospective randomized comparison of fluorouracil versus fluorouracil and high-dose continuous infusion leucovorin calcium for the treatment of advanced measurable colorectal cancer in patients previously unexposed to chemotherapy. J Clin Oncol 8:491 501

68. Colucci G, Maiello E, Giuliani F, Serraveza G, Pezzella G, Leo S et al (1994) Biochemical modulation of 5-fluorouracil (FU) and liver metastases of colorectal cancer patients. Ann Oncol 5(8):53

69. Kunimoto T, Nitta K, Tanaka T, Uehara N, Baba H, Takeuchi M et al (1987) Antitumor activity of 7-ethyl-10-[4-(1-piperidino)-1-piperidino] carbonyloxy-camptothecin, a novel water-soluble derivative of camptothecin, against murine tumors. Cancer Res 47:5944–5947

70. Tsuruo T, Matsuzaki T, Matsushita M, Saito H, Yokokura T (1988) Antitumor effect of CPT-11, a new derivative of camptothecin, against pleiotropic drug-resistant tumors in vitro and in vivo. Cancer Chemother Pharmacol 21:71–74

71. Scheele J, Stang R, Altendorf-Hofmann A, Paul M (1995) Resection of colorectal liver metastases. World J Surg 19:59–71

72. van de Velde CJH, Sugarbaker PH (1984) Liver metastases. Martinus Nijhoff, Amsterdam

73. Fong Y, Cohen AM, Fortner JG, Enker WE, Turnbull AD, Coit DG et al (1997) Liver resection for colorectal metastases. J Clin Oncol 15(3):938–946

74. Schlag P, Hohenberger P, Herfarth Ch (1990) Resection of liver metastases in colorectal cancer – competitive analysis of treatment results in synchronous versus metachronous metastases. Eur J Surg Oncol 16.360–365

75. Haberkorn U, Bellemann ME, Altmann A, Gerlach L, Morr I, Oberdorfer F et al (1997) PET 2-fluoro-2-deoxyglucose uptake in rat prostate adenocarcinoma during chemotherapy with gemcitabine. J Nucl Med 38(8):1215–1221

76. Hughes KS, Simons R, Songhorabodi S, Adson MA et al (1988) Resection of the liver for colorectal carcinoma metastases: a multi-institutional study of indications for resection. Surgery 103:278–288

77. Doci R, Gennari L, Bignami P, Montalto F, Morabita A, Bozzetti F (1991) One hundred patients with hepatic metastases from colorectal cancer treated by resection: analysis of prognostic determinants. Br J Surg 78:797–801

78. Scheele J, Stangl R, Altendorf-Hofmann A, Gall FP (1991) Indicators of prognosis after hepatic resection for colorectal secondaries. Surgery 110:13–29

79. Ekberg H, Tranberg KG, Andersson R, Lundstedt C, Hagerstrand I, Ranstam J et al (1987) Pattern of recurrence in liver resection for colorectal secondaries. World J Surg 11(4):541–547

80. Cunningham JD, Fong Y, Shriver C, Melendez J, Marx WL, Blumgart LH (1994) One hundred consecutive hepatic resections. Blood loss, transfusion, and operative technique. Arch Surg 129(10):1050–1056

81. Jamison RL, Donohue JH, Nagorney DM, Rosen CB, Harmsen WS, Ilstrup DM (1997) Hepatic resection for metastatic colorectal cancer results in cure for some patients. Arch Surg 132:505–511

82. Nguyen KT, Gamblin TC, Geller DA (2008) Laparoscopic liver resection for cancer. Future Oncol 4(5):661–670

83. Buell JF, Thomas MT, Rudich S, Marvin M, Nagubandi R, Ravindra KV et al (2008) Experience with more than 500 minimally invasive hepatic procedures. Ann Surg 248(3):475–486

84. Laurence JM, Lam VW, Langcake ME, Hollands MJ, Crawford MD, Pleass HC (2007) Laparoscopic hepatectomy, a systematic review. ANZ J Surg 77(11):948–953

85. Santambrogio R, Aldrighetti L, Barabino M, Pulitano C, Costa M, Montorsi M et al (2009) Laparoscopic liver resections for hepatocellular carcinoma. Is it a feasible option for patients with liver cirrhosis? Langenbecks Arch Surg 394(2):255–264

86. Zacharias T, Jaeck D, Oussoultzoglou E, Bachellier P, Weber JC (2004) First and repeat resection of colorectal liver metastases in elderly patients. Ann Surg 240(5):858–865

87. Nagano Y, Nojiri K, Matsuo K, Tanaka K, Togo S, Ike H et al (2005) The impact of advanced age on hepatic resection of colorectal liver metastases. J Am Coll Surg 201(4):511–516

88. Brand MI, Saclarides TJ, Dobson HD, Millikan KW (2000) Liver resection for colorectal cancer: liver metastases in the aged. Am Surg 66(4):412–415

89. Figueras J, Ramos E, Lopez-Ben S, Torras J, Albiol M, Llado L et al (2007) Surgical treatment of liver metastases from colorectal carcinoma in elderly patients. When is it worthwhile? Clin Transl Oncol 9(6):392–400

90. Riffat F, Chu F, Morris DL (2006) Liver resection in octogenarians. HPB (Oxford) 8(3):206–210

Section X
Urogenital System

Chapter 77
Invited Commentary

George W. Drach

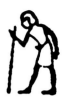

Genitourinary Surgeons Are Mostly Geriatricians

All surgeons in the United States (and indeed other countries) will encounter more elderly patients during future years of practice. Thus, texts like this one serve a very important need by providing references that are valuable in management of such patients. And, for those disciplines that deal with the genitourinary system, the need is greater. Why? Because the average urologist now encounters about 50% of all office patients in the over-65 age (Medicare) category. And, because of the population growth in the older age decades described previously in this text, the urologist will see even more and more elderly patients in his or her office. For example, prostate cancer is now the eighth most common diagnosis amongst Medicare patients, and most of these patients receive their ongoing care from urologists [1]. Added to these activities is the malady of female urinary incontinence which continues to be a major life problem for older women, diagnosed and treated by urologists and gynecologists alike. Independent health surveys of these older women estimate that 9.2–27.6% has some degree of incontinence [2], and most do not mention this to their physicians. Some men also develop incontinence, often related to treatment for that increasing disease condition, prostate cancer. Improvement or cure of incontinence results in significant increases in quality-of-life scores for elderly patients.

Another serious problem for the elderly patient is bladder cancer. As America fought its way through World War II, it gave millions of cigarettes to our soldiers. And, at the same time, millions of women working at factories took "cigarette breaks," under the dubious assumption that a smoke improved alertness and productivity. This WWII cigarette culture passed the habit along to its "Baby Boomer" children, who now reach us in their sixtieth to eightieth decades with fully developed smoking-related invasive bladder cancer. It is of interest that cancer survival data does not even show any significant death rate owing to bladder cancer until after 80 years of age. But, if we take this over-80 group only, cure often requires radical cystectomy and fashioning of some type of urinary diversion, perhaps the most serious and challenging operation performed by urologists [3]. Urologic oncologists must, therefore, have a much more precise understanding of the challenges of treating these elderly surgical patients if they are to have successful outcomes.

Carcinoma of the kidney represents another problem encountered more often in the elderly patient, as does ovarian carcinoma [4]. In both instances, surgical intervention is noted to be less likely than if these diseases occur in a younger patient. It is unclear if this decrease in rate of surgery is related to degree of invasiveness of the disease at time of discovery or simply due to unwillingness to operate on the older patient, a prejudice known as agism. Perhaps part of the reluctance to remove a kidney from or operate on geriatric patients rests in the well-known loss of renal function with aging. At age 85, the average patient has lost 40% of overall renal function so that removal of one kidney could cause them to approach the margin of renal failure. One result of this risk of renal failure is the recent trend toward treatment of smaller renal carcinoma lesions by partial resection only [5].

So where does the genitourinary system fit into the overall provision of care system for our older surgical patients? According to 2005 Medicare statistics, the most active surgical specialty is ophthalmology, having provided over 60 million "allowable" Medicare services during that year. Orthopedics followed with 38 million and urology with 32 million. Gynecology had a much lower number at about 17 million [6]. But, as noted, gynecology and urology share the large geriatric population with incontinence, so their combined provision of services could approach a total of 49 million, second only to ophthalmology. Like it or not, we are evaluating and managing many geriatric patients.

G.W. Drach (✉)
Department of Surgery/Urology, Hospital of the University of Pennsylvania, 3400 Spruce Street, Philadelphia, PA 19104, USA
e-mail: George.Drach@uphs.upenn.edu

The point is this: those of us involved in the care of the elderly genitourinary patient will be exposed to the multiple problems that they bring with them, and we must learn the basic geriatric principles necessary to lead to excellent outcomes when we treat them, either medically or surgically, within the milieu of these problems.

References

1. Hing E, Cherry DK, Woodwell DA (2006) National Ambulatory Medical Care Survey: 2004 summary. Advance data from vital and health statistics; no 374. National Center for Health Statistics, Hyattsville, MD

2. Littford KL, Townsend MK, Curhan GC, Resnick NM, Grodstein F (2008) The epidemiology of urinary incontinence in older women: incidence, progression, and remission. J Am Geriatr Soc 56: 1191–1198

3. Hollenbeck BK, Miller DC, Taub D et al (2004) Aggressive treatment for bladder cancer is associated with improved overall survival among patients 80 years old or older. Urology 64:292–297

4. Chan JK, Urban R, Cheung MK et al (2006) Ovarian cancer in younger vs older women: a population-based analysis. Br J Cancer 95:1314–1320

5. Miller DC, Schonlau M, Litwin MS, Lai J, Saigal CS, Urologic Diseases in America Project (2008) Renal and cardiovascular morbidity after partial or radical nephrectomy. Cancer 112: 511–520

6. Medicare Part B Physician/Supplier National Data. http://www.cms. hhs.gov/MedicareFeeforSvcPartsAB/Downloads/Specialty05.pdf. Accessed 17 Dec 2008

Chapter 78
Change in Renal Function, Fluids, and Electrolytes

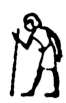

Juan F. Macías-Núñez and Manuel Martínez-Maldonado

Renal Structure and Function

Renal aging is not a pathological process since the aging kidney is able to maintain the homeostasis of the internal medium in conditions of health despite the fact that its resources and ability to adapt to challenges of restriction or overload are limited. It should be understood by the reader that we have based the findings in this chapter mostly on the relatively few studies carried out in healthy aged persons in whom biochemical and clinical findings, including holistic geriatric evaluation, have been done before inclusion in the study protocol. The majority of published studies have been, unfortunately, performed in "apparently healthy" aged individuals in home care institutions, aged persons attending outpatient clinics, or hospitalized individuals whose baseline status was not well evaluated.

In this chapter, we describe the structural and functional changes that occur in the kidney with aging. We also review the senescent kidney's mechanisms for handling fluid, electrolyte, and acid–base derangements, especially during the perioperative period. Clearly, successful management of the elderly patient requires a knowledgeable appreciation of the changes occurring in the senescent kidney that result in: (1) increased tendency for volume depletion and dehydration; (2) decreased ability to tolerate a volume load; (3) increased propensity for potassium disturbances (hypo- and hyperkalemia); (4) diminished production of renin and blunted physiologic response to the effects of aldosterone, and antidiuretic hormone (ADH); (5) increased tendency to lower the levels of phosphate; (6) tendency for the development of hypocalcemia and hypomagnesemia. A brief assessment of the role of extracellular fluid volume (ECFV) depletion and other factors contributing to acute renal failure in the elderly is also presented.

J.F. Macías-Núñez (✉)
Department of Nephrology, Chief Section of Nephrology, University Hospital, Salamanca, Spain
e-mail: jfmacias@usal.es

Histopathology of the Aging Kidney

Autopsy material, biopsy material from kidney donation, and nephrectomy for tumor and trauma from elderly subjects have revealed the presence of glomerular sclerosis [1], a condition that leads to a loss of filtration capacity.

The cause of sclerosis of the aged glomerulus is confusings. It is sometimes difficult to distinguish whether the changes are due from the aging process itself or from common diseases of the elderly, such as hypertension, diabetes, and atherosclerosis. It appears that even in the absence of these diseases such changes occur. Probably the cause of the changes is intraglomerular hypertension resulting from afferent arteriole vasoconstriction in an attempt to raise the glomerular filtration rate (GFR) [2].

Elderly individuals who have hypertension or diabetes may have more deterioration of renal function than elderly people who do not have these underlying medical problems. Glomerular senescence may begin during the fourth decade of life and progresses linearly with age, reducing the GFR by ~1 ml/min for every year over 40 years of age [3]. This predictable reduction of the GFR is one of the main factors responsible for morbidity in the elderly surgical patient.

In addition to glomerular changes, tubular senescence occurs with advancing age [4]. Tubular length decreases, interstitial fibrosis between tubules occurs, and the properties and anatomy of the tubular basement membrane change. Atherosclerosis of nutrient peritubular capillaries contributes in part to these changes. The consequence of tubular senescence is reduced tubular reabsorption and secretion.

Renal Plasma Flow

Healthy Young Individuals

The kidneys only represents 0.5% of the body mass, yet they receive about 20% of the cardiac output, approximately 1,200 ml/min on average at a rate of 4 ml/min/g which is considerably greater than that received by other organs such as the brain, heart, or liver. Renal plasma flow (RPF) is the amount of blood going to the kidneys minus the hematocrit (Hct). Therefore, assuming an Hct of 45%, humans have a RPF of approximately 660 ml/min, which leads to a GFR of 125 ml/min and a filtration fraction (the ratio of GFR to RPF) of 0.19. This means that 19% of the plasma entering the kidney every minute is filtered. RPF in young people (below 30 years old) averages 592 ± 153 ml/min/1.73 m^2 in woman and 654 ± 153 ml/min/1.73 m^2 in man [5]. After the age of 30, RBF progressively decreases [6].

Aged Healthy Individuals

Diodrast clearance (a measure of RBF) decreases from a mean of 613–290 ml/min in the ninth decade of life [7], a fall of over 50% [8]. An exhaustive analysis of the available literature has revealed that the rate of reduction in RPF is approximately 10% per decade of life. Prospective PAH clearance (another measure of RBF) studies confirmed the drop (361 ml/min/1.73 m^2 in the aged vs. 618 in the young) [9]. Filtration fraction increases with age [7], indicating that more filtrate in milliliter per minute is formed (suggesting that, indeed, the increase in glomerular pressure that would result is the cause of sclerosis). Radioactive xenon wash-out curves reveal that the largest drop in renal blood flow occurs in the cortex, while medullary blood flow is relatively well preserved [10].

Glomerular Filtration Rate

Inulin clearance (the gold standard for GFR measurement) increases from approximately 20 ml/min at birth to 120 ml/min by age 30. Thereafter it begins a slow descent reaching a mean of 65 ml/min at 90 years of age [7]; however, the lower limit of inulin clearance (mean $\pm$ 2SD) for a population of apparently healthy 80 years old individuals is 40 ml/min/1.73 m^2. Moreover, the difference between the sexes seen in the young disappears for those 75 years or older [11]. Inulin clearance is inconvenient for routine clinical use because its measurement in blood and urine is cumbersome, requires 3–4 h to perform, and is available in very few institutions. As a result, endogenous creatinine clearance has become the most widespread technique for GFR estimation in clinical practice.

Renal Handling of Creatinine

Creatinine is derived from the metabolism of creatinine in skeletal muscle and from dietary meat intake. It is freely filtered across the glomerulus, reabsorbed, and secreted by the renal tubule. Studies of the tubular secretion of creatinine

in humans are controversial, some indicating that secretion is negligible, yet others suggesting that 15–30% of the creatinine present in the urine derives from tubular secretion. Studies of dehydration have shown that humans can reduce creatinine clearance by approximately 30% and rehydration can raise it back to normal and by as much as 20% above the baseline normal values [11]. This dramatic increase upon rehydration may represent increase in tubular secretion and decrease in tubular reabsorption of creatinine. Thus, low extracellular volume resulting from any maneuver in conjunction with (vide infra) reduced renal capacity to regulate sodium reabsorption and the low-thirst sensation of the elderly will almost certainly imperil renal function.

In studies comparing creatinine and inulin clearances, the ratio of creatinine clearance to inulin clearance reached 1.4 suggesting that 28% of the total creatinine collected in the urine is secreted by the tubules [12]. We have evaluated the difference in GFR between young (<65 years) and old (>65 years) healthy persons of either sex [13] by the clearance of creatinine or Cr^{51}-EDTA and found them to be lower in the aged than in the young. In addition, the ratio of creatinine clearance to Cr^{51}-EDTA is higher in nine out of ten tested healthy young individuals, whereas this is the case in only one subject, and lower than one in five, out of 13 healthy aged individuals, indicating that tubular handling of creatinine differs among healthy young and aged individuals and its clearance is not always a reliable measure of GFR [13, 14].

GFR in Healthy Aged Persons

GFR ranges between 95 ± 20 ml/min in healthy adult female and 120 ± 25 ml/min in young healthy males, but it declines with age (around 40 years of age), regardless of the marker used to assess it. However, the decline in GFR is neither universal nor inevitable since longitudinal studies have revealed some individuals whose GFR remains constant with age, even though the mean GFR of the aging population falls. Importantly, nutritional status of the subjects at the time of measuring GFR influenced the results, particularly when using creatinine clearances. Elderly subjects eating more than 1 g/day of protein per kilogram had a creatinine clearance in the range of 90–100 ml/min/1.73 m^2 while those with a lower protein intake had a lower creatinine clearance [15, 16]. In cross-sectional data [7], inulin clearance in aging subjects fell from a mean of 122 ml/min to a mean of 65 ml/min between ages 30 and 90.

The Cockroft–Gault and Other Formulae

The urinary elimination of creatinine diminishes with age [13]. Therefore, attempts have been made to estimate GFR without the need for urine collection. Cockroft and Gault in deriving their formula to measure GFR used hospital patients that included individuals from 18 to 92 years old regardless of the level of renal function [15]. Others have conducted cross-sectional, except for some data in the study of Rowe et al. [17], rather than longitudinal studies. In an important extended longitudinal study, some patients were followed with repeat measurements for more than 30 years [18]. Despite a mean calculated reduction in creatinine clearance of 0.75 ml/min/year for the whole group, 92 of the 254 subjects showed no reduction in creatinine clearance; a few evidenced increased clearances. Larsson et al. [19] also found no decline in GFR in individuals between the ages of 70 and 79, although plasma creatinine increased from 0.91 to 96 mg/dl in women and from 1.00 to 1.07 mg/dl in men. Despite this evidence of falling GFR as a function of age, there are no dramatic or clear cut increases in plasma creatinine with age. Thus, the normal value of plasma creatinine is statistically the same at the ages of 30 and 90 years.

Because of the uncertainties in the assessment of GFR using creatinine clearance, formulas and nomograms have been developed that theoretically allow a better estimation of GFR in clinical practice. Using plasma creatinine concentration, age, gender, body weight, and height, Cockroft and Gault's [14, 16] formula is the most used, although it may overestimate the decline in GFR, at least in persons older than 80 years. However, a good correlation in 18 individuals aged 66–82 years between GFR calculated by the Cockroft–Gault formula $[(GFR) = ((140 - Age) \times Weight (kg))/72]$ and the clearance of $[^{99}Tc^m]$ diethylenetriamine penta-acetic acid (DTPA) has been found [19]. The simplest formula to estimate the expected mean creatinine clearance in milliliter per minute from 25 to 100 years of age in persons with normal blood creatinine (≤ 1.3 mg/dl) is: $[130 - Age$ (in years)] [20].

Other formulas have been developed to predict GFR based on blood creatinine level including those of the modified diet in renal disease (MDRD) group [21, 22], but have not been formally validated for persons aged over 70 years, diabetic nephropathy or pregnancy, and the very ill and healthy individuals. Formula-calculated GFR may provide a reasonable estimate of renal function compared with clearance of markers such as creatinine and Cr^{51}-EDTA, the variation may be considerable [22] (Table 78.1).

Clinical Implications

Despite the controversy surrounding GFR measurement or calculation, it is clear that "normal" values of serum creatinine do not represent a normal GFR in the vast majority of healthy aged persons. An effort must be made to adjust drugs regime to estimate GFR in the case of all drugs primarily handled by the kidney (vide infra). On the other hand, low GFR in the aged does not automatically means renal disease since it is influenced by many factors.

Two such factors, reversible and common, are depletion of ECFV and poor nutrition (particularly poor protein intake). Aged persons with low GFR (compared with younger adults) in the absence of clear signs of renal insufficiency should be tested for these two reversible findings. Measurement of urine sodium will show low concentrations despite patient-provided history or self-assessment of "normal intake" unless the patient is on diuretic therapy. In that case, other clinical tests, such as postural hypotension and rapid feeble pulse, may be present. Low serum albumin, and a very low (<10 mg/dl) blood urea nitrogen, and a BUN to creatinine ratio of <10 will be clues to the presence of malnutrition. These findings have an important role in the presurgical evaluation of the elderly patient and must be taken into consideration for fluid replacement during and after surgery. Isotonic (0.9%) saline is the fluid of choice for all patients, since it provides the most physiological and metabolically sound approach to the problem of ECFV depletion. Even if the immediate cause of ECFV depletion is corrected in the elderly, it is still wise to adjust drugs regime to the calculated GFR until a new post surgical steady state has been achieved.

Drug Dose Modification in the Elderly

Drugs that are eliminated from the body by renal excretion require dose modifications in the aged. Because the serum creatinine does not accurately reflect reduced renal functioning in the elderly, the doses of toxic drugs, such as the aminoglycosides, require adjustments based on creatinine clearance and calculated by the 24-h urine collection or by the estimate of creatinine clearance using the urine-free

TABLE 78.1 GFR in young and old healthy people measured by CrCl and Cr^{51}-EDTA, and estimated by the MDRD formula

	Age [mean $\pm$ SD (years)]	Blood creatinine [mean $\pm$ SD (mg/dl)]	Urine creatinine [mean $\pm$ SD (mg/dl)]	GFR CrCl [mean $\pm$ SD (mg/dl)]	GFR Cr^{51}-EDTA [mean $\pm$ SD (mg/dl)]	GFR MDRD equation [mean $\pm$ SD (mg/dl)]
Young ($N = 10$)	35.8 ± 11.8	0.81 ± 0.08	122 ± 83	127 ± 25	101.6 ± 13.4	114 ± 15.6
Old ($N = 13$)	74.4 ± 3.7	0.86 ± 0.1	84.4 ± 25.4	91.7 ± 29	81.3 ± 11.3	83 ± 12.8

Source: Modified from [46]

formula described above. The dose interval (DI) can be calculated from the following:

$$DI = \left(\frac{100}{\text{Estimated creatinine clearance}} \right) \times \text{Usual interval.}$$

In a 68-year-old woman with a calculated creatinine clearance of 17 ml/min and requiring a course of gentamicin, a loading dose would be given at the usual 2 mg/kg. Then 1 mg/kg would be given every (100/17)×8 h. Thus, the interval would be every 47 h, a regimen that would lessen the likelihood of an elevated trough level, which has been associated with aminoglycoside toxicity in several studies [23, 24].

Tubular Functions

Proximal Tubule

Over 60–80% of the filtered sodium and water, bicarbonate and other electrolytes, glucose, uric acid, phosphate, amino acids, and small molecular weight proteins are reabsorbed in this segment.

Healthy Aged

No differences have been detected in proximal tubule function when young (<60) are compared with elderly healthy aged individuals (older than 60) in clearance studies performed in healthy persons [25]. Moreover, the handling of lithium, a well-known marker of proximal tubule sodium reabsorption and general function [26] does not differ between young and old. Nevertheless, although the renal reabsorption threshold for most compounds handled by the proximal tubule is not different between young and old, the maximal tubular reabsorption capacity (Tm) is diminished in aged persons, a finding that may be important in the postsurgical period in patients receiving glucose solutions.

Glucose

A lower Tm for glucose will lead to persistent glucosuria and osmotic diuresis resulting in ECFV depletion. Since, as already mentioned, a normal glucose threshold of reabsorption exists in elderly people normal levels by much, at which time the reduced $Tm_{glucose}$ will become apparent and large amounts of glucose may appear in the urine. Tm has been demonstrated to fall in parallel with the reduction in GFR [27]. The apparent $Tm_{glucose}$ averaged 359 mg/min/1.73 m² in the third decade, and only 219 mg/min/1.73 m² in the ninth.

It is therefore critical to follow closely for the presence of glucosuria and the levels of plasma electrolytes to assess the state of homeostasis in the postsurgical elderly patient receiving glucose solutions [28].

Thick Ascending Limb of Henle's Loop

This water and urea impermeable segment sustains the transport of Na^+ from the lumen to the interstitium; thus, resulting in dilute urine emerging into the early portion of the distal nephron. Since it is also responsible for increasing the tonicity of the interstitium, in the presence of ADH, it is also responsible for the reabsorption of water from the urine as it traverses the collecting duct and determines the excretion of concentrated urine (low volume and high osmolality) as fluid ascends in the thick ascending limb, electrolytes pass to the interstitium, but water remains in the lumen. In essence, the ascending limb and the early part of the distal convoluted tubule (DCT) is the site in the nephron where solutes are reabsorbed without water in a process leading to "free water formation," and thus have been named the diluting segment [26].

Healthy Aged

The diluting segment loses some of its capacity to reabsorb Na^+ leading to a higher delivery of Na^+ to the most distal segments of the nephron, which has been shown to be statistically higher in the healthy elderly than in the healthy young [26]. This reduction in Na^+ reabsorb in the thick ascending limb of Henle's loop found in all tested subjects in situations of normal salt diet or salt restriction and at any age [29] does not seem to be the result of obvious structural changes, but results from the normal aging process and, particularly, the fall in GFR [29, 30].

Clinical Implications (see Table 78.2)

Loss of sodium reabsorptive capacity in the thick portion of Henle's loop leads to Na^+ and water spillage make the aged very sensitive to easily becoming dehydrated and desalinated. It is common to find elderly patients in everyday practice who exhibit copious natriuresis and diuresis leading to Na^+ depletion and/or hyponatremia. Particularly vulnerable to these Na^+ abnormalities are aged subjects on low salt diet plus diuretics. Failure of awareness of this effect of aging on renal function and failure of timely replenishment of Na^+ and water deficits may lead to instauration of acute renal failure [31, 32]. It is clinically incorrect to routinely restrict salt intake in the aged unless they suffer from illnesses managed in part by

TABLE 78.2 Key parameters of renal function in healthy adults, old, and very old individuals

	Adult (18–64 years) (mean ± SD) N = 22	Old (>65 years) (mean ± SD) N = 30	Very old (>80 years) (mean ± SD) N = 22
Hemoglobin (g/l)	14.7 ± 1	14.1 ± 0.8	14.3 ± 1
Erythropoietin (U/l)	14 ± 2.7	13 ± 4.8	17 ± 9.4
Creatinine clearance (ml/min)	111 ± 14.4	71 ± 19.8	47 ± 13
Fractional excretion of sodium (%)	0.5 ± 0.1	1.3 ± 0.6	1.4 ± 1
Fractional excretion of urea (%)	30 ± 2	59 ± 3	61 ± 6

Erythropoietin is an indirect measure of functional renal mass. It did not differ statistically in any of the groups
Source: Modified from [46]

salt restriction such as liver, heart, and renal diseases in which edematous syndromes (other than malnutrition) and/or hypertension are manifest. Even under those circumstances, it is advisable to periodically monitor plasma electrolytes, particularly if diuretics are a mainstay of the therapeutic regime. Both hypo- and hypernatremia are dangerous situations in the elderly and should be avoided at all costs.

Despite the reduction in sodium reabsorptive capacity by the loop of Henle with aging, the aged take much longer to eliminate sodium overloads than the young, most likely due to the diminution of GFR. Because of these differences in sodium handling by the elderly kidney, it is important to be cautious in describing hypertension in the aged as "salt dependent" or "salt sensitive." The elderly hypertensive patient may retain a larger portion of an amount of salt, compared with younger individuals, not because their hypertension is salt dependent but because of the low GFR that, despite the reabsorptive defect in more distal segments of the nephron, leads to salt retention.

Collecting Duct

The amount of Na^+ reabsorbed in the collecting duct is approximately 3% of the sodium filtered (plasma sodium concentration multiplied by the GFR). Yet, despite the apparently low sodium capacity of the collecting duct, its normal function is of paramount importance for overall sodium balance to be kept and for ECFV to remain within normal limits [32, 33]. Under the influence of aldosterone, the collecting duct is also responsible for the final control of urinary Na^+ excretion. The synthesis of aldosterone by the adrenal cortex is controlled by angiotensin II, plasma concentration of Na^+

TABLE 78.3 Blood and urine aldosterone levels in healthy young and aged persons under normal diet conditions and after salt restriction

	Young (N = 10)	Elderly (N = 12)	p Value
Normal diet			
Blood	19.6 (9.6) ng/dl	5.56 (4.2) ng/dl	<0.05
Urine	10.95 (8.8) μg/24 h	4.2 (2.8) μg/24 h	<0.05
Salt restriction			
Blood	30.58 (4.8) ng/dl	8.6 (3.9) ng/dl	<0.05
Urine	29.3 (19.6) μg/24 h	9.6 (3.8) μg/24 h	<0.05

Data is mean (SD)
Source: Modified from [70]

and K^+, and ACTH. The level or plasma Na^+ is the least potent stimulus on aldosterone synthesis. In contrast, aldosterone-secreting cells in the adrenal cortex are very sensitive to the concentration of K^+ in the extracellular fluid. The increase in potassium intake increases extracellular potassium, which directly stimulates the production of aldosterone in the adrenal cortex. The increase in plasma aldosterone concentration stimulates sodium reabsorption and K^+ secretion in the cortical collecting duct (CCD). This affects final control of sodium reabsorption and excretion and helps eliminate potassium excesses and prevent hyperkalemia.

The collecting duct is unable to reabsorb greater quantities of Na^+ delivered to it from previous tubular segments, such as the ascending limb of the loop of Henle. Thus, decreases in sodium reabsorption in prior segments will lead to natriuresis and could enhance potassium secretion into the tubular urine and cause hypokalemia and volume depletion.

Aldosterone in the Healthy Aged (see Table 78.3)

It has been proven that aged persons in unrestricted diets of salt and water have lower aldosterone plasma levels (a result of lower renin production by the juxtaglomerular apparatus, therefore less production of angiotensin II) and respond slower (continue to excrete sodium) to salt restriction than healthy young persons [31, 34, 35]. Therefore, the elderly may be susceptible to having a higher plasma potassium level because of inability to secrete the hormone, partial insensitivity to it, and lower the rates of sodium–potassium exchange.

Clinical Implications

The most common and life threatening clinical consequences is the development of hyperkalemia in circumstances where the aged are treated with aldosterone blocking agents such as spironolacatone, or angiotensin-converting enzyme inhibitors

(ACE inhibitors) and angiotensin receptor blocking (A II RB) agents, which diminish aldosterone secretion by blocking either A II production (ACE inhibitors) or its actions (A II RB). Elderly patients with cardiac failure or other comorbidities treated with antialdosterone agents should be periodically investigated for blood potassium and at least every 3 months if they are simultaneously treated with drugs interfering with the renin–angiotensin system such as ACE inhibitors or Angiotensin II receptors blockers [33, 35].

Metabolic Acid–Base Disturbances in the Elderly Surgical Patient

Alkalosis

The reduced GFR in the geriatric patient reduces the body's ability to excrete an alkaline load [34, 36]. Renal tubular damage during the perioperative period resulting, for example, from hypotension or drug injury may further damage the kidney's ability to excrete bicarbonate. The commonest causes of metabolic alkalosis during the perioperative period are prolonged nasogastric suctioning or vomiting. In patients with prolonged vomiting (e.g., secondary to gastric outlet obstruction), the resultant acid–base disturbance is a hypokalemic hypochloremic metabolic alkalosis. The kidney compensates for the chloride loss by reabsorbing excess amounts of that anion and excreting bicarbonate in the urine. Initially, sodium is the cation that accompanies bicarbonate in the urine, but as fluid loss increases, the body excretes potassium and hydrogen in preference to sodium in order to preserve intravascular volume. This results in paradoxically acidic urine in the presence of a metabolic alkalosis and compounds the disturbance.

The elderly patient is less well able to tolerate metabolic alkalosis and may, in this setting, experience the development of rapid, dangerous hypokalemia, as the body preferentially conserves sodium (under the influence of aldosterone) and hydrogen (which is titrated by the excess bicarbonate to carbon dioxide and excreted by the lungs) [36]. The resultant hypokalemic alkalosis is a risk for cardiac dysrhythmias in the elderly surgical patient, especially in those with coronary artery disease, those taking digitalis, or those who may be taking long-term potassium-losing diuretics.

Lactated Ringer's solution is commonly administered as the maintenance intravenous fluid intraoperatively. This lactate is metabolized to bicarbonate. Because of the impaired renal excretion of alkali in the elderly, the serum bicarbonate may accumulate to an unacceptable level. In this case, it is preferable that a balanced salt solution such as normal saline be used. Potassium chloride can be added to this solution as

needed and the plasma level followed by intraoperative monitoring of potassium levels.

Acidosis

The elderly are prone to metabolic acidosis. Western potash diet leads to the daily production of 1 mEq of hydrogen ion per kilogram of body weight. Buffering of this acid load is accomplished by bicarbonate. This produces CO_2, which is then excreted by the lungs [36, 37]. To correct for this loss of bicarbonate, the distal tubule secretes H^+ formed from the conversion of CO_2 to H_2CO_3 (catalyzed by carbonic anhydrase) and, under the influence of aldosterone, the newly regenerated bicarbonate is delivered with sodium back to the circulation. This makes hydrogen ion available to be pumped into the urine, where it lowers the urinary pH. To enhance hydrogen ion excretion, ammonia, filtered phosphate, and filtered sulfate accept hydrogen ions in the urine and the urine becomes maximally acidified. Ammonia is produced in the renal tubular cell from glutamine, and phosphate and sulfate are generated during metabolism of the potash diet. This releases sulfate and phosphate as sulfuric and phosphoric acids, which promptly release their hydrogen ion, leaving the phosphate and sulfate to be filtered and become part of the composition of urine. In the elderly, these tubular processes are less efficient and have less capacity. Moreover, the lower aldosterone levels lead to decreased ability to excrete an acid load and to regenerate bicarbonate. The ability of the kidney to compensate for metabolic acidosis is thus diminished [36].

Metabolic acidosis in the surgical setting is caused by the accumulation of fixed acids (e.g., lactic acid) or from the loss of bicarbonate (e.g., through diarrhea, pancreatic or small bowel fistulas, or renal tubular damage). Any significant period of circulatory failure results in the accumulation of lactic acid, reflecting anaerobic metabolism. In the geriatric patient, the impaired GFR leads to less direct filtration of lactic acids. In addition, the reduced tubular function and lower aldosterone levels lead to less regeneration of bicarbonate. Thus, the elderly patient is more at risk to develop perioperative disturbances of acid–base balance and, compared with the younger patient, has decreased mechanisms of compensation.

Water Balance

Water balance is controlled by the regulation of thirst, neurohypophyseal function (ADH secretion), and the renal capacity for water excretion [38]. Both perception of thirst and spontaneous intake of liquids diminish with age [39]. When healthy active elderly volunteers were water restricted for

24 h, the threshold for thirst was increased and water intake was reduced in comparison to a control group of younger individuals. Despite the reduction in water intake and thirst, a considerable increase in blood osmolality, plasma sodium concentration, and in circulating vasopressin (ADH) occurred during water deprivation [39]. In fact, osmotic release of ADH in response to intravenous hypertonic saline in elderly people is greater than in the young, but the vasopressin response to volume depletion is blunted [40]. The lack of normal thirst sensation in elderly people despite an increase in plasma tonicity remains unexplained. Dryness of the mouth and a decrease of taste with age may contribute to the diminution of thirst [41]. It has also been suggested that a reduction in the sensitivity of the osmoreceptors responsible for thirst regulation may play a part in water-handling alterations in elderly persons. A contrary view has arisen from studies in which an increase in the sensitivity of the osmoreceptors that regulate the release of vasopressin release was observed. Thirst diminution may also result from an inappropriate response to hypovolemia. Age diminishes the sensitivity of baroreceptors and their capacity to influence the release of vasopressin [41, 42]. Finally, plasma concentration of angiotensin II, a powerful generator of thirst, is diminished in elderly people. Therefore, severe hypovolemia and/or hypotension may be required to trigger stimulation of thirst and overcome water deficits [41]. Since there is no difference in the plasma concentration of vasopressin between young and elderly persons before or after water deprivation, this finding cannot be the explanation of poor water conservation in the elderly [37].

The Healthy Aged

Body Water

Total body water is slightly diminished with age and comprises only 54% of total body weight, probably because old people have a greater proportion of their body weight as fat than the young. The diminution seems to be predominantly of intracellular water [43].

Plasma Volume

Cross-sectional and longitudinal studies have revealed that plasma and blood volume do not change solely as a result of age alone in healthy adults [44]. Some investigators [45] have found that elderly women have a significantly greater plasma volume than young women and, as a consequence, variations in plasma potassium. We have found that plasma and blood volume measurements using radiolabeled albumin do not differ between young and elderly healthy volunteers and that males have a greater volume than females, regardless of age [46]. Thus, a diminished plasma volume in an elderly individual is almost always the result of disease [46].

Clinical Implications

When oral fluid intake is prescribed to aged patient for volume replacement, prevention of dehydration, or with other purposes, it should be realized that the aged lose taste recognition and dislike drinking water; they will never drink the amount prescribed. In fact the clinical experience indicates that one of the most difficult tasks for the geriatric nurse is convincing aged patients to drink water.

Immobility (see Table 78.4)

In 40 elderly nursing-home patients (>64 years old), the 20 that were immobilized had a significantly higher total body water (BW) than aged controls who could move [47, 48].

Clinical Implications

Control of BW influences the distribution volume and the pharmacokinetics of water-soluble drugs. It is essential that this state of BW balance, as inferred from plasma sodium concentration and urine sodium excretion, be known in order to properly design therapeutic regimes of drugs whose solubility in water will determine their action and bioavailability.

Mental impairment, particularly deterioration of verbal learning, in the aged can occur as a result of alterations of BW balance. Yet a recent study found that water metabolism in a group of demented elderly patients was not significantly different from controls [48]. Moreover, acute confusion

TABLE 78.4 Water metabolism in mobile and immobile elderly patients

$N=40$	Mobile [Mean (SD)]	Immobile [Mean (SD)]	p Value
Plasma sodium (mEq/l)	143 (1.28)	140 (5.16)	0.014
Plasma osmolality (mOs/l)	281 (5.22)	270 (10.00)	0.025
Antidiuretic hormone (pg/dl)	4.2 (3.56)	3.4 (2.60)	NS
Body water (%)	50 (9.8)	61 (7.7)	0.0003

Data is mean (SD)
Source: Modified from [48]

syndromes may result from water or electrolyte imbalances that are dissipated by correction of their presence, upon which the confused patients recover the previous mental status. Clearly, measurement of plasma electrolytes and urea is mandatory in confused elderly individuals before other diagnoses are entertained.

Urea

Healthy Aging Kidney

The old healthy aged exhibit a higher fractional excretion of urea than young controls, a phenomenon not clearly understood, but that may result from (less reabsorption) diminished function of urea transporters. Moreover, the elderly eat less protein which contributes to the lower blood and kidney urea.

Clinical Implications

It is possible that the impairment in urinary concentration and dilution observed in the healthy aged may be partly the result of the increased urea excretion rather than its accumulation in the renal interstitium. Low interstitial urea would reduce the favorable osmolar gradient for water reabsorption from lumen to blood. Consequently, the steep interstitial osmolar gradient necessary for urinary concentration cannot be maintained.

Urinary Concentration and Dilution

Healthy Young

The generation and maintenance of the hyperosmolar interstitium is equally necessary for both the concentration and the dilution of urine. The former will occur in the presence of hypertonic interstititum, ADH, and maximal increase in permeability of the collecting duct, while the latter will occur with a hypertonic interstititum in the absence of ADH and ADH-mediated collecting duct water permeability. In both processes, normal function of the thick ascending limb of the loop of Henle is mandatory in order to establish the interstitial to lumen gradient. Transport of electrolytes from the lumen to the interstitium makes it hypertonic. The special loop configuration of the vasa recta, that confer counter current flow of tubule fluid is able to sustain the hyperosmolar profile of the interstitium.

Healthy Aging Kidney

Concentration

Aged persons have a reduced renal capacity to maximally concentrate the urine [49] and lose 5% of this capacity with every 10 years of age [50]. From a maximum urinary specific gravity of 1.030 at 40 years of age, they fall to 1.023 at 89 years of age. Rowe et al. [40] found a mean maximum osmolality of 1,109 mOsm/kg in individuals aged 20–39 years, with a minimum urine flow rate of 0.49 ± 0.03 ml/min; 1,051 mOsm/kg in 40- to 59-year-olds; and only 882 mOsm/kg in those aged 60–79 years. In this group, the minimum urinary flow rate of 1.03 ml/min was more than double that of the young. Other groups have recorded that even healthy individuals aged 60–80 years showed a greater excretion of water, sodium, and potassium during the night than younger individuals [51]. The origin of the decreased concentration ability is multifactorial. It has been related to the decrement in GFR that occurs with age in most studies, although some data do not reveal a close relation between the reduction in the GFR and the capacity to concentrate urine in elderly persons [16]. The relative increase in medullary blood flow is unlikely to contribute to the impairment of renal concentration capacity [10, 51, 52]. As already discussed, inappropriately low ADH does not seem to be a factor in the genesis of the defect since the elderly secrete as much hormone as the young. The defect in sodium chloride reabsorption in the ascending limb of the loop of Henle, which is the basic mechanism for the operation of the countercurrent concentration mechanism, may be the most important factor for the decrease in the capacity to concentrate urine seen in aged individuals.

Clinical Implications

Impaired urine concentration may play some role in the frequency of nocturia in the elderly, although this alteration in circadian rhythm does not depend upon inability to concentrate the urine alone, but also reflects the defects in sodium handling and the decreased aldosterone secretion and sensitivity already discussed.

Dilution

Few data in a few numbers of papers are available to explain the change in the capacity of the aging kidney to dilute urine. Nevertheless, it has been found to be decreased [50, 52]. The minimum urine concentration of only 92 mOsm/kg in elderly individuals is almost half of that (52 mOsm/kg) achieved in

TABLE 78.5 Renal handling of potassium

	Young Mean (SD)	Elderly Mean (SD)	p Value
Plasma potassium	3.6 (0.24)	3.6 (0.16)	NS
Urinary potassium output/24 h	43.2 (9.1)	30.5 (9.7)	<0.05
Fractional excretion of potassium (%)	8.6 (3.1)	9.3 (3.4)	NS

Data is mean (SD)
Source: Modified from [70]

the young. Maximum free water clearance (CH_2O) was also reduced in elderly individuals from 16.2 to 5.9 ml/min. This is, probably, mostly dependent on the reduced GFR, but when CH_2O was factored by GFR to normalize it as a percent of filtration rate, it was still somewhat reduced in the older participants (9.1 vs. 10.2%). Again, the functional impairment of the diluting segment (diminished sodium reabsorption) of the thick ascending limb described above seems to account for the remainder of the diminution in the capacity to dilute urine observed in aged persons.

Potassium (see Table 78.5)

Measurements of total exchangeable body potassium by various isotopic dilution methods all agree that total body potassium is 15% lower in elderly than young people [53, 54]. The reasons for these differences are not altogether clear, but one major factor is that muscle mass, a major site for potassium storage, is diminished in the aged. Despite the spontaneous ingestion of lower amounts of potassium by the elderly (<60 mmol/24 h) because of a low diet in meat, fruit, and vegetables, plasma potassium concentrations in aged persons do not differ from those of the younger population [55]. The basal urinary excretion of potassium is also lower than in the young [53–55]. These results have been postulated to result from physiological changes, such as low aldosterone and tendency to retain K associated with age that predisposes the elderly to hyperkalemia (see Table 78.7 below). However, when diuretics are taken, the elderly develop hypokalemia much more rapidly and frequently than the young.

Renal Handling of Divalent Cations, Phosphate, and Uric Acid (see Table 78.6)

Magnesium

The normal range of serum Mg^{2+} is 1.7–2.3 mg/dl, and no difference between the healthy young and the elderly have been discovered. Magnesium is the main intracellular divalent

TABLE 78.6 Fractional excretion of calcium, phosphorus, magnesium, and uric acid in basal conditions and after hyposaline volume overload in healthy young and old–old volunteers

		Young [mean and (range) (mg/dl)]	Old [mean and (range) (mg/dl)]	p Value
Calcium	Basal	0.8 (0.1–1.3)	0.8 (0.2–1.4)	NS
	Expansion	1.6 (1.3–2.3)	2.3 (1.7–4.1)	0.013
Phosphate	Basal	7.5 (1–10.5)	9.5 (0.3–19)	NS
	Expansion	9.6 (2.3–35)	9.8 (2.4–100)	NS
Magnesium	Basal	4.1 (2.6–5)	2.8 (2–4.6)	NS
	Expansion	3.2 (2.5–6.2)	5.1 (2.2–15)	0.02
Uric acid	Basal	7 (3.5–10.4)	6.2 (3.9–22)	NS
	Expansion	12 (9–14)	10 (1.9–31)	NS

Source: Modifed from [69]

cation and 99% is found in the intracellular space [56]. Under basal conditions, the small intestine absorbs 30–50% of the dietary magnesium, a figure that can rise to 80% in cases of severe magnesium deficit [57].

Renal Handling

Approximately 20% of serum magnesium is bound to albumin, and in spite of the fact that 80% of this cation is filtered at the glomerulus only 3% of it is finally excreted in the urine [58]. Renal excretion is determined largely by filtration and tubular reabsorption rates. Tubular Mg^{2+} secretion does not appear to play a significant role in its balance. Between 10 and 15% of the filtered Mg^{2+} is reabsorbed in the proximal convoluted tubules [59], and between 60 and 70% is passively reabsorbed in the thick ascending limb of the loop of Henle via paracellular channels facilitated by a lumen-positive transepithelial gradient generated by the luminal Na–K–2Cl cotransporter and potassium recycling into the lumen [60]. In addition, this nephronal segment contains calcium sensitive receptors on the basolateral pole sensitive to increased plasma calcium or magnesium concentration. Mg^{2+} is still significantly reabsorbed in the DCT, a mechanism responsible for the final control of its excretion. Urinary Mg^{2+} excretion is increased by high natriuresis, osmotic load, and metabolic acidosis; it is reduced by parathyroid hormone, metabolic alkalosis, and perhaps, calcitonin action. Vitamin D seems to have no influence on its renal handling [57].

Healthy Aged

Fractional excretion of magnesium (FE Mg^{2+}) does not differ from the one in a healthy young population. However, in the setting of volume expansion, old people are prone to develop a significant increase in FE Mg^{2+} leading to a reduction in their serum magnesium level, whose normal values are around 2.1 (1.9–2.3 mg/dl) [60]. Since most of the filtered Mg^{2+} is normally reabsorbed in the thick ascending loop of Henle and this segment shows some degree of incompetence for the reabsorption of Na^+, the handling of Mg^{2+} in the elderly may be less effective than in the young.

Calcium

Healthy Young

Calcium is critical for many metabolic functions. Although 99% of body calcium is found as part of the structure of bone and teeth, the remaining 1% found in plasma and body cells is crucial for many functions such as blood clotting, nerve impulse conduction, and muscle contraction. The homeostasis of calcium is a complex process that integrates the function of the gastrointestinal tract, the bones, and the kidneys, all required for normal calcium balance. The normal total serum calcium concentration oscillates between 9 and 10.5 mg/dl; approximately 50% of serum calcium is bound to albumin. A small amount of it is complexed to anions, and the remainder of serum calcium is in the form of free ionized calcium [61].

Renal Handling

The kidney is critically important for the maintenance of overall Ca^{2+} homeostasis in mammals by partly controlling the excretion of Ca^{2+} and by conversion of vitamin D to its active metabolite, 1,25-dihydroxyvitamin D3 $[1,25(OH)_2D_3]$. To maintain a net Ca^{2+} balance, 98% of the Ca^{2+} filtered at the glomerulus must be reabsorbed along the nephron [62]. The main percentage of Ca^{2+} reabsorption takes place along the proximal tubule and the thick ascending limb of Henle's loop through paracellular pathways. The remaining 15% of Ca^{2+} reabsorption occurs in the DCT, connecting tubules (CNT), and the initial portion of the CCD. The relative contribution of these individual segments to active Ca^{2+} reabsorption appears to differ among species [61].

Healthy Aged

In healthy old people, plasma calcium levels and fractional excretion of calcium (FE Ca^{2+}) do not differ from those of a healthy young population. However, when the healthy aged undergoes volume expansion, they develop a significant increase in their FE Ca^{2+}. This increased FE Ca^{2+} induces a significant reduction in blood calcium levels. Healthy elderly people under the conditions of an adequate diet and sun exposure have normal levels of blood calcium, blood phosphate, vitamin D, PTH, and urinary calcium and phosphate excretion

[63]. However, since this population frequently has a deficient dietary content of Vitamin D, reduced sun light exposure, and low serum levels of sexual hormones, they have a tendency to develop hypercalciuria. The latter phenomenon together with a poor calcium intestinal absorption may account for the senile secondary hyperparathyroidism (reduced serum Ca^{2+} and high levels of PTH) communicated by some authors [64].

Phosphate

Healthy Young

Serum concentration ranges between 2.5 and 5.0 mg/dl. Approximately 1% of total body phosphorus is in the extracellular space. Homeostasis of phosphorus is maintained by the transport of phosphate (Pi) across renal and intestinal epithelia [65]. The majority of body phosphorus is absorbed from the digestive tract, mostly in the duodenum and jejunum. Normally, the amount of phosphate in the diet exceeds 1,000 mg/day and its net absorption is more than 60% of the intake.

Renal Handling

Approximately 80% of renal phosphate reabsorption takes place in the proximal tubule by means of sodium-dependent phosphate transporter [65, 66]. Two transporters [Na-Pi-IIa (SLC34A1) and Pi-IIc (SCL34A3)] are specifically expressed in the brush border membrane of the proximal tubular cells. Both are stimulated by serum phosphate depletion, although severe phosphate depletion can reduce the electrolyte reabsorption capability of the proximal and distal tubules [65]. About 5–10% of filtrated phosphorus is reabsorbed by the distal tubules.

Healthy Aged

There is no significant difference in neither the serum phosphorus level or in its fractional excretion between the young and the healthy aged in basal conditions or following volume expansion.

Uric Acid

Healthy Young

The normal plasma uric acid level is 2.2–7.5 mg/dl in adult males, being slightly lower (2.1–6.6 mg/dl) in premenopausal females [67]. Normally, two-thirds of uric acid is eliminated

TABLE 78.7 The clinical manifestations of the principal functional derangements observed in the aged relate to the anatomical site of dysfunction with advance age

Renal site	Tubular dysfunction	Clinical manifestation
Cortex		
Proximal tubule	$\downarrow$ Reabsorption of glucose Na$^+$, HCO$_3^-$, PO$_4^{-3}$, and urate	Renal glucosuria: osmotic diuresis leading to volume depletion; tendency for acidosis and hyperkalemia; hypophosphatemia (muscle weakness and potential for muscle injury or rhabdomyolysis)
		Hypouricemia
Distal tubule acidosis	$\downarrow$ Secretion of: H$^+$, K$^+$	Distal tubular
	$\downarrow$ Reabsorption of: Na$^+$	Hyperkalemia
		Hypokalemia
		Salt wasting (volume depletion and hyponatremia)
		Hypomagnesemia
Medulla	$\downarrow$ Concentrating ability	Distal tubular
	$\downarrow$ Reabsorption of: Na$^+$	Nocturia (increased water loss: dehydration; salt wasting and volume depletion); hyponatremia or hypernatremia

Source: Data from [32, 36, 69–71]

by the kidney and one-third by the gut [68]. Only 4% of this substance is bound to plasma proteins, thus most of it is freely filterable [67]. Approximately 10% of the filtered urate is finally excreted in the urine [69, 70]. This process is usually greater in males than females: fractional excretion of uric acid (FE UAc) is around 12 and 8%, respectively

Healthy Aged

In healthy old people, serum uric acid levels and FE UAc do not differ from those of a healthy young population. Moreover, when healthy old people undergo volume expansion, they show no significant difference in their renal uric excretion before and after the procedure (Table 78.6).

Acute Renal Failure and Its Prevention in the Elderly

Acute renal failure is a disastrous complication of surgery in the elderly patient. In one series, major surgery was the second most common cause of acute renal failure in the elderly [71]. Mortality rate was 57.3% in this group of 122 patients. The causes of death were pneumonia, myocardial infarction and cardiac arrest, pulmonary embolus, and septicemia in decreasing order of frequency. Infection (bronchopneumonia and septicemia, combined) was the leading cause of mortality in the elderly patient with acute renal failure.

There are several types of acute renal failure in the elderly, but the most common (as in other age groups) is acute tubular necrosis [32]. The tubular necrosis results from ECFV depletion leading to circulatory disturbances and ischemia; it

can also be caused by nephrotoxicity (aminoglycoside antibiotics, chemotherapy drugs, or intravenous contrast agents). The diagnosis is made by microscopic analysis of the urinary sediment in which desquamated tubular cells or their degenerative products are observed. The cells degenerate into pigmented granular casts, often called "dirty brown" casts. In addition, there is evidence of tubular dysfunction in the form of impaired sodium conservation. As already mentioned ECFV depletion and circulatory instability in the elderly must be avoided. Early detection and rapid therapy with physiologic saline is of the essence.

In summary numerous electrolyte and acid–base disturbances can occur in the aged that facilitate the development of volume depletion and conditions that can lead to acute renal failure. Table 78.7 summarizes the disturbances already described above and provides the anatomical site and defect that generates them.

Acknowledgments The authors are grateful to Drs. Joaquin Alvarez Gregori, Paula Scibona, and Carlos Musso for their help in the preparation of the manuscript.

References

1. Bruijn JA, Cottran RS (1992) The aging kidney: pathological alterations. In: Martinez-Maldonado M (ed) Hypertension and renal disease in the elderly. Blackwell, Cambridge, MA, pp 1–9
2. Brenner BM, Meyer GW, Hostetter TH (1982) Dietary protein intake and the progressive nature of kidney disease: the role of hemodynamically mediated glomerular injury in the pathogenesis of progressive glomerular sclerosis in aging, renal ablation, and intrinsic renal disease. N Engl J Med 307:652–659
3. Adler S, Lindeman RD, Yiengst MJ et al (1968) Effect of acute acid loading on urinary acid excretion by the aging human kidney. J Lab Clin Med 72:278–279

4. Darmady EM, Offer J, Woodhouse MA (1973) The parameters of the aging kidney. J Pathol 109:195–209

5. MacCrory WW (1972) Developmental nephrology. Harvard University Press, Cambridge, MA

6. Lindeman RD (1992) Renal hemodynamics and glomerular filtration and their relationship to aging. In: Martinez-Maldonado M (ed) Hypertension and renal disease in the elderly. Blackwell, Cambridge, MA, pp 10–25

7. Davies DF, Shock NW (1950) Age changes in glomerular filtration rate, effective renal plasma flow, and tubular excretory capacity in adult males. J Clin Invest 29:490–507

8. Wesson LG (1969) Renal hemodynamics in physiological states. In: Wesson LG (ed) Physiology of the human kidney. Grune & Stratton, New York, p 96

9. Fuiano G et al (2001) Renal hemodynamic response to maximal vasodilating stimulus in healthy older subjects. Kidney Int 59:1052–1058

10. Hollenberg NK, Adams DF, Solomon HS et al (1974) Senescence and the renal vasculature in normal man. Circ Res 34:305–309

11. Sjostrom PA, Odlind BG, Wolgast M (1988) Extensive tubular secretion and reabsorption of creatinine in humans. Scand J Urol Nephrol 22(2):129–131

12. Berglund F (1961) Urinary excretion patterns for substances with simultaneous secretion and reabsorption by active transport. Acta Physiol Scand 52:276–290

13. Musso CG, Michelangelo H, Vilas M, Reynaldi J et al (2009) Creatinine reabsorption by the aged kidney. Int Urol Nephrol 41(3):727–731

14. Macías-Núñez JF, Garcia-Iglesias C, Tabernero Romo J et al (1981) Estudio del filtrado glomerular en viejos sanos. Rev Esp Geriatr Gerontol 16(2):113–124

15. Cockroft DW, Gault MN (1976) Prediction of creatinine clearance from serum creatinine. Nephron 16:31–41

16. Kimmel PL, Lew SQ, Bosch JP (1996) Nutrition, ageing and GFR: is age-associated decline inevitable? Nephrol Dial Transplant 11:85–88

17. Rowe JW, Shock N, De Fronzo RA (1976) The influence of age on the renal response to water deprivation in man. Nephron 17:270–278

18. Lindeman RD (1990) Overview: renal physiology and pathophysiology of ageing. Am J Kidney Dis 16:275–282

19. Larsson A, Jagenburg J, Landahl S (2005) Renal function in an elderly population. Scand J Clin Lab Invest 65(4):301–305

20. Nicholl SR et al (1991) Assessment of creatinine clearance in healthy subjects over 65 years of age. Nephron 59:621–625

21. Keller F (1987) Kidney function and age (letter). Nephrol Dial Transplant 2:382

22. Levey AS, Bosch JP, Lewis JB et al (1999) A more accurate method to estimate glomerular filtration rate from serum creatinine: a new prediction equation. Ann Intern Med 130:461–470

23. Rule AD, Larson TS, Bergstralh EJ et al (2004) Using serum creatinine to estimate glomerular filtration rate: accuracy in good health and in chronic kidney disease. Ann Intern Med 141(12):929–937

24. Duchin KL (1985) Pharmocodynamics and pharmacokinetics of drugs in the elderly. In: Zawada ET Jr, Sica DA (eds) Geriatric nephrology and urology. PSG, Littleton, MA, pp 215–229

25. Durakovic Z (1986) Creatinine clearance in the elderly: a comparison of direct measurement and calculation from serum creatinine. Nephron 44:66–69

26. Macías-Núñez JF, García Iglesias C, Bondía Román A et al (1978) Renal handling of sodium in old people: a functional study. Age Ageing 7:178–181

27. Miller JH, McDonald RK, Shock NW (1952) Age changes in the maximal rate of renal tubular reabsorption of glucose. J Gerontol 7:196–200

28. Butterfield WJH, Keen H, Whichelow M (1967) Renal glucose threshold variations with age. Br Med J 4:505–507

29. Musso C, López-Novoa JM, Macías Núñez JF (2005) Handling of water and sodium by the senescent kidney. Interpretation of a clearance technique for functional study. Rev Esp Geriatr Gerontol 40(2):114–119

30. Musso CG, Macías-Nuñez JF, Musso CA et al (2000) Fractional excretion of sodium in old-old people on low sodium diet. FASEB J 14:A659

31. Refoyo A, Macías-Ñúñez JF (1991) The maintenance of sodium in healthy aged. Geriatr Nephrol Urol 1:65–68

32. Macías-Núñez JF, López-Novoa JM, Martínez-Maldonado M (1996) Acute renal failure in the aged. Semin Nephrol 16:330–338

33. Macías-Núñez JF, García-Iglesias C, Tabernero-Romo JM et al (1980) Renal management of sodium under indomethacin and aldosterone in the elderly. Age Ageing 9:165–172

34. Sica DA, Centor RM (1985) Tests of glomerular and tubular function in the elderly. In: Zawada ET Jr, Sica DA (eds) Geriatric Nephrology and Urology. PSG, Littleton, MA, pp 33–47

35. Weidmann P, De Myttenaere-Bursztein S, Maxwell MH et al (1975) Effect of aging on plasma renin and aldosterone in normal man. Kidney Int 8:325–333

36. Norris SH, Kurtzman NA (1992) Renal acidification and metabolic acidosis in the elderly. In: Martinez-Maldonado M (ed) Hypertension and renal disease in the elderly. Blackwell, Cambridge, MA, pp 185–199

37. Rodriguez-Puyol D (1998) The aging kidney. Kidney Int 54:2247–2265

38. Phillips PA, Rolls BJ, Ledingham JG et al (1984) Reduced thirst after water deprivation in healthy elderly men. N Engl J Med 311:753–759

39. Shannon RP, Minaker KL, Rowe JW (1984) Aging and water balance in humans. Semin Nephrol 4:346–353

40. Rowe JW, Minaker KL, Sparrow D et al (1982) Age-related failure of volume-pressure-mediated vasopressin release. J Clin Endocrinol Metab 54:661–664

41. Robertson GL (1984) Abnormalities of thirst regulation. Kidney Int 25:460–469

42. Helderman JH, Vestal RE, Rowe JW et al (1978) The response of arginine vasopressin to intravenous ethanol and hypertonic saline in man: the impact of aging. J Gerontol 33:39–47

43. Edelman IS, Leibman J (1959) Anatomy of body water and electrolytes. Am J Med 27:256–260

44. Chien S, Usami S, Simmons RL (1966) Blood volume and age: repeated measurements on normal men. J Appl Physiol 21:583–588

45. Edmonds CJ, Jasani BM, Smith T (1975) Total body potassium and body fat estimation in relationship to height, sex, age, malnutrition and obesity. Clin Sci Mol Med 48:431–440

46. Macías-Núñez JF, López Novoa JM (2008) Physiology of the healthy aging kidney. In: Macías Núñez JF, Cameron JS, Oreopoulos DG (eds) The aging kidney in health and disease. Springer, New York, pp 93–112

47. Musso CG, Maytin S, Fainstein I, et al (1999) Water metabolism in elderly with immobility syndrome. XV International Congress of Nephrology, Buenos Aires, (abstracts); p 169

48. Musso CG, Macías-Núñez JF (2008) Renal handling of electrolytes in the old and old-old healthy aged. In: Macías Núñez JF, Cameron JS, Oreopoulos DG (eds) The aging kidney in health and disease. Springer, New York, pp 141–154

49. Dontas AS, Marketos S, Papanayioutou P (1972) Mechanisms of renal tubular defects in old age. Postgrad Med J 48:295–303

50. Lewis WH, Alving AS (1938) Changes with age in the renal function of adult men. Clearance of urea, amount of urea nitrogen in

the blood, concentrating ability of kidneys. Am J Physiol 123:505–515

51. Takazakura E, Sawabu N, Handa A et al (1972) Intrarenal vascular change with age and disease. Kidney Int 2:224–230

52. Kirkland JL, Lye M, Levy DW et al (1985) Patterns of urine flow and electrolyte secretion in healthy elderly people. Br Med J 285:1665–1667

53. Lye M (1981) Distribution of body potassium in healthy elderly subjects. Gerontology 27.286

54. Burini R, Da Silva CA, Ribeiro MA et al (1973) Concentracão de sodio e de potassio no soro e plasma de individuos normais. Influencia da idade, do sexo e do sistema de colheita do sangue sobre os resultados. Rev Hosp Clin Fac Med S Paulo 28:9–14

55. Biswas K, Mulkerrin EC (1997) Potassium homoeostasis in the elderly. Q J Med 90:487–492

56. Kelepouris E, Agus Z (1998) Hypomagnesemia: renal magnesium handling. Semin Nephrol 18:58–73

57. Graham LA, Caesar JJ, Burgen ASV (1960) Gastrointestinal absorption and excretion of magnesium in man. Metabolism 9:646–659

58. Wen SF, Evanson RL, Dirks JH (1970) Micropuncture study of renal magnesium transport in proximal and distal tubule of dog. Am J Physiol 219:570–576

59. Shareghi GR, Agus ZS (1982) Magnesium transport in the cortical thick ascending limb of Henle's loop of the rabbit. J Clin Invest 69:759–769

60. Rude R (1996) Magnesium disorders. In: Kokko J, Tannen R (eds) Fluids and electrolytes. WB Saunders, Philadelphia, pp 421–445

61. Suki WN, Rouse D (1996) Renal transport of calcium, magnesium and phosphate. In: Brenner BM (ed) The Kidney, vol 1. WB Saunders, Philadelphia, pp 472–515

62. Friedman PA, Gesek FA (1995) Cellular calcium transport in renal epithelia: measurements, mechanism and regulation. Annu Rev Physiol 75:429–471

63. Gallagher JC, Kinyamu K, Fowler S et al (1998) Calciotropic hormones and bone markers in the elderly. J Bone Miner Res 13:475–482

64. Freaney R, McBrinn Y, McKenna MJ (1993) Secondary hyperparathyroidism in elderly people: combined effect of renal insufficiency and Vit D deficiency. Am J Clin Nutr 58:187–191

65. Forster IC, Hernando N, Biber J et al (2006) Proximal tubular handling of phosphate: a molecular perspective. Kidney Int 70:1548–1559

66. Goldfarb S, Westby GR, Goldberg M et al (1977) Renal tubular effects of chronic phosphate depletion. J Clin Invest 59:770–779

67. Hershfield M (1996) Gout and uric acid metabolism. In: Bennett JC, Plum F (eds) Cecil textbook of medicine. WB Saunders, Philadelphia, pp 1508–1515

68. Sorensen LB (1980) Gout secondary to chronic renal disease: studies on urate metabolism. Ann Rheum Dis 39:424–430

69. Musso CG, Alvarez Gregori JA, Macias-Nuñez JF (2008) Renal handling of uric acid, magnesium, phosphorus, calcium and acid base in the elderly. In: Macias Nuñez JF, Stewart Cameron JS, Orepoulos DG (eds) The aging kidney in health and disease. Springer, New York, pp 155–172

70. Macias Nuñez JF, Bondía Roman A, Rodriguez Commes JL (1987) Physiology and disorders of water balance and electrolytes in the elderly. In: Macias Nuñez JF, Cameron S (eds) Renal function and disease in the elderly. Butterworths, London, pp 67–93

71. Kumar R, Hill CM, McGeown MG (1973) Acute renal failure in the elderly. Lancet 1:90–91

Chapter 79
Urinary Incontinence in the Elderly

Pat O'Donnell

Urinary incontinence (UI) is one of the most personally devastating diseases of the elderly. It has humiliating social consequences that touch every facet of the quality of life of the old person. One of the most debilitating consequences of UI in the elderly is a loss of self-esteem, which results in self-imposed social isolation. Elderly incontinent persons become prisoners in their own home due to the behavioral changes that occur from the personal fears and shame of UI. Many elderly people believe they are a victim of a disease without having any control over the personal and social consequences. As a result, they suffer in silence because of the shame and lack of awareness of successful treatment options. Because of the loss of self-esteem, treatment of UI in old people is usually deferred until the disease has become severe and the progressive symptoms have compromised many years of the life of the individual. Personal decisions about the treatment of UI often derive from feelings of desperation and shame rather than a careful consideration of the treatment options that meet the quality-of-life needs of the patient. Many elderly people have a strong reluctance to seek treatment or participate in treatment for incontinence because of personal feelings.

Most treatment programs for UI in the elderly require patient involvement and participation, which is important for long-term success of therapy of UI in old people. The requirement to be personally involved in both surgical and nonsurgical treatment programs gives elderly people a feeling of control over their own lives and control over the devastating personal consequences of UI they experience.

Elderly people experience a feeling of loss of control in all areas of their environment and loss of importance to family and society as they become older. They are no longer essential for "the job to get done" in their occupation or essential to "the existence of the family" as they once were when they were younger. The personal feelings of self-esteem

and value to society they once experienced in their occupation are no longer present and they no longer feel important or needed. Their importance to the family is different because their role has changed drastically, and it does not provide the same feeling of being needed by the family. The many personal and social changes associated with aging have a collective effect of lowering self-esteem. The ultimate loss of self-esteem for the elderly person is the humiliation of loss of bladder control.

Loss of bladder control is the most profound reminder to elderly persons that they are not able to control even the most basic body functions of normal life. Particularly in the elderly population who have lost a personal feeling of value within themselves and in society, UI has an unusual capacity as a disease to render the individual emotionally paralyzed to seek treatment. The greatest obstacle to successful treatment of UI in the elderly is getting the individual to consult a physician and subsequently to become involved in a treatment program. Successful treatment of UI can restore to the patient essential control over a basic normal body function necessary to restore self-esteem, which has an enormous impact in all other areas of their life.

Although UI is not a life-threatening disease, it is one of the most serious "quality of life" threatening diseases of elderly people. The economic, social, medical, and psychological impact on the lives of elderly people who have UI is immense [1]. Among the elderly people who are community dwelling and live independently, approximately 38% of women and 19% of men experience UI. Of the old people who live in chronic care facilities, approximately 55% experience UI. The total direct health care cost of UI in the USA during 1987 was approximately $10.3 billion and is estimated to be more than $15 billion at the present time. The annual cost of managing UI in old people is more than the combined annual cost of all coronary artery bypass surgery and all renal dialysis in the USA. Although the economic cost to old people and to society is enormous, the greatest cost by far is the personal distress of the elderly person through self-imposed social isolation and loss in self-esteem resulting from UI.

P. O'Donnell (✉)
Department of Surgery, University of Arkansas for Medical Sciences, Little Rock, AR, USA
e-mail: pdodonnell@uams.edu

R.A. Rosenthal et al. (eds.), *Principles and Practice of Geriatric Surgery*,
DOI 10.1007/978-1-4419-6999-6_79, © Springer Science+Business Media, LLC 2011

Urinary Incontinence in Elderly Women

Clinical Assessment

Elderly women are twice as likely to be incontinent as elderly men in a similar age group. The assessment of incontinence in an elderly patient is essential to ensure that any therapeutic program is based on an accurate diagnosis of urinary bladder and urethral dysfunction. UI in the elderly is much more complex than UI in younger people; and clinical trial and error treatment programs that are not based on a complete diagnostic evaluation of the patient are unlikely to be successful and can be potentially harmful to the patient. The immense importance of the impact of UI on quality of life of the older person must be a factor in every decision including the complexity of the clinical management of UI. Therefore, the incontinence assessment is important and involves many aspects of the pathophysiology of incontinence and the life style of the individual.

Incontinence History

Many elderly women believe that UI is a normal consequence of aging or of being female. Sometimes the patient has been told by a physician that UI is a normal condition associated with becoming older and that nothing should be done about it. The reluctance by the patient to see a physician about the symptoms of UI may be due to personal embarrassment, lack of knowledge of treatment options, fear of surgery, a sense of hopelessness about UI, and low expectations of treatment success. Therefore, the clinical history of old women with UI should always include direct questions about the occurrence of incontinence episodes, the symptomatic characteristics of urinary incontinence, and the severity of urinary incontinence. Typically, incontinence severity can be estimated by a clinician by asking patients how many times they change pads each day. It is important for the clinician to know if the major component of incontinence is urge urinary incontinence (UUI) or stress urinary incontinence (SUI). Typically, SUI is associated with involuntary loss of urine with coughing, straining, and movement [2]. UUI usually is associated with an intense desire to void with an inability to prevent urine loss voluntarily because the patient cannot physically get to the bathroom in time to prevent an incontinence episode [3].

A urinary diary is an essential part of the initial clinical evaluation of urinary incontinence in old women [4]. The diary helps document the severity of incontinence, determine if associated irritative symptoms are present, establish if there is a pattern to the incontinence, identify precipitating events, and assist in planning the treatment approach.

The assessment of symptom distress and quality of life are increasingly important when evaluating the severity of health conditions, such as UI and the impact of the disease on the daily life of the individual.

Although UI in the elderly is a personally devastating disease, it is not a fatal disease for most patients. Successful treatment of UI in elderly women does not prolong survival, so the goal of treatment of UI is to make the life of the person better. Therefore, quality of life assessment is important when determining the success of treatment. Finally, it is essential to determine the functional status of the older patient. Both mental status and physical status of the patient are important when planning treatment so it is specific to the needs of a particular old person. In addition, comorbid medical conditions may have a significant impact on the treatment decisions of UI in older patients.

Physical Examination

The physical examination of the incontinent elderly woman requires more attention to nuances than in the younger woman. For example, atrophic changes in the vaginal epithelium may indicate that similar changes are present in the urethral mucosa [5]. The general body habitus of the elderly woman is important, as is her agility when planning therapy. A pelvic examination is always performed when possible, including an assessment of the perineal skin, the pelvic floor, and the vaginal wall. It is important for the clinician to identify evidence of anatomic incontinence due to prolapse of the bladder and urethra in old patients. In addition to anatomic changes in the urethra, atrophy of the vaginal epithelium may be associated with poor urethral function, which can contribute to intrinsic sphincter deficiency (ISD) being an etiology of the incontinence. ISD is characterized by the failure of urethra to function properly regardless of the anatomic position of the urethra [6]. ISD can exist in old women who have stress incontinence with an associated anatomic abnormality as well as those who have no evidence of anatomic changes or prolapse. Clinically, it is essential to identify elderly women who have ISD as an etiology of SUI so as to counsel the patient about specific therapy for it. ISD is intrinsic failure of the urethra to function normally and requires a therapeutic approach different from that for anatomic SUI.

Urodynamic Studies

Urodynamic studies of bladder function in elderly patients are necessary for the diagnosis and treatment of UI. Such studies consist of a sequence of bladder and urethral function measurements that often seem confusing to elderly patients and to the referring physician. Because UI in elderly women is considerably more complex than that in young women, the value of complete urodynamic studies is especially important in the old patient. Complete urodynamic studies can be performed in elderly patients with minimal discomfort, and the studies provide invaluable clinical information essential to the diagnosis and treatment of incontinence in this group of patients.

The urinary flow rate is usually the initial bladder function measurement, and it can be performed in the physician's office without significant inconvenience or discomfort to the patient. To perform a urinary flow study, the patient is positioned on a specially designed commode chair, and she voids into a urinary flow unit. The urinary flow rate is inexpensive, relatively easy to interpret, and provides valuable clinical information about bladder function. The uroflow parameters include the voiding time, peak urinary flow, mean urinary flow, and voided volume of urine. Usually, the residual urine volume is measured after the patient voids for the urinary flow rate. The residual urine volume can be measured with an ultrasound scan of the bladder or with a catheterized residual volume determination. Although the uroflow studies are valuable clinically, they alone do not provide the necessary information to establish the presence of such disorders as bladder outlet obstruction; further urodynamic evaluation is required here, including a pressure-flow study.

Cystometrography is one of the most important studies of bladder function in elderly women. It is performed by continuous filling of the urinary bladder using a catheter through the urethra to measure the total capacity of the bladder, the sensation of filling experienced by the patient, the pressure–volume relation of the bladder, and the contractility of the bladder. In many elderly women, the capacity of the bladder is small, the bladder may contract involuntarily causing urinary incontinence, or the bladder may not stretch properly, resulting in an abnormal increase in resting pressure during filling. These abnormalities of bladder function are just some of those that occur in elderly patients with UI that can be found on routine cystometric bladder studies, and they must be identified and treated according to the diagnosis provided by routine cystometry.

Pressure-flow studies measure the pressure inside the bladder during voluntary voiding and simultaneously measure the resulting urinary flow rate. This study is essential for assessing the voiding dynamics of the patient who has a low peak flow rate on routine uroflow studies. The clinician must determine if the cause is a low detrusor pressure or a bladder outlet obstruction. Elderly women who have bladder outlet obstruction or low detrusor pressure during voiding may also have incomplete emptying of the bladder. Either of these problems that result in an elevated postvoiding residual urine volume can cause bladder hyperactivity and may be associated with urinary incontinence. A high detrusor pressure during voluntary voiding with an associated low urinary flow rate is diagnostic of bladder outlet obstruction.

Bladder outlet obstruction in elderly women can have a functional or anatomic etiology; it is usually associated with previous surgical procedures that resulted in obstruction of the urethra. Urethral obstruction that results from previous surgery may produce a fixed outlet obstruction without correcting the etiology of the SUI. In these patients, SUI due to sphincteric dysfunction can coexist with bladder outlet obstruction, as the urethral obstruction is enough to produce bladder obstruction but not enough to produce continence. This is because urethral resistance is a static resistance instead of the normal dynamic functional resistance of the urethra. Bladder outlet obstruction due to fixed resistance within the urethra cannot be identified unless combined bladder pressure and urinary flow rate studies are done simultaneously. The pressure-flow studies represent the most important assessment available to determine the dynamics of bladder and urethral function of elderly women who have UI.

Another critical part of the evaluation of elderly women with UI is the measurement of urethral function [7]. Measuring the pressure of the urethra throughout the functional length is a study called the urethral pressure profile (UPP). The UPP is an important measurement of urethral function, but it is not necessarily a measure of the continence function of the urethra. Simultaneous measurement of urethral pressure and intravesical pressure during coughing provides a differential pressure between the bladder and urethra. This has been called the stress UPP and has added significantly to the clinical applications of the UPP. With the introduction of the concept of ISD, the abdominal leak point pressure (ALPP) measurement has been used much more commonly as a clinical assessment of the continence function of the urethra.

The ALPP is a measurement of the intra-abdominal pressure required to produce leakage of urine from the bladder through the urethra [8]. This study requires fluoroscopic evaluation of the patient during a straining maneuver. Although this study is highly accurate and predictive of the outcome of surgical procedures for SUI in elderly women, the requirement of simultaneous use of fluoroscopy during the study precludes routine use of the test in many clinical environments. ALPP does remain the most clinically important study when evaluating urethral function in elderly women with the symptoms of SUI and is essential for diagnosing intrinsic ISD. In patients who have a low ALPP, a urethral sling procedure is required to correct the symptoms of SUI if a surgical procedure is being considered. The long-term failure rate of any of the numerous bladder suspension procedures in these patients is high, and a urethral sling procedure is the only operative procedure that has a high long-term success rate in these patients. If the ALPP is more than

60 cm H$_2$O, then ISD is not likely to be a significant factor in the etiology of UI; hence a routine bladder suspension procedure is usually successful in correcting the problem of anatomic incontinence and alleviating the symptoms of SUI in the elderly woman.

Electromyography (EMG) of the striated sphincteric muscles is one of the more difficult clinical diagnostic studies [9]. Among elderly women it is especially important for patients in whom neurologic disease is the etiology of the UI or a contributing factor. Neurologic disease in the elderly as a cause of urinary incontinence may originate in the central nervous system (CNS) in those who have such diseases as a previous stroke. Neurologic disease as a cause of UI also may originate in the spinal cord in old patients who have diseases such as intervertebral disc disease, or a neurologic disease that causes UI may originate peripherally with such diseases as diabetes. EMG is especially important in patients with UI who may not be suspected to have associated neurologic disease but have a history of degenerative disc disease of the spine or multiple previous operative procedures for disc disease of the back.

Pathophysiology of UI in Elderly Women

Urinary incontinence is usually considerably more complex in elderly women than in young women. In general, incontinence in old women can be caused by abnormalities of bladder function, abnormalities of urethral function, or combinations of bladder and urethral dysfunction [10]. Close attention to the clinical characteristics of the symptoms of UI in old women from their incontinence history can be helpful for identifying the etiology of the UI. However, a precise description by the elderly patient of her symptoms usually is not nearly as helpful in the diagnosis as is a description of the characteristics of symptoms in young women. For this reason, urodynamic studies along with endoscopic and fluoroscopic studies have a significance in the diagnosis and treatment of UI in old women. Even with extreme attention to every detail of the assessment by the clinician, there is a greater degree of imprecision when determining the pathophysiology of UI in old women compared with young women.

Urge Urinary Incontinence

A common cause of incontinence in elderly women is an overactive bladder, which is characterized by the symptoms of urgency, frequency, nocturia, and episodes of urge UI. Elderly women who have symptoms of urinary urgency usually have associated nocturia.

A significant clinical difference between elderly women and young women regarding the symptom of urge UI is that older women frequently complain that they have no warning of the event [11]. Young women usually describe intense urgency with an inability to control the episode of urgency voluntarily. In contrast, the elderly woman often describes the incontinence event as occurring with little or no warning at all. Although the sensation of urgency exists in elderly women, the duration of the sensation prior to the onset of incontinence is often only a few seconds. The etiology of this clinical observation is unclear, but it appears to be associated with aging. The effects of aging on the lower urinary tract function somehow result in bladder overactivity in many elderly women.

Hyperreflexic Contractility

Incontinence associated with true detrusor hyperreflexia is, by definition, caused by some type of associated neurologic disease [12]. Most commonly in the elderly, detrusor hyperreflexia occurs after a stroke or some other CNS disease, such as Parkinsonism. Detrusor hyperreflexia may result from spinal cord disease related to herniated disc disease or previous back surgery in old people. Urinary symptoms due to neurologic detrusor hyperreflexia in elderly patients usually occur both day and at night with a smaller than normal urine volume in the bladder. The cystometrogram almost always shows a reflex detrusor contractile response associated with filling of the bladder to a relatively small volume. In elderly patients with spinal cord disease, the EMG often shows simultaneous contraction of the external urethral sphincter and contraction of the urinary bladder, resulting in extremely high bladder pressures with failure to empty. It is due to the high outlet resistance of the contracted external urethral sphincter and is called detrusor-sphincter dyssynergia. In most of these patients, neurologic disease that affects urinary bladder function also affects other areas of the body; and the associated functional deficits are usually clinically apparent.

Bladder Compliance

Urinary incontinence associated with abnormal bladder compliance is a critical diagnosis that must be excluded in every elderly woman who has symptoms of an overactive bladder. In a normal person, the increase in volume in the bladder is not associated with a significant increase in pressure within the bladder. However, in patients with abnormal compliance, the pressure within the bladder increases as the volume in the bladder increases. This is a serious intrinsic problem of the urinary bladder, as it can result in obstruction of the kidneys due to a high resting pressure within the bladder that does not allow the ureters from the kidneys to drain properly. Abnormal bladder compliance can result from an injury to the bladder; it can occur following radiation therapy or chemotherapy to the bladder; or it can be associated with systemic diseases such as diabetes. A common clinical etiology of abnormal bladder compliance resulting from injury is due to bladder decentralization caused by peripheral neural injury that occurs at the time of a radical hysterectomy or an abdominoperineal resection. Abnormal bladder compliance can also be induced by prolonged treatment with a Foley catheter or an indwelling suprapubic catheter. Abnormal bladder compliance is diagnosed by cystometrography. Urodynamic studies are essential to the diagnosis and treatment of the elderly woman with UI.

Stress Urinary Incontinence

In a normal person, the pressure within the urethra increases reflexly with increases in intra-abdominal pressure. During episodes of coughing or sneezing, the pressure within the abdomen sharply increases to a high pressure. However, through neurologically mediated reflex mechanisms, the normal resting pressure within the urethra quickly increases to a level higher than the pressure within the abdomen to prevent the leakage of urine from the bladder through the urethra [7]. When this normal compensatory reflex mechanism of the urethra fails to function properly, urine leaks through the urethra from the bladder during episodes of increased intra-abdominal pressure. This condition is called SUI.

In the elderly woman, there is a gradual decrease in the resting pressure within the urethra with advancing age. Part of the change in pressure is due to a loss in the vascularity of the submucosa of the urethra. This soft submucosa in young women serves as a "gasket" by providing a seal within the urethra when changes in abdominal pressure occur. Estrogen-deficient elderly women usually have a large loss of vascularity in the urethral submucosa, resulting in loss of the gasket effect within the urethra. Loss of the gasket effect of the submucosal seal of the urethra results in failure of the compensatory pressure mechanism within the urethra to be effective in containing the urine within the bladder during episodes of increased intra-abdominal pressure. Clinically, this condition results in SUI.

Another effect of aging in women is loss of the normal support of the bladder and urethra. Many elderly women are often told by their physician that their bladder has "fallen down." With increases in intra-abdominal pressure such as coughing and straining, there is often rotation of the base of the bladder and proximal urethra into the vagina. Such prolapse is associated with the loss of reflex compensatory pressure mechanism of the urethra. This type of SUI is called anatomic SUI. When an anatomic abnormality or prolapse of the base of the bladder and urethra is associated with urinary incontinence, a surgical procedure is usually required to correct the abnormality and so prevent the persistent symptoms of SUI.

Intrinsic Sphincter Deficiency

When the compensatory reflex pressure mechanism within the urethra is inadequate because of abnormal function of the intrinsic properties of the urethra itself, it is called intrinsic sphincter deficiency (ISD). In many cases, the cause of ISD is unclear. It is much more common in elderly women due to the loss of intrinsic function of the urethra associated with the vascular submucosa that provides the gasket seal of the urethra. ISD is diagnosed by the ALPP test [6]. Currently, an ALPP less than 60 cm H_2O is considered to reflect abnormal intrinsic urethral sphincter function. It is more complicated to manage elderly women with ISD clinically than those who do not have ISD.

When ISD coexists with anatomic incontinence or prolapse, a pubovaginal sling procedure is usually the only treatment for successful long-term management of these patients. The short-term postoperative morbidity associated with a pubovaginal sling procedure for the treatment of UI in elderly women is significant in some patients. If an anatomic abnormality does not exist, intraurethral bulking agents such as collagen may be used successfully in some cases.

Mixed Incontinence

Mixed incontinence in elderly women refers to an etiology of UI within the same patient that consists of both an overactive bladder and SUI due to urethral dysfunction [13]. Mixed incontinence is considerably more complex to treat than either SUI or UUI. Usually both components must be treated, and they are usually treated separately. There appears to be some interaction between SUI and UUI. For example, successful treatment of SUI usually results in improvement or resolution of UUI. Often successful treatment of UUI alleviates the symptoms of SUI. Generally, successful treatment of mixed incontinence requires combination therapy that manages both components.

Nonsurgical Treatment of UI in Elderly Women

Pharmacologic Therapy

Although pharmacologic therapy has been effective in many young women with urinary incontinence, the efficacy and side effects have limited its use in elderly women. For patients with UUI symptoms, cholinolytic drugs such as oxybutynin (Ditropan) are among the most common agents used. In general, cholinolytic drugs have not been as effective in the elderly patient with symptoms of an overactive bladder as in the younger woman. Side effects of a dry mouth and dryness of the eyes in the elderly have frequently limited the use of oxybutynin, but the occasional elderly patient who experiences confusion associated with that drug causes major concern about the use of this drug in old people.

The first group of new drugs available for clinical use for the treatment of the overactive bladder in the elderly is tolterodine (Detrol). Tolterodine is more highly selective for the bladder than for the salivary glands and has been better tolerated in the elderly. In addition, it does not appear that the problem of confusion is as prevalent with tolterodine as it has been with oxybutynin. Tolterodine appears to be a more effective drug for the treatment of bladder overactivity in elderly patients with considerably fewer side effects than are seen with oxybutynin.

α-Adrenergic drugs have produced clinical improvement in young women with mild SUI. One of the most common drugs used is phenylpropanolamine, usually in doses of 75–150 mg daily. Again, the problem of side effects of this class of drugs in the elderly precludes its routine use for SUI. Cardiac problems, including hypertension, are among the many contraindications for the use of α-adrenergic medications in elderly women.

Behavioral Therapy

The most common behavioral therapy used for both SUI and UUI in elderly women is some modification of the Kegel exercises. The original technique of pelvic muscle exercises (PMEs) described by Kegel was a form of biofeedback therapy. However, since the original description by Kegel, multiple modifications of PME have occurred that do not involve any type of feedback. In fact, PME taught by verbal instruction alone is inadequate for the elderly woman to learn to perform the desired muscle contractions for the training program. PMEs work primarily by a reflex inhibition of bladder contraction when the muscles are contracted.

Biofeedback Therapy

Of the behavioral therapies, the most effective form of training is biofeedback, which is a precise technique for teaching patients to do the PMEs. It provides feedback regarding the performance of PMEs to the patient [14]. The performance is usually displayed to the patient by both visual and auditory feedback signals. The patient learns quickly to perform precise muscle contraction activities that allow maximum return of bladder control. PME therapy is useful for both UUI and SUI, although the efficacy of biofeedback for SUI appears to be less than that for UUI. For the elderly woman with UUI, biofeedback is considered by many to be the therapy of choice. It has the advantages of being effective with no potential side effects.

Timed Voiding

It has been shown that the inability to prevent an involuntary bladder contraction is only part of the aging process affecting bladder function. Another significant symptom is the inability to voluntarily initiate voiding. It is common for elderly women who have UUI to be unable to initiate voiding voluntarily even though a significant amount of urine is present in the bladder. Shortly after an unsuccessful attempt to empty the bladder, the elderly woman may experience an episode of UUI. Although it is unclear that prompted voiding addresses this specific problem associated with aging, a timed voiding schedule usually improves continence in this group. The treatment program is relatively simple. The patient voluntarily voids at fixed time intervals while awake. The interval is usually 2 h during waking hours. This regimen teaches the patient to inhibit the bladder voluntarily during the 2-h interval and to initiate voiding upon command. A timed voiding schedule can be combined with biofeedback therapy as a part of a comprehensive behavioral therapy program.

Surgical Treatment of UI in Elderly Women

Surgical treatment of UI is usually much more complex in elderly women than in young women, primarily because of a component of mixed incontinence exists in many elderly women who have SUI and the unusual complexity of the mixed incontinence that often occurs with aging. The approach to surgical treatment of the elderly woman also depends on the general health of the patient and existing comorbid conditions.

There is no question that UI is a debilitating disease in elderly women, but it is rarely a cause of death. For this reason, it must be recognized that surgical treatment of UI in elderly women has improvement in quality of life, as the major goal of treatment. Therefore, it is not reasonable to risk survival or existing quality of life with a surgical approach for the treatment of UI in these women without reasonable assurance of successful improvement in quality of life resulting from the operative procedure. In properly selected elderly patients, the long-term success of surgery is excellent, but the marked improvement in quality of life resulting from surgery is often denied the older patient on the basis of age alone [15].

Conventional urethral suspension procedures can be used routinely in the elderly woman with uncomplicated SUI [16]. An uncomplicated patient is one who has not failed previous operative procedures for SUI, does not have ISD, does not have significant coexisting UUI, and does not have serious comorbid conditions. In addition, urodynamic studies should demonstrate normal bladder function on cystometry and pressure-flow studies. Transvaginal procedures such as the Raz procedure or the modified Pereyra procedure are often used in the elderly woman because of the low risk of mortality from the surgery. Other considerations for the surgical treatment of uncomplicated SUI in the elderly woman include modifications of the Burch operative technique. However, no operative procedure should be considered in the elderly woman with SUI until a complete evaluation of bladder and urethral function has been accomplished.

For elderly women with ISD and any degree of prolapse of the bladder and urethra, a pubovaginal sling procedure is the only operative technique likely to be successful. This operative technique is slightly more difficult to perform than a urethral suspension procedure and has a slightly higher incidence of associated postoperative morbidity. A pubovaginal sling procedure should not be considered in the elderly woman with SUI unless a complete evaluation is done to determine the status of urethral and bladder function. Assessment of the urethra and bladder allows appropriate selection of the operative procedure and the ability to predict the outcome of the operation.

In the elderly woman with ISD without evidence of bladder or urethral prolapse, intraurethral bulking agents such as collagen can be used [17], which typically works well in these patients. It is common for patients after intraurethral collagen to develop recurrent SUI over a long time; however, requiring repeat intraurethral injections of the collagen material. This problem is usually not significant because the injections can be done in the office with local anesthesia, and the procedure is completed within a few minutes. Complications associated with intraurethral injections are minimal, and the success rate has been particularly good in the elderly woman with SUI due to ISD without an anatomic defect.

Urinary Incontinence in Elderly Men

Clinical Assessment

The assessment of UI in elderly men consists of a precise, complete characterization of the symptoms experienced by the patient. A voiding diary is an important part of the assessment of community dwelling elderly men with UI. Also the American Urological Association symptom score for benign prostate hyperplasia (BPH) can be useful for identifying patients with bladder outlet obstruction [18]. In the chronic care environment, assessment of the severity of incontinence is more difficult. Usually the number of times each day absorbent pads must be changed is an indicator of the severity of incontinence in both community dwelling and chronic care elderly men. The severity of incontinence includes the frequency of episodes and the volume of involuntary urine loss. Unlike elderly women, SUI caused by sphincteric incompetence is rare in men who have not undergone previous prostate or pelvic surgery. Therefore, incontinence in elderly men is almost always associated with involuntary detrusor contractions, which means that bladder contractions occur without the patient being able to prevent the occurrence of the episodes voluntarily [19]. Elderly men with symptoms of UUI almost always experience involuntary detrusor contractions, which are the cause of the UI. In fact, it is reasonable to assume clinically that the etiology of UUI in elderly men is involuntary detrusor contractions even though the cystometrogram may show a stable bladder during filling.

The initial clinically useful study in elderly men with UI is usual measurement of the urinary flow rate by office ultrasonography or catheterized residual urine measurement. A peak urinary flow rate of less than 15 ml/s is usually associated with bladder outlet obstruction. An elevated residual urine volume of more than 50 ml is also usually associated with bladder outlet obstruction.

A common characteristic of the aging bladder function in men is the inability to initiate voiding voluntarily. Therefore, the elderly man may be unable to void for a urinary flow rate test, and ultrasonography may show that the bladder contains more than 100 ml of urine. The elderly man with UI often experiences an episode of UI shortly after being unable to void voluntarily even when the bladder contains an adequate amount of urine for voluntary voiding. When the elderly man is unable to void, a catheterized urine volume at that time does not represent a postvoiding residual urine volume. An accurately performed postvoid residual urine volume may show variation from one voiding episode to another within the same elderly male patient and may need to be repeated for accuracy when possible. The postvoid residual volume can be obtained only after the patient has voided. Also, the postvoid residual volume is useful only if the patient has voided a significant urine volume, usually considered to be 100 ml or more.

Cystometrography is important in elderly men who have UI to determine if bladder compliance is normal. That is, the resting pressure in the bladder should not show a significant rise during filling to the capacity at which the patient feels the urge to void. Unstable detrusor contractions are considered to be a significant finding on filling cystometry studies, although detrusor instability is not necessarily diagnostic of an underlying bladder disorder in elderly men, as the instability is seen in otherwise normal elderly men as well. The most significant finding with filling cystometry is determining the capacity of the bladder and establishing that bladder compliance is normal.

The simultaneous measurement of bladder pressure and urinary flow rate during voluntary voiding is the most important study when evaluating bladder outlet obstruction in elderly men due to BPH. A pressure-flow study in an elderly man that shows a high detrusor pressure and low urinary flow rate during voluntary voiding is the diagnostic of bladder outlet obstruction. Therefore, pressure-flow is one of the most important studies in the urodynamic evaluation of the elderly man with UI. Elderly men who have UI and bladder outlet obstruction should be considered for surgical correction of the obstruction. It usually involves transurethral resection of the prostate (TURP). In many elderly men with significant bladder outlet obstruction and associated UUI, the latter resolves within a few weeks to months following surgical correction of the obstruction. If UUI persists after the bladder outlet obstruction has been surgically corrected, cholinolytic drugs such as tolterodine (Detrol) may be used to treat clinical bladder overactivity.

It is clinically necessary to determine if bladder outlet obstruction is present before using a cholinolytic drug in elderly men with UUI. Cholinolytic medications decrease detrusor contractility, which is contraindicated in patients with existing outlet obstruction of the bladder. Elderly men with bladder outlet obstruction due to BPH usually have high bladder pressure during voiding to empty the bladder considering the degree of bladder outlet resistance. If the bladder pressure is decreased by the cholinolytic medications used to treat overactive bladder symptoms, acute urinary retention may result because of a decrease in bladder pressure resulting from the medication. Therefore, surgical correction of bladder outlet obstruction is necessary before implementing cholinolytic drug therapy for bladder overactivity in elderly men who have UI and coexisting bladder outlet obstruction due to BPH.

Pathophysiology of UI in Elderly Men

Although most continent elderly men experience nocturia, those with UI have a higher number of nocturia episodes than continent men. Most old men awaken completely during these events of nocturia and may complain about having difficulty returning to sleep. Poor-quality sleep in old men is common and may contribute significantly to decreased mental alertness during the daytime. Like elderly women, many elderly men who experience episodes of UUI describe the episode as one in which involuntary voiding occurs with little or no warning of an impending incontinence episode.

The ordered biologic systems regulating micturition in normal young men appears to be impaired in elderly incontinent men, and the normal physiology of voiding is disordered. It may be associated with aging or possible localized CNS deficits. Studies have been performed that carefully measured the exact time of an incontinence episode and the exact volume of involuntary urine loss in elderly incontinent men. It was found that within patients the volume of involuntary urine loss had a wide variation, with no predictability regarding volume of urine loss for any given incontinence episode. In addition, the interval between episodes was measured, and it was found that a wide range of variation in interval between episodes occurred with no predictability of the interval. Also, the residual urine was measured following an incontinence episode. The volumes of the urine loss during the incontinence episode and the residual urine were measured. The total volume at the time of the incontinence episode also showed wide variation within patients. It was apparent from these studies that the occurrence of an incontinence episode in elderly incontinent men was independent of the accumulated volume of urine in the bladder at the time of the incontinence episode.

The same group of patients who demonstrated such irregular bladder activity also demonstrated voluntary voiding without incontinence on a routine basis. These clinical observations suggest that elderly men with UUI have random detrusor contractions resulting in urinary incontinence, whereas the neural pathways required for normal voluntary voiding remain intact. This finding suggests that UI may represent abnormal bladder contractions originating from a neurologic mechanism different from the normal bladder contraction that occurs under voluntary control.

This type of UUI is the most common type of incontinence seen in elderly men. As described previously, SUI is rare in men who have not had previous prostate or pelvic surgery. Elderly men who have undergone radical prostatectomy for adenocarcinoma of the prostate may have SUI resulting from sphincteric incompetence. Failure of the urethral sphincter mechanism following radical prostatectomy is usually due to ISD. Urinary incontinence in elderly men due to an abnormality of the urethral sphincter mechanism following a TURP is uncommon. Patients who have persistent UI after a TURP usually have detrusor dysfunction as the etiology of the UI, with the urethral sphincteric mechanism intact. Elderly men with UI following abdomino-perineal resections for colon carcinoma rarely experience SUI due to sphincteric incompetence. The etiology of sphincteric incompetence following abdominoperineal resection is unclear. Voiding disorders following such a resection are uncommon and are likely due to a problem with the bladder, possibly due to partial denervation of the bladder during the operative procedure. These patients may also experience UI due to abnormal bladder compliance. Therefore, all patients who experienced UI following previous pelvic surgery should have complete urodynamic assessment of both bladder and urethral function before considering therapy.

Nonsurgical Treatment of UI in Elderly Men

If bladder outlet obstruction has clearly been excluded as an etiology of UUI in elderly men, nonsurgical therapies can be implemented. They include pharmacologic and behavioral therapies.

Pharmacologic Therapy

Medical management of the overactive bladder in elderly men is similar to that in elderly women. Oxybutynin (Ditropan) has been used to treat the overactive bladder in elderly men for years, but the side effects are poorly tolerated in this patient population. The side effect of most serious concern is confusion, which is of particular concern in those who operate automobiles. For this reason, oxybutynin has not been routinely used in elderly men with UUI.

Tolterodine (Detrol) is a newer drug used to treat the overactive bladder in elderly men. It is highly effective and well tolerated in this group. Because of the ease of administration and the low incidence of side effects, tolteradine is considered the drug of choice for initial therapy of the overactive bladder in elderly men. Before initiation therapy with tolterodine, the clinician must be certain that there is no bladder outlet obstruction due to BPH.

Behavioral Therapy

PMEs can be used in men with UUI that are similar to those used by women. PME programs are typically variations of the original Kegel exercises. It is important to remember that the original Kegel exercises were done by women using a perineometer, which provided visual feedback of performance to the patient. Over a period of time, modifications of the Kegel exercises became various forms of PMEs. The major problem with PME programs is the instruction of the patient. It is difficult to instruct an elderly man in the PMEs. For this reason, more precise techniques (e.g., biofeedback) are considered more efficacious.

Biofeedback is not commonly used for behavioral therapy in elderly men because it requires complex equipment and trained personnel. However, it is extremely effective for treating those with symptoms of an overactive bladder [14].

It is important to select the proper signal source, which is usually perianal EMG activity displayed as visual and auditory feedback of performance.

Biofeedback therapy depends on the functional status of the patient to some extent. It is important that the patient has adequate mental function and reasonable physical function. Because biofeedback is a training program, it requires a level of mental function that allows training to take place; and enough physical function is required to allow contraction of the appropriate muscle groups. Although biofeedback therapy has been used in chronic care patients, it is generally more suitable for community dwelling patients because of the higher level of functional status usually associated with the latter.

A timed voiding schedule is excellent therapy for elderly men with UUI. In general, the patient is required to void every 2 h while awake. He then attempts to prevent voiding during the 2-h interval and voluntarily initiates voiding on command at the end of the 2 h. This regimen teaches the patient to inhibit the bladder voluntarily and to initiate voiding voluntarily, which improves bladder control. As with women, a PME program (which may be biofeedback-based) can be combined with a timed voiding schedule to improve the efficacy of behavioral therapy.

Surgical Treatment of UI in Elderly Men

Surgical treatment of UI in men depends on the etiology of the UI. In patients who have detrusor hyperactivity and bladder outlet obstruction, the bladder outlet obstruction is treated surgically if possible with a TURP. The patient is then observed for resolution of the symptoms of the overactive bladder, which usually occurs in 2–3 months. If urge UI continues, a cholinolytic drug such as tolteradine should be considered. Behavioral therapeutic treatments may also be considered.

With postprostatectomy incontinence following radical prostatectomy for prostate cancer, the damage to the sphincteric mechanism is something that usually cannot be surgically repaired. Intraurethral injections of a bulking agent such as collagen may be used as an initial therapy. Collagen has typically been beneficial in patients having relatively mild SUI. The overall long-term results of intraurethral collagen for severe postradical prostatectomy incontinence have been disappointing. In most patients who have severe SUI following radical prostatectomy, an artificial urinary sphincter is the best surgical treatment. Results with an artificial sphincter are good overall, but in the elderly patient manual dexterity is an important part of the functional status of the patient that is required for satisfactory results. The artificial urinary sphincter has a silicone pump located within the scrotum and requires manual pumping of the device through the scrotal skin. This activity requires a reasonable level of both mental function and manual dexterity.

Urinary incontinence following TURP is uncommon even in elderly patients. When it does occur, the etiology is likely detrusor hyperactivity. Rarely, sphincteric incompetence due to ISD is the etiology, and in these cases an artificial urinary sphincter is required to achieve continence.

Conclusions

Urinary incontinence in elderly women and elderly men has a devastating impact on the quality of life of the individual. Because UI is rarely fatal in old people and because quality of life issues are profound, treatment of UI must improve quality of life without compromising survival or the existing quality of life.

Urinary incontinence in elderly women and men may have an etiology related to dysfunction of the bladder or of the urethra. In elderly men and women, the age-related abnormalities associated with changes in bladder activity are similar. In elderly women, SUI due to abnormal sphincter function is a common cause of incontinence in this group. ISD is much more common in elderly women than in young women. A combination of urethral function and bladder dysfunction may occur in elderly women and is referred to as mixed incontinence. Mixed incontinence is especially complex and usually much more difficult to treat successfully.

The overactive bladder in elderly men is similar to the overactive bladder in elderly women. Bladder outlet obstruction due to BPH is common in elderly men and can be a cause of bladder overactivity and UUI. If bladder outlet obstruction coexists with UUI in elderly men, surgical management of the obstruction should be considered if feasible. Following surgical management of bladder outlet obstruction, significant symptoms of overactive bladder usually appear but resolve over 2–3 months. If significant symptoms continue, cholinolytic drugs such as tolterodine may be used to control them. These drugs are contraindicated in the presence of existing bladder outlet obstruction due to BPH.

Elderly men who have ISD following radical prostatectomy for the treatment of prostate cancer can be treated with intraurethral bulking agents such as collagen. Intraurethral collagen is usually more successful with patients who experience mild incontinence. An artificial urinary sphincter is usually required for postprostatectomy incontinence that is more severe.

Often elderly patients do not complain about the problem of incontinence because they are embarrassed about it and have lost their self-esteem. It is only after the problem is corrected that patients recover their self-esteem and are released from their self-imposed social isolation. Such isolation seriously compromises quality of life. For this reason, every reasonable treatment option for managing incontinence in elderly patients should be utilized to achieve maximum improvement in their quality of life.

References

1. O'Donnell PD (1993) Geriatric issues in female incontinence. In: Walters MD, Karram MM (eds) Clinical urogynecology. Mosby-Year Book, St. Louis, p 409
2. Baldwin DD, Hadley R (1997) Stress urinary incontinence. In: O'Donnell PD (ed) Urinary incontinence. Mosby-Year Book, St. Louis, p 190
3. Awad SA, Gajewski JB (1997) Urge incontinence. In: O'Donnell PD (ed) Urinary incontinence. Mosby-Year Book, St. Louis, p 202
4. Wyman JF, Colling J, O'Donnell PD (1997) Incontinence assessment. In: O'Donnell PD (ed) Urinary incontinence. Mosby-Year Book, St. Louis, p 399
5. Ganabathi K, Zimmern P, Leach GE (1994) Evaluation of voiding dysfunctions. In: O'Donnell PD (ed) Geriatric urology. Little Brown, Boston, p 203
6. Kennelly MJ, McGuire EJ (1997) Intrinsic sphincter deficiency. In: O'Donnell PD (ed) Urinary incontinence. Mosby-Year Book, St. Louis, p 207
7. O'Donnell PD (1993) Surgical goals and mechanism of continence in treatment of stress incontinence. In: McGuire EJ, Kursh E (eds) Female urology. Lippincott, Philadelphia, p 175
8. O'Connell HE, McGuire EJ (1997) Leak point pressure. In: O'Donnell PD (ed) Urinary incontinence. Mosby-Year Book, St. Louis, p 93
9. O'Donnell PD (1998) Electromyography. In: Nitti VW (ed) Practical urodynamics. Saunders, Philadelphia
10. McGuire EJ (1994) Pathophysiology of incontinence in elderly women. In: O'Donnell PD (ed) Geriatric urology. Little Brown, Boston, p 221
11. O'Donnell PD (1991) The pathophysiology of urinary incontinence in the elderly. In: McGuire EJ (ed) Advances in urology, vol 4. Year Book, Chicago, pp 129–142
12. Karram MM (1993) Detrusor instability and hyperreflexia. In: Walters MD, Karram MM (eds) Clinical urogynecology. Mosby-Year Book, St. Louis, p 263
13. O'Donnell PD (1997) Mixed incontinence. In: O'Donnell PD (ed) Urinary incontinence. Mosby-Year Book, St. Louis, p 93
14. O'Donnell PD (1996) Biofeedback therapy of urinary incontinence. In: Raz S (ed) Female urology. Saunders, Philadelphia
15. O'Donnell PD (1997) Urology in the elderly. In: Atkins RB (ed) Surgical care for the elderly. Lippincott, Philadelphia
16. Nitti VW, Bregg KW, Raz S (1994) Surgical management of incontinence in elderly women. In: O'Donnell PD (ed) Geriatric urology. Little Brown, Boston, p 239
17. Appell RA, Winters JC (1997) Intraurethral injections. In: O'Donnell PD (ed) Urinary incontinence. Mosby-Year Book, St. Louis, p 228
18. (1997) American Urological Association Symptom Index. In: O'Donnell PD (ed) Urinary Incontinence. Mosby-Year Book, St. Louis, p 449
19. O'Donnell PD (1994) Pathophysiology of incontinence in elderly men. In: O'Donnell PD (ed) Geriatric urology. Little Brown, Boston, p 229

Chapter 80
Neoplasms of the Kidney and Bladder

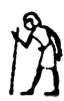

Edward M. Uchio, Juan S. Calderon, and Jonathan J. Hwang

The vast majority of human neoplasms appear to be coupled with the biology of aging. Over 70% of all cancers will occur in individuals over the age of 65 by the year 2030 [1, 2]. The age-specific incidence of many different types of cancer begin to rise steadily as we mature, and neoplasms arising from the kidney and bladder are of no exception. Approximately 88,200 men and 40,500 women developed a malignancy of the kidney or urinary bladder in 2009 [3]. The treatment of these malignancies in the elderly population requires careful consideration of factors such as life expectancy, incidence of treatment complications, and quality of life. This chapter reviews the incidence of kidney and bladder malignancies, the appropriate evaluation in the elderly, surgical and medical treatments available to treat the geriatric patient, and the complications associated with treatment.

Renal Cell Carcinoma

Epidemiology and Etiology

Solid neoplastic lesions of the kidney are comprised of both benign and malignant pathology. Most solid lesions derived from the renal parenchyma are malignant in nature and are predominantly renal cell carcinoma (RCC) (80–90%) [4]. The most common benign solid lesions of the kidney include renal cortical adenoma, metanephric adenoma, oncocytoma, and angiomyolipoma. The latter benign lesion is the only benign tumor that can be readily distinguished by radiographic imaging from its malignant counterpart. These angiomyolipomas are a rare benign clonal neoplasm consisting of adipose tissue, smooth muscle, and blood vessels [5, 6]. The presence of even a small amount of adipose tissue (fat) on computed tomography (CT) is diagnostic of this

tumor and can exclude RCC [7]. Since the majority of solid renal masses are malignant and very few benign lesions can be characterized as noncancerous on imaging, it is the clinical assumption that solid lesions of the kidney are malignant until proven otherwise. RCC accounts for 2–3% of all adult malignancies and is considered the most lethal of all urologic cancers [3]. The majority of RCCs are sporadic in origin with hereditary etiologies (von Hippel–Lindau (VHL), hereditary papillary renal carcinoma syndrome, etc.) accounting for approximately 4% of tumors [8, 9]. RCC is a malignant disease of the elderly, occurring most commonly in the sixth and seventh decades of life [2].

Unlike bladder cancer, there are very few accepted environmental risk factors for RCC. Tobacco exposure is the only accepted factor, with an associated risk as high as 2.5, as compared to controls [10]. In contrast, the hereditary forms of RCC have given us an understanding of the genetic basis of renal carcinogenesis. In many instances, the genes responsible for the hereditary renal cancer syndromes play a role in the more commonly seen sporadic counterparts in the elderly. The most common variant of RCC is clear cell carcinoma. This subtype of RCC is often seen in the autosomal dominant inherited tumor syndrome, VHL disease [11, 12]. Molecular investigations have identified the inactivation of the VHL tumor suppressor gene located on chromosome 3p25 as the genetic cause of renal tumorigenesis in this subtype [13, 14]. A high percentage of sporadic clear cell renal cancer seen in the elderly also demonstrates allelic loss of the VHL locus [15, 16]. In a similar fashion, other hereditary renal syndromes have revealed the genetic etiology of various subtypes of renal cancer (Table 80.1).

Natural History

A thorough understanding of the available knowledge regarding RCC behavior is important for treatment decisions in the elderly population. This special group of patients may have numerous confounding factors such as comorbid disease, which can impact life expectancy not related to their

E.M. Uchio (✉)
Yale University School of Medicine, 800 Howard Avenue, 3rd Floor, New Haven, CT 06519, USA
e-mail: edward.uchio@yale.edu

R.A. Rosenthal et al. (eds.), *Principles and Practice of Geriatric Surgery*,
DOI 10.1007/978-1-4419-6999-6_80, © Springer Science+Business Media, LLC 2011

TABLE 80.1 Hereditary renal cancer syndromes – genetic etiology of RCC subtypes

Disease	Locus	Gene	Protein	Renal manifestations
von Hippel–Lindau disease (VHL)	3p25	VHL	VHL	Clear cell carcinoma, simple and complex cysts
Tuberous sclerosis complex (TSC)	9q34	TSC1	Hemartin	Angiomyelolipoma (most common), renal
	16p13.3	TSC2	Tuberin	cysts, clear cell carcinoma, papillary carcinoma, chromophobe carcinoma
Hereditary leiomyomatosis renal cell cancer (HLRCC)	1q42-q44	FH	Fumarate hydratase	Type II papillary carcinoma
Birt–Hogg–Dubé Syndrome (BHD)	17p11.2	BHD	Folliculin	Chromophobe (34%), chromophobe/oncocytoma(50%), clear cell carcinoma (9%), papillary carcinoma (2%)

TABLE 80.2 2010 AJCC TNM staging for renal cell cancer

TX		Primary tumor cannot be assessed
T0		No evidence of primary tumor
T1		Tumor 7 cm or less in greatest dimension, limited to the kidney
	T1a	Tumor 4 cm or less in greatest dimension, limited to the kidney
	T1b	Tumor more than 4 cm, but not more than 7 cm in greatest dimension, limited to the kidney
T2		Tumor more than 7 cm in greatest dimension, limited to the kidney
	T2a	Tumor more than 7 cm, but less than or equal to 10 cm in greatest dimension, limited to the kidney
	T2b	Tumor more than 10 cm, limited to the kidney
T3		Tumor extends into major veins or perinephric tissues, but not into the ipsilateral adrenal gland and not beyond Gerota's fascia
	T3a	Tumor grossly extends into the renal vein or its segmental (muscle containing) branches, or tumor invades perirenal and/or renal sinus fat, but not beyond Gerota's fascia
	T3b	Tumor grossly extends into the vena cava below the diaphragm
	T3c	Tumor grossly extends into the vena cava above the diaphragm or invades the wall of the vena cava
T4		Tumor invades beyond Gerota's fascia (including contiguous extension into the ipsilateral adrenal gland)

Source: Used with permission of the American Joint Committee on Cancer (AJCC), Chicago, IL, USA. The original source for this material is the AJCC Cancer Staging Manual, Seventh Edition (2010) published by Springer Science and Business Media LLC, http://www.springer.com

diagnosis of RCC. Therefore, it is imperative to understand the natural history of this tumor in the geriatric population. Although most clinical observations of RCC have been in patients in their late decades of life, these investigations do not specifically relate biology of tumor to age [17–19]. Factors such as tumor stage (Table 80.2) and grade are important prognosticators for RCC and can give insight into its clinical behavior [20–22]. Despite these important clinical parameters, the natural history of RCC in a particular patient can be highly variable. The clinical presentation of RCC can vary from an incidentally found solid renal mass seen on imaging only to a large rapidly growing mass with systemic metastasis. Prior to the advent of imaging techniques such as ultrasonography (US), CT, or magnetic resonance imaging (MRI), most of these kidney cancers were detected by clinical symptoms associated with RCC due to local tumor growth, hemorrhage, paraneoplastic syndromes, or metastatic disease. One prominent symptom, flank pain, is usually due to tumor hemorrhage and obstruction of the collecting system from clot. But in advanced disease, the symptom of pain may be the hallmark of local invasion. The classic triad of hematuria, flank pain, and an abdominal mass on physical exam is rarely seen in the modern era of advanced imaging [23]. Prior to CT and US, many of these elderly patients would present with one or more of these symptoms, and most were incurable. Patients with advanced disease also complained of constitutional symptoms, such as weight loss, fever, and night sweats. On physical exam, they were often found to have palpable adenopathy, a nonreducing varicocele, and bilateral lower extremity edema. These tumors were often very large, and up to 25% were associated with metastases. Additionally, half of the patients who appeared to have organ-confined RCC manifest asynchronous metastatic spread following an attempt at curative surgical extirpation [24]. This malignancy preferentially spreads to the lungs, lymph nodes, and bone, although metastatic lesions are also found in less common sites such as brain, gallbladder, epididymis, and skin. The increasing use of noninvasive imaging has shifted the presentation of this disease from a symptomatic course to that of a disease found incidentally in the elderly.

The incidence of RCC has steadily increased during the last 3 decades, mainly due to the use of routine abdominal imaging for renal-related and nonrenal-related indications [25]. Now, most RCCs are detected incidentally as small tumors in patients without symptoms. In the early 1970s, the incidental detection rate was reported as 7–13%; most were for cause, but this percentage has increased to greater than 50% in recent years [19, 26]. The incidence of asymptomatic RCCs detected at autopsy has been reported to be 0.47% [27].

The natural history of these neoplasms has not been investigated adequately, especially that of an incidentally found small renal mass. However, retrospective studies by Bosniak et al. suggest that small solid renal masses <3.5 cm at the time of diagnosis grow slowly (0.36 cm/year) and rarely metastasize [17, 18]. More recently, 32 renal masses in mainly elderly patients (median age 71 years) who refused or were deemed unfit for surgery were followed for a median of 27.9 months. The growth rate of these masses did not differ statistically from zero growth. Only one-third of these presumed RCCs were shown to grow if managed conservatively and followed serially. The growth rate is slow or undetectable in the majority of patients [19, 28]. In other series of active surveillance of renal masses in elderly patients with multiple medical comorbidities, investigators found that 43% of tumors exhibited no tumor growth at a median follow-up of 2 years. At the conclusion of the study, 31% of the patients were deceased, none due to RCC [29]. These data would suggest that conservative management of renal masses may be a possibility, especially for an initial observational period in the elderly population. The optimal duration of this observational period still is not known. Although the previous studies have revealed that conservative management of RCC is possible in select elderly populations, the physician and patient assume a calculated risk when following these tumors. All of the conservative management series with longer follow-up had a small but not insignificant risk of metastatic disease and cancer-associated death. This group of patients who did poorly did not have any characteristic such as tumor size that portended an unfavorable prognosis [30]. Current guidelines for small renal masses <7 cm include active surveillance (AS) as an option, but all require careful counseling between the patient and physician, regarding the risks of this approach and the risk for a future intervention if the tumor shows rapid growth [31].

Management

Management of renal cancer in the elderly may be a very complex decision process. Treatments must incorporate concerns about efficacy, comorbid illnesses, and complications, as well as physiologic effects on renal function and competing causes for future mortality. Surgery remains the mainstay for curative management of localized RCC. The foundation of surgical therapy for renal cancer is complete excision of all neoplastic tissue with an adequate surgical margin. This objective may be obtained by either complete removal of the kidney (radical nephrectomy) or via a nephron-sparing surgical approach (partial nephrectomy). In addition, many newer minimally invasive techniques have gained popularity, such as cryotherapy or radiofrequency ablation (RFA). These new

thermal ablative techniques can be applied during standard open or laparoscopic surgery but are better suited to a percutaneous approach under radiologic guidance (CT or MRI). When performed via the latter technique, a potentially curative treatment can be applied to a completely different patient demographic. Those with significant comorbid illnesses that were previously deemed unsuitable for surgical management can now be given treatment with curative intent, under local anesthetic or minimal sedation. Lastly, as described in the previous section, active surveillance may be an option especially for those elderly individuals with significant competing risk factors for non-RCC-related mortality. Renal biopsy may help delineate the natural history of RCC in this nontreatment group, to help identify aggressive renal cancers from those with minimal growth and metastatic potential [30].

Radiologic Evaluation

The current radiologic modalities used to diagnose and evaluate renal masses include intravenous pyelography (IVP), renal ultrasound (US), CT, and MRI. In the past, the standard IVP was a commonly used test for the evaluation of hematuria. However, due to the lack of sensitivity and specificity for the detection of renal parenchymal tumors, this technology has been supplanted by multidetector computed tomography urography (CTU), for the evaluation of hematuria [32]. Many renal masses found today are detected by the widespread use of US and CT scans, for the evaluation of abdominal and gastrointestinal complaints [25]. More than 70% of these asymptomatic renal masses are found to be simple cysts. The prevalence of benign renal cysts increase with age and are found in over 50% of patients older than 50 years of age, thus a significant finding in the elderly [33]. These lesions are easily characterized by US and CT, and the most common "simple" variety requires no further workup or surveillance [34]. A dedicated renal protocol CT, which entails thin-slice images through the kidney with and without administration of contrast, is the single most important radiologic test to evaluate for RCC. Any renal mass with enhancement characteristics of more than 15 Hounsfield units (HU) after administration of contrast material should be considered an RCC, until proven otherwise (Fig. 80.1) [35]. In the past, gadolinium-enhanced MRI was an excellent modality equal to contrast-enhanced CT that was utilized extensively for patients with renal insufficiency, a significant problem in the elderly population. The gadolinium-based contrast agent (GBCA) used in MRI lacks significant nephrotoxicity [36]. Unfortunately, recent evidence has shown an association of nephrogenic systemic fibrosis (NSF), a debilitating and potentially life-threatening disease, with the use of GBCA in renal failure patients [37]. Due to this finding, many centers

Figure 80.1 Computed tomography (CT) of renal cell carcinoma. (**a**) Axial (**b**) Sagittal (**c**) Coronal (**d**) 3D (**e**) Specimen.

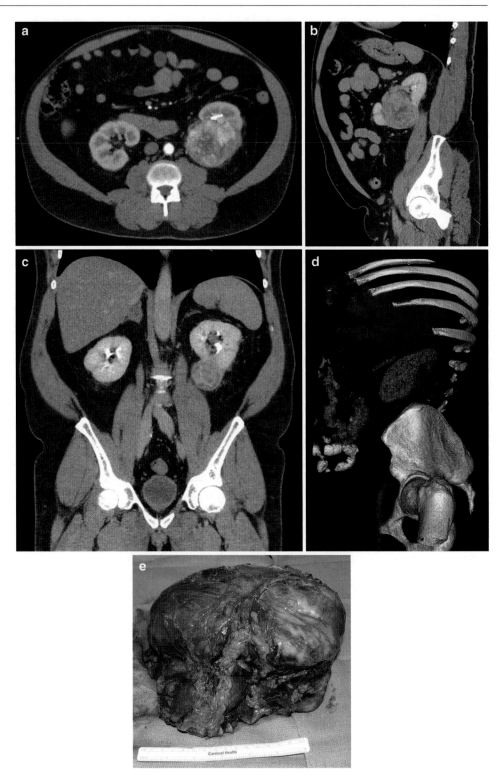

have limited the use of gadolinium-enhanced MRI to patients with a glomerular filtration rate (GFR) >30 mL/min and have avoided gadodiamide, a commonly used type of GBCA [38, 39]. The resulting problem is how to adequately image an elderly patient with poor renal function (GFR<30 mL/min).

Currently, this involves informing the patients regarding the potential risks of gadolinium-enhanced MRI versus performing a standard CT with iodinated contrast media and understanding the risk of contrast medium nephropathy of 5% in patients with a GFR between 15 and 40 mL/min [40].

The use of newer macrocyclic GBCAs may obviate this concern regarding renal function and the development of NSF [41]. These agents by nature of their chemical structure are less likely to release free gadolinium into the tissues, a hallmark of NSF.

Radical Nephrectomy

The radical nephrectomy with en bloc removal of the affected renal unit outside of Gerota's fascia and excision of the ipsilateral adrenal gland, as described by Robson and colleagues, is established as the "gold standard" curative procedure for localized RCC [42]. The procedure also includes removal of the lymphatic tissue in the renal hilar area and immediately adjacent paracaval or paraaortic lymph nodes. Regional lymph node metastasis is an important prognostic factor usually associated with poor survival [43]. The need for a complete regional lymphadenectomy from the crus of the diaphragm to the aortic bifurcation remains controversial. The lymphatic drainage of the kidney is highly variable, and metastasis often occurs through the bloodstream. Only a small percentage (<2–3%) of patients with micrometastatic disease would benefit from this added procedure, and the main benefit is local recurrence without an augment in survival [44–46]. Therefore, the surgeon performing a radical nephrectomy in an elderly patient may consider omission of the extended regional node dissection, to minimize morbidity of the procedure. In addition, another variable in this curative procedure is the choice of surgical incision, which can affect morbidity in the elderly.

The radical nephrectomy can be performed through a variety of surgical incisions. The surgical approach is determined by a variety of factors, which include size and location of the tumor, body habitus, history of previous abdominal surgeries, and morbidity of the patient, which is important in the elderly population. This operation is usually performed through a transabdominal approach, which allows abdominal exploration for metastatic disease and early visualization of the renal vasculature with minimal mobilization of the tumor. The principal disadvantage of this approach is a slightly longer postoperative ileus and possible long-term complications related to adhesions. Other approaches include the flank incision, most commonly at the eleventh and twelfth rib, and a thoracoabdominal incision. The flank incision is an extraperitoneal approach that may be beneficial in the elderly or in patients with poor surgical risk, but exposure of the renal vasculature is limited especially in large tumors. The thoracoabdominal incision extends from the flank anteriorly, involving an incision through the diaphragm. This approach allows excellent visualization of the tumor and vessels but often requires placement of a tube thoracostomy for management of the consequent pneumothorax. Although large RCCs may be removed from this incision, the postoperative morbidity is high and should be avoided in patients with poor pulmonary function, and is rarely indicated in the elderly.

The cancer-specific survival following this procedure is dependent on a number of variables, with pathologic stage proving to be the single most important prognostic factor for RCC [21, 47]. Approximately 70–90% of patients with organ-confined RCC (TNM stage T1-2) are alive without disease at 5 years [21, 48–50]. Survival decreases significantly once the tumor is locally advanced or when lymphatic and systemic metastases are discovered, with a 5-year survival of <20% [50]. Importantly, the absence of effective chemotherapeutic agents in the adjuvant setting for RCC increases the need for complete surgical excision for cure. Oral tyrosine kinase inhibitors (TKI) targeting the mediators in the VHL pathway are currently being studied in the adjuvant setting for high risk disease [51]. The antitumor effects of these targeted agents in metastatic disease may prove to be a benefit in this setting. The side-effect profile is very favorable when compared to classic chemotherapeutic agents which is important when considering use in the elderly.

Laparoscopic Radical Nephrectomy

The first laparoscopic radical nephrectomy (LRN) was performed by Clayman and coworkers in 1991 on an 85-year-old woman with a right renal cancer [52]. Since that initial report, laparoscopic nephrectomy for both benign and malignant disease has become the standard of care at most centers. This minimally invasive surgery is associated with less postoperative discomfort and improved recovery, and costs compare favorably with the open approach [53]. LRN has emerged as a less morbid alternative to open surgery for most tumors (<10 cm) with no local extension. Outcome data for 5- and 10-year cancer-specific survival are comparable with open radical nephrectomy in the treatment of organ confined RCC [54, 55]. These results are not unexpected given the same technique of open radical nephrectomy is emphasized laparoscopically but with the benefits of decreased postoperative morbidity. A variety of approaches are utilized laparoscopically which include transperitoneal, retroperitoneal , and hand-assist approaches, each dependent on the skill and comfort level of the surgeon.

In the elderly population, this technique is attractive due to the decreased convalescence and pain associated with LRN. The latter benefit results in a substantially diminished requirement for narcotic analgesia, and in some patients, its use can be completely avoided with the addition of ketorolac [56]. These benefits have been shown to result in improved pulmonary function among patients treated by LRN as compared to the open counterpart, suggesting that that this procedure may be particularly useful in patients with poor pulmonary reserve [57]. One exception is the patient with severe chronic obstructive pulmonary disease with CO_2 retention. These patients may develop significant hypercarbia or acidosis and will require close monitoring. Some surgeons avoid this situation by using alternate gases such as helium or argon [58]. Lai and coinvestigators attempted to address the comparative morbidity of the LRN in patients of age 70 and over to those under age 70 [59]. In this series, complications rates were the same in both groups, and the only difference was in hospital stay by 1 day (age >70 group). When this procedure was performed purely laparoscopically (no hand-assist), this difference was mitigated.

Nephron-Sparing Surgical Therapy

Postoperative morbidity of radical nephrectomy includes renal dysfunction in the both the short- and long-term setting. This occurrence has prompted surgeons to investigate alternatives to complete removal of the kidney, especially in the patient with a solitary kidney, impaired renal function, or those that present with bilateral renal masses. In the past, parenchymal-sparing partial nephrectomy was performed only for the above reasons due to concerns about incomplete resection and recurrence. In addition, the renal transplant literature concerning donor nephrectomy (patients with a normal contralateral kidneys) have shown that donors do not have a higher rate of kidney failure during their lifetime [60]. However, distinct differences exist between donors and RCC patients. Renal donors tend to be carefully selected for medical comorbidities and are generally young (age 40 or less) [61]. A recent study by Bijol et al. demonstrated a far greater degree of underlying chronic renal disease in RCC patients undergoing surgery than what has been previously appreciated [62]. Only 10% of patients had completely normal adjacent renal tissue in the kidney tumor specimen; most had evidence of significant intrinsic renal abnormalities (diabetic nephropathy, glomerular hypertrophy, mesangial expansion, and diffuse glomerulosclerosis). These changes are reflected in the renal function of RCC patients who choose complete nephrectomy. A landmark study by Huang et al highlighted the impact of radical nephrectomy on future renal function. The incidence of chronic kidney disease (stage 3) was much higher in patients who underwent radical nephrectomy (65%) than after partial nephrectomy (20%) [63]. These data highlight the importance of considering partial nephrectomy even with a normal contralateral kidney.

The classic partial nephrectomy for RCC involves removing the tumor with an adjacent 1 cm margin. A margin this size is easily obtainable for exophytic tumors but is not technically feasible for neoplasms located intraparenchymally or near the renal sinus/vasculature. More contemporary data has shown that a histologic tumor-free margin is more important; the width of the resection margin has no biologic or prognostic significance [64]. Partial nephrectomy is now considered an acceptable therapeutic approach in patients with a single, small T1a (<4 cm) RCC and a normal contralateral kidney. Multiple studies have established that partial nephrectomy for neoplastic lesions <4 cm provides equivalent tumor control compared to radical nephrectomy [65, 66]. In an elderly patient, the choice of a partial nephrectomy is an accepted practice to avoid chronic renal dialysis, as discussed earlier. However, in the setting of a normal contralateral kidney, one must weigh the additional risk of complications unique to this procedure. These include increased bleeding, urinary fistula, positive margins, local recurrence, arteriovenous fistula, and nonfunction of the remaining portion of the kidney. Stephenson et al. attempted to address the issue of comparative morbidity in 1,049 patients who underwent radical nephrectomy or partial nephrectomy [67]. The complication rate when adjusted for other variables was not statistically different between the two groups, but the partial nephrectomy group had more procedural complications due to urinary leak. Overall, the complications of both groups were very minimal. A more recent trend has been to perform partial nephrectomy via the laparoscopic approach. Highly specialized centers have extended this procedure even to the octogenarian population with promising results [68]. The long-term benefit of this more technically demanding procedure for an elderly patient with RCC is uncertain, especially when performed outside centers of excellence.

Thermal Ablative Therapies

In the preceding chapter, nephron-sparing surgery has been shown to be effective in the treatment of RCC while maximally preserving renal function. However, this procedure even when performed laparoscopically requires general anesthesia with its associated risks. Many elderly patients with RCC have significant comorbidities that make them poor surgical candidates. This group of patients is often treated conservatively with active surveillance and not given an option for curative treatment. It is assumed that the patient will most likely have a non-RCC mortality. With improvements in health care, these elderly patients are living longer which would allow a subset of these RCCs to grow and metastasize. In addition, many elderly patients are very anxious about not treating RCC in their kidney, especially for such a chemo-/radiation-resistant tumor. Thermal ablative therapies are a minimally invasive option for curative treatment of RCC. These modalities include renal cryotherapy, RFA, and high-intensity focused ultrasound (HIFU); all are different forms of ablative energy focused on the renal lesion. HIFU is currently not FDA-approved in the United States but has ongoing clinical trials regarding its use, mainly in prostate cancer. Both cryotherapy and RFA use needles to transmit their energy to the tumor and can be placed percutaneously or through laparoscopic exposure. The percutaneous approach can be performed with local anesthetic alone or with intravenous sedation which would allow most patients who are poor surgical risks a chance at curative treatment. These focused thermal ablative therapies allow RCC treatment with minimal morbidity while maximizing posttreatment renal function.

Percutaneous thermal ablative therapies are performed with image guidance: CT, MRI, and ultrasound. The most important principle in all the described therapies is precise localization and treatment application of the energy. In this regard, cryotherapy has an advantage because the treatment area or "iceball" is easily visualized on imaging unlike RFA. In fact, early reports suggested that tumor kill was not as reliable with RFA when compared to cryoablation [69–71]. The authors have experience with both modalities and are now exclusively using cryoablation for the aforementioned benefit in visualization. Between 2005 and 2009, we have treated 33 consecutive renal masses in a total of 29 patients with percutaneous CT-guided cryoablation performed in an outpatient basis with local anesthetic and minimal sedation (Fig. 80.2). All renal masses were able to be treated despite location; novel techniques were utilized to access lesions in close proximity to adjacent vital organs. At a mean follow-up of 22 months, 96% of lesions were successfully treated in one treatment session, as verified by lack of contrast enhancement on postprocedure CTs. There were no major complications;

the only minor complication was postprocedure site pain in one patient which resolved spontaneously. Elderly individuals who are poor surgical candidates or choose not to undergo surgery can safely be treated with renal cryoablation. Although intermediate-term data looks promising regarding the efficacy of this procedure, longer term follow-up is still needed. The elderly must be counseled carefully when choosing thermal ablative therapies.

Management of Advanced RCC

Up to 30% of patients with RCC have metastatic disease at presentation and recurrence develops in approximately 40% of patients treated for localized disease [72]. These elderly individuals with advanced RCC are unlikely to benefit from surgical therapy unless a radical nephrectomy is performed for palliative intent. Therefore, systemic agents offer the most rational treatment options for older patients with this disease. Although categorical recommendations for the therapy of cancers based on chronologic age are neither appropriate nor reasonable, many decisions for or against administration of systemic therapy are often based on the age of the individual. Variability among aging individuals with regard to physiologic senescence and comorbidities suggests that a more practical approach for the clinician is the use of guidelines and performance scores to assess the elderly patient's functional and physiologic tolerability for potentially toxic therapy.

First, it is important to define those who are considered elderly. Without readily usable markers of a patient's physiologic age, Balducci recommended that the clinician consider those individuals over 70 years as elderly and should undergo

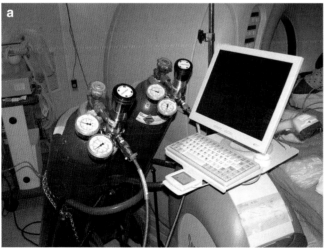
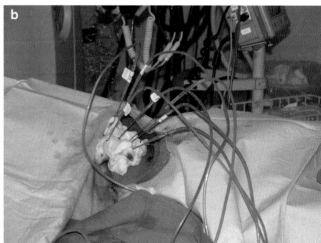

FIGURE **80.2**   Percutaneous cryotherapy. (**a**) Cryotherapy Unit in CT Suite (**b**) Cryotherapy probes in L renal mass.

some form of geriatric assessment [73]. These individuals have an increased occurrence of the following: decreased musculoskeletal mass, functional limitations, geriatric syndromes (dementia, malnutrition, polypharmacy, incontinence, delirium), and multiple comorbidities. Minimizing the occurrence of side effects from chemotherapeutic drugs in the elderly requires careful clinical assessment for functional ability and preexisting neuropathy, cardiac/hepatic/renal function, bone-marrow reserve, nutrition, polypharmacy, and cognitive function. Interventions should include adjusted doses of renally excretable agents to GFR, use of support agents such as growth factors and cytoprotective agents when indicated, appropriate nutritional support, and the preferential use of safer agents when indicated [74].

Traditional cytotoxic chemotherapeutic agents and hormonal therapies have been ineffective in the treatment of metastatic RCC. The overall response rate was very low, usually much less than 15% [75]. Milowsky and Nanus reviewed the chemotherapeutic strategies for RCC; they concluded that most single-agent chemotherapy trials have been disappointing. There was modest enthusiasm for combination chemotherapy, especially with gemcitabine and capecitabine [76]. Recently published trials of their use showed minimal response rates of only 11–16% with significant toxicity [77]. These chemotherapeutic agents likely have no role in the elderly patient in light of these findings.

Until recently, systemic treatment for metastatic RCC was limited to cytokine therapy, which has been the standard of care for over 15 years. The basis of this treatment was built on observations that spontaneous remission of RCC occurred, although infrequently, in individuals with metastatic disease who underwent nephrectomy. Cytokine therapy, or immunotherapy for metastatic RCC consists mainly of two agents, interleukin-2 (IL-2) and interferon-α (IFN). Various combinations and dosages of IL-2 and IFN have been studied in randomized trials for metastatic, recurrent, and unresectable RCC. These studies have suggested that high-dose IL-2 results in higher response rates when compared to low-dose IL-2 and other cytokines [78–80]. The benefit of high-dose IL-2, as compared to even current systemic therapies, is that this drug is the only one shown to produce durable complete remissions [80]. Therefore, in the very select elderly patients with excellent performance status and low volume disease who have undergone a cytoreductive nephrectomy, one may consider the use of high-dose IL-2. The use of immunotherapy for advanced RCC in the aged must be approached cautiously due to the significant toxicities associated with its use.

Improved understanding of the biology of RCC, especially through the VHL pathway [9], has led to the many "targeted therapies" for treatment of metastatic kidney cancer. Over the last few years, systemic treatment options have improved dramatically due to the introduction of broad-spectrum receptor TK, vascular endothelial growth factor (VEGF) antibodies, and mammalian target of rapamycin (mTOR) inhibitors. These agents have shown impressive antitumor activity and improved survival rates when compared to cytokine therapy [72, 81, 82]. Since 2005, two broad-spectrum TKIs (sunitinib malate and sorafenib tosylate), one mTOR inhibitor (temsirolimus), and one VEGF antibody (Bevacizumab) in combination with interferon, have been approved for the treatment of advanced RCC. In addition, another mTOR inhibitor (everolimus) has received FDA approval for patients with advanced RCC after failure of treatment with sorafenib or sunitinib, i.e., second-line therapy [83].

Sunitinib is well tolerated when compared to IFN and has become standard first-line therapy for metastatic RCC. In its phase III trial, treatment-related grade 3 or 4 fatigue was higher with interferon (12% versus 7%), but patients treated with sunitinib had higher rates of diarrhea, vomiting, hypertension, and hand–foot syndrome [72]. In addition, recent data from an expanded access trial has revealed that sunitinib is safe and efficacious in subgroups of patients including those with poor performance status [84]. These findings have made sunitinib standard therapy for metastatic RCC in the elderly. All targeted agents can be used in the elderly metastatic patient with consideration of the caveats mentioned earlier (careful evaluation, GFR dose adjustment, use of growth factors, etc.) to minimize the side effects and improve the tolerability of toxic systemic therapy.

Transitional Cell Carcinoma of the Bladder

Few conditions illustrate the link between cancer and aging better than transitional cell carcinoma of the bladder (TCC). The incidence of bladder cancer peaks at 85 years of age, according to a recent California tumor registry study [85]. As one ages, the risk for higher stage and grade disease increases. This raises the probability of developing invasive cancer and therefore affecting survival [86–88]. The basis for this phenomenon has triggered molecular research aiming to explain the influence of biological changes associated with the aging processes on the development and/or progression of TCC.

Transitional cell carcinoma of the bladder represents a broad spectrum of pathologic processes, extending from indolent low-grade papillomas to invasive poorly differentiated tumors with rapid metastatic capability. Age and performance status play a major role in the election of therapy and outcomes. Therefore, successful management of TCC of the bladder in the elderly patient requires an understanding of the natural history of TCC and the quality-of-life implications of each therapeutic approach.

Diagnosis

Bladder cancer represents an important consideration in the differential diagnosis of voiding complaints in the elderly individual. The presence of a neoplastic lesion within the bladder may be heralded by irritative symptoms such as urinary urgency, frequency, or dysuria. Hematuria, microscopic or gross, may also announce the existence of malignant bladder lesions. It has been estimated that 5–15% of patients, predominantly men, with hematuria harbor unsuspected bladder cancer [89]. Despite this, testing for hematuria cannot be recommended as a screening test for bladder cancer in the elderly population. In a study of 2,356 asymptomatic men aged ≥60 years who underwent dipstick testing for hematuria, only 0.7% of the screened population were found to have a bladder tumor [90]. The 2008 US Preventive Services Task Force found no high quality evidence that screening would impact mortality from bladder cancer. Although screening for TCC specifically is not recommended, many patients do routinely have urinalysis for the above symptoms or by their primary-care physician. Any asymptomatic hematuria (>3 red blood cells per high power field) requires urologic evaluation. A standard workup for TCC includes urinalysis, urine cytology, and cystourethroscopy. Additionally, a radiographic evaluation of the upper urinary tract is also indicated with conventional excretory urography or with the more contemporary computed tomography (CT) urography [91]. The cost implications of this approach, given the incidence of voiding symptoms and hematuria, are obvious. In the absence of a clear etiology such as infection, it is difficult at the present time to identify a subpopulation of patients not requiring a cancer evaluation.

Basic Science and Natural History

Epidemiologic and experimental evidence favors a strong role for environmental exposure as an etiology of bladder cancer in the elderly. However, since many cases arise in patients with no obvious exposure, it is important to understand the molecular basis of this disease. Well-recognized DNA alterations, such as the *p53* tumor-suppressor gene, seem to be responsible for the initiation and promotion of many human cancers including bladder cancer [92]. A recent study showed that the p53 transcriptional activity and p53-dependent apoptosis was significantly decreased in older mice compared to younger mice [93]. In addition to p53, mutational frequency (Mf) studies have also provided new insights on how age-related changes may contribute to the development of bladder cancer later in life. Stuart et al. found a greater rate of Mf in the bladder of old transgenic mice

compared to other tissues examined in the same mouse model [94]. Further analysis revealed that this phenomenon was the result of accumulated mutations through replication during the lifetime of the mouse, rather than repeated insults associated with the aging process. Another mechanism that may be affected in the elderly involves gene transcription. Promoter regions of tumor suppressor genes can be silenced through DNA hypermethylation resulting in unchecked cellular replication [95]. This epigenetic alteration has been intensively studied in the past. CpG hypermethylation has been detected in 43% of aggressive bladder tumors and only seen weakly in normal epithelium which increases with age [96, 97]. Finally, a study by Gu et al. reported that advanced age was associated with decreased expression levels of mRNA of the four major mechanisms assuring genomic stability [98]. The protective mechanisms studied were p53, ataxia telangiectasia mutated (ATM), telomerase reverse transcriptase (hTERT), and telomeric repeat binding factor-2 (TRF2). These studies support the hypothesis that particular regions of the human genome are more susceptible to age-related DNA damage. And, within those regions, important genes, especially those involved with protection of genomic integrity, may be altered which ultimately results in bladder cancer.

The most important epidemiologic risk factors associated with urothelial carcinoma are chemical carcinogens, which are derived from tobacco products or a spectrum of industrial and environmental agents (see Table 80.3). Transitional cell carcinoma of the bladder represents a broad spectrum of pathologic processes, thus preventing a linear description of the natural history of this disease. To better understand the development and progression of TCC, it is important to make a distinction between superficial or nonmuscle invasive bladder cancer and invasive carcinoma. Superficial TCC exhibits an overall low risk of progression (to a life-threatening cancer), but recurrences are very frequent. A minority of these recurrences may eventually progress into high-grade disease,

TABLE 80.3 Identified and potential etiologic agents for transitional cell carcinoma

Established risk factors
Cigarette smoking (black tobacco higher than blond tobacco) [167, 168]
Phenacetin-containing analgesics [169–171]
Aromatic amines (painters, rubber industry workers) [172–174]
Leather workers
Cyclophosphamide (cumulative dose) [175, 176]
Ionizing radiation [177, 178]
Chronic cystitis [179, 180]
Potential risk factors
Coffee drinking (large amounts, 7–10 cups a day) [181, 182]
Hair dyes exposure (hairdressers) [183]
Artificial sweeteners (saccharin, cyclamates, only in rats) [184]
Chlorinated water [185]
Arsenic (in drinking water) [186]

Table 80.4 2010 TMN staging system for carcinoma of the urinary bladder: primary cancer

TX	Primary tumor cannot be assessed
T0	No evidence of primary tumor
Ta	Noninvasive papillary carcinoma
Tis	Carcinoma in situ: flat tumor
T1	Cancer invades subepithelial connective tissue
T2	Tumor invades musclularis propria
	T2a Tumor invades superficial muscularis propria (inner half)
	T2b Tumor invades deep muscularis propria (outer half)
T3	Tumor invades perivesical tissue
	T3a Microscopically
	T3b Macroscopically (extravesical mass)
T4	Tumor invades any of the following: prostatic stroma, seminal vesicles, uterus, vagina, pelvic wall, and abdominal wall
	T4a Tumor invades prostatic stroma, uterus, and vagina
	T4b Tumor invades pelvic wall and abdominal wall

Source: Used with permission of the American Joint Committee on Cancer (AJCC), Chicago, IL, USA. The original source for this material is the AJCC Cancer Staging Manual, Seventh Edition (2010) published by Springer Science and Business Media LLC, http://www.springer.com

Table 80.5 Features associated with an increased risk of recurrence or progression

Multiple papillary recurrences (two or more in a given year)
More than three lesions or any tumor >3 cm in diameter, sessile or with a thick stalk
Invasion of the lamina propria (T1 tumor) or poorly differentiated histology (grade 3)
Incomplete resection due to diffuse bladder involvement and/or unfavorable location
Diffuse Tis alone or in association with papillary tumors

which can then be locally invasive. A retrospective review of 761 patients with superficial bladder cancer treated with endoscopic surgical extirpation alone found that only 7% died of bladder cancer, while 15% died from other causes [99]. The management of high-grade/invasive disease in the elderly is costly and challenging (over $35 million per year) [100]. Treatment options for patients with muscle-invasive disease or recurrent high-grade superficial disease include cystectomy (with or without chemotherapy), radiation and chemotherapy (bladder sparing therapy), and a palliative approach. It is important to understand the difference between a superficial and invasive lesion when considering treatment of a geriatric patient with bladder cancer. The staging system for a primary bladder TCC is shown in Table 80.4 [22].

Superficial Transitional Cell Carcinoma

Approximately 75–80% of all bladders TCCs are classified initially as nonmuscle invasive or superficial. This group of lesions encompasses indolent papillary lesions confined to the urothelium with high recurrence frequency (stage Ta), a poorly differentiated flat cancer called carcinoma in situ (CIS) with higher invasive potential (Tis), and neoplasms invading the lamina propria of the bladder wall (stage T1). Information regarding the recurrence and possible progression of superficial TCC is available after a complete transurethral resection of the bladder tumor (TURBT) has been performed. The pathologic specimen allows incorporation of information regarding the depth of invasion, histologic

grade, and presence or absence of multicentric disease. The remainder of this discussion refers to the biologic behavior of each of these lesions in elderly patients.

Stage and histological grade are central determinants of the disease-specific outcome for superficial TCC [101]. In general terms, a stage Ta lesion exhibits a 50–90% recurrence rate at 5 years with a 2–25% rate of progression to muscle-invasive disease [102–104]. Within this same category (Ta), pathologic grade-1 and 2 cancers exhibit a recurrence rate of approximately 30%, whereas grade-3 lesions recur in over 70% of cases, exemplifying the importance of histologic grade. Many studies have analyzed large retrospective series in an attempt to stratify patients according to their risk of disease recurrence and progression [105–107]. The presence of any feature displayed on Table 80.5 is associated with an increased risk of recurrence or progression. This is encouraging for the geriatric patient with comorbidities who does not present with these risk factors, since they can be managed conservatively. This would involve intermittent resection or even fulguration of recurrent lesions without any additional treatments. In this context, patients who do not develop another tumor within 3 months of the initial resection for TCC have an 80% probability of never demonstrating another tumor in the bladder [102]. However, patients who experience ten or more recurrences exhibit a high rate of progression and death from TCC [108]. Therefore, in this instance, the conservative algorithm for stage Ta TCC with endoscopic resection alone should be complemented by intravesical therapy.

CIS presents as a flat formation of poorly differentiated TCC confined to the mucosal surface of the bladder. This CIS lesion (Tis) may appear as a solitary primary lesion or accompanied by another form of TCC. It has been suggested that the presence of Tis in the mucosa adjacent to a Ta or T1 tumor increases the risk for muscle-invasive disease [109, 110]. Tis may also display a diffuse involvement of the mucosa and extend into the distal ureters or prostatic ducts. This pattern of superficial spread is associated with particularly aggressive disease, with 60–80% progressing to invasive cancer [111, 112]. Common presenting manifestations of CIS include severe irritative voiding symptoms and hematuria. But, many of these patients may be relatively asymptomatic with only an abnormal finding on urine cytology. Tis lesions have demonstrated a recurrence rate ranging from 63 to 92% after resection and intravesical chemotherapy [113]. In addition to recurrence, the literature supports an especially high rate of progression to invasive disease after endoscopic resection [114]. Therefore, patients with primary or concomitant Tis cannot be treated with endoscopic resection alone, regardless of their age. Intravesical therapy should be used in conjunction with TURBT. If this combination therapy fails to control the disease, cystectomy should be considered in the elderly individual with a good performance status [115].

The final type of superficial TCC is a lesion that invades the lamina propria of the bladder wall but not the muscularis propria. This stage T1 lesion exhibits a high rate of recurrence (67–81%) and progression (12–49%). Patients presenting with this stage disease have a cancer-specific mortality ranging from 17 to 71% [114]. Virtually, all of these tumors are of high grade and require therapy beyond standard endosurgical resection due to the risk of progression [116]. T1 tumors are often treated adjuvantly with instillation of chemotherapeutic or immunotherapeutic agents in addition to endoscopic ablation. The intravesical instillation of Bacillus Calmette–Guérin (BCG) has been shown to be efficacious in reducing the recurrence rate by 30–40% [117, 118] and may also reduce progression of T1 tumors [119]. In a series of 86 patients with T1 tumors, a complete response of 91% was demonstrated for the combination of TURBT and intravesical BCG [120]. However, chemotherapy (mitomycin, thiotepa, etc.), on the other hand, has not reliably demonstrated an effect on progression [121]. Elderly individuals with significant comorbidities and solitary T1 disease may comprise a subpopulation of patients for whom endoscopic resection may be adequate. One study evidenced curative rates of 40% for stage T1 TCC, particularly grades 1 and 2, with a single resection and confirmation of complete removal of the lesion on a repeat bladder biopsy [122]. Nevertheless, intravesical immunotherapy in addition to TURBT should be standard practice for T1 lesions in the geriatric population given the high risk for progression and recurrence. One must also verify the lesion to be a true T1 lesion by a repeat resection even when muscle is present in the initial biopsy specimen [123]. Patients who present with recurrent T1 disease within 6 months to 1 year after resection or after one or two courses of BCG should be considered for radical cystectomy [124, 125]. Alternatively, an aggressive approach of early cystectomy for de novo T1 disease has been advocated by one study that compared this approach versus cystectomy for a recurrent T1 lesion. The results suggested that immediate cystectomy at the time of initial diagnosis of a T1 cancer can improve survival [126]. The selection of an adequate therapeutic plan for an elderly patient with T1 TCC must involve performance status, comorbid illness, and impact of the treatment on their quality of life.

Intravesical Therapy

Intravesical therapy permits high local concentrations of a chemotherapeutic or immunotherapeutic agent within the bladder to eradicate residual tumor cells that remain viable after TURBT, thus preventing recurrence. Conceptually, this application is provided after complete resection as a specific strategy against recurrence or progression. Less commonly, intravesical therapy is instituted for residual tumor following incomplete TURBT. These instilled agents may cause symptoms of bladder irritation as a side effect. Furthermore, systemic absorption can occur if the bladder mucosa is damaged and results in systemic toxicity. Treatments, therefore, are generally initiated 2–4 weeks after tumor resection, allowing the reepithelialization of the bladder mucosa.

The most commonly used agent for intravesical therapy is Bacillus Calmette–Guerin (BCG). A number of other agents also have activity, including mitomycin, the anthracyclines, thiotepa, gemcitabine, interferon, and docetaxel [127]. Many prospective trials have compared these other intravesical agents with BCG, but none has been shown to be superior [121, 128–130]. The remainder of this discussion focuses on the application of BCG as an intravesical immunotherapy for Ta, Tis, and T1 TCC. Characteristics of the optimal candidates for intravesical therapy are listed in Table 80.6.

Bacillus Calmette–Guérin is a live attenuated *Mycobacterium* that has been found to incite an immune response within the bladder, which appears to be responsible for its therapeutic efficacy against TCC. The immune activation may persist for a number of months facilitating an ongoing antitumor response. In a systematic review that included 585 patients with Ta or T1 disease, administration of intravesical BCG as prophylaxis has been found to reduce tumor recurrence by approximately 54% compared to transurethral resection alone [131]. This effect is also associated with a decreased incidence of tumor progression [119]. BCG has also demonstrated effectiveness when administered as therapy for CIS of the bladder (Tis), with complete response

TABLE 80.6 Characteristics of candidates for intravesical therapy

Indications
Tumor multiplicity
Recurrent Ta, T1 lesions
Stage Tis
Size >3 cm [187]
Surgically uncontrollable Ta disease
Stage Ta with Tis
Prostatic urethral disease
Relative contraindications
Immunocompromised patient
Hypersensitivity to Bacillus Calmette–Guerin
Severe irritative voiding symptoms
Solitary Ta lesion

rates of 60–79% [132]. The optimal strategy for instillation of BCG consists of a 6-week induction course with maintenance therapy. The largest randomized trial evaluating the effectiveness of BCG induction alone versus induction plus maintenance therapy found a median recurrence-free survival time twice as long in the maintenance arm [133]. Interestingly, only 16% of patients received all eight courses of maintenance therapy over 3 years mainly due to toxicity. One would assume that this strategy represents a challenge for elderly patients who often present with a suboptimal nutritional status and comorbid conditions that may limit their immune response (i.e., diabetes), predisposing them to severe BCG toxicity. At the author's institution, BCG maintenance therapy is the standard intravesical regimen, and the majority of elderly patients complete the full protocol duration with reduction doses if necessary. Lowering the dose of BCG for this population of patients still maintains its efficacy. At a median follow-up of 61 months, one study found no differences between standard or reduced dose BCG with respect to disease recurrence, time to recurrence, need for deferred cystectomy, or disease-specific survival [134]. Severe toxicity rates were lower with the reduced dose. Although these results are encouraging, further confirmatory trials are needed before a reduced dose of BCG can be considered standard therapy in the face of no toxicity. In addition, recent trials have suggested that increased age may confer a less durable response to BCG with earlier recurrences and a shorter cancer-free survival time [135]. These findings highlight the need to investigate the optimal regimen of BCG induction and maintenance in the elderly.

In summary, superficial TCC presents frequently in the aged population often with a protracted natural history and a low risk of progression. Most stage Ta lesions may be managed with endoscopic resection with subsequent outpatient follow-up utilizing cystourethroscopy and urine cytology. Surveillance protocols for such patients often involve cystoscopy every 3 months for 2 years, every 6 months for 2 years, and then every year thereafter. The intensity of this approach may be reduced for individuals in ill health or with favorable lesions at low risk for recurrence and progression. Patients who present with Tis or T1 cancers will benefit from a course of intravesical immunotherapy with BCG, following surgical resection. Again, these patients should be carefully followed with an organized surveillance protocol. Individuals with recurrent or refractory Tis or T1 lesions should be considered for curative radical cystectomy.

Muscle-Invasive TCC of the Bladder

The concept of muscle-invasive disease refers to lesions that have invaded beyond the lamina propria into the muscle wall of the bladder (stage T2). The literature suggests that approximately 50% of individuals who present with stage T2–T4 TCC will develop distant metastasis within 2 years [136]. Most patients who develop T2 lesions of the bladder present initially with this muscle-invasive disease de novo rather than from a previous superficial cancer (Ta-T1). It appears that the proportion of patients with muscle-invasive TCC increases with age. Approximately 18% of patients aged 40–44 years have locally advanced TCC at presentation, whereas 39% of patients over 84 years of age present with this stage disease [137]. As a result, the elderly patient more often faces a life-threatening cancer compared to their younger counterparts. Unfortunately this elderly patient will have a higher surgical risk due to comorbidities. Data extracted from SEER database found that individuals of 75 years of age and older with muscle-invasive bladder cancer had a higher prevalence of cardiac disease, prior cancer diagnosis, chronic anemia and poor American Society of Anesthesiologists Physical Status Classification (ASA) [86]. These factors have a direct impact on treatment choices, especially when surgical options may involve significant morbidity. The evaluation and treatment of this patient with locally advanced TCC will be discussed further.

Locally Advanced Transitional Cell Carcinoma of the Bladder

Radiologic Evaluation

Once the diagnosis of a stage T2 TCC has been established through transurethral biopsy or resection, the patient should be thoroughly examined for evidence of lymphatic or hematogenous spread, as well as invasion into adjacent tissues. The primary sites for the dissemination of TCC include the pelvic lymph nodes (within the obturator and hypogastric regions), lung, liver, and bone. Pertinent radiologic studies include a chest radiograph and an abdominal/ pelvic CT or MRI scan. A bone evaluation with skeletal scintigraphy (bone scan) is indicated in individuals with complaints of musculoskeletal pain or an elevated alkaline phosphatase level [50]. Approximately 5–15% of patients with invasive TCC harbor metastatic bone lesions, which obviate an attempt at curative (surgical) therapy.

Computed tomography is about 80% accurate in differentiating locally advanced tumors involving perivesical fat or surrounding structures from those with less invasive tumors. However, since CT is often performed after a transurethral resection, interpretation of perivesical fat invasion becomes involved. It may be difficult to distinguish inflammatory or postsurgical edematous changes from true extravesical tumor extension. Another important limitation of CT is that it may miss tumors <1 cm in size, particularly those in the bladder trigone or dome. Tumors located in these areas may be better evaluated by gadolinium-enhanced MRI, which may also be superior to CT in detecting extravesical tumor extension and surrounding organ invasion [138–140]. The use of positron emission tomography (PET) in the evaluation of patients with localized TCC remains investigational, largely due to confounding factors from urinary excretion of the glucose-labeled tracers. MRI may ultimately be the preferred study over CT in the older patients since they often present with a suboptimal creatinine clearance. A discussion of contrast-induced nephropathy is detailed in the radiologic section of renal cell cancer.

Treatment

Therapeutic approaches to muscle-invasive TCC of the bladder are determined by the presence or absence of clinically detectable lymphatic or hematogenous metastases. Multimodality curative therapy should be applied only in individuals whose cancers are confined to the bladder wall or associated with minimal-volume regional lymphatic disease. We discuss next the therapeutic alternatives for patients with locally advanced TCC and the use of radical surgery in elderly patients.

Surgical Therapy

The perioperative morbidity associated with radical cystectomy and the substantial impact of urinary diversion on the quality of life has led to the use of less radical approaches for the management of muscle-invasive bladder cancer in the elderly. Alternatives to radical cystectomy include radical transurethral resection (TURBT), partial cystectomy, or chemotherapy/radiation, which combines radical TURBT followed by external-beam radiation therapy with concurrent chemotherapy (cisplatin used as a radiation-sensitizing agent). In general, bladder preservation approaches are considered by many to produce inferior oncologic outcomes compared to radical cystectomy, although this has not been proven in randomized trials. It appears that solitary tumors confined to the muscle wall are ideal candidates for these alternative treatments with intermediate and long-term cancer-specific survival rates approaching that of radical cystectomy. An attempt at complete endoscopic resection of a solid muscle-infiltrating lesion within the bladder represents the most conservative surgical treatment approach. The role of definitive TURBT was illustrated by a retrospective series where 10-year cancer-specific survival rates were similar to those seen with radical cystectomy (76% versus 71%) [141]. However, radical TURBT is applicable only to a small

minority of patients with muscle-invasive disease and demands intensive, long-term cystoscopic follow-up due to local recurrence. This follow-up may represent a challenge for the geriatric population which according to the SEER data has shown suboptimal adherence to surveillance recommendations [142]. Another surgical option, the partial cystectomy, allows complete pathologic staging of the primary tumor with an extended pelvic lymph node dissection. This technique preserves urinary function and avoids the need for diversion, therefore minimizing the impact on the elderly patient's quality of life. As with the radical TURBT, only a few patients are optimal candidates for this partial resection, and the risk of recurrent tumor in the residual bladder remains.

Complete surgical extirpation with radical cystectomy remains the treatment of choice for locally advanced TCC in patients of all age groups. The contemporary surgical approach includes thorough pelvic lymph node dissection followed by complete removal of the bladder, uterus, and anterior vaginal wall in women or bladder with the prostate and seminal vesicles in men. A urinary diversion with either an ileal conduit (noncontinent) or a continent reservoir (orthotopic or nonorthotopic) is constructed following the cystectomy. Skinner and Lieskovsky reported a series of 197 patients in 1984 who had 5-year survival rates of 75% with pT2–T3a disease, 44% with pT3b, and 36% with stage pT4 or positive pelvic lymph nodes [143]. Importantly, the postoperative survival was not affected by application of preoperative radiation therapy. In addition, radiotherapy prior to surgery increases the risk of operative complications and makes the creation of an internal urinary reservoir using irradiated bowel more difficult [144, 145]. Therefore, radical cystectomy alone has become established as satisfactory monotherapy for most patients with locally advanced TCC of the bladder. The impact on survival from a radical cystectomy performed in a healthy surgical patient is clear. The benefit of this extensive surgery, as we age, depends largely on competing risks for death.

In the elderly individual, who typically carries a high burden of comorbid diseases and disability, the benefit of radical cystectomy versus radiation therapy is less dramatic. The largest case series involving contemporary data evaluated the benefit of cystectomy in different age groups (<60, 60–69, 70–79,>79), without correlating outcomes to physiologic measures, such as performance status [146]. A total of 8,034 patients underwent cystectomy, while 2,077 had radiation therapy as their primary treatment for muscle-invasive TCC. They found that older patients were less likely to have a cystectomy and that a sizeable survival advantage was seen with cystectomy in all age groups except for the octogenarian (15 versus 18 months). The small benefit of cystectomy was lost when the elderly patient had a limited or no pelvic node dissection, highlighting the importance of a full lymph node dissection in locally advanced TCC. Another multicenter trial evaluated 888 patients over a 19-year period [147]. Thirty percent of the patients were 70–80 years of age, but only 6% were over 80. Age was an independent predictor for adverse outcomes. Currently, only two small studies have utilized functional geriatric assessment as it relates to radical cystectomy outcomes. Weizer et al. correlated a Karnofsky Performance Status (KPS) score with cystectomy in one hundred and six patients with muscle-invasive disease. Patients with a KPS score below 80 had an overall 4-year survival of 14% versus 33% for those with a KPS score above 80 [148]. This functional assessment tool was validated as the only independent predictor of overall survival in a multi-variable analysis that included age, marital status, treatment type, mobility, and stage. In another retrospective study of 44 patients over 80 years of age, the 6-month rehospitalization rate was higher when accompanied by a drop in KPS score from 70 to 65 at 1 and 3 months following surgery [149]. These findings demonstrate the importance of functional age of the patient in contrast to their chronologic age when deal-ing with muscle-invasive TCC. It is, therefore, not justified to withhold a potentially curative therapy such as radical cys-tectomy on the basis of age alone.

Historically, many individuals are willing to undergo intensive therapy and endure significant morbidity if the like-lihood of cure from a disease is high. As discussed earlier, the ability to eradicate bladder cancer is directly related to the stage at presentation, particularly the presence or absence of lymphatic metastasis. Most reports demonstrate that lymph node metastasis at the time of radical cystectomy is associated with a 6–23% 5-year survival [150]. For the elderly patient with an otherwise asymptomatic stage T2–T4 bladder cancer with borderline nodal enlargement on CT, an accurate identification of lymphatic disease could dissuade them from undergoing radical cystectomy and make more palliative approaches attractive. In this regard, minimally invasive laparoscopic techniques can be employed for accu-rate pelvic lymph node staging. Accumulating evidence has shown that the standard template for pelvic node dissection (distal common iliac, obturator, hypogastric, and external iliac nodes) is inadequate [151]. Lymph nodes proximal to the origin of the inferior mesenteric artery and presacral lymph nodes have been included in an extended template dissection. This minimally invasive technique with an expanded dissection may identify those patients harboring metastatic deposits within the lymphatic drainage of the bladder, thus avoiding the morbidity of radical cystectomy for a cancer with poor prognosis.

Finally, minimally invasive alternatives such as laparo-scopic radical cystectomy or robotic-assisted radical laparo-scopic cystectomy, with the potential for reduced morbidity and more rapid convalescence, are being adopted in many centers worldwide. Reports have demonstrated the technical reproducibility and safety of these techniques, although extensive experience with these procedures is required to achieve optimal results. Advantages include faster reactiva-tion of gastrointestinal motility and shorter hospital length of stay. Although this appears as a promising alternative for the geriatric population, data regarding the long-term oncologic outcomes is lacking at the present time, especially with regard to the adequacy of the pelvic lymph node dissection by these techniques [152, 153].

Multimodality Therapy for Advanced TCC of the Bladder

Chemotherapy is widely used for therapy in advanced or metastatic bladder cancer and remains an area of active research as an adjuvant or neoadjuvant treatment with defini-tive local therapy. Further applications of systemic chemo-therapy include the development of multimodality treatment protocols for curative therapy with bladder preservation. Since Sternberg et al.'s original report of a 72% response rate in metastatic bladder cancer patients using methotrexate/vin-blastine/doxorubicin/cisplatin (M-VAC) [154], the incorpora-tion of newer and highly active agents, such as gemcitabine and paclitaxel, has led to the development of new combination regimens. Multiple randomized studies have demonstrated the superiority of the M-VAC regimen versus other combination regimens positioning M-VAC as the standard first-line regi-men [155–157]. However, the regimen employs agents whose excretion and distribution can be affected by age-related phys-iologic changes. Age alone should not preclude the use of M-VAC; careful evaluation of nutritional state, cardiac and renal function, and screening for underlying neuropathy is paramount to the safe delivery of this combination of drugs.

Gemcitabine has been identified as a highly active single agent in nonrandomized studies for untreated patients with metastatic urothelial carcinoma [158]. This drug was further combined with cisplatin in the GC regimen, showing response rates as efficacious as the ones achieved by the M-VAC regimen. These studies have made GC the new stan-dard first-line therapy especially in regard to tolerability. However, elderly patients may not be fit for intensive cispla-tin-based chemotherapy regimens. A retrospective review of 381 patients with advanced urothelial carcinoma who were treated with one of several platinum-based regimens identi-fied 116 who were ≥70 years of age [159]. The elderly expe-rienced more frequent neutropenia and renal toxicity compared to patients <70 years of age. However, toxic death rates were similar in both age groups, and median survival did not differ significantly. Single-agent regimens with gemcitabine or paclitaxel and various two-drug combina-tions in which carboplatin, whose dose can be adjusted for individual variation in renal function, is substituted for cis-platin have been found to be feasible and have activity in older populations [160–162]. The efficacy of these systemic agents have stimulated investigations into neoadjuvant or adjuvant protocols for locally advanced TCC associated with poor prognostic factors. Multiple large randomized clinical trials and individual patient data meta-analysis have demonstrated a survival benefit for neoadjuvant cisplatin-based regimens, shifting the algorithm of treatment from cystectomy alone [163, 164]. In contrast, definitive recommendations on the use of adjuvant chemotherapy for patients with locally advanced urothelial bladder cancer still require the completion of large randomized trials.

The clinical response of metastatic TCC to systemic chemotherapeutic agents has stimulated the design of investigational protocols with the intention to eradicate locally advanced TCC while preserving bladder function. These bladder-sparing approaches combine the efficacy of an aggressive transurethral resection with external beam radiation therapy and systemic chemotherapy. Although irradiation has demonstrated only modest efficacy as monotherapy, several investigators have advocated its role in a multimodality approach [165]. One study of 94 patients with T2–T4 TCC treated with endoscopic resection followed by two or three cycles of M-VAC or CMV with subsequent 6480 cCy radiation to the bladder was reported in 1995. The 5-year relapse-free survival was 84% for T2, 53% for T3, and 11% for T4 cancers. Importantly, only 18% of the surviving patients had an intact bladder [166]. Bladder preservation is an admirable goal for the healthy individual with an early invasive T2 lesion within the bladder, but it appears that most patients who are cured by this approach ultimately require a radical cystectomy. The older patient must be prepared to submit to the toxicity of the combined therapy while maintaining the potential requirement of a radical cystectomy. Therefore, multimodality therapy for TCC must be considered experimental for patients of all ages, particularly for the person over 70 years of age.

Conclusions

Improvements in diagnostic imaging, surgical techniques, advanced instrumentation, and systemic chemotherapy have been combined to offer older individuals a wide array of treatment options for renal and bladder malignancies. However, the myriad issues confronting these people serve only to complicate the choice of therapy. The literature suggests that aging may affect negatively the treatment response of superficial disease and the outcomes of curative surgery. Comprehensive geriatric assessment tools that incorporate not only age but also physiologic and biologic considerations, such as comorbidities, functional status, renal function, and hemoglobin are necessary to help stratify the elderly into "fit" and "frail" populations, allowing tailoring of appropriate therapy. Clinicians must avoid the unconscious bias against curative treatment for an elderly individual and thoroughly address all potential options and the impact of these in the patient's context of quality of life. Age-specific investigations in conjunction with comprehensive assessment tools are needed before the best treatment options for geriatric patients are identified.

CASE STUDY

Mr. M who initially presented as a 75-year-old male with multiple medical problems including a history significant for coronary artery disease, on ultrasound for right upper quadrant pain, was found to have a 3-cm solid mass in the right lower pole of the kidney. This mass was verified as "enhancing" by a gadolinium-enhanced magnetic resonance imaging (MRI), which was substituted for computed tomography (CT) due to a history of chronic renal insufficiency with a glomerular filtration rate (GFR) of 35 mL/min. All other testing including chest radiograph and blood laboratories were negative for evidence of metastatic disease. Preoperative cardiology evaluation placed him at high risk for a post-surgical event due to his coronary artery disease. The patient was counseled regarding the options for this likely malignant renal mass which included conservative management (surveillance with serial imaging), surgical removal (radical/partial nephrectomy), and new minimally invasive techniques (cryotherapy, radiofrequency ablation). Although the patient was at high risk for open surgery, he was not comfortable following this lesion and wished to have curative treatment. Percutaneous cryotherapy was performed (Fig. 80.2) under local anesthetic with no sedation. The lesion was biopsied during the procedure which revealed a clear cell renal carcinoma – intermediate grade. The procedure was uneventful, and the patient was discharged on the same day.

Mr. M is currently 80 years old with stable coronary artery disease and still very active. All posttreatment imaging since the procedure show "no enhancement" which is consistent with successful treatment. This case highlights the many factors that must be considered when treating genitourinary malignancies in the elderly population.

References

1. Edwards BK, Howe HL, Ries LA et al (2002) Annual report to the nation on the status of cancer, 1973–1999, featuring implications of age and aging on U.S. cancer burden. Cancer 94(10): 2766–2792

2. Pantuck AJ, Zisman A, Belldegrun AS (2001) The changing natural history of renal cell carcinoma. J Urol 166(5):1611–1623

3. Jemal A, Siegel R, Ward E, Hao Y, Xu J, Thun MJ (2009) Cancer statistics, 2009. CA Cancer J Clin 59(4):225–249

4. Dechet CB, Sebo T, Farrow G, Blute ML, Engen DE, Zincke H (1999) Prospective analysis of intraoperative frozen needle biopsy of solid renal masses in adults. J Urol 162(4):1282–1284; discussion 4–5

5. Nelson CP, Sanda MG (2002) Contemporary diagnosis and management of renal angiomyolipoma. J Urol 168(4 Pt 1):1315–1325

6. Bissler JJ, Kingswood JC (2004) Renal angiomyolipomata. Kidney Int 66(3):924–934

7. Bosniak MA, Megibow AJ, Hulnick DH, Horii S, Raghavendra BN (1988) CT diagnosis of renal angiomyolipoma: the importance of detecting small amounts of fat. AJR Am J Roentgenol 151(3):497–501

8. Choyke PL, Glenn GM, Walther MM, Zbar B, Linehan WM (2003) Hereditary renal cancers. Radiology 226(1):33–46

9. Hwang JJ, Uchio EM, Linehan WM, Walther MM (2003) Hereditary kidney cancer. Urol Clin North Am 30(4):831–842

10. Dhote R, Thiounn N, Debre B, Vidal-Trecan G (2004) Risk factors for adult renal cell carcinoma. Urol Clin North Am 31(2): 237–247

11. Iliopoulos O, Eng C (2000) Genetic and clinical aspects of familial renal neoplasms. Semin Oncol 27(2):138–149

12. Maher ER, Yates JR, Harries R et al (1990) Clinical features and natural history of von Hippel–Lindau disease. Q J Med 77(283): 1151–1163

13. Latif F, Tory K, Gnarra J et al (1993) Identification of the von Hippel–Lindau disease tumor suppressor gene. Science 260(5112): 1317–1320

14. Zambrano NR, Lubensky IA, Merino MJ, Linehan WM, Walther MM (1999) Histopathology and molecular genetics of renal tumors toward unification of a classification system. J Urol 162(4): 1246–1258

15. Gnarra JR, Tory K, Weng Y et al (1994) Mutations of the VHL tumour suppressor gene in renal carcinoma. Nat Genet 7(1): 85–90

16. Shuin T, Kondo K, Torigoe S et al (1994) Frequent somatic mutations and loss of heterozygosity of the von Hippel–Lindau tumor suppressor gene in primary human renal cell carcinomas. Cancer Res 54(11):2852–2855

17. Bosniak MA (1995) Observation of small incidentally detected renal masses. Semin Urol Oncol 13(4):267–272

18. Bosniak MA, Birnbaum BA, Krinsky GA, Waisman J (1995) Small renal parenchymal neoplasms: further observations on growth. Radiology 197(3):589–597

19. Volpe A, Panzarella T, Rendon RA, Haider MA, Kondylis FI, Jewett MA (2004) The natural history of incidentally detected small renal masses. Cancer 100(4):738–745

20. Skinner DG, Colvin RB, Vermillion CD, Pfister RC, Leadbetter WF (1971) Diagnosis and management of renal cell carcinoma. A clinical and pathologic study of 309 cases. Cancer 28(5): 1165–1177

21. Thrasher JB, Paulson DF (1993) Prognostic factors in renal cancer. Urol Clin North Am 20(2):247–262

22. Edge SB, American Joint Committee on Cancer, American Cancer Society (2010) AJCC cancer staging handbook: from the AJCC cancer staging manual, 7th edn. Springer, New York

23. Jayson M, Sanders H (1998) Increased incidence of serendipitously discovered renal cell carcinoma. Urology 51(2):203–205

24. Ritchie AW, Chisholm GD (1983) The natural history of renal carcinoma. Semin Oncol 10(4):390–400

25. Chow WH, Devesa SS, Warren JL, Fraumeni JF Jr (1999) Rising incidence of renal cell cancer in the United States. JAMA 281(17):1628–1631

26. Homma Y, Kawabe K, Kitamura T et al (1995) Increased incidental detection and reduced mortality in renal cancer–recent retrospective analysis at eight institutions. Int J Urol 2(2):77–80

27. Carini M, Selli C, Barbanti G, Lapini A, Turini D, Costantini A (1988) Conservative surgical treatment of renal cell carcinoma: clinical experience and reappraisal of indications. J Urol 140(4):725–731

28. Chawla SN, Crispen PL, Hanlon AL, Greenberg RE, Chen DY, Uzzo RG (2006) The natural history of observed enhancing renal masses: meta-analysis and review of the world literature. J Urol 175(2):425–431

29. Abouassaly R, Lane BR, Novick AC (2008) Active surveillance of renal masses in elderly patients. J Urol 180(2):505–508; discussion 8–9

30. Klatte T, Patard JJ, de Martino M et al (2008) Tumor size does not predict risk of metastatic disease or prognosis of small renal cell carcinomas. J Urol 179(5):1719–1726

31. Campbell SC, Novick AC, Belldegrun A et al (2009) Guideline for management of the clinical T1 renal mass. J Urol 182(4): 1271–1279

32. Washburn ZW, Dillman JR, Cohan RH, Caoili EM, Ellis JH (2009) Computed tomographic urography update: an evolving urinary tract imaging modality. Semin Ultrasound CT MR 30(4):233–245

33. Mulholland SG, Stefanelli JL (1990) Genitourinary cancer in the elderly. Am J Kidney Dis 16(4):324–328

34. Bosniak MA (1997) The use of the Bosniak classification system for renal cysts and cystic tumors. J Urol 157(5):1852–1853

35. Davidson AJ, Hartman DS, Choyke PL, Wagner BJ (1997) Radiologic assessment of renal masses: implications for patient care. Radiology 202(2):297–305

36. Trivedi H, Raman L, Benjamin H, Batwara R (2009) Lack of nephrotoxicity of gadodiamide in unselected hospitalized patients. Postgrad Med 121(5):166–170

37. Grobner T (2006) Gadolinium – a specific trigger for the development of nephrogenic fibrosing dermopathy and nephrogenic systemic fibrosis? Nephrol Dial Transplant 21(4):1104–1108

38. Altun E, Martin DR, Wertman R, Lugo-Somolinos A, Fuller ER III, Semelka RC (2009) Nephrogenic systemic fibrosis: change in incidence following a switch in gadolinium agents and adoption of a gadolinium policy – report from two U.S. universities. Radiology 253(3):689–696

39. Thomsen HS (2009) How to avoid nephrogenic systemic fibrosis: current guidelines in Europe and the United States. Radiol Clin North Am 47(5):871–875; vii

40. Thomsen HS, Morcos SK, Barrett BJ (2008) Contrast-induced nephropathy: the wheel has turned 360 degrees. Acta Radiol 49(6):646–657

41. Idee JM, Port M, Dencausse A, Lancelot E, Corot C (2009) Involvement of gadolinium chelates in the mechanism of nephrogenic systemic fibrosis: an update. Radiol Clin North Am 47(5):855–869; vii

42. Robson CJ, Churchill BM, Anderson W (1969) The results of radical nephrectomy for renal cell carcinoma. J Urol 101(3):297–301

43. Pantuck AJ, Zisman A, Dorey F et al (2003) Renal cell carcinoma with retroperitoneal lymph nodes. Impact on survival and benefits of immunotherapy. Cancer 97(12):2995–3002

44. Hellsten S, Johnsen J, Berge T, Linell F (1990) Clinically unrecognized renal cell carcinoma. Diagnostic and pathological aspects. Eur Urol 18(Suppl 2):23

45. Golimbu M, Joshi P, Sperber A, Tessler A, Al-Askari S, Morales P (1986) Renal cell carcinoma: survival and prognostic factors. Urology 27(4):291–301

46. Giuliani L, Giberti C, Martorana G, Rovida S (1990) Radical extensive surgery for renal cell carcinoma: long-term results and prognostic factors. J Urol 143(3):468–473; discussion 73–74

47. Kontak JA, Campbell SC (2003) Prognostic factors in renal cell carcinoma. Urol Clin North Am 30(3):467–480

48. Ramon J, Goldwasser B, Raviv G, Jonas P, Many M (1991) Long-term results of simple and radical nephrectomy for renal cell carcinoma. Cancer 67(10):2506–2511

49. Siemer S, Lehmann J, Loch A et al (2005) Current TNM classification of renal cell carcinoma evaluated: revising stage T3a. J Urol 173(1):33–37

50. Thrasher JB, Crawford ED (1993) Current management of invasive and metastatic transitional cell carcinoma of the bladder. J Urol 149(5):957–972

51. Haas NB, Uzzo R (2008) Adjuvant therapy for renal cell carcinoma. Curr Oncol Rep 10(3):245–252

52. Clayman RV, Kavoussi LR, Soper NJ et al (1991) Laparoscopic nephrectomy: initial case report. J Urol 146(2):278–282

53. Meraney AM, Gill IS (2002) Financial analysis of open versus laparoscopic radical nephrectomy and nephroureterectomy. J Urol 167(4):1757–1762

54. Ono Y, Hattori R, Gotoh M, Yoshino Y, Yoshikawa Y, Kamihira O (2005) Laparoscopic radical nephrectomy for renal cell carcinoma: the standard of care already? Curr Opin Urol 15(2):75–78

55. Portis AJ, Yan Y, Landman J et al (2002) Long-term followup after laparoscopic radical nephrectomy. J Urol 167(3):1257–1262

56. Chacko JK, Koyle MA, Mingin GC, Furness PD III (2007) Minimally invasive open renal surgery. J Urol 178(4 Pt 2):1575–1577; discussion 7–8

57. Eden CG, Haigh AC, Carter PG, Coptcoat MJ (1994) Laparoscopic nephrectomy results in better postoperative pulmonary function. J Endourol 8(6):419–422; discussion 22–23

58. Badger WJ, Gallagher BL, Szeluga DJ, Winfield HN (2008) Hurdles to helium gas laparoscopy and a readily available alternative. J Endourol 22(11):2455–2459

59. Lai FC, Kau EL, Ng CS, Fuchs GJ (2007) Laparoscopic nephrectomy outcomes of elderly patients in the 21st century. J Endourol 21(11):1309–1313

60. Najarian JS, Chavers BM, McHugh LE, Matas AJ (1992) 20 years or more of follow-up of living kidney donors. Lancet 340(8823):807–810

61. Goldfarb DA, Matin SF, Braun WE et al (2001) Renal outcome 25 years after donor nephrectomy. J Urol 166(6):2043–2047

62. Bijol V, Mendez GP, Hurwitz S, Rennke HG, Nose V (2006) Evaluation of the nonneoplastic pathology in tumor nephrectomy specimens: predicting the risk of progressive renal failure. Am J Surg Pathol 30(5):575–584

63. Huang WC, Levey AS, Serio AM et al (2006) Chronic kidney disease after nephrectomy in patients with renal cortical tumours: a retrospective cohort study. Lancet Oncol 7(9):735–740

64. Castilla EA, Liou LS, Abrahams NA et al (2002) Prognostic importance of resection margin width after nephron-sparing surgery for renal cell carcinoma. Urology 60(6):993–997

65. Uzzo RG, Novick AC (2001) Nephron sparing surgery for renal tumors: indications, techniques and outcomes. J Urol 166(1):6–18

66. Lee CT, Katz J, Shi W, Thaler HT, Reuter VE, Russo P (2000) Surgical management of renal tumors 4 cm. or less in a contemporary cohort. J Urol 163(3):730–736

67. Stephenson AJ, Hakimi AA, Snyder ME, Russo P (2004) Complications of radical and partial nephrectomy in a large contemporary cohort. J Urol 171(1):130–134

68. Thomas AA, Aron M, Hernandez AV, Lane BR, Gill IS (2009) Laparoscopic partial nephrectomy in octogenarians. Urology 74(5):1042–1046

69. Michaels MJ, Rhee HK, Mourtzinos AP, Summerhayes IC, Silverman ML, Libertino JA (2002) Incomplete renal tumor destruction using radio frequency interstitial ablation. J Urol 168(6):2406–2409; discussion 9–10

70. Rendon RA, Kachura JR, Sweet JM et al (2002) The uncertainty of radio frequency treatment of renal cell carcinoma: findings at immediate and delayed nephrectomy. J Urol 167(4):1587–1592

71. Matlaga BR, Zagoria RJ, Woodruff RD, Torti FM, Hall MC (2002) Phase II trial of radio frequency ablation of renal cancer: evaluation of the kill zone. J Urol 168(6):2401–2405

72. Motzer RJ, Hutson TE, Tomczak P et al (2007) Sunitinib versus interferon alfa in metastatic renal-cell carcinoma. N Engl J Med 356(2):115–124

73. Balducci L (2009) Supportive care in elderly cancer patients. Curr Opin Oncol 21(4):310–317

74. Balducci L (2009) Pharmacology of antineoplastic medications in older cancer patients. Oncology (Williston Park) 23(1):78–85

75. Yagoda A, Abi-Rached B, Petrylak D (1995) Chemotherapy for advanced renal-cell carcinoma: 1983–1993. Semin Oncol 22(1):42–60

76. Milowsky MI, Nanus DM (2003) Chemotherapeutic strategies for renal cell carcinoma. Urol Clin North Am 30(3):601–609, x

77. Kroog GS, Motzer RJ (2008) Systemic therapy for metastatic renal cell carcinoma. Urol Clin North Am 35(4):687–701, ix

78. Dutcher JP, Fisher RI, Weiss G et al (1997) Outpatient subcutaneous interleukin-2 and interferon-alpha for metastatic renal cell cancer: five-year follow-up of the Cytokine Working Group Study. Cancer J Sci Am 3(3):157–162

79. Negrier S, Escudier B, Lasset C et al (1998) Recombinant human interleukin-2, recombinant human interferon alfa-2a, or both in metastatic renal-cell carcinoma. Groupe Francais d'Immunotherapie. N Engl J Med 338(18):1272–1278

80. Yang JC, Sherry RM, Steinberg SM et al (2003) Randomized study of high-dose and low-dose interleukin-2 in patients with metastatic renal cancer. J Clin Oncol 21(16):3127–3132

81. Hudes G, Carducci M, Tomczak P et al (2007) Temsirolimus, interferon alfa, or both for advanced renal-cell carcinoma. N Engl J Med 356(22):2271–2281

82. Escudier B, Eisen T, Stadler WM et al (2007) Sorafenib in advanced clear-cell renal-cell carcinoma. N Engl J Med 356(2):125–134

83. Motzer RJ, Escudier B, Oudard S et al (2008) Efficacy of everolimus in advanced renal cell carcinoma: a double-blind, randomised, placebo-controlled phase III trial. Lancet 372(9637):449–456

84. Gore ME, Szczylik C, Porta C et al (2009) Safety and efficacy of sunitinib for metastatic renal-cell carcinoma: an expanded-access trial. Lancet Oncol 10(8):757–763

85. Schultzel M, Saltzstein SL, Downs TM, Shimasaki S, Sanders C, Sadler GR (2008) Late age (85 years or older) peak incidence of bladder cancer. J Urol 179(4):1302–1305; discussion 5–6

86. Prout GR Jr, Wesley MN, Yancik R, Ries LA, Havlik RJ, Edwards BK (2005) Age and comorbidity impact surgical therapy in older bladder carcinoma patients: a population-based study. Cancer 104(8):1638–1647

87. Konety BR, Joslyn SA (2003) Factors influencing aggressive therapy for bladder cancer: an analysis of data from the SEER program. J Urol 170(5):1765–1771

88. Briggs NC, Young TB, Gilchrist KW, Vaillancourt AM, Messing EM (1992) Age as a predictor of an aggressive clinical course for superficial bladder cancer in men. Cancer 69(6):1445–1451

89. Mariani AJ, Mariani MC, Macchioni C, Stams UK, Hariharan A, Moriera A (1989) The significance of adult hematuria: 1,000

hematuria evaluations including a risk-benefit and cost-effectiveness analysis. J Urol 141(2):350–355

90. Britton JP, Dowell AC, Whelan P, Harris CM (1992) A community study of bladder cancer screening by the detection of occult urinary bleeding. J Urol 148(3):788–790

91. Vikram R, Sandler CM, Ng CS (2009) Imaging and staging of transitional cell carcinoma: part 1, lower urinary tract. AJR Am J Roentgenol 192(6):1481–1487

92. Sidransky D, Von Eschenbach A, Tsai YC et al (1991) Identification of p53 gene mutations in bladder cancers and urine samples. Science 252(5006):706–709

93. Feng Z, Hu W, Teresky AK, Hernando E, Cordon-Cardo C, Levine AJ (2007) Declining p53 function in the aging process: a possible mechanism for the increased tumor incidence in older populations. Proc Natl Acad Sci U S A 104(42):16633–16638

94. Stuart GR, Oda Y, de Boer JG, Glickman BW (2000) Mutation frequency and specificity with age in liver, bladder and brain of lacI transgenic mice. Genetics 154(3):1291–1300

95. Taylor JA 3rd, Kuchel GA (2009) Bladder cancer in the elderly: clinical outcomes, basic mechanisms, and future research direction. Nat Clin Pract Urol 6(3):135–144

96. Bornman DM, Mathew S, Alsruhe J, Herman JG, Gabrielson E (2001) Methylation of the E-cadherin gene in bladder neoplasia and in normal urothelial epithelium from elderly individuals. Am J Pathol 159(3):831–835

97. Habuchi T, Takahashi T, Kakinuma H et al (2001) Hypermethylation at 9q32-33 tumour suppressor region is age-related in normal urothelium and an early and frequent alteration in bladder cancer. Oncogene 20(4):531–537

98. Gu J, Spitz MR, Zhao H et al (2005) Roles of tumor suppressor and telomere maintenance genes in cancer and aging–an epidemiological study. Carcinogenesis 26(10):1741–1747

99. Koch M, Hill GB, McPhee MS (1986) Factors affecting recurrence rates in superficial bladder cancer. J Natl Cancer Inst 76(6):1025–1029

100. Cooksley CD, Avritscher EB, Grossman HB et al (2008) Clinical model of cost of bladder cancer in the elderly. Urology 71(3):519–525

101. Ro JY, Staerkel GA, Ayala AG (1992) Cytologic and histologic features of superficial bladder cancer. Urol Clin North Am 19(3):435–453

102. Fitzpatrick JM, West AB, Butler MR, Lane V, O'Flynn JD (1986) Superficial bladder tumors (stage pTa, grades 1 and 2): the importance of recurrence pattern following initial resection. J Urol 135(5):920–922

103. Torti FM, Lum BL, Aston D et al (1987) Superficial bladder cancer: the primacy of grade in the development of invasive disease. J Clin Oncol 5(1):125–130

104. Heney NM, Ahmed S, Flanagan MJ et al (1983) Superficial bladder cancer: progression and recurrence. J Urol 130(6):1083–1086

105. Kiemeney LA, Witjes JA, Heijbroek RP, Verbeek AL, Debruyne FM (1993) Predictability of recurrent and progressive disease in individual patients with primary superficial bladder cancer. J Urol 150(1):60–64

106. Allard P, Bernard P, Fradet Y, Tetu B (1998) The early clinical course of primary Ta and T1 bladder cancer: a proposed prognostic index. Br J Urol 81(5):692–698

107. Millan-Rodriguez F, Chechile-Toniolo G, Salvador-Bayarri J, Palou J, Algaba F, Vicente-Rodriguez J (2000) Primary superficial bladder cancer risk groups according to progression, mortality and recurrence. J Urol 164(3 Pt 1):680–684

108. Holmang S, Hedelin H, Anderstrom C, Johansson SL (1995) The relationship among multiple recurrences, progression and prognosis of patients with stages Ta and T1 transitional cell cancer of the bladder followed for at least 20 years. J Urol 153(6):1823–1826; discussion 6–7

109. Pagano F, Garbeglio A, Milani C, Bassi P, Pegoraro V (1987) Prognosis of bladder cancer I. Risk factors in superficial transitional cell carcinoma. Eur Urol 13(3):145–149

110. Althausen AF, Prout GR Jr, Daly JJ (1976) Non-invasive papillary carcinoma of the bladder associated with carcinoma in situ. J Urol 116(5):575–580

111. Wallace DM, Hindmarsh JR, Webb JN et al (1979) The role of multiple mucosal biopsies in the management of patients with bladder cancer. Br J Urol 51(6):535–540

112. Farrow GM, Utz DC, Rife CC, Greene LF (1977) Clinical observations on sixty-nine cases of in situ carcinoma of the urinary bladder. Cancer Res 37(8 Pt 2):2794–2798

113. Bostwick DG (1992) Natural history of early bladder cancer. J Cell Biochem Suppl 16I:31–38

114. Prout GR Jr, Griffin PP, Daly JJ (1987) The outcome of conservative treatment of carcinoma in situ of the bladder. J Urol 138(4):766–770

115. Witjes JA, Mungan NA, Debruyne FM (2000) Management of superficial bladder cancer with intravesical chemotherapy: an update. Urology 56(1):19–21

116. Peyromaure M, Zerbib M (2004) T1G3 transitional cell carcinoma of the bladder: recurrence, progression and survival. BJU Int 93(1):60–63

117. Soloway MS, Sofer M, Vaidya A (2002) Contemporary management of stage T1 transitional cell carcinoma of the bladder. J Urol 167(4):1573–1583

118. Smith JA Jr, Labasky RF, Cockett AT, Fracchia JA, Montie JE, Rowland RG (1999) Bladder cancer clinical guidelines panel summary report on the management of nonmuscle invasive bladder cancer (stages Ta, T1 and TIS). The American Urological Association. J Urol 162(5):1697–1701

119. Sylvester RJ, der MA Van, Lamm DL (2002) Intravesical Bacillus Calmette-Guerin reduces the risk of progression in patients with superficial bladder cancer: a meta-analysis of the published results of randomized clinical trials. J Urol 168(5):1964–1970

120. Cookson MS, Sarosdy MF (1992) Management of stage T1 superficial bladder cancer with intravesical bacillus Calmette–Guerin therapy. J Urol 148(3):797–801

121. Bohle A, Bock PR (2004) Intravesical bacille Calmette–Guerin versus mitomycin C in superficial bladder cancer: formal meta-analysis of comparative studies on tumor progression. Urology 63(4):682–686; discussion 6–7

122. Herr HW (1997) High-risk superficial bladder cancer: transurethral resection alone in selected patients with T1 tumor. Semin Urol Oncol 15(3):142–146

123. Miladi M, Peyromaure M, Zerbib M, Saighi D, Debre B (2003) The value of a second transurethral resection in evaluating patients with bladder tumours. Eur Urol 43(3):241–245

124. Herr HW (1997) Tumour progression and survival in patients with T1G3 bladder tumours: 15-year outcome. Br J Urol 80(5):762–765

125. Oosterlinck W, Lobel B, Jakse G, Malmstrom PU, Stockle M, Sternberg C (2002) Guidelines on bladder cancer. Eur Urol 41(2):105–112

126. Esrig D, Freeman JA, Stein JP, Skinner DG (1997) Early cystectomy for clinical stage T1 transitional cell carcinoma of the bladder. Semin Urol Oncol 15(3):154–160

127. Barlow LJ, McKiernan JM, Benson MC (2009) The novel use of intravesical docetaxel for the treatment of non-muscle invasive bladder cancer refractory to BCG therapy: a single institution experience. World J Urol 27(3):331–335

128. Martinez-Pineiro JA, Jimenez Leon J, Martinez-Pineiro L Jr et al (1990) Bacillus Calmette–Guerin versus doxorubicin versus thiotepa: a randomized prospective study in 202 patients with superficial bladder cancer. J Urol 143(3):502–506

129. Sylvester RJ, van der Meijden AP, Witjes JA, Kurth K (2005) Bacillus Calmette–Guerin versus chemotherapy for the intravesical

treatment of patients with carcinoma in situ of the bladder: a meta-analysis of the published results of randomized clinical trials. J Urol 174(1):86–91; discussion 2

130. Shelley MD, Court JB, Kynaston H, Wilt TJ, Coles B, Mason M (2003) Intravesical Bacillus Calmette–Guerin versus mitomycin C for Ta and T1 bladder cancer. Cochrane Database Syst Rev (3):CD003231

131. Shelley MD, Court JB, Kynaston H, Wilt TJ, Fish RG, Mason M (2000) Intravesical Bacillus Calmette–Guerin in Ta and T1 bladder cancer. Cochrane Database Syst Rev (4):CD001986

132. Lamm DL (1991) Comparison of BCG with other intravesical agents. Urology 37(5 Suppl):30–32

133. Lamm DL, Blumenstein BA, Crissman JD et al (2000) Maintenance bacillus Calmette–Guerin immunotherapy for recurrent TA, T1 and carcinoma in situ transitional cell carcinoma of the bladder: a randomized Southwest Oncology Group Study. J Urol 163(4):1124–1129

134. Martinez-Pineiro JA, Martinez-Pineiro L, Solsona E et al (2005) Has a 3-fold decreased dose of bacillus Calmette–Guerin the same efficacy against recurrences and progression of T1G3 and Tis bladder tumors than the standard dose? Results of a prospective randomized trial. J Urol 174(4 Pt 1):1242–1247

135. Herr HW (2007) Age and outcome of superficial bladder cancer treated with bacille Calmette-Guerin therapy. Urology 70(1):65–68

136. Droller MJ (1992) Treatment of regionally advanced bladder cancer. An overview. Urol Clin North Am 19(4):685–693

137. Silverman DT, Hartge P, Morrison AS, Devesa SS (1992) Epidemiology of bladder cancer. Hematol Oncol Clin North Am 6(1):1–30

138. Tekes A, Kamel I, Imam K et al (2005) Dynamic MRI of bladder cancer: evaluation of staging accuracy. AJR Am J Roentgenol 184(1):121–127

139. Kim B, Semelka RC, Ascher SM, Chalpin DB, Carroll PR, Hricak H (1994) Bladder tumor staging: comparison of contrast-enhanced CT, T1- and T2-weighted MR imaging, dynamic gadolinium-enhanced imaging, and late gadolinium-enhanced imaging. Radiology 193(1):239–245

140. Tanimoto A, Yuasa Y, Imai Y et al (1992) Bladder tumor staging: comparison of conventional and gadolinium-enhanced dynamic MR imaging and CT. Radiology 185(3):741–747

141. Herr HW (2001) Transurethral resection of muscle-invasive bladder cancer: 10-year outcome. J Clin Oncol 19(1):89–93

142. Schrag D, Hsieh LJ, Rabbani F, Bach PB, Herr H, Begg CB (2003) Adherence to surveillance among patients with superficial bladder cancer. J Natl Cancer Inst 95(8):588–597

143. Skinner DG, Lieskovsky G (1984) Contemporary cystectomy with pelvic node dissection compared to preoperative radiation therapy plus cystectomy in management of invasive bladder cancer. J Urol 131(6):1069–1072

144. Reisinger SA, Mohiuddin M, Mulholland SG (1992) Combined pre- and postoperative adjuvant radiation therapy for bladder cancer—a ten year experience. Int J Radiat Oncol Biol Phys 24(3): 463–468

145. Wammack R, Wricke C, Hohenfellner R (2002) Long-term results of ileocecal continent urinary diversion in patients treated with and without previous pelvic irradiation. J Urol 167(5):2058–2062

146. Chamie K, Hu B, Devere White RW, Ellison LM (2008) Cystectomy in the elderly: does the survival benefit in younger patients translate to the octogenarians? BJU Int 3:284–290

147. Nielsen ME, Shariat SF, Karakiewicz PI et al (2007) Advanced age is associated with poorer bladder cancer-specific survival in patients treated with radical cystectomy. Eur Urol 51(3):699–706; discussion 8

148. Weizer AZ, Joshi D, Daignault S et al (2007) Performance status is a predictor of overall survival of elderly patients with muscle invasive bladder cancer. J Urol 177(4):1287–1293

149. Stroumbakis N, Herr HW, Cookson MS, Fair WR (1997) Radical cystectomy in the octogenarian. J Urol 158(6):2113–2117

150. Roehrborn CG, Sagalowsky AI, Peters PC (1991) Long-term patient survival after cystectomy for regional metastatic transitional cell carcinoma of the bladder. J Urol 146(1):36–39

151. Leissner J, Ghoneim MA, Abol-Enein H et al (2004) Extended radical lymphadenectomy in patients with urothelial bladder cancer: results of a prospective multicenter study. J Urol 171(1): 139–144

152. Smith AB, Nielsen ME, Wallen EM, Pruthi RS. Current status of robot-assisted radical cystectomy. Curr Opin Urol. 2009 Oct 28

153. Pruthi RS, Smith A, Wallen EM (2008) Evaluating the learning curve for robot-assisted laparoscopic radical cystectomy. J Endourol 22(11):2469–2474

154. Sternberg CN (1995) The treatment of advanced bladder cancer. Ann Oncol 6(2):113–126

155. Loehrer PJ Sr, Einhorn LH, Elson PJ et al (1992) A randomized comparison of cisplatin alone or in combination with methotrexate, vinblastine, and doxorubicin in patients with metastatic urothelial carcinoma: a cooperative group study. J Clin Oncol 10(7):1066–1073

156. Logothetis CJ, Dexeus FH, Finn L et al (1990) A prospective randomized trial comparing MVAC and CISCA chemotherapy for patients with metastatic urothelial tumors. J Clin Oncol 8(6): 1050–1055

157. Harker WG, Meyers FJ, Freiha FS et al (1985) Cisplatin, methotrexate, and vinblastine (CMV): an effective chemotherapy regimen for metastatic transitional cell carcinoma of the urinary tract. A Northern California Oncology Group study. J Clin Oncol 3(11): 1463–1470

158. Moore MJ, Tannock IF, Ernst DS, Huan S, Murray N (1997) Gemcitabine: a promising new agent in the treatment of advanced urothelial cancer. J Clin Oncol 15(12):3441–3445

159. Bamias A, Efstathiou E, Moulopoulos LA et al (2005) The outcome of elderly patients with advanced urothelial carcinoma after platinum-based combination chemotherapy. Ann Oncol 16(2): 307–313

160. Castagneto B, Zai S, Marenco D et al (2004) Single-agent gemcitabine in previously untreated elderly patients with advanced bladder carcinoma: response to treatment and correlation with the comprehensive geriatric assessment. Oncology 67(1): 27–32

161. Linardou H, Aravantinos G, Efstathiou E et al (2004) Gemcitabine and carboplatin combination as first-line treatment in elderly patients and those unfit for cisplatin-based chemotherapy with advanced bladder carcinoma: Phase II study of the Hellenic Co-operative Oncology Group. Urology 64(3):479–484

162. Bamias A, Lainakis G, Kastritis E et al (2007) Biweekly carboplatin/gemcitabine in patients with advanced urothelial cancer who are unfit for cisplatin-based chemotherapy: report of efficacy, quality of life and geriatric assessment. Oncology 73(5–6): 290–297

163. Grossman HB, Natale RB, Tangen CM et al (2003) Neoadjuvant chemotherapy plus cystectomy compared with cystectomy alone for locally advanced bladder cancer. N Engl J Med 349(9): 859–866

164. Malmstrom PU, Rintala E, Wahlqvist R, Hellstrom P, Hellsten S, Hannisdal E (1996) Five-year followup of a prospective trial of radical cystectomy and neoadjuvant chemotherapy: nordic cystectomy trial I. The Nordic Cooperative Bladder Cancer Study Group. J Urol 155(6):1903–1906

165. Salminen E (1990) Recurrence and treatment of urinary bladder cancer after failure in radiotherapy. Cancer 66(11):2341–2345

166. Given RW, Parsons JT, McCarley D, Wajsman Z (1995) Bladder-sparing multimodality treatment of muscle-invasive bladder cancer: a five-year follow-up. Urology 46(4):499–504; discussion 5

167. Brennan P, Bogillot O, Cordier S et al (2000) Cigarette smoking and bladder cancer in men: a pooled analysis of 11 case-control studies. Int J Cancer 86(2):289–294

168. Morrison AS, Buring JE, Verhoek WG et al (1984) An international study of smoking and bladder cancer. J Urol 131(4): 650–654

169. Piper JM, Tonascia J, Matanoski GM (1985) Heavy phenacetin use and bladder cancer in women aged 20 to 49 years. N Engl J Med 313(5):292–295

170. Fortuny J, Kogevinas M, Zens MS et al (2007) Analgesic and anti-inflammatory drug use and risk of bladder cancer: a population based case control study. BMC Urol 7:13

171. Porpaczy P, Schramek P (1981) Analgesic nephropathy and phenacetin-induced transitional cell carcinoma - analysis of 300 patients with long-term consumption of phenacetin-containing drugs. Eur Urol 7(6):349–354

172. Cole P, Hoover R, Friedell GH (1972) Occupation and cancer of the lower urinary tract. Cancer 29(5):1250–1260

173. Case RA, Pearson JT (1954) Tumours of the urinary bladder in workmen engaged in the manufacture and use of certain dyestuff intermediates in the British chemical industry. II. Further consideration of the role of aniline and of the manufacture of auramine and magenta (fuchsine) as possible causative agents. Br J Ind Med 11(3):213–216

174. Gaertner RR, Trpeski L, Johnson KC (2004) A case-control study of occupational risk factors for bladder cancer in Canada. Cancer Causes Control 15(10):1007–1019

175. Travis LB, Curtis RE, Glimelius B et al (1995) Bladder and kidney cancer following cyclophosphamide therapy for non-Hodgkin's lymphoma. J Natl Cancer Inst 87(7):524–530

176. O'Keane JC (1988) Carcinoma of the urinary bladder after treatment with cyclophosphamide. N Engl J Med 319(13):871

177. Chrouser K, Leibovich B, Bergstralh E, Zincke H, Blute M (2005) Bladder cancer risk following primary and adjuvant external beam radiation for prostate cancer. J Urol 174(1):107–110; discussion 10–11

178. Sella A, Dexeus FH, Chong C, Ro JY, Logothetis CJ (1989) Radiation therapy-associated invasive bladder tumors. Urology 33(3):185–188

179. Delnay KM, Stonehill WH, Goldman H, Jukkola AF, Dmochowski RR (1999) Bladder histological changes associated with chronic indwelling urinary catheter. J Urol 161(4):1106–1108; discussion 8–9

180. Michaud DS (2007) Chronic inflammation and bladder cancer. Urol Oncol 25(3):260–268

181. Sala M, Cordier S, Chang-Claude J et al (2000) Coffee consumption and bladder cancer in nonsmokers: a pooled analysis of case-control studies in European countries. Cancer Causes Control 11(10):925–931

182. Zeegers MP, Dorant E, Goldbohm RA, van den Brandt PA (2001) Are coffee, tea, and total fluid consumption associated with bladder cancer risk? Results from the Netherlands Cohort Study. Cancer Causes Control 12(3):231–238

183. Takkouche B, Etminan M, Montes-Martinez A (2005) Personal use of hair dyes and risk of cancer: a meta-analysis. JAMA 293(20):2516–2525

184. Sontag JM (1980) Experimental identification of genitourinary carcinogens. Urol Clin North Am 7(3):803–814

185. Villanueva CM, Fernandez F, Malats N, Grimalt JO, Kogevinas M (2003) Meta-analysis of studies on individual consumption of chlorinated drinking water and bladder cancer. J Epidemiol Community Health 57(3):166–173

186. Marshall G, Ferreccio C, Yuan Y et al (2007) Fifty-year study of lung and bladder cancer mortality in Chile related to arsenic in drinking water. J Natl Cancer Inst 99(12):920–928

187. Kurth KH, Denis L, Bouffioux C et al (1995) Factors affecting recurrence and progression in superficial bladder tumours. Eur J Cancer 31A(11):1840–1846

Chapter 81
Benign and Malignant Diseases of the Prostate

John A. Taylor III and Peter C. Albertsen

CASE STUDY

An 82-year-old gentleman presents to his urologist with worsening LUTS in spite of combined medical therapy with Flomax and Proscar. His symptoms have become more of an obstructive nature with decreased force of stream, intermittency and need to strain. He is relatively healthy otherwise with only a-fib and HTN managed medically.

His evaluation reveals a flow rate of 6 ml/s with a post-void residual of 250 cc. His rectal exam reveals a very large prostate, which is benign in nature. His PSA, which had been stable at 3.4 ng/ml, has risen in the past year to 5.0 ng/ml. Urodynamic evaluation shows decreased detrusor contractility with borderline obstructive values. He is counseled on options including conservative management or a TURP. He is very concerned about his PSA results and has heard that Proscar can lead to high-grade prostate cancer. Prostate biopsy is discussed, which he chooses to proceed with in light of his desire to pursue aggressive treatment for his urinary symptoms.

He undergoes a 12 core transrectal biopsy which reveals <5% of one core with Gleason 3+3=6 disease. He is counseled on active surveillance, hormone ablation therapy, and external beam radiation in light of his advanced age. He is interested in discussing a robotic prostatectomy as his son just had one at 60. After a long discussion, he agrees to active surveillance. He ultimately undergoes a TURP for his progressive LUTS with good results and all benign tissue found pathologically. He eventually passes from a CVA 10 years later at 92.

Introduction

Benign prostatic hyperplasia (BPH) and prostate cancer are two common neoplastic processes that occur in elderly men. Both of these conditions are rare before the age of 50, but by age 80 more than 80% of men have pathologic evidence of benign hyperplasia and more than 50% have at least microscopic foci of prostate cancer [1, 2]. While BPH associated urinary symptoms will impact quality of life in most elderly men, the likelihood of prostate cancer resulting in significant morbidity remains low [3, 4]. This chapter reviews the incidence of these two diseases, the appropriate evaluation of elderly men and surgical options available to the geriatric patient as well as expected outcomes.

General Anatomical Considerations

The prostate is a glandular organ situated in the pelvis. The base of the prostate is in continuity with the bladder and the apex rests on the pelvic floor. It is composed predominantly of glandular elements with an investing fibromuscular stroma. The latter forms a capsule around the gland which is a unique feature of the human prostate [5]. The urethra runs through the gland with anterior angulation at the veru montanum, representing the exit site of the ejaculatory ducts. The prostate can be defined by anatomical zones (Fig. 81.1) or surgical lobes (Fig. 81.2), which have relevance to both BPH and prostate cancer.

Distinct zones are described based predominantly on the ductal drainage site within the urethra. The transition zone consists of periurethral tissue situated proximal to the veru montanum. The central zone surrounds the ejaculatory ducts, extending posteriorly to the bladder base. The posterior zone encompasses the remainder of tissue posterior to these two

J.A. Taylor III (✉)
Division of Urology, Department of Surgery, University of Connecticut Health Center, 263 Farmington Avenue, Farmingto, CT 06030, USA
e-mail: jtaylor@uchc.edu

R.A. Rosenthal et al. (eds.), *Principles and Practice of Geriatric Surgery*,
DOI 10.1007/978-1-4419-6999-6_81, © Springer Science+Business Media, LLC 2011

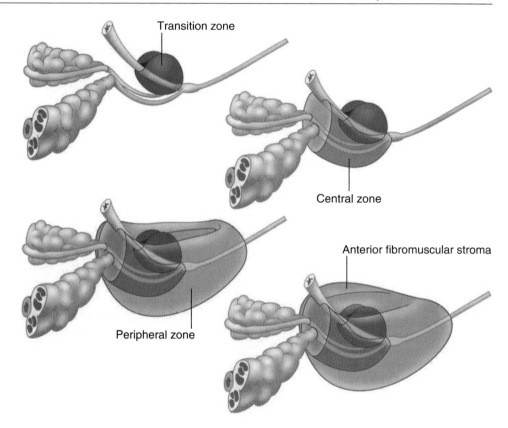

Figure 81.1 Zonal anatomy of the prostate as described by McNeal. (From McNeal JE. Normal histology of the prostate. Am J Surg Pathol 1988;12:619–633).

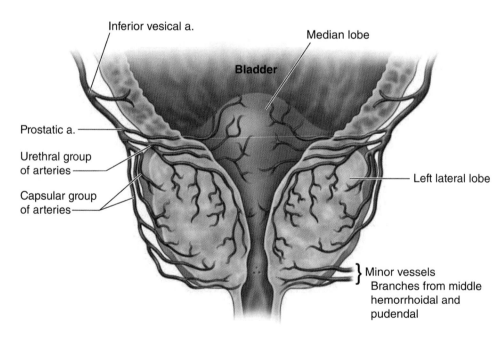

Figure 81.2 Surgical anatomy of the prostate. (Adapted from Gillenwater JY, ed: Adult and Pediatric Urology. St Louis: Mosby Yearbook, 1991:1214).

areas adjacent to the rectal vault and makes up the bulk of the nonpathologic gland. The anterior fibromuscular stroma is devoid of glandular elements and runs from the anterior bladder neck to the pelvic floor.

While BPH arises almost exclusively from the transition zone, 70% of prostate cancers originate in the posterior zone, with approximately 25 and 5% of cases stemming from the transition and central zones, respectively. Surgical lobes have also been described in relation to BPH. Lateral lobes are typically seen on cystoscopy as bilaterally bulging elements impinging on the prostatic urethra. A middle or central lobe represents the hyperplastic component that protrudes superiorly into the floor of the bladder, sometimes creating a perceived ball-valve effect on voiding.

Benign Prostatic Hyperplasia

Terminology

In order to understand the diagnostic and treatment dilemmas facing practitioners caring for the elderly gentleman with BPH, it is important to have working knowledge of the historical terminology used to describe the clinical symptoms. "BPH" represented an acronym for benign prostatic hypertrophy, as the majority of men with urinary symptoms were found to have enlarged prostates. However, from a histologic standpoint, the growth of the gland represents a hyperplastic process with increase in both glandular and stromal elements. Two problems with this new terminology were: (1) hyperplasia has been noted in prostates from men in their third decade of life who exhibit no urinary symptoms and (2) a linear correlation between prostate size and degree of urinary symptoms does not exist. Several other acronyms can be encountered that represent attempts to circumvent these issues. BPE (benign prostatic enlargement) and BOO (bladder outlet obstruction) represent such examples. Although BOO is pathophysiologically correct with regards to the underlying process, it remains a urodynamically defined element thus requiring a semi-invasive and costly test typically not viewed as necessary for treatment or diagnostic purposes. In order to get back to the clinical picture which leads patients to seek treatment yet another acronym was coined being LUTS (lower urinary tract symptoms). This covered the constellation of symptoms (urgency, frequency, hesitancy, intermittency, straining, sense of incomplete emptying, and nocturia) that were associated with the original "BPH." However, LUTS may be resultant from a diverse list of diagnoses not limited to the obstructive processes of an enlarged prostate [6]. Today ICD-9 coding includes both BPH with and BPH without LUTS.

Epidemiology

The prostate is small at birth, enlarges rapidly at onset of puberty, and then remains at a constant size during the next several decades of life. The average weight of the prostate slowly increases after 50 years of age with an associated increase in the incidence of symptomatic BPH (Fig. 81.3). Although the development of pathologic BPH is almost a universal phenomenon in aging men, the cause and

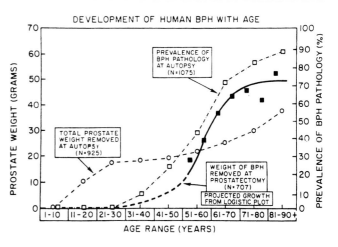

FIGURE 81.3 Development of human benign prostatic hyperplasia (BPH) with age: age-related changes in the weight of the prostate removed at autopsy in 925 men, prevalence of BP hyperplasia at autopsy in 1,075 men, and the weight of the adenoma removed at simple perineal prostatectomy in 707 men. *Long dashed line* indicates the mathematically extrapolated range in this group (From Berry et al. [1] with permission. Copyright Elsevier 1984).

pathogenesis of this disorder are poorly understood. While genetic susceptibility may play a role in younger patients, the relevance dramatically diminishes for those over 60. Androgens are recognized as necessary for the development of pathologic BPH; however, they are not the cause of BPH. While individuals castrated prior to puberty do not develop pathologic BPH, prostate size can continue to increase with age when androgen levels typically decline, suggesting little correlation between the two [7]. Several researchers have suggested that estrogen may contribute to the pathogenesis of BPH, but the alterations in estrogen and androgen production that occur with aging appear to be minor and occur after the onset of this disease [8]. Several other risk factors have been proposed, but to date there is no evidence to suggest that BPH can be attributed to any specific factor [9]. Researchers have investigated sociocultural variables including celibacy, specific blood groups, the use of alcohol or tobacco, and diseases commonly found among geriatric men such as coronary artery disease, peripheral vascular disease, hypertension, and diabetes.

Pathophysiology

The pathophysiology of symptomatic BPH is complex involving both static and dynamic components (Fig. 81.4). BPH is a true hyperplastic process with histologic studies demonstrating an increase in cell numbers throughout the gland. Hyperplasia occurs in the form of nodules that consist of stromal and epithelial elements. In addition, many nodules contain smooth muscle. Prostatic hyperplasia increases

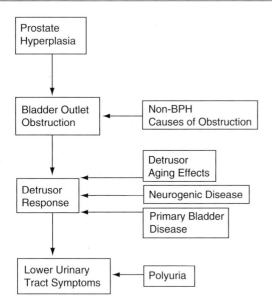

urethral resistance due to mechanical obstruction from tissue expansion. Presumably, the confinement created by the capsule transmits pressure to the urethra leading not only to increased resistance but also compensatory changes in bladder function. How the smooth muscle tissue contributes to symptomatic BPH is unknown, but the muscle fibers are regulated by the adrenergic nervous system. Receptor binding studies indicate that α receptors are the most abundant type of receptor in the human prostate and partially explain the ability of α-blocking medications to relieve BPH-associated LUTS.

In addition, age-related functional changes in the bladder and nervous system have been reported to contribute to LUTS. At the ultrastructural level, normative aging and BOO both result in muscle loss and axonal degeneration with increased collagen deposition [10]. This can lead to both hyperactivity and impaired contractility, which manifest with clinical symptoms associated with symptomatic BPH. It is interesting to note that clinical LUTS are as common in age-matched women as they are in men.

Diagnosis and Evaluation of Prostate Disease

Benign Prostatic Hyperplasia

Physicians evaluating elderly men for obstructive urinary symptoms should begin with a detailed history that focuses on the urinary tract, previous surgical procedures, general health issues, and fitness for possible surgical procedures. Specific areas to discuss include a history of hematuria, urinary tract infection, diabetes, neurologic disorders such as Parkinson's disease or previous stroke, urethral stricture disease, urinary retention, and aggravation of symptoms by cold or sinus medications. Physicians should check all current prescription medications to determine whether the patient is taking any anticholinergic drugs (which impair bladder contractility) or α-sympathomimetics (which increase outflow resistance). A history of lower urinary tract surgery suggests the possibility of urethral or bladder neck stricture.

The etiology of LUTS is multifactorial, and specific symptoms may be a poor indicator of underlying pathophysiology. This is particularly true in the elderly patient. While LUTS are most often attributed to prostatic obstruction, only two-thirds of men with LUTS meet the accepted diagnostic criteria for obstruction. Obstructive symptoms (hesitancy, weakened stream, intermittency, straining, and sense of incomplete emptying) do not reliably predict outlet obstruction. Researchers' have shown that many aspects of detrusor performance decline with aging and progress to detrusor underactivity (DU) in many older individuals [11–14]. DU can influence the clinical picture and may impede the therapy of many LUT disorders including BPH.

Other contributing processes include detrusor overactivity, sensory urgency, sphincteric incontinence, polyuria, or nocturnal polyuria [15]. Nocturia may also result from a wide range of other pathologic conditions, including cardiovascular disease, diabetes mellitus, lower urinary tract obstruction, anxiety, sleep disorders, and other behavioral and/or environmental factors [16]. The use of certain drugs is also associated with increased risk for LUTS. A community-based cross-sectional study that included 2,115 men between 40 and 79 years found that daily use of antidepressants or antihistamines was associated with an increase in symptoms [17].

A tool for symptom assessment has been established and permits objective data for evaluation that can be followed in a longitudinal manner. This is the International Prostate Symptom Score (IPSS) [18] (Table 81.1). This instrument consists of a series of seven questions, correlating to common LUTS that have five-graded responses. Symptoms are considered mild, moderate, and severe with scores between 0 and 7, 8 and 19, and 20 and 35, respectively. The IPSS should not be used to diagnose symptomatic BPH, but rather to evaluate treatment response or disease progression. Symptom scores alone do not capture the morbidity of a prostate problem as perceived by the patient. The impact of symptoms on a patient's life style must be considered as well. Intervening with medical or surgical therapy may make more sense in a patient with moderate symptoms he finds relatively troublesome compared with a patient with severe symptoms who is able to manage them fairly well. Thus, the

TABLE 81.1 International prostate symptom score (I-PSS)

Criterion	Not at all	Less than 1 time in 5	Less than half the time	About half the time	More than half the time	Almost always	Your score
Incomplete emptying: Over the past month, how often have you had a sensation of not emptying your bladder completely after you finished urinating?	0	1	2	3	4	5	
Frequency: Over the past month, how often have you had to urinate again less than 2 hours after you finished urinating?	0	1	2	3	4	5	
Intermittency: Over the past month, how often have you found you stopped and started again several times when you urinated?	0	1	2	3	4	5	
Urgency: Over the past month, how often have you found it difficult to postpone urination?	0	1	2	3	4	5	
Weak stream: Over the past month, how often have you had a weak urinary stream?	0	1	2	3	4	5	
Straining: Over the past month, how often have you had to push or strain to begin urination?	0	1	2	3	4	5	
Nocturia: Over the past month, how many times did you most typically get up to urinate from the time you went to bed at night until the time you got up in the morning?	0	1	2	3	4	5	

Total I-PSS score

critical question for all patients is how much bother these symptoms create and what are they willing to do to improve them. In addition, use of a voiding diary may help to identify patients with polyuria or other nonprostatic disorders.

The physical examination should include a digital rectal examination (DRE) and a focused neurologic examination. The rectal examination establishes the approximate size of the gland and can help to guide which surgical approach is most appropriate should this be warranted. Because prostate size does not correlate with symptom severity or treatment outcomes, and DRE typically underestimates size by 50%, size by DRE should not be used to make a diagnosis and proceed with treatment. The DRE is helpful only for guiding management. A focused neurologic examination can be used to exclude neurologic problems that may cause the presenting symptoms and should include an assessment of rectal sphincter tone.

Diagnostic tools that should be considered when assessing men with moderate or severe urinary symptoms include urinalysis, measurement of serum creatinine, and possibly a prostate specific antigen (PSA) assay. Urinary cytology should be considered in men with severe irritative symptoms and those with hematuria, especially if they have a history of smoking. Patients with renal insufficiency have an increased risk for postoperative complications: 25 versus 17% for patients without renal insufficiency [19]. More important, patients with renal insufficiency have a sixfold increase in

mortality when undergoing surgical treatment for their disease [20]. Although localized prostate cancer typically does not produce urethral obstruction, it can coexist with BPH. Consequently, physicians may wish to consider assessing the serum PSA level should a diagnosis of prostate cancer alter the proposed management. Many patients advised to undergo surgical treatment may have cystoscopy and or a transrectal ultrasound. These examinations are not recommended to determine the need for surgery, but rather to help the surgeon determine the most appropriate technical approach based on prostate size. Finally, formal urodynamic evaluation should be considered in elderly gentlemen who maintain high postvoid residuals, have a known or suspected neurologic disease that may affect the urinary tract or have persistent symptoms after an invasive procedure.

Treatment of Benign Prostatic Hyperplasia

Most men with moderate-to-severe BPH-associated LUTS are advised to consider medical therapy. Those failing medical treatments are then usually offered surgery. Absolute indications for surgery include refractory urinary retention, recurrent urinary infections, recurrent gross hematuria, bladder stones, renal insufficiency caused by obstruction, and the concomitant presence of a large bladder diverticulum.

Urologists have developed several surgical procedures to manage BPH. Open surgical excision, known as a simple prostatectomy, was developed more than 100 years ago. Although surgeons still utilize this approach to remove large glands, most urologists now favor transurethral resection of the prostate (TURP). In 1986, it was reported that 96% of the more than 350,000 men requiring surgical therapy for BPH had a TURP. The advent of medical therapies and less invasive office-based procedures to treat BPH have decreased the frequency of this procedure, so fewer than 200,000 men in the Medicare age group now undergo TURP annually.

Although TURP is considered the standard surgical procedure for treatment of BPH, the associated historical morbidity and related costs of hospitalization have prompted the development of several alternative surgical procedures. The majority involve a form of thermal energy transfer to the tissue which causes necrosis and desiccation with time.

Transurethral Resection of the Prostate

TURP is usually considered the treatment of choice for patients with glands less than 100 g in size. The procedure is typically performed under a spinal or general anesthetic with the patient placed in the lithotomy position. Because urinary tract infections are found in 8–24% of men with symptomatic BPH, many are initially treated with antibiotics and most receive a prophylactic dose prior to initiating surgery. The resection is normally conducted in a fluid medium. Water can be used, but it increases the risk of hemolysis; hence nonhemolytic solutions such as 1.5% glycine, sorbitol, or mannitol are more commonly employed.

The resection technique varies according to the size and configuration of the prostate. The ventral tissue is usually resected first unless the patient has a large median lobe in which case this is done first. Resection is carried out in a circumferential manner from the bladder neck to just proximal to the veru montanum. Resection beyond this point risks damage to the external urinary sphincter. The majority of hyperplastic tissue exists between the 3 and 9 o'clock position with less noted anteriorly. The amount of intraoperative bleeding depends on the size of the prostate, the length of time required to resect the hyperplastic tissue, and the skill of the surgeon. Arterial bleeding is controlled by electrocoagulation. Venous bleeding may be apparent at the end of the procedure, when on irrigating the catheter the returning fluid initially clears but then turns dark red. Venous bleeding can be controlled by inserting a catheter and placing it on traction for several minutes. Extravasation occurs in approximately 2% of patients, usually following capsular penetration. The symptoms associated with extravasation and fluid absorption include nausea, vomiting, and abdominal pain. Most of these patients can be managed simply by

terminating the procedure and placing a urethral catheter. Patients who absorb large amounts of fluid can become severely hyponatremic and may require treatment with hypertonic saline and diuretics.

Over the past 50 years, there has been a steady decline in postoperative complications and mortality associated with TURP. These improvements can be attributed to several factors, including better medical management, better anesthesia, and better surgical equipment including improvements in optics and light sources. Wasson et al. reported that 91% of men undergoing TURP in the Veterans Affairs health care system experienced no complication during the first 30 days after surgery [21]. The mortality rate due to surgery was less than 1%. The most frequent complications reported included the need for catheter exchange (4%), perforation of the prostatic capsule (2%), and hemorrhage requiring transfusion (1%). Long-term complications at 3 years associated with TURP include vesicle neck contracture requiring endoscopic surgery (3%), urethral stricture requiring dilation (3%), and secondary transurethral resection (3%).

Results can be immediate or delayed and are the criteria against which all other treatment options are compared. Improvement in flow rates can be on the magnitude of 120% with decreases in IPSS of 85%. Patients with acute (AUR) or chronic urinary retention (CUR) may not fare as well. TURP can fail to restore spontaneous voiding in 10% of patients with AUR, 38% of those with CUR, and 44% with AUR or CUR. This is of particular concern in the elderly when the presence of DU is known to occur.

Simple Prostatectomy

Open prostatectomy is usually considered when the prostate gland is approximately 100 g or larger. This procedure should also be considered when other concomitant bladder conditions are present, such as a large diverticulum or a large, hard bladder calculus. The advantage of open prostatectomy is a complete removal of the adenomatous tissue under direct vision without the risk of dilutional hyponatremia, which is often associated with a prolonged transurethral resection. The disadvantages include the need for a lower abdominal incision, a longer hospitalization, and an extended convalescence period. In addition, there may be an increased potential for intraoperative hemorrhage from the prostate fossa. Contraindications to this operation include a small prostate gland, a previous prostatectomy, previous pelvic surgery, and prostate cancer.

An open prostatectomy can be accomplished using one of two approaches: retropubic or suprapubic. With the retropubic approach, the anterior prostatic capsule is incised and the hyperplastic adenoma enucleated. Advantages to approach include excellent anatomic exposure of the adenoma, precise transection of the urethra distally, clear and immediate visualization of the prostate fossa to control hemorrhage, and minimal trauma to the urinary bladder. The disadvantages of this approach include the inability to access the bladder and difficulty dealing with a large median lobe.

A suprapubic prostatectomy is accomplished through an extraperitoneal incision in the lower anterior bladder wall. The bladder neck and prostate capsule are scored under direct vision and the adenomatous tissue enucleated. The urethra at the apex of the adenoma is transected sharply under surgeon feel. The major advantage of this procedure over the retropubic approach is that it allows better visualization of the bladder neck and bladder including the ureteral orifices. As a result, this operation is ideally suited for patients with a large median lobe protruding into the bladder, a concomitant symptomatic bladder diverticulum, or a large bladder calculus. It also may be the preferred approach in obese men when it is difficult to gain direct access to the prostate capsule and the dorsal vein complex. The major disadvantage of this approach is the inability to visualize the apical portion of the prostate directly. Contemporary series shows a 60% improvement in obstructive symptoms and approximately 50% improvement in irritative symptoms [22].

Minimally Invasive Surgical Techniques

TUIP

Transurethral incision of the prostate capsule results in significant alleviation of the outflow obstruction, despite the fact that the volume of the prostate remains the same. This involves either unilateral or bilateral incisions, at the 5 and 7 o'clock positions, starting distal to the ureteral orifice ending just proximal to the veru. The depth of the incision is generally described as down to the prostatic capsule. This has been considered an alternative to formal resection in elderly patients who are not deemed medical candidates for more invasive procedures. A meta-analysis of available studies reported similar outcomes as for TURP with a trend toward lower complication and mortality rates [23].

Multiple minimally invasive therapies have been developed. The majority of these involve energy transfer to the prostate causing tissue heating. Treated areas are either vaporized due to high temperatures or develop coagulation necrosis and slough after several days to weeks. Heat generating elements include lasers (Green light, holmium, Nd-Yag, and interstitial), high-intensity focused ultrasound (HIFU), or transurethral microwave thermotherapy (TUMT). Most of these procedures involve delivery of energy through a catheter placed transurethrally or under direct vision cystoscopically. The treatment area can be as long as 40 mm, as wide as 10 mm, and as deep as 10 mm.

Thermotherapy can alleviate voiding symptoms by utilizing a wide range of temperatures. As the intraprostatic temperature rises with the use of higher power devices, more tissue is destroyed, cavities are produced, and more sedation and analgesia are required. Up to 80% of patients experience urinary retention after thermotherapy at high temperature settings. Usually a catheter is placed and may be needed for up to 3 weeks. Patients undergoing these procedures appear to have some reduction in their voiding symptoms, but results are usually less dramatic than are achieved by transurethral resection. Greater symptom improvement usually occurs following treatment with devices delivering higher temperatures. Unfortunately, long-term results are unavailable for many of these procedures. Their role in the treatment of geriatric patients with symptomatic BPH remains to be defined.

Prostate Cancer

Epidemiology

Prostate cancer is now the second most common cancer diagnosed in men. The incidence of this disease increased dramatically following the introduction of testing for prostate-specific antigen (PSA), but has declined somewhat since 1993 to rates that are about twice those recorded prior to the introduction of PSA testing (Fig. 81.5) [24]. Researchers estimated that in 2008, approximately 186,520 men would be diagnosed with this disease and 28,660 men would die from prostate cancer [25]. Prostate cancer is primarily a disease of old men. The probability of developing prostate cancer is about one in seven for men aged 70 and older as compared to one in 15 for men aged 60–69 and one in 39 for men aged 40–59 [25]. The majority of prostate cancer deaths (53%) occur among men age 80 and over [25]. Prostate cancer occurs much more frequently among African-American men than in white Americans. Although the incidence rates are parallel for Whites and African-Americans, the mortality from this disease is almost twice as high for African-American men as for white men.

Despite the significant mortality from prostate cancer, many men never experience symptoms from their disease. Many prostate cancers are indolent. Autopsy data from several countries have confirmed a high incidence of prostate cancer histology, suggesting that less than 1% of men with histologically identifiable cancer die from this disease [26]. There is little geographic or ethnic variability in the rate of small latent carcinomas even when comparing populations with markedly different clinical prostate cancer incidences and mortalities [27, 28]. Numerous studies have demonstrated that as many as 50% of men over the age of 50 years dying of causes other than prostate cancer have microscopic evidence of disease. These studies also demonstrated that the presence of these cancers increases with age. By age 75 years, more than 80% of men have microscopic evidence of prostate cancer at autopsy. Most of these tumors are microscopic foci fulfilling the criterion for prostate cancer, but it is not unusual for an 80-year-old American man dying of heart disease to have an intraprostatic tumor measuring 2–4 cm [29].

The etiology of prostate cancer is unknown. The similar prevalence of latent disease among racial and ethnic groups at autopsy and the vast difference in the incidence of clinically significant disease suggest that the initiation of prostate cancer occurs frequently, but only some groups are susceptible to prostate cancer promoters. Known risk factors include familial inheritance. Several families have been identified with an apparent Mendelian pattern of inheritance, and several prostate oncogenes have been isolated [30]. A man with one first-degree relative with prostate cancer has a two- to threefold risk of being diagnosed with prostate cancer compared with the general population. A man with a first-degree and a second-degree relative may have a sixfold risk of developing prostate cancer [31].

Screening for prostate cancer remains controversial especially among older men. A greater understanding of the

natural history of screen detected prostate cancer suggests that as many as half of the screen detected prostate cancers found among men age 70 and older are not clinically significant [32]. These findings have led the US Preventive services Task Force to recommend against routine PSA testing among men 75 years and older [33].

Pathophysiology

Adenocarcinoma of the prostate is frequently diagnosed as a result of an elevation in PSA. In many cases, tumors cannot be palpated on rectal examination. Among men with clinically localized prostate cancer, the tumor is often multifocal and most of the tumor mass is usually located in a peripheral location near the posterior edge of the prostate [34].

As prostate cancer grows, cancer cells invade the soft tissue surrounding the prostate directly and along the perineural pathways. Penetration of the capsule usually occurs posteriorly and posterolaterally, which may lead to extension into the seminal vesicles. The most frequent sites of metastatic spread are the pelvic lymph nodes and bone, especially the pelvis and vertebral bodies.

In general, the size of a prostate cancer correlates with its extent [35]. Tumors <0.5 ml are usually incidental findings. Capsular penetration is uncommon in tumors <4 ml, whereas larger tumors usually have metastatic elements. The likelihood of developing metastatic prostate cancer depends on the grade of the tumor. The Gleason scoring system is the most common method of estimating malignant potential [36]. The Gleason system is based on the glandular pattern of the tumor as identified at relatively low magnification (Fig. 81.6). The primary (most predominant) and secondary

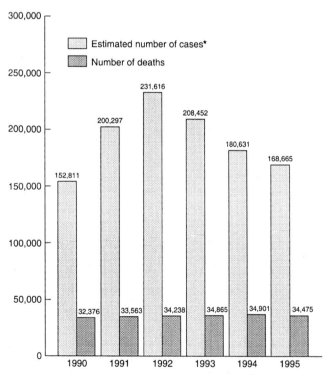

*Estimates obtained by multiplying the age-specific incidence rates for the 11 SEER registries by the U.S. population for each year.

Figure 81.5 Prostate cancer incidence and mortality in the USA, 1990–1995. Estimates were obtained by multiplying the age-specific incidence rates for the 11 SEER registries in the US population for each year (from Stanford et al. [24]).

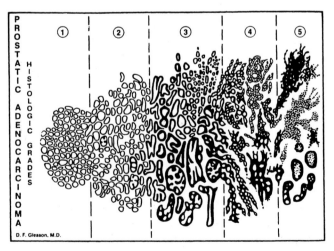

Figure 81.6 Gleason grading system. (From Walsh PC, Retik AM, Vaughan ED JR, Wein AJ (eds) (1998) Campbell's urology, 7th ed. Saunders, Philadelphia, with permission. Copyright Elsevier 1998).

(second most prevalent) architectural patterns are assigned a grade from 1 to 5, with 1 representing the most well differentiated and 5 the most poorly differentiated. A Gleason score is determined by summing the primary and secondary patterns. Men with high-grade disease (Gleason score 8–10) generally have a poor prognosis, whereas men with low-grade disease (Gleason score 6) have an excellent prognosis. Men with Gleason score 7 tumors have a prognosis between these two extremes [37]. Gleason 2–5 scores are rarely assigned to newly diagnosed prostate cancer in contemporary practice [38].

Diagnosis and Evaluation

Unlike BPH, prostate cancer rarely causes symptoms early in the course of the disease because most prostate cancers arise in the periphery of the gland distant from the urethra. Symptoms in men with prostate cancer suggest locally advanced or metastatic disease. Growth of prostate cancer into the urethra or bladder neck can result in obstructive or irritating voiding symptoms. Metastatic disease that involves the bones can cause pain and anemia.

Aggressive screening efforts have reduced the proportion of men with prostate cancer detected because of symptoms suggestive of advanced disease [39]. Because of the significant risk of prostate cancer, transrectal ultrasonography and prostate biopsy are recommended for all men who have an abnormality on DRE regardless of the serum PSA level. Unfortunately, in both screened and nonscreened populations, DRE misses 23–45% of prostate cancers that are subsequently found following prostate biopsy because of elevated serum PSA [40]. Routine use of the serum PSA assay increases the detection of prostate cancer over that achieved by a DRE alone. The use of serum PSA testing increases the lead time for prostate cancer diagnosis and the likelihood of detecting prostate cancers confined to the prostate. Recognizing that PSA elevations are common in aging men because of the high prevalence of BPH, investigators have focused on methods of improving the ability of the PSA test to distinguish between men with BPH and men with cancer. Recommendations include adjusting serum PSA levels for patient age, prostate volume, and the rate of change of PSA values [41–43]. With the advent of specific assays quantifying PSA molecular forms, the measurement of free, unbound PSA has been evaluated as a method of distinguishing between BPH [44].

Imaging studies are frequently employed to evaluate the extent of prostate cancer progression. Bone scans and computed tomography (CT) scans are the most common, but other studies include pelvic magnetic resonance imaging (MRI) and endorectal coil MRI. Unfortunately, most of these studies are insufficiently sensitive to identify microscopic metastases. A prospective analysis of more than 3,600 men demonstrated that imaging studies are positive in fewer than 10% of cases when the serum PSA level is less than 20 ng/ml or the Gleason score is less than 8 [45]. Only men with serum PSA levels higher than 50 ng/ml are likely to have evidence of metastatic disease that can be identified on bone scan, CT scan, or MRI. Unfortunately, more than half of the men with newly diagnosed prostate cancer who have a serum PSA level over 10 ng/ml already have disease extension beyond the confines of the prostate [46]. Men with serum PSA levels over 20 ng/ml are usually poor candidates for surgical therapy because of the high rate of tumor recurrence within 5 years of surgical therapy.

Surgical Treatment of Prostate Cancer

The appropriate treatment of prostate cancer among old men remains controversial. Studies concerning the long-term outcomes of men treated conservatively for their disease have documented the relatively modest disease-specific mortality among men with low and moderate grade tumors [47–49]. A recently published competing risk analysis of men aged 55–74 at diagnosis demonstrated that men with Gleason score 2–4 and five tumors have a 4–7% and 6–11% chance, respectively, of dying from prostate cancer [50]. These data were recently updated to include 20-year outcomes [37]. Older patients had a much greater chance of dying from competing medical hazards (Fig. 81.7). Conversely, men with Gleason score 7 and 8–10 tumors have a 42–70% and 60–87% chance, respectively, of dying from prostate cancer, if it is treated with hormone therapy alone. Men with Gleason score 6 tumors face an intermediate risk (18–30%) of dying from prostate cancer within 15 years, if the tumors are treated with hormone therapy alone. Based on these results, it appears that men over 70 years at diagnosis with Gleason score 2–5 disease face a minimal risk of dying from prostate cancer and therefore may not be good candidates for surgical therapy. Men whose biopsy specimens show Gleason score 7–10 disease face a high risk of death from prostate cancer when treated with hormone therapy alone, even when cancer is diagnosed as late as 74 years. These men may wish to consider surgical treatment in an attempt to cure their disease. Alternatives to surgery include external beam radiation therapy and implantation of radioactive seeds, often referred to as brachytherapy.

When choosing therapy for an individual patient with clinically localized prostate cancer, the age and general health of the patient remain critically important because of the indolent progression of many prostate cancers. Death from a localized cancer left untreated is not likely to occur

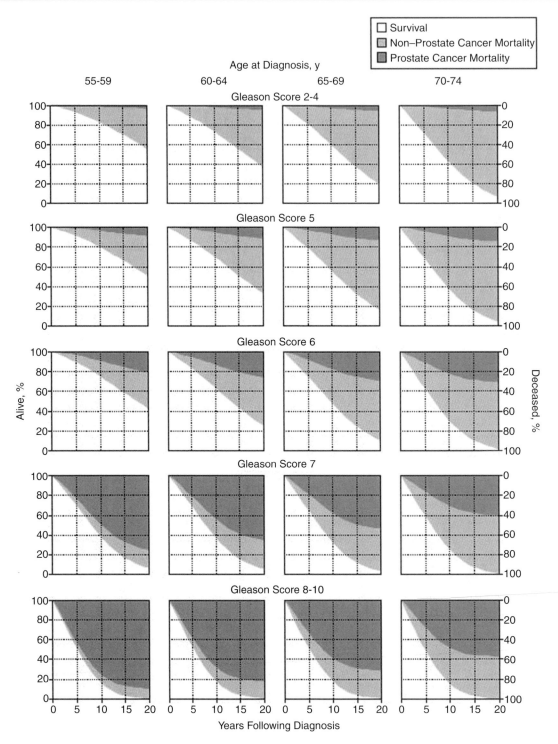

Figure 81.7 Survival (*white lower band*) and cumulative mortality from prostate cancer (*dark gray upper band*) and other causes (*light gray middle band*) up to 20 years after diagnosis stratified by age at diagnosis and Gleason score. Percentage of men alive can be read from the left-hand scale, and percentage of men who have died from prostate cancer or other causes during this interval can be read from the right-hand scale (From Albertsen et al. [37], with permission. Copyright © 2005 American Medical Association. All rights reserved).

for 8–10 years, yet the risk of death from prostate cancer continues to increase for at least 15 years (Fig. 81.7). In 1989, the average life expectancy of a man aged 70 was 12.1 years, and for a 75-year-old man it was less than 10 years

(Table 81.2). Thus, the potential benefits of surgical intervention decreases rapidly as men age.

Chronologic age is only one factor that influences life expectancy. Prostate cancer occurs frequently in elderly men

TABLE 81.2 Life expectancy at single years of age for men, all races

Age (years)	Life expectancy (years)
65	14.6
66	13.9
67	13.3
68	12.7
69	12.1
70	11.6
71	11.0
72	10.5
73	10.0
74	9.5
75	9.0
76	8.6
77	8.1
78	7.7
79	7.3
80	6.9
81	6.5
82	6.1
83	5.8
84	5.5
85	5.2

who have associated comorbid conditions. Conversely, some old patients are in excellent physical condition and have a life expectancy longer than average for their age group. The impact of comorbid conditions on long-term outcomes among men with localized prostate cancer has been assessed [51]. Men with significant comorbid disease, measured using one of several instruments, have a much higher probability of dying from causes other than prostate cancer compared with those men with no or relatively few competing medical hazards (Fig. 81.8). Elderly patients must carefully assess the risks and benefits of surgical management compared with those of conservative management before making a decision concerning which therapy is the appropriate management for their localized prostate cancer.

Radical Prostatectomy

Surgical excision of prostate cancer can be accomplished using one of several surgical approaches: a retropubic approach, a perineal approach, a laparoscopic approach, or a robot assisted approach. Each approach has its advantages and disadvantages, but all appear to offer the same probability of controlling spread of disease. Furthermore, each of these approaches appears to have similar outcomes including length of hospital stay and long-term recovery. The rate of complications associated with each of these techniques appears to be similar.

Radical retropubic prostatectomy done open is performed with the patient in the supine position and laparoscopic or

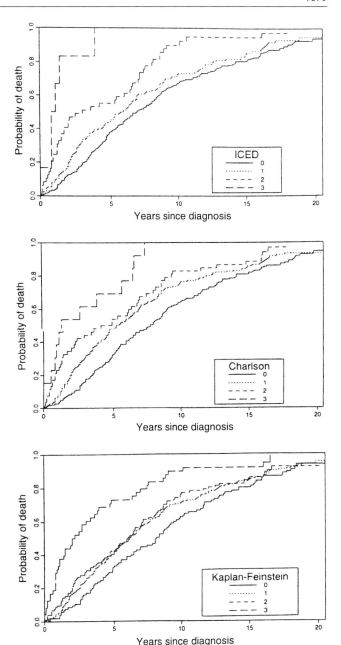

FIGURE 81.8 Cumulative mortality from all causes of death stratified by severity of comorbidities at diagnosis as measured by each of three instruments tested. Data are not adjusted for patient age or Gleason score, ICED, index of coexistent disease (From Albertsen et al. [50], with permission. Copyright Elsevier 1996).

robotic with relatively steep Trendelenberg to increase exposure to the prevesicle space. The procedure is usually performed under general anesthesia, although regional techniques using an epidural catheter are popular because they decrease the need for narcotics during the procedure and the postoperative period. Usually a pelvic lymph node dissection is performed as the first step. The lymphadenectomy is not therapeutic but does provide additional pathology to stage the cancer more accurately. The procedure is performed by entering the prevesicle space either directly through a lower midline incision or transabdominally, when a laparoscope or robot is employed. The open radical retropubic approach begins by incising the endopelvic fascia, controlling the dorsal vein complex, and then dividing the urethra at the level of the prostate apex. The laparoscopic or robotic approach usually approaches the prostate from the posterior, developing the plane between the seminal vesicles and the rectum. The prostate is separated from the bladder neck prior to controlling the dorsal vein complex and dividing the urethra at the level of the prostate apex. In young men, care is taken to preserve the neurovascular bundles that lie on either side of the prostate apex. Unfortunately, among older men, there is a high probability of impotence associated with this procedure. Once the prostate and seminal vesicles have been removed, the bladder neck is repaired and secured to the stump of the urethra. Careful dissection around the apex of the prostate to avoid injury to the pelvic floor musculature should minimize the chance of incontinence.

All techniques for performing a radical prostatectomy are associated with complications, which increase with the patient's age. An analysis of more than 100,000 Medicare claims has demonstrated that approximately one in four patients suffers a major or minor complication associated with these procedures [52]. The radical retropubic approach had higher risks of respiratory complications and miscellaneous medical complications and a lower risk of miscellaneous surgical complications. The perineal approach resulted in a 1–2% incidence of rectal injury, but this appears to be offset by the medical complications of the gastrointestinal tract with the retropubic approach. Short-term mortality following radical prostatectomy is low; approximately 0.5% for men under age 70 and about 1.0% for men aged 75 and older. Table 81.3 demonstrates that the risk of mortality increases sharply with age.

Long-term complications associated with radical prostatectomy include impotence and incontinence. Although modern surgical techniques have decreased the incidence of postsurgical incontinence, reported rates of this complication vary widely. Patient reports of incontinence have been as high as 31%, whereas reports from tertiary medical centers suggest rates under 10% [53–55]. The age of the patient and whether an anastomotic stricture develops influence the recovery of continence. Patients over age 65 have a greater risk of incontinence compared to men under age 65.

Return of erectile function has also been correlated with patient age. Quinlan et al. evaluated 503 potent men between the ages of 34 and 72 who underwent radical retropubic prostatectomy [56]. Among men under the age of 50, about 90% were potent if one or both neurovascular bundles were preserved [57]. Among men age 65–69, only 27% recovered sexual function. Recovery of sexual function is likely to be even lower among men 70 years and older.

Only one randomized trial has been conducted to evaluate the efficacy of radical prostatectomy in the treatment of localized prostate cancer. Recently Bill-Axelson et al. published 11-year outcomes from a randomized trial comparing radical prostatectomy against surveillance for men with clinically localized prostate cancer [58]. They found that all cause survival was not significantly different between the two arms of the study, although there was a modest decrease in prostate cancer mortality from 18% in the watchful waiting arm to 13% in the radical prostatectomy arm. Interestingly, this benefit was only seen in men less than 65 years at the time of diagnosis and was achieved primarily during the first 5 years following treatment.

Conclusions

Prostate diseases cause significant morbidity and mortality among elderly men. Both BPH and prostate cancer are relatively rare before age 50 but become increasingly common as men age into their 60s and 70s. For many patients with mild or moderate symptoms of bladder outlet obstruction, watchful waiting or various medical therapies may be sufficient therapy. As symptoms worsen, however, surgical treatment may offer the best chance of relieving symptoms of urinary frequency, hesitancy, and slow stream. Most patients with symptomatic BPH should be offered therapy with an α-blocker or a 5α-reductase inhibitor before proceeding to transurethral prostatectomy. Only patients with large prostates should be considered for open prostatectomy. Minimally invasive thermal therapies are available but both short- and long-term efficacy appear to be inferior to standard surgical techniques.

Prostate cancer poses a much more difficult problem for elderly men, especially men with well or moderately differentiated tumors. Prostate cancer in these men is frequently a slow-growing tumor, and other medical hazards may become the dominant medical problem long before the cancer metastasizes.

Patients must carefully assess the relative risks and benefits of a surgical approach compared with other less invasive options, such as delayed hormone therapy or irradiation before proceeding with radical prostatectomy. Men with high-grade prostate cancers (Gleason scores 8–10) face a

Table 81.3 Thirty-day mortality following radical prostatectomy by age and surgical approach

Age (years)	30-Day mortality, by surgical approach (%)	
	Retropubic approach	Perineal approach
65–69	0.45	0.22
70–74	0.60	0.36
75+	1.04	0.95
Overall	0.56	0.37

significant risk of dying from their disease even when it is diagnosed as a localized disease as late as age 74. These men may want to consider radical prostatectomy as the preferred treatment option. Fortunately, in 2008, the primary risk associated with radical prostatectomy is impotence. Incontinence is less common, while mortality from surgery is a relatively rare event.

References

1. Berry SJ, Coffey DS, Walsh PC, Ewing LL (1984) The development of human benign prostatic hyperplasia with age. J Urol 132:474
2. Gaynor EP (1938) Zur frage des prostatakrebes. Virchows Arch Pathol Anat 301:602–652
3. Jacobson ST, Jacobson DJ, Girman CJ (1999) et al; Treatment for benign protstatic hyperplasia among community dwelling men: The Olmsted county study of urinary symptoms and health status. J Urol 162:1301–1306
4. Ketchandji M, Kuo YF, Shahinian VB et al (2009) Cause of death in older men after the diagnosis of prostate cancer. J Am Geriatr Soc 57(5):934–935. doi:10.1111/j.1532-5415.2008.02091
5. Caine M, Schuger L (1987) The "Capsule" in benign prostatic hypertrophy. US Department of Health and Human Services, Bethesda, p 221, NIH Publ No. 87-2881
6. Taylor JA 3rd, Kuchel GA (2006) Detrusor underactivity: Clinical features and pathogenesis of an underdiagnosed geriatric condition. J Am Geriatr Soc 54(12):1920–1932
7. Roberts RO, Bergstralh EJ, Cunningham JM et al (2004) Androgen receptor gene polymorphisms and increased risk of urologic measures of benign prostatic hyperplasia. Am J Epidemiol 159:269–276
8. Roberts RO, Jacobson DJ, Rhodes T et al (2004) Serum sex hormones and measures of benign prostatic hyperplasia. Prostate 61:124–131
9. Arrighi HM, Guess HA, Metter EJ et al (1990) Symptoms and signs of prostatism as risk factors for prostatectomy. Prostate 16:253
10. Elbadawi A, Yalla SV, Resnick NM (1993) Structural basis of geriatric voiding dysfunction. I. Methods of a prospective ultrastructural/urodynamic study and an overview of the findings. J Urol 150:1650–1656
11. Malone-Lee J, Wahedna I (1993) Characterisation of detrusor contractile function in relation to old age. Br J Urol 72:873–880
12. Van Mastrigt R (1992) Age dependence of urinary bladder contractility. Neurourol Urodynam 11:315
13. Resnick NM, Yalla SV (1987) Detrusor hyperactivity with impaired contractility: An unrecognized but common cause of incontinence in elderly patients. JAMA 257:3076–3081
14. Resnick NM, Yalla SV, Laurino E (1989) The pathophysiology of urinary incontinence among institutionalized elderly persons. N Engl J Med 320:1–7
15. Chaikin DC, Blaivas JG (2001) Voiding dysfunction: definitions. Curr Opin Urol 11:395–398
16. Weiss JP, Blaivas JG (2000) Nocturia. J Urol 163:5–12
17. Su L, Guess HA, Girman CJ et al (1996) Adverse effects of medications on urinary symptoms and flow rate: a community-based study. J Clin Epidemiol 49:483–487
18. McConnell JD, Barry MJ, Bruskewitz RC et al (1994) Benign prostatic hyperplasia: diagnosis and treatment. clinical practice guideline number 8. Agency for Health Care Policy & Research, Public Health Service, US Department of Health and Human Services, Rockville, MD, AHCPR Publ No. 94-0582
19. Mebust WK, Holtgrewe HL, Cockette ATK, Peters PC, Committee W (1989) Transurethral prostatectomy: immediate and postoperative complications: a cooperative study of 13 participating institutions evaluating 3885 patients. J Urol 141:243–247
20. Melchoir J, Valk WL, Foret JD, Mebust MK (1974) Transurethral prostatectomy in the azotemic patient. J Urol 112:643–646
21. Wasson JH, Reda DJ, Bruskewitz RC et al (1995) A comparison of transurethral surgery with watchful waiting for moderate symptoms of benign prostatic hyperplasia. N Engl J Med 332:75–79
22. Gacci M, Bartoletti R, Figlioli S et al (2003) Urinary symptoms, quality of life and sexual function in patients with benign prostatic hypertrophy before and after prostatectomy: A prospective study. BJU Int 91:196–200
23. Barry MJ, Fowler FJ Jr, O'Leary MP et al (1992) The American Urological Association's symptom index for benign prostatic hyperplasia. J Urol 148:1549–1557, Copyright (c) 1992, Lea & Febiger
24. Stanford JL, Stephenson RA, Coyle LM et al (1999) Prostate cancer trends 1973–1995, SEER program. National Cancer Institute, Bethesda, NIH Pub No. 99-4543
25. Jemal A, Siegel R, Ward E et al (2008) Cancer statistics 2008. CA Cancer J Clin 58:71–96
26. Edwards CN, Steinthorsson E, Nicholson D (1953) An autopsy study of latent prostatic cancer. Cancer 32:498–506
27. Halpert B, Sheehan EE, Schmalhorst WR, Scott R (1963) Carcinoma of the prostate: a survey of 5000 autopsies. Cancer 16:737–742
28. Shimizu H, Ross RK, Bernstein L et al (1991) Cancers of the prostate and breast among Japanese and white immigrants in Los Angeles County. Br J Cancer 63:963–966
29. Yatani R, Chigusa I, Akazaki K et al (1982) Geographic pathology of latent prostatic carcinoma. Int J Cancer 29:611–616
30. Smith JR, Freije D, Carpten JD et al (1996) Major susceptibility locus for prostate cancer on chromosome 1 suggested by a genome-wide search. Science 274:1371–1374
31. Steinberg GS, Carter BS, Beaty TH et al (1990) Family history and the risk of prostate cancer. Prostate 17:337–340
32. Draisma G, Boer R, Otto SJ et al (2003) Lead times and over detection due to prostate specific antigen screening: estimates from the European Randomized Study of Screening for Prostate Cancer. J Natl Cancer Inst 95:868–878
33. U.S. Preventive Services Task Force (2008) Screening for prostate cancer: U.S. Preventive Services Task Force Recommendation statement. Ann Internal Med 149:185–191
34. Byar DP, Mostofi FK (1972) Veterans Administration Cooperative Urologic Research Groups: carcinoma of the prostate: prognostic evaluation of certain pathologic features in 208 radical prostatectomies. Cancer 30:5–13
35. McNeal JE (1992) Cancer volume and site of origin of adenocarcinoma of the prostate: relationship to local and distant spread. Hum Pathol 23:258–266
36. Gleason DF, Mellinger GT (1974) Veterans Administration Cooperative Urological Research Group: prediction of prognosis for prostatic adenocarcinoma by combined histologic grading and clinical staging. J Urol 111:58–64
37. Albertsen PC, Hanley JA, Fine J (2005) 20 year outcomes following conservative management of clinically localized prostate cancer. JAMA 293:2095–2101
38. Albertsen PC, Hanley JA, Barrows GH et al (2005) Prostate cancer and the Will Rogers Phenomenon. JNCI 97(17):1248–1253
39. Gilliland F, Becker TM, Smith A et al (1994) Trends in prostate cancer incidence and mortality in New Mexico are consistent with an increase in effective screening. Cancer Epidemiol Biol Prev 3:105–111
40. Ellis WJ, Chetner MP, Preston SD, Brawer MK (1994) Diagnosis of prostatic carcinoma: the yield of serum prostate specific antigen,

digital rectal examination and transrectal ultrasonography. J Urol 52:1520–1525

41. Oesterling JE, Jacobsen SJ, Chute CG et al (1993) Serum prostate-specific antigen in a community-based population of healthy men: establishment of age-specific reference ranges. JAMA 270:860–864

42. Benson MC, Whang IS, Olsson CA et al (1992) Use of prostate specific antigen density to enhance predictive value of intermediate levels of serum prostate specific antigen. J Urol 147:817–821

43. Carter HB, Pearson JD, Metter JE et al (1992) Longitudinal evaluation of prostate specific antigen levels in men with and without prostate disease. JAMA 267:2215–2220

44. Catalona WJ, Simth DS, Wolfert RL et al (1995) Evaluation of percentage of free serum prostate-specific antigen to improve specificity of prostate cancer screening. JAMA 274:1214–1220

45. Albertsen PC, Hanley JA, Harlan JC et al (2000) The positive yield of imaging studies in the evaluation of men with newly diagnosed prostate cancer: a population-based analysis. J Urol 163:1138–1143

46. Catalona WJ, Smith DS, Ratliff TL, Basler JW (1993) Detection of organ-confined prostate cancer is increased through prostate-specific antigen-based testing. JAMA 270:948–954

47. Johansson JE, Homberg L, Johansson S et al (1997) Fifteen year survival in prostate cancer: a prospective, population-based study in Sweden. JAMA 277:467–471

48. Chodak GW, Thisted RA, Gerber GS et al (1994) Results of conservative management of clinically localized prostate cancer. N Engl J Med 330:242–248

49. Albertsen PC, Fryback DG, Storer BE et al (1995) Long term survival among men with conservatively treated localized prostate cancer. JAMA 274:626–631

50. Albertsen PC, Hanley JA, Gleason DF, Barry MJ (1998) Competing risk analysis of men aged 55 to 74 years at diagnosis managed conservatively for clinically localized prostate cancer. JAMA 280:975–980

51. Albertsen PC, Fryback DG, Storer BE et al (1996) The impact of co-morbidity on life expectancy among men with localized prostate cancer. J Urol 156:127–132

52. Lu-Yao GL, Albertsen PC, Warren J, Yao SL (1999) Effect of age and surgical approach on complications and short-term mortality after radical prostatectomy: a population-based study. Urology 54:301–307

53. Fowler FJ, Barry MJ, Lu-Yao G et al (1993) Patient-reported complications and follow-up treatment after radical prostatectomy. J Urol 149:622–629

54. Eastham JA, Kattan MW, Rogers E et al (1996) Risk factors for urinary incontinence after radical retropubic prostatectomy. J Urol 156:1707–1713

55. Stanford JL, Feng Z, Hamilton AS et al (2000) Urinary and sexual function after radical prostatectomy for clinically localized prostate cancer: The Prostate Cancer Outcomes Study. JAMA 283: 354–360

56. Quinlan DM, Epstein JI, Carter BS, Walsh PC (1991) Sexual function following radical prostatectomy: influence of reservation of neurovascular bundles. J Urol 145:998–1002

57. Murphy GP, Mettlin C, Menck H et al (1994) National patterns of prostate cancer treatment by radical prostatectomy: results of a survey by the American College of Surgeons Committee on Cancer. J Urol 152:1817–1819

58. Bill-Axelson A, Holmber L, Filen F et al (2008) Radical prostatectomy versus watchful waiting in localized prostate cancer: The Scandinavian prostate cancer Group-4 randomized trial. JNCI 100:1144–1154

Chapter 82
Benign Gynecologic Disorders in the Older Woman

Kimberly A. Gerten, W. Jerod Greer, C. Bryce Bowling, Thomas Wheeler II, and Holly E. Richter

Introduction

Nonmalignant genital tract conditions and pelvic floor disorders including pelvic organ prolapse and incontinence are common gynecologic problems encountered by the older woman. With the rapidly increasing population of active older American women, physicians can expect to provide evaluation and treatment of these conditions with increasing frequency. These conditions are typically amenable to both medical and surgical therapies making individualization of treatment approaches important. An anatomically directed survey of nonneoplastic conditions of the lower and upper genital tract conditions is presented along with a discussion of pelvic floor support disorders common in the older woman. Evidenced-based evaluation and treatment suggestions are provided.

Menopause

Menopause is defined as 12 months of amenorrhea secondary to cessation of ovulation. It can also be induced by surgical oophorectomy, chemotherapy, or radiation [1]. The transition into menopause (perimenopause) typically begins 4 years prior to the last period [2] and starts with irregular cycle lengths during which estrogen levels can be normal or elevated. Ultimately, estrogen and progesterone levels decrease with subsequent increase in follicle-stimulating hormone (FSH) levels. Postmenopausal estradiol levels, the most potent estrogen, are typically <20 pg/mL, while FSH is most often >70 mU/mL. Testosterone production, however, is maintained by the ovaries and adrenal glands maintaining

serum levels of testosterone at 2–40 mg/dL. Even though estrogen production declines dramatically with menopause, a small amount of production continues via peripheral conversion of androgens by aromatase in adipocytes [2]. The natural process of aging results in increased fat body mass and decreased lean body mass such that obese postmenopausal women can manifest conditions due to estrogen excess, such as endometrial hyperplasia and carcinoma. In the USA, the mean age of menopause is 51 years [2] with cigarette smoking and low socioeconomic status being risk factors for premature (<40 years old) menopause [1].

Symptoms attributed to menopause include vasomotor symptoms (hot flushes and night sweats), vaginal atrophy symptoms (itching, dryness, and painful intercourse), urinary incontinence, sleeping difficulty, depression, anxiety, mood changes, cognitive decline, and somatic complaints. However, only vasomotor symptoms, atrophy symptoms, and trouble sleeping are consistently related to menopause in longitudinal studies [1–3]. A hot flush is the sudden feeling of warmth of the chest, neck, and/or face. It lasts for about 4 min, usually no longer than 5 min, and may have concurrent perspiration followed by a chill [1, 2]. Hot flushes occur most commonly in the late perimenopause (~65% of women). Symptoms decrease in intensity over time with up to 90% of women having complete resolution in 5 years [1]. The physiology behind hot flashes is poorly understood, but theories center around hypothalamic control in relation to hormonal changes with the transition to menopause [1, 2].

Estrogen therapy is the most effective treatment for vasomotor symptoms [4]. However, use of systemic estrogen has been complicated by results from the Women's Health Initiative (WHI), which found that systemic estrogen alone increased the risk of stroke (relative risk 1.39), while the addition of progestin increased the risk of coronary events (relative risk 1.28), breast cancer (relative risk 1.26), and pulmonary embolism (relative risk 2.13) [2]. The absolute increase in risk for these events is lower in the younger menopausal women [2]. A description of the criticisms and various organizational guidelines regarding hormone replacement therapy is beyond the scope of this chapter.

K.A. Gerten (✉)
Division of Women's Pelvic Medicine and Reconstructive Surgery, Department of Obstetrics and Gynecology, University of Alabama at Birmingham Medical Center, Birmingham, AL, USA
e-mail: kimgerten@hotmail.com

R.A. Rosenthal et al. (eds.), *Principles and Practice of Geriatric Surgery*,
DOI 10.1007/978-1-4419-6999-6_82, © Springer Science+Business Media, LLC 2011

The American College of Obstetricians and Gynecologists and the North American Menopause Society recommend that the lowest effective dose of systemic estrogen (plus progestin if the uterus is present) should be used, and estrogen replacement should not be used for disease prevention [1, 2, 4]. Alternative medicines for the treatment of vasomotor symptoms, especially when estrogen is contraindicated, include paroxetine, clonidine, and gabapentin [1, 2].

Connective tissue, in general, is sex-hormone-sensitive. Therefore, menopause may also be associated with a loss of skin elasticity and strength of bone because of the estrogen sensitive collagen of these structures. Postmenopausal women who are given a combination of estrogen and testosterone have been reported to have greater skin collagen content and greater skin thickness than do untreated women [5]. In untreated women, skin collagen content is inversely proportional to the amount of time since menopause. It also has been shown that oral or transdermal estrogen given together with medroxyprogesterone acetate significantly increases skin collagen content in postmenopausal women [5].

Lower Genital Tract

Vulva

The vulva includes the portions of the genitalia that are externally visible: the mons pubis, labia majora and minora, clitoris, and vestibule. Within the vestibule are the hymen, vaginal orifice, urethral meatus, and the openings of Skene's and Bartholin's ducts [6]. The vulva is covered by keratinized stratified squamous epithelium with the exception of the vestibule which, like the vagina, is not keratinized.

Skin changes that occur with menopause and the accompanying decrease in ovarian estrogen production are evident on the vulva as they are on all skin surfaces. These changes include dryness, roughness, wrinkling, and loss of turgor. Structurally, there is flattening and decreased thickness of the epidermis and dermis, an overall decrease and change in distribution of subcutaneous fat, and loss as well as depigmentation of hair. These changes lead to functional loss of the skin's barrier function, elasticity, mechanical protection, and wound healing [7].

Lichen Sclerosus

Lichen sclerosus is a chronic, benign epithelial condition associated with characteristic skin changes as well as vulvar pain and pruritus. The vulva is the most common site at up to 96% of cases, but lesions can be seen on any skin surface [8].

The condition typically occurs in postmenopausal women, with a mean age of 52.6 years at time of diagnosis in one study, but can also be seen in children, premenopausal women as well as men [9]. The etiology is unknown, but possible mechanisms include genetic and/or local vulvar factors as well as immunologic abnormalities [10, 11].

Patients typically complain of vulvar pruritus, the hallmark symptom of the condition, along with pain or irritation; however, some women are asymptomatic. Other common symptoms include dysuria and painful defecation if fissures are present, and dyspareunia associated with introital stenosis. On physical examination, the classic features of the disease are thin, pale, wrinkled (often described as "parchment paper") skin on the labia (Fig. 82.1). Excoriations may be present secondary to scratching, and fissures can be seen perianally or between the labial folds and around the clitoris. More advanced disease can lead to the destruction of labial and clitoral architecture, with nearly complete midline fusion of the labia. One important distinctive feature of lichen sclerosus is that the vagina and cervix are not involved [12].

Diagnosis is based on high-clinical suspicion and confirmatory 3 mm punch biopsy, as other vulvar dystrophies can have a similar appearance. Women with lichen sclerosus also have an increased risk of invasive squamous cell cancer of the vulva [13]. High-potency topical corticosteroids are the mainstay of therapy for lichen sclerosus, typically with clobetasol or halobetasol propionate 0.05% ointment nightly for at least 4 weeks followed by a slow taper when symptoms resolve. Approximately 95% of patients will have complete or partial resolution of their symptoms with this regimen [14, 15].

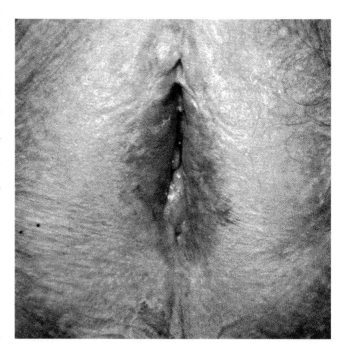

FIGURE 82.1 Lichen sclerosus. Note the destruction of normal architecture and "parchment paper" skin.

Maintenance therapy with twice weekly dosing may decrease flares or recurrent symptoms, though some experts recommend stopping therapy with resolution of symptoms and only retreating for recurrences [16]. It is unclear whether maintenance therapy reduces the chance of malignant evolution, so any recurrent or persistent lesions should be rebiopsied to rule out cancer [17]. Topical immunosuppressants have shown some promise in lichen sclerosus, but are currently considered second-line therapy for disease that is unresponsive to high-potency corticosteroids [12].

Lichen Simplex Chronicus

Lichen simplex chronicus is an eczematoid disease of hyperkeratotic, scaling plaques of varying pigmentation that is associated with severe vulvar pruritus. It may commonly be seen in conjunction with a number of other vulvar skin disorders and is ultimately brought about by chronic scratching and irritation from both environmental and dermatologic processes [18]. Lichen simplex chronicus has been found to be associated with a history of atopic disease in up to 75% of patients, and typically presents later in adult life though it can be seen in children. Initiating events range from chronic heat and excessive sweating to candidal infection or other dermatoses such as lichen sclerosus [12].

Diagnosis of lichen simplex chronicus is based on a history of vulvar irritation, pruritus, and typical hyperkeratotic lesions on examination. Ulcers and excoriations are sometimes seen due to chronic scratching. Biopsy may be done to identify the underlying disease (e.g. lichen sclerosus), and vaginal yeast cultures may also be helpful in this regard [12]. First-line therapy involves treatment of any underlying conditions, and topical corticosteroids may be used for symptomatic relief of inflammation and itching. Additionally, hygiene measures are important in controlling chronic vulvar wetness and avoiding potential irritants (strong soaps, perfumes, or detergents) that might exacerbate or prolong the condition.

Lichen Planus

Lichen planus is another inflammatory disease involving the genital mucosa that is thought to be caused by a cell-mediated autoimmune mechanism [19]. Unlike other vulvar dermatoses, lichen planus is more commonly found on nonvulvar skin or the mucosal membranes, especially the buccal mucosa [20]. Oral lichen planus is present in approximately 1% of the population, and up to one-fourth of women with oral disease will also have genital disease. The condition generally presents from 30 to 60 years, and the typical lesions seen are

white reticulate striae on the buccal mucosal surface (Wickham's striae). Vulvar and skin lesions tend to consist of shiny, pruritic, violaceous papules; vulvar lesions can be less well demarcated and may even appear as white patches that are difficult to distinguish from lichen sclerosus [12]. The erosive form of lichen planus can lead to extremely painful erosions of the posterior vestibule and labia minora, with eventual architectural destruction, scarring and narrowing of the introitus; patients with such advanced disease complain of dyspareunia and difficulty voiding [12].

Diagnostic biopsy specimens are usually nonspecific, but classic findings in lichen planus include liquefactive degeneration of the basal cell layer and a band-like lymphocytic dermal infiltrate [21]. However, biopsy does help to rule out immunobullous diseases as well as cancer. There are a number of treatment options for lichen planus; unfortunately, though, response is typically poor and therapy goals should focus on long-term maintenance of symptoms rather than complete control. Patient education, behavioral modification, and emotional support are all important components of any treatment plan. Medication options include topical and/or systemic high-potency corticosteroids, topical and oral cyclosporine, as well as a number of other immunomodulators [12]. In our experience, Tacrolimus (Protopic) 0.1% ointment applied twice daily has been used with some success.

Bartholin's Cysts and Abscesses

Bartholin's glands are located near the 4 and 8 o'clock positions on the posterolateral aspect of the vaginal opening. The ducts from Bartholin's glands empty into the vestibule, and obstruction of these orifices from chronic inflammation can lead to Bartholin's cysts, which are typically asymptomatic unless they become large. These ducts and cysts may also become infected and evolve into polymicrobial abscesses, which generally present with exquisite pain and swelling. The incidence of Bartholin's cysts or abscesses is up to 2% over a woman's lifetime, but tends to be less common during the postmenopausal years [22]. Due to the possibility of underlying Bartholin's gland carcinoma, cysts and abscesses in women over the age of 40 should be drained and biopsied at the first occurrence, followed by complete excision of the gland for recurrent disease [23].

Vulvodynia

Vulvodynia is defined as chronic pain in the vulvar area lasting at least 3–6 months [24]. In 2003, the International Society for the Study of Vulvovaginal Disease classified vulvar pain into two categories: (1) vulvar pain related to an underlying disorder (infection, inflammation, neoplasm, or neurologic disease) and (2) vulvodynia, defined as vulvar burning or discomfort in the absence of any identifiable cause [25]. The true prevalence is unknown, but has been reported to be between 10 and 16% over a woman's lifetime, and tends to be more common in older patients [26, 27]. The etiology of vulvodynia is also unclear, but is thought to have a neuropathic basis related to long-term tissue damage; it may also be related to changes in hormonal status, possibly explaining its temporal association with menopause [28].

While all patients present with complaints of pain, their descriptions may be widely variable with respect to location, timing, character, and provocations. Many patients believe that they have – and may have been treated for – chronic, recurrent yeast infections. Vulvodynia has been associated with co-existing conditions such as depression, interstitial cystitis, fibromyalgia, irritable bowel syndrome and frequent urinary tract, and yeast infections [27]. The diagnosis of vulvodynia is one of exclusion, and many times vulvar erythema, tenderness to palpation and/or allodynia may be the only physical exam findings; vaginal pH, wet mounts, and yeast cultures may help to exclude other causes.

Vulvodynia can also be a frustrating treatment dilemma, as specific triggers for the pain patients experience are often difficult to identify. General measures should include education, emotional support, hygiene measures, and behavioral therapy; referral to a pain specialist may be helpful, and physical therapy involving pelvic floor muscle rehabilitation can be effective in patients with vaginismus and pelvic floor hypertonicity [29]. First-line pharmacologic therapy consists of tricyclic antidepressants (e.g., amitriptyline 10 mg nightly, increasing by 10 mg weekly until symptoms improve) with or without a topical anesthetic. Topical lidocaine gel may be used on a scheduled basis up to six times a day, or on an as needed basis for intercourse. With the tricyclic antidepressants, care must be taken to watch for anticholinergic side effects as they may be more pronounced in the geriatric population. Other pharmacologic options include gabapentin, duloxetine, and the addition of topical estrogen if atrophy is present. For pain unresponsive to these therapies, local nerve block with a corticosteroid and lidocaine has been found to provide temporary relief, and referral to a pain management specialist may be appropriate in this case [30].

Cervix

In the geriatric patient, the appearance of the cervix changes in comparison to that of premenopausal patients as the transformation zone is usually found high within the endocervical canal. The cervix may also atrophy and become flush with the vaginal vault. While problems arising from the cervix are rare, two of the more common conditions in menopausal women are cervicitis and cervical stenosis.

Cervicitis in postmenopausal females is typically related to atrophic changes rather than an infectious process and can be a common cause of vaginal bleeding in this patient population. If there is no evidence of sexually transmitted or superimposed infection, treatment with vaginal estrogen should be started. A wet mount slide and/or cultures should be performed to evaluate any associated suspicious discharge, and appropriate antibiotics prescribed for any infectious process.

In addition to cervicovaginal atrophy, the menopausal decrease in estrogen also induces changes in the endocervical canal that may lead to the agglutination of the cervix, ultimately resulting in complete stenosis. This can obstruct the outflow of secretions and debris from the atrophic endometrial cavity, leading to hematometria or hydrometria; pyometria can occur if this accumulation of debris becomes infected.

Urogenital Atrophy and Vaginitis

During the menopause, the vagina, in particular, thins and loses elasticity. In addition, the vagina undergoes a decrease in blood flow and secretions. For a third of women, this results in dryness, discomfort, itching, and/or painful intercourse early in menopause and is often referred to as atrophic vaginitis. Unlike vasomotor symptoms, atrophy symptoms continue or worsen and the prevalence increases to about half of women with aging. Additionally, lack of estrogen changes the vagina from an acidic to a more basic environment, which favors colonization with enteric potentially uropathic bacteria [1–3]. Low doses of transvaginal creams, pessaries, tablets, and rings are likely equally effective in treating symptoms of vaginal atrophy and are not associated with significant systemic absorption [3]. Reversing vaginal atrophy before vaginal surgery is often performed (Fig. 82.2).

Other less common forms of vaginal irritation in the older women include bacterial vaginosis (BV) and candidiasis. In the atrophic vagina with a higher pH, lactobacilli, and yeasts are less commonly found likely explaining the decreased incidence of candidiasis [31]. Differentiation between these causes of vaginal irritation is important. Increased vaginal pH is found with both BV and atrophy. The discharge with BV is malodorous, thin, homogenous, grayish, and adherent to the vaginal walls. Candidiasis is odorless and "cottage cheese" like in appearance; the labia

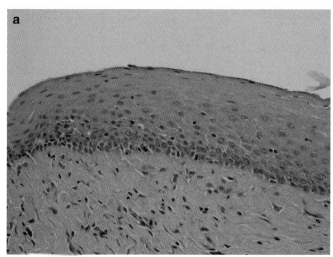

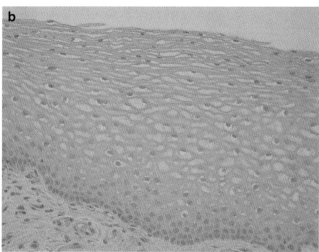

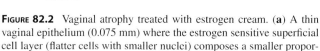

FIGURE 82.2 Vaginal atrophy treated with estrogen cream. (a) A thin vaginal epithelium (0.075 mm) where the estrogen sensitive superficial cell layer (flatter cells with smaller nuclei) composes a smaller propor-

tion of the epithelium. (b) Epithelial changes after nightly treatment with 50 μg of estrogen cream. The thicker epithelium (0.4 mm) contains a larger proportion of superficial cells.

can be erythematous and edematous with satellite lesions. BV also has a characteristic fishy odor with the application of potassium hydroxide. On saline wet mount, BV has clue cells (epithelial cells stippled with bacteria), while candidiasis has pseudohyphae [32]. With atrophy, the wet mount is predominantly intermediate and parabasal epithelial cells with few or no superficial cells [33]. Antibiotic treatment for BV and anticandidal regimens is effective and routinely prescribed by practitioners caring for older women [32].

The lower urinary tract is also estrogen sensitive, as estrogen receptors are found in the bladder and urethra. Symptoms of dysuria, urethral discomfort, overactive bladder (OAB), hematuria, urinary tract infections (UTIs), and urinary incontinence (UI) are associated with aging. Estrogen had been a mainstay of treatment of urinary tract symptoms, generally based on small observational studies [34]. However, a 2003 Cochrane review called into question the routine use of systemic estrogen as a therapeutic agent for UI. Fifteen of the 28 trials in this review favored estrogen use to treat UI, but the results from the Heart and Estrogen/Progestin Replacement Study (HERS) swayed the analysis towards estrogen worsening UI [35]. This review was followed by the negative findings in the Women's Health Initiative which showed increased or worsening of UI in women taking estrogen and progesterone or estrogen alone [34]. It is important to note that the influence of different estrogen formulations and route of delivery, in particular transvaginal estrogen, have yet to be elucidated. However, it is clear that systemic estrogen has not been shown to improve OAB or urinary incontinence and may actually worsen them [1, 34]. There is a role for transvaginal estrogen in preventing recurrent UTIs [36].

Urethra

Urethral Prolapse

The female urethra is typically 4 cm in length and is distally lined by nonkeratinized squamous epithelium. This epithelium and its spongy submucosa are estrogen sensitive and intrinsically remain sealed to each other. Two adherent smooth muscle layers are also present, an inner longitudinal layer and an outer circular layer. A circular disruption in this distal anatomy can result in prolapse out of the external meatus [37].

Urethral prolapse is relatively rare in the menopausal women but is associated with a lack of estrogen as it is found in prepubertal girls and postmenopausal women. Bleeding is the most common symptom, followed by voiding symptoms such as dysuria, urgency, frequency, and nocturia. If strangulated, suprapubic pain can occur. Concurrent infection is common [37].

Since urethral prolapse is rare, careful examination is needed to confirm the diagnosis, as the more common urethral caruncles and rare malignancy are in the differential diagnosis. Urethral prolpase is distinguished by the circumferential prolapse with a central opening, which can be catheterized to confirm the presence of the urethra. Significant swelling can lead to anatomical distortion, strangulation, and potentially necrosis and may necessitate examination under anesthesia to confirm the diagnosis with possible surgical correction. Imaging studies are seldom necessary once the diagnosis has been confirmed with catheterization; otherwise, malignancy should be considered. Histologically, inflammatory infiltrates are seen in the underlying connective tissue.

Treatments include warm sitz baths, transvaginal estrogen cream, topical steroids to reduce inflammation and antibiotics for infection [38, 39]. Estrogen has been reported to resolve the prolapse within 6 weeks [39]. If conservative management fails or if strangulated, surgical excision, and short-term catheterization (less than a week) should be performed [40]. Long-term transvaginal estrogen should be included in the postoperative care.

Urethral Caruncles

Urethral caruncles are benign, usually small, asymptomatic reddish exophytic lesion coming off of the posterior urethra. Often they are an incidental finding but can present with dysuria, tenderness, or bleeding especially if they enlarge to 1–2 cm (Fig. 82.3). The etiology likely starts with incomplete urethral prolapse, which becomes chronically irritated and takes a polypoid form. Like urethral prolapse, its origins are attributed to estrogen deficiency but are more common in older women being rarely found in premenopausal women or prepubertal girls. Cystoscopy is generally unnecessary. Treatment of symptomatic urethral caruncles is conservative and consists of sitz baths, transvaginal estrogen therapy, and anti-inflammatories when necessary. When clinical differentiation from cancer is difficult, such as a large (1–2 cm) lesion, there is a failure of medical therapy, or in the presence of severe symptoms, surgical excision biopsy should be considered [41].

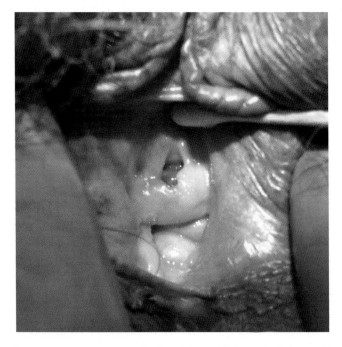

Figure 82.3 Urethral caruncle. Note it is a reddish, exophytic lesion off of the posterior urethra.

Urethral Diverticulum

A urethral diverticulum is an outpouching of the urethra into the anterior vaginal wall and is uncommon past 60 years of age. It is thought to be the result of obstruction of periurethral glands and is most commonly found in the distal urethra. Symptoms include dysuria, dribbling, urgency, frequency, and dyspareunia. On examination, it feels like a suburethral mass that is tender and can be hard if a stone is present. Urine or purulence may be expressed from the meatus when massaged. The differential diagnosis includes vaginal wall cysts from an embryologic remnant or local gland, ectopic ureterocele, and, rarely, malignancy. Magnetic resonance imaging (MRI) is the diagnostic imaging modality of choice to confirm the diagnosis, location, and size. Surgical excision is recommended treatment [42].

Upper Genital Tract

Uterus

Many of the changes evident in the postmenopausal uterus are a direct result of decreasing estrogen levels. There is an estimated 95% decline in blood estrogen concentration from the premenopausal to postmenopausal state [43]. The postmenopausal uterus undergoes involution and gradually becomes smaller with age. Benign abnormalities of the uterus, especially abnormalities of the uterine cavity, may result in postmenopausal bleeding, and endometrial cancer must be ruled out when it occurs in this age group. The primary causes of postmenopausal bleeding include vaginal atrophy with friability, endometrial atrophy, endometrial hyperplasia, endometrial and cervical polyps, and invasive cancer. The workup of all postmenopausal bleeding should consist of an endometrial biopsy either in the office or in the operating room when confronted with cervical stenosis or difficulty with patient discomfort. The use of ultrasound may be a useful first step in determining the existence of a thickened endometrium.

Endometrial Atrophy

Endometrial atrophy is a frequent cause of postmenopausal uterine bleeding. The surface epithelium of the uterine cavity, otherwise known as the endometrial layer, is known to undergo cellular and glandular loss, likely as a result of lowered estrogen levels [44]. This ultimately thinned endometrial surface is subject to bleeding, especially as a result of trauma. The collapsed, atrophic endometrial surfaces contain little or no fluid to prevent intracavitary friction [45]. Microerosions of the surface epithelium then develop that are prone to light bleeding or spotting.

The diagnosis of endometrial atrophy is confirmed by endometrial biopsy or by ultrasound (double layer thickness less than 4 mm). Adequate estrogen therapy is nearly always effective in relieving symptoms of both endometrial and vaginal atrophy. Although many oral preparations are available for the treatment of endometrial atrophy, local vaginal estrogen therapy has also been shown to be effective and well tolerated in the treatment of endometrial atrophy, but should be accompanied by a progestin for doses greater than 50 μg [3, 46].

Endometrial Polyps

Endometrial polyps, which are hyperplastic overgrowths of endometrial glands and stroma, develop from the endometrial basalis layer and are likely the result of estrogenic stimulation. The known association of large endometrial polyps with tamoxifen [47], a selective estrogen receptor modulator, strengthens this likelihood. The incidence peaks in the fifth decade of life; fortunately for most postmenopausal women, the incidence of endometrial polyps greatly decreases after menopause. They may be solitary or multiple and are usually pedunculated. Most are benign, with an estimated 1.5% being malignant [48]. In addition, while most are asymptomatic, they account for 12–25% of cases of postmenopausal bleeding [49, 50].

Endometrial polyps are diagnosed only by microscopic evaluation of the specimen postremoval, although they can be further evaluated and characterized using sonohysterography (Fig. 82.4). Saline infusion sonography has been shown to be more accurate than ultrasound alone in diagnosis, with a sensitivity and specificity of 93 and 94%, respectively, compared to 65 and 76%, respectively, for ultrasound alone [51].

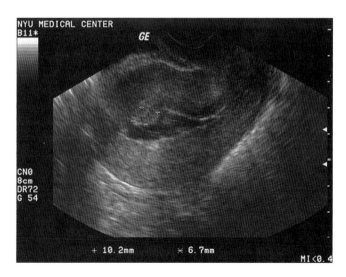

FIGURE 82.4 Saline infusion sonohysterogram of a perimenopausal patient with abnormal uterine bleeding. A polypoid lesion is seen extending near the anterior fundal region. This measures 10.2×6.7 mm (calipers). At the time of D&C with hysteroscopy, a polyp was identified and confirmed by pathology (reprinted with permission from Goldstein SR (2008) Abnormal uterine bleeding. In: Gibbs RS, Karlan BY, Haney RF, Nygaard IE (eds) Danforth's Obstetrics and Gynecology, 10th ed. Lippincott Williams & Wilkins, Philadelphia, p 668).

Treatment is removal by dilatation and curettage (D&C) or hysteroscopic guided polypectomy. Excision is essential to rule out carcinoma. Treatment decisions based on ultrasonography and hysteroscopy provide little utility as neither can adequately distinguish between benign and malignant polyps [48, 52].

Leiomyomas (Fibroids)

Benign uterine leiomyomas, otherwise known as fibroids, are hormonally responsive and typically decrease in size after menopause [53]. Although leiomyomas tend to atrophy as the woman ages, their presence can cause concern during bimanual exams or with their appearance on imaging studies. Medical therapy to decrease fibroid size is generally not indicated in the older postmenopausal woman. Additionally, surgical interventions for simple uterine fibroids in the postmenopausal female usually are not indicated. However, while most uterine masses ultimately prove to be benign fibroids, a rapidly enlarging pelvic mass may represent a uterine leiomyosarcoma. These are relatively uncommon, accounting for only 1–2% of postmenopausal uterine masses [54]. With any enlarging or persistent uterine mass, evaluation in the form of ultrasonography, computed tomography, and referral to a gynecologic specialist is warranted to exclude sarcoma.

Endometrial Hyperplasia and Cancer

Endometrial hyperplasia, or excessive proliferation of the uterine endometrium, can occur from many conditions, almost all associated with long-term unopposed estrogen stimulation. Risk factors for endometrial hyperplasia, other than direct unopposed estrogen stimulation include obesity, nulliparity, diabetes, early menarche, late menopause, polycystic ovarian syndrome, and tamoxifen therapy for greater than 2 years [55].

Endometrial hyperplasia is classified as either atypical hyperplasia or hyperplasia without atypia. These classes are further subdivided into two categories: simple and complex, with complex and atypical classifications having higher risks for malignancy. The diagnosis of endometrial hyperplasia is made from direct tissue sampling in the form of an office endometrial biopsy sampling or D&C. Treatment strategies center around the use of progestins. Progestins can be used for both simple and complex hyperplasia, both with and without atypia. Untreated endometrial hyperplasia can progress to endometrial carcinoma, so early treatment is paramount. Endometrial cancers are covered in Chap. 83.

Ovary

As women progress into menopause, there is a marked depletion of ovarian follicles resulting in decreased synthesis of circulating estrogen. The ovaries become atrophic becoming smaller in size than those of the premenopausal woman and are typically not palpable on bimanual examination. This may present a problem as the gynecologist or primary care physician attempts the examination, however, yearly examinations are paramount for the early detection of ovarian neoplasms. In the older woman, a combined rectovaginal examination may assist with the routine pelvic exam in detecting ovarian abnormalities. The incidence of ovarian neoplasms in the postmenopausal patient rises rapidly and plateaus until the age 70 and then rapidly declines.

Benign ovarian enlargement or benign cysts are rarely found in the postmenopausal female, as the ovary is inactive. Benign teratomas missed at an earlier age are sometimes found, but in general, most postmenopausal ovarian masses are suspect for malignancy. Management of ovarian tumors is discussed in Chap. 83.

Pelvic Floor Disorders

The national prevalence of symptomatic pelvic floor defects including pelvic organ prolapse (POP), urinary incontinence (UI), and fecal incontinence (FI) has been estimated to be 23.7%, regardless of age. Older women are far more affected, with rates up to 49.7% in women 80 years old and older [56]. The prevalence of anatomic stage II–IV POP using the Pelvic Organ Prolapse Quantification (POPQ) [57] (see Table 82.1 and Fig. 82.5) examination in the general population was reported to be 37%; prevalence in an older population of women with a mean age of 68 years was 64.8% [58]. Clearly, these are highly prevalent conditions and contribute significantly to older women's overall quality of life. Despite the availability of effective evaluation and treatment methods, women continue to suffer needlessly, with nearly 50% of affected women neglecting to inform their healthcare providers about their symptoms [59].

The etiology of POP and incontinence is complex, involving potential injury to, or attenuation of the many ligaments, muscles, connective tissue, and innervation of the pelvis. These conditions are associated with several risk factors including age, parity, abdominal circumference, and body mass index. Vaginal support defects as defined by DeLancey include Level I apical support defects (the cardinal–uterosacral ligament complex), Level II defects including cystocele, rectocele, or paravaginal defects (a defect in vaginal support at the level of the arcus tendineous fascia pelvis), or a Level III defect, detachment of the perineal body (Fig. 82.6) [60].

It is common for the older woman to be affected by more than one pelvic floor condition. POP can be associated with urinary as well as bowel dysfunction/incontinence. Women with advanced POP may experience voiding dysfunction, caused by urethral obstruction. Older women are at risk for

TABLE 82.1 Stages of pelvic organ prolapse

Stage 0	No prolapse is demonstrated. Points Aa, Ap, Ba, and Bp are all at −3 cm, and point C is between total vaginal length (TVL) and −(TVL −2 cm)
Stage I	The most distal portion of the prolapse is >1 cm above the level of the hymen
Stage II	The most distal portion of the prolapse is <1 cm proximal or distal to the plane of the hymen
Stage III	The most distal portion of the prolapse is <1 cm below the plane of the hymen but no further than 2 cm less than the total vaginal length
Stage IV	Complete to nearly complete eversion of the vagina. The most distal portion of the prolapse protrudes to >+(TVL −2) cm

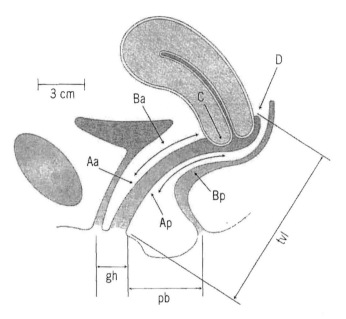

Figure 82.5 Six sites (points Aa, Ba, C, D, Bp, and Ap), genital hiatus (gh), perineal body (pb), and total vaginal length (tvl) used for pelvic organ support quantification (from Bump et al. [57]. Reprinted with permission from Elsevier).

coexisting urinary and fecal incontinence. A thorough history will elucidate these associated symptoms. An evaluation for occult incontinence may be warranted in cases of advanced prolapse, as an incompetent urethra may be masked by the urethral kinking associated with advanced organ descent.

The diagnosis of POP is made during a pelvic examination. The full extent of tissue prolapse may not be appreciated unless the patient stands or uses a strong valsalva force. Bladder and bowel dysfunction may require the use of further diagnostic testing such as urodynamics, anal manometry and ultrasound, or electromyography of the pelvic floor.

Urinary incontinence (UI) is defined as the complaint of any involuntary leakage of urine [61]. Diagnostic categories

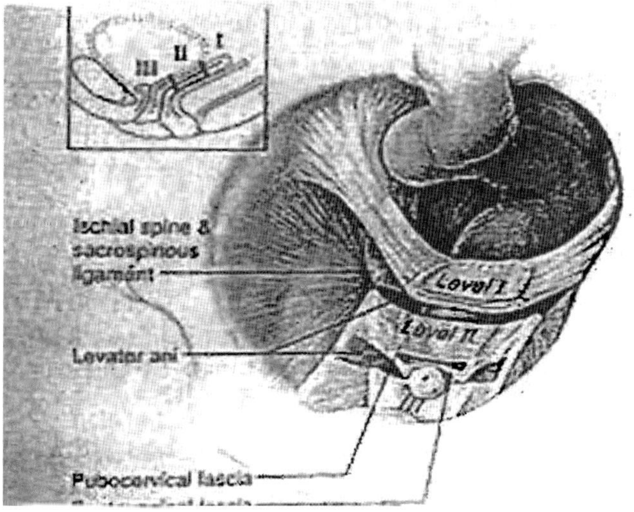

FIGURE 82.6 Vaginal support defects as defined by DeLancey include Level I apical support defects (the cardinal–uterosacral ligament complex). Level II defects including cystocele, rectocele, or paravaginal defects (a defect in vaginal support at the level of the arcus tendineous fascia pelvis), or a Level III defect, detachment of the perineal body (From De Lancey [60]. Reprinted with permission from Elsevier).

of UI include stress incontinence (leakage associated with episodes of increased intra-abdominal pressure), urge urinary incontinence (leakage associated with urgency and involuntary detrusor muscle contractions), overflow incontinence (seen when bladder emptying is insufficient), and mixed incontinence (any combination of the above).

Initial evaluation techniques center on the treatment of reversible causes of UI, for example, infection, inappropriate medication use, and mobility issues. After a thorough history, the examination focuses on pelvic/bladder anatomy and neurologic status. Bladder physiology and function may be further characterized using a stress test or urodynamic assessment, a diagnostic means of observing bladder neurologic and motor/muscle physiologic function.

Medical/Nonsurgical Treatment of POP and UI

Nonsurgical therapy of POP and urinary incontinence includes behavioral management (pelvic floor muscle rehabilitation and for incontinence the teaching of stress and urge incontinence strategies), medications, as well as the use of mechanical devices. A conservative treatment approach is usually considered in older women who do not desire a surgical intervention or where surgery may not be an ideal choice due to medical comorbidities causing increased surgical risk.

Pelvic floor muscle exercises may limit the progression of mild prolapse and related symptoms; however, less response has been noted with prolapse beyond the vaginal introitus

[62]. This method of treatment is often employed to treat accompanying urinary and/or fecal incontinence. Results are generally dependent on patient motivation and adherence to the exercise program.

The use of a mechanical device such as a pessary is an excellent option to nonsurgically treat POP and UI. Several different types of pessaries have been described made with numerous types of material; according to Mylex Products, Inc. (Chicago, IL) brochures, there are six to nine sizes of 13 pessary models used for stress urinary incontinence and/or POP, the majority of which are made of silicone or inert plastic. Pessaries provide pelvic organ support within the vaginal vault. Two categories of pessaries exist for prolapse: support and space filling. The ring pessary (with diaphragm) is a commonly used support pessary and the Gelhorn pessary is a commonly used space-filling pessary. (See Fig. 82.7) The ring and other support pessaries are recommended for Stage 1 and 2 prolapse, whereas the space-filling pessaries are for Stage 3 and 4 prolapse [63].

Possible complications associated with pessary use include vaginal discharge and odor. There may be failure to retain the pessary or conversely, the pessary may be too large, which could lead to excoriation or irritation. There may be de novo or increased stress incontinence [64] with the reduction of vaginal prolapse and in rare instances more severe complications such as fistula development.

The mainstay of treatment for overactive bladder and urge incontinence includes a combination of pelvic floor muscle rehabilitation and use of an anticholinergic medication. Patients refractory to these conservative therapies may be candidates for intra-vesical botulinum toxin A injections or neuromodulation techniques.

Surgical Treatment of POP

The decision for surgical versus conservative intervention for the treatment of pelvic floor disorders should not be based on chronologic age alone. Prior to the selection of a specific treatment or procedure, all existing pelvic floor defects should be evaluated. The older woman can expect similar operative risks as well as subjective and objective anatomic and quality-of-life outcomes as that of younger women undergoing pelvic floor disorder treatment.

Over 200,000 inpatient and outpatient surgeries are performed yearly for the treatment of urinary incontinence (UI) and POP in US women [65]. Demand for the care of pelvic floor disorders has been projected to increase significantly in the coming years due to significant shifting of American age demographics. Women aged 80 years and older are the most rapidly growing segment of the older US population. A woman's lifetime risk of having surgery for either POP or UI up to

a   b

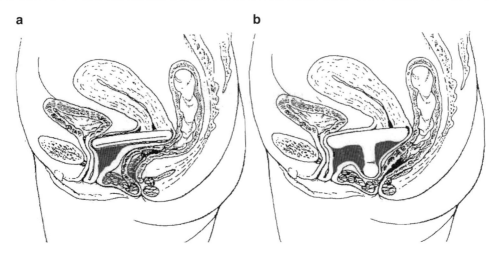

Figure 82.7 (a) Ring pessary without support in place; patient with cervix and uterus. Note that the pessary rests at the level of the bladder neck anteriorly and behind the cervix posteriorly. (b) Gelhorn pessary in place; patient with cervix and uterus. Note that the disk of the Gelhorn pessary rests at the level of the bladder neck anteriorly, and behind the cervix posteriorly (similar to the position of a ring pessary and that the knob rests behind the perineal body) (From Weber and Richter [62]. Reprinted with permission from Lippincott Williams & Wilkins).

the age of 80 years is 11.1% [66]. Women who have undergone a procedure for UI or POP are at risk for recurrence [67].

The ideal procedure in the older woman would robustly repair symptomatic pelvic floor defects, be performed efficiently, allow for rapid postoperative recovery including return to baseline or improved functional status, and conform with the sexual activity desires of the patient. Although many studies have included older women when examining outcomes after pelvic floor surgery, most studies have not specifically addressed POP surgery outcomes in the older woman. However, based on the information we do have, older women undergoing elective pelvic floor surgery face risks similar to patients of all ages undergoing elective general surgery. Pelvic floor surgery is considered an intermediate risk procedure with a perioperative mortality rate <5%. A review of recent studies that examine outcomes of the older woman undergoing pelvic floor surgery show mortality rates from 0.0 to 4.1% and complication rates from 15.5 to 33.0% [68]. Complication rates vary and may be due to the heterogeneous definitions of complications throughout the studies. However, the majority of complications were related to urinary tract infections, febrile morbidity, and blood loss requiring transfusion. Presurgical preparation should include optimization of the urogenital epithelium. In order to prepare the tissue for surgery and optimize healing, vaginal application of estrogen cream several weeks prior to the procedure and in the postoperative period is recommended.

Perioperative management of the older gynecology patient may demand attention to multiple medical considerations. Suggested prophylactic interventions are presented in Table 82.2. Surgery to correct POP and UI should address the specific pelvic floor defects that are present including the anterior vaginal wall (cystocele), posterior vaginal wall (rectocele), and apical vaginal support defects (enterocele) (see Figs. 82.8 and 82.9).

Surgical techniques to address anterior defects are the anterior colporrhaphy and paravaginal repair. Symptomatic anterior wall prolapse repair outcomes were compared at a 21-month average (12 months minimum) follow-up between 31 patients aged 80 years or more and 234 younger patients. They demonstrated similar rates of symptomatic failure between the groups, 6 versus 5%, respectively. Recurrence of any vaginal support defect in the older group was 10% [69].

The most efficacious technique to repair posterior defects is the traditional midline colporrhaphy [62]. Perineorrhaphy should be performed when there is separation of the perineal muscles. The posterior rectovaginal connective tissue should be reattached to the perineal body if separated. However, careful attention should be paid to avoid excessive vaginal narrowing (unless desired) as postoperative dyspareunia is a common complication. Anatomic success is high with this procedure; however, functional success rates may be considerably lower regardless of age.

Surgical techniques to address apical vaginal defects include the abdominal sacrocolpopexy (ASC), uterosacral ligament suspension (USS), ileococcygeus fixation, and sacrospinous fixation. The ASC employs graft material to suspend the anterior and posterior walls of the vagina to the anterior longitudinal ligament of the sacrum. Published ASC apical cure rates range from 78 to 100% [62]. However, this surgery requires a laparotomy, has a longer operative time, a longer recovery period, and higher postoperative complications when compared with vaginal approach surgeries. A recent RCT demonstrated similar perioperative complication rates as well as subjective and objective outcomes in women aged 70 years and older compared to a younger

TABLE 82.2 Perioperative clinical management of the older woman undergoing gynecologic surgery

Issue	Background	Clinical recommendation
Cardiovascular	Perioperative MI associated with 50% morality rate [79]	Perioperative beta-blocker use in the high and moderate risk patient
Delirium	Abrupt change in cognition or consciousness-Post-surgical prevalence estimate 37% [80] At risk for long-term cognitive deficiencies and increased mortality Under diagnosed	Avoid meperidine and anticholinergic agents including promethazine, minimize hospital stay, allow a companion to stay at bedside, maintain circadian pattern
DVT/thromboembolic events	Older patients have 20–40% risk of DVT due to advanced age (>60 years) and length of surgery [82]	Perioperative use of sequential pneumatic compression devices and selective use of heparin prophylaxis, early ambulation
Hypothermia	Decreased immunologic response, prolonged wound healing, [82] increased perioperative cardiac events	Intraoperative forced warm air blanket use, warmed intravenous fluids
Infectious disease	Clean contaminated procedures: mixed flora of the vagina	Perioperative dose of first-generation cephalosporin [83]
Neuropathies	Neurologic injuries due to nerve compression and ischemia as a result of patient positioning	Careful patient positioning with attention to the peroneal, femoral, ulnar, and sciatic nerves with padded stir-ups, avoid hyperflexion or extension of the lower extremities
Pulmonary	Increased perioperative morbidity and mortality rates with development of pneumonia	Pulmonary toilet with deep cough, incentive spirometry, early ambulation
Urinary tract infection	Pelvic floor surgery postoperative rates up to 44% [84]	Screen if new onset bladder/voiding symptoms

Source: Adapted from Gerten et al. [68]. Printed with permission from Elsevier

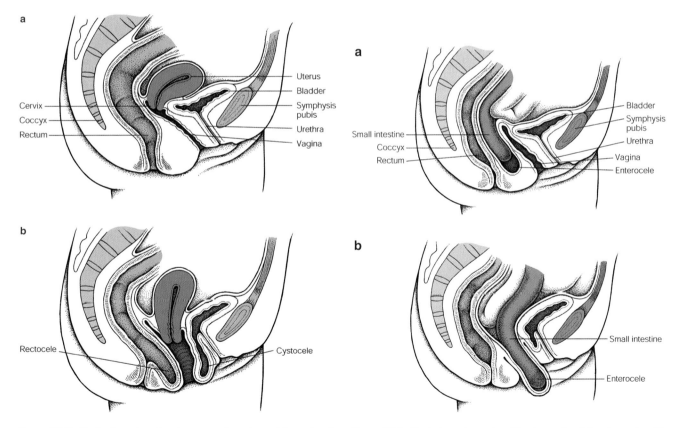

FIGURE 82.8 Sagittal section showing normal anatomy (**a**); cystocele and rectocele (**b**). (Reprinted with permission from Beers and Berkow [7]. Copyright 2000 by Merck & Co, Inc., Whitehouse Station, NJ. Available at: http://www.merck.com/mkgr/mmg/home.jsp. Accessed 22 September 2009).

FIGURE 82.9 Posterior enterocele without eversion (**a**); enterocele with eversion (**b**). (Reprinted with permission from Beers and Berkow [7]. Copyright 2000 by Merck & Co, Inc., Whitehouse Station, NJ. Available at: http://www.merck.com/mkgr/mmg/home.jsp. Accessed 22 September 2009).

group undergoing ASC [70]. ASC may be safely performed laparoscopically, even in the older woman; however, this requires significant surgical skills. Furthermore, there are few studies and no randomized trials looking at outcomes between the open versus laparoscopic approaches, especially in the older woman.

The USS is an intraperitoneal technique that attaches the vaginal vault to the uterosacral ligaments near the ischial spine bilaterally (Fig. 82.10). Published anatomic cure rates range from 65 to 98% depending on the definition of cure and the length of follow-up in an unselected patient population [71]. Sacrospinous fixation and ileococcygeus fixation are extraperitoneal techniques that attach the vaginal vault to the sacrospinous ligament or coccygeus muscle, respectively. Anatomic success for the sacrospinous fixation range from 29 to 98% and 53 to 96% for the ileococcygeus fixation [62].

Colpocleisis or colpectomy (narrowing or closure of the vaginal tissue and introitus) may be offered to the older woman who has no desire for vaginal function. These obliterative procedures have been shown to have shorter operative times and have fewer perioperative complications as compared to reconstructive repair [72]. Patient satisfaction is high and prolapse recurrence is low [73]. Preoperative assessment and operative treatment for occult stress incontinence may help avoid this unwanted postoperative complication.

Little information is available to guide us about which procedure should be considered in the older woman versus the younger woman. The ultimate decision on which approach and which procedure to employ in the treatment of POP in the older woman should take into consideration the patient's overall health and physical activity status, her specific pelvic floor defects and her future sexual activity desires, as well as the surgeon's training, skills, and preference.

Surgical Treatment of Urinary Incontinence

Common surgical approaches for the treatment of stress urinary incontinence include the midurethral sling (retropubic or transobturator), colposuspension, and the pubovaginal sling (autologous, synthetic, or allograft).

Older woman undergoing incontinence surgery can expect continence rates that in general compare favorably to those of younger women. The choice of incontinence surgery will depend upon surgeon experience as well as patient history and whether other concomitant procedures will be performed. Similar favorable short- and long-term outcomes have been demonstrated using the midurethral sling, colposuspension, and pubovaginal sling in the older woman.

Outcomes were compared between 123 women aged 70 years and older (mean 74.8) versus 208 younger women (mean 57.2) undergoing a retropubic midurethral sling (TVT Gynecare). Mean follow-up was 30 months (minimum 12). Persistent SUI was found in 7 versus 6%, respectively, and postoperative complications were similar between groups [74]. Review of current literature demonstrates SUI cure rates in older women who underwent midurethral slings (TVT) range from 45–93% compared to 73–95% in younger cohorts of women in the same studies [68].

A recent secondary analysis of data from the Stress Incontinence Surgical Treatment Efficacy Trial (SISTEr), a randomized trial of Burch colposuspension versus autologous rectus fascial sling addressed 2-year outcomes in older women (≥65 years of age) versus those younger [75]. Older women had a slightly longer time to normal activities (50 days compared with 42 days, $P=0.05$), but there was no difference in time to normal voiding (14 days compared with 11 days, $P=0.42$). Older women were more likely to have a positive stress test at follow-up (odds ratio [OR] 3.7, 95% confidence interval [CI] 1.70–7.97, $P=0.001$), less subjective improvement in stress (eight point lesser decrease, 95% CI 1.5–14.1, $P=0.02$), and urge incontinence (seven point lesser decrease, 95% CI 1.5–12.2, $P=0.01$) as measured by the Medical and Epidemiologic Social Aspects of Aging questionnaire and were more likely to undergo surgical retreatment for SUI (OR 3.9, 95% CI 1.30–11.48). Perioperative adverse events and length of stay did not differ between groups.

Periurethral bulking injections have been employed in the treatment of SUI in the older woman. Regardless of the agent, cure and improvement rates are poor and appear to decline with time. However, given that the risk of the procedure is low and requires no specific anesthesia, this may be a reasonable option in the medically compromised patient or in the patient who has failed other approaches.

Aging is associated with decreased detrusor contractility and decreased urinary flow rates, which may explain the slightly increased occurrence of postoperative voiding dysfunction, irritative urinary symptoms, and UTIs seen in some older women. However, older women who have preoperative irritative lower urinary symptoms demonstrate decreased rates of these symptoms after surgery [76].

Bowel Incontinence

Treatment of bowel or fecal incontinence in the older woman should include evaluation for possible functional, anatomic and neurologic deficiencies in the lower gastrointestinal tract. Behavioral therapies that include diet modification with fluid and fiber balance as well as pelvic floor muscle

Figure 82.10 Diagrams illustrating open vaginal apical area with (**a**) exposure of site for suture placement or lateral pelvic side wall and (**b**) suture placement through ligament then through the posterior and anterior paravaginal tissue where they are locked to enable pulley action to the ligaments when tied. (Reprinted with permission from Berek JS (ed) (2006) Berek and Novak's Gynecology, 14th edn. Lippincott Williams & Wilkins, Philadelphia, pp 923–926.).

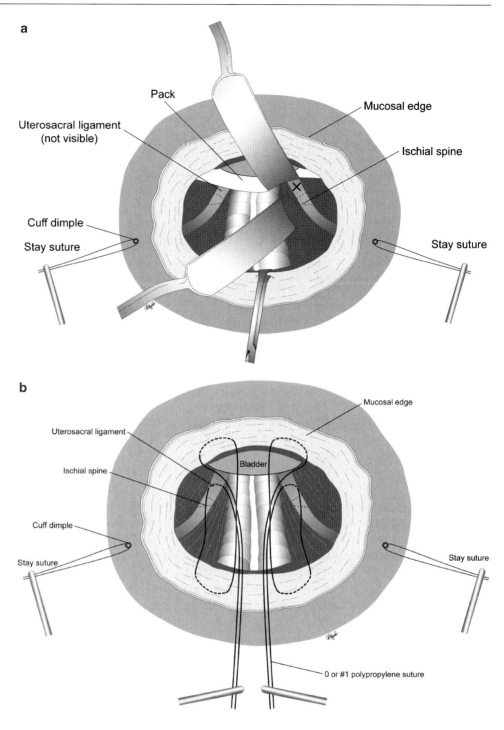

rehabilitation should be considered. If an anatomic defect such as a sphincter disruption is identified, anal sphincter repair could be considered. No specific studies address the efficacy of this approach in the older woman, however "good" short-term outcomes in all age ranges are achieved in approximately 70% of patients. Unfortunately, long-term results may not be as robust, with one study reporting only 23% of patients with "good" results at 10 years follow-up [77]. Other surgical approaches to consider for the treatment of refractory FI include stimulated muscle transposition, artificial anal sphincter implant, sacral nerve neuromodulation, and colostomy.

Research Involving the Older Woman

Given the growing geriatric population along with the high prevalence of pelvic floor disorders, there is a pressing need for information on the nonsurgical and surgical treatment outcomes in this unique population of women. There is a relative paucity of literature that addresses the older woman and the treatment of pelvic floor disorders. In fact, older women have been excluded from many of the trials that have examined the outcomes of pelvic floor surgery. A systematic review found the median percentage of women aged 70 or older who participated in surgical trials for SUI was 3.8%, while the number of surgeries for SUI performed on this population of women is estimated at 16% [78]. As the outcomes of surgery may be different in this population, the older woman should be encouraged to participate in clinical studies. Further investigation is required to understand the impact that surgery for pelvic floor disorders has on anatomic, physiologic, and functional outcomes in older women.

CASE STUDY

Ms RR is a 78-year-old white female from Eastern Europe seen in Urogynecology clinic with her daughter. Both speak English well, however, the daughter did help clarify some issues during the interview. Ms RR complained of an increasing feeling of protrusion and pressure that has markedly worsened over the past 6 months. She does describe problems emptying her bladder and denies significant urinary leakage. She is a widow and not sexually active. The patient had used a pessary for a while and did not wish to continue this nonsurgical treatment approach. Her medical history is significant for a renal transplant approximately 2.5 years previously secondary to a history of polycystic kidney disease; she takes prednisone and Cellcept for this. Other medical conditions include recurrent urinary tract infections, hypertension, coronary artery disease, and hypercholesterolemia. She has had a previous cholecystectomy, back surgery, and a heart catheterization. Other medications include furosemide, amlodipine, augmentin, atenolol, prograf, ASA, and a multivitamin; she has no known drug allergies. Other review of systems was noncontributory.

Physical examination revealed the abdomen to be soft, nontender, no mass effect; genitourinary examination revealed an evident uterine procidentia with total vaginal vault eversion (see Fig. 82.11a). On bimanual examination, there was the appreciation of a mass, just right of midline that was slightly tender to palpation. The urine dip was positive for nitrates and leukocytes and was sent for culture and sensitivities. All surgical options were discussed and it was decided that a vaginal obliterative procedure (colpocleisis, leaving the uterus in situ) would be performed.

The patient was started on some intravaginal estrogen cream to help thicken the vaginal epithelium, an oral antibiotic to treat the urine and dates for a urodynamic evaluation and surgery were set up. A CT scan would be set up to characterize the mass thinking that it may be her pelvic kidney. The urine culture was positive for *E. coli* sensitive to intravenous antibiotics. The renal transplant service subsequently admitted her for treatment and while she was in the hospital, she underwent a noncontrast CT of the abdomen and pelvis. Significant findings included extensive diverticular disease and an air-filled uterus and left fallopian tube. Further evaluation with the placement of transrectal contrast revealed a fistula tract between the sigmoid colon and the left adnexa (Fig. 82.11b). On further discussion with the patient, she did relate a several months history of lower abdominal–pelvic pain and some occasional discharge from the cervix. The patient was transferred to the Urogynecology service, gentle hydration and antibiotic therapy was continued and a colorectal surgery consult obtained. The patient remained afebrile throughout her hospital course. Perioperative medication management was discussed including holding the furosemide and amlodipine the day before surgery; she would take her beta-blocker and receive stress dose steroids the day of surgery. One week after admission, after a gentle bowel preparation and medication management, she underwent a TAHBSO and sigmoid resection. As there was concern about using a mesh to elevate the vagina, the planned colpocleisis was also performed.

Her postoperative course was unremarkable. Her daughter stayed with the patient the majority of the time. Pain was well controlled with initial patient controlled anesthesia, with conversion to oral medications once bowel function was assured. All of her medications

(continued)

CASE STUDY (continued)

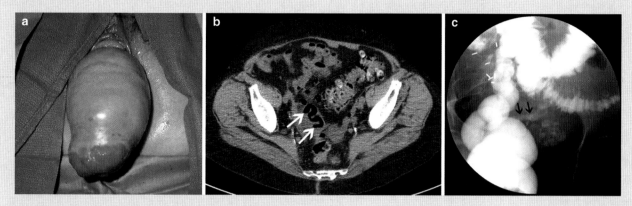

FIGURE 82.11 (a) Total uterine procidentia. (b) CT shows gas in tublar fallopian tube and adjacent stranding. There are numerous diverticula in the sigmoid colon. (c) Water soluble enema shows linear contrast in the tract. The round structure is a calcified fibroid.

were reinstated and she was discharged home with her daughter on POD#4.

This is a case where clinical suspicion for other potential contributing processes resulted in findings that markedly changed the initial surgical plan. Older patients, particularly older patients who are chronically immuno-

suppressed, often do not manifest with typical signs and symptoms of infectious and other pathologic processes. Once the diagnosis was made, careful perioperative planning under nonemergent conditions allowed this complex clinical scenario to be resolved in a very satisfactory manner resulting in markedly improved quality of life.

Acknowledgements Partially supported by the National Institute of Diabetes and Digestive and Kidney Diseases, DK068389.

References

1. Nelson HD (2008) Menopause review. Lancet 371:760–770
2. Grady D (2006) Clinical practice: management of menopausal symptoms. N Engl J Med 355:2338–2347
3. Suckling J, Lethaby A, Kennedy R (2003) Local estrogen for vaginal atrophy in postmenopausal women. Cochrane Database Syst Rev, Issue 4. Art. No.:CD001500. doi:10.1002/14651858. CD001500.pub2
4. Simon J, Snabes M (2007) Menopausal hormone therapy for vasomotor symptoms: balancing the risks and benefits with ultra-low doses of estrogen. Expert Opin Investig Drugs 16: 2005–2020
5. Verdier-Sévrain S (2007) Effect of estrogens on skin aging and the potential role of selective estrogen receptor modulators. Climacteric 10:289–297
6. Netter F. Reproductive system. The Netter Collection of Medical Illustrations, ed. O. E. Vol. 2. 1997, Philadelphia: Elsevier, p 90.
7. Beers M, Berkow R (2000) Aging and the skin. In: Lane K (ed) The Merck manual of geriatrics, 3rd edn. Merck Research Laboratories, Whitehouse Station, NJ, pp 1231–1238
8. Thomas RH et al (1996) Anogenital lichen sclerosus in women. J R Soc Med 89:694–698

9. Goldstein AT et al (2005) Prevalence of vulvar lichen sclerosus in a general gynecology practice. J Reprod Med 50:477–480
10. Meyrick TR, Kennedy C (1986) The development of lichen sclerosus et atrophicus in monozygotic twin girls. Br J Dermatol 114:377
11. Todd P et al (1994) Lichen sclerosus and the Kobner phenomenon. Clin Exp Dermatol 19:262–263
12. ACOG Practice Bulletin No. 93 (2008) Diagnosis and management of vulvar skin disorders. Obstet Gynecol 111:1243–1253
13. Carli P et al (1995) Squamous cell carcinoma arising in vulval lichen sclerosus: a longitudinal cohort study. Eur J Cancer Prev 4:491–495
14. Cooper SM et al (2004) Does treatment of vulvar lichen sclerosus influence its prognosis? Arch Dermatol 140:702–706
15. Lorenz B, Kaufman RH, Kutzner SK (1998) Lichen sclerosus. Therapy with clobetasol propionate. J Reprod Med 43.790–794
16. Neill SM, Tatnall FM, Cox NH (2002) Guidelines for the management of lichen sclerosus. Br J Dermatol 147:640–649
17. Renaud-Vilmer C et al (2004) Vulvar lichen sclerosus: effect of long-term topical application of a potent steroid on the course of the disease. Arch Dermatol 140:709–712
18. Virgili A, Bacilieri S, Corazza M (2001) Managing vulvar lichen simplex chronicus. J Reprod Med 46:343–346
19. Shiohara T (1988) The lichenoid tissue reaction. An immunological perspective. Am J Dermatopathol 10:252–256
20. Scully C, el-Kom M (1985) Lichen planus: review and update on pathogenesis. J Oral Pathol 14:431–458
21. Ramer MA et al (2003) Lichen planus and the vulvovaginal-gingival syndrome. J Periodontol 74:1385–1393
22. Droegemueller W (1992) Comprehensive gynecology, 2nd edn. Mosby, St. Louis, p 637

23. Visco AG, Del Priore G (1996) Postmenopausal bartholin gland enlargement: a hospital-based cancer risk assessment. Obstet Gynecol 87:286–290

24. Bachmann GA et al (2006) Chronic vulvar and other gynecologic pain: prevalence and characteristics in a self-reported survey. J Reprod Med 51:3–9

25. Moyal-Barracco M, Lynch PJ (2004) 2003 ISSVD terminology and classification of vulvodynia: a historical perspective. J Reprod Med 49:772–777

26. ACOG Committee Opinion No. 345 (2006) Vulvodynia. Obstet Gynecol 108:1049–1052

27. Arnold LD et al (2007) Assessment of vulvodynia symptoms in a sample of US women: a prevalence survey with a nested case control study. Am J Obstet Gynecol 196:128 e1–e6

28. Zoubina EV et al (2001) Acute and chronic estrogen supplementation decreases uterine sympathetic innervation in ovariectomized adult virgin rats. Histol Histopathol 16:989–996

29. Haefner HK et al (2005) The vulvodynia guideline. J Low Genit Tract Dis 9:40–51

30. Rapkin AJ, McDonald JS, Morgan M (2008) Multilevel local anesthetic nerve blockade for the treatment of vulvar vestibulitis syndrome. Am J Obstet Gynecol 198:41 e1–e5

31. Hillier S, Lau R (1997) Vaginal microflora in postmenopausal women who have not received estrogen replacement therapy. Clin Infect Dis 25:S123–126

32. ACOG Practice Bulletin Number 72 (2006) Clinical management guidelines for obstetrician – gynecologists. Obstet Gynecol 107:1195–1206

33. McEndree B (1999) Clinical application of the vaginal maturation index. Nurse Pract 24(51–52):55–56

34. Hendrix SL, Cochrane BB, Nygaard IE et al (2005) Effects of estrogen with and without progestin on urinary incontinence. JAMA 293:935–948

35. Moehrer B, Hextall A, Jackson S (2003) Oestrogens for urinary incontinence in women. Cochrane Database Syst Rev, Issue 2. Art. No. CD 001405. doi:10.1002/14651858.CD001405

36. Perrotta C, Aznar M, Mejia R, et al. (2008) Oestrogens for preventing recurrent urinary tract infection in postmenopausal women. Cochrane Database Syst Rev, Issue 2. Art. No.: CD005131. doi:10.1002/14651858.CD005131.pub2

37. Anveden-Hertzberg L, Gauderer MW, Elder JS (1995) Urethral prolapse: an often misdiagnosed cause of urogenital bleeding in girls. Pediar Emerg Care 11:212–214

38. Redman JF (1982) Conservative management of urethral prolapse in female children. Urology 19:505–506

39. Wright M (1987) Urethral prolapse in children – alternative management. S Afr Med J 72:551–552

40. Kleinjan JH, Vos P (1984) Strangulated urethral prolapse. J Urol 132:732–733

41. Park DS, Cho TW (2004) Simple solution for urethral caruncle. J Urol 172:1184–1185

42. Aspera AM, Rackley RR, Vasavada SP (2002) Contemporary evaluation and management of the female urethral diverticulum. Urol Clin North Am 29:617–624

43. Pandit L, Ouslander JG (1997) Postmenopausal vaginal atrophy and atrophic vaginitis. Am J Med Sci 314:228

44. Motta P, Makabe S (2003) An atlas of menopausal aging. Parthenon, New York City

45. Ferenczy A (2003) Pathophysiology of endometrial bleeding. Maturitas 45:1

46. Gerbaldo D, Ferraiolo A, Croce S et al (1991) Endometrial morphology after 12 months of vaginal oestriol therapy in postmenopausal women. Maturitas 13:269–74

47. McGurgan P, Taylor LJ, Duffy SR et al (2006) Does tamoxifen therapy affect the hormone receptor expression and cell prolifera-tion indices of endometrial polyps? An immunohistochemical comparison of endometrial polyps from postmenopausal women exposed and not exposed to tamoxifen. Maturitas 54:252

48. Shushan A, Revel A, Rojansky N (2004) How often are endometrial polyps malignant? Gynecol Obstet Invest 58:212–215

49. Van Bogaert LJ (1991) Clinicopathologic findings in endometrial polyps. Obstet Gynecol 77:954–956

50. Karlsson B, Granberg S, Wikland M et al (1995) Transvaginal Ultrasonography of the endometrium in women with postmenopausal bleeding – a Nordic multicenter study. Am J Obstet Gynecol 172:1488

51. Sylvestre C, Child TJ, Tulandi T et al (2003) A prospective study to evaluate the efficacy of two- and three-dimensional sonohysterography in women with intrauterine lesions. Fertil Steril 79: 1222–1225

52. Ben-Arie A, Goldchmit C, Laviv Y et al (2004) The malignant potential of endometrial polyps. Eur J Obstet Gynecol Reprod Biol 115:206

53. Adams Hillard PJ (2007) Benign Diseases of the Female Reproductive Tract. In: Berek JS (ed) Berek & Novak's gynecology, 14th edn. Lippincott Williams & Wilkins, Philadelphia, PA, pp 431–504

54. Leibsohn S, d'Ablaing G, Mishell DR Jr et al (1990) Leiomyosarcoma in a series of hysterectomies performed for presumed uterine leiomyomas. Am J Obstet Gynecol 162:968–974

55. Herbst AL (2001) Neoplastic diseases of the uterus. In: Stenchever MA, Droegemuller W, Herbst AL et al (eds) Comprehensive gynecology, 4th edn. Mosby, Inc, St. Louis, MO, pp 921–927

56. Nygaard I, Barber M, Burgio K et al (2008) Prevalence of symptomatic pelvic floor disorders in US women. JAMA 300: 1311–1316

57. Bump RC, Mattiasson A, Bo K et al (1996) The standardization of terminology of female pelvic organ prolapse and pelvic floor dysfunction. Am J Obstet Gynecol 175:10–17

58. Nygaard I, Bradley C, Brandt D (2004) Pelvic organ prolapse in older women: prevalence and risk factors. Obstet Gynecol 104: 489–497

59. Harris S, Lind C, Tennstedt S et al (2007) Care seeking and treatment for urinary incontinence in a diverse population. J Urol 177:680–684S

60. De Lancey JO (1992) Anatomic aspects of vaginal eversion after hysterectomy. Am J Obstet Gynecol 166:1717–1724

61. Abrams P, Cardozo L, Fall M et al (2002) The standardization of terminology of lower urinary tract function: Report from the standardization sub-committee of the international continence society. Am J Obstet Gynecol 187:116–126

62. Weber AM, Richter HE (2005) Pelvic organ prolapse. Obstet Gynecol 106:615–634

63. Sulak PJ, Kuehl TJ, Shull BJ (1993) Vaginal pessaries and their use in pelvic relaxation. J Reprod Med 38:919–923

64. Harris TA, Bent AE (1990) Genital Prolapse with and without urinary incontinence. J Reprod Med 35:792–798

65. Nygaard I, Thom DH, Calhoun EA (2007) Urinary incontinence in women. In: Litwin MS, Saigal CS (eds) Urologic diseases in America. US Department of Health and Human Services, Public Health Service, National Institutes of Health, National Institute of Diabetes and Digestive and Kidney Diseases. US Government Printing Office, Washington, DC, pp 71–103, NIH Publication No. 07–5512

66. Olsen AL, Smith VJ, Bergstrom JO et al (1997) Epidemiology of surgically managed pelvic organ prolapse and urinary incontinence. Obstet Gynecol 89:501–506

67. Clark AL, Gregory T, Smith VJ et al (2003) Epidemiologic evaluation of reoperation for surgically treated pelvic organ prolapse and urinary incontinence. Am J Obstet Gynecol 189:1261–1267

68. Gerten KA, Markland AD, Lloyd LK, Richter HE (2008) Prolapse and incontinence surgery in older women. J Urol 179:2111–2118

69. Carey JM, Leach GE (2003) Transvaginal surgery in the octogenarian using cadaveric fascia for pelvic prolapse and stress incontinence: minimal one year results compared to younger patients. Urology 63:665–670

70. Richter HE, Goode PS, Kenton K et al (2007) The effect of age on short-term outcomes after abdominal surgery for pelvic organ prolapse. JAGS 55:857–863

71. Silva WA, Pauls RN, Segal JL et al (2006) Uterosacral ligament vault suspension: five year outcomes. Obstet Gynecol 108: 255–263

72. Sung VW, Weitzen S, Sokol ER et al (2006) Effect of patient age on increasing morbitity and mortality following urogynecologic surgery. Am J Obstet Gynecol 194:1411–7

73. Fitzgerald MP, Richter HE, Bradley CS, et al for the Pelvic Floor Disorders Network. Pelvic support, pelvic symptoms and patient satisfaction after colpocleisis. Intl Urogynecol J 2008;19:1603–1609.

74. Gordon G, Gold R, Pauzner D et al (2005) Tension-free vaginal tape in the elderly: is it a safe procedure? Urology 65:479–482

75. Richter HE, Goode PS, Brubaker L et al (2008) Two-year outcomes after surgery for stress incontinence in older compared with younger women. Obstet Gynecol 112:621–629

76. Friedman WH, Gallup DG, Burke JJ et al (2006) Outcomes of octogenarians and nonagenarians in elective major gynecologic surgery. Am J Obstet Gynecol 195:547–553

77. Madoff RD (2005) Surgery for fecal incontinence in women. In: Abrams P (ed) Incontinence. Health Publications Ltd, France, pp 1585–1588

78. Morse AN, Labin LC, Young SB et al (2004) Exclusion of elderly women from published randomized trials of stress incontinence surgery. Obstet Gynecol 104:498–503

79. Eagle KA, Berger PB, Calkins H et al (2002) ACC/AHA guideline update for perioperative cardiovascular evaluation for noncardiac surgery: executive summary: a report of the American College of Cardiology/American Heart Association Task force on practice guidelines (Committee to update the 1996 guidelines on perioperative cardiovascular evaluation for noncardiac surgery). Circulation 105:1257–1267

80. Bitondo Dyer C, Ashton CM, Teasdale TA (1995) Postoperative delirium. Arch Intern Med 155:461–465

81. Bombeli T, Spahn DR (2004) Updates in perioperative coagulation: physiology and management of thromboembolism and haemorrhage. Br J Anaeth 93:275–87

82. Kurz A, Sessler DI, Lenhardt R (1996) Perioperative normothermia to reduce the incidence of surgical-wound infection and shorten hospitalization. N Engl J Med 334:1209–1212

83. ACOG Practice Bulletin No.74 (2006) Antibiotic prophylaxis for gynecologic procedures. Obstet Gynecol 108:225

84. Schweitzer KJ, Vierhout ME, Milani AL (2005) Surgery for pelvic organ prolapse in women 80 years of age or older. Acta Obstet Gynecol Scand 84:286–289

Chapter 83
Gynecologic Malignancies in the Elderly

Dan-Arin Silasi, Peter E. Schwartz, and Thomas J. Rutherford

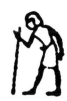

Pelvic reproductive organ cancers include those that arise in the vulva, vagina, cervix, uterus, fallopian tubes, and ovaries. In the United States, the number of persons over 65 years of age has been increasing at a disproportionately higher rate than that of the general population. According to the U.S. Census Bureau, the percentage of women 65 years of age and older has increased from 13.1% in 1980 to 14.6% in 1990.

The risk of gynecological cancers increases with age. It is important that the medical community is aware of the unique aspects of clinical care of older cancer patients.

This chapter presents the epidemiology, presenting symptoms, diagnosis workup, and treatment of pelvic malignancies in elderly women. It also notes the alternative therapies that can be applied to elderly patients when they are unable to tolerate standard treatment due to associated medical comorbidities.

Vulvar Cancer

The vulvar skin can present with a variety of dysplastic and malignant changes that vary from mild dysplasia to carcinoma in situ to invasive cancers involving other pelvic organs or have distant metastases. Vulvar cancer is an uncommon occurrence, representing approximately 4% of genital tract malignancies. Cancer statistics estimated that 3,970 patients were newly diagnosed in the United States in the year 2004 and that 850 deaths occurred [1, 2].

Dysplastic changes of the vulva may be unifocal or multifocal. The disease tends to be unifocal in the elderly population, whereas in women of younger age it tends to be multifocal [3].

Elderly patients, particularly those over 70 years of age, are less likely to have an associated human papilloma virus (HPV) infection [4, 5].

Dysplastic and malignant squamous cell changes are the dominant histologic patterns seen in vulvar neoplasias.

In addition to squamous cell changes, extramammary Paget's disease (EMPD) is most commonly seen in the vulva of postmenopausal Caucasian women but may also be seen in the axilla, male genitalia, eyelid, and ear. It is sometimes associated with an underlying vulvar carcinoma [6]. Patients with EMPD in the anogenital region most commonly present with pruritus, hyperpigmented or hypopigmented lesions, ulceration, and/or areas of leukoplakia and can frequently be mistaken for an inflammatory or infectious process [7].

Squamous cell carcinomas account for approximately 90% of newly diagnosed cancer cases. The second most common malignancy is melanoma [8], and the third most common is adenocarcinoma, arising in a Bartholin's gland or in skin appendages [9].

The etiology of vulvar carcinoma is unknown. The association of vulvar cancer with preceding vulvar intraepithelial neoplasia (VIN) and Human Papillomavirus infection (HPV) is controversial, as is its relationship with vulvar dystrophies. Other authors, however, have reported progression of VIN to invasive cancer [10, 11]. The association of HPV subtypes with oncogenic potential and smoking with invasive vulvar cancers is frequently found in women of relatively younger age [12].

However, vulvar cancer is encountered mostly in elderly patients and appears to be unrelated to smoking and HPV infection, while concurrent VIN is uncommon. This patient population has a high incidence of dystrophic lesions, like lichen sclerosus [13].

Staging of vulvar malignancies is surgical in nature and depends on the extent of the local disease and the presence or absence of inguinal lymph node metastases (Table 83.1).

The diagnosis of vulvar cancer starts with inspection. It is important to distinguish atrophy from dysplasia. Elderly patients often have atrophic changes of the vulva. Lesions that are symmetric in distribution, white, and nonraised are

D.-A. Silasi (✉)
Department of Obstetrics and Gynecology/Gynecologic Oncology,
Yale University School of Medicine/Yale New Haven Hospital,
New Haven, CT, USA
e-mail: dan-arin.silasi@yale.edu

R.A. Rosenthal et al. (eds.), *Principles and Practice of Geriatric Surgery*,
DOI 10.1007/978-1-4419-6999-6_83, © Springer Science+Business Media, LLC 2011

TABLE 83.1 Carcinoma of the vulva [175]

Stage I	Tumor confined to the vulva
IA	Lesions ≤2 cm in size, confined to the vulva or perineum and with stromal invasion ≤1.0 mm[a], no nodal metastasis
IB	Lesions >2 cm in size or with stromal invasion >1.0 mm[a], confined to the vulva or perineum, with negative nodes
Stage II	Tumor of any size with extension to adjacent perineal structures (1/3 lower urethra, 1/3 lower vagina, anus) with negative nodes
Stage III	Tumor of any size with or without extension to adjacent perineal structures (1/3 lower urethra, 1/3 lower vagina, anus) with positive inguino-femoral lymph nodes
IIIA	(i) With 1 lymph node metastasis (≥5 mm), or (ii) 1–2 lymph node metastasis(es) (b5 mm)
IIIB	(i) With 2 or more lymph node metastases (≥5 mm), or (ii) 3 or more lymph node metastases (b5 mm)
IIIC	With positive nodes with extracapsular spread
Stage IV	Tumor invades other regional (2/3 upper urethra, 2/3 upper vagina), or distant structures
IVA	Tumor invades any of the following: (i) Upper urethral and/or vaginal mucosa, bladder mucosa, rectal mucosa, or fixed to pelvic bone, or (ii) Fixed or ulcerated inguino-femoral lymph nodes
IVB	Any distant metastasis including pelvic lymph nodes

Source: Reprinted from FIGO Committee on Gynecologic Oncology [175], with permission

[a]The depth of invasion is defined as the measurement of the tumor from the epithelial–stromal junction of the adjacent most superficial dermal papilla to the deepest point of invasion

usually atrophic in nature. Dysplastic lesions and malignancies tend to be asymmetric in distribution and may be friable.

Most commonly, patients present with the complaint of a vulvar lump or mass. A long history of vulvar burning or pruritus is frequently elicited. Most lesions occur initially on the labia majora and less frequently on the labia minora, clitoris, or perineum. Only approximately 5% of cases are multifocal.

There is little consensus regarding the optimal method of management. There has been a gradual trend toward conservation in the management of dysplastic lesions (vulvar intraepithelial lesion, VIN grade 1–3). Current treatment modalities include carbon dioxide (CO_2) laser vaporization or ablation and surgical excision. Recurrence rates after treatment have been reported to range from 10 to 50% and are thought to be related to the grade of VIN and margin status along with the multifocal nature of the condition and its relationship with HPV [14].

In the elderly, if chosen, surgical excision may be performed under local anesthesia. Generally, a 1-cm margin is adequate for noninvasive lesions. For extramammary Paget's disease of the vulva, however, even 2-cm margins are often insufficient [15, 16].

For extramammary Paget's disease of the vulva, it is sometimes necessary to perform extremely wide local excisions with skin grafts or advancement flaps to cover the defect [17]. Microscopically, positive margins following surgical excision of vulvar Paget's disease is a frequent finding, and disease recurrence is common regardless of surgical margin status. Long-term monitoring of patients is recommended, and repeat surgical excision is often required [18].

The standard surgical management of women with invasive carcinomas of the vulva is a radical vulvectomy with bilateral inguinal–femoral lymphadenectomies [19]. The inguinal lymph nodes are the primary lymphatic drainage for the vulva and lower one-third of the vagina. The lymph node sampling is performed by removing an ellipse of skin in continuity with the underlying fat pad above the cribriform fascia present in the inguinal–femoral subcutaneous tissue. However, the cribriform fascia is difficult to identify in some women or may not be anatomically intact. This treatment can be modified if the tumor is unilateral, in which case a modified radical vulvectomy, effectively a unilateral radical excision of the labia in association with ipsilateral lymphadenectomy, is performed [20].

Data suggest that a woman with a unilateral vulvar cancer having negative ipsilateral inguinal lymph nodes is highly unlikely to have contralateral inguinal lymph node involvement [21].

If the lesion is less than 2 cm in diameter and is associated with minimal invasion (usually <2 mm), the chance of inguinal lymph node metastases being present is virtually nil. For an elderly woman with significant medical problems that presents with a superficial lesion (<2 mm invasion), wide local excision may be adequate management. Such surgery can be accomplished under local anesthesia if the patient is not a candidate for general or regional anesthesia [22–24].

Further modifications in the management of vulvar cancer include inguinal lymph node sampling, rather than a formal inguinal–femoral lymphadenectomy. The sentinel inguinal lymph node is the node most likely to be involved if metastatic disease from the vulvar lesion is present. Inguinal lymph node sampling reduces the likelihood of the postoperative complication of a lymphocyst. Sentinel lymph node technology [25–27] has provided the means for identifying the sentinel lymph node draining a tumor bed, and it can be excised with a minimally invasive approach. Inguinal sentinel lymph node (SLN) dissection in vulvar cancer patients has been shown to be feasible and highly sensitive for the detection of metastatic disease to the inguinal nodal basin. Clinical studies have shown a nearly 100% identification rate of a SLN when lymphatic mapping with a radioactive tracer (Tc-99m sulfur colloid) is used in combination with blue dye. The negative predictive value of a negative sentinel lymph node in these studies has been shown to be 100%.

The utilization of a sentinel node dissection allows for an in-depth pathologic examination of the one or two sentinel lymph nodes. In this approach, pathologic ultrastaging can detect micrometastases [28–30].

If the sentinel lymph node is free of disease, it is unlikely that other lymph nodes would be involved. Particularly in an elderly patient, this technique may reduce the extent of lymphadenectomy [31, 32].

Patients with advanced vulvar cancer (stage III and IV) that are managed with primary surgery tend to be older patients that have smaller lesions but positive lymph nodes, whereas patients treated primarily with chemoradiation are younger and have larger volume disease but fewer lymph node metastases. Despite these differences, patients treated with surgery or primary chemoradiation have no differences in overall survival, progression free survival, or recurrence rates. Age is the most powerful predictor of survival when size, lymph node status, stage, and treatment are accounted for [33].

The combination of postoperative irradiation with or without chemotherapy is used routinely for managing patients with vulvar cancer following a radical vulvectomy and inguinal–femoral lymphadenectomy if lymph node metastases are identified [34]. The most common cytotoxic drug used for concurrent chemoradiation is cisplatin.

The vulvar tissue is supplied with an end-arterial blood supply. The skin and subcutaneous tissue are quite sensitive to the radiation effect. Dry desquamation followed by moist desquamation is a routine problem associated with irradiating the vulva [35].

Nevertheless, relatively low-dose fractions of radiation therapy combined with 5-fluorouracil and mitomycin C have been employed for managing advanced vulvar cancer and cancer in elderly patients who are unable to tolerate a radical vulvectomy [36–40].

Survival of women with vulvar cancer is related to the presence of lymph node metastases. Patients with no lymph node metastasis have approximately an 80% 5-year survival. Those with evidence of lymph node metastasis have a 54% 5-year survival. Patients with unilateral lymph node metastases have a 60% 5-year survival, whereas those with bilateral lymph node metastases have a 23% 5-year survival [41].

Key Points in Vulvar Cancer Affecting Elderly Patients

- It is predominantly a disease of the elderly patient.
- It has a lesser association with HPV infection.
- Squamous cell carcinoma is the most common histology followed by melanoma.
- Vulvar Paget's disease is frequently associated with carcinoma.
- Staging is surgical.
- Tumor size and inguinal lymph node status are the most important predictors.

Vaginal Cancer

Primary cancer arising in the vagina is rare. It constitutes approximately 2% of all gynecologic cancers. It is primarily a disease of older women. Most patients are diagnosed with vaginal cancer in their seventh to eight decade of life [42, 43].

The histology of these lesions is predominantly squamous cell cancer, although adenocarcinoma can arise de novo within the vagina [44].

Less common histologies include melanoma and the rare paravaginal sarcoma [45].

It is appreciated that 84% of vaginal involvement is secondary from cancers of the cervix, uterus, rectum, ovary, vulva, or bladder [46].

The etiology of vaginal cancer is associated with that of cervical cancer, and many of the precancerous changes of the vagina occur after patients have been treated for squamous cell carcinoma in situ of the cervix or invasive cancer of the cervix. However, primary vaginal cancers do occur in elderly women without previous or concurrent cervical disease [47]. Vaginal cancer is associated with HPV infection [48, 49].

By convention, the classification and staging of the International Federation of Gynecology and Obstetrics (FIGO) requires that if a cancer is present in the vagina and reaches the cervix, the cancer is considered a cervical cancer because cervical cancer is much more common than vaginal cancer.

Women with vaginal cancers present with vaginal discharge and sometimes burning or pain. The discharge may be bloody or purulent when the lesion becomes secondarily infected by vaginal flora.

The diagnosis is made by inspection, palpation, and biopsy. Dysplastic changes of the vagina may be confined to the vaginal apex, particularly in women with a history of cervical dysplasia or malignancy. However, multifocal dysplastic lesions of the vagina do occur, usually in association with HPV infection [50–53]. The diagnosis is confirmed by biopsy. The staging of vaginal cancer is presented in Table 83.2.

TABLE 83.2 Carcinoma of the vagina [176]

Stage 0	Carcinoma in situ, intraepithelial neoplasia grade 3
Stage I	The carcinoma is limited to the vaginal wall
Stage II	The carcinoma has involved the subvaginal tissue but has not extended to the pelvic wall
Stage III	The carcinoma has extended to the pelvic wall
Stage IV	The carcinoma has extended beyond the true pelvis or has involved the mucosa of the bladder or rectum; bullous edema as such does not permit a case to be allotted to stage IV
IVA	Tumor invades bladder and/or rectal mucosa and/or direct extension beyond the true pelvis
IVB	Spread to distant organs

Source: Reprinted from Odicino et al. [176], with permission

Management of vaginal cancer is based on the stage of disease, the volume of tumor present, and its location within the vagina. No consensus exists regarding the management of different presentations of vaginal cancer. The low incidence of the disease precludes the organization of large randomized trials and comparison of different treatment modalities. Vaginal cancers that involve the upper one-third of the vagina and are limited in extent (i.e., stage I or stage II) can be treated with a radical hysterectomy in continuity with a radical vaginectomy. Tumors involving the lower third of the vagina can be treated surgically in the form of a wide local excision that includes the adjacent vulvar tissue or by a vulvectomy in continuity with a partial vaginectomy [54, 55].

Most vaginal cancers, however, occur in older age women, and the treatment of choice is radiation therapy. The combination of brachytherapy and external beam radiation therapy is often employed for the management of vaginal cancer. Chemoradiation for vaginal cancer appears appropriate, an approach derived from the treatment of cervical cancer. Reports of experience with chemoradiation in the treatment of vaginal cancer are limited. Most commonly, the cytotoxic drug is cisplatin, administered as a radiation sensitizer concurrently with external beam radiation [56].

Complications of radiation therapy include radiation mucositis and subsequent vaginal stenosis. Vaginal necrosis may occur and lead to vesicovaginal or rectovaginal fistulas, the treatment of which are urinary or colon diversions.

The survival of women with vaginal cancer is based on the stage of the disease at presentation. The overall 5-year survival rate for vaginal cancer is approximately 44% The 5-year survival for stage I disease was 73.4%, stage II, 51.4%, stage III, 32.5%, stage IVA, 20.4%, and stage IVB, 0% [57].

Most recurrences occur in the pelvis. Management of recurrent disease is similar to that for cervical cancer (i.e., exenterative surgery for a centrally localized tumor and chemotherapy for disseminated disease) [54].

Key Points in Vaginal Cancer Affecting Elderly Patients

- It is predominantly a disease of the elderly patient.
- Vaginal involvement with carcinoma is mostly from the surrounding pelvic organs.
- The presenting symptoms are vaginal discharge and sometimes burning or pain.
- The treatment of choice is chemoradiation.

Cervical Cancer

Cervical carcinoma represents the second most common cancer that develops in the female reproductive organs. Data published by the American Cancer Society estimate that 11,070 new cases of cervical cancer were diagnosed in the year 2008 in the United States and that 3,870 deaths occurred as a result of this disease [58].

The median age for cervical cancer is 53 years, which is the lowest median age for all pelvic reproductive organ cancers. Cervical cancer is predominantly a disease of younger age women; nevertheless, 13.1% of all cervical cancers present in women 70 years of age or older.

The most common histology for invasive cervical cancers is the squamous cell variety. The second most common subtype is adenocarcinoma of the cervix [59].

A spectrum of changes can occur in the cervix, from mild dysplasia through carcinoma in situ, all of which may be treated in the office using simple treatments that mechanically destroy the surface epithelium and allow healthy tissue to grow in. However, when a women goes through menopause, the site at which most cervical cancers begin, the transformation zone (i.e., the junction of the exocervical squamous epithelium with that of the endocervical columnar epithelium) recedes into the endocervical canal. Dysplastic changes often cannot be seen within the endocervical canal, especially in elderly women, in whom often there is an associated invasive cancer.

Other invasive cancers that occur in the cervix are adenocarcinomas arising in the glandular epithelium of the endocervix [60].

Adenosquamous carcinomas, a combination of malignant glandular and squamous elements, also arise in the cervix but to a much lesser extent than squamous cell carcinoma and adenocarcinoma [61].

A variety of risk factors have been associated with the development of cervical cancer. They include having multiple sexual partners, sexual intercourse at a young age, cigarette smoking, HPV infections or other sexually transmitted disease infections, immune suppression, genital warts, and multiparity. Human Papillomavirus (HPV) infection is the number one etiologic agent in the development of cervical neoplasia. At least 90% of invasive cervical cancers have evidence of HPV infection [62, 63].

The diagnosis of cervical dysplasia is based on a biopsy of the cervix. It must be remembered that in the elderly patient, the transformation zone is within the canal, so if the elderly patient has an abnormal Pap smear, the endocervical canal must always be biopsied. An office endocervical curetting of the endocervical canal is extremely useful for determining the nature and extent of the lesions. If such a change is present in the endocervical canal, it is the authors' recommendation that the patient should undergo a cone biopsy. A cone biopsy removes a large segment of the cervix and allows the pathologist to determine more accurately the extent and margins of the dysplastic or malignant changes present. Loop electrical excision of the transformation zone (LEETZ) is an alternative method for evaluating the cervix. In the elderly, with the transformation zone in the endocervical canal, the

LEETZ procedure often causes cautery artifacts, so the endocervical and ectocervical margins cannot be interpreted.

In an elderly patient diagnosed with high-grade cervical dysplasia, it is wisest to consider a hysterectomy. If the patient has significant medical comorbidities and is diagnosed with an early cervical cancer, a large cone biopsy of the cervix can be curative [64].

The FIGO (International Federation of Gynecology and Obstetrics) staging system for invasive cervical cancer is presented in Table 83.3. Although advanced imaging modalities are not used when determining the clinical stage of patients

TABLE 83.3 Carcinoma of the cervix uteri [175]

Stage I	The carcinoma is strictly confined to the cervix (extension to the corpus would be disregarded)
IA	Invasive carcinoma which can be diagnosed only by microscopy, with deepest invasion ≤ 5 mm and largest extension ≥ 7 mm
IA1	Measured stromal invasion of ≤ 3.0 mm in depth and extension of ≤ 7.0 mm
IA2	Measured stromal invasion of >3.0 mm and not >5.0 mm with an extension of not >7.0 mm
IB	Clinically visible lesions limited to the cervix uteri or preclinical cancers greater than stage IA[a]
IB1	Clinically visible lesion ≤ 4.0 cm in greatest dimension
IB2	Clinically visible lesion >4.0 cm in greatest dimension
Stage II	Cervical carcinoma invades beyond the uterus, but not to the pelvic wall or to the lower third of the vagina
IIA	Without parametrial invasion
IIA1	Clinically visible lesion ≤ 4.0 cm in greatest dimension
IIA2	Clinically visible lesion > 4 cm in greatest dimension
IIB	With obvious parametrial invasion
Stage III	The tumor extends to the pelvic wall and/or involves lower third of the vagina and/or causes hydronephrosis or nonfunctioning kidney[b]
IIIA	Tumor involves lower third of the vagina, with no extension to the pelvic wall
IIIB	Extension to the pelvic wall and/or hydronephrosis or nonfunctioning kidney
Stage IV	The carcinoma has extended beyond the true pelvis or has involved (biopsy proven) the mucosa of the bladder or rectum. A bullous edema, as such, does not permit a case to be allotted to stage IV
IVA	Spread of the growth to adjacent organs
IVB	Spread to distant organs

Source: Reprinted from FIGO Committee on Gynecologic Oncology [175], with permission

[a]All macroscopically visible lesions – even with superficial invasion – are allotted to stage IB carcinomas. Invasion is limited to a measured stromal invasion with a maximal depth of 5.00 mm and a horizontal extension of not >7.00 mm. Depth of invasion should not be >5.00 mm taken from the base of the epithelium of the original tissue – superficial or glandular. The depth of invasion should always be reported in mm, even in those cases with "early (minimal) stromal invasion" (~1 mm) The involvement of vascular/lymphatic spaces should not change the stage allotment.

[b]On rectal examination, there is no cancer-free space between the tumor and the pelvic wall. All cases with hydronephrosis or nonfunctioning kidney are included, unless they are known to be due to another cause

with cervical cancer, in the developed world, CT, MRI, and 18-F FDG PET scans are routinely ordered and help in planning for the most appropriate treatment modality [65, 66].

Management of invasive cancer of the cervix is by radiation therapy or surgery. Surgery is performed in women with early-stage disease who can tolerate a radical hysterectomy with bilateral pelvic lymph node resection [67].

Patients with microinvasive cancer (<3 mm) can undergo a type II radical hysterectomy in which the tissue that is removed includes the parametria medial to the ureters and the proximal one-third of the vagina. However, if an invasive carcinoma is present, a type III or a Meigs–Wertheim radical hysterectomy is indicated. This procedure removes the parametrial tissue lateral to the ureter and removes approximately one-half of the vagina in continuity with the cervix and uterine corpus. While traditionally these operations have been performed by laparotomy, conventional laparoscopic and robotic techniques are equally effective and carry less morbidity [68–70].

For the elderly patient with more advanced disease or who is unable to tolerate a radical hysterectomy, radiation therapy using intracavitary and external beam techniques is effective for managing an invasive cancer of the cervix. The efficacy of the treatment depends on the stage of the cancer and the tumor volume [71–75].

The overall survival for women with cervical cancers correlates with the stage of the disease. Stage I patients have an 81.6% 5-year survival, stage II 61.3%, stage III 36.7%, and stage IV 12.1% [76].

Treatment of recurrent cervical cancer is based on the extent of the disease present and the primary treatment modality.

Tumor recurrence after surgery for cervical carcinoma is associated with high fatality and morbidity, posing a major therapeutic challenge. Salvage radiotherapy with concurrent chemotherapy for recurrent cervical carcinoma following surgery may result in 40–50% long-term disease-free survival and an acceptable risk of severe treatment complications even in patient with recurrences extending to the pelvic wall [77].

Patients who develop central recurrence (i.e., at the vaginal apex) that does not extend to or reach the pelvic side wall may be treated with exenterative surgery [78–80].

In the past, we used 70 years of age as a cutoff for those eligible for exenterative surgery. As improvements in postoperative care have evolved, we are now able to offer exenterative surgery to women over the age of 70 years if they are otherwise in good health. Exenterative surgery includes anterior pelvic exenteration, which removes the uterus in continuity with the bladder via a radical hysterectomy, radical cystectomy, and urinary diversion. Posterior pelvic exenteration involves a radical hysterectomy in continuity with resection of the sigmoid colon and rectum, and it requires a colostomy. Total pelvic exenteration removes the bladder, uterus, and rectosigmoid colon. The creation of a continent pouch at the time of exenterative surgery avoids the need for continuous collection of urine in an ostomy bag. However, experience at the Yale-New Haven Medical Center suggests that patients who have been heavily pretreated with radiation and are over 65 years of age do poorly with continent pouches and probably are best served by an ileal conduit.

Patients who have extensive recurrent disease not limited to the center of the pelvis are offered chemotherapy. Chemotherapy for the management of recurrent cervical cancer is palliative. Overall response rates to combination chemotherapy of 46.3% have been reported. Responses were higher in patients with disease in nonirradiated sites [81].

Key Points in Cervical Cancer Affecting Elderly Patients

- Only 13% of all cervical cancers occur after the age of 70.
- The evaluation of the endocervical canal can be difficult secondary to stenosis and atrophy.
- Although advanced imaging modalities are not included in the WHO recommended diagnostic workup, MRI, CT, and 18-F FDG PET scans are routinely used.
- Surgery and chemoradiation are equally effective. Surgery is limited to stage IIA and earlier.

Uterine Cancer

In the United States, the uterine corpus is the most common site for cancer in the female reproductive tract, with an estimated 40,100 new cases and 7,470 deaths occurring in the year 2008 [58].

SEER data from 1992 to 2002 state that uterine cancers were diagnosed in 31% of patients between 65 and 74 years of age, 20% between 75 and 84 years of age, and 4% between 85 and 95 years of age [83].

The most common histologic types of uterine cancer arise from the endometrium and are of endometrioid type (Table 83.4). Other subtypes are adenosquamous, clear-cell carcinomas, and uterine serous cancers. Grade 3 endometrioid, clear cell, and serous cancers have an aggressive behavior and require more than a hysterectomy to achieve cure [83, 84].

Uterine sarcomas are a group of rare and usually aggressive soft-tissue cancers. The three major subtypes of uterine sarcomas (listed in decreasing order of incidence) are carcinosarcoma, leiomyosarcoma, and endometrial sarcoma. Most patients with uterine sarcomas are middle- to older-aged women who present with abnormal uterine bleeding or a pelvic mass [85, 86].

Uterine cancers are usually diagnosed after an obvious early signal, postmenopausal bleeding, occurs. Women must be informed that whenever vaginal bleeding occurs after menopause, they must be promptly evaluated [87].

If the vulva, vagina, and cervix appear unremarkable on inspection, an endometrial biopsy should be obtained. Rarely, women are found to have endometrial cells on a routine Pap smear. The presence of such cells from postmenopausal women may be associated with endometrial hyperplasia or malignant changes of the endometrium [88]. This cytologic finding is another indication to perform an endometrial biopsy. An endometrial biopsy can usually diagnose the presence of hyperplasia of the endometrium or carcinoma [89, 90].

Endometrial hyperplasias are categorized into simple and complex hyperplasia. The hyperplasias are further subdivided into those with or without atypia. It is unusual for simple hyperplasia to be associated with cytologic atypia, whereas complex hyperplastic changes are often associated with cytologic atypia. Simple hyperplasia rarely progresses to invasive cancer. Retrospective studies reported that complex hyperplasia without atypia can progress to invasive cancer in approximately 2% of patients over a 12-year period, whereas complex hyperplasia with atypia is associated with an up to 30% chance of developing invasive cancer over an 8-year observation period [91].

Management of simple hyperplasia in the elderly consists of observation. The treatment of complex hyperplasia without atypia is progestin therapy (medroxyprogesterone acetate, megestrol acetate). Repeat endometrial sampling is indicated

TABLE 83.4 Carcinoma of the endometrium [175]

Stage I[a]	Tumor confined to the corpus uteri
IA[a]	No or less than half myometrial invasion
IB[a]	Invasion equal to or more than half of the myometrium
Stage II[a]	Tumor invades cervical stroma, but does not extend beyond the uterus[b]
Stage III[a]	Local and/or regional spread of the tumor
IIIA[a]	Tumor invades the serosa of the corpus uteri and/or adnexae[c]
IIIB[a]	Vaginal and/or parametrial involvement[c]
IIIC[a]	Metastases to pelvic and/or paraaortic lymph nodes[c]
IIIC1[a]	Positive pelvic nodes
IIIC2[a]	Positive paraaortic lymph nodes with or without positive pelvic lymph nodes
Stage IV[a]	Tumor invades bladder and/or bowel mucosa, and/or distant metastases
IVA[a]	Tumor invasion of bladder and/or bowel mucosa
IVB[a]	Distant metastases, including intraabdominal metastases and/or inguinal lymph nodes

Source: Reprinted from FIGO Committee on Gynecologic Oncology [175], with permission
[a]Either G1, G2, or G3
[b]Endocervical glandular involvement only should be considered as stage I and no longer as stage II
[c]Positive cytology has to be reported separately without changing the stage

after 3 months. Persistent hyperplasia is an indication for hysterectomy and bilateral salpingo-oophorectomy. Atypical hyperplasia in an elderly woman should be treated with hysterectomy and adnexectomy [92, 93]. If the patient cannot tolerate surgery, progestin therapy in the form of daily oral medroxyprogesterone acetate or megestrol acetate may be used to revert the endometrium back to an atrophic state.

Uterine cancer is staged surgically (Table 83.3). Patients should routinely undergo a total hysterectomy, bilateral salpingo-oophorectomy, and pelvic and paraaortic lymph node sampling. Omentectomy or omental biopsy is indicated for uterine clear cell and serous carcinomas, and uterine sarcomas [94–97]. Conventional laparoscopic or robotic approaches have less perioperative morbidity [98–101].

Additional therapy is based on the findings of the surgical staging. Patients with histologically low-grade endometrial cancers that do not deeply infiltrate the myometrium require no additional therapy. Patients with high-grade endometrial cancers are usually treated with vaginal apex irradiation alone to prevent local recurrences. Some centers prescribe external beam radiation therapy of the pelvis [102]. Chemotherapy is indicated for clear cell and serous uterine cancers.

Patients with disease that has extended beyond the uterus and cervix are usually treated with chemotherapy in combination with vaginal apex radiation. A Gynecologic Oncology Group Phase III trial has demonstrated that chemotherapy for advanced endometrial carcinoma significantly improves both progression-free survival and overall survival when compared with whole abdominal irradiation. Adverse effects of treatment tended to be more frequent and more severe on the chemotherapy arm, but the majority of acute toxicities were expected and manageable [103–105].

The 5-year survival of women with uterine cancer confined to the uterine corpus (stage I) is approximately 85%. Those who have only superficial invasion without any negative prognostic factors have survivals of 95–100%. Those patients with deep penetration of the uterine wall (i.e., stage IC) have survivals of 70–80%. As the stage of the cancer increases, the likelihood of cure decreases. The 5-year survival for women with stage II disease is 70%, stage III disease is 49%, and stage IV disease is 19% [106].

Elderly patients often are found to have more aggressive histologic types of endometrial cancer and may have medical comorbidities that preclude surgery. Published data show that elderly women with uterine cancers who have severe medical problems can have their cancers controlled with intracavitary radiation therapy administered with or without external beam radiation, particularly if the disease is confined to the uterus [107].

Experience at the Yale-New Haven Medical Center suggests that this approach is effective. Most inoperable patients die of other medical diseases rather than of their

cancer. Fifty-four patients treated at Yale deemed medically inoperable had a significantly shorter overall survival than the 108 control patients with stage I or II disease ($p < 0.0001$). Deaths in the inoperable group were more likely to be due to intercurrent disease (28 of 32 cases) compared to the controls (3 of 15) ($p < 0.0001$). Inoperable patients who did not die of intercurrent disease had a median 5-year survival approaching that of the operable patients. The average age of the stage I patients was 72.0 years (range 44–93 years) and stage II patients 70.0 years (range 51–82 years) [108].

The majority of patients with uterine cancer has disease confined to the uterus and has an excellent overall prognosis. However, some patients present with advanced primary disease. The management of metastatic disease is variable, depending on factors such as medical comorbidities, tumor grade, performance status, and prior treatments. Management options include hormonal therapy, cytotoxic chemotherapy as well as targeted therapies that inhibit angiogenesis and the cellular signaling pathways involved in cell growth and proliferation. Hormonal therapy and cytotoxic chemotherapy have traditionally been used in the treatment of metastatic endometrial cancer. Advances in molecular biology have led to multiple potential targeted therapies to be used in the treatment of metastatic endometrial cancer [109].

Patients with more advanced disease, particularly with extrapelvic disease, may be treated with neoadjuvant chemotherapy [110]. Using this approach, the tumor bulk is reduced, allowing a less extensive surgical procedure with less perioperative morbidity. Patients tend to stop bleeding promptly after the initiation of chemotherapy.

Pelvic irradiation can be administered for elderly patients with multiple medical comorbidities for locoregional control and palliation. Using this approach, vaginal bleeding ceases shortly after the initiation of treatment [111].

Radiation therapy is a regional technique that has no significant impact on overall survival for women with advanced-stage endometrial cancers. In contrast, neoadjuvant chemotherapy may potentially have an impact on overall survival and accomplish the same control of bleeding as that offered by radiation therapy [112].

The management of recurrent uterine cancers is based on the cancer's histology and the extent of disease [113].

Patients with well-differentiated endometrial cancers may respond to progestin therapy. We have used progestin therapy to control recurrent endometrial cancer for prolonged periods of time, although most, but not all, women who have recurrent disease treated with progestin therapy will have further recurrences. Patients with the less well-differentiated or more aggressive histologic subtypes typical in elderly patients are usually treated with chemotherapy to control advanced and recurrent disease.

Three forms of sarcoma involve the uterus: leiomyosarcomas, carcinosarcomas, and endometrial sarcomas [114–117].

Surgery, including hysterectomy and resection of disease, serves as the main treatment modality. Adjuvant therapies, including radiation, chemotherapy, and/or hormonal therapy, have limited benefit on overall survival. Few large randomized controlled trials were conducted because of the uterine sarcomas' rare and aggressive nature. For patients with metastatic or recurrent disease, multimodality therapy is limited by low response rates and limited duration of response [86, 118].

Uterine leiomyosarcomas are treated with hysterectomy. Sarcomas arising within the center of well-delineated leiomyomata and have not penetrated beyond the pseudocapsule of the leiomyoma often are cured with hysterectomy alone [117].

Leiomyosarcomas arising de novo in the muscular wall of the uterus tend to be more aggressive, and surgery alone is insufficient [119]. Currently, a debate remains as to whether such patients should receive chemotherapy at the time of diagnosis or treatment should be delayed until the leiomyosarcoma recurs. The infrequent occurrence of uterine leiomyosarcomas has limited the opportunity for a prospective randomized trial to address this issue. Patients that present with metastatic uterine sarcomas are treated with surgery and chemotherapy. Their prognosis is poor [120–122].

Carcinosarcomas of the uterus histologically contain carcinomatous and sarcomatous elements. The carcinomatous element of a carcinosarcoma is often uterine serous cancer, although poorly differentiated endometrioid carcinoma can also be found or, rarely, a squamous cell carcinoma. The sarcomatous elements have been categorized as homologous elements (tissues normally found in the uterus) and heterologous elements (not normally found in the uterus). An example of a homologous element is a leiomyosarcoma. Heterologous elements include rhabdomyosarcoma, chondrosarcoma, and osteosarcoma.

The management of uterine carcinosarcomas is surgical, including a total hysterectomy, bilateral salpingo-oophorectomy, omentectomy, and pelvic and paraaortic lymphadenectomies. Surgery is followed by combination chemotherapy and irradiation of the vaginal apex or whole pelvis. This approach has been most effective for early-stage disease, but it has not been effective when the disease has spread outside the uterus (i.e., stage III or IV disease) [123–125].

Endometrial stromal sarcomas are low-grade malignancies. They are sensitive to progestin therapy. Following a hysterectomy for a low-grade endometrial stromal sarcoma, patients should be placed on an oral progestin, either megestrol acetate or medroxyprogesterone acetate. Endometrial sarcomas, formerly referred to as high-grade endometrial stromal sarcomas, are high-grade cancers and often are at an advanced stage when diagnosed. Their management is by cytoreductive surgery and postoperative combination chemotherapy [126].

Key Points in Uterine Cancer Affecting Elderly Patients

- The most common presenting symptom is postmenopausal vaginal bleeding.
- Endometrial cells present on a cervical cytology specimen (Papanicolaou smear) require evaluation of the endometrial cavity.
- Uterine cancers in the elderly are frequently of the type II variety: papillary serous carcinomas, clear cell carcinomas, and high-grade endometrioid carcinomas. Even stage I cancers are treated with chemotherapy and radiation following surgery.
- Conventional or robotic laparoscopy is the preferred surgical modality.

Fallopian Tube Cancer

The fallopian tube is the least common site for primary cancers to develop in the female reproductive tract. The age-adjusted incidence rate for fallopian tube carcinoma is 3.72 per million in the United States. The median age for women with fallopian tube carcinomas is 64 years. Fallopian tube cancers are mostly adenocarcinomas, and serous carcinomas are the most common diagnosed histologic type [127]. If the fallopian tube carcinoma involves the ovary, by convention, it is considered to be an ovarian cancer, as ovarian cancer occurs more frequently than fallopian tube carcinoma.

The etiology of fallopian tube carcinoma is unknown. Symptoms associated with fallopian tube carcinoma include lower abdominal pain and pressure and a profuse, clear vaginal discharge (hydrops tubae profluens) [128]. Physical examination often confirms the presence of a mass. Imaging studies may be performed using ultrasonography or computed tomography (CT) scans to identify an adnexal mass. Most fallopian tube carcinomas are found when patients undergo surgery for a pelvic mass or presumed ovarian cancer.

Surgical staging and chemotherapy follow the concepts used in epithelial ovarian cancer (EOC). Surgery consists of total hysterectomy, adnexectomy, pelvic and periaortic lymphadenectomy, omentectomy, and resection of any metastatic disease. The goal of the surgery is to remove all visible and palpable cancer (i.e., cytoreductive surgery) [129].

Postoperative treatment for fallopian tube carcinoma is combination chemotherapy using platinum-based protocols [130]. CA 125 determinations are routinely used for follow-up of patients with fallopian tube cancers [131].

Recurrent disease is managed with combination chemotherapy. Surgery may be employed to resect recurrent tumor if the disease is limited to a few sites rather than diffuse in nature.

The overall survival rate for patients with fallopian tube carcinoma is approximately 30–50%. As in EOC, residual disease after initial surgery is a significant prognostic factor. These figures have not changed significantly with time, indicating the need for further research [132]. Stage of disease at the time of diagnosis is the most important factor affecting prognosis. The calculated 5-year survival rates from six literature series were 62% for stage I, 36% for stage II, 17% for stage III, and 0% for stage IV [133].

Ovarian Cancer

Ovarian cancer is the sixth most commonly diagnosed cancer among women in the world, accounting for nearly 4% of all female cancers. In the United States, ovarian cancer is the eighth most common cancer and the fifth leading cause of cancer death, after lung, breast, colorectal, and pancreatic cancer [134].

Ovarian cancer represents the second leading gynecologic cancer, following cancer of the uterine corpus, and causes more deaths per year than any other cancer of the female reproductive system. An estimated 1 in 70 women in the United States will develop ovarian cancer in their lifetime. In 2007, approximately 22,500 new cases of ovarian cancer were diagnosed, and 15,500 ovarian cancer-related deaths occurred in the United States [135, 136].

Mortality is high with an overall 5-year relative survival rate of 45% because women typically present with late-stage disease. Thus, the public health burden is significant [137]. The incidence of ovarian cancer increases with age, with a median age at diagnosis of 65 years. Over 80% of ovarian cancers occur after 45 years of age.

One of the most significant risk factors for ovarian cancer is a family history of the disease. It is estimated that approximately 7% of women with ovarian cancer have a positive family history for this disease [138–140].

First-degree relatives of ovarian cancer probands have a threefold to sevenfold increased risk, especially if multiple relatives are affected and at an early age at onset [141].

It is clear that a subset of ovarian cancers occur as part of a hereditary cancer syndrome that is inherited in an autosomal dominant pattern. The majority of hereditary ovarian cancers can be attributed to mutations in the *BRCA1* and *BRCA2* genes [142]. According to data from the Breast Cancer Linkage Consortium, the risk of ovarian cancer through 70 years of age is up to 44% in *BRCA1* families and approaches 27% in *BRCA2* families [143–145].

Ovarian cancer lacks early warning symptoms and is not usually diagnosed until it spreads beyond the ovary and the pelvis (i.e., stage III or IV disease). Approximately 70% of women present with advanced disease (Table 83.5) [146].

TABLE 83.5 Carcinoma of the ovary [176]

Stage I	Growth limited to the ovaries
IA	Growth limited to one ovary: no ascites present containing malignant cells. No tumor on the external surface; capsule intact
IB	Growth limited to both ovaries: no ascites present containing malignant cells. No tumor on the external surfaces; capsules intact
IC[a]	Tumor either stage IA or IB, but with tumor on surface of one or both ovaries, or with capsule ruptured, or with ascites present containing malignant cells, or with positive peritoneal washings
Stage II	Growth involving one or both ovaries with pelvic extension
IIA	Extension and/or metastases to the uterus and/or tubes
IIB	Extension to other pelvic tissues
IIC[a]	Tumor either stage IIA or IIB, but with tumor on surface of one or both ovaries, or with capsule(s) ruptured, or with ascites present containing malignant cells, or with positive peritoneal washings
Stage III	Tumor involving one or both ovaries with histologically confirmed peritoneal implants outside the pelvis and/or positive retroperitoneal or inguinal nodes. Superficial liver metastases equal Stage III. Tumor is limited to the true pelvis, but with histologically proven malignant extension to small bowel or omentum
IIIA	Tumor grossly limited to the true pelvis, with negative nodes, but with histologically confirmed microscopic seeding of abdominal peritoneal surfaces, or histologic proven extension to small bowel or mesentery
IIIB	Tumor of one or both ovaries with histologically confirmed implants, peritoneal metastasis of abdominal peritoneal surfaces, none exceeding 2 cm in diameter: nodes are negative
IIIC	Peritoneal metastasis beyond the pelvis >2 cm in diameter and/or positive retroperitoneal or inguinal nodes
Stage IV	Growth involving one or both ovaries with distant metastases. If pleural effusion is present, there must be positive cytology to allot a case to stage IV. Parenchymal liver metastasis equals stage IV

Source: Reprinted from Odicino et al. [176], with permission
[a]In order to evaluate the impact on prognosis of the different criteria for allotting cases to stage IC or IIC, it would be of value to know if rupture of the capsule was spontaneous or caused by the surgeon, and if the source of malignant cells detected, peritoneal washings or ascites

The most common presenting symptoms are abdominal bloating and distension, often in association with vague nonspecific abdominal complaints. Frank pain is unusual. Gastrointestinal dysfunction is seen in about 20% of women with ovarian cancers, and less commonly, postmenopausal bleeding is observed. The diagnosis is based on physical examination and diagnostic imaging, which reveals pelvic and/or abdominal masses and ascites. The tumor marker

CA-125 is frequently elevated especially in patients with metastatic disease.

The ovary forms cancers from a variety of structures. The most common cancer, representing approximately 90% of all ovarian cancers, arises from the surface epithelial cells. These cells give rise to the common epithelial cancers of the ovary, including serous, mucinous, clear-cell, endometrioid, Brenner, transitional, and undifferentiated cancers. Mixed epithelial cancers also occur.

The germ cell is the second most common source for ovarian cancer and represents approximately 5% of all ovarian malignancies [147]. Ovarian germ cell malignancies occur most frequently in teenagers and women in their twenties. They are not found after menopause.

Sex cord-stromal tumors are the third most common cancers developing in the ovary [148]. They may be functional in nature (i.e., produce hormones). The most common functional tumor is the granulosa cell tumor, which produces estrogen. The Sertoli–Leydig cell tumor produces androgens. Mixed tumors and sex cord-stromal tumors are rare and are called gynandroblastomas. Elderly patients, in particular, may present with pure Sertoli cell or pure Leydig cell tumors, and their symptoms are related to the excess hormone production [149–151].

Sarcomas and tumors with sarcomatous elements, such as fibrosarcomas, leiomyosarcomas, and carcinosarcomas, are rare and most often occur in women over 70 years of age. They are a particularly virulent form of ovarian cancer and are usually diagnosed as stage III or IV disease [152].

The ovary is a frequent site of metastasis, particularly from breast and colon cancer. In addition to CT imaging, breast examination, mammograms, and colonoscopy can be useful adjuncts when evaluating women with tumors involving the ovaries [153–156].

The staging of ovarian cancer is surgical (Table 83.5). The conventional treatment for ovarian cancer is maximum cytoreductive surgery followed by combination platinum-based chemotherapy [157, 158]. The surgical treatment consists of total hysterectomy, adnexectomy, pelvic and periaortic lymphadenectomy, total omentectomy, and tumor debulking [159].

Survival is directly related to the stage of the cancer. For women with advanced disease, survival is correlated with the amount of residual tumor left at the time of the initial surgery. Resection of all visible tumors with only microscopic residual disease left at the completion of the procedure confers the best prognosis [160, 161].

In addition to residual tumor volume, age, performance status, and tumor histology are independent prognostic factors in patients with metastatic disease [162].

Surgery is followed by chemotherapy (adjuvant treatment). The most common regimen prescribed is the combination of carboplatin and paclitaxel [163].

The 5-year survival for stage I patients is 81%, stage II patients is 57%, stage III patients is 30%, and stage IV is 14% [164].

While conventional treatment of patients with ovarian cancer consists of cytoreductive surgery followed by chemotherapy, more recently, a shift has occurred in this treatment philosophy. Patients who present with widely metastatic disease and who on preoperative evaluation are not considered candidates for optimal tumor debulking, may be treated with neoadjuvant chemotherapy [165, 166]. The patients eligible for this approach will have a CT scan showing advanced disease and cytologic evidence or biopsy confirming ovarian epithelial cancer. Laparoscopy and biopsies can be used as an alternative approach to determine resectability. Neoadjuvant chemotherapy can also be used to treat patients that are unable to tolerate the lengthy and extensive tumor debulking procedures because of significant medical comorbidities [167, 168]. Patients treated with neoadjuvant chemotherapy have the same survival rates as those treated in a conventional fashion for stage IIIC or IV disease. Retrospective reviews showed no difference in survival [169, 170]. Patients who received neoadjuvant chemotherapy had a much quicker return to their normal status than those women who underwent conventional surgery followed by adjuvant chemotherapy. The rapid improvement in performance status among women who underwent neoadjuvant chemotherapy was impressive despite the fact that their performance status was statistically worse than that of women who underwent conventional treatment. In addition, the median age of patients who were treated with neoadjuvant chemotherapy was significantly older than of those who received conventional treatment [171].

Two-thirds of the women who underwent neoadjuvant chemotherapy for ovarian cancer management also underwent cytoreductive surgery. The survival of the women who underwent cytoreductive surgery was statistically better than the survival of those who did not. More women who underwent cytoreductive surgery after neoadjuvant treatment had no visible residual tumor at the completion of surgery compared to those who underwent conventional therapy [172].

One-third of the neoadjuvant-treated patients were unable to undergo surgery. Chemotherapy alone can be used to palliate women who are elderly and medically unable to undergo surgery. Patients who do not have a complete response to neoadjuvant chemotherapy invariably die of ovarian cancer or intercurrent disease.

Most women who initially present with metastatic ovarian cancer will develop recurrence [173]. Treatment is based on whether the cancer recurs locally or diffusely throughout the abdominal cavity. Isolated recurrent cancers are usually treated by secondary cytoreductive surgery followed by single-agent or combination chemotherapy [174]. Patients whose lesions are optimally cytoreduced at the time of secondary cytoreductive surgery appear to have a longer survival than those whose lesions could not be completely resected. Once ovarian cancer recurs, it acts like a chronic disease that invariably leads to the patient's demise.

Key Points in Ovarian Cancer Affecting Elderly Patients

- It is predominantly a disease of the elderly patient.
- Only 5% of ovarian cancers are caused by inherited mutations, and these patients are affected at younger ages.
- Most patients present with metastatic disease.
- Resection of all visible tumors confers the best prognosis.
- In patients with advanced disease, neoadjuvant chemotherapy increases the rate of optimal tumor debulking and decreases perioperative morbidity without affecting overall survival.

CASE STUDY

MG is an 82-year-old Caucasian patient with medical history significant for well-controlled hypertension who presented to the Emergency Department with sudden onset of palpitations and severe dyspnea. The workup included a CT scan, which showed a massive pulmonary saddle embolus, large ascites, and numerous pelvic and abdominal masses. On further inquiry, the patient stated that she noticed her waist getting wider; however, she attributed this to "getting fat" since she experienced no pain or any changes in her bowel or bladder function. The patient underwent a paracentesis, and the cytologic examination revealed metastatic ovarian adenocarcinoma. She was treated with six cycles of combination neoadjuvant chemotherapy consisting of paclitaxel and carboplatin every 21 days. After two cycles, the ascites resolved; she was able to leave her wheelchair, and she no longer required oxygen therapy. After four cycles, she was her usual self, and the serum levels of CA-125 went from over 1,500 U/mL to normal. Her nutritional status returned to normal. She underwent surgery with successful resection of all visible tumors. The intraoperative findings showed a notable decrease in size of the tumor burden. Her postoperative course was uneventful. Postoperatively, she was treated with six cycles of the same cytotoxic drugs. She remained without evidence of recurrent disease for 12 months after which she was treated with several chemotherapy regimens. Three years after her initial diagnosis, she remains an active person leading a normal life.

Discussion

The concept of neoadjuvant therapy with cytotoxic agents is one of the most important contributions to the treatment of ovarian cancer in the last two decades. Most patients with ovarian cancer have no or minor symptoms until metastases develop. Currently, there is no effective screening test for epithelial ovarian cancer. These factors impede the diagnosis in early stages, and most patients present with stage III or IV disease.

It is well recognized that the best survival is assured when all visible tumors are resected. However, the surgical procedures to accomplish the destruction of all metastatic implants do not carry a trivial morbidity.

Approximately 85% of epithelial ovarian tumors respond when treated with neoadjuvant platinum-based therapy. The results can be dramatic sometimes, with the ascites disappearing and the tumors shrinking or disappearing completely. This effect facilitates a higher rate of optimal tumor debulking, and the perioperative morbidity is much reduced.

This treatment concept is also applicable to patients who are not suitable for an extensive operation because of advanced age, medical comorbidities, or poor nutritional status. The overall survival for patients with ovarian cancer is better when a multimodality approach is used, i.e., chemotherapy and surgery.

References

1. Jemal A, Siegel R, Ward E et al (2007) Cancer statistics, 2007. CA Cancer J Clin 57(1):43–66
2. Saraiya M, Watson M, Wu X et al (2008) Incidence of in situ and invasive vulvar cancer in the US, 1998-2003. Cancer 113(10): 2865–2872
3. Van Beurden M, Kate FJ, Smits HL et al (1995) Multifocal vulvar intraepithelial neoplasia grade III and multicentric lower genital tract neoplasia is associated with transcriptionally active human papilloma virus. Cancer 75:2879–2884
4. Insinga RP, Liaw KL, Johnson LG et al (2008) A systematic review of the prevalence and attribution of human papillomavirus types among cervical, vaginal, and vulvar precancers and cancers in the United States. Cancer Epidemiol Biomarkers Prev 17(7): 1611–1622
5. de Koning MN, Quint WG, Pirog EC (2008) Prevalence of mucosal and cutaneous human papillomaviruses in different histologic subtypes of vulvar carcinoma. Mod Pathol 21(3):334–344
6. Fishman DA, Chambers SK, Kohorn EI et al (1995) Extramammary Paget's disease of the vulva. Gynecol Oncol 56:266–270
7. Lloyd J, Flanagan AM (2000) Mammary and extramammary Paget's disease. J Clin Pathol 53:742–749

8. De Simone P, Silipo V, Buccini P et al (2008) Vulvar melanoma: a report of 10 cases and review of the literature. Melanoma Res 18(2):127–133

9. Lopez-Varela E, Oliva E, McIntyre JF et al (2007) Primary treatment of Bartholin's gland carcinoma with radiation and chemoradiation: a report on ten consecutive cases. Int J Gynecol Cancer 17(3):661–667

10. Jones RW, Baranyai J, Stables S (1997) Trends in squamous cell carcinoma of the vulva: the influence of vulvar intraepithelial neoplasia. Obstet Gynecol 90:448–452

11. Roma AA, Hart WR (2007) Progression of simplex (differentiated) vulvar intraepithelial neoplasia to invasive squamous cell carcinoma: a prospective case study confirming its precursor role in the pathogenesis of vulvar cancer. Int J Gynecol Pathol 26(3):248–253

12. Hussain SK, Madeleine MM, Johnson LG et al (2008) Cervical and vulvar cancer risk in relation to the joint effects of cigarette smoking and genetic variation in interleukin 2. Cancer Epidemiol Biomarkers Prev 17(7):1790–1799

13. van der Avoort IA, Shirango H, Hoevenaars BM et al (2006) Vulvar squamous cell carcinoma is a multifactorial disease following two separate and independent pathways. Int J Gynecol Pathol 25(1):22–29

14. Hillemanns P, Wang X, Staehle S et al (2006) Evaluation of different treatment modalities for vulvar intraepithelial neoplasia (VIN): CO(2) laser vaporization, photodynamic therapy, excision and vulvectomy. Gynecol Oncol 100(2):271–275

15. Hatta N, Yamada M, Hirano T et al (2008) Extramammary Paget's disease: treatment, prognostic factors and outcome in 76 patients. Brit J Dermatol 158(2):313–318

16. DeSimone CP, Crisp MP, Ueland FR et al (2006) Concordance of gross surgical and final fixed margins in vulvar intraepithelial neoplasia 3 and vulvar cancer. J Reprod Med 51(8):617–620

17. Lee PK, Choi MS, Ahn ST et al (2006) Gluteal fold V-Y advancement flap for vulvar and vaginal reconstruction: a new flap. Plast Reconstr Surg 118(2):401–406

18. Black D, Tornos C, Soslow RA et al (2007) The outcomes of patients with positive margins after excision for intraepithelial Paget's disease of the vulva. Gynecol Oncol 104(3):547–550

19. Homesley HD (1995) Management of vulvar cancer. Cancer 76:2159–2170

20. Stehman FB, Bundy BW, Dvoretsky PM et al (1992) Early stage I carcinoma of the vulva treated with ipsilateral superficial inguinal lymphadenectomy and modified radical hemivulvectomy: a prospective study of the Gynecologic Oncology Group. Obstet Gynecol 79:490–497

21. Morris JM (1977) A formula for selective lymphadenectomy: its application to cancer of the vulva. Obstet Gynecol 50:152–158

22. Rouzier R, Haddad B, Atallah D et al (2005) Surgery for vulvar cancer. Clin Obstet Gynecol 48(4):869–878

23. Fanfani F, Garganese G, Fagotti A et al (2006) Advanced vulvar carcinoma: is it worth operating? A perioperative management protocol for radical and reconstructive surgery. Gynecol Oncol 103(2):467–472

24. de Hullu JA, van der Avoort IA, Oonk MH et al (2006) Management of vulvar cancers. Eur J of Surg Oncol 32(8):825–831

25. Moore RG, DePasquale S, Steinhoff MM et al (2003) Sentinel node identification and the ability to detect metastatic tumor to inguinal lymph nodes in vulvar malignancies. Gynecol Oncol 89(3):475–479

26. Levenback C, Coleman RL, Burke TW et al (2001) Intraoperative lymphatic mapping and sentinel node identification with blue dye in patients with vulvar cancer. Gynecol Oncol 83(2):276–281

27. de Hullu JA, Hollema H, Piers DA et al (2000) Sentinel lymph node procedure is highly accurate in squamous cell carcinoma of the vulva. J Clin Oncol 18(15):2811–2816

28. Decesare SL, Fiorica JV, Roberts WS et al (1997) A pilot study utilizing intraoperative lymphoscintigraphy for identification of the sentinel lymph nodes in vulvar cancer. Gynecol Oncol 66(3):425–428

29. Robison K, Steinhoff MM, Granai CO et al (2006) Inguinal sentinel node dissection versus standard inguinal node dissection in patients with vulvar cancer: a comparison of the size of metastasis detected in inguinal lymph nodes. Gynecol Oncol 101(1):24–27

30. Hampl M, Hantschmann P, Michels W, German Multicenter Study Group et al (2008) Validation of the accuracy of the sentinel lymph node procedure in patients with vulvar cancer: results of a multicenter study in Germany. Gynecol Oncol 111(2):282–288

31. Johann S, Klaeser B, Krause T et al (2008) Comparison of outcome and recurrence-free survival after sentinel lymph node biopsy and lymphadenectomy in vulvar cancer. Gynecol Oncol 110(3):324–328

32. Hefler LA, Grimm C, Six L et al (2008) Inguinal sentinel lymph node dissection vs. complete inguinal lymph node dissection in patients with vulvar cancer. Anticancer Res 28((1B):515–517

33. Landrum LM, Skaggs V, Gould N et al (2008) Comparison of outcome measures in patients with advanced squamous cell carcinoma of the vulva treated with surgery or primary chemoradiation. Gynecol Oncol 108(3):584–590

34. Parthasarathy A, Cheung MK, Osann K et al (2006) The benefit of adjuvant radiation therapy in single-node-positive squamous cell vulvar carcinoma. Gynecol Oncol 103(3):1095–1099

35. Micha JP, Goldstein BH, Rettenmaier MA et al (2006) Pelvic radiation necrosis and osteomyelitis following chemoradiation for advanced stage vulvar and cervical carcinoma. Gynecol Oncol 101(2):349–352

36. Landoni F, Maneo A, Zanetta G et al (1996) Concurrent preoperative chemotherapy with 5-fluorouracil and mitomycin C and radiotherapy (FUMIR) followed by limited surgery in locally advanced and recurrent vulva carcinoma. Gynecol Oncol 61:321–327

37. Cunningham MJ, Goyer RP, Gibbons SK et al (1997) Primary radiation, cisplatin and 5-fluorouracil for advanced squamous carcinoma of the vulva. Gynecol Oncol 66:258–261

38. Wagenaar HC, Colombo N, Vergote I et al (2001) Bleomycin, methotrexate, and CCNU in locally advanced or recurrent, inoperable, squamous-cell carcinoma of the vulva: an EORTC gynaecological cancer cooperative group study. European organization for research and treatment of cancer. Gynecol Oncol 81:348–354

39. Han SC, Kim DH, Higgins SA et al (2000) Chemoradiation as primary or adjuvant treatment for locally advanced carcinoma of the vulva. Int J Radiat Oncol Biol Phys 47:1235–1244

40. Mulayim N, Mulayim N, Foster Silver D, Schwartz PE et al (2004) Chemoradiation with 5-fluorouracil and mitomycin C in the treatment of vulvar squamous cell carcinoma. Gynecol Oncol 93(3): 659–666

41. Burger MPM, Hollema H, Emanuels AG et al (1995) The importance of the groin node status for the survival of T1 and T2 vulvar carcinoma patients. Gynecol Oncol 57:334–337

42. Beller V, Sideri M, Maisonneuve P et al (2001) Carcinoma of the vagina: 24th annual report on the results of treatment in gynecological cancer. J Epidemiol Biostat 6:141–152

43. Wu X, Matanoski G, Chen VW (2008) Descriptive epidemiology of vaginal cancer and survival by race, ethnicity, and age in the United States. Cancer 113(10):2873–2882

44. Beller U, Benedet JL, Creasman WT et al (2006) Carcinoma of the vagina. FIGO 6th Annual Report on the Results of Treatment in Gynecological Cancer. Int J Gynaecol Obstet 95:S29–S42

45. Takai N, Kai N, Hirata Y et al (2008) Primary malignant melanoma of the vagina. Eur J Gynaecol Oncol 29(5):558–559

46. Fu YS (2002) Pathology of the uterine cervix, vagina and vulva, 2nd edn. Saunders, Philadelphia

47. Daling J, Madeleine M, Schwartz S et al (2002) A population based study of squamous cell vaginal cancer: HPV and cofactors. Gynecol Oncol 84:263–270

48. Hellman K, Silfversward C, Nilsson B et al (2004) Primary carcinoma of the vagina: factors influencing the age at diagnosis. The Radiumhemmet series 1956-96. Int J Gynecol Cancer 14:491–501

49. Carter JJ, Madeleine MM, Shera K et al (2001) Human papillomavirus 16 and 18 L1 serology compared across anogenital cancer sites. Cancer Res 61:1934–1940

50. Indraccolo U, Chiocci L, Baldoni A (2008) Does vaginal intraepithelial neoplasia have the same evolution as cervical intraepithelial neoplasia? Eur J Gynaecol Oncol 29(4):371–373

51. Schockaert S, Poppe W, Arbyn M et al (2008) Incidence of vaginal intraepithelial neoplasia after hysterectomy for cervical intraepithelial neoplasia: a retrospective study. Am J Obstet Gynecol 199(2):113.e1–113.e5

52. Gonzalez BE, Torres A, Busquets M (2008) Prognostic factors for the development of vaginal intraepithelial neoplasia. Eur J Gynaecol Oncol 29(1):43–45

53. Srodon M, Stoler MH, Baber GB, Kurman RJ (2007) The distribution of low and high-risk HPV types in vulvar and vaginal intraepithelial neoplasia (VIN and VaIN). Am J Surg Pathol 31(9): 1452–1454

54. Stock RG, Chen AS, Seski J (1995) A 30 year experience in the management of primary carcinoma of the vagina: analysis of prognostic factors and treatment modalities. Gynecol Oncol 56:45–52

55. Benedetti PP, Bellati F, Plotti F (2008) Neoadjuvant chemotherapy followed by radical surgery in patients affected by vaginal carcinoma. Gynecol Oncol 111(2):307–311

56. Nashiro T, Yagi C, Hirakawa M et al (2008) Concurrent chemoradiation for locally advanced squamous cell carcinoma of the vagina: case series and literature review. Int J Clin Oncol 13(4): 335–339

57. Beller V, Sideri M, Maisonneuve P (2001) Carcinoma of the vagina: 24th annual report on the results of treatment in gynecological cancer. J Epidemiol Biostat 6:141–152

58. Jemal A, Siegel R, Ward E et al (2008) Cancer statistics, 2008. CA Cancer J Clin 58(2):71–96

59. Smith HO, Tiffany MF, Qualls CR et al (2000) The rising incidence of adenocarcinoma relative to squamous cell carcinoma of the uterine cervix in the United States: a 24 year population-based study. Gynecol Oncol 78:97–105

60. Duggan MA, McGregor SE, Benoit JL (1995) The human papilloma virus status of invasive cervical adenocarcinoma: a clinicopathological and outcome analysis. Hum Pathol 26:319–325

61. dos Reis R, Frumovitz M, Milam MR et al (2007) Adenosquamous carcinoma versus adenocarcinoma in early-stage cervical cancer patients undergoing radical hysterectomy: an outcomes analysis. Gynecol Oncol 107(3):458–463

62. De Vuyst H, Clifford GM, Nascimento MC et al (2009) Prevalence and type distribution of human papillomavirus in carcinoma and intraepithelial neoplasia of the vulva, vagina and anus: a meta-analysis. Int J Cancer 124(7):1626–1636

63. Li W, Wang W, Si M et al (2008) The physical state of HPV16 infection and its clinical significance in cancer precursor lesion and cervical carcinoma. J Cancer Res Clin 134(12):1355–1361

64. Lee SW, Kim YM, Son WS et al (2009) The efficacy of conservative management after conization in patients with stage IA1 microinvasive cervical carcinoma. Acta Obstet Gynecol Scand 88(2): 209–215

65. Yen TC, Lai CH, Ma SY et al (2006) Comparative benefits and limitations of 18F-FDG PET and CT-MRI in documented or suspected recurrent cervical cancer. Eur J Nucl Med Mol Imaging 33(12):1399–1407

66. Mitchell DG, Snyder B, Coakley F et al (2009) Early invasive cervical cancer: MRI and CT predictors of lymphatic metastases in the ACRIN 6651/GOG 183 intergroup study. Gynecol Oncol 112(1):95–103

67. Piver MS, Rutledge F, Smith JP (1974) Five classes of extended hysterectomy for women with cervical cancer. Obstet Gynecol 44:265–272

68. Nezhat FR, Datta MS, Liu C et al (2008) Robotic radical hysterectomy versus total laparoscopic radical hysterectomy with pelvic lymphadenectomy for treatment of early cervical cancer. J Soc Laparoendosc Surg 12(3):227–237

69. Obermair A, Gebski V, Frumovitz M et al (2008) A phase III randomized clinical trial comparing laparoscopic or robotic radical hysterectomy with abdominal radical hysterectomy in patients with early stage cervical cancer. J Minim Invasive Gynecol 15(5):584–588

70. Hosaka M, Watari H, Takeda M et al (2008) Treatment of cervical cancer with adjuvant chemotherapy versus adjuvant radiotherapy after radical hysterectomy and systematic lymphadenectomy. J Obstet Gynaecol Res 34(4):552–556

71. Goksedef BP, Kunos C, Belinson JL et al (2009) Concurrent cisplatin-based chemoradiation International Federation of Gynecology and Obstetrics stage IB2 cervical carcinoma. Am J Obstet Gynecol 200(2):175.e1–175.e5

72. Ohara K, Tanaka YO, Oki A et al (2008) Comparison of tumor regression rate of uterine cervical squamous cell carcinoma during external beam and intracavitary radiotherapy. Radiat Med 26(9): 526–532

73. Huguet F, Cojocariu OM, Levy P et al (2008) Preoperative concurrent radiation therapy and chemotherapy for bulky stage IB2, IIA, and IIB carcinoma of the uterine cervix with proximal parametrial invasion. Int J Radiat Oncol 72(5):1508–1515

74. Zivanovic O, Alektiar KM, Sonoda Y et al (2008) Treatment patterns of FIGO Stage IB2 cervical cancer: a single-institution experience of radical hysterectomy with individualized postoperative therapy and definitive radiation therapy. Gynecol Oncol 111(2): 265–270

75. Walker JL, Morrison A, DiSilvestro P, Gynecologic Oncology Group et al (2009) A phase I/II study of extended field radiation therapy with concomitant paclitaxel and cisplatin chemotherapy in patients with cervical carcinoma metastatic to the para-aortic lymph nodes: a Gynecologic Oncology Group study. Gynecol Oncol 112(1):78–84

76. Kapp DS, Fischer D, Gutierrez E et al (1983) Pretreatment prognostic factors in carcinoma of the uterine cervix: a multivariate analysis of the effect of age, stage, histology and blood counts on survival. Int J Radiat Oncol Biol Phys 9:445–455

77. Haasbeek CJ, Uitterhoeve AL, van der Velden J et al (2008) Long-term results of salvage radiotherapy for the treatment of recurrent cervical carcinoma after prior surgery. Radiother Oncol 89(2):197–204

78. Magrina HF, Stanhope CR, Weaver AL (1997) Pelvic exenterations: supralevator, infralevator and with vulvectomy. Gynecol Oncol 64:130–135

79. Penalven MA, Barreau G, Sevin BU et al (1996) Surgery for the treatment of locally recurrent disease. J Natl Cancer Inst 21: 117–122

80. Vergote IB (1997) Exenterative surgery. Curr Opin Obstet Gynecol 9:25–28

81. Rose PG, Blessing JA, Gershensen DM et al (1999) Paclitaxel and cisplatin as first-line therapy in recurrent or advanced squamous cell carcinoma of the cervix: a Gynecologic Oncology Group study. J Clin Oncol 17:2676–2680

82. Ahmed A, Zamba G, DeGeest K et al (2008) The impact of surgery on survival of elderly women with endometrial cancer in the SEER program from 1992-2002. Gynecol Oncol 111(1):35–40

83. Levy T, Golan A, Menczer J (2006) Endometrial endometrioid carcinoma: a glimpse at the natural course. Am J Obstet Gynecol 195(2):454–457

84. Cirisano FD Jr, Robboy SJ, Dodge RK et al (1999) Epidemiologic and surgicopathologic findings of papillary serous and clear cell endometrial cancers when compared to endometrioid carcinoma. Gynecol Oncol 74(3):385–394

85. Spaziani E, Picchio M, Petrozza V et al (2008) Carcinosarcoma of the uterus: a case report and review of the literature. Eur J Gynaecol Oncol 29(5):531–534

86. Lin JF, Slomovitz BM (2008) Uterine sarcoma 2008. Curr Oncol Rep 10(6):512–518

87. Albert RH, Clark MM (2008) Cancer screening in the older patient. Am Fam Phys 78(12):1369–1374

88. Patel C, Ullal A, Roberts M et al (2009) Endometrial carcinoma detected with SurePath liquid-based cervical cytology: comparison with conventional cytology. Cytopathology 20(6):380–387

89. Leitao MM Jr, Kehoe S, Barakat RR et al (2009) Comparison of D&C and office endometrial biopsy accuracy in patients with FIGO grade 1 endometrial adenocarcinoma. Gynecol Oncol 113(1):105–108

90. Sierecki AR, Gudipudi DK, Montemarano N et al (2008) Comparison of endometrial aspiration biopsy techniques: specimen adequacy. J Reprod Med 53(10):760–764

91. Kurman RK, Kaminski PF, Norris HJ (1985) The behavior of endometrial hyperplasia: a long-term study of "untreated" hyperplasia in 170 patients. Cancer 56:403–412

92. Mittal K, Sebenik M, Irwin C et al (2009) Presence of endometrial adenocarcinoma in situ in complex atypical endometrial hyperplasia is associated with increased incidence of endometrial carcinoma in subsequent hysterectomy. Mod Pathol 22(1):37–42

93. McKenney JK, Longacre TA (2009) Low-grade endometrial adenocarcinoma: a diagnostic algorithm for distinguishing atypical endometrial hyperplasia and other benign (and malignant) mimics. Adv Anat Pathol 16(1):1–22

94. Geisler JP, Geisler HE, Melton ME et al (1999) What staging surgery should be performed on patients with uterine papillary serous carcinoma? Gynecol Oncol 74(3):465–467

95. Bristow RE, Asrari F, Trimble EL et al (2001) Extended surgical staging for uterine papillary serous carcinoma: survival outcome of locoregional (stage I-III) disease. Gynecol Oncol 81(2):279–286

96. Chan JK, Loizzi V, Youssef M et al (2003) Significance of comprehensive surgical staging in noninvasive papillary serous carcinoma of the endometrium. Gynecol Oncol 90(1):181–185

97. Mendivil A, Schuler KM, Gehrig PA (2009) Non-endometrioid adenocarcinoma of the uterine corpus: a review of selected histological subtypes. Cancer Control 16(1):46–52

98. Seamon LG, Cohn DE, Henretta MS et al (2009) Minimally invasive comprehensive surgical staging for endometrial cancer: robotics or laparoscopy? Gynecol Oncol 113(1):36–41

99. Zullo F, Palomba S, Falbo A et al (2009) Laparoscopic surgery vs laparotomy for early stage endometrial cancer: long-term data of a randomized controlled trial. Am J Obstet Gynecol 200(3):296.e1–296.e9

100. Neubauer NL, Havrilesky LJ, Calingaert B et al (2009) The role of lymphadenectomy in the management of preoperative grade 1 endometrial carcinoma. Gynecol Oncol 112(3):511–516

101. Frederick PJ, Straughn JM Jr (2009) The role of comprehensive surgical staging in patients with endometrial cancer. Cancer Control 16(1):23–29

102. Creutzberg CL, van Putten WL, Koper PC et al (2000) Surgery and postoperative radiation versus surgery alone for patients with stage-1 endometrial carcinoma: multicentre randomized trial. Lancet 355:1401–1411

103. Kuoppala T, Mäenpää J, Tomas E et al (2008) Surgically staged high-risk endometrial cancer: randomized study of adjuvant radiotherapy alone vs. sequential chemo-radiotherapy. Gynecol Oncol 110:190–195

104. Fleming GF, Brunetto VL, Cella D et al (2004) Phase III trial of doxorubicin plus cisplatin with or without paclitaxel plus filgrastim

in advanced endometrial carcinoma: a Gynecologic Oncology Group Study. J Clin Oncol 22:2159–2166

105. Randall ME, Filiaci VL, Muss H et al (2006) Randomized phase III trial of whole-abdominal irradiation versus doxorubicin and cisplatin chemotherapy in advanced endometrial carcinoma: a Gynecologic Oncology Group study. J Clin Oncol 24:36–44

106. Linkov F, Taioli E (2008) Factors influencing endometrial cancer mortality: the Western Pennsylvania Registry. Future Oncol 4(6):857–865

107. Shenfield CB, Pearcey RG, Ghosh S et al (2009) The management of inoperable Stage I endometrial cancer using intracavitary brachytherapy alone: a 20-year institutional review. Brachytherapy 8(3):278–283

108. Fishman DA, Roberts KB, Chambers JT et al (1996) Radiation therapy as exclusive treatment for medically inoperable patients with stage I and II endometrioid carcinoma of the endometrium. Gynecol Oncol 61:189–196

109. Temkin SM, Fleming G (2009) Current treatment of metastatic endometrial cancer. Cancer Control 16(1):38–45

110. Homesley HD, Filiaci V, Gibbons SK et al (2009) A randomized phase III trial in advanced endometrial carcinoma of surgery and volume directed radiation followed by cisplatin and doxorubicin with or without paclitaxel: A Gynecologic Oncology Group study. Gynecol Oncol 112(3):543–552

111. Blake P, Swart AM, Orton J, ASTEC/EN.5 Study Group et al (2009) Adjuvant external beam radiotherapy in the treatment of endometrial cancer (MRC ASTEC and NCIC CTG EN.5 randomised trials): pooled trial results, systematic review, and meta-analysis. Lancet 373(9658):137–146

112. Fowler JM, Brady WE, Grigsby PW et al (2009) Sequential chemotherapy and irradiation in advanced stage endometrial cancer: A Gynecologic Oncology Group phase I trial of doxorubicin-cisplatin followed by whole abdomen irradiation. Gynecol Oncol 112(3):553–557

113. Fujimoto T, Nanjyo H, Fukuda J et al (2009) Endometrioid uterine cancer: histopathological risk factors of local and distant recurrence. Gynecol Oncol 112(2):342–347

114. Indraccolo U, Luchetti G, Indraccolo SR (2008) Malignant transformation of uterine leiomyomata. Eur J Gynaecol Oncol 29(5):543–544

115. Wu TI, Hsu KH, Huang HJ et al (2008) Prognostic factors and adjuvant therapy in uterine carcinosarcoma. Eur J Gynaecol Oncol 29(5):483–488

116. Landreat V, Paillocher N, Catala L et al (2008) Low-grade endometrial stromal sarcoma of the uterus: review of 10 cases. Anticancer Res 28(5B):2869–2874

117. Hannigan EV, Gomez LG (1979) Uterine leiomyosarcoma. Am J Obstet Gynecol 134:557–564

118. Hensley ML, Blessing JA, Mannel R et al (2008) Fixed-dose rate gemcitabine plus docetaxel as first-line therapy for metastatic uterine leiomyosarcoma: a Gynecologic Oncology Group phase II trial. Gynecol Oncol 109(3):329–334

119. Reed NS, Mangioni C, Malmstrom H et al (2008) Phase III randomised study to evaluate the role of adjuvant pelvic radiotherapy in the treatment of uterine sarcomas stages I and II: an European Organisation for Research and Treatment of Cancer Gynaecological Cancer Group Study (protocol 55874). Eur J Cancer 44(11):1612

120. Resnik E, Chambers SK, Carcangiu ML et al (1996) Malignant uterine smooth muscle tumors: role of etoposide, cisplatin and doxorubicin (EPA) chemotherapy. J Surg Oncol 63:145–147

121. Kasper B, Dietrich S, Mechtersheimer G et al (2007) Large institutional experience with dose-intensive chemotherapy and stem cell support in the management of sarcoma patients. Oncology 73(1–2):58–64

122. Long HJ 3rd, Blessing JA, Sorosky J (2005) Phase II trial of dacarbazine, mitomycin, doxorubicin, and cisplatin with sargramostim

in uterine leiomyosarcoma: a Gynecologic Oncology Group study. Gynecol Oncol 99(2):339–342

123. Wolfson AH, Brady MF, Rocereto T et al (2007) A gynecologic oncology group randomized phase III trial of whole abdominal irradiation (WAI) vs. cisplatin-ifosfamide and mesna (CIM) as post-surgical therapy in stage I-IV carcinosarcoma (CS) of the uterus. Gynecol Oncol 107(2):177–185

124. Homesley HD, Filiaci V, Markman M et al (2007) Phase III trial of ifosfamide with or without paclitaxel in advanced uterine carcino sarcoma: a Gynecologic Oncology Group Study. J Clin Oncol 25(5):526–531

125. Nemani D, Mitra N, Guo M et al (2008) Assessing the effects of lymphadenectomy and radiation therapy in patients with uterine carcinosarcoma: a SEER analysis. Gynecol Oncol 111(1):82–88

126. Pautier P, Rey A, Haie-Meder C et al (2004) Adjuvant chemotherapy with cisplatin, ifosfamide, and doxorubicin followed by radiotherapy in localized uterine sarcomas: results of a case-control study with radiotherapy alone. Int J Gynecol Cancer 14(6):1112–1117

127. Goodman MT, Shvetsov YB (2009) Incidence of ovarian, peritoneal, and fallopian tube carcinomas in the United States, 1995-2004. Cancer Epidemiol Biomarkers Prev 18(1):132–139

128. Baekelandt M, Kockx M, Wesling F et al (1993) Primary adeno-carcinoma of the fallopian tube: review of the literature. Int J Gynecol Cancer 3:65–71

129. Leath CA 3rd, Numnum TM, Straughn JM Jr et al (2007) Outcomes for patients with fallopian tube carcinoma managed with adjuvant chemotherapy following primary surgery: a retrospective university experience. Int J Gynecol Cancer 17(5):998–1002

130. Arora N, Tewari D, Cowan C et al (2008) Bevacizumab demonstrates activity in advanced refractory fallopian tube carcinoma. Int J Gynecol Cancer 18(2):369–372

131. Rosen AC, Klein M, Rosen HR et al (1994) Preoperative and post-operative CA-125 serum levels in primary fallopian tube carcinoma. Arch Gynecol Obstet 255:665–668

132. Pectasides D, Pectasides E, Economopoulos T (2006) Fallopian tube carcinoma: a review. Oncologist 11(8):902–912

133. Benedet JL, Miller DM (1992) Tumors of fallopian tube: clinical features, staging and management. In: Coppleson M, Monoghan JM, Morrow CP et al (eds) Gynecologic oncology: fundamental principles and clinical practice. Churchill Livingstone, Edinburgh, pp 853–860

134. US Cancer Statistics Working Group. United States Cancer Statistics: 1999–2005 Incidence and Mortality Web-Based Report. http://www.cdc.gov/uscs

135. Permuth-Wey J, Sellers TA (2009) Epidemiology of ovarian cancer. Methods Mol Biol 472:413–437

136. Minino AM, Heron MP, Smith BL (2006) Deaths: preliminary data for 2004. Natl Vital Stat Rep 54(19):1–50

137. Aletti GD, Podratz KC, Moriarty JP et al (2009) Aggressive and complex surgery of advanced ovarian cancer: an economic analysis. Gynecol Oncol 112(1):16–21

138. Barnholtz-Sloan JS, Schwartz AG, Qureshi F et al (2003) Ovarian cancer: changes in patterns at diagnosis and relative survival over the last three decades. Am J Obstet Gynecol 189:1120–1127

139. Nguyen HN, Averette HE, Janicek M (2004) Ovarian carcinoma. A review of the significance of familial risk factors and the role of prophylactic oophorectomy in cancer prevention. Cancer 74: 545–555

140. Stratton JF, Pharoah P, Smith SK et al (1998) A systematic review and meta-analysis of family history and risk of ovarian cancer. Brit J Obstet Gynaecol 105:493–499

141. Sutcliffe S, Pharoah PD, Easton DF et al (2000) Ovarian and breast cancer risks to women in families with two or more cases of ovarian cancer. Int J Cancer 87:110–117

142. Risch HA, McLaughlin JR, Cole DE et al (2001) Prevalence and penetrance of germline BRCA1 and BRCA2 mutations in a popu-

lation series of 649 women with ovarian cancer. Am J Hum Genet 68:700–710

143. Ford D, Easton DF, Bishop DT et al (1994) Risks of cancer in BRCA1-mutation carriers. Breast Cancer Linkage Consortium. Lancet 343:692–695

144. Rebbeck TR, Kauff ND, Domchek SM (2009) Meta-analysis of risk reduction estimates associated with risk-reducing salpingo-oophorectomy in BRCA1 or BRCA2 mutation carriers. J Natl Cancer Inst 101(2):80–87

145. Kauff ND, Domcheck SM, Friebel TM et al (2008) Risk-reducing salpingo-oophorectomy for the prevention of BRCA1- and BRCA2- associated breast and gynecologic cancer: a multicenter, prospective study. J Clin Oncol 26(8):1331–1337

146. Cannistra SA (1993) Cancer of the ovary. N Engl J Med 329:1550–1559

147. Fishman DA, Schwartz PE (1994) Current approaches to the diagnosis and treatment of ovarian germ cell malignancies. Curr Opin Obstet Gynecol 6:98–104

148. Price FV, Schwartz PE (1993) Management of ovarian stromal tumors. Ovarian cancer. McGraw Hill, New York, pp 405–423

149. Nicoletto MO, Caltarossa E, Donach M et al (2006) Sertoli cell tumor: a rare case in an elderly patient. Eur J Gynaecol Oncol 27(1):86–87

150. Oliva E, Alvarez T, Young RH (2005) Sertoli cell tumors of the ovary: a clinicopathologic and immunohistochemical study of 54 cases. Am J Surg Pathol 29(2):143–156

151. Arai M, Jobo T, Iwaya H et al (1999) Androgen-producing ovarian tumors: a clinicopathological study of 3 cases. J Obstet Gynaecol Res 25(6):411–418

152. Silasi DA, Illuzzi JL, Kelly MG et al (2008) Carcinosarcoma of the ovary. Int J Gynecol Cancer 18(1):22–29

153. Jiang R, Tang J, Cheng X et al (2009) Surgical treatment for patients with different origins of Krukenberg tumors: outcomes and prognostic factors. Eur J Surg Oncol 35(1):92–97

154. Young RH (2007) From Krukenberg to today: the ever present problems posed by metastatic tumors in the ovary. Part II. Adv Anat Pathol 14(3):149–177

155. Kiyokawa T, Young RH, Scully RE (2006) Krukenberg tumors of the ovary: a clinicopathologic analysis of 120 cases with emphasis on their variable pathologic manifestations. Am J Surg Pathol 30(3):277–299

156. Cheong JH, Hyung WJ, Chen J et al (2004) Survival benefit of metastasectomy for Krukenberg tumors from gastric cancer. Gynecol Oncol 94(2):477–482

157. Wakabayashi MT, Lin PS, Hakim AA (2008) The role of cytoreductive/debulking surgery in ovarian cancer. J Natl Compr Canc Netw 6(8):803–810

158. Goff BA, Matthews BJ, Wynn M et al (2006) Ovarian cancer: patterns of surgical care across the United States. Gynecol Oncol 103(2):383–390

159. Fader AN, Rose PG (2007) Role of surgery in ovarian carcinoma. J Clin Oncol 25(20):2873–2883

160. Bristow RE, Puri I, Chi DS (2009) Cytoreductive surgery for recurrent ovarian cancer: a meta-analysis. Gynecol Oncol 112(1):265–274

161. Aletti GD, Dowdy SC, Podratz KC et al (2007) Relationship among surgical complexity, short-term morbidity, and overall survival in primary surgery for advanced ovarian cancer. Am J Obstet Gynecol 197(6):676.e1–676.e7

162. Winter WE 3rd, Maxwell GL, Tian C et al (2007) Prognostic factors for stage III epithelial ovarian cancer: a Gynecologic Oncology Group Study. J Clin Oncol 25(24):3621–3627

163. Matulonis UA, Krag KJ, Krasner CN et al (2009) Phase II prospective study of paclitaxel and carboplatin in older patients with newly diagnosed Mullerian tumors. Gynecol Oncol 112(2): 394–399

164. Wethington SL, Herzog TJ, Seshan VE et al (2008) Improved survival for fallopian tube cancer: a comparison of clinical characteristics

and outcome for primary fallopian tube and ovarian cancer. Cancer 113(12):3298–3306

165. Schwartz PE (1995) Neoadjuvant chemotherapy for advanced ovarian cancer. J Gynecol Tech 1:175–180

166. Schwartz PE, Rutherford TJ, Chambers JT et al (1999) Neoadjuvant chemotherapy for advanced ovarian cancer: long-term survival. Gynecol Oncol 72:93–99

167. Markman M (2008) Predictive value of neoadjuvant chemotherapy for the clinical utility of subsequently performed major cancer surgery. Curr Oncol Rep 10(6):447–448

168. Chi DS, Schwartz PE (2008) Cytoreduction vs. neoadjuvant chemotherapy for ovarian cancer. Gynecol Oncol 111(3):391–399

169. Morrison J, Swanton A, Collins S et al (2007) Chemotherapy versus surgery for initial treatment in advanced ovarian epithelial cancer. Cochrane Database Syst Rev 4:CD005343

170. Le T, Alshaikh G, Hopkins L et al (2006) Prognostic significance of postoperative morbidities in patients with advanced epithelial ovarian cancer treated with neoadjuvant chemotherapy and delayed primary surgical debulking. Ann Surg Oncol 13(12):1711–1716

171. Hou JY, Kelly MG, Yu H et al (2007) Neoadjuvant chemotherapy lessens surgical morbidity in advanced ovarian cancer and leads to improved survival in stage IV disease. Gynecol Oncol 105(1): 211–217

172. Moore KN, Reid MS, Fong DN et al (2008) Ovarian cancer in the octogenarian: does the paradigm of aggressive cytoreductive surgery and chemotherapy still apply? Gynecol Oncol 110(2): 133–139

173. Markman M (2008) Pharmaceutical management of ovarian cancer: current status. Drugs 68(6):771–789

174. Tebes SJ, Sayer RA, Palmer JM et al (2007) Cytoreductive surgery for patients with recurrent epithelial ovarian carcinoma. Gynecol Oncol 106(3):482–487

175. FIGO Committee on Gynecologic Oncology (2009) Revised FIGO staging for carcinoma of the vulva, cervix, and endometrium. Int J Gynecol Obstet 105:103–104

176. Odicino F, Pecorelli S, Zigliani L, Creasman WT (2008) History of the FIGO cancer staging system. Int J Gynecol Obstet 101(2): 205–210

Section XI
Nervous System

Chapter 84
Invited Commentary

Dennis Spencer

Prior to the 1980s, advances in neurosurgery were tied to increased surgical competence based on better illumination and magnification of the operative microscope coupled with safer anesthesia and the creation of intensive care units devoted to the special needs of the injured nervous system. Most of the literature in the 1960s and 1970s concentrated on improving outcomes in the most devastating and easily recognized disorders such as those of pediatric development (hydrocephalus and spinal dysraphisms), trauma and, in particular, the vascular anomalies of aneurysms and arteriovenous malformations (AVM). There was little attention applied separately to issues of the elderly since the aforementioned disorders primarily affected a young to middle-aged population.

The most surgically unremediable conditions occurred in the elderly, such as hypertensive intracerebral hematomas and malignant brain tumors, particularly glioblastoma multiforma. The most common diagnostic imaging techniques of pneumoencephalography and arteriography were invasive and held increased risk in the elderly.

The last three decades, however, have seen a revolution in our approach to diseases of the nervous system, primarily because of the computer, which has been the basis of sophisticated noninvasive computerized tomographic (CT) and Magnetic Resonance (MR) imaging of the brain, spinal cord, and bony support elements. Because of the rigid skull, the brain was the first organ precisely navigated utilizing stereotactic coordinates, providing minimally invasive diagnostic and therapeutic potential.

With the continued evolution of high-resolution imaging and intravascular microcatheters, the neurovascular field is changing before our eyes. In a few short years, we have seen the universal application of intracranial aneurysm clipping giving way to endovascular techniques, which are becoming more sophisticated each year and are sure to decrease the morbidity and mortality of aneurysmal subarachnoid hemorrhage in the elderly

MRI scanning delivers anatomically precise and often disease-specific diagnoses and when coupled with stereotactic devices and radiation therapy tools, aids in non-invasive pinpoint destruction of a variety of slow growing tumors (meningiomas, vestibular schwannomas), AVM's and cranial nerves producing drug resistant pain (trigeminal neuralgia). All of these disorders have an increased frequency in the aging population and are much more safely treated with modern technology.

Analyzing the aging brain with techniques other than CT and MRI, such as Positron Emission Tomography (PET), MR Spectroscopy (MRS), functional MR (fMR) and Single Photon Emission Tomography (SPECT), and electrophysiology, may be coupled in the near future with genetically targeted molecules and precise delivery techniques to treat neurodegenerative diseases such as Parkinson's and Alzheimer's. These two diseases, specifically, are increasing in number, as nutrition and cardiovascular advancements have lengthened our life span.

With all of these new techniques, the issue, more than ever, will be the thoughtful and ethical application of therapy, particularly in those individuals over 70 years where there is less systemic reserve and quality of life takes on a different perspective than that of the 40-year old. Some clinical decisions should be obvious, such as the use of endovascular techniques to palliate or cure intracranial vascular disease. The other edge of this sword, however, may be the indiscriminant use of intra-arterial TPA for occlusive vascular disease in the aged brain. There is just no clear data to guide such therapy. Also, common sense should prevail in watchful waiting of incidentally discovered but asymptomatic slow-growing tumors such as the pituitary, meningioma, and schwannoma.

The judicious use of Deep Brain Stimulation (DBS) has already made a major impact on improving the quality of life (QOL) in Parkinsonian patients, and early nonrandomized trials of neurostimulation in medically intractable depression

D. Spencer (✉)
Harvey and Kate Cushing Professor and Chair,
Department of Neurosurgery, Yale University School of Medicine,
Yale New Haven Hospital, New Haven, CT, USA
e-mail: dennis.spencer@yale.edu

R.A. Rosenthal et al. (eds.), *Principles and Practice of Geriatric Surgery*,
DOI 10.1007/978-1-4419-6999-6_84, © Springer Science+Business Media, LLC 2011

show promising effects. As neurostimulation becomes more popular and available, we must develop proper utilization criteria for these devices in the older patients.

We are quickly approaching an era where the declining health of the baby boomers may overwhelm an already strained health-care system. Applying our surgical decisions, tools, and techniques to the elderly in the same manner that we might in young and middle-aged patients may not be the most thoughtful or cost-effective, just as is inappropriate in infants and very young children. Modern medicine has the ability to preserve and prolong life. However, our most important consideration must be the quality of the life that remains. Clinical trials of neuroactive drugs, chemotherapeutic agents, and neurosurgical intervention must include and provide segregated study of older patients. Clinical investigation must carefully examine the physiology and pathophysiology of nervous system disorders before therapies are applied widely or withheld without justification.

Chapter 85
Effects of Aging on the Nervous System

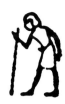

Howard A. Crystal, Pedro J. Torrico, Shefali Gandhi, and Paul J. Maccabee

Anatomic, physiologic, and systems levels changes in the nervous system with age

Parameter	Change with age
Anatomical	
Neuron number	Varies, no change in some brain regions, small decreases in others, possible decrease in number of lower motor neurons in some regions
Synaptic density	Possibly decreased in some regions
Dendritic arborization	Possibly decreased in some regions
Myelin	May be decreased in volume
Muscle mass	Decreased
Muscle fast twitch fibers	Decreased
Neuromodulators	May be decreased
Physiologic	
Speed of conduction over myelinated fibers	Decreased
Synaptic plasticity	Probably decreased
Ability for neuronal assemblies to synchronize and desynchronize	Not known
Neurogenesis	May be decreased
Systems level	
Cognition	
Speed	Decreased
Learning, new episodic memory	Decreased
Recalling old semantic memory	Contradictory data
Recalling old procedural memory	Little data
Learning new procedural memory	Little data
Language	Not decreased
Motor	
Strength	Decreased
Speed	Decreased
Somatosensory perception thresholds	Decreased

An issue in analyzing all human studies of normal aging is separating the effects of highly prevalent diseases such as hypertension and hyperlipidemia from the effects of normal aging. Subjects with chronic degenerative disorders with high prevalence such as Alzheimer's disease that have a very long preclinical phase are often unavoidably included as "normals." The best way to deal with this source of error is to conduct longitudinal studies and only include subjects as "normal" who do not decline over time. Although it is tempting to relate changes on the molecular and cellular level to changes at the system level, correlative data supporting such inferences are rarely available

Source: Data from Hof PR, Morrison JH (2004) The aging brain: morphomolecular senescence of cortical circuits. Trends Neurosci 27(10): 607–613 and Rossini PM, Rossi S, Babiloni C, Polich J (2007) Clinical neurophysiology of aging brain: from normal aging to neurodegeneration. Prog Neurobiol 83:375–400

In this chapter, we will discuss four syndromes that comprise most of the neurological problems encountered by geriatric perisurgical patients: weakness, strokes, seizures, and cognitive impairment.

H.A. Crystal (✉)
Department of Neurology, SUNY Downstate Medical Center,
450 Clarkson Avenue, Box 1213, Brooklyn, NY 11203, USA
e-mail: howard.crystal@downstate.edu

Weakness

Weakness and particularly the inability to wean a patient from a respirator are common neurological problems in critically ill elderly postsurgical patients. Weaning difficulties are often the first sign of weakness as intubated patients do not move out of bed or sit up and eat. Many surgical patients clearly meet criteria for critical illness and systemic inflammatory

CASE STUDY

An 80-year-old man with a 20-year history of hypertension and diabetes is 6 days post-op from an emergency cholecystectomy. He developed pneumonia on the first postoperative day and was never extubated. Neurological consultation was requested on the sixth hospital day when despite recovering from the surgery and pneumonia, it was difficult to wean him from the respirator.

Neurological evaluation showed a drowsy, modestly cooperative man. Mental status testing was done by asking "yes/no" questions and the patient selected the wrong year, month, and hospital name. Facial muscle strength was difficult to assess with the endotracheal tube in place, but eye closure was near normal in strength. Motor exam showed that he was barely able to break gravity in most muscles tested. Reflexes were absent. Sensory exam revealed little useful information.

The neurologist suggested a possible acute neuropathy, most likely critical illness or acute demyelinating and recommended nerve conduction studies and electromyography, but also indicated that the areflexia could have been from his long-standing diabetes, and acute myopathies or neuromuscular junction syndromes needed to be ruled out as well.

This case shows that neurological exam in the ICU is often challenging. Communication may be limited because of intubation, sedation, and/or encephalopathy. These factors influence manual motor and sensory testing. Access may also be limited because of the site and nature of the surgery.

response syndrome (SIRS) and are at risk for critical illness neuropathy and critical illness myopathy. Weakness associated with prolonged neuromuscular blockade from pancuronium or other agents is also not uncommon. The differential diagnosis of weakness in an acute ill postsurgical patient is long (reviewed in Howard et al. [1]). In elderly patients, several diseases may be contributing to motor functional impairment in the same patient.

Critical Illness Polyneuropathy and Myopathy

Critical illness polyneuropathy (CIP) and myopathy (CIM) may be identified in 25–63% of patients who are maintained on artificial respiration for 7 or more days and achieves a 70–100% incidence in the presence of sepsis [2–4]. Factors leading to SIRS, CIP, and CIM are summarized in Fig. 85.1.

CIP is frequently preceded by septic encephalopathy [3]. Perisurgical infection increases the likelihood of SIRS [3]. The use of neuromuscular blocking agents and/or steroids increases the likelihood of CIM. Organ failure increases the likelihood of CIP. Upon successful treatment of SIRS and recovery of encephalopathy, the inability to wean from the respirator is often the initial indication of CIP [5]. SIRS in the context of neuromuscular blocking medications and corticosteroids is further implicated in CIM. Combined CIP and CIM is common, suggesting the designation of critical illness polyneuropathy and myopathy (CIPNM).

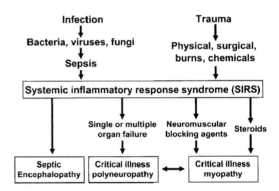

FIGURE 85.1 Factors associated with systemic inflammatory response syndrome (SIRS), critical illness polyneuropathy (CIP), and critical illness myopathy (CIM) (reprinted with permission from Bolton [3]).

Critical Illness Neuropathy

CIP is an acute sensorimotor axonopathy that occurs in patients with multiorgan failure, septic encephalopathy, and systemic inflammatory response syndrome. Hypoalbuminemia and hyperglycemia may further increase risk. Neurological exam typically reveals distal weakness, distal sensory loss, and areflexia, although reflexes may be preserved at the time of the exam, especially early. Facial muscles are usually spared. Weakness is usually more marked than sensory loss. The discrepancy between preserved facial grimace to noxious limb stimuli, with absent or decreased limb movement is "striking" [4]. The main differential diagnosis is preexisting or in-hospital acquired Guillian–Barre syndrome, usually the most common subtype, acute inflammatory demyelinating neuropathy (AIDP). AIDP may be characterized by very slow motor nerve conduction studies and a CSF pattern of high protein with few cells (albumincytologic dissociation). In contrast to CIP, facial weakness may often be present in AIDP. Other important diagnostic possibilities include preexisting decompensated Myasthenia Gravis and Lambert–Eaton Myasthenic syndrome.

Diagnosis may be confirmed by detailed electrophysiological studies, and if possible, nerve biopsy. In general, the sicker the patient the more severe the neuropathy; patients with severe neuropathies may show only limited improvement in strength as long as 4 years later. The etiology is not known and signs of inflammation are not present on postmortem exam.

Appropriate electrophysiologic testing is comprehensive [3]. Studies should include both motor and sensory nerve conductions, F waves, and needle EMG. If respiratory difficulty is present, phrenic nerve conduction studies and needle EMG of respiratory muscles may be critical in establishing the diagnosis [6]. In CIP, the nerve conduction studies indicate a sensorimotor axonal neuropathy, manifest by low amplitude motor and sensory-evoked responses. Decline of motor amplitude responses may be the earliest electrophysiologic finding, following the onset of SIRS but preceding the clinical syndrome [7]. Unlike diffuse axonal sensorimotor neuropathy, demyelinating features in AIDP may include markedly slow motor conduction velocities, extremely prolonged terminal motor and F-wave latencies, absent F waves and H-Soleus reflexes, prolonged distal compound muscle action with potential durations greater than 9 ms, and conduction block. It is important to emphasize that demyelinating abnormalities in AIDP may only be very slight, affecting as few as one or two motor nerves [8, 9].

Neuromuscular Blockade Syndromes

Some patients on neuromuscular blocking agents remain weak for days after the agents are discontinued, long after the blocking agent should have been metabolized and cleared. Several factors increase the likelihood of this syndrome including hypermagnesemia, use of aminoglycoside antibiotics and clindamycin, metabolic acidosis, hepatic or renal failure, and use of high-dose steroids. Hepatic or renal failure will prevent timely metabolism of these agents, resulting in prolongation of neuromuscular block. The syndrome may be distinguished from critical care myopathy by a normal CPK, and a decremental response on repetitive nerve stimulation (see below). This syndrome usually clears over days to 2 weeks, and overall prognosis is good.

It is always necessary to exclude neuromuscular junction disorders by available assays to detect acetylcholine receptor and muscle-specific kinase (MuSK) antibodies. In the presence of significant weakness, neuromuscular junction disorders are electrophysiologically best assessed by repetitive stimulation of single motor nerves (Jolly test) or single fiber EMG (SFEMG). If the patient is paralyzed or uncooperative, stimulation SFEMG will be required. In Myasthenia Gravis, a postsynaptic neuromuscular junction disorder, repetitive stimulation at slow rates typically shows abnormal decremental evoked responses, usually assessed by comparing the first vs. fifth elicited compound muscle action potential amplitude or area. Repetitive stimulation at fast rates in Lambert–Eaton Myasthenic syndrome, a presynaptic junction disorder, reveals abnormal incremental motor-evoked responses. Characteristic abnormalities of SFEMG in Myasthenia Gravis include prolonged jitter (variation in activation time across the same neuromuscular junction to repetitive discharges and blocking of transmission across the same neuromuscular junction to one or more attempted discharges).

Critical Illness Myopathy

The clinical hallmark of CIM is flaccid weakness, usually diffuse, involving limb muscles, neck flexors, often facial muscles and diaphragm, and occasionally extra-ocular muscles [3]. As in CIP, deep tendon reflexes are usually depressed but may be normal. The diagnosis is rarely suspected until it is difficult to wean patient from the respirator. The true incidence of CIM in patients who have difficulty being weaned from a respirator is not known as such studies require extensive electromyography, muscle biopsy, and nerve biopsy (to distinguish from CIP) and cannot rely on physical exam alone. The few studies that have been conducted suggest CIM is as common as CIP [10–14] or more common than CIP [1] Prognosis for CIM is better than for CIP. In over 80% of reported cases of CIM, patients have been exposed to both high-dose steroids and neuromuscular blocking agents, but it can occur in any critically ill patient.

The currently proposed three main subtypes of CIM include (1) myopathy with selective loss of thick filaments, also referred to as "acute quadriplegic" myopathy [15]; (2) rhabdomyolysis; and (3) nonnecrototizing cachectic myopathy, also referred to as disuse atrophy. (1) Myopathy with selective loss of thick filaments is typically seen in the context of acute asthma associated with mechanical respiration, neuromuscular blockade, and administration of high-dose steroids, this disorder is also seen following transplant surgery. Serum CPK can be mildly increased. (2) Rhabdomyolysis is also provoked by the administration of neuromuscular blocking medications and high-dose corticosteroids and may be associated with hyperkalemia, hypocalcemia, myoglobinuria,

TABLE 85.1 Neuromuscular conditions associated with critical illness

Condition	Incidence	Clinical features	Electrophysiologic findings	Serum creatine kinase	Muscle biopsy	Prognosis
Polyneuropathy						
Critical illness polyneuropathy	Common	Flaccid limbs, respiratory weakness	Axonal degeneration of motor and sensory fibers	Nearly normal	Denervation atrophy	Variable
Neuromuscular transmission defect						
Transient neuromuscular blockade	Common with neuromuscular blocking agents	Flaccid limbs, respiratory weakness	Abnormal repetitive nerve stimulation studies	Normal	Normal	Good
Critical illness myopathy						
Thick-filament myosin loss	Common with steroids, neuromuscular blocking agents, and sepsis	Flaccid limbs, respiratory weakness	Abnormal spontaneous activity	Mildly elevated	Loss of thick (myosin) filaments	Good
Rhabdomyolysis	Rare	Flaccid limbs	Near normal	Markedly elevated (myoglobinuria)	Normal or mild necrosis	Good
Necrotizing myopathy of intensive care	Rare	Flaccid weakness, myoglobinuria	Severe myopathy	Markedly elevated, myoglobinuria	Marked necrosis	Poor
Disuse (cachectic) myopathy	Common (?)	Muscle wasting	Normal	Normal	Normal or type II fiber atrophy	Good
Combined polyneuropathy and myopathy	Common	Flaccid limbs, respiratory weakness	Indicate combined polyneuropathy and myopathy	Variable	Denervation atrophy and myopathy	Variable

Source: Adapted with permission from Bolton [3]

and markedly elevated CPK, with resulting renal failure and cardiac irritability. According to Bolton, the acute necrototizing myopathy of intensive care [16] is a further stage in the progression of rhabdomyolysis. (3) Nonnecrototizing cachectic myopathy occurs in the context of malnutrition and starvation, and may be seen in anorexia nervosa and after gastric-bypass surgery. CPK and electrophysiologic testing are normal.

Nerve conduction studies in pure thick filament myopathy and in rhabdomyolysis may typically show preserved sensory nerve action potentials, low amplitude motor-evoked responses, absence of demyelinative findings on nerve conductions, and normal repetitive stimulation at slow and fast rates. Sometimes, it is possible to distinguish CIP from CIM by direct muscle stimulation [17, 18]. In CIP there may be an absent or very low amplitude response to nerve stimulation whereas direct muscle stimulation evokes a significant amplitude response. The hallmark of myopathy on needle EMG is enhanced motor unit recruitment consisting of brief duration, low amplitude polyphasic motor units. Enhancement refers to the demonstration of a full interference pattern often in the presence of weakness; this occurs because in a pure myopathy, the number of voluntarily activated motor units is thought to be full. Active denervation (i.e., the spontaneous presence

of fibrillations and positive sharp waves on needle EMG) may be observed in both CIM and CIP, and therefore does not distinguish either possibility. Another confounding issue is the presence of edema in critically ill patients, which may attenuate sensory nerve action potentials; this can be overcome by direct near nerve recordings at the bedside [19].

Table 85.1 summarizes incidence, clinical features, electrophysiological findings, CPK, muscle biopsy results, and prognosis for the seven neuromuscular syndromes associated with weakness in critical illness.

Strokes and Cerebrovascular Disease

Perioperative stroke is uncommon after general surgery, but incidence can be 8% or higher in patients undergoing heart surgery who also have symptomatic carotid artery disease [20]. Neurologists may be consulted before surgery concerning use or reversal of antiplatelet agents and anticoagulants or management of patients with known or potential carotid artery disease. After surgery, neurologists may be consulted for weakness, difficulty awakening, difficulty weaning from a respirator, or postoperative confusion. A perioperative stroke is one of several causes for any of these problems. We review (1) epidemiology; (2) etiology; (3) management of antiplatelet drugs and of warfarin; (4) management of carotid artery disease in elective surgery; (5) management of acute strokes in the postoperative period; and (6) timing of elective surgery after a stroke.

Epidemiology

The risk of perioperative stroke depends on many factors including patient age, urgency of surgery, co-morbidities, duration of surgery, and most importantly the type of surgery. Table 85.2 from a recent review [20] summarizes incidences for perioperative stroke after different types of surgery.

Brain surgery also has a relative high risk of associated stroke. The risk of stroke for combined CABG and valve surgery in patients with severe carotid artery disease may be as high as 11% [21]. Factors contributing to the risk of stroke are summarized in Table 85.3.

Etiology

Figure 85.2 illustrates mechanisms of perioperative stroke. The figure emphasizes that decreased cerebral perfusion is a relatively uncommon cause of stroke. A distinction should be made between strokes detected in the first 24 h after surgery that comprise around 45% of perioperative strokes, and those that occur in the second surgical day or later. Mechanisms in this latter group include atrial fibrillation, hypercoagulable state, and myocardial infarction [20]. Interruption of antiplatelet [21] and anticoagulant [22–24] therapy may lead to stroke, possibly by inducing a rebound hypercoagulable state.

Patients who are maintained on cardiopulmonary bypass during surgery are at risk for acute strokes because of micro-emboli, macroemboli, and hypotension [25]. Macroemboli

TABLE 85.2 Incidence of stroke after various surgical procedures

Procedure	Risk of stroke (%)
General surgery	0.08–0.7
Peripheral vascular surgery	0.8–3.0
Resection of head and neck tumors	4.8
Carotid endarterectomy	5.5–6.1
Isolated CABG	1.4–3.8
Combined CABG and value surgery	7.4
Isolated value surgery	4.8–8.8
Double- or triple-value surgery	9.7
Aortic repair	8.7

Source: Reprinted with permission from Selim [20] © 2007 Massachusetts Medical Society. All rights reserved

TABLE 85.3 Risk factors for perioperative stroke

Preoperative (patient-related) risk factors

Advanced age (>70 years)[a]

Female sex

History of hypertension, diabetes mellitus, renal insufficiency (creatinine, >2 mg/dl [177 μmol/L]), smoking, chronic obstructive pulmonary disease, peripheral vascular disease, cardiac disease (coronary artery disease, arrhythmias, heart failure), and systolic dysfunction (ejection fraction, <40%)[b]

History of stroke or transient ischemic attack

Carotid stenosis (especially if symptomatic)

Atherosclerosis of the ascending aorta (in patients undergoing cardiac surgery)

Abrupt discontinuation of antithrombotic therapy before surgery

Intraoperative (procedure-related) risk factors

Type and nature of the surgical procedure

Type of anesthesia (general or local)

Duration of surgery and, in cardiac procedures, duration of cardiopulmonary bypass, and aortic cross-clamp time

Manipulations of proximal aortic atherosclerotic lesions

Arrhythmias, hyperglycemia, hypotension, or hypertension

Postoperative risk factors

Heart failure, low ejection fraction, myocardial infarction, or arrhythmias (atrial fibrillation)

Dehydration and blood loss

Hyperglycemia

Source: Reprinted with permission from Selim [20] © 2007 Massachusetts Medical Society. All rights reserved

[a] Age itself does not predict the risk of stroke, and the 70-year cutoff is arbitrary. However, advanced age is a marker of decreased cerebrovascular reserve and multiple coexisting conditions

[b] The effect of systolic dysfunction on the risk of perioperative stroke is particularly pronounced among patients undergoing left-main-stem revascularization and those with atrial fibrillation

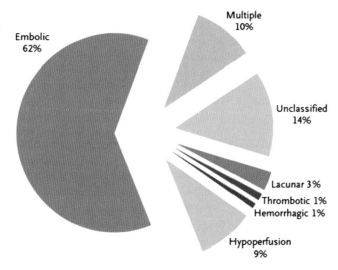

FIGURE 85.2 Mechanisms of perioperative strokes (reprinted with permission from Selim [20] © 2007 Massachusetts Medical Society. All rights reserved).

may come from the aorta or heart. Many heart surgery patients develop atrial fibrillation in the first days after surgery. Microemboli may occur after the release of cross clamping on the aorta, when cardiac ejection is restarting or from the heart-lung machine itself [25]. Post-mortem studies have shown that sometimes millions of microemboli in the brain microvasculature are found.

Hypotension may occur during surgery for several reasons and often it is intentionally induced. If brain cerebral perfusion pressure is kept at 50 mmHg or better hypoxic injury to the brain should not occur [25]. There is no consensus concerning optimal arterial perfusion during surgery, with some experts recommending perfusion pressures around 80 mmHg [20]. Brain regions whose blood supply comes from distal branches of two or more cerebral arteries may suffer borderzone infarction during systemic hypotension. The most common infarcts occur between distal branches of the middle cerebral and anterior cerebral artery (anterior borderzone infarcts), or between branches of the middle cerebral and posterior cerebral arteries (posterior borderzone infarcts). Nonetheless, as indicated above, decreased cerebral perfusion accounts for a small percentage of strokes associated with heart surgery. Indeed, syndromes identical to borderzone infarcts may occur with emboli [26].

Fat emboli can be associated with fractures of long bones. Although most of these emboli usually travel to the lungs and may cause severe hypoxia, in about 2% of cases, the fat emboli enter the arterial circulation and can cause cerebral infarctions [27]. The mechanisms by which the fat emboli enter the arterial circulation are not known. Other uncommon causes of stroke include air emboli from endoscopy, intravascular procedures, or heart-lung bypass, and paradoxical emboli from patients with deep vein thromboses who have a patent foramen ovale [20]. Improper patient positioning may compress or dissect cervical arteries during intubation [21].

Antiplatelets and Anticoagulants in the Perioperative Period

Hundreds of studies have investigated whether antiplatelet agents such as aspirin or clopidigrel should be discontinued prior to surgery so that platelet function returns to normal or whether they can be safely continued up to the time of surgery [28–31]. The risks associated with non-aspirin NSAIDs have also been investigated. In general these studies suggest that although there is a significant increase in bleeding complications associated with these drugs, there is no increase in morbidity or mortality, and that the time to hospital discharge is not prolonged. As discontinuation of antiplatelet agents can be associated with a rebound hyperco-

agulable state and increased risk of infarction, the decision about whether or not to stop antiplatelet agents needs to be weighed carefully. In contrast, there is consensus that antiplatelet agents can be started 6 h after cardiac or carotid artery surgery.

Sixty-five percent of the over 2.3 million patients in the USA with atrial fibrillation are maintained at some time on warfarin. When warfarin is stopped prior to surgery, what is the risk of stroke in these patients? Some surgical procedures have such low risk of major bleeding that it is more risky to stop warfarin. With internal normalized ratios (INRs) of 1.8–2.1, knee or hip replacement, dental procedures, arthrocentesis, and diagnostic endoscopy can proceed without undue risk of major hemorrhage [20]. For surgery with a high risk of bleeding in patients with very high risk of stroke from embolization (such as atrial fibrillation with valvular disease) one expert recommendation is to stop warfarin 4 days prior to procedure, switch to low molecular weight heparin or unfractionated heparin until 12–18 h before the procedure, and restart heparin 6 h after the procedure [32].

In patients who are anticoagulated who require STAT emergency surgery, reversal with fresh frozen plasma, and possibly prothrombin and factor VIII may be indicated. If surgery can be safely delayed for 48–72 h, oral vitamin K supplementation may be sufficient to reduce INR to less than 1.5.

Management of Carotid Artery Disease

Neurological consultation should be considered for presurgical patients with a history of recent TIAs or who have known carotid artery disease. A careful history is required to elicit symptoms of a possible TIA that include unilateral weakness or sensory loss, dizziness, vertigo, language impairment, confusion, diplopia, dysarthria, other visual disturbances, ataxia, and amnesia among others. As these symptoms are not specific, neurological consultation may be useful to assess the likelihood these symptoms were from TIAs in the carotid or vertebral/basilar artery distribution. Prior to elective surgery, imaging of the extracranial arteries with ultrasound, magnetic resonance angiography, or computed tomographic angiography may be indicated. Magnetic resonance imaging of the brain is the most sensitive way to determine whether a patient has had previous strokes. Asymptomatic patients including patients with an audible cervical bruit are at low risk for stroke and probably do not require further evaluation.

A recent study [33] reviewed over 27,000 carotid revascularizations performed between the years 2000 and 2004. Only 3.3% of patients had carotid stenting, and these patients had a lower incidence of stroke or combined stroke and death. Nonetheless, in-hospital death rates were similar. Randomized clinical trials comparing stenting and endartectomy are lacking, and there is no consensus on best management [34, 35].

Evaluation and Management of Acute Infarcts

If a stroke is suspected in a perisurgical patient, a STAT neurological consultation should be requested. Although intravenous tPA is contraindicated within 14 days of major surgery, an interventionist neuroradiologist may be able to offer a thrombectomy [36, 37] or possibly intra-arterial tPA [38]. Most Emergency Departments have worked out the logistics for contacting neurologists for "stroke codes." If a stroke is suspected, it may be most efficient to call the ED physician and tell him or her that you have a stroke code on a hospitalized patient. The stroke team neurologist will then contact the interventionist when appropriate.

How Long Poststroke Is Elective Surgery Permissible?

There are no research studies that address this question, but most stroke experts believe that elective surgery can be scheduled starting 3 months after a moderate- to large-sized acute infarct.

Seizures

In this section, we will discuss four clinical scenarios: (1) patients with epilepsy for years with seizures that are well controlled on antiepileptic drugs (AEDS); (2) patients with known seizures disorder who have poor control or who have stopped taking AEDS; (3) patients with no history of seizures who have seizures in the post-op period; and (4) patients with known epilepsy who have seizures in the post-op period.

Patients with Known Seizure Disorder Stable on AEDs

Seizures disorders are common among geriatric patients with a prevalence of 1–2% [39] and most geriatric patients with seizures are maintained on one or two AEDs with twice or three times a day dosing. In this way, geriatric patients with

epilepsy differ from some younger patients with intractable seizure disorders.

If the duration the patient is expected to have nothing by mouth is 12 h or less, AEDS can be given with a sip of water 2 or more hours before surgery and restarted when clear liquids are permitted. Even if a patient is on three times daily dosing, it is unlikely that AED levels will fall so low that breakthrough seizures will be a problem. If the duration of no oral intake is to be greater than 12 h then either a nasogastric tube can be used or the patient can be maintained on "bridging" therapy with intravenous fosphenytoin/phenytoin, valproic acid, or levetiracetam. If the patient is already on oral monotherapy with these drugs, then the patient should be maintained in intravenous forms of the drug. Measurement of phenytoin and valproic acid levels prior to surgery will be invaluable. Levels of levetiracetam are not available.

It is more complicated for patients who are on gabapentin, carbamazepine, lamotrogine, oxcarbazepine, or topirimate as there are no intravenous forms of these drugs. In these cases, the neurologist will usually recommend temporary monotherapy with intravenous fosphenytoin, valproic acid, and levetiracetam. Fosphenytoin, the proform of phenytoin is completely metabolized to phenytoin within one pass through the liver. Phenytoin has limited solubility in water whereas fosphenytoin is water soluble. Fosphenytoin is preferable to phenytoin for intravenous use because it can be administered more quickly, is less likely to be associated with arrhythmias or hypotension, and is less likely to stick to intravenous tubing. Phenytoin has complicated pharmacokinetics and multiple drug–drug interactions and intravenous forms of valproic acid and levetiracetam are being used more and more for bridging therapies in patients unable to take oral medications.

Patients with Known Seizure Disorders Who Have Stopped Taking Their AEDs

Patients who have gone 2 years without a seizure on AEDs can usually be tapered off their AEDs, particularly if there is no structural lesion on MRI and the EEG does not show epileptiform activity. Accordingly, it becomes a judgment call what to recommend for a patient who has stopped taking AEDs but who has not had a seizure for several months.

Patients with No Previous History Who Have Their First Seizure in the Post-op Period

The first problem is recognizing the seizure. Some movements that are not electrographic seizures may be misinterpreted as seizures. Conversely, some nonconvulsive seizure activity if often missed.

Myoclonus is defined as "brief, shock-like, large amplitude, irregular movement of a muscle or of muscle groups" [40] and may occur with renal or hepatic failure as well as in many different neurological disorders. However, a common setting for myoclonus in a geriatric surgical population is a patient who has suffered an episode of generalized cerebral ischemia leading to coma. Multifocal or generalized myoclonus starts 2–24 h after the arrest [41]. Neurological exam reveals a comatose patient with limited, if any, response to pain, yet stimuli including tracheal suctioning, positioning limbs, and loud noises may elicit the myoclonus. Pupils are usually spared and eye movements may or may not be impaired. The EEG may show little, if any, electrical activity and usually shows no seizure activity. Despite this, when the myoclonus is nearly continuous it is sometimes called myoclonic status epilepticus. The disorder responds poorly to anticonvulsants and has a very poor prognosis.

Conversely, seizures with minimal convulsive or no convulsive features will usually not be suspected by non-neurologists. Clues to nonconvulsive seizures include confusion, personality change, psychosis, coma, abnormal waxing and waning mental status and possibly unidirectional nystagmus [39].

Etiologies to consider for new onset seizures include a new infarct, metabolic disturbances such as hypo or hyperglycemia, hyponatremia, hypocalcemia, hypomagnesemia, withdrawal from alcohol, and withdrawal from AEDs. Occasionally, history that the patient was maintained on AEDs is unavailable. Seizures occurring in patients acutely withdrawn from AEDs may be difficult to stop until the missing AED is restarted. Frequently, workup will reveal an unsuspected old infarct. Cortically based infarcts are more likely to cause seizures than strokes in other sites.

The general rule in neurology that long-term AED should not be started after a single solitary seizure is less clear among geriatric patients. Patients under 40 who have a single seizure of unknown etiology have only a 40–50% risk of having another seizure even if AEDs are never started. In contrast, patients over 70, have about a 70% of having another seizure [39, 42, 43].

In any patient, if a clear-cut reversible, metabolic etiology can be identified, appropriate treatment is correcting the abnormality, not starting AEDs. However, if it appears likely that it will take several days to correct the metabolic abnormality, many experts would use intravenous AED at least until the metabolic abnormality is corrected, and might taper the patient off oral forms of the AED several weeks after surgery.

Patients with Known Epilepsy Who Have Seizures in the Post-op Period

Management of these patients requires a blending of the approaches #1 and #3.

Cognitive Impairment

Three questions about a patient's cognitive function are of special importance to surgeons operating on the elderly: (1) What is the prevalence, clinical course, and prognosis for postoperative cognitive impairment (POCD)? (2) Does surgery in older patients increase their risk for Alzheimer's disease? (3) Special pre-surgical concerns in patients with documented cognitive impairment or dementia.

Postoperative Cognitive Dysfunction

Postoperative cognitive dysfunction (POCD) is extremely common in the elderly with estimates of its prevalence ranging from 10 to 80%. [44–51] Typically, studies distinguish between POCD documented a few days after surgery (typically 5–7 days or around the time of discharge), and POCD present at 3 and 6 months after surgery. The prevalence of POCD at time of discharge or around 7 days post-op ranges from 10 to 80%, with estimates at 3–6 months ranging from 10 to 24% [52, 53]. One study found 80% of post-coronary artery bypass grafting (CABG) patients had abnormal signals on diffusion-weighted MRI sensitive to acute ischemia that were not present prior to surgery [54].

Choice of neuropsychological battery and how change is defined also have big effects on prevalence estimates [55–58]. Many studies used battery of neuropsychological tests covering multiple domains including verbal and nonverbal memory, attention, visuoconstruction, executive function, language, and motor speed [57]. Some data suggest that memory is most likely to be affected [59].

Age, baseline cognitive function, whether surgery was elective or emergency, whether patients are in early stages of Alzheimer's disease or other dementias, co-morbid illness, nature and duration of surgery, choice of anesthesia, and postoperative complications all influence the prevalence of POCD. Finally, cognitive impairment is so prevalent in older subjects – estimates of the prevalence of AD among those in their early 80s range from 10 to 40% [60–63] – that studies lacking appropriate control groups needed to be interpreted with caution.

A few investigators have continued to follow patients and reassessed them at 1–5 years postsurgery. Newman [53] followed 261 patients who had CABGs. POCD was defined by change from presurgical function of greater than 1 standard deviation in at least one cognitive domain. Prevalence of cognitive dysfunction was 53% at discharge, 36% at 6 weeks, 24% at 6 months, and 42% at 5 years. Because most studies end follow-up at 6 months, this delayed deterioration could have been missed. Unfortunately, a control group was not included so it could not be determined whether a similar course would have occurred in comparably ill elderly patients who did not have surgery.

POCD in the first few weeks after surgery influences discharge planning and suitability for rehabilitation [64]. Patients with POCD may require longer time in rehab [65]. Patients with POCD at 1 week are more likely to require help with living independently. Patients with POCD 1 week after surgery are about three times more likely to be cognitively impaired 1 or 2 years after surgery than patients with normal cognition in the immediate postsurgical period.

Patients and families need be advised that in most patients cognitive function will substantially improve in the weeks following surgery. No data are available whether cognitive rehabilitation is useful in such patients. Often neuroleptics, anti-anxiety medications, antidepressants, or hypnotics are prescribed to try to treat some of the behavioral problems associated with POCD. All of these medications are themselves associated with cognitive impairment and need be used especially judiciously.

Several studies have investigated whether POCD is more common after general anesthesia or after regional anesthesia. In a meta-analysis comparing 1,314 patients with regional anesthesia and 1,395 patients with general anesthesia from 18 unique randomized control trials, Bryson et al. [66] found no difference in frequency of POCD which was around 15–25%.

The etiology of POCD is likely to be multifactorial. Inflammatory processes outside of the CNS may be associated with inflammatory markers within the CNS. For example, hip surgery was associated with increase in CSF interleukin 6 and prostaglandin E_2 [67]. Interleukin-8 and RANTES were elevated post-op in CSF from patients with various kinds of non-brain surgeries [68]. Nonetheless, even if "neuroinflammation" has a role in pathogenesis, it remains unclear why it would affect older but not younger patients. Possible explanations include lack of cognitive reserve and a leakier blood–brain barrier in older patients. Growth factors required for repair may be less efficient in older patients. Embolization, particularly if the heart or carotid arteries were manipulated may be a factor. Global ischemia from decreased perfusion or other causes may also have contributed. Alzheimer's disease contributes to some POCD. The relationship between surgery/GA and Alzheimer's disease (AD) is discussed below.

What Is the Risk That Surgery in Elderly Patients "Will Trigger" AD?

> Vignette – Mrs. J is a 73-year-old woman with hypertension. Her daughter said that she handled her finances and travelled independently prior to an elective cholecystectomy. At 1 year after surgery, the patient and her daughter are both concerned about impairment in her recent memory. By 18 months after surgery, she has made mistakes paying bills and gotten lost several times. After reviewing her history, performing a cognitive assessment and neurological exam, and obtaining brain imaging, a dementia specialist diagnoses mild Alzheimer's disease.

Every physician seeing substantial numbers of patients with dementia has encountered the above scenario. Certainly, the data on POCD discussed above would suggest that some patients have sustained cognitive impairment after surgery, but unless the POCD develops a gradually progressive course, there would be no reason to believe there was a relationship between GA/surgery and AD. The findings of Newman et al. [53] are especially provocative because they document such progressive deterioration 5 years after surgery. Nonetheless, the patients in the Newman study had cognitive impairment and did not meet criteria for the diagnosis of AD. Several more years of follow-up would have answered the question of whether they were developing AD.

For years, many dementia specialists maintained with little data that the surgery was only a convenient point in time and that most likely the patient had symptoms of AD for years prior to surgery that went unnoticed by her family. Epidemiological studies have looked at this association with largely negative results. Data from studies with animal models and tissue culture systems have suggested plausible ways that anesthetics might increase the likelihood of AD – although it has to be emphasized that clinical data supporting such an association are equivocal at best.

Epidemiological Studies

In 1991, Breteler et al. [69] performed a meta-analysis of eight case–control studies and found no risk of AD from GA (relative risk = 1.0). In another case–control study involving 252 AD cases and matched controls, Bohnen et al. [70, 71] found positive odds ratios for GA that increased with the duration of anesthetic exposure. However, the confidence intervals were wide and findings were not statistically significant. In a separate analysis, the authors found a significant association between anesthesia exposure before age 50 and earlier onset of AD.

In a study of 502 subjects with vascular dementia and 810 subjects with AD from the California AD centers, Cooper et al. [72] found that GA was overrepresented in the vascular dementia group, a finding confirmed in a larger sample from the same dataset by Corey-Bloom et al. [73]. Both studies lacked a control group to determine whether GA was more frequent in AD than in controls.

Gasparini et al. [74] reviewed hospital records to determine whether GA and surgery up to 5 years earlier were overrepresented in AD. Control groups were patients with Parkinson's disease and patients with nondegenerative neurological diseases – usually peripheral neuropathy or headaches. No association between GA/surgery and AD was found, but the study could not address risks from exposures than occurred more than 5 years earlier.

In a cohort of over 4,000 cognitively normal 65–90-year-olds, Yip et al. [75] studied factors associated with incident dementia at 2 and 6 years after original evaluation. GA was associated with a decrease in risk of dementia (OR 0.6, CI: 0.4–0.9). GA has been associated with both increasing and decreasing apoptosis of brain neurons [76, 77]. If GA actually decreases risk of AD, decreased apoptosis would be one potential mechanism.

In a cohort study involving 9,000 patients, Lee et al. found that the risk of developing AD within 5 years after CABG was 1.7 times higher (CI: 1.02–2.87, $p<0.04$) than after angioplasty [78]. However, using a case–control design that compared the frequency of prior CABG between a group with dementia and cognitively normal control group, Knopman et al. [79] found no association between CABG and dementia. Among patients who already have AD, CABG may be associated with a slower rate of progression [80].

Animal Studies and Tissue Culture Studies

Transient ischemia increased expression of beta (β)-site APP cleaving enzyme in rats [81]. As this enzyme leads to increased ABeta (β) production, and increased brain amyloid is believed by many to be an early step in the pathogenesis of AD, the work provides another theoretical explanation of why hypoxia associated with surgery/anesthesia could lead to AD.

Bianchi et al. [82] exposed adult transgenic and wild-type mice to either isoflurane or halothane. The transgenic mice exposed to halothane had more brain amyloid than those exposed to isoflurane, but neither agent was associated with cognitive impairment in the transgenic mice. On the other hand, isoflurane did cause cognitive impairment in the wild-type mice that was not associated with amyloid deposition.

This study reemphasizes that cognitive impairment associated with anesthetic exposure, need not be due to AD pathology but may occur by an entirely different mechanism.

Tau protein is a microtubule protein needed to stabilize tubulin networks in the axons of neurons. Abnormally increased phosphorylation of tau protein is a consistent finding in AD. Planel et al. [83, 85] exposed wild-type mice to intraperitoneal pentobarbital or chloral hydrate or isoflurane by inhalation. All three agents were associated with hypothermia and hyperphosphorylation of tau mediated by decreased phosphatase activity. They concluded that the hypothermia, not the agents themselves, led to the increase in phosphorylation, which reverted to normal levels with normothermia. Ikeda et al. [85] found that hyperphosphorylation of brain tau could be induced by ether anesthesia or cold water shock.

Palotas et al. [86] administered intraperitoneal propofol or thiopental to rats and then measured levels of amyloid precursor protein (APP) and APP RNA in rat brain. They found these agents caused no changes in APP. In a similar studies, neither midazolam nor propofol was associated with increase in APP [87].

Eckenhoff et al. [88] studied whether anesthetics might increase oligomerization of Aβ in a rat pheochromocytoma tissue culture system. Halothane and isoflurane, but not alcohol or propofol (except at very high concentrations) were associated with increased oligomerization. This finding is important because many investigators believe that oligomers are the most toxic form of Aβ.

Xie et al. [76, 89, 90] exposed human neuroglioma cells that had been genetically engineered to overexpress amyloid to desflurane and hypoxia. Neither desflurane or hypoxia alone were associated with change in amyloid-beta (β)-protein (Aβ) levels, but the combination was. This combination also was associated with increased caspase-3 activation, which can lead to apoptosis and further production of Aβ.

Special Pre-surgical Concerns in Patients with Documented Cognitive Impairment or Dementia

All of this research inevitably leads to the question of which anesthetics to use for elderly patients and especially patients with Alzheimer's disease. An expert NIH panel was convened in [91] 2007 to address this and other issues concerning possible neurotoxicity of anesthetics. The panel concluded that there were not enough data to make any recommendations.

Other issues pertain to patients with dementia who are maintained on acetylcholinesterase inhibitors such as donepezil, galantamine, or rivastigmine. There are no data to suggest these agents are associated with sufficient excess airway secretions to interfere with surgery nor are there data to suggest these agents interfere significantly with the use of succinylcholine [92, 93]. Most anesthesiologists believe that acetylcholinesterase inhibitors do not need to be discontinued prior to elective surgery.

References

1. Howard RS, Tan SV, Z'Graggen WJ (2008) Weakness on the intensive care unit. Pract Neurol 8:280–295
2. Hund E (2001) Critical illness polyneuropathy. Curr Opin Neurol 14:649–653
3. Bolton CF (2005) Neuromuscular manifestations of critical illness. Muscle Nerve 32:140–163
4. Visser LH (2006) Critical illness polyneuropathy and myopathy: clinical features, risk factors and prognosis. Eur J Neurol 13:1203–1212
5. Bolton CF, Young GB, Zochodne DW (1993) The neurological complications of sepsis. Ann Neurol 33:94–100
6. Kumar N, Folger WN, Bolton CF (2004) Dyspnea as the predominant manifestation of bilateral phrenic neuropathy. Mayo Clin Proc 79:1563–1565
7. Tennila A, Salmi T, Pettila V, Roine RO, Varpula T, Takkunen O (2000) Early signs of critical illness polyneuropathy in ICU patients with systemic inflammatory response syndrome or sepsis. Intensive Care Med 26:1360–1363
8. Albers JW, Donofrio PD, McGonagle TK (1985) Sequential electrodiagnostic abnormalities in acute inflammatory demyelinating polyradiculoneuropathy. Muscle Nerve 8:528–539
9. Alam TA, Chaudhry V, Cornblath DR (1998) Electrophysiological studies in the Guillain–Barre syndrome: distinguishing subtypes by published criteria. Muscle Nerve 21:1275–1279
10. Latronico N, Guarneri B (2008) Critical illness myopathy and neuropathy. Minerva Anestesiol 74:319–323
11. Guarneri B, Bertolini G, Latronico N (2008) Long-term outcome in patients with critical illness myopathy or neuropathy: the Italian multicentre CRIMYNE study. J Neurol Neurosurg Psychiatry 79:838–841
12. Latronico N, Bertolini G, Guarneri B et al (2007) Simplified electrophysiological evaluation of peripheral nerves in critically ill patients: the Italian multi-centre CRIMYNE study. Crit Care 11:R11
13. Latronico N, Peli E, Botteri M (2005) Critical illness myopathy and neuropathy. Curr Opin Crit Care 11:126–132
14. Latronico N (2003) Neuromuscular alterations in the critically ill patient: critical illness myopathy, critical illness neuropathy, or both? Intensive Care Med 29:1411–1413
15. Showalter CJ, Engel AG (1997) Acute quadriplegic myopathy: analysis of myosin isoforms and evidence for calpain-mediated proteolysis. Muscle Nerve 20:316–322
16. Zochodne DW, Ramsay DA, Saly V, Shelley S, Moffatt S (1994) Acute necrotizing myopathy of intensive care: electrophysiological studies. Muscle Nerve 17:285–292
17. Rich MM, Pinter MJ, Kraner SD, Barchi RL (1998) Loss of electrical excitability in an animal model of acute quadriplegic myopathy. Ann Neurol 43:171–179
18. Bird SJ, Rich MM (2002) Critical illness myopathy and polyneuropathy. Curr Neurol Neurosci Rep 2:527–533
19. Bolton CF, Laverty DA, Brown JD, Witt NJ, Hahn AF, Sibbald WJ (1986) Critically ill polyneuropathy: electrophysiological studies and differentiation from Guillain-Barre syndrome. J Neurol Neurosurg Psychiatry 49:563–573
20. Selim M (2007) Perioperative stroke. N Engl J Med 356:706–713
21. Naylor AR, Mehta Z, Rothwell PM, Bell PR (2002) Carotid artery disease and stroke during coronary artery bypass: a critical review of the literature. Eur J Vasc Endovasc Surg 23:283–294
22. Charlesworth DC, Likosky DS, Marrin CA et al (2003) Development and validation of a prediction model for strokes after coronary artery bypass grafting. Ann Thorac Surg 76:436–443
23. Likosky DS, Leavitt BJ, Marrin CA et al (2003) Intra- and postoperative predictors of stroke after coronary artery bypass grafting. Ann Thorac Surg 76:428–434, discussion 435
24. Likosky DS, Marrin CA, Caplan LR et al (2003) Determination of etiologic mechanisms of strokes secondary to coronary artery bypass graft surgery. Stroke 34:2830–2834
25. Gottesman RF, Wityk RJ (2006) Brain injury from cardiac bypass procedures. Semin Neurol 26:432–439
26. Belden JR, Caplan LR, Pessin MS, Kwan E (1999) Mechanisms and clinical features of posterior border-zone infarcts. Neurology 53:1312–1318
27. Parizel PM, Demey HE, Veeckmans G et al (2001) Early diagnosis of cerebral fat embolism syndrome by diffusion-weighted MRI (starfield pattern). Stroke 32:2942–2944
28. Merritt JC, Bhatt DL (2004) The efficacy and safety of perioperative antiplatelet therapy. J Thromb Thrombolysis 17:21–27
29. Kitchen L, Erichson RB, Sideropoulos H (1982) Effect of drug-induced platelet dysfunction on surgical bleeding. Am J Surg 143:215–217
30. Michelson EL, Morganroth J, Torosian M, Mac Vaugh HIII (1978) Relation of preoperative use of aspirin to increased mediastinal blood loss after coronary artery bypass graft surgery. J Thorac Cardiovasc Surg 76:694–697
31. Ferraris VA, Swanson E (1983) Aspirin usage and perioperative blood loss in patients undergoing unexpected operations. Surg Gynecol Obstet 156:439–442
32. Management of Warfarin Therapy During Invasive Procedures and Surgery (2004) http://www.bcguidelines.ca/gpac/pdf/warfarin_manage.pdf
33. Timaran CH, Rosero EB, Smith ST, Valentine RJ, Modrall JG, Clagett GP (2008) Trends and outcomes of concurrent carotid revascularization and coronary bypass. J Vasc Surg 48:355–360, discussion 360–361
34. Van der Heyden J, Lans HW, van Werkum JW, Schepens M, Ackerstaff RG, Suttorp MJ (2008) Will carotid angioplasty become the preferred alternative to staged or synchronous carotid endarterectomy in patients undergoing cardiac surgery? Eur J Vasc Endovasc Surg 36:379–384
35. Das P, Clavijo LC, Nanjundappa A, Dieter RS Jr (2008) Revascularization of carotid stenosis before cardiac surgery. Expert Rev Cardiovasc Ther 6:1393–1396
36. Bose A, Henkes H, Alfke K et al (2008) The Penumbra System: a mechanical device for the treatment of acute stroke due to thromboembolism. AJNR Am J Neuroradiol 29:1409–1413
37. Smith WS, Sung G, Saver J et al (2008) Mechanical thrombectomy for acute ischemic stroke: final results of the Multi MERCI trial. Stroke 39:1205–1212
38. Furlan A, Higashida R, Wechsler L et al (1999) Intra-arterial prourokinase for acute ischemic stroke. The PROACT II study: a randomized controlled trial. Prolyse in Acute Cerebral Thromboembolism. JAMA 282:2003–2011
39. Jetter GM, Cavazos JE (2008) Epilepsy in the elderly. Semin Neurol 28:336–341
40. Ropper AH, Brown RH (2005) Tremor, myoclonus, focal dystonias, and tics. In: Adams RD, Victor M, Ropper AH (eds) Principles of neurology. McGraw Hill, New York, p 86
41. Venkatesan A, Frucht S (2006) Movement disorders after resuscitation from cardiac arrest. Neurol Clin 24:123–132

42. Stephen LJ, Brodie MJ (2008) Management of a first seizure. Special problems: adults and elderly. Epilepsia 49(Suppl 1):45–49

43. Berg AT (2008) Risk of recurrence after a first unprovoked seizure. Epilepsia 49(Suppl 1):13–18

44. Abildstrom H, Christiansen M, Siersma VD, Rasmussen LS (2004) Apolipoprotein E genotype and cognitive dysfunction after noncardiac surgery. Anesthesiology 101:855–861

45. Abildstrom H, Hogh P, Sperling B, Moller JT, Yndgaard S, Rasmussen LS (2002) Cerebral blood flow and cognitive dysfunction after coronary surgery. Ann Thorac Surg 73:1174–1178, discussion 1178–1179

46. Abildstrom H, Rasmussen LS, Rentowl P et al (2000) Cognitive dysfunction 1-2 years after non-cardiac surgery in the elderly. ISPOCD group. International Study of Post-Operative Cognitive Dysfunction. Acta Anaesthesiol Scand 44:1246–1251

47. Selnes OA, McKhann GM (2005) Neurocognitive complications after coronary artery bypass surgery. Ann Neurol 57:615–621

48. Selnes OA, Goldsborough MA, Borowicz LM Jr, Enger C, Quaskey SA, McKhann GM (1999) Determinants of cognitive change after coronary artery bypass surgery: a multifactorial problem. Ann Thorac Surg 67:1669–1676

49. Selnes OA, Grega MA, Borowicz LM Jr, Royall RM, McKhann GM, Baumgartner WA (2003) Cognitive changes with coronary artery disease: a prospective study of coronary artery bypass graft patients and nonsurgical controls. Ann Thorac Surg 75:1377–1384, discussion 1384–1386

50. Gottesman RF, Hillis AE, Grega MA et al (2007) Early postoperative cognitive dysfunction and blood pressure during coronary artery bypass graft operation. Arch Neurol 64:1111–1114

51. McKhann GM, Grega MA, Borowicz LM Jr et al (2005) Is there cognitive decline 1 year after CABG? Comparison with surgical and nonsurgical controls. Neurology 65:991–999

52. Newman S, Stygall J, Hirani S, Shaefi S, Maze M (2007) Postoperative cognitive dysfunction after noncardiac surgery: a systematic review. Anesthesiology 106:572–590

53. Newman MF, Grocott HP, Mathew JP et al (2001) Report of the substudy assessing the impact of neurocognitive function on quality of life 5 years after cardiac surgery. Stroke 32:2874–2881

54. Russell D, Bornstein N (2005) Methods of detecting potential causes of vascular cognitive impairment after coronary artery bypass grafting. J Neurol Sci 229–230:69–73

55. Lewis MS, Maruff P, Silbert BS, Evered LA, Scott DA (2006) Detection of postoperative cognitive decline after coronary artery bypass graft surgery is affected by the number of neuropsychological tests in the assessment battery. Ann Thorac Surg 81:2097–2104

56. Lewis MS, Maruff P, Silbert BS, Evered LA, Scott DA (2006) The sensitivity and specificity of three common statistical rules for the classification of post-operative cognitive dysfunction following coronary artery bypass graft surgery. Acta Anaesthesiol Scand 50:50–57

57. Lewis MS, Maruff PT, Silbert BS (2005) Examination of the use of cognitive domains in postoperative cognitive dysfunction after coronary artery bypass graft surgery. Ann Thorac Surg 80:910–916

58. Lewis M, Maruff P, Silbert B (2004) Statistical and conceptual issues in defining post-operative cognitive dysfunction. Neurosci Biobehav Rev 28:433–440

59. Caza N, Taha R, Qi Y, Blaise G (2008) The effects of surgery and anesthesia on memory and cognition. Prog Brain Res 169:409–422

60. Kawas CH (2008) The oldest old and the 90+ study. Alzheimers Dement 4:S56–S59

61. Kawas CH, Corrada MM (2006) Alzheimer's and dementia in the oldest-old: a century of challenges. Curr Alzheimer Res 3:411–419

62. Kawas C, Gray S, Brookmeyer R, Fozard J, Zonderman A (2000) Age-specific incidence rates of Alzheimer's disease: the Baltimore Longitudinal Study of Aging. Neurology 54:2072–2077

63. Corrada M, Brookmeyer R, Kawas C (1995) Sources of variability in prevalence rates of Alzheimer's disease. Int J Epidemiol 24: 1000–1005

64. Hakkinen A, Heinonen M, Kautiainen H, Huusko T, Sulkava R, Karppi P (2007) Effect of cognitive impairment on basic activities of daily living in hip fracture patients: a 1-year follow-up. Aging Clin Exp Res 19:139–144

65. Moncada LV, Andersen RE, Franckowiak SC, Christmas C (2006) The impact of cognitive impairment on short-term outcomes of hip fracture patients. Arch Gerontol Geriatr 43:45–52

66. Bryson GL, Wyand A (2006) Evidence-based clinical update: general anesthesia and the risk of delirium and postoperative cognitive dysfunction. Can J Anaesth 53:669–677

67. Anonymous (2008) Taking the lead in research in postoperative cognitive dysfunction. Anesthesiology 108:1–2

68. Reis HJ, Teixeira AL, Kalman J et al (2007) Different inflammatory biomarker patterns in the cerebro-spinal fluid following heart surgery and major non-cardiac operations. Curr Drug Metab 8:639–642

69. Breteler MM, van Duijn CM, Chandra V et al (1991) Medical history and the risk of Alzheimer's disease: a collaborative re-analysis of case-control studies. EURODEM Risk Factors Research Group. Int J Epidemiol 20(Suppl 2):S36–S42

70. Bohnen N, Warner MA, Kokmen E, Kurland LT (1994) Early and midlife exposure to anesthesia and age of onset of Alzheimer's disease. Int J Neurosci 77:181–185

71. Bohnen NI, Warner MA, Kokmen E, Beard CM, Kurland LT (1994) Alzheimer's disease and cumulative exposure to anesthesia: a case-control study. J Am Geriatr Soc 42:198–201

72. Cooper JK, Mungas D (1993) Risk factor and behavioral differences between vascular and Alzheimer's dementias: the pathway to end-stage disease. J Geriatr Psychiatry Neurol 6:29–33

73. Corey-Bloom J, Galasko D, Hofstetter CR, Jackson JE, Thal LJ (1993) Clinical features distinguishing large cohorts with possible AD, probable AD, and mixed dementia. J Am Geriatr Soc 41:31–37

74. Gasparini M, Vanacore N, Schiaffini C et al (2002) A case-control study on Alzheimer's disease and exposure to anesthesia. Neurol Sci 23:11–14

75. Yip AG, Brayne C, Matthews FE (2006) Risk factors for incident dementia in England and Wales: the Medical Research Council Cognitive Function and Ageing Study. A population-based nested case-control study. Age Ageing 35:154–160

76. Xie Z, Moir RD, Romano DM, Tesco G, Kovacs DM, Tanzi RE (2004) Hypocapnia induces caspase-3 activation and increases Abeta production. Neurodegener Dis 1:29–37

77. Perouansky M (2008) General anesthetics and long-term neurotoxicity. Handb Exp Pharmacol 182:143–157

78. Lee TA, Wolozin B, Weiss KB, Bednar MM (2005) Assessment of the emergence of Alzheimer's disease following coronary artery bypass graft surgery or percutaneous transluminal coronary angioplasty. J Alzheimers Dis 7:319–324

79. Knopman DS, Petersen RC, Cha RH, Edland SD, Rocca WA (2005) Coronary artery bypass grafting is not a risk factor for dementia or Alzheimer disease. Neurology 65:986–990

80. Mielke MM, Rosenberg PB, Tschanz J et al (2007) Vascular factors predict rate of progression in Alzheimer disease. Neurology 69:1850–1858

81. Aarsaether E, Moe OK, Dahl PE, Busund R (2005) Carotid endarterectomy in patients with coronary heart disease. Tidsskr Nor Laegeforen 125:2946–2948

82. Bianchi SL, Tran T, Liu C et al (2008) Brain and behavior changes in 12-month-old Tg2576 and nontransgenic mice exposed to anesthetics. Neurobiol Aging 29:1002–1010

83. Planel E, Richter KE, Nolan CE et al (2007) Anesthesia leads to tau hyperphosphorylation through inhibition of phosphatase activity by hypothermia. J Neurosci 27:3090–3097

84. Planel E, Krishnamurthy P, Miyasaka T et al (2008) Anesthesia-induced hyperphosphorylation detaches 3-repeat tau from microtubules without affecting their stability in vivo. J Neurosci 28: 12798–12807

85. Ikeda Y, Ishiguro K, Fujita SC (2007) Ether stress-induced Alzheimer-like tau phosphorylation in the normal mouse brain. FEBS Lett 581:891–897

86. Palotas M, Palotas A, Bjelik A et al (2005) Effect of general anesthetics on amyloid precursor protein and mRNA levels in the rat brain. Neurochem Res 30:1021–1026

87. Kalman J, Palotas M, Pakaski M, Hugyecz M, Janka Z, Palotas A (2006) Unchanged rat brain amyloid precursor protein levels after exposure to benzodiazepines in vivo. Eur J Anaesthesiol 23: 772–775

88. Eckenhoff RG, Johansson JS, Wei H et al (2004) Inhaled anesthetic enhancement of amyloid-beta oligomerization and cytotoxicity. Anesthesiology 101:703–709

89. Xie Z, Dong Y, Maeda U et al (2006) Isoflurane-induced apoptosis: a potential pathogenic link between delirium and dementia. J Gerontol A Biol Sci Med Sci 61:1300–1306

90. Xie Z, Tanzi RE (2006) Alzheimer's disease and post-operative cognitive dysfunction. Exp Gerontol 41:346–359

91. Kuehn BM (2007) Anesthesia-Alzheimer disease link probed. JAMA 297:1760

92. Ibebunjo C, Donati F, Fox GS, Eshelby D, Tchervenkov JI (1997) The effects of chronic tacrine therapy on d-tubocurarine blockade in the soleus and tibialis muscles of the rat. Anesth Analg 85:431–436

93. Ibebunjo C, Eshelby D, Donati F, Fox GS, Tchervenkov JI (1997) Tacrine does not alter the potency of succinylcholine in the rat. Can J Anaesth 44:1021–1026

Chapter 86
Geriatric Neurosurgical Emergencies

Toral R. Patel and Joseph T. King Jr.

Introduction

Neurologic illnesses are a leading cause of death and disability in the elderly population. Many of these diseases require surgical evaluation. The US Census Bureau estimates that by 2030, 52 million Americans will be over 70 years of age [1]. The presentation, management, and outcomes of neurosurgical emergencies can be quite different in the geriatric population. It is imperative that practitioners are aware of the unique challenges that exist when caring for geriatric patients with neurosurgical emergencies.

Traumatic Brain Injury

Recent studies report that approximately 1.1 million new cases of traumatic brain injury (TBI) are diagnosed and treated in US hospitals each year, approximately 450 cases per 100,000 people. Subgroup analyses demonstrate that the elderly have a significantly higher rate of TBI. In persons over 85 years of age, there were approximately 1,000 cases per 100,000 people [2, 3]. The majority of these injuries are caused by falls [4]. Multiple studies have demonstrated that despite similar injury severity, older patients have worse outcomes than younger patients [5, 6]. Morbidity and mortality from TBI start to increase in the fifth decade of life, but rise sharply after age 70 [7]. It is postulated that elderly patients have worse outcomes due to diminished cardiovascular reserve and fundamental differences in the aging central nervous system (CNS) and its response to injury [6, 7]. Because of this disparity, the literature suggests that age >70 years should be a criterion for full trauma team activation

and that those patients should also be considered for transfer to a certified trauma center, regardless of the severity of the actual event [8, 9].

Extra-Axial Hematomas

Extra-axial hematomas are defined as hemorrhages within the intracranial space, but outside of the brain parenchyma. They occur almost exclusively in the setting of trauma and can be either acute or chronic in nature. Extra-axial hematomas that form under the dura mater are termed subdural hematomas (SDH), while those that form above the dura mater are termed epidural hematomas (EDH).

SDH may be caused by a variety of conditions, but they most commonly occur as a result of trauma. In the elderly population, SDHs occur in 46% of TBIs, while in younger patients, they occur in only 28% of TBIs [7]. This is thought to be due to the increased adherence of the dura mater to the inner surface of the elderly skull, which in concert with general cerebral atrophy, results in continuous stretching of the bridging veins that connect the cerebral cortex to the dural sinuses. With the added insult of a trauma, these stretched veins are easily injured, resulting in hemorrhage between the dura and brain, otherwise known as a SDH. The clinical manifestations of SDHs are the result of focal or diffuse pressure on the brain, or chemical irritation of the underlying cortex. Signs and symptoms include headache, nausea/vomiting, diplopia, altered mental status, pupillary dilatation, seizures, dysphasia, and hemiparesis/hemiplegia. Acute SDHs can become rapidly symptomatic as blood accumulates in the subdural space and presses on the underlying brain. Chronic SDHs can accrue over time as the result of multiple episodes of bleeding from repeated small traumas. Often times, they are larger than acute SDHs, however, their signs and symptoms are usually milder because the chronology of their development allows the brain to accommodate the mass effect. On CT scan, all SDHs appear as crescent-shaped extra-axial collections, which may cross suture lines but do

J.T. King Jr. (✉)
Chief of Neurosurgery, VA Connecticut Healthcare System Chair, VA Neurosurgery Surgical Advisory Board; Associate Professor of Neurosurgery, Director of Outcomes Research, Department of Neurosurgery, Yale University School of Medicine,
950 Campbell Road, West Haven, CT 06516, USA
e-mail: joseph.kingjr@ya.gov

R.A. Rosenthal et al. (eds.), *Principles and Practice of Geriatric Surgery*,
DOI 10.1007/978-1-4419-6999-6_86, © Springer Science+Business Media, LLC 2011

Figure 86.1 Noncontrast axial head CTs demonstrate (**a**) acute subdural hematoma – a hyperdense crescent-shaped extra-axial collection and (**b**) chronic subdural hematoma – a hypodense crescent-shaped extra-axial collection. Both of these lesions are causing significant mass effect and resultant shift of midline brain structures.

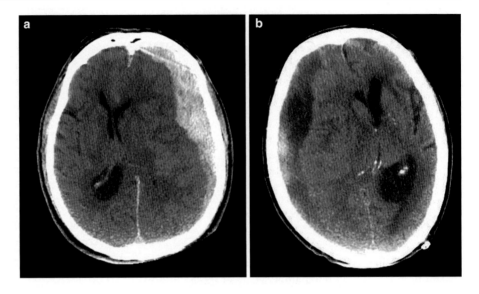

not cross midline. Acute SDHs appear hyperdense to adjacent brain tissue on CT scan, while chronic SDHs are hypodense (Fig. 86.1a, b). Chronic SDHs may also have internal septations visible on the CT scan caused by the formation of membranes. Imaging appearance and symptoms are used to determine the need for surgical evacuation. Any symptomatic acute or chronic SDH needs to be evacuated promptly. In addition, acute SDHs >10 mm in maximal thickness or with >5 mm of midline shift are typically removed, regardless of symptoms [10]. The need for surgical evacuation of large asymptomatic chronic SDHs is less clear. Operative intervention for an acute SDH usually requires a generous craniotomy, evacuation of the hematoma, and control of bleeding. Depending on the degree of underlying parenchymal injury and edema, expansion duroplasty and bone flap removal may be necessary to accommodate swelling of the underlying brain and minimize dangerous increases in intracranial pressure (ICP). Operative intervention for a chronic SDH usually involves burr holes and removal of chronic liquefied hematoma via suction and irrigation, often followed by the placement of temporary postoperative subdural drains. A special consideration in the elderly population is the degree of underlying cerebral atrophy. Because the atrophic brain is often unable to expand and fill the subdural space even after the mass effect has been removed, bridging veins remain under tension and at risk for future traumatic injury, and recurrent chronic SDHs often form. Occasionally, craniotomies are performed for chronic SDHs if there is concern for significant membrane formation and therefore inadequate drainage of the loculated subdural hematoma through one or two burr holes.

EDHs also occur as a result of trauma, but are much less common than SDHs, with an estimated incidence of 2.7–4.1% in TBI patients [10]. The increased adherence of the dura mater to the skull in the elderly serves to tamponade bleeding into the epidural space, thus EDHs are unusual in the geriatric population. When present, EDHs are often associated with skull fractures. Traditionally thought to be of primarily arterial origin, recent studies have indicated that EDHs from venous injuries are quite common as well [10]. Clinically, patients with significant EDHs present with focal and diffuse brain pressure findings similar to those with SDHs. Signs and symptoms include headache, nausea/vomiting, diplopia, altered mental status, pupillary dilatation, seizures, dysphasia, and hemiparesis/hemiplegia. Additionally, some patients present with the classic "lucid interval", an asymptomatic time period immediately following trauma before the onset of symptoms, attributed to the expansion of the hematoma as it slowly dissects between the skull and adherent dura, gradually increasing pressure on the underlying brain. On CT scan, EDHs appear as hyperdense biconvex extra-axial collections, which do not cross suture lines (Fig. 86.2a, b). Surgical evacuation of the hematoma is indicated for symptomatic lesions. EDH evacuation usually requires a craniotomy, with or without expansion duroplasty and bone flap removal, based on the extent of the underlying parenchymal injury and edema.

Intracerebral/Subarachnoid Hemorrhage

In addition to extra-axial hematomas, patients with traumatic brain injuries often have intra-axial hemorrhages, either within the parenchyma of the brain or in the subarachnoid space. The management of traumatic intracerebral hemorrhages is similar to that of nontraumatic intracerebral hemorrhages. These lesions appear as hyperdense intra-axial collections on CT, which can vary in diameter from under a millimeter to several

FIGURE 86.2 Noncontrast axial head CTs demonstrate (**a**) acute epidural hematoma – a hyperdense biconvex extra-axial collection and (**b**) in the same patient, a minimally displaced left frontal skull fracture adjacent to the epidural hematoma, the likely cause of the vascular injury producing the hematoma

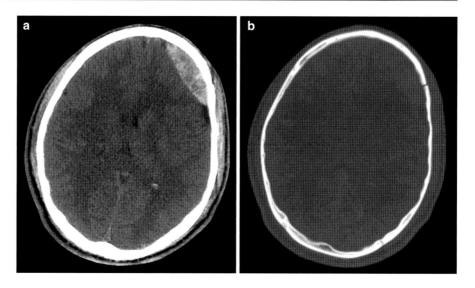

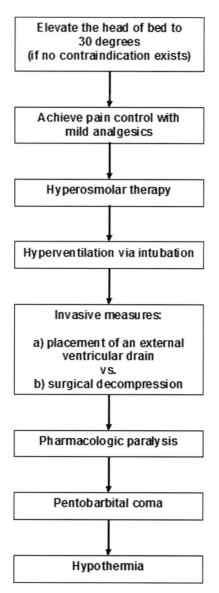

FIGURE 86.3 General schematic for the management of elevated intracranial pressures.

centimeters. Initial treatment should focus on blood pressure control, to prevent rebleeding, and management of ICPs. Frequent neurologic examinations should be performed to assess for acute decompensation and serial imaging studies should be performed to evaluate for rebleeding. In the event of elevated ICPs, medical management should be initiated, and in some cases, surgical decompression is required due to the degree of mass effect (Fig. 86.3) [10, 11].

Subarachnoid hemorrhages are also common sequelae of TBI. Although these hemorrhages seldom require surgical evacuation, they are often associated with seizures, altered mental status, and diffuse axonal injury, all of which can lead to significant morbidity and mortality. On CT, traumatic subarachnoid hemorrhages appear as layered, hyperdense lesions within the subarachnoid spaces, most commonly along the cortical surfaces. Patients with traumatic subarachnoid hemorrhages should be given prophylactic anticonvulsant medications for 7 days posttrauma [12]. Care should be taken in the administration of these medications to the elderly population, as they often have significant side effects including hypotension, cardiac arrhythmias, and confusion. Additionally, for those patients with traumatic subarachnoid hemorrhage and poor neurologic exam in the absence of a focal compressive lesion, placement of an ICP monitor is often required to measure ICPs, which require further management if elevated (Fig. 86.3) [10, 11].

Fractures

The skull is a protective layer meant to absorb high-energy forces and to prevent direct intracranial parenchymal injury. In doing so, the skull is also placed at risk for fracture in the event of a significant trauma. Skull fractures can be loosely categorized into four groups: linear, depressed, skull base, and open, each of which has unique management strategies.

Linear fractures are the most common type of skull fracture and are usually the result of low-energy trauma over a large surface area. These fractures are nondisplaced, seldom require surgical intervention and are treated with observation and expectant management [13].

Depressed skull fractures are usually the result of high-energy trauma over a small surface area. Clinically, depressed skull fractures often manifest with seizures, due to an underlying cortical injury, or as an epidural hematoma, due to laceration of a meningeal artery adherent to the skull. Those fractures that are depressed below the inner table of the adjacent normal bone typically require surgical elevation [13].

Skull base fractures occur in the context of severe trauma and can manifest with a variety of neurologic symptoms [13]. Often, skull base fractures are associated with additional intracranial injuries due to the magnitude of the causative trauma. Most significantly, skull base fractures can cause vascular injuries, commonly to the internal carotid arteries, as well as cerebrospinal fluid (CSF) leaks [14–16]. Therefore, all patients with skull base fractures should undergo computerized tomographic angiography (CTA) to rule out vascular injury [14, 15]. Additionally, they should be monitored closely for the evidence of CSF otorrhea or rhinorrhea. Management of vascular injuries should be deferred to an experienced neurovascular team, which includes both neurosurgeons and neurointerventionalists. Management of CSF leaks includes initial conservative treatment with bed rest and head of bed elevation to reduce the hydrostatic pressure gradient and CSF flow across the dural defect, allowing for the body to seal the breach. If the CSF leak persists despite these conservative measures, CSF diversion using a lumbar drain and/or surgical repair are needed to eliminate the leak to prevent bacterial ingress and subsequent meningitis [16].

Open skull fractures are defined as those lesions with an overlying skin laceration, such that there is a communication between the external environment and the intracranial space. These lesions are at particularly high risk for infection [17]. Open skull fractures often demonstrate significant pneumocephalus on imaging due to the abnormal communication with the external environment. Open skull fractures may be classified as either clean or contaminated. All patients with open skull fractures should receive tetanus toxoid, and those with contaminated fractures should also receive prophylactic antibiotics [17]. In most cases, these injuries require operative exploration for wound cleansing, debridement, and closure [13, 17].

Penetrating Trauma

Penetrating brain injury (PBI) refers primarily to gunshot wounds to the head, although all foreign bodies that invade the cranial vault may be included in this group. The management of PBI has undergone fundamental changes since initial descriptions in the early twentieth century, which were based primarily on military injuries. The current literature includes accounts of both civilian and military experiences. The former contains mostly reports of low-velocity injuries and self-inflicted wounds, while the later includes a higher percentage of high-velocity and shrapnel injuries [18]. Regardless of injury etiology, studies of both groups have derived similar conclusions, and current management recommendations are based on Class III evidence from both civilian and military case series [18].

The primary goals in the treatment of PBIs are infection prevention and ICP management. World War I trauma surgeons advocated extensive exploration and debridement of PBIs, with removal of all foreign bodies and bone fragments to decrease the risk of infections and seizures. Subsequent military and civilian studies have indicated that extensive exploration and debridement of PBIs is unnecessary and leads to higher rates of morbidity and mortality [18, 19]. Modern studies have demonstrated that the primary cause of PBI-related infections is a persistent CSF leak [18–20]. As such, during the initial management of a PBI, care should be taken to achieve good local debridement, followed by a watertight dural and scalp closure. Extensive brain debridement should be avoided to prevent injury to normal tissues. Additionally, prophylactic anticonvulsant medications should be given to prevent seizures [18]. Surgical evacuation of large intracranial hematomas may be necessary to manage elevated ICPs, and earlier surgery is associated with better outcomes [18, 21]. Additionally, intraparenchymal or intraventricular ICP monitors are often needed to follow the response to treatment.

Increasing age is associated with poorer outcomes in patients with PBIs [22]. However, given that PBIs are relatively uncommon occurrences, and even more uncommon in the geriatric population, analyses of this association have been somewhat limited [22]. Of the studies which have examined the role of age in outcome from PBIs, two have demonstrated that increasing age is associated with higher mortality [21, 23]. It is likely that many of the same mechanisms which contribute to poor outcomes in the elderly from general TBIs play a role in PBIs.

Nontraumatic Vascular Lesions

Neurovascular lesions constitute a broad spectrum of pathologies, yet common to each of these disease processes is precipitous neurologic decline from disruption of vital bloodflow to brain tissue. Population studies indicate that neurovascular diseases are more prevalent among the elderly [24]. Moreover, the geriatric population appears to fare worse from neurovascular diseases than their younger counterparts [3]. This finding has significantly affected the treatment strategies for the elderly.

Aneurysms

The accepted prevalence of intracranial aneurysms is 5% of the total population, although the prevalence in autopsy series has ranged from 0.2 to 7.9% [25–27]. It is postulated that most intracranial aneurysms develop as a result of combined hypertension, atherosclerosis, cigarette smoking, and congenital predisposition [27]. Most commonly, these lesions develop in the intracranial anterior circulation arterial blood vessels – carotid, anterior cerebral, middle cerebral, anterior communicating, and posterior communicating arteries – although posterior circulation aneurysms of the vertebrobasilar and posterior cerebral arteries account for approximately 15% of all lesions [25]. Ruptured intracranial aneurysms are one of the most devastating and challenging neurosurgical emergencies.

The majority of ruptured intracranial aneurysms cause sudden-onset of worst headache of life, focal neurologic deficits, and symptoms of increased ICPs (nausea, vomiting, headache, and decreased level of consciousness). Brain imaging shows acute subarachnoid hemorrhage (SAH), although intraventricular and intraparenchymal hemorrhages are not uncommon (Fig. 86.4a, b) [25]. The initial management of these patients focuses on the treatment of elevated ICPs and strict blood pressure control to prevent aneurysm rebleeding [28]. Additionally, the patient must be monitored closely for evidence of neurologic deterioration, which may be indicative of rebleeding, seizures, or hydrocephalus. Systolic blood pressures should be maintained <140 mmHg using short acting, titratable antihypertensive agents, such as labetalol, hydralazine, and nicardipine. However, hypotension must also be avoided as this may lower cerebral perfusion pressure and cause cerebral ischemia. Care should be taken to avoid antihypertensive agents which raise ICPs, such as nitroprusside. If there is clinical evidence for elevated ICPs, these should be treated as previously described (Fig. 86.3) [10, 11].

The incidence of aneurysmal SAH is 6–8 per 100,000 people in most western populations [25]. Approximately 10–15% of patients with aneurysmal SAH incur fatal brain damage and die before reaching medical care [25]. In the early survivors, the initial aneurysm bleeding stops; however, they have a 15–20% risk of rebleeding in the first 2 weeks post-SAH [28, 29]. The 30-day case fatality rate is approximately 50% [30, 31]. Following acute stabilization, decisions must be made regarding aneurysm repair to prevent future bleeding. Several studies regarding the timing of open surgical treatment have been published; however, no definitive conclusions have been drawn [32–34]. Following aneurysmal SAH, patients may develop cerebral vasospasm, during which blood vessels constrict and reduce blood flow to the brain, causing reversible neurologic deficits, stroke, or death. The prevalence of cerebral vasospasm is greatest between days 4 and 10 post-SAH, and patients who undergo aneurysm repair during this interval fare worse than those treated earlier or later [35]. The primary consideration in opting for

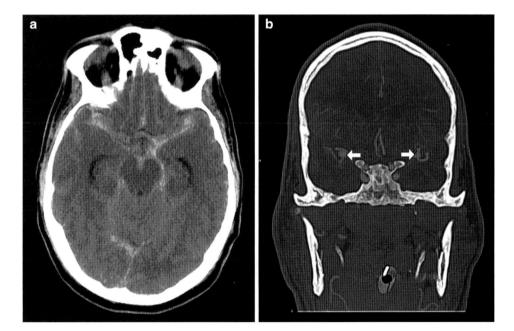

Figure 86.4 (a) Noncontrast head CT demonstrates diffuse subarachnoid hemorrhage throughout the basal cisterns and bilateral Sylvian fissures, from a ruptured intracranial aneurysm and (b) contrast-enhanced cerebral CT angiogram reveals bilateral middle cerebral artery aneurysms (*single arrows*).

early intervention within the first 96 h after aneurysm rupture is to repair the aneurysm and reduce the risk of rebleeding, an event that can cause stroke or death. Many patients are in poor medical and neurological condition after SAH, and may not be stable enough to tolerate aneurysm repair via open surgery or endovascular techniques. Later aneurysm treatment may allow for the improvement of medical and neurological issues, but exposes the patient to a greater risk of rebleeding from the unsecured aneurysm. Currently, the trend is toward early intervention for all patients with aneurysmal SAH, except for those in extremely poor neurological or medical condition.

Intracranial aneurysms may be treated with either open surgical or endovascular techniques [25]. Open surgical treatment involves craniotomy and placement of a small spring-loaded clip across the neck of the aneurysm, isolating the aneurysm from the parent blood vessel while maintaining vital blood flow to the brain. Endovascular treatment involves femoral artery catheterization and deposition of metal coils within the aneurysm, sealing it off from the parent blood vessel. In a randomized trail comparing endovascular treatment with open surgery for patients with aneurysms deemed treatable with either technique, there were 278 patients age 65 or older [36, 37]. Overall neither of the treatments produced better functional outcomes; however, subgroup analyses based on aneurysm location showed that open surgery was superior for middle cerebral artery (MCA) aneurysms and that endovascular treatment was better for internal carotid and posterior communicating artery aneurysms. The generalizability of these findings is limited, since many aneurysms are not equally treatable by open surgery or endovascular techniques. The durability of endovascular repairs has also been questioned [38, 39]. In current practice, the treatment plan is usually decided by a team of neurosurgeons and neurointerventionalists while considering patient condition, aneurysm location, and angioarchitecture. Despite treatment, only ~1/3 of those patients who survive their initial aneurysm rupture will regain a good functional status, while the remaining 2/3 will have significant deficits or die [25]. These outcomes are strongly associated with the patient's admission neurological exam [25, 40].

Historically, patients with aneurysmal SAH and advanced age (>70 years) have been deemed poor candidates for surgical or endovascular treatment [40–44], based on the worse neurological condition of older patients when compared with their younger counterparts [42]. Elderly patients were traditionally treated conservatively, with only medical management of their SAH symptoms. Not surprisingly, this led to very poor outcomes, with the vast majority (>75%) of elderly patients suffering severe morbidity and mortality [40, 43]. Evidence showing improved outcomes in elderly patients who receive surgical or endovascular treatment when compared with medical management [43] has spurred a recent trend toward offering geriatric patients with aneurysmal SAH definitive treatment for their aneurysm. However, it is clear that even with treatment, the geriatric population fares worse than their younger counterparts [42]. Using data from a multicenter randomized trial, it was found that with advancing age, patients have significantly worse admission neurological exams, thicker subarachnoid clots, and higher rates of intraventricular hemorrhage, hydrocephalus, and aneurysm rebleeding [42]. Additionally, older patients have higher incidences of preexisting medical comorbidities [42]. Interestingly, in this study, there were no age-related differences in time to presentation, timing of surgery, aneurysm size and location, or surgical complications. After controlling for the above factors, increasing age was still significantly associated with a poorer outcome [42]. This was thought to be related to the impaired ability of the aging brain to recover from acute stress, as well as the overall diminished cardiovascular reserve in older patients, which can lead to suboptimal cerebral perfusion [6, 42]. As endovascular technology evolves, it is likely that it will be used with increasing frequency in the elderly as a means to mitigate the risk of open surgery while still offering definitive therapy [41]. Regardless, it is clear that geriatric patients have better outcomes with definitive treatment than conservative treatment, although outcomes are worse than those in younger patients.

Vascular Malformations

CNS vascular malformations are congenital vascular lesions that fall into four categories: arterio-venous malformations (AVMs), capillary telangiectasias, venous angiomas, and cavernous malformations [25]. Of these, AVMs are most prone to hemorrhages requiring emergency neurosurgical care and will therefore be the focus of this discussion.

The prevalence of intracranial AVMs is not well known; hospital-based autopsy estimates range from 5 to 613 AVMs per 100,000 persons [45]. Anatomically, AVMs represent abnormal tangles of arteries and veins, with an absence of normal intervening capillary architecture, resulting in high-flow arterio-venous shunting [25, 45]. AVMs are congenital and occur throughout the CNS [45]. Although they may cause a variety of neurologic symptoms, the most common presentation is intracranial hemorrhage (ICH), which is a neurologic emergency (Fig. 86.5a–c) [25, 46].

The management of AVM-related ICHs begins with strict blood pressure control to prevent rebleeding. Subsequently, if there is evidence of increased ICPs, medical management should be initiated, as previously described (Fig. 86.3) [10, 11]. If significant mass effect and concern for herniation exists, surgical evacuation of AVM-related ICHs can be

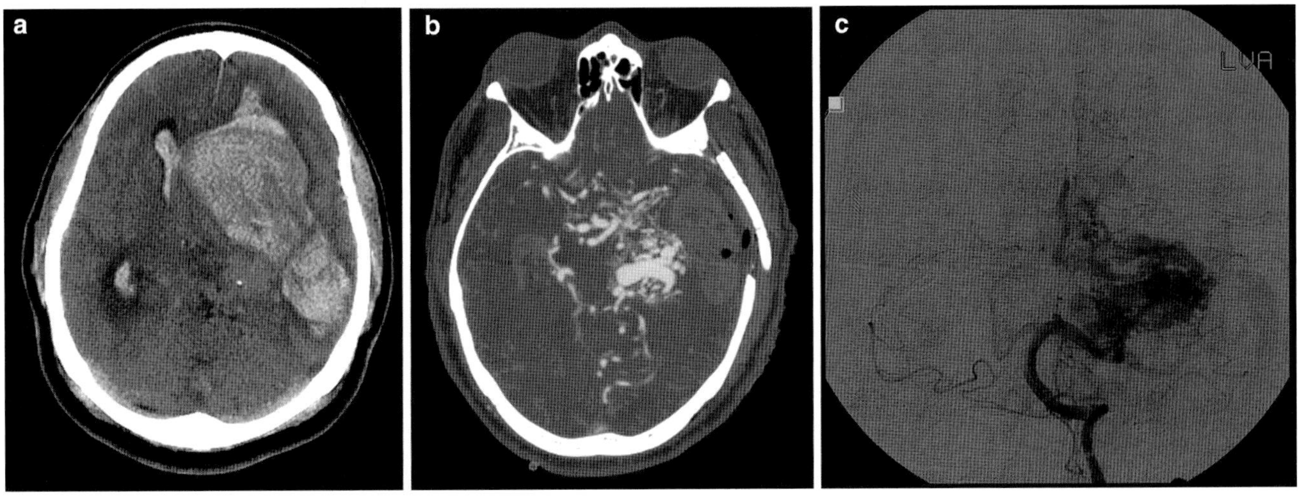

Figure 86.5 (a) Noncontrast head CT demonstrates a large left fronto-temporo-parietal intracranial hemorrhage with associated intraventricular hemorrhage, mass effect, and midline shift, (b) contrast-enhanced cerebral CT angiogram reveals an underlying arterio-venous malformation, and (c) cerebral catheter angiogram confirms the presence of a large arterio-venous malformation.

performed; however, the surgical approach is much different than that for typical ICHs and is beyond the scope of this discussion. If possible, it is preferable to stabilize the patient medically and treat the AVM in a nonacute setting. Treatment options include open surgical resection, radiosurgery, and endovascular embolization.

Most AVMs are diagnosed at an early age (~35 years), and patients who present with hemorrhage are even younger (~31 years) [45, 47]. Prospective data indicate that the patients at highest risk for future hemorrhages are those who have AVMs with deep locations, exclusively deep venous drainage, and a history of previous AVM-related ICH [48]. Additionally, the risk of future hemorrhages increases with age [48]. Given the rarity of this disease, there are no data on specific or different treatment strategies for the elderly population. However, it is likely elderly patients are more often treated with less invasive methods (i.e., radiosurgery and endovascular embolization) when possible, due to the perceived increased risks of open surgery with advanced age.

Stroke

Cerebrovascular accidents, or strokes, are a leading cause of morbidity and mortality, especially among the elderly [3]. Strokes can be either hemorrhagic or ischemic, both of which constitute neurologic emergencies that may require surgical intervention.

Hemorrhagic strokes affect approximately 10–20 per 100,000 people each year [24, 49]. Although these events are less frequent than ischemic strokes, they have much higher rates of associated death and disability [3]. Specifically, the 1-year mortality rate following hemorrhagic stroke is approximately 62% [24]. The most common risk factor for hemorrhagic stroke is hypertension, which is the focus of this discussion [24]. Amyloid angiopathy is also a significant cause of hemorrhagic stroke and will be discussed in detail later in this chapter. Advancing age, male sex, and alcohol and tobacco use are known risk factors for hypertensive hemorrhagic stroke (HHS). Additionally, blacks have an incidence of HHS that is twice that of whites [24].

HHSs most commonly occur from the rupture of small intracranial perforator arteries in deep regions of the brain (e.g., basal ganglia and brainstem), although cortical and cerebellar hemorrhages occur as well (Fig. 86.6) [24, 25, 50]. The initial management of HHS patients focuses on strict blood pressure control and treatment of elevated ICPs (Fig. 86.3) [10, 11]. The INTERACT randomized controlled trial demonstrated that intensive blood pressure control reduces subsequent hematoma growth, although clinical outcome data are lacking [51]. The role of surgical evacuation in the treatment of HHS is controversial. A recent randomized controlled trial (STICH) evaluated the role of early surgical intervention in supratentorial ICHs and determined that there was no overall benefit from early surgery as compared to initial medical management [49]. Given the deep location of many of these hemorrhages and the need to traverse normal intervening brain to evacuate them, it is not surprising that there was no clear benefit with surgical intervention in this study. On the other hand, anecdotal evidence suggests that superficial supratentorial HHSs with significant mass effect

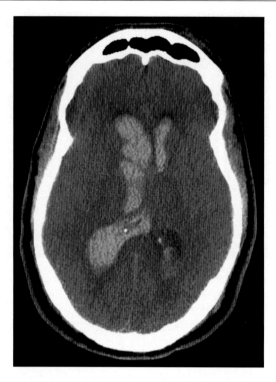

Figure 86.6 Noncontrast head CT demonstrates an acute basal ganglia hemorrhage with mass effect and intraventricular extension.

may respond well to surgical decompression and therefore these patients should be evaluated on a case-by-case basis with the assistance of a neurosurgical team. Alternatively, HHSs in the cerebellum respond much more favorably to surgical evacuation. Cerebellar hemorrhages have a propensity for early hydrocephalus and brainstem compression [24]. Craniotomy and decompression is the definitive treatment for this process and studies have shown that those patients with large cerebellar hematomas (volume greater than 40 mL) have a clear benefit from surgical intervention [24, 52]. Of note, significant research has also been performed to ascertain the role of recombinant-activated factor VIIa (rFVIIa) in the treatment of acute ICHs, including HHSs. The final results of the phase 3 randomized controlled trial (FAST) demonstrated that although rFVIIa reduces the growth of the hematoma, it does not result in any significant improvements in survival or functional outcome, and therefore, the use of rFVIIa for acute ICHs has not become part of standard practice [53].

Ischemic strokes (IS) account for the vast majority of all strokes, with an incidence of 300–500 cases per 100,000 people each year [3]. In general, management of IS should be directed by a neurology team. On rare occasions, IS may require surgical intervention. The role of surgical intervention has been well examined in patients with a "malignant" MCA infarction, where swelling from the damaged brain can cause rapid neurological deterioration and 1-year mortality rates reach up to 80% [54–57]. Several randomized controlled

trials (DESTINY, HAMLET, and DECIMAL) have been performed to evaluate the efficacy of early surgical decompression via hemicraniectomy and durotomy, to relieve the mass effect of the infracted and edematous brain [55–57]. The pooled analysis of these trials demonstrates a significant reduction in mortality; however, overall patient morbidity and functional outcomes remain unchanged despite surgical decompression [54]. It should be noted that these trials did not include patients greater than 60 years of age and therefore, surgical intervention in elderly patients should be considered on a case-by-case basis.

Amyloid Angiopathy

Cerebral amyloid angiopathy (CAA) is an important cause of nontraumatic ICH, comprising approximately 10% of all ICHs and 30% of all lobar ICHs [25, 58]. Moreover, this pathology has a predilection for the elderly population, making its review particularly germane to this discussion [25, 58]. CAA is characterized by the deposition of beta-amyloid, a fibrillar protein, in the media and adventitia of small- and medium-sized arteries [25, 58]. The exact prevalence of CAA is difficult to determine due to the lack of definitive histopathology in most cases; however, it is well known that the prevalence of CAA increases with age and it is rarely identified in those less than 55 years of age [58]. CAA has an equal predilection for both sexes. Approximately 1/3 of people greater than 60 years of age have evidence of CAA on autopsy, and in individuals over 90 years of age, the prevalence of CAA exceeds 60% [58]. Studies have also demonstrated that those individuals who possess the E2 and E4 alleles of the apolipoprotein E gene have a significantly increased risk of developing CAA [25, 58].

Although CAA can cause progressive dementia, transient ischemic attacks, seizures, and ischemic stroke, arguably the most concerning manifestation is ICH, caused by the rupture of amyloid-laden vasculature [25, 58]. These hemorrhages are most frequently lobar and can be multifocal [25, 58].

The management of ICHs due to CAA is not significantly different from the management of hypertensive ICHs. Most hemorrhages do not require surgical intervention; however, if significant mass effect and neurologic deficits exist, craniotomy for evacuation and decompression can be considered. Unlike cerebral aneurysms and AVMs, ICHs due to CAA do not require treatment of a discrete, underlying vascular abnormality. Although the vasculature is altered in patients with CAA, it does not require unique surgical maneuvers to control bleeding. In contrast with ICHs due to hypertension, CAA-associated ICHs are typically more superficial and therefore more amenable to surgical intervention [25, 58]. Although no specific pharmacotherapy exists for the treatment of CAA, there is ongoing research into the development of antiamyloid medications and vaccinations [58]. Additionally, as discussed above, the use of rFVIIa has not resulted in a significant clinical benefit in this patient population [53].

Adverse Drug Reactions

As the population ages, the use of antiplatelet and anticoagulant medications such as aspirin, clopidogrel, and warfarin, has increased dramatically. Protocols for managing patients with acute ischemic stroke using thrombolytic therapies, such as intravenous and intraarterial tissue plasminogen activator (tPA), have become more common [59]. Traditional guidelines recommend administration of tPA within 3 h of onset of stroke symptoms; however, many stroke centers now aim to administer tPA in an urgent fashion, within 60 min of onset of symptoms, for embolic stroke [59]. Given the potency of these medications, it is not surprising that some of their primary side effects include undesired bleeding, including ICHs [60, 61]. Patients who receive tPA and have early hypodensities on CT have significantly higher rates of ICH [62]. Patients who develop ICHs secondary to antiplatelet or anticoagulant therapies should have the offending medications discontinued immediately, followed by reversal of the platelet dysfunction and/or anticoagulation with the appropriate blood products and/or medications. The remainder of their management should follow that of other nontraumatic ICHs; strict blood pressure control should be employed and surgical decompression considered on a case-by-case basis for those patients with significant mass effect. In a study of surgical evacuation of ICH following administration of streptokinase for acute myocardial infarction, surgery was beneficial, although survival was dependent upon the time from the initiation of thrombolytic therapy to onset of stroke symptoms, initial Glasgow coma scale score, volume of ICH, and "baseline clinical characteristics" (defined as age, systolic blood pressure, Killip class, heart rate, infarct location, previous myocardial infarction, height, time to treatment, history of smoking, current smoking, diabetes, weight, history of coronary bypass surgery, type of thrombolytic agent, history of hypertension, and history of cerebrovascular disease) [63]. Importantly, all patients who are started on antiplatelet and anticoagulant medications should be counseled about the potential risk of ICH.

Sinus Thrombosis

Intracranial venous sinus thrombosis (VST) is a relatively rare condition that constitutes a neurologic emergency.

There are several factors which predispose individuals to developing VSTs, including: a hypercoagulable state, dehydration, adjacent tumor or infection, pregnancy, vasculitis, systemic inflammatory disorders, and local trauma [25, 64]. Although most intracranial VSTs become evident through headache and other symptoms of increased ICPs, a significant portion of patients develop seizures, intracranial infarcts, ICHs, or focal motor deficits [25, 64]. VSTs cause venous outflow obstruction and subsequent parenchymal edema and infarction [25, 64]. The primary goal in the treatment of VSTs is the prevention of thrombus propagation while allowing for natural thrombolysis and recanalization of the affected vessel. This is achieved with anticoagulation and is typically managed by a neurology team [25, 64]. However, endovascular thrombolysis of the clot/affected vessel using pharmacologic and mechanical techniques is sometimes indicated, and in cases with large ICHs, surgical decompression and evacuation is occasionally performed [64]. As compared to intracranial arterial thromboses, VSTs have an overall better prognosis [64]. In the largest series to date of patients with VSTs, there was a 13% rate of death or dependence at 6 months after ictus [64]. Risk factors associated with poor outcome include advancing age, male sex, altered mental status on admission, deep cerebral venous system thrombosis, ICH, malignancy, and CNS infection [64].

Infection

Infections of the CNS are neurological emergencies, which must be treated in a timely fashion. Generally, CNS infections can be categorized by their location: meningeal, subdural, epidural, intraparenchymal, and intraventricular. Most CNS infections have bacterial, viral, or fungal etiologies; this discussion will focus on bacterial infections, as these most commonly require surgical intervention. Additionally, this discussion will be limited to intracranial CNS infections; a review of spinal CNS infections can be found in Chap. 87.

Infections of the meninges, also known as meningitis, are the most common intracranial CNS infection [25]. Patients typically develop fever, headache, neck stiffness, photophobia, and malaise. Contrast-enhanced imaging studies often reveal diffuse meningeal enhancement, and CSF analysis demonstrates elevations in the nucleated white blood cell count. As meningitis is most often managed medically, without the need for surgical intervention, further discussion of its management is beyond the scope of this discussion.

Infections of the epidural space, also known as epidural abscesses (EA), comprise approximately 2% of intracranial CNS infections [65]. These infections present with fever, headache, neck stiffness, photophobia, periorbital swelling, scalp tenderness, ear pain, nausea, vomiting, and lethargy. Imaging studies reveal an extra-axial, biconvex lesion with peripheral enhancement. Imaging studies may also reveal evidence of underlying osteomyelitis, sinusitis, or mastoiditis. Cranial EAs typically occur via direct extension of an adjacent sinusitis, although they may also be the result of hematogeneous spread from infections located throughout the body. They most commonly occur in adolescent males, though all age groups may be affected [65]. Treatment of cranial EAs involves surgical evacuation, followed by prolonged antibiotic therapy. If the adjacent bone appears to be involved, it must also be debrided and/or removed [65]. The most commonly isolated organisms in cranial EAs are microaerophilic or hemolytic streptococci; however, staphylococci may also be involved in cases of postoperative or posttraumatic infections [65].

Subdural infections, also known as subdural empyemas (SE), occur in 12–25% of intracranial CNS infections [65]. These infections present similarly to cranial EAs; however, focal neurologic deficits are more common given the direct contact with the cortical surface [65, 66]. Imaging studies reveal extra-axial, crescent-shaped collections with peripheral enhancement. As with cranial EAs, there is often evidence of adjacent osteomyelitis, sinusitis, or mastoiditis. Intracranial SEs typically occur in the setting of sinusitis, via direct extension or hematogenous spread, but may also occur as a result of trauma or neurosurgical intervention [65, 66]. Treatment involves prompt surgical evacuation, followed by prolonged antibiotic therapy [65, 66]. The most commonly isolated organisms in intracranial SEs are aerobic and anaerobic streptococci species, as well as staphylococci species [65, 66].

Intraparenchymal intracranial CNS infections, also known as brain abscesses (BA), are occurring with increasing frequency as the prevalence of immunocompromised individuals rises [65]. These infections cause fevers, headache, meningismus, malaise, seizures, and focal neurologic deficits – and they most often have a rapid progression of symptoms. On contrasted imaging studies, BAs appear as intra-axial lesions with marked peripheral enhancement and restricted diffusion on MRI (Fig. 86.7a–c). They can occur in the setting of sinusitis and mastoiditis, but are also commonly the result of bacteremia in the setting of congenital heart defects, bacterial endocarditis, dental abscesses, pulmonary infections, and acute diverticulitis [65]. Treatment consists of abscess drainage, often with the use of intra-operative stereotactic navigation systems, followed by prolonged antibiotic therapy [65]. The most commonly isolated organisms include aerobic and anaerobic streptococci and bacteroides species, staphylococci species, and fungal organisms in the immunocompromised [65].

Intraventricular CNS infections are rare entities. They commonly cause signs and symptoms of obstructive hydrocephalus: headache, nausea, vomiting, lethargy, and coma [25, 65]. Most often, intraventricular infections are caused by parasites (i.e., neurocysticercosis) [25]. Imaging studies reveal an intraventricular mass with a variable enhancement pattern and evidence of obstructive hydrocephalus. Surgical management of these lesions is usually curative. Medical management using antihelminthics remains controversial and should be discussed with an infectious disease specialist [25]. Of note, bacterial ventriculitis may also develop in the setting of a prolonged intracranial bacterial infection.

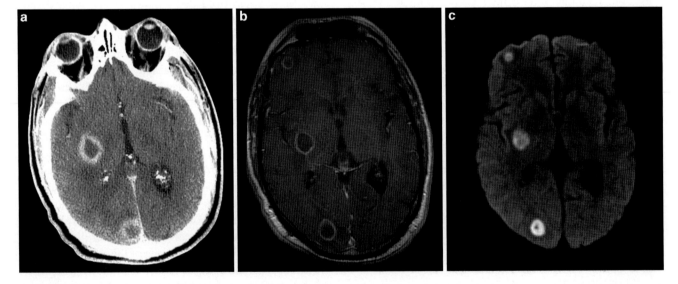

FIGURE 86.7 (a) Contrast-enhanced head CT demonstrates multiple hypodense ring-enhancing lesions, (b) T1-weighted contrast-enhanced brain MRI demonstrates multiple hypodense ring-enhancing lesions with surrounding edema, and (c) diffusion-weighted brain MRI reveals restricted diffusion throughout the enhancing lesions, consistent with multiple brain abscesses.

As with intraventricular parasitic infections, individuals with bacterial ventriculitis typically develop symptoms of hydrocephalus. Imaging studies reveal diffusely enhancing ventricular walls. Management includes CSF diversion for elevated ICPs and prolonged antibiotic therapy.

With the exception of meningitis, most CNS infections require neurosurgical intervention. Risks of prolonged, untreated CNS infections include VST, osteomyelitis, hydrocephalus, seizures, and catastrophic intraventricular BA rupture. Importantly, in the management and initial work-up of CNS infections, lumbar puncture is often considered. Although this can be performed safely in most patients with simple meningitis, for those patients with intracranial mass lesions, lumbar puncture should be deferred due to the risk of causing cerebral herniation [25]. Additionally, significant controversy exists regarding the use of steroids in the context of CNS infections [25]. This issue is best dealt with on a case-by-case basis, after careful review of the particular clinical scenario.

Most CNS infections tend to occur in the young; however, the elderly population deserves special consideration for several reasons. First, geriatric patients often have nonspecific signs and symptoms in the setting of infection [3, 67]. This increases the need for vigilant physical examination and CNS imaging studies in this population. Additionally, the elderly population has a relative immunosenescence, therefore, their clinical course and response to therapy may be worse than a younger counterpart with a similar illness [67]. Finally, the elderly tend to have more frequent and more severe adverse drug effects, especially from antibiotics, and this should be taken into account when choosing the appropriate drug regimen [67].

Peripheral Nerve Injury

Traumatic peripheral nerve injuries (PNIs) are relatively rare occurrences and are treated by a variety of specialists, including neurosurgeons, plastic surgeons, and orthopedic surgeons [68, 69]. Despite their rarity, PNIs can result in devastating functional loss and represent an important neurologic emergency. Clinically, they typically present in the setting of trauma with neurologic deficit confined to a single extremity [70]. PNIs often occur in tandem with bony fractures and peripheral vascular injuries [70]. Traumatic PNIs can be loosely categorized into three broad groups based on mechanism: stretch/avulsion injuries, lacerating injuries, and compressive injuries [71].

Stretch and avulsion injuries are the most common types of PNI [70, 71]. They are usually the result of motor vehicle accidents in which the torsional force of impact results in the movement of an extremity in one direction and the patient's trunk in another [70]. This results in a stretching of nerve roots, which, if severe enough, can cause complete nerve root avulsion from the spinal cord. Spinal imaging studies may reveal pseudomeningoceles indicative of dural nerve root sleeve disruption and adjacent soft tissue injury. Penetrating and lacerating PNIs typically occur as a result of gunshot and knife wounds. They are the second most common type of PNI and are often associated with injuries of adjacent vascular structures [70, 71]. These injuries are usually discovered on physical exam, as the external signs of trauma can be quite obvious. Compressive PNIs often occur as a result of local hematomas, soft tissue swelling, and bony hypertrophy. They cause indirect neural injury via external compression [71].

Operative interventions for PNIs vary widely based on the mechanism of injury, extent of neurologic deficit, presence of additional injuries, and surgeon preference [72, 73]. Surgical interventions may involve decompression, direct repair, removal of neuromas, and nerve grafting or transposition [72, 74]. Nearly all interventions employ the use of pre- and postoperative electromyography, and intraoperative nerve action potential and somatosensory evoked potential recordings [72]. Given the increased incidence of osteoporosis and bony fractures in the elderly, it is likely that they are at increased risk for PNIs in the setting of trauma. Therefore, since early identification of PNIs can maximize the potential for a functional recovery, it is imperative that elderly patients undergo complete neurologic examination as part of their trauma evaluation.

Tumors

Intracranial primary or metastatic tumors can cause medical emergencies via mass effect from tumor growth, edema in the surrounding brain, intratumoral hemorrhage, or seizures. Initial management should focus on the treatment of elevated ICP symptoms, blood pressure control, and seizure cessation. Further discussion of these lesions can be found in Chap. 87.

Conclusions

Geriatric neurosurgical emergencies encompass a broad range of pathologies. Elderly patients have unique treatment challenges that must be accounted for by healthcare providers. The loss of cardiovascular reserve and the fundamental changes within the aging CNS appear to play a significant role in morbidity and mortality and should be carefully considered when treating and counseling geriatric patients with neurosurgical illnesses.

CASE STUDY

History

An 82-year-old male, with multiple medical problems, seeks medical attention after the acute onset of worst headache of life. He also notes nausea, photophobia, and neck pain. He denies trauma, numbness, weakness, tingling, seizures, chest pain, and shortness of breath. A noncontrast head CT (Fig. 86.8a) is obtained and the patient is subsequently transferred to a tertiary care center. During transfer, the patient is noted to become progressively lethargic.

Past Medical History

1. Hypertension
2. Coronary artery disease
3. Chronic renal failure
4. Type II diabetes mellitus
5. Atrial fibrillation

Admission Neurologic Examination

Temp: 99.1 degrees Fahrenheit, HR: 70 beats per minute, BP: 160/70 mmHg, RR: 10 breaths per minute, O_2 Sat: 98% on 4 liters nasal cannula
Lethargic, nonverbal

Opens eyes to noxious stimuli
Pupils equally round and reactive to light, bilaterally
Moving all extremities symmetrically, not following commands
Localizes to noxious stimuli
Unable to assess sensory function
2+ deep tendon reflexes throughout
Toes downgoing, bilaterally

Relevant Admission Laboratory Values

Na: 138
Troponin-I: 0.40
WBC: 8.9 k
PLT: 228 k
INR: 2.8

Clinical Course

Upon arrival to the tertiary care center, the patient is intubated for airway protection. Subsequently, he is treated for hypertension and his systolic blood pressure is maintained below 140 mmHg. He is also given 1 g of IV phenytoin for seizure prophylaxis and 6 U of fresh frozen plasma to normalize coagulation. A cerebral CT angiogram is obtained (Fig. 86.8b), which demonstrates an anterior communicating artery aneurysm. The patient is

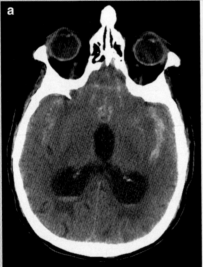 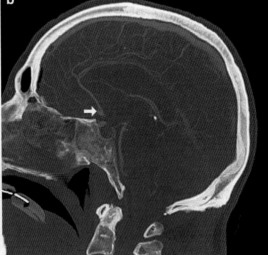

FIGURE 86.8 (**a**) Noncontrast head CT demonstrates diffuse subarachnoid hemorrhage involving the bilateral Sylvian fissures as well as intraventricular hemorrhage and hydrocephalus and (**b**) contrast-enhanced cerebral CT angiogram reveals an anterior communicating artery aneurysm (*single arrow*)

(continued)

CASE STUDY (continued)

transferred to the intensive care unit. His head of bed is elevated to 30°, he is sedated and hyperventilated, and a ventriculostomy catheter is placed to decompress hydrocephalus and manage elevated intracranial pressures. The patient's examination improves over the next 24 h; specifically, he begins to follow commands. An echocardiogram is obtained because of the abnormally elevated cardiac enzymes. The patient is found to have an ejection fraction of 35%. A family discussion is held regarding the risks and benefits of treatment and the decision is made to pursue endovascular therapy. The following day, the patient is taken to the angiography suite where he undergoes successful coil embolization of his intracranial aneurysm. Over the next 2 weeks, he is monitored carefully in the intensive care unit for evidence of vasospasm. His hydrocephalus resolves during this time and the ventriculostomy catheter is discontinued. His neurologic exam slowly improves, although his cognitive function appears somewhat diminished to his family members. He is extubated successfully. His ejection fraction also improves to 45% over this time period. He is later transferred to the floor and subsequently to a rehabilitation facility.

Discussion Questions

1. What are the most important initial measures that should be taken when caring for a patient with a ruptured intracranial aneurysm?
2. What are the possible etiologies of the patient's change in mental status during transfer to the tertiary care facility?
3. What is the clinical and operative significance of the elevated cardiac enzymes on admission?
4. What is the current standard of care for treatment of ruptured intracranial aneurysms in the elderly?

Discussion Answers

1. The most important initial measures to be taken when caring for a patient with a ruptured intracra-

nial aneurysm include: strict blood pressure control, administration of prophylactic anticonvulsant medications, and management of elevated intracranial pressures, if present.
2. Possible etiologies of the patient's change in mental status during transfer include: aneurysm rebleeding, hydrocephalus, and seizure.
3. Elevated cardiac enzymes in the setting of subarachnoid hemorrhage are associated with an increased risk of cardiogenic shock, pulmonary edema, and cerebral vasospasm. Elevated cardiac enzymes are also associated with higher rates of death and severe disability following aneurysmal subarachnoid hemorrhage. Therefore, when caring for patients with elevated cardiac enzymes, careful attention should be paid to optimizing their cardiopulmonary status. Moreover, in the setting of acutely elevated cardiac enzymes, it is often more judicious to treat patients with less invasive procedures (i.e., endovascular treatments) as opposed to maximally invasive procedures (i.e., open surgery), in order to minimize the degree of cardiac stress.
4. The current standard of care for treatment of ruptured intracranial aneurysms in the elderly is definitive surgical or endovascular repair in order to secure the aneurysm and prevent rebleeding. Aneurysm location, size, and configuration will often determine whether open surgery or endovascular techniques are the optimal approach to aneurysm repair. However, the patient's overall systemic health should be evaluated, and if significant comorbidities exist, strong consideration should be given to less invasive endovascular procedures, even if open surgery might provide a more definitive repair. Previously, elderly patients were treated with conservative, medical management without aneurysm repair. However, long-term studies have demonstrated that elderly patients have significantly better outcomes with definitive management and thus, this has become the standard of care. Nonetheless, elderly patients still fare worse than their younger counterparts, and as such, providers should have an open discourse with the patient and their family to discuss the potential need for long-term hospitalization, rehabilitation, and home care, so that treatment plans are made in accordance with the patient's wishes.

References

1. Table 12. Projections of the Population by Age and Sex for the United States: 2010 to 2050 (NP2008-T12) (Accessed 9 February 2009, at http://www.census.gov/)
2. Jager TE, Weiss HB, Coben JH, Pepe PE (2000) Traumatic brain injuries evaluated in U.S. emergency departments, 1992–1994. Acad Emerg Med 7:134–140
3. Kulchycki LK, Edlow JA (2006) Geriatric neurologic emergencies. Emerg Med Clin North Am 24:273–298, v–vi
4. Sterling DA, O'Connor JA, Bonadies J (2001) Geriatric falls: injury severity is high and disproportionate to mechanism. J Trauma 50:116–119
5. Helling TS, Watkins M, Evans LL, Nelson PW, Shook JW, Van Way CW (1999) Low falls: an underappreciated mechanism of injury. J Trauma 46:453–456
6. Vollmer DG, Torner JC, Jane JA et al (1991) Age and outcome following traumatic coma: why do older patients fare worse? J Neurosurg 75:S37–S49
7. Mosenthal AC, Lavery RF, Addis M et al (2002) Isolated traumatic brain injury: age is an independent predictor of mortality and early outcome. J Trauma 52:907–911
8. Demetriades D, Sava J, Alo K et al (2001) Old age as a criterion for trauma team activation. J Trauma 51:754–756, discussion 6–7
9. Meldon SW, Reilly M, Drew BL, Mancuso C, Fallon W Jr (2002) Trauma in the very elderly: a community-based study of outcomes at trauma and nontrauma centers. J Trauma 52:79–84
10. Loftus CM, American Association of Neurosurgeons (2008) Neurosurgical emergencies, 2nd edn. Thieme; American Association of Neurosurgeons, New York Rolling Meadows, IL
11. Rincon F, Mayer SA (2008) Clinical review: Critical care management of spontaneous intracerebral hemorrhage. Crit Care 12:237
12. The Brain Trauma Foundation (2000) The American Association of Neurological Surgeons. The Joint Section on Neurotrauma and Critical Care. Role of antiseizure prophylaxis following head injury. J Neurotrauma 17:549–553
13. Parikh S, Koch M, Narayan RK (2007) Traumatic brain injury. Int Anesthesiol Clin 45:119–135
14. Stengel D, Rademacher G, Hanson B, Ekkernkamp A, Mutze S (2007) Screening for blunt cerebrovascular injuries: the essential role of computed tomography angiography. Semin Ultrasound CT MR 28:101–108
15. Sliker CW (2008) Blunt cerebrovascular injuries: imaging with multidetector CT angiography. Radiographics 28:1689–1708, discussion 709–10
16. Yilmazlar S, Arslan E, Kocaeli H et al (2006) Cerebrospinal fluid leakage complicating skull base fractures: analysis of 81 cases. Neurosurg Rev 29:64–71
17. Bullock MR, Chesnut R, Ghajar J et al (2006) Surgical management of depressed cranial fractures. Neurosurgery 58:S56–S60, discussion Si–iv
18. (2001) Surgical management of penetrating brain injury. J Trauma 51:S16–S25
19. Brandvold B, Levi L, Feinsod M, George ED (1990) Penetrating craniocerebral injuries in the Israeli involvement in the Lebanese conflict, 1982–1985. Analysis of a less aggressive surgical approach. J Neurosurg 72:15–21
20. Gonul E, Baysefer A, Kahraman S et al (1997) Causes of infections and management results in penetrating craniocerebral injuries. Neurosurg Rev 20:177–181
21. Siccardi D, Cavaliere R, Pau A, Lubinu F, Turtas S, Viale GL (1991) Penetrating craniocerebral missile injuries in civilians: a retrospective analysis of 314 cases. Surg Neurol 35:455–460
22. (2001) Part 2: Prognosis in penetrating brain injury. J Trauma 51:S44–S86
23. Kaufman HH, Makela ME, Lee KF, Haid RW Jr, Gildenberg PL (1986) Gunshot wounds to the head: a perspective. Neurosurgery 18:689–695
24. Qureshi AI, Tuhrim S, Broderick JP, Batjer HH, Hondo H, Hanley DF (2001) Spontaneous intracerebral hemorrhage. N Engl J Med 344:1450–1460
25. Greenberg MS, Arredondo N (2006) Handbook of neurosurgery, 6th edn. Greenberg Graphics; Thieme Medical Publishers, Lakeland, FL, New York
26. Wiebers DO, Whisnant JP, Sundt TM Jr, O'Fallon WM (1987) The significance of unruptured intracranial saccular aneurysms. J Neurosurg 66:23–29
27. Sacco RL, Wolf PA, Bharucha NE et al (1984) Subarachnoid and intracerebral hemorrhage: natural history, prognosis, and precursive factors in the Framingham Study. Neurology 34:847–854
28. Inagawa T, Kamiya K, Ogasawara H, Yano T (1987) Rebleeding of ruptured intracranial aneurysms in the acute stage. Surg Neurol 28:93–99
29. Kassell NF, Drake CG (1983) Review of the management of saccular aneurysms. Neurol Clin 1:73–86
30. Sarti C, Tuomilehto J, Salomaa V et al (1991) Epidemiology of subarachnoid hemorrhage in Finland from 1983 to 1985. Stroke 22:848–853
31. Broderick JP, Brott T, Tomsick T, Miller R, Huster G (1993) Intracerebral hemorrhage more than twice as common as subarachnoid hemorrhage. J Neurosurg 78:188–191
32. Milhorat TH, Krautheim M (1986) Results of early and delayed operations for ruptured intracranial aneurysms in two series of 100 consecutive patients. Surg Neurol 26:123–128
33. Disney L, Weir B, Grace M (1988) Factors influencing the outcome of aneurysm rupture in poor grade patients: a prospective series. Neurosurgery 23:1–9
34. Kassell NF, Torner JC, Jane JA, Haley EC Jr, Adams HP (1990) The International Cooperative Study on the timing of aneurysm surgery. Part 2: Surgical results. J Neurosurg 73:37–47
35. Weir B, Grace M, Hansen J, Rothberg C (1978) Time course of vasospasm in man. J Neurosurg 48:173–178
36. Molyneux AJ, Kerr RS, Yu LM et al (2005) International subarachnoid aneurysm trial (ISAT) of neurosurgical clipping versus endovascular coiling in 2143 patients with ruptured intracranial aneurysms: a randomised comparison of effects on survival, dependency, seizures, rebleeding, subgroups, and aneurysm occlusion. Lancet 366:809–817
37. Ryttlefors M, Enblad P, Kerr RS, Molyneux AJ (2008) International subarachnoid aneurysm trial of neurosurgical clipping versus endovascular coiling: subgroup analysis of 278 elderly patients. Stroke 39:2720–2726
38. Thornton J, Debrun GM, Aletich VA, Bashir Q, Charbel FT, Ausman J (2002) Follow-up angiography of intracranial aneurysms treated with endovascular placement of Guglielmi detachable coils. Neurosurgery 50:239–249, discussion 49–50
39. Parkinson RJ, Eddleman CS, Batjer HH, Bendok BR (2008) Giant intracranial aneurysms: endovascular challenges. Neurosurgery 62:1336–1345
40. Asano S, Hara T, Haisa T et al (2007) Outcomes of 24 patients with subarachnoid hemorrhage aged 80 years or older in a single center. Clin Neurol Neurosurg 109:853–857
41. Cai Y, Spelle L, Wang H et al (2005) Endovascular treatment of intracranial aneurysms in the elderly: single-center experience in 63 consecutive patients. Neurosurgery 57:1096–1102, discussion -102
42. Lanzino G, Kassell NF, Germanson TP et al (1996) Age and outcome after aneurysmal subarachnoid hemorrhage: why do older patients fare worse? J Neurosurg 85:410–418
43. Fridriksson SM, Hillman J, Saveland H, Brandt L (1995) Intracranial aneurysm surgery in the 8th and 9th decades of life: impact on population-based management outcome. Neurosurgery 37:627–631, discussion 31–2

44. Elliott JP, Le Roux PD (1998) Subarachnoid hemorrhage and cerebral aneurysms in the elderly. Neurosurg Clin N Am 9:587–594

45. Stapf C, Mohr JP, Pile-Spellman J, Solomon RA, Sacco RL, Connolly ES Jr (2001) Epidemiology and natural history of arteriovenous malformations. Neurosurg Focus 11:e1

46. Drake CG (1979) Cerebral arteriovenous malformations: considerations for and experience with surgical treatment in 166 cases. Clin Neurosurg 26:145–208

47. Stapf C, Mast H, Sciacca RR et al (2003) The New York Islands AVM Study: design, study progress, and initial results. Stroke 34:e29–e33

48. Stapf C, Mast H, Sciacca RR et al (2006) Predictors of hemorrhage in patients with untreated brain arteriovenous malformation. Neurology 66:1350–1355

49. Mendelow AD, Gregson BA, Fernandes HM et al (2005) Early surgery versus initial conservative treatment in patients with spontaneous supratentorial intracerebral haematomas in the International Surgical Trial in Intracerebral Haemorrhage (STICH): a randomised trial. Lancet 365:387–397

50. Brott T, Broderick J, Kothari R et al (1997) Early hemorrhage growth in patients with intracerebral hemorrhage. Stroke 28:1–5

51. Anderson CS, Huang Y, Wang JG et al (2008) Intensive blood pressure reduction in acute cerebral haemorrhage trial (INTERACT): a randomised pilot trial. Lancet Neurol 7:391–399

52. Kobayashi S, Sato A, Kageyama Y, Nakamura H, Watanabe Y, Yamaura A (1994) Treatment of hypertensive cerebellar hemorrhage–surgical or conservative management? Neurosurgery 34: 246–250, discussion 50–1

53. Mayer SA, Brun NC, Begtrup K et al (2008) Efficacy and safety of recombinant activated factor VII for acute intracerebral hemorrhage. N Engl J Med 358:2127–2137

54. Vahedi K, Hofmeijer J, Juettler E et al (2007) Early decompressive surgery in malignant infarction of the middle cerebral artery: a pooled analysis of three randomised controlled trials. Lancet Neurol 6:215–222

55. Vahedi K, Vicaut E, Mateo J et al (2007) Sequential-design, multicenter, randomized, controlled trial of early decompressive craniectomy in malignant middle cerebral artery infarction (DECIMAL Trial). Stroke 38:2506–2517

56. Juttler E, Schwab S, Schmiedek P et al (2007) Decompressive Surgery for the Treatment of Malignant Infarction of the Middle Cerebral Artery (DESTINY): a randomized, controlled trial. Stroke 38:2518–2525

57. Hofmeijer J, Amelink GJ, Algra A et al (2006) Hemicraniectomy after middle cerebral artery infarction with life-threatening edema trial (HAMLET). Protocol for a randomised controlled trial of decompressive surgery in space-occupying hemispheric infarction. Trials 7:29

58. Thanvi B, Robinson T (2006) Sporadic cerebral amyloid angiopathy–an important cause of cerebral haemorrhage in older people. Age Ageing 35:565–571

59. Adams HP Jr, del Zoppo G, Alberts MJ et al (2007) Guidelines for the early management of adults with ischemic stroke: a guideline from the American Heart Association/American Stroke Association Stroke Council, Clinical Cardiology Council, Cardiovascular Radiology and Intervention Council, and the Atherosclerotic Peripheral Vascular Disease and Quality of Care Outcomes in Research Interdisciplinary Working Groups: the American Academy of Neurology affirms the value of this guideline as an educational tool for neurologists. Stroke 38:1655–1711

60. Wardlaw JM, Sandercock PA, Berge E (2003) Thrombolytic therapy with recombinant tissue plasminogen activator for acute ischemic stroke: where do we go from here? A cumulative meta-analysis. Stroke 34:1437–1442

61. Heuschmann PU, Kolominsky-Rabas PL, Roether J et al (2004) Predictors of in-hospital mortality in patients with acute ischemic stroke treated with thrombolytic therapy. JAMA 292:1831–1838

62. Toni D, Fiorelli M, Bastianello S et al (1996) Hemorrhagic transformation of brain infarct: predictability in the first 5 hours from stroke onset and influence on clinical outcome. Neurology 46:341–345

63. Mahaffey KW, Granger CB, Sloan MA et al (1999) Neurosurgical evacuation of intracranial hemorrhage after thrombolytic therapy for acute myocardial infarction: experience from the GUSTO-I trial. Global Utilization of Streptokinase and tissue-plasminogen activator (tPA) for Occluded Coronary Arteries. Am Heart J 138:493–499

64. Ferro JM, Canhao P, Stam J, Bousser MG, Barinagarrementeria F (2004) Prognosis of cerebral vein and dural sinus thrombosis: results of the International Study on Cerebral Vein and Dural Sinus Thrombosis (ISCVT). Stroke 35:664–670

65. Hall WA, Truwit CL (2008) The surgical management of infections involving the cerebrum. Neurosurgery 62(Suppl 2):519–530, discussion 30-1

66. Osborn MK, Steinberg JP (2007) Subdural empyema and other suppurative complications of paranasal sinusitis. Lancet Infect Dis 7:62–67

67. Gavazzi G, Krause KH (2002) Ageing and infection. Lancet Infect Dis 2:659–666

68. Laws ER Jr (2003) Peripheral nerve surgery. J Neurosurg 98: 1157–1158

69. Maniker A, Passannante M (2003) Peripheral nerve surgery and neurosurgeons: results of a national survey of practice patterns and attitudes. J Neurosurg 98:1159–1164

70. Kim DH, Murovic JA, Tiel RL, Kline DG (2004) Mechanisms of injury in operative brachial plexus lesions. Neurosurg Focus 16:E2

71. Burnett MG, Zager EL (2004) Pathophysiology of peripheral nerve injury: a brief review. Neurosurg Focus 16:E1

72. Kim DH, Cho YJ, Tiel RL, Kline DG (2003) Outcomes of surgery in 1019 brachial plexus lesions treated at Louisiana State University Health Sciences Center. J Neurosurg 98:1005–1016

73. Belzberg AJ, Dorsi MJ, Storm PB, Moriarity JL (2004) Surgical repair of brachial plexus injury: a multinational survey of experienced peripheral nerve surgeons. J Neurosurg 101:365–376

74. Kim DH, Murovic JA, Tiel RL, Kline DG (2004) Penetrating injuries due to gunshot wounds involving the brachial plexus. Neurosurg Focus 16:E3

Chapter 87
Benign and Malignant Tumors of the Brain

Andrew D. Norden and Elizabeth B. Claus

Introduction

Data from the Central Brain Tumor Registry of the United States (CBTRUS) indicate that approximately 23,000 Americans were expected to be diagnosed with a primary cancer of the central nervous system (CNS) in 2007 [1]. The incidence rate of all primary malignant CNS tumors in the USA is estimated at 7.3 cases per 100,000 people annually [1]. Brain tumors are increasingly common as people age; approximately 15% of primary malignant brain tumors are diagnosed in individuals aged 70 years or more [2]. Survival rates among patients diagnosed with primary malignant brain tumors vary inversely with age. For example, among patients between the ages of 45 and 54, the 5-year survival rate is 24%, while this rate is only 5% for patients who are at least 75 years old (Table 87.1) [1]. In addition to those with primary brain tumors, up to 150,000 Americans are diagnosed each year with metastatic brain lesions [3], and many of these are elderly patients. This chapter provides a review and discussion of epidemiology and treatment of elderly patients with brain tumors. The focus is on primary tumors, but metastatic lesions will be addressed briefly as well.

Epidemiology and Prognosis

Glioma

Most primary brain tumors among the elderly are thought to be derived from glial cells and are therefore known as gliomas. Glial cells make up the supporting cells of the brain and assist neurons with a variety of structural, protective, and metabolic functions. Subcategories of glioma include astrocytoma, oligodendroglioma, and mixed glioma. According to the World Health Organization (WHO) classification, gliomas receive a histopathologic grade on the basis of microscopic features including cellularity, nuclear atypia, mitotic activity, vascular proliferation, and necrosis [4]. WHO grade I gliomas are typically localized, noninfiltrating lesions that occur predominantly in the pediatric population. Grade II tumors are diffuse, infiltrative neoplasms that usually occur in young adults with a mean age of 39 years [5]. Among elderly patients, the majority of gliomas are high-grade or malignant gliomas (Table 87.2). Subtypes include glioblastomas (GBM; WHO grade IV), anaplastic astrocytomas (WHO grade III), anaplastic oligodendrogliomas (WHO grade III), and anaplastic oligoastrocytomas (WHO grade III).

GBMs are the most common malignant brain tumors in elderly patients; they represent nearly 20% of all brain tumors in adults and have an incidence rate of 3.1 per 100,000 person years. The median age of diagnosis is 64 years, and these tumors are 1.7 times more common in males [1]. Despite a number of recent advances, median survival among newly diagnosed GBM patients *younger* than 70 years who receive optimal therapy is only 14.6 months [6]. Fewer than 4% of patients achieve 5-year survival [1]. Most data suggest that elderly patients with newly diagnosed GBM have a median survival of less than 9 months [7, 8]. Indeed, age is among the most important prognostic factors in GBM [9]. An emerging body of literature suggests that molecular differences in brain tumors may explain prognostic variability between patients of different ages [10]. In one study of 140 GBM specimens, the prognostic significance of *TP53* mutations, epidermal growth factor receptor amplification, *CDKN2A/ p16* alterations, and loss of chromosome 1p depended upon patient age [11].

Meningioma

Meningiomas are the most common primary intracranial tumors diagnosed in adults of all ages [1]. The prevalence

A.D. Norden (⊠)
Department of Neurology, Center for Neuro-Oncology, Dana-Farber Cancer Institute, Brigham and Women's Hospital,
Harvard Medical School, 44 Binney St, Boston, MA 02115, USA
e-mail: anorden@partners.org

R.A. Rosenthal et al. (eds.), *Principles and Practice of Geriatric Surgery*,
DOI 10.1007/978-1-4419-6999-6_87, © Springer Science+Business Media, LLC 2011

TABLE 87.1 Five-year survival rates among patients with primary malignant brain tumors of the CNS

Age (years)	Five-year survival rate (%)
0–19	66.0
20–44	49.2
45–54	24.0
55–64	11.1
65–74	6.7
75 +	4.7

Source: CBTRUS (2008). Statistical Report: Primary Brain Tumors in the United States, 2000–2004. Published by the Central Brain Tumor Registry of the United States [1]

TABLE 87.2 Age-specific incidence rates per 100,000 people per year for selected brain tumor histologies

Histology	Age at diagnosis (years)					
	35–44	45–54	55–64	65–74	75–84	85+
Glioblastoma	1.20	3.70	8.09	12.47	14.13	7.63
Anaplastic astrocytoma	0.48	0.60	0.89	1.07	1.00	0.30
Anaplastic oligodendroglioma	0.22	0.30	0.32	0.34	0.27	Unknown

of meningioma is estimated to be approximately 97.5/100,000 in the USA with over 150,000 individuals currently diagnosed. Data from CBTRUS reveal an age-adjusted incidence rate (per 100,000 person years) of 5.04 and 2.46 for females and males, respectively [1]. The incidence of meningioma increases with age with a median age of diagnosis of approximately 64 years. Although generally considered benign (WHO grade I), approximately 8% of meningiomas display aggressive features such as increased cellularity, high nuclear to cytoplasmatic ratio, increased mitotic activity, patternless growth, and foci of necrosis and are classified as atypical tumors (WHO grade II). Approximately 2–3% of meningiomas exhibit frank malignant histological signs and are classified as anaplastic meningiomas (WHO grade III). Atypical and anaplastic meningiomas account for significant morbidity and mortality. Histology is an important predictor of tumor recurrence rates. Although detailed population-based data are not available, recurrence rates are estimated at 3–20% for benign meningiomas, 30–40% for atypical meningiomas, and 50–80% for anaplastic meningiomas.

Primary Central Nervous System Lymphoma

Primary CNS lymphoma (PCNSL) is an unusual extranodal non-Hodgkin's lymphoma variant that exclusively involves the nervous system and eyes. Only rarely is there spread to the systemic compartment. PCNSL represents 3.1% of CNS tumors, with approximately 2,000 new diagnoses per year in the USA [1]. The reported incidence of PCNSL has increased over the past few decades, primarily due to increases in both immunocompromised individuals and the elderly. Between 1973 and 1984 in the USA, the incidence rate of PCNSL was 0.15 cases per 100,000 person years; between 1985 and 1997, the incidence rate more than tripled to 0.48 cases per 100,000 person years [12]. Reasons for the increase in incidence rates are controversial. Potential explanations include increased use of neuroimaging, changes in disease classification, and delayed response to a putative environmental toxin. Immunodeficiency is the strongest known risk factor for all subtypes of lymphoma, including PCNSL. Most immunocompetent patients with PCNSL are older adults, and there is a slight male preponderance. Although localized extranodal systemic non-Hodgkin's lymphoma is compatible with long-term survival in 70% or more of patients, PCNSL is almost universally fatal. Factors that predict decreased survival among patients with PCNSL include age greater than 60 years, impaired performance status, elevated serum lactate dehydrogenase, increased cerebrospinal fluid protein, and involvement of deep brain structures. Depending upon the number of adverse prognostic factors, 2-year survival rates vary between 24 and 85% [13]. A recent analysis in preparation by our group indicates that survival rates among PCNSL patients are increasing over time, perhaps due in part to advances in the chemotherapeutic management of this disease.

Risk Factors

The only well-validated risk factor for development of a glioma is exposure to ionizing radiation, generally in the form of therapeutic irradiation for cancer [14]. Radiation-induced brain tumors typically develop in young patients. A wide variety of environmental risk factors for primary brain tumors have been proposed [15]. The list of factors includes electromagnetic fields, trauma, occupational and industrial chemicals, medications including anticonvulsants, and viral infections, among others. Recent data show an intriguing association with atopy [16]. In a meta-analysis of 3,450 glioma patients, a history of atopy was associated with a relative risk for glioma diagnosis of 0.61 [17]. A history of an allergic condition or asthma was also protective. The biological basis for this association has yet to be elucidated. At present, no single risk factor has been consistently identified as being associated with cancer risk, particularly within the elderly population.

For meningioma, the evidence for ionizing radiation is even more marked with relative risks as high as 10 [18]. Evidence of an association between hormones and meningioma risk is suggested by a number of findings including the increased incidence of the disease in women versus men (2:1), the presence of estrogen and progesterone receptors on some meningiomas [19], a potential association between breast cancer and meningiomas [20], and an association in some studies between exogenous or endogenous hormones and meningioma risk [21]. These findings warrant consideration in the use of hormone replacement therapy in postmeno pausal women.

Genetics

Glioma

With respect to inherited genetic syndromes for glioma, highly penetrant but relatively rare inherited genes may exist for glioma susceptibility [22]. Some hereditary syndromes such as tuberous sclerosis, neurofibromatosis types 1 and 2, nevoid basal cell carcinoma syndrome, Li-Fraumeni syndrome as well as syndromes involving adenomatous polyps may be associated with a genetic predisposition to glioma. In a population-based study of 500 adults with glioma in San Francisco, less than 1% of cases had a known hereditary syndrome (one had tuberous sclerosis and three had neurofibromatosis) [23]. With respect to familial aggregation, the reported relative risks of brain tumors among family members of brain tumor cases range from nearly one to ten, with a twofold rate seen in larger studies [24]. Not all studies of siblings, and no studies of twins, have supported a simple genetic etiology. Formal segregation analyses have provided evidence for a genetic component but no clear mode of inheritance with approximately 5% of cases estimated to be familial [24]. One linkage study has been reported with statistically significant linkage to 15q23–26.3 for 15 Finnish families with multiple cases of glioma [25]. These data suggest, as for most neoplasms, that glioma development and growth is likely a function of the effects of many genes that are relatively prevalent but not highly penetrant and that interact with environmental exposures to confer risk. An international effort to locate genes for glioma via the collection of families with two or more members affected with glioma is currently underway (GLIOGENE), and results from the first genome-wide association study of glioma are currently in press. Recently, the first examination of DNA repair gene variants and glioma was presented with evidence for such an association [26]. In the most recent and largest study to date of genetic polymorphisms and meningioma risk, Interphone study reported a statistically significant association with meningioma for 12 single nucleotide polymorphisms (SNPs) drawn from DNA repair genes.

These investigators examined 1,127 tagging SNPs selected to capture most of the common variation in 136 DNA repair genes as well as an additional 388 putative functional SNPs (including 69 nonsynonymous coding SNPs that may identify the function of expressed proteins) in 631 cases and 637 controls drawn from five case/control series from the Interphone study. The Interphone study is a case/control project initially designed to examine the relationship between cell phone use and the risk of brain tumors, including meningioma. The group reported a novel and biologically intriguing association between meningioma risk and three variants in the gene that encodes breast cancer susceptibility gene 1-interacting protein 1 (BRIP1) (17q22) [26].

In addition to the study of inherited genes, scientists have attempted to elucidate the somatic genetic changes and pathways associated with the development of a number of primary brain tumors, including most prominently, those associated with the development of GBMs. GBM is considered to be a clinical manifestation of at least two pathways with respect to genetics (Fig. 87.1). One form appears to result from malignant progression of a low-grade astrocytoma. The timing of this transition or progression to a higher grade is variable, and it remains controversial whether aggressive therapy for a low-grade astrocytoma can prevent or delay the subsequent evolution of a GBM. There is evidence to suggest that the progression of tumor grade is associated with a series of genetic changes, similar to those seen for the progression from polyp to carcinoma in colon cancers. The second form of GBM appears to be a tumor that arises de novo in patients with no prior evidence of a low-grade glioma. When survival is measured for the two groups, there does not appear to be an advantage for either type. The latter de novo form is more commonly seen in the elderly population.

Data indicate that the evolution of GBM from a low-grade glioma is genetically distinct from the de novo GBM. Tumors that progress from a low-grade glioma to GBM are associated with p53 mutation. In contrast, de novo glioblastoma does not appear to manifest evidence of a p53 mutation; instead, these tumors have been shown to have amplification and mutation of epidermal growth factor receptor (*EGFR*) and amplification of *MDM2,* as well as loss of heterozygosity of chromosome 10 [27, 28]. Of interest is the fact that epidemiologic data from these studies suggest that advanced age is associated with *EGFR* and *MDM2* amplifications, a condition not present in gliomas arising in younger patients.

Meningioma

Few studies have examined the relationship between a personal diagnosis of meningioma and a family history of menin-gioma although evidence that such a history is

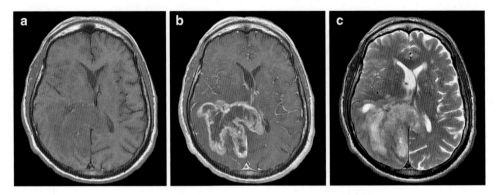

Figure 87.1 Magnetic resonance imaging (MRI) scan of a glioblastoma. (**a**) T1-weighted axial image shows a hypointense lesion involving the right parieto-occipital lobe and corpus callosum, with (**b**) central necrosis and peripheral enhancement following gadolinium administration. (**c**) T2-weighted image shows hyperintense signal and mass effect upon the ventricular system.

associated with risk does exist. Using data from the Swedish Family Cancer Database, Hemminki and Li reported a statistically significant association between meningioma diagnosis and a parental history of meningioma [standardized incidence ratio (SIR): 2.5, 95% CI: 1.3, 4.3] [29]. A recently published hospital-based study found that the risk of meningioma was increased among persons reporting a benign brain tumor (OR: 4.5, 95% CI: 1.2, 15.0) [30]. Population-based surveys suggest that highly penetrant but relatively rare inherited genes may exist for meningioma susceptibility, although it appears at present that these genes may be primarily seen in families with neurofibromatosis 2. Collections of families with multiple family members diagnosed with meningioma and who do not appear to carry inherited mutations in the *NF2* gene are relatively rarely identified despite the fact that up to 1% of the adult population may harbor such a diagnosis, indicating a wide spectrum of phenotypic expression with respect to clinical import. At present no family based linkage studies of meningioma have been reported. Recently, data from Israel provide evidence for genetic predisposition to radiation-associated meningioma [31], highlighting the role of inherited genetic factors in meningioma risk modification. In the most recent and largest study to date of genetic polymorphisms and meningioma risk, investigators from the Interphone study examined that 1,127 tagging SNPs selected to capture common variation in 136 DNA repair genes as well as an additional 388 putative functional SNPs in a combined case/control series of 631 cases and 637 controls drawn from five case/control series from the Interphone study [26]. The group reported a novel association between meningioma risk and the SNP rs496851, which maps to intron 4 of the gene that encodes breast cancer susceptibility gene 1-interacting protein 1 (BRIP1) (mapped at 17q22).

Lymphoma

There is virtually no published data about the potential heritability of PCNSL. Due to the rarity of the disease, there is a limited understanding of its molecular pathogenesis, particularly in comparison to malignant glioma. While p53 mutations are rare, inactivation of the cell cycle regulators p14^{ARF} and p16^{INK4A} is commonly observed [32]. Other abnormalities include translocations of the *BCL6* gene and 6q deletions; both of these appear to have prognostic significance [33].

Symptoms

The presenting symptoms for intracranial lesions vary by tumor location, rate of growth, type of tumor, and age. In elderly patients, the most common presentations are confusion or mental status change, personality change, headache, seizure (often with associated motor or sensory deficits), and aphasia. However, any combination of neurologic symptoms is possible. Symptoms frequently develop over a period of weeks or months. Papilledema and nausea or vomiting are less common features in elderly patients, likely because posterior fossa tumors are uncommon in this age group. In some cases, the symptoms may be confused with more common conditions such as dementia (when cognitive complaints predominate) or cerebrovascular disease (when neurologic deficits develop acutely). The presenting symptoms may be subtle, particularly if the tumor is located in a clinically "silent" area of the brain such as the anterior frontal lobe or if it grows slowly (as is often the case, for example, with meningiomas). Tumor symptoms may present acutely, as with a seizure or hydrocephalus, when the flow of cerebrospinal fluid is suddenly blocked by the tumor.

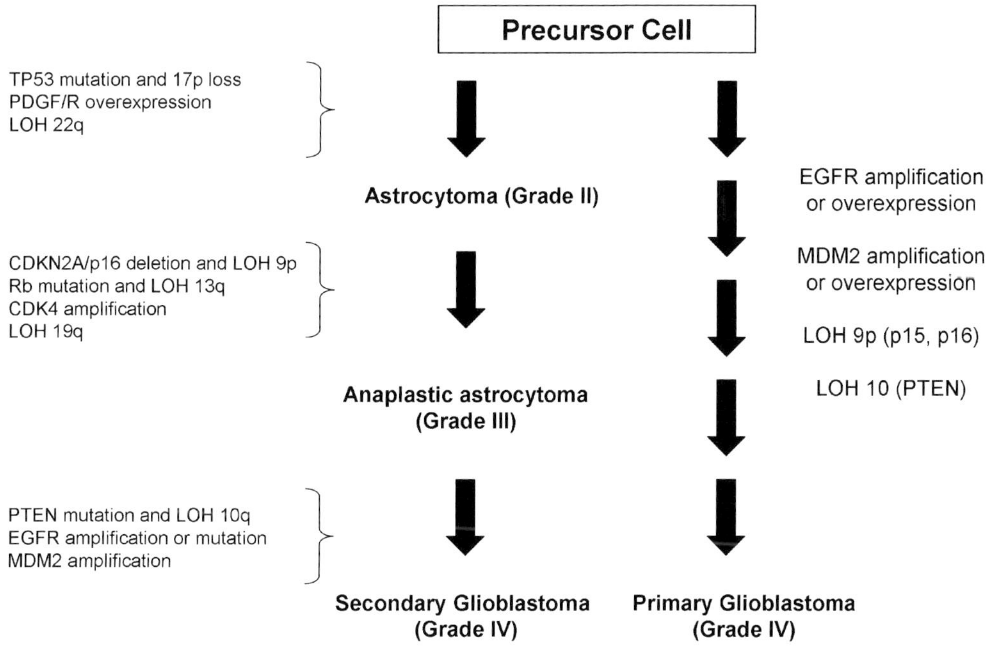

FIGURE 87.2 Molecular changes associated with glioma progression. *PDGF/R* platelet-derived growth factor/receptor, *LOH* loss of heterozygosity, *CDK* cyclin-dependent kinase, *Rb* retinoblastoma, *PTEN* phosphate and tensin homolog deleted on chromosome 10, *EGFR* epidermal growth factor receptor, *MDM2* murine double minute 2 (from Tysnes and Mahesparan [28]. Reprinted with kind permission from Springer Science+Business Media).

Diagnosis

Most brain tumors in the elderly are now identified by neuroimaging with computed tomography (CT) or magnetic resonance imaging (MRI) scans (Fig. 87.2). Although these modalities are critical for tumor detection and often suggest the correct histologic diagnosis, tissue sampling is generally required before treatment can be initiated. These noninvasive tests are usually well tolerated by the elderly patient, but renal function may be adversely affected by iodinated contrast agents used in CT scanning. Elderly patients with impaired renal function may also be at risk for nephrogenic systemic fibrosis when they receive gadolinium-based contrast agents for MRI scanning [34]. In addition to CT and MRI, angiography may play a role in defining the vascular supply of tumors such as meningiomas, although in the elderly patient, the procedural risks may outweigh the benefits of any information gained [35]. In many instances, noninvasive vascular imaging with CT or MR angiography may be sufficient.

The use of diagnostic imaging is of particular interest in the elderly, as its increased use in western countries has been proposed as one of the reasons for the reported increase in brain tumors among the elderly in the 1970s and 1980s. An intriguing population-based study recently reported incidental findings detected on brain MRI scans obtained in nearly 8,000 individuals [36]. Among the abnormalities observed were benign tumors (1.6%), pituitary macroadenomas

TABLE 87.3 Distribution of incidental findings on brain MRI according to age

| Finding | Age (years) | | |
	45–59 (n=750)	60–74 (n=993)	75–97 (n=257)
Meningioma – n (%)	4 (0.5)	10 (1.0)	4 (1.6)
Infarct – n (%)	30 (4.0)	68 (6.8)	47 (18.3)

Source: Data from Vernooij et al. [36]

(0.3%), vestibular schwannomas (0.2%), and one possible low-grade glioma (<0.1%). The benign tumors were mostly composed of meningiomas, and these ranged in diameter from 5 to 60 mm. There was also one case of multiple brain metastases in a patient with a history of lung cancer. The largest proportion of incidental meningiomas was discovered in subjects aged 75–97 years (Table 87.3). A continued examination of the incidence of brain tumors in elderly patients in relation to the proportion diagnosed solely by means of radiology will be of interest in the coming years.

Surgery

Unlike for PCNSL, in which the surgeon's role is limited to biopsy for tissue diagnosis, surgery is a critical component of treatment for gliomas. Surgical options that are frequently considered include gross total resection, partial resection, and stereotactic biopsy. Unfortunately, data to guide surgical decision-making are limited. There are no published studies that examined survival rates and quality of life among elderly patients with brain tumors by type of surgical management. Furthermore, there are no prospective, randomized trials of surgery for this age group. Despite limited data, the standard of care for most patients with GBM involves maximal safe resection followed by radiation and chemotherapy [6]. Some meticulous retrospective data suggest a survival benefit for patients who undergo maximal surgical resection [37], but this result is somewhat controversial. Important issues to consider in deciding between biopsy and resection in all patients include tumor location (and especially proximity to eloquent brain), the patient's general health, and degree of mass effect or midline shift. Stereotactic brain biopsy with a frame or frameless image-guided technique is safe, well tolerated, and typically requires only an overnight hospital stay. An important caveat is that biopsy allows for pathologic evaluation of a small portion of the tumor; according to one study, pathologic diagnosis (more often pathologic grade than histologic type) may change nearly half of the time if surgical resection is performed subsequent to biopsy [38].

The current literature uniformly reports age as the most significant variable correlated with survival, with a less favorable prognosis associated with increased age [39]. For this chapter, we reviewed data from the Connecticut Tumor Registry (CTR), which indicated that the overall 1- and 5-year survival rates for individuals over the age of 70 diagnosed with GBM were 20 and 3%, respectively. This age group, therefore, shows 1- and 5-year death rates that are 1.3- and 1.8-fold higher, respectively, than those of individuals diagnosed prior to 70 years, respectively. Within these CTR data, survival rates for individuals diagnosed with astrocytoma over the age of 70 are somewhat more encouraging, with 59 and 36% of these individuals remaining alive 1 and 5 years, respectively, after diagnosis. These older patients are 1.3 and 2.7 times more likely to succumb to their disease at these time points than are individuals diagnosed prior to age 70, highlighting again the deleterious effect of age on outcome.

Despite the fact that elderly patients have less favorable survival rates, there is limited evidence that surgery benefits these patients if they are selected carefully [40]. For example, the general medical condition and neurologic status must be considered. As would be expected, patients with poor Karnofsky performance status (KPS) scores, a measure of functional status (Table 87.4), do less well with respect to survival [14]. In general, elderly patients who undergo craniotomy for primary brain tumor resection achieve longer survival than those who undergo biopsy [40], but this benefit is complicated by intraoperative and postoperative mortality and morbidity rates, which exceed those in younger individuals [41]. Additionally, most studies that report better outcomes for elderly patients who undergo craniotomy are

Table 87.4 Karnofsky performance status (KPS) score

Score	Interpretation
100	Normal
90	Normal activity; minor signs or symptoms
80	Normal activity with effort; some signs or symptoms
70	Cares for self; unable to do normal activity or active work
60	Requires occasional assistance, but cares for most personal needs
50	Requires considerable assistance and frequent medical care
40	Disabled; requires special care and assistance
30	Severely disabled; hospital admission is indicated but death not imminent
20	Very sick; hospitalization necessary; active supportive treatment necessary
10	Moribund; fatal processes progressing rapidly
0	Dead

susceptible to selection bias, as the patients in these studies often have multiple favorable prognostic factors, age being the sole exception.

The specifics of surgical treatment vary according to histologic subtype and location of the lesion within the CNS. Most primary brain tumors in the elderly are located supratentorially, particularly in the cerebral hemispheres, making a surgical approach feasible. In general, if a tumor is surgically accessible (i.e., not deeply placed in such regions as the brainstem or hypothalamus), surgical resection appears to offer the greatest overall benefit to most patients (both young and old) with respect to survival and quality of life, as measured by the ability to function independently. A study by Kelly and Hunt examined a retrospective, consecutive series of 128 patients diagnosed with GBMs at 65–83 years of age (mean age 71 years) [42]. The study compared survival rates for individuals undergoing stereotactic biopsy with those undergoing stereotactic gross resection. The two groups did not differ significantly with respect to age, KPS score, or presenting symptoms. Individuals with brainstem, callosal, or thalamic tumors were treated primarily by biopsy rather than gross resection. The authors reported that the mean survival times in the biopsy and resection groups were 15.4 and 27.0 weeks ($p=0.01$), respectively. Of note, approximately 20% of elderly patients undergoing resection survived beyond 1 year. As is noted by the authors, patients were not randomly assigned to treatment groups; hence the assignment to treatment group and baseline expected survival are likely to be correlated. In addition, because of the small sample size, more sophisticated multivariate analyses could not sort out the interplay between treatment, irradiation, tumor location, and other variables.

Surgery has long been considered the treatment of choice for most meningiomas, as surgery alone is curative in most cases. In order to achieve cure of a benign meningioma, the tumor must be completely resected in addition to its dural attachment and infiltrated bone [43]. In 1957, Simpson proposed a widely used five-level grading system that is based on the extent of surgical resection; Simpson grade 1 and 2 tumors are synonymous with gross total resection, although classification as grade 2 allows the dura to be left behind with reliable coagulation of the dural attachment. Advanced surgical techniques including image guidance and intraoperative imaging have increased the proportion of gross total resections in recent years [44]. Experimental approaches to optimize surgical resections such as laser-induced fluorescence spectroscopy [45], radioimmunoguidance [46], or intraoperative photodynamic diagnosis with 5-aminolevulinic acid [47] may prove useful in the future.

In an older series of 657 patients with surgically resected benign meningiomas, the recurrence rate at 20 years was 19% [48]. Comparable data have not been published for patients treated with modern neurosurgical techniques. Gross total resection results in a 5-year overall survival of approximately 85% and 5-year progression-free survival of approximately 90% for benign meningiomas [49]. Approximate recurrence rates for benign tumors that are incompletely resected are 30, 60, and 90% at 5, 10, and 15 years, respectively [43]. High recurrence rates are observed when atypical and malignant meningiomas are treated with surgery alone.

Although surgery may be curative, management decisions for patients with meningiomas must account for a variety of factors including patient age, performance status, tumor size and location, history of tumor growth, peritumoral edema, and symptoms. Small retrospective studies have recently attempted to quantify the growth rate of meningiomas during serial radiographic observation, but no large studies are available to allow for the prediction of growth either overall or by age. Many benign meningiomas are slow growing, although there is substantial variability in growth rates that cannot be reliably predicted using clinical factors [50, 51].

Radiation Therapy

Data show that individuals who receive radiation therapy after surgical resection for gliomas have an increased survival time relative to those who undergo surgery alone (with or without chemotherapy). The extent to which radiation therapy is effective, however, is once again dependent on age, with elderly individuals (defined in most studies as more than 60 years) faring less well [7]. Data from the CTR indicate that 44% of individuals diagnosed with all types of primary brain tumors over the age of 69 received radiation therapy. For those over the age of 69 years diagnosed with GBM or astrocytoma, data from the CTR indicate that there is no benefit from radiation therapy with respect to survival time. This differs from what is reported for younger individuals within the registry. For example, among patients

diagnosed with astrocytoma, those under 70 years of age who received radiation therapy had a survival time that was 1.33 times that of individuals who did not receive radiation therapy. Among patients diagnosed with astrocytoma who were 70 years of age or more, those who received radiation were less likely to survive than were those who did not receive such therapy. Although these data are intriguing, the statistics obtained from them must be interpreted with caution because there are insufficient data to explain these results.

The negative influence of age on outcome and survival in GBM patients is so pervasive it has led many clinicians and researchers to adjust treatment protocols for elderly patients in an effort to minimize the time spent in treatment, particularly when survival is estimated to be less than 6 months. For example, standard radiation therapy for a glioma is delivered in 1.8–2.0 Gy fractions with five treatments each week for a period of 6–7 weeks, with a total radiation dose of 60 Gy. A variety of abbreviated radiation schedules have been tested. In an important recent study, 100 newly diagnosed GBM patients who were at least 60 years old were randomized to standard radiation (60 Gy over 6 weeks; $n=51$) or a shorter course (40 Gy over 3 weeks; $n=49$) [52]. The groups were similar with respect to age, KPS, extent of surgical resection, quality-of-life, and time to start of radiation therapy. Median survival from the time of diagnosis was 5.9 months for the standard radiation group and 6.1 months for the abbreviated radiation group ($p=0.61$). Survival at 6 months was also similar. The trial measured health-related quality-of-life and found no difference between the groups. On the basis of these results and similar results obtained from a number of retrospective analyses, we routinely treat elderly GBM patients with abbreviated radiation therapy at our institution.

Given uncertainty about the benefit of radiation therapy for malignant glioma patients 70 years of age or older, a French group recently reported results from a trial in which patients were randomized to supportive care with or without radiation therapy (50 Gy over approximately 6 weeks) [8]. Patients had KPS scores of 70 or higher. The trial was stopped at the first interim analysis after 85 patients were enrolled. Patients in the two treatment groups were similar with respect to age, KPS, type of surgery, and use of corticosteroids. At a median follow-up of 21 weeks, 90% of patients had succumbed to the disease. The hazard ratio for death in the radiation group was 0.47 ($p=0.002$), indicating a 53% relative reduction in the risk of death compared with patients who received supportive care alone. Median overall survival was 29.1 weeks in the radiation group as compared to 16.9 weeks with supportive care alone. Progression-free survival was also significantly prolonged by radiation therapy. After adjusting for other predictors of survival, the hazard ratio for death in the radiation group was 0.42. Another interesting observation was that the extent of surgery (gross total vs. partial resection or biopsy) was associated with survival (hazard ratio for death among patients who underwent gross total resection, 0.49; $p=0.005$). There were no differences in health-related quality-of-life associated with the addition of radiation therapy. These data convincingly demonstrate that elderly patients with good performance can benefit from radiation therapy.

While surgery is often the only treatment modality required for readily accessible meningiomas of the cerebral or cerebellar convexity, meningiomas that occur in many other locations cannot be completely resected without significant morbidity. Parasagittal tumors often abut or invade the sagittal sinus, generally requiring the surgeon to leave behind a margin of tumor tissue [44]. Other technically difficult regions include the cavernous sinus and clivus. Additionally, atypical and malignant meningiomas may have high recurrence rates following even gross total resection. Radiation therapy has a role in meningioma management when gross total resection cannot be safely achieved or when tumors recur following surgery; radiation is routinely provided as adjuvant therapy following resection of atypical and malignant meningiomas [53].

Published data regarding the use of radiation for meningiomas comprise primarily single-institution retrospective series of variable quality. These studies often include heterogeneous patient populations and are susceptible to selection bias. However, there is nearly universal agreement that radiation improves local control. In most modern reports, radiation doses of 50–55 Gy are provided in 1.8–2.0 Gy fractions to the gross tumor volume and a margin of variable size. Five-year progression-free survival for benign meningiomas treated with radiation following incomplete resection is at least 80% and may be higher than 95% [54]. Fractionated radiation with three-dimensional conformal planning or intensity-modulated radiation therapy [55] has reduced radiation dose to normal tissues, and toxicity rates of less than 2% are generally reported [56].

Stereotactic radiosurgery (SRS) is a technique of external irradiation that utilizes multiple convergent beams to deliver a high single dose of radiation to a discrete treatment volume, usually less than 3–4 cm. Radiosurgery can be performed with high energy X-rays produced by a linear accelerator, with gamma radiation, and with charged particles such as protons. All of the stereotactic radiation techniques produce a rapid fall-off of dose at the edge of the target volume resulting in a clinically insignificant radiation dose to normal nontarget tissue. Because many meningiomas are small, well-circumscribed, and easily identified on neuroimaging, they often represent excellent SRS targets.

Using SRS doses of 12–20 Gy to treat meningiomas as primary or adjuvant therapy, 5-year progression-free survival rates of 87–98.5% are reported; treatment-related

complications depend, in part, on the treatment dose and occur in 2.5–13% of cases [57]. Typical toxicities include symptomatic edema following treatment or injury to adjacent cranial nerves. Vascular complications such as internal carotid artery occlusion following SRS for cavernous sinus meningiomas occur rarely. In an effort to reduce toxicity, fractionated stereotactic radiotherapy (FSR) has also been evaluated in meningioma therapy. Potential advantages of FSR include the ability to treat tumors larger than 3–4 cm and tumors that are in close contact with critical structures such as cranial nerves, blood vessels, or the brainstem. At this time, there is no published data to suggest that one stereotactic radiation approach is superior. In the only reported comparative evaluation of FSR and SRS, there was no clear difference with respect to local control, toxicity, and impact on neurologic function [58]. However, interpretation of the results must take into account the differing indications for FSR and SRS treatment. Fractionation should generally be considered for tumors larger than 3–4 cm or those that are in close proximity to critical structures [57].

Chemotherapy

The first randomized clinical trials of chemotherapy for malignant gliomas studied nitrosoureas (carmustine [BCNU] and lomustine [CCNU]), lipid-soluble agents that readily cross the blood–brain barrier (BBB). These studies suggested that chemotherapy prolongs survival to a limited extent [59, 60]. However, they were limited by important methodological issues such as small sample size, failure to stratify patients according to histologic subtypes, and variable response criteria. Subsequent meta-analyses in 1994 and 2002 confirmed that chemotherapy provides a modest survival benefit (a 6–10% increase in 1-year survival) for patients with malignant glioma [61, 62]. In light of these data, most newly diagnosed malignant glioma patients in the USA received adjuvant chemotherapy. Frequently prescribed regimens were BCNU monotherapy or PCV (procarbazine, CCNU, and vincristine).

A new standard of care emerged in 2005 with the publication of a large, randomized, phase III trial that included 573 newly diagnosed GBM patients from 85 centers in Europe and Canada [6]. All patients underwent maximal feasible resection and standard radiation therapy (60 Gy over 6 weeks); they were randomized to receive temozolomide chemotherapy or no chemotherapy. Temozolomide is an orally bioavailable alkylating agent that readily crosses the BBB and in the majority of patients produces only mild adverse effects. Fewer than 10% of patients experience significant myelosuppression. Patients randomized to the chemotherapy arm received radiotherapy with concurrent temozolomide at a dose of 75 mg/m²/day. After a 4-week break, patients received six cycles of adjuvant temozolomide (150–200 mg/m²/day for 5 days during each 28-day cycle). Median survival improved with temozolomide therapy from 12.1 to 14.6 months, and the 2-year survival rate also improved markedly from 10.4 to 26.5% (p=0.001).

Patients included in this landmark study by Stupp et al. were between 18 and 70 years of age (median 56). Therefore, these data leave unanswered the question of whether adding chemotherapy to radiation therapy and surgery is beneficial among elderly patients. No randomized data have been published to date, but some reports are informative. In a recent analysis, patients treated in the study reported by Stupp et al. were classified according to a modified version of the Radiation Therapy Oncology Group recursive partitioning analysis (RPA) classification [63]. The RPA model was developed to help stratify patients into homogeneous groups with similar prognoses for the purposes of comparison between clinical trials [9]. The modified version developed for retrospective analysis of the Stupp et al. trial included age, World Health Organization (WHO) performance status, extent of surgery, and mental status (Table 87.5). Because all patients in the study had GBM as opposed to anaplastic glioma, they were classified into RPA classes III–V. For RPA classes III, IV, and V, survival times were 17, 15, and 10 months, respectively. The benefit of chemotherapy was statistically significant for patients in RPA classes III and IV. For patients in RPA class V, however, the survival difference between the treatment arms was marginal. Median survival was 10 months for patients who received chemotherapy as compared to 9 months for patients who received radiation therapy alone (p=0.054). Since all the patients in class V were 50 years of age or older, this suggests that the benefit of chemotherapy for older patients is uncertain [63].

In a retrospective series, 43 patients 65 years or age or older (median 67) were treated after surgery with radiation and concurrent low-dose temozolomide (50–75 mg/m²). A small subset of patients also received adjuvant temozolomide. Median survival was 11 months and depended on the extent of resection and RPA class. All but five patients (88%)

tolerated radiation and concurrent chemotherapy without significant toxicity. Given that most previous series of elderly GBM patients found median survival rates in the range of 4–9 months, the authors conclude that concurrent chemotherapy is a reasonable consideration in the elderly population. Results from other small retrospective series support this conclusion [64]. Some clinical trial data suggest that temozolomide chemotherapy alone following surgery may also have a role [65]. Because the published data regarding the use of chemotherapy in elderly patients involve small numbers of patients with variable age, performance status, extent of resection, timing and dose of radiotherapy, and dose and schedule of chemotherapy, it is challenging to collate the results and draw definitive conclusions. At present, it seems clear that chemotherapy may be useful for at least a subset of elderly patients. Future work will better define the characteristics of the patients who should be considered for aggressive medical treatment.

Another method of chemotherapy administration is interstitial chemotherapy. This approach involves direct administration of drug into the tumor resection cavity. The primary advantage is the ability to achieve high concentrations of chemotherapeutic agent at the site of the tumor with minimal systemic toxicity. Additionally, interstitial administration eliminates the problem of BBB penetration. Techniques that have been used include catheter implantation and placement of biodegradable polymer wafers impregnated with BCNU. The wafers are designed to release BCNU over several weeks after they have been placed on the surface of the tumor resection cavity. In a double-blind, randomized, phase III trial of 240 newly diagnosed malignant glioma patients, patients received either conventional therapy (surgery followed by radiation therapy) with placement of a BCNU wafer or conventional therapy with placement of an identical placebo wafer [66]. The median survival was significantly increased for the active wafer group (13.9 months) compared with the placebo wafer group (11.6 months). Adverse event rates were similar. Patients in this study were between 18 and 65 years of age.

As is clear from the discussion, elderly patients are excluded from many clinical trials for malignant glioma. Similar exclusion of elderly patients is noted in data from the Connecticut Tumor Registry, which lists only 8% of patients over the age of 70 years as having received chemotherapy for treatment of a CNS tumor. This exclusion reflects an underlying belief that chemotherapy is not beneficial in elderly patients, a belief that may be correct but is not clearly supported by high-quality data.

As opposed to malignant glioma therapy, the role of chemotherapy in meningioma therapy has largely been limited to treatment of tumors that recur after surgery and RT options are exhausted. Data obtained from small clinical trials and

TABLE 87.5 Modified recursive partitioning analysis classes

RPA Class	Criteria
III	Less than 50 years of age and WHO PS 0
IV	Less than 50 years of age and WHO PS 1–2
	or
	At least 50 years of age, at least partial resection, and MMSE score at least 27
V	At least 50 years of age, biopsy only, and MMSE score less than 27

WHO PS World Health Organization performance status, *MMSE* Foley mini-mental status examination
Source: Data from Mirimanoff et al. [63]

case series suggest that most chemotherapeutics have only minimal activity against meningiomas, although promising investigational medical therapies include somatostatin receptor agonists [67] and inhibitors of angiogenesis. In the case of PCNSL, methotrexate-based chemotherapy regimens represent the mainstay of therapy. Blood–brain barrier penetration by methotrexate is limited, so high-dose systemic treatment ($4–8$ g/m^2) is required to achieve cytotoxic levels in the nervous system. When methotrexate-based chemotherapy is combined with whole brain RT, 2-year survival is observed in 43–73% of patients, and median survival is reported in the range of 30–60 months [68]. Because of treatment-related neurotoxicity rates as high as 25%, there has been growing interest in methotrexate-based chemotherapy alone without radiation. Small studies reveal promising results with median overall survival of 4–5 years [69]. At present, most centers that care for patients with PCNSL provide methotrexate-based combination chemotherapy regimens with or without radiation. The use of additional chemotherapeutic agents and intrathecal chemotherapeutics varies from center to center.

Corticosteroids

Steroid therapy is a useful adjunctive therapy for treatment of CNS tumors in patients of all ages. It may be particularly beneficial in older patients when surgical or additional treatments are deemed unwise [70]. The most frequently used steroid, dexamethasone, may be given intravenously or orally. Typically, the initial dose is approximately 10 mg, with maintenance doses of 2–6 mg every 6–12 h thereafter. The medication works by reducing vasogenic edema; clinical response and neurologic improvement are generally seen within 24 h. Although complications do occur (hyperglycemia, impaired wound healing, and gastrointestinal ulcers), the benefits often outweigh the risks, particularly with respect to quality of life.

It is important to note that corticosteroids alone may provoke rapid, dramatic tumor responses in as many as 40% of PCNSL patients [71]. The responses are almost always short-lived, but they can be problematic when they occur prior to definitive diagnosis. Because steroids result in lymphocyte apoptosis, such treatment can dramatically reduce diagnostic yield, regardless of diagnostic modality employed. Even stereotactic biopsy may be nondiagnostic in a patient who has been treated with a single large dose of dexamethasone. Of course, steroid administration may be mandatory in a patient who presents with decreased level of consciousness due to mass effect. In this case, definitive diagnosis may be delayed by weeks or months.

Metastatic Brain Tumors

Secondary, or metastatic, brain tumors represent the majority of brain tumors in the elderly, with intracranial metastases occurring in approximately one-third of individuals initially diagnosed with a systemic malignancy. The prevalence of brain metastases is rising because of improved survival of cancer patients thanks to therapeutic advances, the aging of the population, and enhanced detection of clinically silent lesions. Among the elderly, the most common origins of brain metastasis include lung cancer (50%), breast cancer (15–20%), and melanoma (10%). The next most frequent sources include renal cancer, colorectal cancer, lymphoma, and tumors of unknown primary. Metastases from breast, colon, and renal cell carcinoma are often single, while melanoma and lung cancer have a greater tendency to produce multiple metastases. MRI studies suggest that single metastases account for one-third to one quarter of patients with brain metastases. This is important because SRS is effective only in patients with a limited number of metastases.

Brain metastases are associated with a poor prognosis. Depending on the patient's age, functional status, extent of systemic disease, and number of metastases, median survival ranges from 2 to 14 months. Therapeutic modalities that may be used singly or in combination include surgery, SRS, whole brain RT, and chemotherapy. The optimal combination of therapies for each patient depends on the consideration of various factors including the location, size, and number of brain metastases; patient age, general condition, and neurological status; extent of systemic cancer; and the tumor's response to past therapy and its potential response to future treatments. There are limited data to indicate whether survival differs by age group, although, in general, elderly patients do less well with respect to survival and quality of life.

Surgery

The goals of surgery are to provide immediate relief of neurological symptoms due to mass effect, to establish a histological diagnosis, to provide local control of the metastasis, and if possible, to prolong survival. In general, surgery should be considered for patients with good prognostic factors when there is a single metastasis in an accessible location, especially if the tumor is producing mass effect. This approach is based on the results of two prospective randomized trials [72, 73]. In both studies, reasonably functional patients with a single brain metastasis and well-controlled extracranial disease were randomized to receive stereotactic biopsy of the metastasis followed by whole brain RT versus surgical resection followed by whole brain RT. Patients in the surgery plus radiation group had fewer local recurrences, improved survival (40 versus 15 weeks and 10 versus 6 months), and better performance status than patients who received radiation alone. In addition, patients who had their single metastases removed remained functionally independent longer (38 vs. 8 weeks) and had fewer recurrences at the site of the original metastasis (20 vs. 52%).

Radiation

Patients who are deemed poor surgical candidates because of multiple or inaccessible lesions or poor performance status are best treated with whole brain RT. Recent data indicate that SRS may have an important role in brain metastasis management and may be a viable alternative to surgery in some situations [74]. For example, SRS may be useful for small metastases not producing mass effect. It can also be used to treat lesions in the brainstem or eloquent areas with less risk than surgery. Additionally, because of the noninvasive, outpatient nature of SRS, it is associated with less morbidity and may be a rational consideration in elderly patients. As is the case for conventional surgery, careful selection of patients is critical; patients without good prognostic factors are unlikely to benefit. Although the precise role for SRS remains to be defined by a randomized, prospective trial, many retrospective studies suggest that SRS outcomes for appropriately selected patients are equivalent to those achieved with conventional surgery.

Conclusions

Much of the reason for the poor prognosis noted in elderly patients diagnosed with primary brain tumors is related to the negative impact that neurologic deficits have on survival and the reduced capacity for recovery and adaptation present in the aged patient. Addition of other comorbid conditions (i.e., cardiac, pulmonary, renal, or musculoskeletal disease) associated with advanced age increases the risk of surgical intervention and reduces the systemic tolerance to radiation therapy and chemotherapy. As a result, elderly patients as a group are more likely to be functionally impaired by their disease than are younger patients; and they may have less capacity to withstand the adverse effects of therapy, potentially limiting their treatment options. The negative influence of age on outcome and survival in GBM patients is so pervasive that some have suggested it is not possible to demonstrate any survival benefit from any treatment in patients over the age of 70 years.

Elderly Americans, however, are probably healthier and less disabled than they were perceived to be in the past. This is reflected in all aspects of society including the workplace where mandatory retirement restrictions are beginning to fall and more and more senior citizens enter or reenter the workforce. Although as a group elderly patients may do less well, there may be a significant subset of individuals who benefit from treatment of their CNS tumors. These issues indicate that clinical trials examining the effect of various treatments for primary and metastatic brain tumors in the elderly are needed, including whether survival can be improved with less toxicity and morbidity. This issue remains controversial with respect to the cost/benefit ratio to society. For primary brain tumors, the effort would require multicenter trials, as reports of outcome are relatively rare. For metastatic lesions, the pool of eligible patients is much greater, allowing one or two centers to organize studies. The ability to mount such studies depends greatly on society's willingness to accommodate the medical needs of its aging population within the framework of stressed medical resources.

Summary

- Older individuals are more likely to be diagnosed with primary brain tumors; among elderly patients with GBM, the most common primary malignant brain tumor in adults, median survival is reported to be in the range of 4–9 months.
- The diagnosis of a primary brain tumor in an elderly patient is often suggested by results from a CT or MRI scan, but definitive diagnosis requires tissue confirmation.
- Although outcome data are limited, elderly patients who are healthy enough for surgery and have good performance status may be good candidates for aggressive resection of primary brain tumors.
- Radiation therapy and chemotherapy are important adjuvant treatments for adults with gliomas, and recent data suggest that a subset of elderly patients may benefit from these interventions as well.
- Corticosteroids are useful in managing brain edema related to tumors in patients of any age.
- The molecular pathogenesis of gliomas may differ in young and old patients, suggesting that the optimal therapeutic approaches may also be different between the two populations.
- Metastatic brain tumors are common and are associated with a dismal prognosis in elderly patients.
- In order to improve outcomes for elderly patients with brain tumors, older individuals must be included in clinical trials of surgical, radiation, and medical treatments.

CASE STUDY

An otherwise healthy 81-year-old woman with controlled hypertension presents to her primary care physician at the request of her family because of gait instability and mild confusion over the past 3 weeks. On exam, she is slightly disoriented and has a mild left hemiparesis. Concerned about possible stroke, the physician orders a brain MRI scan (Fig. 87.2). This shows a large, enhancing mass in the right parietal lobe that is interpreted as suspicious for malignant glioma. Given the location of the lesion in the right parietal lobe and involving the corpus callosum, surgical resection is not felt to be the best option. The patient and her family agree to stereotactic biopsy for definitive diagnosis. The procedure is uncomplicated, and the patient is discharged from the hospital after 48 h. High-dose dexamethasone is started immediately after surgery, which results in improved mental status and resolution of hemiparesis.

As expected, the pathology results return as glioblastoma. The patient and her family meet with an oncologist to discuss treatment options. In light of her advanced age and preference to minimize adverse effects to the extent possible, she agrees to an abbreviated course of radiation therapy with concurrent temozolomide chemotherapy. Because she tolerates this treatment well, she goes on to receive four cycles of adjuvant temozolomide. Unfortunately, after this treatment, the patient develops worsening left hemiparesis. A brain MRI scan shows tumor growth. The patient considers palliative surgical debulking and a variety of chemotherapy options, but she ultimately declines further treatment. She enrolls in a home hospice program where she enjoys relatively good quality-of-life for 6 weeks before experiencing a rapid neurologic decline. She dies comfortably at home with multiple family members present.

References

1. CBTRUS (2008). Statistical Report: Primary Brain Tumors in the United States, 2000–2004. Published by the Central Brain Tumor Registry of the United States
2. Parker SL, Tong T, Bolden S et al (1997) Cancer statistics. CA Cancer J Clin 47:5–27
3. Barnholtz-Sloan JS, Sloan AE, Davis FG et al (2004) Incidence proportions of brain metastases in patients diagnosed (1973 to 2001) in the Metropolitan Detroit Cancer Surveillance System. J Clin Oncol 22:2865–2872
4. Kleihues P, Louis DN, Scheithauer BW et al (2002) The WHO classification of tumors of the nervous system. J Neuropathol Exp Neurol 61:215–225, discussion 226–219
5. Claus EB, Black PM (2006) Survival rates and patterns of care for patients diagnosed with supratentorial low-grade gliomas: data from the SEER program, 1973–2001. Cancer 106:1358–1363
6. Stupp R, Mason WP, van den Bent MJ et al (2005) Radiotherapy plus concomitant and adjuvant temozolomide for glioblastoma. N Engl J Med 352:987–996
7. Clarke JW, Chang EL, Levin VA et al (2008) Optimizing radiotherapy schedules for elderly glioblastoma multiforme patients. Expert Rev Anticancer Ther 8:733–741
8. Keime-Guibert F, Chinot O, Taillandier L et al (2007) Radiotherapy for glioblastoma in the elderly. N Engl J Med 356:1527–1535
9. Curran WJ Jr, Scott CB, Horton J et al (1993) Recursive partitioning analysis of prognostic factors in three Radiation Therapy Oncology Group malignant glioma trials. J Natl Cancer Inst 85:704–710
10. Brandes AA, Compostella A, Blatt V et al (2006) Glioblastoma in the elderly: current and future trends. Crit Rev Oncol Hematol 60:256–266
11. Batchelor TT, Betensky RA, Esposito JM et al (2004) Age-dependent prognostic effects of genetic alterations in glioblastoma. Clin Cancer Res 10:228–233
12. Olson JE, Janney CA, Rao RD et al (2002) The continuing increase in the incidence of primary central nervous system non-Hodgkin lymphoma: a surveillance, epidemiology, and end results analysis. Cancer 95:1504–1510
13. Ferreri AJ, Reni M (2005) Prognostic factors in primary central nervous system lymphomas. Hematol Oncol Clin North Am 19:629–649, vi
14. Relling MV, Rubnitz JE, Rivera GK et al (1999) High incidence of secondary brain tumours after radiotherapy and antimetabolites. Lancet 354:34–39
15. Wrensch M, Minn Y, Chew T et al (2002) Epidemiology of primary brain tumors: current concepts and review of the literature. Neuro Oncol 4:278–299
16. Wiemels JL, Wiencke JK, Kelsey KT et al (2007) Allergy-related polymorphisms influence glioma status and serum IgE levels. Cancer Epidemiol Biomarkers Prev 16:1229–1235
17. Linos E, Raine T, Alonso A et al (2007) Atopy and risk of brain tumors: a meta-analysis. J Natl Cancer Inst 99:1544–1550
18. Claus EB, Bondy ML, Schildkraut JM et al (2005) Epidemiology of intracranial meningioma. Neurosurgery 57:1088–1095, discussion 1088–1095
19. Claus EB, Park PJ, Carroll R et al (2008) Specific genes expressed in association with progesterone receptors in meningioma. Cancer Res 68:314–322
20. Lieu AS, Hwang SL, Howng SL (2003) Intracranial meningioma and breast cancer. J Clin Neurosci 10:553–556
21. Claus EB, Black PM, Bondy ML et al (2007) Exogenous hormone use and meningioma risk: what do we tell our patients? Cancer 110:471–476
22. Schwartzbaum JA, Ahlbom A, Lonn S et al (2007) An international case-control study of glutathione transferase and functionally related polymorphisms and risk of primary adult brain tumors. Cancer Epidemiol Biomarkers Prev 16:559–565
23. Wrensch M, Lee M, Miike R et al (1997) Familial and personal medical history of cancer and nervous system conditions among adults with glioma and controls. Am J Epidemiol 145:581–593

24. Malmer B, Adatto P, Armstrong G et al (2007) GLIOGENE an International Consortium to Understand Familial Glioma. Cancer Epidemiol Biomarkers Prev 16:1730–1734

25. Paunu N, Lahermo P, Onkamo P et al (2002) A novel low-penetrance locus for familial glioma at 15q23-q26.3. Cancer Res 62: 3798–3802

26. Bethke L, Murray A, Webb E et al (2008) Comprehensive analysis of DNA repair gene variants and risk of meningioma. J Natl Cancer Inst 100:270–276

27. Ohgaki H, Kleihues P (2005) Epidemiology and etiology of gliomas. Acta Neuropathol (Berl) 109:93–108

28. Tysnes BB, Mahesparan R (2001) Biological mechanisms of glioma invasion and potential therapeutic targets. J Neurooncol 53: 129–147

29. Hemminki K, Li X (2003) Familial risks in nervous system tumors. Cancer Epidemiol Biomarkers Prev 12:1137–1142

30. Hill DA, Linet MS, Black PM et al (2004) Meningioma and schwannoma risk in adults in relation to family history of cancer. Neuro Oncol 6:274–280

31. Sadetzki S, Flint-Richter P, Starinsky S et al (2005) Genotyping of patients with sporadic and radiation-associated meningiomas. Cancer Epidemiol Biomarkers Prev 14:969–976

32. Rubenstein JL, Treseler P, O'Brien JM (2005) Pathology and genetics of primary central nervous system and intraocular lymphoma. Hematol Oncol Clin North Am 19:705–717, vii

33. Cady FM, O'Neill BP, Law ME et al (2008) Del(6)(q22) and BCL6 rearrangements in primary CNS lymphoma are indicators of an aggressive clinical course. J Clin Oncol 26(29):4814–4819

34. Kay J (2008) Nephrogenic systemic fibrosis: a gadolinium-associated fibrosing disorder in patients with renal dysfunction. Ann Rheum Dis 67(Suppl 3):iii66–iii69

35. Dowd CF, Halbach VV, Higashida RT (2003) Meningiomas: the role of preoperative angiography and embolization. Neurosurg Focus 15:E10

36. Vernooij MW, Ikram MA, Tanghe HL et al (2007) Incidental findings on brain MRI in the general population. N Engl J Med 357:1821–1828

37. Lacroix M, Abi-Said D, Fourney DR et al (2001) A multivariate analysis of 416 patients with glioblastoma multiforme: prognosis, extent of resection, and survival. J Neurosurg 95:190–198

38. Jackson RJ, Fuller GN, Abi-Said D et al (2001) Limitations of stereotactic biopsy in the initial management of gliomas. Neuro Oncol 3:193–200

39. Ohgaki H (2009) Epidemiology of brain tumors. Methods Mol Biol 472:323–342

40. Barnholtz-Sloan JS, Williams VL, Maldonado JL et al (2008) Patterns of care and outcomes among elderly individuals with primary malignant astrocytoma. J Neurosurg 108:642–648

41. Roger EP, Butler J, Benzel EC (2006) Neurosurgery in the elderly: brain tumors and subdural hematomas. Clin Geriatr Med 22:623–644

42. Kelly PJ, Hunt C (1994) The limited value of cytoreductive surgery in elderly patients with malignant gliomas. Neurosurgery 34:62–66, discussion 66–67

43. Marosi C, Hassler M, Roessler K et al (2008) Meningioma. Crit Rev Oncol Hematol 67:153–171

44. Black PM, Morokoff AP, Zauberman J (2008) Surgery for extraaxial tumors of the cerebral convexity and midline. Neurosurgery 62:1115–1121, discussion 1121–1113

45. Butte PV, Pikul BK, Hever A et al (2005) Diagnosis of meningioma by time-resolved fluorescence spectroscopy. J Biomed Opt 10:064026

46. Gay E, Vuillez JP, Palombi O et al (2005) Intraoperative and postoperative gamma detection of somatostatin receptors in bone-invasive en plaque meningiomas. Neurosurgery 57:107–113, discussion 107–113

47. Morofuji Y, Matsuo T, Hayashi Y et al (2008) Usefulness of intraoperative photodynamic diagnosis using 5-aminolevulinic acid for meningiomas with cranial invasion: technical case report. Neurosurgery 62:102–103, discussion 103–104

48. Jaaskelainen J (1986) Seemingly complete removal of histologically benign intracranial meningioma: late recurrence rate and factors predicting recurrence in 657 patients. A multivariate analysis. Surg Neurol 26:461–469

49. Johnson WD, Loredo LN, Slater JD (2008) Surgery and radiotherapy: complementary tools in the management of benign intracranial tumors. Neurosurg Focus 24:E2

50. Nakamura M, Roser F, Michel J et al (2005) Volumetric analysis of the growth rate of incompletely resected intracranial meningiomas. Zentralbl Neurochir 66:17–23

51. Zeidman LA, Ankenbrandt WJ, Du H et al (2008) Growth rate of non-operated meningiomas. J Neurol 255:891–895

52. Roa W, Brasher PM, Bauman G et al (2004) Abbreviated course of radiation therapy in older patients with glioblastoma multiforme: a prospective randomized clinical trial. J Clin Oncol 22:1583–1588

53. Yang SY, Park CK, Park SH et al (2008) Atypical and anaplastic meningiomas: prognostic implications of clinicopathological features. J Neurol Neurosurg Psychiatry 79:574–580

54. Rogers L, Mehta M (2007) Role of radiation therapy in treating intracranial meningiomas. Neurosurg Focus 23:E4

55. Milker-Zabel S, Zabel-du Bois A, Huber P et al (2007) Intensity-modulated radiotherapy for complex-shaped meningioma of the skull base: long-term experience of a single institution. Int J Radiat Oncol Biol Phys 68:858–863

56. Debus J, Wuendrich M, Pirzkall A et al (2001) High efficacy of fractionated stereotactic radiotherapy of large base-of-skull meningiomas: long-term results. J Clin Oncol 19:3547–3553

57. Elia AE, Shih HA, Loeffler JS (2007) Stereotactic radiation treatment for benign meningiomas. Neurosurg Focus 23:E5

58. Torres RC, Frighetto L, De Salles AA et al (2003) Radiosurgery and stereotactic radiotherapy for intracranial meningiomas. Neurosurg Focus 14:E5

59. Hildebrand J, Sahmoud T, Mignolet F et al (1994) Adjuvant therapy with dibromodulcitol and BCNU increases survival of adults with malignant gliomas. EORTC Brain Tumor Group. Neurology 44: 1479–1483

60. Walker MD, Green SB, Byar DP et al (1980) Randomized comparisons of radiotherapy and nitrosoureas for the treatment of malignant glioma after surgery. N Engl J Med 303:1323–1329

61. Fine HA, Dear KB, Loeffler JS et al (1993) Meta-analysis of radiation therapy with and without adjuvant chemotherapy for malignant gliomas in adults. Cancer 71:2585–2597

62. Stewart LA (2002) Chemotherapy in adult high-grade glioma: a systematic review and meta-analysis of individual patient data from 12 randomised trials. Lancet 359:1011–1018

63. Mirimanoff RO, Gorlia T, Mason W et al (2006) Radiotherapy and temozolomide for newly diagnosed glioblastoma: recursive partitioning analysis of the EORTC 26981/22981-NCIC CE3 phase III randomized trial. J Clin Oncol 24:2563–2569

64. Minniti G, De Sanctis V, Muni R et al (2008) Radiotherapy plus concomitant and adjuvant temozolomide for glioblastoma in elderly patients. J Neurooncol 88:97–103

65. Chinot OL, Barrie M, Frauger E et al (2004) Phase II study of temozolomide without radiotherapy in newly diagnosed glioblastoma multiforme in an elderly populations. Cancer 100: 2208–2214

66. Westphal M, Hilt DC, Bortey E et al (2003) A phase 3 trial of local chemotherapy with biodegradable carmustine (BCNU) wafers (Gliadel wafers) in patients with primary malignant glioma. Neuro Oncol 5:79–88

67. Chamberlain MC, Glantz MJ, Fadul CE (2007) Recurrent meningioma: salvage therapy with long-acting somatostatin analogue. Neurology 69:969–973

68. Shah GD, DeAngelis LM (2005) Treatment of primary central nervous system lymphoma. Hematol Oncol Clin North Am 19:611–627, v

69. Batchelor T, Loeffler JS (2006) Primary CNS lymphoma. J Clin Oncol 24:1281–1288

70. Laack NN, Ballman KV, Brown PB et al (2006) Whole-brain radiotherapy and high-dose methylprednisolone for elderly patients with primary central nervous system lymphoma: Results of North Central Cancer Treatment Group (NCCTG) 96-73-51. Int J Radiat Oncol Biol Phys 65:1429–1439

71. Ferreri AJ, Abrey LE, Blay JY et al (2003) Summary statement on primary central nervous system lymphomas from the Eighth International Conference on Malignant Lymphoma, Lugano, Switzerland, June 12 to 15, 2002. J Clin Oncol 21:2407–2414

72. Patchell RA, Tibbs PA, Walsh JW et al (1990) A randomized trial of surgery in the treatment of single metastases to the brain. N Engl J Med 322:494–500

73. Vecht CJ, Haaxma-Reiche H, Noordijk EM et al (1993) Treatment of single brain metastasis: radiotherapy alone or combined with neurosurgery? Ann Neurol 33:583–590

74. Norden AD, Wen PY, Kesari S (2005) Brain metastases. Curr Opin Neurol 18:654–661

Chapter 88
Spinal Disorders and Nerve Compression Syndromes

Arash Yaghoobian and John M. Olsewski

Introduction

Spinal disorders and nerve compression syndromes of the elderly are common presenting complaints to both internist and surgeons. In fact, approximately 70% of all patients seeking medical attention have the complaint of back pain at one time in their life. More than 13% have pain lasting more than 2 weeks [1]. A directed history and physical examination and working knowledge of the spinal bony and neural anatomy are key elements for appropriate diagnosis and management. This chapter defines the major disorders affecting the geriatric population and guides the surgeon in the diagnosis and treatment options for each disorder.

Anatomy

The spinal elements, cord and cauda equina are housed by the vertebral column consisting of 33 bony vertebrae. There are normally 7 cervical, 12 thoracic, 5 lumbar, 5 sacral, and 4 coccygeal vertebrae. The sacral and coccygeal vertebrae are fused. When viewed from the front, the spine is straight unless a preexisting or degenerative scoliosis is present. A lateral projection reveals a concave appearance to the cervical and lumbosacral vertebrae from back to front and a convex appearance to the thoracic vertebrae. This arrangement is referred to as cervical and lumbosacral lordosis and thoracic kyphosis [2]. Any reversal of this arrangement (e.g., cervical kyphosis) can be a clue to underlying pathology.

The spinal cord rests within the vertebral canal, which is normally triangular. The canal is guarded in front by the vertebral body, from the side by pedicles, and posteriorly by the laminae and spinous processes (Fig. 88.1). The nerve roots

A. Yaghoobian (✉)
Department of Orthopaedic Surgery, Albert Einstein College of Medicine, Montefiore Medical Center, 210 E. 84th Street, no. 3D, Bronx, New York, NY, USA
e-mail: ayaghoob@hotmail.com

leave the cord to become peripheral nerves through the neural foramen bounded by the pedicles above and below and by facet joints posteriorly. There are four facet joints associated with each vertebral level. The inferior facets lie posterior and medial to their superior counterparts, with which they interlock to provide motion and stability to the spine. In addition, between each vertebral body is a vertebral disc (Fig. 88.2). This structure acts as a shock absorber of the spine [2]. It is made up of an outer fibrocartilaginous ring, called the annulus fibrosis, and an inner gelatinous core; the nucleus pulposus. The intervertebral disc in the adult is avascular. Nutrients are delivered to the cells within the disc by way of diffusion through the central portion of the vertebral endplate. Alterations in any aspect of these structures, be it disc, foramina, or facet joints, can be a cause of pain or nerve compression leading to arm or leg pain depending on where in the spine compression takes place.

Biomechanics

The healthy spine is responsible for protecting the spinal cord and absorbing the forces of axial loading. Tremendous compressive forces act on the spine during everyday activities such as lifting and carrying. The osteoporotic spine often fails under these stresses, leading to compression fractures. Normally, six degrees of freedom are present between each vertebral body and the one below. Flexion, extension, right and left lateral bending, and clockwise and counterclockwise rotations comprise these motions [3]. Processes such as pain, trauma, and previous surgery impede spinal mobility and function.

Pathophysiology

Cadaver studies have shown that more than 70% of spines show signs of degeneration between 60 and 70 years of age. These findings may be localized to the disc, vertebral bodies, or facets; or they may involve combinations of structures [4].

R.A. Rosenthal et al. (eds.), *Principles and Practice of Geriatric Surgery*,
DOI 10.1007/978-1-4419-6999-6_88, © Springer Science+Business Media, LLC 2011

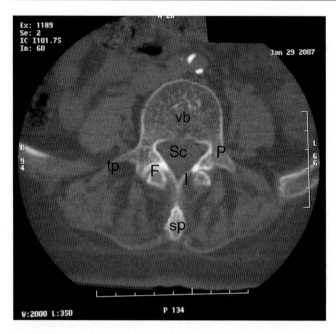

FIGURE 88.1 Bone window axial cut of a computed tomography (CT) scan of the lumbar spine showing the relation of the bony anatomy in the transverse plane. *vb* vertebral body, *p* pedicle, *tp* transverse process, *sc* spinal canal, *f* facet joint, *l* lamina, *sp* spinous process.

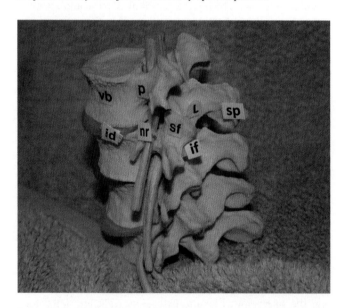

FIGURE 88.2 Model of the motion segment of the lumbar spine in the oblique plane showing the relations of soft tissues and bony elements. *vb* vertebral body, *id* intervertebral disc, *p* pedicle, *nr* nerve root, *sf* superior articular facet, *if* inferior articular facet, *l* lamina.

It is important to note that most patients with such anatomic changes, even when confirmed by radiography, are asymptomatic [5] (Fig. 88.3). The natural history of spinal aging is often related to a degenerative process separated into three distinct stages. The first stage involves degenerative changes to the intervertebral disc, characterized by radial and circumferential tears of the annulus fibrosis. The aging disc loses its ability to retain water and these tears begin to propagate, leading to protrusion of disc material toward the

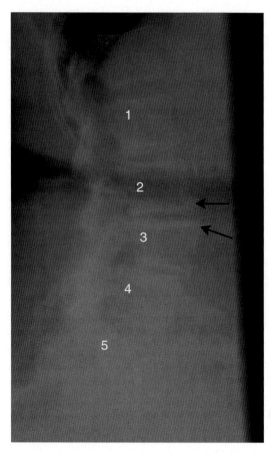

FIGURE 88.3 Seventy-five-year-old female had symptoms of spinal stenosis and degenerative disc disease. This lateral radiograph of the lumbosacral spine shows severe degenerative changes at the L2/L3 disc space, including disc space narrowing, vertebral body endplate sclerosis, neuroforaminal narrowing and traction osteophytes (*arrows*).

spinal canal or neural foramina. Further disc injury can lead to frank extrusion of disc material. As the internal disruption of the disc continues, local instability places increasing stresses on the adjacent facets joints, which hypertrophy in an attempt to provide stability to the spine. When this occurs in the context of a disc herniation, there is an increasing chance of nerve root and/or cord impingement. Furthermore, excessive motion may occur between vertebral bodies, leading to a "slip," or listhesis, of one body on the other. Depending on the extent of intervertebral disc pathology, listhesis, or facet joint hypertrophy, clinical presentation can range anywhere from localized pain and radiculopathy to neurogenic claudication [3, 6, 7]. The clinician must know how to distinguish among these various processes.

Mechanisms of Back Pain

As mentioned, back pain can be related to various pathologic elements of the aging architecture. It may also be related to systemic manifestations such as tumor, infection,

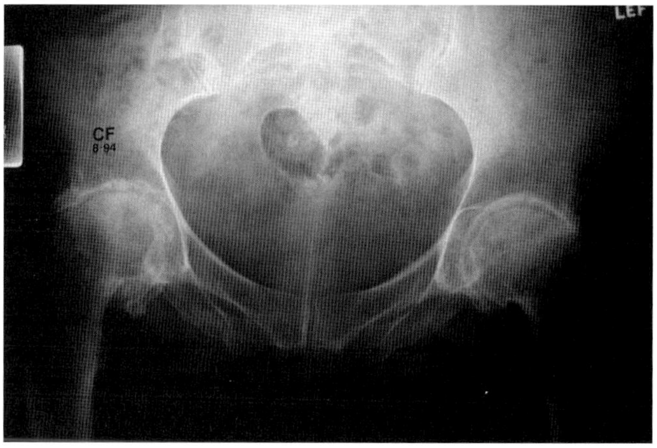

FIGURE 88.4 This 83-year-old female presented with right buttock, groin, and anterior thigh pain. Although an MRI of her lumbar spine showed radiographic evidence of stenosis, her clinical examination was consistent with osteoarthritis of her right hip, as seen on this AP pelvis radiograph, and her symptoms were relieved with total hip arthroplasty.

or ankylosing spondylitis. Patients over age 60 with loss of appetite, fatigue, and night pain must be carefully evaluated for tumor or infection. Although rare, herpes zoster can cause back pain along a unilateral distribution prior to eruption of skin lesions. Back pain may be referred from renal colic, vascular, or splenic pathology. Patients often confuse hip pain and back pain. Similarly, back pain may be a result of a limb length discrepancy or pelvic obliquity. Assessment of hip range of motion, crepitus, and the nature of the complaint can distinguish between the two. We believe that all geriatric patients who warrant radiographic evaluation of their back pain should also undergo anteroposterior (AP) pelvis radiography to detect concomitant hip disease (Fig. 88.4). Lastly, back pain is known to have a large emotional component. Compensation workers and those involved in litigation cases often present with a back complaint for secondary gain [8–10]. Care must be maintained when labeling back pain as psychogenic; however, factors such as depression, especially in the elderly patient, may contribute and must be considered in the differential. A full history and physical examination is warranted to rule out organic pathology.

Specific Pathologic Entities of the Elderly Spine

Cervical Spine Degeneration

Cervical spine degeneration usually begins at age 45–55 and affects men more often than women. Any level of the cervical spine can be involved, but pathologic changes are most often seen at levels C5, C6, and C7. The predominating symptoms depend on the anatomic site of the disease (disc,

facet, neural foramina). The three most common presenting complaints are neck pain (mechanical etiology), radicular pain (nerve root compression), and myelopathic symptoms (cord compromise). A combination of the three elements is often evident [11, 12].

Neck Pain/Mechanical Pain

Patients may present with a complaint of neck pain often exacerbated by motion. Fatigue exacerbates the condition and rest alleviates it. Pain and discomfort may be localized to the midline neck or radiate to the occiput causing headache. It may also radiate to the interscapular region. Patients may feel worse in cold weather, not unlike arthritis in other body areas. Chronic splinting may lead to overuse of surrounding muscles leading to pain in the sternocleidomastoid or deltoid region. Mechanical neck pain can easily be confused with shoulder pathology. A history and physical examination consistent with discomfort with overhead activities is more likely to be related to rotator cuff pathology than cervical degeneration. The patient with rest or night pain, nonmechanical in nature, must be evaluated for the possibility of neoplasm or infection [13].

Physical examination can reveal midline tenderness to palpation. Typically, the examiner notes pain with rotation to the right or left. Strength in the upper extremities is preserved, and reflexes are present in the biceps, triceps, and brachioradialis distributions. Appropriate studies for a patient with mechanical symptoms include AP, lateral, and oblique radiographs. We also order flexion and extension views to detect any dynamic instability (Fig. 88.5). Radiographs typically show loss of disc height and possibly some mild loss of cervical lordosis. Arthritic changes in the facet joints may also be evident. It must be emphasized that such changes may be apparent in the completely asymptomatic patient, and that correlation of clinical and radiographic findings is mandatory.

Treatment of mechanical-type neck pain without neurologic involvement is almost always nonsurgical. First-line therapy involves use of a soft or hard collar in conjunction with a trial of nonsteroidal antiinflammatory drugs (NSAIDs) or a COX-2 inhibitor in an attempt to decrease the inflammatory process. Most patients have considerable relief over a 6-week period. Refractory cases can begin a physical therapy regimen with isometric neck and shoulder exercises followed by active strengthening. If 6 months of therapy does not significantly alleviate symptoms, the patient can be considered for surgery. Any patient considered for surgery for mechanical symptoms should receive an additional study such as magnetic resonance imaging (MRI) or computed tomography (CT) of the neck to delineate the exact nature of the degenerative process. The mainstay of surgical management is fusion via an anterior or posterior approach. The patient

FIGURE 88.5 Eighty-five-year-old male with symptoms of cervical spondylosis and stenosis. Flexion and extension lateral radiographs show evidence of dynamic instability (subluxation) of 4 mm of C7 on T1.

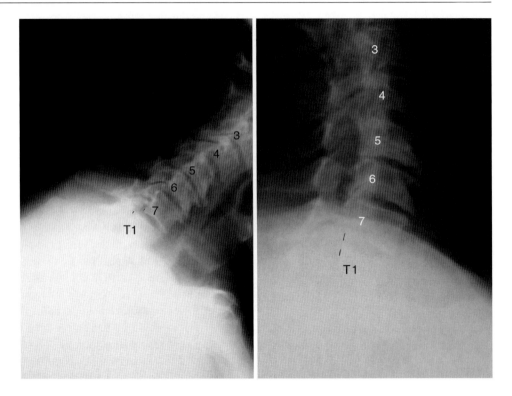

should be cautioned that the results of such surgery for pain relief are variable. In general, surgical management is reserved for all but the most refractory cases [14].

Radicular Neck Pain

Signs and Symptoms

The typical presentation of a patient with cervical radiculopathy is one of neck pain with radiation in the distribution of the affected nerve root. This pain may be acute in nature or develop slowly over time. The geriatric population usually presents with the latter, as the neural compression is related to narrowing of the neural canal from osteophyte formation (hard disc) and generalized loss of disc height rather than an acute disc herniation (soft disc). The patient often describes the pain as a burning or tingling sensation and sensory, motor, or reflex disturbances may or may not be present.

The area of radiation corresponds to the level of the neural compression. C4 compression affects the back of the neck; C5 the lateral shoulder and arm; C6 the lateral forearm, thumb, and index finger; C7 the middle finger; C8 the ring and little finger; and T1 the medial arm and forearm. These distributions are not exact, and there is a considerable amount of dermatomal overlap between the nerve roots. Patients often complain of exacerbation with particular motions: neck rotation and flexion toward the side of the arm pain and hyperextension of the neck. Furthermore, they may present

with motor weakness in the upper extremity. This too, roughly corresponds to the level of neural compression. C5 compression affects deltoid and biceps strength; C6 compression, wrist extension, and biceps; C7 triceps and wrist flexion; C8 finger flexion; T1, grip strength.

Physical examination should assess neck motion, tenderness to palpation along the midline, and the neck muscles. The physician should document the area of burning or tingling down the arm and correlate it with dermatomal distributions. Muscle weakness should be noted in the upper extremity, and this too is correlated with the area of sensory abnormality. Pain in a particular muscle group must also be assessed. Reflex testing with a hammer can reveal diminished reflexes in the biceps, brachioradialis, and triceps. Spurling's test (rotation and lateral bend toward the side of arm pain evokes increased symptoms) may be positive. In addition, holding the head and neck in extension can exacerbate symptoms. Placing the affected extremity with the palm of the hand on top of the head relieves the pain by expanding room for the neural elements [15].

Pathophysiology

As mentioned, radicular pain is secondary to compression of the exiting nerve roots from the neural foramina of the cervical spine. Recent studies have shown that mechanical forces may not be the only factor contributing to the development of pain. Stimulation of nerve roots by proinflammatory cytokines released from the intervertebral disc may also play an important role in this regard. Although not fully understood, these chemical mediators, such as substance P, interleukins 1 (IL-1), IL-6, bradykinin, and prostaglandins can evoke an inflammatory and painful response [16, 17].

Imaging

As with purely mechanical pain, plain radiographs are the first-line study. The oblique film should be studied carefully, as it often demonstrates narrowing of a particular neural foramina and significant osteophyte. MRI or electrodiagnostic studies are reserved for surgical candidates. Axial and sagittal cuts at the level of the neuroforamina can be particularly useful (Fig. 88.6).

Natural History

The natural history of this disease is not as favorable as for purely mechanical neck pain. Despite nonoperative measures it is estimated that 25% of patients with radicular complaints are left with severe symptomatology [18]. These patients may be considerably improved with surgical management [19].

Differential Diagnosis

Cervical radiculopathy can be mimicked by many other conditions affecting the elderly population. Compressive neuropathies (carpal tunnel syndrome or cubital tunnel syndrome) may

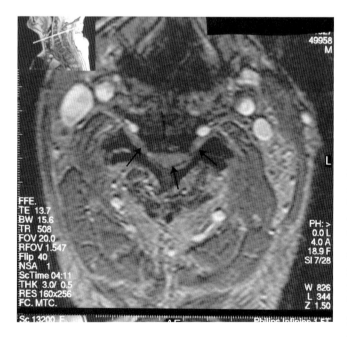

Figure 88.6 Eighty-one-year-old male with symptoms of cervical myeloradiculopathy. Axial cut MRI shows evidence of both central and foraminal stenosis (*arrows*).

lead to radicular-like symptoms. In addition, thoracic outlet syndrome, which represents compression of the brachial plexus or subclavian vessels from a cervical rib or hypertrophic scalene muscles leading to symptoms in the medial arm and forearm may present similarly to cervical radiculopathy [15]. Rotator cuff pathology may mimic a C5–6 radiculopathy. Multiple sclerosis may present with upper extremity sensory symptoms, such as tingling and weakness not following an anatomic distribution. Amyotrophic lateral sclerosis may appear as an upper extremity weakness with preservation of sensation. Finally, spinal tumors occasionally present with radicular symptoms. A careful history concerning systemic signs and night pain or nonmechanical pain must be sought [20].

Nonoperative Management

Nonoperative management of cervical radiculopathy is similar to treatment of mechanical neck pain. Patients are begun on a regimen of antiinflammatory medications, which often decrease the inflammation of affected nerve roots and leads to significant pain relief. Selective Cyclooxygenase-2 (COX-2) inhibitors may decrease the incidence of gastrointestinal side effects, but in controlled studies for osteoarthritis, they do not appear to be any more efficacious than nonselective NSAID [21]. A soft collar can be provided for comfort, followed by a course of passive stretching exercises and active strengthening of the neck, shoulder, and arm when symptoms subside. Patients unresponsive to those measures can receive epidural steroid injections or selective nerve root injections at the level of neural compression. Surgery is reserved for patients who have unremitting pain for 3–6 months despite conservative measures or those with progressive neurologic deficit [22].

Surgical Management

Common indications for surgical management include unrelenting pain that fails to respond to conservative therapy or progressive neurologic deficits, such as weakness or numbness. All patients considered for surgical management should undergo preoperative MRI. This study can confirm the anatomic level of compression based on the location of the patient's radicular symptoms. As mentioned, it is less likely in the geriatric population to have radicular symptoms due to an acute disc herniation than due to slowly evolving nerve root compression from the spondylitic process. Surgery must be aimed at decompression of the affected nerve roots. The most common operation for radiculopathy at a single nerve root level is a diskectomy and fusion from an anterior approach. The affected level of disc degeneration is removed completely, as are any visible osteophytes. Next, a piece of bone graft slightly larger than the original disc height is

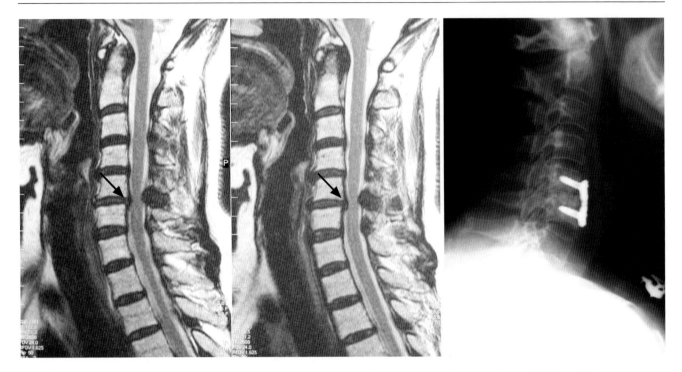

Figure 88.7 Sixty-six-year-old female with symptoms of cervical myelopathy from large central disc herniation at C5/C6 on MRI (*arrow*), treated with anterior cervical discectomy and fusion with plate fixation.

inserted into the former. This provides further enlargement of the neural foramina via distraction. If the graft is well impacted, no instrumentation need be placed; otherwise, a cervical plate can be used. The patient is placed in a postoperative collar for about 6 weeks. The goal here is solid bony fusion, which halts further degeneration and eliminates nerve root compression (Fig. 88.7).

Advantages of anterior discectomy, decompression, and fusion (ACDF) include complete access to the pathologic disc and bony spurring often found at the uncovertebral joint. In addition, the anterior approach is associated with a very low complication rate, the wounds are cosmetically appealing, and there is little postoperative pain. Disadvantages include difficulty with speech and swallowing in the acute postoperative period and an increased pseudarthrosis rate with multilevel decompression and fusion.

Decompression of affected nerve roots can also be accomplished via posterior approaches. With this procedure, small amounts of cervical lamina and facet are removed at the affected level. The surgeon may remove the offending disc material as well. As this procedure is less destabilizing than full diskectomy, no bony fusion is needed. It is important to avoid the posterior approach in a kyphotic cervical spine, as the spinal cord will continue to be tethered anteriorly leading to an inadequate decompression.

Results

The results of surgery for radicular symptoms are encouraging. More than 90% of people can be effectively improved from their pain and discomfort. The best results have been obtained with anterior procedures, making it the recommended choice. Posterior approaches are reserved for foraminal stenosis without a large disc herniation, failed anterior approaches, or for patients unable to undergo anterior procedures for other reasons such as poor skin condition [20, 23].

Cervical Myelopathy

Cervical myelopathy involves compression of the cervical spinal cord (not exiting nerve roots) leading to classic symptomatology in the geriatric population.

Signs and Symptoms

Although neck pain may be present, it is not as constant a feature as with mechanical or radicular compression. In fact, there is a wide spectrum of symptoms from paresthesia to weakness and upper motor neuron signs. Patients can complain of an increasing loss of manual dexterity, typically described as difficulty with handwriting and fastening buttons on clothing. Often they may describe a vague weakness and numbness to the upper extremities. Lower extremity weakness is a frequent complaint; it leads to gait disturbance (wide based) with frequent falling and episodes of instability. When advanced, bowel or bladder function may be affected. Physical examination should begin by noting the patient's gait. A wide-based gait is typical. Patients may be unable to open and close a fist rapidly. Spasticity of the upper extremities is not uncommon. An objective weakness of the upper and lower extremities may be evident. Wasting of the upper extremity is possible in long-standing cases. Reflex changes are important in the myelopathic examination. Typically, the upper extremities are hyporeflexive and the lower extremities hyperreflexive. Bilateral Babinski reflexes are often noted. A positive Hoffman reflex (flexion of the thumb or index finger upon flicking the nail of the middle finger) is a classic test for cervical myelopathy. The "finger escape sign" may be evident. The patient holds his fingers in adduction and extension; if the ulnar two digits drift into abduction in 30–60 s, the test is considered positive [24]. An inverted radial reflex (hyporeflexive brachioradialis with involuntary contraction of the fingers) is another classic sign for C5 myelopathy. Lhermitte's sign (cervical compression with flexion leading to an electric-like sensation in the upper and or lower extremities) is another such sign [20].

Pathophysiology

The etiology of the myelopathy is most often spinal cord encroachment secondary to a single or multilevel degenerative process. The arthritic changes of the facets, bodies, uncovertebral joints, and ligamentum flavum impinge centrally, leading to a reduced space available for the spinal cord. This process is usually slow and evolving, occurring over many years. Patients with a congenitally small spinal canal may develop symptoms more rapidly. A midline disc herniation can lead to the development of acute myelopathy, but this is uncommon except in those with congenitally narrow canals [25]. Pathoanatomic studies show that the degree of compression correlates with ischemia of neural tissue. Chronic histological changes include axonal demyelination, cell necrosis, and gliosis or scarring [26].

Natural History

Cervical myelopathy is a slowly progressive entity. Although most patients' initial complaints do not warrant surgical intervention, once the onset of myelopathy has begun, episodic deterioration is the most common course, and

surgical recommendation should be made. As many as 5% of patients have acute deterioration and require urgent intervention [27].

Imaging

Radiographic changes to the cervical spine associated with myelopathy are degenerative and typically found in patients above the age of 50. Initial studies include AP and lateral plain films of the cervical spine, which may have findings such as sagittal imbalance (kyphosis), coronal imbalance (scoliosis), disc space narrowing, osteophyte formation, and endplate sclerosis. Flexion-extension views are used to rule out instability. The space available for the spinal cord can be estimated on the lateral radiograph. A 13 mm distance between the back of the vertebral body and the back of the lamina at any given level is considered the lower limit of normal. Smaller distances are considered congenitally narrowed and may predispose toward myelopathic symptoms. In some cases, OPLL (ossification of the posterior longitudinal ligament) (Fig. 88.8) can be visualized as a bar of bone posterior to the vertebral bodies. MRI and myelography/CT scans of the cervical spine are invaluable for confirming the myelopathy. Axial cuts demonstrate the available room for the spinal cord as well as evidence of disc or osteophytes leading to canal narrowing. Sagittal MRI cuts can help determine the total number of cervical levels involved, extent of disc herniation, as well as the severity of disease from cord compression; myelomalacia or morbid softening of the spinal cord (Fig. 88.9).

Differential Diagnosis

All of the conditions listed for the differential diagnosis for cervical radiculopathy can mimic myelopathy as well. In particular, intra- or extradural tumors of the spine can lead to myelopathic symptoms. They are easily detected on the MRI scan. Furthermore, cerebellar pathology can lead to gait disturbance, as in myelopathy. Neurologic consultation should be considered if cerebellar pathology is considered the etiology of the gait disturbance [28].

Nonoperative Treatment

Patients can be started on a course of pain medication, physical therapy, and exercise modalities similar to patients with radiculopathy or mechanical symptoms. However, with increasing weakness, gait disturbance, or extremity pain, surgery is indicated. Furthermore, patients with any evidence of bowel or bladder disturbance secondary to cord compression should be considered for emergent decompression [22].

Figure 88.8 Sixty-two-year-old female with cervical myelopathy and findings of OPPL on both sagittal and axial MRI cuts (*arrows*).

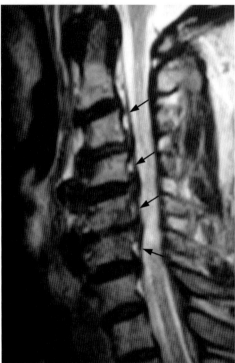

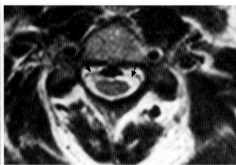

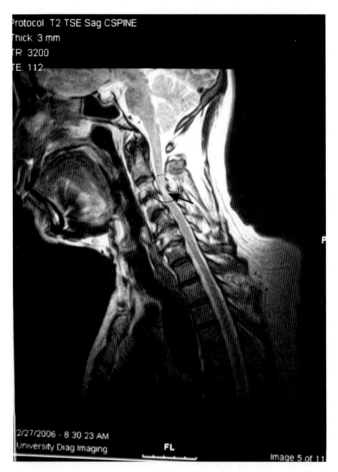

Figure 88.9 Seventy-year-old male with cervical myelopathy and findings of myelomalacia of the spinal cord on T-2 weighted sagittal MRI (*arrow*).

Operative Treatment

Operative treatment of myelopathy focuses on decompression of the spinal canal to expand the space for the spinal cord. The procedure or approach depends on the nature and extent of pathology. If myelopathy is secondary to disc herniation or bony encroachment at one or two levels, the recommendation is anterior discectomy or corpectomy, decompression, and fusion. If the constriction is secondary to a congenitally narrow canal or encroachment at three or more levels, the decompression should be performed posteriorly. This can be done via laminectomies, foraminotomies, or "open door" laminoplasty (Fig. 88.10), depending on the clinical indication. Posterior approaches that do not include stabilization are contraindicated in patients with preexisting cervical kyphosis. While operative indications are based on both radiographic findings and clinical symptoms, rarely a patient may have severe stenosis with minimal deficit. This is a relative indication for decompression as a single hyperextension injury can lead to paraplegia. Counseling is required at a minimum.

Results

Results of surgery for myelopathy are often related to the duration and severity of the disease. If it is secondary to single-level disease without major gait disturbance, about 90% of patients are improved surgically. If symptoms are long-standing, with profound weakness or gait abnormality, the degree of recovery is unpredictable. It is for this reason that myelopathic patients

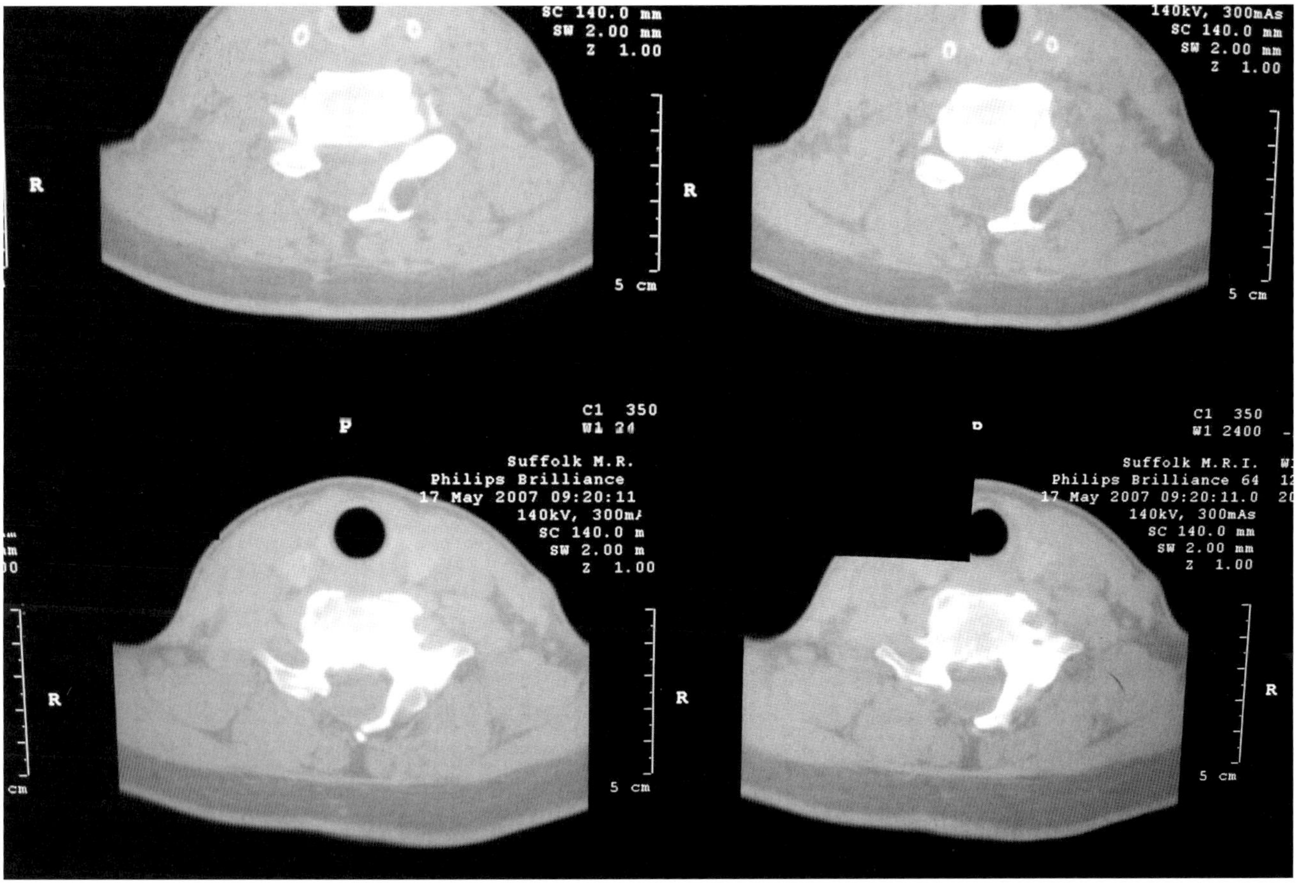

FIGURE 88.10 Axial CT bone window cuts of 60-year-old female with cervical stenosis treated with open door laminoplasty.

should be monitored aggressively and counseled early about the need for surgery with worsening symptoms [29–31].

Thoracic Degenerative Disease

Symptomatic disease in the thoracic spine is relatively uncommon in comparison to disease in the cervical and lumbar levels. The attachment of the ribs to thoracic vertebrae convey an additional stability to the thoracic spine, leading to less bony and soft tissue changes to the thoracic spine with aging. When present, thoracic disc disease can be debilitating and on occasion requires emergent intervention. Additionally, diagnosis may be complicated as there is a high prevalence of incidental thoracic disc degeneration and herniation in the asymptomatic patient population [32–34].

Signs and Symptoms

Pain is the most frequent presenting complaint. The pain may be localized to the involved thoracic vertebrae (axial pain) or radiate in a dermatomal band-like fashion unilaterally or bilaterally around the chest wall. The T10 dermatomal level is the most common reported distribution of pain regardless of the location of disease [33]. Occasionally, the pain radiates to the lower extremity or hip region. Complaints of sensory abnormalities are the second most likely presentation. These may follow chest wall dermatomal patterns or manifest as paresthesias extending to the lower extremities. More concerning is the occasional complaint of weakness, gait disturbance, and loss of bowel and bladder control. These patients must undergo an aggressive workup. The physical examination may be completely normal early in the course of disease. Later, diminished sensation testing to the affected chest wall dermatome may be apparent. Motor weakness, diminished rectal tone, clonus, hyperreflexia, and other upper motor neuron signs (superficial abdominal reflexes or cremasteric reflex) may be noted in long-standing cases or with acute large disc herniations [8].

Pathophysiology

Degeneration in the thoracic spine is secondary to the same processes as in the cervical spine. Water loss to the disc with aging leads to incompetence of bony elements, including

Figure 88.11 Sixty-year-old male with symptoms of thoracic level myelopathy from large central disc herniation obliterating space available for spinal cord at T10/T11.

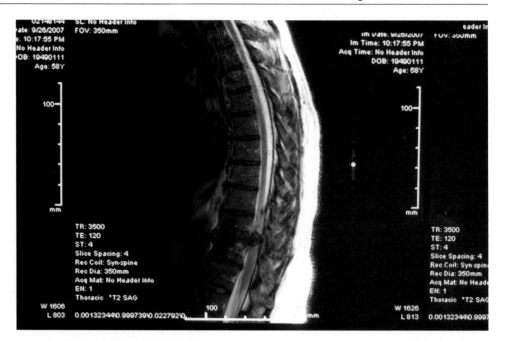

the facets and bodies of affected vertebrae. Osteophytes may form, leading to impingement of nerve roots or if centrally located on the cord itself. With the loss of disc height, the ligamentum flavum may become buckled over time and contribute to central impingement. Acute disc herniations can also occur and often lead to sudden onset of symptomatology [3, 6, 32]. As in the case with cervical or lumbar disease, the location of the disc herniation will dictate clinical presentation. Midline or paramedian herniations have the highest likelihood to precipitate myelopathic symptoms; radicular pain is often the result of lateral herniations.

Natural History

The natural history of thoracic disc disease is variable [32]. In the geriatric population a slow, gradual onset of symptoms is the most likely course. When not accompanied by motor signs or bladder or rectal incompetence, most patients respond well to nonsurgical treatment [35].

Imaging

Diagnostic imaging should begin with AP and lateral projections of the thoracic spine. These are often difficult to interpret because of overlying structures but may show disc narrowing or calcification within an affected disc space. These radiographs may also show evidence of excessive kyphosis in the thoracic spine, a possible predisposition to symptomatic disease. These screening studies should also be used to rule out acute injury (fracture) or potential neoplastic

lesion. MRI of the thoracic spine is currently the premier modality for evaluating suspected thoracic disc disease. Sagittal and axial cuts can determine the site of pathology (disc level, central, or foraminal) and bony vs. disc impingement (Fig. 88.11). It must be stressed that all radiographic findings must be closely correlated to the physical examination and patient complaints because the presence of an asymptomatic radiographic abnormality is quite common [36].

Differential Diagnosis

A number of conditions can mimic thoracic disc disease, including neurologic conditions (amyotrophic lateral sclerosis, multiple sclerosis) and infectious causes of back pain (e.g., discitis, osteomyelitis). Spinal tumors or dural arteriovenous malformations can have similar presentations [32]. Herpes zoster often appears as a unilateral dermatomal chest wall pain band prior to the onset of the classic rash [8]. It is especially prevalent in the geriatric population. Cardiac or pulmonary disease refers to the posterior chest wall on occasion.

Nonoperative Treatment

Avoiding precipitating flexion or extension motions (activity modification) is the first-line therapy. Patients may be begun on NSAIDs for pain relief, which often relieves the occasional pain and discomfort. In the acute phase, the rehabilitation should consist of modalities such as heat, ice, and massage. More aggressive therapy is initiated after this period to promote range-of-motion, flexibility, and strength. A trial of brace immobilization can be suggested in more refractory cases. Patients must be monitored for development of motor weakness or bladder/bowel symptoms. These patients should be seriously evaluated for surgical therapy.

Operative Treatment

Patients manifesting motor weakness, bladder symptoms, and other upper motor neuron signs are candidates for surgical therapy. Patients with pain unresponsive to nonoperative modalities are also appropriate for surgical management. A preoperative MRI scan or myelography followed by CT scan is mandatory in all surgical cases. Surgery involves removing the offending disc, ligament, or bony material. The approach and technique depend on the level of pathology and the surgeon's familiarity with the surgery. Approaches include transternal, transpedicular, costotransversectomy, transthoracic [37], or thoracoscopic [38]. Thoracic spine surgery is among the most challenging operations performed by the spine surgeon. Appropriate intraoperative neural monitoring and consultation with a thoracic or vascular surgeon can ensure a more predictable result.

Results

Results of surgery are often dependent on the severity and duration of the complaint. Acute-onset weakness secondary to thoracic herniation offers a good chance of restoring neurologic function if dealt with emergently. More than 75% of patients are significantly relieved of their pain and discomfort [39]. Surgery for long-standing weakness or bladder dysfunction may halt the progression of the disease but does not restore full, premorbid function.

Lumbar Degenerative Disease

Low back pain in the elderly ranks as one of the most frequent complaints of patients presenting to internists and family practitioners. Attention must be paid to the nature of the pain, its duration, and its aggravating and mitigating factors. Conditions with back pain only, such as degenerative disc disease, must be distinguished from conditions affecting the lower extremities such as sciatica and lumbar spinal stenosis. Referred pain to the back from abdominal, retroperitoneal, or vascular pathology is not infrequently found in the elderly population and must be discerned via an accurate history and physical examination [40].

Degenerative Disc Disease/Mechanical Back Pain

With aging, the lumbar spine alters its original architecture. The aging disc loses height as its water content decreases. Disc space height between adjacent vertebrae diminishes, most commonly at L4–5 [8]. This leads to incompetence of the bony elements of the lumbar spine and increased micromotion between adjacent vertebrae. Osteophytes develop at the facets and along the vertebral body itself [41] (Fig. 88.12). Additionally, the paraspinal musculature becomes affected and may tend toward reflex spasm.

The typical patient with degenerative disc disease offers a history of chronic back pain with pain-free intervals. This point is important for distinguishing this condition from tumor, infection, or other systemic processes. The pain is localized to the lower back with some radiation across the midline or upper buttock, but it does not radiate to the lower extremities. Patients often relate morning stiffness with a decrease in symptoms as the day progresses. Rest or recumbency relieve the pain, and certain activities or motions tend to exacerbate it. Often, sitting in a firm chair that tends to stabilize the spine relieves pain, whereas sitting in a soft cushioned seat sags the lumbar spine and increases discomfort.

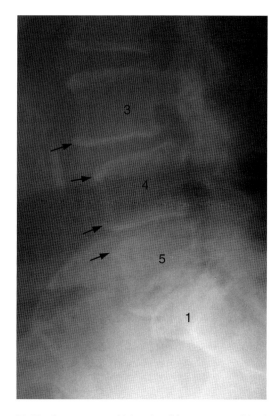

Figure 88.12 Seventy-year-old female with symptoms of lumbar spinal stenosis and evidence of traction osteophytes (*arrows*) present at both L3/L4 and L4/L5 on this lateral lumbosacral spine radiograph.

Pain may be present during exercise but often is more pronounced several hours after activity or the next morning.

The physical examination should note the presence of scoliosis, spinal range of motion in flexion and extension, bending, and lateral rotation. The abdomen should be inspected for muscle tone, which is often diminished, and the presence of any masses, suggestive of intra-abdominal pathology. Tenderness along the affected region of the spinal column is not uncommon. Asking the patient to maintain a semiflexed position often leads to exacerbation, as does asking the patient to drop down on his or her raised heels. Of note, reflexes are normal, full strength of the lower extremities is present, and no clonus or other upper motor neuron signs exist.

First-line imaging studies are AP and lateral radiographs of the lumbosacral spine and an AP view of the pelvis to help distinguish the presence of coexistent hip disease. If symptoms have been of short duration, less than 6 weeks, radiographs need not be obtained, as management will not differ based on their findings. Furthermore, the degree of symptomatology has limited correlation with the radiographic findings. As mentioned, narrowing at the L4–5 level is most common, but patients may also have extensive evidence of multilevel disease with severe arthrosis and little or no symptomatology [42].

Treatment for mechanical back pain is predominantly non-surgical. A short duration of bed rest, 2 days, may be prescribed in conjunction with administration of NSAIDs to decrease the inflammatory component. Exacerbating motions are to be avoided. Next, a physical therapy regimen should be instituted. Strengthening of the abdominal musculature can relieve stress on the paraspinal muscles and vertebral column.

Extension exercises of the lumbar spine are often helpful for pain relief. Flexion exercises in select patients are of benefit but may lead to increased pain. A holistic aerobic reconditioning program should be instituted to ensure a more adequate overall physical profile.

Many patients obtain significant relief from lumbosacral corset or brace wear during symptomatic periods. Other modalities include massage, trigger-point injections, and ultrasound therapy. Most patients obtain significant pain control and improved functional abilities through the use of such nonoperative modalities.

Surgery is only rarely indicated for this condition. Patients with unremitting pain unresponsive to other modalities can be considered. A secondary study, such as MRI or discography, should corroborate the patient's symptomatology. Secondary gain factors such as workmen's compensation or other litigation portends a poor surgical result. The clinician must be sure that a concomitant psychological disorder is not present. The surgical procedure is a solid arthrodesis of the spine most commonly from a posterior approach. Posterior fusion techniques, however, are numerous and can include anything from a posterolateral to interbody approach. The

benefits of interbody techniques include a midline fusion mass and a large bony surface area, which are associated with a decreased incidence of pseudoarthrosis. Interbody fusion can be further broken down to anterior, posterior, lateral, or transforaminal approaches; and which is selected depends on the pathology the surgeon is addressing. It can be accomplished with or without the use of instrumentation. The theory behind this procedure is to stop motion at the level of the degenerated disc. In the appropriately selected patient, pain relief can be expected 50–80% of the time [43–45].

Sciatica

Sciatica is a general term referring to irritation of lumbar or sacral nerve roots (or both) leading to back pain with radiation down the leg. The most common cause is from protrusion, extrusion, or sequestration of an intervertebral disc. The site of pain and numbness depend on the nerve root involved and the site of involvement. Patients are generally 30–50 years old upon presentation, but the elderly can also be affected with this entity.

Signs and Symptoms

If presenting acutely, patients often recall a straining or twisting event to the back, such as lifting a heavy object. Motor vehicle accidents can also lead to acute herniations. The injury leads to intense pain in the back, followed by pain and numbness in the lower extremities. Over the next several days the back pain becomes less intense, and the lower extremity symptoms predominate. Activities such as bending, walking, and exercise exacerbate the symptoms, whereas lying supine tend to relieve the pain. Coughing or sneezing worsens it.

Upon presentation the patient may exhibit "sciatic scoliosis" [45]. This refers to a standing posture where the back and trunk tilt away from the side where painful bending occurs. Examination of range of motion to the spine often reveals restriction, especially to forward flexion, which increases the pressure within the disc. Occasionally, no restriction in motion is present. Examination of the lower extremities is most important in the consideration of sciatica. Midline herniations (less common) may lead to bilateral leg involvement, whereas lateral herniations (more common) produce unilateral symptoms.

Signs and symptoms are dependent on the particular disc and nerve root involved, corresponding to particular sensory and motor dermatomal levels. The most common level for herniation is the L4–5 disc affecting the L5 nerve root. Herniation affecting the L2–3 roots leads to numbness and paresthesias to the anterior thigh and weakness in hip flexion. L4 root involvement leads to medial calf symptoms and knee extension and ankle weakness. L5 root involvement affects sensation along the lateral calf and dorsal foot with weakness to ankle or great toe extension. If the S1 root is affected, the numbness predominates along the posterior calf and the lateral and plantar foot, with weakness to ankle plantar flexion. S2–4 nerve root disease manifests as perianal sensation loss and bowel and bladder dysfunction. It must be emphasized that most patients presenting with a history suggestive of sciatica do not have evidence of motor weakness upon presentation. In fact, the only findings may be subjective numbness and pain in a particular anatomic site of the leg with gross sensation still intact. Reflex testing may reveal abnormalities on examination. Knee jerk is diminished if L4 roots are impinged. Ankle jerk is diminished if S1 is affected. Finally, an absent cremasteric reflex may be present if sacral roots are involved. It must be remembered that symmetric reflex decrease is common in the elderly.

Special nerve root tension signs are helpful for detecting sciatica and nerve root irritation. The femoral stretch test is performed with the patient prone; the affected leg is raised off the table with the knee flexed and the hip extended. Pain or electricity down the anterior thigh or medial calf is suggestive of L2–4 nerve root irritation. The straight leg raise test is performed with the patient supine and the extended knee raised off the table. Pain along the ischial tuberosity radiating down the posterior thigh and lateral foot indicate stretch to the sciatic nerve with irritation to the L5–S1 nerve roots. If pain is present soon after attempting to raise the leg with a tendency toward knee flexion, it is indicative of tight hamstrings and not a positive straight leg raise test. If the pain is accentuated when the foot is quickly dorsiflexed, it is known as a positive Lasegue test. Perhaps the most specific test for sciatica is the contralateral straight leg raise in which the opposite extremity is raised and pain travels down the affected extremity. Digital examination can document rectal tone, and the lower extremity pulses should be noted [46].

Pathophysiology

The mechanism by which herniated disc material leads to pain is a topic of intense research. Mechanical compression of nerve roots by disc material can lead to vascular injury to the nerves and other forms of trauma. However, it does not appear to be enough to induce the syndrome of sciatica. Contents from the nucleus pulposus, such as interleukins and prostaglandins, may induce edema and fibrosis of adjacent nerve roots. In addition, direct channels may form over time between the disc and adherent nerve roots, leading to further inflammatory responses. Hence the most probable explanation for painful sciatica is a combined mechanical and neurotoxic effect of disc material on involved nerve roots [47, 48].

Natural History

The natural history of sciatica is favorable. More than 50% of patients are relieved of symptoms by 1 month, and in 90% of patients the symptoms resolve by the end of 3 months [8, 49]. Hence most patients can be effectively managed without the need for surgery.

Imaging

Standard AP and lateral lumbosacral radiographs are first-line studies. Most cases fail to reveal anything other than degeneration at various levels. L4–5 is most commonly affected. In fact, acute sciatica is more likely to appear in the setting of normal disc height without narrowing than in one with evidence of degeneration. Hence it is less prevalent in the elderly population. Occasionally, plain films demonstrate a transosseous herniation in which the disc carries with it a small part of the vertebral body into the spinal canal. Patients considered for surgical decompression should undergo MRI studies of the lumbosacral spine to confirm the clinical diagnosis (Fig. 88.13). Keep in mind that 35% of patients older than 40 years have MRI or CT evidence of disk herniation in the absence of symptoms [5, 50]. Electromyography (EMG) studies can also be helpful in difficult cases.

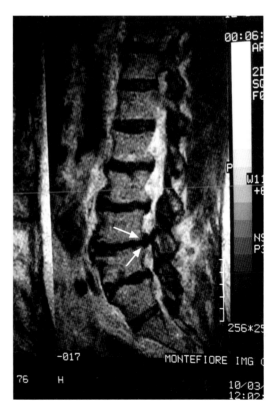

Figure 88.13 Seventy-nine-year-old female with onset of bilateral leg pain from large central disc herniation at L4/L5 (*arrow*) present on this T2-weighted sagittal MRI.

Differential Diagnosis

When an accurate history and physical examination are conducted, sciatica does not present a problem to diagnosis. On occasion, intraspinal tumors present as nerve compression with unremitting pain, which can be easily discerned by MRI. Other neurologic conditions such as multiple sclerosis (MS) or amyotrophic lateral sclerosis (ALS) can be mistaken for sciatica. Vascular claudication can also present with paresthesias to the lower extremities. A good history and neurovascular examination can help discern between the two. One entity that must be immediately recognized is cauda equina syndrome. It presents as a massive midline disc herniation leading to bilateral buttock and leg pain and loss of bladder (urinary retention most common) or bowel control (or both). The patients may also demonstrate diminished rectal tone and decreased perianal sensation. Saddle anesthesia of the buttocks is common. Such patients should undergo urgent MRI to define the site of obstruction and urgent surgery to decompress the neural elements [8, 46, 49].

Nonoperative Treatment

Therapy should begin with a trial of NSAIDs to decrease pain and the inflammatory component of the sciatica. A short course of bed rest, 2 days, can also be helpful. Patients should then be encouraged to ambulate and begin a therapy regimen similar to that for axial back pain. Precipitating activities should be avoided. In particular, flexion exercises may increase symptoms, as they tend to increase pressure within the disc. An aerobic conditioning program must be instituted in the overall therapy scheme. If no relief is achieved after 6 weeks, the patient may benefit from an epidural steroid injection (Fig. 88.14). As mentioned, 90% of patients with sciatica are significantly relieved of symptoms by 3 months [49].

Operative Treatment

Only 10% of patients with sciatica warrant surgical consideration. Patients with bowel/bladder symptoms should warrant consideration immediately upon onset of symptoms. Those with increasing neurologic deficit, particularly motor weakness, should be considered for early surgery. Lastly, patients without relief from nonsurgical therapy should undergo surgical decompression. The standard procedure for disc herniation leading to sciatica is midline decompression with laminotomy and disc excision. It is usually done without fusion. However, if back pain was a source of pain prior to the onset of leg symptoms, some surgeons opt toward fusion in the same surgical sitting. Also, if considerable bone was removed when decompressing the nerve root

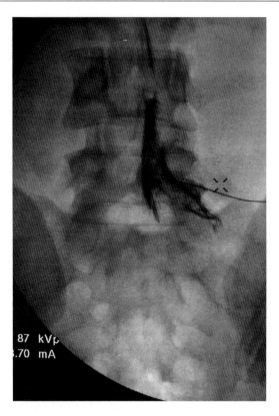

FIGURE 88.14 Epidurogram of 65-year-old female treated for radicular pain with transforminal subpedicular selective nerve root injection of both L5 and S1 nerve roots (Case Courtesy of Sireen Gopal, MD).

and stability is in question, the spine should be fused at that level [51, 52].

Geriatric patients in particular are susceptible to "far lateral herniations." These disc herniations occur outside the spinal canal itself at the level of the neural foramina. Preoperative MRI is helpful for detecting this condition. The surgeon must be careful to ensure that the decompression and disc excision extends laterally into the neural foramina and that the nerve root is free at the end of the procedure. Other surgical procedures available for disk excision include chemonucleolysis and percutaneous discectomy [49]. The indications for these procedures are few, and the results must be weighed against the gold standard of open excision. Recently, arthroscopic spinal procedures have been used in the treatment of disc herniation. More long-term data are needed to assess its usefulness for management of sciatica in the elderly.

Results

If appropriately selected, more than 90% of patients obtain relief from sciatica by surgical disc excision. Patients with long-standing motor weakness may not regain full strength postoperatively. In addition, up to 10% of patients are at risk of having a recurrence of their herniation [49].

Degenerative Lumbar Spinal Stenosis

Lumbar spinal stenosis, also known as spinal claudication, represents narrowing of the overall dimension of the lumbar spinal canal leading to a classic symptomatology. Stenosis may be central, in which the central canal has reduced dimension, or lateral, in which individual nerve roots are encroached by a hypertrophic facet joints, redundant ligamentum, or bulging annulus. Patients are generally elderly, most over age 65, so the geriatric clinician must be intimately familiar with the often subtle presentation of this disease entity.

Signs and Symptoms

Elderly patients with central stenosis usually present with a history of chronic back pain that may have recently improved or worsened. A dull ache across the lumbosacral region is often present, but lower extremity symptoms predominate. A vague or heavy feeling in both legs is described which is slowly progressive. Some patients also have a feeling of the legs giving way. Additionally, the patient states that he or she can only walk several blocks before the pain becomes severe. Pain is positional; sitting relieves the pain, while erect posture and prolonged standing worsens it. Patients often describe relief from leaning forward over a shopping cart, as this tends to widen the overall dimension of the spinal canal. Lying supine with the spine in extension may exacerbate the condition, and as a result night pain is often a feature of this condition. Lateral stenosis patients may present similarly but with unilateral complaints. Physical examination may demonstrate sensory or motor weakness as with sciatica but is most remarkable in most cases for its lack of specific findings. This constellation of symptoms, referred to as neurogenic claudication must be differentiated from vascular insufficiency where leg pain diminishes with cessation of activity rather than a change in position. If radicular pain is present, it is most common in the L5 distribution (91%), followed by S1 (63%), L1–L4 (28%), and S2–S5 (5%) [33]. Straight leg testing, strength, and reflex examination usually are normal [53].

Pathophysiology

The normal young lumbar spinal canal is triangular and has abundant room to house the neural elements. The spinal cord usually ends at approximately the midbody of L1. Below this level the cauda equina nerve roots exit through their respective neural foramina without impingement. The aging process leads to incompetence of the disc, inbuckling of posterior ligamentous structures (particularly the ligamentum flavum), and osteophytes of the facets. All these factors may lead to

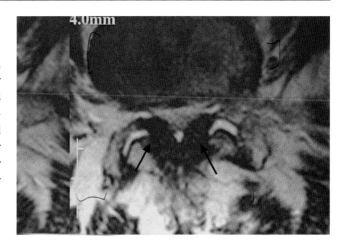

Figure 88.15 Axial MRI cut showing facet joint hypertrophy (*arrows*) resulting in severe spinal stenosis.

medial encroachment into the canal leading to central spinal stenosis. When the absolute area of the lumbar canal is reduced to <100 mm^2, absolute stenosis exists [54]. In dog-based experimentation, when the thecal sac is compressed acutely (45% of original size) there are measurable changes in both motor and sensory function [55]. When the cross-sectional size of the thecal sac is reduced to 65 mm [2], the pressure in the cauda equina can increase to 50 mm Hg, which correlates with decreased nerve conduction [56]. Furthermore, some patients have an abnormally narrow, or trefoil-shaped, canal, which makes them even more susceptible to the development of stenosis. An acute disc herniation may also contribute to stenosis of the canal, although it is less commonly seen. Lateral stenosis is similarly the result of osteophytes of the facets, particularly the superior articular facet, and chronic disc disease leading to stenosis at the level of the neural foramina (Fig. 88.15). A common scenario is spondylolisthesis causing spinal stenosis. Spondylolisthesis refers to the vertebra above slipping in front of the vertebra below. Various causes exist, but the most frequently encountered scenario in the elderly is that of a degenerative spondylolisthesis. Chronic disc degeneration with concomitant arthrosis and incompetence of the facet joints allows vertebral slippage and elongation of the vertebral elements of the upper vertebrae. The slippage most commonly occurs between the L4 and L5 vertebrae. It may lead to signs and symptoms of central stenosis or of L5 nerve root impingement. It may manifest with pain along the lateral calf and with ankle or great toe weakness [45, 49].

Natural History

Spinal stenosis is usually a chronic disease process. Symptoms are often present for many years prior to presentation to a clinician. With continued aging and spinal degeneration, the stenotic spinal canal and neural foramina tend to reduce further in size. Although most patients do not require surgery, 15% have slowly worsening symptoms as the years progress [57].

Imaging

Standard AP and lateral radiographs are first-line studies. Pathology such as fracture, tumor, or infection must be ruled out. X-rays may reveal chronic disc degeneration, arthrosis, scoliosis, and possibly spondylolisthesis. If spondylolisthesis is present, additional flexion and extension views can demonstrate if the slippage increases with those maneuvers and represents a more dynamic and unstable situation. MRI is invaluable for confirming the diagnosis and confirming compression. Axial cuts can give a true measurement of the cross-sectional area of the canal and of stenosis at the foraminal level and lateral recess. CT scans are helpful for determining the contribution of the bony elements and osteophytes to the stenosis. Prior to the advent of MRI, myelographic CT scan had been the gold standard.

Differential Diagnosis

Vascular claudication is the most common entity entering in the differential diagnosis of lumbar spinal stenosis. An accurate history and physical examination can often discern between the two. First, vascular claudication has more severe distal lower extremity pain, whereas neurogenic claudication typically has a proximal to distal pain pattern. Also, with vascular claudication, pain is relieved by ceasing to walk and standing still, whereas neurogenic claudication patients need to sit down and lean forward to relieve the pain. Lastly, vascular patients have significant relief from lying supine, whereas stenosis in the canal may be increased in the supine position. The physical examination in the vascular claudicant is also noteworthy for the trophic skin changes secondary to arterial disease and the lack of peripheral pulses. Nonetheless, the two conditions can coexist in the elderly population, and consultation with a vascular surgeon should be sought in equivocal cases. Any of the previously mentioned neurologic conditions can also mimic lumbar stenosis. Unilateral or foraminal stenosis can present similar to atypical sciatica [8, 45, 53].

Nonoperative Treatment

Nonoperative treatment includes short courses of bed rest, if helpful, and antiinflammatory medications. Physical therapy with an emphasis on aerobic conditioning, and abdominal strengthening should be employed. Weight loss alone can significantly diminish symptoms in the stenotic patients. Flexion exercises are also helpful. A corset or back brace may be worn for support. Epidural steroid injections can be utilized, especially with acute exacerbations. Narcotic analgesics should be avoided as they have addictive properties and fail to target the underlying etiology.

Operative Treatment

Patients unresponsive to nonsurgical measures and those with increasing pain, gait disturbance, or with bowel/bladder dysfunction should be considered for surgical therapy. The cornerstone to surgical management is adequate decompression of all stenotic segments. The preoperative MRI and CT scans must be carefully evaluated for all possible locations of stenosis. Not infrequently the entire length of the lumbar canal must be decompressed to ensure adequate room for the neural elements. The surgeon must be meticulous when addressing the bony, disc, and ligamentous contributions to the narrowed canal. To assure an adequate decompression, nerve roots should be carefully mobilized and the neural foramen probed with the appropriate instrumentation. If no more than 50% of any facet level must be removed and the spine is not unstable for other reasons, fusion is not needed to ensure a good postoperative result. If degenerative spondylolisthesis exists, fusing these segments should be strongly considered in light of the findings of numerous long-term studies [58–60]. Fusion attempts may be supplemented with instrumentation. Studies have shown that while there is a better chance of achieving arthrodesis with instrumentation following posterolateral fusion, clinical outcomes may not differ [33]. Further studies should be done to better understand this issue (Fig. 88.16).

Results

Among appropriately selected patients, more than 75% have significant relief postoperatively [61, 62]. Workmen's compensation patients, secondary gain, and smoking are among the predictors of a poor result [63].

Adult Scoliosis

The normal adult spine when viewed from the front is straight. Any deviation or curvature in the lateral plane is referred to as scoliosis. In actuality, the curvature represents a three-dimensional deformity with rotation of all the vertebral elements and the rib cage. Scoliosis generally affects

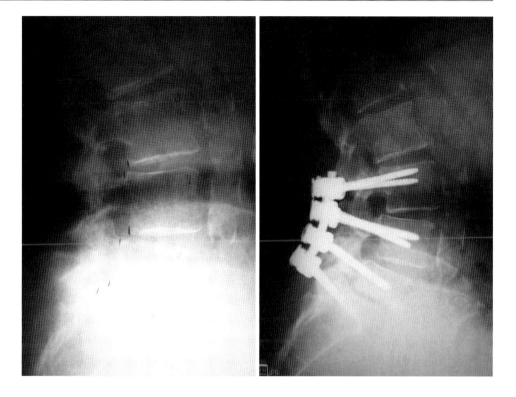

FIGURE 88.16 Seventy-five-year-old female with symptoms of spondylosis and spinal stenosis with multilevel spondylolistheses treated with posterior decompression and instrumented fusion from L3 to S1.

adolescent girls, but the elderly population may also present with scoliosis from various causes.

Pathophysiology

The two major categories of adult scoliosis are the idiopathic and degenerative varieties. Adult idiopathic scoliosis usually is an extension of its adolescent variant and results from a missed or untreated diagnosis. As mentioned, young girls present with this condition during adolescence. The curves are usually in the thoracic spine and are not painful during youth. Curves of less than 40–50° tend not to progress once growth has stopped [64]. Larger curves may progress into adult life. Most are thoracic curves in which the convexity of the curve is to the right. The pathophysiology is unknown, although a hereditary pattern seems to exist. By the same token, there has never been a causal relationship established between osteoporosis and degenerative scoliosis. The recommended treatment of curves of more than 40–50° is fusion during adolescence; bracing and observation are recommended for lesser curves (20–40°). Adult degenerative scoliosis primarily affects the lumbar spine. Disc degeneration, facet arthrosis, degenerative stenosis or listhesis, compression fractures, osteoporosis, and muscle imbalance may contribute to the three-dimensional deformity, yet none have been shown to be directly related [65]. Abnormal rotation of the lumbar vertebral elements is also evident. Why

certain patients with chronic disc degeneration develop a concomitant lumbar scoliosis and others do not is not known [66–68].

Natural History

Degenerative lumbar scoliosis is characterized by minimal structural vertebral deformity, advanced degenerative changes, and a predominance of lower lumbar curves [65]. Adult scoliosis arising from adolescent scoliosis generally does not present a problem with curves <40–50°. For larger curves, pain is often localized to the concavity of the curve (where the facet joints are excessively loaded) [41]. Nerve roots along the concavity may be compressed, and the patients may present with signs of nerve root irritation. Cosmetic concerns such as increasing rib prominence and shoulder asymmetry may be presenting complaints. For extremely large curves (>100°), shortness of breath secondary to diminished lung capacity can be a problem [69, 70] (Fig. 88.17). Degenerative scoliosis usually is less a cosmetic concern, as curves tend to be much smaller. Patients present with nonspecific back pain usually along the concavity of the curve, signs of nerve root irritation, or even spinal stenosis. Progression of deformity is expected in patients with an intercrest line passing through the disc space of L4–5 or below, as well as in cases where the index curve or vertebral rotation is extensive [65].

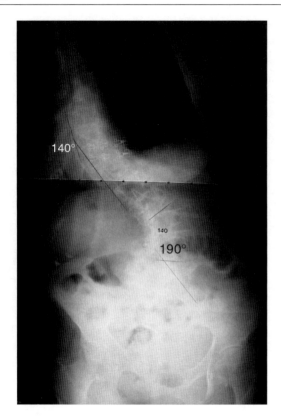

Figure 88.17 Eighty-year-old female with thoracolumbar adult scoliosis measuring 140°.

Nonoperative Treatment

Adult scoliosis should be approached with caution. Nonoperative treatment should be fully exhausted prior to surgical consideration. NSAIDS, bracing, medical management (i.e., bisphosphonates), weight reduction, exercise, and epidural steroids may be employed.

Operative Treatment

Patients with refractory pain, evidence of spinal imbalance, or signs of neural compression can be considered for operative treatment. All patients should undergo full-length radiography of the entire spine in the PA and lateral projection. Bending films can help assess the degree of rigidity to the curve. Additionally, patients with symptoms of nerve root compression or spinal stenosis should undergo MRI or myelography of the affected area.

The operative approach to treatment must be highly individualized. If the presenting problem is back pain without nerve root compression or stenosis, a posterior approach with curve correction, instrumentation, and fusion are recommended. If nerve root compression or stenosis is significant, careful decompression of the affected area must be

included. Lumbar degenerative curves can often be approached anteriorly. Combined anterior and posterior approaches may be needed for difficult rigid curves [68]. If the only symptom is that of a single nerve root compression, simple posterior decompression without curve correction or fusion is reasonable. For patients with pulmonary compromise due to thoracic curves, curve correction to allow increased pulmonary capacity is of paramount importance.

Results

Surgery for adult scoliosis is associated with a high incidence of complications, many of which are medical in nature, including blood loss, infection, pneumonia or atelectasis, inability to achieve fusion, and neurologic injury. Adult curves are stiffer than pediatric curves, and achieving curve correction is limited. Patients must be carefully selected and appraised of these potential complications. Residual back pain may remain despite the presence of a solid fusion [71, 72].

Trauma

Spinal trauma and spinal cord injury represent significant sources of morbidity and mortality. It is estimated that more than 50,000 spine fractures occur yearly, with neurologic injury occurring one-fifth of the time [73]. Most are secondary to significant energy mechanisms such as motor vehicle accidents, falls from heights, and gunshot wounds. The patients generally are young, 20–40 years old, but the elderly are not immune to these injuries. Patients presenting to emergency rooms or practitioners with a history and mechanism suggestive of spinal injury warrant a full evaluation. The elderly often sustain spinal injuries with lesser degrees of energy because of fragility, osteoporosis, or other predisposing conditions of the spine.

Cervical Spine Trauma

Patients sustaining cervical spine trauma present with the complaint of neck pain and or extremity weakness if spinal cord injury has taken place. The mechanism of injury must be carefully ascertained and preexisting medical conditions and any loss of consciousness delineated. The physical examination must be thorough. The cervical spine is examined for evidence of soft tissue contusion as well as tenderness to palpation. Flexion, extension, and rotation are documented. A careful overview of upper extremity motor power, sensation, and reflexes is undertaken.

FIGURE 88.18 Helical CT scan sagittal reconstruction of unilateral facet perch at C6/C7 in 60-year-old male who fell on his head (Case Courtesy of Nathaniel Tindell, MD).

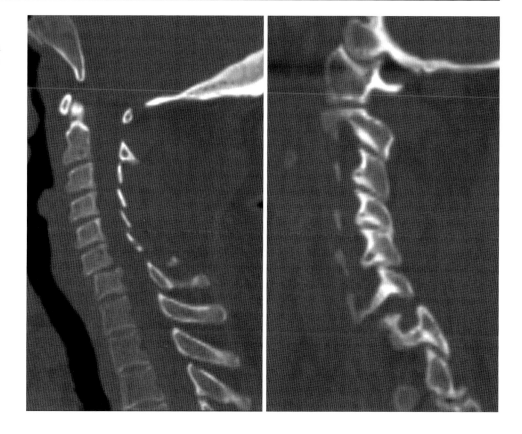

Any abnormality on the examination should prompt the treating physician to obtain cervical spine radiographs. The standard trauma protocol for cervical spine injury includes an AP, lateral, and open-mouth odontoid view. The lateral view must demonstrate C1–T1 to be considered adequate. Recent studies show that helical computed tomography (CT) can be safely used in place of plain radiograph to evaluate the cervical spine for osseous abnormalities such as fracture and dislocations after high-energy trauma (Fig. 88.18). If a pure ligamentous injury is suspected, supervised bending cervical spine films or MRI is recommended [74]. If the mechanism of injury is significant, such as a motor vehicle accident, an AP pelvis and chest radiograph should also be obtained.

A variety of injuries can occur in the cervical spine including flexion-type compression injuries, dislocation of one vertebra on another, burst injuries of the vertebral bodies, spinous process fractures, and lamina fractures. Treatment is affected by the degree of instability present and whether a neurologic injury has occurred. In cases presenting with an acute progressive neurologic injury, urgent MRI, CT or myelogram CT, and surgical decompression with stabilization comprise the treatment of choice once the patient is medically stabilized. Urgent decompression offers the best chance of recovery of neurologic function. Injuries with a static neurologic injury can be addressed on a more elective basis. If an injury has occurred without neurologic injury, the

degree of instability rendered greatly influences further management. Attempts have been made to define criteria for cervical spine instability [3]. The amount of vertebral body destroyed, the angulation and translation at the injury site, and disc space narrowing contribute to the relative instability of the injury.

Certain injuries do not confer instability to the spine. They include isolated lamina fractures, spinous process avulsions or fractures, and simple compression injuries to isolated vertebral bodies. These injuries can be managed with a hard or soft collar depending on the level of patient discomfort. Other injuries are inherently unstable. All dislocations are unstable. They must be reduced regardless of whether neurologic injury has occurred [75] (Fig. 88.19). Difficulty with reduction warrants an MRI to ensure that an entrapped disc fragment is not present [76]. If present, an anterior disc excision should precede the reduction. Following reduction of dislocations, the spine should be stabilized via posterior fusion. When the posterior ligamentous complex is injured, it should be treated by elective posterior fusion [75].

Frequently, patients have negative radiographic and MRI findings despite persistent pain. The severity of these whiplash injuries should not be underestimated. The patient should be placed in a hard collar for support and given adequate muscle relaxant and pain medication. A follow-up appointment with an orthopedic surgeon should take place within 2 weeks. If pain persists, the patient should obtain

FIGURE 88.19 Bilateral facet perch at C7/T1 in 62-year-old male hit by tree branch in the back of head with onset of paraplegia, successfully treated with open reduction and instrumented fusion.

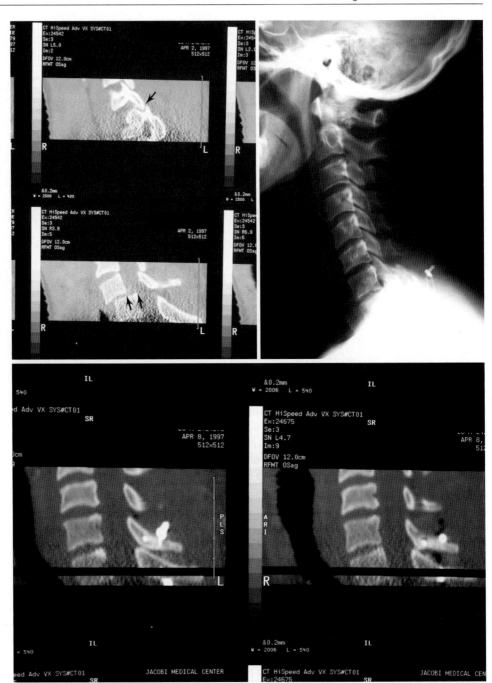

flexion and extension views of the cervical spine to rule out a ligamentous injury [77].

Thoracolumbar/Lumbar Spinal Trauma

As with cervical spinal trauma, thoracolumbar and lumbar spinal trauma is usually the result of high-energy injuries. Timely and appropriate evaluation is crucial to successful management and outcome of these injuries.

Upon presentation to the emergency room, a thorough history and physical examination must take place. Preexisting medical conditions, mechanism of injury, and loss of consciousness at the scene should be ascertained. If secondary to a motor vehicle accident, questioning as to the use of a seat belt or lap belt is important. Assuming the patient maintains stable vital signs, a thorough examination is undertaken. In particular, the presence of bruising to the flank or back suggests a significant injury to the spinal column or retroperitoneum. A thorough examination of all four extremities for motor, sensation, and reflex responses is vital. A rectal examination should be done to document tone. The presence of any neurologic deficit must be noted. Patients noted to have neurologic deficit should be given intravenous steroids. When administered within 8 h after injury, steroids have been shown to be helpful in recovering some neurologic function [78].

Once adequately stabilized, the patient should undergo appropriate radiography. AP and lateral films of the thoracolumbar spine for those with suspected injuries are first-line studies. An AP film of the pelvis, a chest radiograph, and films of the cervical spine complete the trauma series.

There are numerous mechanisms of injury to the thoracolumbar spine leading to various injury patterns, including axial compression, flexion, extension, rotation, and distraction mechanisms. Flexion-distraction injuries are associated with the use of a lap belt without a shoulder strap, which is associated with a high incidence of visceral injuries. They should be suspected in a patient after a motor vehicle accident, particularly with abrasions across the abdomen.

Treatment must be individualized to the patient and the injury pattern. Goals of treatment are rapid mobilization of the elderly patient with the avoidance of further neurologic deterioration. Emergency surgery is indicated only in cases of worsening neurologic deficit. Emergent CT or MRI should be performed in these cases to detect the site of neural compression. A canal or foraminal decompression should take place to remove impinging fragments, and the spine should be stabilized with instrumentation and fusion. The decision to approach the spine from an anterior or posterior approach depends on the injury pattern and the site of neural compression. Generally, more thorough decompression is possible from an anterior approach.

In cases of static neurologic deficit, elective surgery to decompress the canal may be beneficial for regaining neurologic function. Timing of surgical decompression is a topic of debate. We tend to intervene during the first week, although recovery of some neurologic function has been noted with late decompression [79–81].

If no neurologic deficit is present, treatment should be based on the relative stability of the injury and the propensity for satisfactory healing. Certain injuries are stable. Examples include isolated fracture of a spinous process or transverse process secondary to a direct blow. Patients can be managed with a short period of bed rest and pain medication. A brace may be worn for comfort. Compression fractures of the spine are usually secondary to flexion mechanisms (Fig. 88.20). When the height of the anterior vertebral body is compressed less than 50% of the posterior aspect of the body and when no reversal of lumbar lordosis is present, the injury is relatively stable. Treatment can be placement in a thoracolumbosacral orthotic molded in

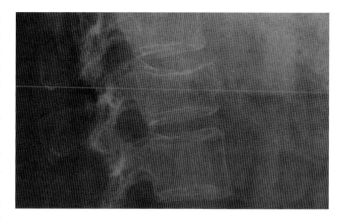

Figure 88.20 Sixty-five-year-old female with sudden onset of pain while opening a window. Lateral lumbosacral spine radiographs shows compression fracture at L1 (Case Courtesy of Nathaniel Tindell, MD).

extension for several months and pain control. In cases of persistent or exaggerated pain that renders the patient incapable of prolonged mobilization, kyphoplasty or vertebroplasty has been shown to improve symptoms allowing for more rapid rehabilitation [82]. These procedures involve percutaneous dilation of the vertebral body with insertion of bone cement. Kyphoplasty utilizes an inflatable balloon tamp which limits the possibility of extravasation of cement to neighboring tissue (Fig. 88.21).

Injuries with anterior compression of more than 50% of the posterior body vertebral height or with reversal of lumbar lordosis are more unstable injuries because they connote injuries to the posterior ligamentous complex of the spine [3]. Surgical stabilization and fusion offer the most predictable healing results. Surgery also allows more predictable restoration of sagittal alignment.

Other injuries further destabilize the spine. They include all fracture-dislocations of the spine and most flexion-distraction injuries. To ensure healing, preservation of neurologic function, and avoidance of postinjury deformity, surgical stabilization and fusion should be undertaken. It is usually done from a posterior approach.

Systemic Disorders of the Spine

Osteoporosis refers to decreased bone mass and increased risk of fracture. The vertebrae are the bones most commonly affected. This condition affects up to 20 million people yearly and represents a significant source of morbidity and cost. This is a condition of the elderly, with postpartum women affected more than twice as frequently as men. An understanding of the pathophysiology and treatment of this entity is essential for the geriatric clinician [83].

Figure 88.21 Sixty-four-year-
old female with low back pain
after fall and radiographic
evidence of compression fracture
at L1 treated with kyphoplasty
(Case Courtesy of Nathaniel
Tindell, MD).

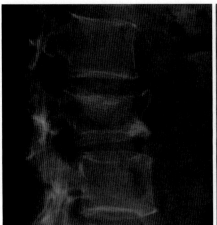
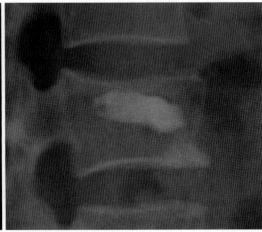

Pathophysiology

Bone is a living tissue constantly undergoing resorption and
formation under the control of osteoblasts and osteoclasts.
Peak bone mass is generally achieved during the third decade
of life. Adequate daily calcium and vitamin D intake as well
as exercise are essential for achieving the highest peak bone
mass possible. Once peak mass is attained, resorption of
bone exceeds formation, leading to a gradual diminution in
bone mass. The rate of resorption is higher for women than it
is for men. Rates of resorption further increase with the onset
of menopause, probably secondary to the absence of estrogen, which acts to increase calcium absorption. Genetics also
plays an important role in the development of osteoporosis.
Fair-skinned individuals of northern European descent have
the highest risk of disease progression. Other associated factors include early menopause, smoking, sedentary life style,
phenytoin use, and excessive alcohol intake [83].

With advancing age, susceptible individuals may experience fragility fractures. The spine and the hip are most commonly affected. These fractures are often seen after minor
trauma such as lifting or tripping.

Evaluation

Evaluation begins with a thorough history with attention to
the aforementioned predisposing factors. The onset of pain
and discomfort must be discerned. A history of long-standing
pain, night pain, or other systemic signs such as fever
or weight loss, should alert the physician to the possibility
of tumor or infection rather than an osteoporotic fracture.
The presentation is usually of local pain to the affected vertebrae without neurologic deficit or radiation to the lower
extremities.

Examination reveals tenderness at the fracture site. Patients
with previous vertebral compression fractures may demonstrate increased kyphosis to the thoracic spine. Radiographs
of the affected area reveal osteopenia, decreased bone mass,
and fracture of the affected vertebrae. In the thoracic spine
this usually takes the form of an anterior compression or
wedged appearance. In the lumbar spine more generalized
flattening of the vertebrae occurs. It is not uncommon for
asymptomatic or minimally symptomatic vertebral compression fractures to be discovered incidentally by radiography.

For first time presenters, laboratory tests should be done
to rule out the reversible causes of osteoporosis, which
include hyperthyroidism and increased cortisol levels.
Otherwise, routine blood values are normal including calcium, hemoglobin, phosphorus, and alkaline phosphatase
levels [84].

More sophisticated methods for evaluating osteoporosis
include dual energy X-ray absorptiometry (DEXA). This test
subjects patients to a low dose of radiation with high accuracy. Bone mass is quantified in terms of density within standard deviations of normal. Individuals with more than two
SD of normal are considered osteoporotic and are at significantly increased risk of fracture [8].

Treatment

The cornerstone of management is prevention. As mentioned,
ensuring adequate calcium and vitamin D intake as well as
exercise during youth are the most reliable methods of
increasing peak bone mass [85]. Patients older than 65 should
maintain a daily intake of 1,500 mg of elemental calcium.
This is especially important in susceptible individuals. Once
fracture has occurred, the goals include pain relief, patient
mobilization, and prevention of further bone loss and deformity. Pain relief can be managed with NSAIDs or a short

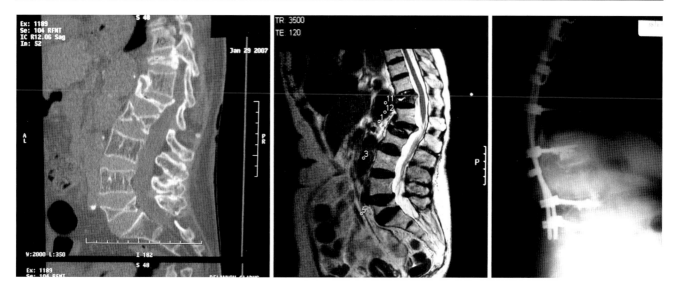

Figure 88.22 Seventy-six-year-old female with multiple compression fractures, kyphosis, and progressive neurologic deficit treated with posterior cement augmented instrumentation and fusion with restoration of sagittal profile and improvement in neurologic status.

course of a narcotic analgesic. Several days of bed rest may be prescribed, after which the patient is encouraged to mobilize. The letter can be aided with the use of a thoracolumbar orthosis molded in extension, which should be worn until pain is resolved and follow-up radiographs show no increase in the deformity. Usually 6–12 weeks suffices.

Pharmacologic treatment of osteoporosis includes administration of supplemental calcium and vitamin D, which can help avoid further bone loss. The use of estrogen in perimenopausal and postmenopausal women has been shown to reduce vertebral compression fractures. Other agents include biphosphonates (Fosamax) [86], which also decrease osteoclastic activity, and fluoride, which stimulates osteoblastic proliferation. The appropriate pharmacologic protocol should be managed by a knowledgeable internist or rheumatologist.

Most of these injuries heal uneventfully. Surgery is rarely indicated for management of osteoporosis of the spine. One indication is an acute fracture with neurologic deficit, which is a rare occurrence. Loss of bowel/bladder control is another indication for surgical decompression. Other indications for surgery include progressive deformity with unremitting pain. The clinician must also be aware of insidious onset of neurologic deficit in the setting of multiple compression fractures with increasing kyphosis or scoliosis (Fig. 88.22). This situation may represent spinal stenosis due to anterior canal compromise. It can occur months to years after injury. Therefore it is recommended that osteoporotic fractures be followed on a regular basis until increasing deformity has definitively stopped. These patients are often risky surgical candidates because of their multiple medical problems. Additionally, poor bone quality makes fixation difficult. The surgical approach depends on the deformity and may be

anterior, posterior, or combined. Patients must be made aware of the significant risk of these surgeries [88].

Studies have shown an association with multilevel compression fractures and a higher risk of death from pulmonary complications in women 65 years and older [88]. Kyphoplasty may be used to stabilize a progressive kyphotic deformity from an osteoporotic compression fracture in the acute or subacute period. In some cases, actual height restoration can be achieved. Long-term complications associated with this procedure include an increased risk of vertebral body fracture from forces exerted by the adjacent cement-injected level [82].

Infections of the Spine

Infections of the spinal column are common in the elderly or the immune compromised population. Diabetes, rheumatoid disease, concurrent urine infection, skin ulceration, and abscesses predispose to spinal infection. Unfortunately, the diagnosis is often missed early in its course, leading to delay in treatment and increased patient morbidity [89].

Vertebral Osteomyelitis: Pyogenic and Mycobacterial

Presentation

The most common presentation of vertebral osteomyelitis is chronic vague back pain. Hematogenous spread is the most common mode of transmission. The lumbar region is most commonly affected followed by the thoracic and cervical regions. Patients relate that the pain is not activity-related and is not relieved with standard measures. Furthermore, it often wakes the patient at night or prevents sleep. Patients may complain of systemic manifestations such as fever, chills, weight loss, and loss of appetite; but these findings are often absent. The physical examination may reveal local erythema and increased temperature over the affected region. The area may be tender to palpation with surrounding muscle spasm. Range of motion is often restricted owing to pain and spasm. Fewer than 10% of patients have neurologic findings upon presentation, although diabetes and a cephalad level of involvement put the patient at increased risk [90].

Laboratory results may indicate an elevated white blood cell (WBC) count but are often normal. The erythrocyte sedimentation rate (ESR) is an extremely sensitive but nonspecific test, with elevated values in more than 90% of cases. It is, however, an excellent method for serial monitoring of the response to treatment.

If fever is present, blood cultures should be obtained but are often negative outside of temperature spikes. Radiographs can be entirely normal early in the disease; later they reveal destruction of the anterior vertebral metaphysis, diminished disc space height, and reactive subchondral bone formation. With mycobacterial infections the disc spaces are remarkably well preserved until late in the disease process [91]. Paraspinal shadows may be prominent owing to soft tissue extension of infection. A technetium bone scan with gallium has a more than 90% accuracy record for infection of the spine, but MRI is currently the modality of choice for confirming the diagnosis of infection; it distinctly reveals decreased signal to the disc and vertebrae on T1-weighted scans and increased signal on T2-weighted scans [92].

Treatment

The key to management of osteomyelitis is identification of the offending agent. *Staphylococcus aureus* causes approximately half of all infections but *Escherichia coli, Staphylococcus epidermidis*, and Pseudomonas are other common organisms [89]. Recently, *Mycobacterium tuberculosis* has made a resurgence among the immune compromised and the elderly. Hence, suspected patients should undergo PPD testing and chest radiography in a search for pulmonary nodules. Thorough evaluation of the MRI scan to look for anterior and paravertebral masses and anterior bony destruction should be undertaken. These are classic findings associated with spinal tuberculosis. Other granulomatous diseases of the spine are also being seen with increasing frequency in this population.

Blood cultures, if positive, can direct antibiotic therapy. Unfortunately, they are positive only 25% of the time. In the absence of positive cultures, biopsy may be attempted via closed technique, CT- or fluoroscopy guided. The yield for closed technique is approximately 75%. If the closed technique fails, open biopsy is mandatory to establish organism identification. Tumor and infection can have similar clinical and radiographic appearances, so all tissues should be sent for pathologic study. Gram staining, aerobic and anaerobic, Mycobacterium, and fungal testing should take place. Once an organism has been identified and its sensitivities established, antimicrobial therapy can be instituted. Six weeks of intravenous therapy followed by oral antibiotics is standard. Additionally, the spine should be immobilized in a brace. Multidrug therapy consisting of isoniazid, rifampin, ethambutol, and pyrazinamide are recommended for tuberculosis infections. Patients are usually treated for 6–12 months. The course of the disease should be monitored by clinical examination, repeat laboratory tests, and repeat MRI at appropriate intervals. When identified early, most infections can be resolved without the need for major surgical procedures [93].

Surgery

Drug therapy is the treatment of choice for spinal infections. Surgery is indicated in specific instances: inability to establish diagnosis; failure of medical management to relieve pain and sepsis; worsening neurologic deficit; or increasing deformity and bony destruction. Additionally, patients with spinal tuberculosis in the cervical region and a neurologic deficit should be treated with surgical débridement because of the high risk of paralysis without surgical intervention. An attempt should be made to delay surgery for 2 weeks to allow the antibiotics to decrease the inflammation and allow an easier surgical approach [94].

If surgery is indicated, the approach and procedure are dictated by the location of the infection. Most of the infections are located anteriorly in the vertebral bodies. The approach therefore is usually anterior via removal of infectious material including the involved vertebral bodies and any soft tissue abscess. Iliac crest bone graft or fibular strut graft should replace the removed bodies. Sometimes a vascularized rib may be utilized with thoracic level infections (Fig. 88.23). If the spine is rendered unstable, an additional posterior fusion can be utilized for further stabilization [90, 95].

Epidural Abscess

Epidural abscesses are foci of infection in the potential space of the spinal canal outside the covering of the cord itself. They occur most commonly in the elderly and are a true medical and surgical emergency. More than 10% of cases are misdiagnosed at the initial visit to a physician.

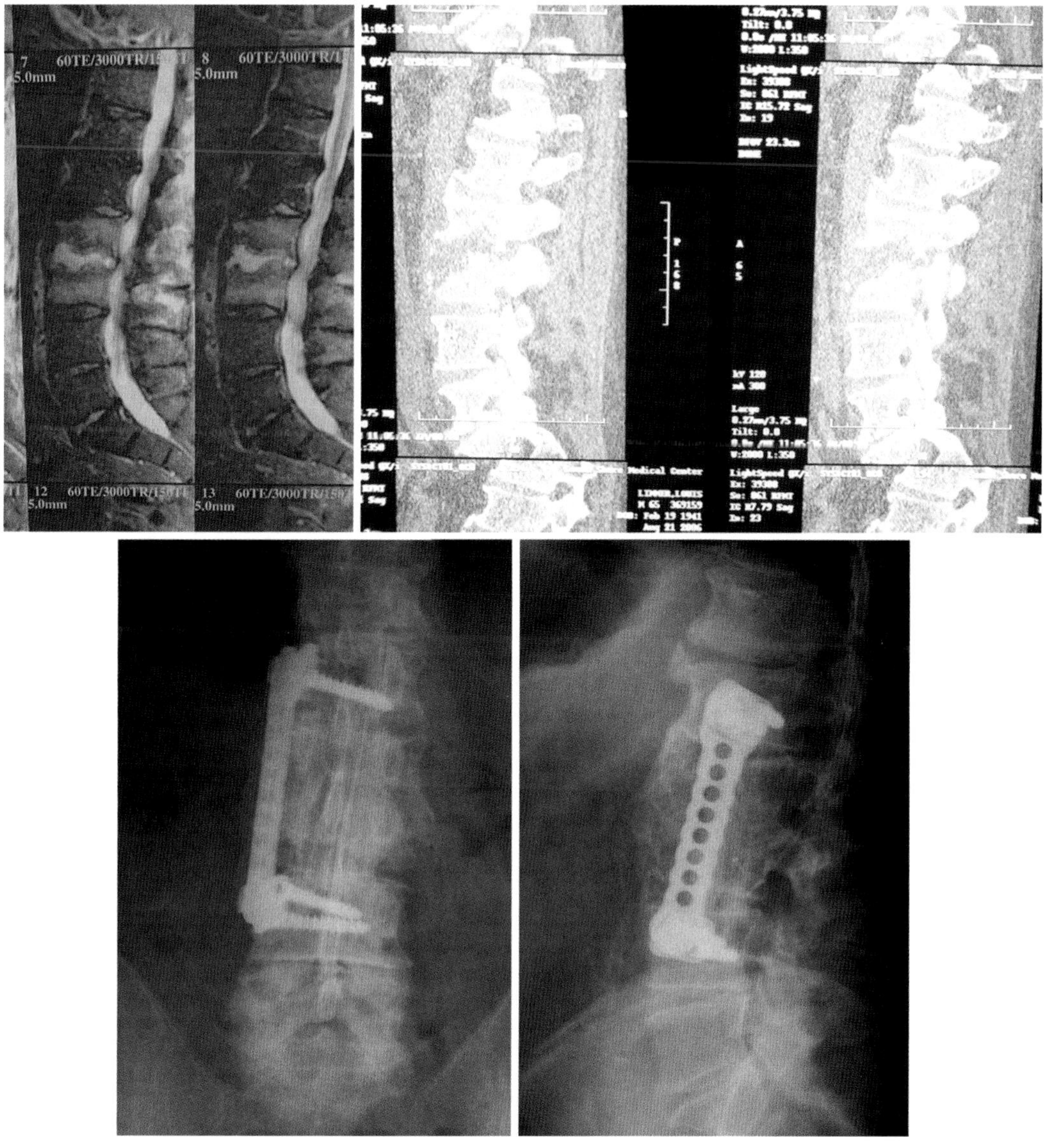

FIGURE 88.23 Seventy-two-year-old male with osteomyelitis, discitis, and psoas abscess at L2/L3 treated with anterior approach, debridement, vascularized rib strut graft fusion and instrumentation.

Predisposing factors are similar to those of osteomyelitis of the spine.

Epidural abscesses may arise via hematogenous spread from a distant site or via direct extension from a focus of vertebral osteomyelitis. Most abscesses are in the lumbar and thoracic region and are located dorsally within the canal. Cervical abscesses are less common but usually represent an extension of vertebral osteomyelitis and are located anteriorly [96].

The most frequent presentation is that of pain localized to the site of the abscess. Patients look and feel ill. More than 50% of patients have increased temperature upon presentation. The examination is otherwise nonspecific and may include spasm, tenderness, and restricted range of motion. Patients may have signs of nerve root irritation. Usually,

neurologic deficit is absent during the first 48 h followed by neurologic dysfunction over the next several days. Frank paresis may evolve if left untreated. Early diagnosis and treatment are essential.

Laboratory values often reveal an increased WBC count and ESR. Radiographs are not usually helpful but may show vertebral endplate erosions or increased soft tissue outlines, especially in the cervical spine. If the diagnosis is suspected, urgent MRI of the affected region is done. The addition of gadolinium further sensitizes the study. Findings are of decreased epidural signal on T1-weighted scans and hyperintensity of the abscess on T2-weighted images [97].

Once the diagnosis is established, broad-spectrum antibiotics to include coverage of Staphylococcus, Streptococcus, and Mycobacterium when indicated, should be administered without delay, followed by urgent surgical decompression. If located in the lumbar or thoracic region simple drainage with laminectomy may suffice. Cervical abscesses necessitate an anterior approach and removal of vertebral bodies with fusion. If the diagnosis is established early, the prognosis is good; delay may lead to mortality rates in excess of 10% [96].

Tumors of the Spine

With the exception of multiple myeloma, primary neoplasms of the spine are rare, especially in the elderly. Metastatic lesions of the spine, however, are common in this population. Other than lung and liver, the spine represents the most frequent site of metastasis and is the most frequent site of skeletal metastasis [98].

Presentation

Patients present most frequently with the complaint of back pain localized to the site of metastases. The pain is slowly progressive and does not respond to standard analgesics, rest, or other modalities. Frequently, night pain is present resulting in an inability to fall asleep. Systemic symptoms such as fever, weight loss, and lethargy are often communicated. Neurologic signs and symptoms may be present, suggesting invasion of the spinal cord or nerve roots by the lesion. The patient may present with chronic progressive back pain, with an acute onset of severe pain, which is often the result of a fracture through a pathologic lesion.

Evaluation

As always, the history and physical examination are the keys to proper evaluation. Back pain in the setting of a current or prior malignancy should alert the physician to the possibility of spinal metastases. Standard laboratory test may reveal anemia, increased alkaline phosphatase, elevated ESR, or in the case of multiple myeloma elevated urine and serum electrophoresis measurements. Standard radiographs of the affected region should be obtained. Close attention should be paid to vertebral body changes and pedicle destruction, as they are the frequent sites of the metastatic deposits. Unfortunately, radiographs are frequently normal, as approximately 50% of marrow replacement must occur to cause findings on plain films [99]. If clinical suspicion exists, an MRI scan should be obtained. MRI is extremely sensitive for the marrow changes seen with malignancy. Metastases appear hyperintense on T2-weighted images.

MRI also enables study of the spinal cord, epidural space, and surrounding soft tissues. This is especially important when evaluating patients with neurologic deficit. Once MRI confirms a lesion, a bone scan is recommended to localize additional bony deposits. Of note, multiple myeloma is frequently cold on bone scans. A chest radiograph may reveal a module suggesting the lung as the site of the primary malignancy.

Management

Once a metastatic lesion to the spine has been established, its pathology must be ascertained. This should be done by correlating the remainder of the workup (laboratory results, radiographs, abdominal or pelvic CT, colonoscopy) or if necessary via biopsy of the lesion. This may be done via a closed technique using CT or fluoroscopic guidance. If this is unsuccessful, an open biopsy must be performed. Once a definitive diagnosis is established, further management must emphasize a team approach, including the help of an internist, oncologist, orthopedic surgeon, and neurosurgeon.

The most sensitive prognostic indicator for survival is not the extent of the spinal lesion but the primary diagnosis. Hence, any treatment must take into account the expected lifetime of the patient. Patients with breast cancer and multiple myeloma have a longer life expectancy, often more than 2 years from the diagnosis. Gastrointestinal and lung malignancies involving the spine have a much shorter life expectancy.

Available modalities include analgesics, bracing, radiotherapy, chemotherapy, and surgery. If no neurologic deficit is present or fracture has not occurred, there is no need for emergent surgery. The radiosensitivity of the lesion should be determined and the effectiveness of chemotherapy. For example, multiple myeloma and lymphoma are extremely radiosensitive. If the tumor is radiosensitive, irradiation can be done. If significant pain relief occurs, it may serve as definitive management. Emergent surgery is indicated for patients with progressive neurologic deficit or fracture of a vertebral element with a propensity for instability, further neurologic injury, or both. All additional lesions must be dealt with on an individual basis. Specifically, surgery may be indicated for unremitting pain unresponsive to other modalities and large lesions suspicious of impending fracture or instability. For highly vascular tumors, such as thyroid and renal cell carcinoma, where irradiation and surgery are planned, surgery should take place prior to initiation of radiotherapy. This is to prevent wound healing complications associated with radiation use. The surgery must be highly individualized. Anterior lesions should be approached anteriorly and posterior legions posteriorly. Generally,

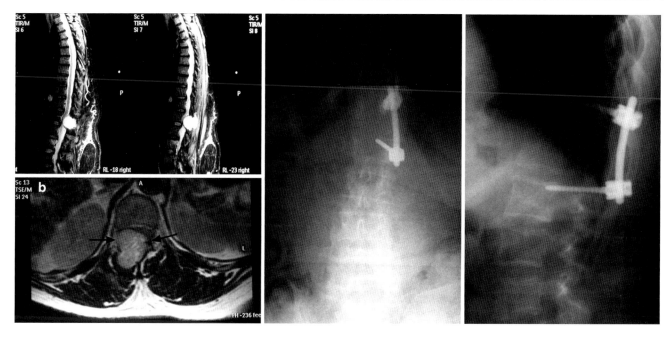

FIGURE 88.24   Sixty-eight-year-old female with metastatic lung carcinoma to posterior elements of T12 with neurologic deterioration treated with posterior decompression, instrumented fusion, and full neurologic recovery.

lesions causing neurologic compromise necessitate an anterior approach. All pathologic tissue should be removed and the spine stabilized with instrumentation. Careful study of the preoperative MRI is necessary. If possible, asymptomatic lesions are included in the stabilization. If life-span is limited, fusion is not mandatory, but if doubt exists as to life expectancy, fusion should be performed [100].

Results

The prognosis for spinal metastases is the same as for the primary lesion. Spinal surgery is never curative, only palliative. However, in patients with unremitting pain and neurologic compromise, surgery enables an improved life style and easier mobilization (Fig. 88.24).

CASE STUDY

Sixty-five-year-old male with history of chronic low back pain and intermittent bilateral lower extremity paresthesia. The patient described worsening lower extremity pain with prolonged standing and walking long distances. He reported a need to sit to relieve symptoms and no difficulty while climbing stairs (see Fig. 88.12).

Neurovascular examination was essentially normal, significant only for loss of lumbar lordosis and a forward flexed gait. Radiographic evaluation was significant for a degenerative lumbar spondyolisthesis at L_3/L_4, degenerative disc disease, and disc desiccation. Spinal stenosis was confirmed by magnetic resonance imaging.

Patient was indicated for posterior lumbar laminectomy, instrumentation, and posterolateral fusion from L_3 to L_5. Postoperatively, the patient had resolution of his symptoms and clinical/radiographic fusion at 3 months time. Rehabilitation was required to restore basic functional capacity.

References

1. Deyo R, Tsui-Wu Y (1987) Descriptive epidemiology of low back pain and its related medical care in the United States. Spine 12:264–268
2. Moore KL (1985) The back. In: Gardner J (ed) Clinically oriented anatomy. Williams & Wilkins, Baltimore, pp 565–625
3. White AA III, Panjabi MM (1990) Clinical biomechanics of the spine, 2nd edn. Lippincott, Philadelphia
4. Miller JA, Schwatz C, Schultz AB (1988) Lumbar disc degeneration: correlation with age, sex, spinal level in 600 autopsy specimens. Spine 13:173–178
5. Boden SD, Davis DO et al (1990) Abnormal magnetic resonance scans of the lumbar spine in asymptomatic subjects: a prospective investigation. J Bone Joint Surg Am 72:403–408

6. Lipson SJ (1990) Aging versus degeneration of the intervertebral disc. In: Weinstein JW, Wiesel JW (eds) The lumbar spine. Saunders, Philadelphia

7. Pritzker KP (1977) Aging and degeneration in the lumbar intervertebral disc. Orthop Clin North Am 8:65–77

8. Miller M (1996) Spine: review of orthopaedics. Saunders, Philadelphia, pp 270–291

9. Rohling ML, Binder LM, Langhinrichsen-Rohling J (1995) Money matters: a meta-analytic review of the association between financial compensation and the experience and treatment of chronic pain. Health Psychol 14:537–547

10. Gatchel RJ, Rolatin PB, Mayer TG (1995) The dominant role of psychosocial risk factors in the development of chronic low back pain disability. Spine 20:2702–2709

11. Jahnke RW, Hart BL (1991) Cervical stenosis, spondylosis and herniated disc disease. Radiol Clin North Am 29:777

12. MacNab I, McCulloch J (1994) Cervical disc degeneration. In: Passano WM III (ed) Neck ache and shoulder pain. Williams & Wilkins, Baltimore, pp 53–62

13. MacNab I, McCulloch J (1994) Classification of shoulder disorders and assessment of shoulder function. In: Passano WM III (ed) Neck ache and shoulder pain. Williams & Wilkins, Baltimore, pp 275–307

14. MacNab I, McCulloch J (1994) Treatment of cervical disc disease. In: Passano WM III (ed) Neck ache and shoulder pain. Williams & Wilkins, Baltimore, pp 79–120

15. Hoppenfeld S (1976) Physical examination of the cervical spine and temporomandibular joint. In: Hoppenfeld S (ed) Physical examination of the spine and extremities. Appleton-Century-Crofts, East Norwalk, CT, pp 105–132

16. Cornefjord M, Olmarter K, Farley DB et al (1995) Neuropeptide changes in compressed spinal nerve roots. Spine 20:670–673

17. Rhee JM, Daniel Riew K (2007) Cervical radiculopathy. J Am Acad Orthop Surg 15:486–494

18. Lees F, Alden Turner JW (1963) Natural history and prognosis of cervical spondylosis. Br Med J 2:1607–1610

19. Bohlman H, Emery SE, Goodfellow DB et al (1993) Robinson anterior cervical discectomy and arthrodesis for cervical radiculopathy: long-term follow-up of one hundred and twenty-two patients. J Bone Joint Surg Am 75:1298–1307

20. An HS (1998) Clinical presentation of discogenic neck pain, radiculopathy, and myelopathy. In: Clark C (ed) The cervical spine, 3rd edn. Lippincott-Raven, Philadelphia, pp 755–763

21. Bensen WG, McMillen JI (1999) Treatment of osteoarthritis with celecoxib, a cyclooxygenase-2 inhibitor: a randomized controlled trail. Mayo Clin Proc 74:1095–1105

22. Kurz LT (1998) Nonoperative treatment of degenerative disorders of the cervical spine. In: Clark C (ed) The cervical spine, 3rd edn. Lippincott-Raven, Philadelphia, pp 779–783

23. Herkowitz HN, Kurz LT, Overholt D (1990) Surgical management of cervical soft disc herniation: a comparison between the anterior and posterior approach. Spine 15:1026–1030

24. Emery SE (2001) Cervical spondylotic myelopathy: diagnosis and treatment. J Am Acad Orthop Surg 9:376–388

25. Benner B (1998) Etiology, pathogenesis, and natural history of discogenic neck pain, radiculopathy and myelopathy. In: Clark C (ed) The cervical spine, 3rd edn. Lippincott-Raven, Philadelphia, pp 735–740

26. Ogino H, Tada K, Okada K et al (1983) Canal diameter, anteroposterior compression ratio, and spondylotic myelopathy of the cervical spine. Spine 8:1–15

27. Clark E, Robinson PK (1956) Cervical myelopathy: a complication of cervical spondylosis. Brain 79:483–570

28. Sachs BL (1998) Differential diagnosis of neck pain, arm pain, and myelopathy. In: Clark C (ed) The cervical spine, 3rd edn. Lippincott-Raven, Philadelphia, pp 741–753

29. Bohlman HH (1977) Cervical spondylosis with moderate to severe myelopathy: a report of 17 cases treated by Robinson anterior cervical discectomy and fusion. Spine 2:151

30. Yonenbou K, Fuji T, Ono K et al (1985) Choice of surgical treatment for multisegmented cervical spondylotic myelopathy. Spine 10:710

31. Garvey TA, Eismont FJ (1991) Diagnosis and treatment of cervical radiculopathy and myelopathy. Orthop Rev 20:595–603

32. Mirkovic S, Cybulishi GR (1997) Thoracic disc herniations. In: Garfin JR, Vaccaro AR (eds) Orthopaedic knowledge update spine. American Academy of Orthopaedic Surgeons, Rosemont, IL, pp 87–96

33. Hilibrand AS, Rand N (1999) Degenerative lumbar stenosis: diagnosis and management. J Am Acad Orthop Surg 7:239–249

34. Wood KB, Garvey TA, Gundry C, Heithoff KB (1995) Magnetic resonance imaging of the thoracic spine. Evaluation of asymptomatic individuals. J Bone Joint Surg Am 11:1631–1638

35. Brown CW, Deffer PA Jr, Akmatijian J et al (1992) The natural history of thoracic disc herniation. Spine 17(Suppl 16):S97–S102

36. Wood KB, Garvey TA, Grundy C (1995) Magnetic resonance imaging of the thoracic spine: evaluation of asymptomatic individuals. J Bone Joint Surg Am 77:631–638

37. Hoppenfeld S, de Boer P (1994) The spine. In: Hannon BC (ed) Surgical exposures in orthopaedics: the anatomic approach, 2nd edn. Lippincott, Philadelphia, pp 216–301

38. Rosenthal D, Rosenthal R, DeSimone A (1994) Removal of a protruded thoracic disc using microsurgical endoscopy: a new technique. Spine 19:1087–1091

39. Simpson JM, Siveri CP, Simeone FA (1993) Thoracic disc herniation: reevaluation of the posterior approach using a modified costotranversectomy. Spine 18:1872–1877

40. MacNab I, McCulloch J (1986) A classification of low back pain. In: Grayson T (ed) Backache, 2nd edn. Williams & Wilkins, Baltimore, pp 22–25

41. Seimon LP. Applied anatomy, pathological anatomy, sources of pain. In: Low back pain: clinical diagnosis and management. East Norwalk, CT: Appleton-Century-Crofts, 1983:3–30

42. Turner JA, Ersch M, Herron L (1992) Patient outcomes after lumbar spinal fusions. JAMA 268:907–911

43. Colhoun E, McCall I, Williams L (1988) Proactive discography as a guide to planning operations on the spine. J Bone Joint Surg Br 70:267–271

44. MacNab I, McCulloch J (1986) Pain and disability (psychogenic back pain). In: Grayson T (ed) Backache, 2nd edn. Williams & Wilkins, Baltimore, pp 26–44

45. Seimon LP. History, examination, special investigations. In: Low back pain: clinical diagnosis and management. East Norwalk, CT: Appleton-Century-Crofts, 1976

46. Hoppenfeld S (1976) Physical examination of the spine and extremities. Appleton-Century-Crofts, East Norwalk, CT

47. O'Donnell JL (1995) Prostaglandin E2 content in herniated lumbar disc disease. Paper No. 266 presented at the 62nd meeting of American Academy of Orthopaedic Surgeons, February 1995

48. Olmarker K (1996) The experimental basis of sciatica. J Orthop Sci 1:230–242

49. MacNab I, McCulloch J (1986) Disc degeneration with root irritation. In: Grayson T (ed) Backache, 2nd edn. Williams & Wilkins, Baltimore, pp 283–334

50. Wiesel SW, Tsourmas N, Teffer HL et al (1984) A study of computer assisted tomography: the incidence of positive CAT scans in an asymptomatic group of patients. Spine 9:549–551

51. Katz JN, Lipson SJ, Larson MG et al (1991) The outcome of decompressive laminectomy for degenerative lumbar stenosis. J Bone Joint Surg Am 73:809–816

52. Hanley EN (1997) The surgical treatment of lumbar degenerative disease. In: Garfin JR, Vaccaro AR (eds) Orthopaedic knowledge update spine. AAOS, Rosemont, IL, pp 127–140

53. Seimon LP. Subacute and chronic low back pain. In: Low back pain: clinical diagnosis and management. East Norwalk, CT: Appleton-Century-Crofts, 1983:89–113

54. Spengler DM (1987) Current concepts review: degenerative stenosis of the lumbar spine. J Bone Joint Surg 69:305

55. Amundsen T, Weber H, Magnaes B (1995) Lumbar spinal stenosis: clinical and radiologic features. Spine 20:1178–1186

56. Antonacci M, Eismont F (2001) Neurologic complications of lumbar spine surgery. J Am Acad Orthop Surg 9:137–145

57. Johnson KE, Rosen I, Uden A (1992) The natural course of lumbar spinal stenosis. Clin Orthop 279:82–86

58. Herkowitz HN, Kurz LT (1991) Degenerative lumbar spondylolisthesis with spinal stenosis: a prospective study comparing decompression with decompression and intertransverse process arthrodesis. J Bone Joint Surg 73:802–808

59. Simmons JC ED, Zheng Y, Munschauer C (1995) Comparative analysis of instrumented and noninstrumented lumbar fusion. Paper No. 454 presented at the 62nd meeting of American Academy of Orthopaedic Surgeons, February 1995

60. Bauchard JA, Aletari H (1995) Degenerative lumbar scoliosis and stenosis: comparison of surgical treatment with and without instrumentation. Paper No. 453 presented at the 62nd meeting of American Academy of Orthopaedic Surgeons, February 1995

61. Lauerman WC, Frame JC, Cain JE et al (1995) A randomized prospective study of lumbar fusion with and without transpedicular instrumentation. Paper No. 455 presented at the 62nd meeting of American Academy of Orthopaedic Surgeons, February 1995

62. Fischgund JS (1995) Degenerative lumbar spondylolisthesis with spinal stenosis: a prospective randomized study comparing arthrodesis with and without instrumentation. Paper No. 456 presented at the 62nd meeting of American Academy of Orthopaedic Surgeons, February 1995

63. MacNab I, McCulloch J (1986) Failure of spinal surgery. In: Grayson T (ed) Backache, 2nd edn. Williams & Wilkins, Baltimore, pp 392–435

64. Weinstein SL, Ponseti IV (1983) Curve progression in idiopathic scoliosis. J Bone Joint Surg Am 65:447–455

65. Tribus C (2003) Degenerative lumbar scoliosis: evaluation and management. J Am Acad Orthop Surg 11:174

66. Perennou D, Marcelli C, Henesson C et al (1994) Adult lumbar scoliosis: epidemiologic aspects in a low back pain population. Spine 19:123–128

67. Bradford DS (1988) Adult scoliosis: current concepts of treatment. Clin Orthop 229:70–87

68. Bradford DS (1995) Adult scoliosis. In: Lonstein JE, Bradford DS, Winter RB, Ogilvie JW (eds) Moe's textbook of scoliosis and other spinal deformities, 3rd edn. Saunders, Philadelphia, pp 369–386

69. Swank S, Winter RB, Moe JH (1984) Scoliosis and cor pulmonale. Spine 7:343–354

70. Stagnara P, Fleury D, Pauchet R et al (1975) Scoliosis majeures de l'adulte superieures a 100–183 cas traites chirurgicalement. Rev Chir Orthop 61:101–122

71. Kostiuk JP (1990) Current concepts review: operative treatment of idiopathic scoliosis. J Bone Joint Surg Am 72:1108–1113

72. Kostiuk JP (1980) Recent advances in the treatment of painful adult scoliosis. Clin Orthop 147:238–252

73. Connolly PJ, Abitbol JJ, Martin RJ et al (1997) Spine: trauma. In: Garfin JR, Vaccaro AR (eds) Orthopaedic knowledge update: spine. AAOS, Rosemont, IL, pp 197–217

74. McCulloch P, France J, Jones D, Krantz W, Nguyen T, Chambers C, Dorchak J, Mucha P (2005) Helical computed tomography alone compared with plain radiographs with adjunct computed tomography to evaluate the cervical spine after high-energy trauma. J Bone Joint Surg Am 87:2388

75. Bucholz RW. Lower cervical spine injuries. In: Skeletal trauma: fractures, dislocations, ligamentous injuries. Philadelphia: Saunders, 1992:699–727

76. Eismont FJ, Arena MJ, Green BA (1991) Extrusion of an intervertebral disk associated with traumatic subluxation or dislocation of cervical facets. J Bone Joint Surg Am 73:1555–1560

77. MacNab I, McCulloch J (1994) Whiplash injury of the cervical spine. In: Passano WM (ed) Neck ache and shoulder pain. Williams & Wilkins, Baltimore, pp 140–159

78. Bracken MB, Shepard MJ, Collins WF et al (1990) A randomized, controlled trial of methylprednisone or naloxone in the treatment of acute spinal cord injury: results of the Second National Acute Spinal Cord Injury Study. N Engl J Med 322:1405–1411

79. Bohlman HH (1985) Treatment of fractures and dislocations of the thoracic and lumbar spine. J Bone Joint Surg Am 67:165–169

80. Bohlman HH, Freehafer A, Dejak J (1985) The results of treatment of acute injuries of the upper thoracic spine with paralysis. J Bone Joint Surg Am 67:360–369

81. Denis F. Thoracolumbar spine trauma. In: Moe's textbook of scoliosis and other spinal deformities, 3rd ed. Philadelphia: Saunders, 1995:431–449

82. Rao R, Singrakhia M (2003) Painful osteoporotic vertebral fractures: pathogenesis, evaluation, and roles of vertebroplasty and kyphoplasty in its management. J Bone Joint Surg Am 85A:2010–2022

83. Lane JM, Riley EH, Wirganowicz PZ (1996) Osteoporosis: diagnosis and treatment. J Bone Joint Surg Am 78:618–632

84. Lane JM, Sandhu HS (1997) Osteoporosis of the spine. In: Garfin JR, Vaccaro AR (eds) Orthopaedic knowledge update spine. AAOS, Rosemont, IL, pp 227–234

85. National Institutes of Health (1994) Optimum calcium intake. NIH Consens Statement 12:1–31

86. Watts NB, Harris ST, Genant HK et al (1990) Intermittent cyclical etidronate treatment of postmenopausal osteoporosis. N Engl J Med 323:73–79

87. Kostuik JP, Heggeness MH (1997) Surgery of the osteoporotic spine. In: Frymoyer JW (ed) The adult spine: principles and practice, 2nd edn. Lippincott-Raven, Philadelphia, pp 1639–1664

88. Schlaich C, Minne HW, Bruckner T (1998) Reduced pulmonary function in patients with spinal osteoporotic fractures. Osteoporos Int 8:261–267

89. Sapico FL (1996) Microbiology and antimicrobial therapy of spinal infections. Orthop Clin North Am 27:9–13

90. Eismont FJ, Bohlman HH, Soni PL et al (1983) Pyogenic and fungal vertebral osteomyelitis with paralysis. J Bone Joint Surg Am 65:19–29

91. Ho EKW, Leong JCY (1994) Tuberculosis of the spine. In: Weinstein SL (ed) The pediatric spine: principles and practice. Raven, New York, pp 837–850

92. Modic MT, Feigh DH, Pirano DW et al (1985) Vetebral osteomyelitis: assessment using MR. Radiology 157:157–166

93. Keenen TL, Benson DR (1997) Differential diagnosis and conservative treatment of infectious diseases. In: Frymoyer JW (ed) The adult spine: principles and practice. Lippincott-Raven, Philadelphia, pp 871–894

94. Keenen TL, Benson DR (1997) Infectious diseases of the spine: surgical treatment. In: Frymoyer JW (ed) The adult spine: principles and practice. Lippincott-Raven, Philadelphia

95. Hodgson AR, Stock FE, Fang HS et al (1960) Anterior spinal fusion: the operative and pathological findings in 412 patients with Pott's disease of the spine. Br J Surg 48:172–178

96. Danner RL, Hartman BJ (1987) Update of spinal epidural abscess: 35 cases and review of the literature. Rev Infect Dis 9:265–274

97. Angtuaco EJ, McConnell JR, Chadduch WM et al (1987) MR imaging of spinal epidural sepsis. AJR Am J Roentgenol 149: 1249–1253

98. Dahlin DC (1978) Bone tumors: general aspects and data on 6221 cases, 3rd edn. Charles C Thomas, Springfield, IL

99. Boriani S, Weinstein JN (1997) Differential diagnosis and surgical treatment of primary benign and malignant neoplasms. In: Frymoyer JW (ed) The adult spine: principles and practice, 2nd edn. Lippincott-Raven, Philadelphia, pp 951–987

100. Harrington KD (1986) Metastatic disease of the spine. J Bone Joint Surg 68:1110–1115

Additional Reading

101. Kirkaldy-Willis WH, Hill RJ (1979) A more precise Diagnosis for Low-Back Pain. Spine 4:102

102. Czerwein J, Olsewski JM (2007) Spine surgery in patients age 80 and older. Proceedings of the 22nd annual meeting of the North American Spine Society, Austin, TX, October 2007

103. Czerwein J, Olsewski JM (2008) Spine surgery in patients age 80 and older. Proceedings of the 75th annual meeting of the American Academy of Orthopaedic Surgeons, San Francisco, CA, March 2008

Chapter 89
Invited Commentary

Roby C. Thompson Jr.

During the past 45 years, the ability to provide expanded care for geriatric patients with soft tissue and musculoskeletal disease and injury has expanded exponentially. As I reflect on the changes experienced in my practice as an orthopedic surgeon from 1963 to now, I am struck by a wide range of opportunities related to advances in either technology or our understanding of the biology of the connective tissues. These advances have fed off each other; in some circumstances, they have been largely dependent on their own merit, whereas in others, they are intimately linked. I have divided this introduction into advances dependent on one or the other – basic biology or technology – and interdependent fields.

Biologic Advances

During the early 1960s, the field of wound healing was just beginning to emerge from the histologic understanding of soft tissue repair and fracture healing to more quantitative understanding of the role of foreign bodies and the cellular response to injury. The advances that have occurred in our understanding of soft tissue healing of tendons and ligaments are responsible for much improved outcomes for patients of all ages with tendon lacerations or ligament tears. We have learned that the temporal relations of repair and reaction to injury dictate the appropriate rehabilitation of these injuries. As a result, rather than external immobilization in a cast for 3–6 weeks to protect a torn ligament or lacerated tendon, those injuries are now treated with early surgical intervention and early controlled motion to enhance the healing and the mobility of the injured part. Likewise, the role of surgical intervention in fracture healing during the 1960s was considered heretical by some because of the complications of

fixation failure and infection. Much of this was due to a lack of appreciation of the concomitant soft tissue injury associated with the fracture and the need for managing the fracture based on the magnitude of the soft tissue injury. This point is best exemplified by the expanded classification systems of "open fractures" to three of four strata depending on the author who has studied these injuries. This has been a great leap forward in managing what were previously described as "compound fractures." It has allowed expanded opportunities for return to function by patients who were previously subjected to prolonged immobilization in casts or traction and for what the great fracture surgeons of the 1960s, such as Harrison L. McLaughlin, Preston Wade, and Reginald Watson-Jones, called "fracture disease."

As a result of our better understanding of the relations between soft tissue injury and fractures, we have been able to modify our treatments to capitalize on early limb function using a variety of techniques. These have spanned "functional bracing," early ambulation in casts for femoral and tibial fractures, and early hand motion for "Colle's fractures," among others. From our expanded understanding of open fractures based on the early classification of Gustilo and Anderson, we learned that a type 1 open fracture with minimal soft tissue injury (e.g., a low-velocity gunshot wound) could be managed with local irrigation and débridement, with conventional fracture management for that fracture. This is in contrast to proceeding to an operating room environment for a type 3 fracture with massive soft tissue damage with or without comminution that demanded meticulous, thorough débridement on an as-necessary basis to provide healthy tissue for wound healing and resistance to infection.

Concomitant with our understanding of fracture repair and bone formation was an expanded understanding of the use of bone grafts largely based on the work of Marshall Urist, C. Andrew Bassett, and others. They pointed out that bone grafts could be osteoproductive, osteoconductive, or even osteoinductive, depending on the characteristic of the graft and how it was applied. We now know that when osteoproduction is required from a bone graft, it can occur only with autogenous cancellous bone that is carefully handled to

R.C. Thompson Jr. (✉)
Department of Orthopaedic Surgery,
University of Minnesota, Minneapolis, MN, USA
e-mail: thomp004@umn.edu

R.A. Rosenthal et al. (eds.), *Principles and Practice of Geriatric Surgery*,
DOI 10.1007/978-1-4419-6999-6_89, © Springer Science+Business Media, LLC 2011

protect the transplanted osteoblasts. Moreover, the graft must be in a viable, receptive environment with adequate well-oxygenated blood supply. In a similar manner, we can rationally expect cancellous allogeneic bone prepared in a way that removes primary cellular antigens and decreases the transplant antigenicity of the residual protein matrix to be comparable to autogenous bone for filling a cavity that requires primary conduction of bone, such as a benign cyst of bone. We have also learned that massive allogeneic bone grafts can be used for reconstructing major skeletal defects, including osteoarticular defects with expectations of 75–80% 10 year function in limbs that were potentially doomed to amputation during the 1960s.

The expanded understanding of tumor biology and the role of surgery of those primary tumors of the musculoskeletal system is a product of the past 35 years. We now know that as sarcomas spread in tissue planes associated with bone and muscle compartments, amputating the limb with a sarcoma is not necessarily the best or the only way to remove the tumor for the best outcome of local control. Thus, with a soft tissue sarcoma of the vastus lateralis muscle in the geriatric patient, it would be unusual today to recommend amputation. Rather, resection of the involved muscle with a fascial envelope surrounding the muscle and reconstruction with muscle transfers and rehabilitation are recommended, following the principles described above for soft tissue healing.

Much of what the surgeon caring for the musculoskeletal system can provide to the geriatric patients of the 2000s is based on generic advances in medicine and on our better understanding of pharmacotherapy. With the advances in antibiotics, chemotherapy, and hormone replacement, we are better able to control the aging process, which is pathologic in certain individuals. The classic example is osteoporosis, and the discoveries of the estrogen dependence of the osteoblast–osteoclast relation for maintenance of skeletal mass. Through the development of a class of drugs called bisphosphonates, we now have the ability to block bone resorption, which holds out major opportunities for better control of osteoporosis. Additional therapies in tumor-related bone resorption are available as well.

Similar advances in the use of blood products and anesthesia have allowed the orthopedic surgeon reasonably to consider surgical intervention in an aging population that would have been unthinkable 35 years ago. For example, it is common today for elective joint replacements to be recommended in octogenarians in reasonably good general health. We are confident that the ability of anesthesiologists to monitor vital signs, oxygenation, and visceral functions allows most unexpected conditions to be corrected quickly, just as we have become accustomed to correcting coagulopathies in our pre- and postoperative patients by defining the problem and replacing the deficit component of the coagulation system.

Technologic Advances

The advancing experience with biomaterials and giant leaps in our understanding of the fundamentals of the biomechanics of the skeletal system have been products of the past 45 years. This time frame has seen many technologic changes; they have not all been advances, and many have subsequently been abandoned. Even those advances that have proved successful have been subject to misapplication as we grope for the appropriate application. If there is one lesson for the future, it would be to enhance our scrutiny of new technology and demand accurate, well-done outcome studies before we embrace the new technology.

With that editorial comment out of the way, I offer the following technologic advances as the most important of the past 35 years for the orthopedic patient. First is our understanding of biomaterials and the biomaterial interface with the biologic and mechanical environment. Biocompatibility was a science well on its way during the 1960s, but it has become a virtual cookbook science during the past few years. Hence, we rarely concern ourselves with the new material and its relation to the biologic environment when it is accepted for market by the U.S. Food and Drug Administration (FDA). In the field of musculoskeletal diseases, we have seen silicone and Teflon arthroplasty wreak havoc at the local level owing to wear product debris in the absence of reaction to an inert material product. Today, the biggest challenge in the field of joint replacement is defining the interface between artificial articulations that have minimal and tolerable wear and yet do not transmit unacceptable forces to the implant–bone interface, which is the link for long-term fixation of the implant. During the past 40 years, we have moved from catastrophic failures with total hips of stainless steel and Teflon articulation, or acrylic replacements of femoral heads, to more successful stainless steel or cobalt-chrome alloy replacements that rely on a press-fit interface with bone, yet frequently, there were only one or two options in size for this interface with articular sizing based on 0.25-in. increments. Today, we have a more than 20-year record of successful experience with the use of polymethylmethacrylate as a bone cement for implant fixation. We have learned new implant skills over the past 30 years that promise a more than 85% 20-year survival of the implants currently in use. Implant manufacturers have responded to competition and demand, and as a result, our patients can expect a large inventory of sizes and shapes for accommodating the individual idiosyncrasies of their anatomy.

The field of internal fixation for fracture care has paralleled the implant development for joint disease. The linked technology of low-exposure intraoperative fluoroscopy and our better understanding of infection control and fracture healing has led to a change in the management of most displaced fractures, which allows early return to function, diminished hospitalization, and lower complication rates with a superior functional outcome.

The midshaft femoral fracture is a good example. If one looks at the standard of care during the 1960s, it was skeletal traction for 6–8 weeks followed by a spica cast for a similar time period, frequently associated limb length discrepancy and, commonly, a stiff knee. This practice was measured against an open reduction and internal fixation with an intramedullary nail or plates and screws that even in skilled hands carried a 10% infection rate. Today, those fractures are most commonly treated with closed intramedullary fixation. Commonly, there is a 3- to 5-day hospital stay with return to full unrestricted weight-bearing in 4 months, with expectations of a normal knee joint in most cases. The common expectation for any intraarticular fracture in the current environment is anatomic restoration of the joint surface through open or semiopen techniques, with early joint motion providing maximum functional return.

Another major technologic advancement of the past 35 years has been the ability to perform semiopen surgery via endoscopic techniques. Arthroscopy was the forerunner of much of the endoscopic surgery that is now common in all fields. Introduction of the Watanabe arthroscope during the 1960s was a major opportunity for orthopedists to see the pathology in the joint, but until the fiberoptic light and hand-held video camera made the arthroscope a practical tool for correcting pathology and removing loose bodies or torn meniscii, the potential went unrecognized. Once again, the 3- to 5-day hospital stay with an open arthrotomy for a meniscus injury has become same-day surgery, with patients returning to active performance in weeks rather than months.

The other technologic advance with dramatic effect in bone and soft tissue surgery has been the ability to perform free vascularized tissue transfers as a result of the introduction of intraoperative microscopy and magnification for microvascular anastomosis. The biologic understanding of the rheology of microvascular flow and reflow has been essential to the successful application of this technology.

The future for soft tissue and skeletal injury and disease management is exciting. Looking back over the past 45 years makes one realize how unpredictable that future may be. The emerging science of biologic manipulation of tissue growth and reconstitution seems real and potentially achievable over the next 30 years. One might eventually resurface a joint with genetically engineered tissue to replace injured or diseased tissue or use a series of linked cytokines or growth factors to reverse a fracture nonunion or reconstitute a skeletal defect.

Chapter 90
Age-Related Changes in Bone and Soft Tissue

David Rispler and Susan M. Day

Introduction

The population of the United States is aging – by 2030, the US Census Bureau estimates that 1 in 5 will be 65 or older. The rapid increase in the size of this population is expected to significantly impact orthopaedic practice especially. The aging process, a normal decline in cell, tissue, and organ function, ultimately leads to progressive changes in the physiology of all the components of the musculoskeletal system: bone, cartilage, muscle, ligament, and tendon. Such change can result in several clinical problems for patients and their treating physicians. Among the most common ailments affecting the geriatric patient are fragility fractures, joint degeneration, and injuries to the aging athlete. The risk of fragility fractures increases as patients suffer from diminished bone mass, osteoporosis, and diminished muscle bulk, which results in weakness that can magnify the effects of neurologic degeneration on gait and posture. Another progressive disabling condition is joint degeneration leading to pain, stiffness, and decreased mobility. As the baby boomer generation matures, but continues to participate in high-impact activities, patients present to physicians with more overuse injuries and traumatic injuries to the muscles, tendons, and ligaments, which function to protect our joints and skeleton.

Physicians, especially orthopaedic surgeons, are the first to document the culmination of these aging processes in elderly individuals, since they are the primary physicians seen when a significant injury, often in the form of a fracture, occurs. Fragility fractures are quite common in the elderly, and they are one of the most important predictors of significant osteoporosis, and risk for further fracture. Orthopaedic surgeons can play a positive role in the management of ongoing aging processes, through diagnosis of underlying disease, treatment, and follow-up, to prevent future injury. The potential importance of this kind of intervention will increase as the US population ages.

In this chapter, we discuss the anatomy and physiology of aging on each part of the musculoskeletal system, as well as current trends in diagnosis, treatment, and management of musculoskeletal ailments related to aging. An overview of these effects is summarized in Table 90.1 for bone and in Table 90.2 for the rest of the musculoskeletal system.

Bone

Bone consists of several cell types, (osteoblasts, osteocytes, and osteoclasts) organic extracellular matrix (Type I collagen), and ground substance (glycosaminoglycans, or GAGs), produced by the cells. Inorganic materials in the form of mineral salts and hydroxyapatite crystals $[Ca_{10}(PO_4)_6 OH_2]$ make the tissue hard and rigid. The organic component gives the bone its flexibility and resilience [1] (Fig. 90.1). A progressive loss of bone density has been observed as part of the normal aging process. The longitudinal trabeculae become thinner, and some of the transverse trabeculae are resorbed [2]. In some patients, this decreased volume of bone tissue and decrease in size is minimal. In others, the decrease becomes pathologic, causing ostopenia or osteoporosis, leading to fragility fractures, deformity, and loss of height (Fig. 90.2).

Bone provides support, movement, protection, and calcium homeostasis. It is a dynamic organ that is constantly remodeled. This remodeling is achieved by the coupling of bone formation, which is the function of osteoblasts, and bone resorption, which is the function of osteoclasts, orchestrated by hormones, growth factors, and cytokines. Early in life, the process of formation and resorption is closely coupled to maintain calcium homeostasis. It is a continuous process throughout life and one that is influenced by genetic and environmental factors including lifestyle choices, gender, pubertal status, physical activity, drugs, and diet [3]. As we

D. Rispler (✉)
Michigan State Orthopedic Residency Program,
Grand Rapids Orthopedic Residency Program,
300 Lafayette Avenue SE Suite 3400,
Grand Rapids, MI 49503, USA
e-mail: rispdt@trinity-health.org

TABLE 90.1 Changes in bone characteristics in the young and old

Property	Young	Old
Blood supply	↑	↓
Osteoblast supply	↑	↓
Osteoclasts	In equilibrium	Increased relative to osteoblasts
Force required to produce fracture	High energy	Low energy
Calcium metabolism	Adequate to maintain bone density	Inadequate to maintain bone density
Remodeling	High, adequate	Low
Bone formation vs. bone resorption	In equilibrium	Bone resorption predominates

age, this process can become easily uncoupled with a reduction in osteoblast activity, increased osteoclast activity, and alterations in hormone stimulation.

Bone mass reaches its peak at around age 25 and is maintained for several years. By age 40, most adults begin losing bone at a rate of 0.5–1.0% per year. For women, menopause differs per individual, but it accelerates bone loss to 1–5% per year. This accelerated phase lasts for 5–10 years and eventually returns to 0.5–1.0% per year [4] (Fig. 90.3). Skeletal regions lose bone at different rates [5] (Fig. 90.4). Cortical bone, found in the diaphysis and the outer envelope of all bones, is composed of concentric lamellae of densely packed mineralized collagen fibers. Cortical bone represents

TABLE 90.2 Characteristic changes in the aging musculoskeletal system

Property	Cartilage	Tendon	Ligament	Muscle
Water content	↓	↓	↓	↓
Collagen	Relatively unchanged	↓	↓	Decreased/disorganized
Collagen structure	Increased Crosslinking	Increased Crosslinking	Increased Crosslinking	Increased Crosslinking
Proteoglycan content (concentration)	↓	↓	↓	↓
Proteoglycan size and molecular weight	↓	↓	↓	↓
Proteoglycan degradation	Outpaces synthesis	Outpaces synthesis	Outpaces synthesis	Outpaces synthesis
Cell size/fiber size	↑	Relatively unchanged	Relatively unchanged	↓
Cell number	↓	↓	Relatively unchanged	↓
Modulus of elasticity (stiffness)	↑	↑	↑	↓
Risk of injury (chondral defect, rupture, sprain, strain)	↑	↑	↑	↑

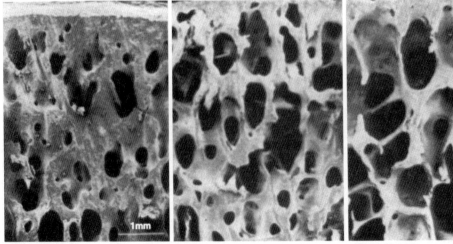

FIGURE 90.1 Age-related trabecular bone loss (reprinted with permission from Keaveny TM and Hayes WC. Mechanical properties of cortical and trabecular bone. In: Bone, a treatise. Bone growth, vol 7, pp 285–344).

24 y.o. Female　　　　　63 y.o. Female　　　　　89 y.o. Female

1mm

Figure 90.2 Appendicular fractures caused by minimal trauma.

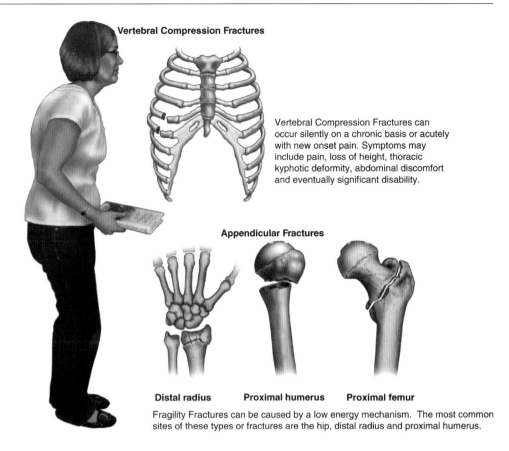

Vertebral Compression Fractures

Vertebral Compression Fractures can occur silently on a chronic basis or acutely with new onset pain. Symptoms may include pain, loss of height, thoracic kyphotic deformity, abdominal discomfort and eventually significant disability.

Appendicular Fractures

Distal radius   Proximal humerus   Proximal femur

Fragility Fractures can be caused by a low energy mechanism. The most common sites of these types or fractures are the hip, distal radius and proximal humerus.

Figure 90.3 Bone mass changes with age (reprinted with permission from Wasnich RD. (1996) Epidemiology of osteoporosis. In: Favus MJ (ed) Primer on the metabolic bone diseases and disorders of mineral metabolism, 3rd edn. Lippincott Raven, Philadelphia.

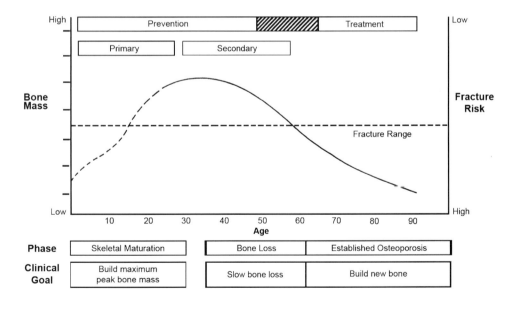

the greatest bone loss that occurs with age. The imbalance in bone remodeling leads to porosity, and long bone cortices become thinner over time [6].

Cancellous bone, in contrast, loses density. Trabeculae decrease in number, and the architecture of cancellous bone changes as a result. In spite of these differences, the loss of

both cortical and cancellous bone with increasing age contributes to bone fragility. Cancellous bone loss is rapid in early menopause, resulting in two clinical issues. First, wrist fractures increase in frequency, and as more cancellous bone deteriorates, the risk of vertebral fractures increase. Second, bone mineral density (BMD) (determined from DEXA scans,

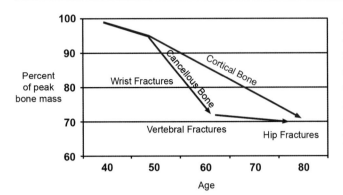

Figure 90.4 Cancellous and cortical bone loss occur at different times and different rates (reprinted with permission from ([5], p 193)).

discussed below) is lost in the vertebral spine before decreases in the hip region are evident. In addition, the cancellous bone of the spine is the earliest measure to determine if interventions are helping to increase BMD.

The Cellular and Molecular Basis of Bone Remodeling

Bone remodeling in adults results in the complete turnover of the skeleton in approximately 10 years and is achieved by tight coupling of osteoblast and osteoclast cell activity [7]. Osteoclast activity removes old bone which is followed by osteoblast activity that deposits new bone. During each remodeling cycle, the amount of bone formed decreases with advancing age [7–9].

Our understanding of bone remodeling at the cellular and molecular level is constantly expanding. A complete review is beyond the scope of this discussion [7], but key players are briefly mentioned here. Bone morphogenetic proteins (BMPs, specifically BMP-2 and -4) maintain the supply of osteoblasts by stimulating differentiation of periosteal mesenchymal cells to osteoblasts. BMP2/BMP4 activates osteoblast specific factor 2/ core binding factor a1 (osf2/cbfa1), which activates osteoblast specific pathway proteins, including osteopontin, bone sialoprotein, type I collagen, and osteocalcin [7]. Recent research suggests that Wnt proteins also play a role in transcriptional activation of osteoblast differentiation [10].

In addition to their role in calcium homeostasis, parathyroid hormone and 1,25 dihydroxyvitamin D3 (1,25 $(OH)_2 D_3$) stimulate osteoclast formation from hematopoietic precursors. Osteoclast formation also relies to an extent upon osteoblast cells, since mice lacking osteoblast cells also lack osteoclast cells [11]. The basis for this dependency stems from the receptor activator of nuclear factor κB (RANK), which is expressed on osteoclast progenitor cell membranes, and RANK-ligand located on committed osteoblastic progenitor cells and T-cells [7]. The binding of RANK-ligand to RANK is essential for

clastogenesis. 1,25 $(OH)_2 D_3$ and PTH, among others, stimulate the production of RANK in osteoblast cells. Osteoprotogerin is a glycoprotein that can bind RANK and inhibit osteoclast development. Further, wnt-3a is implicated in downregulation of RANKL, inhibiting osteoclast formation [10]. Many cytokines either enhance or inhibit production of osteoclasts. Finally, calcitonin, secreted by the C cells of the thyroid, appears to promote osteoclast apoptosis.

The hormone estrogen is widely understood to be important in bone remodeling and considered one of the most important determinants of osteoporosis [12]. Estrogen deficiency leads to a bone remodeling imbalance and decreases bone formation and increases bone degradation. Estrogen appears to exert its effects by decreasing the lifespan or activity of osteoclasts, and increases the lifespan of osteoblasts. The effect of estrogen on osteoblasts is to increase cell proliferation, the synthesis of bone matrix proteins and growth factors such as IGF-1 and TGF-β [13]. Estrogen inhibits bone resorption [14] and production of the cytokines IL-1, IL-6, and TNF [15, 16].

Several growth factors, including transforming growth factor β (TGF-β), affect both bone formation and resorption. TGF-β stimulates osteoclast formation and osteoblast differentiation. The interleukin family (IL-1, IL6, IL-11), TNFs, M-CSF, peroxisome proliferator activated receptor γ2 (PPARγ2), and prostaglandins E_2 and F_2 also affect both processes.

Calcium Homeostasis

PTH and 1,25 dihydroxyvitamin D impact calcium homeostasis. Vitamin D increases absorption of calcium in the GI tract, acting in concert with PTH. Vitamin D deficiency causes lower serum calcium, which stimulates releases of PTH and mobilizes calcium stores from bone. PTH increases calcium reabsorption from the kidney, causes bone to release calcium, and plays a role in GI absorption of calcium. PTH levels increase with age, in part because of lower levels of vitamin D. Lower vitamin D levels in the elderly are well documented and due mainly to decreased synthesis and decreased dietary intake. Hyperparathyroidism, common in elderly women, contributes to bone resorption and bone loss.

Diagnosis: Measurement of Bone Mass

BMD is correlated with bone strength in biomechanical studies of cortical and cancellous bone specimens [17]. Also, BMD is predictive of future fractures in epidemiological studies [18–20]. Bone mass can be measured by several techniques, but the clinical standard is the areal measurement of BMD using dual energy X-ray absorptiometry (DEXA), which is reliable, reproducible, and cost-effective. The T-score, which is a comparison of an individual's BMD via DEXA scan to widely available gender, race, and age standards, is the basis for diagnosis. A T-score greater than −1 is considered normal, while T-scores of −1 to −2.5 are diagnosed as osteopenia, and T-scores lower than −2.5 are consistent with osteoporosis. The presence of fragility fractures indicates greater severity.

The DEXA scan shown in Fig. 90.5 is that of a 44-year-old perimenopausal woman who presented with a third metatarsal stress fracture. She is an avid runner, and her relevant medical and social history included long-term use of birth control medication and a vegetarian lifestyle that she had maintained for more than 20 years. DEXA scan showed a

lumbar spine T-score of −2.5. The total hip T-score was −1.5, and her distal one third radius was −0.7.

This case illustrates important elements of DEXA scan interpretation and diagnosis. First, the pattern and variability of T-scores seen in this scan from different skeletal regions are typical. T-scores in the lumbar spine nearly always show the greatest bone loss since the spine consists mostly of cancellous bone, which is first to show decreases in BMD. Second, in terms of diagnosis, the lowest T-score is used – in this case, −2.5, consistent with a diagnosis of osteoporosis. Although the T-score from the spine is an average, it is not valid to average the T-scores from different skeletal areas (in this example, the average score would be −1.6, which is consistent with osteopenia, not osteoporosis). Third, DEXA

MA Bone Density Dexa Axial Skeleton (GR)-000788450

* Final Report *

* Final Report *

Reason For Exam
Stress Fx--Eval. for Osteopenia

Report
DEXA BONE MINERAL DENSITY STUDY

INDICATION: Stress fracture. Osteopenia.

The findings include the following T-score results, the patient's percentage of normal compared to young adults, and Z-score results:

Site	T-Score	% Peak Reference	Assessment	Z-Score	% Age Matched
Lumbar Spine	-2.5	74%	Osteoporotic	-2.1	77%
Total Hip	-1.5	81%	Osteopenic	-1.2	83%
Distal Radius	-0.7	94%	Normal	-0.2	98%

IMPRESSION: The patient has borderline osteoporosis.

RECOMMENDATIONS:
1. Continue regular weightbearing exercise (30 minutes per day, at least three times per week).
2. Maintain adequate calcium intake (1000 mg per day) and vitamin D (800 to 1000 IU per day).
3. Consider antiresorptives as a preventative measure.
4. A followup study in two years is suggested.

Images and graphical representations of bone mineral density progression are viewable on the Saint Mary's Healthcare PACS and are also available in color hard copy, which can be sent to the referring physician's office upon request (616-685-6209).

Signature Line
********* FINAL REPORT *********
Dictated By: Verde MD, Francis J 05/11/2009 13:17

FIGURE 90.5 DEXA Scan result sheer for a 44-year-old perimenopausal woman who presented with a third metatarsal stress fracture (courtesy of Dr. David Rispler).

Printed by: Wansten , Corinne
Printed on: 5/15/2009 11:44 EDT

scan analysis and diagnosis should be performed by the attending physician. In the example above, the radiologist's interpretation was borderline osteoporosis, with recommendation to continue weight-bearing exercise (30 min per day, at least three times per week), maintain adequate calcium intake (1,000 mg per day) and vitamin D (800–1,000 IU per day), and consider antiresorptives as preventive measure, with follow-up scans in 2 years. Given the patient history, recent fracture, and lumbar T-score of −2.5, a diagnosis of osteoporosis with high risk of recurrent fractures is the appropriate diagnosis. Further, in addition to maintaining calcium and vitamin D intake, 25-hydroxyvitamin D levels should be assessed in this patient to determine whether higher supplementation is required. Finally, while follow-up DEXA scans are helpful to monitor patient BMD, the use of antiresorptives is very controversial given the age of this patient, and the mechanism of action of antiresportives. Because antiresorptives decrease osteoclast activity and bone turnover, they maintain bone, but do not add to bone mass. Recent studies have shown that such adynamic bone can lead to subtrochanteric fractures with long-term use of bisphosphonates [21]. Given this patient's age, an anabolic agent should be considered first if there are no contraindications.

DEXA scans have limitations in that they do not measure bone quality or bone volume. Currently, no single test measures quality of bone. However, the FRAX tool is a mathematical model that predicts the likelihood of fracture in the next 10 years by taking ten risk factors into account (such as smoking and family history of osteoporosis). Knowing the likelihood of fracture, in turn, helps to determine how aggressively to manage bone loss in patients. For instance, although the potential side effects from medications may be great, this may be outweighed by a high risk for fracture and associated morbidity.

Another method of bone assessment is quantitative computed tomography (QCT), which is expensive, but allows greater assessment of bone quality. The use of CT is preferable when differences in size (such as extreme obesity) distort the analysis of bone mineral content [22, 128]. The use of ultrasonography (US) is useful for screening, but this technique is not as reproducible as others. Calcaneal measurements using US are predictive of fracture risk in the hip but are less predictive of fracture risk in the lumbar spine [23].

Management and Prevention

In the elderly, the main result of ongoing changes in bone remodeling physiology is osteoporosis. One of the most important clinical outcomes of osteoporosis is fracture. Fractures heal more slowly and less effectively with advancing age. Over time, the periosteum thins and bone-reforming potential of the periosteal mesenchymal cells decrease

with age, although there is evidence that this is not due to a decrease in the size of the mesenchymal stem cell population [24]. This decline in the rate of fracture repair is probably related to general decrease in bone remodeling, decrease in the expression of cytokines, and a reduction in the inflammatory response to injury [25].

There are a number of treatments currently used to manage bone loss in the elderly. In addition, strategies to reduce the risk of injury are important, as none of the currently available agents can completely reverse bone loss, probably because osteoporosis is so often diagnosed long after significant loss to bone density has occurred. Here, we look at treatments that can reduce the risk of injury (falls) and slow or stop continued bone loss.

Nonpharmacologic

There are several nonpharmacologic methods to reduce the risk of injury resulting from bone loss, including calcium supplementation and vitamin D supplementation, as well as physician counseling on lifestyle choices (tobacco and alcohol use) and fall prevention (via hip protectors, exercise, and balance training). For instance, healthy bone remodeling and mineral density requires adequate calcium intake. Dietary intake of 1,200 mg calcium is the standard recommendation of the National Osteoporosis Foundation in patients 50 years of age and older [26]. While lifestyle choices and fall prevention techniques are beyond the scope of this discussion, we discuss vitamin D supplementation below.

The importance of vitamin D supplementation is clear. Vitamin D supplementation (specifically vitamin D_3, or cholecalciferol) of 400–800 IU is currently recommended in all older patients, although many experts now advise 2,000 IU or more in part because toxicity with overdose is rare [27]. Vitamin D deficiency is commonplace in the elderly, because of decreased absorption in the gut and decreased ability of the skin to produce vitamin D [25]. High doses (800 IU) of vitamin D appear to reduce the risk of vertebral and nonvertebral fractures [28]. Further, 800 IU doses of vitamin D were associated with a lower incidence rate of falls compared to placebo [29].

Pharmacologic Treatment

Currently available treatments for bone loss in the elderly are categorized as antiresorptive or anabolic. Antiresorptive agents decrease the resorption of bone and include bisphosphonates, calcitonin, hormone replacement therapy, and selective estrogen receptor modulators. Anabolic treatments increase bone formation and include parathyroid hormone injection. These treatments are discussed below.

Antiresorptive Agents

Bisphosphonates: Bisphosphonates are nitrogen-containing compounds that bind bone and decrease the activity and lifespan of osteoclasts. They increase BMD by decreasing the rate of bone resorption. They are commonly prescribed, and there are four available in the US: alendronate, risedonate, ibandronate, and zoledronic acid. Each of these bisphosphonates has been shown to increase BMD and to reduce the risk of vertebral fractures [30–36]. Reductions in the rates of hip fractures have also been demonstrated for alendronate, risedonate, and zoledronic acid [31, 37–39]. Overall, bisphosphonate treatment reduces the incidence of vertebral fractures by 40% or more, depending on the study. Common side effects of bisphosphonate treatment are gastrointestinal irritation and ulceration, although the injectable forms of the drug are associated with fewer of these symptoms. These compounds lead in rare instances to osteonecrosis of the jaw, particularly in those undergoing dental procedures (risk is 1/10,000 to 1/100,000) [40].

Long-term treatment of osteoporosis with bisphosphonates has revealed that bone turnover may become oversuppressed, which results in spontaneous nonspinal fractures. These fractures result from the inability of the bone to withstand deformation before breaking and are likely the result of accumulation of microfractures that result from normal wear and tear on the bone that has not been remodeled [41, 42]. A recent study showed that discontinuation of alendronate after 5 years was not associated with a large increase in bone turnover, suggesting a prolonged persistence of the effects of alendronate [43].

Calcitonin

Calcitonin decreases bone resorption by inhibiting the function of osteoclasts [44, 45]. The result is an increase in BMD and decrease in fragility. A large, 5-year, randomized controlled trial showed a 33% reduction in vertebral fractures when 200 IU calcitonin were administered intranasally daily [44].

Selective Estrogen Receptor Modulators

Selective estrogen receptor modulators (SERMs) bind to estrogen receptors and selectively act as agonists or antagonists. Raloxifene is the only SERM that is approved for the prevention and treatment of osteoporosis, and it has been shown to increase BMD, decrease vertebral fractures, and appears to have antiresorptive properties [46–49]. Raloxifene use is associated with an increased risk of stroke and thromboembolism, and thus, benefits and risks must be considered with its use in the treatment of osteoporosis [50]. Other SERMs are currently under development which may have antiresorptive effects without such side effects [51].

Estrogen

Estrogen replacement and estrogen plus progestin replacement therapy have been demonstrated to decrease the number of osteoporotic fractures [52, 53]. However, the associated health risks (increased stroke risk, deep vein thrombosis, and increased rates of breast cancer and uterine cancer) precludes the used of estrogen replacement for those with osteoporosis [52, 54].

Anabolic Agents

Teriparatide (parathyroid hormone), the only anabolic agent available in the treatment of postmenopausal osteoporosis, increases bone turnover rates. Long-term subcutaneous injections of teriparatide are associated with a 9–13% increase in BMD in the lumbar spine and decreased risk of vertebral and nonvertebral fractures [55]. In spite of this, teriparatide use is relatively uncommon because of high cost, inconvenience, and potential side effects. Side effects include swelling, pain, weakness, injection-site erythema, and potential for serum hypercalcemia, although the side effects are reduced with longer treatment [56]. Teriparatide use longer than 2 years is not recommended because evidence suggests that the incidence of osteosarcomas is possible, although only 1 human case history of sarcoma in 300,00 patients has been observed [57, 58].

Summary

The treatments for osteoporosis are not curative, and all have potential risks. However, most treatments can modify the disease and decrease the risk of future vertebral, hip, and distal radius fractures. In spite of this, many patients do not receive treatment. Numerous studies have shown that patients treated for their fragility fractures do not have the proper follow-up treatment of osteoporosis [59, 60]. It is imperative that health professionals involved in the acute care of elderly patients with fractures initiate the process of proper evaluation of their underlying conditions with a DEXA scan and laboratory tests, followed by referral to a physician who is experienced in osteoporosis management. Several studies have shown an improvement in management of osteoporotic patients when using a clinical strategy for management of the disease [61, 62].

Muscle, Tendon, and Ligament

These three types of connective tissues are involved with the movement and protection of the skeleton and joints. Degeneration of these structures in the aging athlete is becoming an increasing problem. As the athlete becomes less flexible, they have an increased incidence of sprains, strains, and overuse injuries. As athletes decrease their BMD and lose the protective effect of these tissues, they become prone to stress fractures [63].

Muscle

Skeletal muscle has a unique skeletal unit, the fiber consisting of a long cylinder cell with hundreds of nuclei. Within each fiber rests a sarcomere composed of actin and myosin filaments that initiate a contraction when the fibers slide past each other. Fibers are encased by endomysium, a loose connective tissue. These fibers are aligned together as fascicles, which are held together by the perimyseum. The complete named muscle is surrounded by the epimysium (Fig. 90.6). The ability of the muscle to provide a forceful contraction is related to the physiologic cross-sectional area of the muscle. With aging, both the number of cells and size of these muscle fibers decrease. This results in a decreased ability to generate maximum contraction [64].

Muscle is a contractile tissue, in which individual cells act in concert to produce and cause a movement. Skeletal muscle is anchored to the bone by tendons. These two structures are attached along the musculotendinous border. This area is

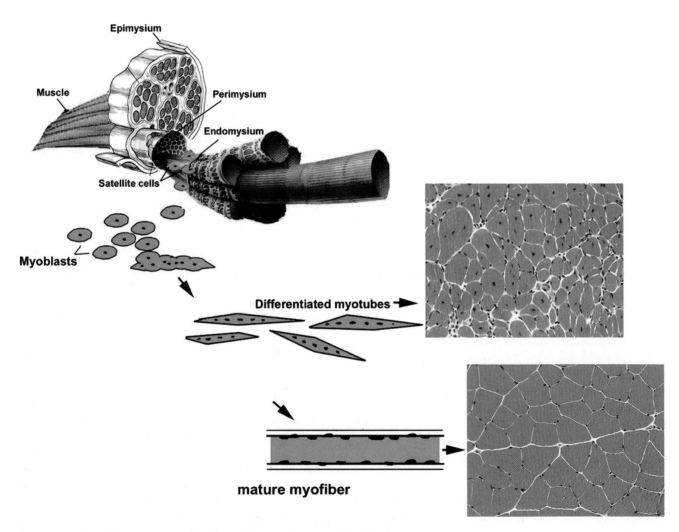

FIGURE 90.6 Skeletal muscle structure (reprinted with permission from [64], Fig. 1).

the most susceptible to injury [65]. Skeletal muscle makes up approximately 40% (females) to 50% (male) of the adult mass. There are two types of fibers, type I, or slow twitch, and type II, or fast twitch [64].

Similar to bone, peak muscle mass is reached by about 30 years of age. Muscle mass is progressively lost after that at a rate of about 4% per decade between the ages 20 and 30, and at 10% per decade after the early 50s [66]. Both the size and number of muscle cells decrease with age, resulting in sarcopenia and decreased muscle strength. Muscle atrophy results from the loss of both type I and type II fibers. Type II muscle fibers lose more size compared with size loss in type I fibers and hence much of the age-related decrease in muscle strength is attributable to loss of these fibers. Muscle loss is accelerated when levels of growth hormone, testosterone, or thyroxine decrease. Further, more muscle is lost in weight-bearing muscles compared to nonweight-bearing muscles. Evidence of these changes are shown in athletic performance as maximal running and swimming velocities for sprint and endurance events decline from the third to eighth decades [67].

These physiologic changes predispose the aging athlete to muscle strain, which results from forcible stretching of a muscle. Histological studies have shown that muscle strain injuries cause a disruption of muscle fibers a short distance from the myotendinous junction. The patient presents with acute pain experienced during intense activity. Muscles that are frequently involved cross two joints, act mainly in an eccentric fashion, and contain a high percentage of fast-twitch fibers. Diagnosis relies on history and exam. Rarely is an MRI indicated. Initial treatment consists of rest, ice, and compression. As pain subsides, physical therapy should be initiated to restore flexibility and strength [65].

Most muscle injuries heal, but some result in incomplete functional recovery. Because of this, the current research is evaluating the use of human recombinant growth factors to regenerate muscle, gene therapy to deliver growth factors to injured muscle, and antifibrotic therapy [64]. Until treatment is developed that restores function in these injuries, prevention is the key. Methods to decrease the risk of injury include decreasing fatigue [68], warming up the muscle [69], and preconditioning the muscle [70]. Also, to prevent injury and improve long-term function, aging patients can benefit from regular weight-bearing exercise to increase strength and muscle mass [71, 72].

Tendons

Tendon connects muscle to bone and functions to withstand tension. It is noncontractile and consists of a tough band of fibrous connective tissue composed mostly of parallel type I

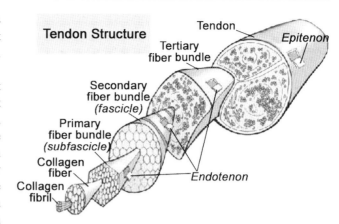

Figure 90.7 Tendon structure (reprinted with permission from ([79], p 188, Fig. 1).

collagen that is cross-linked to fascicles and tertiary bundles [73–75]. Cellular elements of tendon consist of tenocytes and tenoblasts that lie between the collagen fibers along the long axis of the tendon [76], and other cells include chondrocytes at the bone attachment and insertion sites, synovial cells of the tendon sheath, and vascular cells (Fig. 90.7). Elastin, though limited to 2% of the dry mass of tendons, is very important to allow the tendon to adapt to function and to lengthen in response to stress.

After maturation, tendons undergo many changes that bring about a general decline in structure and function beginning in the third decade. There is a decreased vascularity and cellularity leading to reduced collagen turnover, decreased proteoglycan and water content, and an increase in insoluble collagen. Together, these cause the tendon to become stiffer and less compliant. This decline in the aging tendon is characterized by a reduced ability to adapt to environmental stress and loss of function [77]. Among the many changes, part of the tendon insertion becomes hypovascular [78, 79]. Because of this, metabolic pathways shift from aerobic to more anaerobic energy production [80]. Microscopically, older fibroblasts appear flatter and possess fewer protein producing organelles, such as Golgi and endoplasmic reticuli [25]. Tensile strength reaches a plateau and declines with age [81]. This decline is related to decreases in total collagen content [82]. The loss of collagen and its cross-linking, as well as the changes in elastin, leads to an increase in tendon stiffness [83, 84].

These physiologic changes predispose the aging laborer and athlete to several pathologic conditions including tendinopathy and spontaneous, low-energy tendon rupture. When patients present with overuse conditions affecting tendons, clinicians frequently use tendonitis or tendinosis to define the entity. Histological exam of the tissue supports the use of tendinopathy as the proper clinical entity. This disorder shows haphazard healing with an absence of inflammatory cells,

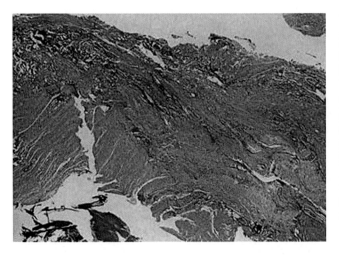

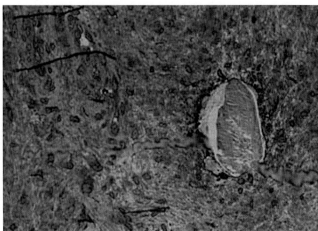

FIGURE 90.8 Photomicrograph of severe tendinopathy (reprinted with permission from [78]).

FIGURE 90.9 Degeneration of tendon structure due to repeated corticosteroid injection (reprinted with permission from [78].

noninflammatory collagen degeneration, fiber disorientation, hypercellularity, scattered vascular ingrowth, and increased interfibrillar glycosaminoglycans [85–87] (Fig. 90.8). In these patients, avoidance of aggravating activities, and conservative treatment is initiated which may include anti-inflammatories, local cortisone injections, and physical therapy. These common modalities can be helpful though no controlled studies have shown Level 1 evidence to support their use. Corticosteroid injections need to be judiciously used because they can inhibit protein synthesis, leading to collagen thinning and can predispose the tendon to rupture [88, 90] (Fig. 90.9). Operative treatment is reserved for patients who fail conservative treatment. Although there are several different techniques depending on the tendon involved, surgery is intended to revitalize, debride, and bypass the area of tendinopathy [78].

Treatment of these tendinopathy conditions is important to avoid tendon rupture. In fact, most laypeople think of tendon ruptures in young healthy athletes, but tendon ruptures generally affect patients as they age [90]. Spontaneous rupture of healthy tendons almost never occurs: preexisting degenerative histologic changes are present almost always. Clinically, tendon ruptures are important injuries to be diagnosed and treated urgently to maintain long-term function. Physical exam by an experienced musculoskeletal physician can detect these ruptures by palpation of structures, loss of active joint motion, and occasionally radiographic findings. If the diagnosis is uncertain or referral to a musculoskeletal physician cannot be arranged quickly, then an MRI can be helpful in confirming the diagnosis. Although the individual timing varies, surgical repair of tendon ruptures need to be performed within an early time frame to provide the best results. For example, rupture of the flexor digitorum profundus to the hand ("Jersey finger") needs to be performed

within the first week. Ruptures of the achilles, patella, quadriceps, and distal biceps need to be performed within the first 3 weeks. Acute rotator cuff repairs can be delayed but still have the most reliable results if performed within the first 3 months.

Ligament

Ligaments are dense connective tissues composed mostly of type I collagen. Their ultrastructure is similar to that of tendons, but their fibers are more variable and have a higher elastin content [91]. Ligaments attach to the bone at both its origin and insertion. They function to provide stability to joints and proprioception. Mechanoreceptors and free nerve endings help ligaments provide feedback to the neuromuscular system to avoid injury.

As ligaments mature, they undergo an increased number and quality of collagen cross-links with a concomitant increase in fibril diameter [92]. After maturation, collagen content decreases which contributes to the gradual decline in the mechanical properties of ligaments. This loss of ultimate tensile strength, increase in stiffness, and inability to withstand deformation make the ligaments and the joint they protect at risk for deformity and injury (Fig. 90.10). Ligament insertions into bone also become weak and can lead to avulsion fractures. In addition, studies have suggested that the number of mechanoreceptors in ligaments decreases with age resulting in the inability to process where the joint is in space [93].

The physiologic changes in ligaments can lead to several different clinic problems. First, the ligament can attenuate, lengthen, and lose its ability to provide stability. For example,

FIGURE 90.10 Grading ligament sprains.

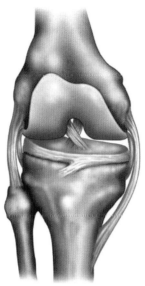
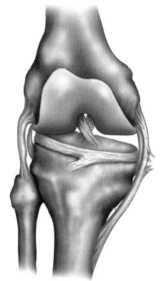
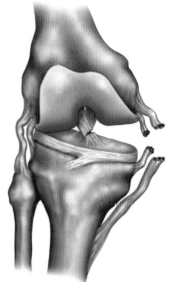

Grade 1
The ligament stretches but does not tear. There will be tenderness to exam but no opening on valgus stress of the knee

Grade 2
The ligament tears but the fibers remain in continuity. There will be swelling, tenderness and a slight increase in joint laxity

Grade 3
The ligament tears and the fibers separate leaving a gap. The exam will show gross instability on provocative stress testing

the loss of ligament integrity can allow the arthritic joint to become more deformed, accelerating degeneration and causing pain. For surgeons, joint replacement, paying attention to rebalance the ligament structures, especially in the knee, is very important to the success of the surgery [94].

Another clinical entity involves acute trauma to the ligament at the ligament–bone interface, causing an avulsion fracture. Ligament tears are described as degrees of sprain. Grade I involves mild stretching of the ligament. Grade II causes the ligament to tear, but still maintains continuity, and Grade III results in tearing and separation of the fiber ends. Treatment and recovery depends on the individual patient and the joint involved.

One interesting example of a ligament tear is the anterior cruciate ligament (ACL) of the knee. If this ligament completely tears, it will not heal or reconstitute itself. This is becoming more common because many older patients are participating in high-impact sports that increase the risk of an ACL tear. Historically, middle-age patients who have sustained ACL tears have been offered conservative treatment with rehabilitation and avoidance of activities that require them to quickly change directions. But, as patients' expectations and lifestyles have changed, many opt for surgical reconstructions. A recent study has confirmed that in carefully selected patients of 50 years of age and older, surgical reconstruction of the ACL can achieve similar results to those in younger patients with no increased complications [95].

Articular Cartilage

Articular cartilage is an amazing structure. It provides pain-free and almost frictionless motion. In fact, the coefficient of friction (0.003–0.006) is significantly less than ice (0.1 at 0°C). Designers of joint replacements have tried to develop bearing surfaces such as metal on metal, ceramic on ceramic, and highly cross-linked polyethylene and metal, but none has been able to come close to the wear properties of healthy articular cartilage. The resiliency and durability of cartilage are due to their histological infrastructure and physical arrangement. However, cartilage is poorly regenerative.

Normal hyaline cartilage consists of a matrix of proteoglycan aggregates, type II collagen and chondrocytes [96]. Like other soft tissues, cartilage is composed mostly of water (80% of wet weight). Large proteoglycans consist of a core structure of hyaluronate (unsulfated glycosaminoglycan). Link proteins branch off of this structure and provide a surface for aggrecan molecules, composed of a core protein and radiating glycosaminoglycan chains. The chains are extremely important because, along with the collagen bundles, they provide compressive strength and load-absorbing properties. The main molecules are chondroitin-4-sulfate, chondroitin-6-sulfate, and keratin sulfate. The relative proportion of each of these glycosaminolgycan chains changes over time and is unique in each individual. The hydrophilic nature and high density of negative charges underlie articular cartilage resiliency (Fig. 90.11).

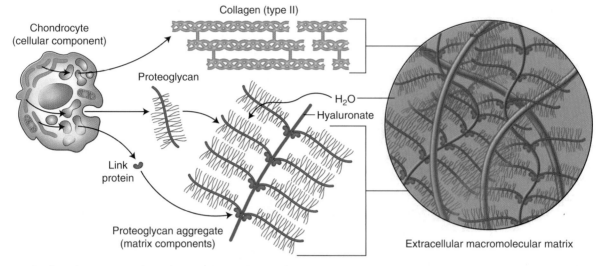

Cartilage is a very complex unique structure able to resist high compressive loads. Early in life, chondrocytes, the cells, produce collagen fibrils and the ground substance, proteoglycans that provide the backbone for cartilage. In aging, the body loses the ability to generate this matrix and repair damage.

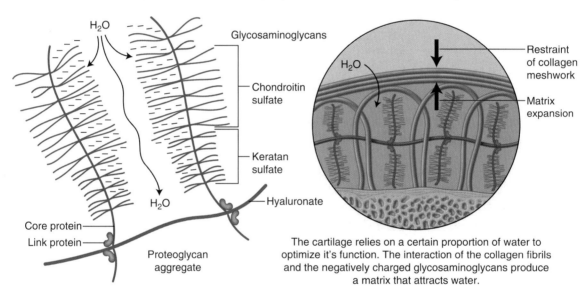

The cartilage relies on a certain proportion of water to optimize it's function. The interaction of the collagen fibrils and the negatively charged glycosaminoglycans produce a matrix that attracts water.

Figure 90.11 Composition of articular cartilage.

This matrix is woven into a complex anatomical structure that provides the unique mechanical properties. These different microscopic structures are orientated differently depending on the depth and layer of the cartilage which changes from the articular surface to the subchondral bone. The organization of these layers includes the superficial zone, the middle zone, the deep zone, the tidemark, and the calcified zone before anchoring to the subchondral bone (Fig. 90.12). The alignment of the chondrocytes differs depending on the layer. The superficial zone, the gliding zone, possesses chondrocytes that are flattened and parallel to the joint with low amounts of proteoglycans. The middle zone shows spherical chondrocytes and large amounts of proteoglycans. The deep layer contains larger spherical chondrocytes and the highest concentration of proteoglycans but the lowest water content. The calcified zone contains collagen fibrils that help anchor the cartilage to the bone by passing from the radial deep zone through the tidemark to the subchondral bone [96].

Despite the resiliency of cartilage, it undergoes age-related changes because chondrocytes do not reproduce themselves. There is a debate concerning the relationship between age-related changes and the development of degenerative arthritis. The biochemical changes differ, and while aging does not always lead to arthritis, it is a risk factor, since more than 50% of those over the age of 65 have radiographic evidence and symptoms of osteoarthritis [97, 98].

FIGURE **90.12** Structure of articular cartilage.

Cell Layers and Architecture of Pristine Articular Cartilage

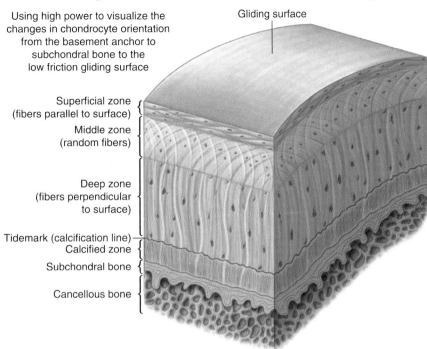

Using high power to visualize the changes in chondrocyte orientation from the basement anchor to subchondral bone to the low friction gliding surface

Gliding surface

Superficial zone (fibers parallel to surface)

Middle zone (random fibers)

Deep zone (fibers perpendicular to surface)

Tidemark (calcification line)
Calcified zone

Subchondral bone

Cancellous bone

In aging, the large proteoglycan structures, chondroitin sulfate and keratin sulfate, which form a compressive hydration gel by binding to hyaluronan via link protein, decrease in the amount present and change in ratio. The amount of chondroitin sulfate decreases, and the amount of keratin sulfate increases [99]. This leads to a decrease in water content and an increase in the stiffness of the tissue. Collagen remains relatively unchanged, but the number and size of chondrocytes decrease. In addition, the levels of advanced glycation end product pentosidine, which are low up to 20 years of age, increase linearly after that. Higher pentoside levels are associated with a stiffer collagen network. The resulting matrix articular cartilage that is lost or damaged is replaced slowly, leading to fraying of articular cartilage [100]. Damage is difficult to repair also, since chondrocytes are not migratory but are bound by lacunae within the tissue.

Arthritis, on the other hand, leads to distinct biochemical changes. The proteoglycans decrease, and their ratio changes. In contrast to aging, chondroitin sulfate increases and keratin sulfate decreases with osteoarthritis. This as well as the damage to the structural integrity of cartilage leads to an increased water content, causing increased permeability, decreased strength, and decreased modulus of elasticity. Collagen content decreases, and collagen becomes disorganized. Hyaluronan and its link proteins fragment and become smaller.

The outward appearance of cartilage changes as the joint deteriorates. The pristine white color darkens. The surface may soften, fissure, and flake off. Eventually, full thickness loss of cartilage occurs, and the subchondral bone becomes eburnated. Radiographically, the joint space narrows, the subchondral bone appears sclerotic, osteophytes form, and the joint deforms (Fig. 90.13). There is some debate as to what to call this process. These kinds of changes have been called osteoarthritis. However, the suffix, "itis," means "inflammation." Most consider this to be wear and tear arthritis and suggest that the term osteoarthrosis might be more appropriate. A new theory based on recent studies is that chondrocytes are actively releasing catabolic enzymes such as interleukin-1, neutral proteases, and metalloproteinases, causing degeneration that *can lead to* inflammation and cause further degenerative changes [101, 102]. In general, aging is different than degenerative arthritis but aging results in the loss of tensile properties of cartilage, leading to a loss of stiffness, fatigue resistance, and strength [96]. Intuitively, these changes cause susceptibility to damage from the daily repetitive microtrauma of the joints and may be the precursor that allows the development of early degenerative changes.

Evaluation of osteoarthritis should begin with history, physical exam, and radiographs. Before obtaining radiographs, it is helpful to have an understanding of the best views for diagnosis. For most patients, weight-bearing views will fully visualize the amount of joint space loss and deformity present, which might not be evident in nonweight-bearing views. There are several grading systems all with some

FIGURE 90.13 Histopathology of osteoarthritis.

Progressive Changes of Osteoarthritis Using the Hip Joint as an Example

Early Degenerative Changes

Loss of normal shiny smooth surface and mild narrowing of the joint space

Minor matrix changes producing changes in biomechanical properties due to increased water content and decreased proteoglycans

Surface fibrillation of articular cartilage

Superficial fissures

Sclerosis

Advanced Degenerative Changes

Loss of cartilage and narrowing of joint space

Release of fibrillated cartilage into joint space

Osteophytes

Enzymatic degradation and thinning of articular cartilage

Pronounced sclerosis of subchondral bone

Reactive synovitis

Fissure penetration to subchondral bone

Joint space narrows with minimal clear space in superior weight bearing portion. Additional changes include further osteophyte formation and bone remodeling.

End Stage Bone on Bone Degenerative Changes

Subchondral cysts

Loss of articular cartilage (bone-on-bone articular surface)

Exposed articular surface of subchondral bone

Capsular fibrosis

Subchondral cartilage

Subchondral sclerosis

Subchondral cysts

Complete loss of articular cartilage in multiple weight bearing zones producing the appearance of no joint space. The size and number of osteophytes and subchondral cysts increase as a reaction to the increased joint reactive forces.

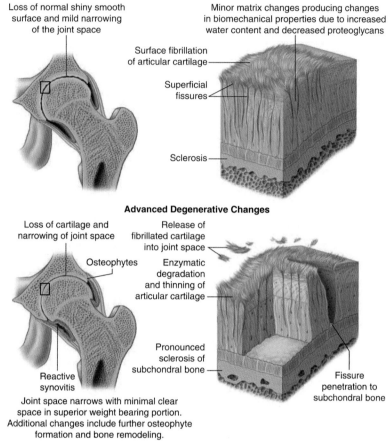
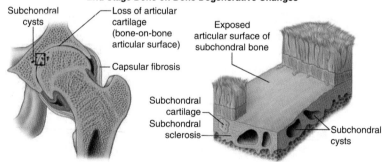

inherent difficulties in intra and interobserver reliability. One of the most common is the Kellegren and Lawrence system using levels I–IV [103, 104]. Grades I and II are considered mild. Grade III is considered moderate, and Grade IV is severe bone-on-bone arthritis. Currently, MRIs are frequently used for assessment of arthritis. However, these tests should be ordered infrequently in elderly patients with arthritis symptoms. Studies have shown that after a certain age, almost every patient – even those that are asymptomatic – will have a surgical lesion on MRI. For instance, knee MRIs are frequently obtained to detect a degenerative meniscus tear even though the patient already has advanced degenerative changes. Such MRIs almost always are read as a meniscus tear, but they really just indicate that the knee is undergoing degeneration. In several studies, asymptomatic patients over the age of 65 underwent an MRI of their knee, and despite a lack of symptoms, 75% had a meniscus tear read by the radiologist on their MRI [105, 106].

Clinical management of degenerative arthritis includes treatment of the symptoms and halting progression. Although a full discussion of the treatment of degenerative arthritis is beyond the scope of this chapter, it involves activity modification, weight reduction, use of non forceful stretching and strengthening, pharmacologic intervention with Tylenol, nonsteroidal anti-inflammatories, nonaddictive pain medications, use of external aids and injections with either cortisone or synovial fluid replacement. Recent attempts to reverse the process and regenerate cartilage have not been successful. Several different types of treatments have been touted to alter the natural history of the disease including glucosamine/chondroitin sulfate [107, 108], electrical stimulation [109, 110], and synovial fluid replacements [111–113]. These treatments have demonstrated efficacy in decreasing pain and improving function. However, none of these adjunctive modalities is supported by Level 1 evidence that they produce changes to aging or degenerative cartilage to produce structurally or biomechanically normal articular hyaline cartilage [111–113].

Surgery can be an option to treat degenerative arthritis, but there are still no surgical options to help the body regrow hyaline cartilage. For instance, the efficacy of arthroscopic procedures of the knee for debridement of arthritis and for degenerative meniscus tears is questionable. Two recent studies comparing arthroscopic and conservative treatment have shown no clinically significant differences at 2 years when treating either degenerative meniscus tears or degenerative arthritis [114, 115]. In addition, Mosely et al. NEJM randomized 180 patients with knee OA into sham surgery, arthroscopic lavage, and arthroscopic lavage and debridement and found no difference in pain and function [116]. Despite these findings, arthroscopy does seem to play a role in treatment of patients with mild degenerative arthritis who present with a degenerative meniscus tear. However, it is important to select only those patients with mild OA and clinical findings consistent with mechanical symptoms of catching and locking with pinpoint pain on the posterior joint line [117].

There have been two procedures claiming to replace cartilage by transplantation, namely, the osteoarticular transplantation system (OATS) and autologous chondrocyte implantation (ACI) (Figs. 90.14 and 90.15). These two procedures cannot reverse global degenerative arthritis and can only be used to treat focal defects in the weight-bearing articular cartilage of joints. The OATs procedure involves taking plugs of bone and cartilage from nonarticular parts of the joint to fill in the defects. In the ACI procedure, cartilage cells are harvested and then grown in vitro. They are then

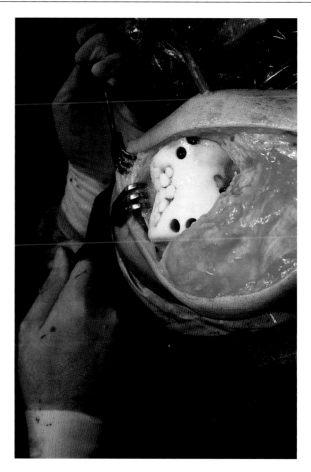

FIGURE 90.14 OATS procedure (osteoarticular transplant system) (reprinted with permission from Hangody L, Fules P (2003) Autologous osteochondral mosaicplasty for the treatment of full-thickness defects of weight-bearing joints: ten years of experimental and clinical experience. J Bone Joint Surg 84-A(Suppl 2):25–32).

placed in the defective area and held in place with a periosteal patch. Both procedures have shown positive results. On follow-up arthroscopy, the areas do seem to be filled with very similar-looking cartilage macroscopically. But, histopathologically, these specimens are not characteristic of hyaline cartilage and are more characteristic of fibrocartilage (scar cartilage) [118–121]. Definitive treatment for degenerative arthritis requires either joint fusion or total joint replacement [122, 123].

Intervertebral Disc

Intervertebral disc is a fibrocartilaginous soft tissue found between the vertebrae which functions to absorb the stress placed on the spine. One of the most common complaints of middle-aged and older patients is back pain, thought to result in part from the changes in intervertebral disc. Fissures and

Figure 90.15 Autologous chondrocyte implantation.

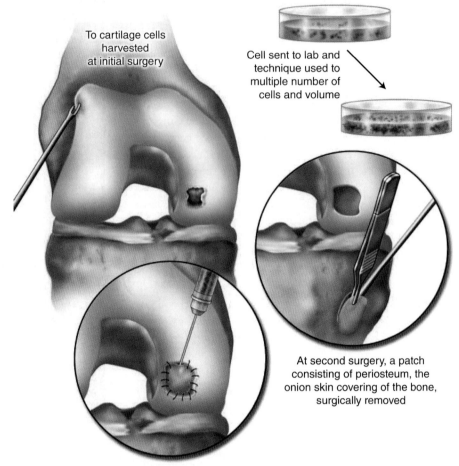

Technique For Autologous Chondrocyte Implantation (ACI)

To cartilage cells harvested at initial surgery

Cell sent to lab and technique used to multiple number of cells and volume

At second surgery, a patch consisting of periosteum, the onion skin covering of the bone, surgically removed

Patch stitched over the cartilage defect and multiplied cells injected into the defect to stimulate growth of cartilage on the articular surface

cracks appear in the intervertebral disc which begin in the periphery (annulus) and extend to the central region (nucleus). During the aging process, the collagen content of the annuli increases both outward in the disc and downward along the levels of the spinal. There is a concomitant decrease in proteoglycan and water content [124]. These changes in chemical composition apparently lead to stiffness and pain in the back [125]. Additionally, these age-related changes may result in disc herniation and nerve compression resulting from spinal stenosis [124].

Treatment options are limited. Degradation of intervertebral disc tissue with enzymatic injections has been a current focus of research and can stimulate regeneration. So far, experiments using such injections show regeneration of intervertebral disc in older animals, but results are not consistent [126]. Also, disc transplantation is an area that is currently under investigation [127].

Conclusion

As the population of elderly people increases, so too will age-related injuries and degenerative disease of the musculoskeletal system. Attempts at regenerative medicine using both traditional and alternative treatments have become popular. In fact, patients spend huge sums of health-care dollars on unproven alternative and complementary products claiming to reverse the aging process. For some treatments, there has been some promising preliminary research, but clinical application is a long way off. The best current advice for patients to decrease age-related degeneration and disease is to stay active, engage in weight-bearing, aerobic, and balance exercise, maintain proper nutrition, and use proven supplements including vitamins such as calcium and vitamin D.

When injury occurs, orthopaedic surgeons may need to adjust current standards of practice in elderly patients.

Traditionally, treatment has been conservative. However, patients are living much longer than previously, and more have active lives. Longitudinal studies on the benefits and risks of choosing conservative or aggressive treatment for injury are needed so that surgeons and patients can be better informed. For instance, the patients in their 70s with a chronic attritional tear of the rotator cuff are traditionally treated conservatively. However, if these patients live well into their 90s, and continue to be healthy and otherwise active, more than likely they will develop a difficult problem of rotator cuff arthropathy. This outcome may be far worse than the results from initially treating the injury aggressively. This kind of issue will play a prominent role in the near future, and surgeons must rethink standard treatment plans in this age group.

References

1. Nordin M, Frankel V (2001) Basic biomechanics of the musculoskeletal system. Lippincott, Williams and Wilkins, Philadelphia, PA
2. Siffert RS, Levy RN (1981) Trabecular patterns and the internal architecture of bone. Mt Sinai J Med 48(3):221–229
3. Raisz LG (1999) Physiology and pathophysiology of bone remodeling. Clin Chem 45(8 Pt 2):1353–1358
4. Warming L, Hassager C, Christiansen C (2002) Changes in bone mineral density with age in men and women: a longitudinal study. Osteoporos Int 13(2):105–112
5. Watts NB (1988) Osteoporosis. Am Fam Physician 38(5):193–207
6. Buckwalter JA, Glimcher MJ, Cooper RR, Recker R (1996) Bone biology. I: Structure, blood supply, cells, matrix, and mineralization. Instr Course Lect 45:371–386
7. Manolagas SC (2000) Birth and death of bone cells: basic regulatory mechanisms and implications for the pathogenesis and treatment of osteoporosis. Endocr Rev 21(2):115–137
8. Melton LJ 3rd, Khosla S, Atkinson EJ, O'Fallon WM, Riggs BL (1997) Relationship of bone turnover to bone density and fractures. J Bone Miner Res 12(7):1083–1091
9. Parfitt AM, Han ZH, Palnitkar S, Rao DS, Shih MS, Nelson D (1997) Effects of ethnicity and age or menopause on osteoblast function, bone mineralization, and osteoid accumulation in iliac bone. J Bone Miner Res 12(11):1864–1873
10. Yavropoulou MP, Yovos JG (2007) The role of the Wnt signaling pathway in osteoblast commitment and differentiation. Hormones (Athens) 6(4):279–294
11. Komori T, Yagi H, Nomura S et al (1997) Targeted disruption of Cbfa1 results in a complete lack of bone formation owing to maturational arrest of osteoblasts. Cell 89(5):755–764
12. Richelson LS, Wahner HW, Melton LJ III, Riggs BL (1984) Relative contributions of aging and estrogen deficiency to postmenopausal bone loss. N Engl J Med 311(20):1273–1275
13. Kuiper GG, Shughrue PJ, Merchenthaler I, Gustafsson JA (1998) The estrogen receptor beta subtype: a novel mediator of estrogen action in neuroendocrine systems. Front Neuroendocrinol 19(4):253–286
14. Qu Q, Harkonen PL, Monkkonen J, Vaananen HK (1999) Conditioned medium of estrogen-treated osteoblasts inhibits osteoclast maturation and function in vitro. Bone 25(2):211–215
15. Manolagas SC, Kousteni S, Jilka RL (2002) Sex steroids and bone. Recent Prog Horm Res 57:385–409
16. Spelsberg TC, Subramaniam M, Riggs BL, Khosla S (1999) The actions and interactions of sex steroids and growth factors/cytokines on the skeleton. Mol Endocrinol 13(6):819–828
17. Jiang C, Giger ML, Kwak SM, Chinander MR, Martell JM, Favus MJ (2000) Normalized BMD as a predictor of bone strength. Acad Radiol 7(1):33–39
18. Cummings SR, Black DM, Nevitt MC et al (1993) Bone density at various sites for prediction of hip fractures. The Study of Osteoporotic Fractures Research Group. Lancet 341(8837):72–75
19. Hui SL, Slemenda CW, Johnston CC Jr (1988) Age and bone mass as predictors of fracture in a prospective study. J Clin Invest 81(6):1804–1809
20. Marshall D, Johnell O, Wedel H (1996) Meta-analysis of how well measures of bone mineral density predict occurrence of osteoporotic fractures. BMJ 312(7041):1254–1259
21. Lenart BA, Neviaser AS, Lyman S et al (2009) Association of low-energy femoral fractures with prolonged bisphosphonate use: a case control study. Osteoporos Int 20(8):1353–1362
22. Johnston C, Slemenda C, Melton L (eds) (1996) Bone density measurements and the management of osteoporosis. Lippincott-Raven, Philadelphia
23. Sone T, Imai Y, Tomomitsu T, Fukunaga M (1998) Calcaneus as a site for the assessment of bone mass. Bone 22(5 Suppl):155S–157S
24. Stenderup K, Justesen J, Eriksen EF, Rattan SI, Kassem M (2001) Number and proliferative capacity of osteogenic stem cells are maintained during aging and in patients with osteoporosis. J Bone Miner Res 16(6):1120–1129
25. Bukata SV, Bostrom MP, Buckwalter JA, Lane J (2005) Physiology of Aging. In: Vaccaro AR (ed) Orthopaedic knowledge update. American Academy of Orthopaedic Surgeons, Rosemont, IL, pp 70–77
26. National Osteoporosis Foundation (2003) Physician's guide to the prevention and treatment of osteoporosis. Excerpta Medica, Inc, Belle Mead, NJ
27. Gehrig L, Lane J, O'Connor MI (2008) Osteoporosis: management and treatment strategies for orthopaedic surgeons. J Bone Joint Surg Am 90(6):1362–1374
28. Bischoff-Ferrari HA, Giovannucci E, Willett WC, Dietrich T, Dawson-Hughes B (2006) Estimation of optimal serum concentrations of 25-hydroxyvitamin D for multiple health outcomes. Am J Clin Nutr 84(1):18–28
29. Broe KE, Chen TC, Weinberg J, Bischoff-Ferrari HA, Holick MF, Kiel DP (2007) A higher dose of vitamin D reduces the risk of falls in nursing home residents: a randomized, multiple-dose study. J Am Geriatr Soc 55(2):234–239
30. Black DM, Cummings SR, Karpf DB et al (1996) Randomised trial of effect of alendronate on risk of fracture in women with existing vertebral fractures. Fracture Intervention Trial Research Group. Lancet 348(9041):1535–1541
31. Black DM, Delmas PD, Eastell R et al (2007) Once-yearly zoledronic acid for treatment of postmenopausal osteoporosis. N Engl J Med 356(18):1809–1822
32. Cummings SR, Black DM, Thompson DE et al (1998) Effect of alendronate on risk of fracture in women with low bone density but without vertebral fractures: results from the Fracture Intervention Trial. JAMA 280(24):2077–2082
33. Harris ST, Watts NB, Genant HK et al (1999) Effects of risedronate treatment on vertebral and nonvertebral fractures in women with postmenopausal osteoporosis: a randomized controlled trial. Vertebral Efficacy with Risedronate Therapy (VERT) Study Group. JAMA 282(14):1344–1352
34. Orwoll E, Ettinger M, Weiss S et al (2000) Alendronate for the treatment of osteoporosis in men. N Engl J Med 343(9):604–610
35. Reginster J, Minne HW, Sorensen OH et al (2000) Randomized trial of the effects of risedronate on vertebral fractures in women

with established postmenopausal osteoporosis. Vertebral Efficacy with Risedronate Therapy (VERT) Study Group. Osteoporos Int 11(1):83–91

36. Reginster JY, Adami S, Lakatos P et al (2006) Efficacy and tolerability of once-monthly oral ibandronate in postmenopausal osteoporosis: 2 year results from the MOBILE study. Ann Rheum Dis 65(5):654–661

37. Lyles KW, Colon-Emeric CS, Magaziner JS et al (2007) Zoledronic acid and clinical fractures and mortality after hip fracture. N Engl J Med 357(18):1799–1809

38. McClung MR, Geusens P, Miller PD et al (2001) Effect of risedronate on the risk of hip fracture in elderly women. Hip Intervention Program Study Group. N Engl J Med 344(5):333–340

39. Papapoulos SE, Quandt SA, Liberman UA, Hochberg MC, Thompson DE (2005) Meta-analysis of the efficacy of alendronate for the prevention of hip fractures in postmenopausal women. Osteoporos Int 16(5):468–474

40. Khosla S, Burr D, Cauley J et al (2007) Bisphosphonate-associated osteonecrosis of the jaw: report of a task force of the American Society for Bone and Mineral Research. J Bone Miner Res 22(10):1479–1491

41. Odvina CV, Zerwekh JE, Rao DS, Maalouf N, Gottschalk FA, Pak CY (2005) Severely suppressed bone turnover: a potential complication of alendronate therapy. J Clin Endocrinol Metab 90(3): 1294–1301

42. Stepan JJ, Burr DB, Pavo I et al (2007) Low bone mineral density is associated with bone microdamage accumulation in postmenopausal women with osteoporosis. Bone 41(3):378–385

43. Ensrud KE, Barrett-Connor EL, Schwartz A et al (2004) Randomized trial of effect of alendronate continuation versus discontinuation in women with low BMD: results from the Fracture Intervention Trial long-term extension. J Bone Miner Res 19(8):1259–1269

44. Chesnut CH 3rd, Silverman S, Andriano K et al (2000) A randomized trial of nasal spray salmon calcitonin in postmenopausal women with established osteoporosis: the prevent recurrence of osteoporotic fractures study. PROOF Study Group. Am J Med 109(4):267–276

45. Munoz-Torres M, Alonso G, Raya MP (2004) Calcitonin therapy in osteoporosis. Treat Endocrinol 3(2):117–132

46. Delmas PD, Bjarnason NH, Mitlak BH et al (1997) Effects of raloxifene on bone mineral density, serum cholesterol concentrations, and uterine endometrium in postmenopausal women. N Engl J Med 337(23):1641–1647

47. Delmas PD, Ensrud KE, Adachi JD et al (2002) Efficacy of raloxifene on vertebral fracture risk reduction in postmenopausal women with osteoporosis: four-year results from a randomized clinical trial. J Clin Endocrinol Metab 87(8):3609–3617

48. Ettinger B, Black DM, Mitlak BH et al (1999) Reduction of vertebral fracture risk in postmenopausal women with osteoporosis treated with raloxifene: results from a 3-year randomized clinical trial. Multiple Outcomes of Raloxifene Evaluation (MORE) Investigators. JAMA 282(7):637–645

49. Siris ES, Harris ST, Eastell R et al (2005) Skeletal effects of raloxifene after 8 years: results from the continuing outcomes relevant to Evista (CORE) study. J Bone Miner Res 20(9):1514–1524

50. Barrett-Connor E, Mosca L, Collins P et al (2006) Effects of raloxifene on cardiovascular events and breast cancer in postmenopausal women. N Engl J Med 355(2):125–137

51. Gennari L, Merlotti D, Valleggi F, Martini G, Nuti R (2007) Selective estrogen receptor modulators for postmenopausal osteoporosis: current state of development. Drugs Aging 24(5):361–379

52. Anderson GL, Limacher M, Assaf AR et al (2004) Effects of conjugated equine estrogen in postmenopausal women with hysterectomy: the Women;s Health Initiative randomized controlled trial. JAMA 291(14):1701–1712

53. Cauley JA, Robbins J, Chen Z et al (2003) Effects of estrogen plus progestin on risk of fracture and bone mineral density: the Women's Health Initiative randomized trial. JAMA 290(13):1729–1738

54. Rossouw JE, Anderson GL, Prentice RL et al (2002) Risks and benefits of estrogen plus progestin in healthy postmenopausal women: principal results from the Women's Health Initiative randomized controlled trial. JAMA 288(3):321–333

55. Neer RM, Arnaud CD, Zanchetta JR et al (2001) Effect of parathyroid hormone (1-34) on fractures and bone mineral density in postmenopausal women with osteoporosis. N Engl J Med 344(19):1434–1441

56. Lindsay R, Miller P, Pohl G, Glass EV, Chen P, Krege JH (2009) Relationship between duration of teriparatide therapy and clinical outcomes in postmenopausal women with osteoporosis. Osteoporos Int 20(6):943–948

57. Vahle JL, Long GG, Sandusky G, Westmore M, Ma YL, Sato M (2004) Bone neoplasms in F344 rats given teriparatide [rhPTH(1-34)] are dependent on duration of treatment and dose. Toxicol Pathol 32(4):426–438

58. Vahle JL, Sato M, Long GG et al (2002) Skeletal changes in rats given daily subcutaneous injections of recombinant human parathyroid hormone (1-34) for 2 years and relevance to human safety. Toxicol Pathol 30(3):312–321

59. Rabenda V, Vanoverloop J, Fabri V et al (2008) Low incidence of anti-osteoporosis treatment after hip fracture. J Bone Joint Surg Am 90(10):2142–2148

60. Rozental TD, Makhni EC, Day CS, Bouxsein ML (2008) Improving evaluation and treatment for osteoporosis following distal radial fractures. A prospective randomized intervention. J Bone Joint Surg Am 90(5):953–961

61. Bogoch ER, Elliot-Gibson V, Beaton DE, Jamal SA, Josse RG, Murray TM (2006) Effective initiation of osteoporosis diagnosis and treatment for patients with a fragility fracture in an orthopaedic environment. J Bone Joint Surg Am 88(1):25–34

62. Miki RA, Oetgen ME, Kirk J, Insogna KL, Lindskog DM (2008) Orthopaedic management improves the rate of early osteoporosis treatment after hip fracture. A randomized clinical trial. J Bone Joint Surg Am 90(11):2346–2353

63. Scherl SA, Templeton K (2003) The aging athlete. In: Bernstein J (ed) Musculoskeletal medicine. American Academy of Orthopaedic Surgeons, Rosemount, IL

64. Huard J, Li Y, Fu FH (2002) Muscle injuries and repair: current trends in research. J Bone Joint Surg Am 84-A(5):822–832

65. Noonan TJ, Garrett WE Jr (1999) Muscle strain injury: diagnosis and treatment. J Am Acad Orthop Surg 7(4):262–269

66. Grimby G, Saltin B (1983) The ageing muscle. Clin Physiol 3(3):209–218

67. Bolin DJ, Stone DA (2002) Overuse injuries. In: Fitzgerald RH, Kaufer H, Malkani AL (eds) Orthopaedics. Mosby, St. Louis, MO, pp 551–564, Section 4: Chapter 5

68. Mair SD, Scaber AV, Glisson RR, Garrett WE Jr (1996) The role of fatigue in susceptibility to acute muscle strain injury. Am J Sports Med 24(2):137–143

69. Noonan TJ, Best TM, Seaber AV, Garrett WE Jr (1993) Thermal effects on skeletal muscle tensile behavior. Am J Sports Med 21(4):517–522

70. Safran MR, Garrett WE Jr, Seaber AV, Glisson RR, Ribbeck BM (1988) The role of warmup in muscular injury prevention. Am J Sports Med 16(2):123–129

71. Alexander JL, Phillips WT, Wagner CL (2008) The effect of strength training on functional fitness in older patients with chronic lung disease enrolled in pulmonary rehabilitation. Rehabil Nurs 33(3):91–97

72. Sullivan DH, Roberson PK, Smith ES, Price JA, Bopp MM (2007) Effects of muscle strength training and megestrol acetate on strength, muscle mass, and function in frail older people. J Am Geriatr Soc 55(1):20–28

73. Astrom M (1997) On the nature and etiology of chronic achilles tendinopathy. University of Lund, Lund, Sweden

74. Jozsa LG, Kannus P (1997) Human tendons: anatomy, physiology and pathology. Human Kinetics, Champaign, IL

75. Movin T, Kristoffersen-Wiberg M, Shalabi A, Gad A, Aspelin P, Rolf C (1998) Intratendinous alterations as imaged by ultrasound and contrast medium-enhanced magnetic resonance in chronic achillodynia. Foot Ankle Int 19(5):311–317

76. Kirkendall DT, Garrett WE (1997) Function and biomechanics of tendons. Scand J Med Sci Sports 7(2):62–66

77. Tuite DJ, Renstrom PA, O'Brien M (1997) The aging tendon. Scand J Med Sci Sports 7(2):72–77

78. Kraushaar BS, Nirschl RP (1999) Tendinosis of the elbow (tennis elbow). Clinical features and findings of histological, immunohistochemical, and electron microscopy studies. J Bone Joint Surg Am 81(2):259–278

79. Sharma P, Maffulli N (2005) Tendon injury and tendinopathy: healing and repair. J Bone Joint Surg Am 87(1):187–202

80. Kvist M, Jozsa L, Jarvinen M, Kvist H (1985) Fine structural alterations in chronic Achilles paratenonitis in athletes. Pathol Res Pract 180(4):416–423

81. Kirkendall DT, Garrett WE (2002) Muscle, tendon, and ligament: structure, function and physiology. In: Fitzgerald RH, Kaufer H, Malkani AL (eds) Orthopaedics. Mosby, St. Louis, MO, pp 168–180, Section 2: Chapter 4

82. Vogel HG (1978) Influence of maturation and age on mechanical and biochemical parameters of connective tissue of various organs in the rat. Connect Tissue Res 6(3):161–166

83. Bailey AJ, Robins SP, Balian G (1974) Biological significance of the intermolecular crosslinks of collagen. Nature 251(5471):105–109

84. Eyre DR, Paz MA, Gallop PM (1984) Cross-linking in collagen and elastin. Annu Rev Biochem 53:717–748

85. Astrom M, Rausing A (1995 Jul) Chronic Achilles tendinopathy. A survey of surgical and histopathologic findings. Clin Orthop Relat Res (316):151–164

86. Khan KM, Maffulli N (1998) Tendinopathy: an Achilles' heel for athletes and clinicians. Clin J Sport Med 8(3):151–154

87. Movin T, Gad A, Reinholt FP, Rolf C (1997) Tendon pathology in long-standing achillodynia. Biopsy findings in 40 patients. Acta Orthop Scand 68(2):170–175

88. Oxlund H (1982) Long term local cortisol treatment of tendons and the indirect effect on skin. An experimental study in rats. Scand J Plast Reconstr Surg 16(1):61–66

89. Best TM, Garrett WE (1994) Muscle and Tendon. In: DeLee J, Drez D (eds) Orthopedic sports medicine: principles and practice. WB Saunders, Philadelphia, PA

90. Clayton RA, Court-Brown CM (2008) The epidemiology of musculoskeletal tendinous and ligamentous injuries. Injury 39(12):1338–1344

91. Brinker MR (2000) Basic Sciences. In: Miller MD (ed) Review of orthopaedics. WB Saunders, Philadelphia, PA

92. Mow VC, Proctor CS, Kelly MA (1989) Biomechanics of Articular Cartilage. In: Nordin M, Frankel V (eds) Basic biomechanics of the musculoskeletal system, 2nd edn. Lea and Febiger, Philadelphia, PA, pp 31–58

93. Aydog ST, Korkusuz P, Doral MN, Tetik O, Demirel HA (2006) Decrease in the numbers of mechanoreceptors in rabbit ACL: the effects of ageing. Knee Surg Sports Traumatol Arthrosc 14(4):325–329

94. Rispler DT (2006) Disorders of Muscles, Tendons, and Ligaments. In: Greene WB (ed) Netter's orthopaedics. Saunders Elsevier, Philadelphia, PA, pp 99–118

95. Dahm DL, Wulf CA, Dajani KA, Dobbs RE, Levy BA, Stuart MA (2008) Reconstruction of the anterior cruciate ligament in patients over 50 years. J Bone Joint Surg Br 90(11):1446–1450

96. Pelligrini VD (2006) Arthritic Disorders. In: Greene WB (ed) Netter's orthopaedics. Saunders Elsevier, Philadelphia, PA, pp 69–98

97. Centers for Disease Control and Prevention (CDC) (2006) Prevalence of doctor-diagnosed arthritis and arthritis-attributable activity limitation – United States, 2003-2005. MMWR Morb Mortal Wkly Rep 55(40):1089–1092

98. Corti MC, Rigon C (2003) Epidemiology of osteoarthritis: prevalence, risk factors and functional impact. Aging Clin Exp Res 15(5):359–363

99. Bayliss MT (1990) Proteoglycan structure and metabolism during maturation and ageing of human articular cartilage. Biochem Soc Trans 18(5):799–802

100. Buckwalter JA, Heckman JD, Petrie DP (2003) An AOA critical issue: aging of the North American population: new challenges for orthopaedics. J Bone Joint Surg Am 85-A(4):748–758

101. Pujol JP, Chadjichristos C, Legendre F et al (2008) Interleukin-1 and transforming growth factor-beta 1 as crucial factors in osteoarthritic cartilage metabolism. Connect Tissue Res 49(3):293–297

102. Ray A, Ray BK (2008) An inflammation-responsive transcription factor in the pathophysiology of osteoarthritis. Biorheology 45(3–4):399–409

103. Lane NE, Kremer LB (1995) Radiographic indices for osteoarthritis. Rheum Dis Clin North Am 21(2):379–394

104. Petersson IF, Boegard T, Saxne T, Silman AJ, Svensson B (1997) Radiographic osteoarthritis of the knee classified by the Ahlback and Kellgren & Lawrence systems for the tibiofemoral joint in people aged 35-54 years with chronic knee pain. Ann Rheum Dis 56(8):493–496

105. Bhattacharyya T, Gale D, Dewire P et al (2003) The clinical importance of meniscal tears demonstrated by magnetic resonance imaging in osteoarthritis of the knee. J Bone Joint Surg Am 85-A(1):4–9

106. Englund M, Guermazi A, Gale D et al (2008) Incidental meniscal findings on knee MRI in middle-aged and elderly persons. N Engl J Med 359(11):1108–1115

107. Rozendaal RM, Uitterlinden EJ, van Osch GJ et al (2009) Effect of glucosamine sulphate on joint space narrowing, pain and function in patients with hip osteoarthritis; subgroup analyses of a randomized controlled trial. Osteoarthritis Cartilage 17(4):427–432

108. Sawitzke AD, Shi H, Finco MF et al (2008) The effect of glucosamine and/or chondroitin sulfate on the progression of knee osteoarthritis: a report from the glucosamine/chondroitin arthritis intervention trial. Arthritis Rheum 58(10):3183–3191

109. Garland D, Holt P, Harrington JT, Caldwell J, Zizic T, Cholewczynski J (2007) A 3-month, randomized, double-blind, placebo-controlled study to evaluate the safety and efficacy of a highly optimized, capacitively coupled, pulsed electrical stimulator in patients with osteoarthritis of the knee. Osteoarthritis Cartilage 15(6):630–637

110. Mont MA, Hungerford DS, Caldwell JR et al (2006) Pulsed electrical stimulation to defer TKA in patients with knee osteoarthritis. Orthopedics 29(10):887–892

111. Caborn D, Rush J, Lanzer W, Parenti D, Murray C (2004) A randomized, single-blind comparison of the efficacy and tolerability of hylan G-F 20 and triamcinolone hexacetonide in patients with osteoarthritis of the knee. J Rheumatol 31(2):333–343

112. Leopold SS, Redd BB, Warme WJ, Wehrle PA, Pettis PD, Shott S (2003) Corticosteroid compared with hyaluronic acid injections for the treatment of osteoarthritis of the knee. A prospective, randomized trial. J Bone Joint Surg Am 85-A(7):1197–1203

113. Petrella RJ, Petrella M (2006) A prospective, randomized, double-blind, placebo controlled study to evaluate the efficacy of intraarticular hyaluronic acid for osteoarthritis of the knee. J Rheumatol 33(5):951–956

114. Herrlin S, Hallander M, Wange P, Weidenhielm L, Werner S (2007) Arthroscopic or conservative treatment of degenerative

medial meniscal tears: a prospective randomised trial. Knee Surg Sports Traumatol Arthrosc 15(4):393–401

115. Kirkley A, Birmingham TB, Litchfield RB et al (2008) A randomized trial of arthroscopic surgery for osteoarthritis of the knee. N Engl J Med 359(11):1097–1107

116. Moseley JB, O'Malley K, Petersen NJ et al (2002) A controlled trial of arthroscopic surgery for osteoarthritis of the knee. N Engl J Med 347(2):81–88

117. Dervin GF, Stiell IG, Rody K, Grabowski J (2003) Effect of arthroscopic debridement for osteoarthritis of the knee on health-related quality of life. J Bone Joint Surg Am 85-A(1):10–19

118. Alford JW, Cole BJ (2005) Cartilage restoration, part 2: techniques, outcomes, and future directions. Am J Sports Med 33(3): 443–460

119. Horas U, Pelinkovic D, Herr G, Aigner T, Schnettler R (2003) Autologous chondrocyte implantation and osteochondral cylinder transplantation in cartilage repair of the knee joint. A prospective, comparative trial. J Bone Joint Surg Am 85-A(2): 185–192

120. Jakobsen RB, Engebretsen L, Slauterbeck JR (2005) An analysis of the quality of cartilage repair studies. J Bone Joint Surg Am 87(10):2232–2239

121. Jones DG, Peterson L (2006) Autologous chondrocyte implantation. J Bone Joint Surg Am 88(11):2502–2520

122. Ethgen O, Bruyere O, Richy F, Dardennes C, Reginster JY (2004) Health-related quality of life in total hip and total knee arthroplasty. A qualitative and systematic review of the literature. J Bone Joint Surg Am 86-A(5):963–974

123. Wright RJ, Sledge CB, Poss R, Ewald FC, Walsh ME, Lingard EA (2004) Patient-reported outcome and survivorship after Kinemax total knee arthroplasty. J Bone Joint Surg Am 86-A(11):2464–2470

124. Buckwalter JA (1995) Aging and degeneration of the human intervertebral disc. Spine 20(11):1307–1314

125. Adams P, Eyre DR, Muir H (1977) Biochemical aspects of development and ageing of human lumbar intervertebral discs. Rheumatol Rehabil 16(1):22–29

126. Deutman R (1992) The case for chemonucleolysis in discogenic sciatica. A review. Acta Orthop Scand 63(5):571–575

127. Ruan D, He Q, Ding Y, Hou L, Li J, Luk KD (2007) Intervertebral disc transplantation in the treatment of degenerative spine disease: a preliminary study. Lancet 369(9566):993–999

128. Favus M (ed) (1996) Primer on the metabolic bone diseases and disorders of mineral metabolism, 3rd edn. Lippincott Raven, Philadelphia

Chapter 91
Common Benign and Malignant Skin Lesions

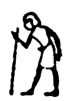

Marcus A. McFerren and David J. Leffell

The elderly patient presents us with a variety of benign and malignant skin lesions. The ability to differentiate various cutaneous neoplasms is especially important in the geriatric population because of the higher incidence of malignant skin tumors that arise in aging skin. The aim of this chapter is to acquaint the surgeon with normal skin anatomy, with changes in skin anatomy during aging, and with the pathophysiology, diagnosis, and treatment of common benign and malignant skin tumors of the elderly.

In general, we recommend an annual total body skin examination for any elderly patient who has any of the following independent risk factors: fair skin color; history of blonde, red, or light-colored hair; green, gray, or blue eye color; a family or personal history of skin cancer; chronic occupational or recreational exposure to the sun; a history of sunburns; or anyone with numerous or atypical nevi. Many patients with a personal history of skin cancer should be seen every 6–12 months.

Basic Skin Anatomy

The skin is composed of two layers: a stratified squamous epithelial layer, or epidermis, and an underlying connective tissue layer, or dermis. The interface between these two layers is termed the dermal–epidermal junction and is characterized by downward folds of the epidermis into the dermis. These folds, called rete ridges, provide mechanical support against shearing forces. Embryologic downgrowths of epithelium into the dermis give rise to epidermal appendages such as hair follicles, sweat glands, and sebaceous glands. Beneath the dermis lies a fatty layer of subcutaneous tissue that serves to insulate and protect the underlying structures.

M.A. McFerren (✉)
Yale New Haven Hospital, Department of Dermatology,
Yale University School of Medicine, New Haven, CT, USA
e-mail: marcus.mcferren@yale.edu

Epidermis

The ectoderm-derived epidermis is comprised of four cell types: keratinocytes, melanocytes, Langerhans' cells, and Merkel cells. Keratinocytes are specialized stratified squamous epithelial cells that make up most of the epidermis. As keratinocytes migrate upward from their origin at the dermal–epidermal junction, they differentiate, forming four morphologically distinct layers. The innermost layer, which contains the germinative keratinocytes, is called the stratum basale. Immediately above the stratum basale, keratinocytes enlarge to form the stratum spinosum, or prickle cell layer. Progressive maturation leads to the accumulation of intracellular keratohyalin granules, giving rise to the next cell layer called the stratum granulosum.

Keratinocytes at the outermost portion of the stratum granulosum lose their nuclei and fuse to form a cornified layer or stratum corneum. These dead keratinocytes function to protect the underlying cells and prevent dehydration. They are eventually exfoliated at a rate that matches the production of cells at the basal layer.

Neuroectoderm-derived melanocytes, which comprise 1% of epidermal cells, are located in the basal layer of the epidermis. They synthesize melanin, which is taken up by nearby keratinocytes and serves to protect the skin from penetration of ultraviolet light, which can damage underlying epidermal and dermal cells. Langerhans cells make up 3–5% of the epidermal cell population. They are derived from cells of the monocyte/macrophage lineage and act as antigen-presenting cells in the skin. Merkel cells are the least abundant cells of the epidermis, comprising less than 1% of all epidermal cells. Their origin is uncertain, either arising from the neural crest or as modified pluripotent amine precursor uptake and decarboxylation (APUD) lineage neuroendocrine keratinocytes. Like melanocytes, they are also located in the basal layer of the epidermis. They function as mechanoreceptors as well as in the induction of the perifollicular nerve plexus during development.

R.A. Rosenthal et al. (eds.), *Principles and Practice of Geriatric Surgery*,
DOI 10.1007/978-1-4419-6999-6_91, © Springer Science+Business Media, LLC 2011

Dermis

The mesoderm-derived dermis sits just below the avascular epidermis, supplying it with a rich neurovascular system. Histologically, the dermis can be divided into two layers. Occupying the space around the rete ridges is the superficial papillary dermis, which is composed of a loosely woven arrangement of connective tissue bundles. Beneath it lies the reticular dermis, so named for its denser, interwoven pattern of connective tissue fibers. The resident cells of the dermis are mostly fibroblasts, which secrete collagen, elastin, and ground substance. Collagen and elastin give the skin its toughness, distensibility, and flexibility. Ground substance, which is comprised of polysaccharides and proteins, provides a supportive matrix for the connective tissue fibers. The overall structure accommodates the network of vascular, lymphatic, and nerve plexi that supply the skin. Other cellular constituents of the dermis include mast cells, macrophages, lymphocytes, and other leukocytes.

Epidermal Appendages

During embryologic development, epidermal cells invaginate and migrate into the dermis forming adnexal structures such as hair follicles, sebaceous glands, and eccrine and apocrine sweat glands collectively termed epidermal appendages. Hair follicles are composed of modified keratinocytes that form a tubular structure enclosed by a collagenous sheath. Each hair follicle is associated with one or more sebaceous glands, which secrete sebum, an oily viscous fluid composed of triglycerides, free fatty acids, wax monoesters, squalenes, and sterols. Sebum functions to help moisturize and waterproof skin and hair. Apocrine glands are modified sweat glands located in the axillae and groin. Like sebaceous glands, they secrete their product into the follicular lumen. In some mammals, they have a demonstrated pheromonal function in territory marking and sexual communication [1]. In humans, their role is uncertain. With the exception of the groin and axillae, the remainder of skin is covered by eccrine sweat glands. These glands are thermoregulatory in their capacity to secrete sweat and immunologic in their capacity to excrete active cytokines [2]. They are independent of the hair follicle having ducts that open directly onto the skin surface.

Skin Function

The basic functions of the epidermis, dermis, and epidermal appendages include that of a physical barrier as well as homeostasis, thermoregulation, immunologic defense,

communication, and sensation. As a physical barrier, the skin protects the body from ultraviolet radiation-associated DNA damage, microorganisms, and toxic chemicals. Far more than simply a sheet of protective wrap, the skin continually regenerates itself by sloughing off damaged cells, and providing a fresh interface for the ever-changing environment. Central to its barrier function is the maintenance of water balance and protection against dehydration. Not all water loss is damaging, however, and eccrine gland-mediated evaporative water loss is critical to thermoregulation. In the battle against microbial invaders, the skin provides the first line of defense. The skin hosts both adaptive and innate immune functions; in the skin itself, circulating lymphocytes and antibodies encounter foreign materials and activate antigen-presenting cells. Cathelcidins, neutrophil-derived polypeptides resident in the skin, also function in antimicrobial defense and cell–cell signaling [3]. Additionally, it is often a fundamental disruption in the immunologic function of the skin that facilitates the development of cutaneous malignancies. In social interaction, the communication and sensory functions of the skin are intertwined. Skin and hair are central to our mechanisms of physical attraction. Neural modulation of the cutaneous blood supply conveys information in interpersonal communication, and the skin is the organ through which touch, temperature, itch, pleasure, and pain are perceived.

Changes in the Skin Associated with Aging

The intrinsic changes that occur in aging skin are important for understanding the pathophysiology of benign and malignant lesions that affect senescent skin.

Epidermis

Between the third and seventh decades, the turnover rate of keratinocytes is reduced by 50% [4]. The slower epidermal turnover rate increases the duration of keratinocyte exposure to carcinogens such as ultraviolet radiation, making the epidermis more susceptible to the development of keratinocytic neoplasms. Decreased proliferative capacity of keratinocytes also prolongs wound healing.

The aging epidermis also undergoes structural alterations. The rete pegs at the dermal–epidermal junction retract, making elderly skin more susceptible to shearing forces. Keratinocytes in the basal layer become increasingly pleomorphic, displaying variations in size, shape, and staining pattern [5]. With age, the stratum corneum increases in thickness due to a slower rate of desquamation. This thicker stratum corneum has reduced intercellular lipid content and reduced water-binding capacity, predisposing aging skin to xerosis, or drying, with cracking, compromised barrier function, and subsequent irritation and inflammation [6, 7].

Melanocytes also undergo age-related decrease in number over time. After age 30, the surviving population of melanocytes drops by 8–20% each decade [8]. As a result, less melanin is produced which allows greater penetration of ultraviolet radiation resulting in an increase in the risk of developing skin cancer. Like melanocytes, Langerhans cells also diminish in number with age. Langerhans cells are especially sensitive to UV radiation and are further functionally impaired by the age-related decrease in protective melanin. This UV-induced immune suppression compromises the cell-mediated immune response in elderly skin, thereby more readily permitting the development of tumors.

Dermis

As the skin ages, the dermis thins and becomes less vascular. Collagen fibers become thickened, less resilient, and the dermis becomes more susceptible to shearing injuries. Elastin fibers display structural degradative changes, resulting in skin laxity and wrinkle formation [5]. The amount of ground substance decreases, reducing the supportive dermal matrix, and so structures such as blood vessels become more susceptible to damage. This manifests clinically as easy bruising in the elderly. Thinning of vessel walls may also contribute to the increased susceptibility to ecchymoses. Other changes in cutaneous vasculature include a decrease in the density of vessels. Diminished cutaneous circulation can lead to impaired clearance of foreign material, delayed wound healing, and diminished thermoregulatory capacity. The aging skin also loses its ability to mount an inflammatory response, leading to muted clinical presentations of cutaneous disease.

Epidermal Appendages

Marked age-related changes also occur in the epidermal appendages. There is an overall reduction in the number and function of eccrine sweat glands, leading to a decrease in thermoregulatory capacity. Apocrine glands attenuate and accumulate lipofuscin with a resultant reduction in secretory function [6]. Sebaceous glands enlarge with age, but their sebum production is paradoxically reduced. These changes in sebaceous glands manifest clinically as sebaceous hyperplasia and xerosis.

Benign Lesions

Epidermal Lesions

Seborrheic Keratoses

Seborrheic keratoses are common, benign, flat-topped papules or plaques that are composed of hyperproliferating keratinocytes. They typically appear during the fifth decade, though early lesions can present in the fourth decade. Early lesions manifest as discrete 1- to 3-cm skin-colored to dark-brown patches that progress to form slightly elevated, warty, greasy plaques. Their exophytic growth pattern makes them appear "stuck on." [9] Although seborrheic keratoses can be found on any part of the body, they are most prevalent on the face and upper trunk (Fig. 91.1). Males and females are equally affected; the lesions occur more frequently in whites.

A histologically identical variant of the seborrheic keratosis, dermatosis papillosa nigra, is commonly found in patients with darkly pigmented skin. Clinically, these lesions present as multiple 0.1–1.0 cm rough brown to black papules of the face. They are especially common on the malar cheeks, forehead, neck, back, and chest.

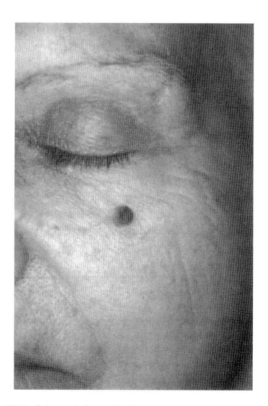

FIGURE 91.1 Seborrheic keratosis, the most common benign cutaneous tumor in the elderly. Its significance lies in its potential to mimic malignant melanoma. Although treatment is not normally indicated, the lesion, which may appear rough or greasy, may be irritated necessitating removal. Alternatively, if there is suspicion about melanoma, biopsy is indicated.

The number of lesions on any given individual can vary from one or two up to hundreds [9], often increasing in number as the patient ages. Once formed, seborrheic keratoses are permanent, remaining in place unchanged for the lifetime of the individual. Seborrheic keratoses are benign and have no malignant potential. However, the eruption of multiple lesions in a short duration of time, known as the sign of Leser–Trelat, has historically been thought to point to internal malignancy, particularly gastrointestinal adenocarcinoma, breast carcinoma, and lymphoma. Despite a large number of case reports and anecdotal evidence in support of an association between widespread eruptive seborrheic keratoses and internal malignancy, the data to support this phenomenon as a true paraneoplastic process is largely lacking [10]. Multiple seborrheic keratoses may, however, occur as a familial trait with autosomal dominant inheritance or may be precipitated by an inflammatory dermatosis.

Histologically, seborrheic keratoses show accumulation of immature keratinocytes with papillomatosis between the basal layer and stratum corneum. Focal keratinization may occur, leading to the formation of horn cysts within the lesion. Melanocytes usually proliferate in the lesion and transfer melanin to immature keratinocytes, accounting for the wide spectrum of color the lesions can acquire.

The diagnosis of seborrheic keratoses is made clinically. Some early lesions may be confused with solar lentigos or pigmented actinic keratoses. Differentiation may be made upon closer inspection with a hand lens, which can reveal a characteristic verrucous appearance and at times the presence of horn cysts. Late lesions may resemble a pigmented basal cell carcinoma (BCC) or malignant melanoma. If a lesion is thought to be a BCC, a shave biopsy is recommended. For lesions suspicious for malignant melanoma, an excisional biopsy should be performed.

Although seborrheic keratoses require no therapy, some patients prefer to have them removed for cosmetic reasons. Treatment should be rapid and nonscarring. This can be accomplished with light curettage, which destroys the superficial layer of the epidermis and minimizes the risk of scarring. The potential for regrowth exists. Should this occur, retreatment may be performed as necessary. Electrodesiccation should be avoided, as it may cause excessive scarring [11]. If the clinical diagnosis is unclear, a shave biopsy should be performed.

Solar Lentigo (Senile Lentigo, Actinic Lentigo)

Chronic sun exposure can induce melanocytes to proliferate locally forming multiple 0.5–2.0 cm brown macules known as solar lentigos, "liver spots" or "age spots." Their presence in more than 90% of individuals over the age of 70 has led to the unflattering descriptive term "senile lentigo," but they are often found on light-skinned persons of any age. These lesions are

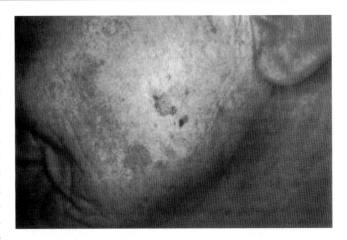

Figure 91.2 Solar lentigo, seen mostly on the face and dorsa of the hands, has tan to brown pigmentation and is flat. They may be of cosmetic concern and occasionally must be biopsied to rule out lentigo maligna.

localized to sun-exposed areas, such as the cheek, forehead, nose, dorsa of hands and forearms, upper back, and chest (Fig. 91.2). They affect males and females equally and are more commonly seen in Caucasians than in Asians.

Solar lentigos can be confused with other benign lesions, such as early seborrheic keratoses, and premalignant lesions such as pigmented actinic keratoses and lentigo maligna. To differentiate solar lentigos from seborrheic keratoses and pigmented actinic keratoses, the lesion must be examined with a hand lens in oblique light. Seborrheic keratoses and pigmented actinic keratoses generally display features of epidermal change, whereas solar lentigos are completely flat. Lentigo maligna, like solar lentigo, may not show epidermal changes. However, it has distinct variations in color from light brown to dark brown with flecks of black. If any lentigo has an irregular border, change in pigment, or focal thickening, a biopsy should be performed to exclude lentigo maligna.

Histologically, solar lentigos display elongated, club-shaped rete ridges containing numerous melanocytes and increased melanin production without cellular atypia or nest formation. Most solar lentigos have virtually no malignant potential. Rarely, a small proportion of lesions occurring on the face slowly develop into lentigo maligna [9]. The incidence of malignant transformation is so rare, however, that most lesions require no treatment. If the patient finds these "age spots" cosmetically unacceptable, treatment can be accomplished in several ways. Topical and physical therapies including cryotherapy, laser, and dermabrasion have been investigated. Cryotherapy and topical retinoids, particularly 0.05% retinoic acid, have demonstrated good effect in randomized controlled trials. Among laser treatments, Q-switched ruby and 532 nm Nd:Yag have been shown effective in controlled trials without randomization [12]. Application of bleaching agents may decrease the pigment, but ongoing treatment is necessary. For those seeking treatment, the use of sunscreen to prevent new lesions should be emphasized.

Melanocytic Nevocellular Nevi (Moles)

Benign nevocellular nevi, or moles, are small, well-circumscribed macules and papules that vary in color from skin-colored to tan and brown (Fig. 91.3). They are composed of nests of melanocytes located in the epidermis, dermis, and rarely subcutaneous tissue. If the cluster of melanocytes is localized to the dermal–epidermal junction, the nevus is classified as a junctional nevus; if the cells are in the dermis, it is called a dermal nevus; and if there are features of both, the lesion is referred to as a compound nevus. Dermal nevi may be pigmented, nonpigmented, smooth, or have a verrucous surface.

Nevocellular lesions are acquired during childhood and early adulthood. They typically increase in number up to the age of 40, following which they begin to involute. With the exception of dermal nevi, most nevocellular nevi disappear by the age of 60. As some junctional and compound nevi age, their melanocytes migrate into the dermis and assume features of dermal nevi. If new nevocellular lesions are acquired after mid-adulthood, they should be regarded with a high degree of suspicion and closely followed to rule out the development of malignancy [13].

Benign Dermal Lesions

Acrochordons (Skin Tags)

Skin tags are soft, pliable, skin-colored to tan-brown pedunculated polyps that occur in intertriginous areas such as the neck and axillae. They are common in middle-aged and elderly individuals, with at least 50% of individuals above the age of 50 having at least one [14]. Over time, they can become larger and more numerous. Skin tags are especially prevalent in postmenopausal women, pregnant women [15], and obese individuals, suggesting a hormonal influence on their development. The exact etiology of skin tags is unknown, though some familial groupings have been noted. Early studies suggested that skin tags could potentially serve as cutaneous markers for colonic polyps [16], but more recently, that association has been largely disproved [17]. The association between diabetes mellitus and multiple skin tags is less clear [18, 19].

Histologically, skin tags consist of protruding loose fibrous tissue covered by a thin epidermis attached to the skin by a narrow stalk. Upon visual inspection they are easily recognized, though they are rarely misdiagnosed as pedunculated seborrheic keratoses, pedunculated melanocytic nevi, neurofibromas, or molluscum contagiosum. Their size offers a clue to their diagnosis: Skin tags tend to be smaller than the average pedunculated melanocytic nevus or neurofibroma.

Skin tags have no malignant potential but tend to be a cosmetic nuisance, especially if they occur in areas exposed to friction such as the belt line. When infarcted, they can cause considerable discomfort. Treatment consists of simple excision requiring no local anesthetic. Lesions can be severed at their base by grasping them with forceps and cutting them with scissors, razors, or scalpels. Skin tags may also be electrodesiccated.

Xanthelasma Palpebrarum (Eyelid Xanthomas)

Xanthelasma palpebrarum is seen mostly in adults in their fourth to fifth decade. They present as yellow velvety plaques confined to the eyelids. The lesions often begin as small yellow spots that initially may be confused with milia or senile closed comedones. They grow over a span of months to form coalescing plaques on the upper eyelids and around the inner canthus (Fig. 91.4). Once their growth stabilizes, these plaques remain permanently.

Histologically, xanthelasma palpebrarum is characterized by lipid-laden macrophages in the superficial dermis.

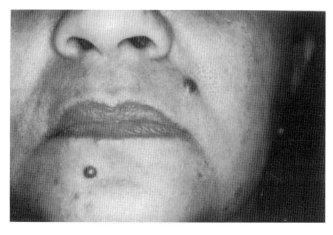

FIGURE 91.3 Nevi of medical significance are uncommon in the elderly, but new pigmented lesions that are not seborrheic keratoses should be evaluated.

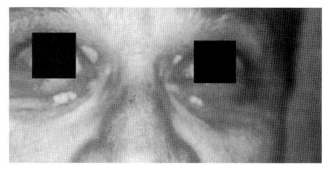

FIGURE 91.4 Xanthelasma. These cholesterol deposits occur on the upper and lower lids and can best be removed surgically. They are yellowish with a smooth surface.

Approximately 50% of patients who present with these lesions have an underlying disorder of lipid metabolism, such as familial hypercholesterolemia or familial dysproteinemia. Patients with these disorders typically have elevated low-density lipoprotein (LDL) and apoprotein E levels and are prone to atherosclerotic cardiovascular disease. Patients who present for the first time with xanthelasma palpebrarum should have their serum lipoproteins and apolipoproteins checked. If the levels are within normal limits, no further testing need be pursued, as nearly half of the patients who present with the lesion have no lipid disturbances. The etiology of xanthelasma palprebrarum in patients with no lipid disorder is unknown.

Systemic therapy with lipid-lowering agents rarely affects the appearance of these lesions. Prior to the advent of laser therapy, excision, cryotherapy, and topical application of 30% trichloroacetic acid were the preferred methods of treatment. With most of these treatments, however, recurrences are common. Excision with primary closure is effective in only 60% of patients and is limited by the location of the lesions [20]. Some authors have advocated excision with secondary intention healing, thereby minimizing the risk of ectropion and complications with skin grafting [21]. Although healing by secondary intention may allow greater margins of resection and therefore minimize the rate of recurrence to as low as 7% [21]. The risk of scarring and infection may make this procedure risky in the hands of the untrained. Recently, various laser modalities including erbium:YAG [22], Argon [23], and 1064 Q-switched Nd:YAG [24] have been utilized in the treatment of xanthelasma with good cosmetic outcomes. Ultrapulse CO_2 laser in only one treatment session has shown excellent results without complications or recurrences at follow-up of up to 1 year [25]. Though promising, the efficacy of these new modalities must be further studied in controlled clinical trials to establish their proper role in therapy.

Sebaceous Hyperplasia

Sebaceous hyperplasia is a benign lesion that is often found on the face of older patients. It typically presents as a cream to yellow umbilicated papule on the forehead, cheeks, eyelids, and nose of individuals over the age of 30 (Fig. 91.5). The incidence of sebaceous hyperplasia increases with age such that about 25% of patients over the age of 65 carry these lesions. Its etiology is unknown, but genetic factors most likely play a role in its pathogenesis as most lesions occur independent of sun exposure and arise in patients of northern European heritage.

Sebaceous hyperplasia often begins as a small, 2- to 3-mm papule with a central depression. This depression represents the opening of a wide sebaceous duct that is surrounded by several enlarged sebaceous gland lobules, lending the lesion its characteristic lobular configuration.

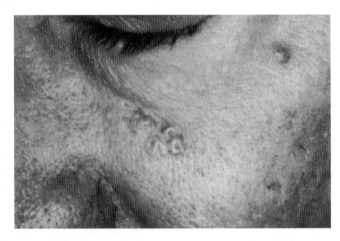

Figure 91.5 Sebaceous hyperplasia. These lesions represent benign hypertrophy of the sebaceous glands. With their central umbilication and rounded edge, they are occasionally confused with basal cell carcinoma.

Some lesions of sebaceous hyperplasia contain central telangiectasias. This feature, combined with the papule's translucent appearance, often leads clinicians to confuse sebaceous hyperplasia with BCC. A clue to the correct diagnosis can be obtained with diascopy (applying pressure on the lesion with a glass slide), which reveals the yellow-white color of sebaceous hyperplasia. Relying on diascopy for diagnosis is not perfect: the yellow-white color sometimes leads to the incorrect diagnosis of xanthomas. Xanthomas can usually be differentiated by their larger size and absence of umbilication [26].

When the clinical diagnosis is uncertain, a biopsy should be performed. In general, no treatment is necessary unless cosmetically desirable. Cryotherapy, in a single freeze–thaw cycle or shave excisions of the elevated portion of the lesion, has been variably successful. Electrodesiccation and curettage should be avoided, as it may result in scarring.

Chondrodermatitis Nodularis Helicis

Chondrodermatitis nodularis helicis (CNH) typically presents as a painful, erythematous nodule on the helices of men over the age of 40. Approximately 30% of cases of CNH occur in young individuals and in women, but the location varies to include the antihelix, tragus, antitragus, and concha [27]. The tender nodule, which often displays central crusting and ulceration, is typically surrounded by hyperemic skin. It enlarges to reach its maximum size of 0.5–2.0 cm within a few months and then remains unchanged indefinitely without evolution to malignancy (Fig. 91.6).

This disorder is thought to be due to compromised local blood supply as a result of pressure or cold temperatures. It often arises in individuals who habitually sleep on one side. Aggravating factors include cold temperatures, pressure from head gear, and trauma. Despite the characteristic

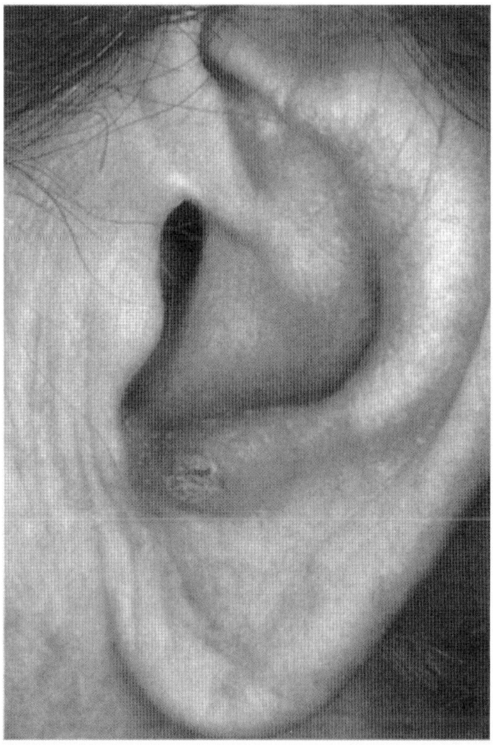

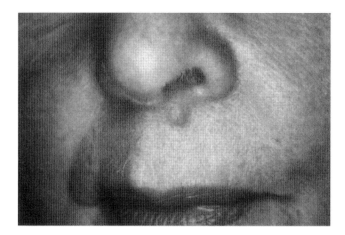

FIGURE 91.7 Hemangioma. This deep-seated hemangioma on the upper lip is benign, but in the absence of the ability to blanch on compression, it should be biopsied to rule out other tumors.

FIGURE 91.6 Chondrodermatitis nodularis helicis. This benign condition of the ear is painful and may present with eroded epidermis. It can be confused with squamous cell cancer of the ear, which usually is not painful.

exquisite tenderness of these lesions, CNH is often mistaken for squamous cell carcinoma (SCC). Biopsy, which is indicated only if there is a degree of suspicion for SCC, characteristically reveals degenerated homogeneous collagen surrounded by vascular granulation tissue with acanthotic overlying epidermis containing a central ulcer. The perichondrium is thickened and shows a lymphocytic infiltrate.

Treatment of CNH may be medical or surgical. Medical therapies include intralesional injection of steroids and collagen [27] and cryotherapy. Conservative management has been advocated in the first instance [28]. Intralesional steroids, such as triamcinolone acetonide administered at a 5–10 mg/ml dose, are generally reserved for first-line treatment of early lesions, as it is successful in only 25% of cases [29]. Higher cure rates, approaching 85% [30], are achieved with surgical approaches, including excision. Electrodesiccation and curettage can be easily performed with adequate margins by allowing the curette to be the guide. Necrotic cartilage, which tends to be soft, is removed easily. Curettage is stopped when healthy, firm cartilage is reached [31]. Techniques for excision vary widely: some advocate removal of abnormal auricular cartilage only [29, 30, 32], whereas others recommend removal of involved cartilage as well as overlying skin [4, 33]. Leaving the overlying skin intact has the advantage of decreasing the deformity of the ear, resulting in a better cosmetic result [34, 35]. A cure rate approaching 100% over a

2-year follow-up period has been reported using CO_2 laser surgery [36, 37], but recent data from large-scale comparative trials are not yet available. To prevent recurrences, the patient should be instructed to minimize pressure and trauma to the ear.

Cherry Hemangioma (Campbell de Morgan Spots)

Cherry angiomas are small, benign, bright red to violaceous, dome-shaped papules that are commonly found in middle-age and older adults. They become more numerous with age. They are distributed over the trunk and proximal extremities and can vary from 2 to 8 mm in diameter (Fig. 91.7). Their etiology is unknown.

Histologically, cherry angiomas are characterized by the presence of numerous dilated capillaries lined by flattened endothelial cells with edematous surrounding stroma and collagen homogenization. The overlying epidermis is frequently thinned with fenestrations.

Cherry angiomas are diagnosed clinically and require no treatment. Occasionally, they are mimicked by angiokeratomas, venous lakes, nodular melanomas, or metastatic carcinomas. If nodular melanoma or metastatic carcinoma is suspected, an excisional biopsy should be performed. If a cherry angioma is at a site of recurrent trauma and therefore prone to ulceration or if it is at a site that is cosmetically unacceptable to the patient, it can be treated by shave excision, cryotherapy, electrodesiccation, or laser ablation.

Venous Lakes

Venous lakes are angiomatous dilations of venules occurring on the face, lips, and ears of patients who are usually above the age of 50. They manifest clinically as dark-blue to violaceous papules with an irregular, cobblestone appearance. After an initial growth phase these lesions stabilize and do not regress. The cause of venous lake formation is unknown. It occurs with equal incidence in both sexes. Microscopically, the lesion reveals small, single-layered interconnected vessels (or one large dilated space) in the upper dermis surrounded by a thin wall of fibrous tissue. A venous lake can resemble a pyogenic granuloma, which should be removed or biopsied, or a nodular melanoma, which requires an excisional biopsy. In most instances, however, venous lakes can be easily distinguished clinically by applying prolonged pressure to the lesion, which causes it to lose its violaceous hue as the venous bed empties.

Treatment of venous lakes is cosmetic. They can be obliterated with electrocoagulation or laser; the long pulse Nd:YAG has recently shown promise [38]. Alternatively, they can be surgically excised, but there is a risk of a cosmetically unacceptable scar.

Premalignant Lesions

Actinic Keratoses (Solar Keratoses)

Actinic keratoses (AKs) are discrete, scaly, pink to red papules that are found on chronically sun-exposed skin of the face, ears, neck, forearms, and dorsal hands. They have a rough quality, allowing them to be more easily felt than seen. Typically, they arise in middle-age individuals, though they may occur at earlier ages in people living in latitudes closer to the equator. Actinic keratoses are generally considered premalignant lesions with a conversion rate to invasive SCC ranging between 0.075 and 0.096% per lesion per year [39]. For the average person with multiple actinic keratoses, the chance of developing invasive SCC has been estimated at 10–20% over a 10 year period if those AKs are left untreated [40]. An alternate viewpoint characterizes actinic keratoses not as premalignant lesions, but rather as malignant lesions akin to SCC in situ [41].

The SCCs that arise from AKs have been considered to be less aggressive than those arising de novo, with a metastatic rate of only 1.6% [39], although there is some doubt about this association.

There are three clinical subtypes of AKs: hypertrophic, pigmented, and lichenoid (Fig. 91.8). The hypertrophic variety develops as a thickened papule that may border on early squamous cell cancer. Pigmented AKs can resemble solar lentigo, seborrheic keratoses, nevi, or in situ melanoma. Lichenoid AK may mimic lichen planus. In general, AKs are relatively easy to recognize clinically and do not require a biopsy unless there is suspicion of malignant transformation.

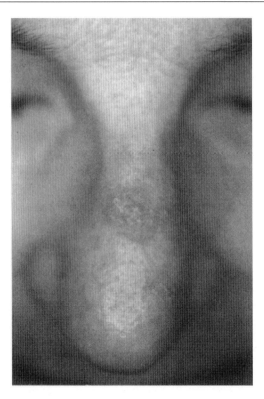

FIGURE 91.8 Actinic keratoses. This is one of the most common sun-related lesions in the elderly. It is biologically and clinically premalignant and should be treated because of the risk of malignant transformation. The lesions can vary in size from 1 to 2 mm up to more than 1 cm and have a rough surface overlying a reddened background.

Biopsy typically reveals large, bright-staining keratinocytes with mild to moderate basal layer pleomorphism that spares follicular units. The abnormal keratinocytes do not invade the dermis.

Because AKs are considered premalignant [41], treatment is ablative and the method determined by the number and location of lesions. If a patient presents with fewer than 10 AKs, cryotherapy is the method of choice. Flat to slightly raised lesions are treated with liquid nitrogen until frosted. For lesions that are thick and hyperkeratotic, 3–5 s of freezing may be necessary. With this technique, cure rates as high as 98% have been reported [41, 42]. Light electrodesiccation and curettage and CO_2 lasers are other effective methods for scattered lesions, but they have the disadvantages of requiring local anesthesia and may increase the risk of scarring.

For numerous lesions, topical fluorouracil (5-FU), which selectively targets abnormal keratinocytes, is one treatment option. It is applied as a 1%, 2%, or 5% cream or solution once or twice daily until the AKs become inflamed and ulcerate. The treatment period can last 2–6 weeks and can cause significant discomfort, which may hamper patient compliance. Inflammation can be minimized with mid-potency topical steroids during the healing phase without affecting the efficacy of the treatment. The recurrence rate with 5-FU is high.

Additional topical methods of treating actinic keratoses include immunologic manipulation with the toll-like receptor-7 agonist imiquimod and the use of the cyclooxygenase inhibitor diclofenac. Clinical investigation of daily topical imiquimod has revealed clinical clearance rates ranging from 45 to 84% [43–45]. Notable side effects include edema, inflammation, and erythema. Three-percent diclofenac in 2.5% hyaluronic acid gel has been investigated and revealed clearance of up to 50% of target lesions with xerosis and rash at the application site cited as adverse events [46, 47].

Exfoliative methods of treatment and lesion reduction include chemical peels with trichloroacetic acid and dermabrasion (by laser or with diamond fraize). Chemexfoliation with 35% tricholoracetic acid, on a repeated basis, can decrease the number of AKs. The advantage of these methods is that their efficacy is not dependent on patient compliance, and they can have the added benefit of improving cosmetic appearance.

Photodynamic therapy, PDT, has been used increasingly to treat actinic keratoses and a variety of other superficial neoplastic lesions. In the process of PDT, a photosensitizing compound, typically the hemoporphyrin derived 5-aminolevulinic acid (5-ALA) or its methyl ester (mALA), is applied directly to diseased skin and incubated for 4–16 h. In the skin cells, ALA is converted to protoporphyrin IX. It is believed that upon illumination with red, blue, noncoherent, or laser light, the photosensitizing compound releases cytotoxic reactive oxygen species leading to overwhelming oxidative stress and cell death.

Growing data support the use of PDT in the treatment of actinic keratoses with response rates comparable to cryotherapy and 5-FU. A number of prospective vehicle-controlled trials have been performed, revealing clearance rates ranging from 77 to 99% with recurrence rates as high as 30% after 1 year [48]. Depending on the duration of incubation and the nature of light activation, transient pain may be a consideration. It is usually manageable with local measures, but post-treatment edema and scaling can be expected depending on the extent of the treatment area.

Patients presenting with AKs usually have a history of chronic sun exposure, which places them at increased risk for developing other skin cancers. Therefore, it is important to follow these patients at regular intervals and to emphasize preventive care by recommending sun protection strategies.

Actinic Cheilitis

Actinic cheilitis is a premalignant disorder of the lip. It usually localizes to the mucosal surface of the lower lip where sunlight exposure is greatest but occasionally occurs on the upper lip (Fig. 91.9). The lesion initially presents as an edematous erythematous patch that progresses to an indurated, scaly plaque with a whitish-gray to brown discoloration. Vertical fissuring and crusting can occur and become painful. Vesicles may arise and burst, giving rise to superficial ulcerations, which may then become secondarily infected. Eventually, warty nodules may form that can undergo malignant transformation to SCC.

The main risk factor for developing actinic cheilitis is chronic sun exposure, as evidenced by a higher incidence of the lesions in people living in sunny regions, outdoor workers, and light-skinned individuals. Its decreased incidence in women may be due to the protective effects of lipstick [4].

Histologically, actinic cheilitis displays regions of flattened, atrophic epithelium adjacent to acanthotic areas. The epidermis may also show disordered maturation without evidence of nuclear atypia. Lymphocytes and plasma cells infiltrate the dermis, which frequently shows signs of solar elastosis such as basophilic degeneration of collagen and elastic fibers.

Actinic cheilitis is often confused with other forms of cheilitis, including lupus erythematosus, lichen planus, and eczematous cheilitis secondary to contact allergies. The occasional blistering may lead to the diagnosis of sunlight-induced herpes simplex virus infection. The propensity for these lesions to develop into SCCs should alert the clinician to look for features associated with malignancy such as ulceration, persistent flaking or crusting, generalized atrophy with focal areas of leukoplakia, and a red and white blotchy appearance with an ill-defined vermilion border. Any lesion with suspicious features should be biopsied.

If the lesion is not indurated, a trial of conservative therapy with opaque zinc oxide or titanium dioxide containing sunscreens and topical steroids may be initiated. Because of the sensitivity of the lip area, ablative treatments can be painful and problematic. Topical agents can be used but can also

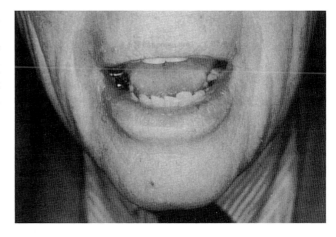

Figure 91.9 Actinic cheilitis. This confluent, hyperkeratotic tumor of the lip is sun-induced. It can be asymptomatic or develop painful fissures. It is premalignant and biologically analogous to actinic keratoses on nonmucosal skin.

cause a painful reaction. In one approach, topical 5% fluo-rouracil can be applied three times daily for 9–15 days result-ing in brisk ulceration followed by a 2- to 3-week period of healing. Even with good compliance, recurrence rates range from 17% at 22 months to 60% at 50 months [49, 50]. Alternative, less aggressive modes of application may be tried. Photodynamic therapy with mALA and red light [51] or ALA and long-pulse pulsed dye laser have been advocated with the latter achieving complete clearance rates of 68% [52]. Imiquimod has been advocated in the treatment of actinic chelitis [53], but high rates of aphthous ulcers have been noted to limit its utility [54]. Diclofenac 3% gel has been used, but there have been no blinded controlled trials to support its efficacy [55]. The most aggressive form of ther-apy is vermilionectomy which involves excision of the ver-milion border down to orbicularis oris muscle with subsequent advancement of a labial mucosal flap [30]. This procedure should be reserved for cases of actinic cheilitis that do not respond to laser, photodynamic, or other therapy.

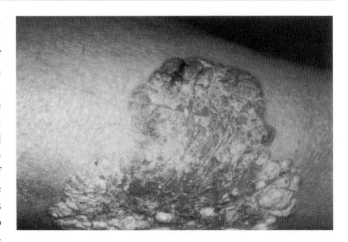

Figure 91.10 Bowen's disease. This large plaque is an extreme exam-ple of squamous cell carcinoma in situ, or Bowen's disease. This nonin-vasive cancer does extend down the hair follicles, so failure to eradicate cells at this level, surgically or otherwise, may result in recurrence of the tumor.

Cutaneous Horn

Cutaneous horn is a clinical term used to describe a hard, yellowish-brown, conical outgrowth of skin, resembling an animal's horn. Cutaneous horns develop on sun-exposed areas such as the scalp, upper part of the face, tips of the ears, and dorsum of hands; they may grow as long as 20 cm [56]. They can arise from benign, premalignant, or malignant epi-dermis. A clue to malignancy can be obtained from close examination of the surrounding epidermis: If the skin sur-rounding the lesion is normal looking or slightly acanthotic, the lesion is more likely to be benign, whereas inflammation or induration of the surrounding skin suggests malignancy. More than 60% of cutaneous horns are derived from benign lesions of epithelial hyperplasia, such as warts, skin tags, seborrheic keratoses, and nevi; 23% arise from premalignant lesions including actinic keratoses, and the remaining 16% arise from mostly squamous cell cancer. Horns arising from basal cell cancer and metastatic and sebaceous carcinomas have been reported [56, 57]. Therefore, all horns should be biopsied with care to preserve their base by performing a deep tangential biopsy.

Bowen's Disease (Squamous Cell Carcinoma In Situ)

Squamous cell carcinoma in situ that localizes to the epider-mis is referred to as Bowen's disease. It typically arises in individuals over the age of 60 and has a slow, indolent course.

Although not invasive into the dermis, it must be considered a variant of squamous cell cancer. Approximately 5% of the lesions progress to invasive SCCs [58]. Bowen's disease ini-tially presents as a slowly enlarging, solitary, erythematous macule with a sharp border that can evolve into a scaling, crusting plaque usually 2–6 cm in diameter (Fig. 91.10). When this lesion develops on the penis, it is known as eryth-roplasia of Queyrat. Its etiology has been associated with chronic exposure to solar radiation, psoralens ultraviolet A (PUVA) therapy, radiation, and environmental toxins such as arsenic, mustard gas, pesticides, and herbicides.

The clinical differential diagnosis for Bowen's disease includes other papulosquamous diseases such as psoriasis and lichen simplex, superficial BCC, actinic keratoses, and dermatitis. If a lesion looks suspicious for Bowen's disease, a biopsy should be performed.

Microscopically, the keratinocytes in Bowen's disease demonstrate full-thickness atypia with hyperchromatic nuclei, loss of polarity, and decreased intracellular adhesions. Giant cells and mitotic figures may be frequent. By definition, tumor cells do not invade the dermis, although the upper der-mis may be infiltrated by mononuclear inflammatory cells.

Bowen's disease can be treated with excision, Mohs microscopically controlled surgery, or with destructive ther-apies such as cryotherapy, electrodesiccation and curettage, topical 5-FU, imiquimod, and photodynamic therapy. Histologic confirmation should be obtained before using one of the destructive modalities. Cryotherapy has had reported cure rates of 90–97% [42, 59]. Retrospective studies support the use of topical imiquimod [60]. Photodynamic therapy with ALA and MAL has increasingly been used in the treatment. On the basis of the evidence of four randomized single- and multicenter-controlled trials [59, 61–63] initial cure rates have been shown to range from 88 to 100% and 1 year recurrence rates range from 0 to 12%. The significant disadvantage of topically applied treatments including photodynamic therapy, however, is that the vehicle often cannot penetrate the epidermal appendages. If the tumor involves the appendages, it may not be fully eradicated. Excision, where feasible, remains the therapeutic method of choice for Bowen's disease. Because of indistinct borders, Mohs surgery is often the treatment of choice.

Lentigo Maligna (Hutchinson's Freckle)

Melanoma In Situ

Lentigo maligna is a noninvasive disorder of atypical melanocytes that is limited to the epidermis. This flat, pigmented lesion, which occurs on sun-exposed skin of elderly fair-skinned individuals, develops into invasive melanoma in about 1 of 750 cases per year [64]. As a result of its malignant potential, most authors view lentigo maligna as a melanoma in situ [65]. The major risk factors for developing lentigo maligna are chronic cumulative sun exposure and light skin color. Additional risk factors include a history of severe sunburn, radiation exposure, estrogen and progesterone therapy, and use of nonpermanent hair dyes [66]. The incidence of lentigo maligna, which is slightly higher in women, peaks during the seventh and eighth decades, with the average age of onset around 65 years.

Clinically, lentigo maligna presents as a uniformly flat macule ranging in size from 3 to 20 cm with intralesional variations in color (Fig. 91.11). The color often appears as a

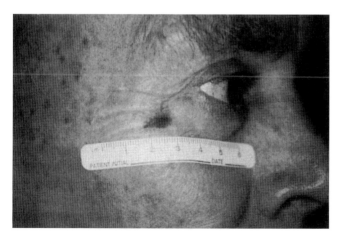

FIGURE 91.11 Lentigo maligna. It is melanoma in situ on sun-exposed skin. Although this lesion is small and easy to excise, these lesions are often long-standing in the elderly and can reach sizes that make excision unfeasible.

disorganized array of dark browns and black on a background of light browns, pinks, and white. The borders of the lesion tend to be irregular with a notched, "geographic" shape.

Biopsy of lentigo maligna reveals cytologically atypical melanocytes proliferating in distinct units throughout the basal layer. These atypical melanocytes can extend far beyond the clinical margin, leading to a high recurrence rate. The black areas of the lesion often display the most advanced histologic changes, whereas the white areas show signs of regression. Regions with surface irregularity may signify invasion.

Several lesions can simulate lentigo maligna, including seborrheic keratoses, solar lentigos, pigmented actinic keratoses, pigmented Bowen's disease, and pigmented BCC. However, these lesions tend to be more uniform in color and rarely contain black pigment. Seborrheic keratoses can usually be distinguished based on their characteristic verrucous surface. Solar lentigos do not exhibit variations in color as seen with lentigo maligna. Pigmented carcinomas tend to be raised. To confirm the diagnosis, an incisional punch or shave biopsy that includes the most darkly pigmented area is recommended.

Complete excision is the treatment of choice for lentigo maligna. Conventional surgery, which provides a 91% cure rate [67], should be performed with 0.5-cm margins if feasible [68]. Depending on the clinical circumstance, mapped serial excision may be required to ensure removal of what can often be very large lesions. This approach is especially helpful for periocular and other cosmetically sensitive areas of the face [69–71]. Mohs surgery has been suggested as a treatment [72], and cure rates as high as 97% have been reported [73]. However, the technical issues related to frozen section interpretation of melanocytic lesions make use of conventional margin analysis preferable at this time, either in a staged fashion or single excision where feasible.

Some lesions of lentigo maligna do not lend themselves to excision because of their size, location, or the patient's comorbid conditions. In such cases, destructive therapies such as CO_2, ruby laser, electrodesiccation and curettage, X-ray therapy, cryotherapy, topical azelaic acid, and topical imiquimod have been used. The major disadvantage of these methods is that they do not provide a specimen to confirm that the cancer has been properly and completely eliminated. These methods may also fail to treat the adnexal melanocytes, which can lead to recurrence. This is suggested by the high recurrence rate of lentigo maligna that occurs with these modalities: 20–25% for electrodesiccation and curettage, 6–36% for cryotherapy, up to 100% for azelaic acid, and up to 38% for irradiation [66]. Small case series utilizing irradiation have, however, demonstrated recurrence rates as low as 0–7% [74, 75]. Topical imiquimod has been advocated [76], but no controlled trials have been performed. A variety of single wavelength and combination laser treatments have been attempted in the treatment of lentigo maligna including argon [77], Q-switched Nd:YAG [78], and Q-Switched ruby [79], but no large controlled trials exist. Laser and imiquimod may be viable therapeutic options in the patient who cannot undergo more aggressive approaches or whose lesion technically precludes excision. Cryosurgery may leave scar tissue that can mask recurrence, especially the development of an invasive desmoplastic melanoma. This is the greatest risk of incomplete treatment of melanoma in situ, and the patient must be aware of this potential problem.

Malignant Lesions

Epidermis

Squamous Cell Carcinoma

Squamous cell carcinoma (SCC) is a malignant tumor of keratinocytes that arises on sun-damaged skin and on mucous membranes. The incidence is higher in men but occurs more frequently on the extremities in women. Individuals over the age of 55 are most frequently affected, with the mean age of onset at 60 years.

The biggest risk factor for SCC is chronic sun exposure. This is evidenced by the fact that SCC occurs most frequently in geographic areas that have sunny climate, such as California and Florida. Also, the incidence of SCC is higher in people who work outdoors. Other predisposing factors include prior trauma, frostbite, ionizing radiation, PUVA therapy, exposure to chemical carcinogens (arsenic, topical hydrocarbons, nitrogen mustards), viruses (human papilloma virus strains 16,18,31,33, and 35), and chronic immune suppression. These tumors may also arise from preexisting pathology, such as the chronic inflammatory lesions of discoid lupus, burn scars (Marjolin's ulcer), osteomyelitis sinuses, lichen planus, and chronic stasis dermatitis. SCC of the lip may additionally be provoked by tobacco use.

SCCs may arise from a premalignant lesion such as actinic keratosis or Bowen's disease. A clue to malignant transformation in these lesions is increased induration and inflammation. Patients often notice that the lesion is growing or changing. Well-differentiated SCC typically presents as an indurated papule, plaque, or nodule with overlying adherent hyperkeratosis. It may become ulcerated or bleed with formation of a central crust and surrounding firm, scaly margin. If the carcinoma is undifferentiated, it may appear as a fleshy, granulating nodule with central ulceration and a necrotic base.

Clinically, SCCs may resemble actinic keratoses, amelanotic melanoma, granulomatous disease, or adnexal tumors.

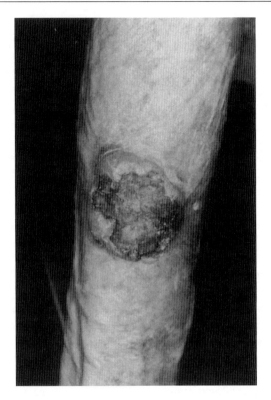

Figure 91.12 Squamous cell cancer. This large lesion was present for many months. Occasionally, when the lesion arises over a 6-week period, keratoacanthoma, a variant of squamous cell cancer, must be considered.

If a lesion appears suspicious for malignancy, it must be biopsied (Fig. 91.12).

Dermatopathologic examination typically reveals masses, strands, or buds of atypical keratinocytes that proliferate downward into the dermis. In well-differentiated tumors, keratin pearls may be present within or on the surface of the tumor. Undifferentiated types display multiple mitoses and little evidence of keratinization.

SCC has the capacity to metastasize. The metastatic potential depends on the location and size. For SCCs arising from actinic keratoses, the metastatic propensity reportedly is low (approximately 0.5%) [80], whereas for those developing de novo, the risk is 7.7–13.7%. Tumors arising from preexisting pathology, such as a burn scar, have a much higher rate of metastasis, estimated to be 20–40%. Patients presenting with an SCC should have regional lymph nodes examined clinically, as regional lymphadenopathy is often the first sign of metastasis. The prognosis for tumors that have spread is poor, with an estimated 5-year survival rate of 26% if the metastasis is localized to regional lymph nodes and 23% if it has spread systemically [81].

The most widely used method for treating SCC is excision. Simple excision with clinically normal-appearing margins is often satisfactory for most lesions up to 0.5 cm. For tumors that are large, deep, recurrent, and have aggressive histology, or are located in areas with high metastatic potential (e.g., lips or ears), the Mohs microscopically controlled technique should be performed. This is a tissue-sparing, office-based method that involves the sequential excision and mapping of the cancer. The final defect can be repaired immediately or allowed to heal by second intention. The Mohs technique has a 3% recurrence rate compared to an 8% recurrence rate with simple excision. As an alternative to excision, small, superficial tumors (<0.5 cm) can be destroyed by electrodesiccation and curettage, which yields a 5-year cure rate of approximately 90% [82]. Radiotherapy can also be effective but is typically reserved for patients who cannot undergo surgery or as adjunctive therapy in high-risk areas with perineural invasion. It is extremely expensive. The treatment regimen can take as much as 4–6 weeks. This method relies on patient compliance; but if used properly, it has a 5-year cure rate similar to that of electrodesiccation and curettage [82]. Topical retinoids have also been shown to be effective for some inoperable lesions [83]. Lymph node dissection is not indicated unless nodes are clinically involved.

Keratoacanthoma

Keratoacanthomas (KAs) are well-differentiated SCCs. Interestingly, in some cases, they have a tendency to resolve spontaneously. KAs most often appear as isolated lesions on sun-exposed areas of middle-age or older individuals. The lesion begins as a small papule that rapidly enlarges over 4–8 weeks to form a painless nodule often containing a central keratin-filled crater. KAs occur twice as often in men as in women and are most commonly found in Caucasians.

The cause of this lesion is unknown. Human papilloma virus has been extracted from some lesions. Others have been associated with carcinogens including UV light, pitch and tar, and other factors such as trauma and immune suppression [84]. Keratoacanthomas are usually solitary, but multiple lesions may arise as part of a syndrome such as Muirr–Torre, Ferguson Smith, or generalized eruptive KAs of Grzybowski [85].

Clinically, KAs appear as well-differentiated SCCs. Unlike most other SCCs, KAs have a history of rapid onset and are not usually associated with regional adenopathy. The history of rapid onset (4–6 weeks) is key to making the diagnosis and distinguishing the KA from other types of SCC. Biopsy of a suspicious lesion is required because KAs can behave like aggressive SCCs, especially when located in the central face. Biopsy can be incisional or excisional so long as it is inclusive of the full depth of the tumor down to the subcutaneous fat. Typically, a biopsy shows a large central crater filled with keratin surrounded by buttressing epidermis. The keratinocytes often display nuclear atypia, mitotic figures, and dyskeratoses. KA-type SCCs can be differentiated from other SCCs histologically based on the presence of epithelial "lips," which surround a central crater, and intradermal abscesses with an accompanying inflammatory infiltrate – both of which are rare features of SCCs.

There remains legitimate controversy regarding the true nature of KAs. Some authorities classify the lesion as a benign epithelial neoplasm [86], whereas others view it as an aborted malignancy [85] or a well-differentiated subtype of SCC [9, 87]. We consider KAs as a form of SCC. Unlike other malignancies, KAs can spontaneously regress, but they have also been shown to metastasize and ultimately be fatal [87]. Therefore, the question of identity becomes more than an academic exercise. KAs should be definitively treated.

Currently, most experts favor early intervention to minimize local tissue destruction because localized scarring can occur with spontaneous healing. Those who favor excision recommend Mohs micrographic surgery because it allows resection with tumor-free margins while maximizing the preservation of normal skin. In a study examining 42 KAs treated by Mohs surgery, the rate of recurrence after 2 years was less than 3% [88]. Other treatment modalities include: curettage and desiccation, which has a recurrence rate of 8% [85]; cryosurgery, which is beneficial for small early KAs; radiation therapy; topical and intralesional 5% 5-FU; interferon-α2a; podophyllin; intralesional steroids; systemic retinoids; and bleomycin [84]. Intralesional methotrexate has been advocated in cases where surgery is not an option and has a reported 92% rate of clearance based on retrospective analysis [89]. Any lesion that does not respond promptly to the above nonsurgical treatments by involuting at least 60% should be excised [30].

Basal Cell Carcinoma

Basal cell carcinoma (BCC) is the most common type of malignant cutaneous neoplasm, constituting 75% of all nonmelanoma skin cancers. BCCs are not thought to be associated with a premalignant lesion. Though they are slow-growing tumors that rarely metastasize, they can be locally invasive and destructive. BCCs most commonly present on habitually sun-exposed skin of the head and neck in fair-skinned individuals over the age of 40. Aside from chronic sun exposure, race, and age, other predisposing factors include genetic defects (basal cell nevus syndrome, xeroderma pigmentosa, Bazex syndrome, Rombo syndrome), radiation exposure, immune suppression, and prolonged contact with chemical carcinogens such as arsenic. The incidence of BCC in the United States has been estimated at approximately 150 cases per 100,000 per year, with men more frequently affected. One exception to this trend is in the lower extremities where the lesion arises three times more commonly in women.

The exact cell of origin of the BCC is unclear. It is thought to be derived from either the pluripotent stem cells of the epidermis or the matrix cells of epidermal appendages. The tumor cells histologically resemble cells in the stratum basale with compact, basophilic nuclei and scant cytoplasm. However, in support of the epidermal appendage derivation, tumor development occurs only in areas of the skin that have the capacity to develop hair follicles. The tumor cells grow in strands or nests into the dermis, displaying little anaplasia and infrequent mitosis. In the more aggressive variants, finger-like strands can extend far into dermal stroma, inducing significant fibrosis. A lymphocytic dermal infiltrate is usually present.

Morphologically, BCCs can be classified into at least five subtypes: noduloulcerative, cystic, pigmented, superficial, and morpheaform. The most common is the noduloulcerative variant, which usually starts as a small papule that slowly enlarges, appearing translucent and pearly with a rolled border and overlying telangiectasias (Fig. 91.13). As the tumor continues to grow, it eventually exceeds its own blood supply and becomes necrotic and centrally ulcerated ("rodent ulcer"). Most lesions are asymptomatic, though some are pruritic. Noduloulcerative BCC may resemble melanocytic nevi, sebaceous hyperplasia, molluscum contagiosum, SCC, verruca vulgaris, keratoacanthoma, amelanotic melanoma, atypical fibroxanthoma, or an adnexal tumor.

Cystic BCC presents as a smooth, pearly, erythematous nodule that rarely ulcerates. The cystic cavity may contain necrotic debris or mucin. This BCC variant can mimic other cystic lesions, such as epidermal inclusion cysts and hidrocystomas.

Excess melanin from epidermal melanocytes can cause BCCs to become pigmented. Pigmented BCCs often occur in dark-skin individuals and can be clinically confused with melanoma. Unlike melanoma, the border of this BCC variant

is often rolled, and the color is browner in contrast to the black–brown hue of malignant melanomas.

The superficial variety of BCC appears as erythematous, scaling, raised plaques with irregular borders. This tumor does not invade beyond the superficial dermis. It is often confused clinically with benign processes (e.g., localized eczema or psoriasis). Superficial BCCs can be differentiated by biopsy.

The most aggressive BCC subtype is the morpheaform, or infiltrative, variety. This locally destructive lesion typically appears as a whitish, sclerotic patch with ill-defined borders. It is firm upon palpation due to the extensive fibrous stroma associated with the tumor. The strands of tumor cells can travel well beyond the clinical margin, making these tumors notoriously difficult to treat without the Mohs technique. Their differential includes morphea and scar.

Rarely, BCC will metastasize with a reported incidence of 0.0028 to 0.5% [91]. Metastatic BCC tends to occur more frequently in Caucasian men, occurs on the head and neck, and has no increased risk with a particular histologic subtype although many so-called metastatic basal cell cancers have had squamous features. In contrast to the relatively benign course of primary BCC, metastatic BCC has a 5-year survival of 10% [91] and commonly affects the lymphatics, lungs, bone, and skin.

Knowledge of the pathology of these five primary BCC subtypes is important when choosing the appropriate method of treatment. In addition to taking the morphologic type into account, the proper treatment modality also depends on the size and location of the tumor, the age and comorbid conditions of the patient, and patient preference. For patients who can undergo surgical procedures, electrodesiccation and curettage, simple excision, and Mohs surgery are the methods of choice. With the exception of the morpheaform subtype, most small, nonrecurrent varieties of BCC can be treated with simple excision, achieving a cure rate exceeding 95% [92]. For large tumors (>1–2 cm), recurrent cancer, infiltrative subtypes, or cancer in the central face, which may invade deeply, Mohs surgery is recommended. It has the added benefit of being tissue-sparing and offers a cure rate approaching 99% for nonrecurrent lesions [93].

Nonsurgical treatment methods include radiotherapy, photodynamic therapy, and topical chemotherapy with agents such as 5-FU and imiquimod. Both topical agents are reserved for the superficial type of BCC because they cannot readily penetrate beyond the dermis. The treatment course can last from 2 to 6 weeks or more, thus requiring high patient compliance. For 5-FU, clinical clearance rates up to 90% have been reported with extended treatment courses of up to 12 weeks [94]. For imiquimod, five times weekly use for 6 weeks has produced 1 year clearance rates as high as 85% and 5-year clearance rates approaching 80% [95]. Photodynamic therapy with ALA and MAL has been used in

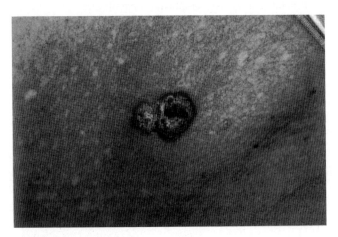

Figure 91.13 Basal cell cancer. The large nodule on the chest is a neglected basal cell cancer. Actinic keratoses and severe solar damage are noted on the rest of the chest.

the treatment of superficial and nodular BCC. Prospective trials comparing standard surgery to MAL in the treatment of nodular lesions have revealed inferior complete responses for MAL-PDT (76–96%) at 5-year follow-up [96]. Amino-levulinic acid PDT has shown response rates of 87% for superficial lesions and 53% for nodular lesions [97]. Increased response rates of nodular BCC to ALA-PDT with adjunctive curetting are controversial. Radiotherapy can also be used to eradicate BCCs but is best reserved for patients who cannot undergo therapy with other destructive modalities. Cutaneous atrophy at the treatment site is a common side effect. The overall cure rate approaches 90%.

Treatment of metastatic BCC relies on aggressive surgery, irradiation, and/or palliative chemotherapy with cisplatin, cyclophosphamide, 5-fluorouracil, bleomycin, and vincristine. A regimen with oral retinoids, imiquimod, and cele-coxib has been disappointing [98].

For patients presenting with a BCC, regular follow-up is essential because a patient with one BCC has a 36% chance of developing a second lesion within 5 years [93]. The protective use of sunscreen should be emphasized.

Melanoma

Melanoma is a malignant tumor of epidermal melanocytes. It is the fifth most prevalent cancer among men and the sixth most prevalent cancer among women in the United States. Its incidence is rising faster than any other cancer [99]. The current lifetime risk of developing melanoma is estimated at 1 in 55. In 2008, it is estimated that 62,480 people will be diagnosed with and 8,420 will die of melanoma. Age-specific incidence rates are highest in elderly patients. Approximately 40% of melanomas are diagnosed in individuals over the age of 65, and these elderly patients seem to have a worse prognosis than their younger counterparts. Specifically, although no comprehensive stage for stage studies have been performed, Austin (1994) notes that among a cohort of 442 patients with stage I and II melanomas, those over age 65 demonstrated a significantly lower 5-year disease-free survival [100].

Nearly 60% of melanoma deaths occur in patients over 65 years of age. Elderly patients have different incidences of melanoma subtypes than younger patients. Men and women are disproportionately affected, and men have a worse prognosis. Male and female incidence rates are 24.6 and 15.6 per 100,000 respectively, and the melanoma death rate in men is more than double that of women (3.9 vs. 1.7 per 100,000) [101].

The main risk factor for melanoma is high exposure to UV radiation, as demonstrated by an increased incidence of the tumor with decreasing latitude. Other predisposing factors include fair skin, blond or red hair, a family history of melanoma, congenital or atypical nevi, an inability to tan,

and an antecedent blistering sunburn. Pigment is a protective factor, as demonstrated by the relative rarity of this tumor in dark-skinned individuals.

Melanoma is traditionally classified into four clinico-pathologic variants: superficial spreading melanoma, nodular melanoma, lentigo maligna melanoma, and acral lentiginous melanoma. Superficial spreading melanoma (Fig. 91.14) is the most common subtype, comprising 40–50% of all cases in patients over age 65 [102]. It typically presents on the trunk in men and on the legs in women in their fourth to fifth decade. The tumor often begins as a small pigmented lesion that develops irregular features such as marked variations in color involving reds, whites, blues, and blacks, as well as notched borders. The tumor is characterized by a radial growth phase, where malignant cells are localized to epidermis, followed by a vertical growth phase, which signifies dermal invasion. The vertical phase is often heralded by elevation, bleeding, and ulceration of the lesion.

The second most common type of melanoma in the elderly is the nodular melanoma. These lesions present as elevated, dome-shaped, reddish-brown nodules most commonly localized on the legs or trunk; they arise more frequently in men. They have a short radial growth phase and therefore rarely grow to more than 2 cm in diameter. As they quickly enter their vertical growth phase, nodular melanomas can easily bleed and ulcerate and develop satellite lesions with surrounding inflammation. The tumors begin to develop during the fifth to sixth decade and peak in incidence during the eighth decade, with men more frequently affected than women. Nodular melanomas must be differentiated from seborrheic keratoses, pyogenic granulomas, and pigmented BCCs. Amelanotic melanoma, considered a subtype of nodular melanoma, displays a similar rapid vertical growth phase. These lesions may lack pigment and prove difficult to diagnose.

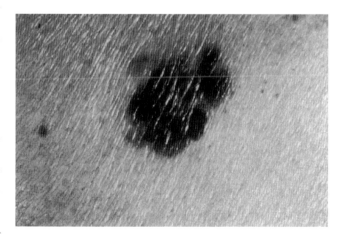

Figure 91.14 Melanoma. This example of superficial spreading melanoma has irregular edges and variable coloration. The elderly have an increased incidence of melanoma relative to other age groups, and early diagnosis is the key to cure.

Lentigo maligna melanoma develops in preexisting lentigo maligna lesions. Although lentigo maligna melanoma represents only 5% of all malignant melanoma cases, it accounts for 10% of melanoma cases in the elderly. Lentigo maligna is, in essence, an in situ melanoma that is in a horizontal growth phase that can last for decades before proceeding to a vertical growth phase. Transformation to lentigo maligna melanoma is defined as invasion of malignant melanocytes into the dermis and is heralded by the formation of an elevated nodule.

Like lentigo maligna melanoma, acral lentiginous melanoma also occurs with a disproportionately greater frequency in the geriatric population. Unlike all other subtypes, these melanomas most commonly affect Blacks, Asians, and Hispanics. Acral lentiginous melanoma appears as a macular, hyperpigmented area with irregular borders and a blue to black color; it arises on the plantar or palmar surfaces of the hands and feet, on mucous membranes, and in the subungual areas of nails. Its location often leads to the mistaken diagnosis of traumatic hematoma. These tumors are therefore often diagnosed at an advance stage. When the tumor becomes invasive, it may appear nodular and ulcerate and may bleed.

Any pigmented lesion that has undergone changes in size, shape, or color or is inflamed, oozing, bleeding, or itching, or is larger than 5 mm in diameter should be considered malignant until proven otherwise by biopsy. The most frequently occurring colors in melanomas are shades of brown, red, white, or blue and black. Pinks and reds signify inflammation. A blue color arises from light scattering from pigment deep within the dermis (Tyndal effect) and is a poor prognostic indicator.

Lesions suspicious for malignant melanoma should undergo elliptical or tangential excisional biopsy. For large tumors or those that cannot be completely excised because of their anatomic location, an incisional biopsy, such as a punch or elliptical biopsy, is recommended.

Although prognosis depends on the type of lesion and the presence or absence of lymphatic invasion, the single strongest prognostic factor is the depth of the melanoma measured in millimeters (Breslow depth) (Table 91.1). Clark's level is sometimes reported but is no longer used as reliably as the Breslow depth. Clinical subtypes of melanoma vary in aggressiveness. For example, lentigo maligna melanoma has a long horizontal growth phase and is usually recognized prior to the development of metastases.

The American Joint Committee on Cancer has devised a classification system for melanomas that not only takes depth into account but also the extent of regional or distant metastasis. The seventh edition was published in 2010 and is currently the system in use [103]. This clinical staging system is designated the TNM classification. The T component is based on Breslow thickness and histologic evidence of ulceration. Newly added was mitotic index for small, T1 lesions,

Table 91.1 Clark and Breslow classification of malignant melanoma

Clark level	
I	Tumor does not invade dermis
II	Tumor invades only papillary dermis
III	Tumor expands into papillary dermis but spares reticular dermis
IV	Tumor invades reticular dermis
V	Tumor invades subcutaneous tissue

Breslow level (mm)	Excision margin	Sentinel node studies
1	1 cm	No
1.0–1.5	1–2 cm	+/–
1.5–4.0	2–3 cm	+
4	3 cm	No

Breslow depth does not correspond precisely to Clark level. It is used for prognostic purposes and to direct therapy.

less than one millimeter in thickness. The N component is based on the extent of regional lymph node involvement and the tumor burden of the nodes. While the sixth addition allowed use of microscopic staging of lymph nodes, newly added in the seventh edition is the immunohistochemical designation of positive lymph nodes using melanoma-associated markers such as HMB-45, Melan-A/MART-1. The M component is based on anatomic site of distant metastases and the serum lactate dehydrogenase level. The TNM classification defines five stages based on prognosis: stage 0 (in situ melanoma), stage II (local disease), stage III (regional nodes, in transit and satellite metastases), stage IV (distant metastases). The stage groupings and clinical/pathologic criteria are described in Table 91.2.

Elderly patients tend to present with poor prognostic features and therefore have increased mortality rates. Malignant melanoma in the elderly tends to present later, be thicker, have histologic ulceration, and be of nodular type. Additionally, elderly patients present more frequently with satellite and in transit metastases and have anatomic localization to areas other than the head and neck [104]. The reasons for this are complex but likely include some combination of decreased vision, increased tolerance for skin lesions, decreased social support, and increased comorbidity.

Patients presenting with malignant melanoma should be thoroughly evaluated. This includes a complete physical examination with special attention to a total body skin examination and lymph node palpation, laboratory studies including a complete blood count with differential, liver function tests, and chest radiography. Treatment of malignant melanoma depends on the depth and stage of the tumor. Though most authorities agree that excision of the primary lesion is the mainstay of treatment for all stages of malignant melanoma, there is controversy surrounding the size of the excisional margin and the method with which the margins are obtained.

TABLE 91.2 American Joint Committee on cancer classification for malignant melanomas

Stage	Classification			Clinical and pathologic criteria
O	Tis	NO	MO	In situ melanoma
IA	T1a	NO	MO	1.0 mm^2 or less in thickness, no ulceration, mitoses less than 1/mm^{2++}
IB	T1b	NO	MO	With ulceration or mitotic rate more than 1/mm^2
	T2a	NO	MO	1.01–2.0 mm^2 in thickness
IIA	T2b	NO	MO	1.01–2.0 mm^2 with ulceration
	T3a	NO	MO	2.01–4.0 mm without ulceration
IIB	T3b	NO	MO	2.01–4.0 mm^2 in thickness with ulceration
	T4a	NO	MO	>4.0 mm^2 in thickness without ulceration
IIIA	T1-4a	N1a	MO	Any invasive T excluding >4 mm^2 in thickness with ulceration, 1 regional node with micrometastases^a
	T1-4a	N2a	MO	Any invasive T excluding >4 mm^2 in thickness with ulceration, 2–3 regional nodes with micrometastases
IIIB	T1-4b	N1a	MO	Any invasive T, 1 regional node with micrometastases
	T1-4b	N2a	MO	Any invasive T, 2–3 regional nodes with micrometastases
	T1-4a	N1b	MO	Any invasive T excluding >4 mm^2 in thickness with ulceration, 1 regional node with macrometastases
	T1-4a	N2b	MO	Any invasive T excluding >4 mm^2 in thickness with ulceration, 2–3 regional macrometastases
	T1-a/b	N2c	MO	In transit or satellite metastases without nodal metastases
IIIC	T1-4b	N1b	MO	Any invasive T, 1 regional node with macrometastases
	T1-4b	N2b	MO	Any invasive T, 2–3 regional macrometastases
	Any T	N3	MO	Any T, >/= 4 regional nodes including in-transit or satellite metastasis with positive metastatic nodes
IV	Any T	Any N	M1	Any lesion with distant skin, subcutaneous, lymph node, or organ metastases

Source: Used with permission of the American Joint Committee on Cancer (AJCC), Chicago, Illinois. The original source for this material is the AJCC Cancer Staging Manual, Seventh Edition (2010) published by Springer Science + Business Media, LLC, www.springlink.com
^{a}Micrometastases now includes those seen on standard H&E staining or with melanoma-specific immunohistochemical markers

In situ lesions (Clark's level I, TNM stage 0) are by definition noninvasive. The goal for treatment of these lesions is to remove all tumor cells locally. If standard excision is the method of choice, usually 0.5-cm margins are adequate for in situ lesions. However, if the tumor is clinically ill-defined, wider margins may be advisable. The tumor margins should be assessed with a Wood's lamp and marked prior to administration of anesthesia. Lesions that have invaded the dermis and that are up to 1 mm in depth require excisional margins of 1 cm. Margins of 2 cm are recommended for lesions with a Breslow depth of 1.0–4.0 mm. Any lesion more than 4 mm thick should undergo wide excision with margins up to 3- to 5-cm.

The role of lymphadenectomy in malignant melanoma is controversial. Prophylactic lymphadenectomy is not indicated for in situ lesions, as they do not show evidence of metastasis. Sentinel lymph node biopsy, a procedure that permits biopsy of the first node that drains a regional lymphatic plexus and is thought to be representative of all nodes in that region, is advocated for all patients with primary melanomas >1 mm thick and for patients with high-risk thin (<1 mm) or stage IB (ulcerated) melanomas. The role of sentinel node biopsy versus clinical observation has recently been addressed by the Multicenter Selective Lymphadenectomy trial-1 [105]. This prospective randomized multicenter trial demonstrated that the result of the sentinel node biopsy is the most powerful independent predictor of survival, but it did not demonstrate that the sentinel lymph node biopsy itself leads to a survival advantage. Contrary to previous speculation, the performance of the sentinel lymph node biopsy was not associated with the development of in-transit metastases. Despite the absence of a clear survival benefit, the sentinel node biopsy does provide valuable staging information and can lead to better management of regional disease. Patients with nodal metastases as demonstrated by the sentinel node biopsy should undergo complete lymph node dissection [106]. Lymph node involvement carries a poorer prognosis, with the 5-year survival dropping to 40%. Because malignant melanoma is considered a radioresistant tumor, the role of irradiation in metastatic disease is mostly palliative.

In the treatment of advanced metastatic disease, immunotherapeutic strategies are a focus of great interest. Specifically, an increasing number of clinical trials with interleukin-2, interferon, allogeneic whole-cell vaccines, recombinant viral vectors, adoptive immunotherapy combined with lymphodepletion, CTLA-4 blockade, allogeneic cell lysates, and dendritic cell manipulation are advancing our understanding of tumor immunology and maybe extending life [107, 108]. The prognosis of patients with widely metastatic disease remains poor, but the full development and refinement of these strategies are progressing.

The perception that aggressive systemic therapy may have unacceptable toxicity in the elderly has limited our understanding of the effect of patient age on chemotherapy efficacy and toxicity. In the treatment of melanoma with isolated limb perfusion, patients of increased age demonstrated similar response rates with no increase in local or systemic toxicity [109]. Similarly, in a small group of elderly patients treated with high-dose IL-2 for melanoma and other tumor types, there was no demonstrated increase in adverse events to warrant their exclusion in future studies [110]. Therefore, while chronological age itself may not affect the efficacy or toxicity of any particular therapy, practical considerations necessitate the careful evaluation of comorbid disease, functional and mental status, support network, and patient willingness to tolerate the difficult side effects of treatment.

Patients who have been diagnosed with melanoma need close follow-up because they may be prone to developing a second primary tumor. Most recurrences arise within the first 18 months but can be delayed for many years. Follow-up should occur four times a year for the first year and at least twice a year thereafter [111]. Early recognition of local or regional disease or new primary melanoma lesions in this population can significantly alter the mortality rate from malignant melanoma.

Atypical Fibroxanthoma

Atypical fibroxanthoma is a spindle-cell neoplasm of mesenchymal origin that develops on the head and neck of elderly, light-skinned individuals. The tumor clinically presents as an asymptotic, solitary, firm nodule less than 2 cm in diameter which may go on to ulcerate or hemorrhage. Grossly, the lesion can resemble a SCC, BCC, epidermoid cyst, or pyogenic granuloma. Risk factors for tumor development include chronic sun exposure, radiation, local trauma, and male gender.

One of the unique features of this tumor is its malignant-appearing histology. Aside from the well-defined tumor margins and absence of deep tissue invasion, the tumor appears histologically indistinguishable from malignant fibrous histiocytoma [112]. It is composed of sheets of polymorphous cells, including spindle cells, large polyhedral cells, and giant multinucleated cells with marked nuclear atypia and numerous mitoses.

Despite its malignant histology, atypical fibroxanthoma has a relatively benign course. Metastases, however, have been reported [113]. This has led some to classify the tumor as a superficial form of malignant fibrous histiocytoma [112], therefore requiring treatment.

Mohs surgery is the treatment for atypical fibroxanthoma. Recurrence rates range from 0 to 6.9% [114, 115]. Electrodesiccation and curettage is not considered adequate treatment because it does not remove the deep tissue, which may be invaded by tumor cells. The recurrence rate with tumors treated by wide excision is estimated to be approximately 10% [114]. Mohs surgery, which has the added advantage of conserving more normal tissue than wide excision, is currently the preferred method of treatment.

Merkel Cell Carcinoma

Merkel cell carcinoma is a rare malignant tumor of the neuroendocrine-derived Merkel cell. This tumor of unknown etiology typically affects persons over the age of 65, though cases of Merkel cell carcinoma developing in individuals as young as 7 years of age have been reported [116]. There have been no documented differences in incidence between men and women.

Merkel cell carcinoma manifests as rapidly growing, solitary, pink to violet nodules on sun-exposed skin. These firm, dome-shaped nodules are most commonly distributed on the head and neck (50% of cases), extremities (40% of cases), and trunk (10% of cases) of elderly Caucasians. Most tumors are less than 2 cm in diameter but can grow to become as large as 15 cm. The overlying epidermis may be shiny and intact with fine telangiectasias, or it may be ulcerated. Because of its nonspecific presentation, Merkel cell carcinoma is often not recognized prior to biopsy. It may be misdiagnosed as an SCC or BCC, a desmoplastic or amelanotic melanoma, a pyogenic granuloma, or a cutaneous metastasis of an oat cell carcinoma. Light microscopy may not be diagnostic because the tumor mimics other poorly differentiated small-cell tumors. The tumor is typically comprised of clusters of small, undifferentiated cells possessing scant cytoplasm that form trabeculae separated by strands of connective tissue. The trabeculae may extend down to the subcutaneous fat but do not invade the epidermis. Frequent mitoses and necrotic cells may be present. Confirmation of the diagnosis may require electron microscopy, which shows the characteristic secretory granules and paranuclear fibrous bodies.

Once the diagnosis of Merkel cell carcinoma is confirmed, a complete physical examination with attention to regional lymphadenopathy and organomegaly and a thorough workup including chest radiography and baseline laboratory tests, with liver function tests, should be performed. Merkel cell carcinoma is an aggressive tumor with a high rate of local recurrence and early lymphatic spread. The treatment protocol for Merkel cell carcinoma is stage-dependent. Stage I or localized disease that has no evidence of lymph node metastases is treated by wide local excision. For localized tumors, adjuvant therapy with irradiation of the primary site is frequently employed, especially if there is angiolymphatic invasion. The role of prophylactic or elective complete lymph node dissection is controversial, but it has been utilized because of the high incidence of lymph node metastases in early disease [117, 118]. Limited studies have advocated a role for lower morbidity sentinel lymph node biopsy in the early detection of regional lymph node metastases, but the overall data to demonstrate its role in predicting survival end points is weak. Sentinel node biopsy may, however, be useful as a tool in determining the appropriate nodal basin for elective radiation therapy [119].

About 55–65% of stage I lesions progress to stage II or locally recurrent disease [120]. Stage II disease is defined by metastases to regional lymph nodes. Treatment involves wide excision of the primary tumor in combination with irradiation and lymph node dissection. Despite aggressive therapy, which may also involve chemotherapy, the mortality rate of stage II disease approaches 66%.

One-third of all patients with Merkel cell carcinoma progress to stage III, or systemic disease involving distant metastases. Stage III disease is managed primarily with chemotherapy. Chemotherapeutic agents similar to those used for treating oat cell carcinoma have been shown to be the most efficacious. The prognosis for stage III disease is grim, with an expected survival of less than 12 months. The average length of survival may increase with the use of in vitro assays that test a tumor's specific drug sensitivities, allowing optimization of the chemotherapeutic regimen [120]. Targeted chemotherapy has recently shown preliminary experimental success with intratumor natural human tumor necrosis factor, systemic imatinib, isolated limb perfusion, and autologous peripheral blood stem cell transplantation receiving attention [119]. Owing to the high recurrence rate of this tumor, patients who initially present should be followed monthly for the first 2 months, every 2–3 months for the next 2 years, and every 6 months thereafter.

Dermis

Angiosarcoma

Angiosarcoma is a rare malignant tumor arising from vascular or lymphatic endothelium. The lesion often starts as a dusky erythematous, painless, "bruise-like" macule with poorly differentiated margins that proceed to ulcerate and hemorrhage as the cancer progresses to involve subcutaneous tissue. This aggressive vascular tumor, which affects men more commonly than women, has a predilection for the scalp and face of patients over the age of 60. Its etiology is unknown, although human herpes virus 8 [121] and environmental toxins such as Thorotrast, vinyl chloride, and insecticides have been implicated [122]. Chronic lymphedema and chronic radiodermatitis are predisposing factors.

Histologically, the early stages of the tumor show endothelial cell-lined intercommunicating vascular channels that appear to dissect through collagen bundles [123]. During the later stages, the tumor loses its organized vascular pattern and develops into large cell aggregates. There is subsequent formation of solid nodules of tumor followed by invasion of vascular channels.

The clinical appearance of this purple, flat, indistinctly bordered tumor often leads to its misdiagnosis as a bruise, hemangioma, or infections such as chronic cellulitis, localized lymphedema, or scarring alopecia [123]. The persistence of a bruise-like lesion, especially in an elderly individual, should warrant a biopsy. Angiosarcomas are frequently recognized late in their course, which partially accounts for their poor prognosis, with an estimated 5-year survival 12–27% [122]. They tend to recur locally and metastasize early in their course. Important prognostic factors include size, grade, and location of the tumor. High-grade tumors >5 cm located on the face tend to carry the worst prognosis [122, 123]. The mainstay of treatment is local excision combined with radiotherapy. Other forms of treatment, such as chemotherapy, have not been shown to alter survival significantly [121] but may be useful for short-term palliation [124].

Conclusions

Common cutaneous neoplasms that afflict the elderly arise from the epidermis or dermis and can be benign, premalignant, or malignant. Recognizing these lesions is important for providing care to a growing geriatric population. A regular, thorough skin examination enables physicians to monitor the elderly patient closely for the development of precancerous and cancerous lesions, which can ultimately be life-threatening. Minimizing the risk of malignant tumor development by avoiding precipitating factors such as UV radiation should be emphasized in this population.

CASE STUDY

Recurrent Basal Cell Carcinoma On The Nose Of A 75-Year-Old Woman

A 75-year-old woman presented with a slowly growing scar-like lesion at the junction of the right nasal ala and cheek. It was present for approximately 3 years. She noted a one-month history of a nonhealing lesion at the same site. Dermatologic history was significant for a BCC of the right nasal ala that was treated by electrodesiccation and curettage 5 years earlier. There was no history of radiation therapy. Her medical history was significant for insulin-dependent diabetes and hypertension. Social history was significant for loss of her husband 2 years ago. She lives alone.

Examination of the right cheek and right nasal ala demonstrated a 1.5 × 1.5 cm irregular, indurated, smooth-surfaced, shiny plaque with an indistinct border. Within this lesion, on the right ala, was a 3-mm crusted telangiectatic papule with hemorrhagic crust.

Laboratory data, including CBC, LFTs, and renal function tests were normal. A biopsy from the edge of the plaque demonstrated irregular, narrow, strand-like proliferations of palisading, basaloid tumor islands in a dense fibrous stroma that extended to the base of the biopsy. These histologic features were consistent with BCC, sclerosing or morpheaform subtype. Mohs surgery was selected as the treatment of choice

The first stage of Mohs surgery revealed a BCC with distinct nodular and morpheaform features. There was a focal area of epidermal ulceration and a nodule of palisading basaloid tumor islands extending from the deep epidermis into the superficial and mid-dermis. In the deeper and lateral sections, there were morpheaform strands of basaloid cells extending to the margins of the specimen. The tumor was cleared after the second stage of Mohs surgery. The postoperative defect extended to the cartilage of the ala and measured 2.5 × 2.3 cm. The wound was repaired under local anesthesia only in the office setting with an auricular cartilage graft and subcutaneous hinge flap. The secondary defect was closed in a linear fashion, and the area over the graft was left to epithelialize by second intention.

Discussion

Morpheaform BCCs and BCCs of mixed type that have morpheaform features are slow-growing, asymptomatic, and resemble scars, making them easily neglected by elderly patients. The clinical borders are indistinct, and the histologic tumor often extends far beyond what the clinical appearance would suggest. These cancers have a propensity for invasion and destruction of adjacent tissues, and they have a higher risk of recurrence than other subtypes of BCC.

Superficially destructive procedures such as cryotherapy, electrodesiccation and curettage, topical imiquimod, or elliptical excision have an increased risk of recurrence as demonstrated in this case. Mohs micrographic surgery is the treatment of choice as it offers the most complete margin evaluation and provides for immediate reconstruction if indicated. Mohs surgery is an office procedure performed using local anesthesia and is generally well tolerated. To facilitate the procedure, there should be proper preoperative consultation that addresses mental status issues, medication use, anticoagulants, the need for prophylactic antibiotics, and comorbid conditions. In the perioperative period, elderly patients often require additional support including attention to positional and emotional comfort as well as monitoring for orthostatic hypotension, hypoglycemia, and cardiovascular events. Anxiety can often be allayed with casual conversation.

Because of the large defects that may result from excision of morpheaform lesions, comorbidities such as diabetes, vascular disease, and the generalized slower wound healing in the elderly must be considered. It must be remembered that complex multistage repairs, while technically possible, may not be advisable in the elderly considering longer operative times and prolonged recovery.

In the postoperative period, pain is most often managed with acetaminophen alone. When more potent analgesics are required, slower drug metabolism, decreased glomerular filtration rates, and potential drug interactions from polypharmacy must be considered. Additionally, the postoperative need for complex or prolonged dressing changes with uncommon materials should be avoided. In general, wound care instructions are discussed with the patient as well as any caregiver present. Before discharge, adequate time is provided for patients to ask questions including concerns for cosmesis and recurrence. As follow-up, we advocate same evening and 24-h phone calls with lesion checks at 1 week.

References

1. Cohn BA (1994) In search of human skin pheromones. Arch Dermatol 130(8):1048–1051
2. Didierjean L, Gruaz D, Frobert Y, Grassi J, Dayer JM, Saurat JH (1990) Biologically active interleukin 1 in human eccrine sweat: site-dependent variations in alpha/beta ratios and stress-induced increased excretion. Cytokine 2(6):438–446
3. Gallo RL (2008) Sounding the alarm: multiple functions of host defense peptides. J Invest Dermatol 128(1):5–6
4. Champion RH, Burton JL, Ebling FJG (1992) Rook/Wilkinson/ Ebling textbook of dermatology, 5th edn. Blackwell Scientific, Oxford
5. Lavker RM, Zheng PS, Dong G (1987) Aged skin: a study by light, transmission electron, and scanning electron microscope. J Invest Dermatol 88:44s–51s
6. Richey ML, Richey HK, Fenske NA (1988) Age-related skin changes: development and clinical meaning. Geriatrics 43:49–64
7. Tagami H (2008) Functional characteristics of the stratum corneum in photoaged skin in comparison with those found in intrinsic aging. Arch Dermatol Res 300(Suppl 1):S1–S6
8. Gilchrest BA, Blog FB, Szabo G (1979) Effects of aging and chronic sun exposure on melanocytes in human skin. J Invest Dermatol 73:141–143
9. Lynch PJ (1994) Dermatology, 3rd edn. Williams & Wilkins, Baltimore
10. Lindelöf B, Sigurgeirsson B, Melander S (1992) Keratoses and cancer. J Am Acad Dermatol 26(6):947–950
11. Epstein E (1995) Treatment of basal cell papillomas. Br J Dermatol 133:492
12. Ortonne JP, Pandya AG, Lui H, Hexsel D (2006) Treatment of solar lentigines. J Am Acad Dermatol 54(5 Suppl 2):S262–S271
13. Beacham BE (1992) Common skin tumors in the elderly. Am Fam Physician 46:138–163
14. Banik R, Lubach D (1987) Skin tags: localization and frequencies according to sex and age. Dermatologica 174:180–183
15. Beitler M, Eng A, Kilgour AB et al (1986) Association between acrochordons and colonic polyps. J Am Acad Dermatol 14:1042–1044
16. Leavitt J, Klein I, Kendricks BS et al (1983) Skin tags: a cutaneous marker for colonic polyps. Ann Intern Med 98:928–930
17. Gould BE, Ellison C, Greene HL et al (1988) Lack of association between skin tags and colonic polyps in a primary care setting. Arch Intern Med 148:1799–1800
18. Rasi A, Soltani-Arabshahi R, Shahbazi N (2007) Skin tag as a cutaneous marker for impaired carbohydrate metabolism: a case-control study. Int J Dermatol 46(11):1155–1159
19. Mathur SK, Bhargava P (1997) Insulin resistance and skin tags. Dermatology 195(2):184
20. Mendelson BC, Masson JK (1976) Xanthelasma: follow-up on results after surgical excision. Plast Reconstr Surg 58:535–538
21. Eedy DJ (1996) Treatment of xanthelasma by excision with secondary intention healing. Clin Exp Dermatol 21:273–275
22. Borelli C, Kaudewitz P (2001) Xanthelasma palpebrarum: treatment with the erbium:YAG laser. Lasers Surg Med 29(3):260–264
23. Basar E, Oguz H, Ozdemir H, Ozkan S, Uslu H (2004) Treatment of xanthelasma palpebrarum with argon laser photocoagulation. Argon laser and xanthelasma palpebrarum. Int Ophthalmol 25(1):9–11
24. Fusade T (2008) Treatment of xanthelasma palpebrarum by 1064-nm Q-switched Nd:YAG laser: a study of 11 cases. Br J Dermatol 158(1):84–87
25. Alster TS, West TB (1996) Ultrapulse CO2 laser ablation of xanthelasma. J Am Acad Dermatol 24:848–849
26. Liu HH, Perry HO (1986) Identifying a common – and benign – geriatric lesion. Geriatrics 41(7):71–76
27. Greenbaum SS (1991) The treatment of chondrodermatitis nodularis chronica helicis with injectable collagen. Int J Dermatol 30:291–294
28. Moncrieff M, Sassoon EM (2004) Effective treatment of chondrodermatitis nodularis chronica helicis using a conservative approach. Br J Dermatol 150(5):892–894
29. Lawrence CM (1991) The treatment of chondrodermatitis nodularis with cartilage removal alone. Arch Dermatol 127:530–535
30. Morganroth GS, Leffell DJ (1993) Nonexcisional treatment of benign and premalignant cutaneous lesions. Clin Plast Surg 20:91–104
31. Coldiron BM (1991) The surgical management of chondrodermatitis nodularis chronica helicis. J Dermatol Surg Oncol 17:902–904
32. de Ru JA, Lohuis PJ, Saleh HA, Vuyk HD (2002) Treatment of chondrodermatitis nodularis with removal of the underlying cartilage alone: retrospective analysis of experience in 37 lesions. J Laryngol Otol 116(9):677–681
33. Ormond P, Collins P (2004) Modified surgical excision for the treatment of chondrodermatitis nodularis. Dermatol Surg 30(2 Pt 1):208–210
34. Long D, Maloney ME (1996) Surgical pearl: surgical planning in the treatment of chondrodermatitis nodularis chronica helicis of the antihelix. J Am Acad Dermatol 35:761–762
35. Rex J, Ribera M, Bielsa I, Mangas C, Xifra A, Ferrándiz C (2006) Narrow elliptical skin excision and cartilage shaving for treatment of chondrodermatitis nodularis. Dermatol Surg 32(3):400–404
36. Taylor MB (1991) Chondrodermatitis nodularis chronica helicis: successful treatment with the carbon dioxide laser. J Dermatol Surg Oncol 17:862–864
37. Taylor MB (1992) Chondrodermatitis nodularis chronica helicis. J Dermatol Surg Oncol 18:641
38. Bekhor PS (2006) Long-pulsed Nd:YAG laser treatment of venous lakes: report of a series of 34 cases. Dermatol Surg 32(9):1151–1154
39. Marks R, Rennie G, Selwood T (1988) The relationship of basal cell carcinomas and squamous cell carcinomas to solar keratoses. Arch Dermatol 124(7):1039–1042
40. Callen JP, Bickers DR, Moy RL (1997) Actinic keratoses. J Am Acad Dermatol 36(4):650–653
41. Ackerman AB, Mones JM (2006) Solar (actinic) keratosis is squamous cell carcinoma. Br J Dermatol 155(1):9–22
42. Graham G (1993) Advances in cryosurgery during the past decade. Cutis 12:365–372
43. Stockfleth E, Meyer T, Benninghoff B et al (2002) A randomized, double-blind, vehicle-controlled study to assess 5% imiquimod cream for the treatment of multiple actinic keratosis. Arch Dermatol 138:1498–1502
44. Lebwohl M, Dinehart S, Whiting D et al (2004) Imiquimod 5% cream for the treatment of actinic keratosis: results from two Phase III, randomized, double-blind, parallel group, vehicle-controlled trials. J Am Acad Dermatol 50:714–721
45. Ulrich C, Bichel J, Euvrard S, Guidi B, Proby CM, van de Kerkhof PC, Amerio P, Rønnevig J, Slade HB, Stockfleth E (2007) Topical immunomodulation under systemic immunosuppression: results of a multicentre, randomized, placebo-controlled safety and efficacy study of imiquimod 5% cream for the treatment of actinic keratoses in kidney, heart, and liver transplant patients. Br J Dermatol 157(Suppl 2):25–31
46. Wolf JE Jr, Taylor JR, Tschen E et al (2001) Topical 3.0% diclofenac in 2.5% hyaluronan gel in the treatment of actinic keratoses. Int J Dermatol 40:709–713
47. Rivers JK, Arlette J, Shear N et al (2002) Topical treatment of actinic keratoses with 3.0% diclofenac in 2.5% hyaluronan gel. Br J Dermatol 146:94–100
48. Stritt A, Merk HF, Braathen LR, von Felbert V (2008) Photodynamic therapy in the treatment of actinic keratosis. Photochem Photobiol 84(2):388–398

49. Robinson JK (1989) Actinic cheilitis: a prospective study comparing four treatment methods. Arch Otolaryngol Head Neck Surg 115:848–852

50. Picascia DD, Robinson JK (1987) Actinic cheilitis: a review of the etiology, differential diagnosis and treatment. J Am Acad Dermatol 17:255–264

51. Berking C, Herzinger T, Flaig MJ, Brenner M, Borelli C, Degitz K (2007) The efficacy of photodynamic therapy in actinic cheilitis of the lower lip: a prospective study of 15 patients. Dermatol Surg 33(7):825–830

52. Alexiades-Armenakas MR, Geronemus RG (2004) Laser-mediated photodynamic therapy of actinic cheilitis. J Drugs Dermatol 3(5):548–552

53. Smith KJ, Germain M, Yeager J, Skelton H (2002) Topical 5% imiquimod for the therapy of actinic cheilitis. J Am Acad Dermatol 47(4):497–501

54. Chakrabarty AK, Mraz S, Geisse JK, Anderson NJ (2005) Aphthous ulcers associated with imiquimod and the treatment of actinic cheilitis. J Am Acad Dermatol 52(2 Suppl 1):35–37

55. Ulrich C, Forschner T, Ulrich M, Stockfleth E, Sterry W, Termeer C (2007) Management of actinic cheilitis using diclofenac 3% gel: a report of six cases. Br J Dermatol 156(Suppl 3):43–46

56. Thappa DM, Garg BR, Tahduea J et al (1997) Cutanous horn: a brief review and report of a case. J Dermatol 24:34–37

57. Yu RC, Pryce DW, MacFarlane AW et al (1991) A histopathological study of 643 cutaneous horns. Br J Dermatol 124:449–452

58. Sober AJ, Burnstein JM (1995) Precursors to skin cancer. Cancer 75:645–650

59. Morton CA, Whitehurst C, Moseley H et al (1996) Comparison of photodynamic therapy with cryotherapy in the treatment of Bowen's disease. Br J Dermatol 135:766–771

60. Rosen T, Harting M, Gibson M (2007) Treatment of Bowen's disease with topical 5% imiquimod cream: retrospective study. Dermatol Surg 33(4):427–431; discussion 431–432

61. Morton C, Horn M, Lehman J, Tack B, Bedane C, Tijoe M et al (2005) A 24-month update of a placebo controlled European study comparing MAL-PDT with cryotherapy and 5-fluorouracil in patients with Bowen's disease. J Eur Acad Dermatol Venereol 19(Suppl 2):237–238

62. Morton CA, Whitehurst C, Moore JV, MacKie RM (2000) Comparison of red and green light in the treatment of Bowen's disease by photodynamic therapy. Br J Dermatol 143:767–772

63. Salim A, Leman JA, McColl JH, Chapman R, Morton CA (2003) Randomized comparison of photodynamic therapy with topical 5-fluorouracil in Bowen's disease. Br J Dermatol 148:539–543

64. Weinstock MA, Sober AJ (1987) The risk of progression of lentigo maligna to lentigo maligna melanoma. Br J Dermatol 116:303–310

65. Somach SC, Taira JW, Pitha JV et al (1996) Pigmented lesions in actinically damaged skin. Arch Dermatol 132:1297–1302

66. Cohen LM (1995) Lentigo maligna and lentigo maligna melanoma. J Am Acad Dermatol 33:923–936

67. Coleman WP, Davis RS, Reed RI et al (1980) Treatment of lentigo maligna and lentigo maligna melanoma. J Dermatol Surg Oncol 6:476–479

68. National Institutes of Health Consensus Conference (1992) Diagnosis and treatment of early melanoma. JAMA 268:1314–1319

69. Demirci H, Johnson TM, Frueh BR, Musch DC, Fullen DR, Nelson CC (2008) Management of periocular cutaneous melanoma with a staged excision technique and permanent sections the square procedure. Ophthalmology 115(12):2295.e3–2300.e3

70. Anderson KW, Baker SR, Lowe L, Su L, Johnson TM (2001) Treatment of head and neck melanoma, lentigo maligna subtype: a practical surgical technique. Arch Facial Plast Surg 3(3):202–206

71. Huilgol SC, Selva D, Chen C, Hill DC, James CL, Gramp A, Malhotra R (2004) Surgical margins for lentigo maligna and lentigo

maligna melanoma: the technique of mapped serial excision. Arch Dermatol 140(9):1087–1092

72. Temple CL, Arlette JP (2006) Mohs micrographic surgery in the treatment of lentigo maligna and melanoma. J Surg Oncol 94(4):287–292

73. Cohen LM, McCall MW, Zax RH (1998) Mohs micrographic surgery for lentigo maligna and lentigo maligna melanoma. A follow-up study. Dermatol Surg 24(6):673–677

74. Farshad A, Burg G, Panizzon R, Dummer R (2002) A retrospective study of 150 patients with lentigo maligna and lentigo maligna melanoma and the efficacy of radiotherapy using Grenz or soft X-rays. Br J Dermatol 146(6):1042–1046

75. Schmid-Wendtner MH, Brunner B, Konz B, Kaudewitz P, Wendtner CM, Peter RU, Plewig G, Volkenandt M (2000) Fractionated radiotherapy of lentigo maligna and lentigo maligna melanoma in 64 patients. J Am Acad Dermatol 43(3):477–482

76. Mahoney MH, Joseph MG, Temple C (2008) Topical imiquimod therapy for lentigo maligna. Ann Plast Surg 61(4):419–424

77. Arndt KA (1986) New pigmented macule appearing 4 years after argon laser treatment of lentigo maligna. J Am Acad Dermatol 14(6):1092

78. Orten SS, Waner M, Dinehart SM, Bardales RH, Flock ST (1999) Q-switched neodymium:yttrium-aluminum-garnet laser treatment of lentigo maligna. Otolaryngol Head Neck Surg 120(3):296–302

79. Thissen M, Westerhof W (1997) Lentigo maligna treated with ruby laser. Acta Derm Venereol 722:163

80. Silverberg N, Silverberg L (1989) Aging and the skin. Postgrad Med 86:131–144

81. Kwa RE, Campana K, Moy RL (1992) Biology of cutaneous squamous cell carcinoma. J Am Acad Dermatol 26:1–20

82. Proper SA, Rose PT, Fenske NA (1990) Non-melanomatous skin cancer in the elderly: diagnosis and management. Geriatrics 45:57–65

83. Lippman SM, Meyskens FL (1987) Treatment of advanced squamous cell carcinoma of the skin with isotretinoin. Ann Intern Med 107:494–501

84. Warner DM, Flowers F, Ramos-Caro FA (1995) Solitary keratoacanthoma (squamous cell carcinoma): surgical management. Int J Dermatol 34:17–19

85. Schwartz RA (1994) Keratoacanthoma. J Am Acad Dermatol 30:1–19

86. Fitzpatrick TB, Johnson RA, Palano MK et al (1992) Color atlas and synopsis of clinical dermatology: common and serious diseases, 2nd edn. McGraw-Hill, New York

87. Hodak E, Jones RE, Akerman AB (1993) Solitary keratoacanthoma is a squamous cell carcinoma: three examples with metastases. Am J Dermatopathol 15:332–342

88. Larson PO (1987) Keratoacanthomas treated with Mohs' micrographic surgery (chemosurgery). J Am Acad Dermatol 16:1040–1044

89. Annest NM, VanBeek MJ, Arpey CJ, Whitaker DC (2007) Intralesional methotrexate treatment for keratoacanthoma tumors: a retrospective study and review of the literature. J Am Acad Dermatol 56(6):989–993

90. Snow SN, Sahl W, Lo JS, Mohs FE, Warner T, Dekkinga JA, Feyzi J (1994) Metastatic basal cell carcinoma. Report of five cases. Cancer 73(2):328–335

91. von Domarus H, Stevens PJ (1984) Metastatic basal cell carcinoma. Report of five cases and review of 170 cases in the literature. J Am Acad Dermatol 10(6):1043–1060

92. Gloster HM, Brodland DF (1996) The epidemiology of skin cancer. Dermatol Surg 22:217–226

93. Keller KL, Fenske NA, Glass LF (1997) Cancer in the older patient. Clin Geriatr Med 13:339–361

94. Gross K, Kircik L, Kricorian G (2007) 5% 5-Fluorouracil cream for the treatment of small superficial basal cell carcinoma: efficacy, tolerability, cosmetic outcome, and patient satisfaction. Dermatol Surg 33(4):433–439

95. Gollnick H, Barona CG, Frank RG, Ruzicka T, Megahed M, Maus J, Munzel U (2008) Recurrence rate of superficial basal cell carcinoma following treatment with imiquimod 5% cream: conclusion of a 5-year long-term follow-up study in Europe. Eur J Dermatol 18(6):677–682

96. Rhodes LE, de Rie MA, Leifsdottir R, Yu RC, Bachmann I, Goulden V, Wong GA, Richard MA, Anstey A, Wolf P (2007) Five-year follow-up of a randomized, prospective trial of topical methyl aminolevulinate photodynamic therapy vs surgery for nodular basal cell carcinoma. Arch Dermatol 143(9):1131–1136

97. Peng Q, Warloe T, Berg K, Moan J, Kongshaug M, Giercksky KE, Nesland JM (1997) 5-Aminolevulinic acid-based photodynamic therapy. Clinical research and future challenges. Cancer 79(12): 2282–2308

98. Soleymani AD, Scheinfeld N, Vasil K, Bechtel MA (2008) Metastatic basal cell carcinoma presenting with unilateral upper extremity edema and lymphatic spread. J Am Acad Dermatol 59(2 Suppl 1):S1–S3

99. Jemal A, Devesa SS, Hartge P, Tucker MA (2001) Recent trends in cutaneous melanoma incidence among whites in the United States. J Natl Cancer Inst 93(9):678–683

100. Austin PF, Cruse CW, Lyman G, Schroer K, Glass F, Reintgen DS (1994) Age as a prognostic factor in the malignant melanoma population. Ann Surg Oncol 1(6):487–494

101. Ries LAG, Melbert D, Krapcho M, Stinchcomb DG, Howlader N, Horner MJ, Mariotto A, Miller BA, Feuer EJ, Altekruse SF, Lewis DR, Clegg L, Eisner MP, Reichman M, Edwards BK (eds). SEER cancer statistics review, 1975-2005. National Cancer Institute, Bethesda, MD. http://seer.cancer.gov/csr/1975_2005/. Accessed November, 2008

102. Mackie RM, Young D (1984) Human malignant melanoma. Int J Dermatol 23:433–443

103. Balch CM, Gershenwald JE, Soong SJ, Thompson JF, Atkins MB, Byrd DR, Buzaid AC, Cochran AJ, Coit DG, Ding S, Eggermont AM, Flaherty KT, Gimotty PA, Kirkwood JM, McMasters KM, Mihm MC Jr, Morton DL, Ross MI, Sober AJ, Sondak VK (2009) Final version of 2009 AJCC melanoma staging and classification. J Clin Oncol 27(36):6199–6206

104. Lasithiotakis K, Leiter U, Meier F, Eigentler T, Metzler G, Moehrle M, Breuninger H, Garbe C (2008) Age and gender are significant independent predictors of survival in primary cutaneous melanoma. Cancer 112(8):1795–1804

105. Morton DL, Thompson JF, Cochran AJ, Mozzillo N, Elashoff R, Essner R, Nieweg OE, Roses DF, Hoekstra HJ, Karakousis CP, Reintgen DS, Coventry BJ, Glass EC, Wang HJ, MSLT Group (2006) Sentinel-node biopsy or nodal observation in melanoma. N Engl J Med 355(13):1307–1317; erratum in: N Engl J Med 2006 355(18):1944

106. Cormier JN, Xing Y, Ding M, Lee JE, Mansfield PF, Gershenwald JE, Ross MI, Du XL (2005) Population-based assessment of surgical treatment trends for patients with melanoma in the era of sentinel lymph node biopsy. J Clin Oncol 23(25):6054–6062

107. Jack A, Boyes C, Aydin N, Alam K, Wallack M (2006) The treatment of melanoma with an emphasis on immunotherapeutic strategies. Surg Oncol 15(1):13–24

108. Fang L, Lonsdorf AS, Hwang ST (2008) Immunotherapy for advanced melanoma. J Invest Dermatol 128(11):2596–2605

109. Noorda EM, Vrouenraets BC, Nieweg OE, van Geel AN, Eggermont AM, Kroon BB (2002) Safety and efficacy of isolated limb perfusion in elderly melanoma patients. Ann Surg Oncol 9(10):968–974

110. Quan W Jr, Ramirez M, Taylor C, Quan F, Vinogradov M, Walker P (2005) Administration of high-dose continuous infusion interleukin-2 to patients age 70 or over. Cancer Biother Radiopharm 20(1):11–15

111. Bernstein SC, Brodland DG (1995) Melanoma in the geriatric patient. J Geriatr Dermatol 3:271–279

112. Fish FS (1996) Soft tissue sarcomas in dermatology. Dermatol Surg 22:268–273

113. Helwig EB, May D (1986) Atypical fibroxanthoma of the skin with metastases. Cancer 57:368

114. Davis JL, Randle HW, Zalla MJ et al (1997) A comparison of Mohs micrographic surgery and wide excision for the treatment of atypical fibroxanthoma. Dermatol Surg 23:105–110

115. Huether MJ, Zitelli JA, Brodland DG (2001) Mohs micrographic surgery for the treatment of spindle cell tumors of the skin. J Am Acad Dermatol 44(4):656–659

116. Ratner D, Nelson BR, Brown MD et al (1993) Merkel cell carcinoma. J Am Acad Dermatol 29:143–156

117. Smith DE, Bielamowicz S, Kagan AR et al (1995) Cutaneous neuroendocrine (Merkel cell) carcinoma: a report of 35 cases. Am J Clin Oncol 18:199–203

118. Victor NS, Morton B, Smith JW (1996) Merkel cell cancer: is prophylactic lymph node dissection indicated? Am Surg 62:879–882

119. Eng TY, Boersma MG, Fuller CD, Goytia V, Jones WE III, Joyner M, Nguyen DD (2007) A comprehensive review of the treatment of Merkel cell carcinoma. Am J Clin Oncol 30(6):624–636

120. Krasagakis K, Almond-Roesler B, Zouboulis CC et al (1997) Merkel cell carcinoma: report of ten cases with emphasis on clinical course, treatment, and in vitro drug sensitivity. J Am Acad Dermatol 36:727–732

121. McDonagh DP, Liu J, Gaffey MJ et al (1996) Detection of Kaposi's sarcoma-associated herpesvirus-like DNA sequence in angiosarcoma. Am J Pathol 149:1363–1368

122. Marc RJ, Poen JC, Tran LM et al (1996) Angiosarcoma: a report of 67 patients and a review of the literature. Cancer 77:2400–2406

123. Jones WE (1990) Some special skin tumors in the elderly. Br J Dermatol 122(Suppl 35):71–75

124. Mendenhall WM, Mendenhall CM, Werning JW, Reith JD, Mendenhall NP (2006) Cutaneous angiosarcoma. Am J Clin Oncol 29(5):524–528

Chapter 92
Surgical Management of Soft Tissue Sarcoma in the Geriatric Population

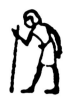

Charlotte E. Ariyan and Murray F. Brennan

Introduction

The management of soft tissue sarcomas in the elderly population requires a multidisciplinary approach. These rare tumors have a wide range of growth patterns and metastatic potential, much of which can be discerned by the pathologic subtype. Increasing age alone has repeatedly been demonstrated to have a negative impact on death from this disease. While surgery continues to be the primary treatment for sarcomas, radiation and chemotherapy have selective utility. The benefits of an aggressive approach must be weighed against the morbidity of treatment, particularly in the geriatric population.

Risk Factors

The majority of soft tissue sarcomas have no defined cause and are secondary to sporadic multiple mutations. However, hereditary forms do exist and are important to recognize (Table 92.1), as the mutation confers a lifelong risk of disease that may be augmented by prior treatments such as chemotherapy or radiation. The retinoblastoma population is an example of this phenomenon. These patients present at a young age for treatment, which often involves radiation. Forty-year follow-up of patients with hereditary retinoblastoma has found secondary malignancy in 36% of the patients, many of which are sarcomas [1, 2].

Additional risk factors for sarcoma include environmental toxins. Radiation predisposes to the development of sarcomas, and can been seen after radiation for any cancer, but particularly breast cancer, Hodgkin's disease, prostate cancer, and cervical cancer [3]. The majority of these radiation-induced sarcomas are high grade, and the ability to com-

pletely remove the new tumor predicts survival [4]. Chronic lymphedema predisposes to lymphangiosarcoma, or Stewart Treves syndrome [5]. Although there has been a suggestion that veterans exposed to Agent Orange have an elevated risk of sarcoma, this has never been shown to be a significant factor in case-controlled studies [6]. Vinyl chloride and poly-vinyl chloride exposure are associated with an increased risk of hepatic angiosarcomas [7].

Staging

Soft tissue sarcomas are classically defined by size, depth, grade, and presence of lymph node or distant metastasis [8]. The presence of lymph node metastasis is rare. There are over 50 different subtypes of sarcoma, with different potential for recurrence and metastasis. More recently, Memorial Sloan-Kettering Cancer Center (MSKCC) has developed a nomogram to predict survival from sarcoma [9]. The factors demonstrated to most accurately predict survival are sarcoma subtype, grade, size, anatomic site, depth, and patient age. This nomogram has been validated with patients at other institutions [9, 10].

Evaluation and Biopsy

Most patients with soft tissue sarcomas present with an asymptomatic mass [11]. The differential diagnosis of a mass includes a hematoma, benign lipoma, lymphoma, germ cell tumor, and sarcoma. A history of an enlarging or changing lesion should raise the suspicion for a malignancy. Physical exam should focus differentiation between a soft, mobile lesion and one that is fixed or invading local structures.

Imaging will assist in determining the features of the mass and its relation to neurovascular structures. An MRI will clearly demonstrate fat and muscle planes and may be more useful in the elderly population that tends to have an increased fat composition. A CT Scan will often clarify intra-abdominal

C.E. Ariyan (✉)
Department of Surgery, Memorial Sloan-Kettering Cancer Center, New York, NY, USA
e-mail: ariyanc@mskcc.org

R.A. Rosenthal et al. (eds.), *Principles and Practice of Geriatric Surgery*,
DOI 10.1007/978-1-4419-6999-6_92, © Springer Science+Business Media, LLC 2011

TABLE 92.1 Risk factors for development of soft tissue sarcoma

Risk factor		Sarcoma
Gene mutation	Gardner's syndrome/ APC mutation	Desmoid
	Li–Fraumeni syndrome/ p53 mutation	Soft tissue, osteogenic
	Neurofibromatosis type 1/ NF-1 mutation	Malignant peripheral nerve sheath tumor
	Retinoblastoma/Rb mutation	Soft tissue, osteogenic
Radiation		Primarily high grade, multiple subtypes
Lymphedema	Postsurgical or parasitic	Lymphangiosarcoma

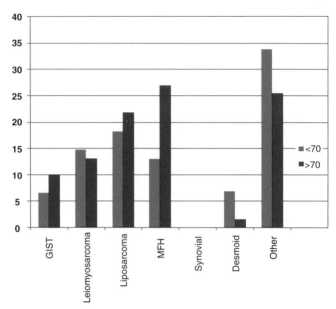

FIGURE 92.1 Incidence of sarcoma subtypes over a 25-year period at Memorial Sloan-Kettering Cancer Center (MSKCC). The data is shown for the geriatric population, and for those patients under 70. The data is expressed as the total number of sarcomas ($n = 7,531$).

lesions with improved clarity. PET scans are rarely used as sarcomas tend not to be FDG avid. Some lesions will be homogeneous and small and can be observed. Any lesion that is changing, heterogeneous on imaging, or large should be considered for biopsy or removal.

Biopsy can be performed by fine-needle aspiration (FNA), core-needle biopsy, incisional biopsy, or excisional biopsy. An FNA rarely provides enough tissue for utility. A core biopsy can be performed easily in the clinic with 95% accuracy [12]. An incisional biopsy provides an abundance of tissue; however, it requires a surgical procedure for the patient and risks the formation of hematoma postoperatively. This procedure must be carefully planned with a longitudinally oriented incision that can be incorporated in a future resection. Small tumors that are less than 5 cm and easily resectable can be removed by an excisional biopsy.

The biopsy grade and histologic subtype will be the most important data gained from the biopsy. Integration of this information with the site, size, and depth will provide important prognostic information. This can be used to derive an optimal treatment plan for the patient.

Surgery for Sarcoma in the Geriatric Population

Of over 7,000 adult sarcomas removed at MSKCC and maintained in our database, there is a difference in the histopathological subtype of soft tissue sarcomas based upon age. As shown in Fig. 92.1, the common subtypes such as malignant fibrous histiocytoma (MFH), liposarcoma, and leiomyosarcoma prevail in both groups; however, there are a few notable differences. Synovial cell sarcoma is classically a tumor of young patients. Desmoids are slow-growing tumors that tend not to metastasize; therefore, the low incidence of these patients seen in our database may reflect a referral bias of older patients. As the designation of MFH is being more

accurately defined in recent years, it is possible that the higher prevalence in the geriatric population reflects the imprecision of earlier diagnoses.

The decision to operate on an extremity sarcoma in an elderly patient is based upon multiple factors. First, there must be an adequate understanding of the natural history of the disease in the absence of treatment. Second, there must be awareness of the additional therapies, namely radiation or chemotherapy. The morbidity of treatments, surgical or medical, must then be balanced with the risk associated with the tumor and the underlying condition of the patient. The major advancement in understanding the natural history of sarcomas comes from the ability to subtype sarcomas based on histopathology and molecular features. With this understanding, a physician can tailor the treatment to the individual patient. This review will focus on treatment of the most common types of sarcomas in the geriatric population.

Extremity/Truncal Sarcomas

The primary treatment of an extremity or truncal sarcoma is surgical excision. The type of surgery is guided by subtype and anatomic location. In the geriatric population, the most common subtypes in the extremity are malignant fibrous histiocytoma (MFH), liposarcoma, and leiomyosarcoma as shown in Fig. 92.2. In the trunk, the most common subtypes are MFH, angiosarcoma, and liposarcoma. This is in contrast to the younger population, where synovial cell is observed more often in the extremity, and desmoids are observed more often in the trunk. Additional therapy includes radiation and chemotherapy, which can be administered in an adjuvant or neoadjuvant fashion.

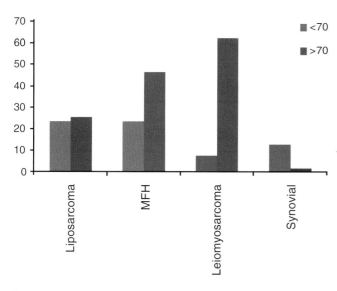

Figure 92.2 Incidence of common extremity subtypes by age for patients. Data shown is percentage of total extremity lesions in the database at Memorial Sloan-Kettering Cancer Center (MSKCC) ($n=3,073$).

Surgical Management

The grade of the tumor and the size are the first items that will guide the treatment algorithm. Both can be obtained from the clinical exam, radiology studies, and possible biopsy. As shown in Fig. 92.3, any lesion less than 5 cm can be primarily removed, if it is in a location where the postoperative field of radiation would not cross a joint or damage a major neurovascular structure. Lesions greater than 10 cm should be biopsied, as some high-grade lesions can be offered neoadjuvant chemotherapy.

Role of Amputation

A prospective, randomized trial published in 1982 did not demonstrate a survival advantage for amputation in patients with extremity sarcoma. Forty-three patients, all undergoing chemotherapy, consented to either amputation or wide excision (WE) with postoperative radiation. Analysis at 5 years demonstrated an increased local recurrence rate in patients with WE; however, there was no difference in disease-specific survival (DSS) at 5 years (71% vs. 78%, $p=0.75$) [13]. The efficacy of

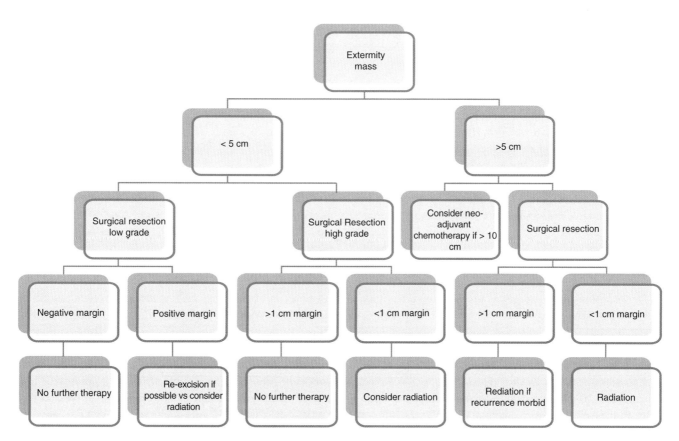

Figure 92.3 Treatment algorithm for extremity sarcoma in the geriatric patient.

Figure 92.4 Incidence of amputations in patients at Memorial Sloan-Kettering Cancer Center (MSKCC) from 1968 to 2006. Note the increase in the number of limb-sparing surgeries performed since the 1980s. While the number of amputations remains relatively stable, the number of amputations per procedure performed has markedly decreased.

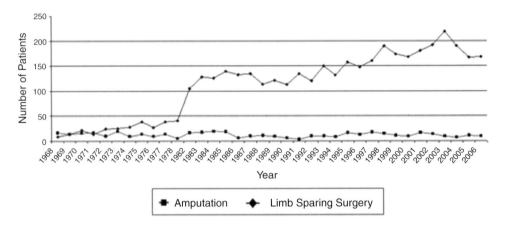

limb-sparing surgery (LSS) in managing sarcomas has been confirmed in follow-up studies from later time periods [14]. The indications for amputation currently are limited to large tumors, where limb-sparing resection would not remove the majority of the disease or would result in a limb with poor function. Over the years, the incidence of amputation has diminished for extremity sarcoma, as shown in Fig. 92.4, and many complicated lesions can be managed with surgery alone or in combination with radiation and chemotherapy.

Low-Grade Extremity Lesions

Atypical lipomatous tumors (ALT) and well-differentiated liposarcomas are similar and should be treated with a wide local excision that preserves function and obtains a negative margin. For those patients with a complete, R0 resection, the risk of recurrence is extremely low. In a study of 91 patients with ALT or well-differentiated liposarcoma, there were no recurrences in 10 years of follow-up for those patients with a negative margin and the absence of a sclerosing component. Distant metastatic disease developed in only one patient who had dedifferentiated sarcoma in the recurrence [15]. Geriatric patients with a microscopic positive margin can either be reexcised or observed, as a recurrence may not happen, or it may take many years to develop. There is no role for adjuvant radiation or chemotherapy in these lesions.

Dermatofibrosarcoma protuberans is a low-grade tumor. Only the fibrosarcomatous variant carries a small risk of metastatic disease [16]. These lesions should also be treated with primary surgical resection. Because DFSP tend to grow along tissue planes that extend beyond the palpable tumor, whenever possible the operation should include a margin of normal subcutaneous tissue around the palpable mass, and the underlying fascia. With surgery obtaining negative margins, the rate of local recurrence is <5% at 5 years; therefore, there is a limited role for adjuvant chemotherapy or radiation [16].

Desmoids are composed of myofibroblasts. The management is complicated, as they do not have metastatic potential yet they can be locally invasive. Extremity desmoids should be treated with a wide excision to obtain negative margins yet preserve functional outcome. In a series of 189 extremity desmoids, the local recurrence rate at 5 years for patients with a negative margin was 22%; in patients with a positive margin the recurrence rate was 24%, yet some of those patients had adjuvant radiation [17]. This provides evidence that debilitating operations should not be performed in an effort to obtain negative margins. The role of radiation therapy for extremity desmoids remains controversial but radiation should be used sparingly. Desmoids are low-grade tumors that never metastasize, and even when they do recur locally they can remain stable for many years even without treatment, as demonstrated in the case at the end of this chapter.

High-Grade Lesions

The common high-grade sarcomas of the extremity and trunk in geriatric patients include leiomyosarcomas, malignant fibrous histiocytoma (MFH), liposarcomas (dedifferentiated, pleomorphic, myxoid round cell), and angiosarcoma. The primary treatment of these lesions is surgery, alone or in combination with radiation or chemotherapy.

Malignant fibrous histiocytoma (MFH) is a term that has been used to characterize high-grade lesions with a fibrohistiocytic pathology over the years. Today, with improved histologic subtyping, many of the lesions originally characterized as MFH can be assigned other high-grade nomenclature, or are referred to as high-grade undifferentiated pleomorphic sarcoma. Therefore, today this term encompasses lesions that are high grade and can not otherwise be placed into another grouping. However, myxofibrosarcomas are one type of MFHs which have a more discernable pattern and characteristic growth pattern.

Myxofibrosarcomas tend to occur in the extremity of elderly patients. These tumors can have satellite nodules or extensions well beyond the primary location of the tumor, which may in part explain the greater than 50% recurrence observed in some series [18–20]. One strategy to minimize recurrence is to carefully review the preoperative CT Scan or MRI for evidence of multifocal lesions as well as sites of distant spread such as lung, bone, soft tissue, and mesentery [21]. These tumors are often relatively resistant to radiation and chemotherapy, making surgery essential to local control.

Angiosarcoma is an aggressive tumor of the blood or lymphatic vessels. Risk factors include a limb with chronic lymphedema (Stewart–Treves Syndrome) [22], as well as radiation. It has been noted in the breast and pelvis after radiation for malignancy [4, 23], and therefore it unfortunately is a near lethal consequence of treatment aimed to reduce local recurrence. This tumor is aggressive and often multifocal at presentation, which challenges the ability to obtain negative margins. The overall survival is poor, with ranges reported between 21% at 2 years [24] and 40% at 5 years [4], so the utility of radiation, a potential causative factor, in reducing a local recurrence needs to be balanced with the risk of development of an aggressive secondary malignancy. In patients with extensive and multifocal angiosarcoma at presentation paclitaxel-based neoadjuvant chemotherapy may be used.

Malignant peripheral nerve sheath tumors (MPNST) can arise sporadically or when associated with NF-1 from neurofibromas. Most MPNST are high grade, and they commonly occur in the trunk or extremity in the geriatric population; however, they can arise from the nerve sheath anywhere in the body. MPNST has an infiltrative, poorly discernable growth pattern that extends beyond the palpable tumor along the fascicles of the nerve root. Surgery should include a 2 cm margin with an additional 2–3 cm of the nerve whenever possible. Preoperatively, the patient needs to be educated and prepared for possible loss of motor function. Patients with acceptable comorbidities and a large (>10 cm) MPNST should be considered for neoadjuvant chemotherapy, while smaller tumors should receive surgical resection and radiation. Survival for MPNST tumors treated aggressively parallels that of other high-grade sarcomas [25].

Role of Radiation

Radiation reduces the risk of local recurrence when used as an adjuvant to surgery, and it can be used in a preoperative fashion to shrink tumor away from vital structures. These benefits of radiation must be balanced with the long-term complications: limb edema, fibrosis, bone fracture, wound complications, and formation of a radiation-associated sarcoma in the future. Fortunately, randomized controlled trials have helped to clarify which patients are most likely to benefit from radiation.

Extremity/truncal radiation is delivered by brachytherapy catheters (BRT) or external beam radiation therapy (EBRT) as a means to improve local control. A prospective randomized trial compared the use of brachytherapy (BRT) catheters, placed at the time of surgical resection, to surgical resection alone. While BRT increased the rate of local control at 5 years in the patients with high-grade tumors (89% vs. 66%, respectively, $p=0.0025$), it had no effect in patients with low-grade tumors [26]. Trials with external beam radiation therapy (EBRT), in contrast, demonstrated improved local control in high-grade and low-grade lesions [27]. Disease-specific survival was not altered by radiation with either brachytherapy or EBRT [28, 29]. Therefore, adjuvant radiotherapy should be considered for patients with large, high-grade sarcomas. Patients with low-grade sarcomas, or high-grade tumors <5 cm, can be treated with primary surgery alone if wide margins (1–2 cm) are obtained, as the recurrence rate is low [29].

An additional randomized trial demonstrated that radiation can be delivered preoperatively or postoperatively, with equal efficacy in decreasing local recurrence but with different complications based on the timing of delivery [27]. Preoperative radiation targets primarily the tumor mass, yet it can make pathological analysis of the specimen more difficult and result in a higher rate of wound complications after surgery. Postoperative radiation encompasses an area around the incision, and therefore it is a larger radiation field. There is increased limb edema and fibrosis over the long term. In an elderly patient, these risks need to be balanced with the comorbidities expected in long-term survival of the patient.

Intensity modulated radiation therapy (IMRT) is a method of delivering radiation to the tumor while minimizing damage to adjacent vital structures such as nerves, arteries, and bone. Therefore, the negative effects of radiation on neighboring nerves, arteries, and bone can be decreased. For example, a large sarcoma resection with periosteal stripping and requiring circumferential radiation is associated with a high risk of bone fractures that reaches 29% at 5 years [30]. This fracture rate can be reduced to 6.4% with the use of IMRT [31].

Chemotherapy in Extremity/Truncal Sarcomas

Multiple attempts have been made to define the role of adjuvant chemotherapy in sarcoma, and unfortunately no one combination has substantially improved survival. The enthusiasm for chemotherapy, in part, began with the use of the anthracycline doxorubicin. In a randomized trial of patients with extremity sarcoma, adjuvant doxorubicin improved overall and disease-specific survival at 3 years [32], but with further follow-up, this survival benefit did not persist [33].. Many additional trials followed attempting to demonstrate a survival advantage with chemotherapy. A meta-analysis of the most vigorous trials failed to reveal an improvement in overall survival with chemotherapy. ($p=0.12$). However, when the analysis was limited to the subgroup of patients with extremity sarcoma, a 7% absolute benefit in overall survival was demonstrated at 10 years ($p=0.029$) [34]. Since 1990, anthracyclines have been combined with alkylating agents such as ifosfamide in an attempt to improve efficacy. However, anthracyclines are cardiotoxic, and therefore the geriatric patient must be carefully assessed prior to administration of anthracyclines.

Ifosfamide is an alkylating agent that delays time to disease progression in patients with advanced, unresectable, or metastatic sarcoma [35].

A recent study utilized ifosfamide in an adjuvant fashion in 104 patients with high-grade extremity sarcoma after surgery. One arm of the study underwent observation, while the other arm underwent treatment with adjuvant epidoxorubicin and ifosfamide. After 2 years, the trial was stopped because, at interim analysis, there was a significant increase in disease-free survival (48 months with chemotherapy vs. 16 months with observation, $p=0.04$) and overall survival (75 vs. 46 months, respectively, $p=0.03$) [36]. However, on longer follow-up the difference in survival no longer persisted [37].

While the role of ifosfamide in an adjuvant manner remains unclear, there has been data to support its role in a neoadjuvant approach. The utilization of neoadjuvant ifosfamide in combination with doxorubicin and mesna resulted in a 21% improvement in disease-specific survival at 3 years in all patients with extremity subtypes of high grade, deep tumors >10 cm. In this study, the most commonly represented subtypes were MFH, liposarcoma, synovial cell, and leiomyosarcoma [38].

Further studies have also supported the role of neoadjuvant chemotherapy in the treatment of liposarcomas. There are three biological groups of liposarcoma, which includes five subtypes: (1) well-differentiated/dedifferentiated, (2) myxoid/round cell, and (3) pleomorphic. The high-grade subtypes with a high risk of systemic recurrence are myxoid/round cell (>5% round cell component) and pleomorphic [39–43]. A retrospective analysis of patients with extremity liposarcoma from MSKCC and UCLA compared patients who received chemotherapy to a similar cohort of patients who did not receive chemotherapy. There was no improvement in survival demonstrated with doxorubicin therapy; however, ifosfamide combined with doxorubicin therapy demonstrated an improved DSS at 5 years compared with no chemotherapy (92% vs. 65%, respectively, $p=0.0003$) [44]. This translates into a 31% survival benefit for lesions >10 cm. Based on the results of this retrospective study, and in the absence of any prospective randomized data, neoadjuvant doxorubicin and ifosfamide chemotherapy can be offered only to elderly patients with large (>10 cm), extremity

round cell or pleomorphic liposarcoma, with an excellent performance status. Dedifferentiated liposarcoma of the extremity is not sensitive to chemotherapy and has a lower risk of metastatic disease; therefore, chemotherapy is not used in this subtype.

Synovial cell sarcoma is very uncommon in the geriatric population. This is a disease of young adults that is associated with a high risk of metastasis and death [45], and therefore, larger lesions are treated with systemic chemotherapy based on retrospective data [46].

Retroperitoneal Sarcoma

Subtypes and Goals of Surgery

The most common subtypes of retroperitoneal sarcomas, regardless of age, are liposarcomas and leiomyosarcomas as shown in Fig. 92.5. Retroperitoneal sarcomas can grow large without specific symptoms; therefore, they are often detected late, at which time they are often large (>10 cm) and encroach on major abdominal structures [47].

Upon presentation, a biopsy is performed when there is concern for a benign process or other malignancy that would not mandate surgical intervention. Additional tumors to consider are lymphomas, angiomyolipomas, pancreatic tail tumors, benign shwannomas, adrenal tumors, and metastatic germ cell tumors. While primary surgical resection obtaining negative margins is associated with improved survival, removal of adjacent organs is not always necessary [47]. If the mass does not encase the renal vessels or invade the renal hilum, a parenchymal-sparing capsular stripping can be performed without compromising disease-specific survival [48].

Surgical management of retroperitoneal liposarcomas must take into account the subtypes, which have been shown to be one of the most important factors in DSS. In a study of 177 patients, the well-differentiated subtype had a very good survival and much lower recurrence rate than the dedifferentiated liposarcoma. The local recurrence rate for patients with well-differentiated liposarcoma was 31% at 3 years compared with 83% at 3 years for dedifferentiated liposarcoma. The dedifferentiated subtype had a 30% risk of distant disease at 3 years. In contrast, well-differentiated liposarcoma rarely developed distant metastasis (1% risk of distant disease at 3 years) [48].

Leiomyosarcomas of the abdomen commonly involve vessels and can involve major structures such as the inferior vena cava. Surgical resection can safely be performed with IVC ligation as long as drainage of the kidneys is preserved [49]. Many abdominal leiomyosarcomas have now been classified as gastrointestinal stromal tumors (GIST) as discussed below.

FIGURE 92.5 Subtypes of sarcoma in the retroperitoneum seen over a 25-year period at Memorial Sloan-Kettering Cancer Center (MSKCC). The majority of retroperitoneal tumors are either liposarcoma or leiomyosarcoma, which do not differ by age.

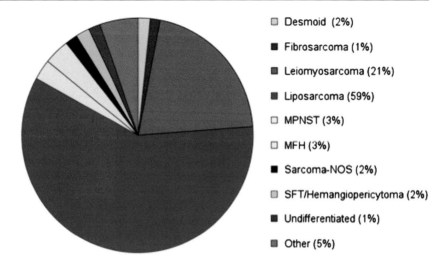

☐ Desmoid (2%)

■ Fibrosarcoma (1%)

■ Leiomyosarcoma (21%)

■ Liposarcoma (59%)

☐ MPNST (3%)

☐ MFH (3%)

■ Sarcoma-NOS (2%)

☐ SFT/Hemangiopericytoma (2%)

■ Undifferentiated (1%)

▨ Other (5%)

Radiation in Retroperitoneal Sarcomas

Retroperitoneal sarcomas have a high local recurrence rate, with prevalence of 20–50% depending on the length of follow-up [47, 50, 51]. Median survival after local recurrence is only 28 months [47]; therefore, consideration has been given to both chemotherapy and radiation in retroperitoneal sarcomas. While there is little data to support the use of chemotherapy, radiation, which addresses the local treatment failure, has been considered.

Radiation of the retroperitoneum is a difficult task as radiation cannot be delivered without risk to the surrounding vessels and intestine. However, small studies suggested that high-dose radiation improves local control [52, 53]. A prospective trial of preoperative radiation in patients undergoing a R0 or R1 resection demonstrated an improvement to 60% local recurrence-free survival in intermediate- or high-grade lesions, at a median follow-up of 40 months, with an associated increased morbidity [54]. Further multi-institutional randomized trials are needed to define the role of preoperative radiation therapy for the treatment of retroperitoneal sarcoma; however, these trials have closed secondary to poor accrual. Newer techniques of external beam radiotherapy such as IMRT may enable administration of radiotherapy with less toxicity to surrounding organs and vital structures.

Locally Recurrent Retroperitoneal Sarcoma

Recurrence in retroperitoneal sarcomas is more difficult to treat, in part secondary to prior contamination and scarring of tissue planes, as well as the aggressive nature of the tumor. Surgical removal must not only remove the mass, but also any tissue plane violated in a previous resection such as drain

tracks or skin flaps. In difficult cases, the surgeon may have to remove the recurrent tumor with an adjacent neurovascular structure, and this should be carefully planned ahead of the operation. An alternative is to give a trial of neoadjuvant radiotherapy or chemotherapy before the tumor is excised to spare a major resection.

Abdominal Desmoid

Abdominal desmoids can arise spontaneously or in association with familial adenomatous polyposis (FAP). Desmoid tumors arising in patients with FAP, commonly present in patients at a younger age, and they are related to the mutation in the adenomatosis polyposis (APC) gene, effecting β-catenin levels [55–58]. Sporadic desmoids have been linked to mutations in the β-catenin gene itself [59–63]. Regardless of the mutation, desmoids do not metastasize and have an unclear natural history. There have been multiple case reports of spontaneous regression of even multifocal tumors [64–67]. Patients on medical therapy fail to have progression of the tumor at least 50% of the time. Whether this is due to the inherent nature of the tumor itself or as a result of the medical therapy has not been clarified by a randomized trial. Most recently, a small clinical trial of abdominal desmoids with the anti-inflammatory suldinac and tamoxifen resulted in a 77% PR/CR [68]. At St. Mark's hospital, all patients with intra-abdominal desmoids first receive medical therapy with suldinac. If there is tumor progression, tamoxifen or other chemotherapies are added. Only patients who fail these conservative measures are then considered for surgical intervention [69]. In the geriatric population, a trial of this more conservative treatment algorithm is warranted.

GIST

Treatment of Primary Disease

Gastrointestinal stromal tumors (GIST) commonly present as asymptomatic pedunculated or submucosal masses arising in the gastrointestinal tract. On imaging, GIST tumors are well-circumscribed, low-density lesions, with possible areas of enhancement or necrosis. A suspected GIST should be removed for diagnosis and treatment if localized and the patient can tolerate the operation. Biopsy risks rupturing the mass and only complete resection offers the best chance of cure.

The important factors of the primary tumor that predict risk of recurrence are the anatomic location of the GIST, size, and mitotic index. For example, a distal small bowel GIST greater than 5 cm with a mitotic index >5 per 50 high-power field (HPF) has an 85% chance of recurrence, while a tumor <2 cm with ≤5 mitoses per HPF has a negligible chance of recurrence regardless of site [70, 71].

A majority (80%) of GIST tumors have an activating mutation of the KIT receptor tyrosine kinase and have therefore been successfully treated with the kinase inhibitor imatinib [72]. Expression of cKit is not enough to predict a response to imatinib, however, and mutation analysis should be performed before considering therapy. For example, exon 11 mutations respond well to imatinib, while exon 9 mutations do not [73, 74]. A small percent (5–10%) of GISTs harbor a mutation in platelet-derived growth factor alpha (PDGFRA) [75], some of which may be resistant to imatinib, but the new multikinase inhibitors such as sunitinib may have efficacy.

The role of imatinib as an adjuvant to surgical resection was evaluated by the ACOSOG intergroup trial. Patients were randomized after complete resection of a tumor >3 cm to 1 year of imatinib at 400 mg daily or placebo. There was a significant improvement in recurrence-free survival with imatinib treatment, although no difference was seen in disease-specific survival [76]. Longer follow-up will help clarify if imatinib prevents, or merely delays, the onset of disease recurrence. It may be that therapy initiated at the time of disease recurrence will be equally effective.

Metastatic GIST

Prior to imatinib, patients with metastatic GIST had a poor survival measured in months. However, recent trials have demonstrated that high-dose imatinib in metastatic disease can result in actual 2-year survival, with 50% of patients alive without disease progression [77]. This raises the question whether surgery should be utilized in conjunction with imatinib therapy to reduce tumor burden, or whether these patients should just be maintained on imatinib therapy. The major downside to imatinib is the development of resistant disease. Studies have demonstrated that resistance develops as soon as 6 months, with a median time to drug resistance of 20 months [77]. A recent study of 40 patients with metastatic GIST supports surgical intervention for those patients with disease that responded to imatinib. Patients with multifocal resistance, however, have a poor 1-year survival (36% alive at 1 year) and should not proceed to surgical debulking but should be considered for a clinical trial with a second line tyrosine kinase inhibitor [78].

CASE STUDY 1

A 73-year-old male with a history of retinoblastoma at age three for which he had eye enucleation and radiation. Past medical history also significant for coronary artery disease, resection of multiple lipomas, a partial nephrectomy for renal cell cancer, as well as an appendectomy. The patient's mother and daughter also had retinoblastoma. The patient presented with a small mass on his face in the field of radiation. Biopsy was consistent with a high grade, <5 cm leiomyosarcoma, and he underwent a wide local excision with negative margins.

Discussion

This patient had childhood retinoblastoma, which is related to a mutation in the retinoblastoma (RB1) gene. In hereditary forms of retinoblastoma, the cumulative risk of developing a secondary malignancy such as sarcoma is 36% [1]. Long-term follow-up of patients such as this with hereditary retinoblastomas has demonstrated that the most common subtype observed is leiomyosarcomas, almost all of which have been observed in patients with prior radiation [2]. Surgical resection is the treatment of this high-grade tumor. There is no role for further radiation. The patient needs continued follow-up for development of recurrence or another sarcoma. This emphasizes the importance of life-long surveillance for such patients with the loss of the Rb tumor suppressor gene.

CASE STUDY 2

A 38-year-old male with an extremity mass. Imaging revealed the mass to extend from the pelvic sidewall to the lower extremity. Biopsy was consistent with a desmoid tumor. The patient had no other comorbidities. He was started on tamoxifen and has had stable disease, with a partial response for 13 years as shown in Fig. 92.6.

Discussion

This case, although not in an elderly patient, demonstrates the importance of cautious observation in patients with desmoid tumors. A surgical option for this patient would be a hemipelvectomy, which would have decreased the quality of life. Stable disease such as this, for more than a decade, is further evidence that many desmoids can be treated without surgery in the geriatric population.

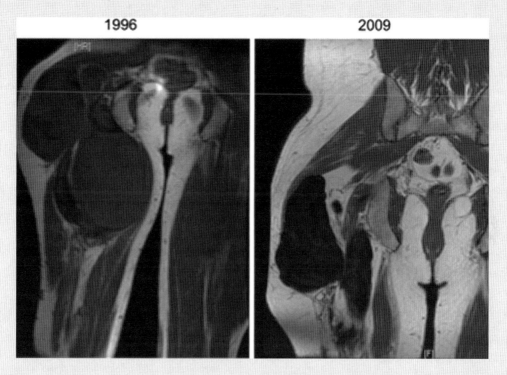

FIGURE 92.6   Thirteen-year follow-up of large extremity desmoids managed with nonoperative therapy.

CASE STUDY 3

85-year-old male with a history of coronary artery disease who underwent a coronary angioplasty and had moderate dementia requiring assistance in a nursing home. The patient presented with a large fungating mass of the thigh that was interfering with ambulation. Biopsy was consistent with a high-grade MFH. After a careful consult with the family and the medical team, a surgical excision was performed. At operation, the mass involved the entire anterior compartment of the thigh down to, but not including, the femoral vessels. Pathology confirmed the high-grade MFH, but margins were microscopically positive. The patient's wound was slow to heal and he underwent careful observation and continued with his functional life. Three years later he had a local recurrence, which was excised without incident. One year later, the patient died of other causes at his nursing home.

Discussion

This case highlights the need to balance the use of medical therapies to maintain the quality of life. The large MFH tumor in this patient could be treated with

(continued)

CASE STUDY 3 (continued)

neoadjuvant chemotherapy, but clearly the morbidity of this treatment with only a marginal potential benefit would not be warranted in this patient. A more aggressive surgical procedure could have been performed, but this would have risked leaving the patient with a functionally compromised or absent limb, and removing all

measurable tumor provided good functional relief for the patient. Postoperative radiation therapy is generally well tolerated, and it could have been utilized in the patient. The decision not to was based on his poor ability to heal his primary wound, and the concern of the patient and family regarding the ability to tolerate weeks of radiation therapy. The expected local recurrence was easily managed with a minor surgical intervention.

Summary

Soft tissue sarcomas represent a heterogeneous group of tumors with varying malignant potential. The decision to operate on a geriatric patient with a sarcoma must be undertaken carefully, with the underlying knowledge that older patients tend to have a decreased disease-specific survival from sarcoma. Surgery remains the mainstay of treatment in patients who can tolerate it. Radiation is generally well tolerated and can be used as an adjuvant to surgery in patients with high-grade tumors. Chemotherapy has yet to show a dramatic improvement in survival and should be used judiciously.

The ability to obtain a complete surgical resection is the primary governor of outcome in patients with retroperitoneal and visceral sarcomas. Many patients will recur locally and this can lead to death from progressive loco-regional disease. The majority of retroperitoneal and visceral sarcomas are poorly responsive to conventional chemotherapy, so chemotherapy is generally only used for palliation of disease in a patient who can tolerate it.

The management of GIST tumors hopefully represents the future of treatment in sarcoma. As characteristic mutations are identified in subtypes, new targeted therapies can be developed. As the population ages, treatment of sarcomas in the geriatric population will continue to involve a multidisciplinary approach to maximize treatment and maintain quality of life.

References

1. Kleinerman RA, Tucker MA, Tarone RE, Abramson DH, Seddon JM, Stovall M, Li FP, Fraumeni JF Jr (2005) Risk of new cancers after radiotherapy in long-term survivors of retinoblastoma: an extended follow-up. J Clin Oncol 23:2272–2279
2. Kleinerman RA, Tucker MA, Abramson DH, Seddon JM, Tarone RE, Fraumeni JF Jr (2007) Risk of soft tissue sarcomas by individual subtype in survivors of hereditary retinoblastoma. J Natl Cancer Inst 99:24–31
3. Brady MS, Gaynor JJ, Brennan MF (1992) Radiation-associated sarcoma of bone and soft tissue. Arch Surg 127:1379–1385
4. Cha C, Antonescu CR, Quan ML, Maru S, Brennan MF (2004) Long-term results with resection of radiation-induced soft tissue sarcomas. Ann Surg 239:903–909, discussion 909–910
5. Stewart FW, Treves N (1948) Lymphangiosarcoma in postmastectomy lymphedema; a report of six cases in elephantiasis chirurgica. Cancer 1:64–81
6. Kang H, Enzinger FM, Breslin P, Feil M, Lee Y, Shepard B (1987) Soft tissue sarcoma and military service in Vietnam: a case-control study. J Natl Cancer Inst 79:693–699
7. Gennaro V, Ceppi M, Crosignani P, Montanaro F (2008) Reanalysis of updated mortality among vinyl and polyvinyl chloride workers: confirmation of historical evidence and new findings. BMC Public Health 8:21
8. AJCC (2002) AJCC cancer staging manual. Lippincott Raven Publishers, Chicago
9. Kattan MW, Leung DH, Brennan MF (2002) Postoperative nomogram for 12-year sarcoma-specific death. J Clin Oncol 20:791–796
10. Mariani L, Miceli R, Kattan MW, Brennan MF, Colecchia M, Fiore M, Casali PG, Gronchi A (2005) Validation and adaptation of a nomogram for predicting the survival of patients with extremity soft tissue sarcoma using a three-grade system. Cancer 103:402–408
11. Lawrence W Jr, Donegan WL, Natarajan N, Mettlin C, Beart R, Winchester D (1987) Adult soft tissue sarcomas. A pattern of care survey of the American College of Surgeons. Ann Surg 205: 349–359
12. Heslin MJ, Lewis JJ, Woodruff JM, Brennan MF (1997) Core needle biopsy for diagnosis of extremity soft tissue sarcoma. Ann Surg Oncol 4:425–431
13. Rosenberg SA, Tepper J, Glatstein E, Costa J, Baker A, Brennan M, DeMoss EV, Seipp C, Sindelar WF, Sugarbaker P, Wesley R (1982) The treatment of soft-tissue sarcomas of the extremities: prospective randomized evaluations of (1) limb-sparing surgery plus radiation therapy compared with amputation and (2) the role of adjuvant chemotherapy. Ann Surg 196:305–315
14. Williard WC, Hajdu SI, Casper ES, Brennan MF (1992) Comparison of amputation with limb-sparing operations for adult soft tissue sarcoma of the extremity. Ann Surg 215:269–275
15. Kooby DA, Antonescu CR, Brennan MF, Singer S (2004) Atypical lipomatous tumor/well-differentiated liposarcoma of the extremity and trunk wall: importance of histological subtype with treatment recommendations. Ann Surg Oncol 11:78–84
16. Bowne WB, Antonescu CR, Leung DH, Katz SC, Hawkins WG, Woodruff JM, Brennan MF, Lewis JJ (2000) Dermatofibrosarcoma protuberans: a clinicopathologic analysis of patients treated and followed at a single institution. Cancer 88:2711–2720
17. Merchant NB, Lewis JJ, Woodruff JM, Leung DH, Brennan MF (1999) Extremity and trunk desmoid tumors: a multifactorial analysis of outcome. Cancer 86:2045–2052

18. Mentzel T, Calonje E, Wadden C, Camplejohn RS, Beham A, Smith MA, Fletcher CD (1996) Myxofibrosarcoma. Clinicopathologic analysis of 75 cases with emphasis on the low-grade variant. Am J Surg Pathol 20:391–405

19. Angervall L, Kindblom LG, Merck C (1977) Myxofibrosarcoma. A study of 30 cases. Acta Pathol Microbiol Scand [A] 85A:127–140

20. Huang HY, Lal P, Qin J, Brennan MF, Antonescu CR (2004) Low-grade myxofibrosarcoma: a clinicopathologic analysis of 49 cases treated at a single institution with simultaneous assessment of the efficacy of 3-tier and 4-tier grading systems. Hum Pathol 35:612–621

21. Waters B, Panicek DM, Lefkowitz RA, Antonescu CR, Healey JH, Athanasian EA, Brennan MF (2007) Low-grade myxofibrosarcoma: CT and MRI patterns in recurrent disease. AJR Am J Roentgenol 188:W193–W198

22. Stewart FW, Treves N (1981) Classics in oncology: lymphangiosarcoma in postmastectomy lymphedema: a report of six cases in elephantiasis chirurgica. CA Cancer J Clin 31:284–299

23. Strobbe LJ, Peterse HL, van Tinteren H, Wijnmaalen A, Rutgers EJ (1998) Angiosarcoma of the breast after conservation therapy for invasive cancer, the incidence and outcome. An unforeseen sequela. Breast Cancer Res Treat 47:101–109

24. Naka N, Ohsawa M, Tomita Y, Kanno H, Uchida A, Myoui A, Aozasa K (1996) Prognostic factors in angiosarcoma: a multivariate analysis of 55 cases. J Surg Oncol 61:170–176

25. Vauthey JN, Woodruff JM, Brennan MF (1995) Extremity malignant peripheral nerve sheath tumors (neurogenic sarcomas): a 10-year experience. Ann Surg Oncol 2:126–131

26. Pisters PW, Harrison LB, Leung DH, Woodruff JM, Casper ES, Brennan MF (1996) Long-term results of a prospective randomized trial of adjuvant brachytherapy in soft tissue sarcoma. J Clin Oncol 14:859–868

27. O'Sullivan B, Davis AM, Turcotte R, Bell R, Catton C, Chabot P, Wunder J, Kandel R, Goddard K, Sadura A, Pater J, Zee B (2002) Preoperative versus postoperative radiotherapy in soft-tissue sarcoma of the limbs: a randomised trial. Lancet 359:2235–2241

28. Yang JC, Chang AE, Baker AR, Sindelar WF, Danforth DN, Topalian SL, DeLaney T, Glatstein E, Steinberg SM, Merino MJ, Rosenberg SA (1998) Randomized prospective study of the benefit of adjuvant radiation therapy in the treatment of soft tissue sarcomas of the extremity. J Clin Oncol 16:197–203

29. Baldini EH, Goldberg J, Jenner C, Manola JB, Demetri GD, Fletcher CD, Singer S (1999) Long-term outcomes after function-sparing surgery without radiotherapy for soft tissue sarcoma of the extremities and trunk. J Clin Oncol 17:3252–3259

30. Lin PP, Schupak KD, Boland PJ, Brennan MF, Healey JH (1998) Pathologic femoral fracture after periosteal excision and radiation for the treatment of soft tissue sarcoma. Cancer 82:2356–2365

31. Alektiar KM, Hong L, Brennan MF, Della-Biancia C, Singer S (2007) Intensity modulated radiation therapy for primary soft tissue sarcoma of the extremity: preliminary results. Int J Radiat Oncol Biol Phys 68:458–464

32. Rosenberg SA, Tepper J, Glatstein E, Costa J, Young R, Baker A, Brennan MF, Demoss EV, Seipp C, Sindelar WF, Sugarbaker P, Wesley R (1983) Prospective randomized evaluation of adjuvant chemotherapy in adults with soft tissue sarcomas of the extremities. Cancer 52:424–434

33. Chang AE, Kinsella T, Glatstein E, Baker AR, Sindelar WF, Lotze MT, Danforth DN Jr, Sugarbaker PH, Lack EE, Steinberg SM et al (1988) Adjuvant chemotherapy for patients with high-grade soft-tissue sarcomas of the extremity. J Clin Oncol 6:1491–1500

34. (1997) Adjuvant chemotherapy for localised resectable soft-tissue sarcoma of adults: meta-analysis of individual data. Sarcoma Meta-analysis Collaboration. Lancet 350:1647–1654

35. Antman KH, Elias A, Ryan L (1990) Ifosfamide and mesna: response and toxicity at standard- and high-dose schedules. Semin Oncol 17:68–73

36. Frustaci S, Gherlinzoni F, De Paoli A, Bonetti M, Azzarelli A, Comandone A, Olmi P, Buonadonna A, Pignatti G, Barbieri E, Apice G, Zmerly H, Serraino D, Picci P (2001) Adjuvant chemotherapy for adult soft tissue sarcomas of the extremities and girdles: results of the Italian randomized cooperative trial. J Clin Oncol 19:1238–1247

37. Frustaci S, De Paoli A, Bidoli E, La Mura N, Berretta M, Buonadonna A, Boz G, Gherlinzoni F (2003) Ifosfamide in the adjuvant therapy of soft tissue sarcomas. Oncology 65(Suppl 2):80–84

38. Grobmyer SR, Maki RG, Demetri GD, Mazumdar M, Riedel E, Brennan MF, Singer S (2004) Neo-adjuvant chemotherapy for primary high-grade extremity soft tissue sarcoma. Ann Oncol 15: 1667–1672

39. Chang HR, Hajdu SI, Collin C, Brennan MF (1989) The prognostic value of histologic subtypes in primary extremity liposarcoma. Cancer 64:1514–1520

40. Gebhard S, Coindre JM, Michels JJ, Terrier P, Bertrand G, Trassard M, Taylor S, Chateau MC, Marques B, Picot V, Guillou L (2002) Pleomorphic liposarcoma: clinicopathologic, immunohistochemical, and follow-up analysis of 63 cases: a study from the French Federation of Cancer Centers Sarcoma Group. Am J Surg Pathol 26:601–616

41. Antonescu CR, Tschernyavsky SJ, Decuseara R, Leung DH, Woodruff JM, Brennan MF, Bridge JA, Neff JR, Goldblum JR, Ladanyi M (2001) Prognostic impact of P53 status, TLS-CHOP fusion transcript structure, and histological grade in myxoid liposarcoma: a molecular and clinicopathologic study of 82 cases. Clin Cancer Res 7:3977–3987

42. McCormick D, Mentzel T, Beham A, Fletcher CD (1994) Dedifferentiated liposarcoma. Clinicopathologic analysis of 32 cases suggesting a better prognostic subgroup among pleomorphic sarcomas. Am J Surg Pathol 18:1213–1223

43. Henricks WH, Chu YC, Goldblum JR, Weiss SW (1997) Dedifferentiated liposarcoma: a clinicopathological analysis of 155 cases with a proposal for an expanded definition of dedifferentiation. Am J Surg Pathol 21:271–281

44. Eilber FC, Eilber FR, Eckardt J, Rosen G, Riedel E, Maki RG, Brennan MF, Singer S (2004) The impact of chemotherapy on the survival of patients with high-grade primary extremity liposarcoma. Ann Surg 240:686–695, discussion 695–687

45. Lewis JJ, Antonescu CR, Leung DH, Blumberg D, Healey JH, Woodruff JM, Brennan MF (2000) Synovial sarcoma: a multivariate analysis of prognostic factors in 112 patients with primary localized tumors of the extremity. J Clin Oncol 18:2087–2094

46. Eilber FC, Brennan MF, Eilber FR, Eckardt JJ, Grobmyer SR, Riedel E, Forscher C, Maki RG, Singer S (2007) Chemotherapy is associated with improved survival in adult patients with primary extremity synovial sarcoma. Ann Surg 246:105–113

47. Lewis JJJ, Leung DD, Woodruff JJM, Brennan MMF (1998) Retroperitoneal soft-tissue sarcoma: analysis of 500 patients treated and followed at a single institution. Ann Surg 228:355–365

48. Singer S, Antonescu CR, Riedel E, Brennan MF (2003) Histologic subtype and margin of resection predict pattern of recurrence and survival for retroperitoneal liposarcoma. Ann Surg 238:358–370, discussion 370–351

49. Hollenbeck ST, Grobmyer SR, Kent KC, Brennan MF (2003) Surgical treatment and outcomes of patients with primary inferior vena cava leiomyosarcoma. J Am Coll Surg 197:575–579

50. Fabre-Guillevin E, Coindre JM, Somerhausen Nde S, Bonichon F, Stoeckle E, Bui NB (2006) Retroperitoneal liposarcomas: follow-up analysis of dedifferentiation after clinicopathologic reexamination of 86 liposarcomas and malignant fibrous histiocytomas. Cancer 106:2725–2733

51. Karakousis CP, Velez AF, Gerstenbluth R, Driscoll DL (1996) Resectability and survival in retroperitoneal sarcomas. Ann Surg Oncol 3:150–158

52. Tepper JE, Suit HD, Wood WC, Proppe KH, Harmon D, McNulty P (1984) Radiation therapy of retroperitoneal soft tissue sarcomas. Int J Radiat Oncol Biol Phys 10:825–830

53. Sindelar WF, Kinsella TJ, Chen PW, DeLaney TF, Tepper JE, Rosenberg SA, Glatstein E (1993) Intraoperative radiotherapy in retroperitoneal sarcomas. Final results of a prospective, randomized, clinical trial. Arch Surg 128:402–410

54. Pawlik TM, Pisters PW, Mikula L, Feig BW, Hunt KK, Cormier JN, Ballo MT, Catton CN, Jones JJ, O'Sullivan B, Pollock RE, Swallow CJ (2006) Long-term results of two prospective trials of preoperative external beam radiotherapy for localized intermediate- or high-grade retroperitoneal soft tissue sarcoma. Ann Surg Oncol 13:508–517

55. Kinzler KW, Nilbert MC, Su LK, Vogelstein B, Bryan TM, Levy DB, Smith KJ, Preisinger AC, Hedge P, McKechnie D et al (1991) Identification of FAP locus genes from chromosome 5q21. Science 253:661–665

56. Kinzler KW, Nilbert MC, Vogelstein B, Bryan TM, Levy DB, Smith KJ, Preisinger AC, Hamilton SR, Hedge P, Markham A et al (1991) Identification of a gene located at chromosome 5q21 that is mutated in colorectal cancers. Science 251:1366–1370

57. Latchford A, Volikos E, Johnson V, Rogers P, Suraweera N, Tomlinson I, Phillips R, Silver A (2007) APC mutations in FAP-associated desmoid tumours are non-random but not 'just right'. Hum Mol Genet 16:78–82

58. Xu W, Kimelman D (2007) Mechanistic insights from structural studies of beta-catenin and its binding partners. J Cell Sci 120:3337–3344

59. Lazar AJ, Tuvin D, Hajibashi S, Habeeb S, Bolshakov S, Mayordomo-Aranda E, Warneke CL, Lopez-Terrada D, Pollock RE, Lev D (2008) Specific mutations in the beta-catenin gene (CTNNB1) correlate with local recurrence in sporadic desmoid tumors. Am J Pathol 173:1518–1527

60. Alman BA, Li C, Pajerski ME, Diaz-Cano S, Wolfe HJ (1997) Increased beta-catenin protein and somatic APC mutations in sporadic aggressive fibromatoses (desmoid tumors). Am J Pathol 151:329–334

61. Shitoh K, Konishi F, Iijima T, Ohdaira T, Sakai K, Kanazawa K, Miyaki M (1999) A novel case of a sporadic desmoid tumour with mutation of the beta catenin gene. J Clin Pathol 52:695–696

62. Tejpar S, Nollet F, Li C, Wunder JS, Michils G, dal Cin P, Van Cutsem E, Bapat B, van Roy F, Cassiman JJ, Alman BA (1999) Predominance of beta-catenin mutations and beta-catenin dysregulation in sporadic aggressive fibromatosis (desmoid tumor). Oncogene 18:6615–6620

63. Miyoshi Y, Iwao K, Nawa G, Yoshikawa H, Ochi T, Nakamura Y (1998) Frequent mutations in the beta-catenin gene in desmoid tumors from patients without familial adenomatous polyposis. Oncol Res 10:591–594

64. Anthony T, Rodriguez-Bigas MA, Weber TK, Petrelli NJ (1996) Desmoid tumors. J Am Coll Surg 182:369–377

65. Bruce JM, Bradley EL 3rd, Satchidanand SK (1996) A desmoid tumor of the pancreas. Sporadic intra-abdominal desmoids revisited. Int J Pancreatol 19:197–203

66. Humar A, Chou S, Carpenter B (1993) Fibromatosis in infancy and childhood: the spectrum. J Pediatr Surg 28:1446–1450

67. Spear MA, Jennings LC, Mankin HJ, Spiro IJ, Springfield DS, Gebhardt MC, Rosenberg AE, Efird JT, Suit HD (1998) Individualizing management of aggressive fibromatoses. Int J Radiat Oncol Biol Phys 40:637–645

68. Hansmann A, Adolph C, Vogel T, Unger A, Moeslein G (2004) High-dose tamoxifen and sulindac as first-line treatment for desmoid tumors. Cancer 100:612–620

69. Latchford AR, Sturt NJ, Neale K, Rogers PA, Phillips RK (2006) A 10-year review of surgery for desmoid disease associated with familial adenomatous polyposis. Br J Surg 93:1258–1264

70. Dematteo RP, Gold JS, Saran L, Gonen M, Liau KH, Maki RG, Singer S, Besmer P, Brennan MF, Antonescu CR (2008) Tumor mitotic rate, size, and location independently predict recurrence after resection of primary gastrointestinal stromal tumor (GIST). Cancer 112:608–615

71. Raut CP, DeMatteo RP (2008) Prognostic factors for primary GIST: prime time for personalized therapy? Ann Surg Oncol 15:4–6

72. Hirota S, Isozaki K, Moriyama Y, Hashimoto K, Nishida T, Ishiguro S, Kawano K, Hanada M, Kurata A, Takeda M, Muhammad Tunio G, Matsuzawa Y, Kanakura Y, Shinomura Y, Kitamura Y (1998) Gain-of-function mutations of c-kit in human gastrointestinal stromal tumors. Science 279:577–580

73. Heinrich MC, Corless CL, Demetri GD, Blanke CD, von Mehren M, Joensuu H, McGreevey LS, Chen CJ, Van den Abbeele AD, Druker BJ, Kiese B, Eisenberg B, Roberts PJ, Singer S, Fletcher CD, Silberman S, Dimitrijevic S, Fletcher JA (2003) Kinase mutations and imatinib response in patients with metastatic gastrointestinal stromal tumor. J Clin Oncol 21:4342–4349

74. Antonescu CR, Sommer G, Sarran L, Tschernyavsky SJ, Riedel E, Woodruff JM, Robson M, Maki R, Brennan MF, Ladanyi M, DeMatteo RP, Besmer P (2003) Association of KIT exon 9 mutations with nongastric primary site and aggressive behavior: KIT mutation analysis and clinical correlates of 120 gastrointestinal stromal tumors. Clin Cancer Res 9:3329–3337

75. Heinrich MC, Corless CL, Duensing A, McGreevey L, Chen CJ, Joseph N, Singer S, Griffith DJ, Haley A, Town A, Demetri GD, Fletcher CD, Fletcher JA (2003) PDGFRA activating mutations in gastrointestinal stromal tumors. Science 299:708–710

76. Dematteo R, Owzar K, Maki R et al (2007) Adjuvant imatinib mesylate increases recurrence free survival (RFS) in patients with completely localized primary gastrointestinal stromal tumor (GIST): North American Intergroup Phase III Trial ACOSOG Z9001. Proc Am Soc Clin Oncol Abstract No 10079

77. Verweij J, Casali PG, Zalcberg J, LeCesne A, Reichardt P, Blay JY, Issels R, van Oosterom A, Hogendoorn PC, Van Glabbeke M, Bertulli R, Judson I (2004) Progression-free survival in gastrointestinal stromal tumours with high-dose imatinib: randomised trial. Lancet 364:1127–1134

78. DeMatteo RP, Maki RG, Singer S, Gonen M, Brennan MF, Antonescu CR (2007) Results of tyrosine kinase inhibitor therapy followed by surgical resection for metastatic gastrointestinal stromal tumor. Ann Surg 245:347–352

Chapter 93
Pressure Sores in the Elderly

Alexander Y. Lin and Mary H. McGrath

Introduction

Capillary perfusion pressure is the source of life for all the cells in our body, and yet, it averages a modest 22 mmHg throughout most systems in the body. Venous capillary closing pressure is about 12 mmHg, and arterial capillary pressure about 32 mmHg [1]. This delicate homeostasis can be upset by something as simple as excessive external pressure on tissue. This situation requires two unyielding surfaces: one an underlying bony prominence and the other an external plane such as a bed, chair, or even a transport gurney. The most common bony surfaces involved, in order of occurrence, are the sacrum, calcaneus, ischium, and greater trochanter [2]. In fact, these areas are subject to pressure exceeding 30 mmHg when lying supine, sitting, or lying on the side, respectively [3]. This situation is usually benign as our autonomic nervous system prompts us to shift our weight frequently to avoid chronic pressure.

Prolonged pressure, as in an elderly patient who is obtunded or with limited mobility, leads to chronic pressures exceeding the capillary perfusion pressure, resulting in compromised oxygenation, ischemia, and eventually tissue necrosis. Studies in models of ischemia have demonstrated that external pressure greater than 60 mmHg for 2 h leads to irreversible tissue damage [4]; clinical studies confirm this range [5, 6]. The sequelae of this damage are pressure sores with ulceration, infection, and exposure of bone. The estimated annual cost of hospital-acquired pressure sores alone is in the $3 billion range [7].

Pressure ulcers are a disease of the elderly: about two-thirds of pressure sores occur in patients over 70 years of age [8]. Most of the remaining are in spinal-cord injury patients. Fourteen percent to 17% of patients in a U.S. acute-care hospital have pressure sores, and the incidence of new hospital-acquired pressure sores is 7–9% [2]. The majority of pressure ulcers occurring in the acute-care hospital setting develop within the first 2 weeks of admission [9], probably because patients are more bed-bound until their acute issues are diagnosed and stabilized. In this elderly population, the presence of multiple comorbidities contributes to the etiopathogenesis of pressure ulcers. Although pressure sores are associated with a twofold increase in mortality [10], they are not usually the immediate cause of death. More commonly, comorbidities that lead to pressure sores such as cardiovascular, neurological, or orthopedic diseases have their own high mortality rates.

The goals in the management of pressure sores are: identification of the etiological factors, elimination of these factors, wound care and debridement to prevent chronic infection from progressing to an acute infection, and consideration for surgical coverage if benefits of repair outweigh risks of anesthesia and recurrence.

Pathophysiology

Both extrinsic and intrinsic factors contribute to the pathogenesis of pressure ulcers. Extrinsic factors include unrelieved pressure as seen in debilitated or spinal-cord injury patients, and also factors that worsen the local wound environment, such as moisture in the perineal area [11], incontinence [12], and shearing forces from patient repositioning. Intrinsic factors include underlying conditions that lead to poor wound healing, such as advanced age [13, 14], diabetes, malnutrition, and edema. Edema may occur in the elderly due to other systemic illnesses and sets up a downward spiral where dependent edema is worsened by pressure exceeding the capillary venous outflow pressure, leading to even worse edema in the dependent regions, compensatory increased arterial pressure, extravasation and worsening edema (Table 93.1).

Extrinsic pressures can also be augmented by positioning, and clinical studies show that some commonplace positions are particularly problematic. In a semirecumbent position with the head of the bed elevated, only friction keeps the

A.Y. Lin (✉)
Former Chief Resident, UCSF Plastic Surgery,
University of California San Francisco, San Francisco, CA, USA
and
Assistant Professor of Surgery, Division of Plastic Surgery, Saint Louis
University Director, St. Louis Cleft-Craniofacial Center, Cardinal
Glennon Children's Medical Center at SLU, St. Louis, MO, USA
e-mail: magicalplastics@gmail.com

R.A. Rosenthal et al. (eds.), *Principles and Practice of Geriatric Surgery*,
DOI 10.1007/978-1-4419-6999-6_93, © Springer Science+Business Media, LLC 2011

Table 93.1 Extrinsic and intrinsic factors contributing to pressure sore formation

Extrinsic	Intrinsic
Limited mobility	Advanced age
Loss of protective sensation	Skin fragility
Abnormal positioning due to spasticity or contracture	Poor nutritional status
Friction and shearing forces	Dependent edema
Chronic moisture	Immunoincompetence
Other mechanical factors that increase pressure	Infection
	Medical conditions

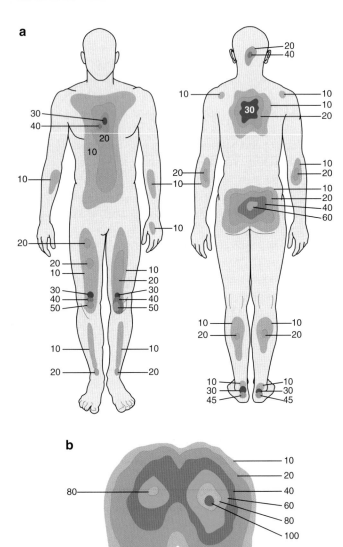

Figure 93.1 Topographic pressure maps of the human body in millimeters of mercury. (**a**) Supine (*left*) and prone (*right*) positions. Note that in the prone position, the highest pressures are centered on the sacrum and heels, exceeding 30 mmHg. (**b**) Seated position reveals pressures much greater than 30 mmHg for the ischii (reprinted from Lindan O (1961) Etiology of decubitus ulcers: An experimental study. Arch Phys Med Rehabil 42:774, with permission from Elsevier).

patient from sliding down. This situation leads to shearing forces on the skin and soft tissue overlying the sacrum which mechanically creates ischemia that predisposes to ulceration [15]. Topographic pressure maps show why certain areas, such as the sacrum, heels, and ischii are prone to ischemic damage (Fig. 93.1) [3].

Malnutrition is prevalent among older patients, with the 2002 Nutritional Screening Initiative estimating the rate of malnutrition among hospitalized elderly as 40–60%, nursing home residents as 40–85%, and home-care elderly patients as 20–60% [16]. Malnutrition increases the likelihood of developing pressure ulcers at least twofold [17].

The Braden Scale for Predicting Pressure Sore Risk is a widely used nursing assessment tool to help predict patients' risk of developing pressure sores. Although there is no clear evidence that risk-assessment scales decrease incidence of pressure ulcers, the Braden scale has reasonable predictive capacity with high interrater reliability [18]. This scale accounts for several extrinsic and intrinsic etiologic factors by scoring six subscales: sensory perception, moisture, activity, mobility, nutrition, and friction/shear. The lower the subscale score, the worse the risk, so the lower the combined Braden score (ranges from 6 to 23), the higher the risk of pressure sore development.

Intrinsically, different tissues can tolerate ischemia at varying levels. Muscle, with its high metabolic requirements, is more sensitive to hypoxia than is skin or subcutaneous fat. Although most pressure sore severity indexes recognize early skin changes as "low-grade," some degree of muscle damage is inevitable by the time the skin shows changes.

Pressure ulcers are some of the most difficult wounds to heal given their dependent positions, relative lack of blood supply, and patient comorbidities that may compromise wound healing in the elderly population. Identifying these causative factors is the first step in the evaluation and management of these wounds.

Evaluation

The evaluation of a pressure sore begins with a careful history and physical exam. The history is essential to establish which of the extrinsic and intrinsic factors contribute to the etiology and chronicity of the wound. Without addressing these factors, therapeutic efforts will fail, whether surgical or nonsurgical. For instance, a sacral pressure sore is bound to recur after surgical coverage if an air mattress and turning schedule are not implemented for an elderly stroke patient with limited mobility.

The most common classification system is the National Pressure Sore Advisory Panel Consensus Development

Conference scale developed in 1989. It is based on which tissue level is exposed in the wound. It is a purely visual scale that does not account for deeper destruction and simply stages according to the four main layers of tissue:

- Does not pass skin
- Does not pass subcutaneous fat
- Does not pass muscle
- Involves bone

Stage I: Skin intact but reddened for more than 1 h after relief of pressure. This stage represents intact skin with various degrees of erythema that does not blanch when compressed. This wound is potentially reversible if extrinsic forces and intrinsic wound healing factors are optimized.

Stage II: Blister or other break in the dermis with or without infection. Here, the skin breaks down which can expose subcutaneous fat. By maintaining coverage over the wound, these wounds often can generate granulation tissue and undergo wound contraction to heal by secondary intention. Because there is violation of skin, the local environment must be monitored even more carefully for moisture and soiling to allow this stage to heal. Stage I and II pressure ulcers are the most prevalent [2].

Stage III: Subcutaneous destruction into muscle with or without infection. Here, bone is not exposed, so theoretically, this can heal and contract over the bony prominence. However, this is usually a short-lived stage as muscle is the most oxygen-sensitive tissue and thus most sensitive to ischemic necrosis, quickly reaching the final stage of exposed bone.

Stage IV: Involvement of bone or joint with or without infection. This is the most common stage that prompts a surgical consultation, as the ulcer is down to the etiologic bony prominence. With bone exposure, there is desiccation and contamination of the surface of the bone, and by definition, there is at least superficial osteitis.

In 2007, the staging system was updated with two new stages [19].

Suspected deep tissue injury. Purple or maroon localized area of discolored intact skin or blood-filled blister due to damage of underlying soft tissue from pressure and/or shear. This new stage allows clinically suspicious deep tissue injury to be identified.

Unstageable. Full-thickness tissue loss in which the base of the ulcer is covered by slough (yellow, tan, gray, green, or brown) and/or eschar (tan, brown, or black) in the wound bed. This new stage points out that eschar or necrosis makes it difficult to determine depth of destruction. These eschars are frequently the superficial aspect of a deep wound, as seen in the example in Fig. 93.2.

In Stage IV pressure ulcers, the most superficial aspect of the exposed bone is desiccated and is therefore necrotic and colonized with the flora of the skin and surrounding areas. This is an osteitis, or inflammation of bone, rather than a hematogenous osteomyelitis that requires long-term systemic antibiotics. If the deep bone has good blood supply, and the patient is not immunocompromised, a patient can tolerate this osteitis for protracted periods as long as good wound care prevents extension of the zone of injury.

Osteomyelitis is infection of the bone. Definitive diagnosis of the extent of osteomyelitis is made during surgical debridement when bone is excised for biopsy and bacterial culture. Imaging modalities to diagnose osteomyelitis have been used, including radiography, tagged white blood cell scans, and magnetic resonance imaging (MRI) [20]. However,

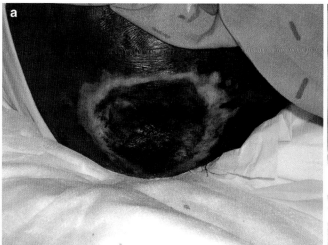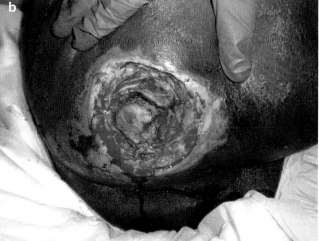

FIGURE 93.2 Elderly homeless man found sitting on the corner of a street, confused. (**a**) Right ischial pressure sore completely covered with eschar, making it unstageable. (**b**) After bedside debridement of necrotic tissue, the wound extends to the ischial tuberosity.

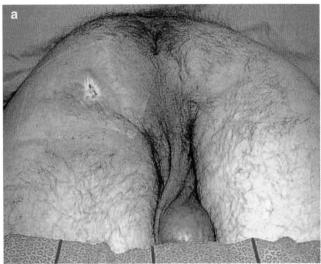

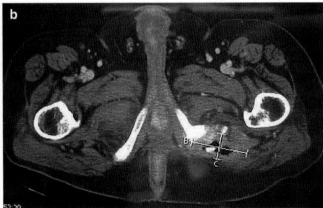

Figure 93.3 The patient presented with a chronic left ischial pressure sore with drainage. (**a**) Patient in prone position with open wound on his left ischium. (**b**) Computed tomography scan of patient (the left ischium is on the *right side* of the scan) revealing a perianal fistula tracking to an ischial abscess. This underlying etiologic factor needs to be addressed before treating the ischial sore.

by the time clinical suspicion, raised by findings such as deep pus not accessible with bedside debridement or systemic infectious symptoms, is high enough to consider imaging, surgical exploration is more appropriate than imaging. Thus, imaging to diagnose osteomyelitis often is not needed. However, appropriate imaging may be useful to evaluate the extent of necrosis in high-risk surgical patients or to help determine the source of infection in atypical pressure sores, such as perianal fistula, or spinal hardware abscesses (Fig. 93.3).

Infections of soft tissue can be polymicrobial due to urine or stool in the area. Thus, *Proteus, Bacteroides, Pseudomonas*, and *Escherichia coli* can accompany the more common staphylococcal and streptococcal species. More than half of long-term care patients harbor methicillin-resistant *Staphylococcus aureus* (MRSA) organisms [21]. Cultures can be sent to determine sensitivities, but swab cultures are invariably positive due to local contamination. Intraoperative cultures are taken from bone deep to the surface of the wound, and deep soft tissue biopsies sometimes provide sensitivity information. In the presence of active infection, the mainstay of initial management is aggressive local and systemic treatment to restore equilibrium between the open wound and the local flora, and then the correction of etiologic factors so that the wound can heal.

Pressure sores always have localized inflammation or infection but uncommonly cause systemic symptoms unless high-stage or neglected. Patients with pressure sores who present for a fever or infection workup almost certainly have comorbidities, such as a urinary tract infection or pneumonia, that must be ruled out as a source of the systemic infection.

Management

The key to management of pressure sores comes down to three principles:

1. *Reduction of pressure* (and other deleterious extrinsic factors)
2. *Restoration of nutrition* (and other intrinsic factors promoting wound healing)
3. *Wound care* (to assess the current wound for active and chronic infection and debride as necessary, and to maintain a clean wound with frequent monitoring for new active infections)

This tripod addresses all of the factors in the etiopathogenesis of pressure sores. Only when these issues are addressed can the benefits of surgical flap coverage be weighed against the probability of either failure to heal or recurrence. High surgical risk or high recurrence risk patients should be offered nonsurgical treatment and maintenance. Notably, this maintenance can have a high nursing care cost with multiple social issues.

Reduction of Pressure and Deleterious Extrinsic Factors

Increased tissue pressure is expected over bony prominences, but prolonged pressure leading to irreversible ischemia is not. In bed-bound patients, as little as 2 h of pressure is sufficient to develop a pressure sore [6]. Elderly patients may be chronically debilitated or acutely obtunded as outpatients or inpatients, and these conditions must be evaluated and optimized to the extent possible. However, even the spinal-cord injury patient, with lack of movement compounded by spasticity and contractures, can have pressure reduced. This requires turning the patient faithfully every 1–2 h to break the cycle of constant pressure and use of a lower pressure air mattress or an air-fluidized chronic pressure-shifting bed. Meta-analysis suggests that higher-specification foam mattresses and other technologic mattresses are better at reducing pressure ulcers than standard hospital foam mattresses [22]. Patients who use wheelchairs must learn to shift their weight constantly and to utilize a lower-pressure seat cushion. Many elderly patients sit in regular household chairs all day long, and even with intact skin sensation, are at risk of pressure ulcer development. In bedridden patients or those who keep their legs elevated on a footstool, heels must be unweighted or padded to reduce pressure. There are commercial products marketed to prevent heel ulcers, but there is insufficient data to determine whether these are better than simple elevation with pillows under the lower legs. Some device-specific clinical trials have suggested that these products, such as waffled foam [23] or cushioned doughnuts [24], can even increase the incidence of heel ulcers. Another way to redistribute pressure on abraded skin or early pressure sores is with thick adhesive dressings and foams marketed for this purpose. Consultation with a physiatrist can be helpful for finding adaptive devices for a patient's individual situation.

Muscle spasms and contractures are more common in patients with spinal cord injury and upper motor neuron defects. Contractures can both contribute to the etiology of the pressure sore by making bony areas more prominent, and they can make positioning and therapeutic efforts to relieve pressure more difficult. Physical therapy and splinting can alleviate the contracture, but sometimes, surgical release by orthopedic and plastic surgeons may be necessary.

Spasticity of large muscles, such as the hip flexors, can impede wound healing and compromise surgical treatment with a flap by placing repeated tension on the incisions and accentuating bony prominences. Spasticity can be addressed pharmacologically with muscle relaxants and antispasmodics, such as benzodiazepenes, baclofen, and cyclobenzaprine. Refractory spasticity may respond to infusion pumps, nerve blocks, rhizotomies, or epidurals [25]. Again, consultation with physiatry for medication, splinting, and physical therapy is useful.

Nursing care plays a major role in achieving reduction of extrinsic factors by regulating the air mattress, frequent turning, physical therapy assistance, reduction of shearing forces during patient transport, and keeping the area clean and dry. The most common pressure sores are in a dependent position where moisture and debris accumulate. Both the elderly population and spinal-cord injury patients can have varying degrees of incontinence of urine and stool, which contribute to the contaminated environment surrounding these wounds. Urinary incontinence may need to be managed with a sheath or indwelling catheter until the pressure sore or surgical flap has healed. For fecal incontinence, a temporary or permanent colostomy may be indicated to increase the likelihood of healing or successful surgical repair.

Restoration of Nutrition and Other Wound-Promoting Intrinsic Factors

The population of patients with pressure sores generally has inadequate nutritional intake. Dietary intake of nutrients and protein is predictive of pressure ulcer development in elderly patients [14, 26]. Serum metabolic panels can help with diagnosis and treatment of malnutrition by monitoring markers such as albumin, prealbumin, C-reactive protein, retinol binding protein, and transferrin. Analysis of nitrogen exchange and food choices helps determine caloric and protein intake, as well as estimate requirements. Other supplements to consider include the vitamins A and C which are implicated in wound healing, zinc, protein shakes, pharmacologic enhancement of appetite (megestrol), tube feeding, and parenteral nutrition [16, 27]. Consultation with a nutritionist can help with the assessment of the above.

Other medical conditions need to be addressed, including anemia and diabetes, HIV, and conditions that lead to edema such as congestive heart failure, kidney disease, liver disease, and other causes of hypoalbuminemia. Patients may require antibiotic treatment as an adjunct to wound care. The duration of antibiotics may be up to 2 weeks for complex soft-tissue infection or 6 weeks for biopsy-proven osteomyelitis, and consultation with an infectious disease specialist is useful.

Wound Care (Active Debridement and Regular Maintenance)

The initial approach to wound care is similar to that for all open wounds: recognizing nonviable tissue and debriding all devascularized tissue. Nonviable tissue can appear as dry gangrene or eschar that is not actively infected and may be amenable to mechanical or chemical debridement. Mechanical debridement relies on irrigation, lavage, whirlpool, and sharp excision. Sharp debridement can be done at the bedside or in the operating room, and often the extent of necrosis is surprisingly extensive due to the greater sensitivity of muscle to ischemia. For this reason, undermining of the wound beyond the skin edges characterizes pressure sores, and the wound may be substantially larger than the opening in the skin. Debriding agents such as proteolytics, fibrinolytics, collagenases, and sterile maggots have been described. Wet gangrene is necrotic tissue that is already superinfected and requires prompt sharp debridement.

In certain areas, such as the heel, pressure sores often are stable and dry. In these wounds, like frostbite injury, local wound care permitting gradual separation of the eschar may be preferable to sharp debridement to maintain as much viable tissue as possible. For these heel sores, dry dressings or topical antibacterials such as silver sulfadiazine are useful.

After debridement, several options are available. The wound can be allowed to heal by secondary intention using a variety of packing materials on a regular basis to allow the wound to heal from the base and prevent premature skin closure and abscess formation. Negative pressure therapy with a vacuum-assisted device can be used to facilitate the secondary wound healing process. These devices stimulate the formation of granulation tissue and encourage wound contraction, but the wound should be free of infection before sealing it under the occlusive vacuum dressing. As with other selected wounds, negative pressure therapy may help to downsize the surface area of a wound so that more complex reconstruction options of local or free flap can be replaced with simpler ones such as skin graft or primary closure.

In a patient with a spinal-cord injury, pressure ulcers in the denervated areas generally are not painful. In nonparaplegic elderly patients, the majority of patients experience pain with pressure ulcers and are particularly uncomfortable during wound care and dressing changes [28, 29]. Pain can be reduced with agents such as topical lidocaine or morphine, or systemic analgesics prior to dressing changes or continuously if necessary.

Surgical Treatment

Once nonsurgical management of a pressure sore addresses the etiology, and the factors that predispose to recurrence are corrected, the risk–benefit ratio of surgery versus the perioperative risks for an individual patient can be weighed. Well-recognized flaps have been developed for the most common pressure sores of the sacrum, ischium, and greater trochanter, but management must begin with adequate debridement of nonviable tissue, sinus tracts, and the bursa-like capsule that lines a chronic wound. Pressure sores that come to surgery almost always track to bone, and ostectomy is done to debride the exposed bone and obtain biopsies for bacterial culture. Ostectomy also serves to reduce the prominence of bone responsible for the sore so that the likelihood of recur-

rence is reduced. It may be helpful to enlist the participation of the primary medical team or infectious disease specialists to obtain special cultures in the setting of immunosuppression or other chronic illnesses. Finally, the cavity is filled with vascularized tissue with enough bulk to cover the bone and close the open wound.

Intraoperative Resection of Soft Tissue

The soft tissue lining a pressure sore cavity is contaminated and generally is poorly vascularized or fibrotic, depending on the duration of the ulcer. At surgery, this tissue is debrided back to normal-appearing, well-vascularized, pliant soft tissue. To accomplish this, a dye such as methylene blue can be used to coat the lining of the wound to identify any pockets or tracts; resection is complete when all the colored surfaces have been removed. It may take more than one operation to complete debridement before definitive flap coverage.

Intraoperative Resection of Bone

If the bone at the base of the wound is exposed, it is colonized with local flora and at least superficially desiccated with a nonviable surface layer. This is superficial osteitis with healthy bone with good blood supply just deep to the desiccated layer. Deeper infection with frank osteomyelitis would have been diagnosed preoperatively, and intraoperative planning for extensive bone resection, sometimes including the participation of an orthopedic surgeon, would have been scheduled.

Intraoperative debridement of the superficial bone is done using visual assessment of avascular bone versus bleeding bone. Using rongeurs and rasps to smooth jutting prominences or to excise heterotopic bone accomplishes the second purpose of bone resection: reducing the physical prominence of bone that causes pressure and predisposes to recurrence of the sore. After adequate bone debridement has been done, a biopsy of the deeper healthy-appearing bone is sent for bone culture. If this were positive, the remaining bone still is infected and the patient will need a long-term course of intravenous antibiotics to treat the osteomyelitis.

Bone resection needs to be approached with the awareness that it is not a benign process. When one of a paired set of pressure points, such as the ischii, is resected, the patient's weight is shifted to the contralateral side, increasing risk of a new pressure sore on the second side. Similarly, resection of both ischii can shift the weight-bearing surface to the perineum, resulting in later perineal or scrotal pressure sores.

Wound Coverage and Closure

For full-thickness ulcers, the basic principle is provision of vascularized tissue to cover bony prominences, lend adequate padding, fill the wound completely, and close the surface with durable soft tissue and skin that is under no tension. The "reconstructive ladder" principle in plastic surgery proposes that the basic, or "lowest rung," options should be considered first, with complex reconstructive options held in reserve in case the wound recurs. However, it is important to recognize when simpler options will be insufficient, and one should choose a more complex option from the outset. In this population of patients, it is also important to consider that using complex muscle flaps at the outset means that they will not be available in the future.

Given the above criteria, where there is a robust vascularized bed over the bone, a select group of ulcers can be repaired by operations on the basic rungs of the reconstructive ladder: delayed primary closure or a skin graft. In general, these options have limited application. Primary closure places the surgical suture line directly over the area of pressure, whereas a flap moves the closure and scar away from the pressure point. A skin graft is a thin and fragile coverage option subject to the shearing forces that created the ulcer in the first place. In addition, a skin graft requires a clean, healthy recipient site with good blood supply and no exposed bone. Only the most superficial of pressure sores meets these requirements for a healthy, well-vascularized base and can be covered successfully with a skin graft.

More often, flap coverage is the surgical choice for pressure sore repair. A flap is different from a graft in that a skin graft has no blood supply and survives by acquiring it from the tissue onto which it is grafted. A flap carries its own blood supply that is preserved while the flap is transferred to a new area. Flaps are often described by their anatomic makeup. Cutaneous flaps are supplied by direct cutaneous vessels and axially oriented perforating vessels ending in a subdermal plexus. Fasciocutaneous flaps include skin, subcutaneous fat, and deep fascia. The blood supply originates from septocutaneous vessels that pass up along fascial septae and fan out at the level of the deep fascia to form a plexus from which smaller perforator vessels supply the subcutaneous fat and skin. Musculocutaneous flaps include muscle, fascia, subcutaneous fat, and skin combined as one unit, based on one or more vascular pedicles, which are musculocutaneous vessels that travel perpendicularly through the muscle into the overlying tissue. Muscle-only flaps have the same blood supply but will require a concurrent skin graft to cover the surface of the muscle.

Previous incisions, whether from trauma or prior surgery, can preclude certain flaps since these incisions and scars are areas where previous blood supply was likely transected. A complete surgical history is mandatory to understand the surgical anatomy when previous flaps were used. Flaps can be designed so that they can be reelevated and readvanced in the future. Since pressure ulcers have a high rate of recurrence [30], another factor in flap selection is choosing one that preserves blood supply for potential future flaps. Finally, the size of the flap usually needs to be much larger than the ulcer, as the wound area enlarges after debridement. A generous flap provides bulk, minimizes tension on the closure, and moves the suture lines to the periphery away from the original ulcer's central pressure point.

Free microvascular flaps are the most complex reconstructive options. They require harvesting a distant flap with its accompanying arteries and veins and transferring it to the recipient bed with microvascular anastomoses to recipient vessels. Elderly patients have comorbidities such as cardiovascular disease and poor general health that can make these lengthy microsurgical tissue transfers problematic.

The elimination of "dead space" is necessary to heal pressure ulcers where there is a soft tissue cavity. After introducing the vascularized flap, this is furthered with surgical drains exerting negative pressure and layered wound closure. Closed surgical drainage systems are used in the recipient bed during the initial phase of healing, and the donor site of a flap with significant dissection also needs a surgical drain to reduce the incidence of postoperative seroma and infection. Drainage should be maintained until the patient is achieving some degree of mobility and the output has tapered to a small volume per day for several days. Layered wound closure is a technique for further elimination of dead space by closing each level of tissue separately, using absorbable sutures to approximate the deep layers and evert the more superficial layers. The surgical wound is dressed carefully with multiple layers of antibiotic ointment and semipermeable dressings to create a barrier against soilage.

Sacral Pressure Sores

Sacral pressure sores develop in supine or semireclining patients with sufficient pressure and shearing over the sacral prominence. This is the most common pressure sore since debilitated, obtunded, or severely ill patients are bedridden and supine much of the time [2]. Given the broad, pointed shape of the sacrum and the thinness of the overlying soft tissues, most ulcers come to the surgeon with bone exposure. This precludes a skin graft in the sacral area, except in the shallowest of ulcers, and even then is useful only in a patient with good sensation and mobility. Chronically ill patients who will remain immobilized have too high a risk of recurrence through a skin graft. In general, flap coverage is a better option in patients who are surgical candidates.

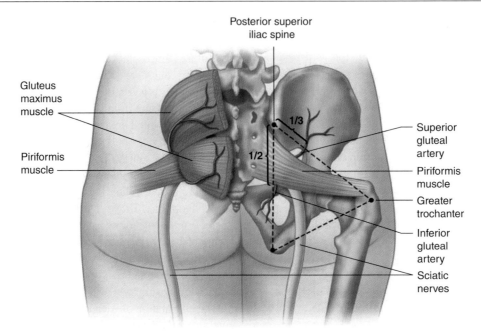

Figure 93.4 The blood supply to the gluteus maximus muscle supplies perforators to the overlying soft tissue surrounding the sacrum. The piriformis muscle marks the midportion of the gluteus maximus muscle, with the superior and inferior gluteal arteries arising above and below the piriformis. The superior gluteal artery can be found one third of the distance from the posterior superior iliac spine to the greater trochanter. The inferior gluteal artery appears halfway between the posterior superior iliac spine and the ischial tuberosity (reprinted from McCarthy J. Current therapy in plastic surgery. WB Saunders. © Elsevier (2005)).

The soft tissues surrounding the sacrum receive their blood supply from perforators from the superior and inferior gluteal arteries, which are also the arteries supplying the gluteus maximus muscles (see Fig. 93.4). Cutaneous, fasciocutaneous, musculocutaneous, and muscle flaps can be developed based on these vessels. The gluteus maximus can survive on either vascular pedicle alone [31]. However, utilizing both pedicles can increase flap reliability and the volume of overlying muscle and soft tissue and also make it easier to readvance the flap in the future if the sacral wound recurs. However, because this muscle extends and rotates the thigh laterally and is required for ambulation, the gluteus maximus is not considered expendable except in the spinal cord injury patient. If the patient has a chance of recovering ambulation, then only the superior or the inferior half of the muscle should be used. For sacral coverage, the superior half of the gluteal muscle is usually used as it is closer to the wound. Alternatively, a cutaneous or fasciocutaneous flap can be used to spare the muscle entirely.

Each half of the gluteus maximus muscle is shaped like a rectangle, originating from the ilium and inserting into the greater tuberosity of the femur. Muscle or musculocutaneous flaps of the superior half of the muscle are constructed and moved in two primary ways: a rotational flap or a V-Y advancement flap. A rotational flap can be as an advancement or with a musculocutaneous skin island. Either way, one end of the muscle is kept in contact with its blood supply, and the other end is detached to advance the entire flap, or to transfer a skin island in a rotational arc to fill the defect.

The V-Y advancement technique involves creating a triangular-shaped skin island over the muscle, with one side being the defect and the other two sides forming a "V." The central "V" is shifted into the open wound and the defect is closed in a "Y" configuration. A V-Y advancement flap can be designed in different ways. If not much bulk is needed, it can be a fasciocutaneous flap based on the gluteal perforators, and it can be advanced over the defect without needing to mobilize the muscle. For greater coverage with a V-Y flap, elevating the gluteus maximus as a musculocutaneous flap provides more bulk and permits more advancement of the overlying soft tissue because the blood supply travels with the muscle. This comes at the expense of a more extensive dissection to mobilize the muscle. Another way to get extended coverage of the sacrum is the use of bilateral V-Y advancement flaps, one based on the right gluteal area and one on the left gluteal area (see Fig. 93.5).

Ischial Pressure Sores

The ischial tuberosities are under high pressure in a seated patient. Unilateral or bilateral ischial sores develop in individuals who are seated for protracted periods of time without

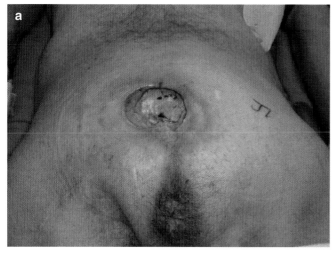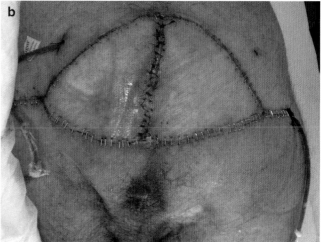

FIGURE **93.5** This male nursing-home patient had a Stage IV sacral pressure sore with exposed sacrum. (**a**) Preoperative view in the prone position. (**b**) Postoperative view after bilateral gluteus maximus musculocutaneous V-Y advancement flaps. Note the use of surgical drains under the flap donor sites.

adjusting their position and weight distribution. Ischial ulcers are challenging for several reasons. The pressure points are bilateral, which means that unweighting one side for pressure-reducing purposes shifts increased pressure onto the contralateral ischium. Resecting bone on both sides runs the risk of shifting weight-bearing onto the perineal soft tissues, which can cause later scrotal or urethral sores. There can be fistulae involving the rectum or urethra, and these may require diversion and control of the fistulae before addressing the ischial ulcers. Finally, because of the strong hip flexors, there can be flexion contractures with varying degrees of deformity which reduce mobility and the capacity for normal weight distribution in either the sitting or the lying position.

Because the ischium has a number of surrounding muscles, a variety of suitable flaps for coverage have been described. These include the inferior gluteus maximus rotational flap, inferior gluteal fasciocutaneous thigh flap, V-Y hamstring advancement flap, gracilis muscle flap, tensor fascia lata rotational flap, and rectus abdominis rotational flap. The first two are considered the most useful flaps and are described in more detail below.

The inferior gluteal fasciocutaneous thigh flap, also called the posterior thigh flap, is a good first choice. This flap is robust, reliable and leaves the gluteus maximus intact to preserve this option for use in case of future recurrence. The posterior thigh region is supplied by perforators from the descending branch of the inferior gluteal artery. This artery descends deep to the gluteal muscles in a midline axis between the ischium and the greater trochanter and courses toward the popliteal fossa. Thus, the flap design is an inverted triangle with its base at the inferior gluteal cleft and its distal point toward the popliteal fossa. The distal limit is about 8 cm proximal to the popliteal fossa [32]. The base of the flap should be about 10–12 cm wide, and the point of rotation is

5 cm superior to the ischial tuberosity (see Fig. 93.6a, b). The dissection is initiated inferiorly by identifying the posterior femoral cutaneous nerve and adjacent descending branch of the inferior gluteal artery. The artery is transected distally and preserved proximally as the flap is raised from inferior to superior up to the gluteus maximus muscle. Now, the flap can be rotated medially to fill an ischial defect (see Fig. 93.6c, d). If there is excess of the length of the flap, the distal end can be the denuded skin and the subcutaneous tissue tucked into the ischial crater to further eliminate dead space (see Fig. 93.7).

The other useful flap is the inferior gluteus maximus rotational flap. Like using the superior half of the gluteus maximus muscle for a sacral wound, the inferior half of the gluteus maximus flap can be rotated into the ischial wound as a rotation advancement (see Fig. 93.8) or a rotational island flap. In the latter case, a skin island over the inferior half of the muscle, lateral to the ischial defect, can be elevated with the muscle and rotated medially (see Fig. 93.9). Rotational flaps have an effective shortening of their pedicles as they rotate, and this must be taken into account when designing the flap. The gluteal muscle will need to be detached from its insertion on the femur as much as necessary to allow complete rotation. An attempt should be made to preserve the descending branch of inferior gluteal artery to allow a future posterior thigh flap.

Greater Trochanter Pressure Sores

Given the mobility of the hip, pressure sores over the greater trochanter characteristically have extensive bursa formation with less skin involvement. After resection of the

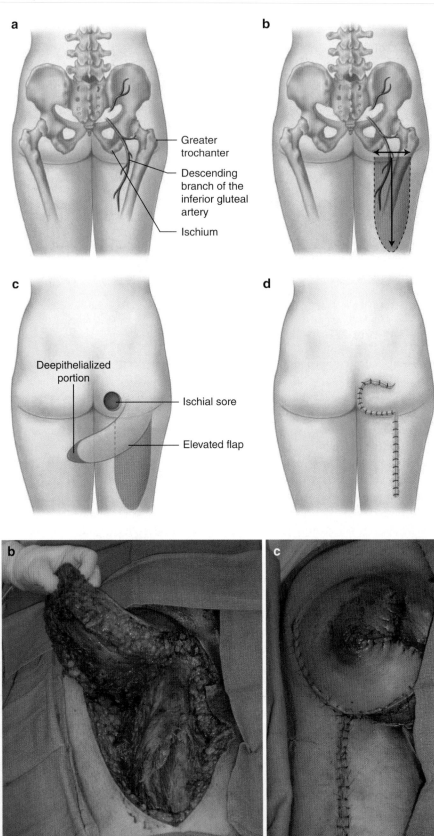

FIGURE 93.6 The inferior gluteal thigh flap. (**a**) The descending branch of the inferior gluteal artery comes off at the midline of the posterior thigh. (**b**) This descending branch supplies the posterior thigh soft tissues, so a flap is designed to allow rotation into the ischial defect and primary closure of the donor site. (**c**) Rotation of the posterior thigh flap medially, inset of the flap into the wound, and primary closure of the donor site. (**d**) Immediate postoperative view after inset of the flap (reprinted from McCarthy J. Current therapy in plastic surgery. WB Saunders. © Elsevier (2005)).

a

Greater trochanter

Descending branch of the inferior gluteal artery

Ischium

b

c

Deepithelialized portion

Ischial sore

Elevated flap

d

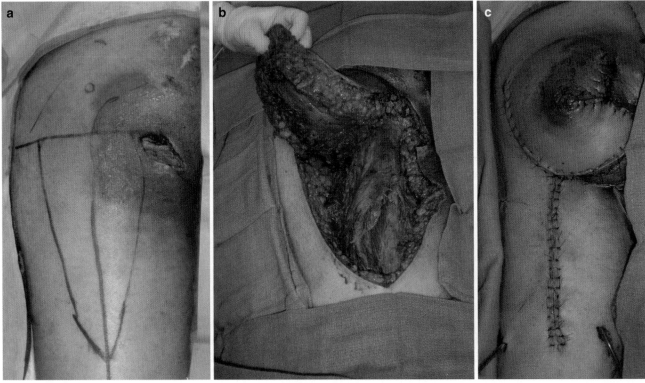

a

b

c

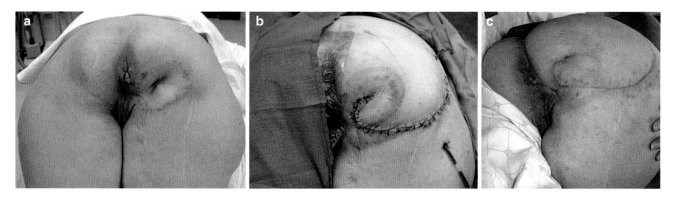

Figure 93.8 This woman had a recurrent right ischial pressure sore. (**a**) On her preoperative view, note the two vertical scars on her posterior thigh, evidence of a previous hamstring advancement flap. These scars preclude the use of a posterior thigh flap. (**b**) After debridement of the wound and rotational advancement flap of the inferior half of the gluteus maximus muscle with its overlying soft tissues, the flap is *inset*, closing the ischial defect. Note the two surgical drains: one superiorly for the donor site, and one inferiorly for the ischial wound recipient site. (**c**) Postoperatively with good healing and intact closure at 3 months.

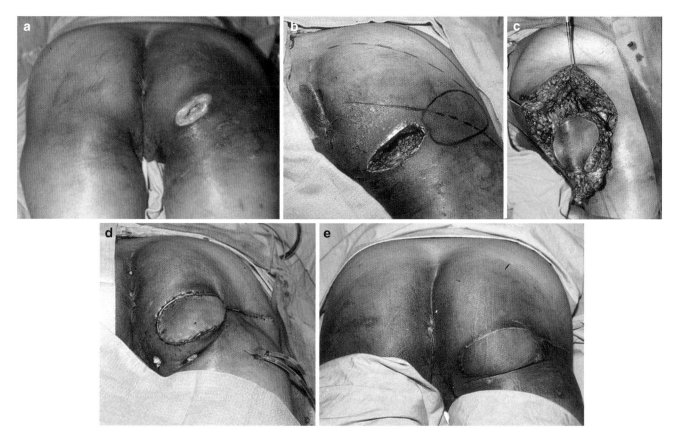

Figure 93.9 This man had a new-onset right ischial pressure ulcer. (**a**) Preoperative view in the prone position shows Stage IV wound that tracks to bone. (**b**) After debridement, the wound is larger, and a musculocutaneous island flap is designed lateral to the wound, overlying the inferior half of the gluteus maximus muscle. (**c**) Elevation of the inferior half of the gluteus maximus muscle maintaining the perforators to the overlying soft tissue island. (**d**) Island flap is rotated medially into the defect and the donor site primarily closed. Note the two surgical drains: one in the donor site and one in the ischial wound recipient site.

Figure 93.7 This man had a chronic left ischial pressure sore that would not heal. (**a**) Preoperative view of ischial pressure with markings for a posterior thigh flap. (**b**) Elevation of the posterior thigh flap, showing it is a fasciocutaneous flap. (**c**) *Inset* of posterior thigh flap to fill the entire defect, obliterate the dead space, and close the ischial pressure sore. Note the two surgical drains: one for the posterior thigh donor site, and one for the ischial recipient site.

trochanter, flaps available for repair of trochanteric pressure sores include local fasciocutaneous rotational flaps, tensor fascia lata (TFL) musculocutaneous flaps, inferior gluteal thigh fasciocutaneous flaps, and muscle flaps incorporating the vastus lateralis, rectus femoris, or rectus abdominis muscles.

The flap often selected for this defect is the tensor fascia lata (TFL) flap. The TFL lies adjacent to the trochanter and originates from the crest of the anterior superior iliac spine and descends to insert into the iliotibial tract of the fascia lata. It is a flap with a single dominant pedicle, the ascending branch of the lateral circumflex femoral artery. The flap can be designed as an inverted triangle with a maximum length of about 20 cm, with the base near the greater trochanter and the distal end towards the knee. The vascular source is about 10 cm below the anterior superior iliac spine along the anterior border of the TFL and must be preserved. The plane of dissection is between the TFL and the vastus lateralis. The pedicle can be identified on the deep medial surface of the TFL. Distally, the flap is detached from its insertion, but the origin proximally is not taken down unless more rotation is needed [33]. Once the TFL flap is elevated, it can be used as a rotational flap, a V-Y advancement, or a V-Y retroposition flap [34]. A V-Y flap places the most reliable portion of the flap over the greater trochanter, which is preferable to the rotational flap, which brings in the distal portion with the most tenuous blood supply (see Fig. 93.10).

Foot Pressure Sores

Pressure sores commonly occur over the heels, malleoli, and the plantar surfaces of the feet. Like other pressure sores, they are initiated by pressure, and most respond favorably to conservative treatment. Since a thick subcutaneous layer is not customary on the feet, most of these ulcers, unlike those in the pelvic girdle, are modest in size and depth. In non-weight-bearing areas where a somewhat less durable surface is necessary, these may be treated conservatively. A scar left by wound contraction and epithelialization may suffice. In larger wounds, debridement and split-thickness skin grafting may be helpful if the bed of the ulcer will support a skin graft. If the ulceration is large, osteomyelitis of the calcaneous may occur, in which event, debridement of any devitalized bone is required. Where flap coverage is mandatory, muscle flaps of the abductor digiti minimi, abductor hallucis, flexor digitorum brevis are described. Fasciocutaneous flaps based on the dorsalis pedis, medial plantar, and lateral plantar arteries can also provide coverage.

Postoperative Care

The postoperative care of surgical flaps includes selected intravenous antibiotics when needed for culture-positive osteomyelitis, protecting the surgical area from body fluids

a

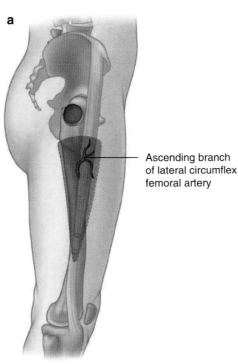

Ascending branch of lateral circumflex femoral artery

Flap design

b

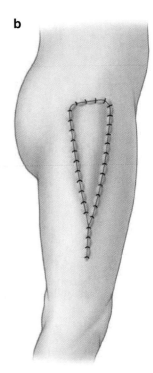

Superior advancement to greater trochanter

Figure 93.10 The tensor fascia lata V-Y advancement flap. (**a**) Design of the flap based on the ascending branch of the lateral circumflex femoral artery. (**b**) Closure after flap advanced and inset (reprinted with permission from Mathes SJ, Nahai F (1997) Reconstructive surgery: principles, anatomy and technique. Quality Medical Publishing, St. Louis).

and soilage, and pressure precautions. The latter is most critical, since a newly transferred flap is susceptible to pressure necrosis in the early postoperative period.

The postoperative protocol is customized depending on the patient, the pressure ulcer, and the flap chosen. It is customary to have 3–6 weeks with strict pressure precautions to allow soft tissue healing. For example, with a sacral or ischial pressure sore, the patient should be positioned prone or on either side with frequent turning, but never supine or sitting.

This may be difficult for the patient, so most often, the alternative is a specialized bed with an air-fluidized mattress. When it is time to begin ambulation, or resume sitting in a chair, the transition is carefully planned and executed with progressive increases in time each day with wound checks in between.

Regardless of the operative and postoperative steps, pressure ulcer flap coverage has a high rate of recurrence of about 40% over the long term [35]. This attests to the difficulty of controlling the etiologic factors of this disease.

CASE STUDY

A 72-year-old man with Alzheimer's dementia is having significant difficulty taking care of himself and performing the activities of daily living (ADLs). He has a history of two myocardial infarctions, congestive heart failure, chronic obstructive pulmonary disease, insulin-depen-

dent diabetes mellitus and is recovering from a colectomy for Stage III cancer, complicated by acute respiratory decompensation requiring ventilatory support. During his convalescence from the colectomy, he developed a 4-cm sacral pressure sore that is fibrinous, foul-smelling, and tracks to bone. Discuss the evaluation and management of this pressure sore.

Elderly patients with dementia and those with severe, acute conditions may be deconditioned and debilitated; being bedridden results in chronic pressure over the sacrum and a resultant pressure sore. Evaluation and treatment of the wound, and correction of the intrinsic and extrinsic factors contributing to the pressure sore are the first steps in taking care of this problem.

Since the wound is foul-smelling, it is assumed to contain necrotic tissue and harbor infection. After evaluation, initial treatment would be debridement. This could involve bedside debridement or operative debridement with cultures of the deep tissue. Wound care with local measures and additional debridement as needed should be ongoing while other evaluations are being done.

Intrinsic factors in his case include stabilizing his cardiopulmonary disease, managing his diabetes, and addressing his nutritional status. Baseline albumin, prealbumin, transferrin, and calorie and protein counts can be used to determine if wound-healing vitamins and protein supplements to maintain caloric intake are needed. Cardiac and pulmonary evaluation for candidacy for further surgery would be obtained.

Extrinsic factors to correct include elimination of pressure over the sacrum with a low-pressure or air-fluidized mattress and frequent turning. These protocols generally are available in the acute care setting and may be available in an extended care facility. His colon cancer should be discussed with his oncologist or colorectal surgeon, and if appropriate,

a diverting colostomy might be considered to eliminate incontinence and soiling of the sacral pressure wound.

If his general condition is deemed unsuitable for pressure sore surgery, a plan for chronic wound care with dressings, possibly negative pressure vacuum dressings, should be initiated. A schedule for intravenous antibiotics could be developed with infectious disease specialists if there were positive bone cultures. The patient's eligibility for placement would be determined with the help of social services. If ineligible for a long-term care facility, arrangements for home care with nursing support and the provision of a low-pressure bed for the home would be necessary.

If he is a good surgical candidate, debridement of the wound followed by a surgical flap would be planned. After the debridement, the wound is 8 cm in diameter. The soft tissues surrounding the sacrum receive their blood supply from the superior and inferior gluteal arteries. Either a rotational or a V-Y advancement flap can be considered, since he has no previous scars. He will be ambulatory, so sparing the gluteus maximus muscle is desirable. Given the size of the wound, bilateral V-Y fasciocutaneous advancement flaps would be a good choice.

His postoperative care would include the use of surgical drains, protective dressings with regular evaluation of the flap, bed rest on an air-fluidized mattress, deep vein thrombosis prophylaxis, antibiotic adjustments as dictated by intraoperative cultures, and management of his medical conditions. Provided the wound is healing satisfactorily, graduated mobilization could begin at about 4 weeks.

Conclusions

Pressure sores are a common problem, with a majority of them affecting the elderly population. The etiopathogenesis is complex, and a multidisciplinary approach is needed to properly evaluate and treat the patient. Extrinsic and intrinsic factors must be addressed before consideration of surgical flap coverage, since the pressure sore will recur postoperatively if they are not. Patients who are at high risk for surgery or recurrence can be treated nonsurgically since an open wound that is clean, even with exposed bone and osteitis, can be maintained with consistent nursing care.

A three-pronged approach summarizes the evaluation and treatment:

1. Reducing deleterious extrinsic factors: reduction of pressure with low-pressure mattress or wheelchair cushion, frequent turning, consultation with physiatry, physical therapy.
2. Improving beneficial intrinsic factors: addressing nutrition and comorbid conditions.
3. Wound care: mechanical or chemical debridement (bedside or operative) and pharmacologic dressings.

For the patient in whom all extrinsic and intrinsic factors are optimized, surgical repair of the pressure sore is undertaken with the understanding that there is typically a long-healing process and a high recurrence rate. The risks related to the operative and postoperative course need to be weighed carefully against potential benefits. Choices for coverage of these wounds can be cutaneous, fasciocutaneous, or musculocutaneous flaps with varying flap designs. These are customized to the patient depending on the location and size of the wound, and the availability of local tissues.

These wounds are some of the most difficult to heal, but with application of these medical and surgical principles, they can be managed, potentially alleviating the physical, emotional, and societal burdens that pressure sores impose.

Acknowledgment The authors wish to thank David S. Chang, MD, for contributing clinical case photographs for the posterior thigh flap.

References

1. Landis E (1930) Micro-injection studies of capillary blood pressure in human skin. Heart 15:209–228
2. Whittington KT, Briones R (2004) National Prevalence and Incidence Study: 6-year sequential acute care data. Adv Skin Wound Care 17(9):490–494
3. Lindan O, Greenway RM, Piazza JM (1965) Pressure distribution on the surface of the human body. I. Evaluation in lying and sitting positions using a "bed of springs and nails". Arch Phys Med Rehabil 46:378–385
4. Kosiak M (1959) Etiology and pathology of ischemic ulcers. Arch Phys Med Rehabil 40(2):62–69
5. Dinsdale SM (1974) Decubitus ulcers: role of pressure and friction in causation. Arch Phys Med Rehabil 55(4):147–152
6. Reuler JB, Cooney TG (1981) The pressure sore: pathophysiology and principles of management. Ann Intern Med 94(5):661–666
7. Beckrich K, Aronovitch SA (1999) Hospital-acquired pressure ulcers: a comparison of costs in medical vs. surgical patients. Nurs Econ 17(5):263–271
8. Allman RM (1989) Pressure ulcers among the elderly. N Engl J Med 320(13):850–853
9. Guralnik JM, Harris TB, White LR, Cornoni-Huntley JC (1988) Occurrence and predictors of pressure sores in the National Health and Nutrition Examination survey follow-up. J Am Geriatr Soc 36(9):807–812
10. Berlowitz DR, Brandeis GH, Anderson J, Du W, Brand H (1997) Effect of pressure ulcers on the survival of long-term care residents. J Gerontol A Biol Sci Med Sci 52(2):M106–M110
11. Bates-Jensen BM, McCreath HE, Kono A, Apeles NC, Alessi C (2007) Subepidermal moisture predicts erythema and stage 1 pressure ulcers in nursing home residents: a pilot study. J Am Geriatr Soc 55(8):1199–1205
12. Schnelle JF, Adamson GM, Cruise PA et al (1997) Skin disorders and moisture in incontinent nursing home residents: intervention implications. J Am Geriatr Soc 45(10):1182–1188
13. Desai H (1997) Ageing and wounds. Part 2: healing in old age. J Wound Care 6(5):237–239
14. Bergstrom N, Braden B (1992) A prospective study of pressure sore risk among institutionalized elderly. J Am Geriatr Soc 40(8):747–758
15. Reichel SM (1958) Shearing force as a factor in decubitus ulcers in paraplegics. J Am Med Assoc 166(7):762–763
16. Langemo D, Anderson J, Hanson D, Hunter S, Thompson P, Posthauer ME (2006) Nutritional considerations in wound care. Adv Skin Wound Care 19(6):297–298, 300, 303
17. Thomas DR, Goode PS, Tarquine PH, Allman RM (1996) Hospital-acquired pressure ulcers and risk of death. J Am Geriatr Soc 44(12):1435–1440
18. Pancorbo-Hidalgo PL, Garcia-Fernandez FP, Lopez-Medina IM, Alvarez-Nieto C (2006) Risk assessment scales for pressure ulcer prevention: a systematic review. J Adv Nurs 54(1):94–110
19. Pressure Ulcer Stages Revised by NPUAP. http://www.npuap.org/pr2.htm. Accessed 18 January 2009
20. Healy B, Freedman A (2006) Infections. BMJ 332(7545):838–841
21. Capitano B, Leshem OA, Nightingale CH, Nicolau DP (2003) Cost effect of managing methicillin-resistant *Staphylococcus aureus* in a long-term care facility. J Am Geriatr Soc 51(1):10–16
22. McInnes E, Bell-Syer SE, Dumville JC, Legood R, Cullum NA (2008) Support surfaces for pressure ulcer prevention. Cochrane Database Syst Rev (4):CD001735
23. Tymec AC, Pieper B, Vollman K (1997) A comparison of two pressure-relieving devices on the prevention of heel pressure ulcers. Adv Wound Care 10(1):39–44
24. Bergstrom N, Bennett MA, Carlson CE, et al (1994) Treatment of pressure ulcers. Clinical practice guideline, no. 15. U.S. Department of Health and Human Services. Public Health Service AHCPR, ed, Rockville, MD
25. McCarthy V, Lobay G, Matthey PW (2003) Epidural anesthesia as a technique to control spasticity after surgery in a patient with spinal cord injury. Plast Reconstr Surg 112(6):1729–1730
26. Stratton RJ, Ek AC, Engfer M et al (2005) Enteral nutritional support in prevention and treatment of pressure ulcers: a systematic review and meta-analysis. Ageing Res Rev 4(3):422–450
27. Bourdel-Marchasson I (2000) Nutritional supplementation in elderly people during the course of catabolic illnesses. J Nutr Health Aging 4(1):28–30
28. Dallam L, Smyth C, Jackson BS et al (1995) Pressure ulcer pain: assessment and quantification. J Wound Ostomy Continence Nurs 22(5):211–215, discussion 217–218

29. Szor JK, Bourguignon C (1999) Description of pressure ulcer pain at rest and at dressing change. J Wound Ostomy Continence Nurs 26(3):115–120

30. Conway H, Griffith BH (1956) Plastic surgery for closure of decubitus ulcers in patients with paraplegia; based on experience with 1,000 cases. Am J Surg 91(6):946–975

31. Ramirez OM, Swartz WM, Futrell JW (1987) The gluteus maximus muscle: experimental and clinical considerations relevant to reconstruction in ambulatory patients. Br J Plast Surg 40(1): 1–10

32. Hurwitz DJ, Swartz WM, Mathes SJ (1981) The gluteal thigh flap: a reliable, sensate flap for the closure of buttock and perineal wounds. Plast Reconstr Surg 68(4):521–532

33. Mathes SJ, Nahai F (1997) Tensor Fascia Lata (TFL) flap. Reconstr Surg 1271–1292

34. Siddiqui A, Wiedrich T, Lewis VL Jr (1993) Tensor fascia lata V-Y retroposition myocutaneous flap: clinical experience. Ann Plast Surg 31(4):313–317

35. Constantian M (1980) Pressure ulcers: principles and techniques of management. Little, Brown, Boston, MA

Chapter 94
Orthopaedic Trauma in the Elderly

William Min, Kenneth A. Egol, and Joseph D. Zuckerman

Introduction

Injuries to the musculoskeletal system in the elderly can be devastating. Many medical and social factors specific to older patients require special consideration when dealing with these injuries both acutely and throughout their rehabilitation. The geriatric segment of the population is rapidly growing and sustains a disproportionate number of fractures compared to others [1–3]. The specific goal of all orthopaedic care is to restore patient function to a preinjury level. Decreased bone stock, muscular weakness, systemic disease, and poor mentation are some challenges that make a return to independent living status difficult following such injuries. Immobilization and the use of devices to assist in ambulation (crutches, walkers, and wheelchairs) may require an elderly patient to be subjected to institutional care for an extended period of time. The following is an overview of the etiology, pathophysiology, and treatment considerations in treating geriatric patients with fractures and associated injuries.

Preinjury Status, Perioperative Risks, and Treatment Considerations

In elderly patients with musculoskeletal injuries, orthopaedic intervention attempts to restore their preinjury level of functioning. Their past medical, functional, and cognitive histories have significant impact on how and if these goals can be reached. Before treatment is initiated for these patients, it remains prudent for the physician to become familiar with the patient's preinjury status.

Systemic diseases and complications can impact injury management. Chronic conditions such as cardiac and pulmonary compromise may diminish a patient's ability to tolerate recumbency, surgery, and rehabilitation. The elderly typically have a higher number of medical comorbidities, and they are also on medications that can affect their health status, injury risks, and response to injuries and treatments [4].

Frequently, elderly patients may have inadequate cardiac and pulmonary reserves, which may not be evident until their physiology is significantly stressed during trauma. In patients over 60 years of age, there is typically a lower cardiac index as well as a lower amount of oxygen delivery and consumption [5]. Furthermore, the elderly also have been found to have a higher risk of developing ARDS following trauma [6]. These findings suggest that, in situations where their physiology is significantly stressed, the elderly may have a higher risk of mortality.

Anesthetic considerations must be taken into account when surgical treatment is selected. The American Society of Anesthesiologists (ASA) has developed a rating system for determining preoperative risks. This rating is considered to be a snapshot of the patient's "acute" medical condition as opposed to the absolute number of medical comorbidities, which portray the patient's "chronic" medical condition. These factors should be considered when planning treatment strategies for patient care. A patient's medical status can affect their intraoperative tolerance and response to surgical intervention and other orthopaedic treatments. For example, patients may develop hypotension during the cementing portion of hip arthroplasty. An elderly patient with little physiologic reserve may not tolerate such stresses, resulting in further cardiac and potential cerebrovascular insults.

Many orthopaedic procedures can be performed with either general or spinal anesthesia. Reports have shown no difference in mortality with either one [7–9]. However, some literature has demonstrated some differences in other outcome measures. Regional anesthesia has been shown to reduce acute postoperative confusion [9]. Covert found that the use of regional anesthesia increases the magnitude and frequency of hypotensive episodes when compared with general anesthesia. Following hip fracture surgery under spinal anesthesia, their patients exhibit better oxygenation in the early postoperative period than that after general anesthesia. These authors also

W. Min (✉)
Department of Orthopaedic Surgery, NYU Hospital for Joint Diseases, 301 E. 17th Street, New York, NY 10003, USA
e-mail: william.min@nyumc.edu

R.A. Rosenthal et al. (eds.), *Principles and Practice of Geriatric Surgery*,
DOI 10.1007/978-1-4419-6999-6_94, © Springer Science+Business Media, LLC 2011

found that the incidence of deep venous thrombosis is reduced following spinal anesthesia as compared with general anesthesia, and that they had less intraoperative blood loss (but, general anesthesia with controlled hypotension also reduced their amount of blood loss). However, they found that their 1-month mortality rate, approximately 8%, was unrelated to anesthetic technique [10].

The presence of diabetes mellitus has been shown to increase the risk of wound complications (dehiscence, infection) and cause delayed fracture union [11]. Additional complications, such as malunion and Charcot arthropathy, are prevalent in this patient population [12]. Peripheral vascular disease can also contribute to wound complications. These medical comorbidities, combined with skin conditions (changes in skin turgor and friability), frequently found in the elderly can result in soft-tissue complications, especially if the patient becomes sedentary or is immobilized in a cast for prolonged periods.

Thromboembolic disease is a significant threat, especially with lower extremity injury and surgery. Coupled with additional cardiopulmonary comorbidities, complications associated with a thromboembolic event can be devastating. Elderly patients may have associated risk factors that may heighten their chance of sustaining a thromboembolic event. It is imperative that either chemoprophylaxis or mechanoprophylaxis (or both) be implemented during the course of patient management. The current recommendations set forth by the American College of Chest Physicians (ACCP) are listed in Table 94.1 [13, 14].

In the elderly, the incidence of deep-vein thrombosis and pulmonary embolism is higher due to the greater frequency of risk factors. With the armamentarium of treatments available, including heparin, low-molecular-weight heparin, oral anticoagulants, consideration for treatment must be guided based on the clinical presentation, risk factors, and social conditions. Older patients may be at increased risk for

TABLE 94.1 Current DVT risk factors and prophylaxis from the ACCP

Risk factor points	Risk factors
1 Point	Minor surgery. Age 41–60, history of major surgery within 1 month. Pregnancy or postpartum within 1 month. Varicose veins. Inflammatory bowel disease. Leg swelling. BMI >25. Oral contraceptive use. Hormone replacement therapy
2 Points	Age >60 years. Malignancy or current chemotherapy or radiation therapy. Major or laparoscopic surgery (>45 min). Confined to bed >72 h. Immobilizing cast <1 month. Central venous access <1 month. Tourniquet time >45 min
3 Points	History of DVT or PE, Family history of thrombosis. Age >75 years. Factor V Leiden/activated protein C resistance. Risk factors of myocardial infarction, congestive heart failure, or chronic obstructive pulmonary disease. Congenital or acquired thrombophilia
5 Points	Major, elective lower extremity arthroplasty TKR, THR, Hip, pelvis or leg fracture within 1 month. Stroke within 1 month. Multiple trauma within 1 month. Acute spinal cord injury with paralysis within 1 month

Risk factor points total	Recommendations
1 or less (low-risk)	Early and aggressive mobilization
2 or less (moderate-risk)	LDUH q12h, LMWH <3,400 U daily, and GCS or IPC
3 or 4 (high-risk)	LDUH q8, LMWH >3,400 U daily, with or without IPC
5 or greater (highest risk)	LMWH >3,400 U daily, fondaparinux, and coumadins (INR 2–3). Dose-adjusted LDUH or LMWH may be used with or without IPC

Additional recommendations	
For elective THA	LMWH 12 h pre-operatively and/or 12–24 h after surgery, or 4–6 h after surgery at one half the dose initially followed by a full dose on the next day. Alternatively, fondaparinux (2.5 mg) started 6–8 h postoperative or coumadin started preoperatively or after surgery (INR target 2.5, range 2–3). Aspirin, dextran or IPC alone not recommended
For elective TKA	LWMH 12–24 h postoperative, fondaparinux 2.5 mg started 6–8 h post-operatively, or adjusted-dose warfarin administered preoperative and/or postoperatively and with INR range of 2–3 (target INR of 2.5). Optional use of IPC devices intraoperatively or immediately postoperatively. LDUH not recommended for sole use as prophylaxis
For hip fractures	LMWH or fondaparinux or adjusted-dose warfarin immediately administered postoperatively, with a target INR of 2.5 (range of 2–3) if bleeding is controlled; LDUH may be alternative (limited data). Aspirin alone is not recommended
For knee arthroscopy	No routine prophylaxis. Early mobilization. LMWH for patients with additional preexisting risk factors for DVT or prolonged tourniquet time
For elective spine surgery	No routine prophylaxis. High-risk patients should be treated with LDUH, LMWH, or perioperative IPC

BMI body mass index; DVT deep venous thrombosis; IPC intermittent pneumatic compression; LDUH low-dose unfractionated heparin; LMWH low molecular weight heparin; PE pulmonary embolism; THA total hip arthroplasty; TKA total knee arthroplasty. Source: Data from Ennis [123]

anticoagulant-related bleeding for several reasons: increased anticoagulant effect of warfarin, increased prevalence of comorbidity, and incidence of adverse drug reactions. The indications for use of an inferior vena cava filter are wider in the older age group, not only for those in whom heparin is contraindicated, or has failed, but also for those who require treatment indefinitely with contraindications to oral anticoagulant [15].

The patient's cognitive status pre- and postinjury is of significant importance when caring for the elderly. Since orthopaedic injuries and treatments usually require protracted physical therapy and rehabilitation, it is necessary for patients to comprehend instructions, clearly communicate, and perform multiple tasks. These requirements are further complicated by the effect of medications on elderly cognition. Individuals with Alzheimer's disease, cognitive deficits from cerebrovascular insults, Parkinson's disease, and other forms of dementia will have difficulty participating in the therapy required to attain preinjury functional status and may lead to a negative outcome in some instances. Their inability to meet rehabilitation goals may result in diminished functional and medical gains. These factors are important considerations when determining the feasibility and appropriateness of operative intervention. A radiographically perfect result does not always translate into a good functional outcome. For example, a comminuted distal radius fracture treated nonoperatively may result in suboptimal radiographic reduction, but their inability to cope with a lengthy rehabilitation course and associated operative complications makes the risks inherent with operative treatment more significant than the functional limitations potentially afforded by nonoperative modalities. In contrast, a patient with preinjury hemiplegia who sustains a humeral shaft fracture may not tolerate long-term immobilization of the functional upper extremity (the standard treatment) and may benefit from surgical intervention to allow earlier weight bearing, with use of the affected extremity for transfers and assisted ambulation.

Decreased bone mass, or osteopenia, is often seen in older patients and is often the result of osteoporosis or osteomalacia. Osteoporosis is a decrease in bone density that does not affect mineralization, while osteomalacia results from decreased bone mineralization with or without changes in bone density. In either situation, less loading and stress are required to cause fractures as compared to normal bone. Factors affecting bone density, such as sedentary life, excessive consumption of alcohol, smoking, certain medications (antiseizure medications such as phenytoin, primidone, and phenobarbital, and certain selective serotonin reuptake inhibitors) and comorbid conditions (i.e., renal disease, malnutrition), also contribute to the patient's overall medical condition [16, 17]. Not only should elderly patients with osteoporotic fractures be treated for those injuries but also with chemoprophylaxis and preventative measures to decrease the risk for future fractures [18]. However, the cornerstone of adequately treating and minimizing the effects of osteoporosis and related conditions is adequate intake of calcium and vitamin D.

Osteopenia presents a problem with fracture stabilization and healing. It is difficult to attain stable fixation in fracture fragments that have decreased bone mass. Stable internal fixation is imperative to allow for early joint range of motion, weight bearing, and therapy without risking fracture displacement. Additionally, osteopenia increases the risk for nonunion since fracture callus in these patients is less dense and poorly organized. Fractures that have tenuous fixation, especially in the lower extremity, may preclude early ambulation, by protracting immobilization; further, "disuse" osteopenia may result.

Bone remodels according to Wolff's law, and the removal of external stresses can lead to significant bone loss. This situation can be reversed to varying degrees upon remobilization and reloading. Additionally, the use of hormone replacement therapy (HRT) is another option in treating bone loss. HRT's effects were investigated by the Women's Health Initiative Study Group. Their investigators found that women taking HRT had 34% fewer hip fractures and 24% fewer fractures than women not receiving hormones. However, the short-term use of HRT to relieve symptoms at the time of menopause does little to prevent fractures in women when they reach 75–80 years of age. Women who take estrogen to maintain bone density must continue taking estrogen because the beneficial effects on bones disappear when it is discontinued. Estrogens are still used to prevent osteoporosis but are not approved to treat a woman who has already been diagnosed with the condition [19].

When presented with osteoporotic patients, orthopaedic surgeons now have certain tools available to aid in the treatment of their injuries. Some of these include: the use of methylmethacrylate (cement) to augment screw fixation and the use of allograft and synthetic bone graft that act in an osteoconductive manner in situations of excessive bone loss [20, 21]. Calcium phosphate implants and cements have also been shown to be another adjuvant to treat these challenging fractures [22]. However, the recent introduction of locked plating technology and its theoretical enhanced fixation in osteoporotic bone has allowed for more secured fracture fixation, which may promote earlier mobilization and ambulation [23, 24].

Minimizing the complications of osteoporosis begins with medical treatment; the mainstay of which is calcium and vitamin D supplementation. In postmenopausal women, calcium supplementation alone can reduce the rate of loss or even increase bone mass. Women with osteoporosis who are older or have low calcium intake show the most benefit from calcium supplementation. The National Institutes of Health Consensus Conference recommends 1,000 mg of calcium a day for women of 65 years of age and younger on estrogen

HRT, and 1,500 mg a day for women younger than 65 and not on estrogen HRT and for women older than 65 years of age. The most commonly used form of calcium supplementation is calcium carbonate, such as OsCal 500 or TUMS. Additionally, vitamin D deficiency is common in the elderly, often from a poor diet, low exposure to sunlight, or aging skin's inability to synthesize vitamin D3. Vitamin D, 400 IU per day, should be added in these cases [25].

Estrogen replacement therapy stimulates bone formation, prevents bone loss, and has been shown to reduce the risk of fractures in various groups of women. For women who have retained their uterus, estrogen must be supplemented with progestin therapy to prevent potential changes in uterine tissue. Estrogen HRT may also alleviate menopausal symptoms and prevent heart disease. However, it may also increase the risk of breast cancer [25].

Bisphosphonates are a class of medications currently utilized to treat osteoporosis. Their mechanism of action is through the inhibition of osteoclasts, which are cells responsible for the resorption of bone. Examples of bisphosphonates include etidronate, pamidronate, and alendronate. Alendronate (Fosamax) has been shown to decrease the rate of bone mineral density loss at all skeletal sites and decrease the rate of fractures. However, the medication must be taken on an empty stomach and may cause gastrointestinal discomfort. It should not be taken by patients with a history of swallowing difficulties or abnormal narrowing of the esophagus [25].

Other pharmacologic treatment options include selective estrogen receptor modulators (SERM), which are used for breast cancer, those seeking alternatives for HRT, and osteoporosis. One type of SERM currently used to treat osteoporosis is raloxifene (Evista). This medication has demonstrated a beneficial effect on bone mineral density and is well tolerated. It is contraindicated in women who are pregnant or have a history of deep venous thromboses. Raloxifene has been found to cause an increase in BMD of the total body and hip similar to estrogen HRT, but has less of an effect on BMD of the lumbar spine. Raloxifene has also been shown to lower LDL cholesterol and is being studied as a way to prevent breast cancer [25].

Alternative medications to treat osteoporosis include calcitonin and parathyroid hormone (PTH) agonists. Approved for the treatment, but not prevention, of osteoporosis, calcitonin has been shown to prevent loss of spinal BMD, decrease the rate of vertebral fractures in women with osteoporosis, and possibly provide pain relief in some patients with fractures [25]. Calcitonin is a potent inhibitor of osteoclastic bone resorption; however, osteoclasts are able to escape from the inhibitory effects of calcitonin following continued exposure. Conversely, PTH agonists function as an anabolic agent to increase bone mass. A recent study has demonstrated that while PTH does decrease vertebral fractures and increase spinal bone density in postmenopausal osteoporosis and glucocorticoid-induced osteoporosis, this occurs at the expense of a decrease in radius bone density [26]. The long-term safety and nonvertebral fracture efficacy are still unknown [26, 27].

The patient's preinjury ambulatory and function status can determine the type or the need for operative intervention. Studies have demonstrated that the ability of a patient to return to their preinjury level of ambulation and function is dependent upon their preexisting functional level, timing and type of operative treatment, and postoperative rehabilitation [28–31]. In Hagino's study, they determined the following factors that significantly affected walking ability at the time of discharge for elderly hip-fracture patients: (1) age, (2) dementia, (3) residence before injury, (4) anemia, (5) electrolyte abnormality, (6) abnormal chest X-ray, and (7) chronic systemic disease. A scoring system based on these factors was able to predict the ambulation prognosis for these patients [32].

While elderly patients may have fractures that appear to be similar to those of younger patients, the comorbidities, physiologic reserves, and functional status make the musculoskeletal injury more than just "a simple fracture." The elderly patient's ability to cope with the metabolic and physiologic demands placed from these injuries is often poorer than their younger counterparts, and as such, treatment must incorporate a multidisciplinary approach. Understanding the preinjury level of function and comorbid status is imperative to work toward the goal of reestablishing the patient's functionality. A multidisciplinary approach must be taken with input from the orthopaedic surgeon, geriatrician, anesthesiologist, physiatrist, therapist, and the caregiver.

Considerations in Elderly Trauma

The treatment of the geriatric trauma patient assumes a more complex role due to the associated comorbidities and functional status impairments seen in the aged. The incidence of geriatric trauma is expected to increase, partly due to the increases in the elderly population and also the increased levels of activity seen in this patient group. Therefore, in treating the elderly traumatic patient, it is important to factor in the following considerations.

While only compromising approximately 12% of the population, elderly patients account for approximately 28% of traumatic deaths. Elderly patients had twice the higher rate of mortality (after adjusting for Injury Severity Score and the Revised Trauma Score), and they were also more likely to succumb later [33].

While earlier literature had stated that the Injury Severity Score did not correlate to mortality in older patients, these studies were from series that included lower energy trauma (such as slips and falls) into their overall study groups. However, if these injuries are excluded and then the actual traumatic mechanisms are examined, it has been conclusively demonstrated that the Injury Severity Scores correlate to mortality [34]. Additionally, Gallagher found that for patients older than sixty with Injury Severity Scores greater than fifteen, there was a 28% morbidity rate, a 36% 2-year mortality rate, and a 60% 2-year complication rate, with mortality rates increasing with patient age [35].

The timing of operative management of the elderly traumatic patient has been the subject of continued controversy. While medical optimization is necessary to minimize perioperative risks for the elderly, delays in operative management have been found to lead to significant increases in morbidity and mortality [28–31, 36]. However, the key to minimizing morbidity and mortality is to perform surgical intervention as soon as the patient is medically stabilized and adequately resuscitated. In the event that patients cannot obtain definitive treatment for their orthopaedic injuries due to underresuscitation, damage-control orthopaedics (by use of temporizing external fixation) may play a significant role.

In the past 30 years, the role of the "trauma center" has played a vital part in the care and treatment of multiply injured patients. Recent studies have also shown that they, along with centers capable of aggressive intensive-care monitoring, have played a significant role in the care of the elderly traumatic patient. Meldon examined the Glasgow Coma Scale, the Injury Severity Score, and the role of acute care in octogenarians in different admission settings. He found that patients with an Injury Severity Score of 21–45 had a 56% survival rate if directly admitted to trauma centers as compared to an 8% survival rate if admitted directly to a community institution [37]. Other studies have also stressed the importance of referring traumatic elderly patients who require adequate resuscitation and monitoring to the appropriate facility initially, as delays in treatment and transfer resulted negatively in mortality rates [38].

Hip Fractures

General Principles

Hip fractures in the elderly can be devastating or fatal, and their effects on the patient's functional and psychological status are significant. Currently, 250,000 hip fractures, at a total medical expenditure of approximately 9 billion dollars, occur annually in the United States. By 2040, 20% of the population will be older than 65 years of age, and the incidence of hip fractures is expected to double by the year 2050 due to aging trends [39–41].

As individuals age, their chance of sustaining a hip fracture greatly increases, doubling every decade after 50 years. Hip fractures occur twice as often in females and are most frequently seen in Caucasian women (followed by Caucasian men, Afro-American women, and Afro-American men). This may be due to differences in bone density between different ethnic groups [42–44]. Institutionalized patients are also more likely to sustain hip fractures [45–47].

Typically, hip fractures in the elderly occur from low-energy trauma (i.e., fall while walking on a flat surface). They can be intracapsular (femoral neck) or extracapsular (intertrochanteric or subtrochanteric). The location of the hip fracture has a significant impact on the healing potential of the fracture, and this has led to different methods of operative fixation. Vascularity is more significantly compromised with intracapsular fractures, and as such, the role of arthroplasty remains an integral treatment option as compared to extracapsular fractures. More than 90% of hip fractures in patients over 65 are femoral neck or intertrochanteric in origin with a slight predominance for intertrochanteric fractures in the octogenarians [48].

Presentation and Management

Patients usually complain of hip and groin pain with an inability to bear weight on the affected extremity after sustaining a relatively low-energy fall. The supine patient will hold the affected extremity externally rotated with slight flexion at the hip; this position will present with a noticeable leg-length discrepancy. This position is one that yields the maximal capsular volume when there is a fracture hematoma, thus providing the most comfort [49].

During the evaluation of the patient, it is imperative that the physician ascertain the length of time from the onset of injury to presentation. Elderly patients who have been in positions of recumbency for prolonged periods will present with significant dehydration and electrolyte imbalance. These factors must be corrected before operative intervention. Additionally, the presence of pressure ulcers, rhabdomyolysis, and deep vein thromboses are likely following prolonged periods of immobilization. Evaluation of bony prominences, creatine phosphokinase, and Doppler ultrasonography, respectively, are warranted in any patient who presents after being "down" for an extended period of time.

A throughout physical evaluation should include a neurovascular exam of the affected extremity, examination of each extremity and the spine for other injuries, documentation of any loss of consciousness, mental status exam, and assessment of skin integrity in appropriate areas. Medical consultation should be obtained to prepare the patient for possible surgery. Injury films, baseline labs, chest radiograph,

Figure 94.1 Intertrochanteric hip fracture visualized on an AP view (**a**) and cross-table lateral view (**b**) of the right hip.

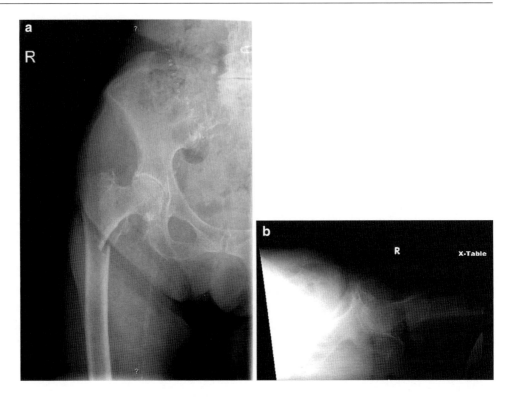

and electrocardiogram (EKG) should be attained at the time of presentation. Care should be taken when acquiring injury films, which must include an AP pelvis, a true AP of the affected hip, and a cross-table lateral of the hip (Fig. 94.1). Obtaining a frog-leg lateral in the case of a suspected hip fracture is detrimental by potentially causing pain, further displacing fracture fragments, and damaging vascular channels. Furthermore, a traction/internal rotation radiograph of the affected hip may aid in the diagnosis and surgical planning of the hip fracture [50].

Many centers have made a policy to acquire a baseline arterial blood gas (ABG) preoperatively, since hip fractures carry an inherent risk of deep venous thrombosis and pulmonary embolus (PE). However, a recent study has demonstrated that ABGs have poor positive predictive value for pulmonary embolism and add little to the positive predictive value or negative predictive value of a careful clinical examination. The study, therefore, concluded that acquisition of baseline ABGs as a routine part of the preoperative evaluation is not warranted [51].

The role of traction in hip fractures is debatable and subject to physician preference. While it may provide significant patient comfort in those with femoral shaft and subtrochanteric fractures, traction forces the hip into a less comfortable position (from its more comfortable flexed and externally rotated position). Therefore, it is not recommended that patients with hip fractures be placed into skeletal traction. To aid in patient comfort, however, a pillow under the affected limb may reduce pain. Furthermore, the

placement of a Foley catheter will eliminate the need for patient transfers to a bedpan, thereby reducing potential discomfort and further fracture displacement.

When the diagnosis of hip fracture is suspected clinically, but not clear with routine radiography, other studies are indicated. As stated before, a traction/internal rotation view will help visualize the entire length of the femoral neck. This view is conducted by shooting an AP hip radiograph as the physician pulls traction at the ankle while internally rotating the hip 15° (the average amount of anteversion seen in the adult femoral neck). Care must be taken to avoid shearing the skin of the lower extremity while performing the maneuver. If question remains, CT scans, technetium bone scans, or MRI may detect presence of an occult hip fracture. However, CT scans have been found to be an inferior modality in detecting these fractures [52]. Both MRIs and bone scans are more sensitive than plain radiography in detecting occult hip fractures, but the bone scan can only detect fractures 2–3 days after injury. On the other hand, the MRI can detect occult fractures that are less than 24 h old [53].

Nonoperative care is reserved for selected patients who are nonambulatory and too ill to undergo anesthesia. Ultimately, the preferred treatment of a hip fracture is surgery. Operative stabilization or arthroplasty will decrease the period of nonweight bearing, risk of malunion/nonunion, cardiopulmonary complications, and mortality. Additionally, operative treatment has been shown to be the most economically advantageous as compared to nonoperative treatment [54].

The risk of deep venous thrombosis (DVT) or pulmonary embolism (PE) is a concern requiring preventive measures. Historically, warfarin has been considered the standard for prophylaxis. Currently, low-molecular-weight heparin (LMWH) has been used subcutaneously with good results, without the need for constant laboratory monitoring (as is required for warfarin). LMWH can be administered within 12–24 h postsurgically. In situations that will not permit the use of pharmacologic prophylaxis, an inferior vena cava filter may be used. Studies evaluating the use of subcutaneous unfractionated heparin for DVT prophylaxis in orthopaedic patients have demonstrated less efficacy as compared to warfarin and LMWH. However, continuous intravenous infusion of unfractionated heparin has been shown to be adequate prophylaxis in patients that are started on warfarin and awaiting therapeutic INR levels [55–58]. Preoperatively, patients should be given pharmacologic and mechanical prophylaxis (i.e., venodyne boots, pneumatic compression stockings, etc.). Twelve hours prior to surgery, pharmacologic prophylaxis should be withheld (to decrease intraoperative and immediate postoperative bleeding complications) while mechanical prophylaxis should be continued.

The duration of DVT prophylaxis is still being debated. Prophylaxis is indicated while in the hospital after major surgery. There is evidence that the prevalence of asymptomatic deep vein thrombosis, detected by routine venography after major orthopedic surgery, is lower at hospital discharge in patients who have received 10 days rather than 5 days of prophylaxis. This observation supports the current ACCP recommendation for a minimum of 7–10 days of prophylaxis after hip and knee replacement, even if patients are discharged from the hospital within 7 days of surgery. As risk of DVT persists for up to 3 months after surgery, patients at high risk for postoperative DVT may benefit from extended prophylaxis (i.e., an additional 3 weeks after the first 7–10 days). Extended prophylaxis with low-molecular-weight heparin (LMWH) reduces the frequency of postdischarge DVT by approximately two-thirds after hip replacement; however, the resultant absolute reduction in the frequency of fatal pulmonary embolism is small (i.e., estimated at 1 per 2,500 patients). Indirect evidence suggests that compared with LMWH, efficacy of extended prophylaxis after hip replacement is greater with fondaparinux, similar with warfarin, and less with aspirin. Extended prophylaxis is expected to be of less benefit after knee than after hip replacement. In keeping with current ACCP recommendations, at a minimum, extended prophylaxis should be used after major orthopedic surgery in patients who have additional risk factors for DVT (i.e., previous DVT, cancer). If anticoagulant drug therapy is stopped after 7–10 days, an additional month of prophylaxis with aspirin should be considered [59].

Outcomes

As previously mentioned, the goal of hip fracture surgery is to restore the patient's functional outcome. One study showed that at 1-year follow-up, 41% of patients regained their pre-injury level of ambulatory function, 40% remained community or household ambulators but required assistive devices, 12% became solely household ambulators, and 8% became nonambulatory. The factors shown to improve the possibility of attaining the preinjury ambulatory status are outlined in Table 94.2 [28].

Initial mortality rates are increased in elderly patients with hip fracture compared to age-matched controls. One-year mortality can be as high as 25% [60, 61]. The highest rate is seen in the first 6 months, and these rates progressively decline to the same as those of age-matched controls by 1 year. Factors shown to negatively affect 1-year mortality rates are outlined in Table 94.1 [29].

Timing from injury to surgical stabilization has been a subject of debate. Multiple studies have cited conflicting recommendations, with some recommending immediate operative stabilization as the key to minimizing mortality [62]. However, other studies have also found no correlation between the delay of surgical intervention and patient mortality [63]. However, the majority of these studies have been based on retrospective reviews of patient records or heterogeneous population databases and were poorly controlled [60, 61, 64]. A prospective study from our institution, controlling for age, sex, and comorbidities, was comprised of 367 hip fracture patients who were not suffering from dementia, were capable of activities of daily living, and had ambulatory abilities prior to injury. The study demonstrated that a delay to surgical stabilization of more than two calendar days doubled mortality [30]. Similar findings were reported in a recent study by Moran that found that delays of greater than 4 days in patients medically fit for surgery led to higher mortality rates at 3 months and 1 year after injury [36]. Furthermore, another study also demonstrated that delays of operative management of hip fractures

TABLE 94.2 Hip fractures: factors influencing outcome

Factors favorable to regaining preinjury ambulatory status	Factors contributing to 1 year mortality
Age below 85 years	Age over 85 years
Preoperative ASA rating of I or II	Preoperative ASA rating of III or IV
Intertrochanteric fracture	Preinjury dependency in activities of daily living
Male sex	History of malignancy (excluding skin cancer)
Absence of dementia	Development of one or more complications during hospitalization

significantly worsened the ability to return to independent living, increased the risk of pressure ulcers, and increased the length of stay [31].

Postoperatively, disparities exist in the rehabilitation protocols outlined for these patients. Protocols range from nonweight bearing to immediate weight bearing as tolerated. Biomechanically, it has been shown that joint reactive forces are greater across the hip when comparing nonweight bearing to toe-touch weight bearing [65].

Additionally, balance and upper extremity strength are important issues to consider when asking the older adult to be limited in their weight bearing. When patients are allowed to weight bear as tolerated immediately postoperatively, they self-regulate the amount of weight on the injured extremity and gradually increase the amount of weight bearing over time [66, 67].

Femoral Neck Fractures

Femoral neck fractures occur between the base of the femoral head and the intertrochanteric line. These fractures are considered intracapsular and, due to the location of the fracture relative to the femoral vascular anatomy, have significant effects on the blood supply to the femoral head. These implications weigh heavily on treatment options and their relative success rates.

The main blood supply to the femoral head comes from branches off the medial and lateral femoral circumflex arteries (medial with much greater contribution). These arteries form an extracapsular ring at the base of the neck with ascending branches that are intracapsular, forming a network ending in bony perforators to the femoral head. The intracapsular extensions represent terminal vessels of the extracapsular ring; the ascending vessels are at significant risk during femoral neck fracture, especially when displaced. Minimal vascular contribution to the femoral head also comes from the ligamentum teres (Fig. 94.2).

Many classifications have been used to describe femoral neck fractures. The most common classification is one derived by Garden in which Types I and II are nondisplaced while types III and IV represent displaced femoral neck fractures [68] (Fig. 94.3). Rates for future osteonecrosis of the femoral head or nonunion of the femoral neck fracture have ranged between 5 and 35%, with significantly higher rates in displaced fractures (5–10% for minimally displaced versus 20–35% for displaced) [68–72]. Nonunion requires reoperation in 75% of cases, while osteonecrosis requires revision surgery in only 30% of cases.

Surgery is the treatment of choice for this injury. In situ pinning should be performed for only minimally displaced/impacted fractures. Although these are inherently stable, they do have an 8–40% chance of displacement without

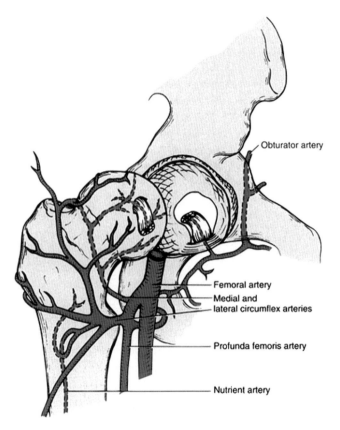

FIGURE 94.2 Contributing vessels to the major sources of blood supply to the proximal femur. Reprinted with permission from Browner, Jupiter, Levine, Trafton (2003) Skeletal trauma: basic science, management and reconstruction, 3rd ed. WB Saunders, Philadelphia. Copyright Elsevier (2003).

operative stabilization [73, 74]. Postoperatively, all patients should be allowed to weight-bear as tolerated with assistive devices, especially due to the difficulty the elderly have in following weight-bearing, gait, and balance guidelines. Furthermore, these patients will regulate their weight bearing based on pain [67].

In displaced fractures, obtaining and maintaining an adequate reduction with pinning is not always possible or advisable. In a physiologically younger patient, all efforts should be made for closed reduction and pinning, but in a physiologically older patient, there is a lower threshold for arthroplasty. This lower threshold is partly due to the lower demands that physiologically older patients would place on the implant, increasing its longevity. In a recent meta-analysis comparing internal fixation and arthroplasty for displaced femoral neck fractures, the authors found that arthroplasty significantly reduces the risk of revision surgery, but at the cost of greater infection rates, blood loss, and operative time [75].

Early reports raised concern for increased operative times and higher dislocation rates for primary total hip arthroplasty when performed for fractures as opposed to degenerative joint disease [56, 76]. However, Blomfeldt determined that a

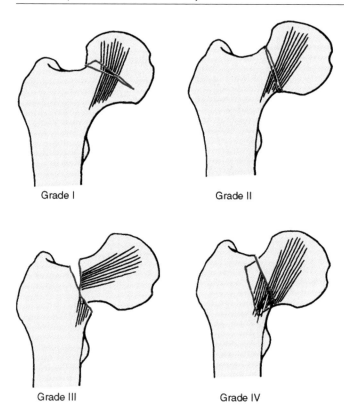

Grade I

Grade II

Grade III

Grade IV

Figure 94.3 Modification of Garden Classification of femoral neck fractures into Displaced (III and IV) and Nondisplaced (I and II) categories. Reprinted with permission from Browner, Jupiter, Levine, Trafton (2003) Skeletal trauma: basic science, management and reconstruction, 3rd ed. WB Saunders, Philadelphia. Copyright Elsevier (2003).

total hip replacement provides better function than a bipolar hemiarthroplasty at 1 year postoperatively without increase the complication rate in the elderly [77]. Before entertaining the option of hip arthroplasty, one must ascertain if the patient can follow postoperative arthroplasty precautions to avoid dislocation. Neurologically impaired or cognitively impaired patients are suboptimal candidates. Currently, total hip arthroplasty is now the treatment of choice in the active elderly and, with improved implants and surgical technique, provides results that exceed those produced by hemiarthroplasty.

In the rare case of nonoperative care for femoral neck fracture, early mobilization to a wheelchair, adequate anesthesia, decubitus precautions, and physical therapy as tolerated are begun as soon as the patient is able to tolerate such activity. However, this option results in poor outcomes and should be avoided in those that can tolerate the surgery and the rehabilitation protocol.

Intertrochanteric Fractures

The intertrochanteric region is extracapsular, distal to the femoral neck between the greater and lesser trochanters. Since this region consists of metaphyseal bone with an abundant

blood supply, there is less danger of healing complications as compared to what is noted for femoral neck fractures. An important area of the intertrochanteric region is the calcar femorale. Located posteromedially, this area is an area of dense cortical bone that acts as an internal strut for the significant forces transmitted through the hip. The disruption of this region creates an unstable fracture pattern, and therefore, the implant of choice for treatment is dependent on the integrity of the calcar femorale. The greater trochanter lies superolaterally and is the insertion site of the hip abductors and short external rotators. The lesser trochanter lies posteromedially and is the insertion site of the iliopsoas (Fig. 94.4).

It is important to determine radiographically if these fractures are stable. The ability to obtain stability is based on cortical continuity of the calcar femorale. On plain radiographs, this stability is gauged by the lesser trochanter's position. If the lesser trochanter is nondisplaced without comminution, then the fracture is termed stable while displacement and comminution represents an unstable fracture. Other markers of instability include fractures that propagate from a superomedial to inferolateral direction (also known as "reverse obliquity" fractures), fractures with excessive posterior sag, and intertrochanteric fractures that extend into the subtrochanteric region. Reduction attempts to establish stability are performed with axial traction, and progression from abduction to adduction. Internal rotation will lock the fracture fragments while axial traction is maintained in adduction [78] (Fig. 94.5).

Surgery is the treatment of choice for almost all intertrochanteric fractures. Indications and goals for nonoperative treatment are similar to those mentioned for femoral neck fractures, but it should be noted that these fractures are often more difficult to manage nonoperatively because of pain and deformity associated with excessive muscle pull and fracture displacement. Closed reduction is attempted after spinal or general anesthesia has been initiated, usually on a fracture table. If reduction is unobtainable by closed means, an open reduction is performed. Commonly, a device incorporating a sliding screw and barrel inserted into the femoral neck with an accompanying side plate (also known as the "sliding hip screw") or intramedullary component is used. The telescoping nature of the implant supplies stability and facilitates compression across the fracture site to stimulate bony healing. The intramedullary devices are currently recommended for more unstable intertrochanteric fracture patterns, while the sliding hip screw design is more appropriate for stable fractures. Currently, lesser trochanteric fractures are not reduced and stabilized with hardware [79].

Rarely, primary prosthetic replacement is indicated in cases of severe comminution. This implant differs from traditional arthroplasty components due to the disruption of the calcar femorale (a necessary structure for traditional arthroplasty components). Implanting these prostheses is associated

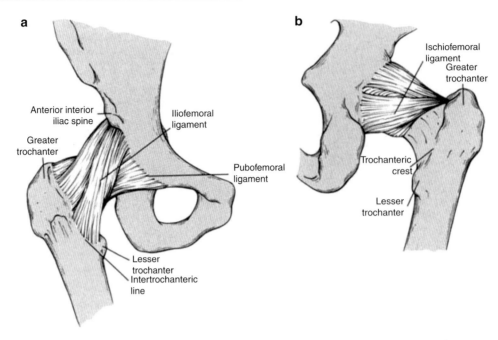

FIGURE 94.4 Hip joint with significant structures and capsule. Anterior (**a**) and Posterior (**b**). Reprinted with permission from Browner, Jupiter, Levine, Trafton (2003) Skeletal trauma: basic science, management and reconstruction, 3rd ed. WB Saunders, Philadelphia. Copyright Elsevier (2003).

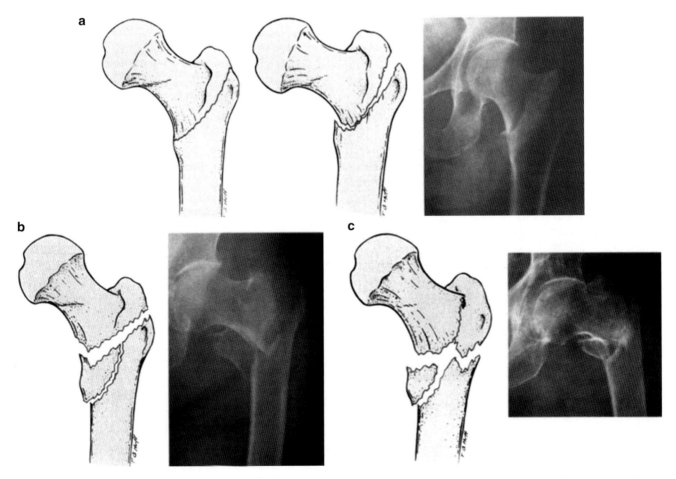

FIGURE 94.5 Nondisplaced and displaced stable (**a**) and unstable (**b**) intertrochanteric fractures. Reprinted with permission from Browner, Jupiter, Levine, Trafton (2003) Skeletal trauma: basic science, management and reconstruction, 3rd ed. WB Saunders, Philadelphia. Copyright Elsevier (2003).

with prolonged operative time, increased blood loss, and higher rates of dislocation as compared to elective total hip arthroplasties [79].

Subtrochanteric Fractures

The subtrochanteric region of the femur lies in the first 5 cm of the femur distal to the lesser trochanter. Fractures in this area are less frequent in the elderly than femoral neck or intertrochanteric fractures. Although these occur with high-energy situations in the young, they may follow a simple fall in aged individuals [43, 80].

Stability in these fractures is also based on the integrity of the posteromedial cortex [81]. Usually, these injuries are treated with an intramedullary nail or fixed angle sliding plate and screw implant. Osteonecrosis is rarely a concern with these extracapsular fractures [82, 83]. The challenge with operative fixation for subtrochanteric fracture lies in obtaining an anatomic reduction prior to implant insertion. The significant amount of displacement is due to the numerous deforming muscle forces in this region of the femur [84] (Fig. 94.6).

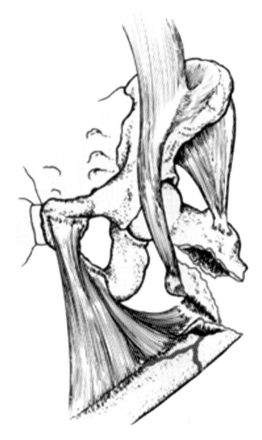

Figure 94.6 Subtrochanteric region of femur. Contributing muscle forces to displacement of fracture fragments. Reprinted with permission from Browner, Jupiter, Levine, Trafton (2003) Skeletal trauma: basic science, management and reconstruction, 3rd ed. WB Saunders, Philadelphia. Copyright Elsevier (2003).

The operative treatment for subtrochanteric fractures requires adequate reduction prior to fixation. Fixation devices include intramedullary nail devices, fixed angle devices (such as blade plates or dynamic condylar screws), and locked plate devices. The use of a sliding hip screw has been found to yield unacceptable failure rates [85, 86].

Ankle Fractures

Ankle fractures are very common fractures and on the rise in the geriatric population. The ankle joint consists of the distal aspects of the tibia and fibula (medial and lateral malleoli) and their articulation with the talar dome. The medial malleolus is connected to the navicular, calcaneus, and talus by the superficial and deep layers of the deltoid ligament. The lateral malleolus is connected to the talus and calcaneus by a three-ligament complex. The tibia and fibula maintain their relationship via a ligamentous complex known as the syndesmosis (which comprises of the anterior-inferior tibiofibular ligament, the interosseous ligament, the posterior tibiofibular ligament, and the transverse ligament) located distally (Fig. 94.7). These ligaments stabilize the ankle joint, or the mortise, by opposing the fibula in the fibular notch (also known as the incisura fibularis tibiae).

Injuries to the ankle can occur by many mechanisms, with the majority being low-energy rotational injuries [87, 88]. Frequently, ligamentous and bony injury can result from a twisting mechanism. Injuries can be bony, ligamentous, or a combination of both. Because bony and/or ligamentous injuries may both produce an unstable ankle joint, negative radiographs do not clearly rule out the presence of an unstable joint. If ligamentous injury is suspected due to signs and symptoms medially in the presence of an isolated fibular fracture, an external rotation stress radiograph should be considered [89].

Patients with ankle injuries often complain of an inability to stand or ambulate along with tenderness around the ankle joint following trauma. The patient may present with swelling and ecchymosis around the ankle. The circumstances of the injury must be elicited to establish the mechanism of injury. Many injuries that may be overlooked during the evaluation of ankle fractures should be excluded through a screening exam. These include fractures of the proximal fibula, lateral process of the talus, anterior process of the calcaneus, and proximal fifth metatarsal [90]. A standard radiographic series includes three views of the ankle joint (AP, lateral, and mortise (15° internal rotation view)) and full-length tibia/fibula films to exclude syndesmotic injury (also known as a Maisonneuve fracture, noticed by a fracture along the proximal fibula). Foot films may also be considered if the physical examination of the foot reveals suspected pathologies.

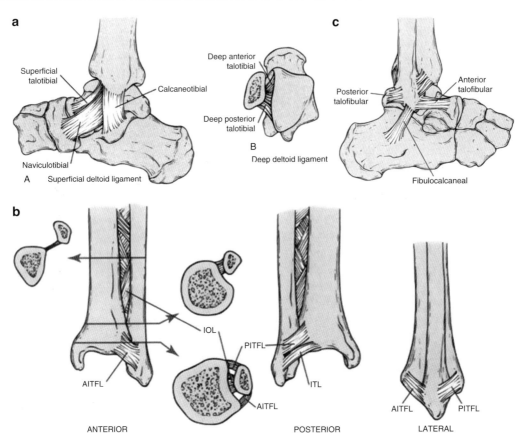

Figure 94.7 Ankle joint with ligamentous restraints: medial (**a**), syndesmosis (**b**), and lateral (**c**). Reprinted with permission from Browner, Jupiter, Levine, Trafton (2003) Skeletal trauma: basic science, management and reconstruction, 3rd ed. WB Saunders, Philadelphia. Copyright Elsevier (2003).

Treatment of ankle fractures depends on the mechanism of injury and stability of the fracture. An isolated fibula fracture occurring at or below the level of the tibia–talus articulation without medial-sided injury is considered stable and may be treated in a short leg cast or brace with early weight bearing. Fractures that are considered unstable are bimalleolar, bimalleolar equivalents, or those with a disruption of the syndesmosis (i.e., high fibula fracture with medial joint line tenderness, widening of the medial clear space of the tibia–talus articulation, or dissociation of the tibia–talus or tibia–fibula articulations). Slight malreduction may result in degenerative arthritis [89]. Surgery provides a stable reduction and allows the patient to begin early joint range of motion to help avoid later stiffness and risk of malreduction. In contrast with nonoperatively treated patients, surgically treated patients do not require long-leg immobilization and can be more easily mobilized with assistive devices.

Operative intervention has been shown to achieve better fracture position and better patient satisfaction, although complications with hardware loosening have been seen in women with osteoporosis [91, 92]. The presence of diabetes, vasculopathy, or history of smoking increases the risk for soft-tissue complications (i.e., infection, wound dehiscence, etc.) with surgery.

Proximal Humerus Fractures

Proximal humerus fractures are frequently encountered in the geriatric population and occur four times more commonly in women [94]. Typically resulting from low-energy falls, the initial treatment of these fractures frequently requires immobilization, which interferes with activities of daily living. The majority of these fractures are stable and are best treated nonoperatively.

The shoulder joint has a complex bony and soft tissue relationship. The round humeral head articulates with the relatively flatter and shallower glenoid to form a joint that, while able to enjoy a relatively larger and more unrestricted range of motion, relies heavily on its soft-tissue connections for its stability. The shoulder capsule envelops this joint to provide static stability. Superficial to the capsule, the rotator

Figure 94.8 Shoulder joint with representation of rotator cuff restraints. Anterior and posterior views (from http://www.nlm.nih.gov/medlineplus/ency/imagepages/19622.htm).

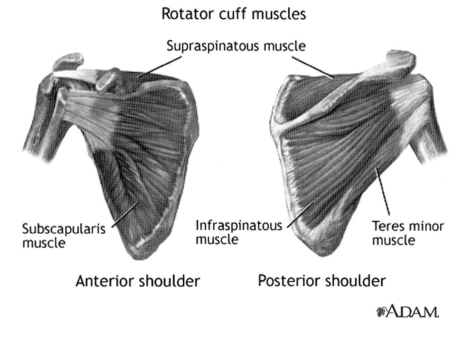

Rotator cuff muscles

Supraspinatous muscle

Subscapularis muscle

Infraspinatous muscle

Teres minor muscle

Anterior shoulder   Posterior shoulder

ADAM.

cuff, composed of the supraspinatus, infraspinatus, teres minor, and subscapularis (Fig. 94.8), with the help of the deltoid and scapular rotators, provide dynamic stability to the shoulder throughout its active range of motion. Each of these rotator cuff muscles insert into specific points on the humeral head, and each provide a direct of motion and stabilization integral for proper shoulder function.

Proximal humeral fractures result in relatively predictable fragments or parts based upon anatomic regions. Typically, they result in fragments that can be separated out as the humeral head, the greater tuberosity, the lesser tuberosity, and the shaft. Because of the typical insertion of the rotator cuff on some of these fragments, the pull of these muscles causes predictable directional displacement of these fracture fragments. As it is obvious to see that these fractures will affect the tension and function of these rotator cuff muscles, poorly treated proximal humerus fractures can significantly affect shoulder function and, therefore, patient outcome.

Patients with proximal humerus fractures complain of an inability to move the arm secondary to pain. During assessment of these fractures, it is imperative that a thorough neurovascular examination documents the presence of intact vascularity (distal pulses may be intact despite vascular injury about the shoulder due to the rich collateral flow) and sensation about the lateral aspect of the deltoid (to rule out damage to the axillary nerve or musculocutaneous nerve). While it will be difficult to assess deltoid strength to document axillary nerve integrity, the patient may be capable of slightly tensing their deltoid to demonstrate the nerve's function.

To adequately assess proximal humerus fractures radiographically, the physician should obtain at minimum three views of the shoulder. The shoulder "trauma series" includes the anteroposterior (AP), scapular "Y," and axillary views. Of particular importance is the axillary view, which is imperative to adequately document the presence of associated dislocations of the humeral head. However, the axillary view, unlike the AP and scapular "Y" views, is not the view used to measure the amount of fracture displacement or angulation [94].

Minimally displaced fractures represent 80–85% of what is seen in the elderly for injuries to the proximal humerus [95]. Provided that the fracture fragments move as "a unit" on clinical examination, it can be assumed that the surrounding soft tissues and periosteum provide stability. As such, these injuries can be treated with a brief period of sling immobilization (for approximately 1 week), followed by range-of-motion exercises (progressing from passive to active-assisted over 4–6 weeks). Minimally displaced proximal humerus fractures usually result in pain-free union [96, 97]. It is important to initiate early mobilization (as early as 72 h to less than 2 weeks) for impacted fracture that are treated nonoperatively, as it has been shown to help with quicker restoration of the physical capability and performance of the injured arm as compared to longer periods of immobilization (prior to commencement of therapy) [98, 99].

The role of surgical intervention has recently changed due to rising patient expectations and the innovation of fixation technologies. In the past, multifragment displaced fractures that do not "move as a unit" on exam were occasionally treated nonoperatively. However, with more emphasis and importance placed on restoring the anatomy of the bony fragments with the appropriate rotator cuff tension and orientation, more of these fractures are undergoing operative treatment. Currently, the role and timing of surgery has been the subject of debate; however, if the patient is medically capable of undergoing operative treatment and will benefit from a function shoulder, then operative intervention is considered. Acute fracture/dislocations of the proximal humerus, however, should be addressed with operative intervention. Past studies had demonstrated that acute hemiarthroplasty is superior to attempting surgical stabilization and conducting delayed hemiarthroplasty [100, 101]. However, a recent study has shown no differences in outcomes associated with pain and patient satisfaction comparing acute versus delayed hemiarthroplasty. All patients had variability in outcomes related to function, and the only difference seen in delayed hemiarthroplasty was increased amounts of scar tissue during the surgical exposure [102]. Overall, low-energy, minimally displaced fractures exhibit better functional outcome compared to high-energy three and four part fractures with associated rotator cuff injuries [103]. Prosthetic replacement results in predictable pain relief, but its ability to result in predictable functional outcomes is more variable [104, 105].

Distal Radius Fractures

Fractures of the distal radius are frequently seen in elderly patients, particularly women, who fall on an outstretched hand. Predisposing factors are osteoporosis, increased incidence of falls in the elderly, dementia, poor eyesight, decreased coordination, medications, and history of strokes or transient ischemic attacks [106].

The wrist is composed of eight carpal bones and the distal radius and distal ulna. The articulations are maintained via a complex ligamentous network on both the dorsal and volar aspects of the wrist. Important factors in predicting a patient's need for surgery and ultimate outcome include the amount of displacement of the fracture fragments (assessed by its amount of angulation, comminution, and shortening), articular surface involvement, and preinjury level of function [107]. While dorsally angulated distal radius fractures that heal in this position can lead to abnormal carpal bone kinematics that may cause significant functional limitations [108], the possibility and clinical significance for the elderly wrist to undergo such changes is questionable.

The presentation of distal radius fractures is pain, swelling, and wrist deformity. The force responsible for a distal radius injury can be transmitted proximally and can result in elbow injury. Radiographic examination should consist of PA, lateral, and oblique views of both wrists. Views of the contralateral wrist help in evaluating the adequacy of reduction.

The ability to determine the stability of a distal radius fracture was initially evaluated by the Lafontaine criteria [109]. Lafontaine suggested five factors to indicate instability: (1) initial dorsal angulation grater than 20°, (2) dorsal comminution, (3) radiocarpal intraarticular involvement, (4) associated ulna fractures, and (5) age greater than 60 years. However, recent studies have demonstrated that age was the only statistically significant risk factor in predicting secondary displacement and instability [110].

If the patient is physiologically active, has higher demands, and has an injury that involves the dominant extremity, treatment should be guided toward an anatomic reduction. Recent studies with the volar fixed-angle plate device for unstable distal radius fractures have shown it to provide stable internal fixation and allow early function [111]. However, in sedentary patients with low demands, functional outcomes are good despite the presence of deformity [112].

Common fracture patterns include: Colles (dorsally displaced articular surface with apex-volar angulation), Smith's (volarly displaced articular surface with apex-dorsal angulation), Barton's (volar or dorsal shear), nondisplaced, and concomitant fracture of the distal ulna [113] (Fig. 94.9). The goal of treatment is to restore function, enable painless range of motion, and maintain grip strength. Whether cast immobilization or surgery is conducted, finger range of motion is encouraged from the onset of injury since finger stiffness can adversely affect outcome.

Acutely, distal radius fractures should be treated with a reduction and splint immobilization to grossly maintain alignment, protect neurovascular structures, and allow for swelling. Nondisplaced or stable, reduced fractures can ultimately be treated with a short-arm cast for 4–6 weeks. When anatomic reduction cannot be obtained or maintained, surgery, with external fixation or open reduction and internal fixation, is required. Implants and devices available to maintain anatomic reduction include plates, external fixators, pins, bone grafting, and calcium phosphate cement. Some of these implants and devices are used concurrently with the other implants or in isolation, depending on the fracture personality, patient factors, and surgeon familiarity.

If an adequate reduction is not obtained and if range of motion exercises are not encouraged, the incidence of pain, stiffness, and decreased grip strength greatly increases. Anatomic reduction (stable fixation) combined with early therapy results in excellent outcomes for up to 90% of patients [114].

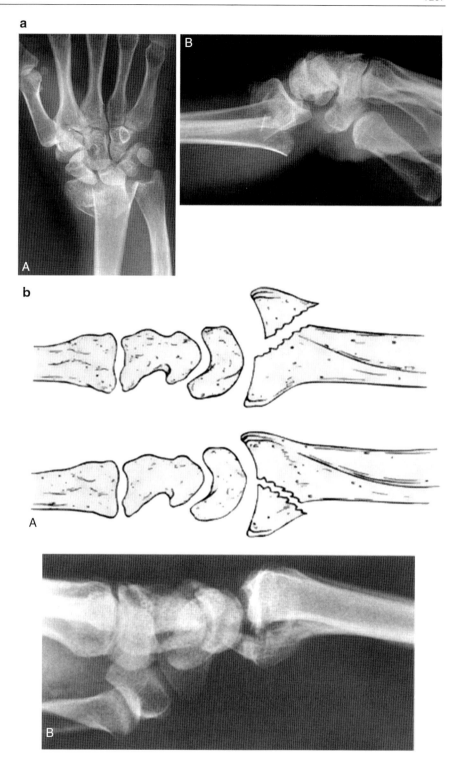

Figure 94.9 Common patterns of distal radius fractures: Colles' (**a**) and Bartons (**b**). Reprinted with permission from Browner, Jupiter, Levine, Trafton (2003) Skeletal trauma: basic science, management and reconstruction, 3rd ed. WB Saunders, Philadelphia. Copyright Elsevier (2003).

Metastatic Pathologic Fractures

As neoplasms are prevalent in the elderly, pathologic or impending fractures are relatively common. With higher rates of survival for patients with cancer, the physician should encounter more skeletal neoplasms than what was initially seen in the past. The most common form of cancer found in bone is a result of metastases [115].

Metastases usually arise from primary neoplasms in the prostate, breast, lung, kidney, and thyroid [116].

Prostate, adenocarcinoma, Hodgkin's lymphoma, and some breast cancers can be osteoblastic ("bone-forming" lesions that are radio-opaque on X-ray). Lung, kidney, thyroid, and some breast cancers are osteolytic ("bone-destroying" lesions that are radio-lucent on X-ray). Both osteoblastic and osteolytic tumors disrupt normal bony architecture and promote fractures. Most metastases affect the axial skeleton and the appendicular skeleton proximal to the knee and elbow. An exception is lung cancer, which is seen to metastasize distally. Multiple myeloma and lymphoma are common primary malignancies in older adults [117].

Nonoperative intervention includes casting and immobilization of the affected bone. Risks of immobilization include pneumonia, decubiti, and thromboembolic phenomena. Thromboembolism is especially a concern in this patient population, as their associated malignancies predispose these patients to a hypercoagulable state. Nonoperative treatment of patients with metastases is associated with higher rates of nonunion.

Operative treatment is preferable in patients with impending and completed pathologic fractures. Internal stabilization with intramedullary rods is frequently used in instances of long-bone involvement. The literature suggests a minimum life expectancy (between 1 and 3 months) for operative intervention [117, 118]. Most importantly, the goal of operative stabilization is to improve the quality of remaining life. This decision should be made following discussion between the surgeon, oncologist, patient, and caregiver. Upper extremity surgery can potentially improve independence with activities of daily living by relieving pain and providing stability. Lower extremity surgery can promote ambulation or transfers in the remainder of life. Most importantly, surgical stabilization, with or without adjunctive chemotherapy and radiotherapy, can alleviate pain.

Prior to undergoing surgery, a full-body bone scan and selected radiographs help determine sites of other metastases. Many authors advocate prophylactic internal fixation of impending pathologic fractures based on size and location of lesions [117]. The decision to proceed with prophylactic stabilization should be made based on the patient's level of function, pain, and life expectancy.

The Role of Rehabilitation

The role of rehabilitation is another important consideration in the treatment of geriatric trauma. Traumatic injuries may limit the patient's ability to ambulate and perform activities of daily living, and these limitations may lead to progressive loss of functionality, associated morbidity and mortality from prolonged recumbency, and increased length of hospital stay [31]. In addition, treatments rendered to these patients have various weight-bearing and functional restrictions, and patients must be instructed and trained within these parameters to optimize their outcomes. As such, specific rehabilitation regimens, degrees of weight-bearing tolerances, and the length of rehabilitation have been extensively discussed in the literature.

These rehabilitation services come in the form of physical and occupational therapists, social workers, case managers, and inpatient versus outpatient rehabilitation centers. The decision to use one or a combination of these services is dependent upon the patient's injury, cognitive, functional, and social support status, the presence of polytrauma, the rendered treatment(s), and the type of rehabilitation desired by the treating physician.

The role and effectiveness of an inpatient rehabilitation program in the geriatric trauma population have been examined in the literature. Kauh et al. performed a retrospective observational pilot study examining the discharge outcomes, postdischarge health care use, and death rates among patients treated in a postacute geriatric rehabilitation unit (GRU) housed within a skilled nursing facility (SNF) with those treated in a traditional SNF [119]. At discharge from the nursing facility, GRU patients showed greater improvement in activities of daily living and mobility, had a significantly shorter length of stay, and were discharged to home more often. At 1 year, GRU patients had significantly fewer hospital readmissions. While GRU patients also had fewer emergency department visits and days in the hospital at 1 year, these results were not significant. The authors concluded that GRU may be an effective means to improve patient outcomes and reduce undesirable health care use after an acute illness.

Logters et al. examined strategies for postoperative care of patients with hip fractures, which included early discharge from the acute-care hospital and inpatient interdisciplinary rehabilitation facilities [120]. This prospective study examined the patient's activities of daily living before, at the end of rehabilitation, and 1 year after trauma. In addition, patient-related variables were correlated with these results. Ninety percent of patients improved their activities of daily living during rehabilitation. However, within 1 year, 40% of patients had deteriorations in their activities of daily living. Fifty-one percent of patients were reintegrated back to their homes, and patients who lived at home before trauma and were reintegrated back to their homes had significantly better activities of daily living at 1 year after trauma than patients who were living in a nursing-care facility before the trauma. The variables of age, level of cognition, and type of fracture had no influence on the long-term outcome. However, the study also noted that an extension of rehabilitation above the mean time period did not improve the sustainable clinical outcome and that their policy for early discharge to geriatric rehabilitation is associated with extension of overall hospital stay. Therefore, the authors concluded that the benefits noted in this study should be weighed against the related increased health care costs.

However, there are other studies that do not demonstrate the benefits of inpatient rehabilitation. Koval et al. assessed the impact of an instituted intensive inpatient rehabilitation on outcomes after femoral neck or intertrochanteric fractures [121]. Comparing patients managed with an instituted inpatient rehabilitation program to those who were not, the authors noted no differences in the hospital discharge status or in the walking ability, place of residence, need for home assistance, or independence in basic and instrumental activities of daily living at the 6 and 12-month follow-up examinations.

CASE STUDY

The patient is an 85-year-old woman with a history of hypertension and coronary artery disease. She is a limited community ambulatory requiring the occasional use of a cane as an assistive device. The patient sustained a closed right distal femoral spiral fracture after a mechanical fall (Fig. 94.10). In the emergency room, the patient was placed into skeletal traction and admitted for treatment.

After the patient was medically cleared for surgical intervention, she was taken to the operating room and treated with a periarticular locked plate. The decision to use this construct was based on the osteoporotic quality of her distal femur. There were no complications intraoperatively, and the patient was kept on antibiotic prophylaxis and initiated on DVT prophylaxis with enoxaparin. A continuous passive motion (CPM) machine was instituted on the first postoperative day to initiate passive range of motion to her right knee (from 0 to 90°). The CPM machine was continued for three days after surgery to maintain knee motion. The patient was kept nonweight bearing on her affected extremity for 6 weeks. Starting on the first postoperative day, the physical therapist assisted the patient with ambulation under these weight-bearing parameters.

The patient was subsequently transferred to an inpatient rehabilitation facility four days after surgery, and progressed well with the therapy program. The patient was discharged from the facility 3 weeks after admission. Radiographic examination of her affected extremity 6 weeks after surgery revealed callus formation along the fracture site (Fig. 94.11). At this point, the patient was permitted to perform partial weight-bearing activities with assistive devices. Three months after the surgery, the patient was nontender at the fracture site, and radiographs demonstrated adequate bony healing. The patient was then allowed to bear weight as tolerated.

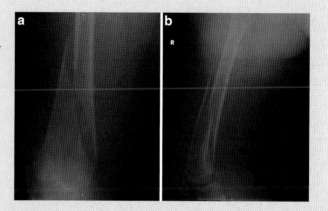

FIGURE 94.10 Right distal femur spiral fracture: AP view (**a**) and lateral view (**b**).

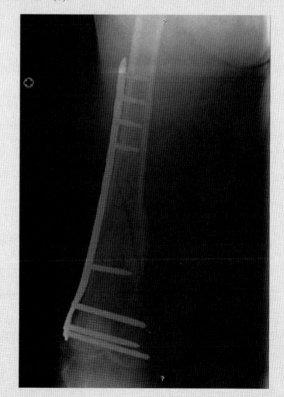

FIGURE 94.11 Right distal femur spiral fracture status-post periarticular locked plate fixation.

Conclusion

Orthopaedic injuries are responsible for significant morbidity and mortality in the geriatric population. With increasing life-expectancy trends, orthopaedic problems are likely to increase. Ideally, treatment should focus on prevention of falls and management of osteoporosis. The primary goals of treatment are to decrease pain, allow mobilization, and return the patient to their prior level of functioning. Treatment must include patient education and rehabilitation. The improvement in functional outcomes borne from these interventions has been shown to result in decreased long-term cost to the health care system [122].

Acknowledgements The authors wish to acknowledge Drs. Frank A. Liporace and Kenneth J. Koval for their work in this chapter.

References

1. Stevens JA, Olson S (2000) Reducing falls and resulting hip fractures among older women. MMWR Recomm Rep 49(RR-2):3–12
2. Kannus P, Parkkari J, Sievanen H, Heinonen A, Vuori I, Jarvinen M (1996) Epidemiology of hip fractures. Bone 18(1 suppl):57S–63S
3. Zuckerman JD (1996) Hip fracture. N Engl J Med 334:1519–1525
4. Vu MQ, Weintraub N, Rubenstein LZ (2006) Falls in the nursing home: are they preventable? J Am Med Dir Assoc 7(3 Suppl):S53–S58, 52
5. Epstein CD, Peerless J, Martin J, Malangoni M (2002) Oxygen transport and organ dysfunction in the older trauma patient. Heart Lung 31(5):315–326
6. Johnson KD, Cadambi A, Seibert GB (1985) Incidence of adult respiratory distress syndrome in patients with multiple musculoskeletal injuries: effect of early operative stabilization of fractures. J Trauma 25(5):375–384
7. Davis FM, Woolner DF, Frampton C, Wikinson A, Grant A, Harrison RT, Roberts MTS, Thakada R (1987) Prospective, multi-centre trial of mortality following general or spinal anaesthesia for hip fracture surgery in the elderly. Br J Anaesth 59:1080–1088
8. Valentin N, Lomholt B, Jensen JS, Hejgaard N, Kreiner S (1986) Spinal or general anaesthesia for surgery of the fractured hip? Br J Anaesth 58:284–291
9. Parker MJ, Handoll HH, Griffiths R (2004) Anaesthesia for hip fracture surgery in adults. Cochrane Database Syst Rev (4):CD000521
10. Covert CR, Fox GS (1989) Anaesthesia for hip surgery in the elderly. Can J Anaesth 36(3 Pt 1):311–319
11. Loder RT (1988) The influence of diabetes on the healing of closed fractures. Clin Orthop 232:210–216
12. Chaudhary SB, Liporace FA, Gandhi A, Donley BG, Pinzur MS, Lin SS (2008) Complications of ankle fracture in patient with diabetes. J Am Acad Orthop Surg 16(3):159–170
13. Geerts WM, Pineo GF, Heit JA, Bergqvist D, Lassen MR, Colwell CW, Ray JG (2004) Prevention of venous thromboembolism: the seventh ACCP conference on antithrombotic and thrombolytic therapy. Chest 126:338S–411S
14. Caprini JA, Arcelus JI, Maksimovic D, Glase CJ, Sarayba JG, Hathaway K (2002) Thrombosis prophylaxis in orthopedic surgery: current clinical considerations. J South Orthop Assoc 11(4):190–196
15. El Kouri D, Chevalet P, Hamidou M, Lemant J, Potel G (1999) Treatment of venous thromboembolic disease in the elderly. J Mal Vasc 24(3):183–188
16. Aaron JE, Gallagher JC, Anderson J et al (1974) Frequency of osteomalacia and osteoporosis in fractures of the proximal femur. Lancet 1:229–233
17. Lane JM, Vigorita VJ (1983) Osteoporosis. J Bone Joint Surg 65A:274–278
18. Gehrig L, Lane J, O'Connor MI (2008) Osteoporosis: management and treatment strategies for orthopaedic surgeons. J Bone Joint Surg Am 90(6):1362–1374
19. Heiss G, Wallace R, Anderson GL, Aragaki A, Beresford SAA, Brzyski R, Chlebowski RT, Gass M, LaCroix A, Manson JE, Prentice RL, Rossouw J, Stefanick ML, for the WHI Investigators (2008) Health risks and benefits 3 years after stopping randomized treatment with estrogen and progestin. JAMA 299(9):1036–1045
20. Jenkins DHR, Roberts JG, Webster D, Williams EO (1973) Osteomalacia in elderly patients with fracture of the femoral neck: a clinico-pathological study. J Bone Joint Surg 55B:575–580
21. Wilton TJ, Hosking DJ, Pawley E, Stevens A, Harvey L (1987) Osteomalacia and femoral neck fractures in the elderly. J Bone Joint Surg 69B:388–390
22. Moroni A, Hoang-Kim A, Lio V, Giannini S (2006) Current augmentation fixation techniques for the osteoporotic patient. Scand J Surg 95(2):103–109
23. Fulkerson E, Egol KA, Kubiak EN, Liporace F, Kummer FJ, Koval KJ (2006) Fixation of diaphyseal fractures with a segmental defect: a biomechanical comparison of locked and conventional plating techniques. J Trauma 60(4):830–835
24. Haidukewych GJ, Ricci W (2008) Locked plating in orthopaedic trauma: a clinical update. J Am Acad Orthop Surg 16(6):347–355
25. Osteoporosis: current evaluation and treatment. http://healthlink.mcw.edu/article/983292666.html. Accessed 27 Dec 2008
26. Crandall C (2002) Parathyroid hormone for treatment of osteoporosis. Arch Intern Med 162:2297–2309
27. Hesp R, Hulme P, Williams D, Reeve J (1981) The relationship between changes in femoral bone density and calcium balance in patients with involutional osteoporosis treated with human parathyroid hormone fragment hPTH (1-34). Metab Bone Dis Relat Res 2:331–334
28. Koval KJ, Skovron ML, Aharonoff GB, Meadows SE, Zuckerman JD (1995) Ambulatory ability after hip fracture: a prospective study in geriatric patients. Clin Orthop Relat Res 310:150–159
29. Aharonoff GB, Koval KJ, Skovron ML, Zuckerman JD (1997) Hip fractures in the elderly: predictors of one year mortality. J Orthop Trauma 11:162–165
30. Zuckerman JD, Skovron ML, Koval KJ, Aharanoff GB, Frankel VH (1995) Postoperative complications and mortality associated with operative delay in older patients who have a fracture of the hip. J Bone Joint Surg 77A:1551–1556
31. Al-Ani AN, Samuelsson B, Tidermark J, Norling A, Ekstrom W, Cederholm T, Hedstrom M (2008) Early operation on patients with a hip fracture improved the ability to return to independent living. A prospective study of 850 patients. J Bone Joint Surg Am 90(7):1436–1442
32. Hagino T, Sato E, Tonotsuka H, Ochiai S, Tokai M, Hamada Y (2006) Prediction of ambulation prognosis in the elderly after hip fracture. Int Orthop 30(5):315–319
33. Perdue PW, Watts DD, Kaufmann CR, Trask AL (1998) Differences in mortality between elderly and younger adult trauma patients: geriatric status increases risk of delayed death. J Trauma 45(4):805–810
34. Tornetta P III, Mostafavi H, Riina J, Turen C, Reimer B, Levine B, Behrens F, Geller J, Ritter C, Homel P (1999) Morbidity and mortality in elderly trauma patients. J Trauma 46(4):702–706

35. Gallagher SF, Williams B, Gomez C, DesJardins C, Swan S, Durham RM, Flint LM (2003) The role of cardiac morbidity in short- and long-term mortality in injured older patients who survive initial resuscitation. Am J Surg 185(2):131–134

36. Moran CG, Wenn RT, Sikand M, Taylor AM (2005) Early mortality after hip fracture: is delay before surgery important? J Bone Joint Surg Am 87(3):483–489

37. Meldon SW, Reilly M, Drew BL, Mancuso C, Fallow W Jr (2002) Trauma in the very elderly: a community-based study of outcomes at trauma and nontrauma centers. J Trauma 52(1):79–84

38. Sugimoto K, Aruga T, Hirata M, Shindo M (1999) Geriatric trauma patients at a suburban level-I trauma center in Japan. Prehosp Disaster Med 14(3):186–190

39. Brody JA (1985) Commentary: prospects for an ageing population. Nature 315:463–466

40. Frandsen PA, Kruse T (1983) Hip fractures in the county of Funen, Denmark. Implications of demographic aging and changes in incidence rates. Acta Orthop Scand 54:681–686

41. Praemer A, Furner S, Rice D (eds) (1992) Musculoskeletal conditions in the United States. The American Academy of Orthopaedic Surgeons, Park Ridge, IL

42. Greenspan SL et al (1994) Fall severity and bone mineral density as risk factors for hip fractures in ambulatory elderly. JAMA 271:128–133

43. Hinton RY, Lennox DW, Ebert FR, Jacobsen SJ, Smith GS (1995) Relative rates of fracture of the hip in the United States: geographic, sex, and age variations. J Bone Joint Surg 77A: 695–702

44. Hinton RY, Smith GS (1993) The association of age, race, and sex with the location of proximal femoral fractures in the elderly. J Bone Joint Surg 75A:752–759

45. Garraway WM, Stauffer RN, Kurland LT, O'Falba WM (1979) Limb fractures in a defined population. I. Frequency and distribution. Mayo Clin Proc 54:701–707

46. Johnell O, Sernbo I (1986) Health and social status in patients with hip fractures and controls. Age Ageing 15:285–291

47. Uden G, Nilsson B (1986) Hip fracture frequent in hospital. Acta Orthop Scand 57:428–430

48. Gallagher JC, Melton LJ, Riggs BL, Bergtrath E (1980) Epidemiology of fractures of the proximal femur in Rochester Minnesota. Clin Orthop 150:163–167

49. Bonnaire F, Schaefer DJ, Kuner EH (1998) Hemarthrosis and hip joint pressure in femoral neck fractures. Clin Orthop Relat Res 353:148–155

50. Koval KJ, Oh CK, Egol KA (2008) Does a traction-internal rotation radiograph help to better evaluate fractures of the proximal femur? Bull NYU Hosp Jt Dis 66(2):102–106

51. Susarla A, Kubiak EN, Egol KA, Karp A, Zuckerman JD, Koval KJ (2006) Predictive value of preoperative arterial blood glass evaluation for geriatric patients with hip fractures. Am J Orthop 35(2):74–78

52. Lubovsky O, Liebergall M, Mattan Y, Weil Y, Mosheiff R (2005) Early diagnosis of occult hip fractures MRI versus CT scan. Injury 36(6):788–792

53. Rizzo PF, Gould ES, Lyden JP, Asnis SE (1993) Diagnosis of occult fractures about the hip. Magnetic resonance imaging compared with bone-scanning. J Bone Joint Surg 75A:395–401

54. Parker MJ et al (1992) Cost-benefit analysis of hip fracture treatment. J Bone Joint Surg 74B(2):261–264

55. Colwell CW, Spiro TE, Trowbridge AA et al (1994) Use of enoxaparin, a low-molecular-weight heparin for the prevention of deep venous thrombosis after elective hip replacement. A clinical trial comparing efficacy and safety. Enoxaparin Clinical Trial Group. J Bone Joint Surg 76A:3–14

56. Geerts WH, Jay RM, Code KI et al (1996) A comparison of low-dose heparin with low-molecular-weight heparin as prophylaxis against venous thromboembolism after major trauma. N Engl J Med 335:701–707

57. Hull R, Delmore T, Genotn E et al (1979) Warfarin sodium versus low-dose heparin in the long-term treatment of venous thrombosis. N Engl J Med 301(16):855–858

58. Merli GJ (1993) Update deep venous thrombosis and pulmonary embolism prophylaxis in orthopaedic surgery. Med Clin North Am 77(2):397–412

59 Kearon C (2003) Duration of venous thromboembolism prophylaxis after surgery. Chest 124:386S–392S

60. Sexson SB, Lehner JT (1988) Factors affecting hip fracture mortality. J Orthop Trauma 1:298–305

61. White BL, Fischer WD, Lauren C (1987) Rates of mortality for elderly patients after fracture of the hip in the 1980s. J Bone Joint Surg 69A:1335–1340

62. Bredahl C, Nyholm B, Hindsholm FB, Mortensen JS, Olesen AS (1992) Mortality after hip fracture: results of operation within 12 h of admission. Injury 23:83–86

63. Office for National Statistics (2008) http://www.statistics.gov.uk. Accessed 9 Sept 2008

64. Kenzora JE, McCarthy RE, Lowell JD, Sledge CB (1984) Hip fracture mortality: relation to age, treatment, preoperative illness, time of surgery and complications. Clin Orthop 186:45–56

65. Frankel VH, Burstein AH, Lygre L, Brown RH (1971) The telltale nail. J Bone Joint Surg 53A:1232

66. Koval K, Friend KD, Aharanoff GB, Zuckerman JD (1996) Weightbearing after hip fracture: a prospective series of 596 geriatric hip fracture patients. J Orthop Trauma 10(8):526–530

67. Koval K, Sala DA, Kummer FJ, Zuckerman JD (1988) Postoperative weightbearing after a fracture of the femoral neck or an intertrochanteric fracture. J Bone Joint Surg Am 80(3):352–356

68. Barnes R, Brown JT, Garden RS, Nicoll EA (1976) Subcapital fractures of the femur. A prospective review. J Bone Joint Surg 58B(1):2–24

69. Schmidt AH, Swiontkowski MF (2002) Femoral neck fractures. Orthop Clin North Am 33(1):97–111

70. Cobb AG, Gibson PH (1986) Screw fixation of subcapital fractures of the femur: a better method of treatment. Injury 17:259–264

71. Garden RS (1971) Malreduction and avascular necrosis in subcapital fractures of the femur. J Bone Joint Surg Br 53B:183–197

72. Stromqvist B, Hansson LI, Nilsson LT et al (1987) Hook-pin fixation in femoral neck fractures: a two-year follow-up study of 300 cases. Clin Orthop 218:58–62

73. Bentley G (1980) Treatment of non-displaced fractures of the femoral neck. Clin Orthop 152:93–101

74. Shuqiang M, Kunzheng W, Zhichao T, Mingyu Z, Wei W (2006) Outcome of non-operative management in Garden I femoral neck fractures. Injury 37(10):974–978

75. Bhandari M, Devereaux PJ, Swiontkowski MF, Tornetta P III, Obremskey W, Koval KJ, Nork S, Sprague S, Schemitsch EH, Guyatt GH (2003) Internal fixation compared with arthroplasty for displaced fractures of the femoral neck. A meta-analysis. J Bone Joint Surg Am 85-A(9):1673–1681

76. Calder SJ, Anderson GH, Jagger C, Harper WM, Gregg PJ (1996) Unipolar or bipolar prosthesis for displaced intracapsular hip fractures in octogenarians. J Bone Joint Surg 78B:391–394

77. Blomfeldt R, Tornkvist H, Eriksson K, Soderqvist A, Ponzer S, Tidemark J (2007) A randomized controlled trial comparing bipolar hemiarthroplasty with total hip replacement for displaced intracapsular fractures of the femoral neck in the elderly patients. J Bone Joint Surg Br 89(2):160–165

78. Evans EM (1949) The treatment of trochanteric fractures of the femur. J Bone Joint Surg 31B:190–203

79. Koval KJ, Zuckerman JD (1994) Hip fractures: II. Evaluation and treatment of intertrochanteric fractures. J Am Acad Orthop Surg 2:150–156

80. Michelson JD, Myers A, Jinnah R et al (1995) Epidemiology of hip fractures among the elderly: risk factors for fracture type. Clin Orthop 311:129–135

81. Kyle RF, Cabanela ME, Russell TA et al (1995) Fractures of the proximal part of the femur. Review. Instr Course Lect 44:227–253

82. Tencer AF, Calhoun J, Miller BB (1985) Stiffness of subtrochanteric fracture of the femur stabilized using a Richards interlocking intramedullary rod or Richards AMBI. Orthop Biomech Lab Report #002. Richards Medical Co., Memphis

83. Tencer AF, Johnson KD, Johnston DWC, Gill K (1984) A biomechanical comparison of various methods of stabilization of subtrochanteric fractures of the femur. J Orthop Res 2:297–305

84. Allis OH (1891) Fracture in the upper third of the femur exclusive of the neck. Med News 59:585–589

85. Miedel R, Ponzer S, Tornkvist H, Soderqvist A, Tidermark J (2005) The standard Gamma nail or the Medoff sliding plate for unstable trochanteric and subtrochanteric fractures. A randomized, controlled trial. J Bone Joint Surg Br 87(1):68–75

86. Haynes RC, Poll RG, Miles AW, Weston RB (1997) An experimental study of the failure modes of the Gamma Locking Nail and AO Dynamic Hip Screw under static loading: a cadaveric study. Med Eng Phys 19(5):446–453

87. Lauge-Hansen N (1948) Fractures of the ankle. Analytic historic survey as basis of new experimental roentgenologic and clinical investigations. Arch Surg 56:259–317

88. Lauge-Hansen N (1950) Fractures of the ankle II. Combined experimental-surgical and experimental roentgenologic investigation. Arch Surg 60:957–985

89. Ramsey P, Hamilton W (1976) Changes in tibiotalar area of contact caused by lateral talar shift. J Bone Joint Surg 58A:356–357

90. Keene JS, Lange RH (1986) Diagnostic dilemmas in foot and ankle injuries. JAMA 256:247–251

91. Beauchamp CG, Clay NR, Thexton PW (1983) Displaced ankle fractures in patients over 50 years of age. J Bone Joint Surg 63B:329–332

92. Ali MS, McLaren AN, Routholamin E, O'Connor BT (1987) Ankle fractures in the elderly: nonoperative or operative treatment. J Orthop Trauma 1:275–280

93. Horak J, Nilsson BE (1975) Epidemiology of fractures of the upper end of the humerus. Clin Orthop Relat Res 112:250–253

94. Simon JA, Puopolo SM, Capla EL, Egol KA, Zuckerman JD, Koval KJ (2004) Accuracy of the axillary projection to determine fracture angulation of the proximal humerus. Orthopedics 27(2):205–207

95. McLaurin TM (2004) Proximal humerus fractures in the elderly are we operating on too many? Bull Hosp Jt Dis 62(1–2):24–32

96. Koval K, Gallagher MA, Marsicano JG, Cuomo F, McShinway A, Zuckerman JD (1997) Functional outcome after minimally displaced fracture of the proximal part of the humerus. J Bone Joint Surg 79A:203–207

97. Court-Brown CM, Garg A, Mc Queen MM (2001) The translated two-part fracture of the proximal humerus: Epidemiology and outcome in the older patient. J Bone Joint Surg Br 83B:799–804

98. Lefevre-Colau MM, Babinet A, Fayad F, Fermanian J, Anract P, Roren A, Kansao J, Revel M, Poiraudeau S (2007) Immediate mobilization compared with conventional immobilization for the impact nonoperatively treated proximal humeral fracture. A randomized control trial. J Bone Joint Surg Am 89(12):2582–2590

99. Koval KJ, Gallagher MA, Marsicano JG, Cuomo F, McShinawy A, Zuckerman JD (1997) Functional outcome after minimally displaced fractures of the proximal part of the humerus. J Bone Joint Surg Am 79-A:203–207

100. Bosch U, Skutek M, Fremerey RW, Tscherne H (1998) Outcome after primary and secondary hemiarthroplasty in elderly patients with fractures of the proximal humerus. J Should Elbow Surg 7:479–484

101. Goldman R, Koval KJ, Cuomo F, Gallagher MA, Zuckerman JD (1995) Functional outcome after humeral head replacement for acute three- and four-part proximal humeral fractures. J Should Elbow Surg 4(2):81–86

102. Prakash U, McGurty DW, Dent JA (2002) Hemiarthroplasty for severe fractures of the proximal humerus. J Shoulder Elbow Surg 11(5):428–430

103. Tejwani NC, Liporace F, Walsh M, France MA, Zuckerman JD, Egol KA (2008) Functional outcome following one-part proximal humeral fractures: a prospective study. J Shoulder Elbow Surg 17(2):216–219

104. Robinson CM, Page RS, Hill RM, Sanders DL, Court-Brown CM, Wakefield AE (2003) Primary hemiarthroplasty for treatment of proximal humeral fractures. J Bone Joint Surg Am 85-A(7):1215–1223

105. Mighell MA, Kolm GP, Collinge CA, Frankle MA (2003) Outcomes of hemiarthroplasty for fractures of the proximal humerus. J Shoulder Elbow Surg 12(6):569–577

106. Alffram P, Bauer G (1962) Epidemiology of fractures of the forearm. J Bone Joint Surg 44A:105–114

107. Fryckman G (1967) Fractures of the distal radius including sequelae. Acta Orthop Scand Suppl 180:1–153

108. Park MJ, Cooney WP III, Hahn ME, Looi KP, An KN (2002) The effects of dorsally angulated distal radius fractures on carpal kinematics. J Hand Surg Am 27(2):223–232

109. Lafontaine M, Hardy D, Delince P (1989) Stability assessment of distal radius fractures. Injury 20:208–210

110. Nesbitt KS, Failla JM, Les C (2004) Assessment of instability factors in adult distal radius fractures. J Hand Surg Am 29A:1128–1138

111. Orbay JL, Fernandez DL (2004) Volar fixed-angle plate fixation for unstable distal radius fractures in the elderly patient. J Hand Surg Am 29(A):96–102

112. Gehrmann SV, Windolf J, Kaufmann RA (2008) Distal radius fracture management in elderly patients: a literature review. J Hand Surg Am 33(3):421–429

113. Colles A (1814) On the fracture of the carpal extremity of the radius. Edinb Med Surg J 10:182–186

114. Villar RN, Marsh D, Righton N, Greatorex RA (1987) Three years after Colles' fracture: a prospective review. J Bone Joint Surg 69B(4):635–638

115. ACS (2008) What is bone metastasis? http://www.cancer.org/docroot/CRI/content/CRI_2_4_1X_What_Is_bone_metastasis_66.asp. Accessed 16 Dec 2008

116. Bhardwaj S, Holland JF (1982) Chemotherapy of metastatic cancer in bone. Clin Orthop Relat Res 169:34

117. Harrington KD (1986) Impending pathological fractures from metastatic malignancy: evaluation and management. Instr Course Lect 35:357–381

118. Harrington KD, Sim FH, Enis JE et al (1976) Methylmethacrylate as an adjunct in internal fixation of pathological fractures. J Bone Joint Surg 58A:1047–1055

119. Kauh B, Polak T, Hazelett S, Hua K, Allen K (2005) A pilot study: post-acute geriatric rehabilitation versus usual care in skilled nursing facilities. J Am Med Dir Assoc 6(5):321–326

120. Logters T, Hakimi M, Linhart W, Kaiser T, Briem D, Rueger J, Windolf J (2008) Early interdisciplinary geriatric rehabilitation after hip fracture: effective concept or just transfer of costs? Unfallchirurg 111(9):719–726

121. Koval KJ, Aharonoff GB, Su ET, Zuckerman JD (1998) Effect of acute inpatient rehabilitation on outcome after fracture of the femoral neck or intertrochanteric fracture. J Bone Joint Surg Am 80(3):357–364

122. Ruchlin HS, Elkin EB, Allegrante JP (2001) The economic impact of a multifactorial intervention to improve post-operative rehabilitation of hip fractures. Arthritis Rheum 45(5):446–452

123. Ennis RS (2008) Deep venous thrombosis prophylaxis in orthopedic surgery. http://emedicine.medscape.com/article/1268573-overview#Table2. Accessed 16 Dec 2008

Chapter 95
Treatment of Degenerative Joint Diseases

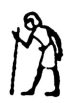

Philip J. Glassner, James Slover, and Joseph D. Zuckerman

If 60 is the new 40, then 80 is the new 60. Nowhere is this more evident than in an adult orthopedic surgery practice. As the population ages, the number of patients developing knee and hip pain is increasing. Patients are living longer and desire, and expect, to maintain high levels of activity and function throughout their lives. There are many causes of knee and hip pain in the elderly, the most common being osteoarthritis. The purpose of this chapter is to review the treatment options for this highly prevalent disease and to briefly discuss the other causes of knee and hip pain that may be encountered in elderly patients.

Osteoarthritis can be treated with nonoperative or operative modalities. Once nonoperative therapies such as nonsteroidal anti-inflammatory medications (NSAIDS), physical therapy, assistive devices, activity modification, weight loss, and injections have been exhausted, operative management should be considered. Total knee arthroplasty (TKA) and total hip arthroplasty (THA) are the most common procedures performed to maintain the quality of a patient's life. In 2004, the number of total knee and total hip arthroplasties being performed annually in the United States was approximately 478,000 and 234,000 [1], respectively. Those numbers are expected to increase dramatically to 3.48 million TKAs and 572,000 THAs by the year 2030 [2].

Excellent outcomes, as defined by pain relief and improvement in quality of life, can be obtained in well over 90% of patients with a multidisciplinary team approach to this elderly population, including internal medicine and its subspecialties, rehabilitation medicine, and the orthopedic surgeon [3–5]. Throughout the course of this chapter, we discuss the underlying pathology of knee and hip pain, the preoperative evaluation, the operation, and the postoperative protocols, along with risks, complications, and outcomes of knee and hip arthroplasty.

P.J. Glassner (✉)
Department of Orthopaedic Surgery, NYU Hospital
for Joint Diseases, New York, NY, USA
e-mail: philip.glassner@nyumc.edu

Causes of Knee and Hip Pain

The most common cause of joint pain in the elderly is osteoarthritis, a disease primarily affecting articular cartilage. Articular cartilage is composed primarily of water (65–80%), collagen (the majority being type II collagen), proteoglycans, and chondrocytes. The function of cartilage is to decrease friction in the joint and to aid in an even distribution of forces to the subchondral bone. Synovial fluid lubricates the articular cartilage and nourishes it via diffusion, as articular cartilage is avascular [6].

Osteoarthritis is characterized by changes in articular cartilage, including an increase in the water content of collagen, alterations in the proteoglycans, and a failure of the chondrocytes ability to repair the cartilage. This degenerative process increases pressure on the subchondral bone, leading to remodeling and sclerosis of the bone, the formation of osteophytes and subchondral cysts, and asymmetric joint space narrowing. These are the most common findings on radiographic evaluation. It is important to note in the evaluation process that there may be little correlation between the amount of joint degeneration seen on radiographs and the symptoms of the patient. That is to say, a patient with advanced degeneration on a radiograph may have very little pain, and vice versa. This pathologic process ultimately leads to complete destruction of the articular cartilage, with bone-on-bone contact, and a stiff, painful joint.

Another important component of the knee joint is the meniscus, which also aids in load distribution. It is a C-shaped fibrocartilaginous structure located between the femur and the tibia. Originally, the meniscus was thought to be an embryological remnant, and if torn a total meniscectomy was performed. However, in 1948, a study by Fairbank demonstrated late radiographic development of osteoarthritis following total meniscectomy [7]. More recent studies have shown a strong correlation between complete meniscectomy and poor outcomes [8,9].

Osteoarthritis is usually idiopathic, but it may be secondary to trauma, infection, ligamentous instability, osteonecrosis, or underlying metabolic and neurologic disorders. The underlying cause of joint pain may also be from a hemorrhagic arthritis, such as from hemophilia or sickle cell disease, or it may be an inflammatory process.

The inflammatory diseases that cause knee and hip arthritis include rheumatoid arthritis (RA), systemic lupus erythematous (SLE), psoriatic arthritis, spondyloarthropathies, and crystalline arthropathies. There are laboratory findings that commonly aid in the diagnosis of these conditions, such as positive rheumatoid factor (RF) in rheumatoid arthritis and SLE, and positive HLA-B27 in ankylosing spondylitis (AS). Further, there are specific physical exam findings, such as morning stiffness in RA, as well as the altered radiographic findings of symmetric joint space narrowing, osteoporosis, and protrusio acetabuli that may suggest an inflammatory arthritis. If, during the evaluation of a patient, there is concern for an inflammatory process, appropriate lab work should be obtained, and referral to a rheumatologist as indicated.

Nonoperative Management

The typical presentation of a patient with degenerative joint disease is that of an insidious onset of pain and stiffness, leading to limitations in function and a decrease in quality of life. The management of a patient depends on the clinical symptoms and findings, as well as on the radiographic stage. Patients with early disease will often have pain after prolonged activity, commonly medial-sided or anterior patellofemoral complaints in the knee, and groin and thigh pain with hip disease. As the process progresses, patients may develop pain at rest, pain that interferes with sleep, or pain that limits activities of daily living, such as the ability to use public transportation or even put on shoes and socks. Pain can be referred from elsewhere, and therefore, it is always important to examine adjacent joints. For example, one should examine a patient's hips when they complain of knee pain, as pain may be referred to the knee from the hip via the obturator nerve. In addition, when evaluating knee or hip pain, one must always examine the spine, as pain may be referred to either location from a lumbosacral spine disorder.

Standard radiographs should be obtained based on the patient's history and physical exam. When imaging the knee, one should obtain a weight-bearing AP view, a lateral view, and a sunrise view to visualize the patellofemoral joint. For the hip, one should obtain an AP pelvis and cross-table lateral radiographs. Spine films can also be ordered as indicated. Review of the images will assist in the management of the patient by assessing the severity of the arthritic changes,

aiding the ability to evaluate other possible causes of pain, including fracture or tumor. Once a diagnosis of degenerative joint disease has been made, a treatment plan can be reached based on the underlying pathology and the severity of patient symptoms.

When a patient presents with joint pain, an attempt is made to relieve the symptoms. Often, the first line of treatment is a nonsteroidal anti-inflammatory medication (NSAID). It is imperative to take a careful medical history to identify contraindications to the use of NSAIDs, such as gastritis, ulcers, or renal disease, before prescribing any medication.

Newer medications, such as the COX-2 inhibitors (coxibs), were initially expected to cause a dramatic decrease in gastrointestinal side effects due to their mechanism of action. There are numerous studies comparing traditional NSAIDS with the coxibs, with some evidence of decreased upper GI complications with coxibs. However, there are other studies that show no statistically significant difference [10–12]. If a patient has a history of ulcers or gastritis, it is often prudent to prescribe a proton pump inhibitor (PPI) in conjunction with the NSAIDs to protect against gastric bleeding [13].

There has also been concern over increased risk of cardiac complications with the use of the COX-2 inhibitors. This began following the results of the VIGOR and APPROVe studies, where rofecoxib (Vioxx) was shown to cause a significant increase in the rate of myocardial infarction or stroke, which led to the removal of rofecoxib from the market. Studies have been performed since that time, on other COX-2 inhibitors, because of concern of a class effect of the drugs. A meta-analysis by Zhang in 2006 showed that a statistically significant increased risk of hypertension, renal dysfunction, ventricular fibrillation, and cardiac arrest were only associated with rofecoxib. There was no significant increase in the events with the use of celecoxib (Celebrex) or ibuprofen (Advil, Motrin) versus placebo [14]. If concerns remain after thorough evaluation, it may be prudent to have the patient consult with their medical physician prior to starting an NSAID.

Acetaminophen can also be prescribed, and it is not associated with GI or kidney problems, but high doses can lead to hepatic dysfunction. Tramadol is another option, as it acts uniquely on the mu-opioid receptor, providing pain relief without the side-effect profile of opioid medications (i.e., dizziness, constipation, respiratory suppression) and without GI or cardiac side effects. However, tramadol use must be monitored closely in patients with impaired renal or hepatic function [12].

If medications do not provide sufficient pain relief, an intra-articular injection may be offered. Options include either a lidocaine and corticosteroid combination or a series of viscosupplementation injections. Viscosupplementation consists of a series of 3–5 weekly injections of hyaluronic acid (HA) products. Knee injections are performed by the physician in the office, but hip injections are typically performed by a radiologist, as they utilize fluoroscopic, ultrasound, or CT scan guidance. In addition to providing pain relief, intra-articular injections can be used as diagnostic tools, to confirm the location of a patient's symptoms. The lidocaine should provide almost immediate relief, and if it does not, one must consider other sources of the pain, such as referred pain from another joint. The corticosteroid may take 7–10 days to take effect and has variable results. A recent meta-analysis of knee injections by Aroll et al. showed consistently significant improvement at 2 weeks, and several studies showed improvement at 16–24 weeks [15]. A Cochrane review of intra-articular knee injections demonstrated no significant difference between corticosteroid and HA at 1–4 weeks but showed improved efficacy of HA at 5–13 weeks [16]. That same review showed triamcinolone hexacetonide to be superior to betamethasone with regard to pain relief at 4 weeks after injection [16]. Subsequent injections of corticosteroids generally provide a shorter period of pain relief (i.e., "diminishing returns"), such that it is uncommon to consider more than three injections in a specific joint.

Physical therapy and the use of assistive ambulatory aids can be used in conjunction with medications. Although patients are often reluctant to use a cane or a walker, as they do not like the stigma of appearing disabled, they should be counseled that assistive devices provide significant relief by decreasing contact forces at the joint and providing greater stability during ambulation [17]. If a patient is willing to use a cane, it should be placed in the hand on the painless side for hips and on the painful side for knees.

The role of formal physical therapy is to strengthen the muscles around the joint, improve or maintain range of motion, and attempt to decrease pain. A recent systematic review of physical therapy for patients with OA of the knee showed that weight loss and exercise are effective at reducing pain and improving function [18]. The same review demonstrated that modalities such as transcutaneous electrical nerve stimulation (TENS) and acupuncture can provide pain relief, but further research is needed in these areas as the quality of evidence is not as high [18]. A recent randomized controlled trial looking at the use of physical agents (i.e., heat packs, TENS, short-wave diathermy) prior to exercise demonstrated improved function and decreased pain as compared to a group who received exercise alone [19].

Physical therapy has also been shown to be beneficial for OA of the hip, although manual therapy may be more beneficial than exercise therapy as demonstrated in a study by Hoeksma. In this randomized trial, the manual therapy group had significantly better outcomes in pain, stiffness,

hip function, and range of motion at 5 weeks, with some benefit lasting as long as 6 months [20]. Furthermore, in both OA of the knee and hip, patients have had significant improvements in pain, range of motion, and quality of life following aquatic physical therapy regimens [21]. This most likely reflects the decreased impact this regimen places on the joints.

If these nonoperative options fail to provide sufficient relief, and a patient's quality of life is declining due to the joint pain and limited function, a discussion of surgical options can be undertaken with the patient.

The role of arthroscopy for degenerative joint disease is controversial. Several studies of arthroscopic debridement of osteoarthritic knees have shown significant improvements in pain relief, with high rates of patient satisfaction at up to 4 years [22–24]. However, a recent randomized controlled trial in *The New England Journal of Medicine*, as well as a Cochrane review, showed no added benefit of arthroscopic lavage and debridement over optimized physical and medical therapy in elderly patients with osteoarthritis [25,26]. There are far fewer studies evaluating the role of arthroscopy for degenerative joint disease in the hip, and most studies are small series of a younger population with early osteoarthritis. These studies did demonstrate good short-term results with debridement or microfracture, and arthroscopy may have a place in delaying the need for THA in young patients [27–29]. At this time, there is no data to support hip arthroscopy in the elderly patient.

If a patient has unicompartmental disease of the knee, one surgical option is a high tibial osteotomy (HTO). This procedure is generally performed on young, active patients without inflammatory disease. Another option for unicompartmental disease is a unicompartmental knee arthroplasty (UKA), in which only the diseased medial or lateral compartment is replaced. This surgery maintains bonestock in the unresurfaced compartments, as well as maintaining the cruciate ligaments. This is also performed in patients without inflammatory disease, those with a mechanical axis of no greater than 10° varus or 5° valgus, and with flexion contractures less than 15°. This surgical option is typically used in younger patients as their first knee surgery with the expectation of needing a later conversion to a TKA, or in elderly patients as their last knee surgery as they may not outlive the prosthesis.

A long-term follow-up study showed a 90 and 76% survival of UKAs versus HTOs respectively at 10 years, which dropped to 88 and 65% at 15 years [30]. Second decade survivorship of UKAs has been shown to be less than 90% in several studies and is often due to degeneration of the opposite compartment [30–32]. If HTO or UKA are not indicated or have been performed and failed, it is time for the patient to consider a total joint arthroplasty.

Once a patient is indicated for surgery, it is essential that they undergo a complete medical evaluation, so that their health is optimized prior to surgery. The patient will require routine labs including CBC, BMP, coagulation panel, and type and screen. An EKG and chest radiograph is also obtained. If there is any abnormality noted on EKG, or the patient has a history of cardiac disease, they should receive a cardiology evaluation, with consideration for a stress test and/or echocardiogram for further evaluation. The patient should also meet with the anesthesia team prior to the day of surgery so that they can address any concerns from their viewpoint.

Patients often donate 1 or 2 units of their own blood prior to surgery, or as an alternative, receive erythropoietin (EPO) preoperatively. The decision on which, if either, method is chosen is currently controversial. The initial impetus for donating autologous blood was a concern over disease transmission in the 1980s and 1990s. This risk has decreased with current testing techniques, but it still estimated to be 1 in 493,000 for HIV; 2 in 63,000 for hepatitis B; and 1 in 103,000 for hepatitis C [33]. Guidelines regarding blood donation or premedication are based on preoperative hemoglobin. Generally, for a Hgb of 14–15 g/dl no intervention is needed; for a Hgb of 10–13 g/dl, preoperative EPO should be considered, as predonating would decrease their Hgb further, thus increasing the need for allogeneic transfusion; and for those with a Hgb<10 g/dl, a hematologic evaluation should be obtained to elicit the underlying cause of anemia. Patients with a Hgb>13 g/dl are often given the option of donating blood preoperatively, although studies have shown that approximately 44% of these units are discarded. These guidelines are for patients undergoing primary joint arthroplasties [34]. When a patient is expected to have an increased blood loss, such as with a revision procedure, those with Hgb>13 g/dl are often encouraged to predonate blood.

Several studies have demonstrated the effectiveness of EPO. The first orthopedic studies were in the mid 1990s and showed a decrease in the risk of postoperative allogeneic blood transfusion from 53% in the controls to 16% in the patients who received EPO, which was statistically significant. When these groups were further stratified to the patients with preoperative Hgb between 10 and 13 g/dl, the results were even more impressive, with controls having a 78% risk of transfusion versus 14% in the EPO group [35–37].

A study in 2007, attempted to elicit postoperative differences in vigor and strength in patients who donated autologous blood compared with those who used EPO (600 IU/kg once weekly for 3 weeks preoperatively and a fourth dose within 24 h postoperatively). The study did not show significant differences in vigor or hand strength, but showed a significant difference in the need for allogeneic transfusion, with only 3% of patients in the EPO group

receiving allogeneic blood versus 14% in the autologous donor group [38].

This debate has lead to the development of patient-specific strategies (PSS) in which algorithms are used to determine the appropriate management of a specific patient. These algorithms are procedure-specific, and even hospital- or individual surgeon-specific, so that operative blood losses may be accurately predicted. These estimates, combined with an evaluation of a patient's hemoglobin, weight, and medical comorbidities have led to preoperative management strategies that have caused decreased transfusion rates of 20–56%, reduced wasted autologous blood by 50%, and increased use of EPO by 11% [39,40]. All patients donating autologous blood or receiving EPO should receive iron supplementation. There are contraindications to the use of EPO, including severe heart disease, vascular disease, or recent myocardial infarction or stroke. Further, the prescribing physician should inquire whether a patient's insurance policy provides coverage of the injections, as this varies by company and by state.

Screening for methicillin-resistant *Staphylococcus aureus* (MRSA) is sometimes performed prior to elective surgery to try to decrease the risk of postoperative infection. This is performed using nasal swab cultures and at times perineal or groin swabs. Studies have shown that up to 5.3% of patients admitted electively to general or orthopedic surgical wards are colonized with MRSA [41]. Risk factors for MRSA infection include male gender, age >70, prior hospital admission, prior antibiotic treatment, and living in a long-term care facility [42]. If a patient has a positive MRSA nasal swab, they can receive mupirocin nasal ointment in an attempt to decrease their postoperative risk of surgical site infection (SSI). For positive skin cultures, triclosan bathing is often used. A study by Sankar compared postoperative infections in patients undergoing elective total joint arthroplasties before and after the implementation of a MRSA screening and treatment protocol. One patient developed a postoperative SSI with MRSA, and this patient was in the preprotocol group. However, there was a significant difference in the overall infection rate between the two groups, with more MRSA lower respiratory infections developing in the preprotocol group. The increased infection rate in the preprotocol group resulted in an increased length of stay and increased cost of care. They concluded that screening elective orthopedic patients for MRSA decreased morbidity and was cost-effective [42]. A similar study was performed by Wilcox, in which pre- and postprotocol MRSA SSI infection rates in orthopedic patients were compared after introducing an MRSA screening and treatment program. Their results were more impressive with a decrease in MRSA SSI from 23/1000 to 3.3/1000 ($p<0.001$) with prescreening and treatment [43]. A prospective, randomized, double-blinded study in the *New England Journal of Medicine* comparing a mupirocin treatment group with a placebo group showed no significant difference in the overall *S. aureus* SSI rate, but did show a significant decrease in SSI among the patients who were *S. aureus* nasal carriers. They also concluded that screening and treatment with mupirocin was beneficial and cost-effective [44]. However, this study did not include orthopedic patients. A prospective, randomized, and double-blinded study from the Netherlands did find a significant decrease in the nasal carriage of *S. aureus* after mupirocin treatment, and a trend toward a decrease in SSI, but the difference was not statistically significant. Treatment also did not decrease the length of hospital stay [45]. Another point of controversy is whether MRSA carriers should receive vancomycin rather than cefazolin for prophylaxis. Many feel this should be done only after infectious disease consultation to avoid increased antibiotic resistance. Hospitals must make individualized decisions at this time, as there is no clear-cut support for screening and treating for nasal MRSA carriers. Assessing local MRSA rates, and individual patient risk factors may contribute to the decision making process. Further, large, multicenter randomized trials will likely be necessary to gain sufficient power to determine the effectiveness of screening and treatment protocols.

A risk assessment for venous thromboembolism, one of the most common complications after knee and hip replacement, is also performed for all patients undergoing surgery at our institution. The decision on which type of medication to be used (i.e., low-molecular-weight heparin, fondaparinux, aspirin, or Coumadin), along with a sequential compressive device for the lower extremities, is based on patient risk factors and type of surgery being performed (Fig. 95.1). This standardization of prophylaxis is important for decreasing postoperative thromboembolism, by ensuring that all patients receive appropriate prophylaxis. However, the best regimen to be used is not known, especially in patients who are at low risk. The American College of Chest Physicians recommends that patients undergoing THA, TKA, or hip fracture surgery receive thromboprophylaxis with LMWH, fondaparinux, or warfarin for at least 10 days postoperatively and that THA and hip fracture patients be considered for prolonged prophylaxis (28–35 days). A prospective cohort study of low-risk patients undergoing THA or TKA who received a 10-day LMWH regimen, by Burnett et al., found a 3.8% rate of symptomatic DVT and 1.3% rate of nonfatal symptomatic PE, which were higher than reported previously. The researchers found a 4.7% rate of wound complications, with 3.4% returning to the OR for drainage of a wound hematoma. This leads to a conclusion that LMWH may not be as effective as prior studies have shown and that wound complications need to be considered when recommending appropriate DVT prohylaxis [46]. A study by Dorr et al. compared the results of low-risk THA and TKA patients receiving aspirin and intermittent pneumatic

compression devices (IPCs) to a high-risk group receiving LMWH and/or warfarin. There were no fatal pulmonary emboli, 0.3% nonfatal PEs in the low-risk group, 0% in the high-risk group, 0.38% symptomatic DVTs in the low-risk group, and 0.75% in the high-risk group. None of the differences were statistically significant. They did, however, find a significant increase in wound hematomas in patients receiving warfarin or LMWH. They concluded that multimodal prophylaxis is safe and effective when patients are stratified based on risk assessment [47]. Two meta-analyses performed in 2000, one for THA and the other for TKA, showed a decreased risk of DVT and PE in patients receiving LMWH or warfarin as compared to aspirin alone [48,49]. However, none of the studies reviewed at that time had a patient group using aspirin and IPCs, making it difficult to draw conclusions from the studies. A more recent meta-analysis by Sharrock looked at all causes of mortality and rates of PE in patients undergoing THA or TKA, dividing them into three groups. Group A included patients receiving potent anticoagulants (i.e., LMWH, fondaparinux), group B included patients on aspirin and IPCs, and group C consisted of patients on warfarin. They found the rates of symptomatic nonfatal PE and all causes of mortality to be significantly higher in group A (LMWH) than in group B (ASA and IPCs), whereas no significant difference was found between groups B and C (warfarin). This led them to conclude that the American College of Chest Physicians may need to reevaluate their recommendations [50]. The difficulty when drawing a conclusion from these studies is the lack of comparison of multimodal prophylaxis with medication options, for example, using ASA, LMWH, or warfarin with the use of IPCs and current regional anesthesia modalities. A large, highly powered, multicenter trial comparing treatment regimens would be needed to identify the best treatment regimen.

Current available data supports that patients should be risk-stratified prior to surgery to determine the appropriate prophylaxis as outlined in Fig. 95.1. Patients who are known to be very high risk, such as those with a recent history of DVT or PE, should be bridged with LMWH to warfarin, and should remain on warfarin for 3–6 months. However, clinicians must understand that none of the interventions discussed above have been shown to decrease the rate of fatal pulmonary embolism.

To optimize outcomes, it is also important for a patient to understand the components of the postoperative restrictions and physical therapy protocol. To facilitate patient understanding, they often attend a preoperative "Total Joint School," where they meet with nurses, social workers, and physical therapists who can explain the protocols and answer any questions. These programs enhance patients' understanding of the procedure, reduce anxiety, and provide them with realistic expectations regarding their recovery.

NYU NYU HOSPITALS CENTER
Medical NYU Hospital for Joint Diseases
Center Department of Orthopaedic Surgery

Lastname [   ]   Firstname [   ]

MRN [   ]   Sex [   ] DOB [   ]

ACCT [   ]   Pt Type [   ]

ADULT VENOUS THROMBOEMBOLISM (VTE) PREVENTION PROTOCOL

Tables 1a and 1b:
Patient Risk Factors for VTE

Table 1a: Major Risk Factors
Hypercoagulable state, inherited or acquired
Prior DVT or PE
Prolonged immobility (> 72 hrs) or paralysis

Table 1b: Non-Major Risk Factors:
Acute myocardial infarction
Central venous access
Heart failure, decompensated Pericarditis
Hormonal replacement therapy, raloxifene
   (Evista) or tamoxifen
Immobilizing cast or splint on the lower extremity
Inflammatory bowel disease
Malignancy
Nephrotic syndrome
Obesity (BMI of 30 or greater)
Oral contraceptive use
Pregnancy or < 1 month postpartum
Stroke, nonhemorrhagic

Table 2:
Contraindications to Pharmacologic VTE Prophylaxis

Active peptic ulcer disease
Acute pelvic or acetabular fracture
Bacterial endocarditis
Current cerebrovascular hemorrhage (not history of)
Current ulcerative GI lesions (not history of)
Dissecting or cerebral aneurysm
Eye, brain or spinal cord surgery within the past 48 hours
Hemorrhagic blood dyscrasias
Hypertension: Severe, uncontrolled
Major, active uncontrollable bleeding
Malignant hypertensive crisis
PT or PTT > 1.5 x Control at baseline
Recent TURP (within several weeks)
Sepsis or infection severe
Severe head trauma
Severe thrombocytopenia (platelet count < 30,000)
Threatened abortion
Contraindications to specific pharmacologic agents:
Heparin, LMW heparins and heparinoids: History of heparin induced thrombocytopenia
IPC's: Open wounds located where devices are worn
Warfarin: Pregnancy

Table 3: Definitions

- **Minor surgery** is defined as a procedure requiring less than one hour of general, neuroaxial or regional anesthesia. Surgery preformed with a local anesthetic never requires VTE prophylaxis, regardless of the patient risk factors.

- **Major surgery** is defined as a procedure requiring 90 minutes or more of general, neuroaxial, or regional anesthesia, excluding total knee and hip replacements and surgery for hip fractures.

- **Outpatient surgery** is defined as a procedure not requiring an overnight hospital stay.

- **Neuroaxial anesthesia** is defined as a subarachnoid block (spinal) or an epidural block.

- **IPC** = Intermittent pneumatic compression devices for lower extremity

Table 4: Procedure and Condition Specific VTE Prophylaxis Options

Check one category and one treatment:

A. Spinal cord injury (SCI) with paralysis: Place IPC's immediately and wait *48 hours after injury* to begin pharmacologic prophylaxis regimen, as per "Major surgery with one or more major patient risk factors" (see F next page).

B. Minor surgery with no patient risk factors or any procedures preformed under a local anesthetic:
No formal VTE prophylaxis is recommended.

ZNYNN0nnnn (Rev. 4/08)

Figure 95.1 NYU Hospital for Joint Diseases Adult Venous Thromboembolism Prevention Protocol.

NYU HOSPITALS CENTER

MRN, Name, DOB:

NYU Hospital for Joint Diseases
Department of Orthopaedic Surgery

VTE Prevention Protocol – Page 2

C. Minoroutpatient surgery with one or more major or non-majorpatient risk factors (See Tables 1a and 1b).

(1)   Enoxaparin 30 mg SC prior toor as soon as circumstances permit* after surgery **OR**

(2)   IPC's worn during surgery.

D. Major surgery with no patient risk factors:

(1)   Enoxaparin 30 mg SC prior toor as soon as circumstances permit* after surgery **OR**

(2)   IPC's worn during surgery.

E. Major surgery with one or more non-major patient risk factorsand no major patient risk factors:

(1)   Enoxaparin 30 mg SC prior toor as soon as circumstances permit* after surgery; continued twice daily until patient is ambulatory **OR**

(2)   Warfarin started preoperatively or immediately after surgery,witha target INR range of **2.0 to 3.0**, until patient is ambulatory **OR**

(3)   Fondaparinux 2.5 mg started 6 to 8 hours after surgery; continueduntil patient is ambulatory **OR**

(4)   In patients with contraindications to pharmacologic VTE prophylaxis **(See Table2),** IPC's should be used intraoperatively.

F. Major surgery with one or more major patient risk factors:

(1)   Enoxaparin 30 mg SC prior toor as soon as circumstances permit* after surgery; continued twice daily until patient is ambulatory **OR**

(2)   Warfarin started preoperatively or immediately after surgery, with a target INR range of **2.0 to 3.0**, until patient is ambulatory **OR**

(3)   Fondaparinux 2.5 mg started 6 to 8 hours after surgery; continued until patient is ambulatory **OR**

(4)   In patients with contraindications to pharmacologic VTE prophylaxis **(See Table 2)**, IPC's should be used intraoperatively and a vena caval filter should be placed prior to surgery.

G. Total hip arthroplasty (THA), total knee arthroplasty (TKA), and hip fracture:

(1)   Enoxaparin 30 mg SC twice daily: starting 6 to 12 hours after surgery performed under a general anesthetic or subarachnoid block [in those patients with an indwelling epidural catheter, the standard dose is started after the catheter is removed; dose is decreased to 30 mg daily in patients with a creatinine clearance of less than 30 mg per day] and IPC's placed in the recovery room **OR**

(2)   Fondaparinux 2.5 mg started 6 to 8 hours after surgery (except in those patients with an indwelling epidural catheter in whom the first dose is given immediately after the catheter is removed) and IPC's placed in the recovery room **OR**

(3)   Warfarin started preoperatively or immediately after surgery, with a target INR range of 2.0 to 3.0; IPC's placed in the recovery room **OR**

(4)   Aspirin and IPC's (foot pumps or SCD's) in patients who receive neuroaxial anesthesia and who do not have any pre-existing patient risk factors for developing VTE **(See Table 1)**. [these therapies must be continued for 10 days after surgery, after which time aspirin should be used for an additional 28 days] **OR**

(5)   In patients who present a significant risk of postoperative bleeding or have a known contraindication to pharmacologic VTE prophylaxis **(see Table 2)**, IPC's should be used and consideration given to placement of a preoperative vena caval filter.

*See detailed recommendations for enoxaparin under category G, Total hip arthroplasty, item 1.

ZNYNN0nnnn (Rev. 4/08)

Figure 95.1 (continued)

Total Knee Arthroplasty

History of TKA

"Total knee arthroplasty is a safe and reliable procedure in the very aged patient for the management of pain and deformity secondary to arthritis of the knee." [51] This statement by Tankersley and Hungerford is the result of more than 135 years of research and development related to biomechanical concepts, prosthetic materials and designs, and surgical techniques. The history of knee replacement surgery is extensive and is only briefly outlined to document the progression of events that have unfolded to reach the successful designs and techniques of today.

Knee replacement surgery is a resurfacing procedure and is most effective when the principal cause of knee pain is related to pathologic bone contact. Based on this concept, resection arthroplasty (removal of the diseased joint surfaces) was an early attempt to treat these disease processes. The first results of resection knee arthroplasty were reported in 1861 by Ferguson as "satisfactory" at 5 years [52]. Verneuil went a step further and performed what is believed to be the first interpositional knee arthroplasty in 1863. He used flaps of joint capsule to cover the resected articular surfaces. Other tissues, including fat, fascia lata, bursal tissue, skin , and materials including cellophane and nylon were also utilized for interpositional arthroplasty [53]. No material proved to be effective in relieving pain in the diseased knee, and all proved to be less successful than knee arthrodesis (fusion), which relieved pain and provided stability, but did not improve function.

The first documentation of metal being used as resurfacing material in the knee was by Campbell in 1938. He performed two hemiarthroplasties (replacing only one side of the joint) with replacement of the distal femur using an inert metallic alloy mold designed by Boyd [54]. Campbell concluded that "the use of vitallium (an alloy of Co–Cr–Mb) in the reconstruction of a new joint is in the experimental stage and that the ultimate outcome of these cases is at present doubtful." [54] Variations of the distal femoral mold were created and expanded to include a medullary stem, which improved fixation. Hemiarthroplasty eventually crossed the knee joint in the form of a tibial plateau resurfacing. Overall, the general consensus was that hemiarthroplasty of the knee was not successful and frequently failed secondary to loosening and continued pain from the nonresurfaced joint surfaces [53].

The first total knee replacement, where both sides of the joint were resurfaced, was a hinged prosthesis design. One of the first hinged total knee replacements was performed by Magoni in 1949. The procedure was limited to patients who suffered from advanced degenerative joint disease,

rheumatoid arthritis or patients who required reconstruction following tumor resection or trauma. The hinged prosthesis dictated the amount of flexion and extension of the knee while providing stability. It was these advances that made it a viable alternative to knee fusion [53].

The advancements in total knee arthroplasty were directly related to the success obtained with hip replacement surgery. Major gains were made with the use of polymethylmethacrylate (bone cement) for prosthetic fixation, and with the development of materials for prosthetic use, including stainless steel, cobalt-chrome, and ultrahigh-molecular-weight polyethylene. Gunston designed the first nonhinged prosthesis in 1968. It included a metal femoral component and a tibial component designed from high-density polyethylene fixed to the tibia with polymethylmethacrylate. This design was the first to allow near-physiologic knee motion. It also was the first prosthesis that relied on the patient's own ligaments for stability.

In 1978 Scott et al. reported on the use of patella replacements and found a decrease in patients' patellofemoral pain and overall improvement in the quality of life with the addition of patellar resurfacing [55]. Further advances continue to focus on joint stability, prosthetic fixation, and implant material characteristics to optimize the long-term survival of the implant.

The inherent stability of a total knee prosthesis is based on its design. The typical primary TKA is performed with an unconstrained prosthesis, which relies exclusively on the patient's own ligamentous restraints for stability. These include posterior cruciate retaining and posterior cruciate sacrificing prostheses, both of which remove the anterior cruciate ligament. This progresses to the semiconstrained knee, with a large tibial post to provide improved varus and valgus stability, followed by the constrained (hinged) prosthesis which are most often used in complex revision or tumor cases. Prosthetic fixation is accomplished with bone cement in most patients, although a press-fit technique with the use of screws and without the use of cement is occasionally used in younger patients.

The history of knee replacement surgery documents a stepwise progression to the development of today's prostheses. These efforts have made total knee arthroplasty a successful treatment option for patients with degenerative joint disease.

The Operation

On the day of surgery, the patient will have any final questions answered by the surgeon as well as the anesthesiologist. The operative limb is initialed by the surgeon in the holding room, which is formally documented, to avoid wrong site surgery. This method of surgical site identification has become a standard part of all surgical procedures. The patient is brought to the operating room, and either general or spinal/epidural anesthesia is induced, followed by prepping of the operative limb and draping. A final "time-out" is performed prior to beginning the surgery, during which the attending surgeon, anesthesiologist, and circulating nurse reconfirm the correct operative site and appropriate administration of antibiotics. Often, a thigh tourniquet is applied and used during the procedure to decrease blood loss. The decision to use a tourniquet is often based on the presence or absence of strong, palpable distal pulses.

The incision is drawn out with a marker on the skin midline from approximately 3 cm above the superior pole of the patella to just medial to the tibial tubercle. The incision is made with a scalpel and carried down to the fascia. A medial flap of tissue is raised for exposure, using an electrocautery to coagulate any obvious bleeding. A smaller lateral flap is also raised. The type of deep approach/arthrotomy performed is based on surgeon preference. The options include a quadriceps tendon splitting approach, a mid vastus approach, and the subvastus approach. The proponents of the midline approach cite the ease of everting the patella and obtaining exposure. The midvastus approach turns the arthrotomy medially, creating an oblique split in the vastus medialis obliquus parallel with its fibers. The proponents of this technique cite a quicker return of quadriceps function as the muscle is not detached from the quadriceps tendon as it is in the midline approach. The subvastus approach takes this concept one step further by elevating the muscle directly off bone, without incising it.

Outcome studies comparing the approaches have shown mixed results. Two randomized studies were performed on patients undergoing primary bilateral TKA's, one knee having the median parapatellar approach, and the other the midvastus. The study by Dalury found a significantly earlier return of straight leg raise in the midvastus group (1.7 days MV, 5.2 days MP), whereas the study by Keating found no significant difference. Further the study by Dalury found improved quadriceps strength at 6 weeks in the midvastus group, but this equalized at 3-month follow-up [56,57]. A prospective, randomized study comparing the median parapatellar approach and the subvastus approach found an earlier return of straight leg raise in the subvastus group (3.2 SV vs. 5.8 MP), with greater knee flexion at 1 week, but range of motion at 4 weeks and 3 months were not different between the groups [58]. A retrospective study comparing subvastus and median parapatellar approaches found significantly better patellar tracking and patellar stability in the subvastus group, but no difference in ROM, Knee Society scores, or stair-climbing ability [59].

Following the arthrotomy, a medial release is performed beginning with removal of peripheral osteophytes and subperiosteal elevation of the deep medial collateral ligament. Further releases may be progressively performed later if needed to balance the knee. The infrapatellar fat pad is often excised to enhance visualization of the joint. The knee is then gently flexed to 90°, while subluxing the patella laterally. The femur is generally addressed first as resecting the femur provides enhanced exposure of the tibia. A starting hole is made in the distal femur to open the femoral canal, followed by an opening reamer and placement of an intramedullary jig for femoral sizing. Once the appropriate size has been determined, a jig is applied to make the distal femoral resection. This is followed by placement of the femoral cutting block, which has been sized previously, to complete the posterior and anterior resections, followed by the oblique (chamfer) resections. These resections are made with an oscillating saw and the soft tissues are protected with retractors.

The tibia is then subluxed anteriorly, and any remaining ACL and medial and lateral menisci are excised. The PCL can be retained, recessed, or sacrificed based on surgeon preference and patient factors. This decision will determine whether a cruciate retaining (CR) or posterior stabilized (PS) knee is used. The PS knee has a box cut in the femoral component into which a short post on the tibial polyethylene articulates to substitute for the ligaments.

An extramedullary or intramedullary guide is placed anteriorly to assess the appropriate amount of bone to be resected from the tibia. This is also used to assure the proper alignment of the cut, keeping it parallel to the floor, and dialing in the desired posterior tibial slope. Again, retractors are used to protect the soft tissues and ligaments while using the oscillating saw. The tibial trials are then used to assess the proper size. At this point, the trial femoral and tibial components, with the trial tibial insert, may be placed to assess ligamentous stability and balancing. A sizing block may be used prior to this step for a similar assessment. If the balance in the medial–lateral plane is not correct, further medial or lateral releases may need to be performed. If the knee is tight or loose in flexion or extension, at times, it is necessary to recut the tibia or femur. Once proper balancing is obtained, the tibial component rotation is set.

Attention is then turned to the patella, where a saw or a reamer is used to remove the sclerotic bone leaving a remaining thickness of 12–15 mm. One or three holes (based on manufacturer) are then drilled into the patella so that the polyethylene patellar button can be placed. With the appropriate size patella in place, a final check of stability and range of motion is performed with all trial components in place. The typical parameters evaluated are limb alignment, extension, flexion, stability in flexion and extension, coronal balancing, component rotation, and patellar tracking. When the surgeon is satisfied with these parameters, an extensive irrigation of the knee joint is performed.

After drying the bony surfaces, polymethylmethacrylate (PMMA), i.e., bone cement, is mixed and applied to the components and to the bone surfaces. The components are placed and impacted into place on the femur and tibia, while using a clamp for the patella. After the cement hardens, the knee is irrigated again, and the tourniquet may be released based on surgeon preference.

The knee is then closed in layers, beginning with the arthrotomy and working up to the skin. A deep drain may be placed based on surgeon preference. There have been several recent studies of patients undergoing primary TKA and THA in which patients were randomized to a group with a deep suction drain or a group with no drain. The overall conclusions were that use of a drain in associated with a higher risk of postoperative transfusion, whereas lack of a drain is associated with an increased need to reinforce dressings. There has been no statistical difference in regard to wound infection, hematoma, wound dehiscence, range of motion, rate of DVT, or length of hospital stay [60–63]. A sterile dressing and ACE bandage is applied. AP and lateral radiographs may be obtained in the operating room to evaluate proper component positioning, prior to taking the patient to the recovery room.

Postoperative Course

Standard postoperative protocols have the goal of mobilizing the patient as early as possible. This typically occurs on the same day or on postoperative day (POD) #1 (i.e., the day after surgery). This is facilitated by the discontinuation of intravenous fluids and epidural or PCA pumps, as well as by removal of foley catheters and hemovac drains if appropriate. Patients are often started on continuous passive motion (CPM) machines for 60 min, three times per day while progressively increasing motion daily. Studies have shown the benefit of an earlier return of range of motion, but by 1 year, the knee motions of patients who did not use CPM were equivalent. This earlier return of range of motion may be important as studies have shown a significant decrease in length of stay and in need for knee manipulation under anesthesia in patients receiving CPM combined with traditional physical therapy [64–68].

Ambulation training is also started POD #1, with the use of a walker and assistance of a physical therapist. Mobilizing the patient early also helps to prevent medical complications such as atelectasis, pneumonia, decubiti, and venous thromboembolism. Other preventative measures taken include 24 h of IV antibiotics (usually ancef, with clindamycin as an alternative if the patient has a penicillin allergy), the use of an incentive spirometer, and appropriate DVT prophylaxis.

The typical hospital length of stay is 3–4 days in the acute setting, followed by discharge to home with home therapy or transfer to rehab facility. This is determined based on each patient's needs, and performance in the perioperative period.

Most patients will have a gradual increase in range of motion and activity level, while their pain will steadily decrease. The ultimate range of motion that a patient will obtain has been shown to be generally within 10° of their preoperative range of motion, and this goal is typically achieved by 6 weeks. However, patients may have some smaller gains in ROM for the first 2 years postoperatively [69]. If ROM is not progressing as expected or has begun to decrease despite aggressive physical therapy, a manipulation under anesthesia may be performed.

The greatest success of manipulation is obtained if performed within the first 3 months following surgery. Studies have shown improvement in range of motion of >30° at 1–2 year follow-up [70,71]. Prior to manipulation, the alignment and rotation of the components should be carefully assessed as it could be a factor in poor range of motion. If there is any concern for infection, this should also be evaluated. This is discussed in detail later in the chapter. If a manipulation is unsuccessful, or >3 months have passed since surgery, and the prior concerns have been addressed, an arthroscopic or open lysis of adhesions may be performed. The success rates of these procedures have been variable, with improvements between 16 and 62° reported [72,73].

Overall, 95% of TKA patients have excellent satisfaction and improvement in lifestyle [3]. There are, however, several important complications such as infection, VTE, PE, prosthetic loosening, and periprosthetic fracture, which is discussed later in combination with THA, as the evaluations are quite similar. Follow-up appointments at 6 weeks, 3,6 months, 1 year, and every 1–2 years thereafter (with radiographs obtained at each visit) are an essential part of patient management.

CASE STUDY

The patient is a 78-year-old female who presented for evaluation of bilateral knee pain, left greater than right. The pain had been present for 5 years and had been worsening recently. The knee pain was worse with activity. She used a cane for ambulation and could ambulate only six blocks before needing to rest secondary to her knee pain. She denied low back or hip pain and denied numbness or tingling in the lower extremities. She had received visco-supplementation injections to the knee in the past, which provided 1 year of relief, but the pain had now worsened. She had been treated with a course of physical therapy with limited benefits, and she utilized NSAIDs in the past, but they were discontinued due to peptic ulcer disease. Her medical problems included hypertension, urinary incontinence, and hypercholesterolemia. Medications included Lipitor, Foltx, Monopril, and hydrochlorothiazide.

Physical examination revealed a healthy appearing elderly female in no acute distress. She walked with an antalgic gait referable to the left lower extremity. Examination of the left knee showed a moderate effusion and tenderness to palpation over the medial joint line and distal medial femoral condyle. There was no ligamentous laxity, and range of motion was 5–130°, with pain on extreme flexion. She had 5/5 strength of her quadriceps and hamstrings. Distally motor and sensory function was intact, and distal pulses were palpable. Examination of the right knee did not show significant findings; range of motion was from 0 to 125°. Screening examination of both hips was unremarkable. Examination of the lumbosacral spine showed painless range of motion, and a negative straight leg raise bilaterally.

Radiographs of the left knee showed an area of osteonecrosis of the medial femoral condyle with secondary osteoarthritis of the medial compartment (Figs. 95.2–95.4). Right knee radiographs showed moderate osteoarthritis, primarily in the lateral compartment, but less pronounced than the changes noted in the left knee.

Left total knee arthroplasty was recommended, and after extensive discussion, the patient decided to proceed. During preoperative medical evaluation, cardiac problems were identified, for which she underwent angioplasty and placement of two stents without complications. Her surgery was postponed until she was able to temporarily discontinue anticoagulation (Plavix), and final clearance was obtained from her cardiologist.

She underwent left TKA without complication (Figs. 95.5–95.7). Initial postoperative monitoring was in the surgical intensive care unit, due to her medical history.

She was placed on lovenox and SCDs postoperatively for DVT prophylaxis. She received one unit of packed red blood cells for postoperative anemia, to which she responded appropriately. She started physical therapy on postoperative day 1 for weight bearing as tolerated ambulation and range of motion, with the assistance of a CPM machine. Postoperative day 4, she was transferred to the inpatient rehab facility at our institution. She continued to progress well and was discharged to home 1 week later.

At 6-week follow-up, she was doing very well, ambulating with a single cane. Knee ROM was from 0 to 105°. She had regained good strength, and a straight leg raise could be performed without extensor lag. She continued to progress well. At 2 year follow-up, she had painless ROM of 0–115° (Fig. 95.8). She had been able to perform her daily activities, including using public transportation and going to the theater. Her right knee pain, however, had slowly worsened for which she had received intra-articular steroid injections with good relief. If the pain continues to worsen, she will likely become a candidate for a right total knee replacement.

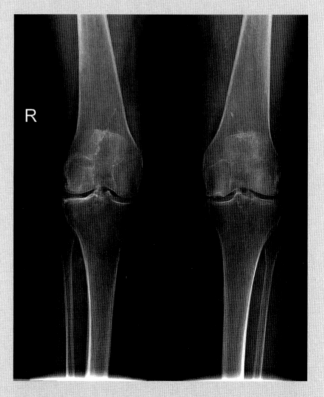

FIGURE 95.2 Bilateral weight-bearing AP knee radiograph of a 78-year-old female with bilateral knee pain, left greater than right. It shows an area of osteonecrosis in the left medial distal femoral condyle, with secondary osteoarthritis. Osteoarthritis is also seen in the right knee, more pronounced in the lateral compartment.

(continued)

CASE STUDY (continued)

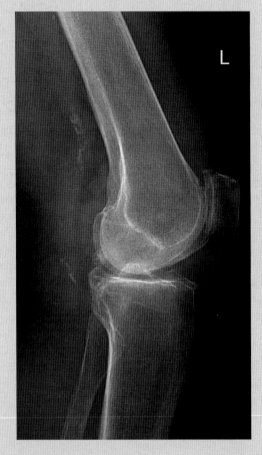

FIGURE 95.3 Lateral radiograph of the left knee showing osteoarthritis and vascular calcifications.

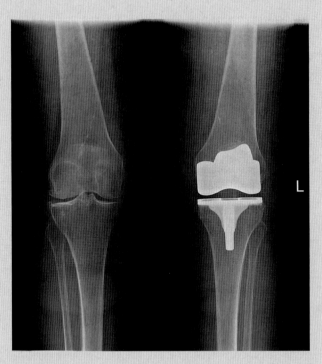

FIGURE 95.5 Postoperative bilateral AP knee radiograph showing a *left cruciate* retaining total knee arthroplasty.

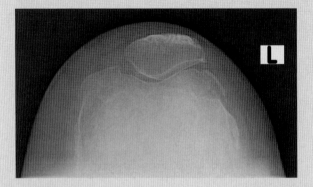

FIGURE 95.4 Sunrise radiograph of the left knee, showing osteoarthritis of the patellofemoral articulation, with large medial and lateral osteophytes.

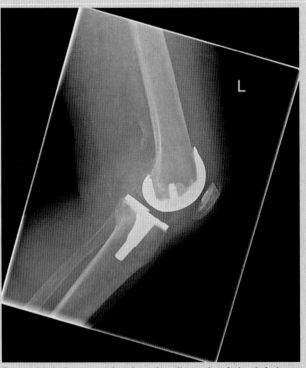

FIGURE 95.6 Postoperative lateral radiograph of the left knee, showing cruciate retaining total knee arthroplasty, with a resurfaced patella.

(continued)

CASE STUDY (continued)

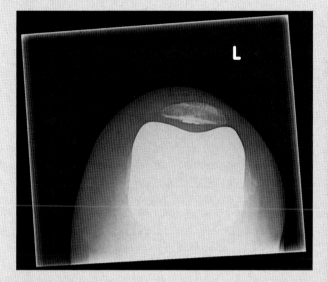

FIGURE 95.7 Postoperative sunrise radiograph of the left knee which shows proper positioning of the resurfaced patella within the trochlear groove.

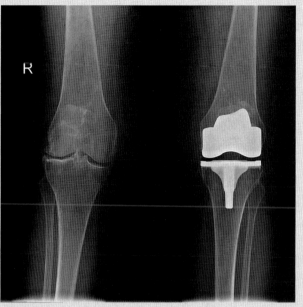

FIGURE 95.8 Bilateral weight-bearing AP radiograph, 2 years after left TKA which shows excellent component alignment, and worsening right knee osteoarthritis.

Total Hip Arthroplasty

History of THA

Total hip arthroplasty is one of the most successful operations performed today. This is only possible due to the extensive work that was performed to develop the modern day prosthesis, beginning in the late 1800s and early 1900s. As with the knee, early attempts at relieving pain and preserving motion in the hip utilized interpositional biologic or inorganic materials such as autologous fascia lata grafts and even gold. The initial attempts were by Sir Leopold Ollier in the late 1800s, but did not have much success until the early 1900s when Sir Robert Jones reported its long-term outcomes [74–76]. As these methods were largely unsuccessful, Smith-Peterson developed the "mold arthroplasty" in which glass, and later materials such as Pyrex, was applied over the bleeding cancellous bone of the femoral head and acetabulum. While patients did have some initial pain relief, the molds failed within a few months due to their brittle nature. In 1937, the development of vitallium (a metal alloy) provided a material with better durability, thus improving patient outcomes [74–76].

In addition to the interpositional arthroplasties, the Judet brothers in France performed early attempts at hip arthroplasty. They developed an acrylic femoral head replacement, which, unfortunately, failed rapidly due to high wear rates [74]. These efforts did provide a stepping-stone for the development of stemmed, metallic endoprostheses, which are similar to those used today. The problem with these metallic prostheses was an increased wear rate within the acetabulum, leading to persistent and worsening pain. Attempts were made to resurface the acetabulum with metal as well, but due to the high friction between the surfaces, abundant metallic debris was produced, leading to osteolysis and loosening.

Some of the most important contributions to total hip arthroplasty were made by Sir John Charnley. He was able to take all of the lessons learned by his predecessors and develop the low-frictional torque arthroplasty. This decrease in friction was obtained by using a 22-mm metallic head with a polytetrafluoroethylene acetabular cup, which lowered the coefficient of friction to near that of the native total hip. This procedure was further improved by his use of PMMA to cement both the stem and the cup in place, allowing adequate fixation and a more uniform load distribution. An important change was made when the polytetrafluoroethylene was replaced by high-density polyethylene, and later ultrahigh-molecular-weight polyethylene, greatly decreasing wear rates [74–77].

The prevalence of total hip arthroplasties being performed began to increase steadily in the 1970s, as Charnley's patients were experiencing good results. Continued modifications in cementing techniques further improved outcomes. However, concerns over component loosening, especially in younger individuals, led to the development of prosthetic designs that could be inserted without the use of cement. This has been quite successful, largely due to improvements in materials, component design, and the use of hydroxyapatite, providing successful bony ingrowth and stability of the prostheses.

The search for the ideal materials for total hip arthroplasty is ongoing. This is evident by the more recent developments of highly cross-linked polyethylene, ceramic femoral head, and acetabular shell components, as well as a return to resurfacing with metal components. These newer components are being developed due to advances in material properties and the machining/processing of these materials. Recent studies have shown improved wear rates and improved hip stability, which may lead to better long-term survival of the prostheses. This continual research will likely maintain the reputation of total hip arthroplasty as one of the most successful operations performed.

The Operation

Prior to the surgery, the standard protocols discussed for the TKA apply regarding the preoperative discussion with the surgeon and anesthesiologist, as well as regarding surgical site verification. After induction of general or spinal/epidural anesthesia, the patient is most commonly placed in the lateral position with the operative limb up. The patient is maintained in this position by the use of a well-padded hip positioner that keeps the pelvis fixed and stable. This is used for the posterior and anterior-lateral approaches, which are the most common. The patient is at times placed supine for the direct lateral or direct anterior approach. We discuss the posterior approach with placement of press-fit metal on polyethylene components, as this is the most common. There is a brief discussion of the advantages and disadvantages of the other surgical approaches and components later in the chapter. The exact use of retractors and steps can vary, but here, we describe a common approach used at our institution.

The limb is sterilely prepped and draped, followed by drawing out the skin incision with a marker, centered over the posterior 1/3 of the greater trochanter. From the tip of the greater trochanter it extends proximally about 4–6 cm and distally 4–6 cm in line with the shaft of the femur. The incision is made with a scalpel through the skin and subcutaneous tissues, down to the level of the deep fascia. Any bleeding is coagulated with an electrocautery. An incision centered over the trochanter is made with a scalpel through the fascia. Proximally, the gluteus maximus muscle belly is split bluntly. A Charnley retractor is now placed beneath the fascial edges,

and perpendicular to the wound for exposure. The bursa over the greater trochanter is now visualized, and gently peeled off with the use of a long-tipped electrocautery. This exposes the short external rotators of the hip. A cobra retractor is placed beneath the gluteus minimus tendon, and the piriformis tendon is visualized. The knee of the patient is now on a sterile bump, keeping the femur parallel to the floor. An assistant begins to internally rotate the limb, placing tension on the short external rotators. They are detached directly from bone, beginning with the piriformis tendon proximally, then distally through the superior gemellus, obturator internus, inferior gemellus, and a portion of the quadratus femoris. This is carried distally until the lesser trochanter is visualized. Prior to taking down the rotators, the sciatic nerve is palpated and carefully protected to avoid injury. The external rotators may be released separate from the hip joint capsule, or the capsule and rotators may be released together. A T-shaped capsular incision is made exposing the femoral head and rim of the acetabulum. The external rotators and capsule are then tagged with sutures, so that they can be repaired at the end of the procedure. The hip is then dislocated by gentle flexion, adduction, and internal rotation. The bump is then repositioned beneath the patient's knee, keeping the femur level.

A trial broach is used to mark the correct angle of the femoral neck osteotomy. The level of the cut is determined from preoperative templating and measured with a ruler from the lesser trochanter. An oscillating saw is used to make the osteotomy, carefully protecting the soft tissues. The femoral head is then removed, exposing the acetabulum.

A cobra or Hohmann retractor is used to retract the femur anteriorly for visualization. Steinman pins are placed superiorly and posteriorly, with a cloverleaf retractor placed inferior. This provides excellent acetabular exposure. The remaining labrum is excised from the rim of the acetabulum, followed by removal of the ligamentum teres from the acetabular floor.

Reaming is performed to reshape the acetabulum to match the implant. Initial reaming is performed with a small size, often 43 mm, removing the degenerative floor of the acetabulum and medializing. The size is sequentially increased by either 1 or 2 mm until the appropriate size is reached based on the preoperative templating and intraoperative assessment. During reaming, one must carefully position the reamers to obtain appropriate anteversion (15–20°) and coronal tilt (35–45°). The last reamer used is typically 1–2 mm smaller than the final implant size, for noncemented components (cemented acetabular components are rarely used during hip arthroplasty). A trial acetabular cup is then placed to assess proper fit. If the fit is correct, the acetabular component is then placed, using an antenna on the impactor handle to confirm proper positioning. With the appropriate version aligned, the cup is impacted. If there is concern over cup stability, screws may be placed to augment fixation. The polyethylene liner is then placed within the cup and impacted into place.

Attention is turned to the femur after the acetabulum is completed. The limb is internally rotated, placing the lower leg perpendicular to the ground. A retractor is placed beneath the proximal femur, allowing visualization of the femoral canal. Soft tissues remaining anterior to the greater trochanter and superior to the remaining femoral neck are removed. A box osteotome is used to open the femur proximally, followed by a starting broach that is placed down the femoral canal. The canal is then sequentially enlarged with reamers and broaches until the appropriate fit is obtained. This is also guided by the preoperative templating. One must maintain proper version of the stem throughout the process.

A trial femoral neck and head are then placed on the femoral broach, with the size and offset determined preoperatively to give the patient appropriate soft tissue tension and leg length. The hip is reduced and taken through range of motion testing to assess stability of the hip. Further verifications of appropriate size are made intraoperatively and compared with preoperative templating. When appropriate stability and length have been obtained, the trials are removed and the final stem is impacted into place. A trial femoral head is again placed for a final check of stability and limb length before placing the head.

The wound is extensively irrigated with sterile saline. Two drill holes are then placed through the greater trochanter to allow reattachment of the piriformis, capsule, and the other external rotators. The deep fascia is repaired with interrupted sutures, followed by a similar closure for the deep and subcutaneous layers. The skin may be closed with staples, sutures, or a subcuticular absorbable stitch with Dermabond. A sterile dressing is applied.

The drapes and hip positioner are removed, and the patient is placed supine on the table, with special care to maintain the hip abducted and externally rotated, as the most common position of dislocation is flexion, adduction, and internal rotation. This is assisted by the use of an abduction pillow. Clinical limb length is assessed, followed by obtaining an AP pelvis radiograph to assess final component placement, and assure that the hip is reduced prior to moving the patient to the recovery room.

Postoperative Course

The initial postoperative course is quite similar to the TKA, in which IV fluids, foley catheters, hemovac drains, and epidural/PCA pain pumps are discontinued, with a goal of early mobilization. At least, the patient should be out of bed to a hip chair (an elevated chair to prevent flexion of the hip beyond 90°), and an incentive spirometer is used to prevent atelectasis on POD #1. Routine labs, including BMP and CBC, are drawn and addressed as needed. If a patient's hematocrit is less than 27 and the patient is symptomatic (i.e., tachycardic, hypotensive, weak, dizzy), the patient may require a blood transfusion. In a patient with medical comorbidities, such as CAD or history of MI, the goal hematocrit is often 30 or greater, based on the preoperative recommendations of the medical team.

Ambulation is begun with a walker and instruction by a physical therapist. The patient will be weight bearing as tolerated (WBAT) unless there is a concern over initial stability of the components, or a complication such as a fracture occurred. The therapist will also review hip precautions and demonstrate basic exercises such as dorsi/plantar flexion of the ankles and heel slides in the bed. This routine will continue, usually twice per day, until POD 3 or 4, when the patient is cleared for transfer to home or to a rehab center.

A home nurse will remove skin staples, or sutures, at 2 weeks postoperatively, and the patient will continue home therapy. The first follow-up visit is at 6 weeks, followed by visits at 3, 6 months, and 1 year. Evaluation of gait, range of motion, and strength will be performed at each visit with radiographs obtained annually unless there are symptoms that necessitate radiographic evaluation. By the 6th week visit, the patient will often have progressed to the use of a cane.

The overall success rate of THA is >95%, making it one of the most successful surgeries performed. This is based on outcome studies regarding the relief of pain and return of function. A patient may progress from being wheelchair-dependent due to pain to ambulating and returning to work. The longevity of the prostheses is excellent as well, with 95% lasting 10–15 years [4,5,78]. The use of alternate bearing surfaces, and advancing technologies, may continue to improve these results. These alternate bearings include ceramic and all metal surfaces. They are primarily used in the younger population. In the elderly population, the components are routinely a cobalt-chrome metal head with a highly cross-linked polyethylene liner within a metal acetabular shell. The femoral stem may be cemented in place if there are concerns over obtaining adequate fixation, while minimizing the risk of fracture, in brittle, osteoporotic bone. Based on a review of the literature, currently, the NIH recommends a hybrid THA in the elderly with a cemented femoral stem and a press-fit acetabular component. This is due to the excellent long-term outcomes obtained and the fact that when both components are cemented the acetabulum is usually the site of early loosening [79–81]. However, at our institution, we routinely press-fit both components with excellent results, which has been supported in several studies [82–85].

Complications

The complications after THA are very similar to those after TKA (including VTE, PE, MI, UTI, fracture, loosening, infection), the main difference being stiffness in TKA and dislocation and limb-length discrepancy in THA. It is possible to dislocate a TKA with extreme flexion in a ligamentously loose or unbalanced knee, but this is very rare. The dislocation rate after a primary THA has been shown to range between 0 and 7% across different studies [86–91]. The high variability is related to the type of surgical approach used. The highest rate of dislocation has been shown with the posterior approach, but with improved technique, including repair of the posterior soft tissues, these rates have decreased from 4% to less than 1% in several studies [86–91]. A further improvement has been obtained with the use of larger femoral heads, 32 mm and greater, which provide increased stability by increasing the head to neck ratio. This provides a larger arc of motion before impingement and levering of the femoral head [88,92]. The anterolateral and direct lateral approaches have had traditionally lower dislocation rates but may have higher risk of a postoperative abductor lurch [87,93]. These two factors have led to the development of new approaches, such as the direct anterior approach, with the goal of eliminating these two complications.

This approach to THA was first described in 1947 but has been recently modified by Joel Matta. In this approach a small, 10-cm incision is made anteriorly over the hip, in which the hip joint may be exposed without the release of any musculature. The surgical window is between the tensor fascia lata and sartorius superficially, and the gluteus medius and rectus femoris in the deep layer. The technique is performed in the supine position on a specially designed fracture table, which allows free, independent movement of the limbs. Intraoperative fluoroscopy is also used to assist in appropriate component positioning, as well as in obtaining equal leg lengths. In Matta's series of 494 consecutive THA, the dislocation rate was 0.61%, with leg lengths being within 3 mm on average. Further, as no muscles are detached, no postoperative hip precautions are needed, and patients often progress to independent ambulation at a faster rate [95]. While the early results of this technique are quite impressive, there is a steep learning curve, and it must be used in carefully selected patients.

Morbidity from medical complications is best prevented by appropriate preoperative medical evaluations and postoperative regimens including VTE prophylaxis, early removal of indwelling catheters, and early mobilization. However, in spite of these measures, they are not all preventable. The more common, yet still rare, medical complications are myocardial infarctions/cardiac arrhythmias, VTE, PE, urinary tract infection, pneumonia, and *Clostridium difficile* infection. In a study by Parvizi et al., 1,636 patients undergoing TJA had 104 major life-threatening complications, including: one cardiac arrest, 33 tachyarrythmias, 6 myocardial infractions, 10 cases of congestive heart failure/pulmonary edema, 14 cases of acute renal failure, and 1 death (.06%) during the initial hospital stay. Most of the minor complications were anemia, but they did have 50 urinary tract infections, 20 mental status changes (which all resolved), 4 pneumonia, and 5 cases of *C. difficile* infection. They found that increased age, high BMI (>30.5), and preexisting medical comorbidities were all risk factors for complications. However, they note that 58% of the patients who developed a complication had no predisposing risk factors. Further, greater than 90% of the complications occurred in the first 4 postoperative days. These last two points lead to the conclusion that all patients need careful postoperative monitoring and that early discharge (i.e., prior to postoperative day 4) may lead to greater overall morbidity and mortality [95]. In 2008, Parvizi conducted a more detailed study of *C. difficile* infection, finding a 0.16% incidence in 9,880 TJA, with increased risk associated with increased ASA score, receiving more than one postoperative antibiotic, and a prolonged hospital stay [96]. A study of over 10,000 patients who underwent TJA from the Mayo Clinic found similar results with the incidence of myocardial infarction 0.4%, PE 0.7%, VTE 1.5%, and death 0.5%. They also found a correlation with increasing age [97]. This is not to say that increasing age should be considered a contraindication to TJA, but rather to assure that appropriate preoperative evaluation is obtained and that any postoperative problems are treated aggressively with early involvement of the medical team. Two recent studies of TJA in patients in the 9th and 10th decades of life did find an increased risk of complications as compared to younger patients but had an overall low event rate with significant improvements in pain score and overall outcomes. The authors of both studies concluded that with careful patient selection, total joint arthroplasty could be an excellent option for elderly patients [98,99].

Complications related to the prostheses include aseptic loosening, periprosthetic fracture, and infection. Any patient with a TKA or THA who presents with pain following surgery must have all of these possibilities considered. Based on the history and physical examination, the physician should be able to narrow down these possibilities. If the patient did not have a fall or acute injury, then fracture is unlikely, and usually can be ruled out with routine radiographs. Patients with aseptic loosening may report start-up pain that is worse during the first few steps and then decreases. The pain is typically located about the groin, thigh, or knee. Radiographs assist in the evaluation by the detection of radiolucencies around the prosthesis. Whenever there is a concern of loosening, an infection must be ruled out, as the treatment protocols are quite different.

Infection should be considered if a patient reports a dull pain that has been persistent since the time of surgery. A history of fevers, chills, warmth or erythema of the operative site provoke obvious concern, as does a recent history of illness or surgical procedure in a potentially contaminated area, such as oral, vaginal, or lower GI procedures.

There is a risk of seeding a prosthetic joint after any surgical procedure, but as the risk is increased following dental procedures, a protocol has been developed. The recommendation of the American Dental Association and the American Academy of Orthopaedic Surgeons is that for the first 2 years after joint arthroplasty, all patients undergoing high-risk dental procedures (i.e., tooth extractions, implantations, root canals, etc.) should receive prophylactic antibiotics. After 2 years, patients who have had previous infection of the artificial joint, inflammatory arthritis, type-1 diabetes mellitus, hemophilia, immunosuppression, history of prior or present malignancy, dental extractions, periodontal procedures, dental implantation, root canal work, cleaning if bleeding is anticipated, certain specialized local anesthetic injections, or placement of orthodontic bands should still receive prophylaxis. The standard is 2 g of oral amoxicillin 1–2 h before the procedure or 600 mg clindamycin for those with a penicillin allergy [100]. There have been several studies of infected TJA in association with dental procedures [101,102]; however, a recent literature review has found little scientific data to support the need for routine prophylaxis [103]. We feel that prophylaxis should be continued at this time due to the morbidity and cost associated with a total joint infection.

Concern of infection should initially be evaluated with routine labs, including a CBC with differential, an erythrocyte sedimentation rate (ESR), and a C-reactive protein (CRP). These are used as markers for infection as CRP should return to normal, after transient postoperative elevation, in 2–3 weeks, and ESR by 1–2 months. The normal values for these markers depend on normalized values that vary by hospital but are ESR < 30 mm/h and CRP < 10 mg/dl at our institution. If the values are somewhat elevated, but not definitive, it is often prudent to aspirate the suspected joint, prior to undergoing an extensive surgical procedure. A recent study of patients undergoing revision THA found that an elevated ESR (>30) and CRP (>10) with a hip aspiration cell count >3,000 had the highest combined sensitivity, specificity, positive and negative predictive values, and accuracy for an infection [104]. This coincided with a recent study by Della Valle, in which a level of >3,000 white blood cells/ml in aspirated fluid from a TKA was most predictive of infection [105].

Information can also be gathered from a Technitium-99 3-phase bone scan, followed by an indium-111/sulfur colloid scan as indicated. Technitium-99 scans are sensitive, but not specific for infection. The addition of indium-111 and sulfur colloid scans greatly increase specificity to 97% [106].

A study evaluating the effectiveness of Indium-111-labeled WBC scans alone found that the sensitivity and specificity alone decreased, but they had a 95% negative predictive value, such that a negative scan is highly predictive of a joint not being infected [107].

If an infection is confirmed or strongly suspected, surgery is indicated. The most common organisms involved are S. aureus and S. epidermidis. The type of surgery performed depends on the acuteness of the infection. Infections have been classified by Coventry as acute (<6 weeks), subacute (6–24 months), and chronic-hematogenous (>2 years). Currently, many consider an acute infection being <4 weeks from index event or surgery. The time frame for an acute infection is from the index surgery or from a postoperative procedure that likely seeded the joint. In an acute infection, good results have been obtained with extensive irrigation and debridement of the joint, with exchange of the polyethylene liners in the hip or knee. This is possible, as the bacteria usually cannot form a protective glycocalyx (which shields the bacteria from the immune system on the implant) by this point, allowing the infection to be eradicated from the metal and bone. The debridement is followed by 6 weeks of intravenous antibiotics, based on the results of intraoperative cultures and recommendations of an infectious disease specialist. Success rates of 71% have been obtained for THA when performed within 4 weeks of the onset of symptoms [108]. For TKA, success rates have varied, with some studies having 80% success, but several studies show only a 30% success rate. Importantly, failure of this procedure has been significantly associated with a S. aureus infection. A study by Deirmengian of acute TKA infections showed a success rate of only 8% for knees infected with S. aureus, while 56% of all other infections were treated successfully [109].

In more long-standing infections, it is necessary to perform a two-stage revision with removal of the entire prosthesis, followed by the placement of an antibiotic cement spacer. The diagnosis is confirmed intraoperatively by frozen section (>10 PMNs per high power field is positive) and intraoperative cultures [110,111]. The spacer remains in place for at least 3 months while the patient receives intravenous antibiotics. The levels of ESR and CRP will be monitored to assess response to the treatment. At the 3-month point, once antibiotics have been discontinued for approximately 6 weeks, and the ESR and CRP have normalized, the patient returns to the OR for the second stage of the procedure. This includes removal of the antibiotic spacer, extensive irrigation and debridement, and the evaluation of intraoperative frozen sections, gram stains, and cultures. If the frozen section is negative for infection (less than 10 PMNs per high power field), then a new prosthesis can be placed [112,113].

The type of prosthesis used is based on the remaining bone stock and ligamentous stability. In a revision THA, it may be necessary to use long-stemmed, modular femoral components so that distal fixation is obtained; or metallic augments for the acetabulum. In the knee, stemmed tibial and femoral components are often needed for adequate fixation with metal augments for areas of bone loss. The overall complication rates are higher than after a primary replacement, but two-stage revisions for infection have success rates of 85–90% for THA [108,114] and 90% for TKA [115].

The revision components used for a noninfected revision are similar, with good results obtained, but with an increased risk of postoperative complications and infections when compared with primary procedures. Excellent outcomes have been obtained in the elderly as demonstrated by Parvizi et al. who showed significant functional improvement following revision THA performed in octogenarians with no increase in medical comorbidities as compared to a younger cohort [116]. For revision of TKA, successful outcomes have been obtained in 74–88% of patients [117–119].

Another significant complication is fracture. Periprosthetic fractures occur at a rate of approximately 2.3% for THA and 2% for TKA over the long term, with a slightly higher increased risk of fracture in the elderly [120,121]. Fractures around a THA are commonly described by the Vancouver classification, with the type of fracture guiding treatment. They are classified as A, B, or C as follows: Type A are proximal fractures of the trochanters, B are at the level of the stem, and C are below the tip of the prosthesis. Type A fractures can often be treated nonoperatively with modified weight bearing, type B fractures by a plate with cables and screws if the stem is well fixed or with conversion to a long-stemmed prosthesis, and type C fractures by a plate with cables and screws [122,123].

The treatment of fractures around a TKA also depends on the location of the fracture. One classification describes fractures proximal to the femoral component, to the level of the component, or to within the area of the component [124]. A determining factor in treatment is whether the prosthesis is loose or well fixed which determines if it will be retained or removed. If the fracture is quite distal, the standard of care is open reduction with internal fixation (ORIF) using a plate and screw construct. If it is more proximal, there is some debate whether a plate or a retrograde intramedullary nail is better suited with good outcomes shown with both fixation constructs [125,126]. Fractures involving the acetabular component of a THA or the tibial component of a TKA are less common, as they tend to require a higher level of energy such as from a motor-vehicle accident or fall from height.

An interesting recent development is the use of THA for the treatment of femoral neck fractures in the elderly. These were traditionally treated with a hemiarthroplasty or internal fixation using screws, unless a patient reported significant hip pain prior to the fracture, which suggested preexisting degenerative joint disease in which case a THA was preferred. However, several recent studies comparing hemiarthroplasty or ORIF to total hip arthroplasty in the active elderly patient have shown superior results in patients undergoing THA with respect to functional outcomes, relief of pain, and need for further surgery [127–130].

CASE STUDY

The patient is 70-year-old male who presented for evaluation of left-hip pain. He reports a history of left femoral neck fracture 3 months prior to presentation, which was treated by internal fixation with three screws. Since the surgery, he has been ambulating with a walker, weight bearing as tolerated, but with significant pain in the groin and laterally about the hip. He denies any low back pain or neurological symptoms. His medical history is significant for hypertension, for which he is treated with Dyazide.

Physical examination revealed a healthy-appearing older man, in no acute distress. Evaluation of the left lower extremity showed a healed incision about the lateral aspect of the left hip. There was tenderness to palpation over this region and pain with hip ROM. ROM was flexion to 90°, internal rotation to 0°, external rotation to 10°, and abduction to 10°. Quadriceps and hamstring strength were 4/5, limited by pain. Distal neurovascular function was intact. There was a limb length discrepancy of 1 cm with the left shorter than the right. Straight leg raise testing was negative bilaterally. He ambulated with an antalgic gait and obvious pain about the left hip.

Radiographs revealed a vertically oriented left femoral neck fracture, which was treated with three cannulated screws. There was limited evidence of healing of the fracture with overall shortening, varus alignment, and backing out of the screws (Figs. 95.9 and 95.10). These findings suggested loss of fracture alignment and delayed healing. Based on these findings and the clinical exam, he was indicated for a removal of hardware from the left hip and conversion to left THA.

(continued)

CASE STUDY (continued)

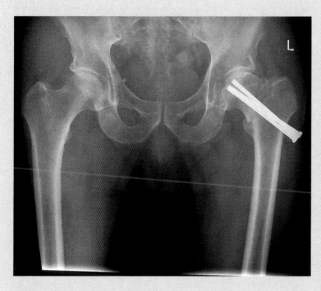

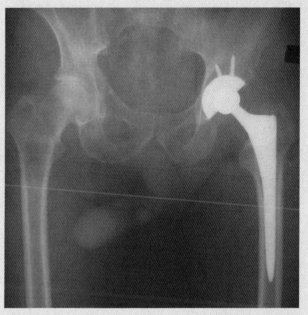

FIGURE 95.9 AP pelvis radiograph of a 70-year-old man which shows a vertically oriented left femoral neck fracture, which was treated with cannulated screws. There is limited evidence of healing of the fracture with overall shortening, varus alignment, and backing out of the screws.

FIGURE 95.11 Postoperative AP pelvis radiograph, showing a noncemented left total hip arthroplasty, with two screws in the acetabular component for additional fixation.

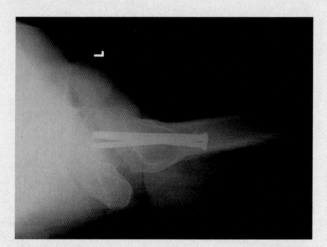

FIGURE 95.10 Cross-table lateral radiograph of the left hip, showing a left femoral neck fracture after fixation with cannulated screws.

complications (Fig. 95.11). He did well postoperatively and was placed on Arixtra and SCDs for DVT prophylaxis. He started physical therapy on postoperative day 1 and ambulated weight bearing as tolerated with a walker. He was discharged to home on POD 5 with home physical therapy.

At the 6-week follow-up visit, he was doing very well, ambulating with part-time use of a single cane and often without assistive devices. He was participating in an outpatient physical therapy program walking on a treadmill. The incision was well healed, and limb lengths were clinically equal. Hip ROM was flexion to 90°, internal rotation to 10°, external rotation to 20°, and abduction to 30°. He was able to straight leg-raise without discomfort, and distal neurovascular function was intact. Radiographs showed the components to be in good position without signs of changes at the bone–prosthesis interface.

He continued to progress well and at 1-year follow-up was ambulating without assistive devices and was pain-free. Radiographs showed good alignment of the implant without complication (Figs. 95.12 and 95.13).

After appropriate medical clearance, the patient underwent removal of the screws and conversion to a noncemented left THA with a metal head and polyethylene liner via a posterior approach, without

(continued)

CASE STUDY (continued)

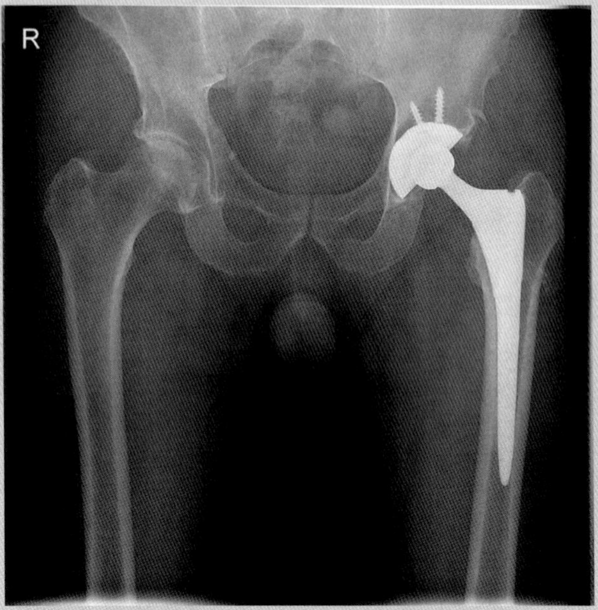

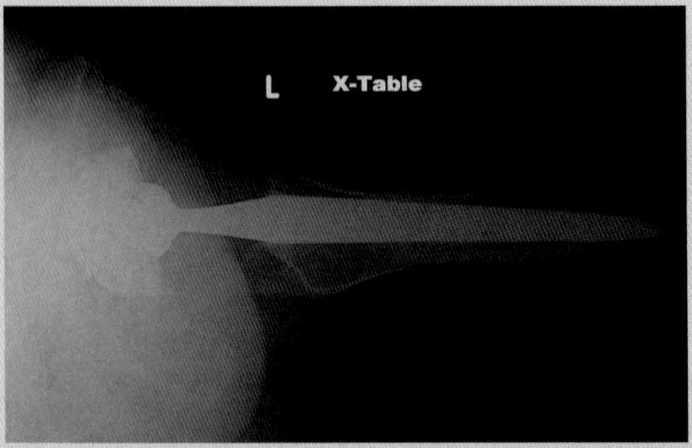

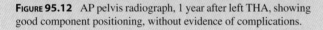

FIGURE **95.13** Cross-table lateral radiograph of the left hip, 1 year after left THA, showing good component positioning, without evidence of complications.

FIGURE **95.12** AP pelvis radiograph, 1 year after left THA, showing good component positioning, without evidence of complications.

Conclusions

As the elderly population continues to grow and stay active, the demand for total knee and total hip arthroplasty will grow along with it. Projections indicate that by 2030, these numbers are expected to grow to the staggering figures of 3.48 million TKAs and 572,000 THAs annually [2]. Modern surgical techniques and a multidisciplinary approach with close involvement of medical specialists will enable excellent outcomes in over 90% of patients. Orthopedic surgeons will continue to refine surgical techniques and implant design, while minimizing complications and carefully evaluating patient outcomes, to ensure that the success of TKA and THA is maintained and improved upon in the future.

References

1. DeFrances CJ, Podgornik MN (2004) National Hospital Discharge Survey. Advance Data from Vital and Health Statistics. National Center for Health Statistics, Hyattsville, MD, May 4 2006
2. (2006) 73rd annual meeting of the American Academy of Orthopaedic Surgery, Chicago, IL
3. Khaw FM, Kirk LM, Gregg PJ (2001) Survival analysis of cemented Press-Fit Condylar total knee arthroplasty. J Arthroplasty 16(2):161–167
4. Gaffey JL, Callaghan JJ, Pedersen DR et al (2004) Cementless acetabular fixation at fifteen years. A comparison with the same surgeon's results following acetabular fixation with cement. J Bone Joint Surg Am 86-A:257–261
5. Klapach AS, Callaghan JJ, Goetz DD et al (2001) Charnley total hip arthroplasty with use of improved cementing techniques: a minimum twenty-year follow-up study. J Bone Joint Surg Am 83-A:1840–1848
6. Buckwalter JA, Einhorn TA, Simon SR (eds) (2000) Orthopaedic basic science: biology and biomechanics of the musculoskeletal system, 2nd edn. American Academy of Orthopaedic Surgeons, Rosemont
7. Fairbank T (1948) Knee joint changes after meniscectomy. J Bone Joint Surg Br 30:664–670
8. Johnson RJ, Kettelkamp DB, Clark W, Leaverton P (1974) Factors effecting late results after meniscectomy. J Bone Joint Surg Am 56:719–729
9. Roos EM, Ostenberg A, Roos H, Ekdahl C, Lohmander LS (2001) Long-term outcome of meniscectomy: symptoms, function, and performance tests in patients with or without radiographic osteoarthritis compared to matched controls. Osteoarthritis Cartilage 9:316–324
10. Jüni P, Rutjes AW, Dieppe PA (2002) Are selective COX-2 inhibitors superior to traditional non steroidal anti-inflammatory drugs? Br Med J 324:1287–1288
11. Simon LS (2007) The COX-2 selective inhibitors. What the newspapers have not told you. Bull NYU Hosp Jt Dis 65:229–241
12. Kean WF, Rainsford KD, Kean IRL (2008) Management of chronic musculoskeletal pain in the elderly: opinions on oral medication use. Inflammopharmacology 16:53–75
13. Lai K-C, Chu K-M, Hui W-M et al (2005) Celecoxib compared with lansoprazole and naproxen to prevent gastrointestinal ulcer complications. Am J Med 118:1271–1278
14. Zhang J, Ding EL (2006) Song, Y Adverse effects of cyclooxygenase 2 inhibitors on renal and arrhythmia events: meta-analysis of randomized trials. JAMA 296(13):1619–1632

15. Arroll B, Goodyear-Smith F (2004) Corticosteroid injections for osteoarthritis of the knee: meta-analysis. Br Med J 328(7444):869
16. Bellamy N, Campbell J, Robinson V, Gee T, Bourne R, Wells G (2006) Intraarticular corticosteroid for treatment of osteoarthritis of the knee. Cochrane Database Syst Rev (2):CD005328. doi:10.1002/14651858.CD005328.pub2.
17. Blount WP (1956) Don't throw away the cane. J Bone Joint Surg Am 38 A(3):695–708
18. Jamtvedt G, Dahm KT et al (2008) Physical therapy interventions for patients with osteoarthritis of the knee: an overview of systematic reviews. Phys Ther 88(1):123–136
19. Cetin N, Aytar A et al (2008) Comparing hot pack, short-wave diathermy, ultrasound, and TENS on isokinetic strength, pain, and functional status of women with osteoarthritic knees: a single-blind, randomized, controlled trial. Am J Phys Med Rehabil 87:443–451
20. Hoeksma H, Dekker J et al (2004) Comparison of manual therapy and exercise therapy in osteoarthritis of the hip: a randomized clinical trial. Arthritis Rheum 51(5):722–729
21. Hinman R, Heywood S, Day A (2007) Aquatic physical therapy for hip and knee osteoarthritis: results of a single-blind randomized control trial. Phys Ther 87(1):32–43
22. Steadman JR, Ramappa AJ et al (2007) An arthroscopic treatment regimen for osteoarthritis of the knee. Arthroscopy 23(9):948–955
23. van den Bekerom MPJ, Patt TW et al (2007) Arthroscopic debridement for grade III and IV chondromalacia of the knee in patients older than 60 years. J Knee Surg 20:271–276
24. Bin S, Lee S et al (2008) Results of arthroscopic medial meniscectomy in patients with grade IV osteoarthritis of the medial compartment. Arthroscopy 24(3):264–268
25. Laupattarakasem W, Laopaiboon M, Laupattarakasem P, Sumananont C (2008) Arthroscopic debridement for knee osteoarthritis. Cochrane Database Syst Rev (1):CD005118. doi:10.1002/14651858.CD005118.pub2
26. Kirkley A, Birmingham TB et al (2008) A randomized trial of arthroscopic surgery for osteoarthritis of the knee. N Engl J Med 359(11):1097–1107
27. Jerosch J, Schunck J, Khoja A (2006) Arthroscopic treatment of the hip in early and midstage degenerative joint disease. Knee Surg Sports Traumatol Arthrosc 14(7):641–645
28. Philippon M, Schenker M et al (2008) Can microfracture produce repair tissue in acetabular chondral defects? Arthroscopy 24(1):46–50
29. Byrd JWT (2006) Hip arthroscopy. J Am Acad Orthop Surg 14:433–444
30. Weale A, Newman J (1994) Unicompartmental knee arthroplasty and high tibial osteotomy for osteoarthrosis of the knee: a comparative study with a 12 to 17-year follow-up period. Clin Orthop Relat Res 302:134–137
31. Squire M, Callaghan J et al (1999) Unicompartmental knee replacement: a minimum 15-year follow-up study. Clin Orthop Relat Res 367:61–72
32. Marmor L (1988) Unicompartmental knee arthroplasty: ten to 13-year follow-up study. Clin Orthop Relat Res 226:14–20
33. Keating EM (2000) Hemoglobin management in hip arthroplasty. Semin Arthroplasty 11:174
34. Keating EM, Ritter MA (2002) Transfusion options in total joint arthroplasty. J Arthroplasty 17(4 Suppl 1):125–128
35. Faris PM, Ritter MA, Abels RI (1996) The effects of recombinant human erythropoietin on perioperative transfusion requirements in patients having a major orthopaedic operation. J Bone Joint Surg Am 78:62
36. de Andrade JR, Jove M, Landon G et al (1996) Baseline hemoglobin as a predictor of risk of transfusion and response to epoetin alfa in orthopedic surgery patients. Am J Orthop 25:533
37. Goldberg MA, McCutchen JW, Jove M et al (1996) A safety and efficacy comparison study of two dosing regimens of epoetin alfa in patients undergoing major orthopedic surgery. Am J Orthop 25:544
38. Keating EM, Callaghan J et al (2007) A randomized, parallel-group, open-label trial of recombinant human erythropoietin vs preoperative autologous donation in primary total joint arthroplasty: effect on postoperative vigor and handgrip strength. J Arthroplasty 22(3):325–333
39. Stulberg B, Zadzilka J (2007) Blood management issues using blood management strategies. J Arthroplasty 22(4 Suppl 1):95–98
40. Martinez V, Monsaingeon-Lion A et al (2007) Transfusion strategy for primary knee and hip arthroplasty: impact of an algorithm to lower transfusion rates and hospital costs. Br J Anaesth 99:794–800
41. Shams W, Rapp R (2004) Methicillin-resistant staphylococcal infections: an important consideration for orthopedic surgeons. Orthopedics 27(6):565–568
42. Sankar B, Hopgood P, Bell KM (2005) The role of MRSA screening in joint-replacement surgery. Int Orthop 29:160–163
43. Wilcox MH, Hall J et al (2003) Use of perioperative mupirocin to prevent methicillin-resistant *Staphylococcus aureus* (MRSA) orthopaedic surgical site infections. J Hosp Infect 54:196–201
44. Perl T, Cullen J et al (2002) Intranasal mupirocin to prevent postoperative *Staphylococcus aureus* infections. N Engl J Med 346:1871–1877
45. Kalmeijer MD, Coertjens H et al (2002) Surgical site infections in orthopedic surgery: the effect of mupirocin nasal ointment in a double-blind, randomized, placebo-controlled study. Clin Infect Dis 35:353–358
46. Burnett R, Clohisy J et al (2007) Failure of the American College of Chest Physicians-1A protocol for lovenox in clinical outcomes for thromboembolic prophylaxis. J Arthroplasty 22(3):317–324
47. Dorr L, Gendelman V et al (2007) Multimodal thromboprophylaxis for total hip and knee arthroplasty based on risk assessment. J Bone Joint Surg Am 89:2648–2657
48. Westrich G, Haas S et al (2000) Meta-analysis of thromboembolic prophylaxis after total knee arthroplasty. J Bone Joint Surg Br 82-B:795–800
49. Freedman K, Brookenthal K et al (2000) A meta-analysis of thromboembolic prophylaxis following elective total hip arthroplasty. J Bone Joint Surg Am 82-A(7):929–938
50. Sharrock N, Gonzalez Della Valle A et al (2008) Potent anticoagulants are associated with a higher all-cause mortality rate after hip and knee arthroplasty. Clin Orthop Relat Res 466:714–721
51. Tankersley WS, Hungerford DS (1995) Total knee arthroplasty in the very aged. Clin Orthop 316:45–49
52. Ferguson M (1861) Excision of the knee joint: recovery with a false joint and useful limb. Med Times Gaz 1:601
53. Hungerford DS, Krackow KA et al (1984) Total knee arthroplasty: a comprehensive approach. Williams & Wilkins, Baltimore
54. Campbell WC (1940) Interposition of vitallium plates in arthroplasties of the knee: preliminary report. Am J Surg 47:639–641
55. Scott WN, Rosbruch JD et al (1978) Clinical and biomechanical evaluation of patella replacement in total knee arthroplasty. Orthop Trans 2:203
56. Dalury D, Jiranek W (1999) A comparison of the midvastus and paramedian approaches for total knee arthroplasty. J Arthroplasty 14(1):33–37
57. Keating EM, Faris P et al (1999) Comparison of the midvastus muscle-splitting approach with the median parapatellar approach in total knee arthroplasty. J Arthroplasty 14(1):29–32
58. Roysam GS, Oakley MJ (2001) Subvastus approach for total knee arthroplasty: a prospective, randomized, and observer-blinded trial. J Arthroplasty 16(4):454–457
59. Matsueda M, Gustillo R (2000) Subvastus and medial parapatellar approaches in total knee arthroplasty. Clin Orthop 371:161–168
60. Parker MJ, Livingstone V, Clifton R, McKee A (2007) Closed suction surgical wound drainage after orthopaedic surgery. Cochrane Database Syst Rev (3):CD001825. doi:10.1002/14651858.CD001825.pub2

61. Parker MJ, Roberts CP et al (2004) Closed suction drainage for hip and knee arthroplasty: a meta-analysis. J Bone Joint Surg Am 86-A(6):1146–1152

62. Walmsley PJ, Kelly MB et al (2005) A prospective, randomised, controlled trial of the use of drains in total hip arthroplasty. J Bone Joint Surg Br 87-B(10):1397–1401

63. Kumar S, Penematsa S et al (2007) Are drains required following a routine primary total joint arthroplasty? Int Orthop 31:593–596

64. Milne S, Brosseau L et al (2003) Continuous passive motion following total knee arthroplasty. Cochrane Database Syst Rev (2):CD004260. doi:10.1002/14651858.CD004260

65. Lensen T, Steyn M et al (2008) Effectiveness of prolonged use of continuous passive motion (CPM), as an adjunct to physiotherapy, after total knee arthroplasty. BMC Musculoskelet Disord 9:60

66. Bennett L, Brearly S et al (2005) A comparison of 2 continuous passive motion protocols after total knee arthroplasty. J Arthroplasty 20(2):225–233

67. Denis M, Moffet H et al (2006) Effectiveness of continuous passive motion and conventional physical therapy after total knee arthroplasty: a randomized clinical trial. Phys Ther 86(2):174–185

68. Brosseau L, Milne S et al (2004) Efficacy of continuous passive motion following total knee arthroplasty: a metaanalysis. J Rheumatol 31:2251–2264

69. Schurman DJ, Parker JN et al (1985) Total condylar knee replacement: a study of factors influencing range of motion as late as two years after arthroplasty. J Bone Joint Surg Am 67:1006–1014

70. Daluga D, Lombardi AV Jr et al (1991) Knee manipulation following total knee arthroplasty: analysis of prognostic variables. J Arthroplasty 6:119–128

71. Esler CN, Lock K et al (1999) Manipulation of total knee replacements: is the flexion gained retained? J Bone Joint Surg Br 81:27–29

72. Bong M, Di Cesare P (2004) Stiffness after total knee arthroplasty. J Am Acad Orthop Surg 12:164–171

73. Jerosch J, Aldawoudy A (2007) Arthroscopic treatment of patients with moderate arthrofibrosis after total knee replacement. Knee Surg Sports Traumatol Arthrosc 15:71–77

74. St. Clair S, Higuera C et al (2006) Hip and knee arthroplasty in the geriatric population. Clin Geriatr Med 22:515–533

75. Learmonth I, Young C et al (2007) The operation of the century: total hip replacement. Lancet 370(9597):1508–1520

76. Canale S, Beaty J (eds) (2008) Campbell's operative orthopaedics, 11th edn. Mosby Elsevier, Philadelphia

77. Charnley J (1961) Arthroplasty of the hip: a new operation. Lancet 1:1129–1132

78. Levy R, Levy C et al (1995) Outcome and long-term results following total hip replacement in elderly patients. Clin Orthop Relat Res 316:25–30

79. Buckwalter A, Callaghan J et al (2006) Results of charnley total hip arthroplasty with use of improved femoral cementing techniques. A concise follow-up, at a minimum of twenty-five years, of a previous report. J Bone Joint Surg Am 88:1481–1485

80. Firestone D, Callaghan J et al (2007) Total hip arthroplasty with a cemented, polished, collared femoral stem and a cementless acetabular component: a follow-up study at a minimum of ten years. J Bone Joint Surg Am 89-A(1):126–132

81. Klapach A, Callaghan J et al (2001) Charnley total hip arthroplasty with use of improved cementing techniques: a minimum twenty-year follow-up study. J Bone Joint Surg Am 83-A(12):1840–1848

82. Meading J, Keating M et al (2004) Minimum ten-year follow-up of a straight-stemmed, plasma-sprayed, titanium-alloy, uncemented femoral component in primary total hip arthroplasty. J Bone Joint Surg Am 86-A(1):92–97

83. McLaughlin J, Lee K (2008) Total hip arthroplasty with an uncemented tapered femoral component. J Bone Joint Surg Am 90-A(6):1290–1296

84. Keisu K, Orozco F et al (2001) Primary cementless total hip arthroplasty in octogenarians: two to eleven year follow-up. J Bone Joint Surg Am 83-A(3):359–363

85. Lettich T, Tierney M et al (2007) Primary total hip arthroplasty with an uncemented femoral component: two- to seven-year results. J Arthroplasty 22(7 Suppl 3):43–46

86. Kwon MS, Kuskowski M et al (2006) Does surgical approach affect total hip arthroplasty dislocation rates? Clin Orthop Relat Res 447:34–38

87. Masonis JL, Bourne RB (2002) Surgical approach, abductor function and total hip arthroplasty dislocation. Clin Orthop Relat Res 405:46–53

88. Sierra RJ, Raposo JM et al (2005) Dislocation of primary THA done through a posterolateral approach in the elderly. Clin Orthop Relat Res 441:262–267

89. Tsai SJ, Wang CT et al (2008) The effect of posterior capsule repair upon post-operative hip dislocation following primary total hip arthroplasty. BMC Musculoskelet Disord 9:29

90. Pellicci PM, Bostrom M et al (1998) Posterior approach to total hip replacement using enhanced posterior soft tissue repair. Clin Orthop 355:224–228

91. Jolles BM, Bogoch ER (2006) Posterior versus lateral surgical approach for total hip arthroplasty in adults with osteoarthritis. Cochrane Database Syst Rev (3):CD003828.doi:10.1002/14651858. CD003828.pub3

92. Peters C, McPherson E et al (2007) Reduction in early dislocation rate with large-diameter femoral heads in primary total hip arthroplasty. J Arthroplasty 22(6 Suppl 2):140–144

93. Baker AS, Bitounis VC (1989) Abductor function after total hip replacement – An electromyographic and clinical review. J Bone Joint Surg Br 71-B:47–50

94. Matta J, Shahrdar C et al (2005) Single-incision anterior approach for total hip arthroplasty on an orthopaedic table. Clin Orthop Relat Res 441:115–124

95. Parvizi J, Mui A et al (2007) Total joint arthroplasty: when do fatal or near-fatal complications occur? J Bone Joint Surg Am 89:27–32

96. Kurd M, Pulido L et al (2008) *Clostridium difficile* infection after total joint arthroplasty: who is at risk? J Arthroplasty 23(6):839–842

97. Mantilla C, Horlocker T et al (2002) Frequency of myocardial infarction, pulmonary embolism, deep venous thrombosis, and death following primary hip or knee arthroplasty. Anesthesiology 96:1140–1146

98. Kreder H, Berry G et al (2005) Arthroplasty in the octogenarian: quantifying the risks. J Arthroplasty 20(3):289–293

99. Berend M, Thong A et al (2003) Total joint arthroplasty in the extremely elderly: hip and knee arthroplasty after entering the 89th year of life. J Arthroplasty 18(7):817–821

100. American Dental Association; American Academy of Orthopaedic Surgeons (1997) Advisory statement: antibiotic prophylaxis for dental patients with total joint replacements. J Am Dent Assoc 128:1004–1007

101. Waldman BJ, Mont MA, Hungerford DS (1997) Total knee arthroplasty infections associated with dental procedures. Clin Orthop 343:164–172

102. LaPorte D, Waldman B et al (1999) Infections associated with dental procedures in total hip arthroplasty. J Bone Joint Surg Br 81-B(1):56–59

103. Uckay I, Pittet D et al (2008) Antibiotic prophylaxis before invasive dental procedures in patients with arthroplasties of the hip and knee. J Bone Joint Surg Br 90B:833–838

104. Schinsky M, Della Valle C et al (2008) Perioperative testing for joint infection in patients undergoing revision total hip arthroplasty. J Bone Joint Surg Am 90:1869–1875

105. Della Valle C, Sporer S et al (2007) Preoperative testing for sepsis before revision total knee arthroplasty. J Arthroplasty 22 (6 Supp 2): 90–93

106. Palestro CJ, Kim CK et al (1990) Total-hip arthroplasty: periprosthetic indium-111-labeled leukocyte activity and complementary technetium-99m-sulfur colloid imaging in suspected infection. J Nucl Med 31(12):1950–1955

107. Scher DM, Pak K et al (2000) The predictive value of indium-111 leukocyte scans in the diagnosis of infected total hip, knee, or resection arthroplasties. J Arthroplasty 15(3): 295–300

108. Tsukayama D, Estrada R et al (1996) Infection after total hip arthroplasty: a study of the treatment of one hundred and six infections. J Bone Joint Surg Am 78A(4):512–523

109. Deirmengian C, Greenbaum J et al (2003) Open debridement of acute gram-positive infections after total knee arthroplasty. Clin Orthop Relat Res 416:129–134

110. Lonner JH, Desai P, Dicesare PE et al (1996) The reliability of analysis of intraoperative frozen sections for identifying active infection during revision hip or knee arthroplasty. J Bone Joint Surg Am 78A(10):1553–1558

111. Della Valle C, Zuckerman J et al (2004) Periprosthetic sepsis. Clin Orthop 420:26–31

112. Della Valle CJ, Bogner BA, Desai P et al (1999) Analysis of frozen sections of intraoperative specimens obtained at the time of reoperation after hip or knee resection arthroplasty for the treatment of infection. J Bone Joint Surg Am 81A(5): 684–689

113. Banit D, Kaufer H et al (2002) Intraoperative frozen section analysis in revision total joint arthroplasty. Clin Orthop Relat Res 401:230–238

114. Haddad FS, Muirhead-Allwood S et al (2000) Two-stage uncemented revision hip arthroplasty for infection. J Bone Joint Surg Br 82(5):689–694

115. Hofman A, Goldberg T et al (2005) Treatment of infected total knee arthroplasty using an articulating spacer: 2- to 12-year experience. Clin Orthop Relat Res 430:125–131

116. Parvizi J, Pour A et al (2007) Revision total hip arthroplasty in octogenarians: a case-control study. J Bone Joint Surg Am 89A(12):2612–2618

117. Peters C, Erickson J et al (2005) Revision total knee arthroplasty with modular components inserted with metaphyseal cement and stems without cement. J Arthroplasty 20(3):302–308

118. Bertin KC, Freeman MAR, Samuelson KM et al (1985) Stemmed revision arthroplasty for aseptic loosening of total knee arthroplasty. J Bone Joint Surg Br 67B:242

119. Peters CL, Hennessy R, Barden RM et al (1997) Revision total knee arthroplasty with a cemented posteriorstabilized or constrained condylar prosthesis. J Arthroplasty 12:896

120. Cook R, Jenkins P et al (2008) Risk factors for periprosthetic fractures of the hip: a survivorship analysis. Clin Orthop Relat Res 466:1652–1656

121. Berry DJ (1999) Periprosthetic fractures after major joint replacement. Epidemiology: hip and knee. Orthop Clin North Am 30:183–190

122. Brady OH, Garbuz DS, Masri BA et al (2000) The reliability and validity of the Vancouver classification of femoral fractures after hip replacement. J Arthroplasty 15:59–62

123. Masri B, Meek R et al (2004) Periprosthetic fractures evaluation and treatment. Clin Orthop 420:80–95

124. Su E, DeWal H et al (2004) Periprosthetic femoral fractures above total knee replacements. J Am Acad Orthop Surg 12:12–20

125. Kim K, Egol K et al (2006) Periprosthetic fractures after total knee arthroplasties. Clin Orthop Relat Res 446:167–175

126. Haidukewych GJ (2007) Periprosthetic distal femur fracture: plate versus nail fixation. J Orthop Trauma 21(3):219–221

127. Blomfeldt R, Tornkvist H et al (2005) Comparison of internal fixation with total hip replacement for displaced femoral neck fractures. J Bone Joint Surg Am 87A(8):1680–1688

128. Johansson T, Bachrach-Lindström M (2006) The total costs of a displaced femoral neck fracture: comparison of internal fixation and total hip replacement: a randomised study of 146 hips. Int Orthop 30:1–6

129. Klein G, Parvizi J et al (2006) Total hip arthroplasty for acute femoral neck fractures using a cementless tapered femoral stem. J Arthroplasty 21(8):1134–1140

130. Mouzopoulos G, Stamatakos M et al (2008) The four-year functional result after a displaced subcapital hip fracture treated with three different surgical options. Int Orthop 32:367–373

Section XIII
Transplantation

Chapter 96
Invited Commentary

Khalid M.H. Butt

When asked to comment on organ transplantation in senior citizens, I reflected on the evolution of this restorative therapy over the past four decades, during which I have been a student of the subject while actively performing kidney transplants.

End-stage failure of vital organs inevitably results in death unless function is replaced either by artificial means, as in the case of the kidney with dialysis therapy, or when a transplant is accomplished and the graft works (liver, heart, and lung). In the latter case, the quality of life is markedly improved and longevity may be nearly doubled with a successful kidney transplant. Justifiably then, if an organ is available and the patient is judged to have enough physiologic reserve to be able to withstand the vicissitudes of anesthesia, surgery, and the immunosuppressive regimen, transplantation remains the best therapy.

Drawing on the steady advances in anesthesia and surgical technique (especially vascular) during the first half of the twentieth century, Joseph Murray and colleagues launched a new era by successfully performing the first kidney transplant between identical twins in 1954. This revolutionary life-preserving new therapy had to be applied cautiously. First, it was imperative to ascertain that no long-term harm was done to the donor, whose rights had to be vigorously protected. Our obligation to protect the donor's interests had to be clearly enunciated. Second, the recipients needed to be observed for quite some time to determine any unforeseen complications and the durability of this treatment. Initially, only end-stage renal disease patients between the ages of 15 and 45 years with no significant involvement of any other organ system were offered kidney transplantation. During the sixties and seventies, broadening acceptance of the determination of death by neurologic criteria offered increased opportunities for recovery of organs from "heart-beating" cadavers. Extending transplantation horizons, Starzl successfully transplanted liver in 1963, and in 1967, Barnard transplanted a heart.

Incomplete understanding of the pathogenic mechanisms of immunologic allograft rejection, and our limited ability to halt and reverse this process continued to be the major concern into the eighties. Infections and malignancies as complications of immunosuppression took a heavy toll. With the discovery of cyclosporine, a calcineurin inhibitor and somewhat more specific immunosuppressive drugs, transplant outcomes started to improve. The introduction of other agents into our immunosuppressive armamentarium, and the evolution of more efficacious and safer combination regimens extended the spectrum of candidates for organ replacement at both ends, i.e., from infancy to the elderly (seventies and eighties). Age by itself, as a consideration of candidacy for organ transplantation, is no longer an overwhelming concern. Needless to say, age-associated maladies, like coronary and carotid artery disease, malignancy, general nutritional status and viability of the patient must be properly assessed. Results of kidney transplantation in the elderly (≥65 years) are now comparable to those of younger adults.

There still remains a societal concern. With little increase in the numbers of deceased-donor organs recovered over the past many years, paired with an ever-increasing demand, society, not the doctors, must decide how these precious resources are to be utilized. Allocating the organs in a manner that employs the best mix of justice (equality to all the patients waiting) and utility (getting the most value) continues to challenge the minds and hearts of all concerned. Family members of deceased donors, potential recipients and their families and friends, transplant doctors, other health-care workers, scientists and researchers, lawyers and judges, politicians and public officials, social scientists, philosophers and ethicists all grapple with the task of developing the best schema. When the name of a criminal on death row pops up for heart transplantation, no amount of rational debate can overcome the strong emotions aroused. Elderly patients often garner a similar, though usually not as visceral, response.

Eurotransplant, an organization of six European countries (covering a population of 118 million) collaborating in recovery and allocation of deceased donor organs, as well as

K.M.H. Butt (✉)
Department of Surgery – Transplant Section,
Westchester Medical Center, 95 Grasslands Road, Valhalla,
NY 10595, USA
e-mail: buttk@wcmc.com; khalidmhbutt@att.net

R.A. Rosenthal et al. (eds.), *Principles and Practice of Geriatric Surgery*,
DOI 10.1007/978-1-4419-6999-6_96, © Springer Science+Business Media, LLC 2011

transplant research, developed a Eurotransplant Seniors Program (ESP) about 10 years ago. They rapidly allocate a kidney recovered from a ≥65-year-old donor to a ≥65-year-old recipient who is not sensitized and is ready to receive a first transplant. Cold ischemia time is thus cut short, resulting in decreased incidence of delayed graft function, and survival results comparable to those of adults <65 years of age. Equally important, this program significantly contributes to better utilization of deceased donor kidneys; Eurotransplant has a discard rate of one in twenty (1/20), compared to that of the US of one in seven (1/7). This seems a step in the right direction.

There are some rudimentary efforts to predict the "additional quality-adjusted life years" gained by an organ transplant and the projected cost per year. This imperfect and imprecise future casting is an attempt to maximize the utilitarian aspect of organ allocation. While the dilemma of resource allocation awaits resolution, perhaps success in in vitro generation of organs from autologous stem cells or developments allowing clinical application of xenotransplantation from animals used for food will emerge. In the meantime, we can surely take the position today that denying seniors this vital therapy on the basis of age alone is ethically and morally reprehensible, and may be illegal.

Chapter 97
Elderly Donors in Transplantation

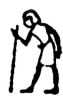

Manuel Mendizabal, John W. Hsu, and Abraham Shaked

Introduction

At the time of the writing of this chapter the number of candidates on the waiting list, as designated by the United Network for Organ Sharing (UNOS), totals just over 100,000 [1]. A closer look at yearly tabulations of patients transplanted and patients newly listed shows that for about every two patients added to the transplant list, one patient is actually transplanted. Because the waiting list continues to grow, there has been increased interest in the use of expanded criteria donors (ECD). While there are many different ways to define the ECD, one universal attribute of ECD that makes it germane to the topic of this textbook is increased donor age. The aims of this chapter are to (1) examine the elderly donor evaluation and screening process in this patient population; (2) discuss the predonation management of these older patients as well as the donor procedure and technical complications that may be encountered in the procurement operation, and (3) discuss the allocation process and examine the results and outcomes in the use of these elderly organs.

How Old Is Old?

The definitions of the ECD are based on the premise of increased risk of poorer outcomes in the usage of these organs when compared with the ideal or standard criteria donor (SCD). One aspect that is constant in all organ types is increased donor age; assuming that geriatric organs would portend to a higher risk of worsened recipient outcomes. Organ specific and nonspecific risk factors that determine allograft outcomes are shown in Table 97.1.

In kidney transplantation, the ECD is defined as a donor greater than 60 years of age or donor greater than 50 years of

age with two of the three following attributes: donor with terminal creatinine greater than 1.5 mg/dL; donor whose death resulted from a cerebrovascular accident; and donor with history of hypertension [2–4]. In general, despite an increase in delayed graft function (DGF), long-term graft function of the older allograft and patient survival are acceptable when compared to SCDs, and mortality decreased when compared to those on the waiting list, thereby justifying the use of such organs [5].

In a recent consensus meeting on liver transplantation, the ideal donor was defined according to the following criteria: trauma as the cause of death, donation after brain death, age below 40 years, hemodynamic stability at the time of procurement, no steatosis or any other underlying chronic liver lesion, and no transmissible disease [6, 7]. Certainly the elderly liver donor would has a significant impact on allograft function as advanced age have been attributed to a liver with impaired regenerative capacity and an increased severity of hepatitis C virus (HCV) recurrence. Despite documented increased donor risk as related to age, there is no absolute limit to donor age for liver transplantation, and indeed, successful transplantation has occurred even with octogenarian donor organs [8].

There are no clearly defined criteria for ECD for pancreas transplantation. In general only, 20–25% of pancreata is procured from donors due to the strict criteria defining the acceptable pancreatic donor. This, in part, is due to the high rate of complications associated with pancreatic transplant, which has led to the use of mostly pristine organs. In one series of simultaneous pancreas–kidney transplants, ECD was defined as donors <10 and ≥40 years or donor after cardiac death (DCD) status. However, outcome studies demonstrate similar graft survival when compared with a cohort of SCD [9].

In lung transplantation, many programs consider a donor who fulfill any of the following criteria as an ECD: age 55 years or older, donor smoking history 20 pack-years or more, purulent secretions or inflammation at bronchoscopy, evidence of significant chest trauma, a pulmonary infiltrate on chest radiograph, duration of ventilation longer than 5 days, and PaO_2/FiO_2 ratio less than 300 mmHg just before donor pneumonectomy [10]. Recipients of these organs had an

A. Shaked (✉)
Division of Surgery, University of Pennsylvania Transplant Institute, Hospital of the University of Pennsylvania, Philadelphia, PA, USA

R.A. Rosenthal et al. (eds.), *Principles and Practice of Geriatric Surgery*,
DOI 10.1007/978-1-4419-6999-6_97, © Springer Science+Business Media, LLC 2011

TABLE 97.1 Proposed donor variables for extended criteria donors

Donor variables	Kidney[a]	Liver[b]	Lung[b]	Heart[b]
Age (years)	≥60 or >50	N/A	≥55	>55
Cause of death	CVA	N/A	N/A	CVA
Cold ischemia time	N/A	>12 h	N/A	>5 h
Past medical history	• Hypertension • Cr>1.5 mg/dL	Hepatitis C	≥20 pack/year smoking history	• Hepatitis C • CAD • Cocaine abuse • Alcoholism
Graft	N/A	• Macrovesicular steatosis>30% • Vasopressor at time of procurement	• Ventilation>5 days • PaO$_2$/FiO$_2$<300 mmHg • Pulmonary infiltrate on CXR • Purulent secretions	• Under sizing (<30% mismatch) in recipients with PHT • Over sizing (>30% mismatch) in recipients with LVADs for acute MI or multiple reoperations

N/A non applicable; *CVA* cerebrovascular accident; *Cr* creatinine; *CAD* coronary artery disease; *CXR* chest X-ray; *PHT* pulmonary hypertension; *LVADs* left ventricular automated devices; *MI* myocardial infarction

[a] ≥60 or >50 and at least two other variables

[b] At least one variable present

increased mortality rate; however, the transplanted lungs exhibited adequate posttransplant function. Interestingly, a recent series of transplants with donors aged 50 and older found no difference in survival and functional reserve between the ECD recipients and a cohort of SCD recipients [11]. In addition, a subanalysis of those donors over 50 showed no difference in 1-year survival. It is concluded that the true cutoff for a potential lung donor is yet to be vigorously studied, and it may be at a different borderline than that currently defined.

Once, the upper limit of donor age for transplantation of the heart was 35 years of age; nowadays, it is common for cardiac donors to be greater than 50 years of age. Nevertheless, the current definition of ECD for heart donors includes donors older than 55, as well as other variables such as prolonged ischemia times (>5 h), HCV infection, alcohol abuse, cocaine abuse, atraumatic intracranial hemorrhage, under- and oversizing, and preexisting coronary artery disease (CAD) [12]. Despite data indicating increased initial posttransplant mortality risk, a review of the UNOS registry shows that mortality of patients on the waiting list is higher.

As organs continue to remain a scarce resource for transplantation, it is predictable that the utilization of organs of older donors will continue to increase. Despite what some deem as the inferior outcomes of extended criteria transplantation, the unacceptable sequelae of end-stage disease will compel continuous redefinition of the extended criteria.

Determination of Brain Death

As with most cadaveric donors, the evaluation of the geriatric donor begins with the declaration of brain death. A review of the Scientific Registry of Transplant Recipients (SRTR) data shows that most brain deaths occur secondary to stroke, with the second most prevalent diagnosis occurring with trauma (41.9 and 38.1%, respectively) [13]. When a brain-injured patient presents with coma and evidence of irreversible structural brain injury, the screening process for organ donation is begun. In general, the physician or medical team taking care of this individual is responsible for notifying the area organ procurement organization (OPO) to start the process. Once the process is initiated, the OPO will dispatch field coordinators who are then responsible for facilitating declaration of brain death, family counseling, and consent for donation, as well as completing the screening process with review of medical and social histories, and the completion of laboratory and serologic tests. Once all information is acquired, communication with the transplant center and transplant center physician will lead to an appropriately matched recipient with arrangements made for eventual procurement of the organs.

The declaration of brain death is mandatory prior to proceeding with evaluation for procurement. The current brain death criteria in the USA is outlined in a set of guidelines published in 1981 entitled the President's Commission for the Study of Ethical Problems and adopted under the Uniform Determination of Death Act. This act states that death has occurred once there is irreversible cessation of brain function including the brainstem. Each state government has adopted these guidelines in legislating local criteria for determining brain death. Usually there are variations in the necessity and type of confirmative testing required, how many examinations are required to determine brain death, and how many physicians are required to make that determination. Most hospitals will then establish their own protocols for determining brain death for potential donors under their care.

Symptoms that support the diagnosis of brain death include the absence of brainstem reflexes, cortical activity, and demonstration of irreversibility of the injury. All reversible causes of a coma must then be ruled out, including hypothermia, hypoxia, hypoglycemia, hyperglycemia, uremia, hepatic failure, Reye's syndrome, hyponatremia, hypercalcemia, myxedema, adrenal failure, and CNS depressants. When reversible causes are ruled out and symptoms of brain death exist, then brain death is initially confirmed with apnea testing. The patient should be warm, maintaining a blood pressure greater than 90 mmHg, preoxygenated with 100% FiO_2 for 10 min, and eucapnia must be confirmed with initial pretest blood gas. The test is commenced by disconnecting the patient from the ventilator. During this time, high-flow oxygen is delivered into the trachea via catheter at the level of the carina. The patient is monitored for respiratory activity; if any is present, the patient is immediately reconnected to the ventilator. A standard waiting time of 8 min is instituted if the patient remains apneic and hemodynamically stable. If a repeat blood gas yields a $PaCO_2$ of 60 mmHg or greater then brain death is declared. The test can be repeated with 10-min duration if 60 mmHg is not attained. Confirmatory tests include the EEG, and tests that confirm lack of cerebral blood flow (cerebral angiography, duplex ultrasound, radionuclide cerebral blood flow scanning).

Donor Management

The physiology of brain death has been delineated over the years by animal models and observations in human case series. Brain death proceeds as ischemia in a rostral-caudal fashion. This progression causes initially an increased vagal activation followed by the Cushing reflex due to a mixed vagal/sympathetic stimulation. Continued progression of ischemia down the brainstem produces an autonomic surge causing extreme elevation of heart rate and blood pressure, followed by sympathetic deactivation as the spinal cord is eventually affected. In general, this results in a hemodynamically unstable patient. The initial goal of donor management, therefore, is an assessment and maintenance of hemodynamic stability. This is achieved via echocardiography and resuscitation via crystalloid, colloid, and blood product infusions. Vasoactive support could be added via use of dopamine and dobutamine infusions. Finally, hormone replacement therapy (i.e., thyroxine, methylprednisolone, insulin, and vasopressin) may be instituted in a donor with persistent hemodynamic lability. The goal is maintenance of blood pressure above 100 mmHg, CVP around 10 mmHg, and urine output above 40 mL/h. There may be benefit in maintaining urine outputs greater than 100 mL/h, however detriment in outputs greater than 300 mL/h. When donors

develop diabetes insipidus, hypotonic replacement to keep up with hypotonic urine loss becomes necessary combined with desmopressin. When urine output drops below 40 mL/h the addition of diuretics and mannitol may be helpful in donor management.

Previous studies have shown shortened time to graft failure in donors with terminal serum creatinine levels greater than 1.5 mg/dL. In a separate analysis of donor factors that predispose to decreased graft survival, it has been reported that the goal in donor management of keeping serum creatinine levels under 2 mL/dL seems to exert favorable effect on graft function in recipients [14]. The likelihood of impaired renal function in the older donor mandates donor management that is aimed to optimize serum creatinine levels.

Much consideration has been given to renal biopsy and correlation with function and level of glomerulosclerosis (GS). However, there have been mixed results, and no consistent correlation has been observed between increased GS and graft survival and function. In general, worse outcomes were demonstrated with GS greater than 20% [15]. In theory, the transfer of more nephron mass via transplanting two same donor ECD allografts may improve posttransplant glomerular filtration rate (GFR) [16]. Further improvements may be achieved by using pulsatile perfusion to improve ECD outcomes. Ex vivo perfusion of ECD kidneys did not show definite survival advantage; however, there are indications that pumped kidneys have increased final use of ECD kidneys as well as decreased DGF [17].

In the elderly donor, advanced age impairs regenerative capacity of the liver and therefore injury due to ischemia and subsequent recovery from injury could be exaggerated. Occasionally, a liver biopsy can be used to assess other variables that may increase the rate of primary nonfunction; the presence of steatosis > 30% is considered as extremely high-risk, as is periportal fibrosis [18]. A short cold ischemia CIT (< 6 h) is imperative in optimizing outcomes of ECD liver allograft. Consequently, acceptance of ECD liver should consider donor age and the ability to transplant the allograft within short time after procurement.

In the evaluation of cardiac donors, a consensus conference report on the maximization of use of organs from cadaveric donors recommended angiography for all donors aged greater than 55 years [19]. Donors with mild coronary artery disease (CAD) can be used for high-risk recipients. Some centers are performing backbench bypass grafting and valve repair with acceptable results of graft patency and function [20]. To reduce the ill effects of contrast nephrotoxicity, a left-sided ventriculography can be avoided if a quality echocardiogram was performed. One series reported successful implementation of backbench coronary angiography to avoid exposing the kidneys to contrast [21].

Since all brain-dead donors are mechanically ventilated, special consideration must be taken in the management of the lung donor. In consideration of the optimization of the lung donor, judicious fluid management with aggressive maintenance of euvolemia is key. High tidal volumes and use of PEEP are traditional management practices. Volutrauma is kept at a minimum by careful titration of PEEP as well as keeping peak pressures at less than 35 cmH$_2$O and increasing minute ventilation [22]. In a recent series evaluating lungs from donors older than 50 years or older, lungs were assessed by bronchoscopy, lab work, and medical history. Aggressive pulmonary toilet was instigated, and those with difficult-to-clear airways as well as evidence of physical lung injury were rejected for transplant. Selection of donors was also predicated on a PF ratio greater than 300 upon donor resuscitation and optimization with ventilator adjustments and bronchoscopy. Optimization of the lung donors with these maneuvers resulted in the use of extended criteria lungs with acceptable posttransplant function [11].

The Procurement Procedure

In order to avoid potential complications, elderly donors should undergo a thorough evaluation, prior to the procurement procedure (Table 97.2). The fate of recipient outcomes is greatly influenced by the procurement operation. Careful dissection and tissue handling are important, and usability of the graft depends on the viability of critical anatomic structures. This multifaceted procedure requires coordination between thoracic and abdominal procurement team, aiming at a speedy recovery of the organ, as factors such as warm and cold ischemia gravely affect transplant outcomes and ultimately influences the success of the recipient procedure.

TABLE 97.2 Elderly donor considerations

Comorbidities

- Coronary artery disease
- Valvular disease
- Diabetes
- Peripheral vascular disease
- Renal dysfunction
- CMV positive
- Malignancy
  - Melanoma
  - Renal cell carcinoma
  - Choriocarcinoma
- Prior surgeries

Technical difficulties

- Atherosclerosis
- Vascular stents
- VAD
- Radiotherapy

VAD ventricular assist device

The patient is prepped from chin to groin and laterally, table to table. It is our practice to drape about two to three inches on either side of our midline incision which is then carried out from sternal notch to pubis. In the elderly donor, one must be mindful of prior surgeries and the need of an extensive exploration to rule out the presence of malignancies. Donor-related malignancies can be either due to direct transmission of tumor or due to tumor arising in cells of donor origin. Kauffman et al. analyzed UNOS data for donor-related malignancies during 1994–2001 [23]. During this time, 108,062 patients underwent a solid transplant, and only a total of 21 donor-related malignancies in transplant recipients were reported [23]. The most frequently reported transmission of non-CNS tumor after solid organ transplant has been renal cell carcinoma followed by melanoma and choriocarcinoma [24].

Removal of Thoracic Organs

Concomitant to the procurement operation by the intra-abdominal team, the chest is opened via a median sternotomy. The chest team then proceeds to expose the heart and examine the lungs. The heart is mobilized and superior vena cava (SVC) exposed. The pleura are opened by incising through the pleura behind the sternum. The pleural spaces are examined along with all lobes of the lung. The posterobasal bases are often atelectatic and should be reexpanded by bronchoscopy and vigorous hand bagging. The thoracic organs are then kept moist until completion of mobilization of the intra-abdominal organs. Once this is done, heparinization is commenced and standard cardioplegia cannula is placed in the ascending aorta and a large-bore cannula is placed in the proximal pulmonary artery. The SVC is ligated and divided, and the lower trachea is encircled by a nylon tape. Hypotension is then induced via infusion of medications or exsanguination. The ascending and descending aorta are then clamped, and cardioplegia solution infusion is begun. At the same time, the pulmonary artery, abdominal aorta, and portal vein flush are begun as well. Ice slush or cold saline is then placed in the cardiac well and around all organs. Once cold perfusion has been achieved, the heart is elevated out of the pericardium, and the pulmonary veins are divided individually and the pulmonary artery is divided at the level of its bifurcation. The aorta is divided at the level of the innominate artery and the heart is removed and packaged. The pericardium is then incised vertically on both sides to expose the lung hilum. The inferior pulmonary ligaments are taken down. Dissection continues up the back of the trachea in an obvious plane immediately anterior to the esophagus. This is continued on the right side until the nylon tape is encountered. Dissection continues on the left at the level of the aortic arch until meeting up with the nylon tape. After the hilum is free the anesthetist is instructed to reinflate the lungs to approximately three quarters the total lung capacity. The trachea is then stapled after withdrawal of endotracheal tube. The lung block is then removed and packaged.

Procurement of Abdominal Organs

A midline laparotomy incision is made from the xyphoid to the pubis. The ligamentum teres is isolated and divided between clamps and ties, and the falciform ligament is taken down toward the suprahepatic inferior venous cava (IVC). The left lateral segment is freed from its lateral triangular ligament attachments and folded medially to divide the pars flaccida. It is lifted with forceps and a hole is made in it. Using gentle palpation, the rest of the ligament is palpated for a replaced left hepatic artery, taking care to preserve a replaced or accessory left hepatic artery.

The abdomen is retracted bilaterally providing ample exposure to the entire intra-abdominal cavity. A Cattell–Braasch maneuver is then performed with kocherization of the duodenum to expose the infrahepatic IVC and the junctions of the left and right renal veins. To secure perfusion of the abdominal organs, portal and aortic flush sites are isolated and secured. The aorta just proximal to its bifurcation can be skeletonized quickly by spreading with the Metzenbaum scissors along each side taking care not to spread into lumbar branches, not to injure the inferior mesenteric artery (IMA), and to preserve take-off of lower pole renal arteries. In older donors, one must survey this region and find a suitable noncalcified area for proximal control. Once a suitable area of the aorta is designated, two umbilical tapes are passed underneath the aorta with the use of a long right-angle clamp. Access to the portal system is achieved by isolating the inferior mesenteric vein (IMV), which is skeletonized and prepared for the insertion of a flush cannula.

With the portal and aortic flush sites isolated and ready, the supraceliac aorta is isolated after dividing the crura of the diaphragm. Skeletonizing the aorta can be achieved by gentle spreads of surrounding tissue. The aorta is cross-clamped once preservation solution is infused via the portal and aortic cannulas. Dissection of hepatic vessels at the porta hepatis is limited, since injury may deem the organ to be inappropriate for transplant. The aims are to divide the common bile duct, to expose the portal vein, and identify the anatomy of the arterial blood supply. If the pancreas is being procured, the lesser sac is entered to evaluate the pancreas along its entire length. The pancreas is palpated to feel that it is soft, without induration and calcifications. The right and left gutters are exposed; however, the kidneys are not dissected until after perfusion with preservation solution.

When the thoracic and abdominal teams are ready, cannulas are inserted into the IMV and aorta, the donor is heparinized, and the supraceliac aorta is clamped. The aortic cannulation can be difficult especially if the donor has had a graft, severe atherosclerotic disease, or a stent.

The right pericardium is opened so that the exsanguinated blood can flow into the chest cavity and evacuate. Ice slush is placed on the liver, behind the liver, on the pancreas, and over the kidneys. In general, the aortic flush is ran for three liters of chilled University of Wisconsin solution, and two liters usually suffice for the portal flush.

The hierarchy in the extraction of abdominal organs proceeds by removing individual organs, liver, pancreas, kidneys, or by block removal of all organs with dissection of individual organs on the backbench. The organs are removed taking care to pressure appropriate inflow and outflow vessels, length of ureters and bile duct, and loop of duodenum when the pancreas is used for transplant. The iliac vessels are then procured along with nodes for tissue typing. The vessels may be used for arterial or venous reconstruction when needed. The abdomen is then closed with a running nylon suture with full thickness bites.

Procurement of Living Donors

The donor nephrectomy technique varies among different centers. Open surgical technique has been the traditional method for removing a kidney from a living donor; however, since the mid-1990s many centers have embarked on laparoscopic living donor nephrectomy. If an open approach is to be used, the donor is placed in the lateral position and a modified flank incision is made, just above or below the twelfth rib. Most surgeons avoid entering the pleural and peritoneal cavities. The kidney is carefully dissected to preserve all renal arteries, renal veins, and the periureteral blood supply. During the procedure, mannitol and furosemide plus adequate crystalloid solutions are administered to the donor to ensure brisk diuresis. The kidney is removed once the renal vessels are securely ligated and divided. The excised kidney is then perfused with cold heparinized electrolyte solution.

For a laparoscopic-assisted procedure, the patient is placed in the flank position and a pneumoperitoneum is established through a Veress needle. The instruments and the video camera are manipulated through four ports established through small incisions in the abdominal wall. The whole procedure is visualized on a video monitor. First, the colon is mobilized and reflected medially, which exposes Gerota's fascia. Subsequently, the liver (for right-sided procedures) and spleen (for left-sided procedures) are retracted away from the upper pole of the kidney. The ureter and periureteral tissues are freed from the perinephric tissues. Next, the renal vein and artery are carefully dissected. The kidney is placed in a plastic bag and is removed through a Pfannenstiel incision.

Finally, the kidney is then flushed with heparinized solution as for open nephrectomy.

In general, elderly liver donors are not accepted. The upper age limit for living liver donation varies from center to center and is usually between 50 and 65 years. Since the incidence of unknown medical diseases and postoperative morbimortality increases with age, acceptance of elderly donors must be exercised with caution.

Elderly Living Donors

Living donation is an ideal modality for transplantation and optimizes patient selection, ischemia times, and survival outcomes. The desire to extend criteria for suitable organs extends into this population of donors as well. Central to this goal of optimizing availability of living donor organs is the juxtaposition of the notion of *primum nocerum*, in which the assurance of donor safety becomes a priority in the evaluation process. This is then heightened as considers the use of older donors where aging physiology and more brittle general health contribute to less margin of safety. A prerequisite for performing live donor transplantation is assessing an acceptable risk–benefit ratio for both donor and recipient. A detailed evaluation of a potential donor in order to minimize the donor risks and assurance of a completely voluntary donation should be addressed.

Living donor renal transplant (LDRT) is a robust and prevalent modality in transplant. In the USA, the number of LDRTs has exceeded that of deceased donor kidney transplants, while in Japan 80% of the kidney transplants are dependent on LDRT [25, 26]. Donor safety and lifetime risk was ascertained in a large, long-term study that included 3,698 patients [27]. In this study, survival of kidney donors was similar to that of controls in the general population with end-stage renal disease (ESRD) developing in 11 patients, which is a rate of 180 per million persons per year. This is compared with a rate of 268 per million persons in the white population of the USA. In addition, a subanalysis of 255 donors revealed better health-related quality of life than those in the general population. In a subsequent Japanese study, survival of LDRT is slightly better than the age- and gender-matched general population with the causes of donor death being similar to that of the general population [26]. The perioperative morbidity and mortality of living kidney donation is well documented by an US survey that included 171 transplant centers [28]. This study looked at 10,828 living donor nephrectomies: 52% were open, 21% hand-assisted laparoscopic, and 27% total laparoscopic procedures. Two donors died from surgery complications and one other remained in a vegetative stage. Reoperation was necessary in 0.4% of open surgery patients, 1% in hand-assisted patients,

and 0.9% in the totally laparoscopic patients. Bleeding and incisional hernia were the most common indications for reoperation in the laparoscopic group and in the open and hand-assisted group, respectively. Readmission rate was higher in the laparoscopic group (1.6%) than in the open nephrectomy group (0.6%), mostly because of gastrointestinal complications. This data shows that living donor nephrectomy carries a low incidence of morbidity and mortality in US transplant centers.

Among the options for decreasing time on the waiting list, elderly donors have emerged as a potential alternative. A survey performed among all US kidney transplant programs revealed that 21% of the programs excluded candidates over 65 years old. Meanwhile, the percentage of programs without a set upper age limit has now more than doubled to 59% when compared to a similar survey performed 12 years ago [29]. Furthermore, the number of LDRTs from donors >55 years has increased from 1,133 in 1996 to 1,491 in 2004 [30]. This observational cohort study using data from OPTN/UNOS compared the outcomes of LDRT in recipients older than 60 years receiving either kidney from old donors (>55 years) or young donors (≤55 years). Similar graft and patient survival rates were found after 4 years in both groups: 78 and 82% in the old donor group and 81 and 84% in the young donor group, respectively. Thus, LDRT from the older donor appears to be a suitable option to decrease time on the waiting list, especially in elderly recipients.

Living donor liver transplantation (LDLT) was first performed in 1989 with transplantation of a left hepatic lobe of an adult into a child [31]. Ten years later, adult-to-adult LDLT was introduced attempting left-hepatic lobe transplantation, but dismal results due to small-to-size graft syndrome discouraged this approach [32]. Consequently, the larger right-hepatic lobe grafts have replaced them in routine use at many centers. Recently, the Adult-to-Adult Living Donor Liver Transplantation Cohort Study (A2ALL) investigated the rate and severity of complications in right-lobe living donors [33]. A 38% complication rate was reported, with infection (12.5%), biliary leak (9.2%), and incisional hernias (6%) being the most common ones; overall mortality was 0.8%. Certain donor characteristics were associated to significant higher risk of postoperative complications. Intraoperative transfusion of more than 1 unit of blood and alkaline phosphatase ≥86 IU/L were associated to increased risk of developing complications after LDLT. Patel et al. reported an overall complication rate after left- and right-lobe LDLT of 29% [34]. Interestingly, they described donors older than 50 years as a risk factor for major complications. Decreased capacity of regeneration in older donors has been hypothesized as possible explanation for this finding [35]. In other studies, diminished early graft regeneration from older donors was shown to affect graft survival as well [36, 37]. It is well established that donors can experience severe psychiatric complications [38]. In an A2ALL retrospective study including 392 patients, one or multiple psychiatric complications were presented in 4% of the patients including three severe psychiatric complications like suicide, accidental drug overdose, and suicide attempt. These tragic events may be prevented with careful psychiatric assessment and monitoring of liver donors. Presumably, quality of life should be affected after LDLT, but a recent meta-analysis evaluating adult LDLT outcomes reported that the donors rated higher on quality-of-life scales than the general population and one study even reported some improvements in their psychosocial measures [39].

Organ Allocation Policies

UNOS is a private not-for-profit organization created in 1987 that nucleates all transplant hospitals' waiting lists and links all OPOs. In order to optimize the distribution and allocation of organs, different organ allocation systems were created to assure maximal utility, justice, and transparency of this scarce resource. The efficacy of any organ allocation system is measured by patient and graft survival rates and patient survival rates can be divided into survival on the waiting list and survival after transplantation.

Liver allocation is now based on the Model for End-Stage Liver Disease (MELD) that predicts 3-month mortality on the waiting list and benefit from transplantation. MELD is based on logarithmic transformation of the recipient's bilirubin, creatinine, and international normalized ratio (INR) into a validated mathematical model. After 1 year of introducing the MELD score, a 3.5% reduction in waiting list mortality, a 12% reduction of new candidates to the liver transplant waiting list, and identical posttransplant survival were reported [40]. Despite the positive effect the MELD score had on organ allocation, there is still potential room for improvement such as incorporation of new parameters (i.e., sodium) and donor factors, which are now not taken into consideration.

The kidney allocation system has evolved over the past 20 years. Currently, patients are ranked according to an allocation algorithm based on their waiting time, degree of HLA matching, pediatric candidates, and panel-reactive antibodies. However, the waiting time on the kidney transplant list continues to increase, largely due to the increase of the number of new registrants aged 50 years or older. Consequently, the criteria for accepting kidneys for transplantation were extended and organs from donors ≥ 55 years of age are used with increasing frequency. An Italian group reported similar long-term graft survival in those recipients who received a kidney from donors older than 60 years when compared with donors ≤ 60 years [41]. In order to improve the distribution of the scarce resource of cadaveric kidneys the current allocation policy is being reviewed by UNOS Kidney Transplant Committee.

Since May 2005, the order of candidates on the waiting list for lung transplantation has been based on the Lung Allocation Score (LAS). LAS is defined as the transplant benefit measure minus the waiting list urgency measure, which are calculated using a statistical model and candidate's clinical and physiological characteristics. The factors used in calculating each factor are described elsewhere [42]. LAS is represented by a continuous scale from 0 to 100, higher scores represent higher urgency and greater potential transplant benefit. Since LAS was implemented, waiting time has decreased from 681 to 446 days ($p < 0.001$) [43] and the annual number of transplants has increased. However, 1-year survival after transplantation remained unchanged [43].

UNOS heart allocation policy prioritizes time on the waiting list, the candidate medical urgency and, given that the duration of ischemic time is a limiting factor, distance between the donor hospital and the transplant center is also taken into consideration. In 2006, the heart allocation policy was modified prioritizing the sickest patients (status 1A and 1B) over local status 2 patients. The outcomes of this new system were recently analyzed showing a decreased mortality of patients on the waiting list, from 469 deaths in 2005 to 374 in 2007, while 1-year survival across the status groups remained unchanged [44]. Regardless of these promising results, there are still several groups of patients who may not benefit from this allocation system, especially those patients who are not listed as status 1A or 1B. Ongoing evaluation of the allocation policy and utilization of marginal donors hopefully will promote a more equitable distribution of organs.

The different allocation systems aforementioned dramatically changed the way in which deceased organs are allocated in the USA. However, donor organ shortage remains one of the foremost causes of death on the waiting list. As described earlier in this chapter, ECD arises as a viable option to increase the donor pool and, subsequently, diminish mortality on the waiting list.

One allocation scheme that deserves special mention is that of the Eurotransplant Senior Programme (ESP). Eurotransplant is an organ exchange organization in which transplant centers, donor hospitals, and tissue-typing centers in Austria, Belgium, Germany, Luxembourg, the Netherlands, and Slovenia collaborate. In 1999, it developed the ESP as an allocation scheme based solely on the concept of matching between metabolic demand of the graft recipient and excretory capacity of the donor organ [45–47]. The aim of ESP is to match donors with recipients of the same age group (i.e., donors > 65 years to recipients > 65 years), with the goal of kidney grafts outliving the recipients. HLA matching is disregarded, kidneys are allocated to local transplant candidates to decrease the CIT as much as possible, and only nonimmunized (panel reactive antibodies <5%) first-transplant recipients are included [47]. Three years after collecting data, the ESP showed similar kidney graft survival rates between recipients of kidneys ESP donors and recipients of donor kidneys obtained through the usual standardized HLA-matched allocation schemes, 64% vs. 67%, respectively ($p=0.4$). When graft loss was censored, survival rates were 70% for the ESP group and 71% for the SCD group. ESP data suggest that if care is taken to avoid the accumulation of such additional risk factors as extended CIT, retransplantation, and damage to the kidney during surgery, an allocation scheme using older kidney donors for transplantation into older recipients can be operated successfully.

Is the Older Recipient the Appropriate Candidate for ECD Organs?

Traditionally, worse results with an ECD kidney than a non-ECD kidney were reported (Tables 97.3 and 97.4); however, older patients may particularly benefit from ECD kidney transplantation because they have a higher death rate while waiting for an SCD kidney, and longer time on dialysis therapy is more detrimental for older than younger patients. Ojo et al. [5] showed that the average increase in life expectancy for recipients of "marginal" kidneys (defined as one of the following variables: donor age > 55 years, nonheart beating donor, CIT > 36 h, and donor hypertension or diabetes) compared favorably with the waiting list dialysis cohort that did not undergo transplantation was 5 years [5]. To deter-

mine whether accepting an ECD kidney is the right choice for an individual recipient, the critical issue is how much longer the patient would have to wait before the poorer outcomes and increased costs of waiting on dialysis therapy would outweigh the benefits of receiving an SCD kidney [48]. Interestingly, Merion et al. compared the relative risk of mortality for ECD kidney recipients versus those receiving standard therapy [49]. Because of the increased ECD recipient mortality in the perioperative period, cumulative survival did not equal that of standard dialysis therapy patients until 3.5 years of kidney transplantation. Consequently, recipient survival longer than 3.5 years justifies ECD kidney transplantation. The subgroups with significant ECD survival benefit included both sexes, patients >40 years, non-Hispanics, unsensitized patients, and those with diabetes or hypertension. Importantly, survival benefits are demonstrated in centers with long median waiting times, where ECD recipients had a 27% lower risk of death when compared to staying on dialysis ($p<0.001$) [49].

Despite the necessary use of older donors, these organs have an increased risk of failure [50, 51]. Kidney allografts from older patients not only present with histologic changes and decline in renal function associated with age but, they are also more susceptible to drug toxicity, ischemia, and reduced capacity for repair. Kauffman et al. [50] analyzed early mortality rates in older recipients with and without comorbid conditions (history of CAD, cerebrovascular disease, peripheral vascular disease, chronic obstructive pulmonary disease, and previous malignancy). They noted that patients 60 years or older who received an ECD kidney transplant presented a higher 1-year mortality rate than an SCD kidney transplant, 14% vs. 9%, respectively. When analyzing those patients aged 60 years or older with comorbidities, transplantation with an ECD kidney presented a greater 1-year mortality than patients with the same comorbidities who remained on the waiting list. It was concluded that only patients aged ≥60 and without comorbidities will benefit from an ECD kidney over remaining on the waiting list; thus, utility may be poorly served by allocating ECD kidneys to older patients with comorbidities [50]. This approach is not universally accepted; Rao et al. [52] reported that transplant recipients older than 70 years, including those with diabetes and hypertension, benefit from ECD kidney transplantation, with lower mortality compared with waiting list patients on dialysis.

Identifying the most appropriate candidates for ECD kidneys remains an open question. It is critical to balance the survival benefit against the reduced graft survival associated with ECD. It has been suggested that ECD kidneys should be preferentially directed toward candidates older than 60, diabetic candidates older than 40, candidates with failing vascular access, and candidates whose expected waiting time exceeds their life expectancy on the waiting list without a

Table 97.3 Patient survival for expanded criteria donor kidney transplants

Age (years) at Tx	Years posttransplantation			
	3 Months	1 Year	3 Years	5 Years
18–34	98.4%	96.9%	93.1%	87.6%
35–49	98.5%	95.4%	86.3%	77.8%
50–64	95.4%	89.5%	76.7%	63.5%
≥65	93.8%	85.8%	63.8%	55.5%

Source: Adapted from Metzger et al. [2], with permission of Wiley-Blackwell

Table 97.4 Patient survival for nonexpanded criteria donor kidney transplants

Age (years) at Tx	Years posttransplantation			
	3 Months	1 Year	3 Years	5 Years
18–34	99.2%	97.9%	96.3%	90.4%
35–49	98.5%	96.6%	92.5%	84.8%
50–64	96.4%	92.3%	86.2%	74.7%
≥65	94.6%	88.7%	77.6%	59.0%

Source: Adapted from Metzger et al. [2], with permission of Wiley-Blackwell

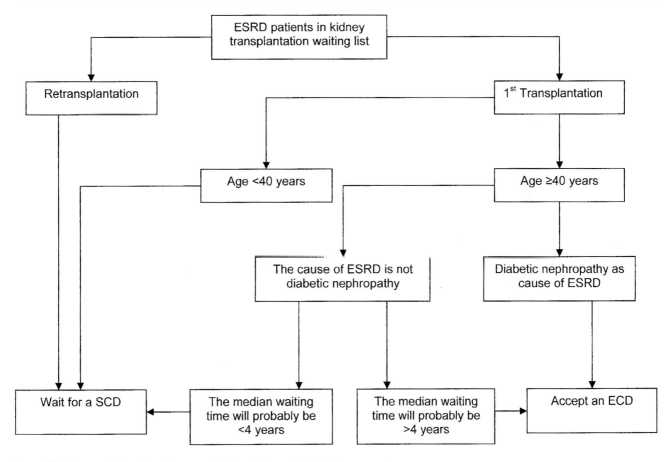

Figure 97.1 Proposed algorithm for expanded criteria donor (ECD) kidney transplant acceptance. *ESRD* end-stage renal disease, *SCD* standard criteria donor (from Pascual et al. [3] Reprinted with permission from Elsevier).

transplant [2]. An algorithm for ECD kidney transplant has been proposed (Fig. 97.1).

In the liver setting, the impact of ECD criteria on liver graft function and recipient survival is still under investigation. Similar results regarding graft function and patient survival after transplantation of ECD versus SCD were reported by some investigators. However, there is increasing awareness of the potential impact of aggressive utilization practices on graft and patient outcomes. Donor age has been clearly identified as an important risk factor for poor outcome after liver transplantation [7, 53, 54]. Feng et al. [7] analyzed more than 20,000 transplants from the SRTR and developed a donor risk index (DRI) that identified seven donor characteristics and two transplant variables that independently predicted significant increase in risk of graft failure. These included donor older than 40 years (and particularly over 60 years), less donor height, DCD, African-American race, split/partial grafts, cerebrovascular accident or other cause of death (except trauma, stroke, or anoxia), CIT and sharing outside the local donor service area. They described that high-DRI grafts have been preferentially transplanted into older candidates (>50 years of age) with low disease

severity [model for end-stage liver disease (MELD) score of 10–14] and without HCV. The reason why high-DRI grafts were allocated to candidates with lower MELD scores can be explained by the concept that most ill patients may have disproportionately poorer outcomes with high-risk grafts. However, several studies demonstrated that patients with a MELD score ≥ 20 experienced significant survival benefits even when they received a high-DRI organ [55–57]. The unpredictable underlying course of the liver disease makes timing of liver transplantation a more complex problem; therefore, ECD should be proposed for patients with higher risks of dying such as those with MELD scores ≥ 20. The survival benefit of high-DRI organ allocation to older candidates requires further assessment.

Old Organ Function

In kidney transplantation, the goal of the special allocation procedure is to reduce the time associated with placement by matching ECD grafts with patients previously designated as being willing to accept them. In assessing the potential impact of these allocation procedures, the sensitivity of ECD grafts to cold ischemia time became of great importance. ECD transplant recipients have a greater DGF prevalence than non-ECD kidney transplant recipients, in part related to CIT [58]. A European multicenter study described transplants performed with kidneys retrieved from elderly donors: CIT was associated with greater incidence of DGF and decreased graft survival when censored for death [59]. Most analyses suggest that ECD kidneys should be used locally to minimize any detrimental effect of CIT on graft function and survival. Currently, ESP and OTPN/UNOS organ allocation policy for ECD kidneys favors reducing CIT over HLA matching.

A great concern has been raised about the effect of donor age on long-term outcome. A review from UNOS data confirms that cadaveric kidneys from donors older than 60 years are associated with a 50% survival at 5 years, compared with the graft survival rate of 70% in patients receiving cadaveric donor kidneys from donors aged 19–45 years [60]. Interestingly, living donors older than 55 years have been reported to represent a significant risk of allograft failure [61]. However, as it was mentioned earlier, a recent review from OTPN/UNOS database suggested that recipients older than 60 years might benefit from living donors aged 65 years or older. These data support that donor age has turned to be a powerful predictor of long-term renal allograft function.

The main reason for kidney allograft loss in ECD recipients is death with a functioning kidney. Gill et al. [30] described cardiovascular disease and infection as the most common identifiable causes of death in ECD recipients (28.6 and 19.8%, respectively). These are expected findings reflecting the current trend to allocate ECD grafts to older recipients. With conventional immunosuppressive regimens, the risk of infectious death in older recipients increases exponentially because of higher infectious vulnerability in the elderly population, and it can be decreased by lowering immunosuppression [60]. Reduction of immunosuppression may be better tolerated in the elderly population since the incidence and severity of acute rejections is lower than in younger recipients, possibly because of the immune impaired aging [62, 63]. Nevertheless, kidneys from older donors are more likely to undergo acute rejection episodes in the early posttransplantation period when compared with kidneys from younger donors [64, 65] and may be related to a more intense proinflammatory response, increased expression of HLA in epithelial and endothelial cells, and the recruitment of antigen-presenting cells [51]. Consequently, it has been suggested that immunosuppression individualization and adequate patient selection, together with better HLA-matching, tend to decrease infection and rejection risk in ECD kidney transplant recipients [46, 66].

In liver transplantation, immediate and long-term function of liver allograft procured from older donors is affected by the exposure to cold ischemia with an increased rate of primary and delayed nonfunction [53, 67, 68]. Grafts with more than 14 h of cold ischemia have been associated with a twofold increase in preservation damage resulting in prolonged postoperative course, biliary stricture, and decreased graft survival [67–69]. The European Liver Transplant Registry survey showed that 5-year recipient survival was 57% with CIT > 15 h versus 64% with CIT between 12 and 15 h and 67% with CIT < 12 h [70]. Elderly donors' liver grafts and donors with steatosis are even more affected by prolonged CIT and preservation injury [71]. These results emphasize the need to shorten CIT as much as possible in the case of ECD.

Recently, Burroughs et al. [53] described that those who received allografts from donors older than 60 years presented an increased 3- and 12-month mortality of 12 and 22%, respectively. Different recipient factors can have a major impact on ECD graft function – fulminant hepatic failure as the indication for transplantation and hepatorenal syndrome are associated with higher incidence of primary nonfunction [69, 72]. Recipient obesity (body mass index > 30 mg/m^2) has been reported to increase the risk of postoperative complications after ECD liver transplantation, such as respiratory failure and infections [73]. Furthermore, transplantation of livers from donors older than 40 years of age is associated with increased severity of HCV recurrence and fibrosis rates [74]. It is debatable whether old livers should be allocated to recipients with HCV infection [75].

Ethics

Ethical allocation priorities are a topic of ongoing discussion [76]. Disclosing the risk and benefits of solid-organ transplantation and obtaining inform consent from patients might occur at any moment of the transplant process, when the patients are placed on the waiting list and/or when an organ is offered. Candidates willing to accept an ECD organ should be specifically informed about the potential risks a marginal graft can carry. A distinction between the risk of disease transmission and graft failure should be emphasized as part of the informed consent process. In all cases, patients should be informed to whether declining ECD will delay their receipt of an organ, and provide reasonable assessment of the potential of death before SCD becomes available. Candidates, who did not consider ECD as an option, should be offered the chance to reassess their decision, especially when their clinical condition is changed. In such circumstances, transplant physicians' clinical judgment plays a key role to establish risk and benefits of providing a particular organ to a particular patient. Transplant teams are therefore ethically obliged to look carefully into the principles, rules, or preferences they use to allocate ECD organs.

CASE STUDY

A 69-year-old male with history of smoking, hypertension, coronary artery disease, and atrial fibrillation on coumadin presented to the ER with headache, nausea, and vomiting. Initial workup including head CT scan demonstrated large intracranial hemorrhage and significant brain edema. The patient continued to experience neurological deterioration with evidence of brain herniation and hemodynamic instability requiring multiple vasopressors. The family was notified and expressed interest in organ donation.

1. *Determination of brain death*: All reversible causes of a coma were ruled out (i.e., hypothermia, hypoxia, hypoglycemia, etc.). An apnea testing was consistent with brain death, and that was later confirmed by a radionuclide cerebral blood flow scan.
2. *Donor management*: Hemodynamic stability was achieved via resuscitation with crystalloids and vasoactive support. Hormone replacement therapy with thyroxine was instituted, helping to wean-off vasopressors. Blood pressure was maintained >100 mmHg, CVP >10 mmHg, urine output >40 mL/h. Finally, reversal of diabetes insipidus was achieved with desmopressin.
3. *Procurement procedure*: The presence of abdominal donor malignancies was excluded after an extensive abdominal exploration, and the thoracic and abdominal organs were evaluated for transplantation.

   • Heart and lung were discarded because of advanced donor age and comorbidities.
   • *Liver allocation*: liver function tests revealed a total bilirubin 1.2 mg/dL, AST 35 IU/mL, ALT 51 IU/mL and viral hepatitis serologies were negative. In order to exclude fibrosis and steatosis, a liver biopsy was performed showing macrosteatosis <5% and no significant fibrosis.
   • *Kidney allocation*: renal function was preserved, creatinine 1.1 mg/dL and BUN 33. For evaluation of the kidney, a biopsy was obtained that showed glomerulosclerosis <10%.

4. *Recipient procedure and outcome*: the risk and benefits of an extended criteria allograft were carefully explained to the potential recipients who consented to go forward with the transplant procedure.

   • *Liver recipient*: A 53-years-old male with alcoholic cirrhosis with refractory ascites, recurrent episodes of hepatic encephalopathy, a low MELD score of 18, and no previous abdominal surgeries received the ECD liver. Given the fact that elderly donors are even more affected by prolonged cold ischemia time (CIT) and preservation injury, the liver allograft was reperfused within 4.4 h after procurement. The recipient required two units of blood during surgery; his postoperative course was uneventful except for a bile leak that resolved without endoscopic intervention after 2 weeks. One year later the patient presents a totally functioning liver with no major events and performing his daily activities with no restrictions.
   • *Kidney recipient*: A 54-years-old female with diabetic nephropathy who had been on hemodialysis for the last 6 years accepted the ECD kidney. In order to minimize any detrimental effect of prolonged CIT on graft function and survival the organ was allocated locally, prioritizing CIT over HLA matching. Postoperative course was significant for acute tubular necrosis requiring hemodialysis for 3 weeks. One month later the patient presented with an acute cellular rejection episode that was successfully treated with methylprednisolone. After 1 year the graft function is well preserved with a creatinine of 1.7 mg/dL.

Conclusion

The shortage of organs has led transplant centers to expand their criteria for the acceptance of marginal donors. UNOS and ESP have addressed this problem implementing an allocation scheme for organ allocation with improvement in survival rate, and standard definitions of ECD organs were established. A better understanding of the impact of ECD on outcome improved allocation pathways, and identifying the appropriate recipients should result in more efficient utilization and improved graft and patient survival. Graft and patient survival data on transplant recipients aged 50 years or older suggest that there should not be an absolute upper age limit at which transplantation of any organ should be contraindicated. Candidate's biological, rather than chronological age, and careful evaluation of the overall health and quality of life of the transplant candidate should be deciding factors of whether transplantation would be beneficial or not. The recipient must be educated and informed of the risk and benefits when transplanted with an ECD organ.

Summary

- Extended criteria donation emerges as a good option to reduce the gap between the number of patients needing a transplant and the number of donors.
- Careful selection of ECD organs and potential recipients should be done.
- Elderly patients who received ECD kidney transplant will enjoy improved survival than those who remain on dialysis.
- Future studies assessing ECD outcomes on liver, heart, pancreas, and lung patients are warranted.
- Transplant candidates willing to accept an ECD organ should be informed about the potential risks a marginal graft can carry.

References

1. United Network for Organ Sharing. http://www.unos.org. Accessed April 2009
2. Metzger RA, Delmonico FL, Feng S, Port FK, Wynn JJ, Merion RM (2003) Expanded criteria donors for kidney transplantation. Am J Transplant 3(Suppl 4):114–125
3. Pascual J, Zamora J, Pirsch JD (2008) A systematic review of kidney transplantation from expanded criteria donors. Am J Kidney Dis 52:553–586
4. Port FK, Bragg-Gresham JL, Metzger RA et al (2002) Donor characteristics associated with reduced graft survival: an approach to expanding the pool of kidney donors. Transplantation 74:1281–1286
5. Ojo AO, Hanson JA, Meier-Kriesche H et al (2001) Survival in recipients of marginal cadaveric donor kidneys compared with other recipients and wait-listed transplant candidates. J Am Soc Nephrol 12:589–597
6. New York State Department of Health (2005) Workgroup on expanded criteria organs for liver transplantation. Liver Transpl 11:1184–1192
7. Feng S, Goodrich NP, Bragg-Gresham JL et al (2006) Characteristics associated with liver graft failure: the concept of a donor risk index. Am J Transplant 6:783–790
8. Nardo B, Masetti M, Urbani L et al (2004) Liver transplantation from donors aged 80 years and over: pushing the limit. Am J Transplant 4:1139–1147
9. Singh RP, Rogers J, Farney AC et al (2008) Outcomes of extended donors in pancreatic transplantation with portal-enteric drainage. Transplant Proc 40:502–505
10. Pierre AF, Sekine Y, Hutcheon MA, Waddell TK, Keshavjee SH (2002) Marginal donor lungs: a reassessment. J Thorac Cardiovasc Surg 123:421–427, discussion 427–428
11. Fischer S, Gohrbandt B, Struckmeier P et al (2005) Lung transplantation with lungs from donors fifty years of age and older. J Thorac Cardiovasc Surg 129:919–925
12. John R (2004) Donor management and selection for heart transplantation. Semin Thorac Cardiovasc Surg 16:364–369
13. 2007 Annual Report of the Organ Procurement and Transplantation and U.S. Scientific Registry of Transplant Recipients. http://www.optn.org. Accessed January 2009
14. Lucas BA, Vaughn WK, Spees EK, Sanfilippo F (1987) Identification of donor factors predisposing to high discard rates of cadaver kidneys and increased graft loss within one year posttransplantation – SEOPF 1977–1982. South-Eastern Organ Procurement Foundation. Transplantation 43:253–258
15. Nyberg SL, Matas AJ, Kremers WK et al (2003) Improved scoring system to assess adult donors for cadaver renal transplantation. Am J Transplant 3:715–721
16. Stratta RJ, Rohr MS, Sundberg AK et al (2006) Intermediate-term outcomes with expanded criteria deceased donors in kidney transplantation: a spectrum or specter of quality? Ann Surg 243:594–601, discussion 601–593
17. Moers C, Smits JM, Maathuis MH et al (2009) Machine perfusion or cold storage in deceased-donor kidney transplantation. N Engl J Med 360:7–19
18. Zamboni F, Franchello A, David E et al (2001) Effect of macrovesicular steatosis and other donor and recipient characteristics on the outcome of liver transplantation. Clin Transplant 15:53–57
19. Zaroff JG, Rosengard BR, Armstrong WF et al (2002) Consensus conference report: maximizing use of organs recovered from the cadaver donor: cardiac recommendations, March 28–29, 2001, Crystal City, Va. Circulation 106:836–841
20. Musci M, Pasic M, Grauhan O et al (2004) Orthotopic heart transplantation with concurrent coronary artery bypass grafting or previous stent implantation. Z Kardiol 93:971–974
21. Weng CF, Chang CY, Lee YT et al (2008) Extending donor source with bench coronary angiography: a case report. Transplant Proc 40:2846–2847
22. Gabbay E, Williams TJ, Griffiths AP et al (1999) Maximizing the utilization of donor organs offered for lung transplantation. Am J Respir Crit Care Med 160:265–271
23. Kauffman HM, McBride MA, Cherikh WS, Spain PC, Delmonico FL (2002) Transplant tumor registry: donors with central nervous system tumors1. Transplantation 73:579–582
24. Gandhi MJ, Strong DM (2007) Donor derived malignancy following transplantation: a review. Cell Tissue Bank 8:267–286
25. Cecka JM (2005) The OPTN/UNOS Renal Transplant Registry. Clin Transpl 1–16
26. Okamoto M, Akioka K, Nobori S et al (2009) Short- and long-term donor outcomes after kidney donation: analysis of 601 cases over a 35-year period at Japanese single center. Transplantation 87:419–423
27. Ibrahim HN, Foley R, Tan L et al (2009) Long-term consequences of kidney donation. N Engl J Med 360:459–469
28. Matas AJ, Bartlett ST, Leichtman AB, Delmonico FL (2003) Morbidity and mortality after living kidney donation, 1999–2001: survey of United States transplant centers. Am J Transplant 3:830–834
29. Mandelbrot DA, Pavlakis M, Danovitch GM et al (2007) The medical evaluation of living kidney donors: a survey of US transplant centers. Am J Transplant 7:2333–2343
30. Gill J, Bunnapradist S, Danovitch GM, Gjertson D, Gill JS, Cecka M (2008) Outcomes of kidney transplantation from older living donors to older recipients. Am J Kidney Dis 52:541–552
31. Strong RW, Lynch SV, Ong TH, Matsunami H, Koido Y, Balderson GA (1990) Successful liver transplantation from a living donor to her son. N Engl J Med 322:1505–1507
32. Soejima Y, Taketomi A, Yoshizumi T et al (2006) Feasibility of left lobe living donor liver transplantation between adults: an 8-year, single-center experience of 107 cases. Am J Transplant 6:1004–1011
33. Ghobrial RM, Freise CE, Trotter JF et al (2008) Donor morbidity after living donation for liver transplantation. Gastroenterology 135:468–476
34. Patel S, Orloff M, Tsoulfas G et al (2007) Living-donor liver transplantation in the United States: identifying donors at risk for perioperative complications. Am J Transplant 7:2344–2349
35. Olthoff KM (2003) Hepatic regeneration in living donor liver transplantation. Liver Transpl 9:S35–S41

36. Abt PL, Mange KC, Olthoff KM, Markmann JF, Reddy KR, Shaked A (2004) Allograft survival following adult-to-adult living donor liver transplantation. Am J Transplant 4:1302–1307

37. Yoshizumi T, Taketomi A, Soejima Y et al (2008) Impact of donor age and recipient status on left-lobe graft for living donor adult liver transplantation. Transpl Int 21:81–88

38. Trotter JF, Hill-Callahan MM, Gillespie BW et al (2007) Severe psychiatric problems in right hepatic lobe donors for living donor liver transplantation. Transplantation 83:1506–1508

39. Middleton PF, Duffield M, Lynch SV et al (2006) Living donor liver transplantation – adult donor outcomes: a systematic review. Liver Transpl 12:24–30

40. Freeman RB, Wiesner RH, Edwards E, Harper A, Merion R, Wolfe R (2004) Results of the first year of the new liver allocation plan. Liver Transpl 10:7–15

41. Remuzzi G, Cravedi P, Perna A et al (2006) Long-term outcome of renal transplantation from older donors. N Engl J Med 354:343–352

42. Davis SQ, Garrity ER Jr (2007) Organ allocation in lung transplant. Chest 132:1646–1651

43. Kozower BD, Meyers BF, Smith MA et al (2008) The impact of the lung allocation score on short-term transplantation outcomes: a multicenter study. J Thorac Cardiovasc Surg 135:166–171

44. Vega JD, Moore J, Murray S, Chen JM, Johnson MR, Dyke DB (2009) Heart transplantation in the United States, 1998–2007. Am J Transplant 9:932–941

45. Cohen B, Smits JM, Haase B, Persijn G, Vanrenterghem Y, Frei U (2005) Expanding the donor pool to increase renal transplantation. Nephrol Dial Transplant 20:34–41

46. Fritsche L, Horstrup J, Budde K et al (2003) Old-for-old kidney allocation allows successful expansion of the donor and recipient pool. Am J Transplant 3:1434–1439

47. Smits JM, Persijn GG, van Houwelingen HC, Claas FH, Frei U (2002) Evaluation of the Eurotransplant Senior Program. The results of the first year. Am J Transplant 2:664–670

48. Schnitzler MA, Whiting JF, Brennan DC et al (2003) The expanded criteria donor dilemma in cadaveric renal transplantation. Transplantation 75:1940–1945

49. Merion RM, Ashby VB, Wolfe RA et al (2005) Deceased-donor characteristics and the survival benefit of kidney transplantation. JAMA 294:2726–2733

50. Kauffman HM, McBride MA, Cors CS, Roza AM, Wynn JJ (2007) Early mortality rates in older kidney recipients with comorbid risk factors. Transplantation 83:404–410

51. Schratzberger G, Mayer G (2003) Age and renal transplantation: an interim analysis. Nephrol Dial Transplant 18:471–476

52. Rao PS, Merion RM, Ashby VB, Port FK, Wolfe RA, Kayler LK (2007) Renal transplantation in elderly patients older than 70 years of age: results from the Scientific Registry of Transplant Recipients. Transplantation 83:1069–1074

53. Burroughs AK, Sabin CA, Rolles K et al (2006) 3-month and 12-month mortality after first liver transplant in adults in Europe: predictive models for outcome. Lancet 367:225–232

54. Ioannou GN (2006) Development and validation of a model predicting graft survival after liver transplantation. Liver Transpl 12:1594–1606

55. Amin MG, Wolf MP, TenBrook JA Jr et al (2004) Expanded criteria donor grafts for deceased donor liver transplantation under the MELD system: a decision analysis. Liver Transpl 10:1468–1475

56. Maluf DG, Edwards EB, Kauffman HM (2006) Utilization of extended donor criteria liver allograft: Is the elevated risk of failure independent of the model for end-stage liver disease score of the recipient? Transplantation 82:1653–1657

57. Schaubel DE, Sima CS, Goodrich NP, Feng S, Merion RM (2008) The survival benefit of deceased donor liver transplantation as a function of candidate disease severity and donor quality. Am J Transplant 8:419–425

58. Johnston TD, Thacker LR, Jeon H, Lucas BA, Ranjan D (2004) Sensitivity of expanded-criteria donor kidneys to cold ischaemia time. Clin Transplant 18(Suppl 12):28–32

59. Sola R, Alarcon A, Jimenez C, Osuna A (2004) The influence of delayed graft function. Nephrol Dial Transplant 19(Suppl 3):iii32–iii37

60. Morrissey PE, Gohh R, Yango A, Gautam A, Monaco AP (2004) Renal transplant survival from older donors: a single center experience. Arch Surg 139:384–389, discussion 389

61. Bunnapradist S, Daswani A, Takemoto SK (2003) Graft survival following living-donor renal transplantation: a comparison of tacrolimus and cyclosporine microemulsion with mycophenolate mofetil and steroids. Transplantation 76:10–15

62. Humar A, Denny R, Matas AJ, Najarian JS (2003) Graft and quality of life outcomes in older recipients of a kidney transplant. Exp Clin Transplant 1:69–72

63. Wick G, Grubeck-Loebenstein B (1997) The aging immune system: primary and secondary alterations of immune reactivity in the elderly. Exp Gerontol 32:401–413

64. de Fijter JW, Mallat MJ, Doxiadis II et al (2001) Increased immunogenicity and cause of graft loss of old donor kidneys. J Am Soc Nephrol 12:1538–1546

65. Waiser J, Schreiber M, Budde K et al (2000) Age-matching in renal transplantation. Nephrol Dial Transplant 15:696–700

66. Carter JT, Chan S, Roberts JP, Feng S (2005) Expanded criteria donor kidney allocation: marked decrease in cold ischemia and delayed graft function at a single center. Am J Transplant 5:2745–2753

67. Briceno J, Lopez-Cillero P, Rufian S et al (1997) Impact of marginal quality donors on the outcome of liver transplantation. Transplant Proc 29:477–480

68. Piratvisuth T, Tredger JM, Hayllar KA, Williams R (1995) Contribution of true cold and rewarming ischemia times to factors determining outcome after orthotopic liver transplantation. Liver Transpl Surg 1:296–301

69. Ploeg RJ, D'Alessandro AM, Knechtle SJ et al (1993) Risk factors for primary dysfunction after liver transplantation – a multivariate analysis. Transplantation 55:807–813

70. Durand F, Renz JF, Alkofer B et al (2008) Report of the Paris consensus meeting on expanded criteria donors in liver transplantation. Liver Transpl 14:1694–1707

71. Yersiz H, Shaked A, Olthoff K et al (1995) Correlation between donor age and the pattern of liver graft recovery after transplantation. Transplantation 60:790–794

72. Farmer DG, Anselmo DM, Ghobrial RM et al (2003) Liver transplantation for fulminant hepatic failure: experience with more than 200 patients over a 17-year period. Ann Surg 237:666–675, discussion 675–666

73. Nair S, Verma S, Thuluvath PJ (2002) Obesity and its effect on survival in patients undergoing orthotopic liver transplantation in the United States. Hepatology 35:105–109

74. Berenguer M, Prieto M, San Juan F et al (2002) Contribution of donor age to the recent decrease in patient survival among HCV-infected liver transplant recipients. Hepatology 36:202–210

75. Mutimer DJ, Gunson B, Chen J et al (2006) Impact of donor age and year of transplantation on graft and patient survival following liver transplantation for hepatitis C virus. Transplantation 81:7–14

76. Halpern SD, Shaked A, Hasz RD, Caplan AL (2008) Informing candidates for solid-organ transplantation about donor risk factors. N Engl J Med 358:2832–2837

Chapter 98
Elderly Transplant Recipients

Aaron M. Winnick, Ilhan Karabicak, and Dale A. Distant

CASE STUDY

SN is an 84-year-old African-American male who developed renal failure after undergoing a triple-vessel coronary artery bypass graft (CABG) following a myocardial infarction in 2004. He has a history of hypertension and has been stable on hemodialysis via an AV fistula. He has excellent exercise tolerance, a normal ejection fraction on cardiac catheterization, and was asymptomatic with regard to his coronary artery disease. He is fully functional and living independently since he retired from his job as a bus operator. He was placed on the waiting list for renal transplant in 2007. He received a zero mismatch offer from a 75-year-old deceased donor in August 2008. The donor was a 125 lb woman with no significant

medical history who died from a cerebrovascular attack (CVA). Her serum creatinine was 0.7 mg/dL and postprocurement biopsy revealed minimal glomerulosclerosis. Both kidneys were pumped and then implanted ipsilaterally in a 4½-h operation. He exhibited good immediate function and mild troponin elevation, but no other complications. He received induction therapy with three doses of thymoglobulin (1.5 mg/kg/dose), Prograf, and steroids. He was discharged to home 5 days later with a creatinine of 2.0 mg/dL. No hospital readmissions occurred, and 1 year following transplantation, his creatinine level was 1.2 mg/dL. He is currently being maintained on Prograf 2 mg twice daily and prednisone 5 mg daily. He remains quite active working as a producer for a local radio station, and he travels extensively visiting family.

While the total number of organs transplanted in this country has increased over the years, there is still an ever-widening gap between the need for organs and our capacity to meet that need as the overall waiting list continues to grow. This is due in part to significant advances in transplant techniques and outcomes such that Americans with organ failure now seek transplants in greater numbers. Additionally, life-expectancy gains in the United States are creating an aging population who are more likely to suffer organ failure than younger Americans. The national transplant waiting list has continued to shift toward older candidates. The Scientific Registry of Transplant Recipients (SRTR) reported that at the end of 2007, 59.7% of all 97,248 candidates on the waiting list for all organs were 50 years old or older, and 14.9% were 65 years or older. These percentages are substantially higher than they were in 1998 (41.5 and 8.1%, respectively) [1].

In the United States, there is no upper age limit above which patients can no longer receive a transplanted organ. Over the past 10 years, there has been a significant increase in the number of transplants performed on patients over 60 years of age. The annual number of recipients transplanted rose from 21,518 in 1998 to 28,345 in 2007, a 32% increase. In contrast, the number of patients over the age of 65 has more than doubled, from 1,470 (6.8% of total) to 3,498 (12.3% of total). According to this data, the only age groups demonstrating an annual increase in the number of recipients every year over the 10-year period were those aged 50–64 and those over 65 [1].

Among solid organs transplanted in the United States, approximately 59% are kidney, 21% liver, 7% heart, and 5% lung [1]. There are several aspects of transplanting elderly patients that deserve discussion, including ethical issues, differences in pretransplant evaluation, mechanisms of graft

D.A. Distant (✉)
Department of Transplant Surgery, SUNY Downstate
Medical Center, Brooklyn, NY, USA

R.A. Rosenthal et al. (eds.), *Principles and Practice of Geriatric Surgery*,
DOI 10.1007/978-1-4419-6999-6_98, © Springer Science+Business Media, LLC 2011

loss and death, and the degree and type of immunosuppressive therapy. This discussion focuses primarily on deceased-donor organ transplants into the elderly, since fewer live-donor transplants are performed in the aged (670 transplants in 2008). The kidney being the most frequently transplanted solid organ offers the most data in older patients and is therefore a primary focus of this chapter. No consensus exists as to what age defines "elderly" or "geriatric" within the transplant literature, and therefore, no attempt is made to offer such a definition; rather, the studies and data are examined with regard to the issues to be examined and the principles to be applied to older transplant candidates.

Kidney Transplantation

Older Americans are an increasingly important consumer of End Stage Renal Disease services in the United States. The U.S. Renal Data System (USRDS) collects and provides national demographic information about patients with kidney disease treated with either dialysis or transplantation. The average age of the dialysis patient continues to increase each year, with nearly half of patients undergoing regular dialysis now over 65 years of age, and the mean age of those beginning treatment is now greater than 60 years [2]. There are currently 48,773 patients on the waiting list for a kidney, with 7,800 (16%) over the age of 65. In 2007, nearly 17,000 kidney transplants were performed in the United States, with 2,377 (14%) going to patients over the age of 65 [1].

Kidney transplantation has been shown to improve quality of life and length of life compared with those remaining on dialysis [3]. In one longitudinal study of mortality, investigators evaluated data collected over 6 years on 228,552 patients who were receiving dialysis as treatment for their end-stage renal disease. Of these, 46,164 were deemed healthy enough to be placed on the waiting list for transplantation, and 23,275 received a first deceased-donor kidney transplant. The mortality ratio for the patients on dialysis who were awaiting transplantation was 38–58% lower than that for all patients on dialysis (annual death rates of 6.3 and 16.1 per 100 patient-years, respectively). The long-term mortality rate was 48–82% lower among transplant recipients than patients on the waiting list (annual death rate 3.8 per 100 patient-years). Recipients over the age of 60 demonstrated significant benefit in mortality after transplantation, with annual death rates per 100 patient-years at risk for all patients on dialysis, patients on the waiting list, and transplant recipients being 23.2, 10, and 7.4, respectively. It is estimated that, among those over the age of 60, projected remaining years of life are approximately 6 and 10 years for those who remain on a waiting list or undergo renal transplant, respectively [4]. Multiple studies over the past

10 years have confirmed that patients older than 60 years of age have longer life expectancy with deceased-donor kidney transplantation when compared to patients of the same age group on the waiting list. Post-kidney transplant recipients report a better quality of life, from mental well-being to physical functionality and social functioning. In addition, after adjusting for comorbidities, there is no significant difference in graft failure compared to younger patients [5–8]. As with all organ transplants, the risks and benefits must be carefully weighed, especially in the elderly. Will this organ improve the patients' overall survival and quality of life? Will an older patient be able to survive the operation, manage the medications, endure the potential side effects of immunosuppression, and have the social and financial support necessary to recover and maintain rigorous doctor appointments?

Current success in transplanting kidneys into older recipients has quieted misconceptions within medical communities and the general public, among them the erroneous belief that advanced age alone prevents a successful surgical outcome, that the elderly patient with ESRD has a very limited life expectancy, and thus cannot receive a transplant, and that older recipients have poor results based upon outdated information from the previous era of transplantation and immunosuppression. Older recipients, however, do have a higher risk of cardiovascular events, infection, and malignancy after kidney transplantation compared to younger patients [9]. Also, they are more prone to drug side effects and toxicity [10]. The absolute gain in survival provided by a donor kidney varies considerably depending on recipient factors, such as age and comorbid illnesses.

Although overall graft failure rates are not higher for elderly recipients, death with a functioning graft does occur more often which shortens the lifespan of the donated kidney (especially from a young donor) [10]. Clearly, a younger recipient would more likely experience more years of allograft function with the same kidney. With ever-increasing organ shortages, the ethical dilemma of including age as a potential allocation factor has been raised. The argument pits the increased survival and quality of life for the older transplant recipient against the population gain in allograft survival by transplanting kidneys preferentially into younger recipients. What is the best way to deal with these competing allocation philosophies, namely, giving everyone an equal chance to receive an organ vs. getting the maximum benefit from each organ transplanted? In the U.S., the United Network for Organ Sharing (UNOS) provides regulatory oversight and balances these ethical principles in an effort to achieve socially acceptable allocation policy.

An alternate strategy to maximize the benefit of donor organs matches kidneys with lower expected graft survival time (principally older donors) to patients with lower expected longevity (principally older recipients). The current allocation of expanded criteria donor (ECD) kidneys attempts to do this. These kidneys are procured from donors older than 60 years of age or donors aged 50–59 years with at least two of the following conditions: cerebrovascular accident as cause of death, a history of hypertension, or a serum creatinine > 1.5 mg/dL [11]. While ECD kidneys carry a relative risk of graft failure greater than 1.7 compared to a reference group of donors aged 10–39 years without any of the above three conditions, elderly recipients of ECD kidneys were found to have a survival benefit compared with waiting-list candidates (RR = 0.75; 95% CI 0.65–0.86; $p < 0.0001$) [8]. The benefits (shortening of waiting time) and risk (impaired long-term graft function) associated with the use of ECD kidneys should be addressed on an individual basis. As with all recipients, elderly patients do best with an ideal donor kidney; however, the ECD policy achieves a compromise that enhances the donor pool and provides good alternative to dialysis.

Another option for increasing the number of organs and decreasing the waiting period for renal transplantation is to perform a dual kidney transplant. Both kidneys from an older donor, which individually would be considered marginal or inadequate for transplantation, are transplanted into a single recipient. This expands the use of kidneys that otherwise would not be used. There is a misconception that dual kidney transplantation involves the transferring of an inferior organ; on the contrary, it is just a different type of organ transplant. For all kidneys being evaluated for donation, the creatinine clearance is calculated. If it is greater than 65 mL/min, each individual kidney may be transplanted into two different recipients. If it is below 40 mL/min both kidneys are usually deemed unsuitable for transplant. The area in between, 40 and 65 mL/min, constitutes the range to use two kidneys together to give recipients the function of one kidney. This allows for the transplantation of as much kidney function as, if not more than, a standard single transplant from a nonexpanded criteria donor. With careful selection, the amount of kidney function that is being transplanted with dual kidney is comparable to a single kidney transplant [12].

Patient Selection

Prior to transplantation of any organs, the prospective recipient has to be carefully evaluated to detect and treat any coexisting illnesses that may affect patient and graft survival after transplantation. In the elderly, this is imperative for two reasons: graft loss in the elderly is related primarily to patient death, and the main causes of morbidity and mortality following transplantation are infection and cardiovascular disease [13, 14].

Regardless of the age of the recipient, a thorough medical, surgical, and psychosocial history needs to be obtained, along with a detailed physical examination. Careful examination of the abdomen for previous operations is important, as is the presence or absence of peripheral arterial pulses. Initial laboratory testing includes blood type, HLA typing and a panel reactive antibody assay to detect for previous sensitization, complete blood count (CBC), blood urea nitrogen, creatinine, electrolytes, calcium, phosphorous, albumin, liver function tests, prothrombin time, and partial thromboplastin time. Serologic studies for cytomegalovirus (CMV), hepatitis B and C viruses (HBV, HCV), human T cell leukemia virus (HTLV-1), and human immunodeficiency virus (HIV) are routine. One element of the evaluation process includes baseline age-appropriate screening tests. It is also important and appropriate to maintain a higher index of suspicion for malignancy in patients of this age group. In women, this consists of gynecologic examination and Papanicolaou smear, breast examination, and in those over the age of 40 without a family history of breast cancer in the premenopausal years, mammography. In men, testicular examination, prostate examination, and for those over age 50, prostate-specific antigen (PSA) assay should be performed. All patients over the age of 50 should undergo screening colonoscopy. A screening purified protein derivative (PPD) test may be used depending on the patient population and patient history. Radiologic studies include chest X-ray and electrocardiogram as routine and can include ultrasound or computed tomography (CT) scan of the abdomen to evaluate anatomy if indicated. Estimation of urine output preoperatively is important because it determines the significance of postoperative urine output and helps determine the need for any urologic evaluation. A history of claudication warrants a workup for peripheral vascular disease and may also point towards a higher chance of ischemic heart disease. The presence of strong femoral and peripheral pulses indicates that the pelvic vessels will likely be adequate for the transplant vascular anastomosis. Assessment of cardiac risk is critical in the evaluation process of elderly patients. Cardiovascular disorders, such as hypertension, coronary artery disease, congestive heart failure, and arrhythmias are common in elderly transplant recipients and account for most of the deaths in this population. Blood pressure, blood glucose, and cholesterol control is of particular concern because this patient population frequently have or develop these complications. The prevalence of ischemic heart disease is very high in patients with end-stage renal disease, and almost half of the deaths that occur during the first 30 days posttransplant are due to ischemic heart disease [15]. The current guidelines from the American Society of Transplantation recommend assessing ischemic heart disease risk factors in any patient with a prior history, men over the age of 45 or women over the age of 55 years, cardiac disease in a first-degree relative, current cigarette smoking, diabetes, hypertension, fasting total cholesterol > 200 mg/dL, high-density lipoprotein cholesterol < 35 mg/dL, and left ventricular hypertrophy. Any patient at high risk, including those with renal disease from diabetes, prior history of ischemic heart disease, or more than two of the above risk factors, should undergo an echocardiogram and cardiac stress test. Angiography with possible revascularization, if indicated, should be performed prior to any transplantation. Asymptomatic patients can also undergo noninvasive tests first that may help determine the risk for posttransplant complications, in the form of chemical stress echocardiography or scintography [15].

Based on an initial evaluation, the 2005 Canadian Society for Transplantation Guidelines suggested that the following patients with coronary heart disease may be eligible for kidney transplantation: asymptomatic low-risk patients; asymptomatic patients in whom noninvasive testing is negative; patients on appropriate medical therapy with angiographic results showing noncritical disease; and those patients in whom successful interventions have been performed [16].

Currently, there is no strong evidence to suggest a benefit to the routine screening of asymptomatic renal transplant candidates for cerebrovascular disease. Risk factors for posttransplant cerebrovascular disease include a history of prior disease, age, smoking, diabetes, hypertension, and hyperlipidemia [15]. Patients who have already suffered from a cerebrovascular event and have significant deficits may be poor operative candidates due to their poor operative risk and rehabilitative potential. Patients with recent transient ischemic attacks need to be adequately evaluated by a neurologist.

Pulmonary risks associated with surgery for transplantation include infection, fluid overload, and ventilator dependency. Pretransplant evaluation of elderly patients with respiratory disease should be consistent with that for the general population who undergo a preoperative pulmonary assessment [17]. The 2005 Canadian Transplant guidelines suggest that patients should not be considered candidates for kidney transplantation if they require home oxygen therapy, have uncontrolled asthma, severe cor pulmonale, or severe COPD, pulmonary fibrosis, or restrictive disease. The latter is defined by FEV1 < 25% predictive value, room air pO_2 < 60 mmHg with exercise desaturation SaO_2 < 90%, or more than four lower respiratory tract infections in the last 12 months [16].

The transplant candidate must be free of all active infections before transplantation could be considered. Whenever possible, all treatable infections should be dealt with appropriately. Chronic infection precludes transplantation and the subsequent use of immunosuppressive therapy. Infectious complications occur frequently in the transplanted patient, with pneumonia being one of the most common infections seen in elderly hospitalized patients. As such, elderly patients must be immunized against influenza and pneumococcus.

Not too long ago, most centers considered patients who tested positive for HIV inappropriate for transplantation secondary to immunosuppressant-induced opportunistic infection and the suspected short life span. With the advancement in antiretroviral therapy, more centers now are willing to transplant patients who are HIV positive, but the general recommendation is to evaluate on a case-by-case basis.

Patients with a malignancy prior to receiving an organ may still be a suitable candidate for transplantation depending on the tumor type, stage, and response to therapy. The concern is that malignancies are common after transplantation, possibly due to immunosuppression favoring the growth of malignant cells and/or viral infection. This part is addressed in a later section on postoperative issues. While it has been reported that patients with ESRD on dialysis have a higher rate of cancer compared to the general population, this relative risk has been shown to be higher in younger patients [18]. Most patients previously treated for cancer benefit from a waiting period prior to renal transplantation to decrease the risk of recurrence. Depending on tumor characteristics, recommendations range from no wait time to 5 years. No waiting time is required for basal cell carcinoma of the skin, in situ cancer of the bladder or cervix. A 2-year waiting time is proposed for lymphoma, leukemia, cancers of the prostate, lung, breast (early stage), testicle, thyroid, uterine body, bladder, Wilm's tumor, renal cell carcinoma (<5 cm), or Kaposi's or other sarcoma. Patients with localized, successfully treated carcinoma of the uterine cervix may benefit from waiting 2 years, and in some cases 5 years, prior to transplantation. A 5-year waiting time is recommended for colorectal, invasive breast, and renal cell carcinoma (>5 cm), and malignant melanoma [15, 16, 19].

While some contraindications to kidney transplantation are absolute, many are relative and determined by individual centers. Absolute contraindications to receiving a renal transplant include: recent or metastatic malignancy; active substance abuse; severe extrarenal disease with life expectancy of less than 1 year; untreated current infection; psychiatric or other illness impairing adherence to regimen. Relative contraindications include: morbid obesity; active heavy tobacco use; acute coronary or cerebrovascular event; HIV infection if untreated or poorly monitored [13, 15].

The actual surgery for transplanting a kidney is the same for the elderly patients as for any adult, with the caveat that careful attention must be paid to fluid maintenance and monitoring in the elderly, depending on the cardiac and pulmonary history. The standard incision for adult kidney transplantation is an oblique incision from the symphysis in the midline, curving in a lateral and superior direction to the iliac crest. The donor renal artery and vein are anastomosed to the recipient external iliac artery and vein, respectively, and the donor ureter anastomosed to the recipient bladder. The kidney is placed in the iliac fossa where it is easily accessible if an ultrasound, biopsy, or other intervention is required.

Immunosuppression and Prophylaxis

While the benefit of renal transplantation in the elderly has already been established, there is a paucity of data evaluating the safety and efficacy of immunosuppression regimens. Most centers use traditional principles and their transplant protocols with modifications when considering the factors unique to the elderly. Analysis of registry data suggests that while the risk of acute rejection decreases with age, the impact of rejection on long-term graft function in this elderly population is greater when compared to younger groups. It is of no surprise that posttransplant mortality is greater in the elderly; however, censoring graft survival data for patient death demonstrates no significant difference between outcome in older and younger patients [5, 6, 20, 21].

The goal of an immunosuppression protocol should be to maintain a level necessary for a reduced risk of infection without increasing the risk for rejection. The elderly have less immunocompetence, and the therapy has to be adjusted in the elderly transplant recipient. This may result in a decreased likelihood of immunologic rejection but increased risk of infection. Immunosuppressive therapy also has to be adjusted to account for the different pharmacokinetics and altered effects of drugs in the elderly. The aging process results in physiological changes that affect drug absorption, distribution, and metabolism. In addition, due to the many comorbid conditions in the elderly, they often take many medications which may have drug–drug interactions with immunosuppressive medications [22].

There are currently no prospective multicenter trials that specifically evaluate immunosuppressive medication protocols in the elderly in a randomized fashion. Most of the time, the elderly are excluded from trials. As such, most of the data is from single-center, observational studies or retrospective database analyses [23]. Any approach should be based on the risks of acute rejection, infections, malignancy, and comorbid conditions.

There is no set immunosuppression protocol that has been universally accepted in the elderly or any patient population. Although acute rejection decreases with recipient age, chronic allograft nephropathy seems to increase with age, and this phenomenon is further confounded by increased death from infectious disease and drug-related causes. This has led to some protocols that support less-intensive immunosuppressive drug therapy in elderly recipients [24].

Current treatments consist of triple therapy with corticosteroids, a calcineurin inhibitor (cyclosporine or tacrolimus), and an antimetabolite, but these regimens may be replaced by substitution or addition of newer antiproliferative agents. Treatment with mycophenolate mofetil (MMF), which inhibits purine synthesis, has been found to result in a longer time to the first episode of acute rejection but had significantly greater rates of opportunistic infection and graft loss and mortality [25]. One study comparing MMF to azathioprine evaluated over 5,000 patients over the age of 65 and showed improved patient and graft survival with lower rates of late acute rejection with MMF. The most prescribed immunosuppressive protocol is a combination of MMF with calcineurin inhibitor, and there appears to be no contraindication to use this protocol in the elderly [26, 27].

An alternative or supplement to standard triple therapy is the use of augmented immunosuppression with antilymphocyte antibodies, commonly termed "induction immunotherapy." These cytolytic agents have been found to reduce the risk of early rejection but tend to increase the risk of infection. Induction therapy in the form of Atgam® (equine antithymocyte globulin) or OKT3® (muromonab-CD3) was the mainstay but now has been largely replaced by the use of Thymoglobulin® (rabbit anti-lymphocyte globulin) or monoclonal antibody therapy directed against the IL-2 receptor – Zenapax® (daclizumab) or Simulect® (basiliximab) [1].

In addition to the immunosuppression and steroids making the elderly more susceptible to infection, fractures, weight gain, and other side effects, they are at a 30% higher risk of developing new-onset diabetes posttransplant per decade of life [28]. This has led to a movement in recent years for the avoidance or early withdrawal of calcineurin inhibitors and/or corticosteroids. Multiple studies demonstrated appropriate patient and graft survival, as well as excellent graft function, after using induction agents and minimizing the use of calcineurin inhibitor [29–31].

Considering the elderly's increased risk for adverse affects and infection, and the limited prospective data available, any protocol must consider that decreasing the risk of acute rejection may augment the morbid consequences of rejection. As such, protocols are currently tailored based on donor type and immunologic status of the elderly recipient. The low-risk recipient of a kidney from a young donor may be a candidate for rapid steroid withdrawal or steroid minimization strategies due to the lower risk of rejection and increased risk of steroid-induced adverse effects. The low-risk recipient of a kidney from an older donor may have an enhanced risk of chronic allograft nephropathy and nephrotoxicity from the calcineurin inhibitors, so it may be appropriate to use a calcineurin inhibitor minimization strategy. As already mentioned, interleukin-2 receptor antibodies or antilymphocyte antibodies may be used as induction agents with a calcineurin inhibitor, with the interleukin-2 receptor antibody showing a superior safety profile. Minimizing immunosuppression is not appropriate in an elderly patient with high immunologic risk, so a regimen consisting of antibody induction, corticosteroids, calcineurin inhibitors, and/or MMF is more reasonable [23].

Since there is potential for severe consequences with acute graft rejection in the elderly, a biopsy should be performed in all unexplained cases of allograft dysfunction. Treatment should be based on histologic findings, whenever possible, with empiric steroid use for treatment of presumed acute rejection used sparingly due to the increased risk of adverse events in the elderly.

Patient and Graft Outcomes

Renal allograft and patient survival in the elderly transplant recipient are currently excellent, when looked at as a group and compared to younger recipients. Patient survival at 1, 5, and 10 years ranges from 80 to 90, 70, and 50%, respectively [1, 5, 6, 32]. This is based in part on the type of allograft. Based on the 2008 SRTR analyzing transplants from 1998 to 2007, 3-month, 1-, and 5-year patient survival rates for those 65 years of age and older receiving a renal transplant are: 98, 96, and 78% for recipients of living-donor kidney transplants, respectively; 96, 92, and 66% for recipients of deceased-donor nonextended criteria donor kidneys, respectively; and 95, 87, and 58% for recipients of deceased-donor extended criteria donor kidneys, respectively [1].

Graft survival has increased in parallel, averaging 85% at 1 year and 70% at 5 years [5, 6]. Allograft survival at 3 months, 1, and 5 years for those 65 years of age or older are: 97, 94, and 74% for recipients of living-donor kidney transplants, respectively (Fig. 98.1); 94, 88, and 59% for recipients of deceased-donor nonextended criteria donor kidneys, respectively; and 90, 81, and 48% for recipients of deceased-donor extended criteria donor kidneys, respectively (Fig. 98.2) [1].

Patient death with a functioning graft accounts for the majority of reported "graft loss" in the elderly patients. Nearly 50% of graft loss is due to death in the elderly recipient compared to 15% in the younger recipient. Acute rejection is reported to occur less often in elderly recipients, but there is an increased risk of chronic allograft nephropathy, especially if the allograft is from the older donor [33].

The predominant causes of death in elderly transplant recipients are cardiovascular disease and infection. Most infectious episodes occur in the first 6 months posttransplant, likely due to the degree of immunosuppression. The risks of overimmunosuppression and cardiovascular disease are related to the natural effects of aging and factors having to do with end-stage renal disease. Overimmunosuppression will increase infectious complications in all patients, regardless of age. However, the elderly are less immunocompetent, leading them to be more susceptible to infection at lower lev-

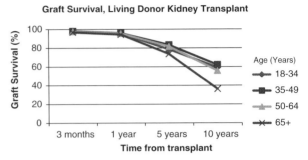

2008 OPTN/SRTR Annual Report 1998-2007.

Figure 98.1 Adjusted graph survival, living-donor kidney transplants, data from 1998 to 2007; 2008 SRTR Annual Report.

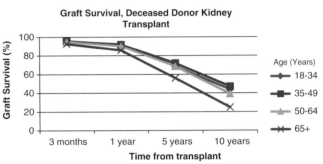

2008 OPTN/SRTR Annual Report 1998-2007.

Figure 98.2 Adjusted graph survival, deceased-donor kidney transplants, data from 1998 to 2007; 2008 SRTR Annual Report.

els of immunosuppressive therapy. Most likely to contribute to this are high-dose corticosteroids and antilymphocyte antibodies at induction. Other causes of death in the elderly recipient include malignancy and gastrointestinal hemorrhage. Death due to malignancy has been reported to increase disproportionately with time after transplantation in the elderly recipient [22]. Despite the mortality risks, there is still a better life expectancy and quality of life afforded by kidney transplantation compared to dialysis. With careful selection and responsible follow-up, advanced age alone is not a contraindication to successful transplantation. Age should not be the primary determinant of donor allocation; rather, the focus should be on baseline comorbidity or functional status [10].

Liver Transplantation

End-stage liver disease (ESLD) results from many etiologies and eventually leads to complications including bleeding, ascites, infection, renal failure, fluid and electrolyte disturbances, hepatic encephalopathy, hepatocellular carcinoma, and eventually, liver failure. Currently, the only definitive treatment for patients with ESLD is liver transplantation. There were 6,223 deceased-donor liver transplants performed in the U.S. in 2007, of which 619 (9.9%) were in patients 65 years or older. 3,445 (55%) deceased-donor liver transplants were allocated for recipients between the ages of 50–64. There were 266 living-related liver transplants, of which only 27 were for older recipients. Of the approximately 16,500 patients on the waiting list for liver transplant, 1,450 (11.6%) are over the age of 65. This is a dramatic increase from the 4,424 liver transplants in 1998, with only 322 (7.3%) going to patients over the age of 65. As is seen with other organs, far fewer livers are available than patients who need them [1].

Indications

The most common diagnoses in elderly patients waiting for liver transplantation are cirrhosis, alcoholic liver disease, hepatitis, primary biliary cirrhosis, and hepatocellular carcinoma. Elderly patients should only be considered for transplantation if they are thought to be capable of surviving the perioperative period and complying with the intense chronic medical regimen and follow-up [34].

Older patients are frequently seen as higher risk recipients due to their comorbidities and increased mortality to both hepatic and nonhepatic causes [35]. Liver transplantation in patients over the age of 55 was discouraged as recently as 20 years ago. However, since that time, there have been many studies demonstrating success in patients over the age of 60, encouraging more centers to list and operate on older patients [36–41]. More recent data suggest that patients over the age of 70 may successfully undergo liver transplantation; however, it has to be at a less-severe level of disease to have a good outcome [42].

Most contraindications for liver transplantation relate to comorbid conditions. Relative contraindications include alcohol or illicit drug use in past 6 months in a patient with a history of abuse, severe extrahepatic disease, adverse psychosocial factors, anatomic difficulties resulting from previous abdominal trauma or surgery, and age. Absolute contraindications generally include uncontrolled infection or sepsis, extrahepatic malignancy, advanced hepatic malignancy, and irreversible brain injury [39, 43]. HIV infection had previously been considered to be an absolute contraindication for liver transplantation. However, with the significant improvements with antiretroviral therapy and improved monitoring methods, it is no longer a sufficient reason to refuse surgery. While some centers may still list it as a relative contraindication, many will no longer restrict recipients as long as attention is paid to the comorbid conditions.

Criteria for Transplantation

For more than 30 years, the Child–Pugh classification system was used to predict morbidity and mortality in patients with liver disease. While useful in stratifying patients for transplantation, it does not provide an adequate method of prioritizing patients on the liver transplant waiting list [44]. As a result, organ allocation in adults is now based on the Model for End-Stage Liver Disease (MELD), which is a logarithmic transformation of the recipient's bilirubin level, creatinine level, and international normalized ratio (INR) into a mathematical model. It allows for an objective assessment of need for transplantation and short-term prognosis while waiting for a transplant. It does not, however, necessarily correlate with posttransplant survival [45].

Preoperative assessment of all liver transplant candidates includes abdominal ultrasound, thoracic and abdominal computed tomography, and upper gastrointestinal endoscopy in addition to routine blood studies. Patients older than 50 years must undergo screening colonoscopy, and in male patients older than 55 years, the serum prostate-specific antigen concentration must be studied with digital rectal examination. In female patients, cervical and breast cancer screening must be done as indicated before listing.

Age-related morbidity is one of the main causes of mortality after liver transplantation.

Older patients have to be evaluated by specialists in the field of cardiology and pulmonary disease [46]. The cardiovascular workup for patients over the age of 60 years includes a routine history and physical examination, EKG, and two-dimensional echocardiography. A history of coronary artery disease (CAD) or symptoms of exceptional angina are clear indications for performing cardiac catheterization prior to transplantation. A negative stress test is not sufficient to exclude cardiac disease in patients with clinical history strongly suggestive of CAD. In this situation, the clinician may elect to proceed directly to cardiac catheterization [47]. Doppler studies of the carotid, vertebral, and peripheral limb arteries are performed on these patients if clinically warranted. Revascularization strategy must be performed prior to listing for liver transplantation if there is extensive coronary heart disease [38]. Diabetes mellitus may be the most important risk factor for the presence of CAD in patients with liver disease and must be assessed and managed appropriately in the perioperative setting [44, 48]. Older patients with end-stage liver disease, particularly those with cholestatic liver disease, are also at risk for osteopenia or osteoporosis. Postoperative corticosteroid therapy will also contribute to bone loss, increasing the risk of sustaining compression fractures. For all elderly patients, determination of vitamin D serum levels and baseline bone densitometry is encouraged [44]. Any patient over the age of 60 with a history of encephalopathy, seizures, or ischemic event should have an MRI of the brain prior to being listed. Older patients also have to be routinely screened for malignancy. Patients waiting for liver transplants need to be evaluated for hepatocellular carcinoma (HCC) in particular, as well as for colon, skin, prostate, and breast neoplasms.

For liver transplant recipients, the pretransplant status has been found to be associated with survival, and this is seen more in elderly patients. In a retrospective review of 1,446 liver transplant recipients, of which 241 were over the age of 60, the elderly patients were found to be especially at risk for lower survival if they had a bilirubin level of 10 mg/dL or greater, an albumin level of less than 3 g/dL, a markedly prolonged (>20 s) prothrombin time, or generalized poor nutrition. The authors recommended forgoing transplantation in a patient over the age of 60 who is an inpatient in the hospital or in the intensive care unit with any of the above values [49].

Immunosuppression

The immunosuppression protocol and dose of immunosuppressive drugs do not drastically differ between older and younger liver transplant patients [43]. Immunosuppressive strategies vary from center to center in the selection of specific agents, the number of agents, and the duration of use of each agent. The combinations used have evolved to predominantly tacrolimus, mycophenolate mofetil/mycophenolic acid, and steroids. Triple drug therapy remains the predominant drug regimen; however, many centers are attempting to minimize or eliminate long-term steroid use. The key is to tailor the regimen to the patient to best prevent cellular rejection, have no associated morbidity with respect to opportunistic infections, have no nephrotoxicity, and preclude the development of infection, which continues to be a leading cause of death in the year after transplantation.

Results

Although there are some studies reporting that the long-term survival of patients older than 60 years was lower than younger recipients [50–53], most studies report similar [38, 54, 55] or even better [43, 56] survival in recipients older than 60 years old.

One study evaluating the survival rates of elderly liver transplant recipients found that the short-term survival of the elderly is comparable to those younger adults, but the longer survival was not encouraging. The long-term survival was significantly lower in elderly recipients, with a 5-year patient survival of 52% in the elderly group and 75% in the younger patients ($p < 0.05$). The study period was divided into two eras; 1984–1991 and 1992–1997. In both eras, recipient survival in those older than 60 years was significantly lower than younger recipients, lending support to the idea that older recipients are not good candidates for liver transplantation [50].

A different study showing better survival rates in elderly patients looked at 240 liver transplant recipients, of which 23 were over the age of 60. They reported 87.5 and 83.3% 1- and 3-year patient survival in the elderly, respectively, compared to 77.8 and 73.5% in the younger group. Graft survival rates at 1 and 3 years were found to be 79.2 and 75% in the older group and 76.5 and 71% in the younger group, respectively. Neither set of data showed any statistical significance [52].

Some studies divided older recipients into two groups to show the effect of age more clearly: recipients between 60 and 65 years of age and those older than 65 years. One study reported that the patient survival in the older than 65 years of age group was 99%, 82 and 73% in 3 days, 1, and 5 years, respectively [38].

A different study found a lower survival rate in patients older than 65 years than in patients between 60 and 65 years, although there was no statistical significance. Overall, patients older than 60 years had lower survival rates than younger patients, which could possibly be explained since that group had a higher rate of HCC as the reason for transplantation [47].

Similar results can be found in smaller studies for recipients over the age of 70. One study found a 58% 3-year survival in 33 patients, while another has 1- and 3-year survival rates of 78.8 and 71.4%, respectively [39, 53]. Data is limited in this age group, but transplantation in septuagenarians is definitely feasible if the patient is otherwise healthy.

There are few studies looking at the survival in older patients after a living-donor liver transplant (LDLT), and the results have been mixed. Some investigators reported that recipient age had an influence on allograft failure [48], while others found that older recipient age and prolonged cold ischemia time increased the risk of graft failure [49]. One of the larger studies investigated the impact of age in living-donor liver transplantation by following recipients over 60 years of age over a 10-year period. They found the following parameters as risk factors influencing survival rate in patients after LDLT: MELD score equal to or greater than 25; Child's classification C; preoperative status of the recipient being in an intensive care unit; and blood type incompatibility. Recipient age of 60 years of age or older had no influence on the survival. 1-, 3-, and 5-year survival of the recipients older than 60 years were 81.9, 78.7, and 78.7%, respectively. Interestingly, their results in older patients were better than in younger patients (1-, 3-, and 5-year survivals in patients younger than 60 years is 75, 70.8, and 69.3%, respectively). A possible explanation for this better survival is that the selection criteria of older recipients were more stringent. The MELD score for older group recipients was significantly lower, and high-risk older patients were not considered for LDLT as a treatment option for their advanced liver disease in that study [43].

It is evident that after 5 years, survival of patients aged 65 years and older begins to diminish [38]. The 10-year survival of recipients older than 60 years was found to be 48%, which is significantly lower than the 72% survival rate of recipients younger than 60 [47, 57]. One study evaluated 91 transplant recipients over the age of 60 over a 13-year span and reported a 10-year patient survival of 35% in the elderly group and 60% in the younger patients ($p < 0.05$). The most common cause of late mortality in elderly liver recipients was malignancy (35%), whereas most of the young adult deaths were the result of infectious complications (24%) [50].

Based on the 2008 SRTR analyzing transplants from 1998 to 2007, 3-month, 1-, 5-, and 10-year patient survival rates for those 65 years of age and older receiving a liver transplant are 91, 81, 64, and 42% for recipients of deceased-donor liver transplants, respectively and 93, 85, 71, and 54% for recipients of living-donor livers, respectively. Allograft survival at 3 months, 1-, 5-, and 10-years for those 65 years of age or older are 94, 84, 68, and 53% for recipients of living-donor livers, respectively (Fig. 98.3) and 89, 78, 61, and 40% for recipients of deceased-donor liver transplants, respectively (Fig. 98.4). The results at all intervals were comparable to those of younger age groups [1].

When evaluating a patient's risk for rejection after liver transplant, younger age has been found to be an independent risk factor [58]. Older patients usually have a lower incidence of episodes and severity of graft rejection, possibly a result of immune senescence [46, 51, 59]. One study noted that liver recipients over the age of 65 tended to have lower rates of rejection, although there was no statistical significance [38]. Some centers have reported no difference in episodes of acute rejection among older or younger recipients [56, 60].

Most studies report no statistical differences in the incidence of complications in terms of hospitalization, infection (surgical or opportunistic), repeat operation, readmission, or repeat transplant between the patients older or younger than 60 years [56]. Older patients are more prone to having higher incidence of osteoporosis, nontraumatic bone fractures, coronary artery disease, and malignancy after liver transplantation, with skin cancer being the most common [43, 47].

The most prevalent cause of death in recipients older than 60 years is malignancy (both recurrent and de novo) and sepsis [38, 43, 47]. In one study, investigators reported that seven of ten recipients died secondary to sepsis in the early phase after LDLT within 3 months. In patients younger than 65 years of age, most causes of death are related to cardiovascular (myocardial infarction, congestive heart failure, cerebrovascular accident, intracranial hemorrhage) and sepsis. A possible explanation for not having the cardiac problems as a leading cause of death in older patients may be that the older recipients are more rigorously assessed for comorbidities that could be detrimental to outcome.

Well-selected patients over the age 60 or 65 have a comparable survival after liver transplantation to younger

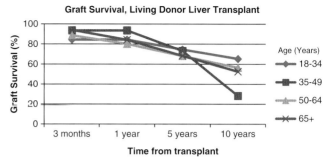

2008 OPTN/SRTR Annual Report 1998-2007.

Figure 98.3 Adjusted graph survival, living-donor liver transplants, data from 1998 to 2007; 2008 SRTR Annual Report.

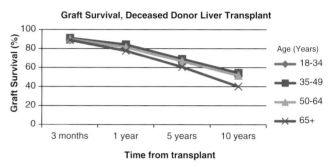

2008 OPTN/SRTR Annual Report 1998-2007.

Figure 98.4 Adjusted graph survival, deceased-donor liver transplants, data from 1998 to 2007; 2008 SRTR Annual Report.

recipients at 1-, 3-, and 5-years posttransplant. Advances in surgical technique, improved intensive care, and standardized immunosuppressive therapy all contribute to the good survival results. Unfortunately, long-term results have not been as promising, possibly explained by older patients having fewer years of life remaining. Nonetheless, this should not preclude liver transplantation in elderly patients deemed strong and otherwise healthy enough to undergo the procedure [38].

Heart Transplantation

Chronic heart failure remains one of the most common diseases affecting the population. With increases in life expectancy and improvements in medical care, more elderly patients are being seen by cardiologists and cardiac surgeons for end-stage heart failure. Cardiac transplantation is the treatment of choice for many patients with end-stage heart failure who remain symptomatic despite optimal medical therapy. The 2007 report from the Registry of the International Society for Heart and Lung Transplantation (ISHLT) estimated that slightly more than 5,000 heart transplants are performed annually worldwide [61]. The SRTR estimates that anywhere from 2,000 to 2,400 heart transplants were performed in the

United States yearly over the past decade, with 2,207 transplanted in 2007. Of this, 44–52% of the recipients are 50–64 years of age, and 8–11% are 65 years of age or older. The most recent data list 1,408 active patients on the waiting list, with 168 (12%) being over the age of 65. The median time to transplant in this elderly group is 103 days [1].

Older patients have been excluded from consideration for heart transplantation in the past, typically due to the supposed adverse effect of increased age on long-term survival and the shortage of donor organs. However, advances in posttransplant care have improved outcomes in older patients, and several centers have demonstrated results comparable to younger patients. The criteria regarding the recipient's older age limit continue to be expanded, and older patients are increasingly being considered as potential heart transplant candidates [62–65].

Indications

Over the past decade, there has been a significant decrease in mortality in patients with advanced heart failure treated aggressively with medical and device therapy, leading to a reassessment of the role of cardiac transplantation [66, 67]. The ideal heart transplant candidate is a person with end-stage heart disease for whom conventional therapy is not likely to provide acceptable symptomatic benefit or satisfactorily improve life expectancy. The Clinical Practice Committee of the American Society of Transplantation published recommendations in 2001 for considering heart transplantation in patients with cardiac conditions that have not responded to maximal medical management [13]. Although severe heart failure refractory to medical therapy is the most common indication for transplantation, other circumstances warranting transplant include severely limiting ischemia not amenable to interventional or surgical revascularization, recurrent symptomatic ventricular tachyarrhythmia refractory to medical therapy, an implantable cardioverter-defibrillator (ICD), or surgery and rarely, for the management of cardiac tumors. Nonischemic cardiomyopathy accounts for approximately 45% of cases, and coronary artery disease accounts for about 38% of cases. Nonischemic conditions include systolic heart failure, defined by left ventricular ejection fraction < 35% (Ischemic and dilated cardiomyopathy, valvular heart disease, and hypertensive heart disease); intractable arrhythmia uncontrolled with implantable cardioverter-defibrillator; and hypertrophic cardiomyopathy with persistent heart failure despite valve replacement, pacemaker, or medical therapy.

There are a few absolute contraindications to cardiac transplantation. Fixed pulmonary hypertension or any systemic illness that will limit survival despite heart transplant, such as high-grade neoplasm, AIDS, multisystem or active systemic lupus erythematosus or sarcoid preclude transplantation. HIV infection has been considered to be an absolute contraindication to transplant, primarily due to concerns about the increased frequency of infectious and malignant complications and the previously poor survival of such patients. The prognosis of HIV has changed since the advent of highly active antiretroviral therapy (HAART), and guidelines are being amended so that HIV infection itself is not a sufficient reason to refuse heart transplantation [68]. Age greater than 70 years was an absolute contraindication in previous guidelines, but the ISHLT has recently modified their recommendations in 2006 to state that "carefully selected patients > 70 years of age may be considered for cardiac transplantation. For centers considering these patients, the use of an alternate-type program (i.e., use of older donors) may be pursued." [63] The guidelines regarding neoplasm were also modified, with new consideration being given to tumors with low recurrence rate, response to therapy, and negative metastatic workup.

Criteria for Transplantation

In general, the most objective assessment of functional capacity in patients with heart failure, and what may be the best predictor of when to list a patient for transplantation, is measurement of peak oxygen consumption (VO_2max). This can be measured using exercise testing with ventilatory gas analysis. Several studies have demonstrated that peak VO_2 independently predicted mortality, which is highest for patients with values <10 mL/kg/min, and significantly improved if between 10 and 15 mL/kg/min [69–71].

Although peak VO_2 is an important factor used to guide the selection of heart transplant candidates, it does not provide an optimal risk profile. One model that has been validated prospectively is the Heart Failure Survival Score (HFSS), derived from a multivariable analysis of 268 patients referred for consideration of cardiac transplantation form 1986–1993 at one institution and validated in 199 similar patients from 1993 to 1995 at another institution. It incorporated noninvasive parameters, including the following seven variables and their pathophysiological constructs: presence or absence of coronary artery disease (myocardial ischemia), resting heart rate (activation of sympathetic nervous system), left ventricular ejection fraction (the degree of systolic dysfunction), mean arterial blood pressure, presence or absence of intraventricular conduction defect on baseline ECG (the extent of myocardial fibrosis), serum sodium (the degree of activation of the renin–angiotensin system), and peak VO_2 [72].

The Seattle Heart Failure Model is another model that, in contrast to the HFSS, incorporated the impact of newer heart failure therapies on survival, including ICDs (implantable cardioverter-defibrillators) and CRT (cardiac resynchronization therapy) [73].

Immunosuppression

As with other organs, there is no general consensus regarding a preferred immunosuppressive protocol in this age group. Treatment with mycophenolate mofetil/mycophenolic acid, a purine analog, has been shown to reduce the rate of rejection and improve survival, but it did have a higher incidence of nonfatal, opportunistic infections as compared with azathioprine therapy [74]. The two most common regimens in 1997, which was used for 75% of transplant recipients, consisted of cyclosporine with mycophenolate mofetil/mycophenolic acid or another antimetabolite and steroids. Over the years, these combinations have evolved to be predominantly tacrolimus, mycophenolate mofetil/mycophenolic acid, and steroids (49% of transplant recipients), and to a lesser extent cyclosporine, mycophenolate mofetil/mycophenolic acid, and steroids (29% of transplant recipients). At 1-year posttransplantation, triple drug therapy remains the predominant drug regimen [1].

The ideal immunosuppressive regimen will prevent cellular rejection, have no associated morbidity with respect to opportunistic infections, have no nephrotoxicity, and preclude the development of coronary allograft vasculopathy, which affects 50% of patients at 5 years. This immunosuppressive therapy used to prevent rejection predisposes patients to infection, which continues to be the leading cause of death in the year after cardiac transplantation [58].

A notable trend over the past 10 years has been the declining number of recipients who needed treatment for rejection episodes in the first year after heart transplantation, decreasing from 36% in 1996 to 25% in 2005. This could reflect the improved efficacy of newer immunosuppression medication and regimens, as well as earlier recognition and prompt treatment [1].

Results

Multiple studies have demonstrated comparable survival rates in elderly cardiac transplant recipients compared to younger recipients [59–62, 75–78]. Included in this is a multi-institutional study of the UNOS database where it was found that there was a satisfactory but lower 5-year survival between elderly (>60 years) and young (18–59 years) recipients (69% vs. 75%, respectively). The elderly group, however, had more infections, renal failure, and longer postoperative length of stay and were at increased risk of malignancy [62].

One retrospective study showed no statistically significant difference in 1- and 4-year survival (1-year survival: 93.3% vs. 88.3%; 4-year survival: 73.5% vs. 69.1%), length of intensive-care unit stay, incidence of rejection, and incidence of cytomegalovirus infection between patients over the age of 70 and younger patients [59]. A 10-year follow-up of cardiac transplant recipients >65 years of age (*n*=66) demonstrated survival rates comparable to those of younger patients (<60 years: *n*=679; 60–64 years: *n*=137) [60].

The adjusted graft survival for recipients over the age of 65 at 3 months (90%), 1 year (85%), 5 years (66%), and 10 years (44%) were all found to be comparable within a few percentage points to various younger age groups (Fig. 98.5) [1].

The increased risk of renal failure has been consistent in various studies over the years and may be attributed to the already known preexisting renal disease in elderly, as suggested by elevated preoperative creatinine. Another consideration is the nephrotoxic effects of immunosuppression. Tailoring therapy for the elderly may be beneficial, and some data support minimizing the use of calcineurin inhibitors and azathioprine in exchange for using mycophenolate mofetil and mammalian target of rapamycin inhibitors (mTOR inhibitors, sirolimus) [79].

Transplant patients have been the subject of extensive investigation into the increased risk of malignancy, especially in the elderly. Increased age has been independently associated with increased risk of malignancy in nontransplanted controls, and heart transplant recipients have been shown to have a 7.1-fold increase in incidence of malignancy [80]. Among all solid-organ transplant recipients, skin cancer is the most common malignancy. Heart and/or lung transplant recipients have a 26.2-, 21-, and 9.3-fold increased risk of developing lymphoproliferative disorders, head and neck cancer, and lung cancer, respectively. Malignancy does not necessarily shorten survival in older recipients, but one may surmise that it does affect quality of life [75].

The demand for heart transplantations is unlikely to ever be fully met, and more resources are needed to slow down the progression of heart failure and prevent the need for

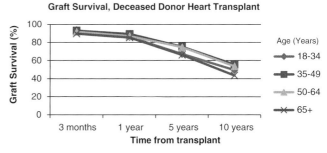

2008 OPTN/SRTR Annual Report 1998-2007.

FIGURE 98.5 Adjusted graph survival, deceased-donor heart transplants, data from 1998 to 2007; 2008 SRTR Annual Report.

transplant surgery in the first place. As ventricular assist device technology improves, it may be used to complement heart transplantation to avoid immunosuppression and its side effect of malignancy in older patients with advanced heart failure.

Lung Transplantation

Lung transplantation should be considered for patients with advanced lung disease whose clinical status has progressively worsened despite optimal medical or surgical therapy.

One thousand four hundred sixty-five lung transplants from deceased donors were performed in the United States in 2007, increased from 840 in 1998 and 941 in 2000. Of these, 223 were for recipients over the age of 65, representing 15% of all lung transplant recipients and dramatically increased from 30 (3.6%) in 1998 and 30 (3.2%) in 2000. The percentage of patients 50–64 years of age receiving lung transplants has not changed substantially over the past few years, with 54% of deceased-donor lungs going to these patients in 2007, up slightly from 48% in 1997. The most recent data list 1,005 active patients on the waiting list, with 91 (9%) being over the age of 65. The median time to transplant in this elderly group is 57 days. Donor lung shortage has been the major limiting factor to the number of lung transplants performed. The procurement rate of lung from deceased donors has consistently been lower than those for kidney, liver, and heart. While kidneys and livers are harvested from more than 85% of all cadaveric donors, and hearts from 30% of deceased donors, lungs are harvested from only 15% of all cadaveric donors [1]. This discrepancy may be attributed to the lung's vulnerability to potential complications that arise before and after donor death such as aspiration, pneumonia, ventilator-associated lung injury, and neurogenic pulmonary edema. Over the past several years, the number of single lung transplants performed annually in the United States has remained stable, while the number of bilateral transplants has consistently increased and even surpassed the number of single lung procedures [81].

The most common indications for lung transplantation, accounting for 85% of procedures worldwide, are advanced chronic obstructive pulmonary disease (COPD), idiopathic pulmonary fibrosis, cystic fibrosis, emphysema due to alpha-1 antitrypsin deficiency, and idiopathic pulmonary arterial hypertension. Survival benefit has been demonstrated for both single and double lung transplants in patients with cystic fibrosis, pulmonary fibrosis, and primary pulmonary hypertension. There have been less convincing and reproducible results regarding the benefit of transplantation in patients with emphysema or Eisenmenger's syndrome [82, 83].

Absolute contraindications for lung transplantation include malignancy within the last 2 years (excluding cutaneous squamous and basal cell tumors); significant chest wall deformity; noncurable chronic extrapulmonary infection (active Hepatitis B,C, HIV); untreatable advanced dysfunction of another major organ (e.g., heart, liver, kidney); known noncompliance or inability to follow medical regimen, especially if related to an untreatable psychiatric or psychological condition; absence of a consistent or reliable social support system; and substance addiction within the last 6 months [84]. Coronary artery disease not amenable to percutaneous intervention or bypass grafting, or associated with significant impairment of left ventricular function, is an absolute contraindication to lung transplantation, but heart–lung transplantation could be considered in highly selected cases.

Relative contraindications to lung transplantation include: Age older than 65 years; critical or unstable clinical condition; severely limited functional status with poor rehabilitation potential; colonization with highly resistant or virulent bacteria, fungi, or mycobacteria; severe obesity (Body Mass Index exceeding 30 kg/m^2); severe or symptomatic osteoporosis; and poorly controlled or managed medical conditions (diabetes mellitus, systemic hypertension) [81].

Immunosuppression

As with other organ transplantation, induction therapy has become a major part of the immunosuppression regimen with lung transplantation. Induction therapy was used in the first 5–7 days after transplantation for 57% of all lung transplants performed in 2006, up from only 22% of lung transplants in 1997. Among the most common were antilymphocyte antibodies (antithymocite globulin or OKT3) or monoclonal IL-2 receptor antagonists (basiliximab or daclizumab). Baseline therapy prior to discharge at most centers included corticosteroids, calcineurin inhibitor (tacrolimus 83%, cyclosporine), and an antimetabolite (azathioprine 39% or mycophenolate mofetil 52%). Maintenance immunosuppression administered for the first year following transplantation was essentially the same. Steroids are typically tapered to a low dosage or even discontinued in some protocols. Acute rejection within the first year was treated most commonly with corticosteroids, used in 95% of acute rejection cases [85, 86].

Despite the multitude of medications available, no drug has been found to be consistently superior in delaying rejection or bronchiolitis obliterans or in prolonging long-term survival. Protocols vary widely between lung transplant centers

Results

The adjusted graft survival for recipients over the age of 65 at 3 months (92%), 1 year (79%), 5 years (42%), and 10 years (13%) are all comparable within a few percentage points to

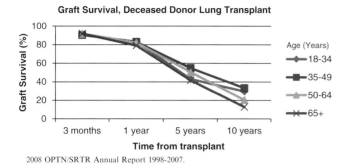

Graph Survival, Deceased Donor Lung Transplant

2008 OPTN/SRTR Annual Report.

Figure 98.6 Adjusted graph survival, deceased-donor lung transplants, data from 1998 to 2007; 2008 SRTR Annual Report.

various younger age groups (Fig. 98.6) [1]. The average death rate in the first year after transplantation decreased steadily from 290 per 1,000 patient-years at risk in 1997 to 169 deaths per 1,000 patient-years at risk in 2004, a 10-year low. According to the 2007 ISHLT Registry report, the median survival for all adult recipients is 5 years, but bilateral lung recipients have a better median survival than single lung recipients (5.9 vs. 4.4 years, respectively) [78]. It is not delineated if this survival advantage is related to the underlying patient characteristics or choice of operation. The impact of underlying diagnosis on survival after lung transplantation has often been linked to age, with older recipients having a significantly shorter survival than younger ones. Recipients with COPD have the best 1-year survival, but a lower 10-year survival when compared to those with cystic fibrosis and alpha-1 antitrypsin deficiency. In contrast, patients with idiopathic pulmonary arterial hypertension have the lowest 1-year survival, but their 10-year survival approaches those with cystic fibrosis and alpha-1 antitrypsin deficiency [87].

This data is significantly different when evaluating patients over the age of 70. An analysis of UNOS data of lung transplants from 1999 to 2006 showed that patients 70 years and older had substantially increased risks of 30-, 90-day, and 1-year mortality when compared to younger groups. The authors' recommendation was that lung transplantation may be used with caution in older patients over the age of 60, but should not be performed in patients older than age 70 [88].

Management strategies have been more effective at reducing early complications than later ones, which may be due to refinements in surgical technique and postoperative care. However, beyond the first year of transplantation, survival is mostly affected by infections and chronic rejection, and the incidence of these complications has not changed substantially since 1988 [84].

The leading cause of death in the first 30 days after lung transplantation is graft failure, a form of Acute Respiratory Distress Syndrome (ARDS), accounting for almost 30% of deaths [78]. The leading cause of mortality after the first year, typically accounting for 40% of deaths, is chronic

allograft rejection (e.g., chronic graft dysfunction), which usually manifests as bronchiolitis obliterans syndrome (BOS) [89]. Survival 3 years after the onset of BOS is only 50% and drops to 30–40% at 5 years [90].

Infectious complications remain a leading cause of rejection and death at any point after lung transplantation, in any age group. It has been attributable to up to 35% of deaths in the first year and 20% of deaths thereafter. Bacterial bronchitis and pneumonia are most common, but cytomegalovirus, mycobacteria, fungi, and community-acquired respiratory viruses all contribute to morbidity and mortality [84, 87].

Malignancy accounts for 7–10% of deaths beyond the first year after lung transplantation. Nonmelanoma skin cancer is most common overall, but posttransplant lymphoproliferative disease (PTLD) is the most common malignancy in the first year after transplant [78]. Other malignancies include colon, breast, Kaposi's sarcoma, and transitional cell carcinoma of the bladder [91].

Combined Organ Transplantation

Often times, there are patients with multiple organ failure that may benefit from dual organ transplantation. Examples include kidney–pancreas and heart–lung. While there has been success with these combined organ transplantations over the years, its use has been limited in the elderly population. From 1998 to 2007, there were a total of 14 kidney–pancreas transplants in patients over the age of 65, while none were reported for heart–lung for a patient over the age of 65 [1]. As with individual organs, the overall risk–benefit of the surgery needs to be weighed, considering the overall health of the patient and potential survival benefits of transplantation. While age is often considered a significant factor in determining candidacy, it should not be the limiting factor.

Conclusion

The elderly population is on the rise in this country, and older patients comprise the fastest growing segment of the population. This trend is mirrored in the transplantation population. The discipline of organ transplantation has grown remarkably over the last half-century and has evolved from infrequent, highly dangerous procedures with very high mortality to complex operations performed regularly across the country and world. Data from centers across the country clearly indicate that patients over the age of 65 can undergo kidney, liver, heart, or lung transplantation with excellent results (Fig. 98.7). The limiting factor, however, is the shortage of organs and excess of patients on the waiting list; which raises many ethical and social concerns regarding transplanting

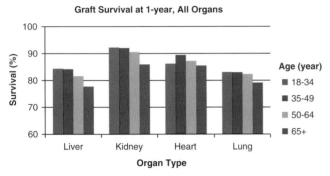

Graft Survival at 1-year, All Organs

2008 OPTN/SRTR Annual Report 1998-2007.

FIGURE 98.7 Graph survival at 1 year, all organs. Data from 1998 to 2007; 2008 SRTR Annual Report.

healthy organs into older patients who may not have as much of a survival benefit as a younger patient. Although the allocation of organs according to age may be a simple approach to satisfying the goal of social justice, the inclusion of patient comorbidity and potential for survival benefit in the elderly must also be considered.

Kidney and liver transplantation has been successfully performed and results substantiated in patients over the age of 70. The results depend on the selectivity used to identify those elderly candidates on the waiting list for transplant. Cardiac and lung transplants have shown some promising results in patients over the age of 65, but not over the age of 70. It is important to note that with cardiac and lung transplantation, there is a slight discrepancy with the proportion of elderly patients on the waiting list and with overall survival rates. This is likely due to patient selection more than the overall results. This patient population is a highly selective group of elderly patients with cardiac and lung disease, who are often not placed on the waiting list until they worsen clinically. All things being equal, discrimination against older candidates for organ transplantation on age-related grounds alone is not warranted. Despite potential utilitarian gains to be made limiting transplantation in the elderly recipients, the sense of fairness in the system will be harmed. Elderly patients who are healthy will be the ones who suffer. Older patients already face huge hurdles to get on the waiting list for transplantation, and they are already such a small number. There already is enough discrimination against the elderly, and we ought not to add to that injustice by further limiting their access.

References

1. 2008 Annual Report of the U.S. Organ Procurement and Transplantation Network and the Scientific Registry of Transplant Recipients: Transplant Data 1998–2007. U.S. Department of Health and Human Services, Health Resources and Services Administration, Healthcare Systems Bureau, Division of Transplantation, Rockville, MD

2. U.S. Renal Data System, USRDS 2008 Annual Data Report: Atlas of Chronic Kidney Disease and End-Stage Renal Disease in the United States, National Institutes of Health, National Institute of Diabetes and Digestive and Kidney Diseases, Bethesda, MD

3. Cameron JI, Whiteside C, Katz J et al (2000) Differences in quality of life across renal replacement therapies: a meta-analytic comparison. Am J Kidney Dis 35(4):629–637

4. Wolfe RA, Ashby VB, Milford EL et al (1999) Comparison of mortality in all patients on dialysis, patients on dialysis awaiting transplantation, and recipients of a first cadaveric transplant. N Engl J Med 341(23):1725–1730

5. Oniscu GC, Brown H, Forsythe JL (2004) How old is old for transplantation? Am J Transplant 4(12):2067–2074

6. Fabrizii V, Winkelmayer WC, Klauser R et al (2004) Patient and graft survival in older kidney transplant recipients: does age matter? J Am Soc Nephrol 15(4):1052–1060

7. Albrechtsen D, Leivestad T, Sodal G et al (1995) Kidney transplantation in patients older than 70 years of age. Transplant Proc 27(1):986–988

8. Rao PS, Merion RM, Ashby VB et al (2007) Renal transplantation in elderly patients older than 70 years of age: results from the Scientific Registry of Transplant Recipients. Transplantation 83(8):1069–1074

9. Palomar R, Ruiz JC, Zubimendi JA et al (2002) Acute rejection in the elderly recipient: influence of age in the outcome of kidney transplantation. Int Urol Nephrol 33(1):145–148

10. Wu C, Shapiro R, Tan H et al (2008) Kidney transplantation in elderly people: the influence of recipient comorbidity and living kidney donors. J Am Geriatr Soc 56(2):231–238

11. Port FK, Bragg-Gresham JL, Metzger RA et al (2002) Donor characteristics associated with reduced graft survival: an approach to expanding the pool of kidney donors. Transplantation 74(9):1281–1286

12. Moore PS, Farney AC, Sundberg AK et al (2007) Dual kidney transplantation: a case-control comparison with single kidney transplantation from standard and expanded criteria donors. Transplantation 83(12):1551–1556

13. Steinman TI, Becker BN, Frost AE et al (2001) Guidelines for the referral and management of patients eligible for solid organ transplantation. Transplantation 71(9):1189–1204

14. Bunnapradist S, Danovitch GM (2007) Evaluation of adult kidney transplant candidates. Am J Kidney Dis 50(5):890–898

15. Kasiske BL, Cangro CB, Hariharan S et al (2001) The evaluation of renal transplantation candidates: clinical practice guidelines. Am J Transplant 1(Suppl 2):3–95

16. Knoll G, Cockfield S, Blydt-Hansen T et al (2005) Canadian Society of Transplantation: consensus guidelines on eligibility for kidney transplantation. CMAJ 173(10):S1–S25

17. Smetana GW (1999) Preoperative pulmonary evaluation. N Engl J Med 340(12):937–944

18. Maisonneuve P, Agodoa L, Gellert R et al (1999) Cancer in patients on dialysis for end-stage renal disease: an international collaborative study. Lancet 354(9173):93–99

19. Penn I (1993) The effect of immunosuppression on pre-existing cancers. Transplantation 55(4):742–747

20. Danovitch G, Savransky S (2006) Challenges in the counseling and management of older kidney transplant candidates. Am J Kidney Dis 47(4 Suppl 2):S86–S97

21. Oniscu GC, Brown H, Forsythe JL (2004) How great is the survival advantage of transplantation over dialysis in elderly patients? Nephrol Dial Transplant 19(4):945–951

22. Martins PN, Pratschke J, Pascher A et al (2005) Age and immune response in organ transplantation. Transplantation 79(2):127–132

23. Danovitch GM, Gill J, Bunnapradist S (2007) Immunosuppression of the elderly kidney transplant recipient. Transplantation 84(3):285–291

24. Bradley BA (2002) Rejection and recipient age. Transpl Immunol 10(2–3):125–132

25. Johnson DW, Nicol DL, Preston JM et al (2003) Use of mycophenolate mofetil in immunosuppressive protocols in elderly renal transplant recipients. Transplantation 76(3):619

26. Meier-Kriesche HU, Morris JA, Chu AH et al (2004) Mycophenolate mofetil vs. azathioprine in a large population of elderly renal transplant patients. Nephrol Dial Transplant 19(11):2864–2869

27. Meier-Kriesche HU, Li S, Gruessner RW et al (2006) Immunosuppression: evolution in practice and trends, 1994 2004. Am J Transplant 6(5 Pt 2):1111–1131

28. Shah T, Kasravi A, Huang E et al (2006) Risk factors for development of new-onset diabetes mellitus after kidney transplantation. Transplantation 82(12):1673–1676

29. Arbogast H, Huckelheim H, Schneeberger H et al (2005) A calcineurin antagonist-free induction/maintenance strategy for immunosuppression in elderly recipients of renal allografts from elderly cadaver donors: long-term results from a prospective single centre trial. Clin Transplant 19(3):309–315

30. Emparan C, Wolters H, Laukotter M et al (2004) Long-term results of calcineurin-free protocols with basiliximab induction in "old-to-old" programs. Transplant Proc 36(9):2646–2648

31. Segoloni GP, Messina M, Squiccimarro G et al (2005) Preferential allocation of marginal kidney allografts to elderly recipients combined with modified immunosuppression gives good results. Transplantation 80(7):953–958

32. Kauffman HM, McBride MA, Cors CS et al (2007) Early mortality rates in older kidney recipients with comorbid risk factors. Transplantation 83(4):404–410

33. Bentas W, Jones J, Karaoguz A et al (2008) Renal transplantation in the elderly: surgical complications and outcome with special emphasis on the Eurotransplant Senior Programme. Nephrol Dial Transplant 23(6):2043–2051

34. Kemmer N, Safdar K, Kaiser TE et al (2008) Liver transplantation trends for older recipients: regional and ethnic variations. Transplantation 86(1):104–107

35. Hoshida Y, Ikeda K, Kobayashi M et al (1999) Chronic liver disease in the extremely elderly of 80 years or more: clinical characteristics, prognosis and patient survival analysis. J Hepatol 31(5):860–866

36. Stieber AC, Gordon RD, Todo S et al (1991) Liver transplantation in patients over sixty years of age. Transplantation 51(1):271–273

37. Pirsch JD, Kalayoglu M, D'Alessandro AM et al (1991) Orthotopic liver transplantation in patients 60 years of age and older. Transplantation 51(2):431–433

38. Bromley PN, Hilmi I, Tan KC et al (1994) Orthotopic liver transplantation in patients over 60 years old. Transplantation 58(7):800–803

39. Bilbao I, Balsells J, Lazaro JL et al (1995) Liver transplantation in patients over 60 years of age. Transplant Proc 27(4):2337–2338

40. Garcia CE, Garcia RF, Mayer AD et al (2001) Liver transplantation in patients over sixty years of age. Transplantation 72(4):679–684

41. Cross TJ, Antoniades CG, Muiesan P et al (2007) Liver transplantation in patients over 60 and 65 years: an evaluation of long-term outcomes and survival. Liver Transpl 13(10):1382–1388

42. Safdar K, Neff GW, Montalbano M et al (2004) Liver transplant for the septuagenarians: importance of patient selection. Transplant Proc 36(5):1445–1448

43. Lucey MR, Brown KA, Everson GT et al (1997) Minimal criteria for placement of adults on the liver transplant waiting list: a report of a national conference organized by the American Society of Transplant Physicians and the American Association for the Study of Liver Diseases. Liver Transpl Surg 3(6):628–637

44. Wiesner RH, McDiarmid SV, Kamath PS et al (2001) MELD and PELD: application of survival models to liver allocation. Liver Transpl 7(7):567–580

45. Desai NM, Mange KC, Crawford MD et al (2004) Predicting outcome after liver transplantation: utility of the model for end-stage liver disease and a newly derived discrimination function. Transplantation 77(1):99–106

46. Kuramitsu K, Egawa H, Keeffe EB et al (2007) Impact of age older than 60 years in living donor liver transplantation. Transplantation 84(2):166–172

47. Keswani RN, Ahmed A, Keeffe EB (2004) Older age and liver transplantation: a review. Liver Transpl 10(8):957–967

48. Carey WD, Dumot JA, Pimentel RR et al (1995) The prevalence of coronary artery disease in liver transplant candidates over age 50. Transplantation 59(6):859–864

49. Levy MF, Somasundar PS, Jennings LW et al (2001) The elderly liver transplant recipient: a call for caution. Ann Surg 233(1):107–113

50. Herrero JI, Lucena JF, Quiroga J et al (2003) Liver transplant recipients older than 60 years have lower survival and higher incidence of malignancy. Am J Transplant 3(11):1407–1412

51. Abt PL, Mange KC, Olthoff KM et al (2004) Allograft survival following adult-to-adult living donor liver transplantation. Am J Transplant 4(8):1302–1307

52. Olthoff KM, Merion RM, Ghobrial RM et al (2005) Outcomes of 385 adult-to-adult living donor liver transplant recipients: a report from the A2ALL Consortium. Ann Surg 242(3):314–323

53. Collins BH, Pirsch JD, Becker YT et al (2000) Long-term results of liver transplantation in older patients 60 years of age and older. Transplantation 70(5):780–783

54. Emre S, Mor E, Schwartz ME et al (1993) Liver transplantation in patients beyond age 60. Transplant Proc 25(1 Pt 2):1075–1076

55. Filipponi F, Roncella M, Boggi U et al (2001) Liver transplantation in recipients over 60. Transplant Proc 33(1–2):1465–1466

56. Rudich S, Busuttil R (1999) Similar outcomes, morbidity, and mortality for orthotopic liver transplantation between the very elderly and the young. Transplant Proc 31(1–2):523–525

57. Adam R, McMaster P, O'Grady JG et al (2003) Evolution of liver transplantation in Europe: report of the European Liver Transplant Registry. Liver Transpl 9(12):1231–1243

58. Gomez-Manero N, Herrero JI, Quiroga J et al (2001) Prognostic model for early acute rejection after liver transplantation. Liver Transpl 7(3):246–254

59. Zetterman RK, Belle SH, Hoofnagle JH et al (1998) Age and liver transplantation: a report of the Liver Transplantation Database. Transplantation 66(4):500–506

60. Shaw BW Jr (1994) Transplantation in the elderly patient. Surg Clin North Am 74(2):389–400

61. Taylor DO, Edwards LB, Mohacsi PJ et al (2003) The registry of the International Society for Heart and Lung Transplantation: twentieth official adult heart transplant report – 2003. J Heart Lung Transplant 22(6):616–624

62. Blanche C, Blanche DA, Kearney B et al (2001) Heart transplantation in patients seventy years of age and older: a comparative analysis of outcome. J Thorac Cardiovasc Surg 121(3):532–541

63. Zuckermann A, Dunkler D, Deviatko E et al (2003) Long-term survival (>10 years) of patients >60, years with induction therapy after cardiac transplantation. Eur J Cardiothorac Surg 24(2):283–291

64. Demers P, Moffatt S, Oyer PE et al (2003) Long-term results of heart transplantation in patients older than 60 years. J Thorac Cardiovasc Surg 126(1):224–231

65. Weiss ES, Nwakanma LU, Patel ND et al (2008) Outcomes in patients older than 60 years of age undergoing orthotopic heart transplantation: an analysis of the UNOS database. J Heart Lung Transplant 27(2):184–191

66. Mehra MR, Kobashigawa J, Starling R et al (2006) Listing criteria for heart transplantation: International Society for Heart and Lung Transplantation guidelines for the care of cardiac transplant candidates – 2006. J Heart Lung Transplant 25(9):1024–1042

67. Costanzo MR, Augustine S, Bourge R et al (1995) Selection and treatment of candidates for heart transplantation. A statement for health professionals from the Committee on Heart Failure and Cardiac Transplantation of the Council on Clinical Cardiology, American Heart Association. Circulation 92(12):3593–3612

68. Halpern SD, Ubel PA, Caplan AL (2002) Solid-organ transplantation in HIV-infected patients. N Engl J Med 347(4):284–287

69. Szlachcic J, Massie BM, Kramer BL et al (1985) Correlates and prognostic implication of exercise capacity in chronic congestive heart failure. Am J Cardiol 55(8):1037–1042

70. Likoff MJ, Chandler SL, Kay HR (1987) Clinical determinants of mortality in chronic congestive heart failure secondary to idiopathic dilated or to ischemic cardiomyopathy. Am J Cardiol 59(6):634–638

71. Cohn JN, Johnson GR, Shabetai R et al (1993) Ejection fraction, peak exercise oxygen consumption, cardiothoracic ratio, ventricular arrhythmias, and plasma norepinephrine as determinants of prognosis in heart failure. The V-HeFT VA Cooperative Studies Group. Circulation 87(6 Suppl):VI5–VI16

72. Aaronson KD, Schwartz JS, Chen TM et al (1997) Development and prospective validation of a clinical index to predict survival in ambulatory patients referred for cardiac transplant evaluation. Circulation 95(12):2660–2667

73. Levy WC, Mozaffarian D, Linker DT et al (2006) The Seattle Heart Failure Model: prediction of survival in heart failure. Circulation 113(11):1424–1433

74. O'Neill JO, Taylor DO, Starling RC (2004) Immunosuppression for cardiac transplantation – the past, present and future. Transplant Proc 36(2 Suppl):309S–313S

75. Morgan JA, John R, Mancini DM et al (2004) Should heart transplantation be considered as a treatment option for patients aged 70 years and older? J Thorac Cardiovasc Surg 127(6):1817–1819

76. Forni A, Faggian G, Chiominto B et al (2007) Heart transplantation in older candidates. Transplant Proc 39(6):1963–1966

77. Nagendran J, Wildhirt SM, Modry D et al (2004) A comparative analysis of outcome after heart transplantation in patients aged 60 years and older: the University of Alberta experience. J Card Surg 19(6):559–562

78. Marelli D, Kobashigawa J, Hamilton MA et al (2008) Long-term outcomes of heart transplantation in older recipients. J Heart Lung Transplant 27(8):830–834

79. Villar E, Boissonnat P, Sebbag L et al (2007) Poor prognosis of heart transplant patients with end-stage renal failure. Nephrol Dial Transplant 22(5):1383–1389

80. Roithmaier S, Haydon AM, Loi S et al (2007) Incidence of malignancies in heart and/or lung transplant recipients: a single-institution experience. J Heart Lung Transplant 26(8):845–849

81. Christie JD, Edwards LB, Aurora P et al (2008) Registry of the International Society for Heart and Lung Transplantation: twenty-fifth official adult lung and heart/lung transplantation report – 2008. J Heart Lung Transplant 27(9):957–969

82. Charman SC, Sharples LD, McNeil KD et al (2002) Assessment of survival benefit after lung transplantation by patient diagnosis. J Heart Lung Transplant 21(2):226–232

83. De Meester J, Smits JM, Persijn GG et al (2001) Listing for lung transplantation: life expectancy and transplant effect, stratified by type of end-stage lung disease, the Eurotransplant experience. J Heart Lung Transplant 20(5):518–524

84. Orens JB, Estenne M, Arcasoy S et al (2006) International guidelines for the selection of lung transplant candidates: 2006 update – a consensus report from the Pulmonary Scientific Council of the International Society for Heart and Lung Transplantation. J Heart Lung Transplant 25(7):745–755

85. Wain JC, Wright CD, Ryan DP et al (1999) Induction immunosuppression for lung transplantation with OKT3. Ann Thorac Surg 67(1):187–193

86. Brock MV, Borja MC, Ferber L et al (2001) Induction therapy in lung transplantation: a prospective, controlled clinical trial comparing OKT3, anti-thymocyte globulin, and daclizumab. J Heart Lung Transplant 20(12):1282–1290

87. Trulock EP, Christie JD, Edwards LB et al (2007) Registry of the International Society for Heart and Lung Transplantation: twenty-fourth official adult lung and heart-lung transplantation report – 2007. J Heart Lung Transplant 26(8):782–795

88. Weiss ES, Merlo CA, Shah AS (2009) Impact of advanced age in lung transplantation: an analysis of United Network for Organ Sharing data. J Am Coll Surg 208(3):400–409

89. Meyers BF, de la Morena M, Sweet SC et al (2005) Primary graft dysfunction and other selected complications of lung transplantation: a single-center experience of 983 patients. J Thorac Cardiovasc Surg 129(6):1421–1429

90. Boehler A, Estenne M (2003) Post-transplant bronchiolitis obliterans. Eur Respir J 22(6):1007–1018

91. Amital A, Shitrit D, Raviv Y et al (2006) Development of malignancy following lung transplantation. Transplantation 81(4):547–551

Index

R.A. Rosenthal et al. (eds.), *Principles and Practice of Geriatric Surgery*,
DOI 10.1007/978-1-4419-6999-6, © Springer Science+Business Media, LLC 2011